High School Edition of EMERGENCY CARE

14TH EDITION

DANIEL LIMMER • MICHAEL F. O'KEEFE

MEDICAL EDITOR: EDWARD T. DICKINSON, MD, NRP, FACEP

High School Edition of EMERGENCY CARE

14TH EDITION

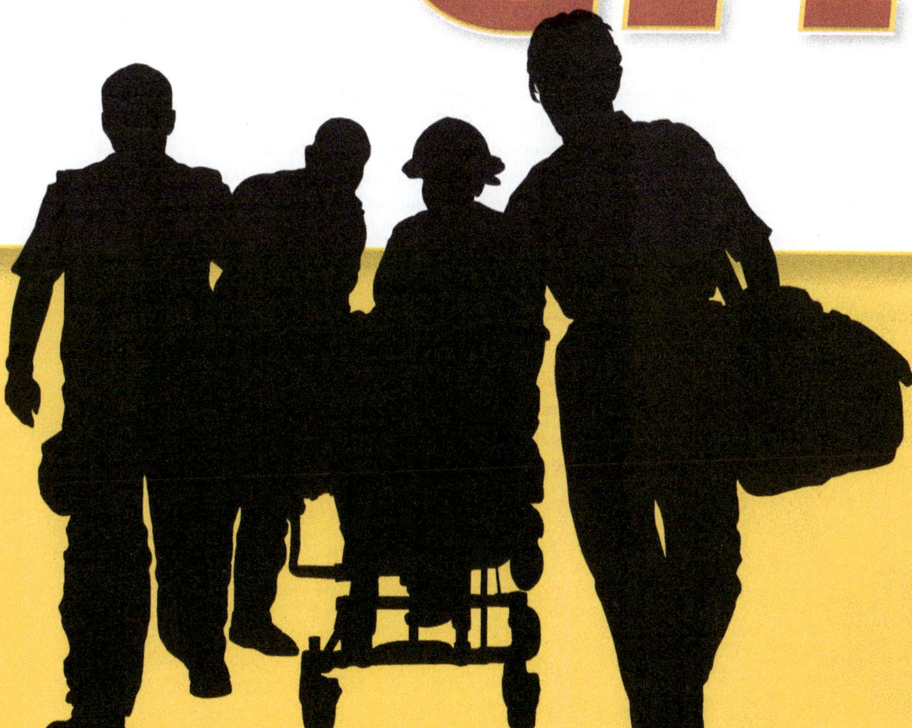

LEGACY AUTHORS
HARVEY D. GRANT
ROBERT H. MURRAY, JR.
J. DAVID BERGERON

Please contact https://support.pearson.com/getsupport/s/ with any queries on this content

Cover Art: Pearson photo by Michal Heron

Notice on Care Procedures: It is the intent of the authors and publisher that this text be used as part of a formal Emergency Medical Technician (EMT) education program taught by qualified instructors and supervised by a licensed physician. The procedures described in this textbook are based on consultation with EMT and medical authorities. The authors and publisher have taken care to make certain that these procedures reflect currently accepted clinical practice; however, they cannot be considered absolute recommendations.

The material in this text contains the most current information available at the time of publication. However, federal, state, and local guidelines concerning clinical practices, including (without limitation) those governing infection control and universal precautions, change rapidly. The reader should note, therefore, that the new regulations may require changes in some procedures.

It is the reader's responsibility to familiarize himself or herself with the policies and procedures set by federal, state, and local agencies as well as the institution or agency where the reader is employed. The authors and the publisher of this text and the supplements written to accompany it disclaim any liability, loss, or risk resulting directly or indirectly from the suggested procedures and theory, from any undetected errors, or from the reader's misunderstanding of the text. It is the reader's responsibility to stay informed of any new changes or recommendations made by any federal, state, or local agency as well as by his or her employing institution or agency.

Notice on Gender Usage: The authors in the fourteenth edition have made great efforts to eliminate gender-preferential language in all general discussions. However, in case studies in which a patient is identified as a man or a woman, the applicable pronoun is used.

Notice Regarding "Street Scenes" and "Scenarios": The names used and situations depicted in the Street Scenes and Scenarios throughout this text are fictitious.

Notice on Medications: The authors and the publisher of this text have taken care to make certain that the equipment, doses of drugs, and schedules of treatment are correct and compatible with the standards generally accepted at the time of publication. Nevertheless, as new information becomes available, changes in treatment and in the use of equipment and drugs become necessary. The reader is advised to carefully consult the instruction and information material included in the page insert for each drug or therapeutic agent, piece of equipment, or device before administration. This advice is especially important when using new or infrequently used drugs. Prehospital care providers are warned that use of any drugs or techniques must be authorized by their Medical Director, in accordance with local laws and regulations. The publisher disclaims any liability, loss, injury, or damage incurred as a consequence, directly or indirectly, of the use and application of any of the contents of this text.

---

37 2025

Pearson

ISBN-10: 0-13-662617-3
ISBN-13: 978-0-13-662617-6

Dedication

This edition is dedicated to Stephanie, Sarah and Margo. I am fortunate to be surrounded by your love and support. And to my buddy, Lulu.

– D.L.

To the memory of my parents, Mike and Noreen, and to my family.

– M.O'K.

To my wife Debbie for her endless patience and support for this 14th edition, and to all the EMS providers of PennStar and the Malvern, Berwyn, and Radnor Fire Companies who keep me grounded in the prehospital environment.

– E.T.D.

Acknowledgments

This 14th edition of *Emergency Care*, like others, has left your authors feeling grateful for the dynamic and talented team we have worked with. It is also a time for change, so as we give our thanks, we must sadly say goodbye to some people very dear to us.

First on this list is Michal Heron. Since the 6th edition of Emergency Care, Michal has been our photo editor and photographer extraordinaire. Her talent, vision, and attention to detail have been a foundation not only for the visuals, but for the book itself, creating a bright and welcoming appearance with accurate images to learn from. Michal–there will never be another you and we will miss you acutely.

Sandy Breuer was the editor of Emergency Care, also since the 6th edition. She came onboard with Michal and changed the way books were done at Brady. Her talent and sense of humor were limitless. Her dedication is legendary. We didn't get to work with Sandy on this edition but her legacy lives on in the book you see before you today.

Faye Gemmellaro is a gentle giant behind the scenes. If books had air traffic controllers, Faye would be ours. Guiding this edition to a safe landing with skill and aplomb, Faye manages multiple tasks effortlessly and coordinates pieces that, while unseen to many who write and read these books, are so necessary. Faye has moved to another part of Pearson. It won't be the same without you, Faye.

Editors come and go over the years. This edition saw several members of the editorial team leave the fold. Marlene Pratt, Executive Editor, is no longer with the team. Marlene was the editor for this product for many years, including the Pearson award-winning

10th edition. She later oversaw all of Brady. Derril Trakalo was with us for the kick-off of this edition and got us started on a solid course before relocating to another corner of Pearson. Our sincere thanks to both Marlene and Derril for their dedication to this book and our best wishes to you. Julie Alexander was a Vice President over Brady for many, many years and also no longer with us. Julie was always personable and approachable while at the helm. We are sad knowing you aren't there.

When we say so many goodbyes, there are many people to introduce to you. Katrin Beacom is the new Director of Product Management. She is a familiar and friendly face to us as the former marketing manager for Brady years ago. Kat, it is good to have you back. Kevin Wilson recently replaced Derril Trakalo. We still call him an editor even though Pearson calls him Content Manager. Kevin comes from the sales force and has brought much to the table bringing this edition to fruition. We look forward to working with you.

Our editor this edition is Rachel Bedard. Rachel had tough shoes to fill but did so admirably. Rachel and her team tracked content and schedules, edited manuscript, made sure photos were placed and referenced, and perhaps the most difficult task, dealt with busy authors. Your authors know EMS and EMS education, but putting together a textbook is something totally different and sometimes foreign. We are grateful for Rachel and her team for artfully assembling the book you have before you now.

There are so many people to thank including Pearson's editorial assistants, the sales reps who help get the book out to you and your instructors, Beth Muniz who directs our sales force, magician and problem solver Lenny Losacco, marketing professionals like our old friends Brian Hoehl, Rachele Strober, and more. We're sorry we can't name you all.

We thank our families who put up with the schedule of writing and publishing a textbook and support us in this labor of love.

We are grateful for the educators who put their trust in us to provide the book which serves as a foundation for their course. We salute the current EMRs, EMTs, AEMTs, and paramedics who make EMS what it is today. Finally, we welcome the students who enter EMS through their EMT course. You give us hope for the future. We wish you the joys, successes and lasting friendships we have gained over the years we have been in EMS.

– D.L.

BRIEF CONTENTS

CONTENTS

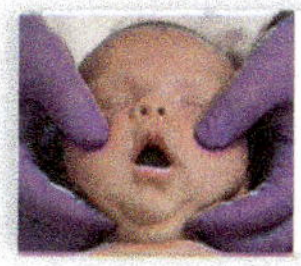

SECTION 1

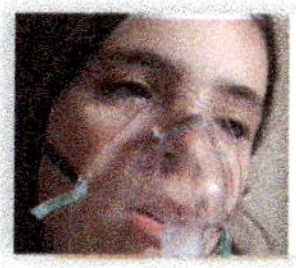

SECTION 2

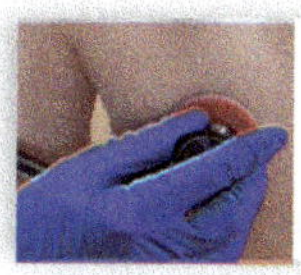

SECTION 3

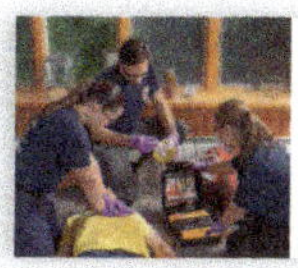

SECTION 4

Medical Emergencies 493

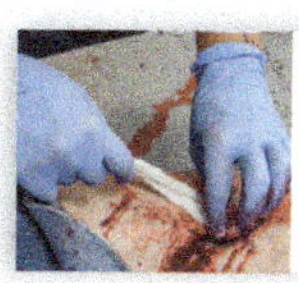

SECTION 5

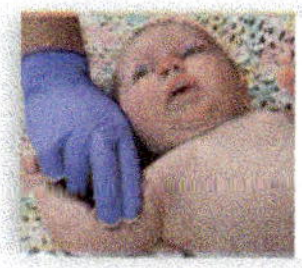

SECTION 6

PHOTO SCANS

VISUAL GUIDES

Letter to Students

Dear Student:

Welcome to the exciting world of EMS.

We are pleased that your instructor has chosen *Emergency Care* as your classroom textbook. We believe our textbook will serve you well in class, on your certification exam, and long into your experience as an EMT, whether you are seeking your first job in EMS or looking to serve your community as a volunteer.

We would like to offer some advice to you as you begin your program—advice likely given to you by your instructor as well. Please be sure to keep up on your reading and assignments, pay attention in class, and engage fully in your skills during labs. Teachers will teach, but true *learning* is driven by you, the student. Take notes and make flash cards. Pay particular attention to the pathophysiology material in this text. Understanding pathophysiology is the difference between understanding a disease process and simply memorizing the signs and symptoms.

This is a very exciting time in EMS. EMTs are using new and exciting technologies. You may have opportunities to take additional classes such as Advanced EMT (AEMT) and paramedic in the future. We have seen growth in the critical care and flight paramedic roles and a relatively new area called community paramedic, which bridges EMS with primary, in-home medical care.

We hope you share our excitement about the class you are beginning. Our sincerest best wishes to you for success in your class—and wherever EMS takes you.

Daniel Limmer
AS, LP, I/C
danlimmer@mac.com

Michael F. O'Keefe
NRP
MikeOKVT@aol.com

Edward T. Dickinson, MD, NRP, FACEP
edward.dickinson@uphs.upenn.edu

PREFACE

EMERGENCY CARE has set the standard for EMT training for more than thirty-five years. We strive to stay current with new research and developments in EMS, and this new edition is no exception. The text meets the current American Heart Association guidelines for CPR and ECC to prepare your students for testing and practice today and beyond.

The foundation of *Emergency Care* is the National EMS Education Standards. While using the Standards as our base, *Emergency Care*, fourteenth edition, has been written to go beyond the Standards to provide the most current reflection of EMS practice and show readers what EMS systems and EMTs are actually doing around the country today. The caveat "follow local protocols," of course, appears frequently–whenever the equipment or practice described has been adopted in some but not all systems.

In addition, the text was developed taking into account the years of experience that the authors have had with EMS curricula and practice, with the input of countless instructors and students. The result is a proven text with outstanding readability and a level of detail that instructors have found more appropriate for their classrooms than any other.

The content of the fourteenth edition is summarized in the following text, followed by brief details on "what's new" in each section of this edition.

What's New in the Fourteenth Edition?

The fourteenth edition has undergone extensive development and change.

This edition boasts more new professional photos than any previous edition. The author and photographic team worked together to supply a combination of realistic and real-life emergency images that are unrivaled in EMT literature. The resulting artwork in *Emergency Care* 14e is a powerful teaching tool for students.

The Patient Care feature that appears in clinical chapters has been fine-tuned to address Fundamental Principles of Care first, followed by actions that the EMT may need to employ in caring for the patient. In this edition, actions are not numbered, because there is no one correct sequence for patient care. The EMT must continually base decisions and priority actions on the evolving condition of the patient.

All chapters throughout the text have been updated to conform to the *most current American Heart Association Guidelines for Cardiopulmonary Resuscitation and Emergency Cardiovascular Care.*

The *Operations* section of the book has been updated and expanded to include new triage procedures and updated guidelines for handling incident scenes.

There is significant **organizational change** in this edition.

- This edition has integrated the assessment, care, and treatment of children into all parts of the text. We take the approach that children, while having some physiological differences from adults, do not constitute a distinct and separate population. Their needs and functions are generally like those of adults. We provide clear information about the differences while providing the overall continuity of care for patients from neonates to older adults.
- Likewise, the care of older adults is no longer discussed separately. Our text provides chapters with patient scenarios that cover a range of ages, so that students have continuous practice considering age as a factor in their overall information gathering and assessment.
- The Secondary Assessment chapter was reworked into three more focused chapters that address specific aspects of the EMT's role and care of patients. Details are provided below under Section 3.
- *Cardiac Emergencies* and *Resuscitation* are two distinct chapters in the fourteenth edition. *Infectious Diseases and Sepsis* is a new chapter in this edition, as you will see under Section 4.
- *Special Populations,* Section 6 of the fourteenth edition, has been changed significantly, with pediatric and geriatric care integrated throughout the text, and updates to remaining chapters.

SECTION 1

Foundations: Chapters 1-8

The first section sets a framework for all the sections that follow by introducing some essential concepts, information, and skills. The section introduces the EMS system and the EMT's role within the system. The section then covers issues of EMT safety and well-being, including safe techniques of lifting and moving patients. Legal and ethical issues are then discussed. Basic medical terminology, anatomy, physiology, pathophysiology, and lifespan development round out this first section.

What's New in the Foundations Section?

- *In Chapter 2, Well-Being of the EMT,* there is new text on Invisible Wounds—Preventing Psychological Trauma and discussion of eSCAPe, a mnemonic for dealing with posttraumatic stress. There are also updated sections on Realities of Well-Being and self-protection in a violent event.
- *Chapter 3, Lifting and Moving Patients,* has new text on bariatric patients and provides new images of the "no lift-at-all" stretcher. It also updates information on the use of long spine boards
- *Chapter 7, Principles of Pathophysiology,* has new text on the regulation of homeostasis and the fight-or-flight response, plus new information about pediatric vascular response and pediatric compensation.

SECTION 2

Airway Management, Respiration, and Artificial Ventilation: Chapters 9-10

There are only two chapters in Section 2, but it may be the most important section in the text, because no patient will survive without an adequate airway, adequate respiration, and adequate ventilation.

As mentioned, the chapters in this section and throughout the text have been updated to conform to the *current American Heart Association Guidelines for Cardiopulmonary Resuscitation and Emergency Cardiovascular Care.*

What's New in the Airway Management, Respiration, and Artificial Ventilation Section?

- *In Chapter 9, Airway Management* has new text on the head-elevated, sniffing position; providing an airway; manual airway maneuvers; obstructed airways; conscious choking adults and children; and unconscious choking. It also includes Scan 9-5 Insertion of a King Airway and Scan 9-6 Insertion of an i-gel™ Airway, and covers using gravity to clear an airway. There are new pediatric text sections on pediatric airway physiology and suctioning in pediatrics.
- *Chapter 10, Respiration and Artificial Ventilation,* has added new text: Face Mask Ventilation—Core Principles, and Ventilation Rates and Volume. There is also new pediatric text in the form of a Pediatric Note about providing supplemental oxygen.

SECTION 3

Patient Assessment: Chapters 11-17

Key elements of the EMT's job are the ability to perform a thorough and accurate assessment, treat for life-threatening conditions, and initiate transport to the hospital within optimum time limits. This section explains and illustrates all of the assessment steps and their application to different types of trauma and medical patients. In addition, it focuses on the skills of measuring vital signs, using monitoring devices, taking a patient history, communicating, and documenting.

What's New in the Patient Assessment Section?

- *In Chapter 11, Scene Size-Up,* there is a new Think Like an EMT section (Should I or Shouldn't I stay or retreat from a scene?) There is also additional text on airbag deployment.
- *Chapter 12, Primary Assessment,* includes updated text on spinal motion restriction.
- *Chapter 13, Vital Signs and Monitoring Devices,* has new text on capnography.
- *Chapter 14, Principles of Assessment,* pulls together assessment processes for adults and children. It also discusses critical thinking skills that EMTs can develop to improve their work in the field.
- *Chapter 15, Secondary Assessment,* drills down on the secondary assessment needs of patients with medical emergencies and traumatic emergencies. A section of this chapter covers important considerations for caring for children who are experiencing trauma.
- *Chapter 16, Reassessment,* focuses on the need for continual review of patient status until patient care has been transferred to the Emergency Department or health care facility.
- *Chapter 17, Communication and Documentation,* has updated forms and equipment as well as new text on completion of the Prehospital Care Report.

SECTION 4

Medical Emergencies: Chapters 18-28

The Medical Emergencies section begins with a chapter on pharmacology that introduces the medications the EMT can administer or assist with under the current curriculum. The section continues with chapters on respiratory emergencies, cardiac emergencies, resuscitation, diabetic/altered mental status (including seizure and stroke) emergencies, allergic emergencies, infectious diseases and sepsis emergencies, poisoning/overdose emergencies, abdominal emergencies, behavioral/psychiatric emergencies, and hematologic/renal emergencies.

What's New in the Medical Emergencies Section?

- *Chapter 18, General Pharmacology,* has updated text on naloxone plus new photos of nasal naloxone administration.
- *Chapter 19, Respiratory Emergencies,* has new text on the pressures of the respiratory system, a Pediatric Note on

bronchiolitis, as well as content on pediatric respiratory distress and croup.

- *Chapter 20, Cardiac Emergencies*, includes more information on 12 lead ECG and special information for helping pediatric patients. This chapter focuses on the needs of the incipient medical cardiac patient.
- *Chapter 21, Resuscitation*, focuses on patients who require life-restoring procedures. In particular, the updated *Resuscitation* chapter provides procedures and requirements for high-performance CPR.
- *Chapter 22, Diabetic Emergencies and Altered Mental Status*, has new content on pediatric patients with seizures. It also describes thrombectom, and advances in the treatment of patients with stroke.
- *Chapter 23, Allergic Reactions*, includes pediatric as well as adult epinephrine devices.
- *Chapter 24, Infectious Diseases and Sepsis*, is a **new chapter** in Emergency Care's fourteenth edition. It provides an overview of common infectious diseases that EMTs may encounter. It also describes conditions that lead to sepsis and signs that sepsis may be occurring.
- *Chapter 25, Poisoning and Overdose Emergencies*, includes a new Scan 25-6 Absorbed Poisons—HAZMAT—Illegal Meth Lab.
- *Chapter 26, Abdominal Emergencies*, now includes text on abdominal pain associated with the female reproductive system.

SECTION 5

Trauma: Chapters 29-35

The Trauma Emergencies section begins with a chapter on bleeding and shock and continues with chapters on soft-tissue trauma; chest and abdominal trauma; musculoskeletal trauma; trauma to the head, neck, and spine; multisystem trauma; and environmental emergencies.

What's New in the Trauma Section?

- *Chapter 29, Bleeding and Shock*, has had an extensive rewrite with information on progression of actions in response to extensive bleeding. New content includes junctional tourniquets and methods of preventing or coping with the development of shock.
- *Chapter 30, Soft-Tissue Trauma*, has numerous new images to prepare students for events they may encounter in the field.
- *Chapter 31, Chest and Abdominal Trauma*, includes sections on the pathophysiology of the chest and abdomen and on rib fracture, plus additional material on occlusive and flutter-valve dressings.
- *In Chapter 33, Trauma to the Head, Neck, and Spine*, there is continued updating on methods of spinal motion restriction and new text on the rigid spine board and scoop stretcher.
- *Chapter 34, Multisystem Trauma*, includes new content on multiple trauma in the pediatric patient.
- *Chapter 35, Environmental Emergencies*, has updated information on scuba and water accidents and a new section on high-altitude emergencies.

SECTION 6

Special Populations: Chapters 36-37

Special populations discussed in this section include those with emergencies related to the female reproductive system, pregnancy, or childbirth; and to patients with certain disabilities or those who rely on advanced medical devices at home. As mentioned, pediatric and geriatric information has been integrated into appropriate chapters throughout the book. The chapters in this section emphasize how to serve all of these patients by applying the basics of patient assessment and care that the student has already learned.

What's New in the Special Populations Section?

- *Chapter 36, Obstetric and Gynecologic Emergencies*, contains updated text on neonatal resuscitation.
- *Chapter 37, "Emergencies for Patients with Special Challenges*, has new text addressing an emergency involving a home ventilator and a new section stressing the need for awareness of vulnerable populations (including child, elder, and domestic abuse and human trafficking).

SECTION 7

Operations: Chapters 38-41

This section deals with nonmedical operations and special situations, including EMS operations, hazardous materials, multiple-casualty incidents and incident management, highway safety, vehicle extrication, and the EMS response to terrorism.

What's New in the Operations Section?

- *Chapter 38, EMS Operations*, has updated images and procedures required by EMTs.
- *Chapter 39, Hazardous Materials, Multiple-Casualty Incidents, and Incident Management.* Includes a new swxtion on SALT (Sort, Assess, Lifesaving Interventions, Treatment/Transport), a triage method used at MCIs that is gaining popularity and acceptance in EMS systems.
- *Chapter 40, Highway Safety and Vehicle Extrication*, includes new text on alternative fuel vehicles.
- *Chapter 41, EMS Response to Terrorism*, has been updated to address "homegrown" terrorist attacks and strategies for providing care safely during such events.

APPENDIX AND REFERENCES

The Appendix in this edition provides a basic cardiac life support review. References include a listing of medical terms along with root prefixes and suffixes; anatomy and physiology illustrations; and the answer key, glossary, and index. All have been reviewed and updated.

OUR GOAL

Improving Future Training and Education

Some of the best ideas for better training and education methods come from instructors who can tell us what areas of study caused their students the most trouble. Other sound ideas come from practicing EMTs who let us know what problems they faced in the field. We welcome any of your suggestions. If you are an EMS instructor who has an idea on how to improve this book or EMT training in general, please write to us at:

Brady/Pearson Health Sciences
c/o EMS Editor Pearson Education
221 River Street
Hoboken, NJ 07030

You can also reach the authors through the following email addresses:

danlimmer@mac.com

MikeOKVT@aol.com

edward.dickinson@uphs.upenn.edu

Visit Brady's web site:

http://www.bradybooks.com

About the People

CONTENT CONTRIBUTORS

Becoming an EMT requires study in a number of content areas ranging from airway to medical and trauma emergencies to pediatrics and rescue. To ensure that each area is covered accurately and in the most up-to-date manner, we have enlisted the help of several expert contributors. We are grateful for the time and energy they have put into their contributions.

14th Edition:

Dan Batsie, BA, NRP
Chief of Emergency Medical Services
Vermont Department of Health
Burlington, VT

Brooke Beck, OMS III, UNTHSC
Texas College of Osteopathic Medicine
Ft. Worth, TX

Edward T. Dickinson, MD, NRP, FACEP
Professor
Department of Emergency Medicine
University of Pennsylvania School of Medicine
Philadelphia, PA

Ben Esposito EMT-P
Lieutenant/Hazardous Materials Specialist
Youngstown Fire Department
Youngstown, OH

Jake Freudenberger, OMS III, EMT-B, UNTHSC
Texas College of Osteopathic Medicine
Ft. Worth, TX

Robert Kronenberger
Fire Chief
Middletown Fire Department
Middletown, CT

David Lambert MD FACEP
Department of Emergency Medicine
Perelman School of Medicine
University of Pennsylvania
Philadelphia, PA

Steven J. Salengo, MEd, NRP
EMS Faculty
Hillsborough Community College
Tampa, FL

Eric Steffel, NRP, BSEMSA
Northwest EMS
Tomball, TX

REVIEWERS

We wish to thank the following reviewers for providing invaluable feedback and suggestions in preparation of the 14th edition of *Emergency Care.*

Andrew Appleby
Instructor of Paramedics and EMS
Western Wyoming Community College
Rock Springs, WY

Randall W. Benner
Instructor in the Department of Health Professions
Youngstown State University
Youngstown, OH

Sarah Clark
Program Director
ENTPKY, Inc.
Lexington, KY

Robert Cormier
Instructor
Centauri High School
La Jara, CO

Kenneth Crank
Instructor
Cincinnati State Tech and Community College
Cincinnati OH

James Dinsch
Program Director, Department Chair & EMS Assistant Professor
Indian River State College
Fort Pierce, FL

Robert Farnum
EMS Instructor
Department of Public Health and Human Services
Big Timber, MO

David Fifer M.S., NRP, FAWM
Assistant Professor & Program Coordinator
Eastern Kentucky University
Richmond, KY

Scott Gano
Associate Professor
Columbus State University
Columbus, OH

Jonathan Hockman
EMS Outreach Representative
Detroit Medical Center
Detroit, MI

Mark Hornshuh
Program Specialist
Portland Community College
Portland, OR

Michael Hunter
Education Coordinator
Harrison County Hospital
Corydon, IN

Jennifer Kline
Program Manager
Gateway Community College
Phoenix, AZ

Kurt Larson
EMT Instructor
George Stone Technical Center
Pensacola, FL

Marisa Laurent
Fire Science Assistant Instructor
Community College of Rhode Island
Warwick, RI

David Leclair
EMS Instructor
Otsego County EMS
Cooperstown, NY

Mike McDonough
EMT Faculty
Santa Barbara City College
Santa Barbara, CA

Dean C. Meenach, RN, BSN, CEN, CCRN, CPEN, EMT-P
Director of EMS Education
Mineral Area College
Park Hills, MO

Margaret Mittelman
EMT Basic and Advanced Program Coordinator
Utah Valley University
Orem, UT

Jeff Orphal
EMS Faculty
Apollo Career Center
Lima, OH

Robert Preshong
United States Army Medical Department Center and School
San Antonio, TX

Branson K. Ratsep, EMT-P
Lead EMT Instructor
Monterey Peninsula College
Salinas, CA

Gates Richards, MEd, WEMT-I, FAWM
EMT Director
NOLS Wilderness Medicine Institute
Lander, WY

James Robertson
EMT Instructor
Van Buren Intermediate School District
Lawrence, MI

Steven J. Salengo, MEd, NRP
EMS Faculty
Hillsborough Community College
Tampa, FL

Laurie Sheldon
EMT Faculty
Union County College
Cranford, NJ

Jennifer Stout
EMS Faculty
Howard College
San Angelo, TX

Joshua Tilton, NR-P, CCEMTP, EMS I, F I
EMS Instructor
City of Columbus Division of Fire
Columbus, OH

Jeremiah Underwood
Program Director, Emergency Medical Science
Guilford Technical Community College
Jamestown, NC

Tim Williamson
Program Director, EMS/Paramedic
Gateway Technical College
Burlington, WI

ORGANIZATIONS

We wish to thank the following organizations for their assistance in creating the photo program for this edition:

Essex Rescue (Essex Junction, VT)
Will Moran, Executive Director, EMT-P
Colleen Nesto, Deputy Executive Director, EMT-P
Sean McCann, A-EMT

Malvern Fire Company (Malvern, PA)
Keith Johnson, EMS Chief
Rich Constantine, Deputy EMS Chief

Sarasota County Fire Department (Sarasota, FL)
Chief Michael Regnier

Suncoast Technical College (Sarasota, FL)
Scott Kennedy, ARNP–Health and Public Safety Program Manager
Brian Kehoe, EMT-P–EMS Program Director
Mark Tuttle, EMT-P–Human Simulation Coordinator/Lead EMT Instructor
Dustin Martinez, EMT-P–EMT Instructor

Vermont Hazardous Materials Response Team

Dave Patneaude, VHMRT and Derby Line Fire Dept.
Paul Snider, VHMRT and Derby Line Fire Dept.
Harry Fell, VHMRT, Colchester Rescue and Vergennes Rescue
Kaitlyn Armstrong, VHMRT and VT DMV Detective
William Irwin, VHMRT, Bakersfield Vol. Fire/Rescue and VT Department of Health
Todd Cosgrove, VHMRT and Bakersfield Vol. Fire/Rescue

SUBJECT MATTER EXPERTS/PHOTO COORDINATORS

Thanks to the following for valuable assistance directing the medical accuracy of the shoots and coordinating models, props, and locations for our photo shoots:

Dan Batsie,
Chief of Emergency Medical Services, Vermont Department of Health (Burlington, VT)

Dustin Martinez,
EMT-P, Sarasota County Fire Department (Sarasota, FL)

Sean McCann,
Advanced EMT, Essex Rescue (Essex Junction, VT)

Mark Tuttle,
PMD BS, EMS Program Director, EMT-P, Suncoast Technical College (Sarasota, FL)

Rodney Van Orsdol,
EMT-P, Sarasota County Fire Department (Sarasota, FL)

CREDITS

All photos not credited here, or under the photograph, are Pearson-owned assignment photos.
Detail of Section Two photo on Page xi © Daniel Limmer
Section Opener Two: © Daniel Limmer
Section Opener Three: © Daniel Limmer
Chapter Opener for all chapters in Section Three: © Daniel Limmer
Chapter Opener for all chapters in Section Four © Ed Effron
Chapter Opener for all chapters in Section Seven © Ed Effron

Models

Thanks to the following people who portrayed patients and EMS providers in our photographs:

Grace Batsie
Margo Batsie
Addyson Brown
Aubrey Brown
Ava Brown
Jude Brown
Seth Bueno
Natalie Corapi
Davian Craddock
Caera Crosby
Bambi Dame
Emily Danis
Hillary Danis
Arianna Franzen
Jennifer Franzen, EMT
Jackie Goss, EMT-P
Duncan Higgins, AEMT
Timothy Kinville
Scott Kramer
Amelia Lamberty
Margo Limmer
Sarah Limmer
Jacy Lunna
Tyler Lyke
Alex McCarthy
McKenna Martin
Mairead McCann
Sean McCann, EMT
William Mitchell
Colleen Nesto, EMT-P
Andrew Rychlak
Mark Scanlon
Makayla Shanahan
Ashton Stewart
Victoria Stokes
Matthew Thompson
Lillian Turner
Michelle Turner
Jordan Tuttle, EMT/FF
Mark Tuttle, PMD BS, EMS Program Director, EMT-P
Hadley Warner, EMT
Leo Wermer
Deborah Williams
Joshua Williams, EMT
Michael Wheeler
Peter Withbroe

Photographers

Michal Heron
Kevin Link
Maria Lyle
Isaac Turner

Digital Post-Production

Maria Lyle, Maria Lyle Photography

About the Authors

AUTHOR

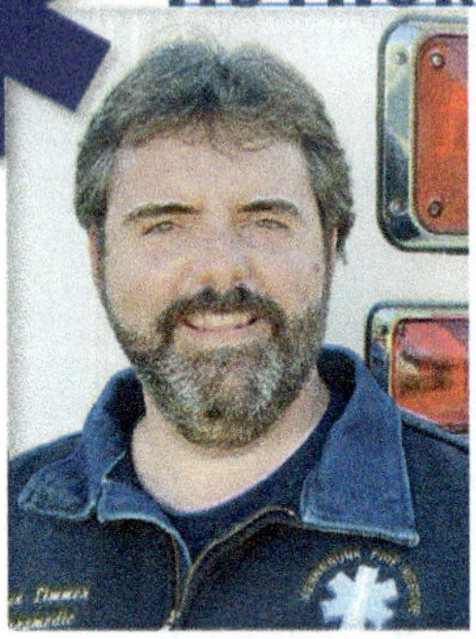

DANIEL LIMMER

- Began EMS in 1978. Became an EMT in 1980 and a Paramedic in 1981.
- Is a Lecturer at Central Washington University in Ellensburg, Washington, and an Adjunct Faculty member at Eastern Maine Community College in Bangor, Maine.
- Especially enjoys teaching patient assessment, and believes critical thinking and decision-making skills are the key to successful clinical practice of EMS.
- Works part-time as a freelance photojournalist and is working on a documentary project photographing EMS people and agencies throughout the United States.
- In addition to his EMS experience, was a dispatcher and police officer in upstate New York.
- Lives in Maine with his wife, Stephanie, and daughters Sarah and Margo.
- Is a Jimmy Buffett fan (Parrothead) who attends at least one concert each year.

AUTHOR

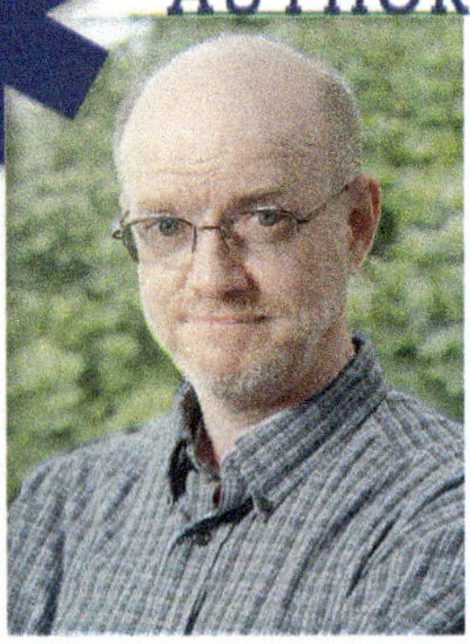

MICHAEL F. O'KEEFE

- EMT Provider Level Leader for National EMS Education Standards.
- Expert writer for 1994 revision of EMT-Basic curriculum.
- EMS volunteer since college in 1976.
- Member of development group for the National EMS *Education Agenda for the Future: A Systems Approach* and *The National EMS Scope of Practice Model.*
- Has a special interest in EMS research, and got a master's degree in biostatistics.
- Past chairperson of the National Council of State EMS Training Coordinators.
- Interests include science fiction, travel, foreign languages, and stained glass.

MEDICAL EDITOR

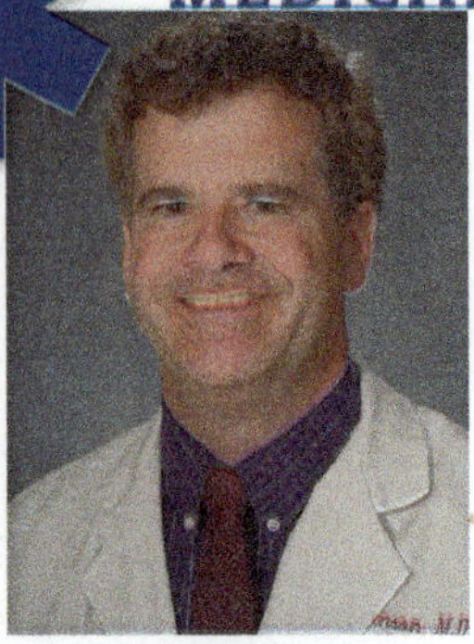

EDWARD T. DICKINSON

- In 1985, was the first volunteer firefighter to receive the top award from *Firehouse Magazine* for heroism for the rescue of two elderly women trapped in a house fire.
- Is the Medical Director of the Malvern, Berwyn, and Radnor Fire Companies in Pennsylvania.
- Has been continuously certified as a National Registry Paramedic since 1983.
- First certified as an EMT in 1979 in upstate New York.
- Has a full-time academic emergency medicine practice at Penn Medicine in Philadelphia, where he also serves as the Medical Director for PENNStar Flight.
- Is board-certified in both Emergency Medicine and Emergency Medical Services.
- Has served as medical editor for numerous Brady EMT and First Responder texts.
- Lives in Chester County, Pennsylvania, where he is married to Debbie and has two sons, Steve and Alex.

A Guide to...

KEY FEATURES

9

Airway Management

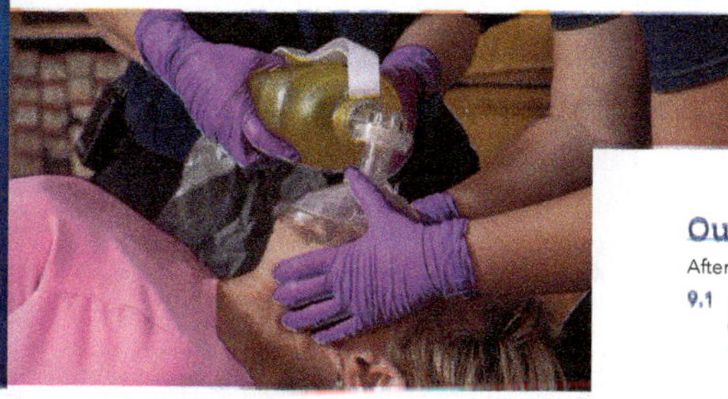

Related Chapters

The following chapters provide additional information re discussed in this chapter:

- 3 Lifting and Moving Patients
- 6 Anatomy and Physiology
- 7 Principles of Pathophysiology
- 10 Respiration and Artificial Ventilation
- 19 Respiratory Emergencies

Standard

Airway Management, Respiration, and Artificial Vent Management)

Competency

Applies knowledge (fundamental depth, foundational bre anatomy and physiology to patient assessment and manag a patent airway, adequate mechanical ventilation, and respir of all ages.

Core Concepts

- Physiology of the airway
- Pathophysiology of the airway

Outcomes

After reading this chapter, you should be able to:

9.1 Describe the structure and function of the normal airway. (pp. 203-206)
- Differentiate the structures of the upper airway from those of the lower airway.
- Match airway structures to their functions.

9.2 Explain concepts of airway pathophysiology. (pp. 206-210)
- List causes of obstruction of the upper and lower airway.
- List the steps to airway assessment in the primary assessment.
- Distinguish between signs that indicate absent breathing, inadequate airway, and adequate airway.
- List signs of inadequate airway that are more likely in children than in adults.
- Explain how to determine whether a patient's airway status may worsen.

9.3 Describe the use of manual maneuvers to open the airway. (pp. 210-216)
- Given a scenario, provide a rationale for selecting the type of manual maneuver that is best for the patient in the scenario.

9.4 Explain the use of adjunctive equipment to manage a patient's airway. (pp. 216-234)
- State the importance of having a suction device immediately available during airway management procedures.
- Given scenarios, identify adherence to general rules for using airway adjuncts.
- Describe how the features of an oropharyngeal airway allow it to provide an air passage in patients who cannot maintain their own airways.
- List the sequence of steps used in the insertion of an oropharyngeal airway.
- Identify instances when a nasopharyngeal airway offers benefits over an oropharyngeal airway.
- List the sequence of steps used in the insertion of a nasopharyngeal airway.
- Describe the minimum features required of suction units.
- Match the components and attachments of suction devices with their designed purposes.
- Suggest responses to complications encountered when suctioning a patient's airway.

201

CORE CONCEPTS Highlight the key points addressed in each chapter. The topics not only help students anticipate chapter content, but also guide their studies through the textbook and supplements.

Core Concepts

- Physiology of the airway
- Pathophysiology of the airway

CORE CONCEPT
Components of the secondary assessment

OBJECTIVES Objectives form the basis of each chapter and were developed around the Education Standards and Instructional Guidelines.

Outcomes

After reading this chapter, you should be able to:

9.1 Describe the structure and function of the normal airway. (pp. 203-206)
- Differentiate the structures of the upper airway from those of the lower airway.
- Match airway structures to their functions.

9.2 Explain concepts of airway pathophysiology. (pp. 206-210)
- List causes of obstruction of the upper and lower airway.
- List the steps to airway assessment in the primary assessment.
- Distinguish between signs that indicate absent breathing, inadequate airway, and adequate airway.
- List signs of inadequate airway that are more likely in children than in adults.
- Explain how to determine whether a patient's airway status may worsen.

VISUAL GUIDES Visually present patient assessment in a series of flow charts.

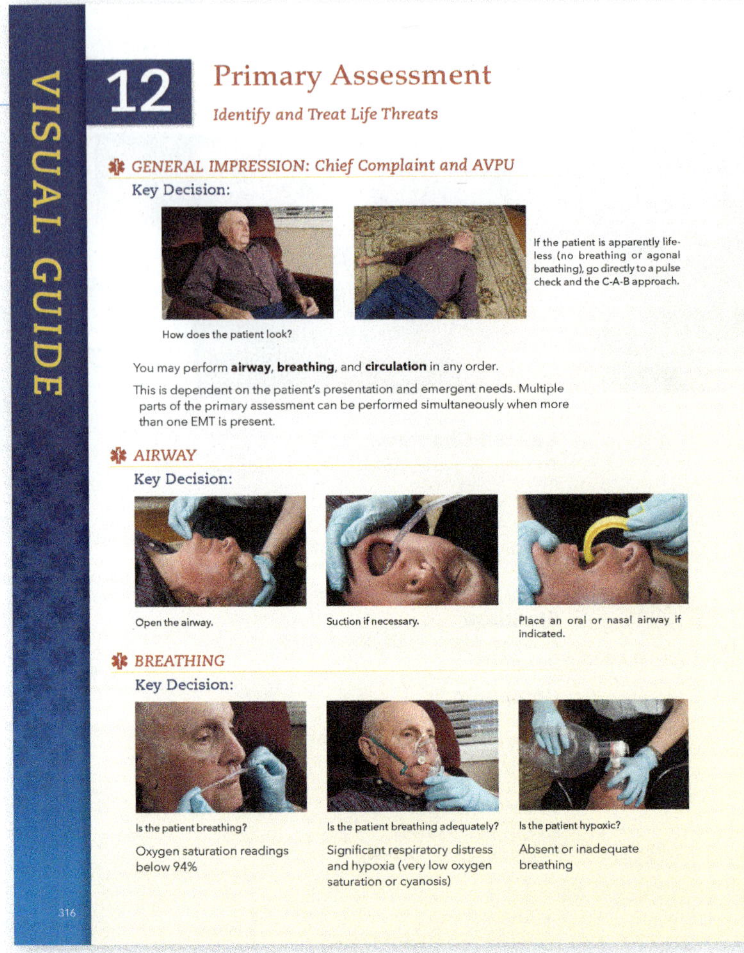

VISUAL GUIDE

12 Primary Assessment

Identify and Treat Life Threats

GENERAL IMPRESSION: *Chief Complaint and AVPU*

Key Decision:

How does the patient look?

If the patient is apparently lifeless (no breathing or agonal breathing), go directly to a pulse check and the C-A-B approach.

You may perform **airway**, **breathing**, and **circulation** in any order.

This is dependent on the patient's presentation and emergent needs. Multiple parts of the primary assessment can be performed simultaneously when more than one EMT is present.

AIRWAY

Key Decision:

Open the airway.

Suction if necessary.

Place an oral or nasal airway if indicated.

BREATHING

Key Decision:

Is the patient breathing?

Oxygen saturation readings below 94%

Is the patient breathing adequately?

Significant respiratory distress and hypoxia (very low oxygen saturation or cyanosis)

Is the patient hypoxic?

Absent or inadequate breathing

316

"The most important things we can do for our patients are in the A-B-Cs."

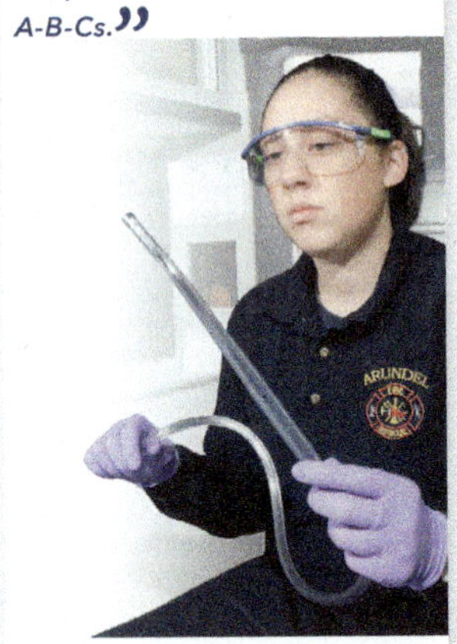

(© Daniel Limmer)

VOICES Insights or facts from EMTs in the field.

Point of View

"It happened so fast. I knew I was allergic to bees, but I never had a reaction that bad. It was like all of a sudden, I just couldn't breathe. I was fine just a few moments earlier, then my voice started to get real raspy and I could barely take a breath. I thought I was going to die. I remember the EMTs arriving, but not much more. I know they helped me with a dose of epinephrine, but by the time I regained consciousness, I was at the hospital. That medicine saved my life."

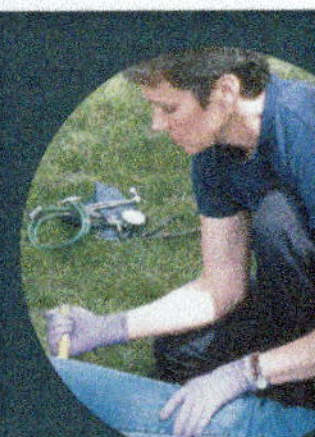

POINT OF VIEW Tells stories of EMS care from the patient's perspective and includes photos that illustrate the patient's viewpoint.

PATIENT CARE SECTIONS Provide descriptions of the fundamental principles and critical actions needed for various patient care scenarios.

Patient Care

Care of the Patient with Severe Choking

Fundamental Principles of Care

Severe choking implies that the airway is completely blocked by a foreign body. It is indicated (and differentiated from nonsevere choking) by an inability to move air. Here the patient is not breathing, coughing, or speaking. This situation requires immediate intervention.

In patients with signs and symptoms indicating severe choking, take the following steps:

- Call for advanced life support assistance.
- Immediately assess for air movement. If no air movement is found, begin foreign-body airway maneuvers.
- For conscious adults and children (patients over the age of 1 year), initiate abdominal thrusts.
- For conscious infants (patients 1 year old or younger), initiate back slaps and chest thrusts.
- For any unconscious choking patient, or a patient who becomes unconscious due to choking, begin CPR.

THINK LIKE AN EMT A scenario-based feature that offers practice in making critical decisions.

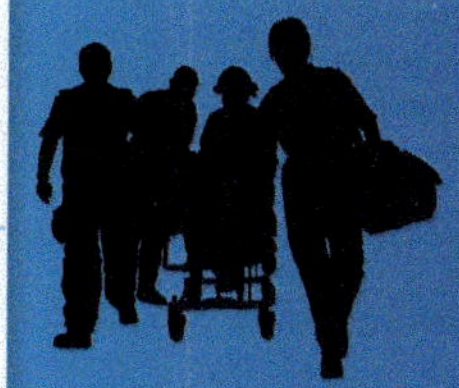

Think Like an EMT

Will the Airway Stay Open?

You have learned about the signs of an unstable airway. Use this information to consider whether the following patients have airways that will stay open.

1. A 16-year-old asthma patient who tells you he is tired and seems to be nodding off to sleep
2. A 72-year-old female who was recently diagnosed with pneumonia. Today she has called you because her breathing is much worse. She is breathing rapidly and has diminished lung sounds on the left side.
3. A 35-year-old male who tells you he is having trouble breathing. You notice he is drooling and is sitting bolt upright. When you attempt to lean him back on the stretcher, he coughs, gags, and repositions himself in a sniffing position.
4. A 16-month-old whose mother tells you the child has had a cold for two days and woke up with a cough tonight. The child is awake and alert but barking like a seal when coughing.

CHAPTER REVIEW Includes a summary of key points, key terms and definitions, review questions, and critical-thinking exercises that ask students to apply knowledge, case studies, and more.

Chapter Review

Key Facts and Concepts

- The primary assessment is a systematic approach to quickly finding and treating immediate threats to life.
- The general impression, although somewhat subjective, can provide extremely useful information regarding the urgency of a patient's condition.
- The determination of mental status follows the AVPU approach.
- Evaluating airway, breathing, and circulation quickly but thoroughly will reveal immediate threats to life that must be treated before the EMT proceeds further with assessment.
- Your approach to a patient will vary depending on how the patient presents. The American Heart Association recommends a C-A-B approach for patients who appear lifeless and apparently are not breathing or have only agonal respirations. This begins with a pulse check and chest compressions if there is no pulse.
- If your patient shows signs of life (e.g., moving, moaning, talking) and is breathing, you will take a traditional A-B-C approach.
- Remember that the mnemonic *A-B-C* is a guide to interventions that may be taken. You will choose your interventions based on the patient's immediate needs. They may be done in any order that fits the patient's needs.
- The patient's priority describes how urgent the patient's need to be transported is and how to conduct the rest of your assessment.

Key Decisions

- Is this patient medical or trauma; responsive or unresponsive; adult, child, or infant?
- Does this patient have any signs of life?
- Does this patient require a C-A-B approach (likely in cardiac arrest)? Does the patient therefore require chest compressions and defibrillation as the first priority?
- Do I need to stop and suction the airway, insert an artificial airway, administer oxygen, or ventilate the patient?
- Is the patient's condition stable enough to allow further assessment and treatment at the scene?

Chapter Glossary

A-B-Cs airway, breathing, and circulation.

AVPU a memory aid for classifying a patient's level of responsiveness or mental status. The letters stand for alert, verbal response, painful response, unresponsive.

chief complaint in emergency medicine, the reason EMS was called, usually in the patient's own words.

general impression impression of the patient's condition that is formed on first approaching the patient, based on the patient's environment, chief complaint, and appearance.

interventions actions taken to correct or manage a patient's problems.

manual stabilization using one's hands to prevent movement of a patient's head and neck until a cervical collar can be applied.

mental status level of responsiveness.

primary assessment the first element in a patient assessment; steps taken for the purpose of discovering and dealing with any life-threatening problems. The six parts of primary assessment are: (1) forming a general impression, (2) assessing mental status, (3) assessing airway, (4) assessing breathing, (5) assessing circulation, and (6) determining the priority of the patient for treatment and transport to the hospital.

priority the decision regarding the need for immediate transport of the patient versus further assessment and care at the scene.

spinal motion restriction a procedure for limiting movement of the head, neck, and spine when spinal injury is possible or likely.

Preparation for Your Examination and Practice

Short Answer

1. List factors you will take into account in forming a general impression of a patient.
2. Explain how to assess a patient's mental status with regard to the AVPU levels of responsiveness.
3. Explain how to assess airway, breathing, and circulation during the primary assessment. Explain the interventions you will take for possible problems with airway, breathing, and circulation.
4. Explain the C-A-B approach to the primary assessment, and explain the circumstances in which the C-A-B approach would be appropriate.

335

STUDENT RESOURCE

WORKBOOK FOR EMERGENCY CARE, 14TH EDITION This self-paced workbook contains updated and revised matching exercises, multiple-choice questions, short-answer questions, labeling exercises, skills checklists, and case studies that promote critical decision making, and a NEW Grey Zone feature with real-life practice scenarios. This workbook is available for purchase at www.bradybooks.com.

MyLab BRADY

www.mybradylab.com

What Is MyLab Brady?

Part of the world's leading collection of online homework, tutorial, and assessment products, Pearson **MyLab BRADY** is designed with a single purpose in mind: to improve the results of all higher education students, one student at a time.

With input from more than 11 million student users annually, **Pearson MyLab** creates online learning experiences that are truly personalized and continuously adaptive. **MyLab** reacts to how students are actually performing, offering data-driven guidance that helps them better absorb course material and understand difficult concepts.

Pearson also provides **Learning Management System (LMS) integration services** so you can easily access **MyLab BRADY** from Blackboard Learn, Brightspace by D2L, Canvas, or Moodle. From a single course section to delivery across an entire institution, we offer the integration, support, and training you need.

Understand How Your Students Make Decisions

Decision-Making Cases take EMT students through typical real-world scenarios. These branching cases give students practice with critical thinking, gathering patient data, and making decisions for care and treatment. Access all of the multimedia resources for your text in one place.

Multimedia Library

Each MyLab BRADY course comes with a Multimedia Library full of supporting visual and audio media, and other resources. Use it to build assignments, supplement your lectures, or give your students access to a wealth of related material. Support the learning needs of individuals and the entire class.

Results

Instructors can view students' results by chapter, outcome, homework, and more—to identify where more classroom time is needed. Digital access anytime, anywhere.

Pearson eText

The Pearson eText gives students access to their textbook anytime, anywhere, **on the device of their choice, including PC, tablet, or smartphone**. In addition to note taking, highlighting, and bookmarking, the Pearson eText offers interactive and sharing features. Rich media options let students watch lecture and example videos as they read or do their homework. Instructors can share their comments or highlights, and students can add their own, creating a tight community of learners in your class.

Where Can Instructors Get More Information?

Contact us at **www.mybradylab.com/contactus** for more information.

BRIEF CONTENTS

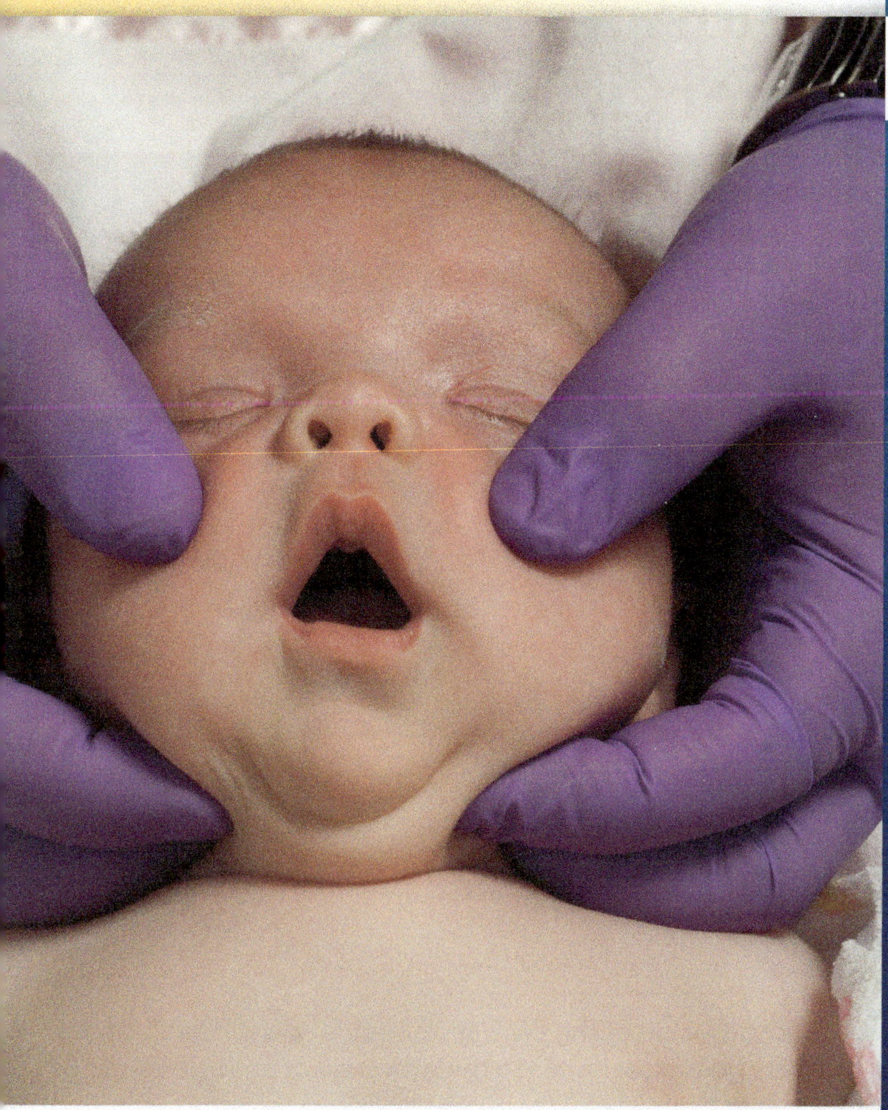

SECTION 1

Foundations

The "Foundations" section details essential concepts and skills you will need as an Emergency Medical Technician.

Chapter 1 gives an overview of the Emergency Medical Services and the health care system. Chapter 2 emphasizes how to keep yourself safe and well. Chapter 3 explains techniques for safe lifting and moving. Chapter 4 discusses legal and ethical issues you will face as part of your career.

Chapter 5 provides basic information about how medical terms are constructed. Chapter 6 offers an overview of the structure (anatomy) and function (physiology) of the human body. Chapter 7 introduces principles of pathophysiology: how illness and injury affect the body. Finally, Chapter 8 concerns life span development: physical and mental patterns common to the different age groups who will be your patients.

1

Introduction to Emergency Medical Services

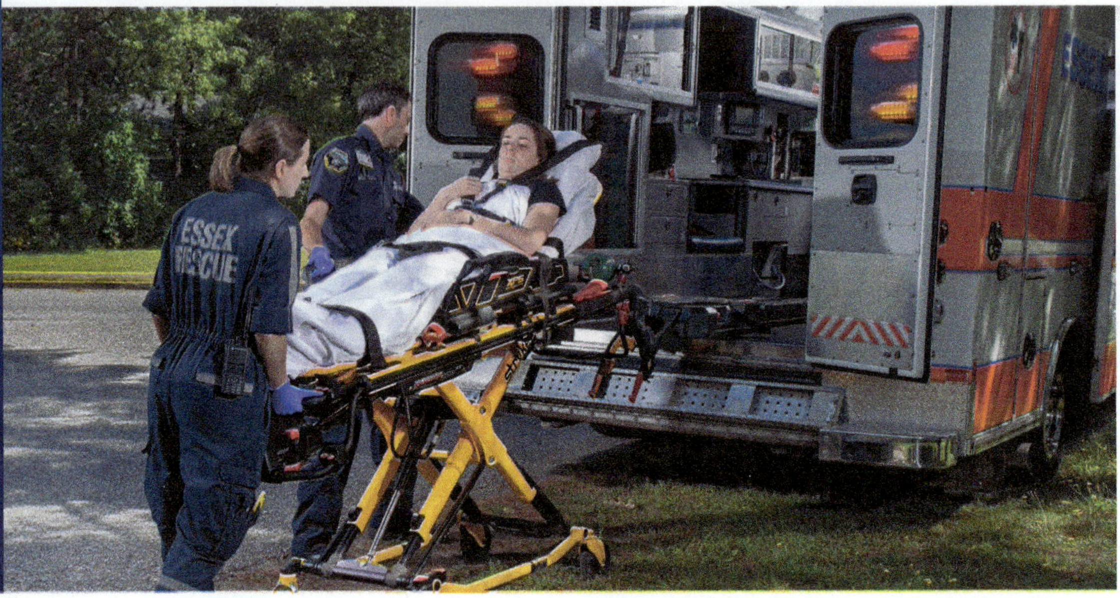

Standard

Preparatory (EMS Systems; Research); Public Health

Competency

Applies fundamental knowledge of the EMS system, safety/well-being of the EMT, and medical/legal and ethical issues to the provision of emergency care.

Core Concepts

- The chain of human resources that forms the EMS system
- How the public activates the EMS system
- Your roles and responsibilities as an EMT
- The process of EMS quality improvement

Outcomes

After reading this chapter, you should be able to:

1.1 Describe the components of the EMS system. (pp. 3–8)
- Describe the connections between EMS history and EMS today.
- Recognize components that make up EMS systems.
- Diagram the chain of human resources in EMS systems.
- Describe the communications systems by which the public can access EMS.

1.2 Summarize the roles and responsibilities of EMTs. (pp. 9–15)
- Explain the different levels of EMS training.
- Describe the tasks within the roles and responsibilities of an EMT.

- Explain the traits of an EMT that convey professionalism.
- Explain the EMT's role in quality improvement.
- Explain the role of an EMS system physician Medical Director.

1.3 Describe the connection between public health and EMS systems. (pp. 16–17)

- List ways that EMS systems can support public health.

1.4 Summarize the role of evidence-based research in EMS. (pp. 17–19)

- Identify ways research impacts EMS.
- Explain the evidence-based process for EMTs.
- Compare the different methods of medical research.
- Explain how to evaluate medical research.

Key Terms

evidence-based techniques, *17*
medical direction, *14*
Medical Director, *14*
911 system, *7*
off-line medical direction, *15*
on-line medical direction, *15*
patient outcomes, *17*
peer reviewed, *19*
protocols, *14*
quality improvement, *13*
standing orders, *14*

When a person is injured or becomes ill, it rarely happens in a hospital with doctors and nurses standing by. In fact, some time usually passes between the onset of the injury or illness and the patient's arrival at the hospital, time in which the patient's condition may deteriorate, or the patient may even die. The modern Emergency Medical Services (EMS) system has been developed to provide what is known as *prehospital* or *out-of-hospital* care. Its purpose is to get trained personnel to the patient as quickly as possible and to provide emergency care on the scene, en route to the hospital, and at the hospital until care is assumed by the hospital staff. The Emergency Medical Technician (EMT) is a key member of the EMS team.

As you begin to study for a career as an EMT, you will want to answer some basic questions, such as "What is the EMS system?" "How did it develop?" and "What will my role be in the system?" This chapter will help you begin to answer these questions.

The Emergency Medical Services System

How It Began

In the 1790s the French began to transport wounded soldiers away from the scene of battle so they could be cared for by physicians. This is the earliest documented Emergency Medical Service. However, no medical care was provided for the wounded on the battlefield. The idea was simply to carry the victim from the scene to a place where medical care was available.

Other wars inspired similar emergency services. For example, Clara Barton began such a service for the wounded during the American Civil War and later helped establish the American Red Cross. During World War I, many volunteers joined battlefield ambulance corps. And during the Korean Conflict and the Vietnam War, medical teams

> *"Where else can you work with great people, have fun, and make a difference? Welcome to EMS."*

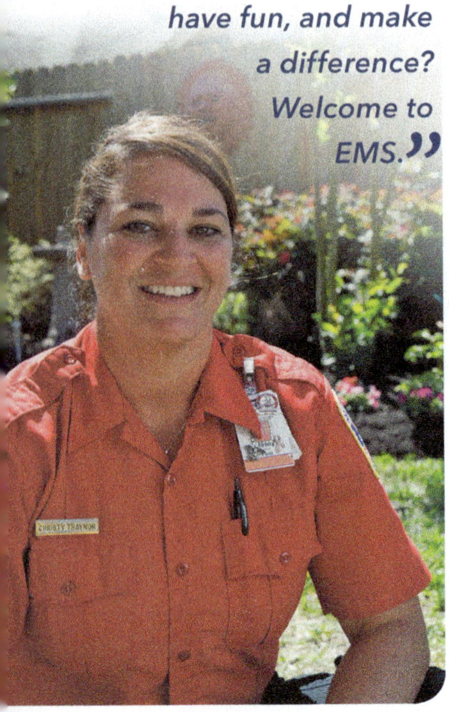

produced further advances in field care, many of which led to advances in the civilian sector, including specialized emergency medical centers devoted to the treatment of trauma (injuries). Lessons from military settings continue to provide new information for improving emergency care.

Nonmilitary ambulance services began in some major American cities in the early 1900s—again as transport services only, offering little or no emergency care. Smaller communities did not develop ambulance services until the late 1940s, after World War II. Often the local undertaker provided a hearse for ambulance transport. In locations where emergency care was offered along with transport to the hospital, the fire service often was the responsible agency.

The importance of providing hospital-quality care at the emergency scene—that is, beginning care at the scene and continuing it, uninterrupted, during transport to the hospital—soon became apparent. The need to organize systems for such emergency prehospital care and to train personnel to provide it also was recognized.

EMS Today

During the 1960s, the development of the modern EMS system began. In 1966 the National Highway Safety Act charged the U.S. Department of Transportation (DOT) with developing EMS standards and assisting the states to upgrade the quality of their prehospital emergency care. Most EMT courses today are based on models developed by the DOT.

In 1970 the National Registry of Emergency Medical Technicians was founded to establish professional standards. In 1973 the U.S. Congress passed the National Emergency Medical Services Systems Act as the cornerstone of a federal effort to implement and improve EMS systems across the United States.

Since then, the states have gained more control over their EMS systems, although the federal government continues to provide guidance and support. For example, the National Highway Traffic Safety Administration (NHTSA) Technical Assistance Program has established an assessment program with a set of standards for EMS systems. The categories and standards set forth by NHTSA, summarized in the following list, will be discussed in more detail throughout this chapter and the rest of this textbook.

- **Regulation and policy.** Each state EMS system must have in place enabling legislation (laws that allow the system to exist), a lead EMS agency, a funding mechanism, regulations, policies, and procedures.
- **Resource management.** There must be centralized coordination of resources so that all victims of trauma or medical emergencies have equal access to basic emergency care and transport by certified personnel, in a licensed and equipped ambulance, to an appropriate facility.
- **Human resources and training.** At a minimum, all those transporting prehospital personnel (those who ride the ambulances) should be trained to the EMT level using National EMS Education Standards that are taught by qualified instructors.
- **Transportation.** Safe, reliable ambulance transportation is a critical component. Most patients can be effectively transported by ground ambulances. Other patients require rapid transportation, or transportation from remote areas, by helicopter or airplane.
- **Facilities.** The seriously ill or injured patient must be delivered in a timely manner to the closest appropriate facility.
- **Communications.** There must be an effective communications system that encompasses the universal system access number (911) and dispatch-to-ambulance, ambulance-to-ambulance, ambulance-to-hospital, and hospital-to-hospital communications.
- **Public information and education.** EMS personnel may participate in efforts to educate the public about their role in the system, their ability to access the system, and prevention of injuries.

FIGURE 1-1 Some methods of delivering Emergency Medical Services: (A) By bicycle. (B) By mobile EMS unit.

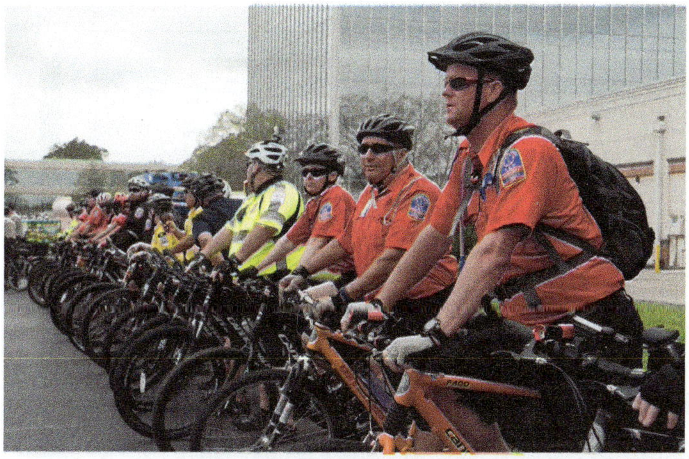

A

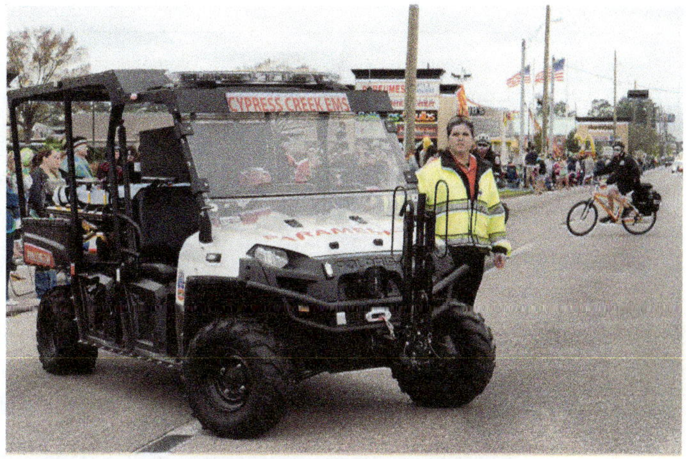

B

- **Medical direction.** Each EMS system must have a physician as a Medical Director who is accountable for the activities of EMS personnel within that system. The Medical Director must be involved in all aspects of the patient-care system, including protocol development, training, and quality improvement.
- **Trauma systems.** In each state, enabling legislation must exist to develop a trauma system including one or more trauma centers, triage and transfer guidelines for trauma patients, rehabilitation programs, data collection, mandatory autopsies (examination of a body to determine cause of death), and means for managing and ensuring the quality of the system.
- **Evaluation.** Each state must have a program for evaluating and improving the effectiveness of the EMS system, known as a quality improvement (QI) program, a quality assurance (QA) program, or total quality management (TQM).

With the development of the modern EMS system, the concept of ambulance service as a means merely for transporting the sick and injured passed into oblivion. No longer could ambulance personnel be viewed as people with little more than the strength to lift a patient into and out of an ambulance. Instead, the EMS system extended the hospital emergency department to reach the sick and injured at the emergency scene. "Victims" became patients, receiving prehospital assessment and emergency care from highly trained professionals. The "ambulance attendant" was replaced by the Emergency Medical Technician.

Becoming an EMT now offers even more possibilities for advancement in EMS (Figure 1-1). In addition to the traditional path to Advanced Emergency Medical Technician (AEMT) and paramedic, opportunities exist in tactical EMS, Mobile Integrated Healthcare (community paramedicine), and employment in emergency departments. Many colleges and universities have degrees specifically focused on EMS majors such as paramedic and EMS leadership programs.

Components of the EMS System

To understand the EMS system, you must look at it from the patient's viewpoint rather than from that of the EMT (Figure 1-2). For the patient, care begins with the initial phone call to the Emergency Medical Dispatcher (EMD). The EMS system responds to the call for help by sending to the scene available responders, including Emergency Medical Responders, EMTs, and advanced life support providers (Advanced EMTs and paramedics). An ambulance will transport the patient to the hospital.

CORE CONCEPT

The chain of human resources that forms the EMS system

FIGURE 1-2 The chain of human resources making up the EMS system. *(Emergency Department staff, Allied health staff photos: © Edward T. Dickinson, MD)*

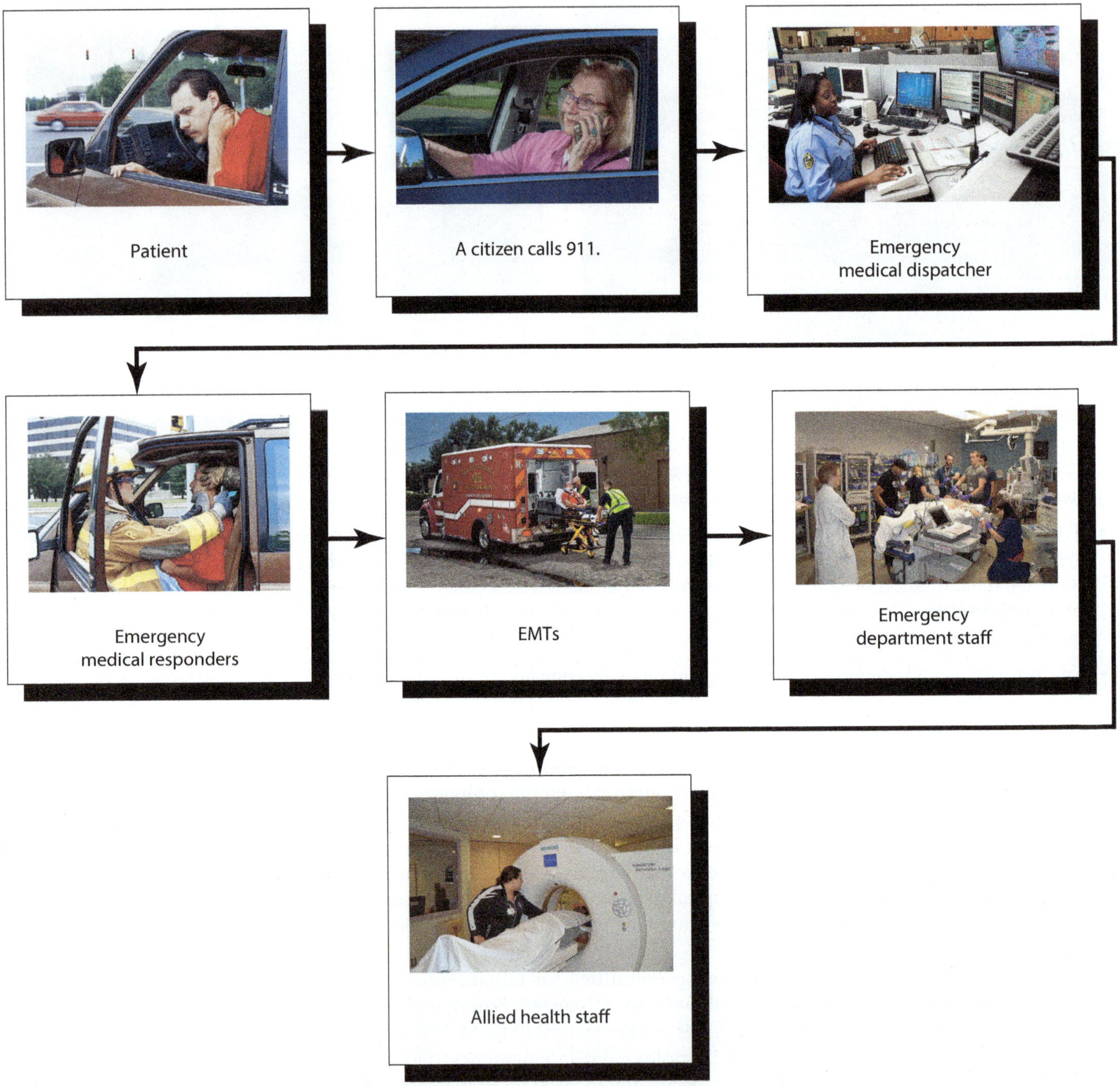

From the ambulance, the patient is received by the emergency department. There, the patient receives laboratory tests, diagnosis, and further treatment. The emergency department serves as the gateway for the rest of the services offered by the hospital. If a patient is brought to the emergency department with serious injuries, care is given to stabilize the patient, and the operating room is readied to provide further lifesaving measures.

Some hospitals handle all routine and emergency cases but have a specialty that sets them apart from other hospitals. One specialty hospital is the trauma center. In some hospitals a surgery team may not be available at all times. In a trauma center, surgery teams capable of the comprehensive treatment of trauma patients are available 24 hours a day.

In addition to trauma centers, there are also hospitals that specialize in the care of certain conditions and patients, such as burn centers, pediatric centers, cardiac centers, and stroke centers.

As an EMT, you will become familiar with the hospital resources available in your area. Many EMS regions have specific criteria for transporting patients with special needs. Choosing the right hospital may actually be a lifesaving decision. Of course, it is important to weigh the patient's condition against the additional transport time that may be required to reach a specialized facility. On-line medical direction (discussed later) may be available to help with this decision.

Dispatchers and EMTs are key members of the prehospital EMS team. (The levels of EMS training will be discussed later in the chapter.) Many others make up the hospital portion of the EMS system. They include physicians, nurses, physician's assistants, respiratory and physical therapists, technicians, aides, and others.

Accessing the EMS System

For 99% of the population, a ***911 system*** provides telephone access to report emergencies. A dispatcher answers the call, takes the information, and alerts EMS, the fire department, and law enforcement as needed. According to the National Emergency Number Association, about 240 million calls are received by 911 centers each year, and more than 80% of those calls come from mobile devices. Wireless carriers and 911 centers are working together on two phases of development so that emergency dispatchers can see the number the mobile caller is calling from (phase 1) and identify the actual physical location of the mobile device (phase 2). Success in developing this capacity will have a huge impact on locating and providing care to ill or injured callers. VoIP (Voice over Internet Protocol) also poses challenges for communication centers in locating callers. Technological solutions are in the works for this issue as well.

911 system
a system for telephone access to report emergencies. A dispatcher takes the information and alerts EMS or the fire or police department as needed. *Enhanced 911* also identifies the caller's phone number and location automatically.

CORE CONCEPT
How the public activates the EMS system

Enhanced 911 centers have the capability of identifying the caller's landline phone number and location automatically, and some have the additional capability of locating wireless callers. This enables the dispatcher to send emergency personnel to the scene even if the phone is disconnected or the patient loses consciousness.

Another development in the communication and dispatch portion of the EMS system is the training and certification of emergency medical directors (EMDs). Not only do these specially trained dispatchers obtain the appropriate information from callers, but they also provide medical instructions for emergency care. These include instructions for CPR, artificial ventilation, bleeding control, and more. Research has consistently pointed to the importance of early access and prompt initiation of emergency care and CPR. The EMD is one example of the EMS system providing emergency care at the earliest possible moment.

Levels of EMS Training

There are four general levels of EMS training and certification (described in the following list). These levels may vary slightly from place to place. Your instructor will explain any variations that exist in your region or state.

1. **Emergency Medical Responder (EMR).** This level of training is designed for the person who is often first at the scene. Many police officers, firefighters, and industrial health personnel function in this capacity. The emphasis is on activating the EMS system and providing immediate care for life-threatening injuries, controlling the scene, and preparing for the arrival of the ambulance.

2. **Emergency Medical Technician (EMT).** In most areas, EMT certification is considered the minimum level of training for ambulance personnel. EMTs provide basic-level medical and trauma care and transportation to a medical facility and frequently work with advanced-level EMS providers.

3. **Advanced Emergency Medical Technician (AEMT).** The AEMT, like the EMT, provides basic-level care and transportation but also provides some advanced-level care. Advanced care may include use of advanced airway devices and administration of some fluids or medications via intravenous (IV) and intraosseous (IO) routes.
4. **Paramedic.** The paramedic performs all of the skills of the EMT and AEMT plus additional advanced-level assessment, decision making, and skills. The paramedic provides the most advanced level of prehospital care.

In some states, specially trained registered nurses and physicians can also hold prehospital certification and provide even more advanced patient care as part of the prehospital EMS system (Figure 1-3).

FIGURE 1-3 (Left) As an EMT, you will work with patients of many ages, from older adults to newborns. (Right) Specially trained physicians and RNs may provide advanced care as part of the prehospital care in some EMS systems. Some states have a prehospital EMS system that can provide more advanced patient care at the scene. *(Right photo: © Edward T. Dickinson, MD)*

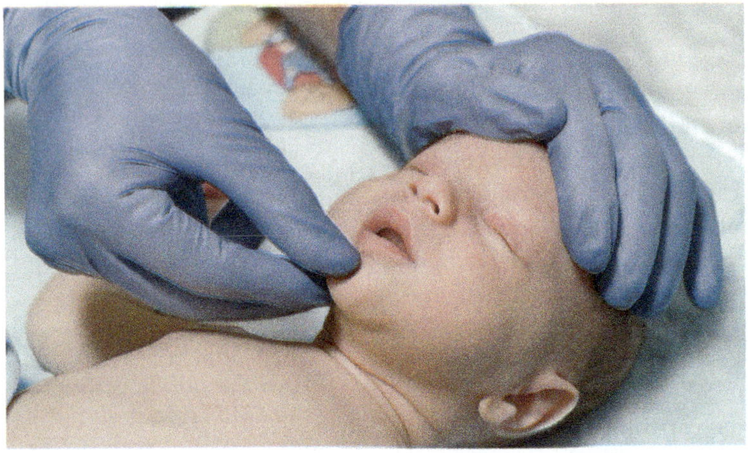

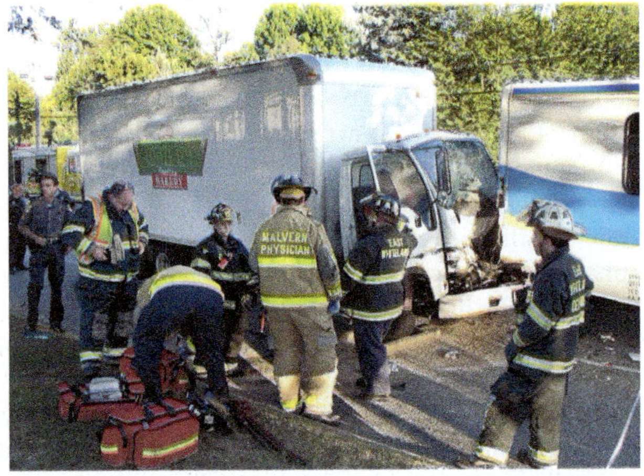

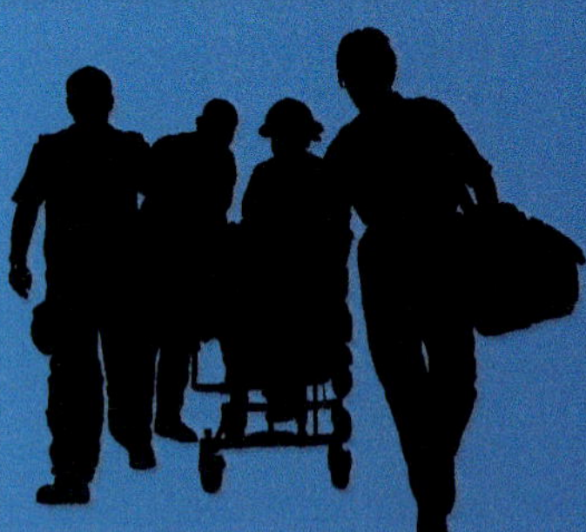

Think Like an EMT

A Key Concept

Critical decision making is a very important concept. It essentially means that an EMT takes in information from the scene, the patient assessment, and other sources and makes appropriate decisions after synthesizing—or interpreting—all the information. There are times when the information you obtain initially won't be enough to be a basis for decision making. When this happens, you will need to ask more questions and perform additional examinations to get everything you need to make a decision.

It may be difficult to see how this all fits together now. Before long, however, you'll be learning and practicing patient assessment and care. Some examples of critical decision making that will be a part of the assessment and care you will perform include:

1. *Deciding which hospital to transport someone to.* Should you take your patient to the closest hospital or to a more distant specialty hospital?
2. *Deciding whether you should administer a medication to a patient.* Will it help the patient's current condition? Could it make the condition worse?

When you begin to work with more experienced EMTs, you will come across many who are smart and know what to do and how to treat patients (both clinically and personally). These are the EMTs you would want to take care of you or your family should EMS be needed. These EMTs are good critical decision makers.

Roles and Responsibilities of the EMT

As an EMT, you will be responsible for a wide range of activities. In addition to patient assessment and emergency care, your responsibilities will include preparation, safe response to the scene, safe transportation to the hospital, and transferring the patient to hospital personnel for continuity of care. The following are specific areas of responsibility for the EMT.

CORE CONCEPT
Your roles and responsibilities as an EMT

- **Personal safety.** It is not possible to help patients if you are injured before you reach them or while you are providing care, so your first responsibility is to keep yourself safe. Safety concerns include dangers from other human beings, animals, unstable buildings, fires, and more. EMTs may be called to respond to incidents where mass violence has occurred, including shootings, explosions, and attacks with vehicles. Though emergency scenes are usually safe, they also can be unpredictable. You must take care at all times to stay safe.
- **Safety of the crew, patient, and bystanders.** The same dangers you face will also be faced by others at the scene. As a professional, you must be concerned with their safety as well as your own.
- **Working with other public safety professionals.** As an EMT you will work closely with advanced EMS providers, firefighters, police officers, specialty rescue teams, and others.
- **Patient assessment.** As an EMT, one of your most important functions will be assessment of your patient, or finding out enough about what is wrong with your patient to be able to provide appropriate emergency care. Assessment *always* precedes emergency care.
- **Patient care.** The actual care required for an individual patient may range from simple emotional support to life-saving CPR and defibrillation. Based on your assessment findings, patient care is an action or series of actions that your training will prepare you to take to help the patient deal with and survive illness or injury.
- **Lifting and moving.** Since EMTs are usually involved in transporting patients to the hospital, lifting and moving patients are important tasks. You must perform them without injury to yourself and without aggravating or adding to the patient's existing injuries.
- **Transport.** It is a serious responsibility to operate an ambulance at any time, but even more so when there is a patient on board. Safe operation of the ambulance and securing and caring for the patient in the ambulance will be important parts of your job as an EMT.
- **Transfer of care.** Upon arrival at the hospital, you will turn the patient over to hospital personnel. You will provide information on the patient's condition, your observations of the scene, and other pertinent data so that there will be continuity in the patient's care. Although this part of patient care comes at the end of the call, it is crucial. You must never abandon care of the patient at the hospital until transfer to hospital personnel has been properly completed.
- **Patient advocacy.** As an EMT, you are there for your patients. You are an advocate, the person who speaks up for your patients and pleads their cause. It is your responsibility to address each patient's needs and to bring patients' concerns to the attention of the hospital staff. You will have developed a rapport with the patient during your brief but very important time together, a rapport that gives you an understanding of the patient's condition and needs. As an advocate, you will do your best to transmit this knowledge to help the patient continue through the EMS and hospital systems. In your role as an advocate, you may perform a task as important as reporting information that will enable the hospital staff to save the patient's life or as simple as making sure a relative of the patient is notified. Actions that may seem minor to you often provide major comfort to your patient.

EMTs may also be involved in community health initiatives such as injury prevention. The EMT is in a position to observe situations where injuries are possible and to help correct them before injuries, or further injuries, are sustained. Hospital personnel do not see the scene and cannot offer this information. An example might be a call to the residence of a senior citizen who has fallen. You make observations about improper railings or slippery throw rugs and bring this to the attention of the patient and the family. Another instance where injury prevention may be beneficial is with children. If you respond to a residence where there are small children and you observe potential for injury (e.g., poisons the child can access or unsafe conditions such as a loose railing), your interventions can make a difference. These community health issues are discussed throughout the book and in the chapter *Poisoning and Overdose Emergencies*.

Traits of a Good EMT

Certain physical traits and aspects of personality are desirable for an EMT.

Physical Traits

Physically, you should be in good health and fit to carry out your duties. If you are unable to provide needed care because you cannot bend over or catch your breath, then all your training may be worthless to the patient who is in need of your help.

You should be able to lift and carry up to 125 pounds (57 kg). Practice with other EMTs is essential so you can learn how to carry your share of the combined weight of the patient, stretcher, linens, blankets, and portable oxygen equipment. For such moves, you need coordination and dexterity as well as strength. You will have to perform basic rescue procedures, lower stretchers and patients from upper levels, and negotiate fire escapes and stairways while carrying patients.

Your eyesight is very important in performing your EMT duties. Make certain that you can clearly see distant objects as well as those close at hand. Both types of vision are needed for patient assessment, reading labels, controlling emergency scenes, and driving. Any eyesight problems must be corrected (as with prescription eyeglasses or contact lenses) in order to provide safe patient care.

Be aware of any problems you may have with color vision. Not only is this important when driving, but it could also be critical for patient assessment. Color of the patient's skin, lips, and nail beds often provides valuable clues to the patient's condition.

You should be able to give and receive oral and written instructions and communicate with the patient, bystanders, and other members of the EMS system. Eyesight, hearing, and speech are important to the EMT, so any significant problems must be corrected if you are going to be an EMT.

Personal Traits

Good personal traits are very important in an EMT (Figure 1-4). You should be:

- *Pleasant* to inspire confidence and help to calm the sick and injured.
- *Sincere* to be able to convey an understanding of the situation and the patient's feelings.
- *Cooperative* to allow for faster and better care, establish better coordination with other members of the EMS system, and bolster the confidence of patients and bystanders.
- *Resourceful* to be able to adapt a tool or technique to fit an unusual situation.
- *A self-starter* to show initiative and accomplish what must be done without having to depend on someone else to start procedures.
- *Emotionally stable* to help overcome the unpleasant aspects of an emergency so that needed care may be given and any uneasy feelings that exist afterward may be resolved.
- *Able to lead* to take the steps necessary to control a scene, organize bystanders, deliver emergency care, and, when necessary, take charge.
- *Neat and clean* to promote confidence in both patients and bystanders and to reduce the possibility of contamination.

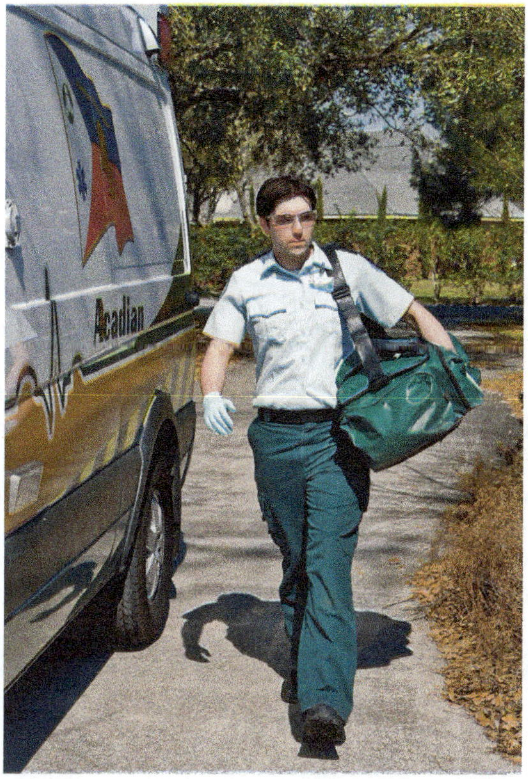

FIGURE 1-4 A professional appearance inspires confidence.

- *Of good moral character and respectful of others* to allow for trust in situations when patients cannot protect their own bodies or valuables and to convey all information truthfully and reliably.
- *In control of personal habits* to reduce the possibility of rendering improper care and to prevent patient discomfort. This includes never consuming alcohol within eight hours of duty and not smoking when providing care. (Remember: Smoking can contaminate wounds and is dangerous around oxygen delivery systems.)
- *Controlled in conversation and able to communicate properly* to inspire confidence and avoid inappropriate conversation that may upset or anger the patient or bystanders or violate patient confidentiality.
- *Able to listen to others* to be compassionate and empathetic, to be accurate with interviews, and to inspire confidence.
- *Nonjudgmental and fair*, treating all patients equally regardless of race, religion, lifestyle, or culture. You will encounter many cultural differences among patients. Figure 1-5 highlights one example of the cultures you may encounter in EMS. You will find additional features involving cultural issues throughout the book.

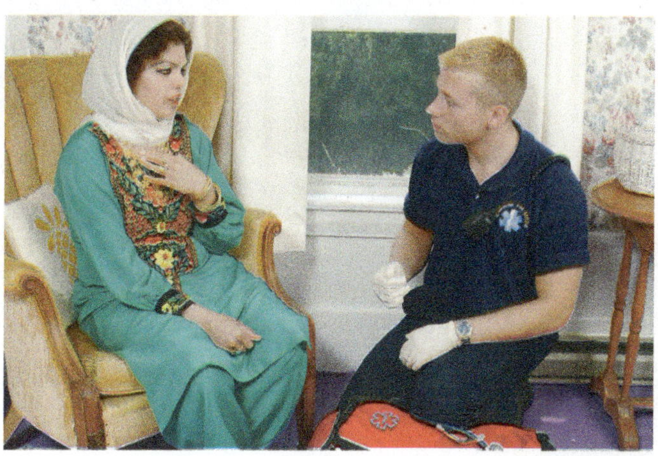

FIGURE 1-5 Your patients may come from a wide variety of cultures. As an example, Muslims such as this woman from Afghanistan have standards of modesty that may require examination by an EMT of the same sex.

Education

An EMT must maintain up-to-date knowledge and skills. Since ongoing research in emergency care causes frequent changes in procedure, some of the information you receive while you are studying to become an EMT will become outdated during your career—and sometimes during your course! You must always be prepared to update your understanding and practice with newer, evidence-based procedures.

There are many ways to stay current. One way is through refresher training. Most areas require recertification at regular intervals. Refresher courses present material to the EMT who has already been through a full course but needs to receive updated information. Refresher courses, which are usually shorter than original courses, are required at two- to four-year intervals.

Continuing education is another way to stay current. This type of training supplements the EMT's original course. It should not take the place of original training. For example, you may wish to learn more about pediatric or trauma skills or driving techniques. You can obtain this education in conferences and seminars and through lectures, classes, videos, or demonstrations.

It is important to realize that education is a constant process that extends long past your original EMT course.

Where Will You Become a Provider?

As an EMT, you will have a wide variety of opportunities to use the skills you will learn in class. EMTs are employed in public and private settings—such as fire departments, ambulance services, and in urban/industrial settings as well as rural/wilderness settings (Figure 1-6). In fact, most fire departments require their firefighters to be cross-trained as both firefighters and EMTs.

You may be taking this course as a volunteer. A large portion of the United States is served by volunteer fire departments and Emergency Medical Services. Your willingness to participate in training to help others is both necessary for and appreciated by your community.

National Registry of Emergency Medical Technicians

The National Registry of Emergency Medical Technicians (NREMT), as part of its effort to establish and maintain national standards for EMTs, provides registration to EMRs, EMTs, AEMTs, and paramedics. Registration is obtained by successful completion of NREMT practical and computer-based knowledge examinations. Holding an NREMT registration may help in reciprocity (transferring to another state or region). It is usually considered favorably when you apply for employment, even in areas where NREMT registration is not required (Figure 1-7).

FIGURE 1-6 There are many career opportunities for EMTs, including work in (A) urban/industrial settings and (B) rural/wilderness settings. *(Photo B: © Edward T. Dickinson, MD)*

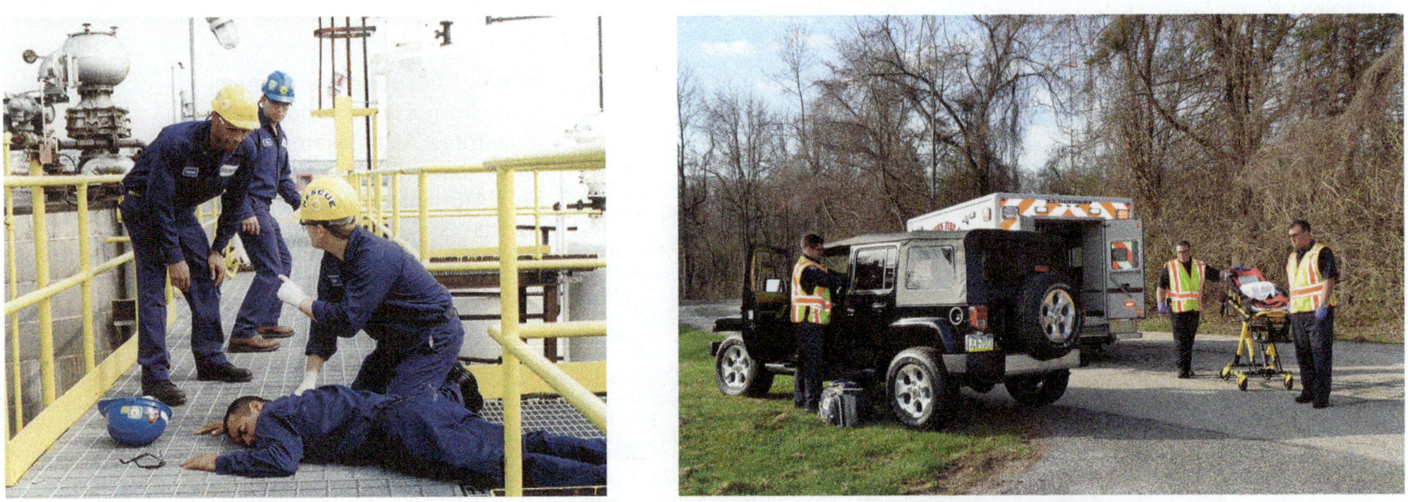

A B

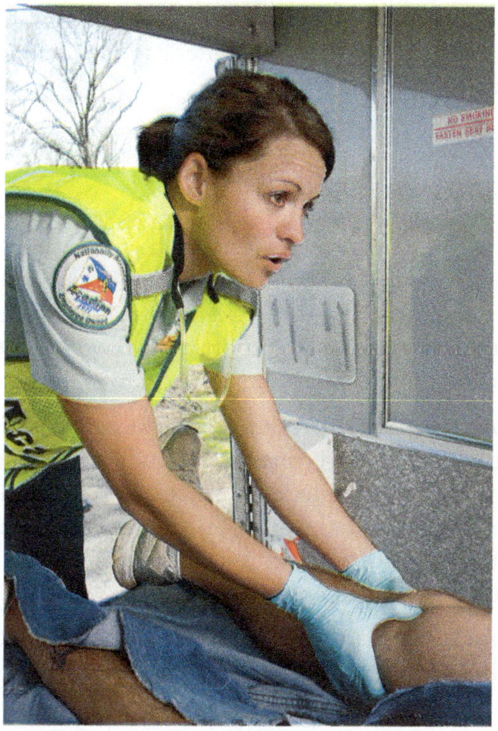

FIGURE 1-7 In many states an EMT candidate must have passed the NREMT exam to be licensed and certified by the state. This EMT practices in Louisiana, one state that requires NREMT registration.

Most states use the National Registry examinations as their certification exams. If your state or region does not use the registry exam, ask your instructor how you can sit for the examination. Upon passing the exam and obtaining registry, you will be entitled to wear the NREMT patch.

The National Registry is also active in EMS curriculum development and other issues that affect EMS today. For information, contact:

National Registry of Emergency Medical Technicians
6610 Busch Boulevard
P.O. Box 29233
Columbus, OH 43229
614-888-4484
www.nremt.org

Quality Improvement

Quality improvement, an important concept in EMS, consists of continuous self-review with the purpose of identifying aspects of the system that require improvement. Once a problem is identified, a plan is developed and implemented to prevent further occurrences of the same problem. As implied by the name, quality improvement is designed and performed to ensure that the public receives the highest-quality prehospital care.

quality improvement a process of continuous self-review with the purpose of identifying and correcting aspects of the system that require improvement.

A sample quality improvement review might go as follows:

As part of a continuous review of calls, the Quality Improvement (QI) committee has reviewed all of your squad's run reports that involve trauma during one particular month. The committee has noted that the time spent at the scene of serious trauma calls was excessive. (You will learn in later chapters that time at the scene of serious trauma should be kept to a minimum because the injured patient must be transported to the hospital for care that cannot be provided in the field.)

The QI committee has brought this fact to the attention of the Medical Director and the leadership of the ambulance squad. As a result, better protocols have been instituted. Monthly squad training is developed that covers topics such as how to identify serious trauma patients and that requires skill practice to reinforce techniques of trauma care. (Later in the year, the QI committee will review the same criteria to ensure that the extra training has been effective in improving the areas that were found to be deficient.)

CORE CONCEPT
The process of EMS quality improvement

During the review, the QI committee has also identified calls during which the crews followed procedures and performed well. A letter has been sent to these EMTs commending them for their efforts.

As an EMT, you will have a role in the quality improvement process. In fact, a dedication to quality can be one of the strongest assets of an EMT. There are several ways you can work toward quality care. These include:

- **Carefully preparing written documentation.** Call reviews are based on the prehospital care reports that you and other crew members write. If a report is incomplete, it is difficult for a QI team to assess the events of a call. If you are ever involved in a lawsuit, an inaccurate or incomplete report may also be a cause for liability. Be sure the reports you write are neat, complete, and accurate.
- **Becoming involved in the QI process.** As you gain experience, you may wish to volunteer for assignment to the QI committee. In addition, quality improvement can be implemented on every call. An individual ambulance crew can perform a critique after each call to determine things that went well and others that may need improvement. You can have another EMT or advanced EMT look over your report before turning it in to ensure it is accurate and complete.
- **Obtaining feedback from patients and the hospital staff.** This may be done informally or, in some cases, formally. Your organization may send a letter to patients that asks for comments on the care they were given while you were attending them. Hospital staff may be able to provide information that will help strengthen your care-giving skills.
- **Maintaining your equipment.** It will be difficult to provide quality care with substandard, damaged, or missing equipment. Although the ingenuity of EMTs should never be underestimated, it could be dangerous to administer oxygen or provide cardiac defibrillation without proper, functional equipment. Check and maintain equipment regularly.
- **Continuing your education.** An EMT who was certified several years ago and has never attended subsequent training will have a problem providing quality care. Seldom-used skills deteriorate without practice. Procedures change. Without some form of regular continuing education, it is difficult to maintain standards of quality.

Quality improvement is another name for providing the care that you would want to have provided to you or a loved one in a time of emergency. That is the best care possible. Maintaining continuous high quality is not easy; it requires constant attention and a sense of pride and obligation. Striving for quality—both in the care you personally give to patients and as a collective part of an ambulance squad—is the way to uphold the highest standards of the EMS system.

Medical Direction

Each EMS service or agency has a ***Medical Director***, a physician who assumes the ultimate responsibility for ***medical direction***, or oversight of the patient-care aspects of the EMS system. *Off-line medical direction* consists of standing orders issued by the Medical Director that allow EMTs to give certain medications or perform certain procedures without speaking to the Medical Director or another physician. *On-line medical direction* consists of orders from the on-duty physician given directly to an EMT in the field by radio or telephone.

The Medical Director also oversees training, develops ***protocols*** (lists of steps for assessment and interventions to be performed in different situations), and is a crucial part of the quality improvement process. Presence of a physician who is actively involved in an EMS system is one sign of a high-quality EMS agency.

The physician obviously cannot physically be at every call. This is why EMS systems develop ***standing orders***. The physician issues a policy or protocol that authorizes EMTs

Medical Director
a physician who assumes ultimate responsibility for the patient-care aspects of the EMS system.

medical direction
oversight of the patient-care aspects of an EMS system by the Medical Director. Direction can be either off-line or on-line.

protocols
lists of steps, such as assessments and interventions, to be taken in different situations. Protocols are developed by the Medical Director of an EMS system.

standing orders
a policy or protocol issued by a Medical Director that authorizes EMTs and others to perform particular skills in certain situations.

and others to perform particular skills in certain situations. An example may be the administration of naloxone. Naloxone is used to reverse opioid overdoses when the patient has a decreased respiratory drive. The Medical Director issues a standing order that allows EMTs to give naloxone in certain circumstances without speaking to the Medical Director or another physician. This kind of "behind the scenes" medical direction is called ***off-line medical direction***.

off-line medical direction standing orders issued by the Medical Director that allow EMTs to give certain medications or perform certain procedures without speaking to the Medical Director or another physician.

Certain other procedures that are not covered by standing orders or protocols require the EMT to contact the on-duty physician by radio or telephone prior to performing a skill or administering a medication. For example, EMTs carry aspirin, which is beneficial to many—but not all—patients who have possible cardiac symptoms. Prior to administering aspirin, you may be required to consult with the on-duty physician. You would use a radio or cell phone from the ambulance to provide patient information to the physician. After receiving your information, the physician would instruct you on whether and how to administer the aspirin. Orders from the on-duty physician given by radio or phone are called ***on-line medical direction***. On-line medical direction may be requested at any time you feel that medical advice would be beneficial to patient care.

on-line medical direction orders from the on-duty physician given directly to an EMT in the field by radio or telephone.

Protocols and procedures for on-line and off-line medical direction vary from system to system. Many have protocols available online or in an application that is accessible from a smartphone or tablet. Your instructor will inform you what your local policies are and where to locate your protocols. Always follow your local protocols.

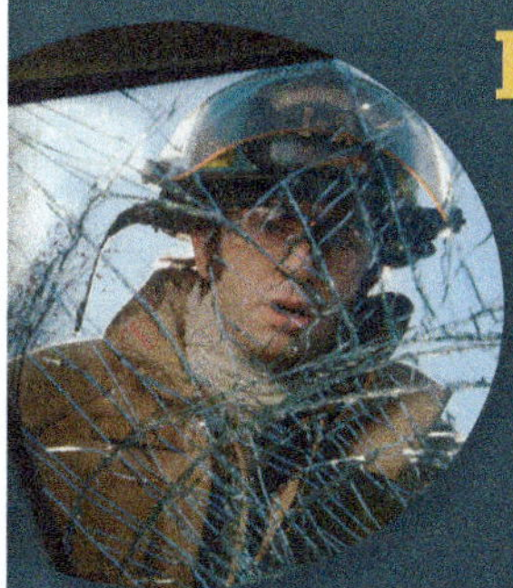

Point of View

"I was driving along, not a care in the world, when all of a sudden this car pulled out from a side street–and pulled right in front of me. I couldn't brake in time. I couldn't steer in time. The crash made thunder seem like a whisper. I didn't just hear it. I felt it. The next thing I knew I was sitting in my car and it was smoky. I thought it was on fire. Then I noticed the air bag, which must've gone off. People were running up to my window to ask if I was OK. I felt so foggy, I didn't even know what to say.

"A fireman came up to my window and asked how I was doing. By then I had a minute to think and compose myself. It felt like I'd cry if I opened my mouth to say anything. The ambulance came in, and the EMTs and firefighters worked to get me out of the car. The fireman who came to my window must've climbed into the backseat. I could feel hands alongside my head.

"The collar felt like it was going to choke me. And everything was so, so loud. But what I remember most, more than the crash or the hospital or the bills, were the kind words the fireman said from behind me. In spite of everything going on that day, his reassuring, kind voice is my best memory from the whole miserable day. It was like an angel being there for me."

As you begin your training as an EMT, you will learn many clinical skills. For this patient, you will perform an assessment, restrict motion of the neck and spine, take vital signs, and transport the patient–perhaps to a trauma center.

You will also provide emotional reassurance and support in this time of crisis. It has been said that you should treat your patients as you would want your family to be treated. This is a good rule.

"Point of View" features such as this one will appear throughout the text. Their purpose is to present an emergency from the patient's perspective because understanding how the patient feels is a critical element in developing people skills. The clinical skills you learn are vital to your success in becoming an EMT. However, people skills are essential for you to thrive as an EMT.

The EMS Role in Public Health

From clean drinking water and sewage systems to the decline of infectious diseases through vaccination, we have reaped the benefits of public health. Although public health has many definitions, it is generally considered to be the system by which the medical community oversees the basic health of a population. Additional efforts by the public health system include prenatal care, reducing injury in children and geriatric patients, campaigns to reduce the use of tobacco, and campaigns to reduce the incidence of obesity through better diet choices.

EMS has a role in many public safety issues, including:

- **Injury prevention for geriatric patients.** When on a call to a patient's home, the EMT can identify things that may cause falls, such as loose-fitting footwear or throw rugs (Figure 1-8). EMS may also run blood pressure clinics and offer methods for older adults to present medications and medical history to EMTs in the event of emergency (e.g., File of Life).
- **Injury prevention for youth.** EMS is frequently involved in car-seat clinics, distribution of bicycle helmets, and other programs for youth.
- **Public vaccination programs.** More and more EMS providers are being trained and allowed to provide vaccination clinics for the public. Seasonal flu and variations such as H1N1 are examples of vaccinations that are frequently offered by EMS providers. Some regions allow specially trained EMS providers to take routine vaccinations (e.g., routine childhood vaccinations) out to the public—especially in areas where many children do not have routine well care and are at risk.
- **Disease surveillance.** On the front lines, EMS reports may serve as an indication that a trend in injury or disease is beginning. Such trends may range from flu to opioid overdose to terrorist attacks.

Programs are being developed around the country that use EMS providers in different and innovative public health roles. These programs vary from location to location according to need but are collectively referred to as Mobile Integrated Health Care. Unlike hospital- or office-based medicine, EMS is always in the field, in patients' homes, and in the public eye. This visibility and access are vital to bringing health services

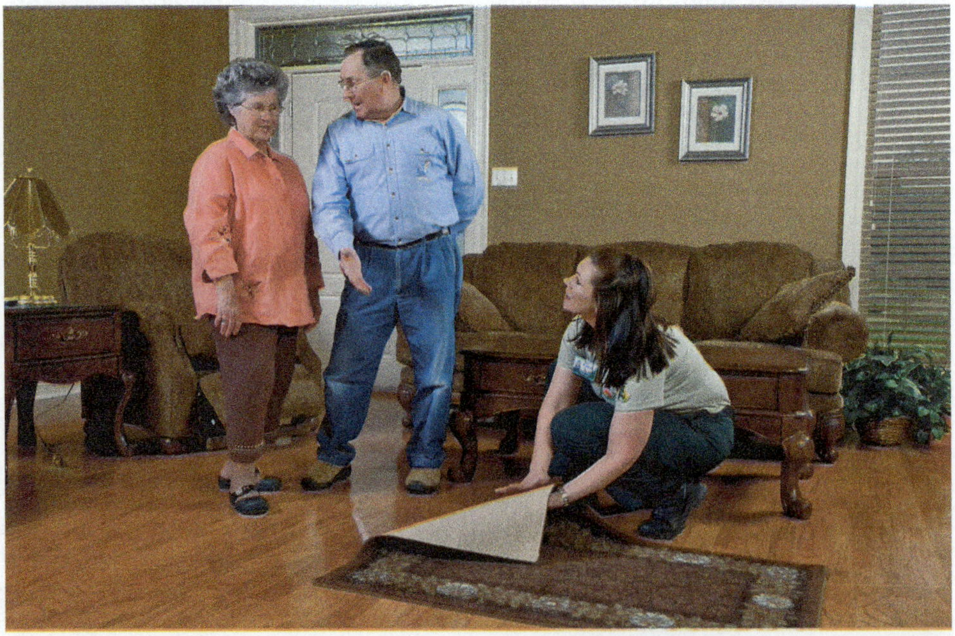

FIGURE 1-8 EMTs play important roles in public safety issues, such as providing fall-prevention advice to older patients.

to points where they are needed and to identifying areas where injuries and disease may be prevented.

One thing is certain: EMS does more than just respond to emergencies. In your future as an EMT, you will likely play an even greater role in public health.

Research

Medicine is based on research. Some—but not all—of the procedures you will be trained to perform have been developed as a result of research. Experts universally agree that research must play a greater role in EMS for it to continue to evolve as a respected profession. Many of the things we do are based on tradition—meaning they are done because that is how we have always done them. Other techniques have been developed from hospital procedures and applied to the field.

Although teaching how to perform or even interpret research is beyond the scope of your EMT class, it is important for you to know the importance of research and how it will shape the future of EMS.

Two ways research affects EMS are through a focus on improving ***patient outcomes*** and through ***evidence-based techniques***.

patient outcomes the long-term survival of patients.

evidence-based techniques techniques or practices that are supported by scientific evidence of their safety and efficacy, rather than merely on supposition and tradition.

Although our concern may seem to be whether patients make it to the hospital alive, we must remember that EMS is part of a larger system. What we do also affects the patient's long-term survival. If something appears to help in the short term but has no effect in the long term, it is not useful. Reasearch into long-term results (patient outcomes) allows us to make the best decisions for the patient's overall care.

Evidence-based decision making means that the procedures and knowledge we use in determining what care works are based on scientific evidence. A scenario involving evidence-based decision making might go like this:

> You are at the ambulance bay when an experienced member of your crew is talking with your Medical Director about adding a new medication to the EMT scope of practice. This member has heard that the new drug has been successful in other local squads and has seen it in magazines for EMS providers.
>
> Your Medical Director finds it interesting but asks the member for evidence. "Check the literature," she says. "If we can find evidence that this makes a difference in outcomes and doesn't have a significant risk, we'll take a look at it."

The evidence-based process here demonstrates the general procedures needed to make these decisions. It includes:

- **Forming a hypothesis.** In this case, the experienced provider felt that a new medication would be safe to use and beneficial.
- **Reviewing literature.** The provider searches medical literature to determine if the new medication has been studied—especially for use by EMTs (Figure 1-9).
- **Evaluating the evidence.** The provider meets with the Medical Director to review the literature. If there was no literature, they could decide to create a research project to study it in the organization or region.
- **Adopting the practice if evidence supports it.** It turns out that the medication has been studied and appears safe. The Medical Director is convinced that the medication should be brought into the EMT scope of practice. Training sessions are scheduled prior to implementation.

The Basics of EMS Research

Moving to evidence-based medicine is not simple. EMS is not an easy field in which to gather research, and serious challenges exist. As a provider, you should understand the value of research not only to your profession but to your everyday practice. There are

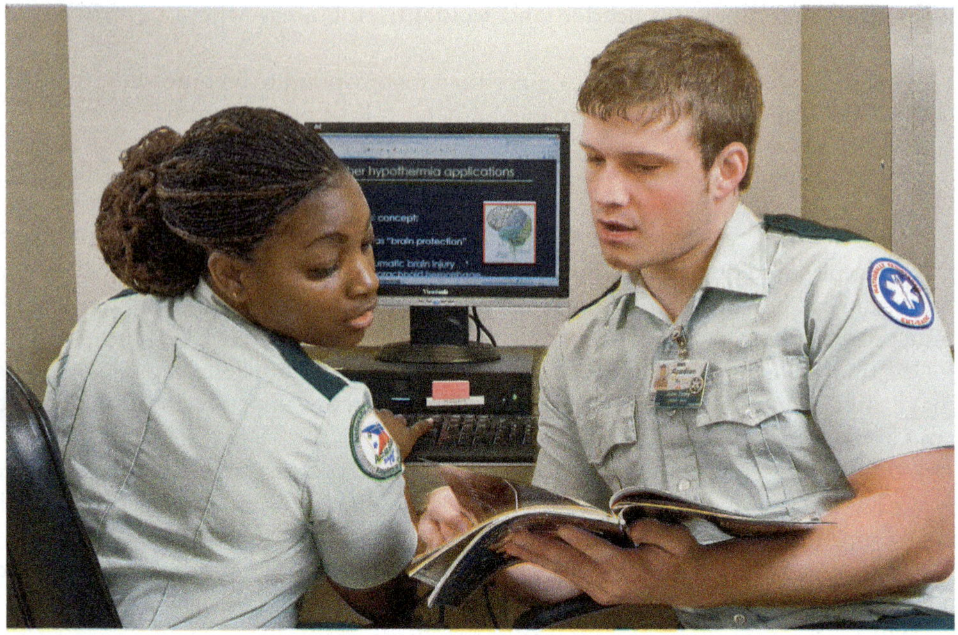

FIGURE 1-9 Many EMS/rescue operations adopt new procedures and equipment on the basis of research providing evidence that they are effective.

simple steps you can take to improve your understanding and to help move EMS toward a more evidence-based approach.

Here is an example of how research affects your practice as an EMT:

It was not long ago that EMTs gave oxygen—a lot of oxygen—to almost every patient. Oxygen was nicknamed the "wonder drug" because it was needed by humans to live—and EMTs could administer it. However, oxygen use turns out to be a bit more complicated than that.

Oxygen, given at the wrong time or in excess, can cause harm. Research showed that raising the oxygen levels of patients with certain conditions (e.g., heart attack and stroke) can make their condition worse. While some patients who need it will still receive oxygen, EMTs have learned that it is not the "wonder drug" anymore and that *all* medications should be administered wisely and according to the patient's needs.

The dynamic nature of our treatment setting makes research difficult at best. We encounter many obstacles to research that simply do not exist in other areas of the health care field. Often our work environment is unstable, our encounters are brief, and our data collection is disjointed and lacks centralization. Furthermore, we face many ethical dilemmas. Obtaining consent from patients in critical condition is challenging at best. We do have many opportunities to create valid and important studies on prehospital care, but to do so we must promote the best practices of research so our outcomes can truly guide us to high-quality care.

Not all research is created equal. There are good studies, and there are bad studies. As we evolve in an evidence-based environment, we should embrace the best practices of conducting and evaluating research (Figure 1-10). The finer points of medical research are by no means a simple topic, and a thorough examination of how to evaluate research is beyond the scope of this text. However, a few broad concepts can be helpful to consider.

Remember that the process of research is the same whether you are an EMS researcher or a scientist in a laboratory. We all rely on the *scientific method*, a process of experimentation for answering questions and acquiring new knowledge that was developed by Galileo about four hundred years ago. In this method, general observations are turned into a *hypothesis* (or unproven theory). Predictions are then made, based on the hypothesis, and these predictions are tested to help prove or disprove the hypothesis.

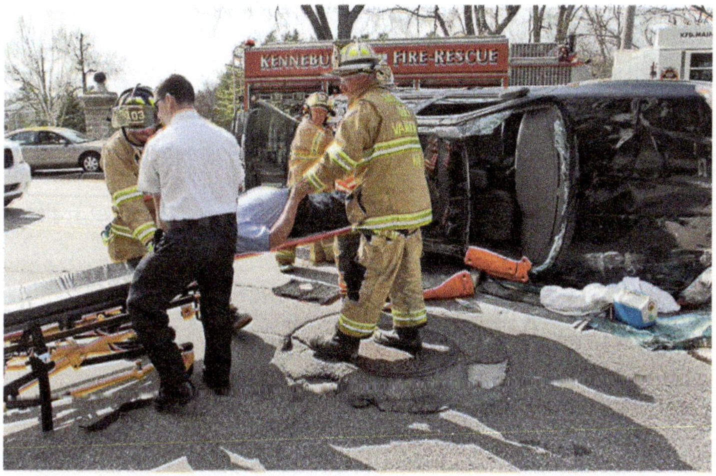

FIGURE 1-10 EMS must strive to embrace best practices of conducting and evaluating research to provide high-quality care for our patients. *(© Daniel Limmer)*

For example, you might note that applying a bandage seems to control minor external bleeding. To use the scientific method, you might hypothesize that bandages do indeed control bleeding better than doing nothing at all. You could conduct a randomized control study to test your hypothesis by randomly assigning patients to the "bandage group" or to the "do-nothing group." You could then measure the amount of bleeding in each group and compare your results. Although there are some ethical issues with your study, this experiment would help you prove or disprove the value of bandaging. Furthermore, if your experiment were done properly, your results would hold up if the study were repeated, regardless of who conducted the experiment. That is the value of quality research.

The research that is published in medical journals is ***peer reviewed***. This means that the research was submitted to a professional journal and reviewed by several of the researcher's peers. This process helps to ensure that the research methods and results are accurate and high quality. This research is published in peer-reviewed journals.

peer reviewed submitted to a professional journal and reviewed by several of the researcher's peers.

Not all the sources you will find are peer reviewed. It is very common to have EMS magazines around the station. These magazines contain articles written by EMTs, paramedics, and physicians. They are designed to educate and inform you, but they usually do not present original research, and they are not peer reviewed.

The importance of research in bringing EMS to the point where it is now—and to where it will go in the future—cannot be overstated.

Special Issues

EMTs are people, and people make mistakes. You may have seen stories in your local news about errors that have occurred in the hospital and have resulted in lawsuits. All of medicine—including EMS—recognizes this as a serious issue. The chapter *Medical/Legal and Ethical Issues* will address this topic in detail.

In the coming weeks and through the chapters that follow in this textbook, you will be studying to become an EMT. As part of your course, your instructor will advise you on local issues and administrative matters, such as a course description, class meeting times, and criteria including physical and mental requirements for certification as an EMT. They will also inform you of specific statutes and regulations regarding EMS in your state, region, or locality.

The Americans with Disabilities Act (ADA) has set strict guidelines to preserve the rights of Americans with disabilities. If you have a disability or have questions about the ADA, ask your instructor for more information.

Chapter Review

Key Facts and Concepts

- The EMS system has been developed to provide prehospital as well as hospital emergency care.
- The EMS system includes 911 or another emergency access system, dispatchers, EMTs, the hospital emergency department, physicians, nurses, physician's assistants, and other health professionals.
- The EMT's responsibilities include safety; patient assessment and care; lifting, moving, and transporting patients; transfer of care; and patient advocacy.
- An EMT must have certain personal and physical traits to ensure the ability to do the job.
- Education (including refresher training and continuing education), quality improvement procedures, and medical direction are all essential to maintaining high standards of EMS care.

Key Decisions

Making accurate decisions in patient care is the hallmark of a competent EMT. This feature will be used throughout this text to help you identify these significant decisions and to relate their importance in emergency care.

Since this is a nonclinical chapter, picture yourself applying for a job or being interviewed for membership in a volunteer squad. How would you answer the following questions asked in the interview?

- Why do you think EMS makes a difference?
- If EMS is about helping people, how do you anticipate helping people as an EMT?
- Can EMS have a role in injury prevention or public health?
- What will EMS look like in the future?

Chapter Glossary

evidence-based techniques techniques or practices that are supported by scientific evidence of their safety and efficacy, rather than merely by supposition and tradition.

medical direction oversight of the patient-care aspects of an EMS system by the Medical Director. Direction can be either off-line or on-line.

Medical Director a physician who assumes ultimate responsibility for the patient-care aspects of the EMS system.

911 system a system for telephone access to report emergencies. A dispatcher takes the information and alerts EMS or the fire or police department as needed. *Enhanced 911* also identifies the caller's phone number and location automatically.

off-line medical direction standing orders issued by the Medical Director that allow EMTs to give certain medications or perform certain procedures without speaking to the Medical Director or another physician.

on-line medical direction orders from the on-duty physician given directly to an EMT in the field by radio or telephone.

patient outcomes the long-term survival of patients.

peer reviewed submitted to a professional journal and reviewed by several of the researcher's peers.

protocols lists of steps, such as assessments and interventions, to be taken in different situations. Protocols are developed by the Medical Director of an EMS system.

quality improvement a process of continual self-review with the purpose of identifying and correcting aspects of the system that require improvement.

standing orders policies or protocols issued by a Medical Director that authorize EMTs and others to perform particular skills in certain situations.

Preparation for Your Examination and Practice

Short Answer

1. What are the primary components of the Emergency Medical Services system?
2. What are some of the special designations that hospitals may have? Name the specialty centers in your region.
3. What are the four national levels of EMS training and certification?
4. What are the roles and responsibilities of the EMT?
5. What are desirable personal and physical attributes of the EMT?
6. What is the definition of the term *quality improvement*?
7. What is the difference between on-line and off-line medical direction?

Critical Thinking Exercises

Of course you want to be the best EMT you can be. The purpose of this exercise will be to consider some ways to accomplish that goal.

1. What qualities would you like to see in an EMT who is caring for you? How can you come closer to being this kind of EMT?
2. You are devoting a considerable amount of time to becoming an EMT. How do you plan to refresh your knowledge and stay current once you are out of the classroom?

Street Scenes

As a new EMT, you are assigned to Station 2 to ride with Susan Miller, a seasoned EMS veteran with seven years on the job. You have heard that she is a good EMT, and you remember that she helped teach some of your skill sessions. She was a good instructor–patient, understanding, and considerate.

When you arrive at the station, you find out she has been delayed and you will be riding with Chuck Hartley instead. When you are introduced to Chuck, you see that his uniform is unkempt. He tells you to sit until he needs you.

Your first call of the day is a 70-year-old woman with abdominal pain. As you approach the ambulance, Chuck tells you to get in the back. He'll let you know when you can help. At the scene, after ensuring scene safety, you both enter the patient's home. Chuck doesn't bother to introduce himself and proceeds to ask the patient, "What's wrong, hon?" She describes her symptoms. Chuck tells you to put her on a nasal cannula. As you hook up the O_2, Chuck says in a loud voice, "Didn't you learn anything in EMT class? That liter flow rate is too high."

As the patient is being loaded onto the stretcher, she tries to tell Chuck something that she obviously believes is urgent. Chuck tells her that if it's that important, she can tell the doctor at the hospital.

Street Scene Questions

1. **What would have been a more appropriate action for Chuck to suggest when the shift started?**
2. **What behavioral characteristics of Chuck's would be considered unprofessional?**
3. **What would you expect from someone providing initial field training?**

When you return to the station, Susan Miller has arrived. This time, when you are introduced, you notice that her uniform is pressed and neat. She asks you about your background and when you finished training. She remembers you from class, she says. Then she tells you there are some things you both need to do. "First let's go to the ambulance and check the equipment. Next, I want to explain how we operate on calls. You need to know what equipment we always take to the patient and what the responsibilities of the crew members are."

Just as you are completing your orientation, a call comes in for a 55-year-old man with chest pain. While en route, Susan briefly goes over the routine that she and her partner use. She asks you to take the automatic defibrillator. When you enter the patient's house, Susan introduces herself and the members of the crew. She asks the patient, "Sir, why did you call 911?" He tells you that he had chest pain but he took a nitroglycerin tablet and now most of the pain is gone. He apologizes for calling.

While you get the vital signs, Susan tells the patient that he did just the right thing by calling EMS. He is reassured and agrees to be transported for further evaluation.

Street Scene Questions

4. **What did Susan Miller do that was appropriate and professional?**
5. **How was Susan's behavior beneficial to you as a new EMT?**
6. **What personal traits are the professional standards for EMTs?**

During the trip to the hospital, Susan continues to reassure the patient. In fact, she tells you to talk to the patient about his medical history. When you arrive at the hospital, Susan sees that the oxygen tank is getting low, so she asks you to switch "bottles" before moving the patient, but you forget to turn off the tank being replaced. Susan turns it off, sets it aside, looks you in the eyes, and gives you a smile. You both know that you will not forget the next time.

After the call, Susan gives a short critique and discusses the prehospital care report. When you call back in service (tell the dispatcher you are ready to take another run), you realize that to be a good EMT, you not only need to have good technical skills but, just as important, you also must act professionally with your patients and with your colleagues.

2

Well-Being of the EMT

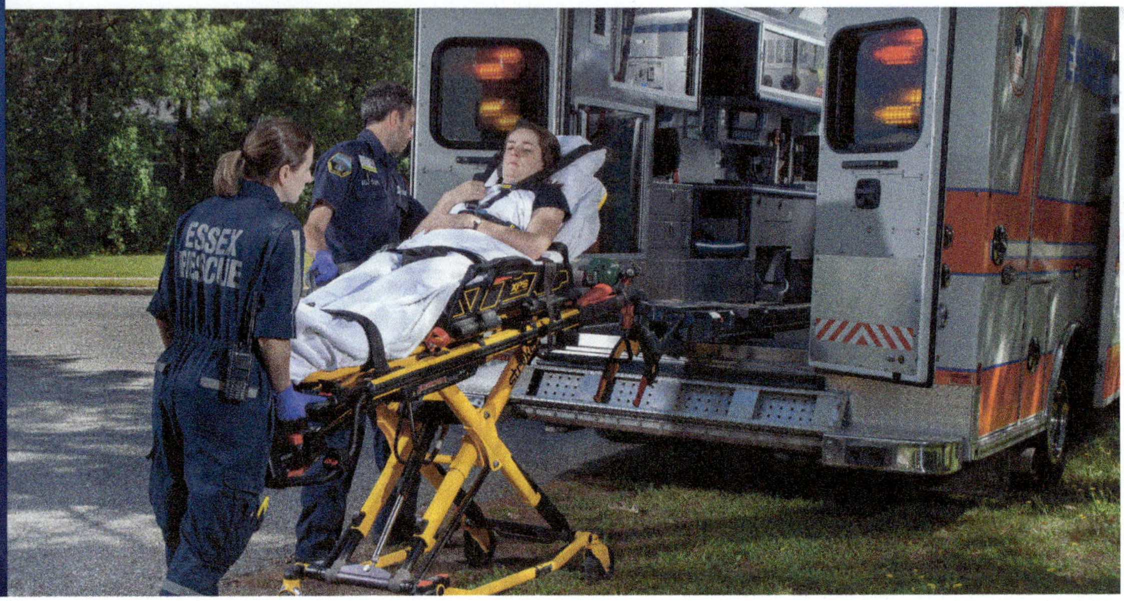

Related Chapters

The following chapters provide additional information related to topics discussed in this chapter:

Standard

Preparatory (Workforce Safety and Wellness)

Competency

Uses fundamental knowledge of the EMS system, safety/well-being of the EMT, and medical/legal and ethical issues to the provision of emergency care.

Core Concepts

- Standard Precautions, or how to protect yourself from transmitted diseases
- The kinds of stress caused by involvement in EMS and how they can affect you, your fellow EMTs, and your family and friends

- The impact that dying patients can have on you and others
- How to identify potential hazards and maintain scene safety

Outcomes

After reading this chapter, you should be able to:

2.1 Describe how specific healthy habits can affect the EMT's well-being. (pp. 24–38)
- Identify the role of a support system in maintaining well-being.
- Recognize the health benefits of an exercise program.
- Relate the importance of sleep to performance as an EMT.
- Identify the health benefits of eating right.
- List the negative impacts of excess consumption of alcohol and caffeine.
- Recognize the importance of regular visits to your physician, including keeping current on vaccines.
- Explain the concepts of personal protection from communicable diseases.

2.2 Explain why EMS can be a particularly stressful job. (pp. 38–45)
- Describe what happens in each stage of stress.
- Contrast acute, delayed, and cumulative stress reactions.
- Give examples of types of situations in EMS that have a higher probability than routine circumstances of causing a stress reaction in EMS providers.
- Recognize when an EMT is exhibiting signs and symptoms of stress.
- Identify the components of an employer's comprehensive system for stress management.
- Interpret the statements and behaviors of a dying patient or that patient's family members in terms of emotional stages of grief.
- Given a scenario, translate generic approaches for dealing with death and dying patients into actions specific to the situation.

2.3 Summarize concepts of scene safety in EMS. (pp. 46–51)
- State the rationale for the priority given to scene safety in EMS.
- List the most common causes of EMS line-of-duty deaths (LODD).
- State the primary actions expected of EMTs upon encountering a potential hazardous materials situation.
- State actions EMTs can take in advance to plan for encountering violence on an EMS call.
- Explain specific observations EMTs should make on every call to detect potential indications of violence.
- Given a scenario, translate the generic approach to reacting to danger to situation-specific actions.

Key Terms

contamination, *26*
critical incident stress management (CISM), *44*
decontamination, *47*
hazardous material incident, *46*
multiple-casualty incident (MCI), *41*
pathogens, *25*
personal protective equipment (PPE), *25*
resilience, *39*
Standard Precautions, *25*
stress, *39*

At no point in the history of modern EMS have we been more concerned about our safety on EMS calls. It seems that there has been an unprecedented amount of violence and an unprecedented number of emerging diseases to deal with–and EMS has been asked to take a greater role in tactical response to these incidents. This chapter will discuss threats to EMTs and other EMS providers and provide ways to assess and respond to them.

Stress is also at the forefront of our thoughts when we think of incidents we may be called to. You will be exposed to situations that are stressful, including those involving death and dying.

This may seem like a discouraging way to begin a chapter, but it is important to be realistic. Although most calls are safe, as an EMT you will face dangers and stressors. There are successful ways to deal with these threats and stressors that will protect your health and success now and in years to come.

Finally, this material is important not only to make sure you remain safe and healthy, but also to protect you from harm and allow you to care for patients rather than becoming a patient yourself.

Well-Being

Prevention is a hot topic. Our physicians stress this when we see them. Eat right, lose weight, exercise. This advice—and this chapter—are designed to promote your overall well-being. This section begins the well-being chapter with some important concepts designed to help you obtain and maintain a state of well-being.

If you were faced with a dangerous situation, would you respond better if you were in good physical shape? If you were faced with a challenging situation in which you had to drag or carry a patient several hundred feet to safety, would you do better if you were in shape? If you were faced with a call that hit you hard emotionally, would you get through it better if you were in a better physical and mental place?

The answer to all these questions is yes. And the concepts of well-being aren't difficult if you start and maintain some healthful habits. These include:

- **Maintaining solid personal relationships.** If you have a difficult call, you will do better dealing with it if you have a support system. Family, EMS colleagues, and friends who are there for you every day and in difficult times are vital for well-being.
- **Exercise.** An exercise program helps you in many ways. A well-designed program helps you build strength and improve flexibility and also promotes cardiovascular fitness. An exercise regimen is also an important part of a weight-loss program.
- **Sleep.** Rest is important. Lack of sleep can be a significant factor in medical errors and improper decision making. Fatigue also increases the potential for motor-vehicle collisions, harms personal relationships, and can lead to frequent illnesses by decreasing immune system function.
- **Eating right.** Eating provides fuel for the body—especially during long EMS shifts and with strenuous activities. Eating the right foods rather than wolfing down junk foods is critical.
- **Limiting alcohol and caffeine intake.** Although alcohol may be enjoyable in moderation, excess intake reduces performance and brings on personal, medical, and social issues. Caffeine may seem like a pick-me-up at the moment, but as the saying goes, what goes up must come down. Your body will take only so much artificial stimulation before it crashes. Plus, even though you feel more awake with caffeine in your system, your decision making and reaction times can still be impaired.

- **Seeing your physician regularly and keeping up to date on vaccines.** Bringing this well-being section full circle: Regular check-ups help ensure we are well—and can help prevent or catch any serious issues before they arise.

The topics that follow in this book involve safety and response to danger, decision making, lifting and moving, and others—all of which will be better performed if you are well. Furthermore, if well performed, they can help keep you well. The section on dealing with stress addresses all of the items just listed. It is reasonable to expect that practicing wellness daily can eliminate or significantly reduce stress. Why not do it now?

Personal Protection

Standard Precautions

Diseases are caused by ***pathogens***, organisms such as viruses and bacteria that cause infection. Pathogens may be spread through the air or by contact with blood and other body fluids. *Bloodborne pathogens* can be contracted by exposure to the patient's blood and sometimes other body fluids, especially when they come in contact with an open wound or sore on the EMT's hands, face, or other exposed parts, including mucous membranes of the nose, mouth, or eyes. Even minor breaks in the skin, such as those found around fingernails, can provide a pathway for a pathogen to enter your body. *Airborne pathogens* are spread by tiny droplets sprayed during breathing, coughing, or sneezing. These particles can be absorbed through your eyes or when you inhale.

pathogens
the organisms that cause infection, such as viruses and bacteria.

CORE CONCEPT
Standard Precautions, or how to protect yourself from transmitted diseases

Since it is impossible for an EMT or other health care professional to identify patients who carry infectious diseases just by looking at them, all body fluids must be considered infectious, and appropriate precautions should be taken for all patients at all times.

Equipment and procedures that protect you from the blood and body fluids of the patient—and protect the patient from your blood and body fluids as well—are referred to as ***Standard Precautions***. For each situation you encounter, it is important to apply the appropriate precautions. Taking too few will clearly increase your risk of exposure to disease. Too many can potentially alienate the patient and reduce your effectiveness.

Standard Precautions
a strict form of infection control that is based on the assumption that all blood and other body fluids are infectious; also known as Standard Precautions.

Your selection of which Standard Precautions to use is one of the most important decisions you will make on any call. You will make this decision initially upon seeing the patient and reconsider it throughout the call as the patient's condition changes.

The Occupational Safety and Health Administration (OSHA) has issued strict guidelines about precautions against exposure to bloodborne pathogens. Under the OSHA guidelines, employers and employees share responsibility for these precautions. Employers must develop a written exposure control plan and must provide emergency care providers with training, immunizations, and proper ***personal protective equipment (PPE)*** to prevent transmission of disease. (Volunteer organizations are also required to provide these services for their members.) The employee's responsibility is to participate in the training and to follow the exposure control plan.

personal protective equipment (PPE)
equipment that protects the EMS worker from infection and/or exposure to the dangers of rescue operations.

There is also a requirement for all agencies to have a written policy in place in the event of an exposure to infectious substances. Any contact such as a needlestick or contact with a potentially infectious fluid must be documented. Refer to your local policy for reporting an exposure incident. Most plans call for baseline testing of the exposed person immediately following the exposure and periodic follow-up testing. In addition, federal legislation has made it possible for emergency care providers to be notified if a patient with whom they have had potentially infectious contact turns out to be infected by a disease or virus such as tuberculosis (TB), hepatitis B, or HIV (the virus associated with AIDS).

Although deciding on and taking Standard Precautions may seem intimidating—especially if you are just beginning your training—remember that by following the proper precautions, it is possible to have a long and safe career in EMS free from infection and disease.

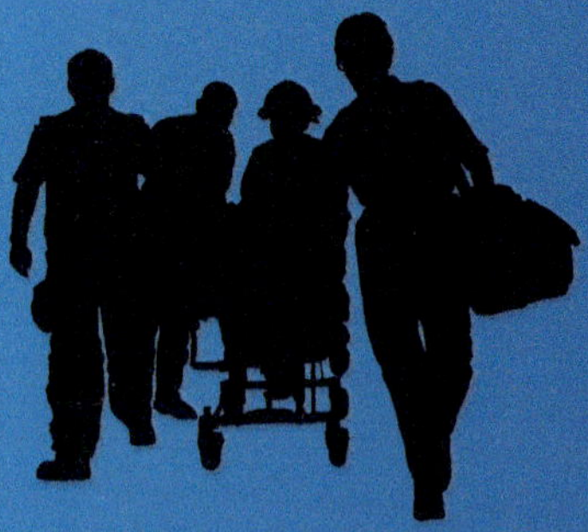

Think Like an EMT

Standard Precautions

Although you may be thinking that the most important decisions you will make as an EMT have to do with clinical situations affecting your patient, some of the most important decisions you will make actually have to do with routine things such as Standard Precautions.

Be sure you always carry gloves on your person and have face protection immediately available in kits (e.g., first-in bags) and suction units. Your decision about the level of precautions to take will initially be determined as part of the scene size-up (the first part of the patient assessment process you will learn about in the *Scene Size-Up* chapter). Take precautions against anything you see *or anything you reasonably expect to encounter*. Some examples include:

1. When called to a motor-vehicle collision where you observe broken glass, you should expect broken skin and the potential for contact with blood—even if you don't see wounds. It is wise to wear nonlatex gloves to protect you from blood as well as heavy-duty gloves to protect you from the broken glass.
2. When called to a nursing home for an interfacility transfer, you must reach under the patient to move the person to your stretcher. Because of the possibility of contact with urine, feces, or bedsores, you should wear protective gloves.
3. You are called to a patient with a sprained ankle. There are no open wounds. Guidelines indicate that no precautions are necessary, although many routinely wear gloves on all calls.
4. You are working with an advanced life support crew treating a patient with chest pain. Although there are no open wounds, the paramedic started an IV, and some blood is present on the patient's forearm from the IV start. In addition, a small amount is seen on the IV tubing. Gloves are required.

Your decisions about Standard Precautions do not end at the scene size-up. In fact, you should be alert for changes throughout the call. For example:

5. You are treating a patient with chest pain who suddenly becomes unresponsive. The patient requires suction. In addition to the gloves you may already be wearing, you will now need to protect your face from spatter encountered in airway and suction procedures.

Personal Protective Equipment

contamination the introduction of dangerous chemicals, disease, or infectious materials.

Protect yourself from all possible routes of ***contamination***, or introduction of disease or infectious materials. Follow Standard Precaution guidelines and wear the appropriate personal protective equipment on every call (Figure 2-1).

Protective Gloves

Vinyl or other nonlatex gloves should be used whenever there is the potential for contact with blood and other body fluids. This includes actions such as controlling bleeding,

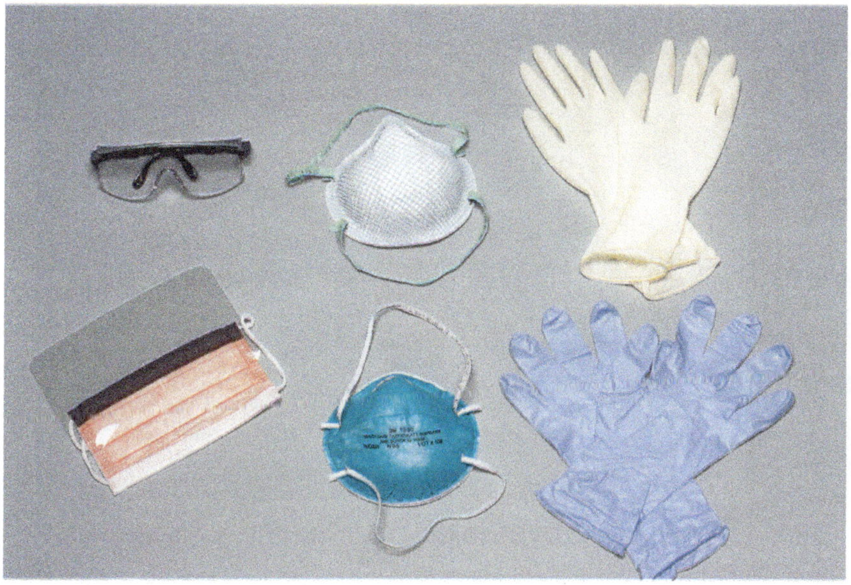

FIGURE 2-1 Always wear personal protective equipment to prevent exposure to contagious diseases.

"Everyone thinks to wear gloves. Remember to protect your eyes and face as well."

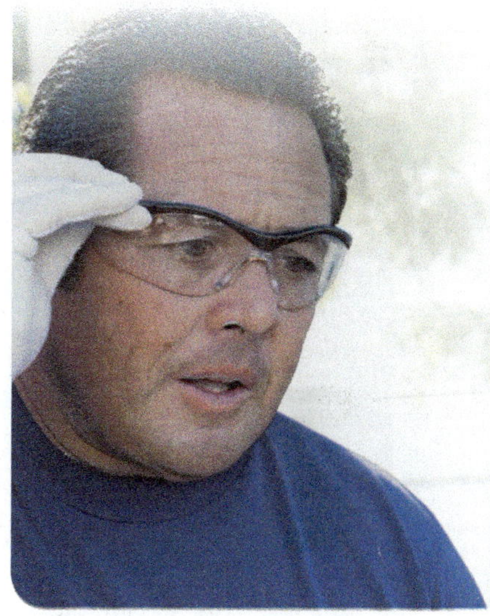

suctioning, artificial ventilation, and CPR. Make sure that you have the gloves on or available before you come in contact with a patient. Otherwise, you might get distracted and forget the gloves, and may accidentally become contaminated. Be sure to change gloves between patients. See Scan 2-1, which shows how to remove contaminated gloves safely.

In many years of using latex in health care—in both hospital and prehospital environments—many patients and providers developed allergies to latex. The gloves you will see in the ambulance are now latex free, as are oxygen delivery devices and other supplies.

A different type of glove must be worn when you clean the ambulance and soiled equipment. This glove should be heavyweight and tear resistant. The force and type of movements involved in cleaning can cause lightweight gloves to rip, exposing your hands to contamination.

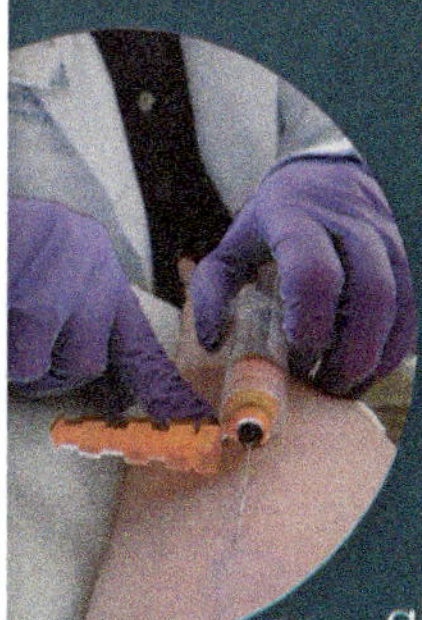

Point of View

"I consider myself careful. I wear gloves on every call. But here I am getting blood drawn because I had an exposure to a patient's blood.

"I'm really not sure when or how it happened. I guess I put on gloves and then was on autopilot. I didn't notice they had a rip in them. Making things worse, I had a cut on my finger. Murphy's Law–the cut was right near the tear in the glove. It didn't even seem like a lot of blood at the scene. I looked at my glove. Saw the tear. Took off the glove and saw the blood on my open skin. My heart sank.

"Now the nurse will draw blood. Then I have to talk with a counselor. I'll get more blood drawn every so often. I already dread waiting to get the results–wondering if I'll get sick.

"Trust me. Never take Standard Precautions lightly. Think about them during the call. If I did, I would've seen that tear in my gloves. And my life would be very different. I'd give anything not to be sitting here right now."

SCAN 2-1 Glove Removal

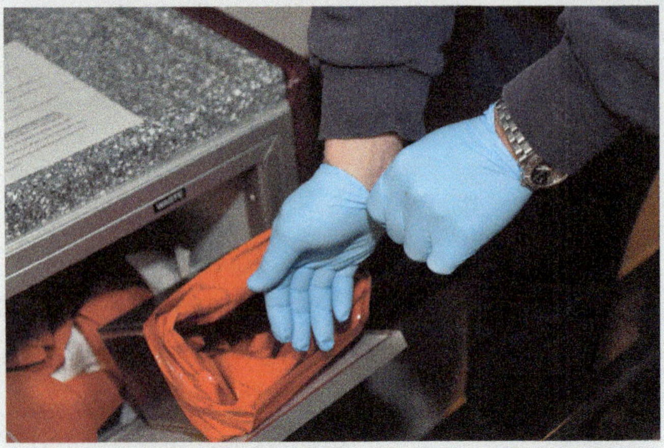

1. **PULL AT TOP OF GLOVE #1.** *(© Edward T. Dickinson, MD)*

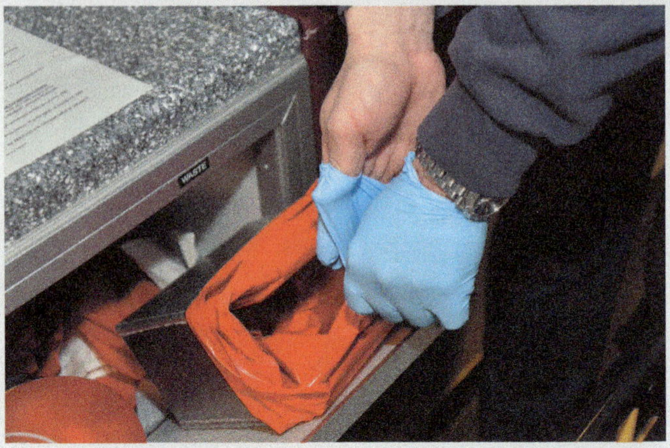

2. **PULL GLOVE #1 INSIDE OUT.** *(© Edward T. Dickinson, MD)*

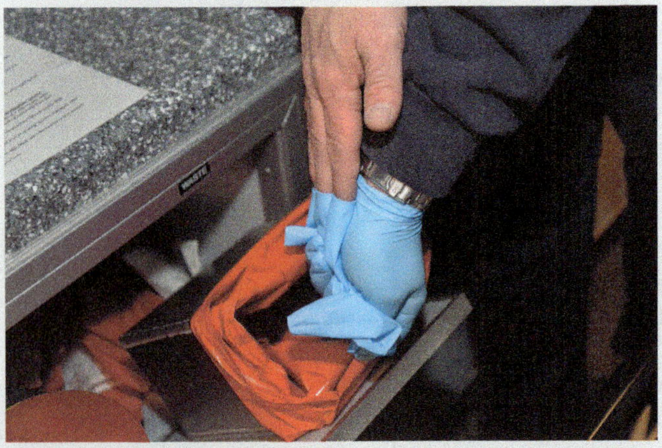

3. **PULL GLOVE #1, USING HAND INSIDE GLOVE #2.** This move ends with the first glove inside the second. *(© Edward T. Dickinson, MD)*

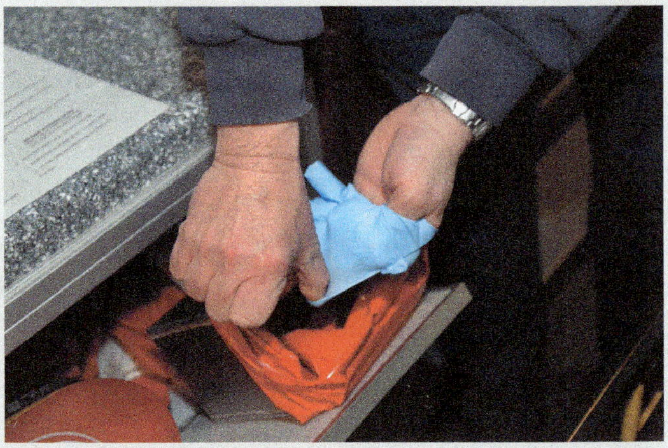

4. **PUT UNGLOVED THUMB FROM HAND #1 INSIDE CUFF OF GLOVE #2 TO PULL GLOVE #2 OFF.** Do not touch the contaminated outer surface of glove #2. *(© Edward T. Dickinson, MD)*

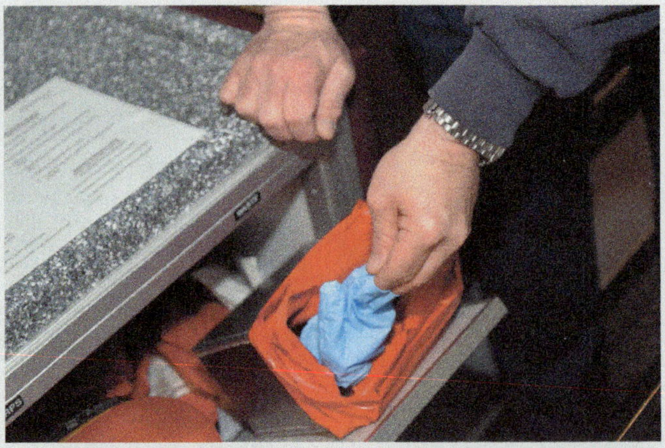

5. **DISPOSE OF GLOVE IN BIOHAZARD CONTAINER.** *(© Edward T. Dickinson, MD)*

Hand Cleaning

Even though you wear gloves when assessing and caring for patients, you must still wash your hands after patient contacts when gloves are removed. There are two methods of hand cleaning (Figure 2-2):

- **Hand washing.** When soap and water are available, vigorous hand washing is recommended. Wash your hands after each patient contact (even if you were wearing gloves) and whenever they become visibly soiled.
- **Alcohol-based hand cleaners.** These cleaners are considered effective by the Centers for Disease Control and Prevention (CDC)—except when hands are visibly soiled or when anthrax is present—and are often available when soap and water are not. The alcohol helps kill microorganisms. Place the amount of hand cleaner recommended by the manufacturer in one palm and rub it so it covers your hands. Rub until dry.

Eye and Face Protection

The mucous membranes surrounding the eyes are capable of absorbing fluids. Wear eye protection to prevent splashing, spattering, or spraying fluids from entering the body through these membranes. Protective eyewear should provide a guard from the front and the sides. Various types of eyewear are on the market. If you wear prescription eyeglasses, clip-on side protectors are available. Some companies offer protective eyewear that resembles eyeglasses.

FIGURE 2-2 (A) Careful, methodical hand washing is effective in reducing exposure to contagious diseases. (B) Use a paper towel to turn off the faucet. (C) Alcohol-based hand cleaners are effective and often available when soap and water are not.

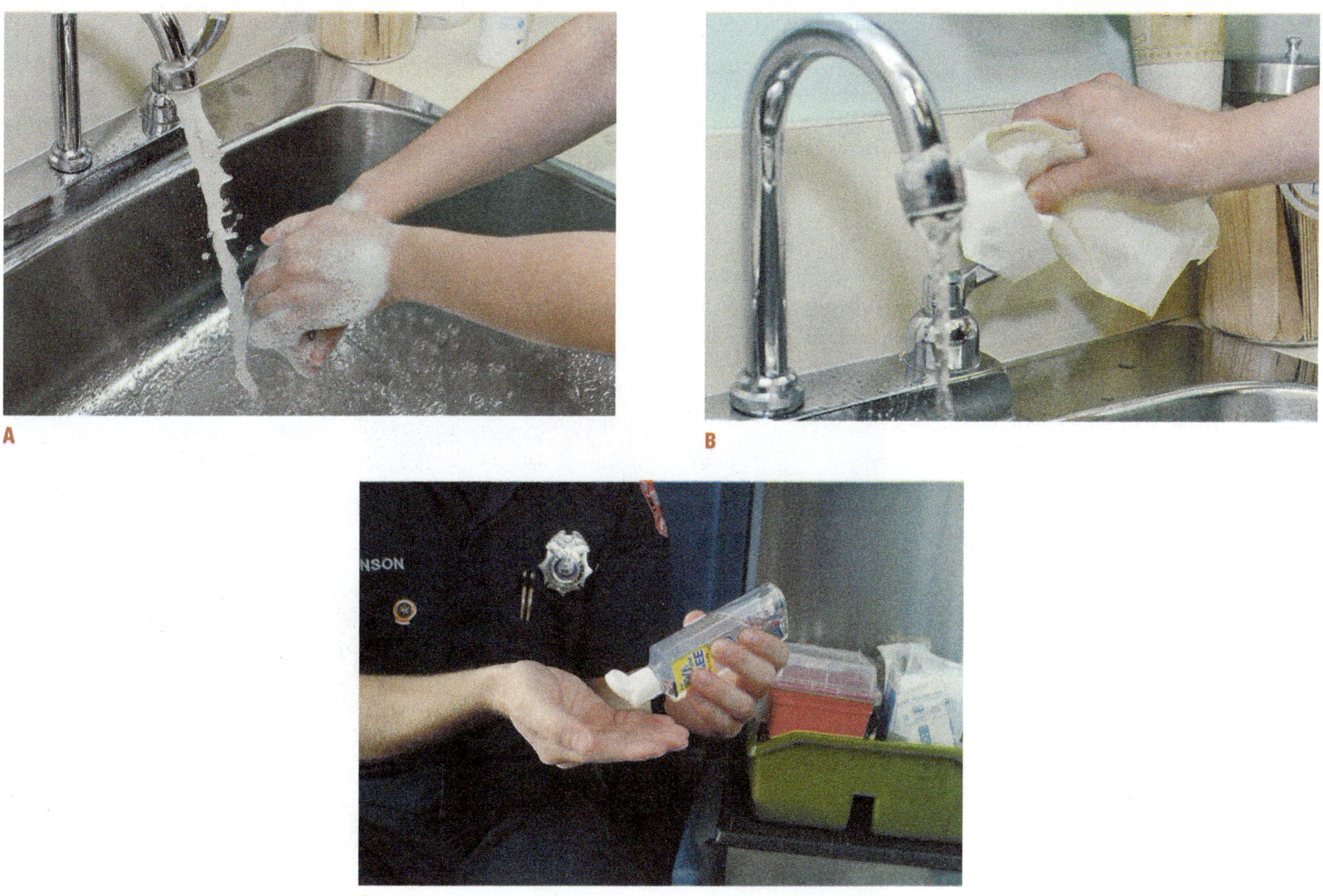

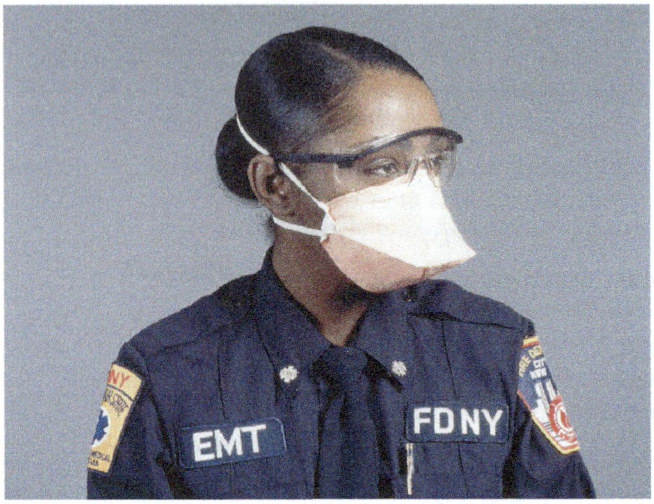

FIGURE 2-3 Wear a NIOSH-approved respirator when you suspect a patient may have tuberculosis.

Masks

In cases when there will be blood or fluid spatter, wear a surgical-type mask. In cases where tuberculosis (a disease carried by fine particles in the air) is suspected, an N-95 or a high-efficiency particulate air (HEPA) respirator approved by the National Institute for Occupational Safety and Health (NIOSH) is the standard (Figure 2-3). Face shields offer protection of the entire face by use of a mask with an attached see-through shield that covers the eyes (Figure 2-4).

In some jurisdictions, when a patient is suspected of having an infection spread by droplets (such as flu or measles), a surgical-type mask may be placed on the patient if the patient is alert and cooperative.

NOTE: *When you cover a patient's mouth and nose with a mask of any kind, use caution. The mask reduces your ability to visualize and protect the airway. Monitor respirations and be prepared to remove the mask and use suction to clear the airway if necessary. (See the chapters titled* Airway Management *and* Respiration and Artificial Ventilation.*)*

Gowns

Gowns and aprons are worn to protect clothing and bare skin from spilled or splashed fluids. Arterial (spurting) bleeding is an indication for a gown. Childbirth and patients with multiple injuries also often produce considerable amounts of blood. Any situation that would call for the use of a gown would also require gloves, eye protection, and a mask.

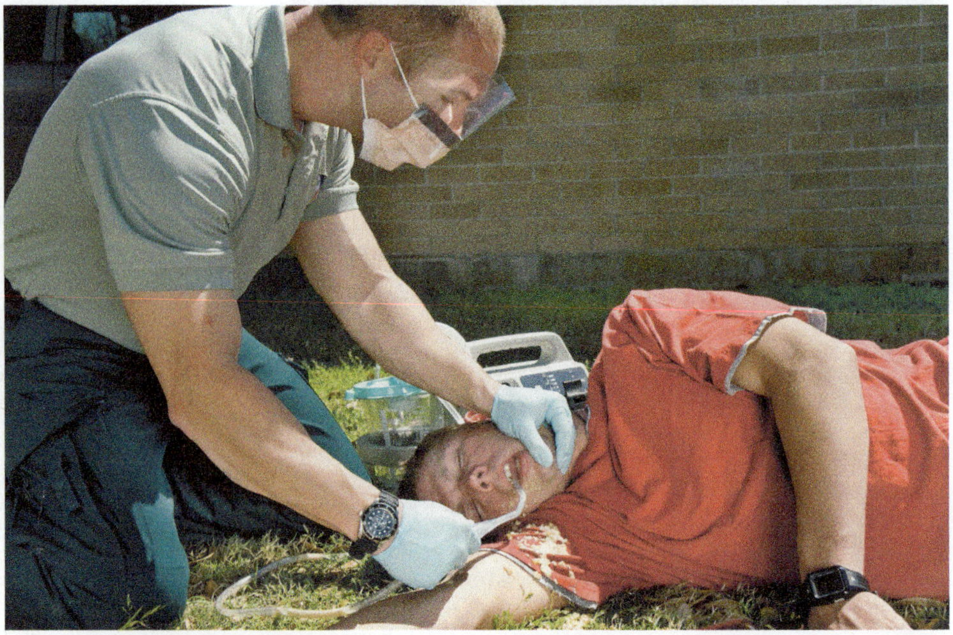

FIGURE 2-4 Wear a protective mask and face shield when suctioning a patient.

It is a good idea not only to use personal protective equipment yourself but also to be an advocate for its use—that is, to encourage members of your crew and others to use appropriate protective equipment. In addition to the moral and ethical obligation to do so, you will be helping to keep your crew in good health.

Always properly remove and discard protective garments after use, carry out disinfection and cleaning operations, and complete all reporting documentation regarding infection control. You will learn more about these procedures in the *EMS Operations* chapter.

NOTE: *When you finish your EMT training and begin in the field, you will observe differences in the methods and levels of Standard Precautions taken by those around you. You will likely notice that some EMTs don gloves and protective eyewear before exiting the ambulance and wear them throughout the call. Others will go through an entire call without even wearing gloves.*

In the 1980s, an increased emphasis was placed on body substance isolation. Diseases such as AIDS and hepatitis brought a startling reality to the health care profession. As a result, gloves, protective eyewear, and masks were used with increasing frequency. These items were worn as a "precaution," even when not technically necessary.

Today, providers have a more realistic attitude about Standard Precautions. Think back to your last physical examination, for example. Your physician most likely examined your eyes and ears, palpated your abdomen, and performed other examinations without gloves. This is because it is not necessary to wear gloves if your skin and the skin of your patient are intact. In addition, wearing gloves while you exit the ambulance, carry equipment, and enter a scene may cause the gloves to rip before you reach the patient, rendering them ineffective.

Common sense should be the rule. To protect yourself from disease:

- *Follow Standard Precaution guidelines as outlined in this chapter and in the rules and policies of your organization.*
- *Always have personal protective equipment immediately available on your person and in kits.*
- *Carry two sets of gloves–one to put on when you encounter infectious substances and another in the event your gloves tear or become soiled.*
- *If in doubt, take Standard Precautions.*

Diseases of Concern

As humans, we are concerned about communicable diseases like dangerous strains of flu that travel the world and gastrointestinal illnesses that happen on cruise ships. As an EMT, you will have an additional set of concerns. You will need to protect yourself from communicable diseases caused by bloodborne and airborne pathogens such as viruses, bacteria, and other harmful organisms. Bloodborne pathogens are contracted by exposure to an infected patient's blood, especially exposure through breaks in the noninfected person's skin. Airborne pathogens are spread by tiny droplets sprayed when a patient breathes, coughs, or sneezes. These droplets are inhaled or are absorbed through the noninfected person's eyes, mouth, or nose.

Whether you think about catching the flu or getting a stomach virus off duty or about contracting a disease from a patient in EMS, the methods to protect yourself are the same.

Although there are many communicable diseases (Table 2-1), four are of particular concern: hepatitis B, hepatitis C, tuberculosis, and HIV/AIDS.

- *Hepatitis*, an infection that causes an inflammation of the liver, comes in several forms, including hepatitis A, B, C, and other strains. Hepatitis A is acquired primarily through contact with food or water contaminated by stool (feces). The other forms are acquired through contact with blood and other body fluids. The virus that causes hepatitis is especially hardy. Hepatitis B has been found to live for many days in dried blood spills, posing a risk of transmission long after many other viruses would have died. For this reason, it is critical for you to assume that any body fluid in any form, dried or otherwise, is infectious until proven otherwise. Hepatitis B can be deadly. Before hepatitis B vaccine was available, the virus (HBV) killed hundreds of health care

TABLE 2-1 Communicable Diseases

DISEASE	MODE OF TRANSMISSION	INCUBATION
AIDS (acquired immune deficiency syndrome)	HIV-infected blood via intravenous drug use, unprotected sexual contact, blood transfusions, or (rarely) accidental needlesticks. Mothers also may pass HIV to their unborn children.	Several months or years
Chicken pox (varicella)	Airborne droplets. Can also be spread by contact with open sores.	11-21 days
Ebola	Blood and body fluids (e.g., urine, saliva, feces, vomit, sweat, and semen)	2-21 days (most commonly 8-10 days)
German measles (rubella)	Airborne droplets. Mothers may pass the disease to unborn children.	10-12 days
Influenza (flu–various strains including swine and avian)	Respiratory droplet	1-7 days
Hepatitis	Blood, stool, or other body fluids, or contaminated objects	Weeks to months, depending on type
Meningitis, bacterial	Oral and nasal secretions	2-10 days
Mumps	Droplets of saliva or objects contaminated by saliva	14-24 days
Pneumonia, bacterial and viral	Oral and nasal droplets and secretions	Several days
Staphylococcal skin infections	Direct contact with infected wounds or sores or with contaminated objects	Several days
Tuberculosis (TB)	Respiratory secretions, airborne or on contaminated objects	2-6 weeks
Whooping cough (pertussis)	Respiratory secretions or airborne droplets	6-20 days

workers every year in the United States, more than any other occupationally acquired infectious disease. There is no cure, but an effective vaccine that prevents contracting HBV is available. (See *Immunizations* in this chapter.) Today, hepatitis C infects many EMS providers in the same way as hepatitis B; there is as yet no vaccine against hepatitis C.

- *Tuberculosis (TB)* is an infection that sometimes settles in the lungs and that in some cases can be fatal. It was once thought to be largely eradicated, but in the late 1980s it made a comeback. TB is highly contagious. Unlike many other infectious diseases, it can spread through the air. Health care workers and others can become infected even without any direct contact with a carrier. Because it is impossible for the EMT to determine why a patient has a productive cough, it is safest to assume that it could be the result of TB and to take the necessary respiratory precautions. This is especially true in institutions such as nursing homes, correctional facilities, or homeless shelters where there is an increased risk of TB.
- *AIDS (acquired immune deficiency syndrome)* is a set of conditions that results when the immune system has been attacked by HIV (human immunodeficiency virus) and becomes unable to combat certain infections adequately. Although advances are being made in the treatment of HIV/AIDS, no cure has been discovered at the time of publication of this text. HIV/AIDS presents far less risk to health care workers than hepatitis and TB because the virus does not survive well outside the human body. This limits the routes of exposure to direct contact with blood by way of open wounds, intravenous drug use, unprotected sexual contact, blood transfusions, and puncture wounds into which HIV is introduced, such as an accidental needlestick. However, less than half of 1 percent of such incidents result in infection, according to the U.S. Occupational Safety and Health Administration (OSHA), compared with 30 percent for the hepatitis B virus (HBV). The difference is due to the quantity and strength of HBV compared with those of HIV.

Hepatitis B, hepatitis C, TB, and HIV/AIDS are the communicable diseases of greatest concern because they are potentially life threatening. However, there are many communicable diseases to which emergency response and other health care personnel may be exposed. Review Table 2-1 for common communicable diseases, their modes of transmission, and their incubation periods (the time between contact and the first appearance of symptoms).

Detailed coverage of infectious diseases can be found in the chapter, *Infectious Diseases and Sepsis*.

Specific Diseases of Concern

In recent years some diseases have worsened and new ones have been discovered. Ebola is a viral disease that first appeared in Africa in 1976. In 2014, for the first time, Ebola infected people in the United States. This disease is of particular concern because of the high rate of deaths and the lack of a definitive vaccination or treatment.

Ebola causes initial symptoms that include fever, chills, and weakness. These progress to watery diarrhea, vomiting, and abdominal pain. Ebola is a hemorrhagic fever. Therefore, late signs may include bruising as well as internal and external bleeding.

Refer to the most recent recommendations from the CDC and your EMS protocols for information on patient screening, preventing transmission of Ebola, and methods of decontamination. These will differ from those for many other diseases. Screening by dispatchers for the patient's travel history or potential contacts with other symptomatic Ebola patients is important. Consideration of Ebola early in the call is crucial for preventing transmission of the disease to EMS personnel (Figure 2-5).

People get respiratory infections quite commonly. In most cases these are mild, causing runny nose, sore throat, and fever, and are limited to a few days. However, more severe respiratory illnesses have been found around the world. You may have heard about two of these in the news. MERS (Middle Eastern respiratory syndrome) is one of the more recent syndromes. It has been found primarily on the Arabian Peninsula, although cases have been found in more than a dozen other countries and regions. Severe acute respiratory syndrome (SARS) caused concern worldwide when it emerged in 2003. It infected more than eight thousand people around the world and caused almost eight hundred deaths. It was spread through respiratory droplets, by coughing, sneezing, or touching something contaminated, then touching the nose or eyes. Protection against MERS and other respiratory infections in a patient-care setting includes frequent hand washing and the use of gloves, gowns, eye protection, and an N-95 respirator.

Avian flu is a disease found in poultry that can also affect humans. Outbreaks have been seen in Asia, the Near East, and Africa, and have been fatal in about half the reported cases. The virus has not shown to be easily transmissible from human to human. Symptoms

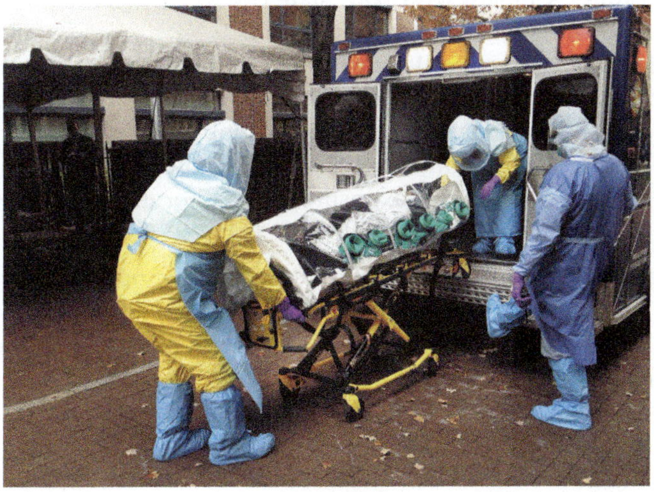

FIGURE 2-5 Care and transport for patients with diseases like Ebola require a high level of personal protective equipment and preparation of the ambulance prior to transport. *(Edward T. Dickinson, MD)*

include traditional flulike symptoms that progress to more severe conditions such as pneumonia and acute respiratory distress syndrome. Precautions are the same as for SARS.

Influenza has been around for hundreds of years. The influenza pandemic of 1918 killed between 30 million and 50 million people around the world. There are many strains of flu, including each year's seasonal flu. The avian and swine flu viruses have caused widespread illness and some panic. EMS can help prevent the spread of flu by recognizing flu symptoms and placing a mask on any potential flu patient before entering the hospital.

One additional effect of these diseases has been to quicken the pace at which EMS becomes involved in public health endeavors. EMS is on the front lines of care for any acute disease or condition like Ebola or the flu. EMS, hospitals, and public health agencies work closely together to assure high-quality care for the patient while preventing contamination of the public and health care providers.

Some diseases are on the decline. For example, vaccines have significantly reduced chickenpox and epiglottitis in children. Diseases of concern will change while you are an EMT. Health agencies will issue warnings and advisories on these diseases, as will the CDC.

Infection Control and the Law

Scientists have identified the main culprits in the transmission of many deadly infectious diseases: blood and body fluids. EMTs and other health care workers have been recognized as having a higher-than-usual exposure and, therefore, a higher risk of contracting these unwanted infections.

Congress and federal agencies have responded by taking several steps to ensure the safety of people who are in high-risk positions. In particular, OSHA and the CDC have issued standards and guidelines for the protection of workers whose jobs may expose them to infectious diseases. The Ryan White CARE Act and the Ryan White HIV/AIDS Treatment Extension Act of 2009 establish procedures by which emergency response workers may find out whether they have been exposed to life-threatening infectious diseases. These legal protections are described in more detail in the next sections.

Occupational Exposure to Bloodborne Pathogens

OSHA has created a standard for bloodborne pathogens. It mandates employers of emergency responders take certain measures to protect employees who are likely to be exposed to blood and other body fluids. One of the basic principles behind the standard is that infection control is a joint responsibility between employer and employee. The employer must provide training, protective equipment, and vaccinations to employees who are subject to exposure in their jobs. In return, employees must participate in an infection exposure control plan that includes training and proper workplace practices.

Without the active participation of both the employer and the employee, any workplace infection control program is destined to fail. Be sure your system has an active and up-to-date infection exposure control plan and that you and your fellow EMTs follow it carefully at all times. Consult with your state OSHA representative to make sure that specific hazards are identified and corrected.

Contact the U.S. Department of Labor to request the booklet *Occupational Exposure to Bloodborne Pathogens: Precautions for Emergency Responders—OSHA 3106 1998*, an overview of the standard. For details regarding how to develop an infection control plan, request Title 29 Code of Federal Regulation 1910.1030 for the complete text of the standard and all requirements regarding occupational exposure to bloodborne pathogens. Critical elements of the standard are summarized in the following list:

- **Infection exposure control plan.** Each emergency response employer must develop a plan that identifies and documents job classifications and tasks in which there is the possibility of exposure to potentially infectious body fluids. The plan must outline a schedule of how and when the bloodborne pathogen standards will be implemented. It also must include identification of the methods used for communicating hazards to employees, postexposure evaluation, and follow-up.

- **Adequate education and training.** EMTs must be provided with training that includes general explanations of how diseases are transmitted, uses and limitations of practices that reduce or prevent exposure, and procedures to follow if exposure occurs.
- **Hepatitis B vaccination.** Employers must make the hepatitis B vaccination series available free of charge and at a reasonable time and place.
- **Personal protective equipment.** This equipment must be of a quality that will not permit blood or other infectious materials to pass through or reach an EMT's work clothes, street clothes, undergarments, skin, eyes, mouth, or other mucous membranes. This equipment must be provided by the employer to the EMT at no cost and include, but not be limited to, protective gloves, face shields, masks, protective eyewear, gowns, and aprons, plus bag-valve masks, pocket masks, and other ventilation devices.
- **Methods of control.** Engineering controls remove potential infectious disease hazards or separate the EMT from exposure. Examples include pocket masks, disposable airway equipment, and puncture-resistant needle containers. Work practice controls improve the manner in which a task is performed to reduce risk of exposure. Examples include the proper and safe use of personal protective equipment; proper handling, labeling, and disposal of contaminated materials; and proper washing and decontamination practices.
- **Housekeeping.** The EMT and the employer are both responsible for maintaining clean and sanitary conditions of the emergency response vehicles and work sites. Procedures include the proper handling and proper decontamination of work surfaces, equipment, laundry, and other materials.
- **Labeling.** The standard requires labeling of containers used to store, transport, or ship blood and other potentially infectious materials, including the use of the biohazard symbol (Figure 2-6).
- **Postexposure evaluation and follow-up.** EMTs must immediately report suspected exposure incidents—including mucous membrane or broken-skin contact with blood or other potentially infectious materials—that result from the performance of an employee's duties. (See Figure 2-7 for a model plan based on the Ryan White CARE Act and the Ryan White HIV/AIDS Treatment Extension Act of 2009, which are described next.)

FIGURE 2-6 The biohazard symbol must be included with warning labels for containers used to ship blood or other potentially infectious materials.

Ryan White CARE Act

The Ryan White Comprehensive AIDS Resources Emergency (CARE) Act (also called the Ryan White CARE Act) was enacted by the U.S. Congress in 1990. It was named for Ryan White, a teenager who contracted AIDS from a tainted hemophilia treatment in 1984, became an advocate for AIDS research and awareness, and died from the disease in 1990. In 1994, the CDC issued the final notice for the Ryan White CARE Act Regarding Emergency Response Employees. This federal act, which applies to all 50 states, mandates a procedure by which emergency response personnel can seek to find out if they have been exposed to potentially life-threatening diseases while providing patient care. The procedures for exposure follow-up by emergency response personnel denoted in the act remain in force under its most recent extension as the Ryan White HIV/AIDS Treatment Extension Act of 2009. Emergency response personnel referred to in this act include firefighters, law enforcement officers, EMTs, and other individuals who provide emergency aid on behalf of a legally recognized volunteer organization.

The CDC has published a list of potentially life-threatening infectious and communicable diseases to which emergency response personnel can be exposed. The list includes airborne diseases such as TB, bloodborne diseases such as hepatitis B and HIV/AIDS, and uncommon or rare diseases such as diphtheria and rabies.

The Ryan White CARE Act requires every state's public health officer to designate an official within every emergency response organization to act as a "designated officer."

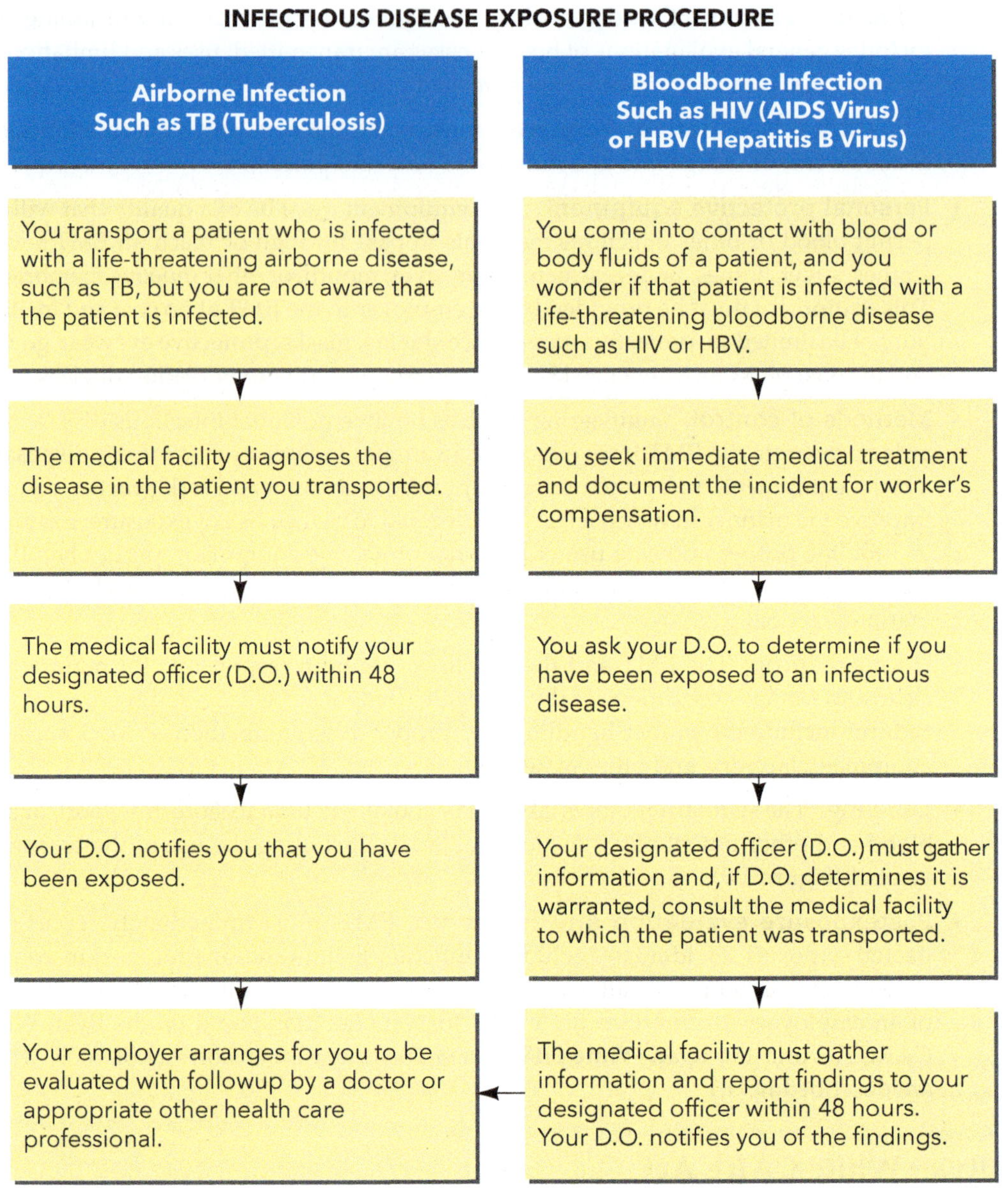

FIGURE 2-7 Under the Ryan White CARE Act and the Ryan White HIV/AIDS Treatment Extension Act of 2009, there is a procedure for finding out whether and following up if you have been exposed to a life-threatening disease.

The designated officer is responsible for gathering facts surrounding possible emergency responder airborne or bloodborne infectious disease exposures. Take time to learn who is the designated officer within your organization.

Two different notification systems for infectious disease exposure are defined in the act:

- **Airborne disease exposure.** You will be notified by your designated officer when you have been exposed to an airborne disease.
- **Bloodborne or other infectious disease exposure.** You may submit a request for a determination as to whether you were exposed to a bloodborne or other infectious disease.

The differences between the two procedures results from the differences in how an exposure is most likely to be detected. With an airborne disease such as TB, you may not realize that the patient you have cared for and transported was infected. However, a disease such as TB will be diagnosed at the hospital. Therefore, the Ryan White CARE Act states that for airborne diseases such as TB, the hospital will notify the designated officer, who will notify you.

A bloodborne disease such as hepatitis B or HIV/AIDS may or may not be diagnosed at the hospital, but you will know if you have had contact with a patient's blood or body fluids. If so, you can submit a request to your designated officer, who will gather the information necessary to request a determination from the hospital on whether you have been exposed and who will notify you of the result.

In either case, once you have been notified of an exposure, your employer will refer you to a doctor or other health care professional for evaluation and follow-up.

Consider how the Ryan White CARE Act would apply in the following example of exposure to an airborne pathogen.

> As an EMT, you treat and transport a patient who complains of weakness, fever, and chronic cough. The next day, you receive a phone call from your organization's designated officer, who informs you that you have been exposed to a patient with TB. The designated officer helps you arrange an appointment with a doctor who can determine whether you have contracted the disease and arrange for early treatment if you have.

According to CDC guidelines, exposure to airborne pathogens may occur when you share "air space" with a tuberculosis patient. So if a medical facility diagnoses that patient as having the airborne infectious disease, it must notify the designated officer within 48 hours. The designated officer must then notify the emergency care workers of disease exposure. Finally, the employer must schedule a postexposure evaluation and follow-up.

Consider a possible exposure to a bloodborne pathogen.

> As an EMT, you are called to treat an unconscious woman. Pink, frothy sputum trickles from her mouth. Her breathing is labored. A hypodermic needle lies beside her. While you are suctioning the patient, your eye shield slips and fluids from her mouth splash into your eyes. You immediately flush your eyes and report the incident as soon as the call is completed. Your designated officer follows up, and you learn that you have not been exposed to a life-threatening bloodborne disease.

Under CDC guidelines, after contact with the blood or body fluids of a patient you have transported, you may submit a request for a determination to your designated officer. The designated officer must then gather information about the possible exposure. If the information indicates a possible exposure, the officer forwards the information to the medical facility where the patient is being treated. If the patient can be identified, medical records are reviewed to determine if the patient has a life-threatening disease. The medical facility then must notify your designated officer of their findings in writing within 48 hours after receiving the officer's request. The designated officer must notify you, and you will be directed by your employer to a health care professional for a postexposure evaluation and follow-up as appropriate.

It is important to note that the Ryan White CARE Act does not empower hospitals to test patients for bloodborne diseases at the request of the emergency worker or designated officer. Rather, they can only review the patient's medical records to see if evidence of a bloodborne or other disease exists. Thus, a patient could be infected, but if the records reveal no testing or known indication of the presence of such an infection, the hospital can report only that "no evidence of bloodborne infection could be detected."

Tuberculosis Compliance Mandate

Thousands of new cases of TB are reported in the United States each year. Hundreds of health care workers have been infected or exposed. Of particular concern is multidrug-resistant TB (MDR-TB), which does not respond to the usual medications. In 1994 the CDC issued guidelines for treating a suspected or confirmed TB patient. OSHA has announced it will enforce those guidelines as if they were OSHA rules and will also require employers of health care workers to follow OSHA's respiratory standard (1910.134). This standard describes the selection and proper use of different kinds of respirators, including those classified as N-95 or HEPA.

Study the guidelines as summarized in the following text. Learn to recognize situations in which the potential of exposure to TB exists. Those at greatest risk of contracting and transmitting TB are people who have suppressed immune systems, including people with HIV/AIDS and elderly patients such as those living in nursing homes. Patients who have

TB may have the following signs and symptoms: productive cough (coughing up mucus or other fluid) and/or coughing up blood, weight loss and loss of appetite, lethargy and weakness, night sweats, and fever. It is safest to assume that any person with a productive cough may be infected with TB.

> **NOTE:** *If you are actually exposed to a bloodborne pathogen (e.g., by a needlestick or splashing of fluids to a mucous membrane), you must seek medical attention immediately. It is important that you receive care for the wound, obtain baseline blood work including determining hepatitis B immunity, evaluate the need for a tetanus shot, and document the incident for worker's compensation or insurance. You may also be asked to consider taking an antiviral drug or combination of drugs to attempt to counteract the effects of HIV if it is present. This is a personal issue and a very serious decision. It is important to know that current research indicates that waiting 48 hours for the requested Ryan White information to determine whether the patient whose blood you were exposed to may be HIV infected may reduce the effectiveness of the drugs. Even a few hours may make a significant difference in treatment outcome. Do not delay seeking care. Each situation is different. You will wish to seek the advice of the attending physician where you are being treated as well as that of your Medical Director.*

When the potential exists for exposure to exhaled air of a person with suspected or confirmed TB, OSHA requires that you wear a NIOSH-approved N-95 or HEPA respirator. You are required to wear an N-95 or HEPA respirator when you are:

- **Caring for patients suspected of having TB.** High-risk areas include correctional institutions, homeless shelters, long-term care facilities for the elderly, and drug treatment centers.
- **Transporting an individual from such a setting in a closed vehicle.** If possible, keep the windows of the ambulance open and set the heating and air conditioning system on the nonrecirculating cycle.
- **Performing high-risk procedures such as endotracheal suctioning and intubation.**

Remember to take all recommended infection control precautions, including hand washing and using personal protective equipment and barrier devices such as pocket masks or bag-valve masks for rescue breathing. Properly dispose of contaminated equipment and materials, and decontaminate all surfaces, clothing, and equipment.

Immunizations

Immunizations against many diseases are available. Most people receive tetanus immunizations either routinely or after certain injuries. There is currently an immunization available to prevent hepatitis B. It will be provided by your EMS agency, usually through a local physician or your Medical Director.

Although there is no immunization against tuberculosis used in the United States, a tuberculin skin test (TST) can detect exposure. (The CDC now uses the term *tuberculin skin test (TST)* rather than the older but synonymous term *purified protein derivative (PPD) test*.) EMTs are often given this test during routine or employment screening physicals. If the test determines that you have been exposed to tuberculosis, seek treatment and follow-up from a doctor or other health care professional. EMS workers should be checked for exposure to TB on a regular basis (usually yearly).

Some EMS agencies and medical facilities may require immunizations for measles, influenza, and other common communicable diseases. Consult your instructor, your Medical Director, or your personal physician for more information on your current status and local protocols for immunizations.

Emotion and Stress

Take a minute to think about the last time you told someone that you felt "stressed out." How did you feel? Did you feel tense, as if every muscle were tight, every nerve on edge? Were your palms sweaty and your stomach in knots? Was your heart pounding, and did you have a lump in your throat? Did you have trouble sleeping or always feel exhausted no matter how much sleep you had the previous night? What was going on in your life at that time? Were you preparing for a big exam? Was a family member's illness causing you to worry? Did you feel torn between the demands of family, work, and school? Were you worried about your financial state, wondering how you would cover some large unexpected expense? Were you about to change jobs, or were you going through a divorce? How you manage these and other stressors is critical to your well-being.

A term that has come to prominence is ***resilience***. Resilience means "toughness" or an ability to overcome tough situations. It is used as a strategy to help prepare EMS providers to deal with difficult things they may experience, with minimal lasting psychological trauma. Components of resilience include understanding stress, being physically and mentally prepared, and using certain actions and techniques immediately after an incident to help mentally "process" difficult scenes.

CORE CONCEPT

The kinds of stress caused by involvement in EMS and how they can affect you, your fellow EMTs, and your family and friends

resilience
toughness; an ability to recover quickly from difficult situations.

Physiologic Aspects of Stress

During the Middle Ages and for much of the next two hundred to three hundred years, people viewed the mind and body as separate entities. In the last third of the twentieth century, however, medical science began to give increasing scrutiny to how the mind and body work together and influence each other. In fact, today it would be hard to find anyone who denies that there is a connection between mind and body or that stress plays a role in illness.

Stress is a widely used term in today's society. It is derived from a word used in the 1600s (*stresse*, a variation of *distresse*), which meant acute anxiety, pain, or sorrow. Today doctors and psychologists generally define stress as a state of physical and/or psychological arousal to a stimulus. Any stimulus is capable of being a stressor for someone, and stressors vary from individual to individual and from time to time.

stress
a state of physical and/or psychological arousal to a stimulus.

Many agree that stress poses a potential hazard for EMS personnel. However, it is important to recognize that stress is a normal part of life and, when managed appropriately, does not have to pose a threat to your well-being. As an EMT, you will be routinely exposed to stress-producing agents or situations. These stressors may be environmental factors (e.g., noise, inclement weather, unstable wreckage), your dealings with other people (e.g., unpleasant family or work relationships, abusive patients or bystanders), or your own self-image or performance expectations (e.g., worry over your expertise at specific skills or guilt over poor patient outcomes).

Ironically, these stress-causing factors may be some of the same things that first attracted you to EMS, such as an atypical work environment, an unpredictable but varied workload, dealing with people in crisis, or the opportunity to work somewhat independently. How you manage these stressors is critical to your survival as an EMS provider as well as in life.

Dr. Hans Selye, a Canadian physician and educator who was born in Austria, did a great deal of research in this area and found that the body's response to stress (*general adaptation syndrome*) has three stages:

- **First stage: alarm reaction.** During the first stage, your sympathetic nervous system increases its activity in what is known as the fight-or-flight syndrome. Your pupils dilate, your heart rate increases, and your bronchial passages dilate. In addition, your blood sugar increases, your digestive system slows, your blood pressure rises, and blood flow to your skeletal muscles increases. At the same time, the endocrine system produces more cortisol, a hormone that influences your metabolism and your immune response. Cortisol is critical to your body's ability to adapt to and cope with stress.
- **Second stage: stage of resistance.** In the second stage, your body systems return to normal functioning. The physiologic effects of sympathetic nervous system stimulation and the excess cortisol are gone. You have adapted to the stimulus, and it no longer produces stress for you. You are coping. Many factors contribute to your ability to cope; these include your physical and mental health, education, experiences, and support systems, such as family, friends, and coworkers.

- **Third stage: exhaustion.** Exhaustion occurs when exposure to a stressor is prolonged or the stressor is particularly severe. During this stage, the physiologic effects described by Selye include what he called the stress triad: enlargement (hypertrophy) of the adrenal glands, which produce adrenaline; wasting (atrophy) of lymph nodes; and bleeding gastric ulcers. At this point the individual has lost the ability to resist or adapt to the stressor and may become seriously ill as a consequence. Fortunately most individuals do not reach this stage.

Types of Stress Reactions

Three types of stress reactions are commonly encountered: acute stress reactions, delayed stress reactions, and cumulative stress reactions. Any of these may occur as a result of a *critical incident,* which is any situation that triggers a strong emotional response. An *acute stress reaction* occurs simultaneously with or shortly after the critical incident. A *delayed stress reaction* (also known as posttraumatic stress disorder) may occur at any time, days to years, following a critical incident. A *cumulative stress reaction* (also known as *burnout*) occurs as a result of prolonged recurring stressors in our work or private lives.

Acute Stress Reaction

Acute stress reactions are often linked to catastrophes, such as a large-scale natural disaster, a plane crash, or a coworker's line-of-duty death or injury. Signs and symptoms of an acute stress reaction will develop simultaneously or within a very short time following the incident. They may involve any one or a combination of the following areas of function: physical, cognitive (the ability to think), emotional, or behavioral. These are signs that this particular situation is overwhelming your usual abilities to cope and to perform effectively. It is important to keep in mind that they are ordinary reactions to extraordinary situations. They reflect the process of adapting to challenge. They are normal and are not a sign of weakness or mental illness.

Some of these signs and symptoms require immediate intervention from a physician or mental health professional, whereas others do not. As a rule, any sign or symptom that indicates an acute medical problem (such as chest pain, difficulty breathing, or abnormal heart rhythms) or an acute psychological problem (such as uncontrollable crying; inappropriate behavior; or a disruption in normal, rational thinking) indicates the kind of problem that demand immediate corrective action. These are the same signs that alert us to a potentially dangerous situation when we see them in a patient, and they should trigger the same response when exhibited by us or our coworkers. Helping people is not just about taking care of your patient; it is also always about taking care of each other and yourself.

As previously mentioned, some signs and symptoms associated with an acute stress reaction may not require intervention. For instance, you may feel nauseated, tremulous, or numb after working with a patient in cardiopulmonary arrest, particularly if your patient is close to your age. You may feel confused, or have trouble concentrating or difficulty sleeping, after working at a particularly bloody crash scene or a prolonged extrication. You may find that you have no appetite for food or cannot get enough to eat. If not too severe or long lasting, these responses are uncomfortable but probably not dangerous, since they pose no immediate threat to your health, safety, or well-being.

Remember that you are not losing your mind if you exhibit signs and symptoms of stress after a critical incident. You are merely reacting to an extraordinary situation. Remember, too, that there is nothing wrong with you if you do *not* experience any symptoms after such an incident. This, too, is common. In other words, a wide range of responses is normal and to be expected.

Delayed Stress Reaction

Like an acute stress reaction, a delayed stress reaction, also known as posttraumatic stress disorder (PTSD), can be triggered by a specific incident. However, the signs and symptoms may not become evident until days, months, or even years later. This delay in presentation may make it harder to deal with the stress reaction, since the individual has seemingly moved past the incident and moved on with life. Signs and symptoms may include flashbacks, nightmares, feelings of detachment, irritability, sleep difficulties, self-harm behaviors or habits, or problems with concentration or interpersonal relationships occurring for a month or longer.

PTSD is not new. The syndrome was first identified in soldiers and called "battle fatigue" or "shell shock." Many combat veterans experience PTSD. It may also be seen in victims of natural disasters, those who have been violently assaulted or abused, and those who have witnessed unusually violent events.

It is not uncommon for persons suffering from PTSD to seek solace through drug and alcohol abuse. Because of the delay and the apparent disconnect between the triggering event and the response, the patient with PTSD may not understand what is causing the problems. PTSD requires intervention by a mental health professional.

Cumulative Stress Reaction

Cumulative stress reaction, or burnout, is not triggered by a single critical incident, but instead results from sustained, recurring low-level stressors—possibly in more than one aspect of one's life—and develops over a period of years.

The earliest signs are subtle. They may present as a vague anxiety, progressing to boredom and apathy, and a feeling of emotional exhaustion. If problems are not identified and managed at this point, the progression will continue. Now the individual will develop physical complaints (such as headaches or stomach ailments), significant sleep disturbances, loss of emotional control, irritability, withdrawal from others, and increasing depression. Without appropriate intervention, the person's physical, emotional, and behavioral condition will continue to deteriorate, with manifestations such as migraines, increased smoking or alcohol intake, loss of sexual drive, poor interpersonal relationships, deterioration in work performance, limited self-control, and significant depression.

At its worst, cumulative stress may present as physical illness, uncontrollable emotions, overwhelming physical and emotional fatigue, severe withdrawal, paranoia, or suicidal thoughts. Long-term psychological intervention is critical at this stage if the individual is to recover.

The ultimate key to preventing or managing cumulative stress lies in seeking balance in our lives.

Causes of Stress

Emergencies are stressful by nature. Although most EMS calls are considered "routine," some calls seem to have a higher potential for causing excess stress on EMS providers (Figure 2-8). They include the following:

- **Multiple-casualty incidents.** A ***multiple-casualty incident (MCI)*** is a single incident in which there are multiple patients. Examples range from a motor-vehicle crash in which two drivers and a passenger are injured to a hurricane that causes injuries to hundreds of people.
- **Calls involving infants and children.** Involving anything from a serious injury to sudden infant death syndrome (SIDS), these calls are known to be particularly stressful to all health care providers.
- **Severe injuries.** Expect a stress reaction when your call involves injuries that cause major trauma or distortion to the human body. Examples include amputations, deformed bones, deep wounds, and violent death.
- **Abuse and neglect.** Cases of abuse and neglect occur in all social and economic levels of society. You may be called to treat infant, child, adult, or elder abuse victims.
- **Death of a coworker.** A bond is formed among members of the public services. The death of another public-safety worker—even if you do not know that person—can cause a stress response.

multiple-casualty incident (MCI)
an emergency involving multiple patients.

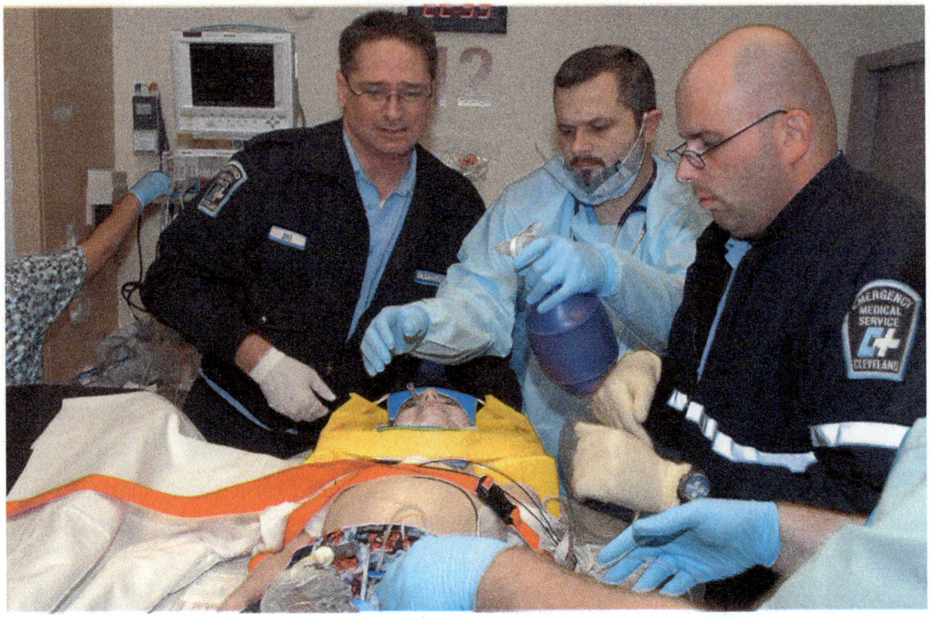

FIGURE 2-8 Emergencies involving infants and children are often stressful for EMS providers. *(© David Effron, MD)*

Stress may be caused by a single event, or it may be the cumulative result of several incidents. Remember that any incident may affect you and your coworkers differently. Two EMTs on the same call may have opposite responses. Never make negative judgments about another person's reaction.

Stress may also stem from a combination of factors, including problems in your personal life. One common cause of stress is people who "just don't understand" the job. For example, your EMS organization may require you to work on weekends and holidays. Time spent on call may be frustrating to friends and family members. They may not understand why you cannot participate in certain social activities or why you cannot leave a certain area. You might get frustrated, too, because you cannot plan around the unpredictable nature of emergencies. Then, after a very trying or exciting call, for instance, you may wish to share your feelings with a friend or someone you love. You find instead that the person does not understand your emotions. This can lead to feelings of separation and rejection, which are highly stressful.

Signs and Symptoms of Stress

There are two types of stress: eustress and distress. *Eustress* is a positive form of stress that helps people work under pressure and respond effectively. *Distress* is negative. It can happen when the stress of a scene becomes overwhelming. As a result, your response to the emergency will not be effective. Distress also can cause immediate and long-term problems with your health and well-being.

The signs and symptoms of stress include irritability with family, friends, and coworkers; inability to concentrate; and changes in daily activities, such as difficulty sleeping or nightmares, loss of appetite, loss of interest in sexual activity, anxiety, indecisiveness, guilt, isolation, and loss of interest in work.

Dealing with Stress

Lifestyle Changes

There are several ways to deal with stress. They are called *lifestyle changes* and offer a benefit in both preventing stress and dealing with it when stress occurs. They include:

- **Develop more healthful and positive dietary habits.** Avoid fatty foods and increase your carbohydrate intake. Also reduce your consumption of alcohol and caffeine, which can have negative effects, including an increase in stress and anxiety and disturbance of sleep patterns.

- **Exercise.** When performed safely and properly, exercise helps to "burn off" stress. It also helps you deal with the physical aspects of your responsibilities, such as carrying equipment and performing physically demanding emergency procedures.
- **Devote time to relaxing.** Try relaxation techniques too. These techniques, which include deep-breathing exercises and meditation, are valuable stress reducers.

In addition to the changes you can make in your personal life to help reduce and prevent stress, there also are changes you can make in your professional life. If you are in an organization with varied shifts and locations, consider requesting a change to a different location that offers a lighter call volume or different types of calls. You may also want to change your shift to one that allows more time with family and friends.

Invisible Wounds—Preventing Psychological Trauma

It's no secret that you can see some bad things in EMS. You and your patients can be profoundly affected by psychological trauma. Some people see a tragic scene involving a death and are relatively unaffected, while others experience long-term effects. There are ways to help yourself, your patients, and your partners. This section will provide concrete solutions to help in the moments, hours, and days after a traumatic incident.

On an average day—or even a bad day—the body takes in the stimulus from the environment and those in it. Whether it is work or family or recreation, the brain is constantly working to evaluate this input and "file" it properly.

In a traumatic incident, this filing system may malfunction. The input is overwhelming and the brain has trouble processing something so out of the ordinary. It is believed that this faulty processing is at the root of the ongoing posttraumatic issues faced by those who are involved in these incidents.

Consider the following situations:

- Your team has been attempting to resuscitate a man who was found unresponsive by his wife. There is no hope for recovery, and efforts to save the man are terminated. You are charged with telling the wife that her husband has died.
- You have been attempting to care for a teenage boy who is trapped in a car. The extrication was prolonged, and you watch the patient deteriorate from shock. You arrive to find him responsive and talking, but during the time you are with him you watch him fade and die. You were unable to help him because he was pinned in the car.
- You are called to a collision involving an ambulance. A passenger in the other car is critically injured. The operator of the ambulance is uninjured but pale and sweaty. She keeps repeating, "I hope I didn't kill him. I hope I didn't kill him."

Whether it is a patient, a family member, you, or another EMS provider, there will be times that specific care will help prevent or reduce long-term stress as a result of a traumatic incident. The Northeast Resilience Consortium and LaGuardia Community College in New York City developed the eSCAPe curriculum (Figure 2-9) to help patients and EMS providers deal with posttraumatic stress.

Patients who have experienced a traumatic incident but have reported less stress than others in the aftermath had a few things in common. The first was social support. The belief that they are being cared for, that they are not alone, and that they are part of a team or system had significant benefit in reducing posttraumatic stress.

The second factor that reduces stress is the belief in one's ability to manage one's own problems (self-efficacy). If people feel less helpless and more in control, it is believed they will experience less long-term stress as a result of the incident. The "filing system" in the brain has the ability to function more normally.

Note that in the two examples (social support and self-efficacy) that we used the term "believed." The patients *believed* they had some control and they *believed* they were being cared for. In a tragic or violent scene, the actual control over the situation may be minimal, but creating an environment where patients believe they have choices and control is still very important.

FIGURE 2-9 The eSCAPe mnemonic for dealing with posttraumatic stress.

e = Every Patient
S = provide Social support
C = give the patient Choices
A = help the patient Anticipate what will happen next
P = help the patient Plan and organize
e = Every time

This is where the eSCAPe curriculum applies. Consider each of the following steps. The first "e" stands for every patient—even on calls that seem routine to us. The second "e" refers to every time. The remaining concepts are applied as follows:

S: Social Support—Prevent feelings of isolation. Tell patients you are there to take care of them. Let them know they are not alone. Let a calm, clear, and compassionate voice reassure them.

C: Choice and Control—Replace hopelessness with hope and structure. Choices help provide patients with some sense of control. Even simple choices (when possible) such as asking which arm they prefer the BP cuff on can give patients some sense of control. Other choices might include asking whether they want someone to come with them to the hospital or whether someone needs to lock up the house.

A: Anticipate—Reduce anxiety and prevent unexpected events. Explain to patients what happens next at each step along the way. Simple things like stretcher movements, whether a procedure may hurt, and how long the trip to the hospital will take should be explained. Patients should never have to wonder what happens next.

P: Plan and Organize—Reduce bewilderment and loss. Encourage patients to consider each of the preceding steps and recognize that there is a plan. Continue to help and anticipate patient needs. Offer to make any calls or notifications. Help them lock the house and secure a pet so they won't add that worry to the current problem.

Remember that this process can be applied equally and effectively to patients, family members, and emergency personnel. Consider a situation where your partner just performed CPR on a child the same age as hers, or a situation caring for a police officer involved in a shooting. How would you apply eSCAPe to them?

Critical Incident Stress Management

critical incident stress management (CISM) a comprehensive system that includes education and resources to prevent stress and to deal with stress appropriately when it occurs.

Critical incident stress management (CISM) is a comprehensive system that includes education and resources both to prevent stress and to deal with stress appropriately when it does occur. EMS systems and organizations have different systems for dealing with stress prevention, critical incident stress, and chronic stress, including wellness incentives, professional counseling, and peer support.

Medical professionals and EMS leaders agree that the best course of action for an EMT who is experiencing significant stress from a serious call or experience is to seek help from a mental health professional who is experienced in treating these issues.

Everyone responds to these stresses differently. Remember that seeking care is an act of strength, not a sign of weakness. Many professionals can help you deal with stress, and much of the care may be covered by health insurance policies or employee assistance programs.

The critical incident stress debriefing (CISD) model is a process in which a team of trained peer counselors and mental health professionals meet with rescuers and health care providers who have been involved in a major incident. The meetings are generally held 24–72 hours after the incident. The goal is to assist emergency care workers in dealing with the stress related to that incident.

Sometimes a "defusing session" is held within the first few hours after a critical incident. Although CISD includes all personnel involved in the incident, a defusing session is usually limited to the people who were most directly involved with the most stressful aspects. It provides them an opportunity to vent feelings and receive information before the larger group meets.

The CISD (debriefing/defusing) model is now used less frequently and is not recommended by many in EMS and mental health professions.

Stress can take a toll on EMS providers at all levels. Not everyone experiences it—it affects everyone differently. The Code Green Campaign (codegreencampaign.org) is focused on ways of preventing stress and creating awareness of PTSD and suicide among EMS providers.

Understanding Reactions to Death and Dying

As an EMT, you will undoubtedly be called to patients who are in various stages of a terminal illness. Understanding what the families and the patients go through can help you deal with the stress they feel as well as your own.

CORE CONCEPT
The impact that dying patients have on you and others

When patients find out that they are dying, they go through emotional stages that vary in duration and magnitude. These sometimes overlap, and all affect both patients and family.

- **Denial or "Not me."** The patient denies that the patient is dying. This puts off dealing with the inevitable end of the process.
- **Anger or "Why me?"** The patient becomes angry at the situation. This anger is commonly vented upon family members and EMS personnel.
- **Bargaining or "OK, but first let me . . . "** In the mind of the patient, bargaining seems to postpone death, if only for a short time.
- **Depression or "OK, but I haven't . . . "** The patient is sad, depressed, and despairing, often mourning things not accomplished and dreams that will not come true. The patient retreats into a world of the patient's own and is unwilling to communicate with others.
- **Acceptance or "OK, I'm not afraid."** The patient may come to accept death, although not welcoming it. Often the patient may come to accept the situation before family members do. At this stage, the family may need more support than the patient.

Not all patients go through all these stages. Some may seem to be in more than one stage at the same time. Some reactions may not seem to fit any of the described stages. Those who die rapidly are likely not to have such a predictable response to their own mortality. However, a general understanding of the process can help you to communicate with patients and families effectively.

As an EMT, you will also encounter sudden, unexpected death—for example, as a result of a motor-vehicle collision. In cases of sudden death, family members are likely to react with a wide range of emotion.

You can take several steps or approaches in dealing with the patient and family members who are confronted with death or dying:

- **Recognize the patient's needs.** Treat the patient with respect and do everything you can to preserve the patient's dignity and sense of control. For example, talk directly to the patient. Avoid talking about the patient to family members in the patient's presence, as if the patient were incompetent or no longer living. Be sensitive to how the patient seems to want to handle the situation. For example, allow or encourage the patient to share feelings and needs, rather than cutting off such communications because of your own embarrassment or discomfort. Respect the patient's privacy if the patient does not want to communicate personal feelings.
- **Be tolerant of angry reactions from the patient or family members.** There may be feelings of helpless rage about the death or prospect of death. The anger is not personal. It would be directed at anyone in your position.
- **Listen empathetically.** Although you cannot "fix" the situation, just listening with understanding and patience will be very helpful.
- **Do not falsely reassure.** Avoid saying things such as "Everything will be all right," which you, the patient, and the family all know is not true. Offering false reassurance can be irritating and can give the impression that you do not really understand the situation.
- **Offer as much comfort as you realistically can.** Comfort both the patient and the family. Let them know that you will do everything you can to help or to get them whatever help is available from other sources. Use a gentle tone of voice and a reassuring touch, if appropriate.

Scene Safety

CORE CONCEPT
How to identify potential hazards and maintain scene safety

Scene safety is perhaps the most important concept in your EMT training—and whether the scene is safe is the most important decision you will make on a call. Unless you stay safe, you will not be able to help your patient and you may suffer serious injury or death.

When watching the news, it doesn't take long to see a violent incident on the street or the ravages of drug abuse. Mass incidents of violence have placed EMTs in a position where they may be called to chaotic and unpredictable situations—and have a front row seat.

While violence is on our minds, it is important to look at what kills and injures EMS providers. In a review of EMS provider deaths over the past several years, few EMS providers were killed by violence. Heart attack, motor-vehicle collisions, and air-medical crashes were greater risks by far. People are more likely to leave EMS because of back injuries than because of injuries caused by violence.

The remainder of this chapter will discuss several ways to remain safe in EMS. You will learn more on safety in the *Scene Size-Up* chapter.

Hazardous Material Incidents

hazardous material incident the release of a harmful substance into the environment.

Many chemicals are capable of causing death or lifelong complications even if they are only briefly inhaled or in contact with a person's body. Many of these materials are commercially transported, often by truck or rail. Such materials are also often stored in warehouses and used in industry. When there is an accident or when containers begin to leak, a ***hazardous material incident*** may occur, which will pose serious dangers for you as an EMT as well as for others who are in the vicinity. When you face an emergency involving such materials, remember you will not be able to help anyone if you are injured. Exercise caution.

The primary rule is to maintain a safe distance from the source of the hazardous material. Make sure your ambulance or other emergency vehicle is equipped with binoculars. They will help you identify placards, which are placed on vehicles, structures, and storage containers when they hold hazardous materials (Figure 2-10). These placards use coded colors and identification numbers that are listed in the *Emergency Response Guidebook* developed by the U.S. Department of Transportation, Transport Canada, and the Secretariat of Communications and Transportation of Mexico. This reference book should be placed in every vehicle that responds to, or may respond to, a hazardous material incident. It provides important information about the properties of the dangerous substance as well as information on safe distances, emergency care, and suggested procedures in the event of spills or fire. The *Emergency Response Guidebook* is available online from the U.S. Department of Transportation Pipeline and Hazardous Materials Safety Administration at www.phmsa.dot.gov.

FIGURE 2-10 (A) Using binoculars to identify hazardous materials before approaching an emergency site. (B) Placards with coded colors and identification numbers must be used on vehicles and containers to identify hazardous materials.

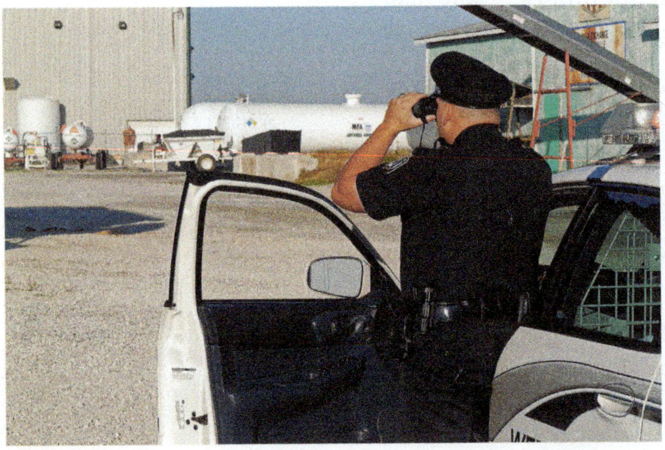
A

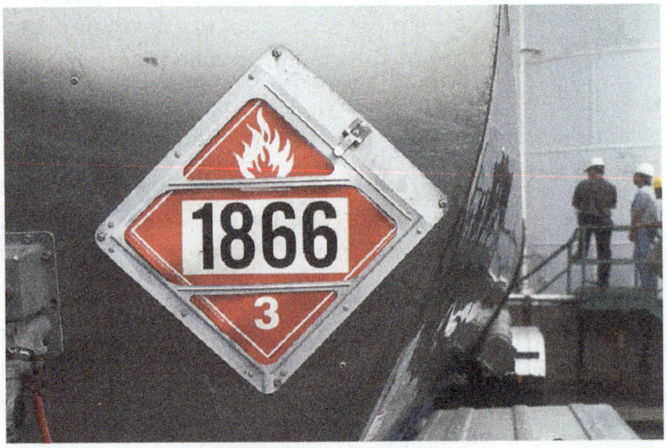

B

Your most important roles at the scene of a hazardous material incident are recognizing potential problems, taking initial actions for your personal safety and the safety of others, and notifying an appropriately trained hazardous material response team. Do not take any actions other than those aimed at protecting yourself, patients, and bystanders at the scene. An incorrect action can cause a bigger problem than the one that already exists.

The hazardous material response team is made up of specially trained technicians who will coordinate the safe approach to and resolution of the incident. Each wears a special suit that protects the skin. A self-contained breathing apparatus (SCBA) is also required, because of the strong potential for poisonous gases, dust, and fumes at a hazardous material incident. You will generally not be required to wear personal protective equipment of this sort unless you have been specially trained to be part of a hazardous material response team. Instead, you will remain at a distance until the team has made the scene safe.

As an EMT, you should not be treating patients until after they have undergone ***decontamination*** (cleansing of dangerous chemicals and other materials). If you take a contaminated patient into your ambulance, it will be considered contaminated and cannot be used again until it is thoroughly decontaminated. Furthermore, if you bring a contaminated patient to the emergency department of a hospital, you could effectively close that hospital down. (See the chapter titled *Hazardous Materials, Multiple-Casualty Incidents, and Incident Management* for more information on hazardous material incidents.)

decontamination the removal or cleansing of dangerous chemicals and other dangerous or infectious materials.

Terrorist Incidents

As an EMT, you may be called to respond to a terrorist incident. This incident may be small or large in scale and may include chemical agents, biological agents, radiation, weapons, and/or explosive devices (Figure 2-11).

Although these topics are covered in other areas of this text—including the *EMS Response to Terrorism* chapter—it is important to consider this type of incident and its effect on your personal safety in the general context of scene safety.

As part of your initial and subsequent training, you will likely be made aware of any specific threats or targets in your area in addition to any specific protocols relating to potential chemical, biological, nuclear, or explosive incidents.

Rescue Operations

Rescue operations include rescuing or disentangling victims from fires, auto collisions, explosions, electrocutions, and more. As with hazardous materials, it is important to evaluate each situation and ensure that appropriate assistance is requested early in the call. Depending on the emergency, you may need the police, fire department, power company, or other specialized personnel. Never perform acts that you are not properly trained to do.

FIGURE 2-11 Your first responsibility at the scene of a terrorist incident is to remain safe so that you will be able to assist when the scene has been secured. (A) Memorial to 17 victims of Parkland, FL, school shooting. (B) People fleeing the scene of the Las Vegas shooting of 2018. *(A: ZUMA Press, Inc./Alamy Stock Photo; B: David Becker/Getty Images)*

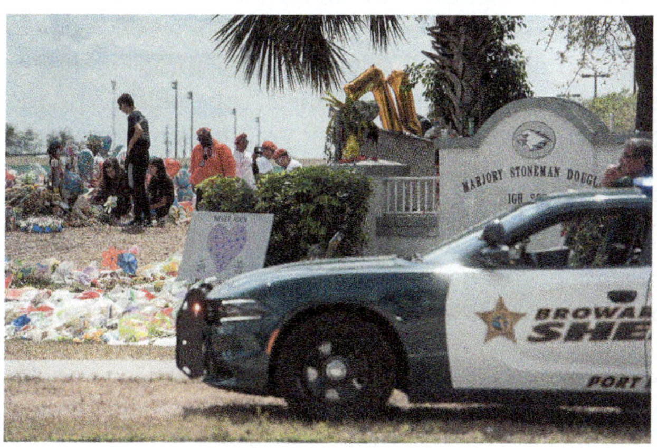

A

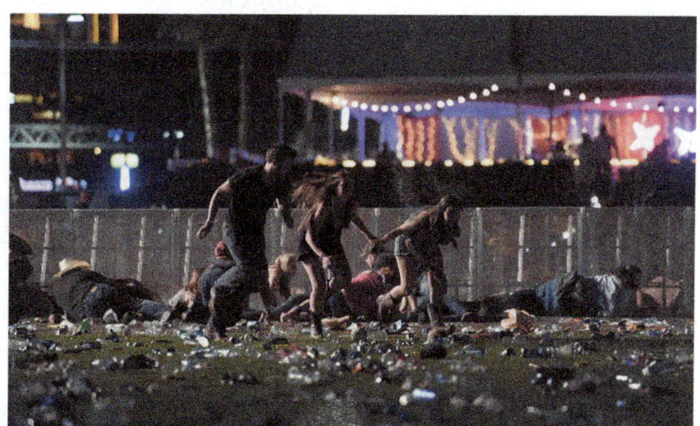

B

Do your best to secure the scene. Then stand by for the specialists. (You will learn more about rescue operations in the *Highway Safety and Vehicle Extrication* chapter.)

As you work in rescue operations or on patients during a rescue operation, you will need personal protective equipment that includes turnout gear (coat, pants, and boots), protective eyewear, helmet, and puncture-proof gloves.

The Realities of Well-Being

This chapter explains concepts that are very important to know, like how to protect yourself from diseases and dangers you may encounter at an emergency scene. Things seem straightforward, almost clear-cut, but they are not. Strict advice like "Don't touch anything that might cause you to catch a disease" or "Never go into an unsafe scene" is prudent, but is it practical? Consider the following situations:

- You are off duty at a shopping mall where a shooting has just occurred. The shooter has been killed by police. You observe a woman bleeding badly from a wound in the thigh. You don't have gloves on you. Do you let her bleed to death or help her?
- You are on the ambulance and were dispatched to a collision. You were nearby, and you arrive first to find a car with the engine fully engulfed in flames. The driver is unresponsive behind the wheel. The passenger compartment is filled with smoke. The fire will reach the patient soon. Do you attempt to rescue the driver or wait for the fire department?
- You are a firefighter assisting the ambulance at the scene of a "man down." An apparently unresponsive man is loaded into the ambulance. He suddenly jumps up, forcefully strikes the paramedic, places her in a headlock, and tries to choke her. Do you jump in and help the paramedic, or do you retreat and call for the police?

EMS curricula and standards generally say that the correct action is to call for help and not get into a dangerous situation. Some may choose to do that. Others may decide to take a calculated risk to save a life. The fire service has a saying that applies here: "Risk a little to save a little. Risk a lot to save a lot."

The list of possible situations cannot all be discussed here. In the examples above—all of them real-life situations—the EMS providers decided to take a risk and act. The EMT at the shooting scene used what he could to create a barrier between himself and the blood. The EMT and paramedic at the crash scene pulled the man from the burning car. Firefighters jumped into the back of the ambulance to help the paramedic who was being assaulted.

As part of building resilience, it is important to know that despite your best efforts, some patients will die. The woman who was shot in the mall died despite the heroic actions of the EMT. Happily, the firefighter who was assaulted and the man in the burning car recovered from their injuries.

You must also recognize that some scenes are just too dangerous to enter, and that this may result in the death of a patient. An example is a worker who has become unresponsive from toxic gases in a confined space. If even a brief exposure to the gases would result in death, it would be pointless for any provider to enter the environment until it was made safe.

Recounting these situations is not an attempt to tell you that you should or should not take risks. Doing so is a personal decision based on your beliefs, capabilities, and the dynamics of a scene. These situations are presented here to tell you that ensuring your well-being at a scene isn't about rules. *Scene safety and well-being are determined by the decisions you make under pressure.* To do this, it is best to have a realistic set of guidelines.

The "plan, observe, react" sections that follow provide a decision-making framework to handle a wide variety of situations. Safety begins now, in your EMT course, as you learn about what to do—and when to do it. It continues as you begin to practice with a mind toward safety, work as part of a team, and learn how to make good decisions.

Violence

Three words sum up the actions required to respond to danger: *plan*, *observe*, and *react*.

Plan

Many EMTs work together to prevent dangerous accidents and know what to do as a team when danger strikes. Scene safety begins long before the actual emergency. Plan to be as safe as possible under all circumstances. The following factors should be addressed:

- **Wear safe clothing.** Nonslip shoes and practical clothing will not only help you provide emergency care more efficiently, but they also help you to respond to danger without unnecessary restrictions. For personal protection, have ANSI-approved reflective clothing available if you will be near traffic or in areas where it is important for you to be visible. Some EMTs wear body armor (bulletproof vests) when working in high-risk areas or situations.
- **Prepare your equipment so it is not cumbersome.** You will be carrying your first-response kit into emergencies. If it is too heavy or bulky, it will take your attention away from the careful observation of the scene as you approach and will slow you down if retreat becomes necessary. Many practical containers of reasonable size and weight are available.
- **Carry a portable radio whenever possible.** A radio allows you to call for help if you are separated from your vehicle.
- **Decide on safety roles.** If there will be more than one EMT on any call, tasks should be split up. For example, one EMT can obtain vital signs while another prepares the stretcher. One role that is frequently underused is that of observer. The EMT directly involved in patient care should always be aware of, but will have trouble constantly monitoring, the surroundings. The EMT who is not directly involved with patient care will be better able to actively observe for such things as weapons, mechanisms of injury, medications, and other important information.

Observe

Remember that it is always better to prevent a dangerous situation than to deal with one. If you observe or suspect danger, call the police. Do not enter the scene until they have secured it.

Observation begins early in the call. Observe the neighborhood as you look for house or building numbers. As you near the scene, turn off your lights and sirens to avoid broadcasting your arrival and attracting a crowd.

As you approach an emergency scene, notice what is going on. Emergencies are very active events. In situations where you notice an unusual silence, a certain amount of caution is advisable (Figure 2-12). In addition, observe for the following:

- **Violence.** Any indication that violence has occurred or may take place is significant. Signs include broken glass or overturned furniture, arguing, threats, and other violent behavior.

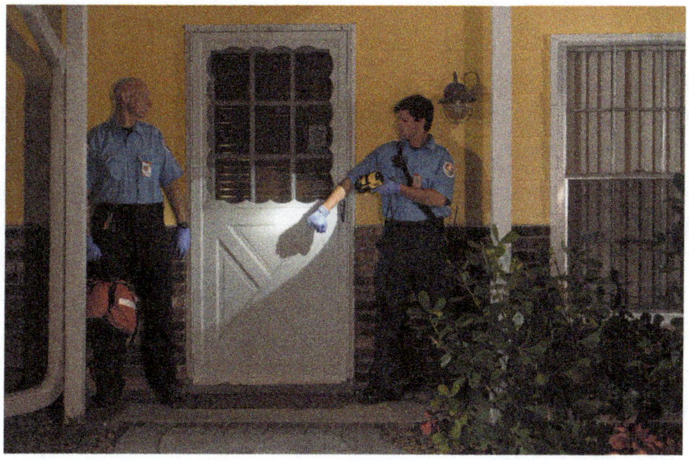

FIGURE 2-12 As a safety precaution, do not stand directly in front of a door when knocking or ringing the bell.

- **Crime scenes.** Try not to disturb a crime scene except as necessary for patient care. Make every effort to preserve evidence. You will learn more about these aspects of emergency care at a crime scene in the chapter titled *Medical/Legal, and Ethical Issues.*
- **Alcohol or drug use.** When people are under the influence of alcohol and other drugs, their behavior may be unpredictable. You also may be mistaken for the police because you drove up in a vehicle with lights and sirens.
- **Weapons.** If anyone at the scene (other than law enforcement officers) is in possession of a weapon, your safety is in danger. Even weapons that are only in view of a hostile person are a potential problem. Remember that almost any item may be used as a weapon. Weapons are not limited to knives and guns. If you observe or suspect the presence of any kind of weapon, notify the police immediately.
- **Family members.** Emotional or overwrought family members are often capable of violence or unpredictable behavior. Even though you are there to take care of a loved one, the violence may be directed at you.
- **Bystanders.** Many people gather at the scene of a collision (or anywhere an emergency vehicle parks). Sometimes you will find a bystander or group of bystanders beginning to show aggressive behavior. If this happens, call for the police. In some settings, it may be necessary to place the patient in the ambulance and leave the scene rather than wait for the police.
- **Perpetrators.** A perpetrator of a crime may still be on the scene—in sight or in hiding. Do not enter a crime scene or a scene of violence until police have secured it and told you it is safe to do so.
- **Pets.** Although most domestic animals are not dangerous in ordinary circumstances, the presence of an animal at the emergency scene poses problems. Even friendly animals may become defensive when you begin to treat the owner. Animals also can be very distracting, interfere with patient care, and cause falls while you are lifting and moving the patient. No matter what the pet owner says ("He won't hurt you. He's very friendly."), it is usually best to have pets placed securely in another room.

Keep in mind that the vast majority of EMS calls will resolve uneventfully. As an EMT, you are a vital part of the EMS system. Nothing in this text is intended to create fear or paranoia. However, when a call does pose some kind of threat, you must be prepared to recognize the subtle and not-so-subtle signs that can warn you before danger strikes.

React

Observation has provided the critical information needed about the danger. The next step involves knowing how to react. The three Rs of responding to danger are respond, radio, and reevaluate.

It is not part of your responsibilities as an EMT to subdue a violent person or wrestle a weapon away from anyone. You may make a decision to react to help or rescue a patient, but this is a personal decision—and done strategically, only when there is a high likelihood of success. To retreat from dangers is also a clear and justifiable course of action in situations that are too dangerous or that you cannot handle by yourself (e.g., armed or barricaded suspect, hazardous material incident with a man down). Note that some ways of retreating are safer than others:

- **Flee.** Get far enough away so you will have time to react should the danger begin to move toward your new position. Place two major obstacles between you and the danger. If the dangerous person gets through one of the obstacles, you have a built-in buffer with the second.
- **Get rid of any cumbersome equipment.** In the event you must flee from the scene, do not get bogged down by your equipment. Discard all of it if this will enhance your ability to get away. Use equipment to your benefit. For example, if you are being pursued, wedge your stretcher in a doorway to slow down the aggressor.

FIGURE 2-13 (A) Concealing yourself is placing your body behind an object that can hide you from view. (B) Taking cover is finding a position that protects your body from projectiles. The best position is one that both conceals and protects.

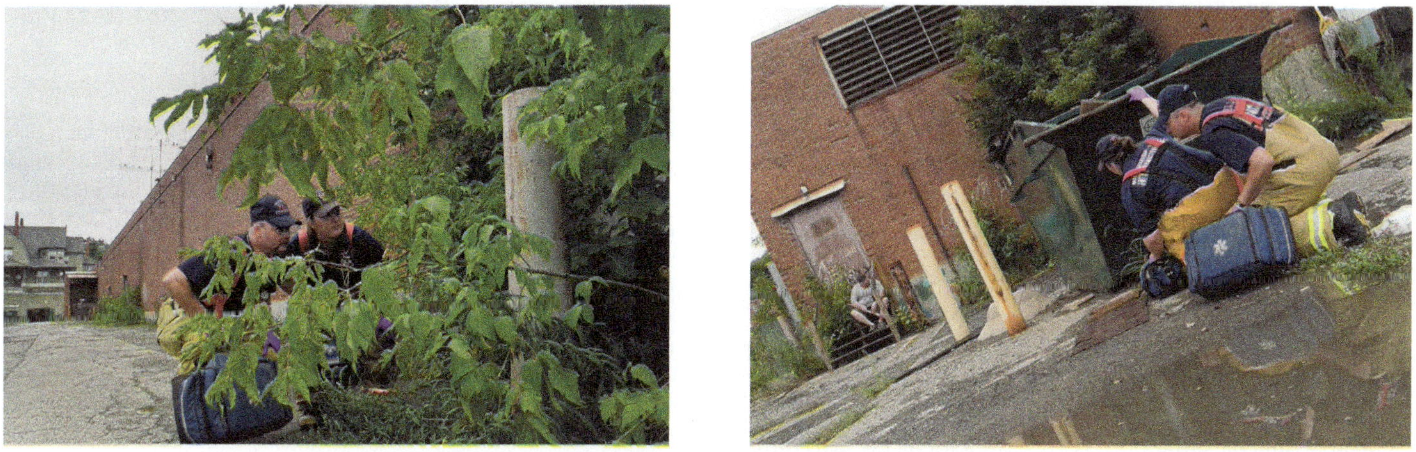

A

B

- **Take cover and conceal yourself.** Taking cover means finding a position that protects your body from projectiles, such as behind a brick wall. Concealing yourself is hiding your body behind an object that cannot protect you, such as a shrub. Find a position that will both conceal and protect you (Figure 2-13).

The first R of responding to danger is to *respond*, using distance, cover, and concealment to protect yourself. Do not return to the scene until the police have secured it.

The second R of reacting to danger is *radio*. The portable radio is an important piece of safety equipment. Use it to call for police assistance and to warn other responding units of the danger. Speak into it clearly and slowly. Advise the dispatcher of the exact nature and location of the problem. Specify how many people are involved and whether weapons were observed. Remember, the information you have about the scene must be shared as soon as possible to prevent others from encountering the same danger.

Finally, the third R of reacting to danger is *reevaluate*. If you've retreated from a scene, do not reenter it until it has been secured by the police (Figure 2-14). Even then, be aware that where violence has been, it may begin again. Emergencies are situations packed with stress for families, patients, responders, and bystanders. Maintain a level of alert observation throughout the call. Occasionally you may find weapons or drugs while you are assessing the patient. If that happens, stop what you are doing and radio the police immediately. After the call, document the situation on your run report. Occasionally the danger may cause delays in reaching the patient. Courts have held this delay acceptable, provided there has been a real and documented danger.

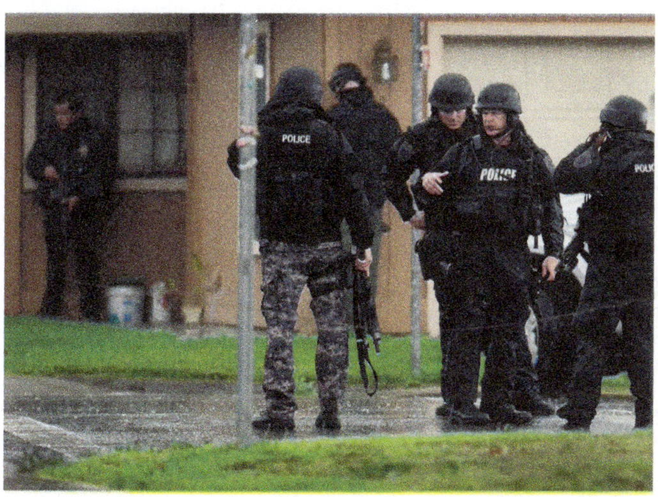

FIGURE 2-14 Never enter a scene that is potentially violent until the police have secured it and told you it is safe. *(Randy Pench/ The Sacramento Bee/ ASSOCIATED PRESS)*

Chapter Review

Key Facts and Concepts

- Your well-being is an important concept. This chapter has provided several ways to protect and maintain it.
- You should never take safety or Standard Precautions lightly. Each yields an important decision you will make at least once at each scene you respond to—always.
- Protect yourself from violence and scene hazards at all costs.
- Protect yourself from disease. Do not be paranoid about catching a disease, but take appropriate precautions.
- Resilience means "toughness" or ability to recover quickly from a difficult situation. It is important for all EMTs to remain physically and mentally strong.
- Stress may be an immediate reaction from a particular call or cumulative from a combination of life and EMS. Both kinds are bad for you. Seek help if you need it.
- You will see death and reaction to death. Each is very personal to those involved. The stages of death are denial, anger, bargaining, depression, and acceptance.
- Treat people who are under stress fairly and compassionately, even if it is difficult to do so.

Key Decisions

- Is the scene safe? Should I enter or not?
- What Standard Precautions must I take? What PPE should I use?
- Is stress getting the best of me? Is it hurting me, my work, or my family and friends?

Chapter Glossary

contamination the introduction of dangerous chemicals, disease, or infectious materials.

critical incident stress management (CISM) a comprehensive system that includes education and resources to both prevent stress and deal with stress appropriately when it occurs.

decontamination the removal or cleansing of dangerous chemicals and other dangerous or infectious materials.

hazardous material incident the release of a harmful substance into the environment.

multiple-casualty incident (MCI) an emergency involving multiple patients.

pathogens the organisms that cause infection, such as viruses and bacteria.

personal protective equipment (PPE) equipment that protects the EMS worker from infection and/or exposure to the dangers of rescue operations.

resilience toughness; an ability to recover quickly from difficult situations.

Standard Precautions a strict form of infection control that is based on the assumption that all blood and other body fluids are infectious; also known as body substance isolation (BSI).

stress a state of physical and/or psychological arousal to a stimulus.

Preparation for Your Examination and Practice

Short Answer

1. Differentiate between acute stress, delayed stress, and cumulative stress. Give an example of each.
2. Name some of the causes of stress for an EMT and explain some ways the EMT can alleviate job-related stress.
3. Explain the eSCAPe concept and how it can be used to help patients and fellow EMTs.
4. What are the stages a person may express when confronted with death and dying? Why is it important for the EMT to understand these reactions? How should the EMT deal with these emotions?
5. List the types of personal protective equipment used in Standard Precautions. Identify a condition or patient with which each one should be used.

Thinking and Linking

Body substance isolation is an important concept to protect you from disease. Linking with the roles and responsibilities of an EMT in Introduction to Emergency Medical Services *and the material covered in this chapter, list the types of Standard Precautions you would use in each of the following circumstances:*

1. A patient who has severe bleeding from his arm
2. A patient who is vomiting
3. A patient who is spitting up blood

Critical Thinking Exercises

Many emergency calls pose dangers to EMS personnel. The purpose of this exercise is to consider actions you should take at a dangerous scene.

- You are called to an unknown emergency at a tavern. As you approach the scene, you see a man lying supine in the parking lot, apparently bleeding profusely. Two other men are scuffling, and one seems to have a gun. What actions must you take?

Pathophysiology to Practice

The following questions are designed to assist you in gathering relevant clinical information and making accurate decisions in the field.

1. How do you think you caught your last cold or stomach "bug"?
2. What is your body's response to stress? What does it do to your pulse, respiration, and blood pressure?
3. How is "good stress" different than "bad stress" to your body?

Street Scenes

While you are en route to a motor-vehicle collision, the dispatcher gives your responding ambulance an update. "Ambulance Charlie 7, you have one patient with bad facial injuries." After judging the scene safe to enter, you immediately start to assess the patient. Just as you open the airway and your partner provides oxygen, the paramedic unit arrives and takes over care of the patient.

As you are finishing loading the patient into the back of the paramedics' ambulance, one of them asks where your gloves are. You don't think much of it and start to clean up your equipment. As you get into the ambulance, your partner tells you that not only is it against the ambulance service's standard operating procedure for you not to wear gloves on this type of call, but it is foolish. You reluctantly agree to tell your supervisor.

Later, you enter the supervisor's office, describe the call and the amount of blood, and then tell her that you did not wear any protective gloves. You also point out that you may have had a partially healed cut on your hand. She tells you that you are out of service.

Street Scene Questions

1. **Why wear protective gloves on this type of call?**
2. **What is the impact of an occupational exposure on you, your family, and your fellow EMS workers?**
3. **What can you expect after exposure?**

Your supervisor explains that you need to go to the emergency department for an occupational evaluation. There is an arrangement with the hospital, and they will have a member of their infection control staff go through your evaluation and counseling.

When you get to the hospital, the infection control nurse interviews you and asks many specific questions about the call, your health, and what immunizations you have had. She examines your hands for breaks in the skin, and a number are identified. When the interview is over, she recommends that you get some baseline blood tests; one is for HIV. All of a sudden you realize the seriousness of this situation. She recommends that you take some medications and gives you information on precautions that you need to take when having intimate relations with your spouse. It hits you again how serious this has become.

Street Scene Questions

4. **How will stress be a factor in your life for the next few months?**
5. **How important is hand washing?**
6. **What type of Standard Precautions should EMTs always be ready to use on all EMS calls?**

You try to take your mind off the situation but you can't. It affects your sleep. You are irritable around your family. When you try to talk to your partner, you find you're too embarrassed.

Quite some time later, the infection control nurse tells you that your latest blood tests are back. They're all negative. A personal tragedy has been avoided. As you start to leave her office, the nurse tells you to remember gloves and hand washing are very important. With a big smile, you look back and say, "I get it!"

3 Lifting and Moving Patients

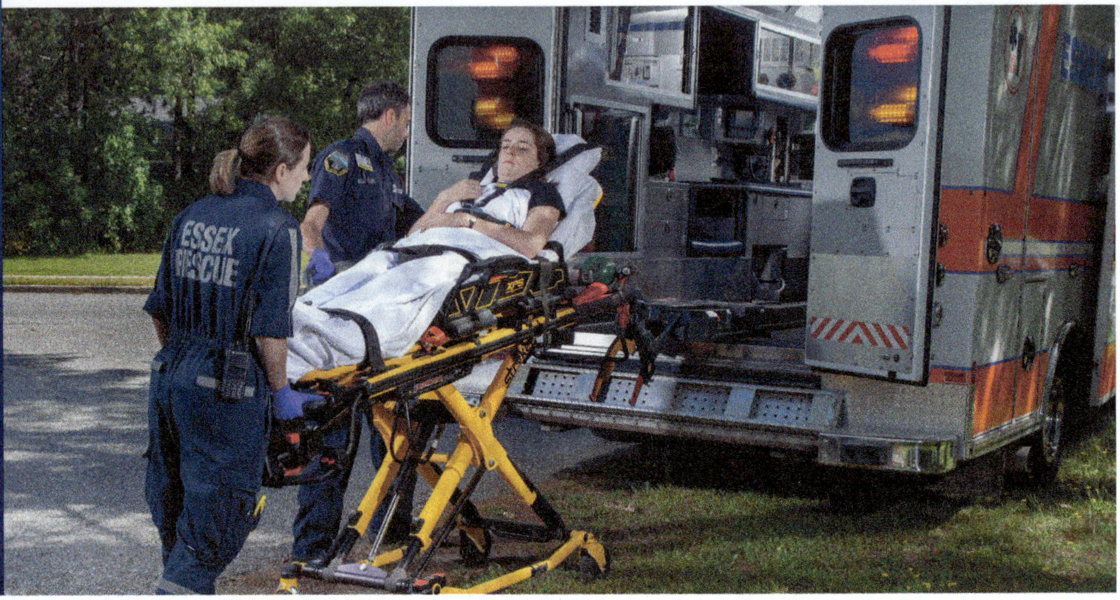

Related Chapters

The following chapters provide additional information related to topics discussed in this chapter:

12 Primary Assessment

15 Secondary Assessment

33 Trauma to the Head, Neck, and Spine

Standard

Preparatory (Workforce Safety and Wellness)

Competency

Uses fundamental knowledge of the EMS system, safety/well-being of the EMT, and medical/legal and ethical issues to the provision of emergency care.

Core Concepts

- How using body mechanics to lift and move patients can help prevent injury
- When it is proper to move a patient and how to do so safely
- The various devices used to immobilize, move, and carry patients

Outcomes

After reading this chapter, you should be able to:

3.1 Describe the considerations in preventing injury to the EMS crew when lifting and moving patients. (pp. 56–58)

- Given descriptions of situations, estimate whether it is safe to attempt to lift the patient.
- Distinguish between proper use of body mechanics and improper lifting and moving technique.

3.2 Summarize the considerations in moving patients. (pp. 58–76)

- Given a selection of descriptions, categorize the need to move the patients as emergent, urgent, or nonurgent.
- Recognize the specific techniques used for each method of moving a patient.
- Identify patient-carrying devices.
- Given a description of a situation, select the most appropriate patient-carrying device.
- Contrast the general considerations for moving a patient with a suspected spine injury and one with no suspected spine injury.
- Distinguish between techniques for moving a patient without suspected spine injury onto a carrying device.
- Match descriptions of patient problems with considerations for positioning the patient.

Key Terms

bariatric, *67*
body mechanics, *56*
direct carry, *75*
direct ground lift, *71*
draw-sheet method, *75*
extremity lift, *71*
power grip, *57*
power lift, *57*

Speed is a major objective on many of the calls you will make as an EMT. At dangerous scenes, for example, you must move the patient rapidly to a safe place. When there is a life-threatening medical problem or a serious injury, getting the patient to a hospital quickly can mean the difference between life and death.

Doing things fast, however, can mean doing them wrong. You can be so focused on the need to hurry as you lift and carry the patient that you make careless moves. These can injure your patient. They can also injure you. Back injuries are serious and have the potential to end an EMS career as well as to cause lifelong problems. With the proper techniques, however, you can lift and move patients safely. Proper lifting and moving must be practiced on every call.

Protecting Yourself: Body Mechanics

body mechanics
the proper use of the body to facilitate lifting and moving and to prevent injury.

CORE CONCEPT
How using body mechanics to lift and move patients can help prevent injury

Body mechanics refers to the proper use of your body to prevent injury and to facilitate lifting and moving. Consider the following before lifting any patient:

- **The object.** What is the weight of the object? Will you require additional help in lifting?
- **Your limitations.** What are your physical characteristics? Do you (or your partner) have any physical limitations that would make lifting difficult? Although it may not always be possible to arrange, EMTs of similar strength and height can lift and carry together more easily.
- **Communication.** Make a plan. Then communicate the plan for lifting and carrying to your partner. Continue to communicate throughout the process to make the move comfortable for the patient and safe for the EMTs.

When it comes time to do the lifting, there are rules that must be followed to prevent injury:

- **Position your feet properly.** They should be on a firm, level surface and positioned shoulder-width apart.
- **Use your legs.** Do not use your back to do the lifting.
- **Never turn or twist.** Attempts to make any other moves while you are lifting are a major cause of injury.
- **Do not compensate when lifting with one hand.** Avoid leaning to either side. Keep your back straight and locked.
- **Keep the weight as close as possible to your body.** This allows you to use your legs rather than your back while lifting. The farther the weight is from your body, the greater your chance of injury.
- **Use a stair chair when carrying a patient on stairs whenever possible.** Keep your back straight. Flex your knees and lean forward from the hips, not the waist. If you are walking backward down stairs, ask a helper to steady your back (Figure 3-1).

There are many kinds of patient-carrying devices, including stretchers, backboards, and stair chairs. (Specifics are offered later in this chapter.) When possible, it is almost always safer, as well as more efficient, to move patients over distances on a wheeled device such as a wheeled stretcher or a stair chair. These devices allow the patient to be rolled along instead of carried.

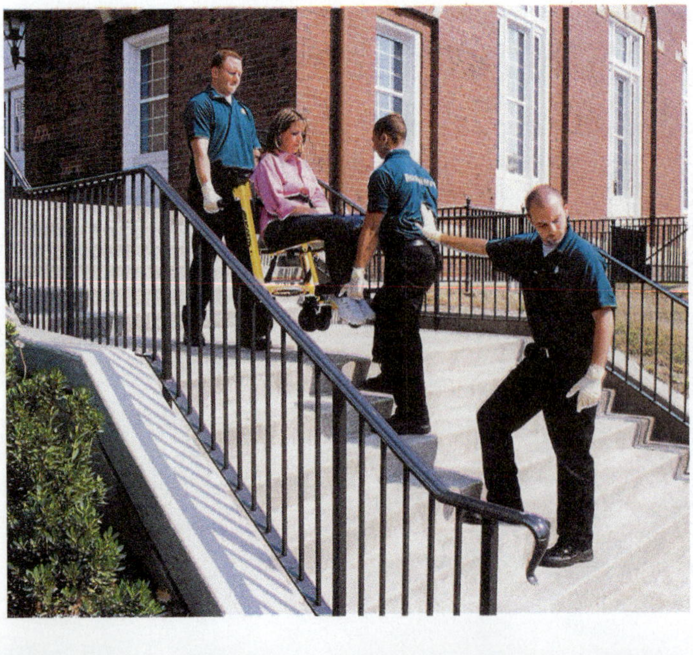

FIGURE 3-1 Moving a stair chair down steps.

When lifting a patient-carrying device, it is best to use an even number of people. For a stretcher or backboard, one EMT lifts from the end near the patient's head, the other from the feet. If there are four rescuers available, one person can take each corner of a stretcher or board. If there are only three people available, however, never allow the third person to assist by lifting one side. This can cause the device to be thrown off balance, resulting in the stretcher's tipping over and injuring the patient.

To prevent injury when lifting a patient-carrying device, the general rules of body mechanics mentioned earlier apply. Two more methods also can help to prevent injury. The first is the ***power lift*** (Figure 3-2A), so named because it is used by power weight lifters. It is also known as the *squat-lift* position. In this position, you will squat rather than bend at the waist, and you will keep the weight close to your body, even straddling it if possible. When rising, your feet should be a comfortable distance apart, flat on the ground, with the weight primarily on the balls of the feet or just behind them. Your back should be locked in. When you are lowering a patient, use the reverse order of this procedure.

The second method is the ***power grip*** (Figure 3-2B). Remember that your hands are often the only portion of your body actually in contact with the object you are lifting, making your grip a very important element in the process. As great an area of your fingers and palms as possible should be in contact with the object. All of your fingers should be bent at the same angle. When possible, keep your hands at least 10 inches apart.

There are situations in which you will find yourself reaching for patients or using a considerable amount of effort to push and pull a weight. These are moves that must be performed carefully to prevent injury. In general:

power lift
a lift from a squatting position with weight to be lifted close to the body, feet apart and flat on the ground, body weight on or just behind the balls of the feet, and the back locked in. The upper body is raised before the hips. Also called the *squat-lift position*.

power grip
gripping with as much hand surface as possible in contact with the object being lifted, all fingers bent at the same angle, and hands at least 10 inches apart.

When reaching:

- Keep your back in a locked-in position.
- Avoid twisting while reaching.
- Avoid reaching more than 20 inches (about 50 cm) in front of your body.
- Avoid prolonged reaching when strenuous effort is required.

FIGURE 3-2 (A) The power lift and (B) the power grip.

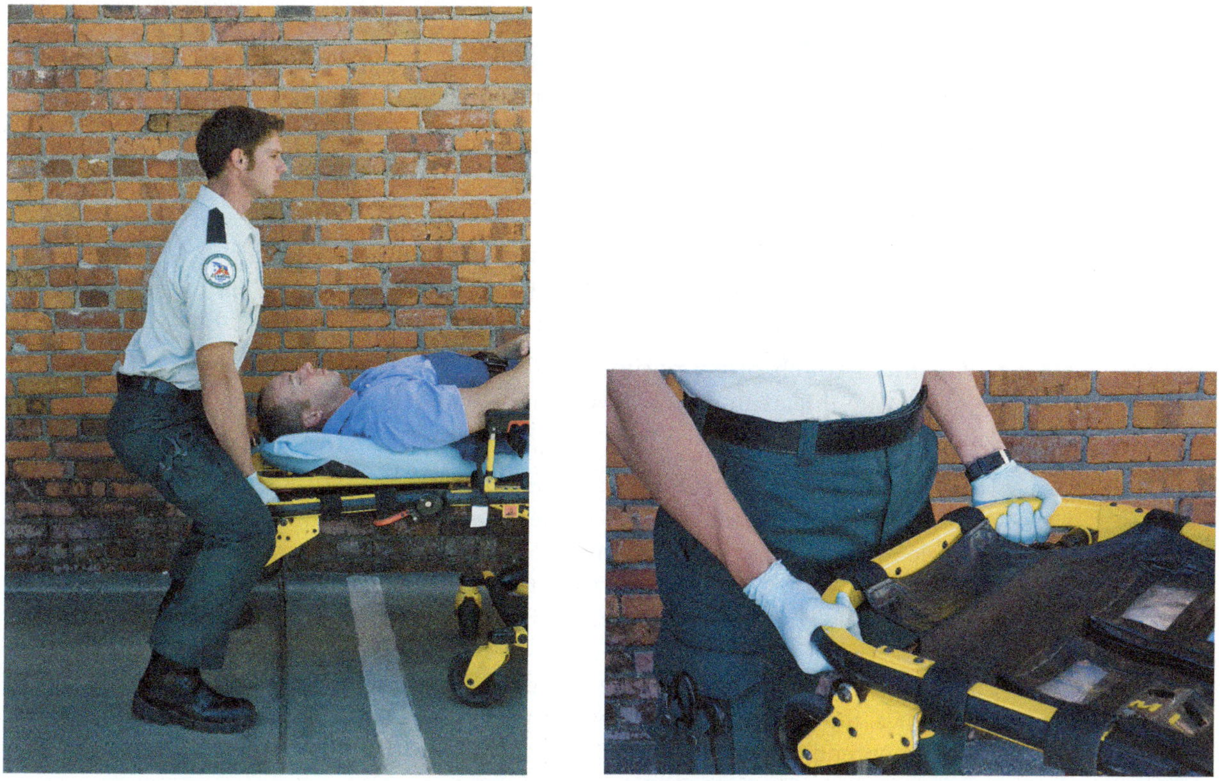

A B

When pushing or pulling:

- Push, rather than pull, whenever possible.
- Keep your back locked in.
- Keep the line of pull through the center of your body by bending your knees.
- Keep the weight close to your body.
- If the weight is below your waist level, push or pull from a kneeling position.
- Avoid pushing or pulling overhead.
- Keep your elbows bent and arms close to your sides.

Protecting Your Patient: Emergency, Urgent, and Nonurgent Moves

CORE CONCEPT

When it is proper to move a patient and how to do so safely

How quickly should you move patients? Must you complete your assessment before moving them? How much time should you spend on spinal precautions and other patient-safety measures? The answer is: It depends on the circumstances.

If the patient is in a building that is in danger of collapse or a car that is on fire, speed is the overriding concern. The patient must be moved to a safe place, probably before you have time to complete or even begin an assessment, consider possible spinal injuries, or move a stretcher into position. In this situation you would use what is known as an *emergency move.*

Sometimes the situation is such that you have time to carry out an abbreviated assessment. For example, consider the patient who has been trapped in wreckage, possibly incurring serious injuries. When the patient is extricated, you would place the patient on a spine board (if indicated by protocols) or other carrying device, working quickly to perform the proper assessments and patient care. This move is called an *urgent move.*

Most of the time, you will be able to complete your on-scene assessment and care procedures then move the patient onto a stretcher or other device in the normal way. This would be called a *nonurgent move.*

Emergency Moves

Three situations may require the use of an emergency move:

- **The scene is hazardous.** Hazards may make it necessary to move a patient quickly to protect you and the patient. This may occur when there is uncontrolled traffic, fire or threat of fire, possible explosions, electrical hazards, toxic gases, or radiation.
- **Care of life-threatening conditions requires repositioning.** You may have to move a patient to a hard, flat surface to provide CPR, or you may have to move a patient to reach the wound area to stop life-threatening bleeding.
- **You must reach other patients.** When there are patients at the scene requiring care for life-threatening problems, you may have to move another patient to access them.

The greatest danger to the patient in an emergency move is that an injury may be aggravated. Since the move must be made immediately to protect the patient's life, you may not be able to protect the patient's spine or other injured areas. In this case, to minimize or prevent aggravation of the injury, *move the patient in the direction of the long axis of the body when possible.* The long axis is the line that runs down the center of the body from the top of the head and along the spine.

There are several rapid moves called drags. In this type of move, the patient is dragged by the clothes, the feet, or the shoulders, or while on a blanket. These moves are reserved only for emergencies because they do not provide protection for the neck and spine.

Most commonly a long-axis drag is made from the area of the shoulders. This causes the remainder of the body to fall into its natural anatomic position, with the spine and all limbs in normal alignment.

Drags and other emergency moves known as carries and assists are illustrated in Scan 3-1, Scan 3-2, and Scan 3-3.

NOTE: *For a majority of emergency and urgent moves, you will not have time for a full spinal assessment before moving the patient, so you won't know whether you will use spinal motion restriction. In this case, make every effort to prevent additional injury until a full assessment can be performed in a safe location. You will learn more about spinal immobilization and spinal motion restriction in the chapter titled* Trauma to the Head, Neck, and Spine.

"Before you lift, think and plan. The back you save will be your own."

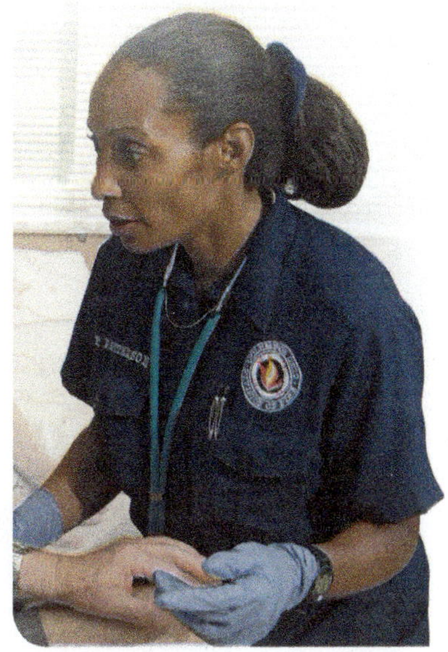

Urgent Moves

Urgent moves are required when the patient must be moved quickly for treatment of an immediate threat to life. However, unlike emergency moves, urgent moves are performed with precautions for spinal injury when necessary. Examples in which urgent moves may be required include the following:

- **The required treatment can be performed only if the patient is moved.** A patient must be moved to support inadequate breathing or to treat for shock or altered mental status.
- **Factors at the scene cause patient decline.** If a patient is rapidly declining because of heat or cold, for example, the patient may have to be moved.

Moving the patient to a backboard is often performed as part of an urgent move. The backboard is used to transport the patient safely to the stretcher. It is also useful as a firm surface for performing CPR, should that become necessary. Current thinking has changed the role of the backboard to more of a transportation device than a long-term immobilization device, because of the discomfort and other problems seen with long-term immobilization. There will be times you will immobilize a patient because of a specific concern for spinal injury.

There are many ways to move a patient to a backboard. One of these is the log roll, which is shown in Figure 3-3.

Nonurgent Moves

When there is no immediate threat to life, the patient should be moved when ready for transportation, using a nonurgent move. On-scene assessment and any needed on-scene treatments, such as splinting, should be completed first. Nonurgent moves should be carried out in such a way as to prevent injury or additional injury to the patient and to avoid discomfort and pain.

In a nonurgent move, the patient is moved from the site of on-scene assessment and treatment (perhaps a bed or sofa, perhaps the floor or the ground outdoors) onto a patient-carrying device.

CORE CONCEPT
The various devices used to immobilize, move, and carry patients

Patient-Carrying Devices

A patient-carrying device is a stretcher or other device designed to carry the patient safely to the ambulance and/or to the hospital. Devices described on the following pages are pictured in Scan 3-4.

Patient-carrying devices are mechanical devices, and all EMTs must be familiar with how to use them. Errors in the use of these devices may result in injuries to the patient and to you. For example, a stretcher that is not locked in position may collapse, and untended stretchers may simply roll away. Such incidents may be cause for a lawsuit if the patient is injured as a result of improper practices or faulty equipment. The devices must be regularly maintained and inspected. You should know the rating of each piece of equipment (how much weight it will hold safely). Have alternatives available if the patient is too heavy or too large for a device.

(Text continues on p. 62.)

SCAN 3-1 Emergency Moves, One-Rescuer Drags

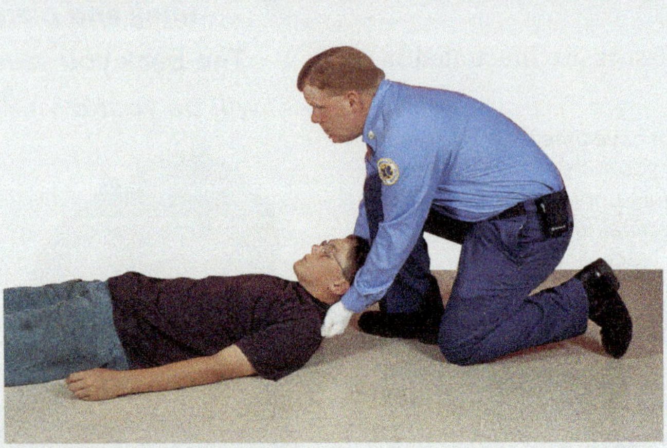

CLOTHES DRAG.

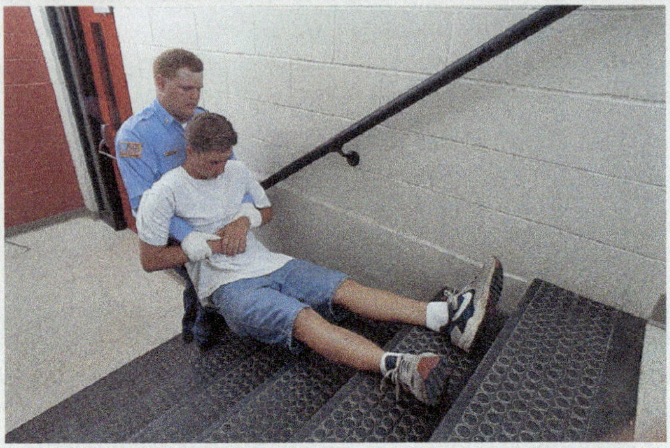

INCLINE DRAG. *Always* head first.

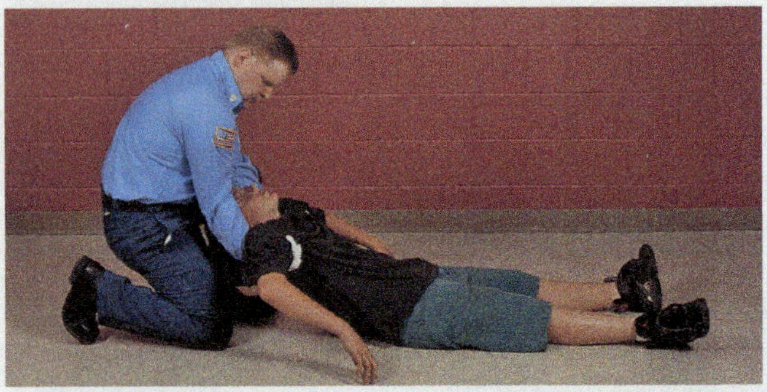

SHOULDER DRAG.

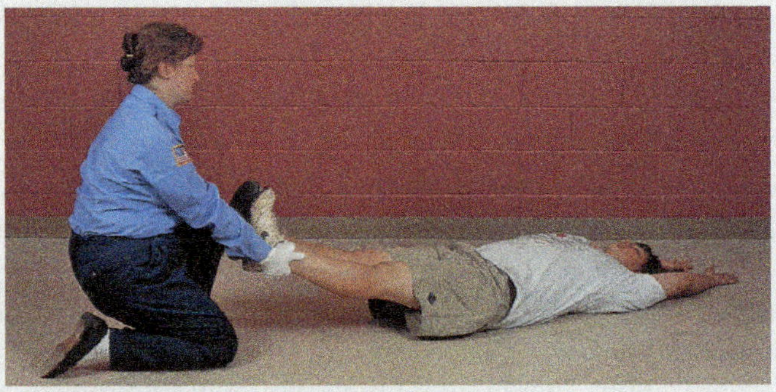

FOOT DRAG. Do not bump the patient's head.

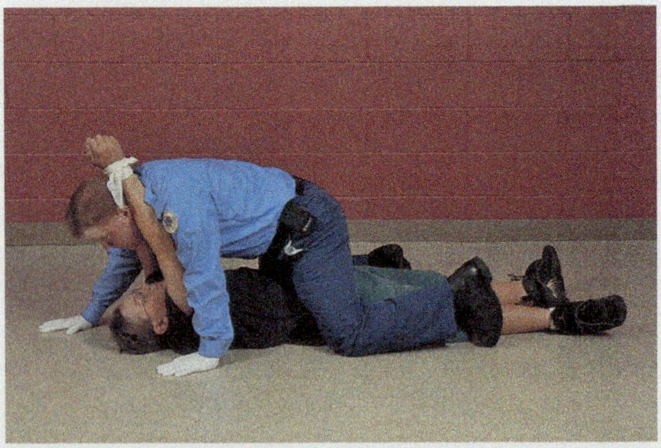

FIREFIGHTER'S DRAG. Place patient supine and tie the patient's hands together. Straddle the patient, crouch, and pass your head through the patient's trussed arms. Raise your body and crawl on your hands and knees. Keep the patient's head as low as possible.

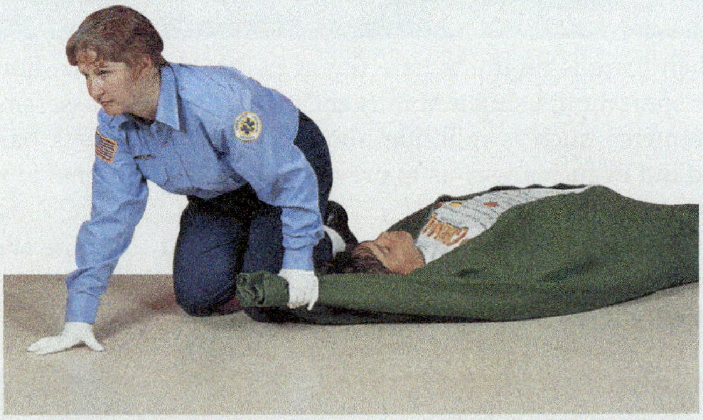

BLANKET DRAG. Gather half of the blanket material up against the patient's side. Roll the patient toward your knees, place the blanket under the patient, and gently roll the patient onto the blanket. During the drag, keep the patient's head as low as possible.

SCAN 3-2 Emergency Moves, One Rescuer

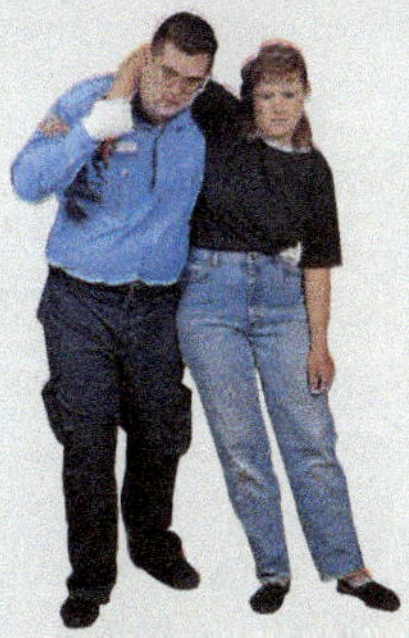

ONE-RESCUER ASSIST. Place the patient's arm around your neck, grasping the patient's hand in yours. Place your other arm around the patient's waist. Help the patient walk to safety. Be prepared to change your movement technique if the level of danger increases. Be sure to communicate with the patient about obstacles, uneven terrain, and so on.

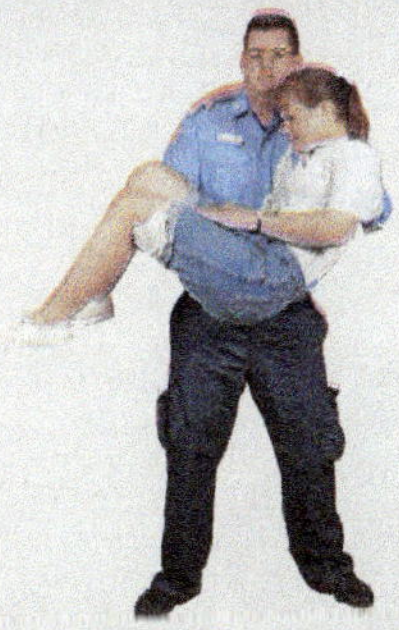

CRADLE CARRY. Place one arm across the patient's back with your hand under the patient's arm. Place your other arm under the patient's knees and lift. If the patient is conscious, have the patient place the near arm over your shoulder.

NOTE: *This carry places a lot of weight on the carrier's back. It is usually appropriate for only very light patients.*

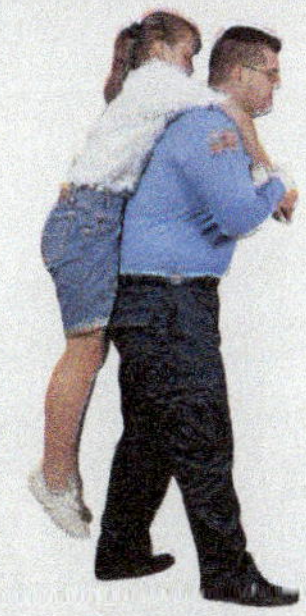

PACK STRAP CARRY. Have the patient stand. Turn your back to the patient, bringing the patient's arms over your shoulders to cross your chest. Keep the patient's arms as straight as possible, with the patient's armpits over your shoulders. Hold the patient's wrists, bend, and pull the patient onto your back.

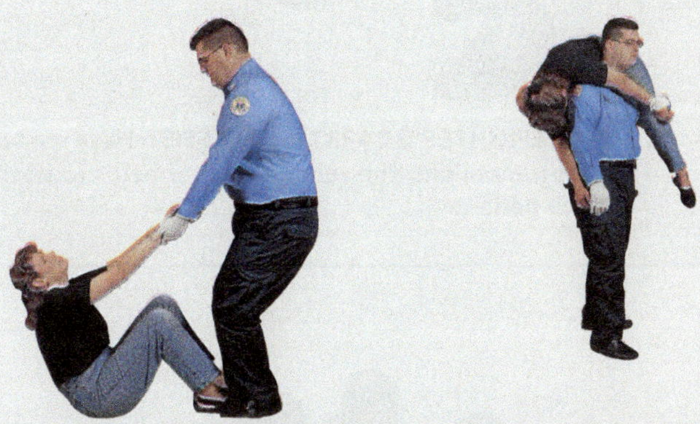

FIREFIGHTER'S CARRY. Place your feet against the patient's feet and pull the patient toward you. Bend at your waist and flex your knees. Duck and pull the patient across your shoulder, keeping hold of one of the patient's wrists. Use your free arm to reach between the patient's legs and grasp the patient's thigh. This way, the weight of the patient falls onto your shoulders. Stand up. Transfer your grip on the patient's thigh to the patient's wrist.

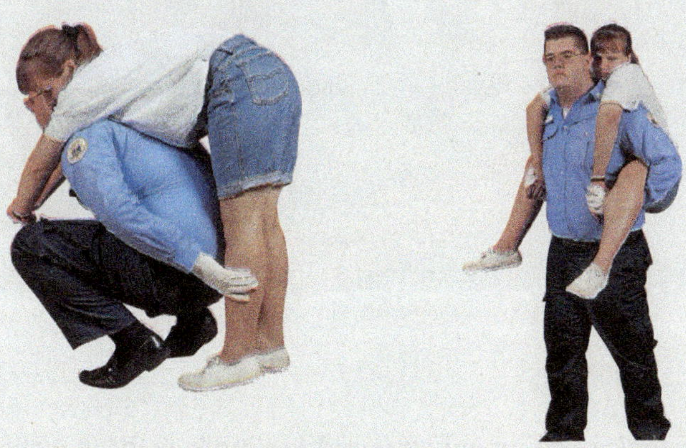

PIGGYBACK CARRY. Assist the patient to stand. Place the patient's arms over your shoulder so they cross your chest. Bend over and lift the patient. While the patient holds on with the arms, crouch and grasp each leg. Use a lifting motion to move the patient onto your back. Pass your forearms under the patient's knees and grasp the patient's wrists.

SCAN 3-3 Emergency Moves, Two Rescuers

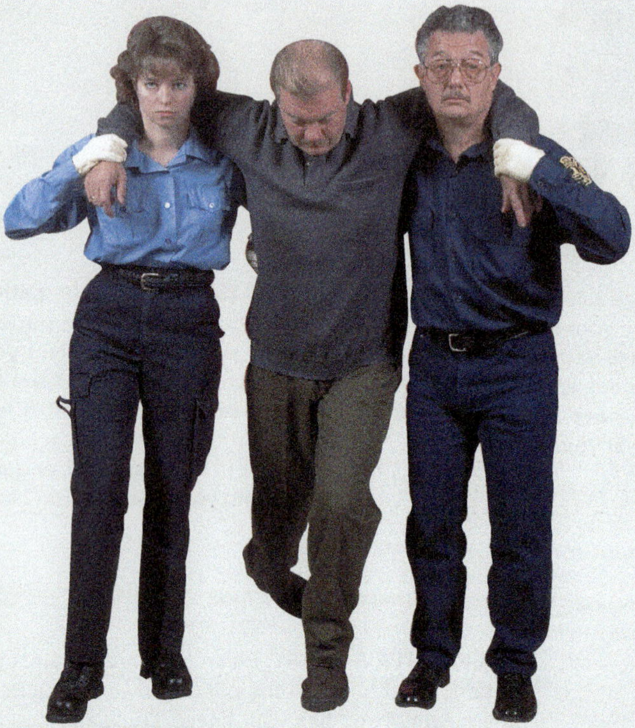

TWO-RESCUER ASSIST. Place the patient's arms around the shoulders of both rescuers. They each grip a hand, place their free arms around the patient's waist, and help the patient walk to safety.

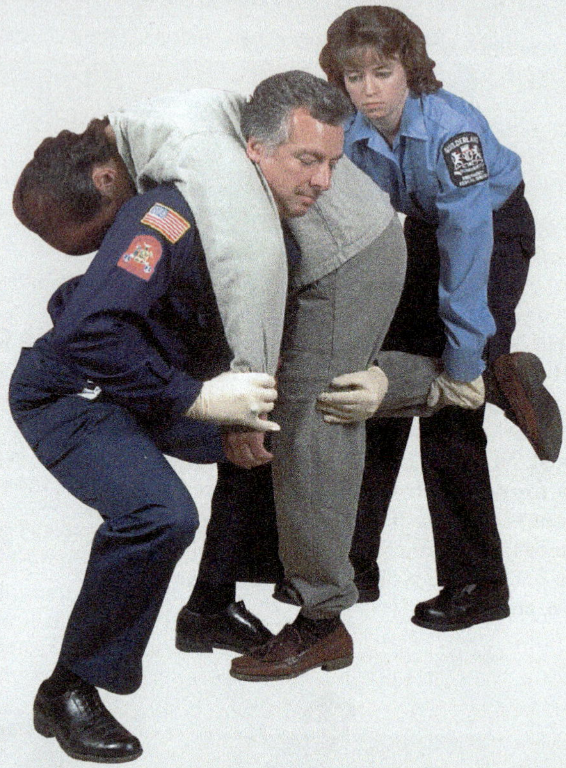

FIREFIGHTER'S CARRY WITH ASSIST. Have someone lift the patient. The second rescuer helps to position the patient.

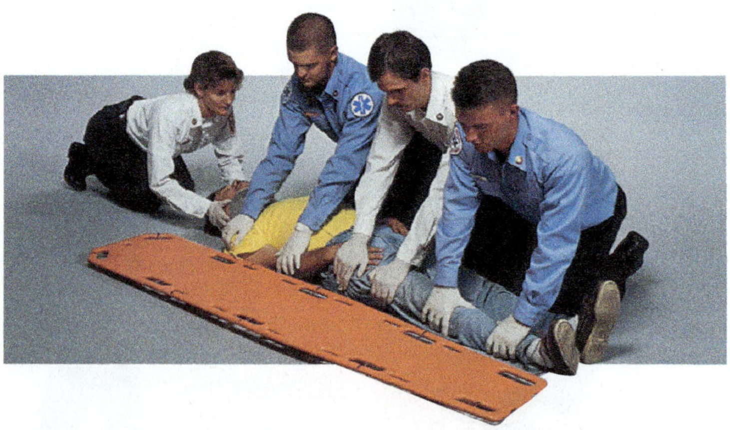

FIGURE 3-3 When doing a log roll, keep your back straight, lean from the hips, and use your shoulder muscles.

Wheeled Stretchers. This device—commonly referred to simply as the stretcher, cot, or litter (Figure 3-4)—is in the back of all ambulances. There are many brands and types of wheeled stretcher, but their purpose is the same: to safely transport a patient from one place to another, usually in a reclining position. The head of the stretcher can be elevated, which will be beneficial for some patients—including cardiac patients—who have no suspected neck or spinal injuries.

Depending on the model, the stretcher will have variable levels. When moving the patient, the safest level is closest to the ground. Wheeling the stretcher in the elevated position raises the center of gravity, making it easier for the stretcher to tip over. The stretcher is ideal for level surfaces. Rough terrain and uneven surfaces may cause the stretcher to tip.

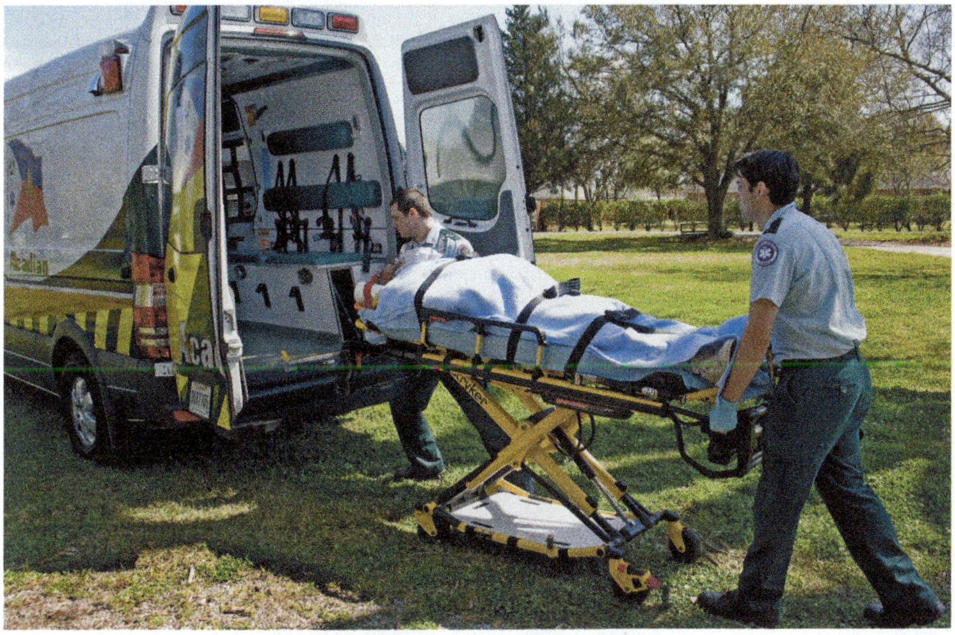

FIGURE 3-4 A wheeled stretcher is carried on every ambulance.

Make sure to use proper body mechanics while placing the stretcher into or taking it out of the ambulance. Proper body mechanics are also important while wheeling the stretcher from place to place. Remember, as discussed earlier in the chapter, odd numbers of EMTs may cause the stretcher to become off balance. When the stretcher is lifted, two EMTs should lift at opposite ends of the stretcher—head and foot. Scan 3-5 shows procedures for loading two types of wheeled stretchers into an ambulance.

SCAN 3-4 Patient-Carrying Devices

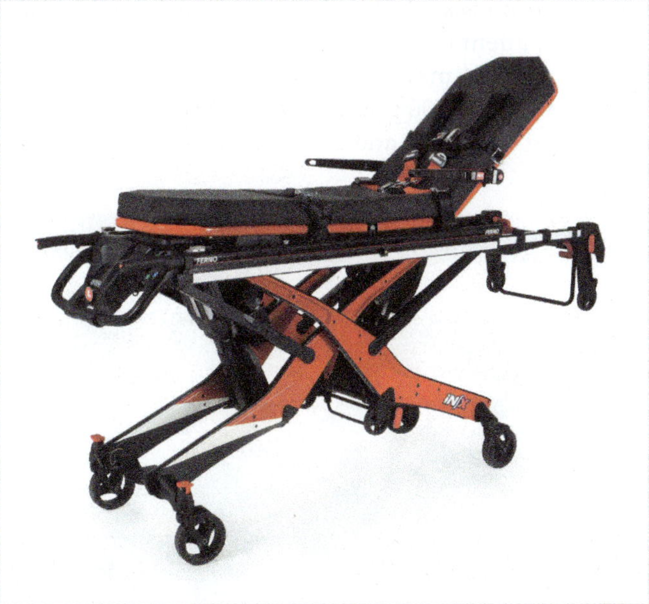

Power stretcher. *(© Ferno–Washington, Inc.)*

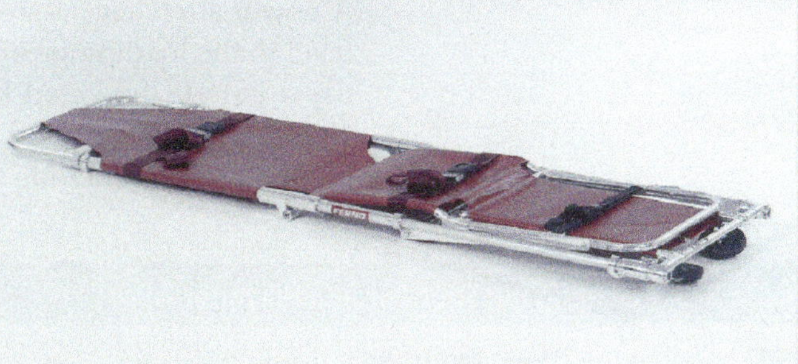

Portable stretcher. *(© Ferno–Washington, Inc.)*

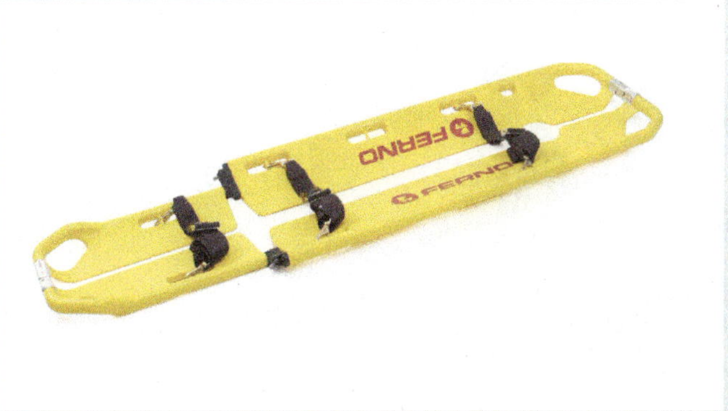

Scoop (orthopedic) stretcher. *(© Ferno–Washington, Inc.)*

(continued)

SCAN 3-4 Patient-Carrying Devices *(continued)*

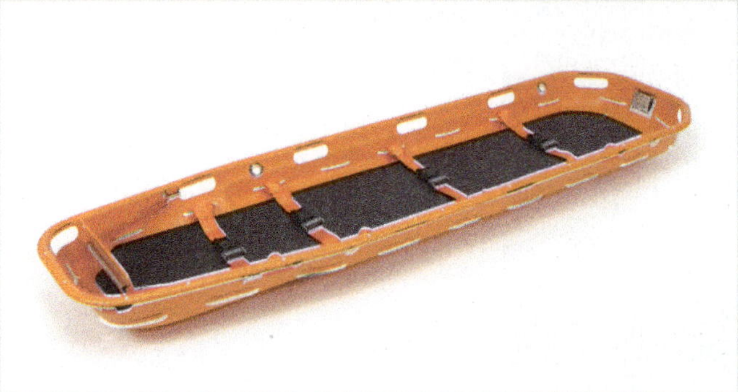

Basket stretcher. *(© Ferno–Washington, Inc.)*

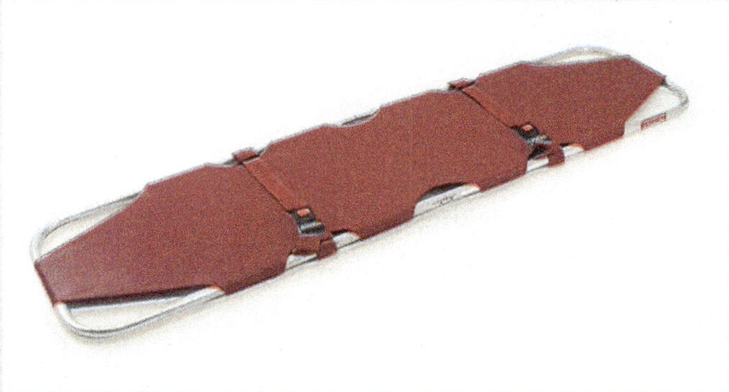

Flexible stretcher. *(© Ferno–Washington, Inc.)*

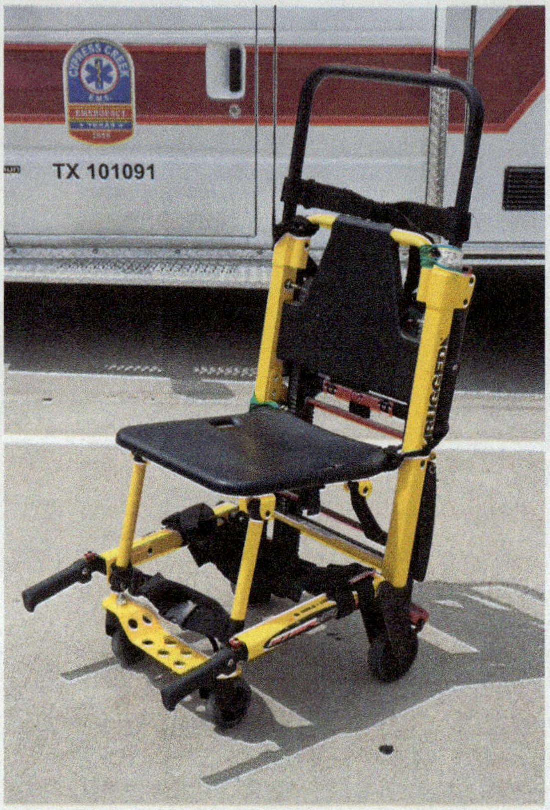

Stair chair.

There are two basic types of stretchers: power stretchers and manual stretchers. A power stretcher (as shown in Scan 3-4 and Scan 3-5) will lift a patient from the ground level to the loading position or lower a patient from the raised position. These stretchers use a battery-powered hydraulic system that manufacturers state will lift patients on 20 consecutive runs and will lift patients up to 700 pounds. Manual stretchers are lifted by EMTs. These include the "self-loading" stretcher and the standard stretcher.

SCAN 3-5 Loading the Stretcher into the Ambulance

EMT Loading the Power Stretcher

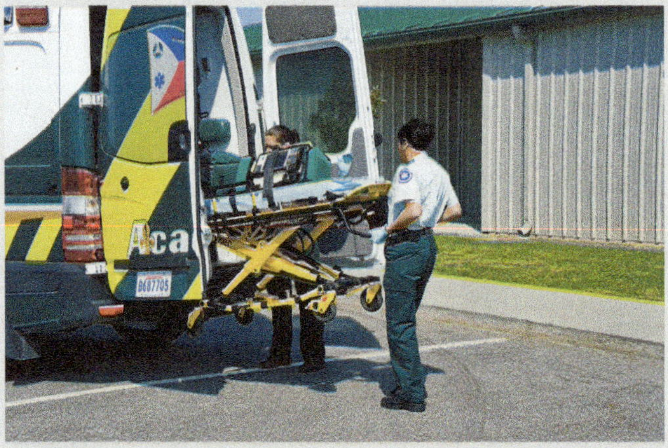

1. Remove the power stretcher from the ambulance. Equipment that will be needed is loaded on top of the stretcher.

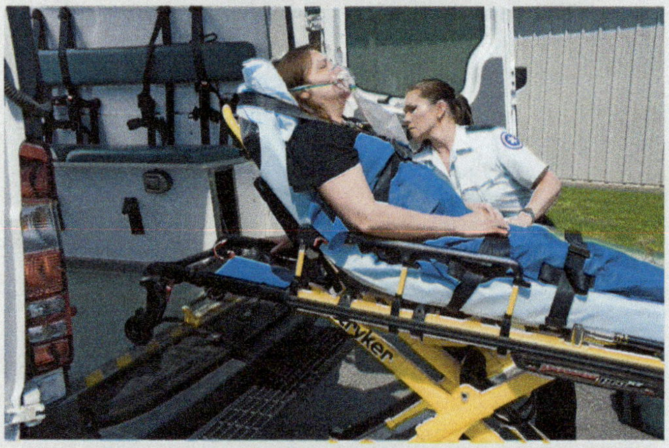

2. Check that the stretcher is properly supported as the patient is loaded into the ambulance.

SCAN 3-5 Loading the Stretcher into the Ambulance *(continued)*

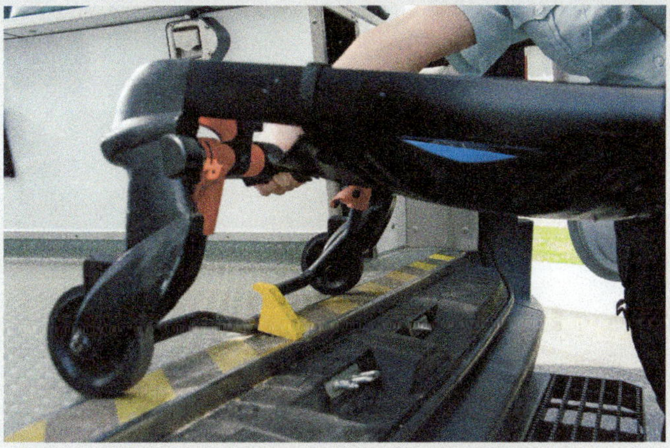

3. Make sure the locking mechanism is secured.

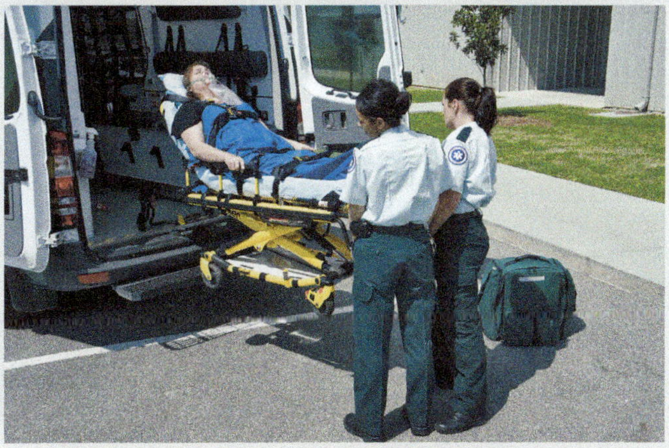

4. Once the head of the stretcher is supported inside the ambulance, raise the stretcher legs.

Loading the "No-lift-at-all" Power Stretcher

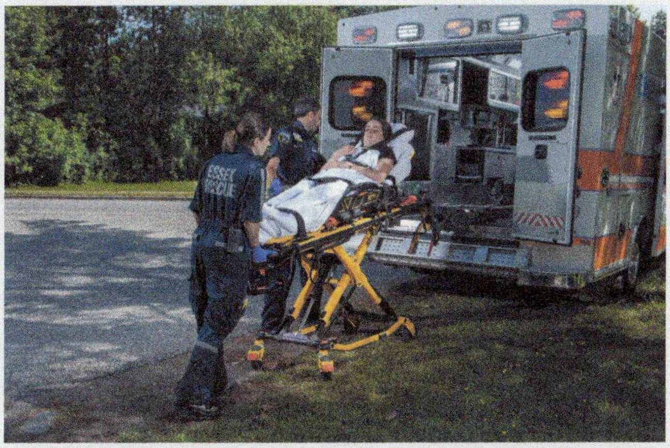

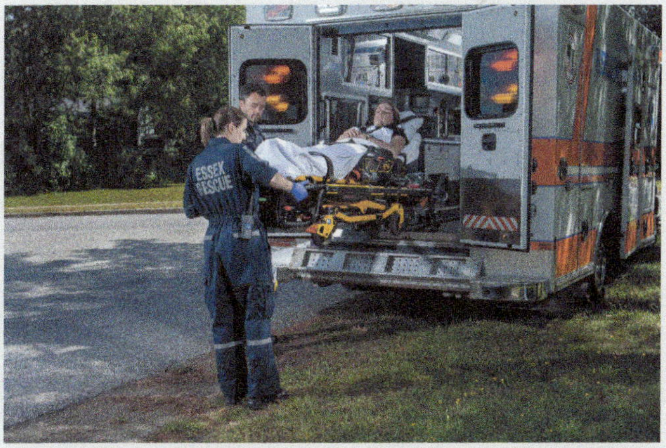

1. "No-lift-at-all" stretcher engaged with the ambulance (*left*) and folded up for moving patient horizontally into the cabin (*right*).

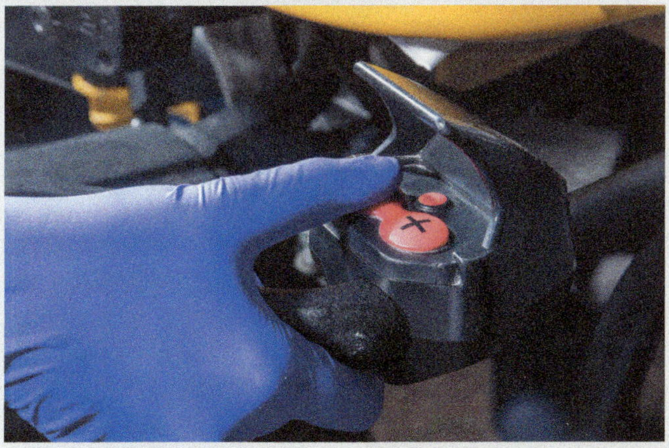

2. Hand pressing power control button.

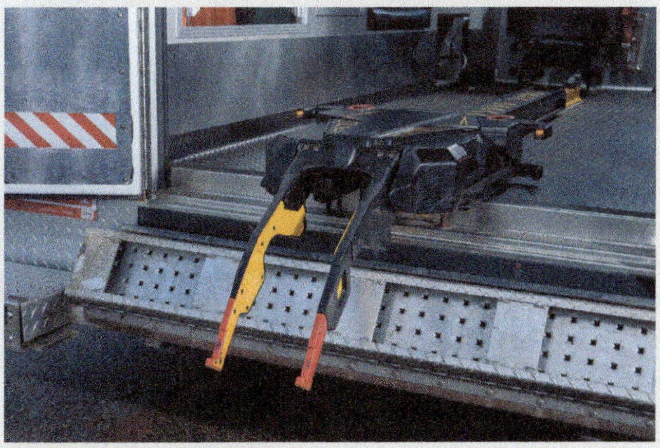

3. Mechanism that pulls the stretcher.

(continued)

SCAN 3-5 Loading the Stretcher into the Ambulance *(continued)*

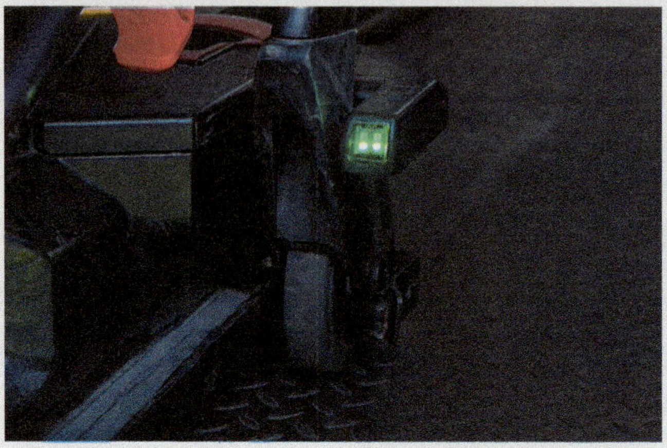

4. A green light indicating stretcher engagement with the ambulance.

Self-Loading (Manual) Stretcher

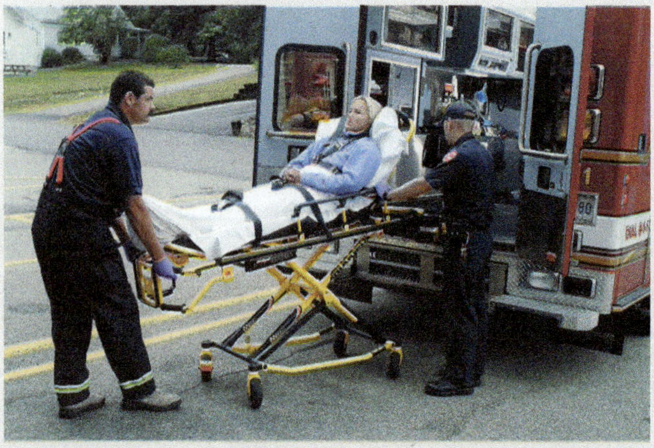

1. Position the wheels closest to the patient's head securely on the inside floor of the ambulance.

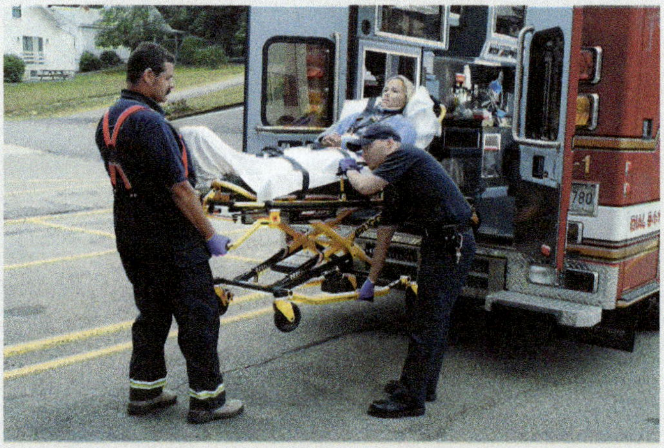

2. Once the wheels are securely on the ambulance floor, the rescuer at the rear of the stretcher activates the lever to release the wheels. (This may require a slight lift to get weight off the wheels.) The second rescuer should guide the collapsing carriage into the ambulance, if necessary.

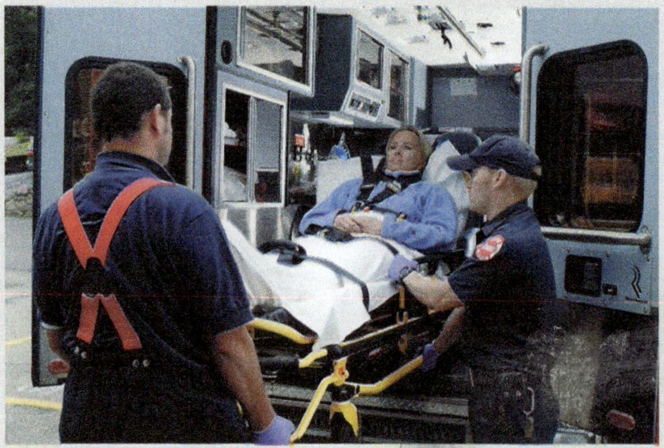

3. Move the stretcher into the securing device and secure the stretcher in the front and rear.

Power stretchers undoubtedly help prevent back injuries. However, anytime a patient is on your stretcher, it is vital to follow the manufacturer's guidelines for their use, to maintain the stretcher properly, and to use safe techniques as discussed in this chapter.

Many services use ***bariatric*** stretchers. These are stretchers that are constructed to transport obese patients (Figure 3-5A). Some stretchers are rated for 800 pounds or more. Many ambulance services have ambulances specially equipped for the loading and transport of the bariatric patient. These ambulances have oversized equipment for patient assessment and care as well as ramps or hydraulic lifts to raise the loaded stretcher into the ambulance (Figure 3-5B). In addition, an increasing number of emergency departments are equipped with hydraulic lifts to transfer obese patients onto the hospital cot (Figure 3-5C).

bariatric
having to do with patients who are significantly overweight or obese.

A stretcher can be carried by four EMTs, one at each corner. This method can be useful on rough terrain because it helps keep the wheels from touching the ground and provides greater stability. It is also beneficial when carrying a patient a long distance because it divides the weight among four EMTs instead of two.

Make sure that the stretcher is always used in accordance with manufacturer's recommendations. Secure the patient to the stretcher before lifting or moving. After placing the

FIGURE 3-5 (A) Challenges occur when patients with a very high BMI need safe transfer to an ambulance. (B) Many EMS services are now equipped with specially constructed stretchers and loading equipment for bariatric patients. (C) An increasing number of emergency departments are being equipped with hydraulic lifts to transfer obese patients onto the hospital cot. *(Photo C: © Edward T. Dickinson, MD)*

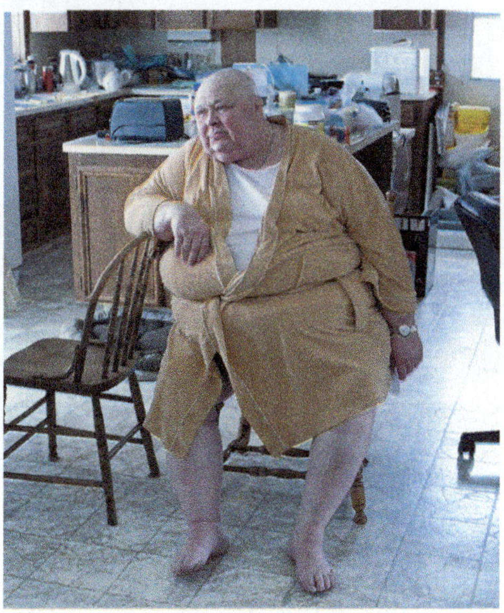
A

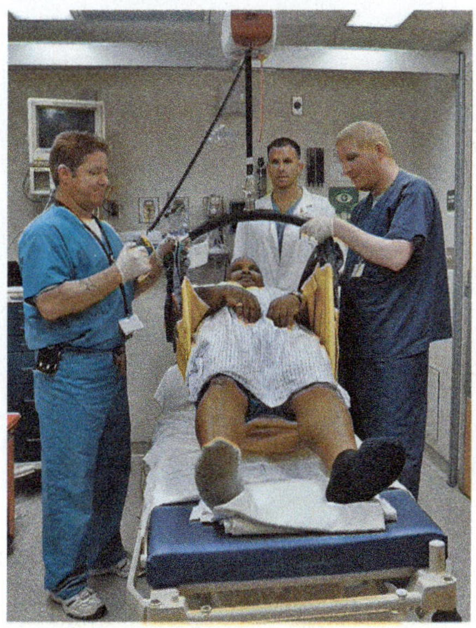
C

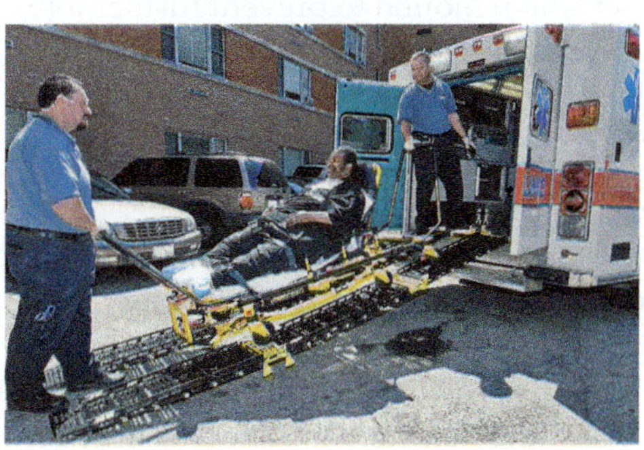
B

patient into the ambulance, secure the stretcher to the ambulance. The patient will remain on the stretcher during transport to the hospital. Ambulances have hardware installed for keeping the stretcher secured while the ambulance is moving. Failure to secure the stretcher properly will allow it to shift during transit, causing an unsafe condition for the EMTs as well as the patient.

Stair Chairs. The stair chair has many benefits for moving patients from the scene to the stretcher. The first benefit, as the name implies, is that it is excellent for use on stairs. Large stretchers often cannot be carried around tight corners or up and down narrow staircases. The stair chair transports the patient in a sitting position, which greatly reduces the length of patient and device, allowing the EMT to maneuver around corners and through narrow spaces. It also has a set of wheels that allows the device to be rolled like a wheelchair over flat surfaces, lessening the strain on the EMT.

Many stair chairs that have wheels to roll the patient along a floor or level ground also have a tracklike system that allows EMTs to gently slide the patient down a staircase instead of lifting the patient (Figure 3-6). The patient's weight increases the friction along the track, which helps to control the rate of descent. You will still need at least two rescuers to use the tracks down stairs, as well as a spotter when available.

Point of View

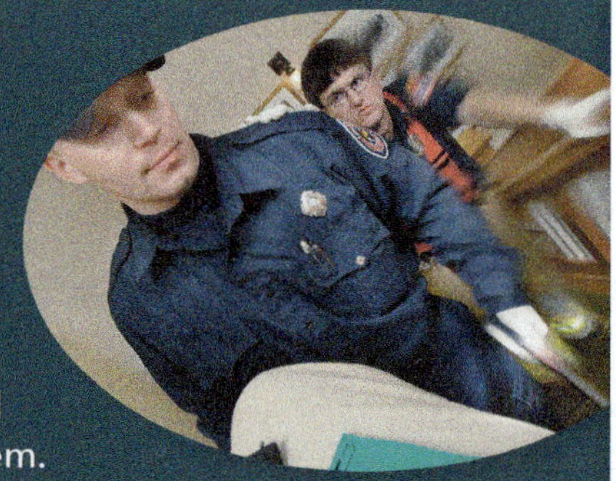

"I just wanted to ask, 'Have you ever dropped anyone before?'

"I really thought I could just walk down the stairs but they said no. They put me in that chair, strapped me in, and off we went.

"'Are you sure it isn't better for me to walk down?' They told me the chair had treads—like a tank—and it wouldn't be a problem. Problem for whom?

"I remember feeling like I should be holding on to something so I kept trying to grab the railing to help. Or maybe to save myself. They were very polite but were getting frustrated when I kept trying to grab.

"Maybe they don't know what it is like to be on stairs with absolutely no control. It was almost as scary as not being able to breathe."

As with all devices in this chapter, there are times when the stair chair should be used and times when it should not. The device is often ideal for patients with difficulty breathing. These patients usually find that they must sit up to breathe more easily, which the stair chair allows them to do. The stair chair must not be used for patients with neck or spine injury, because of the need to restrict spinal motion to prevent further injury. Unresponsive patients, those with a severely altered mental status, or patients who require airway care may not be transported on the stair chair.

Spine Board. There are two types of spine boards, or backboards: short and long (Figure 3-7). They are used to transport patients from the scene to the stretcher and, in some cases, to immobilize a patient with a suspected spine injury. Wooden boards are no longer recommended. Boards today are made of a material that resists absorbing blood and body fluids.

Short spine boards and other extrication devices are rarely used in EMS practice. Most protocols recommend that patients seated in a vehicle with potential spine injuries who cannot extricate themselves from the vehicle be rotated in the seat and moved to a long backboard for transport to the stretcher. Again, these devices are rarely used in EMS practice but are still included on some skills exams, so they will be covered briefly in this text. You will learn more about extrication and care of the patient with potential spine injuries in the chapter titled *Trauma to the Head, Neck, and Spine*.

FIGURE 3-6 (A) A modern stair chair has wheels to roll the patient along a floor or level ground. (B) It also has a track that can be lowered that (C and D) allows EMTs to gently slide the patient down a staircase.

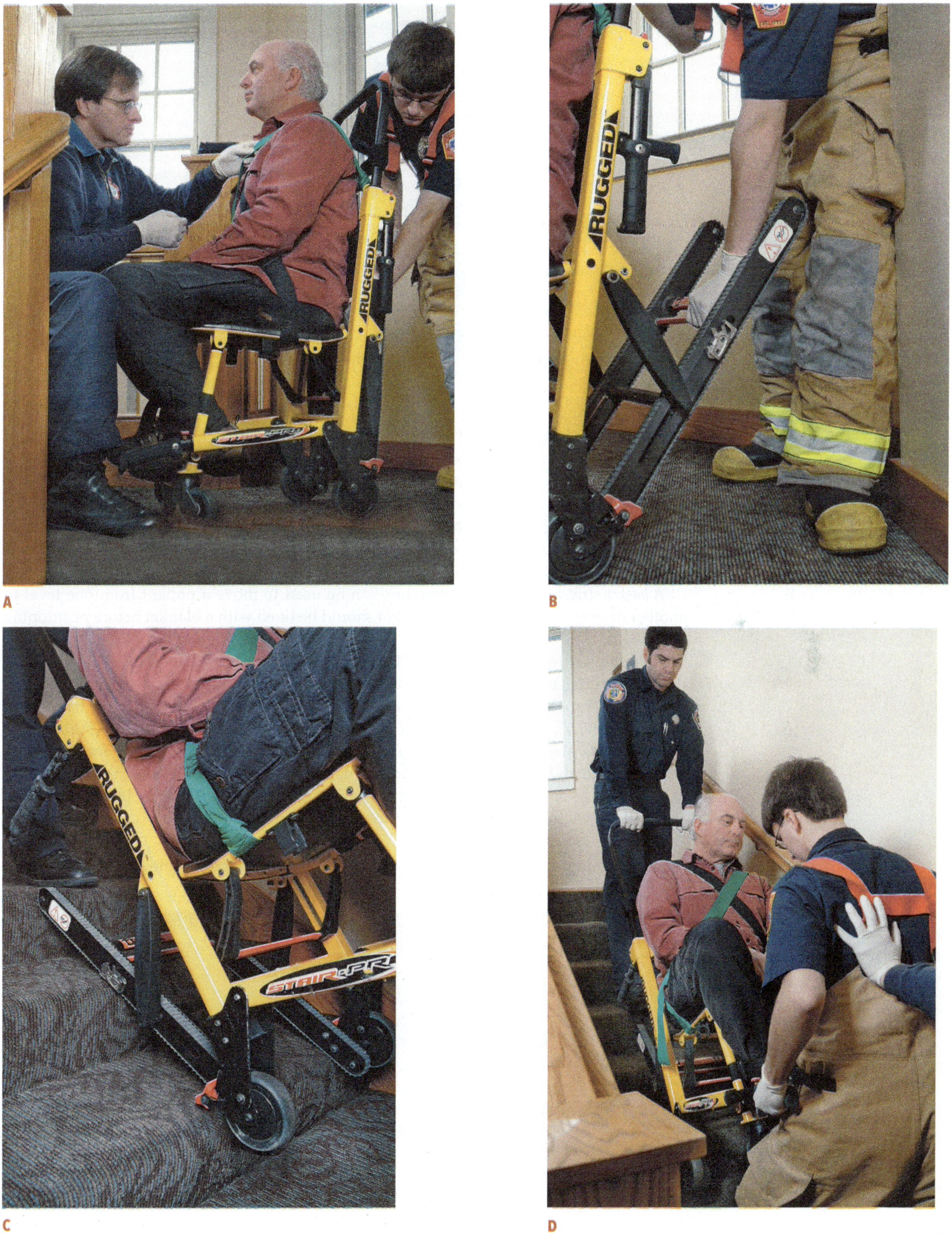

FIGURE 3-7 Long spine boards.

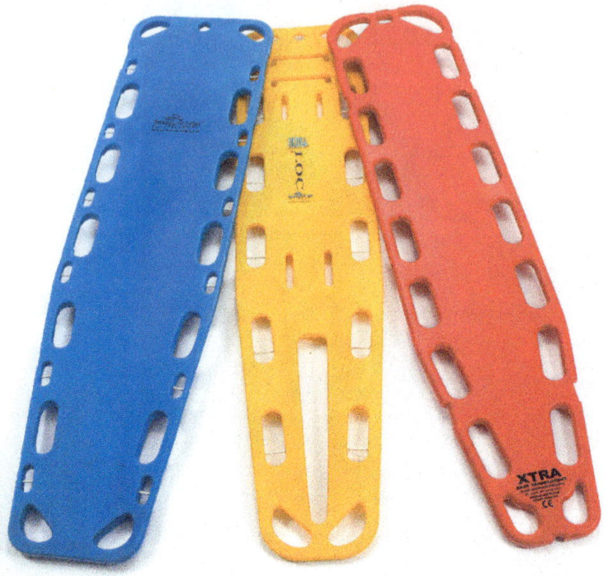

Other Types of Stretchers. The *portable stretcher*, or folding stretcher, may be beneficial in multiple-casualty incidents (incidents with many patients). These stretchers may be canvas, aluminum, or heavy plastic, and usually fold or collapse.

The *scoop stretcher*, or orthopedic stretcher, splits into two pieces vertically, allowing the EMTs to "scoop" and push the halves together under the patient. The scoop stretcher does not offer any support directly under the spine, so it is not recommended for patients with suspected spinal injury. Follow your local protocols on the use of this device.

A *basket stretcher*, or Stokes stretcher, can be used to move a patient from one level to another or over rough terrain. The basket should be lined with a blanket before positioning the patient.

A *flexible stretcher*, or Reeves stretcher, is made of canvas or some other rubberized or flexible material, often with wooden slats sewn into pockets and three carrying handles on each side. Because of its flexibility, it can be useful in restricted areas or narrow hallways.

Some services now use a *vacuum mattress* when transporting patients (Figure 3-8). The patient is placed on the device, and air is withdrawn by a pump. The mattress then becomes rigid and conforming, padding voids naturally for greater comfort. Vacuum mattresses reduce some of the discomfort associated with rigid backboards. In later chapters, you will see vacuum splints that use the same principle.

FIGURE 3-8 (A) A vacuum mattress may be used to transport a patient. (B) When the patient is placed on the device and air is withdrawn, the mattress becomes rigid and conforming, automatically padding voids.

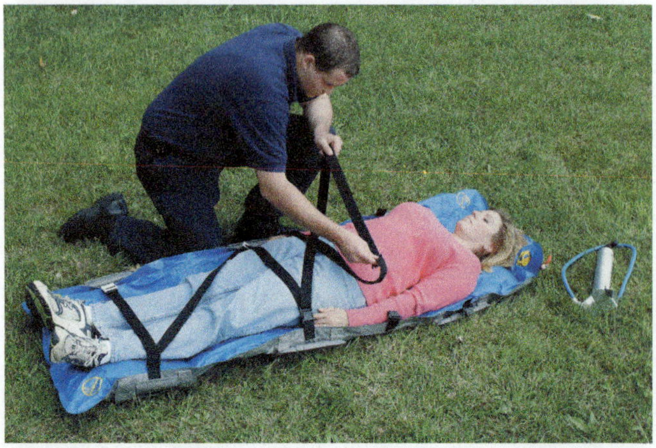

A

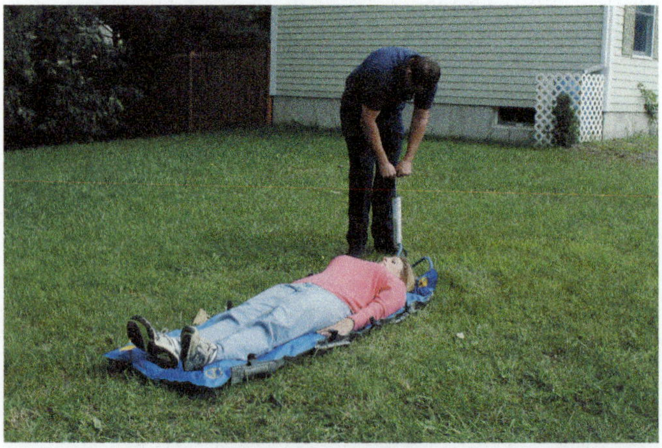

B

Think Like an EMT

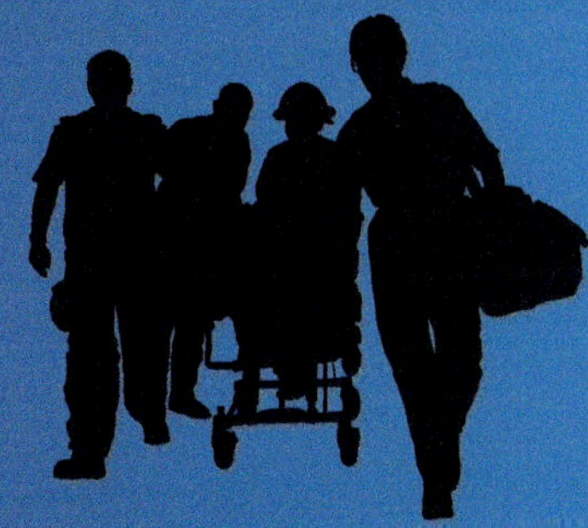

Choosing a Patient-Carrying Device

The process of lifting and moving patients requires more than just muscles. Decisions made in patient transportation have a significant impact on the patient's condition–and the EMTs' well-being. For each of the following patients, choose a carrying device to get the patient from the scene to the ambulance stretcher:

1. A patient complaining of severe respiratory distress who is in an upstairs back bedroom
2. A patient thrown from an ATV several hundred yards into the woods
3. A patient who fell down several stairs from the back deck to the concrete landing who complains of neck and back pain
4. An unresponsive medical patient found down a narrow hallway on the first floor

Moving Patients onto Carrying Devices

There are several ways to move patients onto a carrying device. Choose a move based on the position of the patient when it is time to move the patient to a carrying device and whether the patient is suspected of having a spine injury.

Patient With Suspected Spinal Injury. Patients with suspected spinal injury must have movement of the head, neck, and spine restricted to prevent further injury. This involves performing manual stabilization, placing a rigid cervical collar, and restricting movement of the neck and spine. If patients are able to move under their own power, they may be assisted to the stretcher and secured with straps. Many believe that assisting patients to move under their own power causes less strain on the spine than lifting, rolling, or otherwise manipulating them. For patients seated in a vehicle, first achieve manual stabilization, then either assist them out of the vehicle under their own power or transfer them directly to a long backboard, preventing unnecessary movement of the spine. Then move patients to the wheeled stretcher and remove them from the backboard for transport. A patient who, after a careful spinal assessment, appears to have a spine injury may remain on the backboard for transport.

For patients who are standing, first achieve manual stabilization, then move patients directly to the ambulance stretcher and secure them with the straps or belts on the stretcher. If patients are seated and unable to move under their own power, you will move them to a long backboard and then to the ambulance stretcher. You will learn more about manual stabilization in the chapter *Primary Assessment*, about spinal assessment and cervical collars in the chapter *Secondary Assessment*, and about spinal motion restriction and immobilization for possible spine injury in the *Trauma to the Head, Neck, and Spine* chapter.

Patient With No Suspected Spinal Injury. The extremity lift, direct ground lift, draw-sheet method, and direct carry, described in the following list, are methods of moving a patient to a stretcher. All are appropriate only for a patient with no suspected spine injury. See Scan 3-6 for pictures and detailed descriptions of these methods.

- An ***extremity lift*** is used to carry a patient with no suspected spine or extremity injuries to a stretcher or a stair chair. It can be used to lift a patient from the ground or from a sitting position.
- A ***direct ground lift*** is performed when a patient with no suspected spine injury needs to be lifted from the ground to a stretcher.

(Text continues on p. 75.)

extremity lift
a method of lifting and carrying a patient in which one rescuer slips hands under the patient's armpits and grasps the wrists, while another rescuer grasps the patient's knees.

direct ground lift
a method of lifting and carrying a patient from ground level to a stretcher in which two or more rescuers kneel, curl the patient to their chests, stand, then reverse the process to lower the patient to the stretcher.

SCAN 3-6 Nonurgent Moves, No Suspected Spine Injury

Extremity Carry

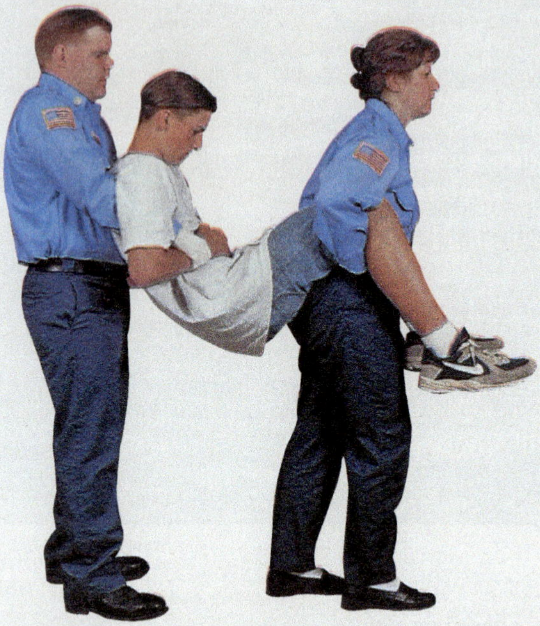

The extremity carry may be used as an emergency move or a nonurgent move for patients with no suspected spine injury.

Place the patient on the patient's back with knees flexed. Kneel at the patient's head. Place your hands under the patient's shoulders. The second EMT kneels at the patient's feet, grasps the patient's wrists, and lifts the patient forward. At the same time, slip your arms under the patient's armpits and grasp the patient's wrists. The second EMT can grasp the patient's knees while facing, or facing away from, the patient. Direct the second EMT, so you both move to a crouch, and stand at the same time. Move as a unit when carrying a patient.

If the patient is found sitting, crouch and slip your arms under the patient's armpits and grasp the patient's wrists. The second EMT crouches then grasps the patient's knees. Lift the patient as a unit.

Draw-Sheet Method

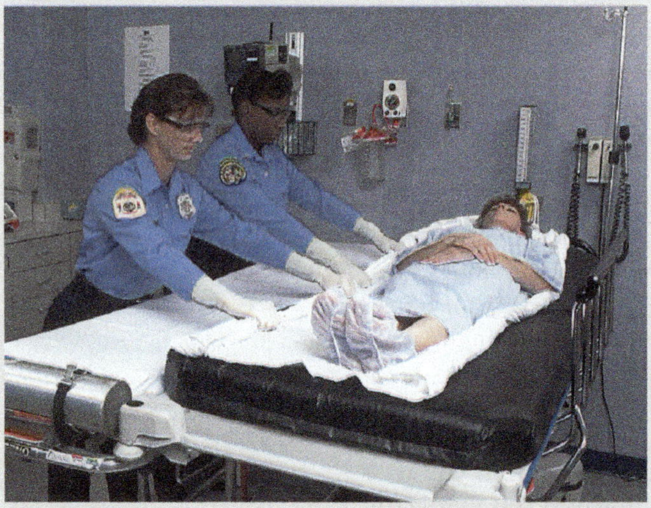

1. Loosen the bottom sheet of the bed and roll it from both sides toward the patient. Place the stretcher, rails lowered, parallel to the bed and touching the side of the bed. EMTs use their bodies and feet to lock the stretcher against the bed.

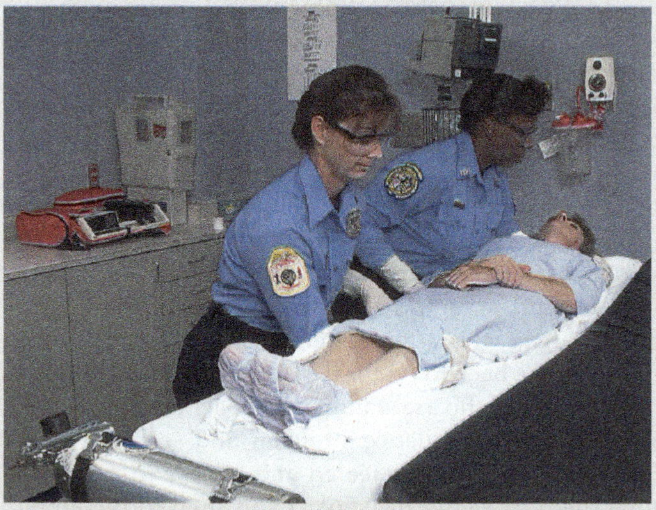

2. EMTs pull on the draw sheet to move the patient to the side of the bed. Both use one hand to support the patient while they reach under the patient to grasp the draw sheet. Then they simultaneously draw the patient onto the stretcher.

SCAN 3-6 Nonurgent Moves, No Suspected Spine Injury *(continued)*

Direct Ground Lift

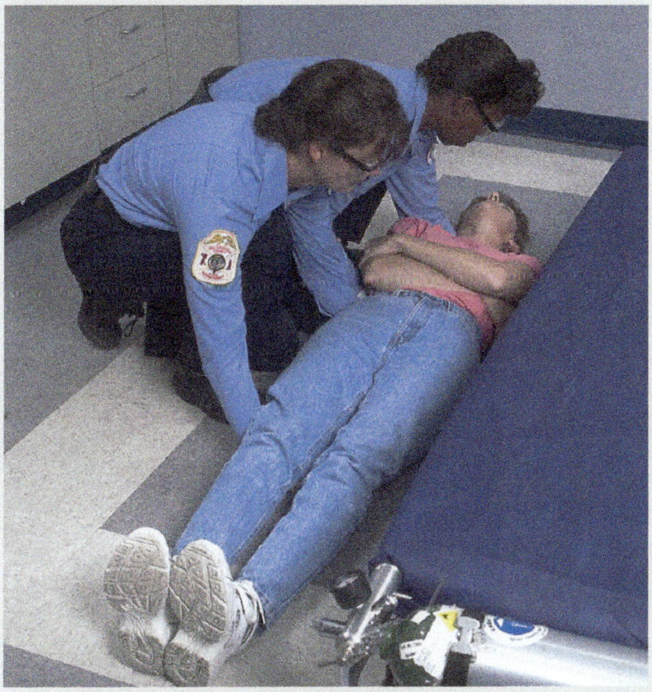

1. The stretcher is set in its lowest position and placed on the opposite side of the patient. The EMTs face the patient, drop to one knee, and if possible, place the patient's arms on the patient's chest. The head-end EMT cradles the patient's head and neck by sliding one arm under the neck to grasp the shoulder, moving the other arm under the patient's back. The foot-end EMT slides one arm under the patient's knees and the other arm under the patient above the buttocks.

NOTE: *If a third rescuer is available, that rescuer should place both arms under the patient's waist while the other two slide their arms up to the mid-back or down to the buttocks, as appropriate.*

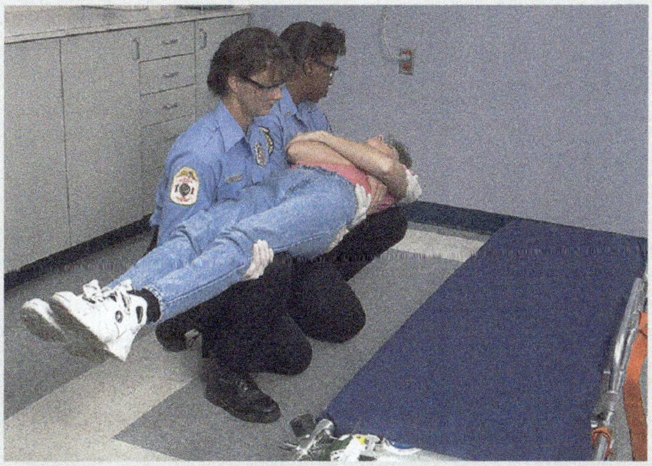

2. On signal, the EMTs lift the patient to their knees.

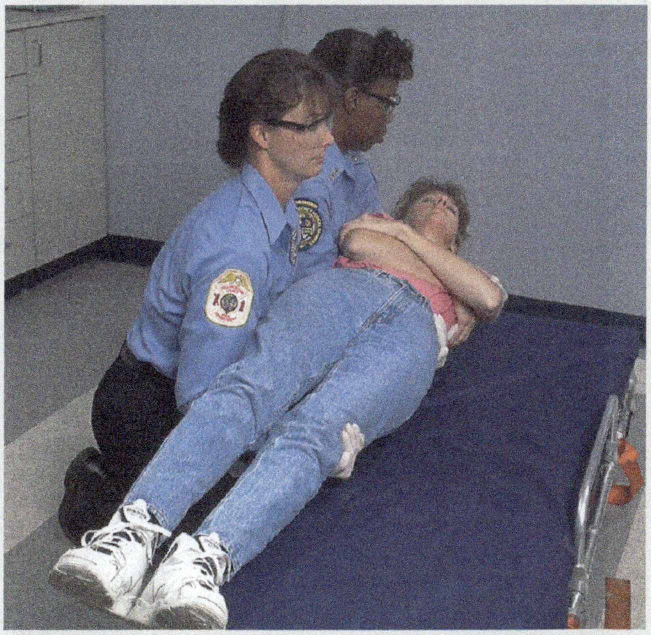

3. On signal, the EMTs stand and carry the patient to the stretcher, drop to one knee, and roll forward to place the patient onto the mattress.

(continued)

SCAN 3-6 Nonurgent Moves, No Suspected Spine Injury *(continued)*

Direct Carry

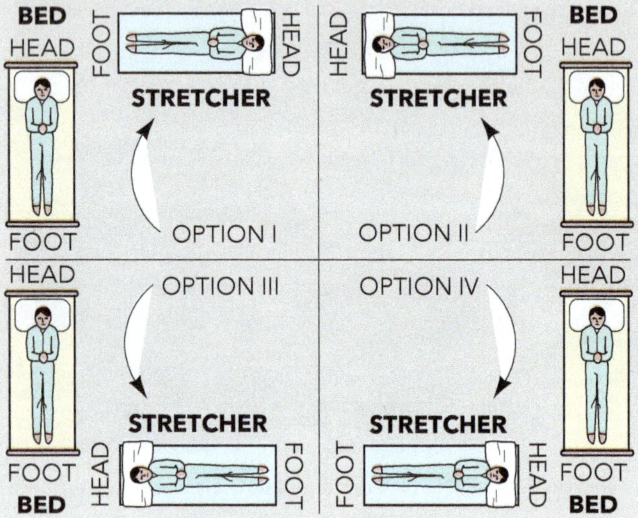

Place the stretcher at a 90-degree angle to the bed, depending on the room configuration. Prepare the stretcher by lowering the rails, unbuckling straps, and removing other items. Both EMTs stand between the stretcher and bed, facing the patient.

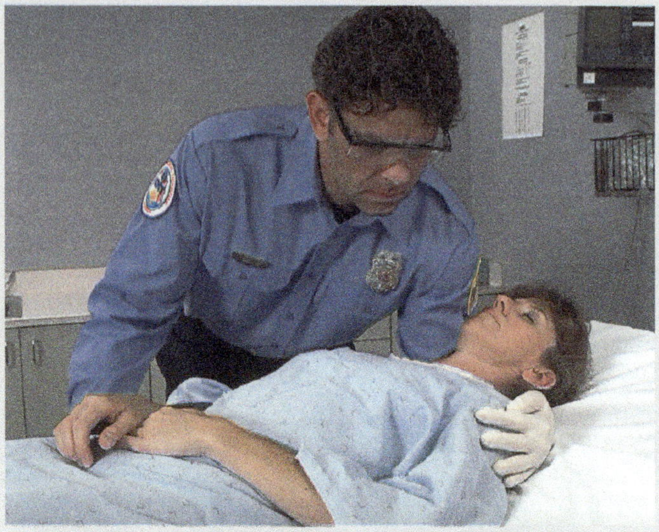

1. The head-end EMT cradles the patient's head and neck by sliding one arm under the patient's neck to grasp the shoulder.

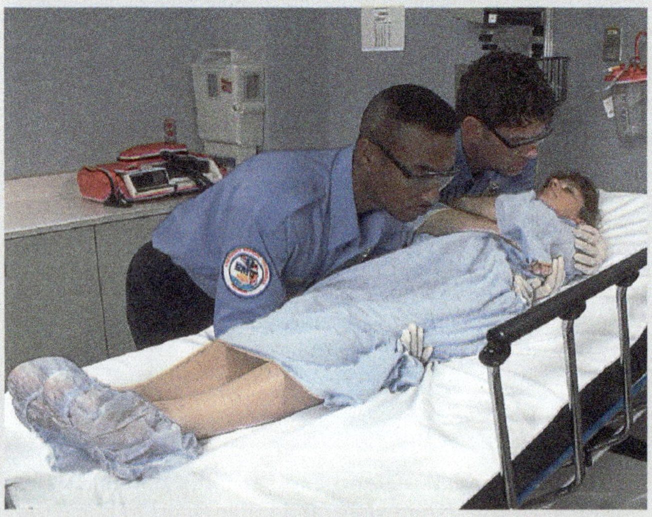

2. The foot-end EMT slides a hand under the patient's hip and lifts slightly. The head-end EMT slides the other arm under the patient's back. The foot-end EMT places arms under the patient's hips and calves.

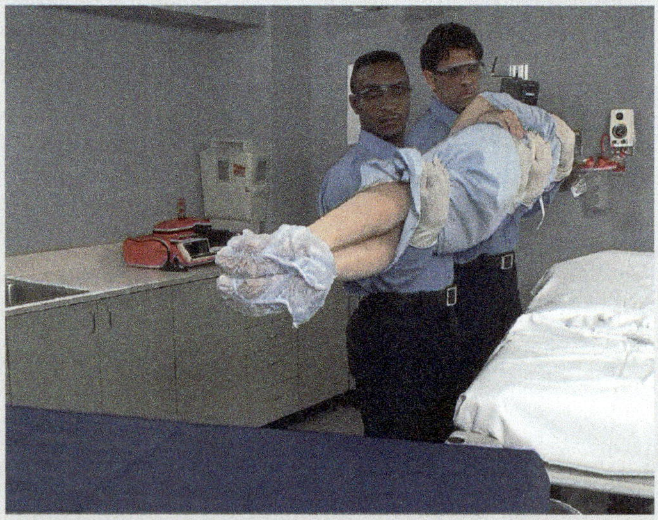

3. EMTs slide the patient to the edge of the bed and bend toward the patient with their knees slightly bent. They lift and curl the patient to their chests and return to a standing position. They rotate, then slide the patient gently onto the stretcher.

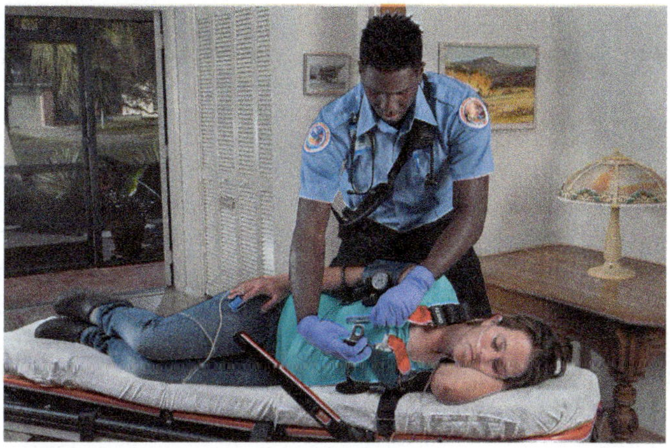

FIGURE 3-9 A patient in the recovery position.

- The ***draw-sheet method*** is one of two methods (along with the direct carry method) that is performed during transfers between hospitals and nursing homes, or when a patient must be moved from a bed at home to a stretcher. It is used for a patient with no suspected spine injury.
- A ***direct carry*** is performed to move a patient with no suspected spine injury from a bed or from a bed-level position to a stretcher.

draw-sheet method
a method of transferring a patient from bed to stretcher by grasping and pulling the loosened bottom sheet of the bed.

direct carry
a method of transferring a patient from bed to stretcher, during which two or more rescuers curl the patient to their chests, then reverse the process to lower the patient to the stretcher.

Patient Positioning

Positioning the patient during transfer to the ambulance and during transportation is a very important part of your care. Lifting, moving, and transport must be performed as an integral part of your total patient-care plan. The position in which the patient is transported depends on the patient's medical condition and the device best designed to help this condition.

Unresponsive patients with no suspected spine injury should be placed in the recovery position (Figure 3-9). The patient should be on one side to aid drainage from the mouth and to help prevent breathing vomitus into the lungs if vomiting occurs. This can be accomplished on a wheeled stretcher. You should avoid transporting the unresponsive patient in a chair-type device, since the airway cannot be properly maintained in this device.

Many patients who have no suspected spine injuries may be transported in a position of comfort. This includes many patients with medical complaints such as chest pain, nausea, or difficulty breathing. In this situation, allow the patient to choose a comfortable position. Breathing is often aided by raising the back of the stretcher so the patient is in a semi-sitting position, also called the Fowler or semi-Fowler position (Figure 3-10). The position must be safe and must not prohibit the proper use of any transportation device.

FIGURE 3-10 For many patients, the position of comfort is a semi-sitting (semi-Fowler or Fowler) position.

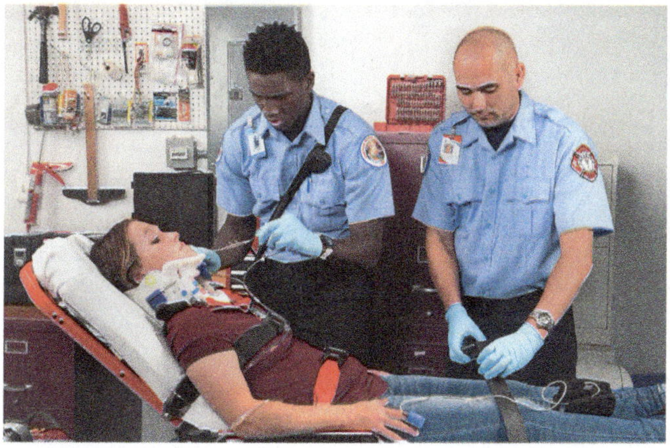

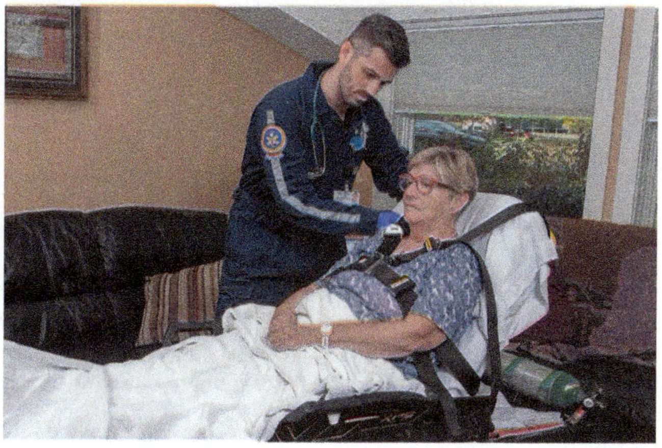

The position of comfort must be used cautiously, in case the patient vomits. Always monitor the patient's airway and level of responsiveness. Place the patient in the recovery position at the first sign of a decreased level of responsiveness.

Positioning for Shock. Patients who are believed to be in shock are placed in a supine position. This allows maximum blood flow throughout the body with minimal resistance from gravity. It is important that all parts of the body—especially vital organs such as the brain—remain perfused.

Patients who have experienced trauma (injury) may require positioning to restrict motion and prevent further injury to the spine. Do not lower the head (which may cause difficulty breathing) or raise the legs (which may aggravate injury and make transportation more difficult). In this case, the risks of raising the legs outweigh the benefits. Recent research has shown there is minimal or no benefit to elevating the legs.

Transferring the Patient to a Hospital Stretcher

When you arrive at the hospital, you will move the patient from the ambulance stretcher to the hospital stretcher. You will probably use a modified draw-sheet method to transfer the patient (Scan 3-7).

SCAN 3-7 Transfer to A Hospital Stretcher

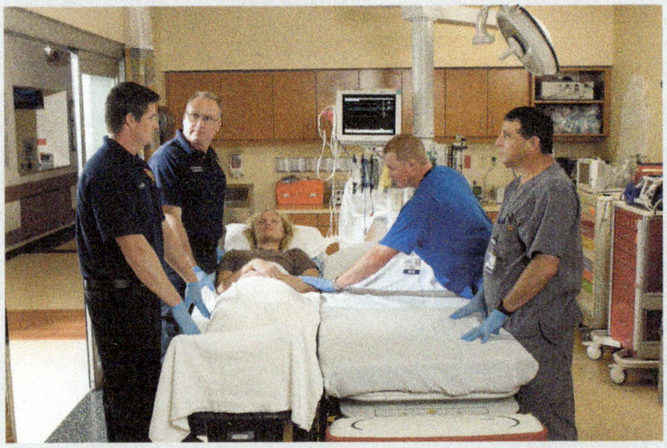

1. Position the raised ambulance cot next to the hospital stretcher. Hospital personnel then adjust the stretcher (raise or lower the head) to receive the patient.

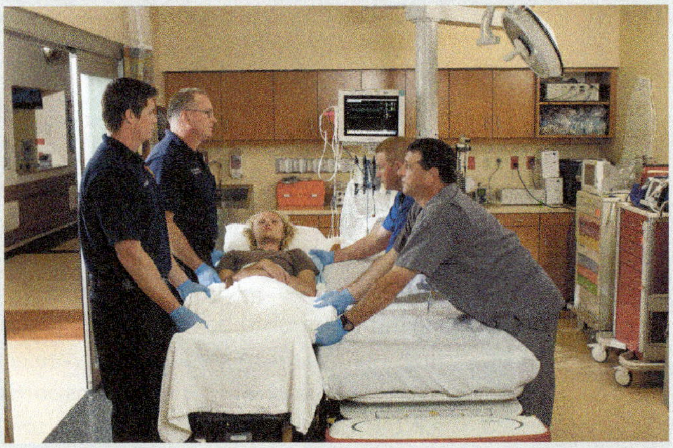

2. You and the hospital personnel gather the sheet on either side of the patient and pull it taut to transfer the patient securely.

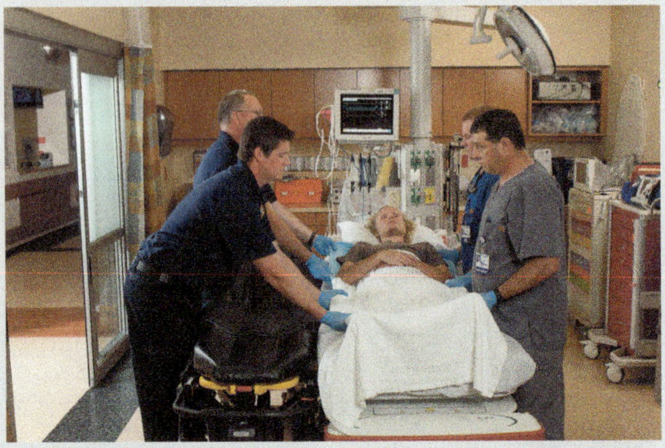

3. Holding the gathered sheet at support points near the patient's shoulders, mid-torso, hips, and knees, you and the hospital personnel slide the patient in one motion onto the hospital stretcher.

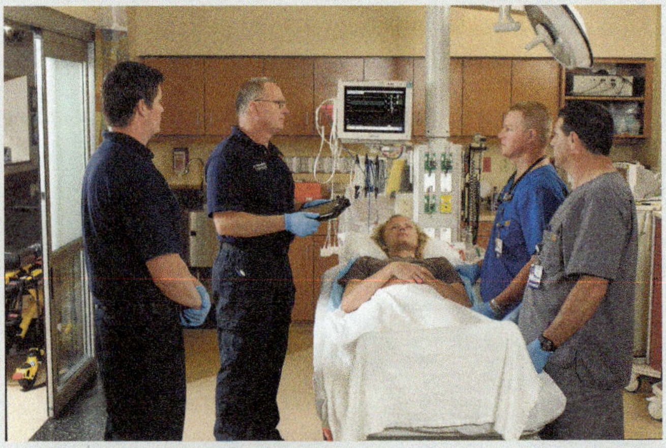

4. Make sure the patient is centered on the stretcher and the stretcher rails are raised before turning the patient over to the emergency department staff.

Chapter Review

Key Facts and Concepts

- The process of lifting and moving patients is a task that requires planning, proper equipment, and careful attention to body mechanics to prevent injury to your patient and to yourself.
- The most important rule in lifting is to lift with your legs, not your back. Keep your feet shoulder-width apart and keep your knees bent. Rules for lifting are for patients as well as equipment.
- Emergency moves are those that may aggravate spine injuries and, therefore, are reserved for life-threatening situations.
- Urgent moves are used when the patient must be moved quickly but there is time to provide quick, temporary consideration toward preventing or aggravating spinal injury.
- Nonurgent moves are normal ways of moving a patient to a stretcher after performing a complete on-scene assessment and restricting movement of the spine when necessary.
- Positioning the patient for transport should take into account the patient's comfort, medical needs, and safety.
- Remember the importance of correct lifting and moving techniques on every call. Protect your patient and protect yourself from injury to maintain a long and positive EMS experience.

Key Decisions

- How quickly must I move this patient?
- Is the patient at risk where the patient is?
- Do I need to move this patient to provide care?
- Will moving the patient cause further harm?
- Is there a way to move or position the patient that will improve the current condition?
- Can I move this patient with the personnel and equipment available on scene?
- What can I do to make my patient comfortable?

Chapter Glossary

bariatric having to do with patients who are significantly overweight or obese.

body mechanics the proper use of the body to facilitate lifting and moving and prevent injury.

direct carry a method of transferring a patient from bed to stretcher, in which two or more rescuers curl the patient to their chests then reverse the process to lower the patient to the stretcher.

direct ground lift a method of lifting and carrying a patient from ground level to a stretcher in which two or more rescuers kneel, curl the patient to their chests, stand, then reverse the process to lower the patient to the stretcher.

draw-sheet method a method of transferring a patient from bed to stretcher by grasping and pulling the loosened bottom sheet of the bed.

extremity lift a method of lifting and carrying a patient during which one rescuer slips hands under the patient's armpits and grasps the wrists, while another rescuer grasps the patient's knees.

power grip gripping with as much hand surface as possible in contact with the object being lifted, all fingers bent at the same angle, and hands at least 10 inches apart.

power lift a lift from a squatting position with weight to be lifted close to the body, feet apart and flat on the ground, body weight on or just behind the balls of the feet, and the back locked in. The upper body is raised before the hips. Also called the *squat-lift position*.

Preparation for Your Examination and Practice

Short Answer

1. Define the term *body mechanics*. Then describe several principles of body mechanics related to safe lifting and moving.
2. List several situations that may require an emergency move of a patient.
3. Name the most common lifts and drags used by the EMT.
4. Define a long-axis drag and explain its importance.

Thinking and Linking

Use your knowledge from the chapter titled *Well-Being of the EMT* along with the material learned in this chapter to answer the following question.

1. How could infectious diseases be spread to patients and/or EMTs while using the following devices or procedures?

    One-rescuer assist

    Firefighter's carry

    Transporting the patient on the wheeled stretcher

    Applying a vest-type extrication device

Critical Thinking Exercises

For each of the following patients, use the knowledge gained in this chapter to identify the appropriate procedure or device for lifting and moving that patient:

1. A patient who has fallen 18 feet (about 5.5 meters) and has suspected spinal injuries
2. A patient with chest pain who lives on the fifth floor of a building with no elevator
3. A patient who is found in an environment with a risk of immediate explosion

Street Scenes

You are having a discussion with a group of your EMS colleagues about the role of the EMT. You focus on direct patient care and the need to do thorough assessments. Another person argues that EMS focuses on doing airway, breathing, and circulation care really well. Kim, an EMT who has been doing EMS for more time than anyone else in the room, says that EMTs must know how to do all those things well "but don't forget that moving and transporting patients is significant too." When you hear that, you silently disagree. "That's really not an important part of patient care," you say to yourself.

Well, the discussion ends–at least for you–when dispatch sends you and your partner to a single-occupant motor-vehicle crash. When you reach the scene, the police tell you that the patient is conscious and alert but is complaining of neck pain, that the crash appears to be low impact with significant front-end damage, and that the patient was wearing a lap belt but the torso part of the restraint was tucked behind her back.

You introduce yourself to the patient, who is still sitting in the driver's seat of her car, and begin your assessment. The patient states that she ran into a parked car. At impact, her head hit the steering wheel, but she denies any loss of consciousness. You continue with the primary assessment and determine the patient is alert and having no difficulty breathing. You observe no signs of bleeding.

Street Scene Questions

1. **What device should be used to remove the patient from the vehicle?**
2. **What patient-care issues are important when using an extrication device?**
3. **What is the next thing to consider when actually moving the patient from the vehicle?**

Since the patient wasn't ambulatory, your local protocol requires that a patient with this mechanism of injury–a car crash resulting in the head's impacting the steering wheel–gets a cervical collar and spinal motion restriction. Your partner, who has been stabilizing the patient's head and neck since shortly after making contact, asks the emergency medical responder unit from the fire department for assistance and suggests to you that a quick neuro exam be done to check for pulses, motor function, and sensation in all extremities. After the neuro exam and palpation of the spine for pain or tenderness, you size a cervical collar and apply it to the patient. You ask the patient if it is causing any additional pain, and she responds that it is uncomfortable but that there's "no additional pain." Next, while your partner still maintains manual stabilization, you position a long backboard on the seat next to the patient. You carefully press the backboard into the seat to help get it under the patient's buttocks. With the help of additional responders, and upon the direction of the rescuer holding cervical-spine (c-spine) stabilization, the patient is rotated onto the long board and lowered into a supine position on the board. The patient is carefully moved to the ambulance stretcher, where she is gently slid from the board onto the stretcher and carefully secured with instructions to limit movement of her neck. As you tighten the straps on the stretcher, you ask if it is causing any difficulty with breathing. The patient responds again, "No."

Street Scene Questions

4. **What emergency-care equipment was used for this patient? Why?**
5. **Why wasn't the patient transported on the backboard?**
6. **By the time this patient is at the ED on a hospital bed, how many times will the EMTs have moved the patient?**

The patient is moved into the ambulance. The patient is comfortable on the stretcher and the cervical collar is not causing any additional pain.

After placing the stretcher in the ambulance, you recheck the stretcher locking device. During transport to the hospital, you take the patient's vital signs and obtain a patient history. At the hospital, the crew moves the stretcher from the ambulance and raises it onto its wheels. You take the patient to an examination room in the emergency department and, with assistance, transfer the patient to the hospital gurney.

After the call, you return to the station. The folks are still in the ready room having the same discussion about the role of an EMT. You pipe in and say, "You know, after this last call, I have to agree with Kim. EMS has a lot to do with knowing how to properly, effectively, and safely move patients."

Medical, Legal, and Ethical Issues

4

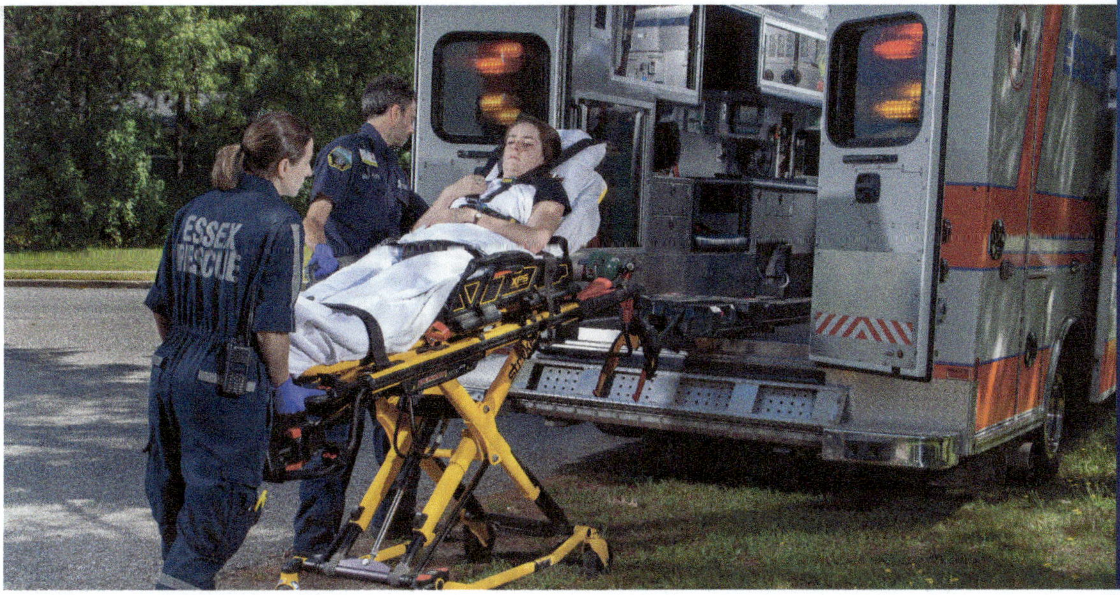

Related Chapters

The following provide additional information related to topics discussed in this chapter:

1 Introduction to Emergency Medical Services
2 Well-Being of the EMT
3 Lifting and Moving Patients
27 Behavioral and Psychiatric Emergencies and Suicide

Standard

Preparatory (Medical/Legal and Ethics)

Competency

Applies fundamental knowledge of the EMS system, safety/well-being of the EMT, and medical/legal and ethical issues to the provision of emergency care.

Core Concepts

- The scope of practice of an EMT
- How a patient may consent to or refuse emergency care
- The legal concepts of torts, negligence, and abandonment
- What it means to have a duty to act
- The responsibilities of an EMT at a crime scene

Outcomes

After reading this chapter, you should be able to:

4.1 Summarize the relationship between scope of practice and standard of care. (pp. 81-82)

- Classify tasks and procedures as either within or outside of an EMT's scope of practice.
- Give examples of ways an EMT can maintain the expected standard of care.

4.2 Give a synopsis of concepts of patient consent to and refusal of care and ethical challenges that arise in the EMT's work. (pp. 82-90)

- Describe when each of the types of consent applies.
- Recognize the criteria that must be met when a patient refuses emergency medical care.
- Given scenarios, derive specific actions from the general steps for interacting with a patient who refuses emergency medical care.
- Describe the EMT's obligations when confronted with different types of Physician's Orders for Life-Sustaining Treatment (POLST).
- Recognize the presence of an ethical challenge.
- Explain various actions that could be taken to address an ethical challenge.
- Predict how various decisions about ethical challenges might play out.

4.3 Outline concepts associated with legal issues that affect EMTs. (pp. 90-99)

- Given a scenario in which a patient makes a claim of negligence against an EMT, determine whether the elements required to prove negligence are present.
- Differentiate between a tort and a criminal act.
- Summarize what Good Samaritan laws are.
- Identify ways in which EMTs may inadvertently violate a patient's confidentiality.
- Describe how the Health Insurance Portability and Accountability Act (HIPAA) impacts the legality of what patient information can be shared by EMTs.
- Identify situations with potential for slander or libel.
- State how medical identification devices and organ donor status identification can guide the decisions of EMTs.
- Describe the purpose of "safe haven" laws.
- Give examples of observations EMTs should make and document at crime scenes.
- Given scenarios, translate the general list of actions EMTs should take at crime scenes into specific actions.

Key Terms

Every time you respond to a call, you will be faced with some aspect of medical/legal or medical/ethical issues. The issue may be as simple as making sure that the patient will accept help or as complex as a terminally ill patient who refuses all care. You may also be faced with decisions such as "Should I stop and help even though I am off duty?" or "Can I get sued if I stop to help outside of my ambulance district?" Understanding of medical, legal, and ethical issues is an essential foundation for all emergency care. This knowledge may also reduce or prevent the legal liability that you may face as a result of calls.

Scope of Practice

The EMT is governed by many medical, legal, and ethical guidelines. This collective set of regulations and ethical considerations may be referred to as a ***scope of practice***, which defines the extent and limits of an EMT's job. The skills and medical interventions the EMT may perform (what you do to help the patient) are defined by legislation that varies from state to state. Sometimes different regions within the same state may have different rules and guidelines for their EMTs. Be sure you understand the rules and guidelines that govern your area.

scope of practice a set of regulations and ethical considerations that define the scope, or extent and limits, of the EMT's job.

CORE CONCEPT
The scope of practice of an EMT

For example, an EMT in one area may be able to perform certain basic procedures and levels of care. In the adjoining region, EMTs may provide that care and also perform special advanced procedures. Your duty is to provide for the well-being of the patient by rendering necessary and legally allowed care as defined under the scope of practice in your area.

Falling within your scope of practice are certain ethical responsibilities. The primary ethical consideration is to make patient care and well-being a priority, even if this requires some personal sacrifice. For example, there may be times when a patient feels cold, even in a hot climate. You may want to turn on the air conditioner in the ambulance, but you refrain out of consideration for your patient. Actions such as this may seem small but mean a lot to the patient.

The scope of practice, as the name indicates, describes the scope of the EMT's job but does not define the ***standard of care***, which is usually defined as the care that would be expected to be provided by an EMT with similar training when caring for a patient in a similar situation. Standard of care will be discussed again later in this chapter with regard to the concept of negligence. In general, scope of practice refers to what you should be

standard of care for an EMT providing care for a specific patient in a specific situation, the care that would be expected to be provided by an EMT with similar training when caring for a patient in a similar situation.

able to do, while standard of care refers to what you should do in a particular situation and how you should do it.

To be an effective EMT, you must maintain your skills and knowledge. This includes practicing until you have obtained confidence and mastery of the skills. After that, continuing education and recertification are necessary to maintain mastery. Every patient deserves the best care.

Emergency care can be improved on the crew and agency levels as well as on an individual level. After a call, constructively critique both yourself and the crew. Accept suggestions from others to improve your skills, communication, and patient outcome. Participation in this kind of mutual critique is part of the process known as *quality improvement*. It should be practiced with the aim of maintaining the standards you would wish to have provided for yourself or someone in your family.

During the rest of this chapter, you will learn about some specific aspects of the scope of practice.

Patient Consent and Refusal

Consent

consent
permission from the patient for care or other action by the EMT.

CORE CONCEPT
How a patient may consent to or refuse emergency care

Consent, or permission from the patient, is required for any treatment or action taken by the EMT. Most patients or their families will have called for your assistance and will readily accept it. A simple statement such as "I'm Karla Maguire, an EMT from the ambulance. I'd like to help you. OK?" is enough to request consent. Most patients will respond positively. Expressed consent must be obtained from every conscious, mentally competent adult before providing care and transportation.

The principle of consent may seem simple, but it often brings up complex issues in patient care. There are three types of consent: expressed, implied, and consent to treat minors or incompetent patients.

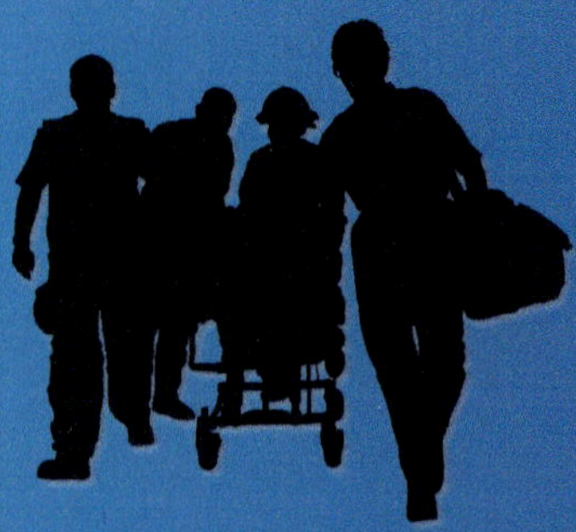

Think Like an EMT

Ethical Dilemmas

Not all critical or difficult decisions you make will be clinical in nature. You may be faced with an ethical dilemma that will test your decision-making skills. For each of the following situations, describe how you would handle the situation. It may be helpful to list the options available to you in each case, then choose the course you think best.

1. You are driving the ambulance to the hospital and listening to the conversation in the back between a paramedic and an EMT. You hear the paramedic say, "Oh, no! I can't believe I just did that. I gave her 10 times the dose I was supposed to." You hear the paramedic ask the EMT not to tell anyone. What do you do?
2. You are on the way home from a sporting event. While there, you had two drinks. You come across a crash with injury. What do you do?
3. A patient tells you that he received the injury you are treating while climbing a fence after being involved in a break-in at a local business. The patient swears he was just the lookout, and if anyone knows he told, he may be killed. What do you do?

Expressed Consent

Expressed consent, the consent given by adults who are of legal age and are mentally competent to make a rational decision with regard to their medical well-being, must be obtained from all patients who are physically and mentally able to give it. Expressed consent must be *informed consent*. That is, patients must understand the risks associated with the care they will receive. It is not only a legal requirement but also appropriate emotional care to explain all procedures to the patient.

expressed consent
consent given by adults who are of legal age and are mentally competent to make a rational decision with regard to their medical well-being.

Children and Mentally Incompetent Adults

Children and mentally incompetent adults are not legally allowed to provide consent or refuse medical care and transportation. The parents and guardians of these patients have the legal authority to give consent, so it must be obtained before care can be given. There are times, however, when care may be given without this direct consent from a parent or guardian.

One situation where care may be given without direct consent from a parent or guardian involves a child care provider or school authority who may act ***in loco parentis*** (in place of a parent) when the parents are not physically present. Parents may provide written documentation to these individuals allowing them to act in their absence.

in loco parentis
literally 'in place of a parent,' indicating a person who may give consent for care of a child when a parent is not present or able to give consent.

In cases of life-threatening illness or injury when a parent or guardian is not present, care may be given based on implied consent. The law provides that it is reasonable to believe that a responsible parent or guardian would consent to care if the parent or guardian were present. In some states, statutes allow emancipated minors—those who are married or of a certain age—to provide consent. Finally, minors who themselves have children and those who serve in the armed forces may also be able to provide consent for their own care. Find out the laws where you will practice as an EMT in reference to consent of minors.

Implied Consent

In the case of an unconscious patient (or one who may be physically or mentally incapacitated but in need of emergency care), consent may be assumed. The law states that rational patients would consent to treatment if they were conscious. This is known as ***implied consent***. In this situation, the law allows EMTs and other health care providers to provide treatment, at least until the patient becomes conscious and able to make rational decisions.

implied consent
the consent it is presumed patients or their parents or guardians would give if they could, such as for an unconscious patient or a child whose parents cannot be contacted when care is needed.

Involuntary Transportation

There will be times when patients are going to the hospital involuntarily (against their will). This is frequently the result of a decision made by police officers or mental health workers when they believe patients pose a threat of harm to themselves or others. Patients may also be transported against their will as a result of a court order.

In some of these cases, you will be transporting patients who are physically restrained. This is a significant legal responsibility. Many lawsuits alleging negligence are brought against EMS providers for improper restraint or for harm caused to patients during restraint or transport. When a patient has been denied the ability to move freely, it is a great responsibility for the EMT to ensure the patient's health and well-being during this time. It is essential to frequently and thoroughly monitor the patient's mental status and vital signs while the patient is in your care.

Restraint is discussed in two other places in this text: the chapter titled *Lifting and Moving Patients* and the chapter titled *Behavioral and Psychiatric Emergencies and Suicide*.

When a Patient Refuses Care

You may think that all patients who need medical care will accept it. Most do. However, you will find that some patients who require treatment and transportation to the hospital will refuse care. Many reasons exist for this, including denial, fear, failure to understand the seriousness of the situation, and intoxication.

Although patients generally have the right to refuse care, it is your responsibility as an EMT to be sure that patients are fully informed about their situation and the implications of refusing care.

In order for patients to refuse care or transport, several conditions must be fulfilled:

- **Patients must be legally able to consent.** They must be of legal age or emancipated minors.
- **Patients must be awake and oriented.** They must not be affected by any disease or condition that would impair judgment. These conditions include unstable vital signs, alcohol intoxication or the influence of drugs, and altered mental status.
- **Patients must be fully informed.** They must have the mental capacity to understand their situation and the potential consequences of refusal of care.
- **Patients will be asked to sign a "release" form (Figure 4-1).** Such a form is designed to release the ambulance agency and individuals from ***liability*** (legal responsibility) arising from the patient's informed refusal.

liability
being held legally responsible.

Even carefully following these steps will not guarantee that you will be free from liability if a patient refuses care or transport. Leaving a patient who will not accept care or transport is a leading cause of lawsuits against EMS agencies and providers, even though it was the patient who refused. Occasionally the patient's condition deteriorates to the point of unconsciousness, which leaves the patient unable to summon help, leading to a severely worsened condition or even death.

In addition to the liability factor, there is also an ethical issue. You would undoubtedly feel guilty if a patient were found unconscious or deceased after refusing care and you felt that transportation would have prevented the circumstance.

If in doubt, do everything possible to persuade the patient to accept care and transport. Take all possible actions to persuade a patient you feel should go to the hospital but who refuses to go. These actions may include:

- **Spend time speaking with the patient.** Use principles of effective communication. It may take reasoning, persistence, "dealing" ("We'll call a neighbor to take care of your cat, but then you go to the hospital"), or another strategy.
- **Listen carefully to try to determine why the patient is refusing care.** Often the patient has a fear of the hospital, procedures, prolonged hospitalization, or even death. Refusal to go to the hospital may be a form of denial or unwillingness to accept the idea of being ill. If you identify the cause of the refusal, you may be able to develop a strategy to persuade the patient to accept your care and transportation to the hospital. Listening to the patient is the key to determining why the patient is refusing.
- **Inform the patient of the consequences of not going to the hospital. This is an essential component of every refusal-of-care situation.** For example, in the case of patients who you believe may be having a heart attack or other potentially life-threatening condition refusing transport, it is appropriate to tell the patients that they may get very ill or die without treatment. If these patients still refuse, you should stress the importance of transport to an emergency department and tell the patients that death may result without treatment.
- **Consult medical direction.** If you are in a residence, use a phone to contact medical direction. If the on-line doctor is willing, let the doctor speak to the patient when all else fails. Many services require physician contact before accepting a refusal under these circumstances.
- **Ask the patient if it is all right if you call a family member—or advise the patient that you would like to call a family member.** Often family members can provide the patient with reasons to go to the hospital. An offer from a loved one to meet the patient at the hospital may be very helpful. *Note, however, that notifying others and sharing protected information against a patient's wishes may constitute a violation of privacy laws.* If you ask for permission or if you advise the patient of your intention to call a

family member and the patient either agrees or does not object, this constitutes consent. As part of your call's documentation, you should document that this permission to speak to family was verbally granted to you by the patient. Be sure you understand your agency's policy on how to handle this issue.

- **Call law enforcement personnel if necessary.** Police may be able to order or force patients who refuse care to go to the hospital. This is done under the premise that patients might be temporarily mentally incompetent, as demonstrated by refusal of potentially lifesaving care. Be very sure that there is evidence of incompetence because you are assuming possible legal liability if you are wrong. Remember that a patient is not mentally incompetent just because they refuse lifesaving care. Again, be sure you understand your agency's policies on this issue.
- **Ask the patient to sign the refusal of care form used by your agency.** Sometimes a patient will refuse to sign these forms. If the patient refuses to sign the form, you should specifically document in your patient care report that you carefully explained the risks and consequences of refusal to the patient and that the patient had the capacity to understand your warnings but still declined to sign the form.

Always bear in mind that you do not have the right in most cases to force patients with appropriate mental capacity to go to the hospital against their will. Subjecting patients to unwanted care and transport has actually been viewed in court as ***assault*** (placing a person in fear of bodily harm) in some instances and ***battery*** (causing said harm or restraining) in others.

assault
placing a person in fear of bodily harm.

battery
causing bodily harm to or restraining a person.

If all efforts fail and the patient does not accept your care or transportation, it becomes vital to document the attempts you made—to make your efforts a part of the official record—in order to prevent liability. Write into your records every step you took to persuade the patient to accept care or to go to the hospital. Include the names of any witnesses to your attempts and the patient's refusal. (See the sample EMS patient refusal procedures checklist shown in Figure 4-1.)

In all cases of refusal, you should advise patients to call back at any time if they have a problem or wish to be cared for or transported. It is advisable to call a relative or neighbor who can stay with the patient in case problems develop. If the local emergency number is not 911, make sure the patient knows the number to call. You should also recommend that the patient or a relative call the family physician to report the incident and arrange for follow-up care. Document all actions you have taken for the patient.

Although there may be patients who legitimately refuse care (for minor wounds, unfounded calls, and the like), a patient with any significant medical condition should be transported and seen at a hospital.

Point of View

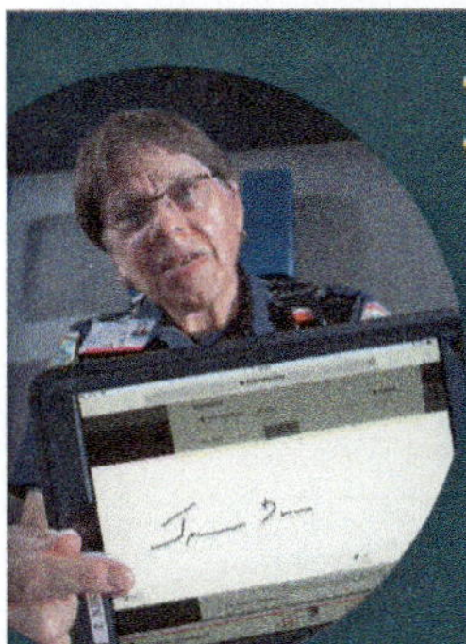

"My wife said I passed out. I don't remember passing out. To be honest, I don't remember much about it at all. I woke up and the ambulance was there. They said they'd take me to the hospital if I wanted. Who wants to go to the hospital? Not me, that's for sure. My parents died in the hospital. My brother died at the hospital. The best thing I could do was stay out of the hospital.

"My wife looked so nervous. She almost convinced me to go. And the boys on the ambulance. No, one of them was a girl. Nice kids. They put a computer in front of me. Wanted me to sign in a little box on the screen. Not sure what. I can't hear much anymore anyway. They were telling me all kinds of things in big medical words. At my age, what difference does it make anyway?

"So I signed it."

FIGURE 4-1 Certain procedures should be followed when a patient refuses care or transport.

EMS PATIENT REFUSAL CHECKLIST

PATIENT'S NAME: ______________________ AGE: ________

LOCATION OF CALL: ______________________ DATE: ________

AGENCY INCIDENT #: __________ AGENCY CODE: __________

NAME OF PERSON FILLING OUT FORM: ______________________

I. ASSESSMENT OF PATIENT (Check appropriate response for each item)

1. Oriented to:
   - Person? ☐ Yes ☐ No
   - Place? ☐ Yes ☐ No
   - Time? ☐ Yes ☐ No
   - Situation? ☐ Yes ☐ No
2. Altered level of consciousness? ☐ Yes ☐ No
3. Head injury? ☐ Yes ☐ No
4. Alcohol or drug ingestion by exam or history? ☐ Yes ☐ No

II. PATIENT INFORMED (Check appropriate response for each item)

- ☐ Yes ☐ No Medical treatment/evaluation needed
- ☐ Yes ☐ No Ambulance transport needed
- ☐ Yes ☐ No Further harm could result without medical treatment/evaluation
- ☐ Yes ☐ No Transport by means other than ambulance could be hazardous in light of patient's illness/injury
- ☐ Yes ☐ No Patient provided with Refusal Information Sheet
- ☐ Yes ☐ No Patient accepted Refusal Information Sheet

III. DISPOSITION

- ☐ Refused all EMS assistance
- ☐ Refused field treatment, but accepted transport
- ☐ Refused transport, but accepted field treatment
- ☐ Refused transport to recommended facility
- ☐ Patient transported by private vehicle to ______________________
- ☐ Released in care or custody of self
- ☐ Released in care or custody of relative or friend

  Name: ______________ Relationship: ______________
- ☐ Released in custody of law enforcement agency

  Agency: ______________ Officer: ______________
- ☐ Released in custody of other agency

  Agency: ______________ Officer: ______________

IV. COMMENTS: ______________________

____

____

____

Do Not Resuscitate Orders and Physician's Orders for Life-Sustaining Treatment

It will only be a matter of time before you come upon a patient who has a ***do not resuscitate (DNR) order*** (Figure 4-2A). This is a legal document, usually signed by the patient and patient's physician, which states that the patient has a terminal illness and does not wish to prolong life through resuscitative efforts. A DNR order may be part of an ***advance directive***, because it is written and signed in advance of any event where resuscitation might be undertaken. It is more than the expressed wishes of the patient or family.

(Text continues on p. 90.)

do not resuscitate (DNR) order
a legal document, usually signed by both patient and physician, which states that the patient has a terminal illness and does not wish to prolong life through resuscitative efforts.

advance directive
a DNR order; instructions written in advance of an event.

FIGURE 4-2A Example of a do not resuscitate (DNR) order. *(Adapted from Mistovich, Joseph, J. Prehospital Emergency Care, (11ed). Chapter 3 Medical, Legal, and Ethical Issues. Pages 50-51, Figure 3-1.)*

DNR COMFORT CARE

DNR IDENTIFICATION FORM

Patient Name:		
Address:		
City:	State:	Zip:
Birthdate:	Gender: ❑ M ❑ F	
Signature: (optional)		

Printed name of physician*:	
Signature:	Date:
Address:	Phone:

DO NOT RESUSCITATE COMFORT CARE PROTOCOL

After the protocol has been activated for a specific DNR Comfort Care patient, the protocol specifies that emergency medical services and other health care workers are to do the following:

WILL:

- Suction the airway
- Administer oxygen
- Position for comfort
- Splint or immobilize
- Control bleeding
- Provide pain medication
- Provide emotional support
- Contact other appropriate health care providers, such as hospice, home health, attending physicians, CNPs, and CNSs

WILL NOT:

- Administer chest compressions
- Insert artificial air way
- Administer resuscitative drugs
- Defibrillate or cardiovert
- Provide respiratory assistance (other than that listed above)
- Initiate resuscitative IV
- Initiate cardiac monitoring

If you have responded to an emergency situation by initiating any of the WILL NOT actions prior to confirming that the DNR Comfort Care protocol should be activated, discontinue them when you activate the protocol. You may continue respiratory assistance, IV medications, etc., that have been part of the patient's ongoing course of treatment for an underlying disease.

If family or bystanders request or demand resuscitation for a person for whom the DNR Comfort Care protocol has been activated, do not proceed with resuscitation. Provide comfort measures as outlined above and try to help the family members understand the dying process and the patient's choice not to be resuscitated.

(continued)

FIGURE 4-2B Example of a Physician's Order for Life-Sustaining Treatment (POLST). *(Physician Orders for Life Sustaining Treatment (POLST) Form by the California Emergency Medical Services Authority, http://www.emsa.ca.gov//Media/Default/PDF/Final-2014-ENG-CA-POLST-Form-1.pdf.)*

HIPAA PERMITS DISCLOSURE OF POLST TO OTHER HEALTH CARE PROVIDERS AS NECESSARY

Physician Orders for Life-Sustaining Treatment (POLST)

EMSA #111 B
(Effective 4/1/2011)

First follow these orders, then contact physician. This is a Physician Order Sheet based on the person's current medical condition and wishes. Any section not completed implies full treatment for that section. A copy of the signed POLST form is legal and valid. POLST complements an Advance Directive and is not intended to replace that document. Everyone shall be treated with dignity and respect.

Patient Last Name:	Date Form Prepared:
Patient First Name:	Patient Date of Birth:
Patient Middle Name:	Medical Record #: *(optional)*

A Check One

CARDIOPULMONARY RESUSCITATION (CPR): ***If person has no pulse and is not breathing. When NOT in cardiopulmonary arrest, follow orders in Sections B and C.***

☐ **Attempt Resuscitation/CPR** (Selecting CPR in Section A **requires** selecting Full Treatment in Section B)

☐ **Do Not Attempt Resuscitation/DNR** (Allow Natural Death)

B Check One

MEDICAL INTERVENTIONS: ***If person has pulse and/or is breathing.***

☐ **Comfort Measures Only** Relieve pain and suffering through the use of medication by any route, positioning, wound care and other measures. Use oxygen, suction and manual treatment of airway obstruction as needed for comfort. ***Transfer to hospital only*** *if comfort needs cannot be met in current location.*

☐ **Limited Additional Interventions** In addition to care described in Comfort Measures Only, use medical treatment, antibiotics, and IV fluids as indicated. Do not intubate. May use non-invasive positive airway pressure. Generally avoid intensive care.

☐ ***Transfer to hospital only*** *if comfort needs cannot be met in current location.*

☐ **Full Treatment** In addition to care described in Comfort Measures Only and Limited Additional Interventions, use intubation, advanced airway interventions, mechanical ventilation, and defibrillation/cardioversion as indicated. ***Transfer to hospital*** *if indicated. Includes intensive care.*

Additional Orders ______________________________

____

C Check One

ARTIFICIALLY ADMINISTERED NUTRITION: ***Offer food by mouth if feasible and desired.***

☐ No artificial means of nutrition, including feeding tubes. Additional Orders: ______________

☐ Trial period of artificial nutrition, including feeding tubes. ______________

☐ Long-term artificial nutrition, including feeding tubes. ______________

D

INFORMATION AND SIGNATURES:

Discussed with: ☐ Patient (Patient Has Capacity) ☐ Legally Recognized Decisionmaker

☐ Advance Directive dated _______ available and reviewed→
☐ Advance Directive not available
☐ No Advance Directive

Health Care Agent if named in Advance Directive:
Name: ______________
Phone: ______________

Signature of Physician

My signature below indicates to the best of my knowledge that these orders are consistent with the person's medical condition and preferences.

Print Physician Name:	Physician Phone Number:	Physician License Number:
Physician Signature: *(required)*		Date:

Signature of Patient or Legally Recognized Decisionmaker

By signing this form, the legally recognized decisionmaker acknowledges that this request regarding resuscitative measures is consistent with the known desires of, and with the best interest of, the individual who is the subject of the form.

Print Name:		Relationship: *(write self if patient)*
Signature: *(required)*		Date:
Address:	Daytime Phone Number:	Evening Phone Number:

SEND FORM WITH PERSON WHENEVER TRANSFERRED OR DISCHARGED

FIGURE 4-2B Example of a Physician's Order for Life-Sustaining Treatment (POLST). *(continued)*

HIPAA PERMITS DISCLOSURE OF POLST TO OTHER HEALTH CARE PROVIDERS AS NECESSARY

Patient Information

Name (last, first, middle):	Date of Birth:	Gender: M F

Health Care Provider Assisting with Form Preparation

Name:	Title:	Phone Number:

Additional Contact

Name:	Relationship to Patient:	Phone Number:

Directions for Health Care Provider

Completing POLST

- Completing a POLST form is voluntary. California law requires that a POLST form be followed by health care providers, and provides immunity to those who comply ingood faith. In the hospital setting, a patient will be assessed by a physician who will issue appropriate orders.
- POLST does not replace the Advance Directive. When available, review the Advance Directive and POLST form to ensure consistency, and update forms appropriately to resolve any conflicts.
- POLST must be completed by a health care provider based on patient preferences and medical indications.
- A legally recognized decisionmaker may include a court-appointed conservator or guardian, agent designated in an Advance Directive, orally designated surrogate, spouse, registered domestic partner, parent of a minor, closest available relative, or person whom the patient's physician believes best knows what is in the patient's best interest and will make decisions in accordance with the patient's expressed wishes and values to the extent known.
- POLST must be signed by a physician and the patient or decisionmaker to be valid. Verbal orders are acceptable with follow-up signature by physician in accordance with facility/community policy.
- Certain medical conditions or treatments may prohibit a person from residing in a residential care facility for the elderly.
- If a translated form is used with patient or decisiomaker, attach it to the signed English POLST form.
- Use of original form is strongly encouraged. Photocopies and FAXes of signed POLST forms are legal and valid. A copy should be retained in patient's medical record, on Ultra Pink paper when possible.

Using POLST

- Any incomplete section of POLST implies full treatment for that section.

Section A:

- If found pulseless and not breathing, no defibrillator (including automated external defibrillators) or chest compressions should be used on a person who has chosen "Do Not Attempt Resuscitation."

Section B:

- When comfort cannot be achieved in the current setting, the person, including someone with "Comfort Measures Only," should be transferred to a setting able to provide comfort (e.g., treatment of a hip fracture).
- Non-invasive positive airway pressure includes continuous positive airway pressure (CPAP), bi-level positive airway pressure (BiPAP), and bag valve mask (BVM) assisted respirations.
- IV antibiotics and hydration generally are not "Comfort Measures."
- Treatment of dehydration prolongs life. If person desires IV fluids, indicate "Limited Interventions" or "Full Treatment."
- Depending on local EMS protocol, "Additional Orders" written in Section B may not be implemented by EMS personnel.

Reviewing POLST

It is recommended that POLST be reviewed periodically. Review is recommended when:

- The person is transferred from one care setting or care level to another, or
- There is a substantial change in the person's health status, or
- The person's treatment preferences change.

Modifying and Voiding POLST

- A patient with capacity can, at anytime, request alternative treatment.
- A patient with capacity can, at any time, revoke a POLST by any means that indicates intent to revoke. It is recommended that revocation be documented by drawing a line through Sections A through D, writing "VOID" in large letters, and signing and dating this line.
- A legally recognized decisionmaker may request to modify the orders, in collaboration with the physician, based on the known desires of the individual or, if unknown, the individual's best interests.

This form is approved by the California Emergency Medical Services Authority in cooperation with the statewide POLST Task Force. For more information or a copy of the form, visit **www.caPOLST.org**.

SEND FORM WITH PERSON WHENEVER TRANSFERRED OR DISCHARGED

Physician's Order for Life-Sustaining Treatment (POLST) physician order that states not only the patient's wishes regarding resuscitation attempts but also the patient's wishes regarding artificial feeding, antibiotics, and other life-sustaining care if the patient is unable to state those desires later.

It is an actual legal document. A DNR order may also be part of a ***Physician's Order for Life-Sustaining Treatment (POLST)*** (Figure 4-2B), which typically include not just whether patients wish resuscitation attempts but also whether patients wish artificial feeding or antibiotics if unable to express their desires later. These forms will often specify on the front page whether patients wish resuscitation attempts. Some states may have variations on this form that allow a provider or clinician such as a physician assistant or advanced practice nurse to validate the form. This is an area that is evolving, so keep an eye on what is occurring in your state.

There are varying degrees of DNR orders, expressed through a variety of detailed instructions that may be part of the order. Such an instruction might stipulate, for example, that resuscitation be attempted only if cardiac or respiratory arrest is observed, but not attempted if the patient is found already in arrest (to avoid the possibility of resuscitating a patient who may already have sustained brain damage).

Many states also have laws governing living wills, which are statements signed by the patient, usually regarding use of long-term life support and comfort measures such as respirators, intravenous feedings, and pain medications. Other states require naming a *proxy*—a person whom the signer of the document names to make health care decisions in case the signer is unable to make those decisions. Living wills and health care proxies usually pertain to situations that will occur in the hospital, rather than in the prehospital situation.

Become familiar with the laws regarding DNR orders, living wills, and health care proxies for your region or state, and the laws and rules governing their implementation. It is important to know the forms and policies before you go to the call, since often the patient is in cardiac arrest (heart and breathing have stopped) or near death. These are stressful times for the family and for you, occasions when the window of time for making a resuscitation decision may be only a few moments.

A legal DNR order prevents unwanted resuscitation and awkward situations. In most cases the oral requests of a family member are not reason to withhold care. If the family requests you to not resuscitate the patient, and if there are no legal DNR orders available, it is a legal and ethical dilemma that is usually best resolved by providing care. It is better to be criticized or sued for attempting to save a life than for letting a patient die. At times, a family under duress may ask that a DNR order be ignored and resuscitation be initiated despite the DNR. In such a situation, contact medical direction for advice and, if necessary, ask the medical direction physician to speak directly to the family.

Other Legal Issues

CORE CONCEPT

The legal concepts of torts, negligence, and abandonment

Negligence

To the layperson, ***negligence*** means that something that should have been done was not done or was done incorrectly. The legal concept of negligence in emergency care is not that simple. A finding of negligence, or failure to act properly, requires that *all* of the following circumstances be proved:

negligence a finding that there was failure to act properly in a situation in which there was a duty to act, that needed care as would reasonably be expected of the EMT was not provided, and that harm was caused to the patient as a result.

- The EMT had a duty to the patient (duty to act—see the next section).
- The EMT did not provide the standard of care (committed a breach of duty). This may include the failure to act—that is, the EMT did not provide needed care as would be expected of an EMT in the relevant locality. Failure to act is a major cause of legal actions against EMS systems or EMTs.
- There was *proximate causation* (the concept that the damages to the patient were the result of action or inaction by the EMT). This means that by not providing the standard of care, the EMT caused harm to the patient. The harm can be physical or psychological. An example of proximate causation would be injuries caused when EMTs dropped the stretcher carrying a patient.

This concept cannot be applied to patients who are seriously injured and cannot be saved. If you perform CPR according to guidelines and the patient dies, there is no proximate causation between your actions and the patient's death.

Negligence is the basis for a large number of lawsuits involving prehospital emergency care. If the previously listed circumstances are proved, the EMT may be required to pay damages if the court considers the harm to the patient to be a loss that requires reimbursement (compensable). The negligent EMT may be required to pay for medical expenses, lost wages (possibly including future earnings), pain and suffering, and various other factors as determined by the court.

The proceedings or lawsuits against EMTs are usually classified as torts. A ***tort*** is a civil offense (as opposed to a criminal offense resulting in arrest). A tort may be defined as an action or injury caused by negligence from which a lawsuit may arise.

tort
a civil, not a criminal, offense; an action or injury caused by negligence from which a lawsuit may arise.

A concept used in tort law is ***res ipsa loquitur***, a Latin term meaning 'the thing speaks for itself.' This is a foundational concept in negligence because it allows a finding of negligence even when there is no specific evidence of a negligent act. Looking back at the stretcher-drop example in which the patient was injured, the plaintiff would not have to prove specific intent or negligence on the part of the EMTs or even that the EMTs were the ones who caused the stretcher to drop. Because the EMTs had exclusive control over the stretcher when it was dropped, there is a reasonable assumption that the EMTs caused the accident and that without negligence of some sort, the accident would not have happened.

res ipsa loquitur
a Latin term meaning 'the thing speaks for itself.'

Two of the most common and significant causes of lawsuits against EMTs are patient refusal and ambulance collisions (Figure 4-3). In patient refusal situations, EMTs are sued because the patient's condition deteriorated after the ambulance left the scene. This makes it critical to follow your agency's guidelines when a patient refuses care.

Collisions are dangerous in any vehicle. When an ambulance is involved, collisions become serious because of the size and weight of the vehicle, the number of occupants (including the patient), and the nature of emergency driving. It is important to remember that most collisions are preventable. (This is why they are no longer referred to as "accidents.") Emergency driving must be done responsibly.

Lawsuits against EMTs are uncommon, especially in light of the number of calls that are dispatched each day in this country. Although liability and negligence should be important considerations, you should not live or work in fear of a lawsuit. When you perform proper care that is within your scope of practice, and you document that care properly, you will prevent most, if not all, legal problems.

"Follow your protocols. Treat people well. Ask for help when you need it. That is how to stay legally safe."

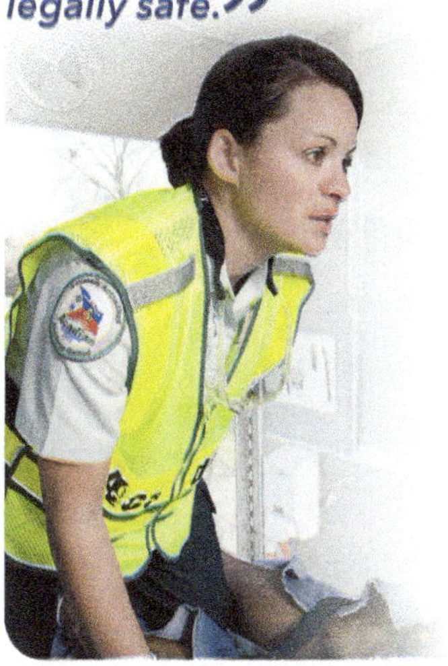

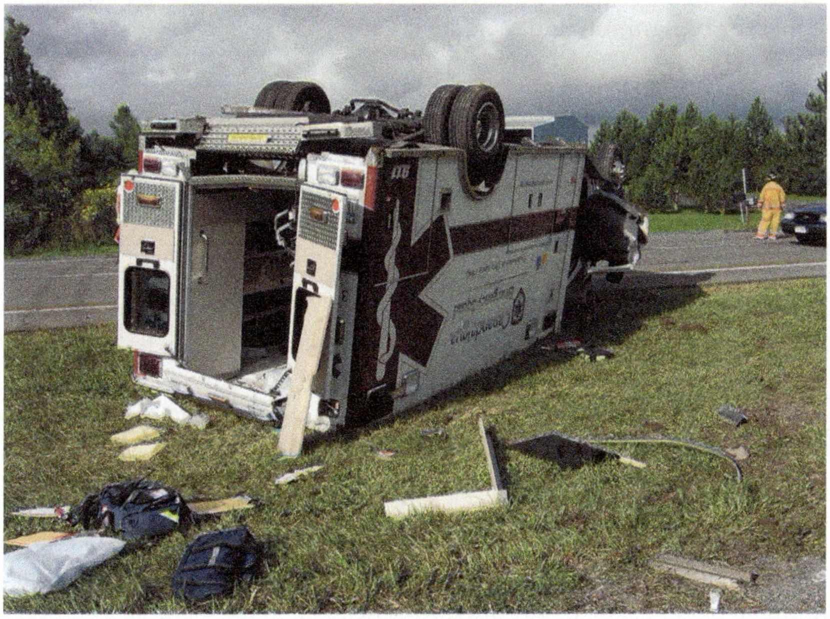

FIGURE 4-3 Ambulance collisions cause injuries and may prompt lawsuits. *(Canandaigua Emergency Squad)*

duty to act
an obligation to provide care to a patient.

CORE CONCEPT
What it means to have a duty to act

abandonment
leaving a patient after care has been initiated and before the patient has been transferred to someone with equal or greater medical training.

moral
regarding personal standards or principles of right and wrong.

ethical
regarding a social system or social or professional expectations for applying principles of right and wrong.

Good Samaritan laws
a series of laws, varying by state, designed to provide limited legal protection for citizens and some health care personnel when they are administering emergency care.

confidentiality
the obligation not to reveal information obtained about a patient except to other health care professionals involved in the patient's care or under subpoena or in a court of law or when the patient has signed a release of confidentiality.

Duty to Act

An EMT in certain situations has a ***duty to act***, or an obligation to provide emergency care to a patient. An EMT who is on an ambulance and is dispatched to a call clearly has a duty to act. If there is no threat to safety, the EMT must provide care. This duty to act continues throughout the call.

If an EMT has initiated care, then leaves a patient without ensuring that the patient has been turned over to someone with equal or greater medical training, ***abandonment*** has occurred. Similarly, if a paramedic has begun advanced care and then turns the patient over to an EMT for transport, abandonment (on the part of the paramedic) may exist.

The duty to act is not always clear. It depends on your state and local laws. In many states, an off-duty EMT has no legal obligation to provide care. However, you may feel a ***moral*** or ***ethical*** obligation to act; for example, if you observe a motor-vehicle collision while off duty, you may feel morally bound to provide care, even if no legal obligation exists. If you are off duty, you decide to begin care, and then you leave before other trained personnel arrive, you may still be considered to have abandoned the patient.

Other situations are even more confusing. If you are an EMT in an ambulance but you are out of your jurisdiction, the laws are again often unclear. In general, if you follow your conscience and provide care, you will incur less liability than if you do not act. Always follow your local protocols and laws. Your instructor will provide information about local issues.

Good Samaritan Laws

Good Samaritan laws have been developed in all states to provide immunity to individuals trying to help people in emergencies. Most of these laws will grant immunity from liability if the rescuers act in good faith to provide care to the level of their training and to the best of their ability. These laws do not prevent someone from initiating a lawsuit, nor will they protect rescuers from being found liable for acts of gross negligence or other violations of the law.

You must familiarize yourself with the laws that govern your state. Good Samaritan laws may not apply to EMTs in your locality. In some states, the Good Samaritan laws apply only to volunteers. If you are a paid EMT, different laws and regulations may apply.

Some states have specific statutes that authorize, regulate, and protect EMS personnel. Typically, to be protected by such laws, you must be recognized as an EMT in the state where care was provided. Some states have specific licensing and certification requirements that must be met for recognition under Good Samaritan laws.

Confidentiality

When you act as an EMT, you obtain a considerable amount of information about a patient. You also are allowed into homes and other personal areas that are private and contain much information about people.

Any information you obtain about a patient's history, condition, or treatment is considered confidential and must not be shared with anyone else. This principle is known as ***confidentiality***. Such information may be disclosed only when a written release is signed by the patient. Your organization will have a policy on this. Patient information should not be disclosed based on verbal permission, nor should information be disclosed over the telephone.

However, you may be subpoenaed, or ordered by a legal authority into court, where you may legally disclose patient information (Figure 4-4). If you have a question about the validity of a legal document, contact a supervisor or your agency's attorney for advice.

Patient information also may be shared with other health care professionals who will have a role in the patient's care or in quality improvement. It is appropriate to turn over information about the patient to the nurse and physician at the receiving hospital. This is necessary for continuity in patient care. It may also be necessary and permissible to supply certain patient-care information for insurance billing forms.

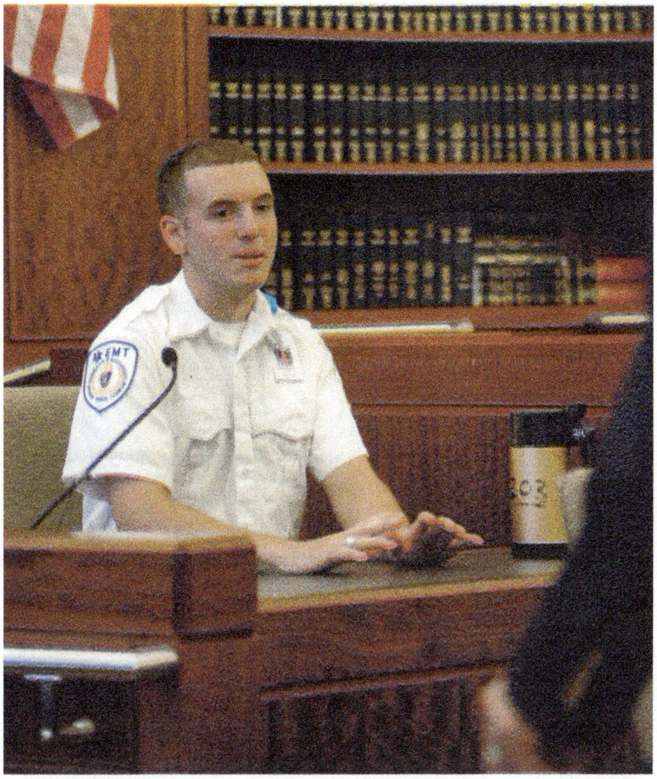

FIGURE 4-4 An EMT may be required to testify in court in a variety of legal settings.

Although confidentiality has always been a part of health care, federal regulations give it even greater emphasis. The Privacy Rule of the Health Insurance Portability and Accountability Act (***HIPAA***) has specific requirements for record keeping, storage, access, and discussion of patient-specific medical information. EMS agencies that bill for services (electronically or by employing a private company that does this work) are mandated to have policies, procedures, and training in place to deal with these privacy issues. Box 4-1 summarizes key points about HIPAA and how it will impact your work as an EMT.

HIPAA
the Health Insurance Portability and Accountability Act, which includes the Privacy Rule protecting the privacy of patient-specific health care information and providing the patient with control over how this information is used and distributed.

Special Situations

Libel and slander are two legal terms that may apply when information is shared inappropriately or falsely. ***Libel*** is when information that is false and injurious to another is spread in written form. ***Slander*** is when the information is shared verbally.

libel
false, injurious information in written form.

slander
false, injurious information stated verbally.

BOX 4-1 The Privacy Rule of the Health Insurance Portability and Accountability Act (HIPAA)

When you go through ambulance orientation, or when you begin to work or volunteer, you will likely hear much about HIPAA regulations. These federal regulations are designed to limit access to records by unnecessary personnel as well as to provide patients the right to review their information and have a greater say in its use and distribution. How will this affect you as an EMT?

- You will discuss patient-specific information only with those with whom it is medically necessary to do so.
- Your EMS agency will have specific privacy policies and procedures in place.
- You will get a printed copy of these policies and procedures, as will the patients in your care. You will ask your patients to sign a form indicating they have received this information. This form may be combined with your insurance-release form.
- Your EMS agency will have a Privacy Officer to oversee HIPAA issues and deal with the documentation required by law.

Remember that you will be provided information about your agency's specific privacy policies and procedures.

Medical Identification Devices

Patients may wear a medical identification device (Figure 4-5) to alert EMTs and other health care professionals that they have a particular medical condition. Then, if a patient is found unconscious, the device provides important medical information. The device may be a necklace, bracelet, or card. The medical identification jewelry available today is quite stylish and may not always look like the traditional oval bracelets many are familiar with. Medical identification devices may indicate a number of conditions, including:

- Heart conditions
- Allergies
- Diabetes
- Epilepsy

It is becoming increasingly common to see patients with tattoos that identify their medical condition (Figure 4-6). If you see a tattoo that appears to identify a medical condition, you should treat it like a medical identification device and explore how that condition relates to the patient's presentation. Tattoos do have a few issues. Unlike medical identification devices, tattoos cannot be removed if a medical condition changes or is cured. Also, EMTs may not think to look for tattoos as they would for medical identification jewelry. Remember to be alert for medical tattoos as you assess patients.

Finally, some organizations distribute systems for medical identification that are stored in the patient's residence. Sometimes called File of Life or Vial of Life, these systems ask a patient—often a senior citizen—to affix a sticker to the outside of the residence indicating that the medical information is stored inside, often on the refrigerator or in another specific and clear location. This system is dependent on the patient or family members' keeping the information up to date. Be sure to verify the information found with the patient or family members.

FIGURE 4-5 (A) Example of a medical identification device (front and back). (B) Sports-style medical identification bracelet (front and back).

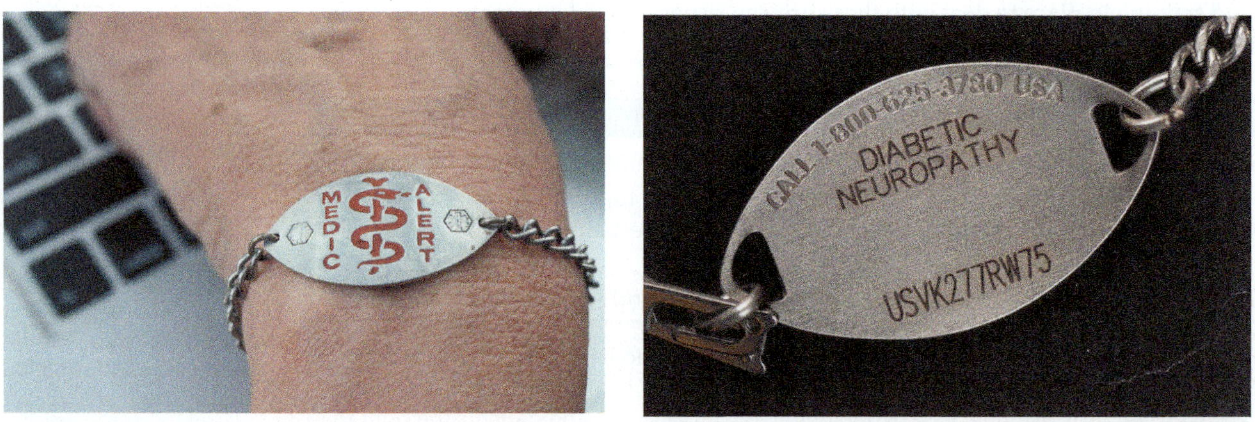

A

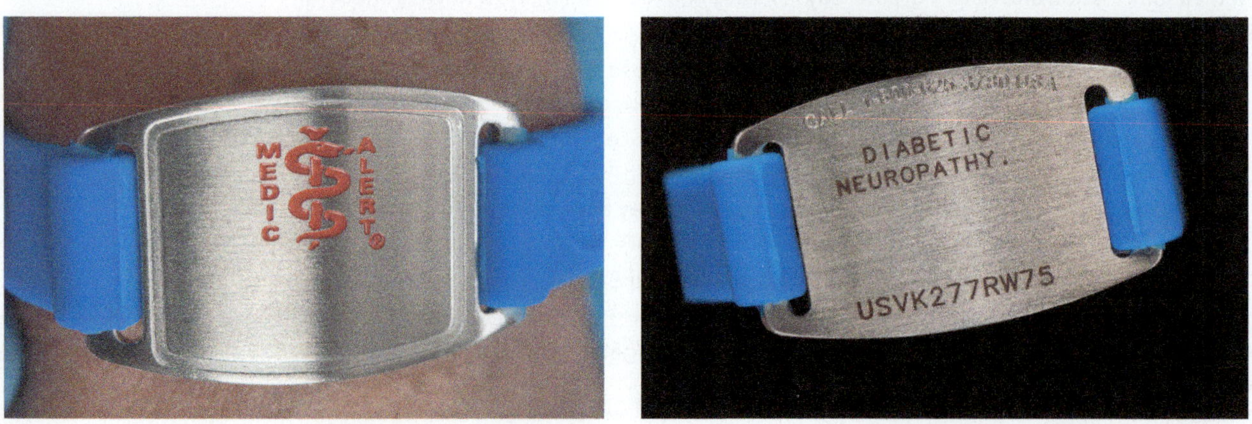

B

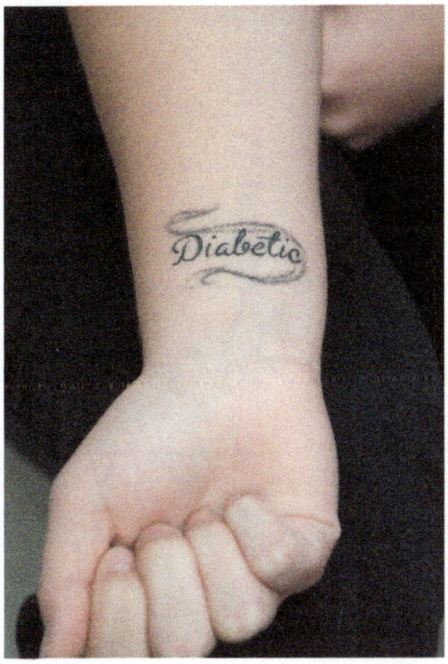

FIGURE 4-6 Example of a tattoo that identifies a medical condition.

Organ Donors

You may respond to calls where a patient is critically injured—perhaps near death—and is an ***organ donor***. An organ donor is a patient who has completed a legal document that allows for donation of organs and tissues in the event of death. Many people have benefited from the donation of organs by persons who have completed this paperwork (Figure 4-7).

You may learn that the patient is an organ donor when told so by a family member. Often an organ donor card is kept in a patient's wallet. The patient's driver's license may also contain an indication that the patient wishes to donate organs at the time of death.

The emergency care of a patient who is an organ donor must not differ from the care of a patient who is not a donor. All emergency care measures must be taken. If a patient is recognized as an organ donor, contact medical direction. The on-line physician may order you to perform CPR on a patient when you might normally not resuscitate due to fatal injuries. Oxygen delivered to body cells by CPR helps preserve organs until they can be harvested for implantation in another person.

organ donor
a person who has completed a legal document that allows for donation of organs and tissues in the event of death.

Safe Haven Laws

Most states have implemented some sort of ***"safe haven" law***. Under such a law, a person may permanently leave an infant or child at any police, fire, or EMS station or deliver the infant or child to any available public safety personnel. Each state has different guidelines for the ages of children included under the act—usually infants to young children.

"safe haven" law
a law that permits a person to drop off an infant or child at a police, fire, or EMS station or to deliver the infant or child to any available public safety personnel. The intent of the law is to protect children who may otherwise be abandoned or harmed by parents who are unable or unwilling to care for them.

Crime Scenes

A ***crime scene*** is defined as the location where a crime has been committed or any place where evidence relating to a crime may be found. Many crime scenes involve crimes against people. These crimes cause injuries that are often serious. Once police have made the scene safe, the EMT's priority at a crime scene is to provide patient care (Figure 4-8).

crime scene
the location where a crime has been committed or any place that evidence relating to a crime may be found.

While you are providing care at the crime scene, there are actions that you can take to help preserve evidence. To preserve evidence, you must first know what evidence is, as described in the following list:

- **Condition of the scene.** The condition in which you find the scene is important evidence to the police. If you arrive first, make a mental note of the exterior of the scene. Remember how you gained access. Doors found ajar, pry marks, and broken windows are signs of danger for you and important evidence for the police. Make note of whether the lights were on or off and of the condition of the TV and radio.

FIGURE 4-7 Example of an organ donor form.

Valley General Hospital
Permission for
Organ Donation/Anatomical Gift
by an Individual Prior to Death

PATIENT IDENTIFICATION PLATE

I, ______________________, currently residing at ______________________
______________________, being eighteen (18) years of age or older, do hereby make the following organ donation/anatomical gift to take effect upon my death:

1. I give, if medically acceptable:
   - ☐ My body
   - ☐ Any needed organs or parts
   - ☐ The following organs or parts: ______________________

   ____

   ____

2. I make this gift to Valley General Hospital or to physicians or institutions designated by them for the following purposes:
   - ☐ Any purpose authorized by law
   - ☐ Transplantation
   - ☐ Therapy
   - ☐ Medical Research and/or Education

3. I acknowledge that I have read this document in its entirety and that I fully understand it and that all blank spaces have either been completed or crossed off prior to my signing.

4. I understand that Valley General Hospital and its authorized designees will rely upon this consent.

____
SIGNATURE DATE

____
PRINT NAME

____
ADDRESS

____
TELEPHONE NUMBER

____
WITNESS TO SIGNATURE DATE
(PRINT NAME and ADDRESS BELOW)

____

____

____
WITNESS TO SIGNATURE DATE
(PRINT NAME and ADDRESS BELOW)

____

____

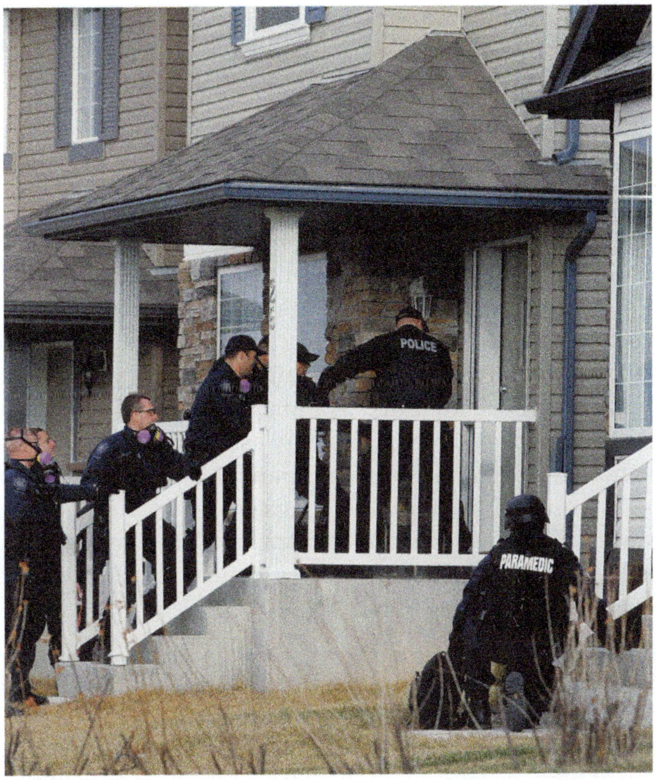

FIGURE 4-8 Paramedic and police at a crime scene.
(Kevin Link/Science Source)

- **The patient.** The patient often will provide valuable information. The position, condition of clothing, and injuries of the patient are all valuable pieces of evidence.
- **Fingerprints and footprints.** Fingerprints are perhaps the most familiar kind of evidence. They may be obtained from almost any surface. It is important for you to avoid unnecessarily touching anything at the scene, in order to preserve prints. Wearing gloves at the scene will prevent you from leaving your fingerprints on objects. If you touch these objects, however, even while wearing gloves, you may smudge fingerprints that were left by someone else.
- **Microscopic evidence.** Microscopic evidence is a wide range of evidence that is usually invisible to the naked eye. It consists of small pieces of evidence such as dirt and carpet fibers. To the eye, there may be no way to distinguish one from another. Under a microscope, scientists can develop valuable information. From just a few fibers, the materials and sometimes the brand name of carpets or clothes can be determined. Traces of blood may be enough to determine blood type or to be used for DNA comparison.

CORE CONCEPT
The responsibilities of an EMT at a crime scene

To preserve evidence at the crime scene, the following actions will be helpful to the police. Remember that your first priority is always patient care.

- **Remember what you touch.** It may be necessary to move the patient or furniture to begin CPR or other patient care. Although this cannot be avoided, it is helpful to tell the police what you have touched or moved. Once you leave, if they find furniture moved or bloodstains in two locations, they may think that a scuffle took place when in fact it did not. If you are forced to break a window to get to the patient and do not tell the police, they will think that a breaking-and-entering has occurred.
- **Minimize your impact on the scene.** If you are forced to move the patient or furniture to begin care, move as little as possible. Do not wander through the house or go to areas where it is not necessary to go. Avoid using the phone, which otherwise would prevent the police from using the redial button to determine the person the victim called last.

Do not use the bathroom, since this may also destroy evidence. Do not cut through holes left in clothing by bullets or knives, which will also destroy evidence. Cut at least 6 inches (about 15 cm) away from these holes.

- **Work with the police.** The police may require you to provide a statement about your actions or observations at the scene. Although it may not be possible to make notes while patient care is ongoing, after you arrive at the hospital, make notes about your observations and actions at the scene.

You may also wish to critique the scene—both with your crew and, if possible, with the police. Invite a member of your local or state police department to your agency for an in-service drill on crime scenes. Evidence-recovery methods and procedures vary from area to area. The police officer who comes to your station will brief you on local procedures.

Interestingly enough, police are often as unfamiliar with EMS procedures as you are with police evidence procedures. The police may ask you to delay your work at the scene so they can take photographs or interview the patient. They may do this because they do not understand—as you will learn in later chapters—that in the case of serious injury, the time that elapses before on-scene care and transport to the hospital must be kept to a minimum for the patient to have the best chance of survival. Education and critiques can be beneficial to both EMTs and police officers.

Special Reporting Requirements

Many states require EMTs and other health care professionals to report certain types of incidents. Hotlines exist in many areas for reporting crimes such as child, elder, or domestic abuse, or suspicion of human trafficking. These topics are discussed in the chapter *Emergencies for Patients with Special Challenges*.

Reporting may be mandatory in your area, and failure to report certain incidents may actually be a crime. Beyond this, there is a strong moral obligation to report crimes against vulnerable, at-risk populations. Many states offer immunity from liability to people who report such incidents in good faith.

Other crimes may also require reports. Violence (such as gunshot wounds or stabbings) and sexual assaults often fall into this category. If you are required by law to report such incidents, you are usually exempt from confidentiality requirements. You may also be required to notify police of other situations, such as cases where restraint may be necessary, where intoxicated persons have been found with injuries, or where mentally incompetent people have been injured.

Other Ethical Responsibilities

Many of the topics discussed in this chapter have both legal and ethical implications, but there are a few topics that still need to be addressed. Morality refers to personal opinions and beliefs about what is right and wrong. Ethics, when speaking about a profession, refers to standards of behavior for those who practice that profession. Some of the ethical expectations for an EMT include:

- Being honest in reporting.
- Refraining from actions that cause harm to a patient. ("First, do no harm.") This sounds obvious, but another way to think of this is to say that if you are going to make a mistake, make it a reversible one. For example, when in doubt about whether to start CPR, it is generally better to start and then stop after more information is available than to refrain initially and start CPR later, when it is much less likely to be effective.
- Working to help the patient, which includes putting the patient's interests above your interests and comfort.
- Respecting the right of adult patients to make decisions on their own behalf when they are informed and able to make decisions.
- Treating all patients fairly and justly without regard to sex, race, ability to pay, and other conditions as described by law and ethical codes.

- Assisting others, as appropriate, to learn your profession. This does not mean you have to become an EMT instructor or preceptor, but once you become an EMT, you should deal with EMT students in a fair and respectful manner.
- Reporting misconduct that affects or may affect patient care.
- Making sure, if you participate in research, that it is approved by the appropriate authorities and that you understand it well enough to avoid inflicting harm.

Chapter Review

Key Facts and Concepts

- Medical, legal, and ethical issues are a part of every EMS call.
- Consent may be expressed or implied. If patients who are awake and oriented and have the capacity to fully understand their situation refuse care or transport, you should make every effort to persuade them, but you cannot force them to accept care or go to the hospital.
- Negligence is failing to act properly when you have a duty to act. As an EMT, you have a duty to act whenever you are dispatched on a call. You may also have a legal or moral duty to act even when off duty or outside your jurisdiction.
- Abandonment is leaving a patient after you have initiated care and before you have transferred the patient to a person with equal or higher training.
- Confidentiality is the obligation not to reveal personal information you obtain about a patient except to other health care professionals involved in the patient's care, under court order, or when the patient signs a release.
- As an EMT, you may be sued or held legally liable on any of these issues. However, EMTs are rarely held liable when they have acted within their scope of practice and according to the standard of care, and have carefully documented the details of the call.
- At a crime scene, care of the patient takes precedence over preservation of evidence; however, you should make every effort not to disturb the scene unnecessarily and to report your actions and observations to the police.

Key Decisions

- Does the care I wish to give fall into my scope of practice?
- Does this patient consent to my care? Can this patient consent to my care?
- Does this patient need to go to the hospital? How can I convince the patient to go if the patient doesn't want to go?
- Is the DNR order valid? Does it apply to this patient?
- How should I act on each call, and what can I do to prevent lawsuits?
- Do I have a duty to act in this situation?
- Is this confidential information? Can I tell anyone or share the information?
- Is this a crime scene? If so, how do I preserve evidence while taking care of the patient?
- Is this a crime that I am required to report?

Chapter Glossary

abandonment leaving a patient after care has been initiated and before the patient has been transferred to someone with equal or greater medical training.

advance directive a DNR order; instructions written in advance of an event.

assault placing a person in fear of bodily harm.

battery causing bodily harm to or restraining a person.

confidentiality the obligation not to reveal information obtained about a patient except to other health care professionals involved in the patient's care or under subpoena or in a court of law or when the patient has signed a release of confidentiality.

consent permission from the patient for care or other action by the EMT.

crime scene the location where a crime has been committed or any place that evidence relating to a crime may be found.

do not resuscitate (DNR) order a legal document, usually signed by both patient and physician, which states that the patient has a terminal illness and does not wish to prolong life through resuscitative efforts.

duty to act an obligation to provide care to a patient.

ethical regarding a social system or social or professional expectations for applying principles of right and wrong.

expressed consent consent given by adults who are of legal age and mentally competent to make a rational decision with regard to their medical well-being.

Good Samaritan laws a series of laws, varying by state, designed to provide limited legal protection for citizens and some health care personnel when they are administering emergency care.

HIPAA The Health Insurance Portability and Accountability Act, a federal law protecting the privacy of patient-specific health care information and providing the patient with control over how this information is used and distributed.

implied consent the consent it is presumed a patient or patient's parent or guardian would give if they could, such as for an unconscious patient or a child whose parents cannot be contacted when care is needed.

in loco parentis literally 'in place of a parent,' indicating a person who may give consent for care of a child when the parents are not present or able to give consent.

liability being held legally responsible.

libel false, injurious information in written form.

moral regarding personal standards or principles of right and wrong.

negligence a finding that there was failure to act properly in a situation in which there was a duty to act, that needed care as would reasonably be expected of the EMT was not provided, and that harm was caused to the patient as a result.

organ donor a person who has completed a legal document that allows for donation of organs and tissues in the event of death.

Physician's Orders for Life-Sustaining Treatment (POLST) physician orders that state not only the patient's wishes regarding resuscitation attempts but also the patient's wishes regarding artificial feeding, antibiotics, and other life-sustaining care if the person is unable to state the person's desires later.

res ipsa loquitur a Latin term meaning 'the thing speaks for itself.'

safe haven law a law that permits a person to drop off an infant or child at a police, fire, or EMS station or to deliver the infant or child to any available public safety personnel. The intent of the law is to protect children who may otherwise be abandoned or harmed.

scope of practice a set of regulations and ethical considerations that define the scope, or extent and limits, of the EMT's job.

slander false, injurious information stated verbally.

standard of care for an EMT providing care for a specific patient in a specific situation, the care that would be expected to be provided by an EMT with similar training when caring for a patient in a similar situation.

tort a civil, not a criminal, offense; an action or injury caused by negligence from which a lawsuit may arise.

Preparation for Your Examination and Practice

Short Answer

1. Explain the difference between expressed and implied consent.
2. What are the components required to prove negligence?
3. What is your first priority at a crime scene: evidence preservation or patient care? Why?
4. You bring a patient to the hospital and the nurse tells you, "Put the patient in bed 5; I'll be right there." The nurse doesn't come over, and you leave. Is this abandonment? Why or why not?
5. You have a patient who weighs 400 pounds. You want other EMTs at your squad to know this so they can be prepared. Can you leave a copy of your patient care report on the bulletin board at the station to notify the others?

Thinking and Linking

As you work on this exercise, think back to what you have learned in the chapters Introduction to Emergency Medical Services, Well-Being of the EMT, *and* Lifting and Moving Patients. *Combine those concepts with concepts explained in this chapter.*

1. What roles and responsibilities of an EMT are important in preventing lawsuits?
2. What can I do when lifting and moving patients to help prevent injury to patients and the lawsuits that may result?

Critical Thinking Exercises

Many aspects of EMS require moral or ethical decisions. The purpose of this exercise will be to apply these considerations to several situations you might encounter.

1. You and your partner are in your ambulance on the way back from a call when you come upon a motor-vehicle crash. It is in an adjoining ambulance district. Do you have a duty to act? Do you have a moral or ethical obligation?
2. You have transported a patient who was seriously injured when he was ejected from his vehicle in a high-speed collision. The next day you talk to another member of your crew, who tells you the patient died. That crew member is worried about getting sued over the death. Do you think that a lawsuit against you is likely? Why or why not?
3. You respond to a motor-vehicle crash and find a seriously injured patient. You find he has no pulse, and you are about to begin CPR when someone tells you, "He's got cancer and a DNR. Don't do that, man!" No one has the DNR order at the scene. Do you do CPR and transport the patient?

Street Scenes

On a hot summer day, you receive a call for a 37-year-old woman with general body weakness. After your primary assessment, you ask the patient about her medical history. She informs you that she has AIDS. You continue to take vital signs, find it appropriate to provide oxygen, and package her for transport. Your partner makes the radio report to the hospital, and you notice that he makes no reference to AIDS. When you arrive at the hospital, your partner gives the patient report in the hallway leading to the examination room. He provides all the patient information but does not tell the doctor that the patient reported she has AIDS until he can do it discreetly in the room. He asks the patient to sign a form that allows release of information for insurance billing and acknowledges receipt of the Notice of Privacy Practices in place at your agency.

Street Scene Questions

1. **Was it appropriate not to include the information that the patient has AIDS during the radio report to the hospital?**
2. **What is the obligation of EMTs concerning the confidentiality of patient information?**
3. **Would you have handled the transfer of information differently?**

After the call is over, you discuss with your partner issues of confidentiality. He tells you that he felt the fact the patient had AIDS did not need to be part of the radio report. He was concerned that it might breach the patient's confidentiality if it was said over the radio. But your partner was quick to add that AIDS was definitely a pertinent part of the medical history and that he made sure it was conveyed in a discreet manner at the hospital. Although you may not believe that having HIV or AIDS is as sensitive a topic as it was in the past, it is still a cause of discrimination and a source of fear to uninformed people. For this reason, being discreet about the client's AIDS was probably the right approach.

Street Scene Question

4. **Would it be appropriate to tell all the hospital staff about the patient's AIDS so they would know to take infection-control precautions?**

As you and your partner further discuss the issue, you tell him that alerting the hospital staff so they would know to use infection-control precautions would be appropriate. He responds by saying that all emergency medical personnel, whether EMS or in-hospital, should routinely be taking infection-control precautions, but that this should not be a reason for being careless with patient information and possibly breaching a patient's confidentiality.

Street Scene Questions

5. **Should the information that this patient has AIDS be shared with other EMS providers in case they get a call for this patient?**
6. **What are the principles for confidentiality that EMTs should always maintain?**

As you pull into the garage, you suggest to your partner that you should alert the other crews about this patient's having AIDS. Your partner tells you that this would be a breach of the patient's confidentiality. It would be very inappropriate to do this. He reminds you that patient information is always to be kept confidential unless it needs to be shared for the purpose of giving care. "For example," he says, "the patient's information on the report to the hospital included the fact that she told us she had AIDS. Also, the physician needed to know because it was part of the medical history that we obtained. Unless there is another reason to share this information that I haven't thought of, no one else needs to hear from us that this patient has AIDS. Confidentiality is an EMS standard that pertains to the history, condition, and treatment of all the patients we see." As he gets out of the ambulance at the station, he adds, "Remember, confidentiality is a professional responsibility."

5

Medical Terminology

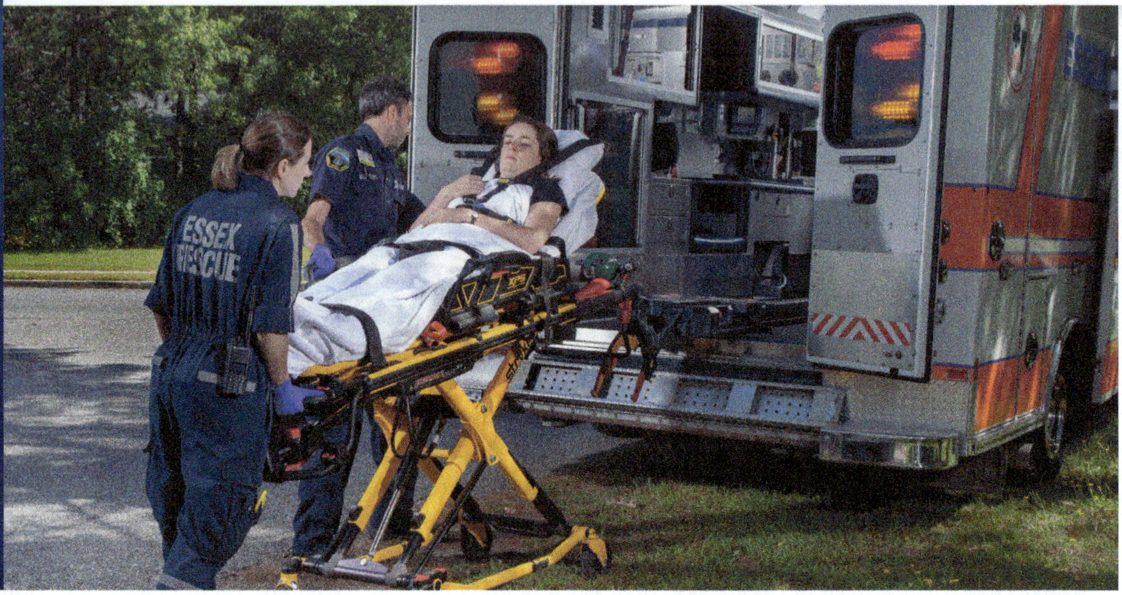

Related Chapters

The following chapter provides additional information related to topics discussed in this chapter:

6 Anatomy and Physiology

References:

Medical Terms
Anatomy and Physiology Illustrations

Standard

Medical Terminology

Competency

Uses foundational anatomical and medical terms and abbreviations in written and oral communication with colleagues and other health care professionals.

Core Concepts

- Medical terminology and how terms are constructed
- Directional terms
- Positional terms

Outcomes

After reading this chapter, you should be able to:

5.1 Demonstrate communication in the language of medicine. (pp. 104–107)

- Analyze the meanings of medical terminology components.
- Recognize the meanings of common acronyms, mnemonics, and abbreviations used in the language of medicine.
- Distinguish between circumstances in which an EMT should use medical terminology, abbreviations, and acronyms; and situations in which plain language is a better choice.

5.2 Apply terms of position and direction to describe a location on the human body. (pp. 107–112)

- Identify the anatomic regions of the body.
- Match anatomic terms of position and direction to their definitions.

Key Terms

abdominal quadrants, *110*
anatomic position, *107*
anatomy, *107*
anterior, *109*
bilateral, *109*
combining form, *104*
compound, *104*
distal, *109*
dorsal, *109*
Fowler position, *111*
inferior, *109*
lateral, *109*
medial, *109*
midaxillary line, *109*
midclavicular line, *110*
midline, *109*
palmar, *110*
physiology, *107*
plane, *107*
plantar, *110*
posterior, *109*
prefix, *104*
prone, *111*
proximal, *109*
recovery position, *111*
root, *104*
suffix, *104*
superior, *109*
supine, *111*
torso, *109*
unilateral, *109*
ventral, *109*

As you embark on your journey through the world of health care, be prepared to discover an entirely new language. As you enter this world, you will find ideas described very differently than you may be used to seeing. Patients are no longer "sweaty," they are "diaphoretic." You don't say a patient is "short of breath,"; instead you note the patient has "dyspnea." When a patient stretches out an arm, you now say it is "extended" or "abducted."

At first, these new terms may seem too complicated, but you will find that medical terminology allows a precision that common terms do not. Much of what you do as an EMT will require clear-cut and exact communication. Whether you are describing a patient over the radio to medical direction or documenting your findings in a prehospital care report, being specific matters. Health care professionals use terminology designed to be precise and explicit because ambiguity can make proper care more difficult.

Learning medical terminology can be frustrating at first, but you will soon find that common concepts run through medical language and show up again and again in medical terms. By understanding these common concepts, you will quickly see the relationships among root words, prefixes, and suffixes that make it easier to decode and comprehend medical terms.

This chapter will review key medical terminology relevant to life as an EMT. We will further describe techniques used to form common medical words.

Medical Terminology

CORE CONCEPT
Medical terminology and how terms are constructed

Although you may be just getting started with your EMT course, you have probably already seen some sizable words and heard a few more from your instructors. You will encounter more as you begin the patient assessment and care sections of this text. Some say medicine has a language of its own. As with any language, understanding some of the basics will make it easier to understand this special language and use it correctly when communicating with other medical professionals.

The Components of Medical Terms

Medical terms are composed of words, and medical words may be composed of roots, prefixes, and/or suffixes—each with its own definition. (See the examples in Table 5-1.)

compound
a word formed from two or more whole words.

Some medical words are ***compounds***, made up of two or more whole words. For example, the word *small* is joined with the word *pox* to form the medical term *smallpox*, the name of a disease.

root
foundation of a word that is not a word that can stand on its own.

combining form
a word root with an added vowel that can be joined with other words, roots, or suffixes to form a new word.

Roots are the foundations of words and are not usually used by themselves. *Therm* is a root that means "heat." Used alone, it would make no sense. But when a vowel is added to the end of the root (in this case, the added vowel is *o*) it becomes a ***combining form***, *therm/o*, which can be joined with other words, roots, or suffixes. For example, *therm/o* and *meter* combine to form *thermometer*, an instrument for measuring heat or temperature.

Some medical terms combine more than one root or combining form. *Electrocardiogram* is a good example. The combining forms *electr/o* (electric) and *cardi/o* (heart) are joined to *gram* (a written record) to form the term. An electrocardiogram is a written record of the heart's electrical activity.

prefix
word part added to the beginning of a root or word to modify or qualify its meaning.

Prefixes are added to the beginnings of roots or words to modify or qualify their meaning. They usually tell the reader what kind of, where, in what direction, or how many. The root *pnea* relates to breathing but says nothing about the quality or kind of breathing. Adding the prefix *dys-* (painful; difficult) makes it *dyspnea*, or difficult breathing. The prefix *tachy-* (rapid; fast) when combined with *pnea* creates *tachypnea*, or rapid breathing.

Abdominal pain is a broad term. Adding the prefix *intra-* (within; inside) narrows the meaning. *Intraabdominal pain* is pain within the abdomen.

Plegia refers to paralysis of the limbs. The prefix *quadri-* (four) tells the reader how many limbs are paralyzed. *Quadriplegia* is paralysis of all four limbs.

suffix
word part added to the end of a root or word to complete its meaning.

Suffixes are word parts added to the ends of roots or words to complete their meaning. A number of suffixes have specialized meanings. The suffix *-itis* means inflammation, and the root *arthr* refers to a joint; thus, *arthritis* is inflammation of a joint. The suffix *-iac* forms a noun indicating a person afflicted with a certain disease—for example, *hemophiliac*, a patient suffering from the bleeding disorder hemophilia.

Some suffixes are joined to roots to form terms that indicate a state, quantity, condition, procedure, or process. *Pneumonia* and *psoriasis* are examples of medical conditions, whereas *appendectomy* and *arthroscopy* are examples of medical procedures. (Suffixes in each case are underlined.)

Some suffixes combine with roots to form adjectives, words that modify nouns either by indicating quality or quantity or by distinguishing one thing from another. *Gastric, cardiac, fibrous, arthritic,* and *diaphoretic* are all examples of adjectives formed by adding suffixes (underlined) to roots.

Some suffixes are added to roots to express reduction in size, such as *-iole* and *-ule*. An *arteriole* is smaller than an artery, and a *venule* is smaller than a vein.

When added to roots, *-e* and *-ize* form verbs. *Excise* and *catheterize* are examples. Given the definitions of the word's root and suffixes, you can tell that a *cardiologist* is one who specializes in the study of the heart, as shown in Figure 5-1.

This text will help you understand medical terminology by providing definitions in the margins and in a glossary.

TABLE 5-1 Common Roots, Prefixes, and Suffixes

EXAMPLE	WORD PART	MEANING
Broncho/pulmo	Root	Lungs
Cardi	Root	Heart
Gastro	Root	Stomach
Hepat	Root	Liver
Neur	Root	Nerve
Nas	Root	Nose/nasal
Or	Root	Mouth/oral
Pneumo	Root	Air or lungs
Ab-	Prefix	Away from
Ad-	Prefix	Toward or near
Ante-	Prefix	Before
Brady-	Prefix	Slow/below normal
Contra-	Prefix	Against
Dys-	Prefix	Difficult or painful
Hyper-	Prefix	Above normal, high
Hypo-	Prefix	Below normal, low
Inter-	Prefix	Between
Intra-	Prefix	Within, inside
Peri-	Prefix	Around
Poly-	Prefix	Many
Post-	Prefix	After
Pre-	Prefix	Before
Sub-	Prefix	Below, under
Super/Supra-	Prefix	Above or in excess
Tachy-	Prefix	Above normal, rapid
Uni-	Prefix	One
-ac	Suffix	Pertaining to
-algia	Suffix	Pain
-emesis	Suffix	Vomiting
-itis	Suffix	Inflammation
-ology	Suffix	Study of
-plegia	Suffix	Paralysis
-pnea	Suffix	Breathing
-rrhea	Suffix	Discharge
-spasm	Suffix	Contraction
-al	Suffix	Pertaining to
-ist	Suffix	One who specializes in

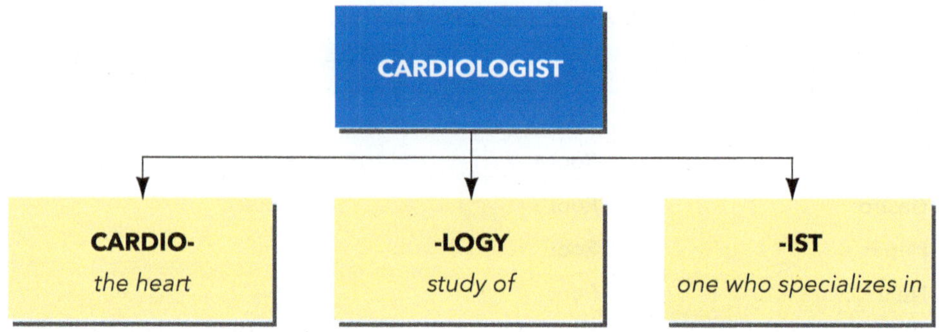

FIGURE 5-1 *Cardiologist*: An example of root and suffixes.

Abbreviations and Acronyms

Abbreviations and acronyms also abound in the world of EMS. (An acronym is an abbreviation made up of initials that can be pronounced as a word, such as *CPAP*, pronounced "SEE-pap," for continuous positive airway pressure, which will be discussed in the chapter *Respiratory Emergencies*.) You will encounter many abbreviations and acronyms in your class and in the field. Until you know them well, it may be helpful to keep a list of acronyms you are learning.

Although abbreviations and acronyms are commonly used as a sort of "shorthand" in EMS, they have downsides. Abbreviated words can lead to communication errors, especially when you use more obscure or local abbreviations—and particularly when you use them in written documentation, where clarification is more difficult. (The person reading your report can't look up and say "What do you mean by that?") For example, some practitioners use the abbreviation WNL to mean "within normal limits," but a reader who isn't familiar with that usage might think it means "we never looked."

This is not to say that abbreviations are uniformly "evil." In fact, many abbreviations and acronyms are well accepted and commonly used, but you should always take care about when and how you use them. One of the most common problems in medicine is faults and omissions in communication during patient handoff—especially in the report you give when transferring care of a patient to the emergency department. Research has shown that the use of acronyms and abbreviations is a common cause of medical errors. Although it may be appropriate to use abbreviations such as CPR or EMS, we should do our best to use plain language and to spell out terms, avoiding abbreviations and acronyms, especially in high-risk situations such as patient handoff and in patient-care documentation.

Dissecting A Compound Word—Cholecystitis

Like the intricacies of the human body, complicated compound words can be examined and better understood by looking carefully at their component parts. Looking at the meanings of prefixes, roots, and suffixes can help you quickly understand even some of the most complicated medical terms.

Cholecystitis is a big word and a challenge to understand if you are new to health care. Breaking this compound word into its three component parts can help you understand its meaning. The first part of the word is *Chol/e*, meaning bile; the second component is *cyst*, which refers to a closed sac; and finally its suffix, *-itis*, pertains to inflammation. If you then assemble the word with the parts' common meanings, you get "bile-sac-inflammation." *Cholecystitis* means inflammation of the gallbladder (which stores bile).

Although *cholecystitis* is a large and complex word, its meaning is quite precise. That one word names both the specific organ and the problem associated with that organ. As an EMT, you will learn to recognize key roots, prefixes, and suffixes that occur frequently in medical terms. For example, *-itis*, meaning inflammation, is used to indicate a wide variety of inflammatory conditions, from cholecystitis (inflammation of the gall bladder) to hepatitis (inflammation of the liver), as well as familiar conditions such as appendicitis (inflammation of the appendix) and tonsillitis (inflammation of the tonsils).

Thinking of breaking down compound words as similar to dissecting the human body can be very helpful as you learn this new language.

When and When Not to Use Medical Terms

Naturally you want to avoid making errors when you use medical terms, but there are also situations when using complex medical terminology may not be the best practice, even if you are using it correctly.

You should avoid using any type of obscure medical terminology, jargon, abbreviations, or acronyms when you are talking to patients and families. For example, if you ask a female patient if she has ever had "an MI" (for myocardial infarction—a heart attack), the patient will not be able to provide the correct answer if she is not familiar with the term you used. Children also often have difficulty understanding complex terms. Occasionally complex terms used in messages can cause confusion even among trained health care professionals. If there is a potential for ambiguity or if the person you are speaking to may not understand, it is better to use simple terms.

The language of medicine, like any other language, must be applied appropriately and practically in any given situation.

The Language of Anatomy and Physiology

There will be much more detailed discussion in the next chapter, *Anatomy and Physiology*; however, you should first understand that describing body systems and functions requires a working knowledge of the associated terms and phrases.

Anatomy is the study of body structure. When talking about anatomy, you will use terms to describe particular organs and organ systems. These organs and systems usually have associated prefixes and roots such as *cardi-*, referring to the heart. Anatomy also requires language that describes location and position. ***Physiology*** is the study of body function. The terminology of physiology describes the actions of organs and organ systems. For example, *diffusion* describes the movement of a solute from an area of low concentration to an area of high concentration. Understanding this term and concept will help you conceptualize, for example, how oxygen is moved from the alveoli in the lungs into the bloodstream.

anatomy
the study of body structure.

physiology
the study of body function.

Anatomic Terms

As an EMT, you will often have to describe where an injury is located or where a patient describes feeling pain. So you will need to know terms for direction and position. These terms will be discussed in the next sections.

Directional Terms

CORE CONCEPT
Directional terms

For clear communication among health care professionals, there must be a standardized way of referring to places on the body when describing illness or injury. For this purpose, the body is divided into regions (Figure 5-2), and standardized anatomic directional terms are used (Figure 5-3). For example, the directions *left* and *right* always refer to the patient's left and right.

A universal reference when discussing human anatomy is called ***anatomic position***. All descriptions of the body use anatomic position as their starting point. Anatomic position is a person standing, facing forward, with palms forward. (Review Figure 5-2.) When describing locations on the body, you will use anatomic position as a reference even if your patient is not in this position. For example, your patient's face would be referred to as anterior (at the front) because the face is anterior in anatomic position, even if the patient you are describing is lying facedown. The importance of always referring to this standardized position is that all health care providers, everywhere, will use the same anatomic starting point when describing the body and will understand each other's references.

anatomic position
the standard reference position for the body in the study of anatomy. In this position, the body is standing erect, facing the observer, with arms at the sides and the palms of the hands forward.

For direction and spatial relationships, we divide the body into planes. A ***plane*** is a flat surface, the kind that would be formed if you sliced straight through a department store dummy or an imaginary human body. Cutting through from top to bottom, you could slice the body either into right and left halves or into front and back halves. Slicing the body

plane
a flat surface formed when slicing through a solid object.

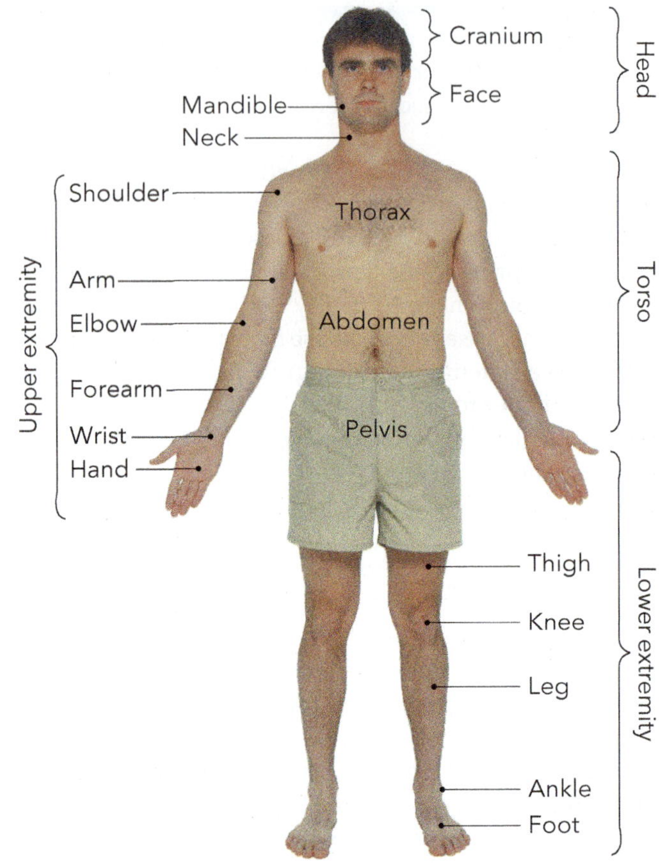

FIGURE 5-2 Body regions and anatomic position.

FIGURE 5-3 Directional terms.

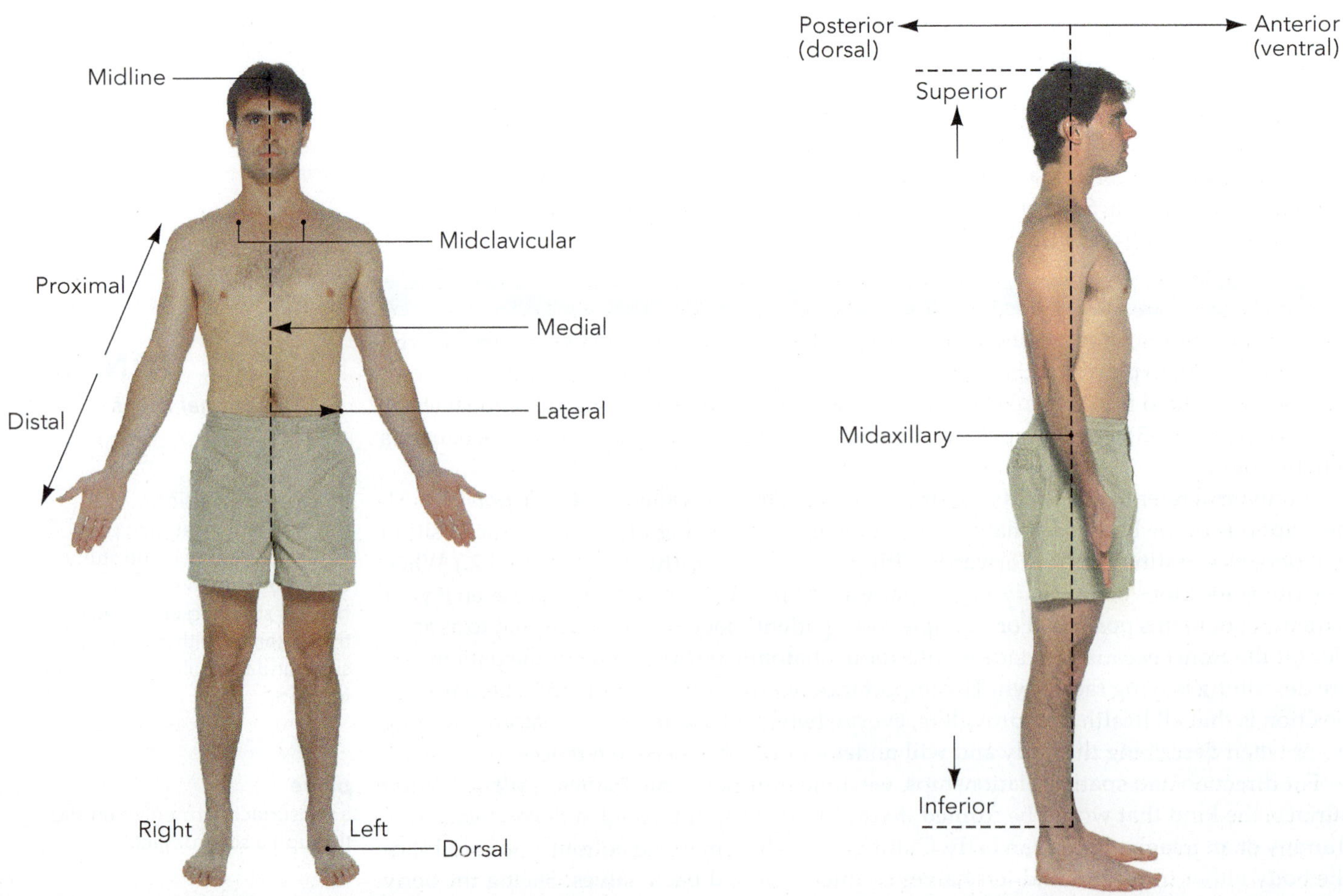

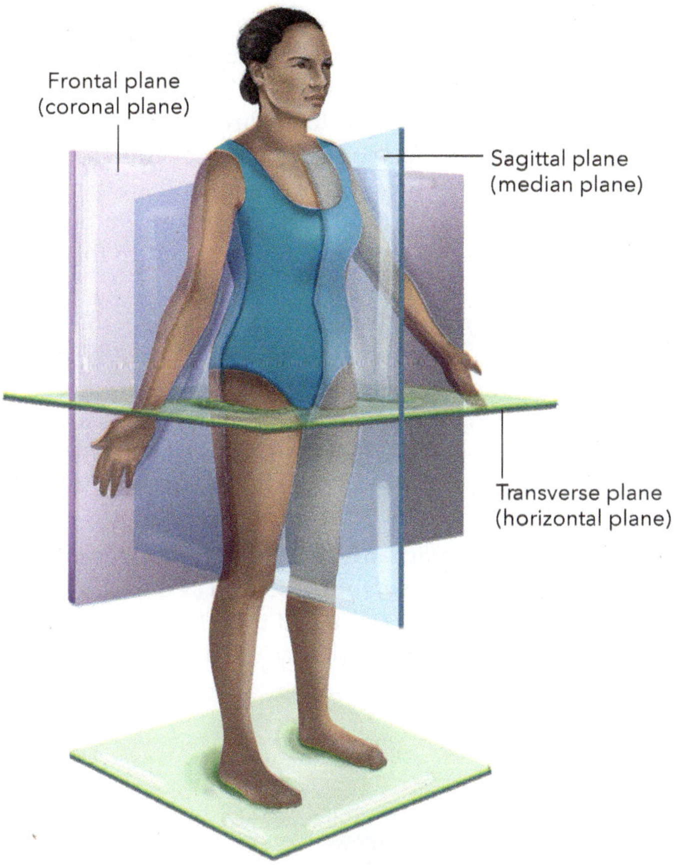

FIGURE 5-4 The planes of the body.

down the middle to create two side-by-side halves would create *sagittal* or *median planes*. Slicing the body into two halves, front and back, would create *frontal* or *coronal planes*. Finally, slicing the body into two halves near the waist, top and bottom, would create *transverse* or *horizontal planes* (Figure 5-4). Note that although it is good to understand the meanings of terms referring to planes of the body, terms referring to planes are not usually used in communications among health care providers.

The ***midline*** of the body is created by drawing an imaginary line down the center of the body, passing between the eyes and extending down through the umbilicus (navel). (Refer again to Figure 5-3.) Slicing through the imaginary body at the midline divides the body into right and left halves.

The term ***medial*** refers to a position closer to the midline (with regard to anatomic position). The term ***lateral*** refers to a position farther away from the midline. For example, you would say "The bridge of the nose is medial to the eyes." You also can say that an arm has a medial side (close to the body) and a lateral side (the outer arm, away from the body).

The term ***bilateral*** refers to "both sides" of anything. Patients may have diminished lung sounds on both sides when you listen with a stethoscope. This would be reported as "The patient has diminished lung sounds bilaterally." The term ***unilateral*** refers to one side.

The ***midaxillary line*** extends vertically from the middle of the armpit to the ankle. (The anatomic term for the armpit is *axilla*, so midaxillary means "middle of the armpit.") This line divides the body into front and back halves. The term for the front is ***anterior***. The term for the back is ***posterior***. For example, you would say, "The patient has wounds to the posterior arm and the anterior thigh." A synonym for anterior is ***ventral*** (referring to the front of the body). A synonym for posterior is ***dorsal*** (referring to the back of the body or back of the hand or foot). Remember that these terms always reference anatomic position regardless of the current position of the patient.

The terms ***superior*** and ***inferior*** refer to vertical, or up-and-down, directions. Superior means above; inferior means below. An example of this would be "The nose is superior to the mouth."

The terms ***proximal*** and ***distal*** are relative terms. Proximal means closer to the ***torso*** (the trunk of the body, or the body without the head and the extremities). Distal means

midline
an imaginary line drawn down the center of the body, dividing it into right and left halves.

medial
toward the midline of the body.

lateral
to the side, away from the midline of the body.

bilateral
on both sides.

unilateral
limited to one side

midaxillary (mid-AX-uh-lair-e) ***line***
a line drawn vertically from the middle of the armpit to the ankle.

anterior
the front of the body or body part.

posterior
the back of the body or body part.

ventral
referring to the front of the body. A synonym for *anterior*.

dorsal
referring to the back of the body or the back of the hand or foot. A synonym for *posterior*.

superior
toward the head (e.g., the chest is superior to the abdomen).

inferior
away from the head, usually compared with another structure that is closer to the head (e.g., the lips are inferior to the nose).

proximal
closer to the torso.

distal
farther away from the torso.

torso
the trunk of the body, or the body without the head and the extremities.

palmar
referring to the palm of the hand.

plantar
referring to the sole of the foot.

midclavicular (mid-clah-VIK-yuh-ler) ***line***
the line through the center of each clavicle.

abdominal quadrants
four divisions of the abdomen used to pinpoint the location of a pain or injury: the right upper quadrant (RUQ), the left upper quadrant (LUQ), the right lower quadrant (RLQ), and the left lower quadrant (LLQ).

farther away from the torso. For example, think of an elbow. It is proximal to the hand because it is closer to the torso than the hand is. The elbow also is distal to the shoulder, since the elbow is farther away from the torso than the shoulder is. The terms are usually used when describing locations on extremities. For example, to be sure circulation has not been cut off after splinting an arm or leg, you must feel for a distal pulse. This is a pulse found in an extremity, a pulse point that is farther away from the torso than the splint is. When using relative terms such as *proximal* and *distal*, it is helpful to give a point of reference. For example, you might say a laceration is proximal to the elbow. In this case, the elbow is your point of reference.

Two other terms you may sometimes hear are ***palmar*** (referring to the palm of the hand) and ***plantar*** (referring to the sole of the foot).

The ***midclavicular line*** divides the chest into regions. It runs through the center of a clavicle (collarbone) and extends inferiorly. Since there are two clavicles, there are two midclavicular lines. When you use a stethoscope to listen for breath sounds, you will place the stethoscope at the midclavicular lines to listen to each side of the chest and assess the function of both lungs.

The abdomen is divided into four parts, or quadrants, by drawing horizontal and vertical lines through the navel. The ***abdominal quadrants*** are described as the right upper quadrant, the left upper quadrant, the right lower quadrant, and the left lower quadrant (Figure 5-5). These are often abbreviated as, respectively, RUQ, LUQ, RLQ, and LLQ.

FIGURE 5-5 Abdominal quadrants.

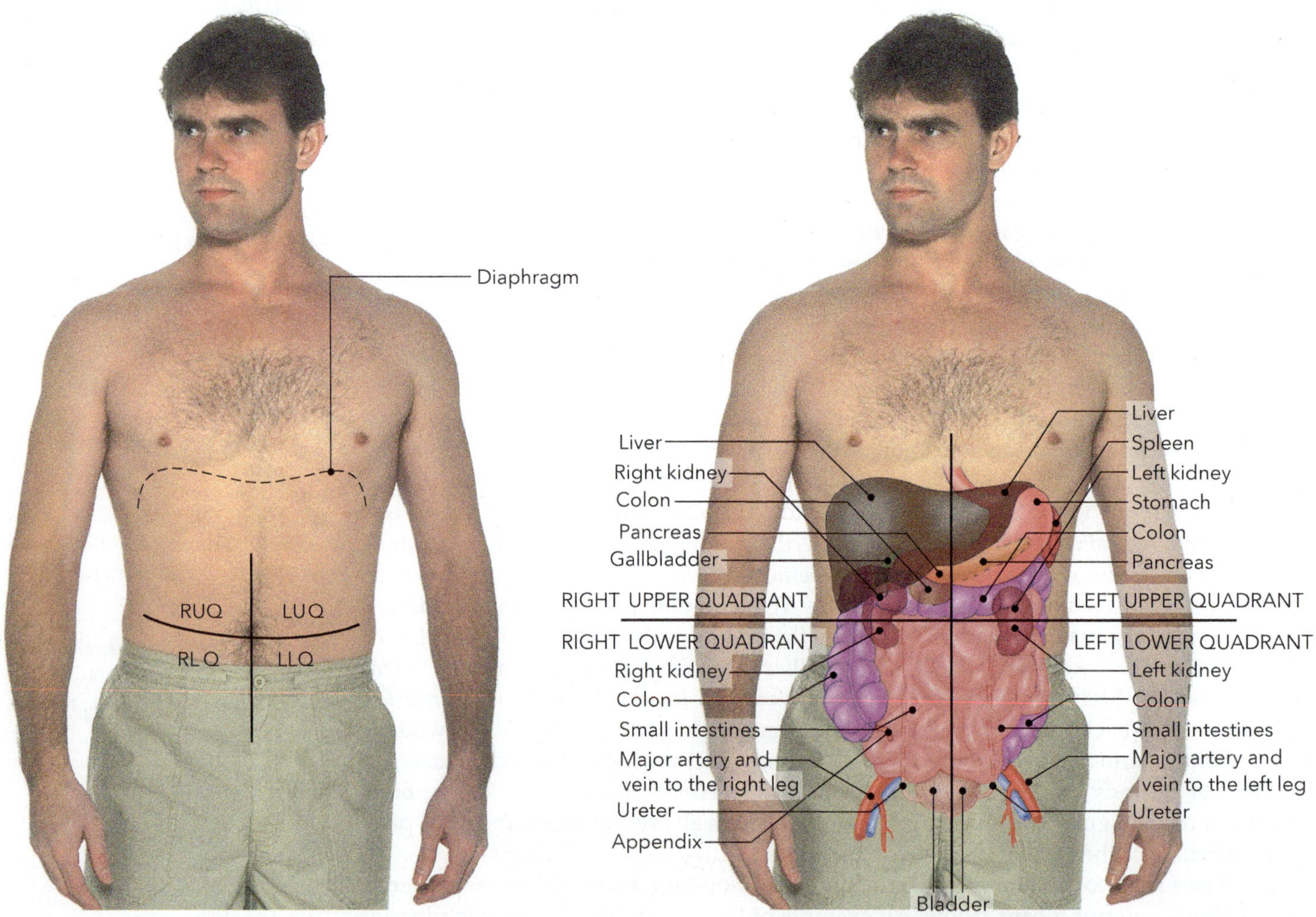

Positional Terms

Four terms describe specific patient positions: *supine*, *prone*, *recovery*, and *Fowler*.

A ***supine*** patient is lying on the patient's back. A ***prone*** patient is lying on the abdomen. A person may also be lying on one side, a position traditionally called the ***recovery position***. The recovery position is the preferred position for any unconscious nontrauma patient because it is a position in which fluids or vomitus can drain from the mouth and be less likely to be aspirated (inhaled) into the lungs. Because the patient is lying on one side, this position is also called the *lateral recumbent position*. If the patient's right side is in contact with a surface, the patient is in the *right lateral recumbent position*; if the left side is in contact with the surface, the patient is in the *left lateral recumbent position* (Figure 5-6).

When patients are transported on a stretcher, they may be placed in one of several positions. In the ***Fowler position***, the patient is seated. This is usually accomplished by raising the head end of the stretcher so the body is at a 45- to 60-degree angle. The patient may be sitting straight up or leaning slightly back. Leaning back in a semi-sitting position is sometimes called *semi-Fowler position* (Figure 5-7). In a Fowler position, the legs may be straight out or bent.

CORE CONCEPT
Positional terms

supine
lying on the back.

prone
lying facedown.

recovery position
lying on the side. Also called *lateral recumbent position*.

Fowler position
a sitting position.

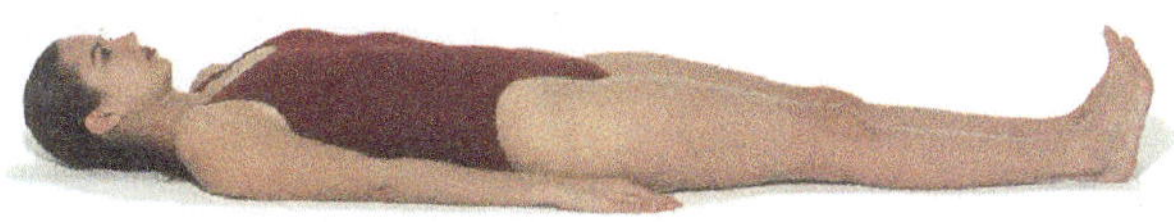

Supine

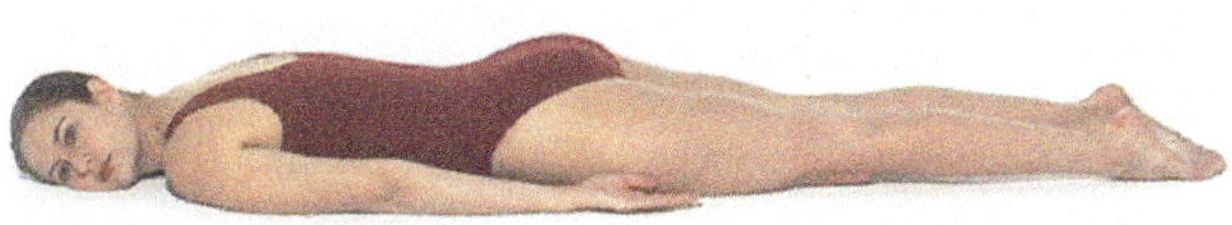

Prone

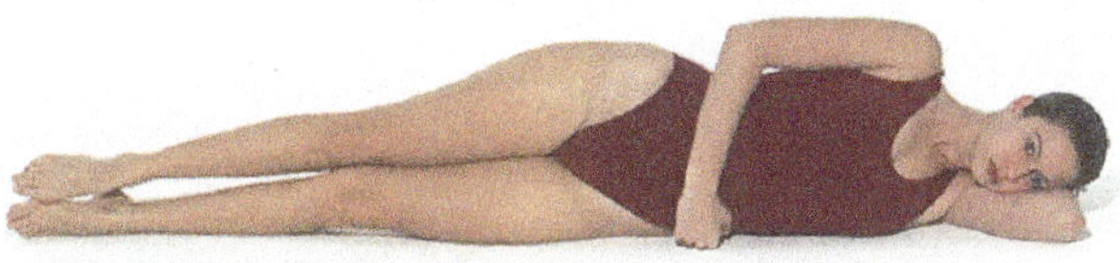

Lateral recumbent (recovery)

FIGURE 5-6 Anatomic positions.

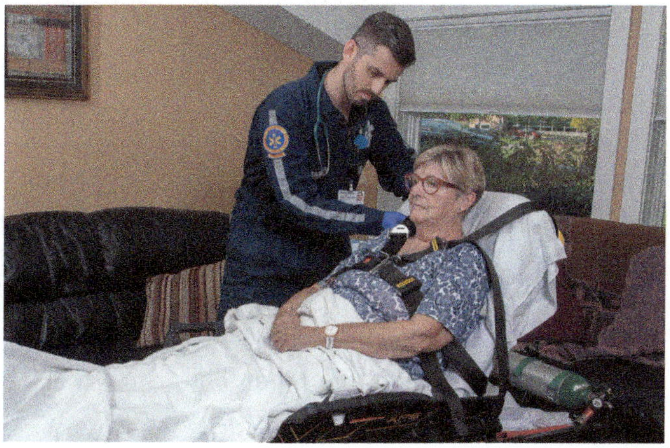

FIGURE 5-7 Semi-Fowler position.

Point of View

"I really thought that all of the chapters before the cool medical stuff was just fluff. You know, nice but not important. I wanted to learn about oxygen and suction and trauma and defibrillation—not medical terminology.

"Whoa. Was I wrong! One of my first calls was a transfer from the emergency department to a long-term facility. The hospital was busy. The nurse handed me these orders. Then she asked if I had any questions. I'm not sure if I looked as pale as I felt. They stared at me until I took the orders and read them. They actually made sense—but only because my instructor made us pay attention to the medical terms. She said, 'You can't be a professional unless you think—and talk—like one.'

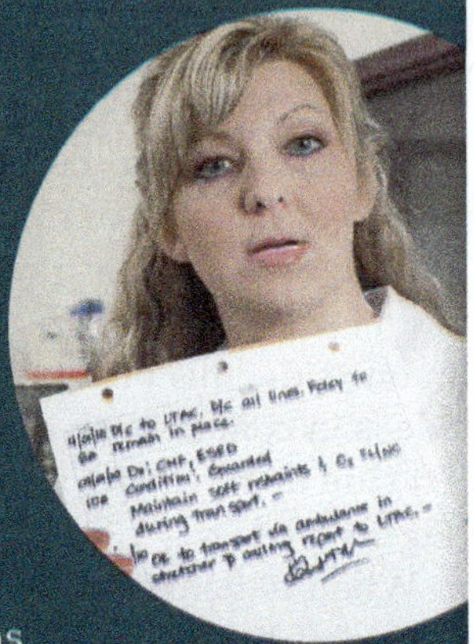

"If anyone ever tells you medical terminology isn't important, they are wrong. Way wrong."

Chapter Review

Key Facts and Concepts

- Medicine has a language of its own. As an EMT, you will frequently communicate with medical professionals who speak this language.
- Medical terms generally consist of a root with a prefix and/or suffix.

Key Decisions

- Are my medical terms accurate and descriptive?
- Do I understand when and when not to use medical terminology?
- Can I identify by direction the area where a patient has a complaint or traumatic injury?
- Can I identify the position a patient is in when found or the position in which the patient will be placed?

Chapter Glossary

abdominal quadrants four divisions of the abdomen used to pinpoint the location of a pain or injury: the right upper quadrant (RUQ), the left upper quadrant (LUQ), the right lower quadrant (RLQ), and the left lower quadrant (LLQ).

anatomic position the standard reference position for the body in the study of anatomy. In this position, the body is standing erect, facing the observer, with arms down at the sides and the palms of the hands forward.

anatomy the study of body structure.

anterior the front of the body or body part.

bilateral on both sides.

combining form a word root with an added vowel that can be joined with other words, roots, or suffixes to form a new word; for example, the combining form *therm/o* added to *meter* makes the new word *thermometer*.

compound a word formed from two or more whole words; for example, the compound *smallpox* formed from *small* and *pox*.

distal farther away from the torso. *See also* proximal.

dorsal referring to the back of the body or the back of the hand or foot. A synonym for *posterior*.

Fowler position a sitting position.

inferior away from the head, usually compared with another structure that is closer to the head (e.g., the lips are inferior to the nose).

lateral to the side, away from the midline of the body.

medial toward the midline of the body.

midaxillary (mid-AX-uh-lair-e) ***line*** a line drawn vertically from the middle of the armpit to the ankle.

midclavicular (mid-clah-VIK-yuh-ler) ***line*** the line through the center of each clavicle.

midline an imaginary line drawn down the center of the body, dividing it into right and left halves.

palmar referring to the palm of the hand.

physiology the study of body function.

plane a flat surface formed when slicing through a solid object.

plantar referring to the sole of the foot.

posterior the back of the body or body part.

prefix word part added to the beginning of a root or word to modify or qualify its meaning; for example, the prefix *bi-* added to the word *lateral* forms the word *bilateral*.

prone lying facedown.

proximal closer to the torso. *See also* distal.

recovery position lying on the side. Also called *lateral recumbent position*.

root foundation of a word that is not a word that can stand on its own—for example, the root *cardi*, meaning "heart," in words such as *cardiac* and *cardiology*.

suffix word part added to the end of a root or word to complete its meaning; for example, the suffix *-itis* added to the root *laryng* forms the word *laryngitis*.

superior toward the head (e.g., the chest is superior to the abdomen).

supine lying on the back.

torso the trunk of the body, or the body without the head and the extremities.

unilateral limited to one side.

ventral referring to the front of the body. A synonym for *anterior*.

Preparation for Your Examination and Practice

Short Answer

1. Define the following pairs of anatomic terms:

medial	lateral
anterior	posterior
proximal	distal

2. List two prefixes that mean "below."
3. List two suffixes that mean "pertaining to."
4. Describe the difference between the prone and supine positions.
5. Describe the anatomic location of the midaxillary line.
6. Describe how the abdomen is divided into quadrants.
7. What does the term *palmar* refer to?

Thinking and Linking

Linking your knowledge of medical terminology and anatomy with common diseases will help you to understand the diseases and communicate about them. For each of the following diseases, use word parts (root, prefix, and/or suffix as appropriate) to determine what organs the disease affects. Refer to Table 5-1 and the discussion under "The Components of Medical Terms" for assistance.

Gastritis
Neurology
Hepatitis
Postnasal
Tachycardia
Bradypnea
Neuritis

Critical Thinking Exercises

Understanding medical terminology and knowing how to use it is important in your practice as an EMT. The purpose of this exercise will be to consider how you might appropriately use medical terminology in your radio report about a patient's injuries.

- As an EMT, you are called to respond to a teenage boy who has taken a hard fall from his dirt bike. He has a deep gash on the outside of his left arm about halfway between the shoulder and the elbow, and another on the inside of his right arm just above the wrist. His left leg is bent at an odd angle about halfway between hip and knee, and when you cut away his pants leg, you see a bone sticking out of a wound on the front side. You take the necessary on-scene assessment and care steps, and are on the way to the hospital in the ambulance. How do you describe your patient's injuries on the phone or over the radio to the hospital staff?

Street Scenes

"Unit 144, respond to a motor-vehicle collision multiple vehicles at the intersection of route 690 and 81. Be advised you will be reporting to 81 command." You and your partner are excited to be finally called to this crash, as you have been listening to multiple other ambulances responding to what seems to be a big, multi-casualty scene. You switch on the emergency lights and travel to the scene.

"Unit 144 to 81 command, where do you want us?" your partner asks over the radio as you pull up. Your heart beats just a little faster as you see for the first time the debris and severe damage of what appear to be several wrecked cars strewn across the highway.

"Command to 144, pull up behind the rescue, you will be reporting to the treatment area."

Your partner stays with the unit as you briskly walk to an area marked with a red tarp. You are met by a familiar person dressed in a vest that reads *TREATMENT* in bold letters. She points to a patient lying on a backboard and gives you the following report: "Forty-six-year-old male driver of car 3. High speed, severe damage to the car. Patient complains of dyspnea. Secondary triage noted medial tenderness to the chest wall and pain in the upper left quadrant of the abdomen. He also has a possible proximal humerus fracture and possible bilateral tibia/fibula fractures. He's all yours."

Street Scene Questions

1. **As you assess your patient, how does a knowledge of medical terminology impact your process?**
2. **Specifically where does this patient's chest hurt?**
3. **Would pain in the upper left quadrant of the abdomen be located above or below the belly button?**
4. **What part of the humerus has sustained a traumatic injury? Where would the fracture be located?**

You begin a more comprehensive assessment. Your primary assessment finds the patient to have shortness of breath but adequate breathing. When you listen to his chest, you hear lung sounds on only one side. You also find a penetrating wound in the patient's armpit on the left side of his chest. You seal the wound and immediately let the treatment officer know that you will need advanced life support (ALS). As you continue your assessment, a paramedic approaches you.

Street Scene Questions

5. **Use medical terminology to describe to the paramedic the location of the penetrating wound.**
6. **What term would be useful in describing lung sounds heard on only one side of the chest?**

The paramedic quickly checks the penetrating wound and finds that you have already sealed it with an occlusive dressing. She listens to the chest while you assess a blood pressure–72/40. "That's no good," says the paramedic as she grabs the chest decompression kit. You watch as she inserts a needle into the patient's chest along the midclavicular line. You hear a slight rush of air and a sigh from the patient. "Good job, kid, you caught this problem in time."

Anatomy and Physiology

6

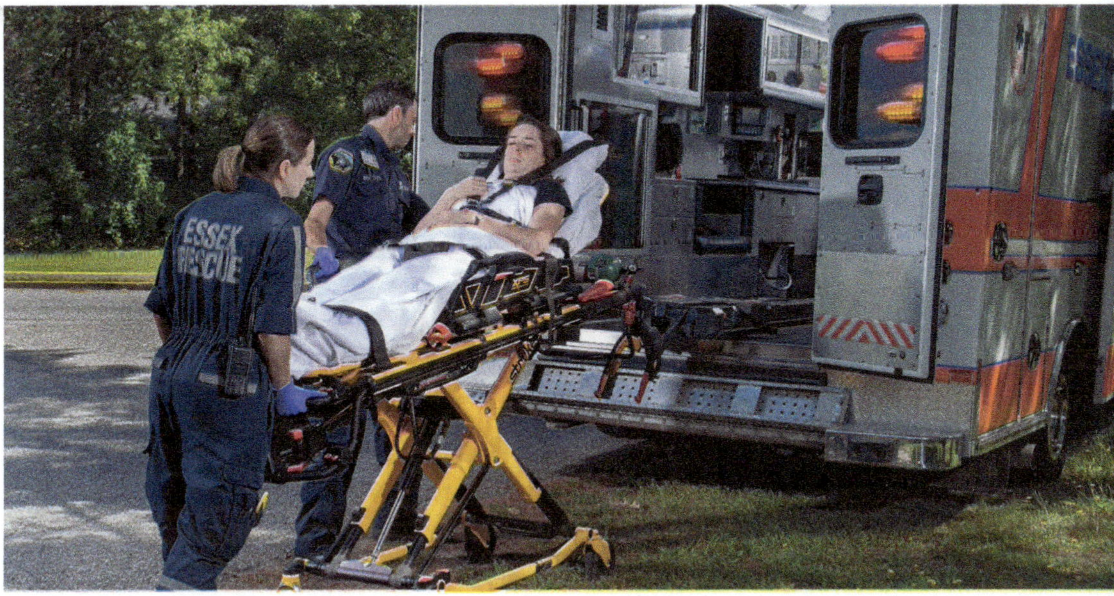

Related Chapters

The following chapters and reference sections provide additional information related to topics discussed in this chapter:

- **5** Medical Terminology
- **7** Principles of Pathophysiology
- **9** Airway Management
- **10** Respiration and Artificial Ventilation
- **19** Respiratory Emergencies
- **20** Cardiac Emergencies
- **22** Diabetic Emergencies and Altered Mental Status
- **26** Abdominal Emergencies
- **28** Hematologic and Renal Emergencies
- **29** Bleeding and Shock
- **30** Soft-Tissue Trauma
- **31** Chest and Abdominal Trauma
- **32** Musculoskeletal Trauma
- **33** Trauma to the Head, Neck, and Spine
- **36** Obstetric and Gynecologic Emergencies

References:

- Medical Terms
- Anatomy and Physiology Illustrations

Standard

Anatomy and Physiology

Competency

Applies fundamental knowledge of the anatomy and function of all human systems to the practice of EMS.

Core Concept

The structure and function of major body systems

Outcomes

After reading this chapter, you should be able to:

6.1 Explain the locations of the major systems in the body. (pp. 118–149)

- Relate topographic landmarks to the locations of underlying body structures.
- Identify the structures in various diagrams of organs.
- Given a description of how a patient was injured, predict internal organs that may be harmed.

6.2 Analyze the overall roles of each organ system in maintaining normal body functions. (pp. 118–149)

- Recognize how each organ system in the body contributes to that system's function.
- Relate observable signs to potential dysfunctions of internal organs.

Key Terms

acetabulum, *125*
acromioclavicular joint, *126*
acromion process, *126*
alveoli, *129*
anatomy, *118*
aorta, *133*
appendix, *143*
arteriole, *134*
artery, *133*
atria, *130*
automaticity, *126*
autonomic nervous system, *142*
bladder, *147*
blood pressure, *136*
brachial artery, *133*
bronchi, *127*
buffer system, *130*
calcaneus, *126*
capillaries, *134*
cardiac conduction system, *132*
cardiac muscle, *126*
cardiovascular system, *130*
carotid arteries, *133*
carpals, *126*
central nervous system (CNS), *139*
central pulses, *136*
clavicle, *126*
coronary arteries, *133*
cranium, *118*
cricoid cartilage, *127*
dermis, *143*
diaphragm, *129*
diastolic blood pressure, *136*
digestive system, *142*
dorsalis pedis artery, *134*
endocrine system, *144*
epidermis, *143*
epiglottis, *127*
epinephrine, *144*
exhalation, *129*
femoral artery, *133*
femur, *125*
fibula, *125*
gallbladder, *143*
humerus, *126*
hypoperfusion, *136*
ilium, *125*
inhalation, *129*
insulin, *144*
involuntary muscle, *126*
ischium, *125*
joint, *126*
kidneys, *144*

The sciences of anatomy and physiology are like the owner's manual to the body. When mechanics work on your car, they often refer to the manual to help them better understand where the specific parts are placed and what those parts do. As an EMT, you will use a knowledge of the body's anatomy and physiology to better understand where vital structures are located, how the body functions, and how injuries and illnesses affect the body in general.

Anatomy is the study of body structure. A working knowledge of anatomy will help you understand where organs and organ systems are located and also how external injuries may impact internal systems. ***Physiology***, the study of body function, will give you a baseline idea of how the body should work normally. Understanding this will help you identify abnormal function and predict the impact of challenges to normal function.

Anatomy and physiology will be helpful guides to decision making throughout your experience as an EMT. You should use basic understanding to help you assess and treat ill or injured patients. As you assess, ask yourself, "What organs and organ systems could be affected, and what does affecting these organs do to normal body function?" Think of it as referring to the owner's manual. While studying this chapter, also refer to *Reference: Anatomy and Physiology Illustrations* at the back of this book.

anatomy
the study of body structure.

physiology
the study of body function.

thyroid (THI-roid) ***cartilage***
the wing-shaped plate of cartilage that sits anterior to the larynx and forms the Adam's apple.

CORE CONCEPT
The structure and function of major body systems

Locating Body Organs and Structures

There are two ways to help locate organs and structures of the body. The first is visualizing, or being able to picture, the organs and structures that are inside the body as you look at the outside of the body. The second is topography, or external landmarks, such as notches, joints, and "bumps" on bones. Some external landmarks are obvious (e.g., the navel, the nipples), some you know by other names but will learn their medical terms (e.g., the "Adam's apple," which is properly called the ***thyroid cartilage***), and some will probably be new to you (e.g., the *xiphoid process*—the inferior part of the sternum, or breastbone, as described later in this chapter). It is important to learn where internal organs and structures are in relation to landmarks that you can easily see or feel on the outside of the body.

Body Systems

Refer to Table 6-1 as you read the following sections about the various body systems.

musculoskeletal (MUS-kyu-lo-SKEL-e-tal) ***system***
the system of bones and skeletal muscles that support and protect the body and permit movement.

skeleton
the bones of the body.

muscles
tissues that can contract to allow movement of a body part.

ligaments
tissues that connect bone to bone.

tendons
tissues that connect muscle to bone.

skull
the bony structure of the head.

cranium
the top, back, and sides of the skull.

Musculoskeletal System

Unlike many other systems, the ***musculoskeletal system*** extends into all parts of the body. The ***skeleton*** consists of the skull and spine, ribs and sternum, shoulders and upper extremities, and the pelvis and lower extremities (Figure 6-1). Interacting with the skeletal system are ***muscles***, ***ligaments*** (which connect bone to bone), and ***tendons*** (which connect muscle to bone).

The musculoskeletal system has three main functions:

1. To give the body shape
2. To protect vital internal organs
3. To provide for body movement

In addition to these functions, the marrow inside the bone produces blood cells and stores certain nutrients.

Skull

To list the parts of the skeleton from top to bottom, you would begin with the skull (Figure 6-2). The ***skull*** is the bony structure of the head. A main function of the skull is to enclose and protect the brain. The ***cranium*** consists of the top, back, and sides of the skull. The face is the front of the skull.

Point of View

"I had a stroke. It wasn't a big stroke, but it sure scared me. Of all the memories from my medical care–and I got a lot of it that day–the one that stands out the most is the EMTs who came to my house. I'll never forget how kind and caring they were. They checked all kinds of things: my face, my speech, and they shone a light in my eyes. I'm a diabetic so I thought it might be that. Somehow. they seemed to know it was a stroke pretty early and told the hospital so they could be ready. I recovered fully, thanks to them. I always respected the EMTs, but I guess now I am just amazed at how much they need to know to do what they do."

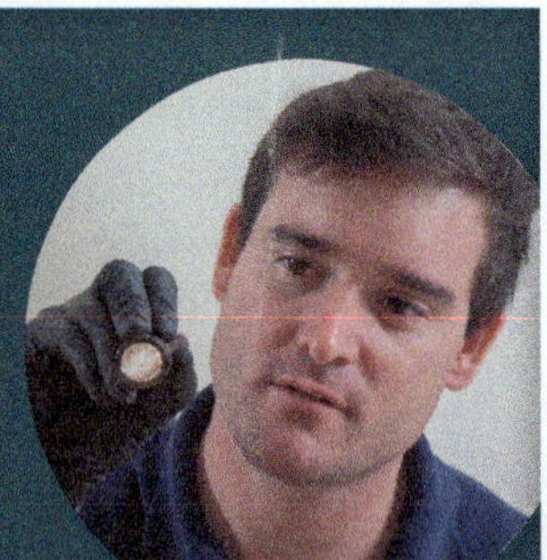

TABLE 6-1 Systems and Structures of the Human Body

SYSTEM	STRUCTURES	FUNCTIONS
Musculoskeletal	• Bones • Joints • Muscles 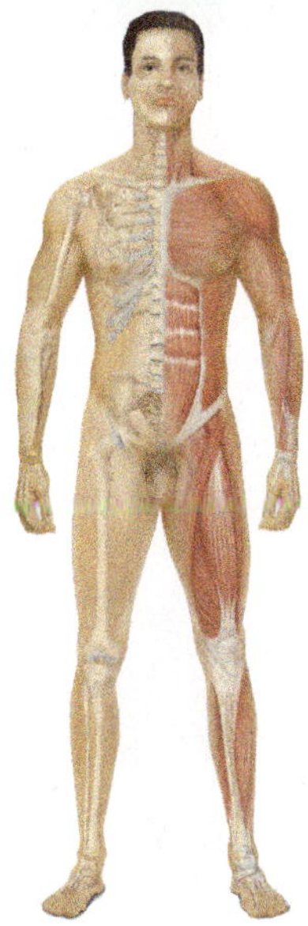	Skeleton supports and protects the body, forms blood cells, and stores minerals. Muscles produce movement.
Respiratory	• Nasal cavity • Pharynx • Larynx • Trachea • Bronchial tubes • Lungs 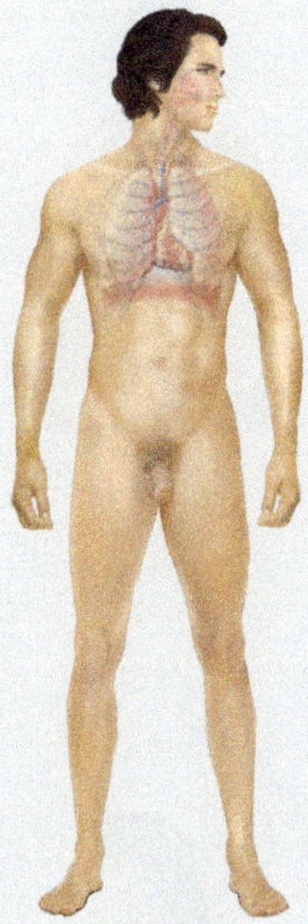	Obtains oxygen and removes carbon dioxide from the body.
Cardiovascular	• Heart • Arteries • Veins 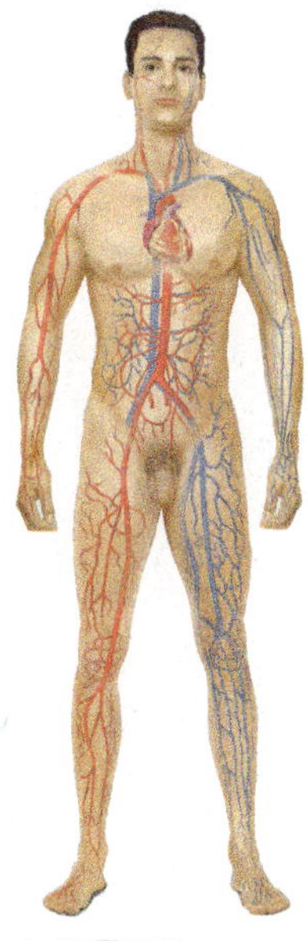	Pumps blood throughout the entire body to transport nutrients, oxygen, and wastes.

(continued)

TABLE 6-1 Systems and Structures of the Human Body (*continued*)

SYSTEM	STRUCTURES	FUNCTIONS
Blood	• Plasma • Red blood cells • White blood cells • Platelets 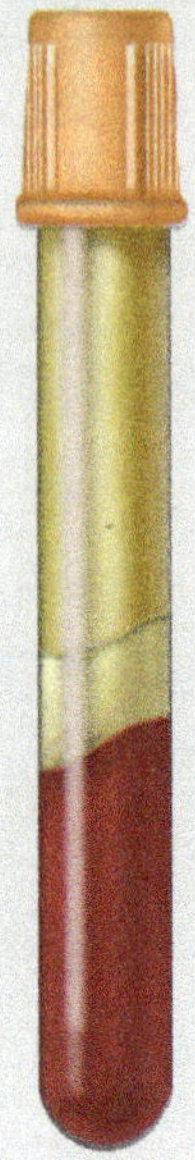	Transports oxygen, protects against pathogens, and promotes clotting to control bleeding.
Lymphatic	• Tonsils/adenoids • Thymus gland • Spleen • Lymph nodes • Lymphatic vessels 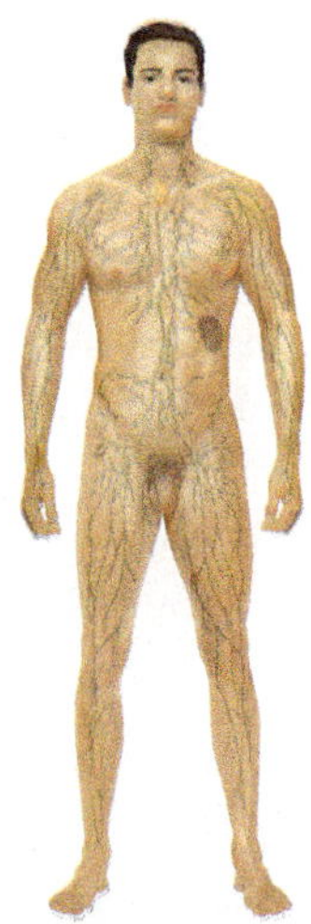	Helps to maintain the fluid balance of the body and contributes to the body's immune system.
Nervous	• Brain • Spinal cord • Nerves 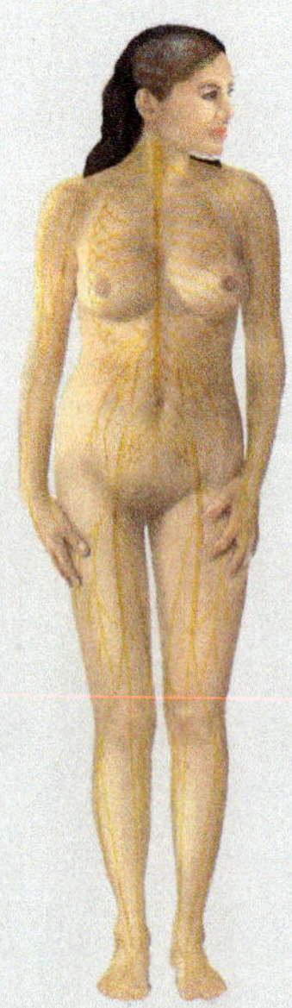	Receives sensory information and coordinates the body's response.

TABLE 6-1 Systems and Structures of the Human Body (*continued*)

SYSTEM	STRUCTURES	FUNCTIONS
Digestive	• Oral cavity • Pharynx • Esophagus • Stomach • Small intestine • Large intestine (colon) • Liver • Gallbladder • Pancreas 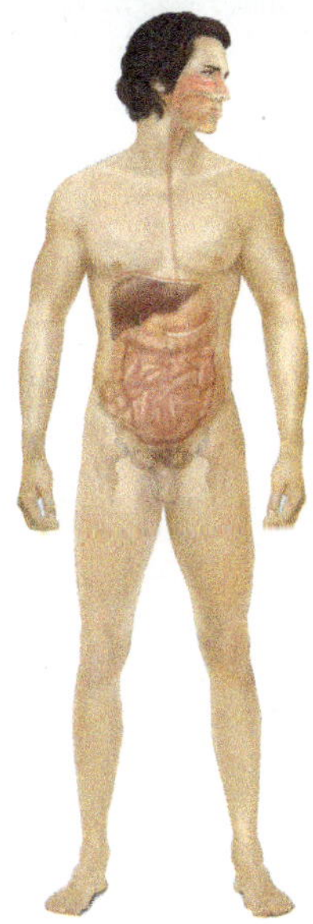	Ingests, digests, and absorbs nutrients for the body.
Integumentary	• Skin • Hair • Nails • Sweat glands 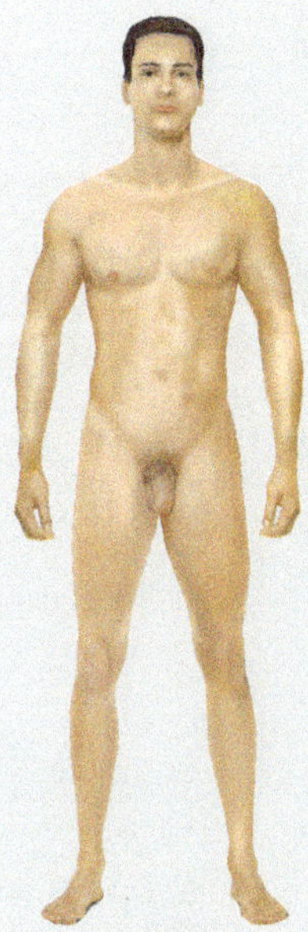	Forms protective barrier and aids in temperature regulation.
Endocrine	• Pituitary gland • Pineal gland • Thyroid gland • Parathyroid glands • Thymus gland • Adrenal glands • Pancreas • Testes • Ovaries 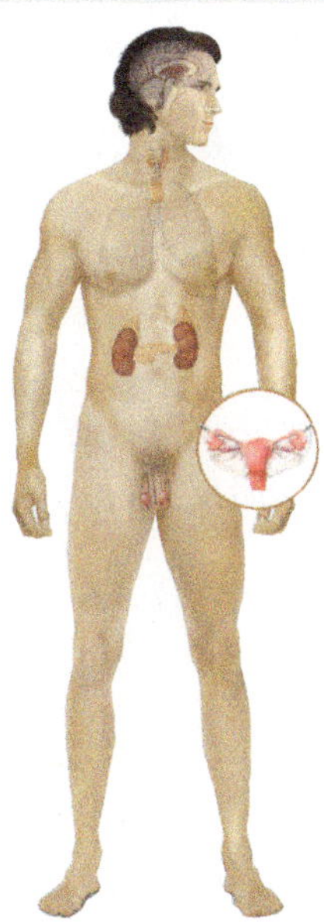	Regulates metabolic/hormonal activities of the body.

(*continued*)

TABLE 6-1 Systems and Structures of the Human Body (*continued*)

SYSTEM	STRUCTURES	FUNCTIONS
Renal/Urinary	• Kidneys • Ureters • Urinary bladder • Urethra 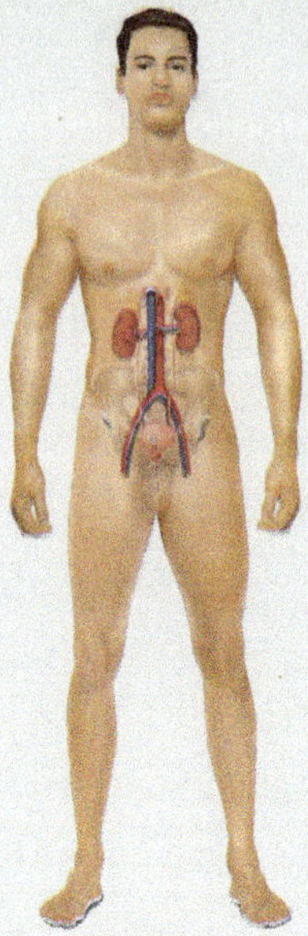	Filters waste products out of the blood and removes them from the body.
Male Reproductive	• Testes • Epididymis • Vas deferens • Penis • Seminal vesicles • Prostate gland 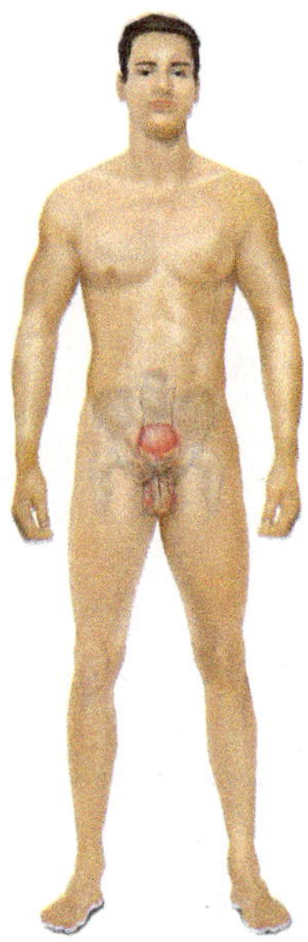	Produces sperm for reproduction.
Female Reproductive	• Ovaries • Fallopian tubes (oviducts) • Uterus • Vagina • Vulva • Breasts 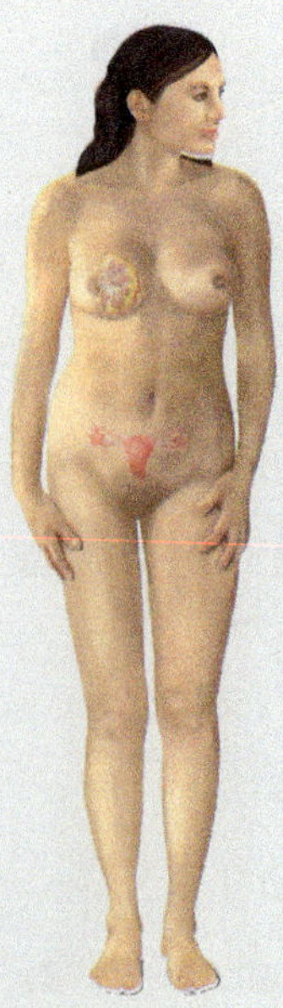	Produces eggs for reproduction and provides an environment and nutrients for growing baby.

FIGURE 6-1 The skeleton.

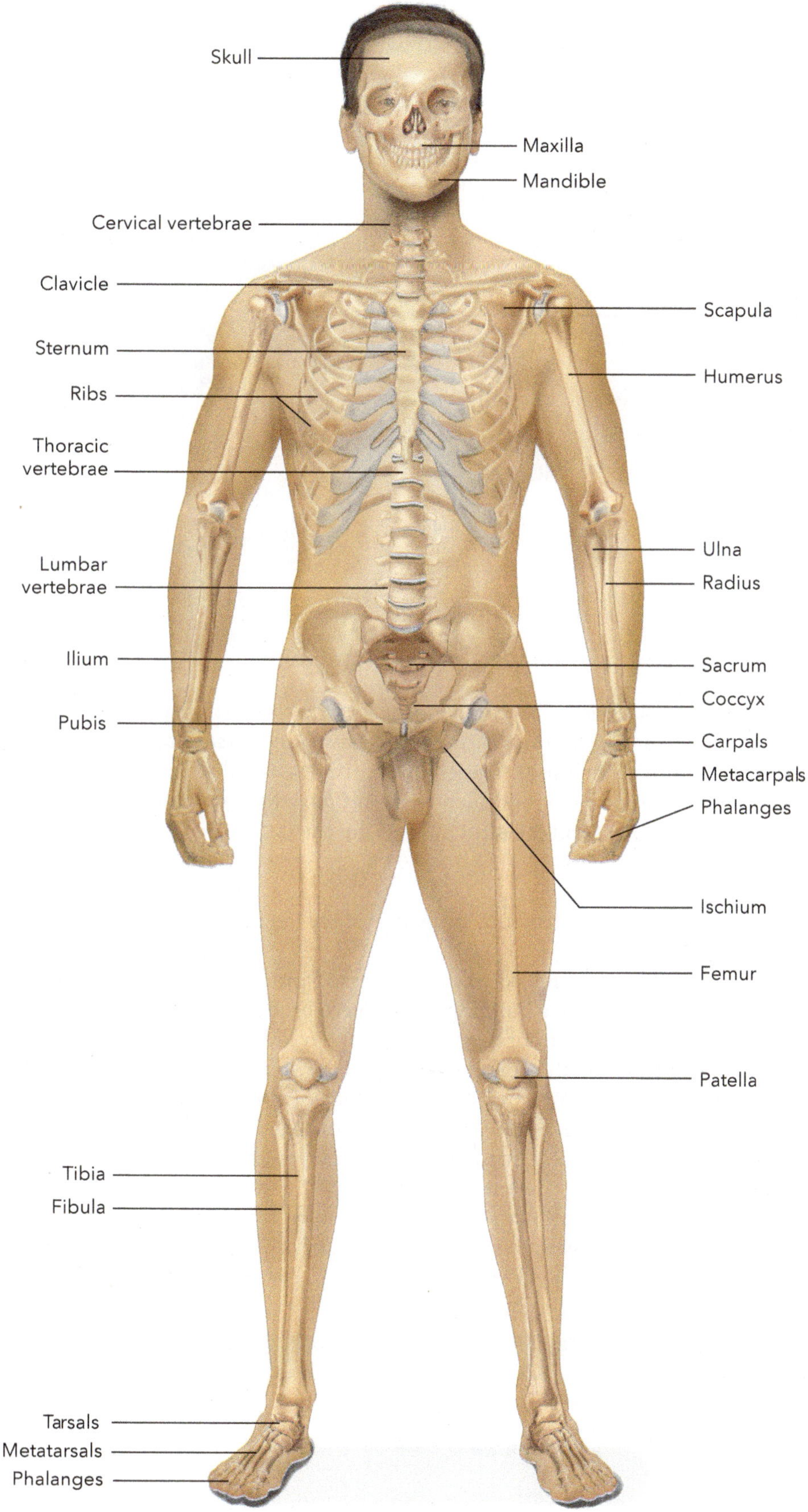

FIGURE 6-2 The skull consists of the cranium and face.

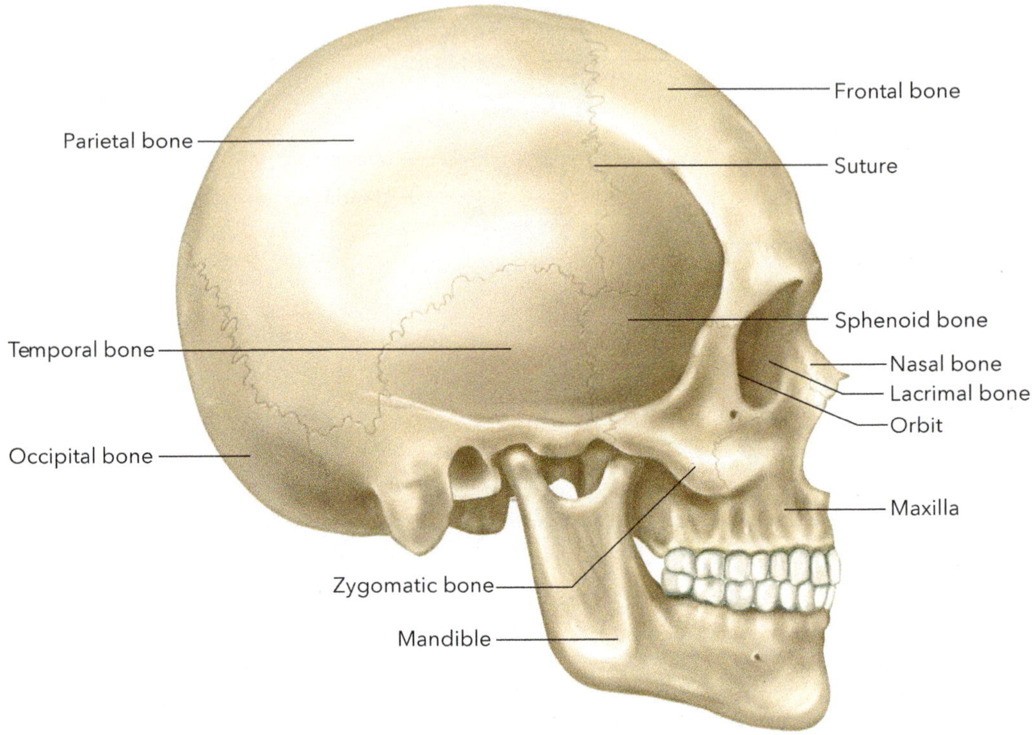

mandible (MAN-di-bul)
the lower jawbone.

maxillae (mak-SIL-e)
the two fused bones forming the upper jaw.

nasal (NAY-zul) ***bones***
the nose bones.

orbits
the bony structures around the eyes; the eye sockets.

zygomatic (ZI-go-MAT-ik) ***arches***
the bones that form the structure of the cheeks.

vertebrae (VER-te-bray)
the 33 bones of the spinal column.

The bones of the anterior cranium connect to facial bones, including the ***mandible*** (lower jaw), ***maxillae*** (fused bones of the upper jaw), and ***nasal bones*** (which provide some of the structure of the nose). These bones form the facial structures. Some of these structures consist of multiple bones, such as the ***orbits***, which surround the eyes, and the ***zygomatic arches***, which form the structures of the cheeks.

Spinal Column

The spinal column provides structure and support for the body and houses and protects the spinal cord.

The spinal column (also referred to simply as the spine) consists of 33 ***vertebrae***, the separate bones of the spine. Like building blocks, vertebrae are stacked one upon the other to form the spinal column. Vertebrae are open in the middle, somewhat like doughnuts, creating a hollow center for the spinal cord. Since the spinal cord is essential for movement, sensation, and vital functions, injuries to the spine have the potential to damage the cord, possibly resulting in paralysis or death. For this reason, you will see references throughout this text to "spinal precautions" for some patients.

The five divisions of the spine are listed in Table 6-2 and shown in Figure 6-3.

The anatomy of the body allows some vertebrae to be injured more easily than others. Since the head is large and heavy, resting on the slender neck, incidents such as car crashes

TABLE 6-2 The Divisions of the Spine

DIVISION	CORRESPONDING ANATOMY	NUMBER OF VERTEBRAE
Cervical	Neck	7
Thoracic	Thorax, ribs, upper back	12
Lumbar	Lower back	5
Sacral	Back wall of pelvis	5
Coccyx	Tailbone	4

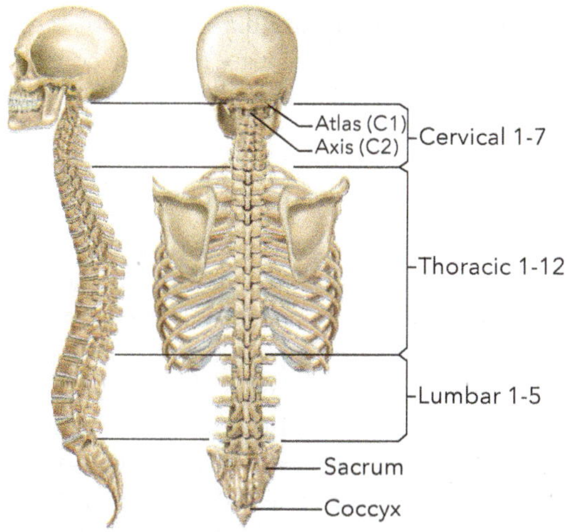

FIGURE 6-3 The divisions of the spine.

may cause the head to whip back and forth or strike an object such as the windshield. This frequently causes injuries to the cervical spine. An injury to the spinal cord at this level may be fatal because control of the muscles of breathing, such as the diaphragm and the muscles between the ribs, arises from the spinal cord in the cervical region. The lumbar region is also subject to injury because it is not supported by other parts of the skeleton. The thoracic spine, to which the ribs are attached, and the sacral spine and coccyx, which are supported by the pelvis, are less easily injured.

Thorax

The ***thorax*** is the chest. The bones of the thorax form an internal space called the thoracic cavity. This cavity contains the heart, lungs, and major blood vessels. An important function of the thorax is to protect these vital organs. This is accomplished by the 12 pairs of ribs that attach to the 12 thoracic vertebrae of the spine. In the front, 10 of these pairs of ribs are attached to the ***sternum*** (breastbone) and 2 are called "floating ribs," since they have no anterior attachment. You will remember the sternum from your CPR training. This flat bone is divided into three sections: the ***manubrium*** (superior portion), the body (center portion), and the ***xiphoid process*** (inferior tip).

Pelvis

The ***pelvis*** is sometimes referred to by laypeople as the hip, although the hip is actually the joint where the femur (thigh bone) joins the pelvis. The pelvis contains bones that are fused together. The ***ilium*** is the superior bone that contains the iliac crest, which is the wide, bony wing that can be felt near the waist. The ***ischium*** is the inferior, posterior portion of the pelvis. The ***pubis*** is formed by the joining of the bones of the anterior pubis. The pelvis is joined posteriorly to the sacral spine.

The hip joint consists of the ***acetabulum*** (the socket of the hip joint) and the ball at the proximal end of the femur.

Lower Extremities

The pelvis and hip joint, described previously, may be considered part of the lower extremities. Moving downward from the hip, the large thigh bone is the ***femur***. The femur, the largest long bone in the body, has a slight bend at its proximal end where it attaches to the pelvis. This bend is a frequent site of fractures and is commonly what breaks when a patient "breaks a hip." Progressing down the leg, the ***patella***, or kneecap, sits anterior to the knee joint. The knee connects superiorly with the femur and inferiorly with the bones of the lower leg, the tibia and fibula. The ***tibia*** is the medial and larger bone of the lower leg, also referred to as the shinbone. The ***fibula*** is the lateral and smaller bone of the lower leg.

The ankle connects the tibia and fibula with the foot. Two distinct landmarks are the *malleoli* at each side of the ankle: the *lateral* ***malleolus*** (at the lower end of the fibula) and

thorax (THOR-ax)
the chest.

sternum (STER-num)
the breastbone.

manubrium (man-OO-bre-um)
the superior portion of the sternum.

xiphoid (ZI-foid) ***process***
the inferior portion of the sternum (breastbone).

pelvis
the basin-shaped bony structure that supports the spine and is the point of proximal attachment for the lower extremities.

ilium (IL-e-um)
the superior and widest portion of the pelvis.

ischium (ISH-e-um)
the lower, posterior portions of the pelvis.

pubis (PYOO-bis)
the medial anterior portion of the pelvis.

acetabulum (AS-uh-TAB-yuh-lum)
the pelvic socket into which the ball at the proximal end of the femur fits to form the hip joint.

femur (FEE-mer)
the large bone of the thigh.

patella (pah-TEL-uh)
the kneecap.

tibia (TIB-e-uh)
the medial and larger bone of the lower leg.

fibula (FIB-yuh-luh)
the lateral and smaller bone of the lower leg.

malleolus (mal-E-o-lus)
protrusion on the side of the ankle. The *lateral malleolus*, at the lower end of the fibula, is seen on the outer ankle; the *medial malleolus*, at the lower end of the tibia, is seen on the inner ankle.

tarsals (TAR-sulz)
the ankle bones.

metatarsals (MET-uh-TAR-sulz)
the foot bones.

calcaneus (kal-KAY-ne-us)
the heel bone.

phalanges (fuh-LAN-jiz)
the toe bones and finger bones.

clavicle (KLAV-i-kul)
the collarbone.

scapula (SKAP-yuh-luh)
the shoulder blade.

acromion (ah-KRO-me-on) ***process***
the highest portion of the shoulder.

acromioclavicular (ah-KRO-me-o-klav-IK-yuh-ler) ***joint***
the joint where the acromion and the clavicle meet.

humerus (HYU-mer-us)
the bone of the upper arm, between the shoulder and the elbow.

radius (RAY-de-us)
the lateral bone of the forearm.

ulna (UL-nah)
the medial bone of the forearm.

carpals (KAR-pulz)
the wrist bones.

metacarpals (MET-uh-KAR-pulz)
the hand bones.

joint
the point where two bones come together.

voluntary muscle
muscle that can be consciously controlled.

involuntary muscle
muscle that responds automatically to brain signals but cannot be consciously controlled.

cardiac muscle
specialized involuntary muscle found only in the heart.

automaticity
(AW-to-muh-TISS-it-e)
the ability of the heart to generate and conduct electrical impulses on its own.

the *medial malleolus* (at the lower end of the tibia). These are the protrusions that you see on the lateral and medial aspects of your ankles. The ankle consists of bones called ***tarsals***. The foot bones are called ***metatarsals***. The heel bone is called the ***calcaneus***. The toe bones are the ***phalanges***.

Upper Extremities

Each shoulder consists of several bones: the clavicle, the scapula, and the proximal humerus. The ***clavicle***, or collarbone, is located anteriorly. The ***scapula***, or shoulder blade, is located posteriorly. The ***acromion process*** of the scapula is the highest portion of the shoulder. It forms the ***acromioclavicular joint*** with the clavicle and is a frequent area of shoulder injury.

The upper arm and forearm consist of three bones connected at the elbow. The bone between the shoulder and the elbow is the ***humerus***. The ***radius*** and ***ulna*** are the two bones between the elbow and the hand. The radius is the lateral bone of the forearm. It is always aligned with the thumb. (The radial pulse is taken over the radius.) The ulna is the medial forearm bone.

The wrist consists of several bones called ***carpals***. The bones of the hand are the ***metacarpals***. The finger bones, like the toe bones, are called *phalanges*.

By this point in the chapter, you are realizing the importance of anatomical terms such as *superior*, *inferior*, *medial*, *lateral*, *anterior*, and *posterior*. These terms will be used throughout the text, and you will need to use them correctly to document and report your patient's injuries and complaints properly.

Joints

Joints are formed when bones connect to other bones. There are several types of joints, including ball-and-socket joints and hinge joints. The hip is an example of a ball-and-socket joint, in which the ball of the femur rotates in a round socket in the pelvis. The elbow is an example of a hinge joint in which the angle between the humerus and ulna—which are connected by ligaments—bends and straightens, as the name suggests, like a hinge.

Muscles

Like the skeleton, the muscles protect the body, give it shape, and allow for movement. There are three types of muscle (Figure 6-4): voluntary muscle, involuntary muscle, and cardiac muscle.

Voluntary muscle, or skeletal muscle, is under conscious control of the brain via the nervous system. Attached to the bones, the voluntary muscles form the major muscle mass of the body. They are responsible for movement. Voluntary muscle can contract upon voluntary command of the individual. For example, if you want to, you can reach to pick up an item, or walk away. These are examples of voluntary muscle use.

Involuntary muscle, or smooth muscle, is found in the gastrointestinal system, lungs, blood vessels, and urinary system, and controls the flow of materials through these structures. Involuntary muscles respond automatically to orders from the brain. You do not have to consciously think about using them to breathe, digest food, or perform other functions that occur under their control. In fact, we have no direct control over involuntary muscles. Involuntary muscles do respond to stimuli such as stretching, heat, and cold.

Cardiac muscle, a specialized form of involuntary muscle, is found only in the heart. Cardiac muscle is extremely sensitive to decreased oxygen supply and can tolerate an interruption of its blood supply for only very short periods. The heart muscle has its own blood supply through the coronary artery system.

The heart also has a property called ***automaticity***. This means that the heart has the ability to generate and conduct electrical impulses on its own. The heartbeat (contraction) is controlled by these electrical impulses.

FIGURE 6-4 Three types of muscle.

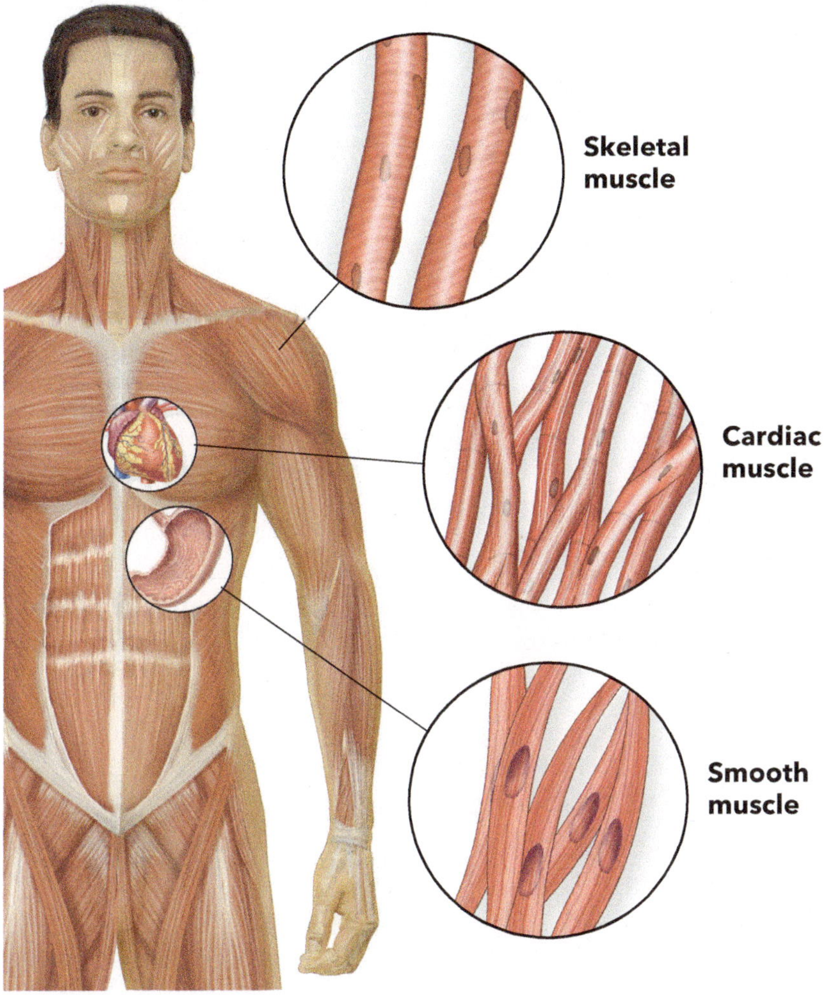

Respiratory System

The purposes of the ***respiratory system***, also known as the pulmonary system, are ventilation and oxygenation. Oxygen (O_2) is moved into the bloodstream through inhalation, and carbon dioxide (CO_2) is picked up by the blood and excreted from the body through exhalation.

Respiratory Anatomy

A number of structures make up the respiratory system (Figure 6-5). Air enters the body through the mouth and nose. It moves through the ***oropharynx*** (the area directly posterior to the mouth) and the ***nasopharynx*** (the area directly posterior to the nose). The ***pharynx*** is the area that includes both the oropharynx and the nasopharynx.

From the pharynx, air moves on a path toward the lungs. A leaf-shaped structure called the ***epiglottis*** closes over the *glottis*, the opening to the trachea, to prevent foods and foreign objects from entering the trachea during swallowing. The ***larynx***, or voice box, contains the vocal cords. The ***cricoid cartilage***, a ring-shaped structure, forms the lower portion of the larynx.

The ***trachea***, or windpipe, is the tube that carries inhaled air from the larynx down toward the ***lungs***. It is formed and protected by 16 C-shaped (incomplete) rings of cartilage. At the level of the lungs, the trachea splits (bifurcates) into two branches called the ***bronchi***. One "mainstem" bronchus goes to each lung. Inside each lung, the bronchi continue to branch and split like the branches of a tree (the branches are called *bronchioles*),

respiratory (RES-pir-ah-tor-e) ***system***
the system of nose, mouth, throat, lungs, and muscles that brings oxygen into the body and expels carbon dioxide. Also called the *pulmonary system*.

oropharynx (OR-o-FAIR-inks)
the area directly posterior to the mouth.

nasopharynx (NAY-zo-FAIR-inks)
the area directly posterior to the nose.

pharynx (FAIR-inks)
the area directly posterior to the mouth and nose. It is made up of the oropharynx and the nasopharynx.

epiglottis (EP-i-GLOT-is)
a leaf-shaped structure that prevents food and foreign matter from entering the trachea.

larynx (LAIR-inks)
the voice box.

cricoid (KRIK-oid) ***cartilage***
the ring-shaped structure that forms the lower portion of the larynx.

trachea (TRAY-ke-uh)
the "windpipe"; the structure that connects the pharynx to the lungs.

lungs
the organs where exchange of atmospheric oxygen and waste carbon dioxide takes place.

bronchi (BRONG-ki)
the two large sets of branches that come off the trachea and enter the lungs. There are right and left bronchi. *Singular* bronchus.

FIGURE 6-5 The respiratory system.

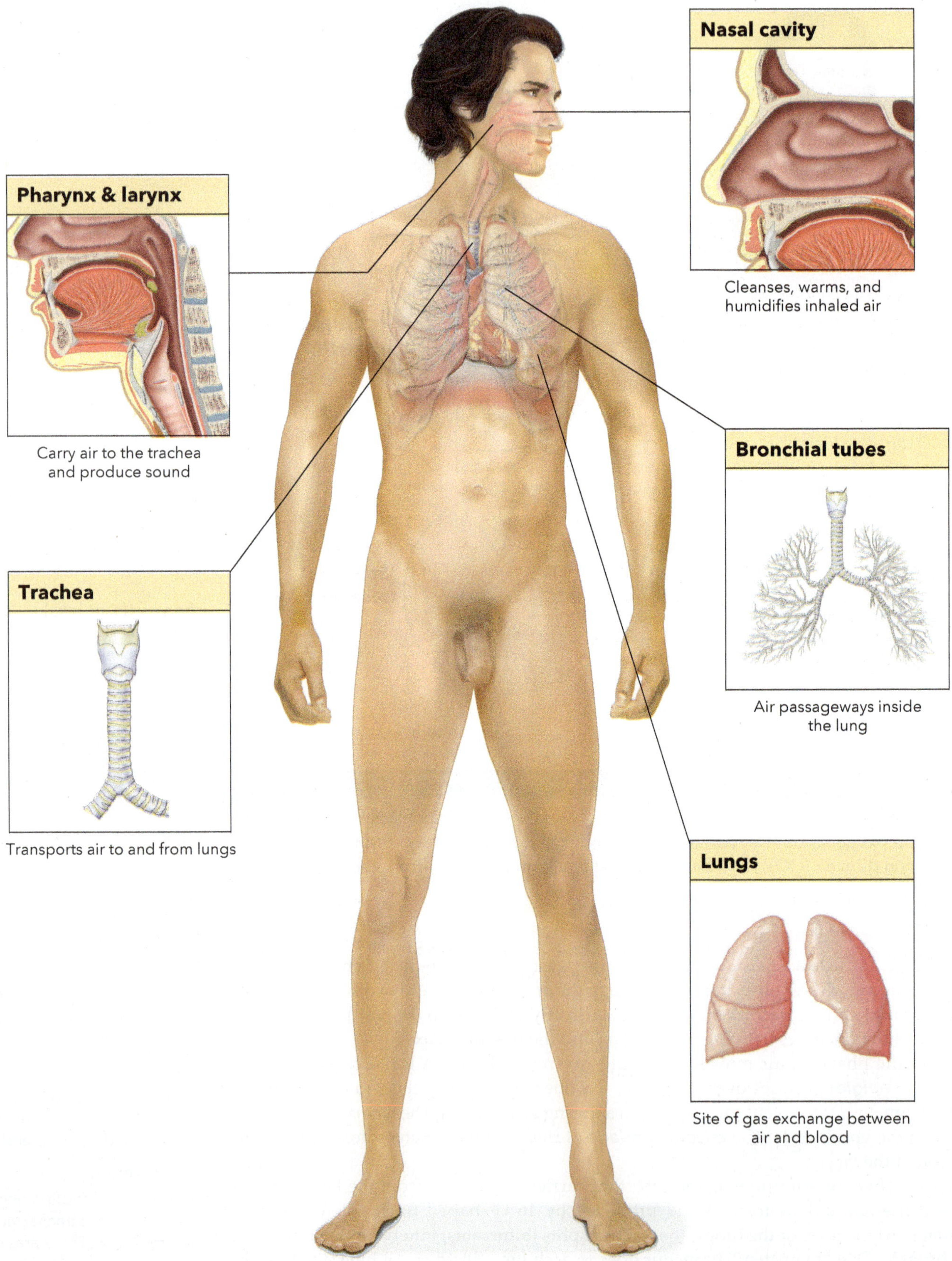

and the air passages get smaller and smaller. Eventually each branch ends at a group of alveoli. The ***alveoli*** are the small sacs within the lungs where gas exchange—the exchange of oxygen and carbon dioxide—takes place with the bloodstream.

alveoli (al-VE-o-li)
the microscopic sacs of the lungs where gas exchange with the bloodstream takes place.

The ***diaphragm*** is a structure that divides the chest cavity from the abdominal cavity. It is a large muscle that is primarily controlled by the *phrenic nerve*. During a normal respiratory cycle, the diaphragm and other parts of the body work together to allow the body to inhale and exhale. The role of the diaphragm and other muscles in the respiratory cycle is described next.

diaphragm (DI-uh-fram)
the muscular structure that divides the chest cavity from the abdominal cavity; a major muscle of respiration.

Respiratory Physiology

Inhalation is an active process. The muscles of the rib cage (*intercostal muscles*) and the diaphragm contract. The diaphragm lowers, and the ribs move upward and outward. This expands the size of the chest and thereby creates a negative pressure inside the chest cavity. This negative pressure pulls air into the lungs.

inhalation (IN-huh-LAY shun)
an active process in which the intercostal (rib) muscles and the diaphragm contract, expanding the size of the chest cavity and causing air to flow into the lungs.

Exhalation is a passive process during which the intercostal muscles and the diaphragm relax. The ribs move downward and inward, while the diaphragm rises. This movement causes the chest to decrease in size and positive pressure to build inside the chest cavity. This positive pressure pushes air out of the lungs.

exhalation (EX-huh-LAY-shun)
a passive process in which the intercostal (rib) muscles and the diaphragm relax, causing the chest cavity to decrease in size and air to flow out of the lungs.

During inhalation, air is moved through the airway and into the alveoli. These tiny sacs in the lungs are the site of gas exchange between air and blood. Each single alveolus is surrounded by pulmonary capillaries. The pulmonary capillaries bring circulating blood to the outside of the alveoli. Through the very thin walls of the alveoli and the capillaries, oxygen is transferred from the air inside the alveoli to the bloodstream, and carbon dioxide is moved from the bloodstream into the air within the alveoli. This movement of gases to and from the alveoli is called ***ventilation***.

ventilation
the process of moving gases (oxygen and carbon dioxide) between inhaled air and the pulmonary circulation of blood.

Oxygenated blood is carried from the lungs to the heart so it can be pumped into the body's circulatory system. As the blood leaves the heart, it travels through a branching series of arteries that gradually become smaller and finally connect to capillaries. Just as happened with the capillaries that pass by the alveoli of the lungs, the capillaries that pass by the cells throughout the body's tissues conduct a gas exchange. At a cellular level, oxygen that was picked up from the lungs and carried by the blood is now transferred

Pediatric Note

There are a number of special aspects of the respiratory anatomy of infants and children (Figure 6-6). In general, all structures in a child are smaller than in an adult. A child's tongue takes up proportionally more space in the pharynx than does an adult's. The trachea is relatively narrower than in adults and, therefore, more easily obstructed by swelling or foreign matter. The trachea is also softer and more flexible in infants and children, so more care must be taken during any procedure when pressure might be placed on the neck, such as in applying a cervical collar. The cricoid cartilage is also less developed and less rigid in infants and children. The rib cage of an infant or small child is not as curved inward at the bottom as is an adult's. This makes generating that negative pressure used to breathe a bit more difficult. The chest wall is also softer and more flexible, so infants and children tend to rely more on the diaphragm when they are having breathing difficulty. This causes a visible "see-saw" breathing pattern in which the chest and abdomen alternate movement.

Special procedures that take into account the respiratory anatomy of infants and children will be discussed in later chapters on the airway and respiration.

FIGURE 6-6 Comparison of child and adult respiratory anatomies.

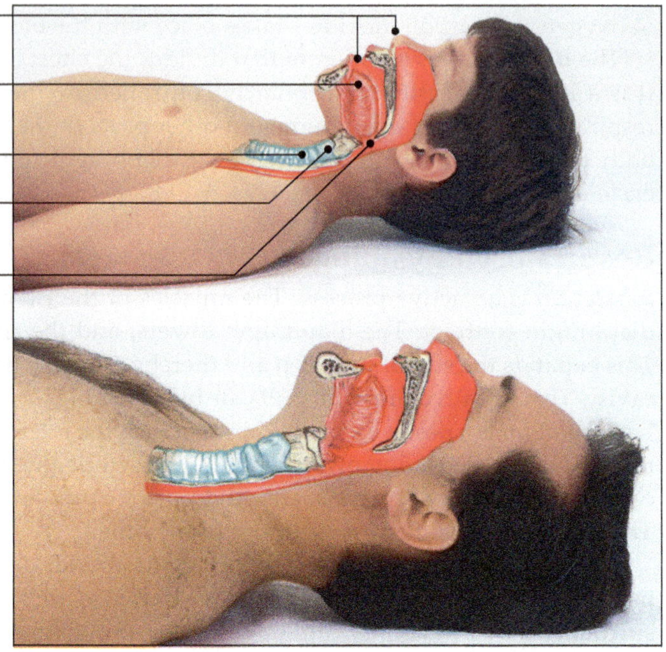

respiration
the process of moving oxygen and carbon dioxide between circulating blood and the cells.

buffer system
a system that helps manage the pH of the body to maintain it at a normal level.

cardiovascular (KAR-de-o-VAS-kyu-ler) ***system***
the system made up of the heart (cardio) and the blood vessels (vascular); the *circulatory system*.

atria (AY-tree-ah)
the two upper chambers of the heart. There is a right atrium (which receives unoxygenated blood returning from the body) and a left atrium (which receives oxygenated blood returning from the lungs). *Singular* atrium.

ventricles (VEN-tri-kulz)
the two lower chambers of the heart. There is a right ventricle (which sends oxygen-poor blood to the lungs) and a left ventricle (which sends oxygen-rich blood to the body).

venae cavae (VE-ne KA-ve)
the superior vena cava and the inferior vena cava. These two major veins return blood from the body to the right atrium. *Singular* vena cava.

through the capillary walls and across cell membranes into the cells. Waste carbon dioxide from the cells moves in the opposite direction, out of the cells and into the capillaries. Capillaries then connect to veins and veins return blood to the heart, where it can be pumped to the lungs to get rid of the waste carbon dioxide and pick up more oxygen, completing the cycle of gas exchange. The process of moving gases (and other nutrients) between the cells and the blood is called ***respiration***.

The exchange of gases, both in the lungs and at the body's cells, is critical to support life. Oxygen is essential to sustain normal cellular function, and the removal of carbon dioxide helps regulate the body's pH, or relative acidity. In general, the body regulates its pH through the ***buffer system***, and the removal of carbon dioxide is an extremely important element of this system.

Breathing (the process of inhaling and exhaling air) may be classified as adequate or inadequate. Simply stated, adequate breathing is sufficient to support life. Inadequate breathing is not. Adequate and inadequate breathing, and how you as an EMT should assess and care for breathing problems, will be discussed in detail in the *Respiratory Emergencies* chapter.

Cardiovascular System

The ***cardiovascular system*** consists of the heart, the blood, and the blood vessels. It is also called the *circulatory system*.

Anatomy of the Heart

The human heart is a muscular organ about the size of a fist, located in the center of the thoracic cavity. The heart has four chambers: two upper chambers called ***atria*** and two lower chambers called ***ventricles*** (Figure 6-7A).

Blood is circulated through the heart and out to the body via a very specific pathway (Figure 6-7B). This pathway is governed by the chambers of the heart, as follows:

- **Right atrium.** The ***venae cavae*** (the superior vena cava and the inferior vena cava) are the two large veins that return blood to the heart. The right atrium receives this blood and, upon contraction, sends it to the right ventricle.
- **Right ventricle.** The right ventricle receives blood from the chamber above it, the right atrium. When the right ventricle contracts, it pumps this blood out to the lungs via the pulmonary arteries. Remember, this blood is very low in oxygen and

FIGURE 6-7(A) Cross-section of the heart showing chambers, layers, valves, and major associated blood vessels.

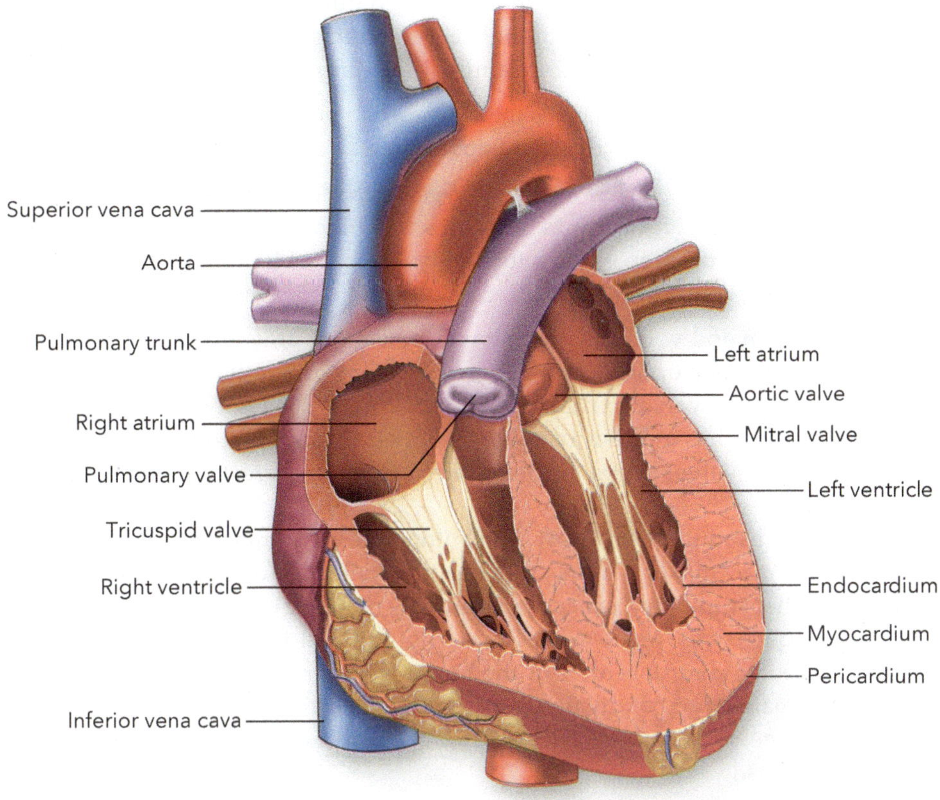

FIGURE 6-7(B) The path of blood flow through the heart.

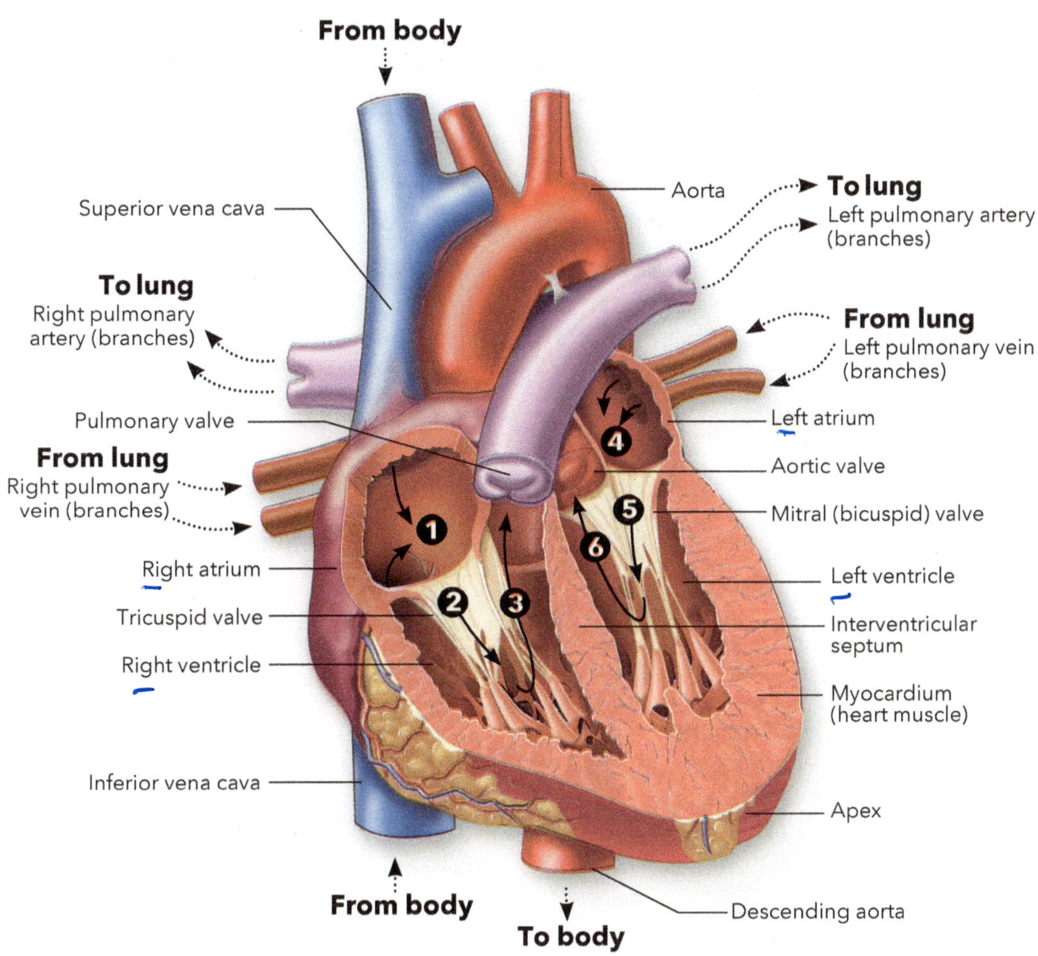

is carrying waste carbon dioxide that was picked up as the blood circulated through the body. While this blood is in the lungs, the carbon dioxide is excreted (taken out of the blood and, when the person exhales, carried out of the body), and oxygen is obtained (taken into the blood from air the person has inhaled). The oxygen-rich blood then returns to the left atrium via the pulmonary veins.

- **Left atrium.** The left atrium receives the oxygen-rich blood from the lungs. When it contracts, it sends this blood to the left ventricle.
- **Left ventricle.** The left ventricle receives oxygen-rich blood from the chamber above it, the left atrium. When it contracts, it pumps this blood into the aorta, the body's largest artery, for distribution to the entire body. Since the blood must reach all parts of the body, the left ventricle is the most muscular and strongest part of the heart.

valve
a structure that opens and closes to permit the flow of a fluid in only one direction.

Between each atrium and ventricle is a one-way ***valve*** that prevents blood in the ventricle from being forced back up into the atrium when the ventricle contracts. The pulmonary artery has a one-way valve so that blood in the artery does not return to the right ventricle. The aorta also has a one-way valve to prevent backflow to the left ventricle. This system of one-way valves keeps the blood moving in the correct direction along the path of circulation.

cardiac conduction system
a system of specialized muscle tissues that conducts electrical impulses that stimulate the heart to beat.

The contraction, or beating, of the heart is an automatic, involuntary process. The heart has its own natural "pacemaker" and a system of specialized muscle cells that conduct electrical impulses that stimulate the heart to beat. This network is called the ***cardiac conduction system*** (Figure 6-8). Regulation of rate, rhythm, and force of heartbeat comes, in part, from the cardiac control centers of the brain. Nerve impulses from these centers are sent to the pacemaker and conduction system of the heart. These nerve impulses and chemicals (epinephrine, for example) released into the blood control the heart's rate and strength of contractions.

Circulation of the Blood

When the blood leaves the heart, it travels throughout the body through several types of blood vessels. Blood vessels are described by their function, their location, and whether they carry blood away from or to the heart.

FIGURE 6-8 The cardiac conduction system.

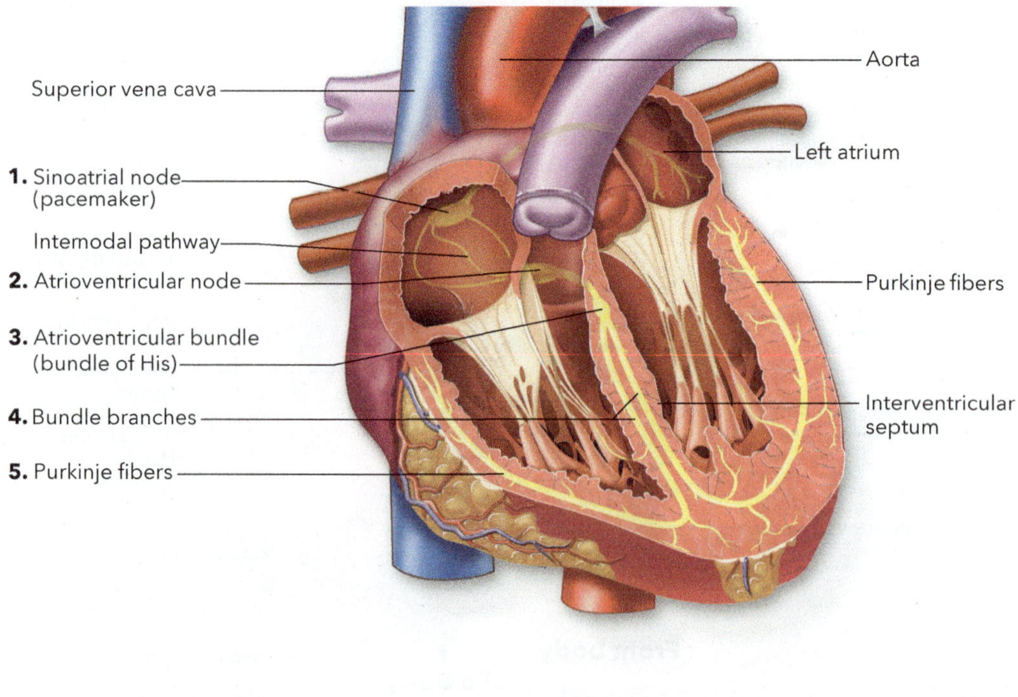

The kind of vessel that carries blood away from the heart is called an ***artery***. There are several arteries that are important to know:

- **Coronary arteries.** The ***coronary arteries*** (Figure 6-9) branch off from the aorta and supply the heart muscle with blood. Although the heart has blood constantly moving through it, it receives its own blood supply from the coronary arteries. Damage, severe narrowing, or blockage to these arteries usually results in chest pain.
- **Aorta.** The ***aorta*** is the largest artery in the body. It begins at its attachment to the left ventricle, travels superiorly, then arches inferiorly in front of the spine through the thoracic and abdominal cavities. At the level of the navel, it splits into the iliac arteries.
- **Pulmonary artery.** The ***pulmonary artery*** begins at the right ventricle. It carries oxygen-poor blood to the lungs. You may notice that this is an exception to the rule that arteries carry oxygen-rich blood and veins carry oxygen-poor blood. It does, however, follow the rule that arteries carry blood away from the heart while veins carry blood to the heart.
- **Carotid arteries.** The ***carotid arteries*** are the major arteries of the neck. You will be familiar with these vessels from your CPR class. The carotid artery is the artery that is palpated during CPR pulse checks for adults and children. It carries the main supply of blood for the head. There is a carotid artery on each side of the neck. Never palpate both at the same time, because of the danger of interrupting the supply of blood to the brain.
- **Femoral artery.** The ***femoral artery*** is the major artery of the thigh. You can relate the name *femoral* to the bone in the thigh, the femur. Pulsations for this artery can be felt in the crease between the abdomen and the groin. This artery is the major source of blood supply to the thigh and leg.
- **Brachial artery.** The ***brachial artery*** in the upper arm is the pulse checked during infant CPR. Its pulse can be felt anteriorly in the crease over the elbow and along the medial aspect of the upper arm. It is also the artery that is used when determining blood pressure with a blood pressure cuff and a stethoscope.
- **Radial artery.** This artery travels through, and supplies, the lower arm. The ***radial artery*** is the artery felt when taking a pulse at the thumb side of the wrist. Again, you can relate the name *radial* to the radius, a bone in the forearm that the radial artery is near.

artery
any blood vessel carrying blood away from the heart.

coronary (KOR-o-nar-e) ***arteries***
blood vessels that supply the muscle of the heart (myocardium).

aorta (ay-OR-tah)
the largest artery in the body. It transports blood from the left ventricle to begin systemic circulation.

pulmonary (PUL-mo-nar-e) ***artery***
the vessel that carries deoxygenated blood from the right ventricle of the heart to the lungs.

carotid (kah-ROT-id) ***arteries***
the large neck arteries, one on each side of the neck, that carry blood from the heart to the head.

femoral (FEM-o-ral) ***artery***
the major artery supplying the leg.

brachial artery
artery of the upper arm; the site of the pulse checked during infant CPR.

radial artery
artery of the lower arm; the artery felt when taking the pulse at the thumb side of the wrist.

FIGURE 6-9 The coronary arteries.

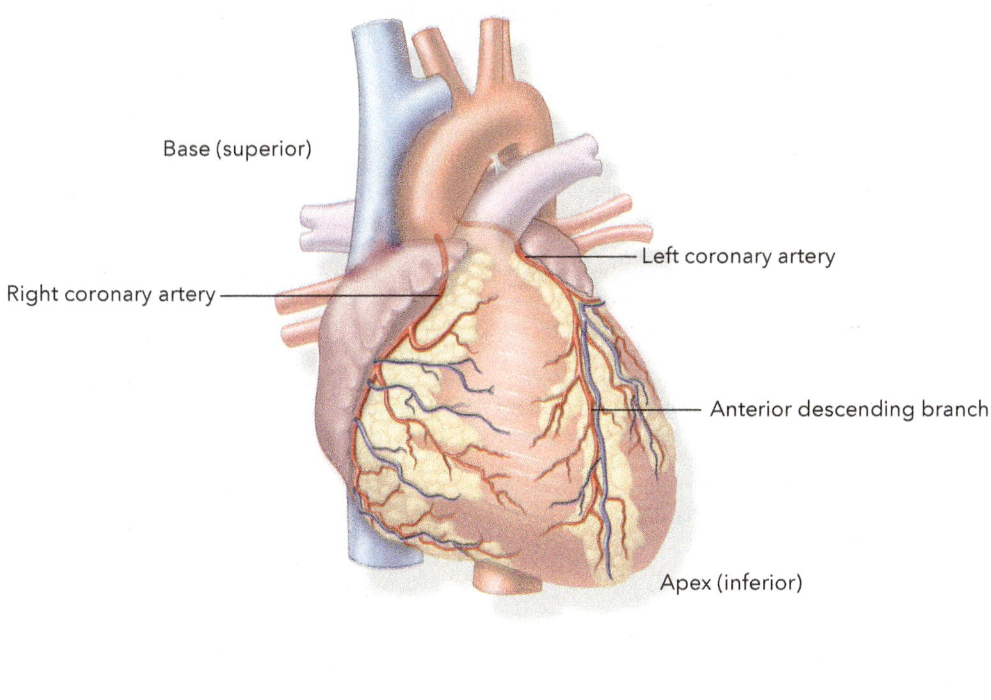

- **Posterior tibial artery.** This artery is often used when determining the circulatory status of the lower extremity. The ***posterior tibial artery*** may be palpated on the posterior aspect of the medial malleolus.
- **Dorsalis pedis artery.** The ***dorsalis pedis artery*** lies on the top (dorsal portion) of the foot, lateral to the large tendon of the big toe.

Arteries begin with large vessels, like the aorta. They gradually branch into smaller and smaller vessels. The smallest branch of an artery is called an ***arteriole***. These small vessels lead to the capillaries. ***Capillaries*** are tiny blood vessels found throughout the body. As explained earlier, the capillaries are where gases, nutrients, and waste products are exchanged between the body's cells and the bloodstream. From the capillaries, the blood begins its return journey to the heart by entering the smallest veins. One of these small veins is called a ***venule*** (Figure 6-10).

The kind of vessel that carries the blood from the capillaries back to the heart is called a ***vein***. Remember that the blood flow from the heart started in the largest arteries and moved into smaller and smaller arteries until it reached the capillaries. The blood takes an opposite course through the veins back to the heart. Immediately after leaving the capillaries, the blood enters venules, the smallest veins. Blood then travels through increasingly larger veins until it reaches the venae cavae.

There are two *venae cavae*. The superior vena cava collects blood that is returned from the head and upper body. The inferior vena cava collects blood from the body below the heart. The superior and inferior venae cavae meet to return blood to the right atrium, where the process of circulation begins again.

posterior tibial (TIB-ee-ul) ***artery***
artery supplying the foot, behind the medial ankle.

dorsalis pedis (dor-SAL-is PEED-is) ***artery***
artery supplying the foot, lateral to the large tendon of the big toe.

arteriole (ar-TE-re-ol)
the smallest kind of artery.

capillaries (KAP-i-lair-e)
thin-walled, microscopic blood vessels where the oxygen/carbon dioxide and nutrient/waste exchange with the body's cells takes place.

venule (VEN-yul)
the smallest kind of vein.

vein
any blood vessel returning blood to the heart.

FIGURE 6-10 Arteries, capillaries, and veins.

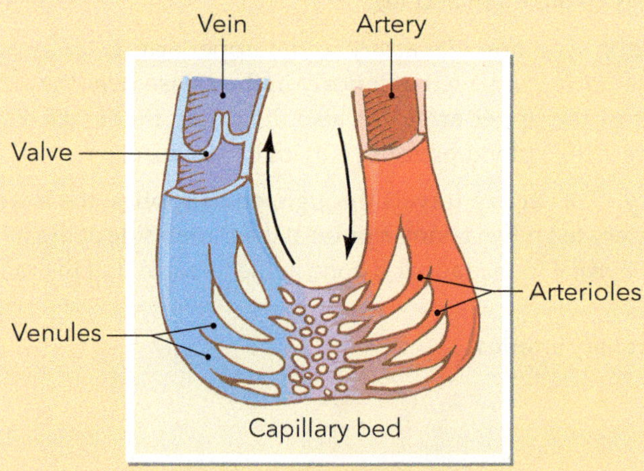

From the heart, oxygen-rich blood is carried out into the body by arteries. The arteries gradually branch into smaller arteries called arterioles. The arterioles gradually branch into tiny vessels called capillaries.

In the capillaries, the blood gives up oxygen and nutrients, which move through the thin walls of the capillaries into the body's cells. At the same time, carbon dioxide and other wastes move in the opposite direction, from the cells and through the capillary walls, to be picked up by the blood.

On its return journey to the heart, the oxygen-poor blood, now carrying carbon dioxide and other wastes, flows from the capillaries into small veins called venules which gradually merge into larger veins.

The ***pulmonary vein*** carries oxygenated blood from the lungs to the left atrium of the heart. This is an exception to the rule that veins carry oxygen-poor blood. However, it does follow the rule that arteries carry blood away from the heart while veins return blood to the heart.

pulmonary vein
vessel that carry oxygenated blood from the lungs to the left atrium of the heart.

Composition of the Blood

The blood is made up of several components: plasma, red and white blood cells, and platelets (Figure 6-11).

- **Plasma.** ***Plasma*** is a watery, salty fluid that makes up more than half the volume of the blood. The red and white blood cells and platelets are carried in the plasma. Waste carbon dioxide from the cells also dissolves in plasma to be transported back to the lungs.
- **Red blood cells.** ***Red blood cells*** are also called *RBCs*, *erythrocytes*, or *red corpuscles*. Their primary function is to carry oxygen to the tissues. The hemoglobin molecules on these cells also provide the red color to the blood.
- **White blood cells.** ***White blood cells*** are also called *WBCs*, *leukocytes*, or *white corpuscles*. They are involved in destroying microorganisms (germs) and producing substances called antibodies, which help the body resist infection.
- **Platelets.** ***Platelets*** are membrane-enclosed fragments of specialized cells. When these fragments are activated, they release chemical *clotting factors* needed to form blood clots.

plasma (PLAZ-mah)
the fluid portion of the blood.

red blood cells
components of the blood. They carry oxygen to and carbon dioxide away from the cells.

white blood cells
components of the blood. They produce substances that help the body fight infection.

platelets
components of the blood; membrane-enclosed fragments of specialized cells.

FIGURE 6-11 Blood consists of plasma, red and white blood cells, and platelets.

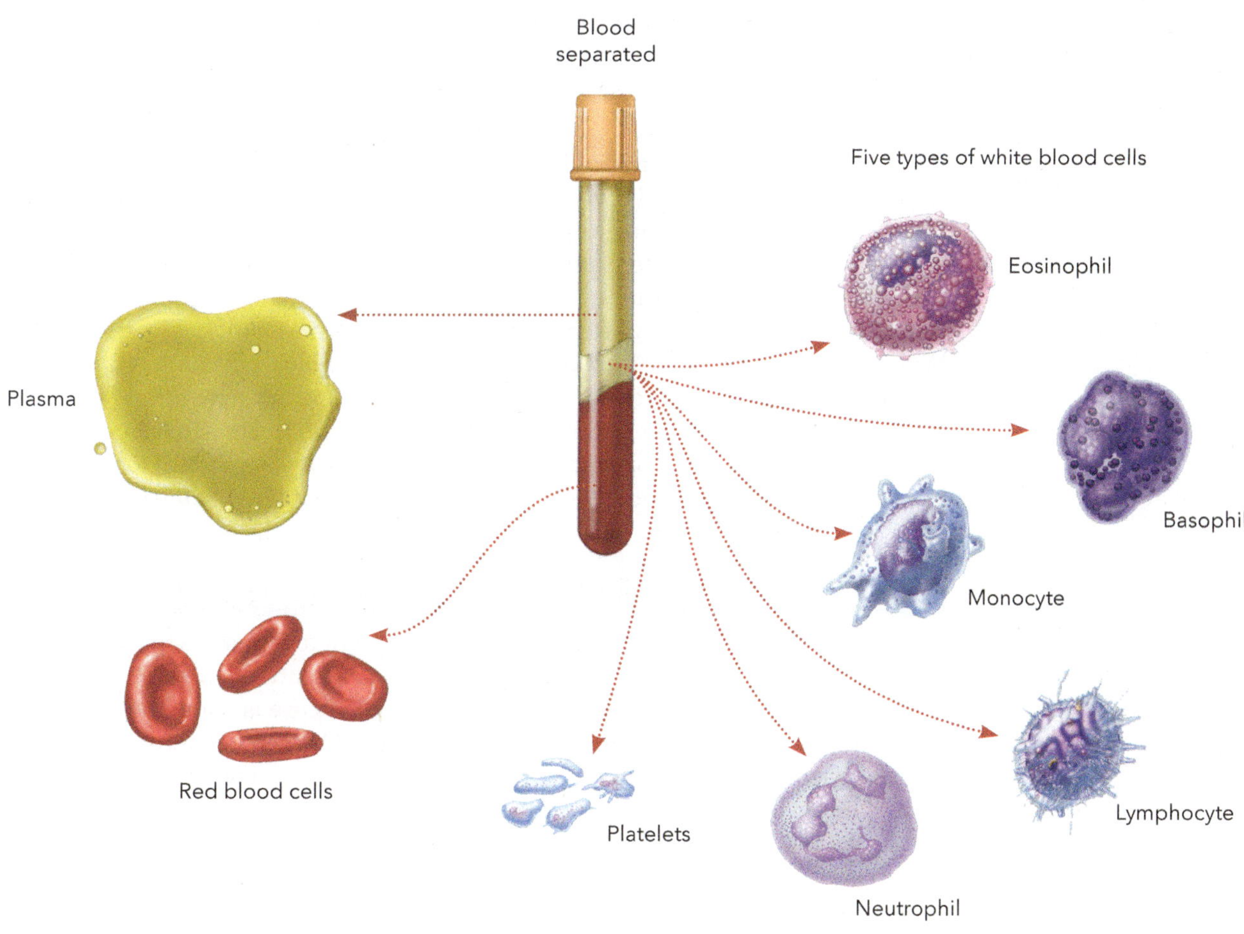

As you can see, the blood has a variety of functions. It is used to transport gases such as oxygen and carbon dioxide and also can serve as a reservoir for oxygen dissolved in its plasma. Blood also plays a role in fighting infection and the production of clotting factors. Other functions include the regulation of body pH through chemicals transported in the blood (otherwise known as the *blood buffer*).

Pulse

A ***pulse*** is formed when the left ventricle contracts, sending a pressure wave of blood through the arteries. The pulse is felt by compressing an artery over a bone. This allows you to feel the wave of blood, or pulse, as it comes through the artery.

Earlier in this chapter, several arteries were named. Among them were the primary arteries where a pulse is taken for vital signs or CPR: the carotid, brachial, and radial arteries. You will also use the pulses at the ankles and feet (posterior tibial and dorsalis pedis) to check for adequate circulation to the lower extremities.

The radial, brachial, posterior tibial, and dorsalis pedis pulses are called ***peripheral pulses*** because they can be felt on the periphery, or outer reaches, of the body. The carotid and femoral pulses are called ***central pulses*** because they can be felt in the central part of the body. Because they are larger vessels closer to the heart, the carotid and femoral pulses can be felt even when peripheral pulses are too weak to be felt.

pulse
the rhythmic beats caused as waves of blood move through and expand the arteries.

peripheral pulses
the radial, brachial, posterior tibial, and dorsalis pedis pulses, which can be felt at peripheral (outlying) points of the body.

central pulses
the carotid and femoral pulses, which can be felt in the central part of the body.

Blood Pressure

The force blood exerts against the walls of blood vessels is known as ***blood pressure***. Usually arterial blood pressure (pressure in an artery) is measured.

Each time the left ventricle of the heart contracts, it forces blood out into circulation. The pressure created in the arteries by this blood is called the ***systolic blood pressure***. When the left ventricle of the heart is relaxed and refilling, the pressure remaining in the arteries is called the ***diastolic blood pressure***. The systolic pressure is reported first, the diastolic second, as in "120 over 80," which is written as *120/80*.

blood pressure
the pressure caused by blood exerting force against the walls of blood vessels. Usually arterial blood pressure (the pressure in an artery) is measured. There are two parts: *diastolic blood pressure* and *systolic blood pressure*.

systolic (sis-TOL-ik) ***blood pressure***
the pressure created in the arteries when the left ventricle contracts and forces blood out into circulation.

diastolic (di-as-TOL-ik) ***blood pressure***
the pressure in the arteries when the left ventricle is refilling.

Perfusion

The movement of blood through the heart and blood vessels is called circulation. In healthy individuals, circulation is adequate—that is, there is enough blood within the system and there is a means to pump and deliver it to all parts of the body efficiently (Figure 6-12). The adequate supply of oxygen and nutrients to the cells of the body, with the removal of waste products, is called ***perfusion***.

Hypoperfusion (inadequate perfusion), also known as ***shock***, is a serious condition. With hypoperfusion, there is inadequate circulation of blood through one or more organs or structures. Blood is not reaching and filling all the capillary networks of the body, which means that oxygen will not be delivered to, and waste products will not be removed from, all the body's tissues. Hypoperfusion can lead to death. It is important to understand what hypoperfusion is, how it occurs, and how to recognize it. This will be discussed in more depth in the chapter titled *Bleeding and Shock*.

perfusion
the supply of oxygen and nutrients to and removal of wastes from the cells and tissues of the body as a result of the flow of blood through the capillaries.

hypoperfusion
inability of the body to adequately circulate blood to the body's cells to supply them with oxygen and nutrients. A life-threatening condition. Also called *shock*. *See also* perfusion.

shock
See *hypoperfusion*.

Life Support Chain

The respiratory system and the cardiovascular system together make up the *cardiopulmonary system*. The interaction of these two systems is essential to life.

Oxygen and glucose are necessary to the cells. Glucose is converted by the cells into energy in the form of adenosine triphosphate (ATP). Oxygen is a necessary component of this conversion process. When oxygen is present, glucose is converted in a process called *aerobic metabolism*. This process produces efficient amounts of energy and minimal waste products, such as carbon dioxide and water. If oxygen is not present in sufficient supply, the process will shift to *anaerobic metabolism*. This process produces less energy and more waste products, such as *lactic acid*. Waste products, in turn, make the body more acidotic. Acidosis injures the body's cells and limits the blood's ability to carry oxygen.

FIGURE 6-12 (A) The major arteries of the body.

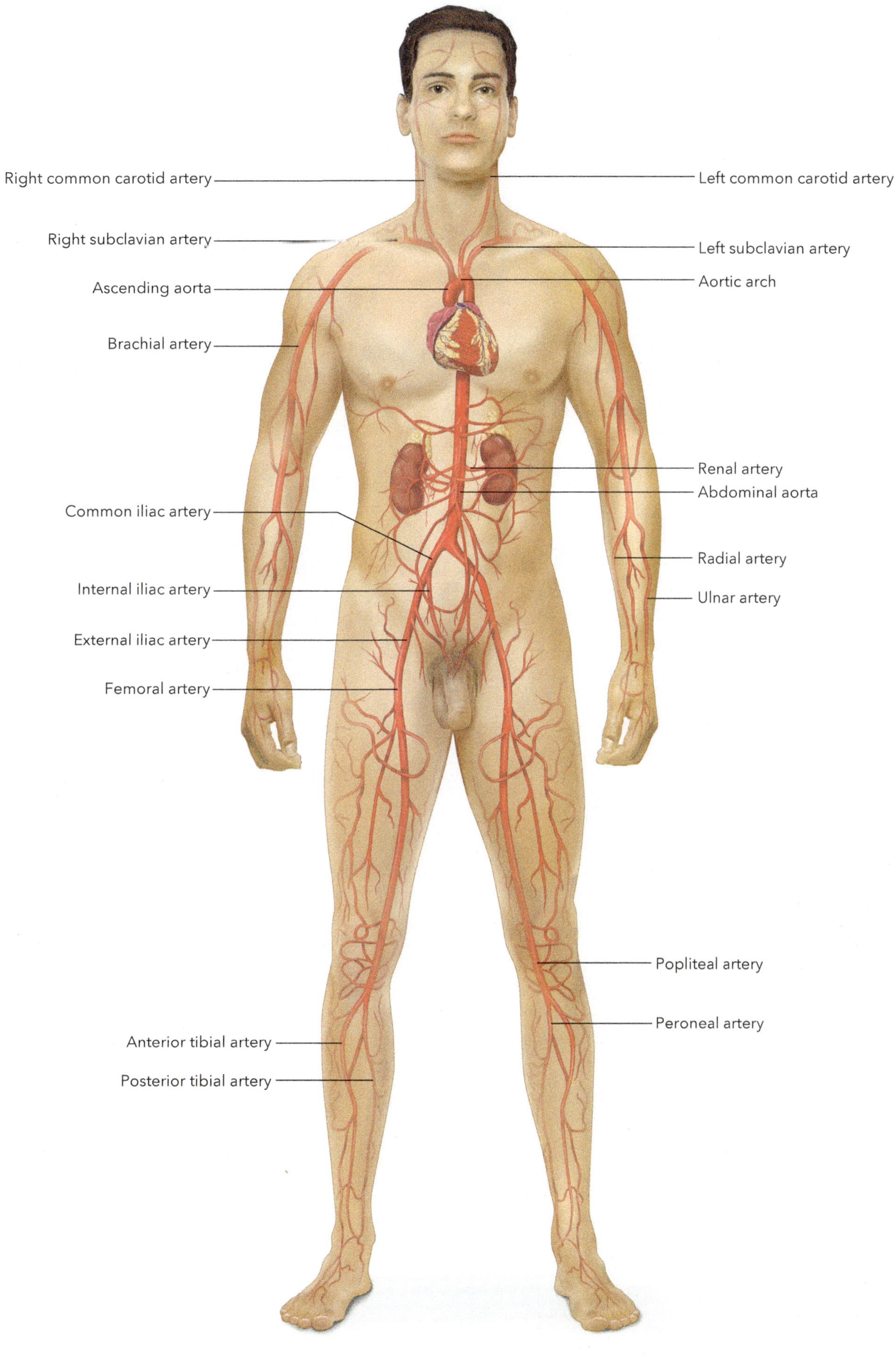

FIGURE 6-12 (B) The major veins of the body.

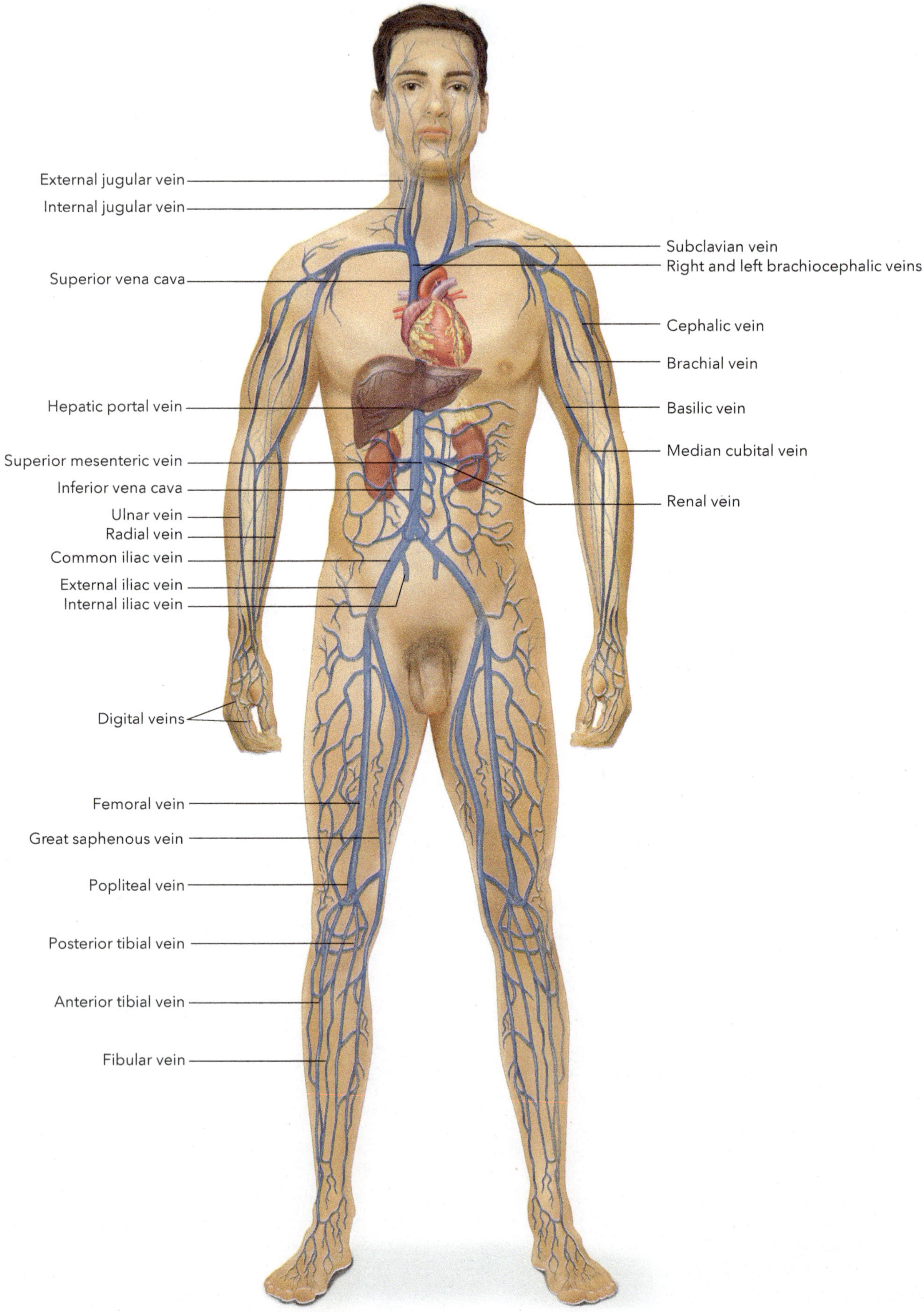

The movement of oxygen from the blood into the cells, coupled with the removal of waste products, is referred to as perfusion. As stated previously, perfusion is essential to normal cell function. Perfusion depends on the cardiopulmonary system, as described next.

In order for cells to be oxygenated and carbon dioxide to be removed, a variety of factors must be working properly. First and foremost, oxygen-containing air must be reaching the alveoli of the lungs and, once there, must be matched up with a sufficient supply of blood in the pulmonary capillaries. If, for example, air is obstructed from getting to the alveoli, as in a foreign body obstruction, gas exchange cannot occur. Similarly, if there is not enough blood passing through the pulmonary capillaries, as in the case of severe external bleeding, gas exchange cannot occur. This coupling of a sufficient amount of air with a sufficient amount of blood is called a ventilation perfusion match and abbreviated as a V/Q match.

Other elements are also critical to normal perfusion. The heart must pump effectively. If the pump fails, blood will not move. There must be sufficient oxygen in the air that is breathed. The blood must be capable of carrying enough oxygen to cells. (Anemia is a condition that reduces the number of oxygen-carrying red blood cells.) Furthermore, if the mechanics of respiration are disrupted, air will not move into and out of the lungs. All of these elements are critical to the process of perfusion.

There are other potential perfusion problems. To simplify things, consider anything that threatens the normal function of the cardiopulmonary system to be a threat to quality perfusion. Threats to perfusion will be discussed in greater detail in the chapter titled *Principles of Pathophysiology*.

Lymphatic System

The ***lymphatic system*** (Figure 6-13) is a collaboration of organs, tissues (nodes), thin-walled vessels, and fluids that are found throughout the entire body. One chief function of the lymphatic system is to capture fluid (called lymph) that escapes from cells and tissues and return it to the bloodstream. In this way, the lymphatic system functions to maintain a balance of fluids within the body. The associated lymphoid organs also have an immune function, producing lymphocytes and other white blood cells that fight infection. In fact, the lymphatic system is a critical part of the body's immune system.

lymphatic (lim-FAT-ik) ***system*** the system composed of organs, tissues, and vessels that helps to maintain the fluid balance of the body and contributes to the body's immune system.

Lymphoid organs include the adenoids, tonsils, spleen, and thymus. Some sources include the appendix as a lymphoid organ because of the density of lymph tissue found there. The lymphatic system also consists of lymph nodes that are normally soft and round or irregularly shaped. These nodes filter lymphatic fluid, removing bacteria and foreign cells as well as making lymphocytes and other infection-fighting cells. You may recall your physician feeling the lymph nodes in your neck. The physician was examining for enlargement and tenderness of the lymph nodes, which may be a sign of infection.

Women who have had a breast removed (total mastectomy) because of breast cancer will often be instructed not to allow a blood pressure to be taken on the arm on the same side as the mastectomy. This is because a mastectomy often includes removal of lymphatic tissue from the armpit area. The compression of an inflated blood pressure cuff on the upper arm can potentially damage the fragile remaining lymphatic tissue. As an EMT, you must avoid taking a blood pressure on the side of a woman's body where a mastectomy has been performed.

Nervous System

The ***nervous system*** (Figure 6-14) consists of the brain, spinal cord, and nerve tissue. It transmits impulses that govern sensation, movement, and thought. It also controls the body's voluntary and involuntary activity. It is subdivided into the central and peripheral nervous systems.

nervous system the system of brain, spinal cord, and nerves that governs sensation, movement, and thought.

The ***central nervous system (CNS)*** is composed of the brain and the spinal cord. The brain could be likened to a powerful computer that receives information from the body and, in turn, sends impulses to different areas of the body to respond to internal and external changes. The spinal cord rests within the spinal column and stretches from the brain to the lumbar vertebrae. Nerves branch from each part of the cord and reach throughout the body.

central nervous system (CNS) the brain and spinal cord.

FIGURE 6-13 The lymphatic system. *("The Lymphatic and Immune Systems Illustrated," from* Medical Terminology: A Living Language, *5E, by Bonnie F. Fremgen and Suzanne S. Frucht. Published by Pearson Education, Inc., © 2013.)*

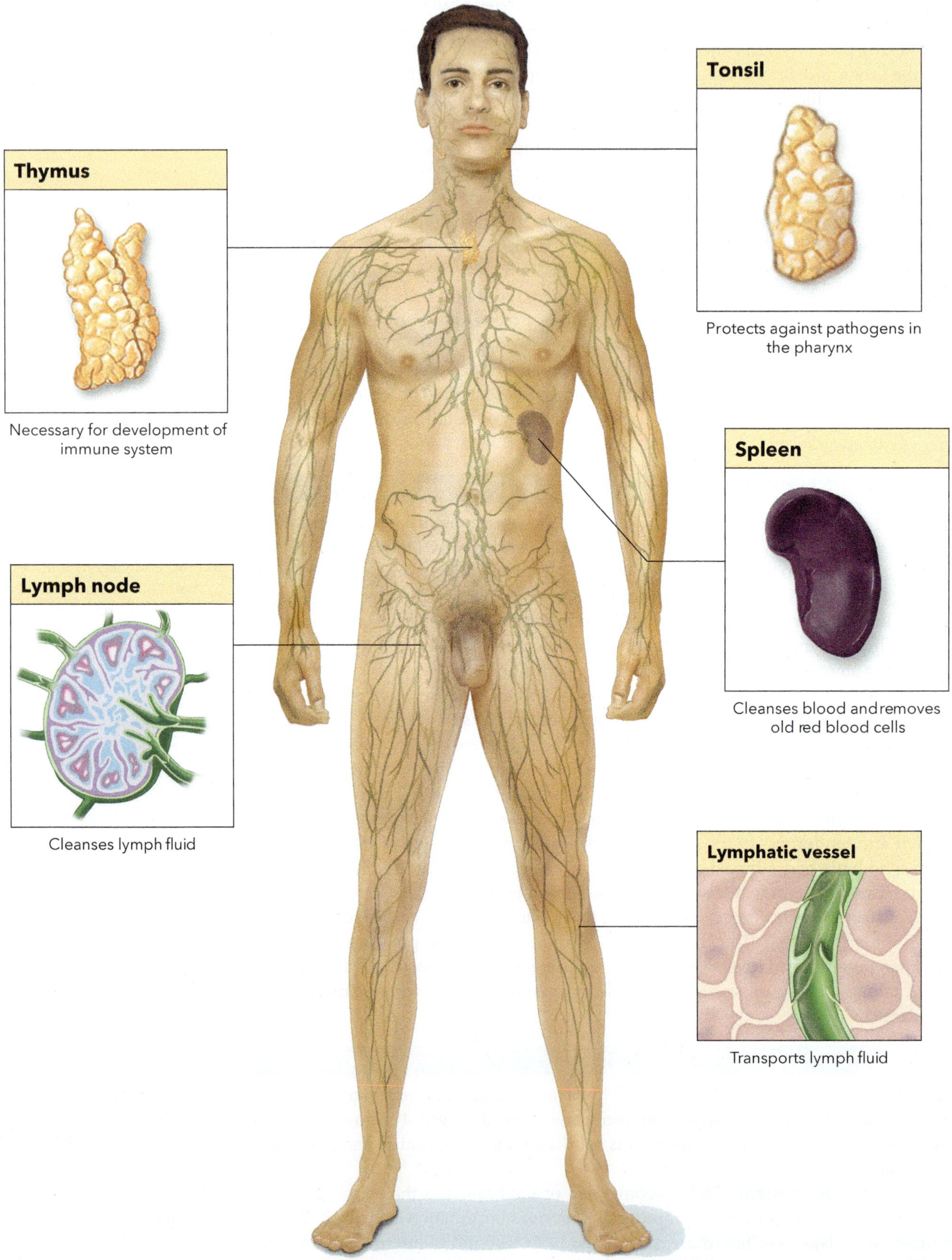

FIGURE 6-14 The nervous system.

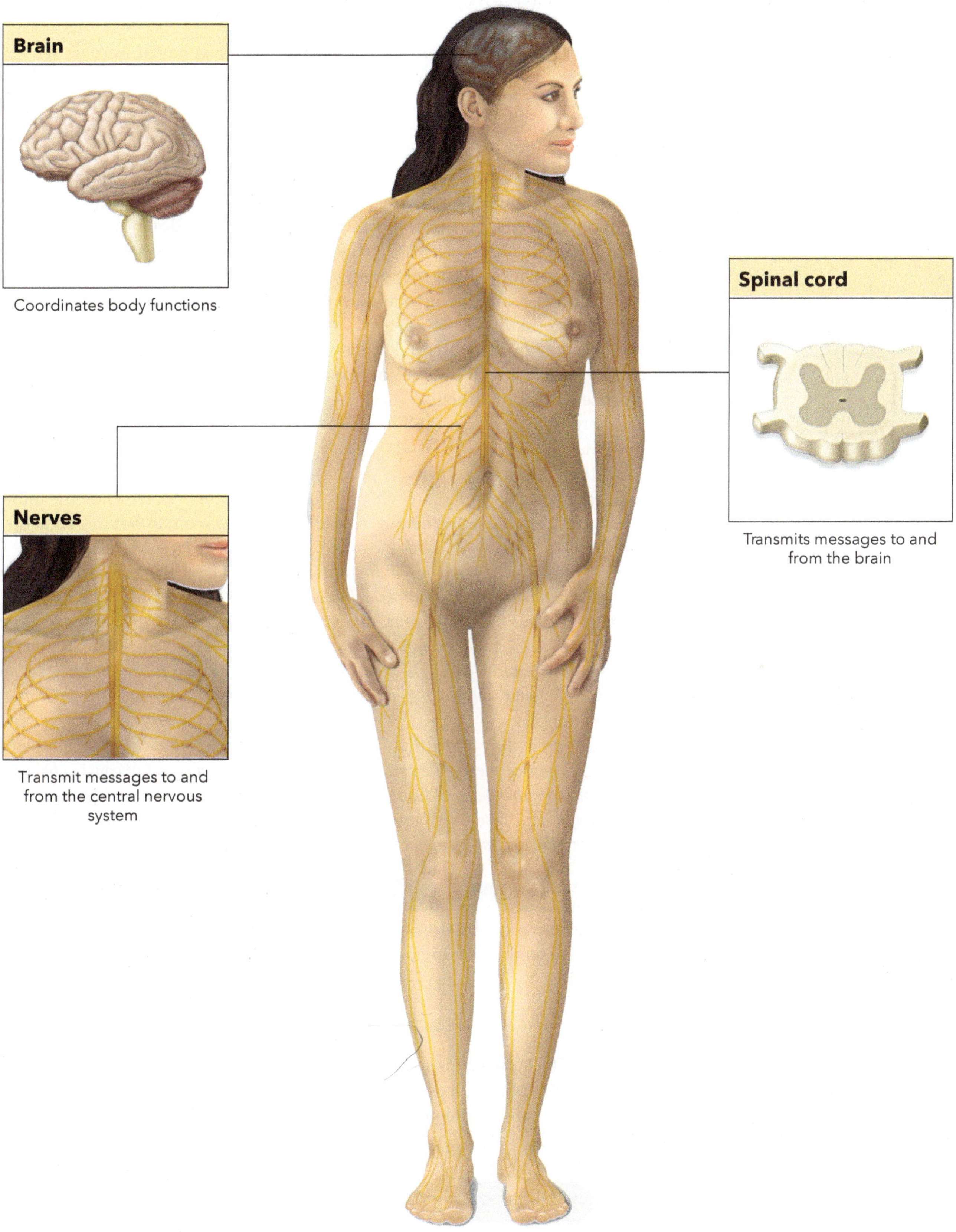

A key function of the central nervous system is consciousness. The reticular activating system is a series of nerve pathways in the brain and is essentially responsible for keeping a person awake.

peripheral nervous system (PNS)
the nerves that enter and leave the spinal cord and travel between the brain and organs without passing through the spinal cord.

autonomic (AW-to-NOM-ik) ***nervous system***
the division of the peripheral nervous system that controls involuntary motor functions.

The ***peripheral nervous system (PNS)*** consists of two types of nerves: sensory and motor. The sensory nerves pick up information from throughout the body and transmit it to the spinal cord and brain. If you touch something hot, your sensory nerves transmit this to the spinal cord and brain so immediate action may be taken. The motor nerves carry messages from the brain to the body.

The ***autonomic nervous system*** is the division of the peripheral nervous system that controls involuntary motor functions and affects such things as digestion and heart rate. The autonomic nervous system can be further broken down into the *sympathetic and parasympathetic nervous systems*. The sympathetic nervous system function is often referred to as the fight-or-flight response. This system is engaged when the body is in crisis. Stimulation of sympathetic tone causes the heart to beat faster, the lungs to breathe deeper, and the blood vessels to constrict. Imagine all the responses you might need if you had to run away from a potential threat. The *parasympathetic nervous system* asserts an opposite effect. It is engaged in times of relaxation and is often referred to as the feed-or-breed response. Parasympathetic tone causes increased blood flow to the digestive tract and to the reproductive organs. It also can cause the heart to slow down and the blood vessels to dilate.

Often a patient's sympathetic nervous system will be activated as the result of injury or illness. Recognizing its signs can help alert you to a problem even when the immediate cause is unknown. Let's use the example of a 72-year-old woman having an acute myocardial infarction.

Something very wrong is happening in this patient. A coronary artery is blocked, and her heart is not getting the oxygen supply it desperately needs. In most people this will cause chest pain, but in this case, no chest pain is present. This happens in quite a few patients, especially older women. The woman does, however, feel weak and nauseated. Despite the obscure symptoms, her body is reacting. Her brain engages the sympathetic nervous system to respond to the challenge. Her heart beats a bit faster, she breathes a bit more quickly. Her blood vessels constrict and divert blood away from the skin.

Although she is presenting atypically—that is, in an unusual fashion—your assessment reveals a few red flags. You notice she is pale and sweaty (diaphoretic as a result of constricted blood vessels). You also observe the elevated heart rate and respiratory rate. By noticing these signs, you recognize a "sympathetic discharge" and know that the body is responding to a serious problem. This may be more than an upset stomach.

digestive system
system by which food travels through the body and is digested or broken down into absorbable forms.

stomach
muscular sac between the esophagus and the small intestine where digestion of food begins.

small intestine
the muscular tube between the stomach and the large intestine, divided into the duodenum, the jejunum, and the ileum, that receives partially digested food from the stomach and continues digestion. Nutrients are absorbed by the body through its walls.

large intestine
the muscular tube that removes water from waste products received from the small intestine and moves anything not absorbed by the body toward excretion from the body.

Digestive System

The ***digestive system*** provides the mechanisms by which food travels through the body and is digested, or broken down into absorbable forms. Food enters the mouth and is broken down by both saliva and chewing. The food passes from the mouth through the oropharynx and into the esophagus, where it is transported to the stomach. Except for the mouth and the esophagus, all of the organs of digestion are contained in the abdominal cavity.

- **Stomach.** The ***stomach*** is a hollow organ that expands as it fills with food. In the stomach, acidic gastric juices begin to break food down into components that the body will be able to convert into energy.
- **Small intestine.** The ***small intestine*** is divided into three parts: the *duodenum*, the *jejunum*, and the *ileum*. This organ receives food from the stomach and continues to break it down for absorption. Nutrients are absorbed by the body through the wall of the small intestine.
- **Large intestine (colon).** The ***large intestine*** removes water from waste products as they move toward elimination from the body. Anything not absorbed from this point is moved through the colon and excreted as feces.

Several organs located outside of the stomach–intestines continuum assist in the food breakdown process.

- **Liver.** The ***liver*** produces bile, which is excreted into the small intestine to assist in the breakdown of fats. The liver has many additional functions, including detoxifying harmful substances, storing sugar, and assisting in production of blood products.
- **Gallbladder.** The ***gallbladder*** serves as a storage system for bile from the liver.
- **Pancreas.** Perhaps best known for production of the hormone insulin, which is involved in the regulation of sugar in the bloodstream, the ***pancreas*** also secretes juices that assist in breaking down proteins, carbohydrates, and fat.
- **Spleen.** Acting as a blood filtration system, the ***spleen*** filters out older blood cells. It has many blood vessels, and at any given time holds significant quantities of blood reserves the body can use in case of significant blood loss.
- **Appendix.** Located near the junction of the small and large intestines, the ***appendix*** is made up of lymphatic tissue. Its exact function is not well understood, but it is often considered part of the digestive system because an infected appendix (appendicitis) is a common cause of abdominal pain.

liver
the largest organ of the body, which produces bile to assist in breakdown of fats and assists in the metabolism of various substances in the body.

gallbladder
a sac on the underside of the liver that stores bile produced by the liver.

pancreas
a gland located behind the stomach that produces insulin and juices that assist in digestion of food in the duodenum of the small intestine. The pancreas also functions as part of the endocrine system.

spleen
an organ located in the left upper quadrant of the abdomen that acts as a blood filtration system and a reservoir for reserves of blood.

appendix
a small tube located near the junction of the small and large intestines in the right lower quadrant of the abdomen, the function of which is not well understood. Its inflammation, called appendicitis, is a common cause of abdominal pain.

Integumentary System

The integumentary system consists primarily of the skin. The ***skin*** performs a variety of functions, such as protection, water balance, temperature regulation, excretion, and shock absorption.

- **Protection.** The skin serves as a barrier to keep out microorganisms, debris, and unwanted chemicals. Underlying tissues and organs are protected from environmental contact. This helps preserve the chemical balance of body fluids and tissues.
- **Water balance.** The skin helps prevent water loss and stops environmental water from entering the body.
- **Temperature regulation.** Blood vessels in the skin can dilate (increase in diameter) to carry more blood to the skin, allowing heat to radiate from the body. When the body needs to conserve heat, these vessels constrict (decrease in diameter) to prevent heat loss. The sweat glands found in the skin produce perspiration, which will evaporate and help cool the body. The fat layer beneath the skin also serves as a thermal insulator.
- **Excretion.** Salts and excess water can be released through the skin.
- **Shock (impact) absorption.** The skin and its layers of fat help protect the underlying organs from minor impacts and pressures.

skin
the layer of tissue between the body and the external environment.

The skin has three major layers: the epidermis, dermis, and subcutaneous layers (Figure 6-15). The outer layer of the skin, the ***epidermis***, is composed of four layers (strata) everywhere except at the palms of the hands and soles of the feet. These two regions have five skin layers. The outermost layers of the epidermis are composed of dead cells, which are rubbed off or sloughed off and replaced. The pigment granules of the skin and living cells are found in the deeper layers. The cells of the innermost layer divide, replacing the dead cells of the outer layers. Note that the epidermis contains no blood vessels or nerves. Except for certain types of burns and injuries due to cold, injuries of the epidermis present few problems in EMT-level care.

epidermis (ep-i-DER-mis)
the outer layer of skin.

The layer of skin below the epidermis is the ***dermis***, which is rich with blood vessels, nerves, and specialized structures such as sweat glands, sebaceous (oil) glands, and hair follicles. Specialized nerve endings are also found in the dermis. They are involved with the sense of touch and reactions to cold, heat, and pain. Once the dermis is opened to the outside world, contamination and infection become major problems. These wounds can be serious, accompanied by profuse bleeding and intense pain.

dermis (DER-mis)
the inner (second) layer of skin, rich in blood vessels and nerves, found beneath the epidermis.

FIGURE 6-15 The layers of the skin.

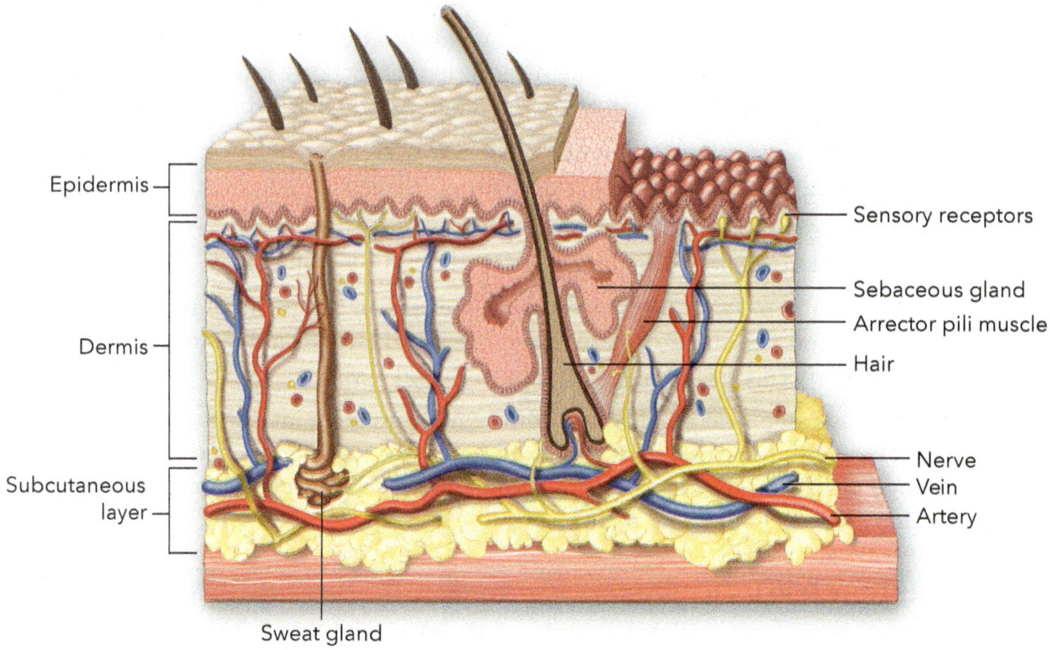

subcutaneous (SUB-ku-TAY-ne-us) ***layers***
the layers of fat and soft tissues found below the dermis.

endocrine (EN-do-krin) ***system***
system of glands that produce chemicals called hormones that help to regulate many body activities and functions.

insulin (IN-suh-lin)
a hormone produced by the pancreas or taken as a medication by many people with diabetes.

epinephrine (EP-uh-NEF-rin)
a hormone produced by the adrenal glands. As a medication, it dilates respiratory passages and is used to relieve severe allergic reactions.

renal system
the body system that regulates fluid balance and the filtration of blood. Also called the *urinary system*.

kidneys
organs of the renal system used to filter blood and regulate fluid levels in the body.

The layers of fat and soft tissue below the dermis make up the ***subcutaneous layers***. Shock absorption and insulation are major functions of this layer. Again, tissue and bloodstream contamination, bleeding, and pain are problems when these layers are injured or exposed.

Endocrine System

The ***endocrine system*** (Figure 6-16) produces chemicals called hormones that help to regulate many body activities and functions.

The pancreas is a key organ of the endocrine system. Among other functions, it secretes the hormone ***insulin***. Insulin is critical to the body's use of glucose, a sugar that fuels the body. (Insulin will be discussed in greater detail in the chapter titled *Diabetic Emergencies and Altered Mental Status*.)

The adrenal glands are also an essential component of the endocrine system. They secrete ***epinephrine*** (also known as adrenaline) and norepinephrine. These chemicals serve as neurotransmitters (chemical messengers) and engage the sympathetic nervous system through a series of chemical receptors located in specific organ systems. For example, when the fight-or-flight response is engaged, norepinephrine is released. It activates receptors in the lungs (called *beta 2 receptors*), which stimulate the bronchioles to dilate and therefore move more air. Receptors in the heart (called *beta 1 receptors*) are activated to increase the heart's rate and force of contraction.

Renal System

The ***renal system***, also called the *urinary system* (Figure 6-17), helps the body regulate fluid levels, filter chemicals, and adjust body pH. Fluid balance is essential to a healthy body. An average adult excretes roughly a liter and a half of urine per day. The renal system can adjust this fluid movement to account for changes in fluid intake or fluid loss such as bleeding.

The ***kidneys*** are the principal organs of the renal system. They help filter a waste product called urea from the blood and provide fluid balance by regulating the uptake of sodium and the excretion of urine. The kidneys also assist the buffer system with production of bicarbonate for the blood. Bicarbonate is an essential substance used to help regulate acidity or pH in the body.

FIGURE 6-16 The endocrine system

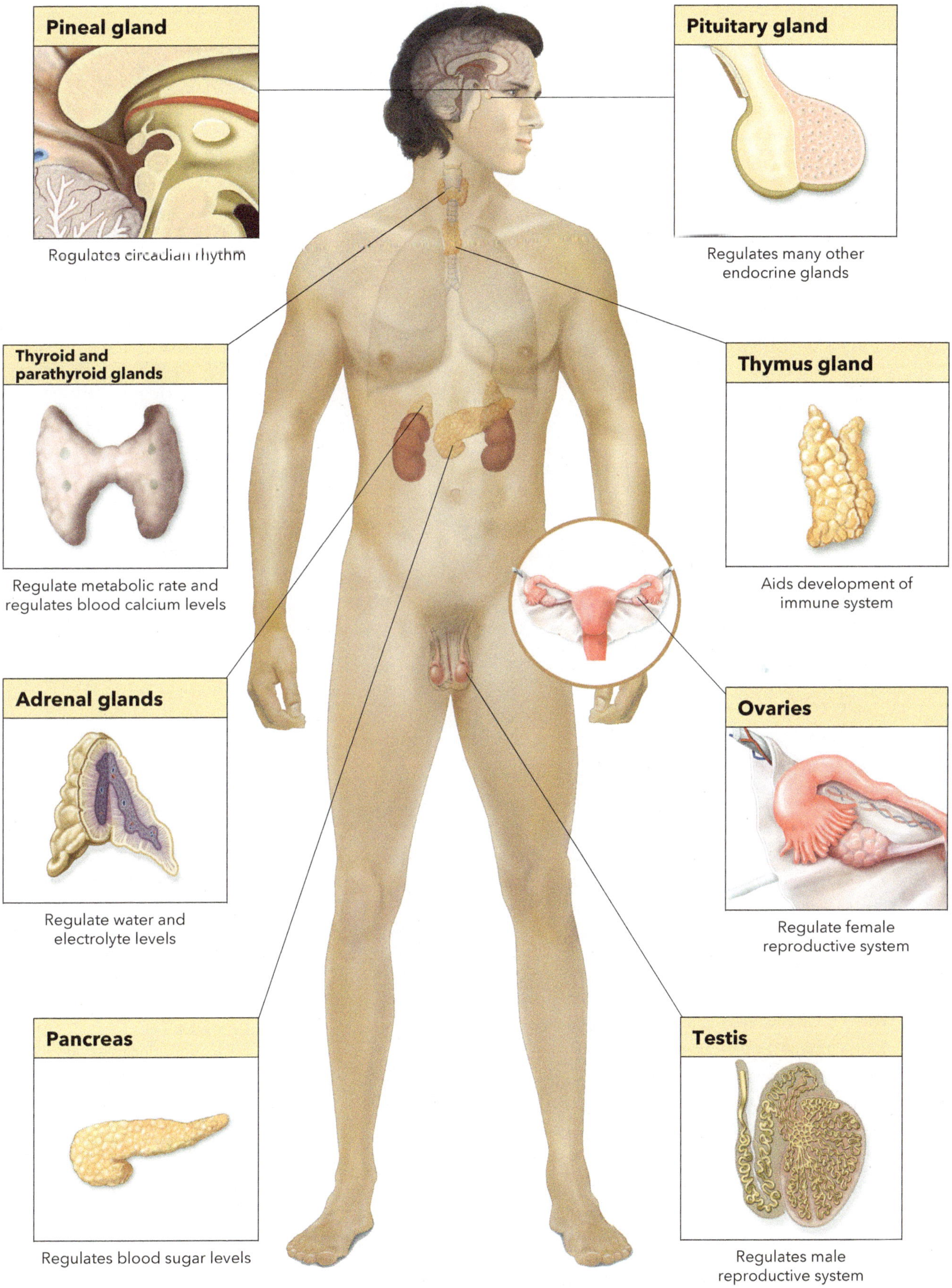

FIGURE 6-17 The renal/urinary system.

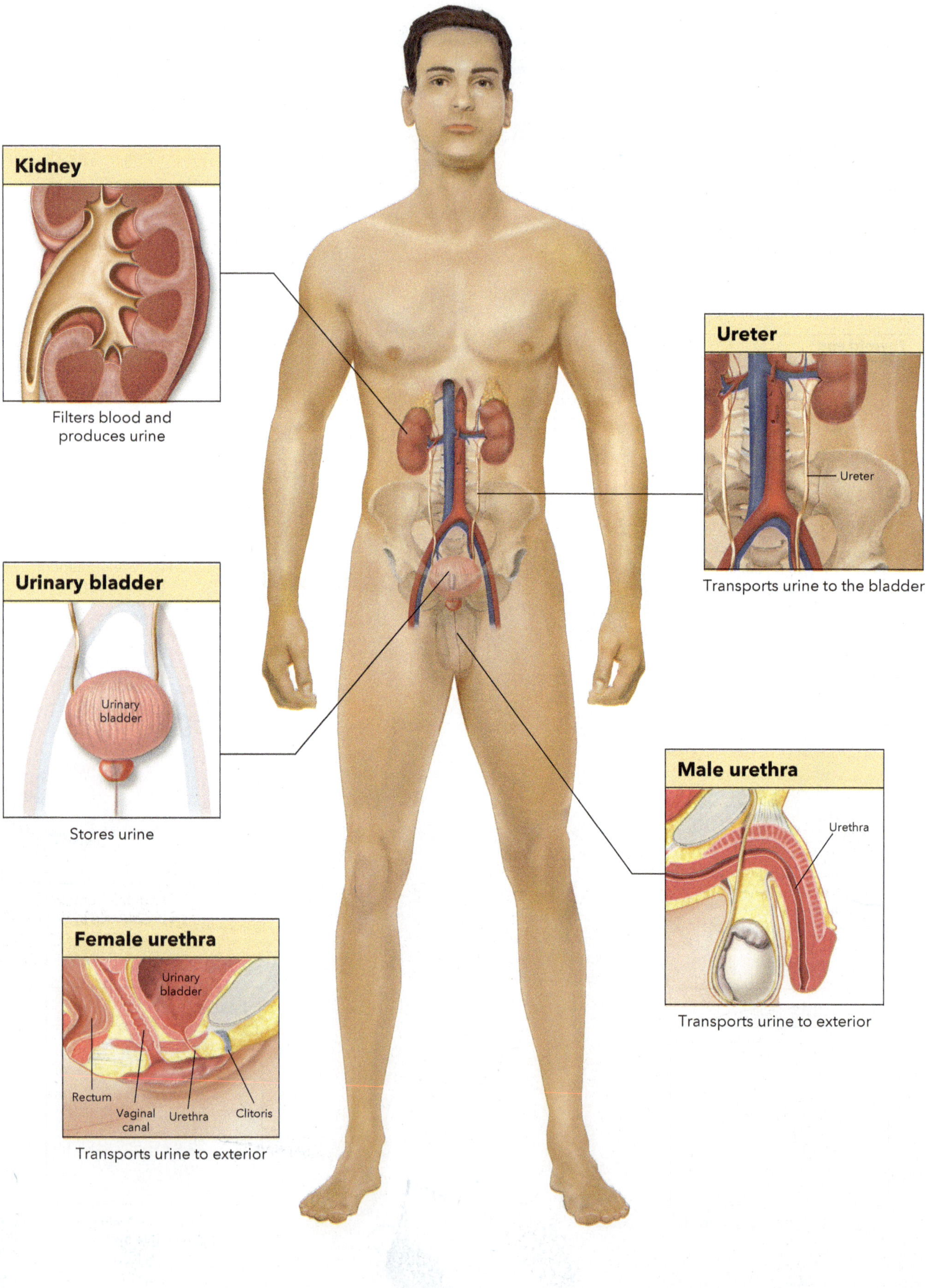

The renal system also includes the ***bladder*** and its connecting passages. The bladder is a round, hollow sac that serves as a fluid reservoir for urine. It receives urine from the kidneys via small tubes called ***ureters***. Urine is excreted from the bladder to the outside world through a tube called the ***urethra***. In males, the urethra passes through the penis. In females, the urethra is shorter and emerges from the body just above the vaginal opening.

Reproductive System

The ***reproductive system*** is a group of organs and glands designed for the specific purpose of reproduction. As you undoubtedly know, the reproductive systems of men and women vary greatly and contain different organs. The female reproductive system will be discussed in more detail in the *Obstetric and Gynecologic Emergencies* chapter.

Male Reproductive System

The primary organs of the male reproductive system (Figure 6-18A) are the testes and the penis. The ***testes*** produce sperm, the male component of reproduction, and are housed outside the body in the *scrotum*. The testes are connected to the penis through a small tube called the *epididymis*. The ***penis*** is the external reproductive organ of the male and is used for both sexual intercourse and urination.

Female Reproductive System

The primary organs of the female reproductive system (Figure 6-18B) are the ovaries, the uterus, and the vagina. The ***ovaries*** are located bilaterally in the lower quadrants of a female's abdomen and serve to develop and release ova (eggs) for reproduction. The ovaries are connected to the uterus via the *fallopian tubes*, also called the *oviducts*. The fallopian tubes are the site where sperm fertilizes the descending ovum. The ***uterus*** is a muscular organ located along the midline in the lower quadrants of a female abdomen. The uterus is designed to contain the developing fetus through the 40 weeks of pregnancy. Although it is a small organ, it has a huge potential to grow as pregnancy develops. It is also highly vascular and at times of pregnancy can be prone to serious bleeding. The uterus connects to the ***vagina***, or birth canal. The vagina serves not only as the exit route for the fetus but also as the female reproductive organ and site of sexual intercourse.

bladder
the round, saclike organ of the renal system used as a reservoir for urine.

ureters (YER-uh-terz)
the tubes connecting the kidneys to the bladder.

urethra (you-RE-thra)
tube connecting the bladder to the vagina or penis for excretion of urine.

reproductive system
the body system that is responsible for human reproduction.

testes (TES-tees)
the male organs of reproduction used for the production of sperm and hormones.

penis
the organ of male reproduction responsible for sexual intercourse and the transfer of sperm.

ovaries
egg- and hormone-producing organs within the female reproductive system.

uterus (YOU-ter-us)
female organ of reproduction used to house the developing fetus.

vagina (vuh-JI-na)
the female organ of reproduction used both for sexual intercourse and as an exit from the uterus for the fetus.

Think Like an EMT

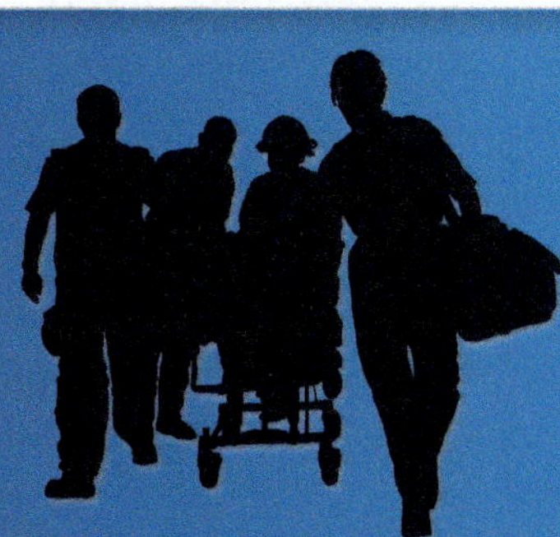

Identifying Possible Areas of Injury

Your knowledge of anatomy is a critical foundation for making solid clinical decisions in the field. For each of the patients in the following list, identify which organ or body system may be involved in that patient's complaint. This exercise requires no knowledge of diseases or conditions—just of the anatomy of the body.

1. Your patient falls in an icy parking lot. She tries to catch herself and breaks the bones of the arm just above the wrist. What are these bones called?
2. Your patient was the driver of a car that was hit in a "T-bone," or side-impact, crash. He was the driver. He complains of pain in the left upper abdominal quadrant. What solid organ is located in this area that can cause severe internal bleeding?
3. Your patient was riding a motorcycle and was thrown over the handlebars in a crash. She has broken the large bone in her right thigh. What bone is this, and would you expect blood loss from the fracture?

FIGURE 6-18(A) The male reproductive system.

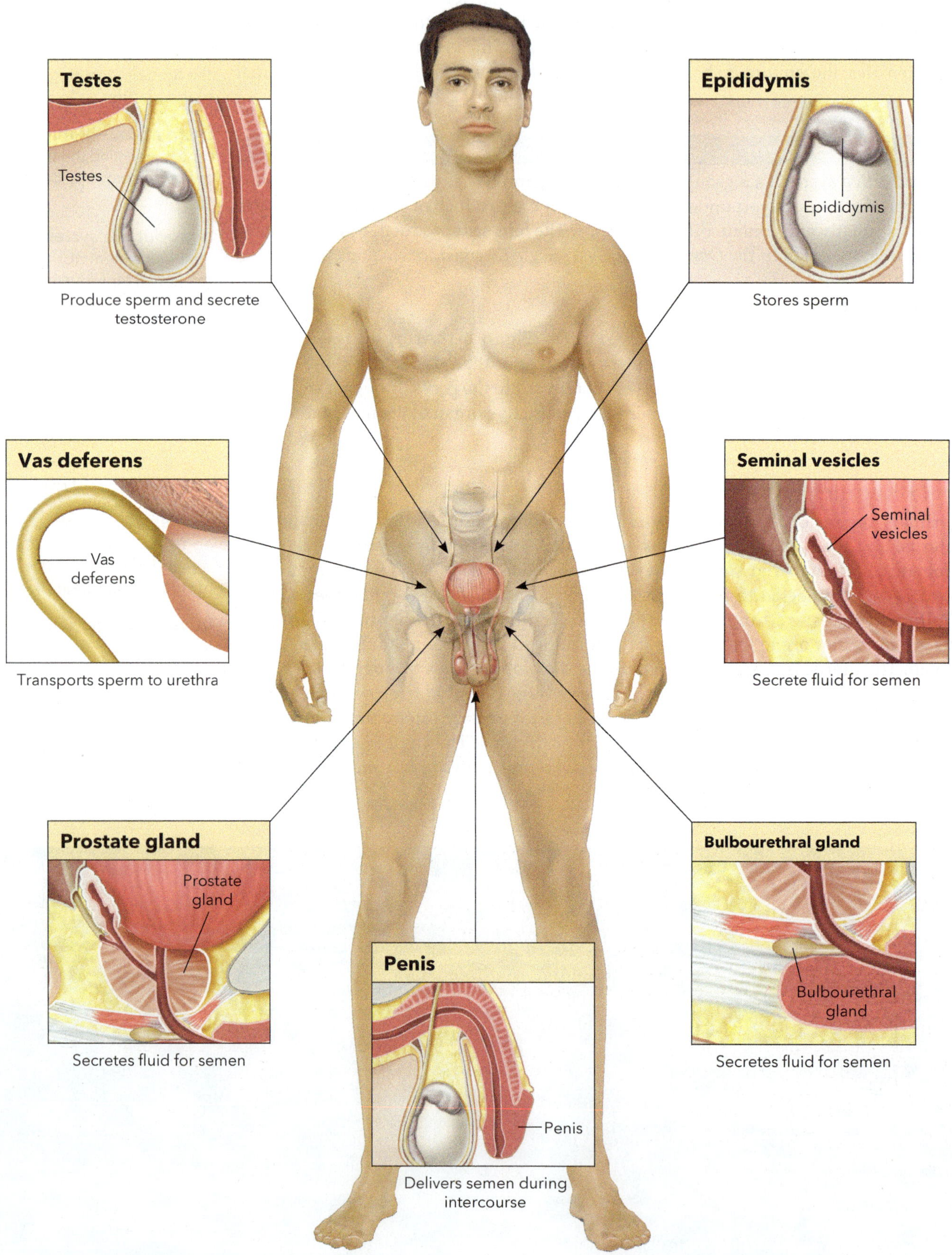

FIGURE 6-18(B) The female reproductive system.

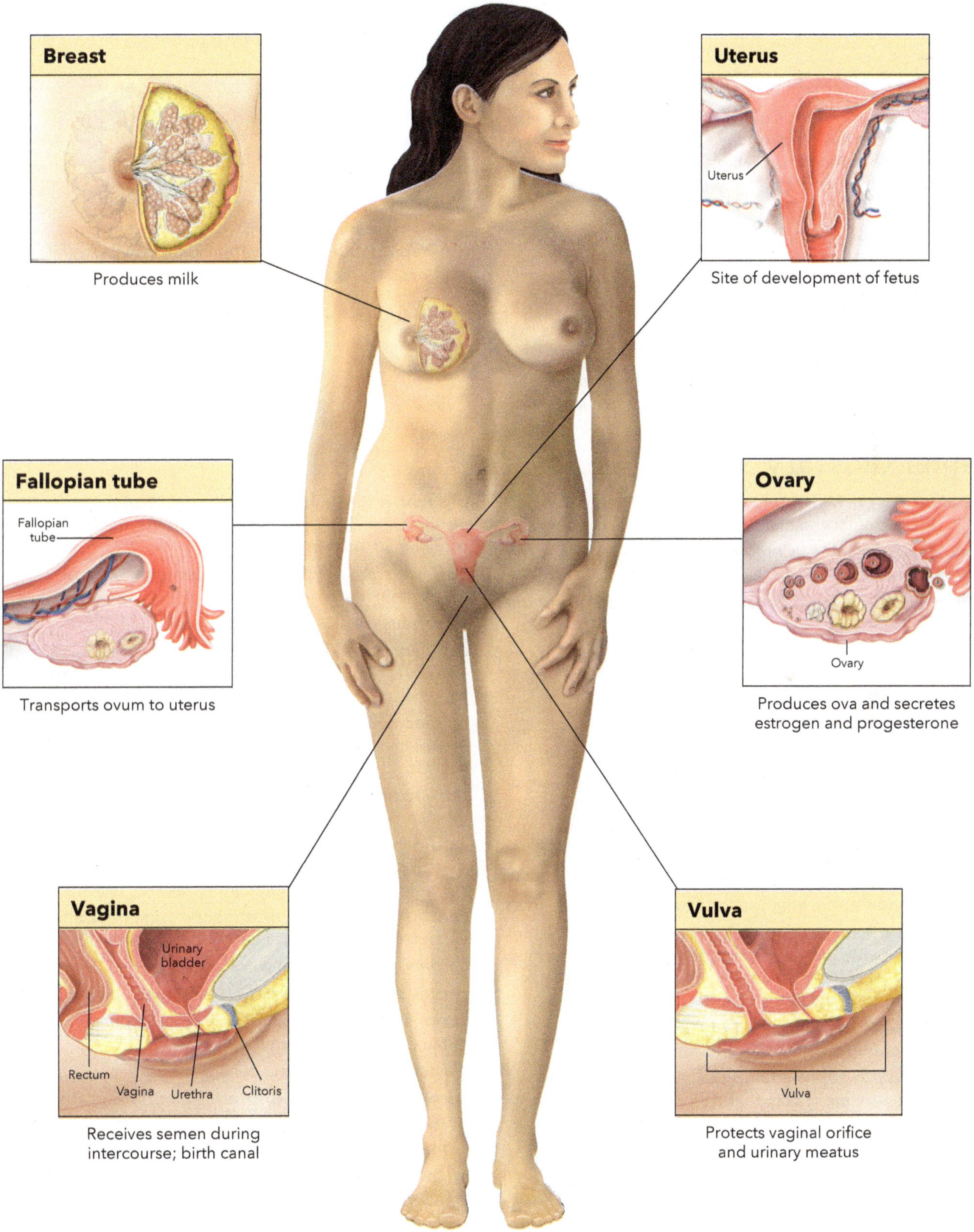

Chapter Review

Key Facts and Concepts

- As an EMT, your knowledge of the anatomy, or structure, and the functions, or physiology, of the body will be important in allowing you to assess your patient and communicate your findings accurately and efficiently to other EMS personnel and hospital staff.
- Major body systems with which you should be familiar:
  - Musculoskeletal system
  - Respiratory system
  - Cardiovascular system
  - Nervous system
  - Digestive system
  - Integumentary system
  - Endocrine system
  - Renal system
  - Reproductive systems (male and female)

Key Decisions

- Can I identify critical organs and structures that reside in an area where a patient has a complaint or traumatic injury?

Chapter Glossary

acetabulum (AS-uh-TAB-yuh-lum) the pelvic socket into which the ball at the proximal end of the femur fits to form the hip joint.

acromioclavicular (ah-KRO-me-o-klav-IK-yuh-ler) ***joint*** the joint where the acromion and the clavicle meet.

acromion (ah-KRO-me-on) ***process*** the highest portion of the shoulder.

alveoli (al-VE-o-li) the microscopic sacs of the lungs where gas exchange with the bloodstream takes place.

anatomy the study of body structure.

aorta (ay-OR-tah) the largest artery in the body. It transports blood from the left ventricle to begin systemic circulation.

appendix a small tube located near the junction of the small and large intestines in the right lower quadrant of the abdomen, the function of which is not well understood. Its inflammation, called appendicitis, is a common cause of abdominal pain.

arteriole (ar-TE-re-ol) the smallest kind of artery.

artery any blood vessel carrying blood away from the heart.

atria (AY-tree-ah) the two upper chambers of the heart. There is a right atrium (which receives unoxygenated blood returning from the body) and a left atrium (which receives oxygenated blood returning from the lungs). *Singular* atrium.

automaticity (AW-to-muh-TISS-it-e) the ability of the heart to generate and conduct electrical impulses on its own.

autonomic (AW-to-NOM-ik) ***nervous system*** the division of the peripheral nervous system that controls involuntary motor functions.

bladder the round, saclike organ of the renal system used as a reservoir for urine.

blood pressure the pressure caused by blood exerting force against the walls of blood vessels. Usually arterial blood pressure (the pressure in an artery) is measured. *See also* diastolic blood pressure; systolic blood pressure.

brachial artery artery of the upper arm; the site of the pulse checked during infant CPR.

bronchi (BRONG-ki) the two large sets of branches that come off the trachea and enter the lungs. There are right and left bronchi. *Singular* bronchus.

buffer system a system that helps manage the pH of the body to maintain it at a normal level.

calcaneus (kal-KAY-ne-us) the heel bone.

capillary (KAP-i-lair-e) a thin-walled, microscopic blood vessel where the oxygen/carbon dioxide and nutrient/waste exchange with the body's cells takes place.

cardiac conduction system a system of specialized muscle tissues that conducts electrical impulses that stimulate the heart to beat.

cardiac muscle specialized involuntary muscle found only in the heart.

cardiovascular (KAR-de-o-VAS-kyu-ler) ***system*** the system made up of the heart (cardio) and the blood vessels (vascular). Sometimes called the circulatory system.

carotid (kah-ROT-id) ***arteries*** the large neck arteries, one on each side of the neck, that carry blood from the heart to the head.

carpals (KAR-pulz) the wrist bones.

central nervous system (CNS) the brain and spinal cord.

central pulses the carotid and femoral pulses, which can be felt in the central part of the body.

clavicle (KLAV-i-kul) the collarbone.

coronary (KOR-o-nar-e) ***arteries*** blood vessels that supply the muscle of the heart (myocardium).

cranium the top, back, and sides of the skull.

cricoid (KRIK-oid) ***cartilage*** the ring-shaped structure that forms the lower portion of the larynx.

dermis (DER-mis) the inner (second) layer of skin, rich in blood vessels and nerves, found beneath the epidermis.

diaphragm (DI-uh-fram) the muscular structure that divides the chest cavity from the abdominal cavity; a major muscle of respiration.

diastolic (di-as-TOL-ik) ***blood pressure*** the pressure in the arteries when the left ventricle is refilling.

digestive system system by which food travels through the body and is digested, or broken down, into absorbable forms.

dorsalis pedis (dor-SAL-is PEED-is) ***artery*** artery supplying the foot, lateral to the large tendon of the big toe.

endocrine (EN-do-krin) ***system*** system of glands that produce chemicals called hormones that help to regulate many body activities and functions.

epidermis (ep-i-DER-mis) the outer layer of skin.

epiglottis (EP-i-GLOT-is) a leaf-shaped structure that prevents food and foreign matter from entering the trachea.

epinephrine (EP-uh-NEF-rin) a hormone produced by the body. As a medication, it dilates respiratory passages and is used to relieve severe allergic reactions.

exhalation (EX-huh-LAY-shun) a passive process in which the intercostal (rib) muscles and the diaphragm relax, causing the chest cavity to decrease in size and air to flow out of the lungs.

femoral (FEM-o-ral) ***artery*** the major artery supplying the leg.

femur (FEE-mer) the large bone of the thigh.

fibula (FIB-yuh-luh) the lateral and smaller bone of the lower leg.

gallbladder a sac on the underside of the liver that stores bile produced by the liver.

humerus (HYU-mer-us) the bone of the upper arm, between the shoulder and the elbow.

hypoperfusion inability of the body to adequately circulate blood to the body's cells to supply them with oxygen and nutrients; a life-threatening condition. Also called *shock*. *See also* perfusion.

ilium (IL-e-um) the superior and widest portion of the pelvis.

inhalation (IN-huh-LAY-shun) an active process in which the intercostal (rib) muscles and the diaphragm contract, expanding the size of the chest cavity and causing air to flow into the lungs.

insulin (IN-suh-lin) a hormone produced by the pancreas or taken as a medication by many diabetics.

involuntary muscle muscle that responds automatically to brain signals but cannot be consciously controlled.

ischium (ISH-e-um) the lower, posterior portions of the pelvis.

joint the point where two bones come together.

kidneys organs of the renal system used to filter blood and regulate fluid levels in the body.

large intestine the muscular tube that removes water from waste products received from the small intestine and moves anything not absorbed by the body toward excretion from the body.

larynx (LAIR-inks) the voice box.

ligament tissue that connects bone to bone.

liver the largest organ of the body, which produces bile to assist in breakdown of fats and assists in the metabolism of various substances in the body.

lungs the organs where exchange of atmospheric oxygen and waste carbon dioxide takes place.

lymphatic (lim-FAT-ik) ***system*** the system composed of organs, tissues, and vessels that helps to maintain the fluid balance of the body and contributes to the body's immune system.

malleolus (mal-E-o-lus) protrusion on the side of the ankle. The *lateral malleolus*, at the lower end of the fibula, is seen on the outer ankle; the *medial malleolus*, at the lower end of the tibia, is seen on the inner ankle.

mandible (MAN-di-bul) the lower jawbone.

manubrium (man-OO-bre-um) the superior portion of the sternum.

maxillae (mak-SIL-e) the two fused bones forming the upper jaw.

metacarpals (MET-uh-KAR-pulz) the hand bones.

metatarsals (MET-uh-TAR-sulz) the foot bones.

muscle tissue that can contract to allow movement of a body part.

musculoskeletal (MUS-kyu-lo-SKEL-e-tal) ***system*** the system of bones and skeletal muscles that support and protect the body and permit movement.

nasal (NAY-zul) ***bones*** the nose bones.

nasopharynx (NAY-zo-FAIR-inks) the area directly posterior to the nose.

nervous system the system of brain, spinal cord, and nerves that governs sensation, movement, and thought.

orbits the bony structures around the eyes; the eye sockets.

oropharynx (OR-o-FAIR-inks) the area directly posterior to the mouth.

ovaries egg-producing organs within the female reproductive system.

pancreas a gland located behind the stomach that produces insulin and juices that assist in digestion of food in the duodenum of the small intestine.

patella (pah-TEL-uh) the kneecap.

pelvis the basin-shaped bony structure that supports the spine and is the point of proximal attachment for the lower extremities.

penis the organ of male reproduction responsible for sexual intercourse and the transfer of sperm.

perfusion the supply of oxygen to and removal of wastes from the cells and tissues of the body as a result of the flow of blood through the capillaries.

peripheral nervous system (PNS) the nerves that enter and leave the spinal cord and travel between the brain and organs without passing through the spinal cord.

peripheral pulses the radial, brachial, posterior tibial, and dorsalis pedis pulses, which can be felt at peripheral (outlying) points of the body.

phalanges (fuh-LAN-jiz) the toe bones and finger bones.

pharynx (FAIR-inks) the area directly posterior to the mouth and nose. It is made up of the oropharynx and the nasopharynx.

physiology the study of body function.

plasma (PLAZ-mah) the fluid portion of the blood.

platelets components of the blood; membrane-enclosed fragments of specialized cells.

posterior tibial (TIB-ee-ul) ***artery*** artery supplying the foot, behind the medial ankle.

pubis (PYOO-bis) the medial anterior portion of the pelvis.

pulmonary (PUL-mo-nar-e) ***arteries*** the vessels that carry deoxygenated blood from the right ventricle of the heart to the lungs.

pulmonary veins the vessels that carry oxygenated blood from the lungs to the left atrium of the heart.

pulse the rhythmic beats caused as waves of blood move through and expand the arteries.

radial artery artery of the lower arm; the artery felt when taking the pulse at the thumb side of the wrist.

radius (RAY-de-us) the lateral bone of the forearm.

red blood cells components of the blood. They carry oxygen to and carbon dioxide away from the cells.

renal system the body system that regulates fluid balance and the filtration of blood. Also called the *urinary system*.

reproductive system the body system that is responsible for human reproduction.

respiration the process of moving oxygen and carbon dioxide between circulating blood and the cells.

respiratory (RES-pir-ah-tor-e) ***system*** the system of nose, mouth, throat, lungs, and muscles that brings oxygen into the body and expels carbon dioxide.

scapula (SKAP-yuh-luh) the shoulder blade.

shock *See* hypoperfusion.

skeleton the bones of the body.

skin the layer of tissue between the body and the external environment.

skull the bony structure of the head.

small intestine the muscular tube between the stomach and the large intestine, divided into the duodenum, the jejunum, and the ileum, that receives partially digested food from the stomach and continues digestion. Nutrients are absorbed by the body through its walls.

spleen an organ located in the left upper quadrant of the abdomen that acts as a blood filtration system and a reservoir for reserves of blood.

sternum (STER-num) the breastbone.

stomach muscular sac between the esophagus and the small intestine where digestion of food begins.

subcutaneous (SUB-ku-TAY-ne-us) ***layers*** the layers of fat and soft tissues found below the dermis.

systolic (sis-TOL-ik) ***blood pressure*** the pressure created in the arteries when the left ventricle contracts and forces blood out into circulation.

tarsals (TAR-sulz) the ankle bones.

tendon tissue that connects muscle to bone.

testes (TES-tees) the male organs of reproduction used for the production of sperm.

thorax (THOR-ax) the chest.

thyroid (THI-roid) ***cartilage*** the wing-shaped plate of cartilage that sits anterior to the larynx and forms the Adam's apple.

tibia (TIB-e-uh) the medial and larger bone of the lower leg.

torso the trunk of the body; the body without the head and the extremities.

trachea (TRAY-ke-uh) the "windpipe"; the structure that connects the pharynx to the lungs.

ulna (UL-nah) the medial bone of the forearm.

ureters (YER-uh-terz) the tubes connecting the kidneys to the bladder.

urethra (you-RE-thra) tube connecting the bladder to the vagina or penis for excretion of urine.

uterus (YOU-ter-us) female organ of reproduction used to house the developing fetus.

vagina (vu-JI-na) the female organ of reproduction used for both sexual intercourse and as an exit from the uterus for the fetus.

valve a structure that opens and closes to permit the flow of a fluid in only one direction.

vein any blood vessel returning blood to the heart.

venae cavae (VE-ne KA-ve) the superior vena cava and the inferior vena cava. These two major veins return blood from the body to the right atrium. *Singular* vena cava.

ventilation the process of moving gases (oxygen and carbon dioxide) between inhaled air and the pulmonary circulation of blood.

ventricles (VEN-tri-kulz) the two lower chambers of the heart. There is a right ventricle (which sends oxygen-poor blood to the lungs) and a left ventricle (which sends oxygen-rich blood to the body).

venule (VEN-yul) the smallest kind of vein.

vertebrae (VER-te-bray) the 33 bones of the spinal column.

voluntary muscle muscle that can be consciously controlled.

white blood cells components of the blood. They produce substances that help the body fight infection.

xiphoid (ZIF-oid) ***process*** the inferior portion of the sternum (breastbone).

zygomatic (ZI-go-MAT-ik) ***arches*** bones that form the structure of the cheeks.

Preparation for Your Examination and Practice

Short Answer

1. List the three functions of the musculoskeletal system.
2. Name the five divisions of the spine and describe the location of each.
3. Describe the physical processes of inhalation and exhalation.
4. List four places a peripheral pulse may be felt.
5. Describe the central nervous system and peripheral nervous system.
6. List three functions of the skin.

Thinking and Linking

Linking your knowledge of medical terminology with anatomy not only will help you better understand body systems but will provide practice for better understanding some compound terms. Identify the following organs and structures, and list their associated body system.

The hepatic vein
The pulmonic valve
The gallbladder
The coronary arteries
The renal artery
The esophagus
The aorta

Critical Thinking Exercises

Understanding anatomy and physiology is one thing, but applying it to patient care is another. Use the lessons of this chapter to apply anatomic structure to the injuries described below. Use the locations of key organs to predict the likely damage that has been inflicted.

- A 31-year-old male was involved in a shooting. You arrive to find him lying on the ground unconscious. After ensuring a patent airway and adequate breathing, you visualize his chest and abdomen and observe three penetrating wounds. The first wound is found at the nipple line at the intersection of the midclavicular line. The second wound is found just below the rib cage in the upper right abdominal quadrant. The third wound is found in the center of the left upper quadrant of the abdomen. All three penetrations have corresponding exit wounds on the posterior side of the patient. Use your knowledge of anatomy to describe the organs and organ systems that are likely involved with these three wounds.

Street Scenes

"Respond to Elm Street near the intersection of Central Avenue for a report of a motor-vehicle crash. Third-party call from a passerby on a cell phone. The time is now 1505 hours." Your response time is relatively fast, and you arrive before the dispatcher can provide any additional information. As you approach the scene, you see that two vehicles are involved in the crash. It appears a truck rear-ended a four-door sedan. A police officer on-scene has already taken charge of traffic control. You ask him, "How many patients?" He replies, "Three." You find an open area to place the ambulance. Once assured that the scene is safe, you begin your assessment.

The driver of the truck is walking around the scene. The other vehicle had two occupants—a mother and her son, who was belted in the backseat. The mother is tending to the child, who appears to be unresponsive. It doesn't look as if the impact speed was great, but the child hit his head fairly hard on the headrest and you can still see the dent. An Emergency Medical Response unit is also on-scene, and they tell you they will check on the driver of the truck. You turn your attention to the child.

The mother tells you she is fine. "Just take care of Peter. He's only six years old." You get into the vehicle next to the child and hear that he has snoring respirations. You remember that the tongue is the most likely cause, so provide manual cervical spine motion restriction to the head and neck to help minimize any further injury to his head and cervical spine that may be present. As you do so, you push Peter's jaw forward to move the tongue in the direction of the mandible. The maneuver works and the snoring sound stops. Your partner prepares for extrication of the child to the backboard.

Street Scene Questions

1. As you assess your young patient, how does his anatomy impact the process?
2. What should you be alert to when examining the child's abdomen?

Before rotating Peter onto the backboard, you apply a cervical collar. Then you rotate him onto the board. Remembering that a child's head is larger in proportion to the rest of the body than an adult's, you place a folded towel under Peter's shoulders in order to keep his head in a neutral position with the airway open. Your partner calls out to Peter to see if his mental status has changed. Peter responds to painful stimuli only.

Once Peter has been moved into the ambulance, you perform a head-to-toe exam. When you get to the abdomen, you palpate all four quadrants and observe a bruise, probably caused by the lap portion of the seat belt. Peter reacts as if in pain when you touch the left upper quadrant, and you think that his spleen may have been injured.

En route to the hospital, you find the patient is breathing at a rate of 32 and has a pulse of 150. You call out to Peter, and this time he responds to your voice.

Street Scene Questions

3. What are the significant findings based on the assessment and your knowledge of the human body?
4. Do you have any concerns about additional injuries to this patient? If so, what are they?

You take another set of vital signs and find that Peter has an increase in pulse and respiration rates. You perform a reassessment and find there is still pain in the left upper quadrant of the abdomen. As you run your hands over the patient's back, you are concerned by his apparent pain in the lumbar region of the spine, which may have been caused by the force of the crash.

Your partner tells you the ETA to the hospital is 10 minutes and notifies emergency department personnel by radio. The transmission gives an overview of the injuries and the vital signs, noting the change in the last 10 minutes. He mentions how the patient's mental status has changed and describes the abdominal and lumbar pain and location.

While the patient is being wheeled into the trauma room, the staff do a quick assessment and check the abdomen. The emergency department physician tells you that because of assessment findings given in the radio report, she has a surgeon on the way to check Peter.

"You did good!" she adds.

7 Principles of Pathophysiology

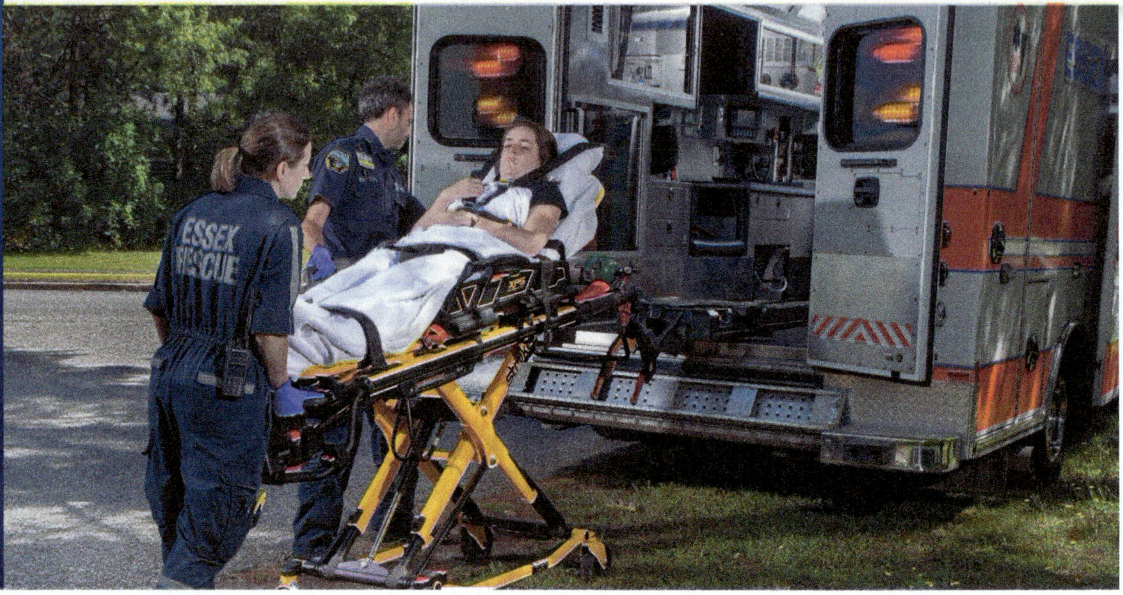

Related Chapters

The following chapters provide additional information related to topics discussed in this chapter:

Standard

Pathophysiology

Competency

Uses fundamental knowledge of the pathophysiology of respiration and perfusion for patient assessment and management.

Core Concepts

- The cell, cellular metabolism, and results of the alteration of cellular metabolism
- The cardiopulmonary system and its combined respiratory and cardiovascular functions

- The respiratory system and the importance of oxygenation and ventilation
- The cardiovascular system and the movement of blood
- The principles of perfusion, hypoperfusion, and shock
- Disrupted physiology of major body systems

Outcomes

After reading this chapter, you should be able to:

7.1 Summarize the structures and functions of body cells. (pp. 157–159)

- Describe the influence of water on cells.
- Describe the role of glucose in cells.

7.2 Summarize the coordinated processes required of the cardiopulmonary system to maintain perfusion. (pp. 159–174)

- Contrast the processes of aerobic and anaerobic metabolism in cells.
- Relate the composition of air with the demands of the cardiopulmonary system.
- Distinguish between the processes of ventilation, respiration, and perfusion.
- Identify the structures of the airway.
- Explain the impact on the body of changes in the tidal volume, minute volume, and dead air space.
- Explain circumstances that lead to respiratory dysfunction.
- Describe the mechanism by which the body attempts to compensate for disruptions of respiration.
- Describe the functions of the various components of blood.
- Describe the consequences of reduction of blood volume, red blood cells, and water-retaining proteins.
- Distinguish the functions of arteries, veins, and capillaries.
- Outline the process of gas (oxygen and carbon dioxide) exchange in the body.
- Explain how the nervous system can correct low and high blood pressure.
- Given a change in the balance of sympathetic and parasympathetic components of the nervous system, predict the impact on heart function.
- Analyze how loss of blood vessel tone, increased permeability, and increased systemic vascular resistance affect blood pressure.
- Illustrate the interaction of stroke volume, cardiac preload, cardiac contractility, and cardiac output.
- Predict the consequences of mechanical and electrical dysfunctions of the heart.
- Explain the concept of V/Q (ventilation-perfusion) match.

7.3 Summarize the pathophysiology of shock. (pp. 174–176)

- Describe the mechanism which underlies all forms of shock.
- Contrast hypovolemic, distributive, cardiogenic, and obstructive shock.
- Given descriptions of patient presentations, categorize them as being in either compensated or decompensated shock.

7.4 Summarize fluid balance in the body. (pp. 176–178)

- Recall the distribution of water throughout the spaces of the body.
- Explain the distribution of water throughout the spaces of the body.
- Identify the structures that regulate fluid distribution throughout the spaces of the body.
- Describe disruptions of fluid balance.

7.5 Give a synopsis of general concepts of nervous system dysfunction. (p. 179)

- Explain how trauma can result in nervous system dysfunction.
- Explain how medical problems can result in nervous system dysfunction.
- Given a scenario, predict whether a patient has nervous system dysfunction.

7.6 Describe the mechanism by which the endocrine system contributes to control of body functions. (p. 180)

- Recall the structures primarily at the root of endocrine dysfunction.
- Explain the general categories of endocrine disorders.

7.7 Describe the relationship between perfusion and the gastrointestinal system. (p. 180)

- Describe the anatomy that can contribute to the severity of gastrointestinal bleeding.
- Recall potential causes of nausea and vomiting.
- Describe the consequences of ongoing loss of blood or fluid through the gastrointestinal tract.

7.8 Summarize the mechanism by which a response by the immune system can lead to shock. (p. 181)

- Give examples of types of substances that may provoke a hypersensitivity reaction.
- Compare normal immune response to foreign substances with allergic reactions.
- Describe the impact on body tissues of excess release of histamine.

Key Terms

aerobic metabolism, *159*
anaerobic metabolism, *159*
cardiac output, *173*
chemoreceptors, *165*
dead air space, *164*
dehydration, *178*
diaphoresis, *175*
edema, *178*
electrolyte, *159*
FiO_2, *163*
hydrostatic pressure, *169*
hypersensitivity, *181*
hypoperfusion, *174*
metabolism, *159*
minute volume, *164*
patent, *163*
pathophysiology, *157*
perfusion, *174*
plasma oncotic pressure, *168*
shock, *175*
stretch receptors, *170*
stroke volume, *173*
systemic vascular resistance (SVR), *172*
tidal volume, *164*
V/Q match, *174*

Officer Walker did not hear the first gunshots. His mind was in pure reaction mode as a man emerged from the back room with a pistol. Walker saw the muzzle flashes as he and his partner drew their weapons and returned fire. Years of training replaced momentary panic and, in an instant, the gunfight was over. The assailant was down and the threat was neutralized. That's when Officer Walker realized that he had been shot.

The first bullet entered Walker's shoulder just to the right of his body armor. The second struck him in the right leg just below his groin. He reached down and felt the blood. When he took a breath, he coughed and felt pain in his chest. He felt his heart race. Officer Walker knew he was in trouble.

The body is an amazing system. Its capacity to adapt to its environment and its ability to overcome challenges are seemingly limitless. Even with the most extreme injuries, such as the situation detailed above, the systems of the body immediately collaborate in an elaborate effort to adjust to the insult and to preserve life. To take on even the simplest challenges, the body has a few core requirements.

To fuel its most basic functions and to respond to life-threatening challenges, the body requires a balance of glucose, oxygen, and water. Every day, dozens of body systems work together to provide feedback and make adjustments to ensure that each of these elements is in its proper proportion. When threatened with major challenges, such as blood loss or inadequate oxygen supply, the body systems work together to recognize the threat and take immediate corrective action. These adjustments the body makes to correct imbalances—known as *compensation*—create a steady-state environment—called *homeostasis*—that allows the body to grow, heal, and carry out the normal functions necessary to live life.

This delicate balancing act is not a simple process. Compensation relies on a constant supply of energy, an energy demand that increases when the body faces its most difficult challenges. Energy creation requires a consistent delivery of nutrients and oxygen to the body's cells. Without a steady and adequate supply of oxygen and nutrients, energy production fails. When injury or disease interferes with energy production, the body cannot compensate for imbalances, and when the body cannot compensate, cells, organs, and organ systems die.

Understanding the body's quest for homeostasis and recognizing compensation are fundamental to the practice of excellent medical care. When we understand these basic concepts, we can readily identify problems and, more importantly, support the body's efforts to stay alive. To support the body's compensation efforts, we first have to recognize that compensation is happening. Fortunately, compensation commonly produces telltale signs that can be recognized with thorough patient assessment. These warning signs allow the astute EMT to identify the onset of specific problems and anticipate declines in body function. Well-prepared EMTs will use the signs of compensation as guideposts toward the most appropriate treatment steps.

Pathophysiology is the study of how disease processes affect the function of the body. It is an essential foundation for almost every problem discussed within this text. You will use pathophysiology to understand how a particular challenge affects the body's most essential functions and how the body will react to an injury or illness in an effort to restore those necessary functions. Although pathophysiology may be a very broad concept now, as you learn more about specific disorders and injuries, core concepts will emerge and begin to make more sense. More importantly, you will find consistent patterns among these concepts that cross over and apply among very different body challenges. As a result, pathophysiology will help you simplify otherwise complex disorders. By the time you have progressed to the end of your course, you should see how an understanding of pathophysiology will not only help you identify changes that are occurring in your patient

pathophysiology (path-o-fiz-e-OL-o-je) the study of how disease processes affect the function of the body.

as a result of illness or injury but also help you recognize the needs of the body in its most vulnerable state, needs that you can help to fill by providing knowledgeable care for your patient.

NOTE: *Throughout this chapter, we attempt to simplify topics that are just not simple. We do not attempt to cover every aspect of human pathophysiology but rather provide a basic understanding of its most important principles. Covering all the topics pertaining to pathophysiology in this short chapter would be both impossible and beyond the scope of the EMT.*

Maintaining professionalism requires you, the EMT, to undergo constant self-improvement and to obtain ongoing education beyond your EMT course. There are many available informative resources and courses in pathophysiology. Learning more will make you a better provider.

The Cell

CORE CONCEPT

The cell, cellular metabolism, and results of the alteration of cellular metabolism

The basic building block of the body is the cell. A normal cell incorporates a series of structures designed to accomplish specific functions. These structures occupy the space within a cell and are surrounded by a *cell membrane* that protects and selectively allows water and other substances into and out of the cell (Figure 7-1).

Although some types of cells, such as cardiac muscle cells, are specialized to serve specific purposes, some important components and functions are common to most cells. For example, the cell nucleus contains DNA, the genetic blueprint for cellular reproduction, and the endoplasmic reticulum plays a key role in synthesizing proteins. Energy for the cell is produced largely by the mitochondria, the structures that are responsible for the conversion of glucose and other nutrients into energy in the form of *adenosine triphosphate (ATP)*. ATP, essentially the cell's internally created fuel, is responsible for powering all the other cellular functions. Without ATP, many of the cell's specialized structures cannot function. For example, without ATP, a specialized mechanism called the *sodium potassium pump* cannot actively move ions back and forth across the cell

FIGURE 7-1 The cell.

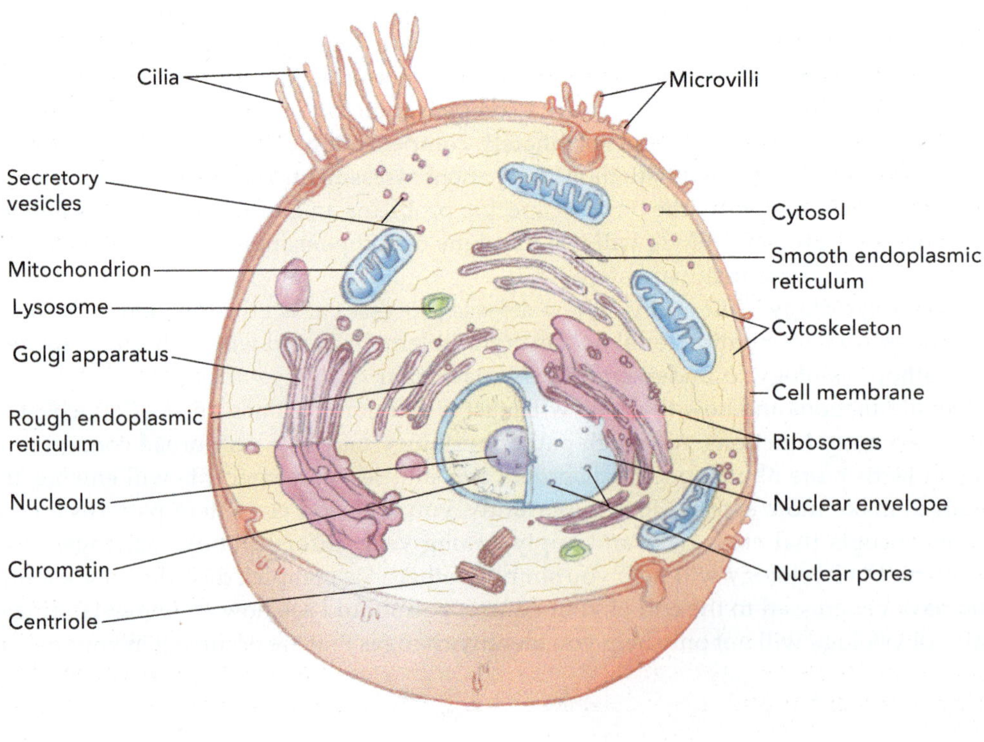

membrane. This movement of ions is responsible for generating an electrical charge to cause depolarization, which is the stimulus for muscle contraction, including contractions of the heart. The conversion of glucose into ATP is an essential process of ***metabolism***.

The most essential functions of cells rely on some basic requirements, principally water, glucose, and oxygen.

Water and the Cell

A cell needs the correct balance of water between its inside and its outside. Water moves into a cell from the environment around the cell. Without enough water, the cell will dehydrate and die. By contrast, too much water will interrupt basic cellular function. Water levels also influence the concentrations of important chemicals called ***electrolytes***. Electrolytes are substances that, when dissolved in water, separate into charged particles. The movements of these charged particles enable the electrical functions of cells, such as nerve transmission and cardiac muscle depolarization. Important electrolytes in the body include potassium, sodium, and magnesium.

Levels of water in the body are controlled by the circulatory and renal systems, and the proper function of these systems maintains a balance to provide cells a healthy environment. Absorption and elimination of water not only provide balance to the cells but also affect the body as a whole.

Glucose and the Cell

Glucose, a simple sugar obtained from the foods we eat, is the basic nutrient of the cell. It is the building block for energy in the form of ATP. During metabolism, glucose is broken down inside the cell and combined with oxygen to create energy that is used to perform cellular functions. Without glucose, normal energy production within the cell and normal cell function cease. Most of the body's cells require the presence of insulin in the blood to help move glucose from the blood into the cells. Therefore, a consistent supply of insulin must match the body's glucose requirements and be present to ensure that the energy needs of the cells are met.

Levels of glucose and insulin in the body are controlled by the digestive and endocrine systems.

Oxygen and the Cell

Healthy metabolism requires oxygen. Oxygen is used by the cell to metabolize glucose into energy. When oxygen enters the cell in the correct quantity, metabolism is very efficient and yields a high quantity of energy in the form of ATP. This oxygen-supplied process also produces heat and helps regulate body temperature. Metabolism that occurs in the presence of sufficient oxygen is called ***aerobic metabolism*** (Figure 7-2A). All cellular metabolism produces waste products, including carbon dioxide and hydrogen ions, which cause the body to form acids. Aerobic metabolism produces energy with a minimal amount of waste products, which are easily managed and removed by the body.

Anaerobic metabolism occurs when glucose is metabolized without oxygen, or without enough oxygen. In this situation, energy is produced inefficiently and in a much smaller quantity compared with aerobic metabolism (Figure 7-2B). In fact, aerobic metabolism yields roughly 16 times more energy than anaerobic metabolism. Without oxygen, metabolism also produces many more waste products. Excess carbon dioxide is produced, and hydrogen ions are released and create lactic acid. Resulting hypothermia can affect blood clotting and many other essential body functions.

With anaerobic metabolism, the body must shift energy to the removal of waste products. Carbon dioxide is typically removed by exhaling. When the level of carbon dioxide is too high, the body adapts by increasing the respiratory rate to increase the rate of carbon dioxide elimination. Acid in the body is converted into more carbon dioxide and water and, again, the body must expend energy to remove these by-products. Waste products also have other harmful effects. High levels of acid in the body affect the oxygen-carrying

"When you understand how things work on the inside, you'll understand better what you see on the outside."

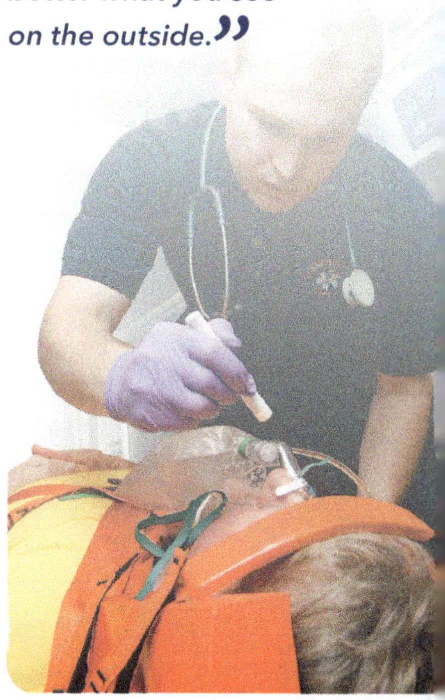

(© Daniel Limmer)

metabolism (meh-TAB-o-lizm) the cellular function of converting nutrients into energy.

electrolyte (e-LEK-tro-lite) a substance that, when dissolved in water, separates into charged particles.

aerobic (air-O-bik) ***metabolism*** the cellular process in which oxygen is used to metabolize glucose. Energy is produced in an efficient manner, with minimal waste products.

anaerobic (AN-air-o-bik) ***metabolism*** the cellular process in which glucose is metabolized into energy without oxygen. Energy is produced in an inefficient manner, with many waste products.

FIGURE 7-2 (A) Aerobic metabolism. Glucose broken down in the presence of oxygen produces a large amount of energy (ATP). (B) Anaerobic metabolism. Glucose broken down without the presence of oxygen produces acidic by-products and only a small amount of energy (ATP).

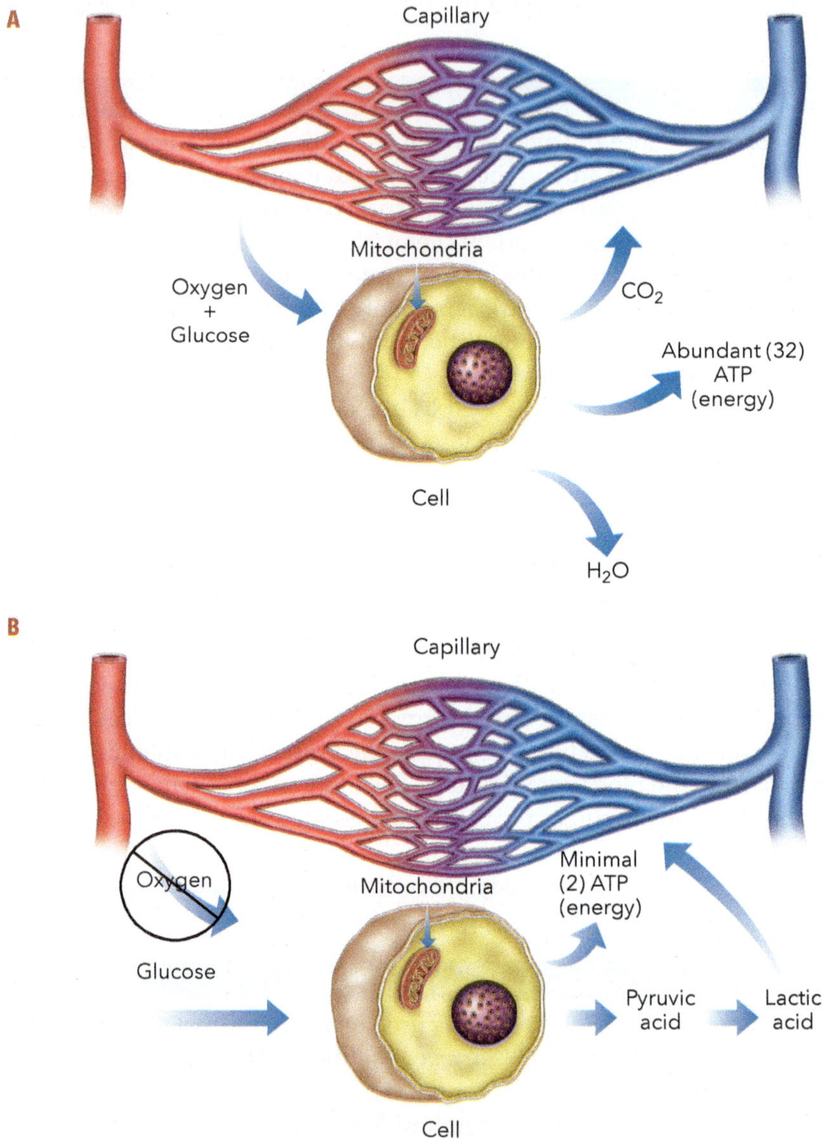

molecules in the blood, called hemoglobin. Hemoglobin's attraction to oxygen is diminished in acidotic states. As a result, less oxygen can be transported by the blood, making it even more difficult to oxygenate tissues. The result is a downward spiral of events in which lack of oxygen creates an acidotic state, decreasing the ability of the blood to carry oxygen to the cells and causing an even more severe acidotic state.

As these discussions of aerobic and anaerobic metabolism make clear, the levels of oxygen and carbon dioxide in the body are controlled by the respiratory and cardiovascular systems. To summarize: The oxygen necessary for aerobic metabolism is supplied by the respiratory system and carried to the cells by the cardiovascular system. To provide adequate quantities of oxygen, inhaled air must reach the alveoli of the lungs, and blood must reach the capillaries that surround the alveoli. The process of *diffusion* moves oxygen across the thin membrane from the alveoli to the capillaries. Within the capillaries, the oxygen is loaded onto the hemoglobin in the blood for transport to the cells. The cardiovascular and respiratory systems also facilitate removal of the waste products of cellular metabolism. Carbon dioxide follows an opposite pathway to oxygen, being transferred from the cells to the blood in the adjacent capillaries, then being off-loaded from the capillaries into the alveoli of the lungs by a similar process of diffusion, then being exhaled. The removal of carbon dioxide also helps regulate acid levels in the body.

Officer Walker slumps to the ground as his partner radios for help. He can see the pool of blood forming on the ground and he recognizes he is having a hard time breathing. The bullet that entered his shoulder has collapsed his lung, and the damage has significantly impaired his gas exchange. He is becoming hypoxic.

At a cellular level, changes are occurring in Officer Walker's body. Red blood cells are flowing rapidly out of the cardiovascular system and spilling onto the ground. Although his respiratory system is working hard to deliver air to his alveoli, the collapsed lung has minimized the amount of lung tissue available for gas exchange. The remaining red blood cells delivered to the lungs find little oxygen available. The blood delivered to Officer Walker's cells becomes low in oxygen. Aerobic metabolism can no longer be supported. Large numbers of Walker's cells shift to anaerobic metabolism. Carbon dioxide and acids begin to build up. Heat production is impaired. Officer Walker's ability to produce ATP is failing.

The Vulnerability of Cells, Organs, and Organ Systems

The cell membrane is a vulnerable element of the cell. Many disease processes alter its *permeability*, or its ability to effectively transfer fluids, electrolytes, and other substances in and out of the cell. An ineffective cell membrane can allow substances into the cell that should not be there (such as toxins) and interfere with the regulation of water.

Thus far we have been discussing the structure and function of one cell. Remember, however, that many cells work together to form organs and organ systems, and just as a single cell's function can be disturbed by illness or injury, so can the function of an entire organ system.

The Regulation of Homeostasis

Homeostasis is regulated in the brain and is maintained through a delicate balance of nervous system feedback and messaging. Key brain structures, such as the hypothalamus and the medulla oblongata, receive sensory input and recognize challenges such as increasing carbon dioxide levels, hypoxia, and blood loss. It is in these structures that compensation begins.

When challenges are recognized, the brain and spinal cord signal the body to make the appropriate adjustments. Once again, the nervous system is essential to transmitting these messages to the distal areas of the body. Chemical messages, regulated by the endocrine system, are also key to enacting compensatory changes.

The Fight or Flight Response

Hormones and the endocrine system will be discussed in further detail in *Respiratory Emergencies*. However, understanding the basic principles of the sympathetic nervous system is important to any discussion on compensation.

The central nervous system can be divided into two basic categories. The parasympathetic nervous system controls "feed or breed" functions. Here chemical messengers called *neurotransmitters* regulate functions such as digestion and reproduction. The parasympathetic nervous system dominates when the body is at rest, and is typically responsible for slowing down the heart and reducing blood pressure. Conversely, the sympathetic nervous system responds in "fight or flight" situations and has evolved over time to offer protection in times of danger (Figure 7-3). Neurotransmitters such as epinephrine (sometimes called adrenaline) and norepinephrine are produced by the adrenal glands and secreted out to enhance the body's ability to protect itself. These neurotransmitters play a vital role in compensation.

Epinephrine and norepinephrine cause bronchial tubes in the lungs to dilate, enabling better gas exchange. They cause the heart to pump harder and faster, thereby increasing

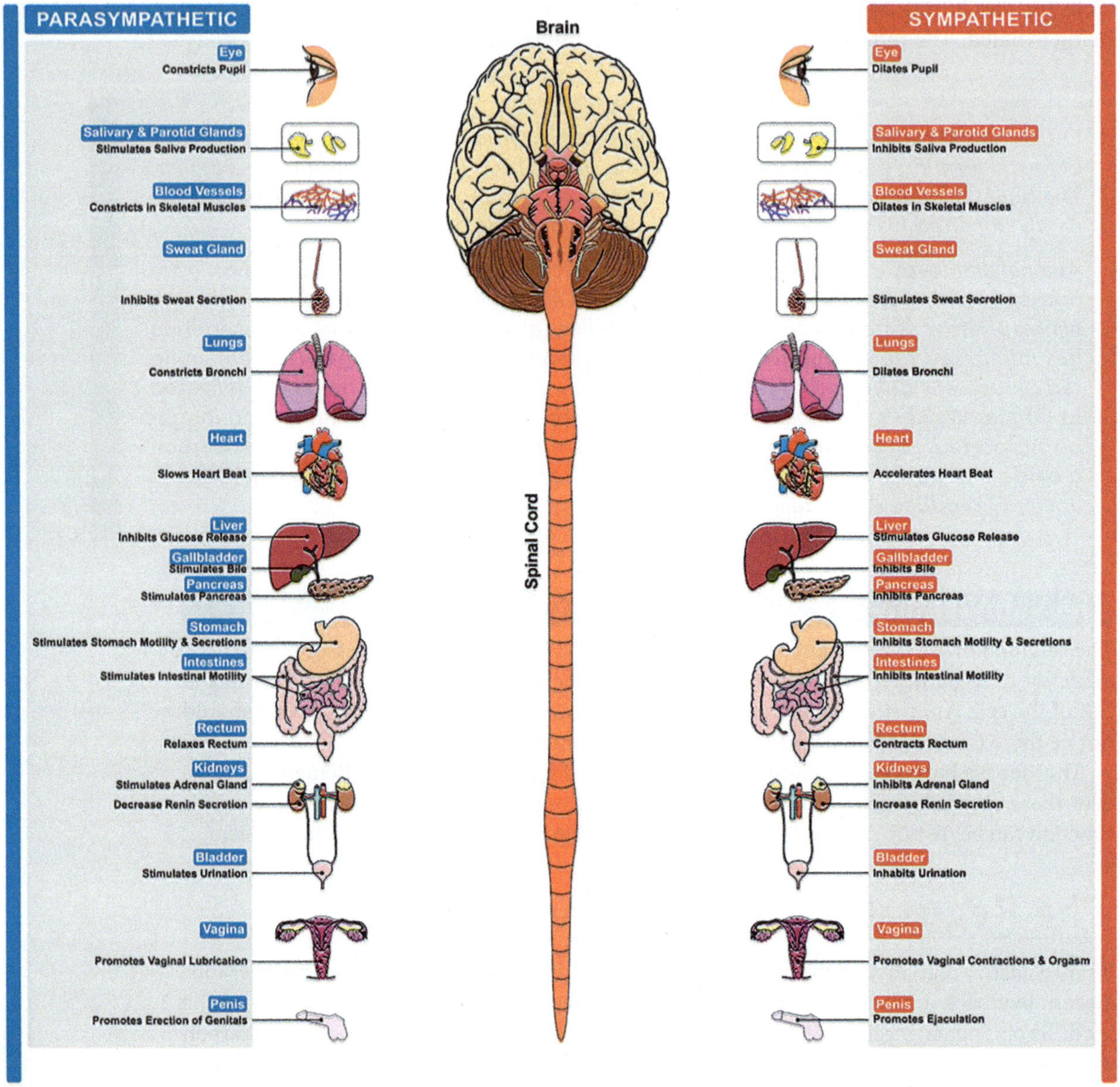

FIGURE 7-3 The autonomic nervous system. *(udaix/ Shutterstock.)*

blood flow to skeletal muscle and vital organs. Finally, epinephrine and norepinephrine have potent effects on the circulatory system, causing blood vessels to constrict. These effects have profound impact with regard to compensation but can also become problems themselves if the body fails to regulate them properly. Certain conditions and medications can limit the body's production of epinephrine and norepinephrine and alter the ability to mount sympathetic responses. Without sufficient quantities of these important neurotransmitters or of the hormones that signal their release, parasympathetic effects can dominate. For example, a condition such as Addison's disease can cause a state of adrenal insufficiency in which the body essentially lacks sympathetic response. The net result can be crisis states of vasodilation and shock. Poorly regulated sympathetic response can also affect the body's ability to compensate for injury. Many patients take medications that regulate or block the effects of the sympathetic nervous system. For example, beta blockers are a classification of medication that reduces the effects of epinephrine and norepinephrine on the body. Many people take these medications to help regulate high blood pressure, but their presence can impair compensation in times of need.

CORE CONCEPT

The cardiopulmonary system and its combined respiratory and cardiovascular functions

The Cardiopulmonary System

Air goes in, air goes out, and blood goes round and round. This is an old saying in EMS, referring to the proper function of the respiratory system and the cardiovascular system.

The functions and effects of these two systems are so intertwined that they are often referred to as a single system: the *cardiopulmonary system.* That old saying is an oversimplification of a complicated process, but it sums up the importance of some of the body's most basic—cardiopulmonary—functions.

We have already noted that cells need oxygen for the efficient production of energy. As humans, we obtain oxygen from the air we breathe. Typically, inhaled air contains mostly nitrogen (79 percent) but also oxygen (21 percent). The concentration of oxygen in the air we breathe in is referred to as the fraction of inspired oxygen, or ***FiO_2***. The lungs (pulmonary system), heart, blood vessels, and the blood itself (cardiovascular system) work in concert to deliver oxygen and nutrients to the cells and to remove waste products from the cells. These basic operations rely on the coordinated movements of blood and air. Interruption of any part of this balance results in a compromise to, or even a failure of, the system. (See *Visual Guide: Ventilation, Respiration, and Perfusion.*)

FiO_2
fraction of inspired oxygen; the concentration of oxygen in the air we breathe.

The Airway

CORE CONCEPT
The respiratory system and the importance of oxygenation and ventilation

The respiratory system begins at the airway. The airway is made up of the structures from the mouth and nose to the alveoli of the lungs. Air follows a path from the openings of the mouth and nose into the pharynx and/or nasopharynx, travels to the rear of the throat (or hypopharynx), then enters the larynx, below which the trachea begins. Air travels down the trachea to the point where it branches into two large tubes called the mainstem bronchi, one leading to each lung. Air follows the paths of the bronchi as they subdivide repeatedly, like branches of a tree (Figure 7-4), until they reach their endpoints at the multitude of tiny air pockets in the lungs called alveoli (Figure 7-5A). The alveoli are where the exchange of oxygen and carbon dioxide with the blood takes place (Figure 7-5B).

Moving air in and out of the chest requires an open pathway. In EMS, we refer to this open pathway as a ***patent*** airway. Although a healthy person with a normal mental status should have no problem keeping the airway open, there are a number of potential airway challenges that occur with disease and trauma.

patent (PAY-tent)
open and clear; free from obstruction.

Upper-airway (above the trachea) obstructions are common. These obstructions can be caused by foreign bodies (as in a person choking), by infection (such as in a child with croup), or even by trauma or burns causing the soft tissue of the larynx to swell. Any of these obstructions can seriously and significantly inhibit the flow of air and interrupt the process of moving oxygen in and carbon dioxide out.

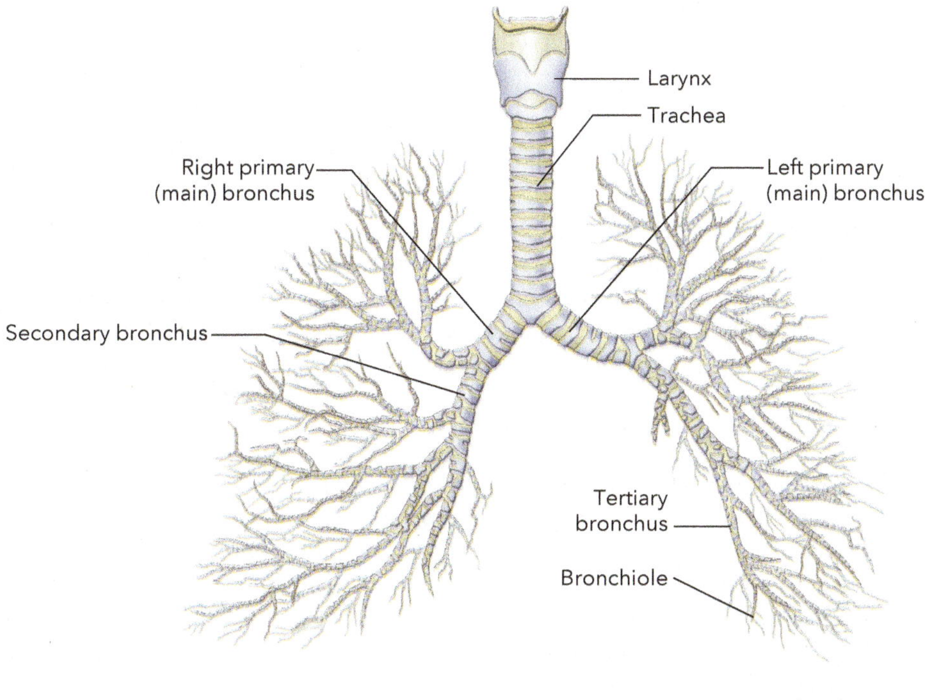

FIGURE 7-4 The bronchial tree. Each mainstem bronchus enters a lung, then branches into smaller and smaller bronchi, ending in the smallest bronchioles.

FIGURE 7-5 (A) Each bronchiole terminates in a tiny air pocket called an alveolar sac. (B) The alveoli are encased by networks of capillaries; oxygen and carbon dioxide are exchanged between the air in the alveoli and the blood in the capillaries.

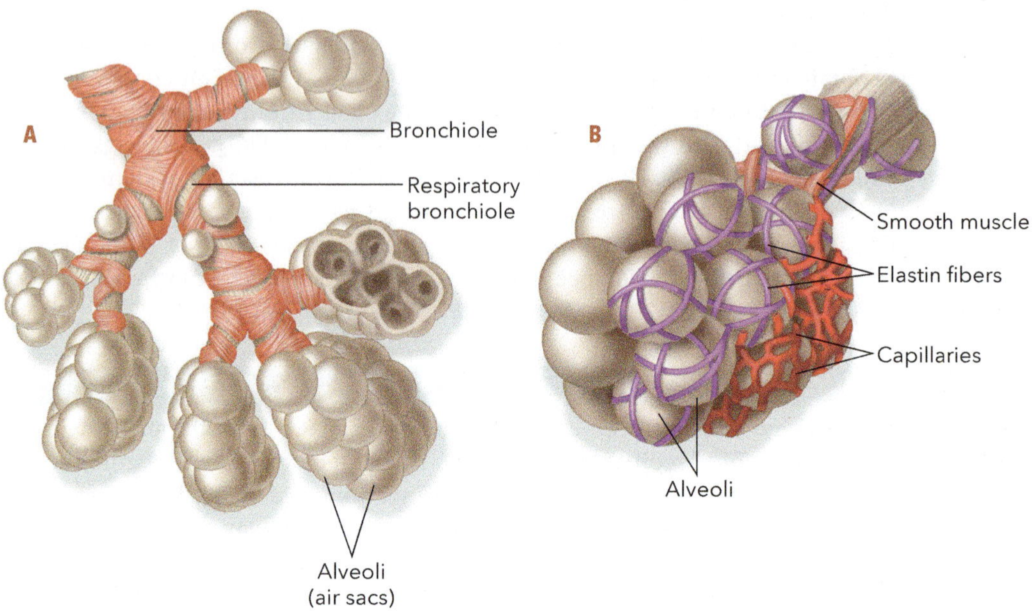

The Lungs

tidal volume
the volume of air moved in one cycle of breathing.

minute volume
the amount of air breathed in during each respiration multiplied by the number of breaths per minute.

dead air space
air that occupies the space between the mouth and alveoli but that does not actually reach the area of gas exchange.

The lungs are part of the lower airway (below the opening of the trachea). The lungs, together with the diaphragm and the muscles of the chest wall, change their internal pressures to pull air in or push air out. The volume of air moved in one in-and-out cycle of breathing is called the ***tidal volume***. We multiply tidal volume by the respiratory rate to obtain ***minute volume***, the amount of air that gets into and out of the lungs in one minute. Obviously minute volume can be affected by changes in either tidal volume or rate (or both). Here are two examples of how minute volume can be impacted by very different mechanisms:

- A 25-year-old male has a normal minute volume of 5000 mL (tidal volume of 500 mL × 10 breaths per minute). He overdoses on heroin. Because heroin is a narcotic, it interferes with the respiratory center in his brain, and his breathing rate slows to 4 breaths per minute. He is breathing the same tidal volume as he was before, but because his rate has become so slow, his minute volume has significantly decreased (tidal volume of 500 mL × 4 breaths per minute = 2000 mL minute volume).
- A 30-year-old woman has a normal minute volume of 6000 mL (tidal volume of 500 mL × 12 breaths per minute). She has an asthma attack and, as the attack grows more severe, her tidal volume decreases to 250 mL. Even though her breathing rate has not changed, she is taking in less air with each breath, so her minute volume has significantly decreased (tidal volume of 250 mL × 12 breaths per minute = 3000 mL minute volume).

Remember also that not all of the minute volume of air reaches the alveoli. About 150 mL of a normal tidal volume occupies the space between the mouth and alveoli but does not actually reach the area of gas exchange. We refer to this as ***dead air space***. *Alveolar ventilation* occurs only with the air that reaches the alveoli.

The .40-caliber bullet that entered Officer Walker's shoulder ricocheted off his scapula and sent a large fragment into his chest wall. Traveling just below the second rib on the right side, the bullet fragment crossed the pleura and punctured the underlying lung tissue. With each breath Officer Walker takes, air escapes from the lung and enters the pleural space. The elastic lung cannot maintain pressure, and collapses under the weight of escaping air and blood.

Respiratory Dysfunction

Specific lung diseases and dysfunctions will be discussed later, in the *Respiratory Emergencies* chapter. However, in general, a respiratory dysfunction occurs any time minute volume is interfered with.

Disruption of Respiratory Control. A section of the brain called the medulla oblongata is the seat of respiratory control. From time to time, disorders that affect this portion of the brain can interfere with respiratory function. Medical events such as stroke and infection can disrupt the medulla's function and alter the control of effective breathing. Toxins and drugs such as narcotics can also affect the medulla's capabilities and adversely impact minute volume. Brain trauma and intracranial pressure can physically harm the medulla and disrupt its function. Even with an intact brain, messages must make their way to the muscles of respiration. Spinal cord injuries and other neurologic disorders can interrupt these transmissions.

Disruption of Pressure. The thorax is essentially a vault. The large muscle called the diaphragm forms its lower boundary just below the rib cage. The lungs are encased by the chest walls, where ribs are separated by intercostal muscles that contract and relax to create the motion of breathing. The lungs are in direct contact with the inner walls of the chest. Although they are in contact, there is a slight space between the lung tissue and chest wall called the pleural space. Here a slight negative pressure keeps the lungs adhered to the chest wall as it moves. There is typically a small amount of fluid in this space to lubricate and to reduce the friction of movement. The area between the lung and the chest wall is also a potential space where blood, fluid, and/or air may accumulate as a result of chest trauma or other medical conditions.

Ventilation is activated by changing pressures within this vault. Inhalation is an *active* process. To inhale, the diaphragm contracts, the muscles of the chest expand, and a negative pressure is created in the chest cavity and lungs. This negative pressure pulls air in through the trachea. By contrast, exhalation is a *passive* process. To exhale, those same muscles relax to make the chest contract, creating a positive pressure that pushes air out. These changing pressures rely on an intact chest compartment. If a hole is created in the chest wall and air is allowed to escape or be drawn in, the pressures that are needed for breathing and that keep the lungs adhered to the chest wall can be disrupted. Lung function can be impaired. Furthermore, if bleeding develops within the chest, blood can accumulate in the pleural space and force the lung to collapse away from the chest wall. This can also occur if a hole in either the lung or the chest wall (or both) allows air to accumulate between the lung and the chest wall.

Disruption of Lung Tissue. In addition to changing the actual amount of air moved per minute, disruption of lung tissue can also interfere with lung function. Trauma is obviously the chief culprit. When lung tissue is displaced or destroyed by mechanical force, it cannot exchange gas.

However, medical problems can also disrupt lung tissue. For example, problems such as congestive heart failure and severe sepsis change the ability of the alveoli to transfer gases across their membranes. The permeability of the thin wall that separates the alveoli from the capillary changes, resulting in impaired diffusion. When this happens, the blood in the alveolar capillaries can neither receive oxygen nor offload carbon dioxide normally.

The net result of any of these challenges is low oxygen (hypoxia) and high carbon dioxide (hypercapnia) within the body. The more the challenge interferes with the movement of air, the more significant the disruption in oxygenation and ventilation.

Respiratory Compensation

When the respiratory system is affected by any of the challenges we have just discussed, the body attempts to compensate for the gas exchange deficits. Specific sensors in the brain and vascular system register low oxygen levels and high carbon dioxide levels. These ***chemoreceptors*** send messages to the brain that assistance is required. Normally respiration or the need to breathe is triggered in the brain by changing carbon dioxide levels. When carbon dioxide levels are increased, the brain stimulates the respiratory system to breathe at

(Text continues on page 168.)

chemoreceptors (kee-mo-re-cept-erz) chemical sensors in the brain and blood vessels that identify changing levels of oxygen and carbon dioxide.

7 Ventilation, Respiration, and Perfusion

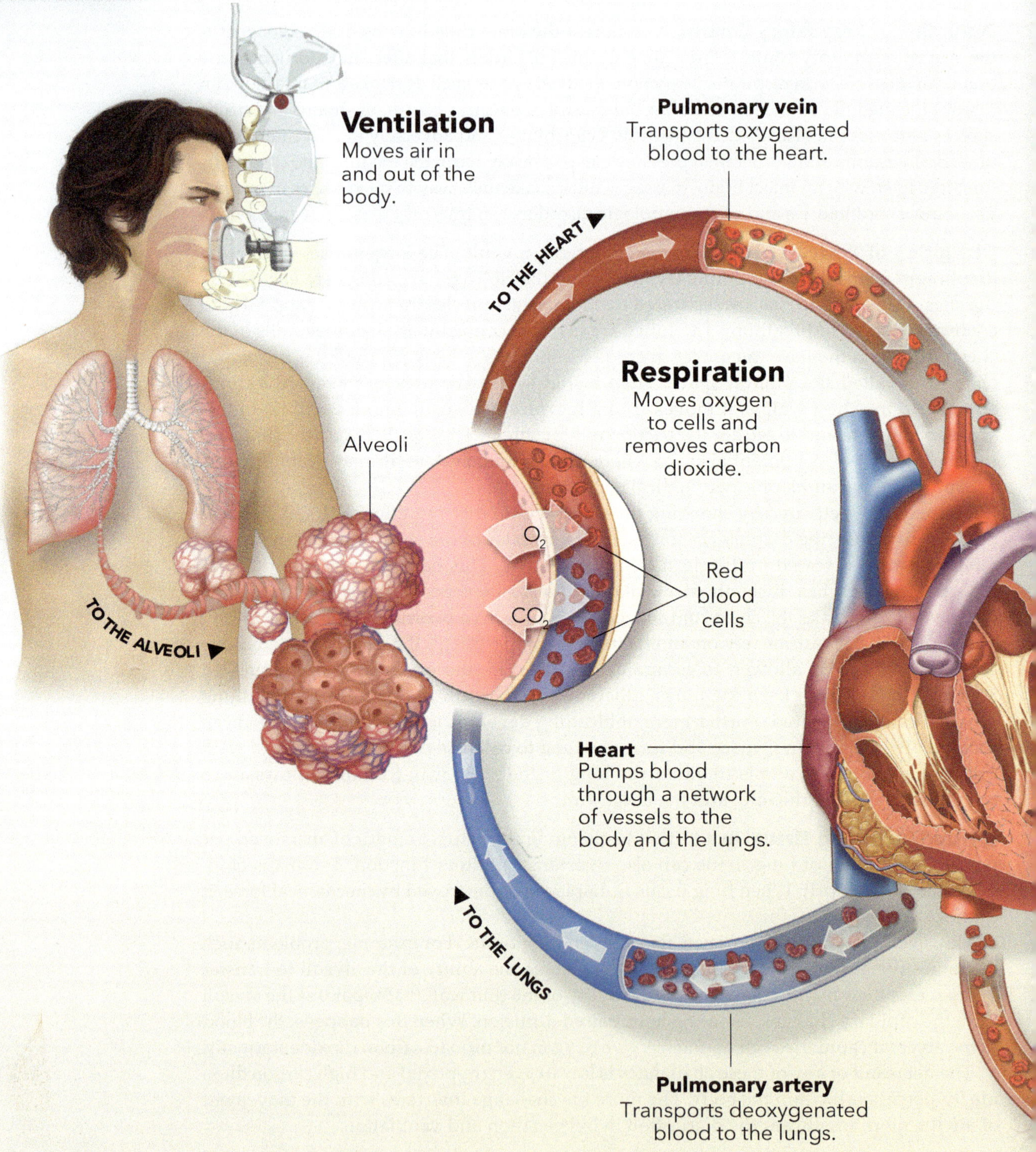

The ultimate goal of emergency care is to move air into the body and ensure adequate circulation so that all cells are perfused with oxygen.

Cells die when they don't receive oxygen. People die when too many cells die.

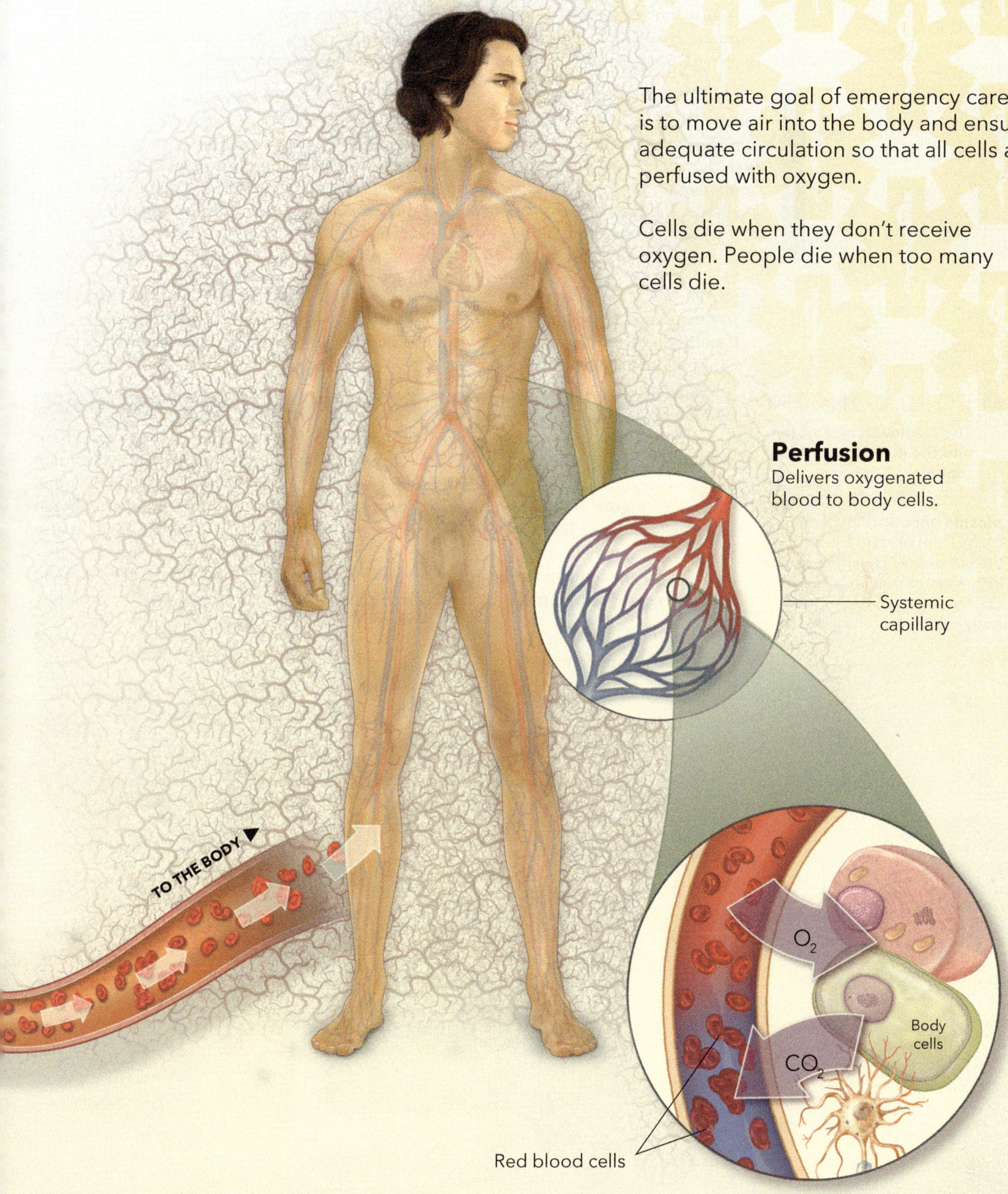

an increased rate to expel the excessive carbon dioxide. In a similar fashion, when the respiratory system is challenged, chemoreceptors sense changing gas levels and send messages to the brain. The brain then stimulates the respiratory system to increase rate and/or tidal volume. When a patient feels the sensation of shortness of breath, or dyspnea, it usually results from a need for gas exchange that cannot be met by current breathing levels (i.e., minute ventilation). From a patient-assessment standpoint, the most obvious sign of these changes is an evident increase in respiratory rate and respiratory effort.

Officer Walker's cells are becoming hypoxic. Chemoreceptors in his cardiovascular system sense the buildup of carbon dioxide and acids due to anaerobic metabolism. His brain unconsciously recognizes the problem and begins countermeasures. The medulla oblongata signals the respiratory system to compensate. Officer Walker's respiratory rate increases. The brain also signals the adrenal glands to secrete adrenaline. Epinephrine and norepinephrine enter the blood stream, and the "fight or flight" response begins.

The respiratory system moves air in and out, but to *perfuse* cells, the air that is breathed in must be matched up with blood. The cardiovascular system moves blood that has been oxygenated as it passed by the alveoli to the cells, to provide the second half of the cardiopulmonary equation.

CORE CONCEPT

The cardiovascular system and the movement of blood

The Blood

plasma oncotic (PLAZ-ma on-KOT-ik) ***pressure*** the pull exerted by large proteins in the plasma portion of blood that tends to pull water from the body into the bloodstream.

Blood is the vehicle by which oxygen and carbon dioxide are transported. The liquid portion of blood is called plasma. Other components include red blood cells that contain oxygen-carrying hemoglobin, white blood cells that fight infection, and platelets that form clots (Figure 7-6). Blood transports oxygen by binding it to the hemoglobin in red blood cells and, to a lesser extent, by dissolving it into the *plasma*. Carbon dioxide is also dissolved into the plasma.

Blood plasma contains large proteins that tend to attract water away from the area around body cells and pull it into the bloodstream. This force is called ***plasma oncotic pressure***.

FIGURE 7-6 Blood components.

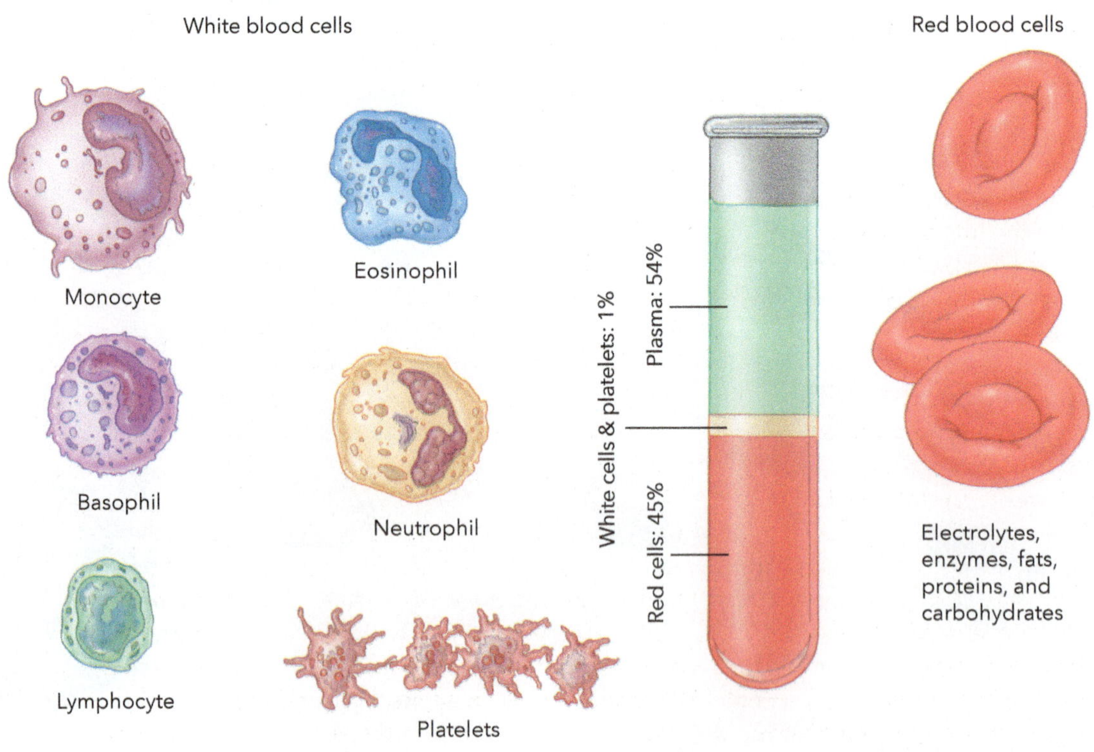

It is counterbalanced by the pressure created inside the vessels when the heart beats. This pressure tends to push fluid back out of the blood vessels toward the cells, and is called ***hydrostatic pressure***.

hydrostatic (HI-dro-STAT-ik) ***pressure***
the pressure within a blood vessel that tends to push water out of the vessel.

The balance between the pulling-in force of plasma oncotic pressure and the pushing-out force of hydrostatic pressure is critical to regulating both blood pressure and cell hydration. A loss or disruption of either of these pressures can be devastating. For example, albumin, one of the large proteins in plasma, is created in the liver. Liver-failure patients often do not produce enough albumin. Without the pulling-in force of albumin, water freely leaves the bloodstream and accumulates around the body cells and even in cavities, leading to dehydration of the blood and edema (swelling) in the patient as fluid accumulates outside the bloodstream.

Blood Dysfunction

The most common blood dysfunctions relate to volume. You simply have to have enough blood to accomplish the goals of moving oxygen and carbon dioxide. Bleeding obviously defeats this goal, as does dehydration.

Other blood dysfunctions are caused by conditions that affect the components of the blood. Anemia is a decrease in the number of red blood cells. When severe, anemia decreases the blood's ability to carry oxygen. Other conditions, such as liver failure, affect water-retaining proteins in the blood (such as albumin), causing a decrease in volume.

Officer Walker is also bleeding. The gunshot to his right leg has perforated the femoral vein, and blood pours from the wound. Vital red blood cells are lost from circulation, and pressure within the vascular system falls. Luckily, though, Officer Walker's partner sees this massive blood loss and takes immediate action. Direct pressure followed by the rapid application of a tourniquet stems the flow of blood. Seconds pass but feel like minutes. "When will that ambulance arrive?" they wonder.

The Blood Vessels

Blood is distributed throughout the body, thanks to the pumping action of the heart, then returned to the heart by a network of blood vessels. Arteries, veins, and capillaries form this network of blood vessels (Figure 7-7). Arteries carry blood away from the heart. Artery walls are composed of layers, and arteries can change diameter by contracting their middle layer of smooth muscle. Veins carry blood back to the heart and also can change diameter with a layer of smooth muscle. Arteries carry oxygenated blood while veins carry deoxygenated blood. The only exceptions to this rule are the pulmonary arteries (they carry deoxygenated blood from the heart to the lungs) and the pulmonary veins (which carry oxygenated blood from the lungs to the heart).

As blood leaves the heart, it travels through arteries, whose diameter decrease as they approach the cellular level, eventually reaching the smallest arteries, known as arterioles. Arterioles then feed the *oxygenated* blood into tiny vessels called capillaries. Capillaries have thin walls, like cell membranes, that allow for movement of substances into and out of the bloodstream. Through these thin capillary walls, oxygen is offloaded and carbon dioxide is picked up from the cells of the body. Capillaries then connect to the smallest veins, called venules. Venules turn into veins as they grow larger, and veins transport blood back to the heart.

A similar process takes place in the lungs, but it is reversed from the process that happened at the level of the body cells. *Deoxygenated* blood that has been returned to the right side of the heart is pumped to the lungs via the pulmonary arteries and arterioles. The pulmonary arterioles connect with pulmonary capillaries that surround the alveoli, the tiny air pockets in the lungs. Carbon dioxide is offloaded from the capillaries across the alveolar membrane to the alveoli to be exhaled from the lungs. Oxygen is transferred from the air in the alveoli across the alveolar membrane and into the surrounding capillaries.

FIGURE 7-7 The network of arteries, veins, and capillaries.

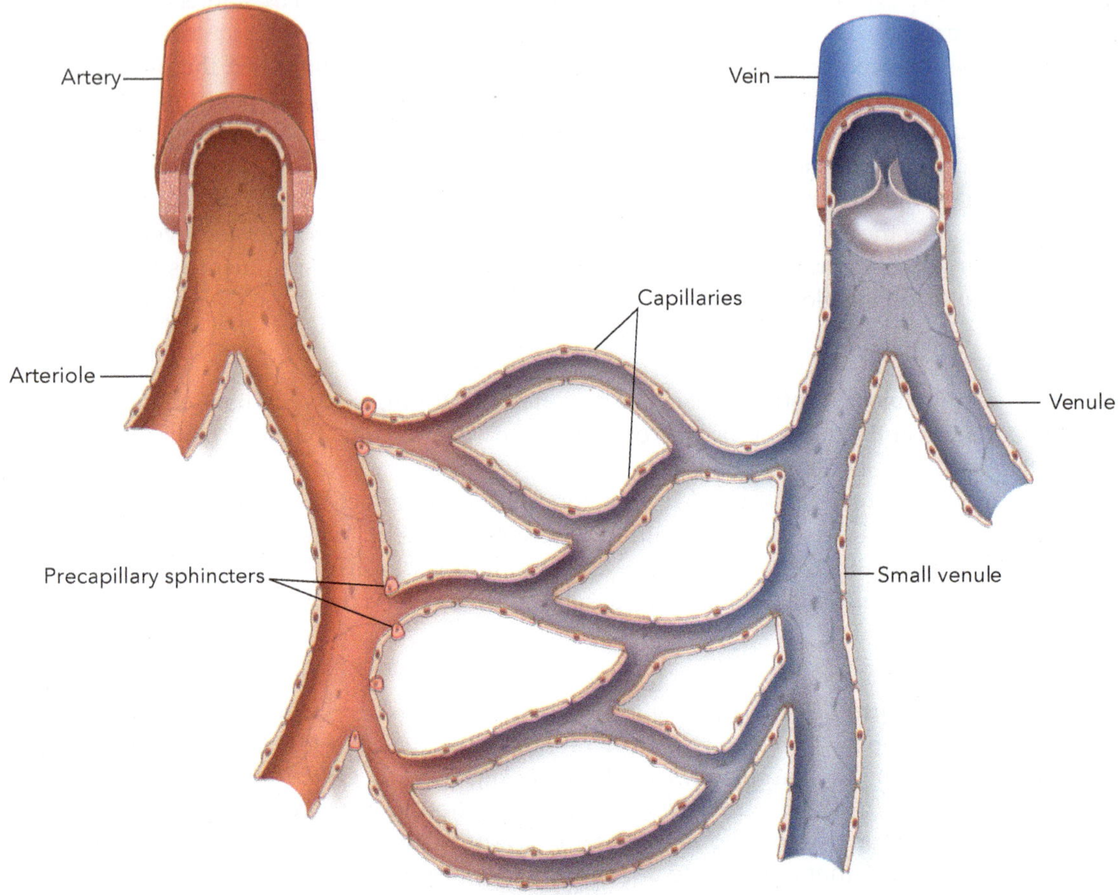

The newly oxygenated blood then continues on its way from the pulmonary capillaries to the pulmonary venules and into the pulmonary veins. The pulmonary veins return the oxygenated blood to the left side of the heart, which pumps it out to the body.

The movement of blood through the blood vessels depends on pressure in the system. For the leading blood molecule to get where it is going, it must have other molecules behind it, pushing it along (normal pressure). If the molecules are too spread out, there is no push on that leading molecule, and it does not move (low pressure). We will discuss the heart's role in creating the needed pressure later in the chapter, but one factor besides the heart that helps determine pressure within a blood vessel is its size or, more specifically, the vessel's diameter.

stretch receptors sensors in blood vessels that identify internal pressure.

We noted earlier that most vessels can change their diameter by using a layer of smooth muscle in the vessel wall. Depending on the circumstances, vessels will frequently change size to adjust for changes in pressure. In fact, certain blood vessels contain specialized sensors called ***stretch receptors*** that detect the level of internal pressure and transmit messages to the brain via the nervous system. When pressure in the circulatory system drops, the medulla oblongata processes the information and begins the steps of compensation. The sympathetic nervous system is engaged, and the adrenal glands are signaled to secrete epinephrine and norepinephrine. These chemical neurotransmitters tell the blood vessels to constrict and the heart to beat faster and harder. In most cases, these actions cause the pressure in the circulatory system to increase. When pressure normalizes, those same vascular stretch receptors will signal the brain once again and compensatory measures will be regulated. Circulatory pressure may need to be adjusted for a variety of reasons, including loss of volume (blood) in the system or too much volume in the system. For example:

- A 3-year-old boy has a gastrointestinal virus. For the last three days he has had vomiting and diarrhea. Although he isn't actively bleeding, the vomiting and diarrhea have robbed his cells of vital body water, and the pressure within the circulatory system has fallen. His blood has a difficult time moving. Stretch receptors in his aorta sense the falling pressures. Messages are transmitted to the central nervous system, and the blood vessels are stimulated to contract. Because this decreases the container size, the pressure within the system normalizes (for now).

- A 30-year-old woman experiences a spike in blood pressure after a frightening near-collision on the highway, as her sympathetic nervous system causes her heart rate to increase and her blood vessels to constrict. When she realizes that she has averted the collision and everything is all right, her parasympathetic nervous system causes her heart rate to slow and her blood vessels to relax, bringing her blood pressure back to normal.

The autonomic nervous system plays a major role in controlling vessel diameter. In particular, the sympathetic nervous system in its fight-or-flight response stimulates blood vessels to constrict. By contrast, the parasympathetic nervous system stimulates blood vessels to relax.

Pediatric Note

Pediatric Vascular Response

Infants and children respond to circulatory challenges in the same manner adults do. However, vasoconstriction in pediatric patients is a powerful response. Vasoconstriction in this population is effective and often sustained through massive volume loss. This means we must take care not to wait for drops in blood pressure to recognize hypovolemia. In many cases, blood pressure can be normal even though circulatory volume is very low (such as in internal bleeding or dehydration).

Capillary refill time is also an important indicator of compensation in pediatric patients. When blood vessels constrict, blood is commonly shunted away from the small vessels in the skin. This is what causes pale skin, otherwise known as *pallor*, in shock patients. Shunting also slows the filling of blood vessels in areas of skin that are compressed. The capillary refill test can be performed by pressing down on a patient's fingernail bed (or skin of the hand, if the patient is small). The pressure should cause the area to become pale as blood is compressed out. When pressure is released, the blood should return rapidly. For pediatric patients, color should be restored in less than two seconds. Longer times would suggest vasoconstriction and compensation. This finding is less reliable in the adult population. This test will be discussed in more detail in the chapter *Vital Signs and Monitoring Devices*.

Blood Vessel Dysfunction

Loss of Tone. A major problem with blood vessels occurs with their inability to control their diameter. If blood vessels are unable to constrict when necessary—or, worse, if they are forced into an uncontrolled dilatation—internal pressure can drop seriously (Figure 7-8). Many conditions can cause this loss of tone. Injuries to the brain and spinal cord can cause uncontrolled dilation of the blood vessels (vasodilation). Severe systemic infections (sepsis) can also cause vessel dilation. Systemic allergic reactions can cause similar problems.

Excessive Permeability. Certain conditions cause capillaries to become overly permeable, or "leaky," allowing too much fluid to flow out through their walls (Figure 7-9). Sepsis, high altitude, and certain diseases can frequently cause increases in capillary permeability. Leaky capillaries can lead to volume loss from the bloodstream. In the lungs, increased permeability allows the plasma in the blood to cross the membrane and occupy space in the tissues in and around the alveoli. If fluid occupies this space, airflow can be restricted, causing significant gas-exchange problems.

FIGURE 7-8 Dilated blood vessel. (A) Normal vessel. (B) Partially occluded vessel.

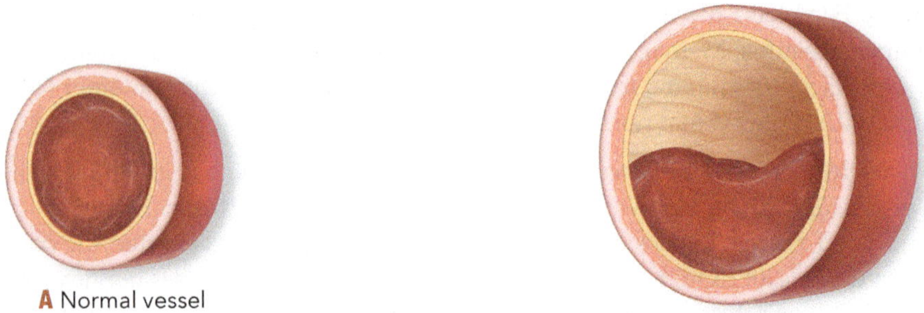

FIGURE 7-9 Increased permeability allows too much fluid to escape through capillary walls.

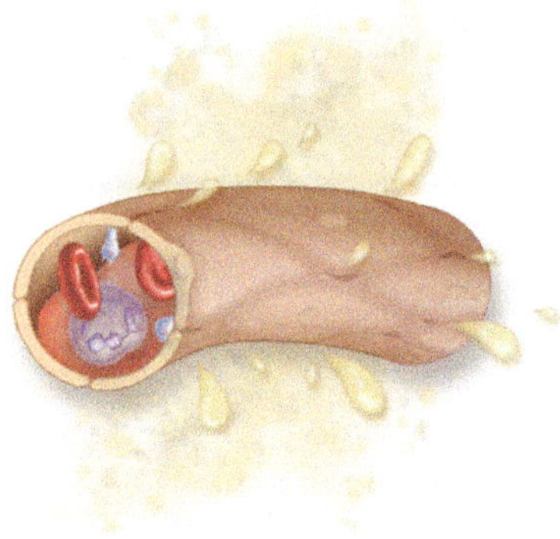

systemic vascular resistance (SVR)
the pressure in the peripheral blood vessels that the heart must overcome to pump blood into the system.

Hypertension. The pressure inside the vessels that the heart has to pump against is called ***systemic vascular resistance (SVR)***. Normally, this pressure is an important factor in moving blood. However, in some patients, the pressure is abnormally increased. Chronic smoking, certain drugs such as cocaine, and even genetics can cause an abnormal constriction of the peripheral blood vessels, and therefore an unhealthy, high pressure level. This increased pressure can be a major risk factor in heart disease and stroke.

Loss of Regulation. Blood vessels rely on chemical messengers to know when to dilate and constrict. If these signals are blocked or are not available, problems can arise. For example, spinal injuries can cause a break in nervous system pathways and therefore block important compensation messages. A lack of sympathetic response in these injuries can lead to dropping circulatory system pressure and profound shock.

Officer Walker's partner is scared. Although the tourniquet has stopped the bleeding from the leg, the puddle of blood beneath Officer Walker is very big. He sees his friend becoming pale and sweaty. "Where is that ambulance?"

Inside Officer Walker's body, profound changes are occurring. Because of the blood loss, pressure within his circulatory system has dropped. The stretch receptors in his aorta are sending signals to his brain that action is necessary. The medulla responds by signaling the adrenal glands to begin the fight-or-flight response. Epinephrine and norepinephrine surge into the bloodstream, and Officer Walker's blood vessels respond with vasoconstriction. His pulse increases, and small vessels in the skin contract to move blood to vital organs. The paleness of his skin demonstrates this effect. The pressure is holding steady, but these actions require energy. The question now is how long Officer Walker can hold out with so many of his cells in anaerobic metabolism.

The Heart

The heart is the key to cardiovascular function. The movement of blood and the resulting transportation of oxygen and carbon dioxide depend on the heart's working properly.

At its most basic level, the heart is a pump. Its job is very straightforward: to move blood. To do this, it mechanically contracts and ejects blood. The volume of blood ejected in one squeeze is known as the ***stroke volume***. An average person ejects roughly 70 mL of blood per contraction. Stroke volume depends on a series of factors:

stroke volume
the amount of blood ejected from the heart in one contraction.

- *Preload* is how much blood is returned to the heart prior to the contraction; in other words, how much it is filled. The greater the filling of the heart, the greater the stroke volume.
- *Contractility* is the force of contraction—that is, how hard the heart squeezes. The more forcefully the muscle squeezes, the greater the stroke volume.
- *Afterload* is a function of systemic vascular resistance. It is how much pressure the heart has to pump against to force blood out into the system. The greater the pressure in the system, the lower the stroke volume.

When we discussed the lungs, we determined the *minute volume* by multiplying the tidal volume (amount of air breathed in per respiration) by the respiratory rate (number of respirations in one minute). ***Cardiac output***, like minute volume, is a per-minute measurement and is calculated in a similar fashion. Cardiac output is determined by examining the stroke volume (amount of blood ejected in one beat) and the heart rate (number of beats in one minute). In other words, to calculate cardiac output, you would multiply the stroke volume by the heart rate.

cardiac output
the amount of blood ejected from the heart in one minute (heart rate · stroke volume).

Cardiac output can be affected by changes to either part of the equation. Either slowing the heart rate or decreasing the stroke volume will decrease cardiac output. Cardiac output can also be impacted by heart rates that are too fast. Although increasing heart rate would normally increase cardiac output, very fast rates (usually > 180 in adults) limit the filling of the heart and in fact *decrease* stroke volume. Some examples of impaired cardiac output include:

- Officer Walker has lost a large volume of his blood. This results in a decreased stroke volume. In an effort to maintain his cardiac output in the face of the falling stroke volume, his body releases epinephrine and norepinephrine to raise his heart rate to maintain cardiac output.
- A 46-year-old woman has a tachycardia (rapid heartbeat) at a rate of 220. Her cardiac output has dropped, even though she has increased her heart rate. As a result of the tachycardia, her ventricles have little time to fill and her stroke volume has decreased.
- An 82-year-old woman has a bradycardia (slow heartbeat) at a rate of 38. Her heart rate has decreased and, because of this, so has her cardiac output.
- A 90-year-old male is having his fourth heart attack. In this case, the muscle wall of the left ventricle is no longer working. Because his heart is having difficulty squeezing out blood, his cardiac output has dropped.

The autonomic nervous system also plays a large role in adjusting cardiac output. The sympathetic nervous system's fight-or-flight response increases heart rate and the strength of heart muscle contraction. The parasympathetic nervous system slows the heart down and decreases contractility.

On an ongoing basis, it is the heart that creates the pressure in the cardiovascular system. Without its pumping force, blood does not move.

Pediatric Compensation

Infants and young children rely a great deal on heart rate to compensate for poor perfusion. Very young hearts lack contractile muscle cells and therefore cannot regulate the force of the squeeze as much as adults can. Therefore, they increase cardiac output principally by increasing heart rate. Always be wary of a child with a fast heart rate, as this sign is often an accurate indicator of compensation.

Heart Dysfunction

Heart dysfunctions can be either mechanical or electrical. That is, they can be a result of a structural/muscle problem or the result of a problem with the electrical stimulation of that muscle.

Mechanical problems include physical trauma (such as bullet holes and stab wounds), squeezing forces (such as when the heart is compressed by bleeding inside its protective pericardial sac), and loss of cardiac muscle function from cell death (as in a heart attack).

Electrical problems typically occur from diseases such as heart attacks or heart failure that damage the electrical system of the heart. The conduction system in the heart can also be disrupted by hypoxia and external influences like toxins or medications. These cardiac electrical problems include unorganized rhythms, such as ventricular fibrillation, and rate problems, such as bradycardias (too slow) and tachycardias (too fast). In infants and children, bradycardia is often the result of acute hypoxia from inadequate ventilation rather than from a primary cardiac cause.

(For more information on cardiac dysfunctions, see the *Cardiac Emergencies* chapter.)

The Cardiopulmonary System: Putting It All Together

Air goes in, air goes out, and blood goes round and round. Now that you have had an opportunity to explore what really happens in the cardiopulmonary system, you may see just how important that old saying is to understanding the big picture. (Review *Visual Guide: Ventilation, Respiration, and Perfusion*.) See the following discussion of the term *perfusion* and the discussion in the following section on shock.

For the system to do its job, all of the components must be doing theirs. In the respiratory system, air movement must bring oxygen all the way to the alveoli and move carbon dioxide all the way back out; there must be a significant quantity of air moving, and the alveoli must be capable of exchanging gas. In the cardiovascular system, there must be enough blood; the heart must adequately pump the blood, and there must be enough pressure in the system to provide perfusion throughout the body—that is, to move the blood between the alveoli and the body cells, and between the body cells and the alveoli. Furthermore, the blood must be capable of carrying oxygen and carbon dioxide.

V/Q match
ventilation/perfusion match. This implies that the alveoli are supplied with enough air and that the air in the alveoli is matched with sufficient blood in the pulmonary capillaries to permit optimum exchange of oxygen and carbon dioxide.

When all these functions are in place, we have what is called a ventilation/perfusion match, otherwise known as a ***V/Q match***. What this implies is that the alveoli have sufficient air and that air is matched up with sufficient blood in the pulmonary capillaries. V/Q matching is rarely perfect. In fact, even in healthy lungs, a force as simple as gravity can mean that alveoli in the upper areas of the lungs may not be matched with as much blood as are alveoli in the lower areas. As a result, we often express the V/Q match as a ratio rather than a true match.

In Officer Walker's case, two problems exist. He has a severe lung injury in the form of a collapsed lung (otherwise known as a pneumothorax). Blood may be reaching the lungs, but in its collapsed state, the lung is not moving air to the alveoli. Therefore, he cannot match ventilation to the blood supply (perfusion). Officer Walker also has sustained a large loss of blood due to the injured blood vessel in his leg. If enough blood has been lost, there simply may not be enough red blood cells to support perfusion. Blood may not be reaching the lungs for gas exchange.

perfusion (per-FEW-zhun)
the supply of oxygen to and removal of wastes from the cells and tissues of the body as a result of the flow of blood through the capillaries.

hypoperfusion (HI-po-per-FEW-zhun)
inability of the body to adequately circulate blood to the body's cells to supply them with oxygen and nutrients. A life-threatening condition. Also called *shock*.

The V/Q ratio can be disrupted by any challenge that interferes with any element of the cardiopulmonary system. Minute volume problems, cardiac output problems, and structural damage to the lungs all can disrupt the match between air and blood.

Shock

Shock will be discussed again in the chapter titled *Bleeding and Shock*, but it is important to discuss here, since many medical and traumatic conditions can cause shock. As we noted previously, all cells require regular delivery of oxygen and nutrients, and removal of waste products. This is a function of a regular supply of blood and is referred to as ***perfusion***. Shock occurs when perfusion is inadequate. Inadequate perfusion is referred to as ***hypoperfusion***, which is considered to be a synonym for ***shock***. In other words, shock occurs when the regular delivery of oxygen and nutrients to cells, and the removal of their waste products, are interrupted. Without a regular supply of oxygen, cells become hypoxic and must rely on anaerobic metabolism. When this type of metabolism occurs, lactic acid and other waste products accumulate and harm the cells. Without the removal of carbon dioxide, the buildup of harmful waste products is accelerated. Unless it is reversed, shock will kill cells, organs, and eventually the patient.

CORE CONCEPT

The principles of perfusion, hypoperfusion, and shock

shock
See *hypoperfusion*.

Dozens of injuries and illnesses can cause shock, but in fact, the pathophysiology of shock is often quite similar regardless of its origin. Although shock can be caused by either medical conditions or traumatic injuries, the disorder of shock is commonly categorized into four distinct groupings:

1. **Hypovolemic shock**—Hypovolemia, or low blood volume, occurs when blood is lost from the cardiovascular system (as in severe bleeding) or when the volume portion of the blood is lost (as in dehydration). In this case, too little volume leads to reduced pressure in the cardiovascular system. Without adequate pressure, the heart has great difficulty pumping blood to all the necessary regions of the body, and cells become hypoperfused. Lost blood also leads to lost oxygen-carrying capacity, furthering the oxygen deficit in the cells.
2. **Distributive shock**—In distributive shock, blood vessel tone is lost. The smooth muscle in the vessels loses its ability to maintain a normal diameter. Conditions such as anaphylaxis or sepsis cause normally constricted vessels to dilate, and as a result, pressure within the system is reduced. With low pressure, the blood cannot efficiently be pumped, and blood flow to the cells is diminished. Hypoperfusion is the net result.
3. **Cardiogenic shock**—In this form of shock, the heart fails in its ability to pump blood. Conditions such as myocardial infarction or trauma can lead to either an electrical problem, such as a dysrhythmia, or a mechanical problem, such as damage to the heart muscle itself. In either case, the pump fails and cardiac output suffers. Hypoperfusion occurs when the heart can no longer maintain the pressure in the cardiovascular system and blood fails to be pumped to the cells.
4. **Obstructive shock**—Occasionally blood is physically prevented from flowing. In conditions such as tension pneumothorax, pericardial tamponade, and pulmonary embolism, large quantities of blood are prevented from reaching essential organs and vital areas. Hypoperfusion occurs as these organs and vital areas go without the blood they need.

Shock causes the body to adjust rapidly and attempt to compensate for the hypoperfusion. Although the body responds differently depending on the nature of the shock state, there are some common and predicable responses. Most commonly, the brain will signal the sympathetic nervous system to engage the fight-or-flight response and take steps to enhance perfusion and conserve blood. Heart rate will most commonly increase, and blood vessels will constrict and direct blood flow to the most vital organs. Breathing rate will also increase as the body attempts to introduce more oxygen into the system. The body will also release hormones that signal the kidneys to stop eliminating fluid and the bone marrow to begin producing more red blood cells. In many cases these adjustments will provide the body necessary time to self-correct the challenge and sustain normal function (at least temporarily). We refer to these steps as *compensated shock*, and in many cases they are recognizable in patient assessment. The following are signs and symptoms commonly associated with compensated shock:

- Slight mental status changes, including anxiety and feeling of impending doom
- Increased heart rate
- Increased respiratory rate
- Delayed capillary refill time
- Pale skin that is cool and moist to touch (***diaphoresis***)
- Sweating

diaphoresis (DI-uh-for-EE-sis)
sweating; condition of cool, pale, and moist/sweaty skin.

NOTE: *These findings will be discussed in depth in the* Bleeding and Shock *chapter.*

Unfortunately, not every type of shock state can be compensated for in the manner outlined above. Cardiogenic shock, for example, may not allow the heart rate to increase, and septic shock may not allow blood vessels to constrict. Further, many of the problems that cause shock will rapidly overcome the body's ability to compensate. If massive bleeding is not corrected, it will soon not matter how constricted blood vessels become. An empty cardiovascular system cannot adequately perfuse tissues. Decreased delivery of oxygenated blood to the cells causes them to shift to anaerobic metabolism. When cells begin producing energy without enough oxygen, compensating for shock becomes even more difficult. As previously discussed, anaerobic metabolism produces far less energy than aerobic metabolism. This deficit occurs now at a time when the body's energy requirements are increased.

Compensation for shock demands that muscles work harder, and harder-working muscles of the respiratory system, the heart, and even the smooth muscles of constricting blood vessels require more energy and oxygen to maintain their struggle to keep the body alive. Anaerobic metabolism frequently falls short of necessary energy delivery. As a result, these muscles tire faster, leading to failed compensation. Anaerobic metabolism also leads to increased production of waste products. As oxygen levels drop and more acids are produced, the hemoglobin begin to carry less oxygen, and gas exchange is further affected. Of course, this occurs at a time when compensating muscles are demanding more and more oxygen, and theoretically at a time when the body may not have enough oxygen to begin with. Compensation fails as a result.

When compensatory measures fail, we call it *decompensated shock* (or hypotensive shock). This term implies that compensatory mechanisms have not been successful or have subsequently failed in their effort to sustain perfusion. Decompensated shock is commonly characterized by decreased blood pressure and altered mental status. If this condition is not rapidly reversed, it will lead to *irreversible shock*, as inadequately perfused organ systems begin to die. Patient death commonly follows.

At last the ambulance has arrived. Officer Walker struggles to speak, and the EMT sees he is coughing up blood. The second EMT places an occlusive dressing over the shoulder wound and listens to lung sounds. "No movement on the right," he says, and signals his partner that this is a load-and-go situation. Advanced life support is on the way, but they will have to meet them in route. This patient has no time to spare.

On the way to the hospital, oxygen is administered, and Officer Walker's blood-soaked clothing is removed. The EMT wraps him up in heavy blankets, trying to preserve body temperature. The tourniquet is holding, and Officer Walker's breathing is okay. Time for a full set of vital signs.

Pathophysiology of Other Systems

CORE CONCEPT
Disrupted physiology of major body systems

Fluid Balance

About 60 percent of the body is made up of water, and without this fluid, the functions of the cells would cease. Water is distributed throughout the body, both inside and outside the cells, and balancing this distribution is an important part of maintaining normal cellular function.

Normally water is divided among three spaces in the body, with the following percentages representing averages (Figure 7-10):

- Intracellular (70 percent)—This is water that is inside the cells.
- Intravascular (5 percent)—This is water that is in the bloodstream.
- Interstitial (25 percent)—This is water that can be found between cells and blood vessels.

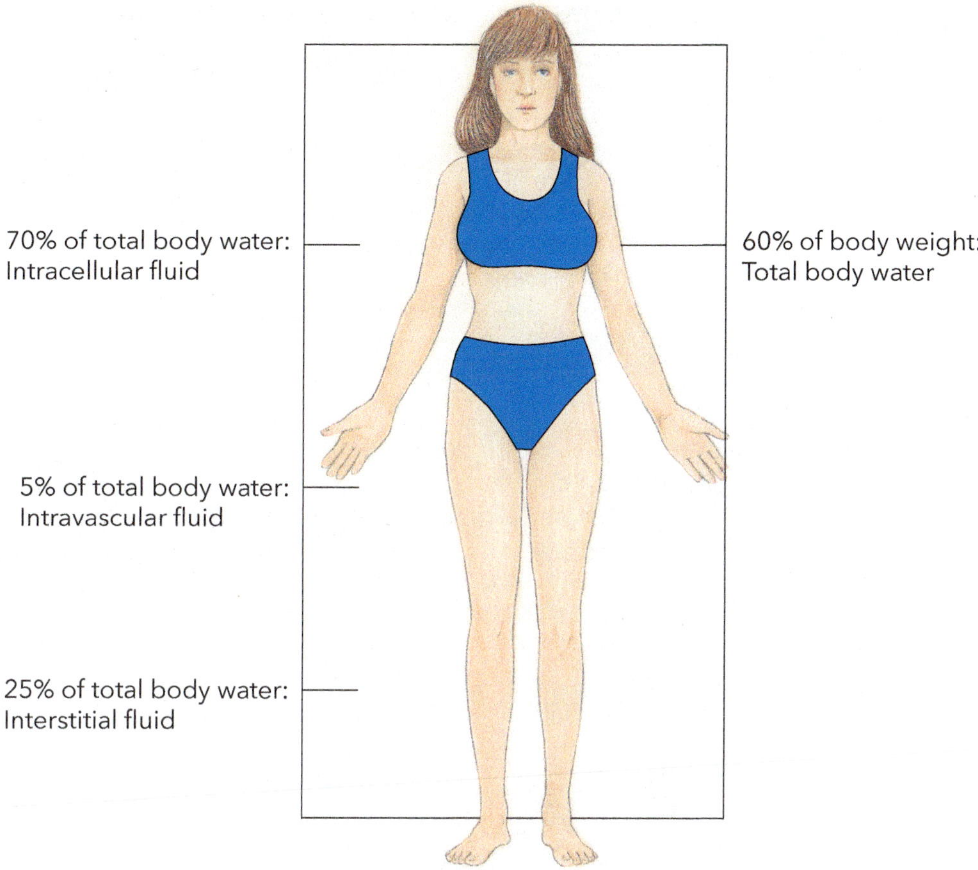

FIGURE 7-10 Water comprises approximately 60 percent of body weight. The water is distributed into three spaces: intracellular, intravascular, and interstitial.

We regulate the levels of water in our body by drinking fluids and making/excreting urine. This allows us to constantly adjust our hydration based on our levels of activity. Inside our bodies, fluid is distributed appropriately through a number of factors:

- The brain and kidneys regulate thirst and elimination of excess fluid.
- The large proteins in our blood plasma pull fluid into the bloodstream.
- The permeability of both cell membranes and the walls of capillaries helps determine how much water can be held in and pushed out of cells and blood vessels.

Each of these factors helps us regulate the amount and distribution of fluid. If these factors were to be interfered with, fluid levels and distribution could become problematic.

Recognizing Compensation

When a V/Q mismatch occurs, the body compensates in predictable ways. Commonly the autonomic nervous system engages the fight-or-flight mechanism of its sympathetic arm. This causes blood vessels to constrict and the heart to beat faster and stronger. The sympathetic nervous response also causes pupils to dilate and decreases blood flow to the skin, which results in diaphoresis (cool, moist, and pale skin). Chemoreceptors in the brain and blood vessels sense increasing carbon dioxide and hypoxia, and stimulate the respiratory system to breathe faster and more deeply.

The signs and symptoms of these changes are often readily apparent. Look for increased pulse and respirations. You may note delayed capillary refill and pale, diaphoretic skin. Pupils may be dilated, and the patient may be sweaty even in cool environments.

Although you may not know exactly what the nature of the V/Q mismatch is, recognizing these common signs of compensation will help you identify that the mismatch exists. Each of these signs should serve as a red flag when you assess your patient. Learn to recognize the signs of compensation as a warning that the body is dealing with a challenge. Consider that these findings point out that something important and dangerous may be taking place.

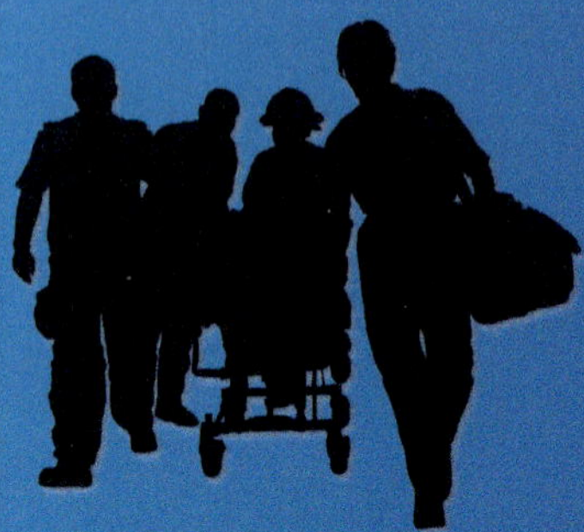

Think Like an EMT

Why Is Her Heart Beating Rapidly?

You and your partner respond to a 10-year-old female who has crashed her bicycle. When you arrive, her mother is with the child, and says, "Everything is fine. She's just a little upset." The child is crying but is able to tell you she fell off her bike and "hurt her belly on the handlebars." Mom allows you to examine the child. She is awake and alert. She is crying, so she seems to be moving air and breathing without any problems. Her radial pulse is present, but you note it to be 128. You double-check your pediatric vital sign chart and find that the rate is faster than it should be for her age group.

In your head, you are facing an important question. Why is her heart beating rapidly? The easy answer is that the rate is caused by her crying and emotional response to the situation. This may very well be the correct answer. However, you also must consider that she has a mechanism of injury–that is, a force that you would expect to cause injury (striking the handlebars)–and she has pain as a result of that force. You recall that a rapid heart rate can be a sign of compensation.

You think, *"This is a red flag. Could her heart be beating fast because she is bleeding into her belly and going into shock? Maybe I need to err on the side of caution and assume this is the case. After all, if it turns out that she just is upset and I've taken this call too seriously, then the little girl is still OK and no harm has been done. On the other hand, if I treat it like it's nothing and the girl really has internal bleeding . . . "*

Clues to your assessment come in many forms. Learn to recognize the important ones.

Disruptions of Fluid Balance

dehydration (de-hi-DRAY-shun) an abnormally low amount of water in the body.

Fluid Loss. ***Dehydration*** is an abnormal decrease in the total amount of water in the body. This may be caused by a decreased fluid intake or a significant loss of fluid from the body by one or more of a variety of means. Remember, however, that maintaining a balance of water relies on a healthy gastrointestinal system. Severe vomiting or diarrhea can significantly alter the amount of water in the body. Fluid can be lost, as well, through rapid breathing (as with a patient in respiratory distress) and profuse sweating. The plasma portion of blood can be lost with injuries such as burns. Substantial fluid volume loss can lead to hypovolemic shock.

Poor Fluid Distribution. Sometimes the body has enough water but cannot get it to where it needs to go. Certain disease processes interfere with the body's mechanisms of moving fluid. We discussed previously the loss of proteins in blood from liver failure and the changes in capillary membrane permeability that occur with severe infections. In these cases, water migrates out of the bloodstream and cells and into the interstitial space (where it is much less useful). Often this can be seen in the form of edema. ***Edema*** is swelling associated with the movement of water.

edema (eh-DEE-muh) swelling associated with the movement of water into the interstitial space.

Edema can be seen best in *dependent* parts of the body—that is, those parts most subject to gravity, such as the hands, feet, and legs. Edema can also occur because of an injury (for example, when your thumb swells up after you hit it with a hammer). In this case, the injury has altered the permeability of local capillaries and fluid has shifted. The larger the injury, the more the fluid shifts. Occasionally fluid can be shifted by changing pressures inside the blood vessels. When pressure is high, the tendency will be to move the fluid portion of the blood out. This can be seen in disorders such as acute pulmonary edema.

The Nervous System

The brain and spinal cord will be discussed in greater detail in the chapter titled *Trauma to the Head, Neck, and Spine*. However, it is important to note here that almost all body functions are regulated by the brain and the spinal cord. The brain is the control center, and the spinal cord is the messenger. Trauma or disease to either of these organs can be devastating to body functions.

The brain and spinal cord are well protected by bone and muscle. In addition, they are covered by protective layers called meninges. They are further defended by a layer of shock-absorbing fluid called cerebrospinal fluid.

Although they are well protected, brain and spinal cord function can be damaged by trauma or disease.

Nervous System Dysfunction

Trauma. Despite all their defenses, occasionally the brain and spinal cord are subjected to forces that injure them. Motor-vehicle crashes, falls, and diving accidents all can cause injury to these systems. In the brain, mechanical damage will interrupt the function of the area that has been harmed. For example, injuries to the area that controls speech can result in an inability to speak or to speak normally.

Because the brain is enclosed in the cranial vault, bleeding and swelling also are concerns. Since the skull is a closed container, blood or edema takes up space where brain tissue would otherwise be, and presses on the brain. Blood pressure inside the vault (intracranial pressure) can also be increased, and this pressure can damage additional structures and alter functions as well.

Mechanical damage to the spine and other nervous pathways results in disruption of nervous system communication. When we think of severing the spinal cord, paralysis comes to mind. However, remember that beyond motor function, the patient also loses sensory and autonomic messaging. That means that when a nervous pathway is destroyed, movement, sensation, and even automatic functions such as breathing and blood vessel dilation may be altered. As in the brain, bleeding and edema are also threats in the closed container of the spinal column.

Medical Dysfunction. Medical problems, both acute and chronic, can alter nervous system function. Strokes result from clots in or bleeding from the arteries that perfuse the brain. In these cases, brain cells are deprived of oxygen and die. As with trauma, the net result of the damage will depend on the affected area's function. Diseases can also affect the brain and spinal cord. Meningitis, an infection of the protective layers of the brain and spinal cord; encephalitis, an infection of the brain itself; and a variety of diseases that affect the nerves, such as Lou Gehrig's disease and multiple sclerosis, all can impair the transmission of messages in the nervous system. General medical problems can also affect normal brain function; for example, diabetics with low blood sugar (hypoglycemia) will become confused and eventually unresponsive when the brain is deprived of the glucose it needs for proper functioning.

Signs of neurologic impairment include:

- Altered mental status
- Seizures
- Inability to speak or difficulty speaking
- Visual or hearing disturbance
- Inability to walk or difficulty walking
- Paralysis (sometimes limited to one side)
- Weakness (sometimes limited to one side)
- Loss of sensation (sometimes limited to one side or area of the body)
- Pupil changes.

The Endocrine System

The endocrine system is made up of a variety of glands that secrete chemical messages in the form of hormones. These hormones dictate and control a variety of body functions, such as glucose transfer and water absorption in the kidneys, among many others. As previously discussed, the adrenal glands play an important role in regulating the fight-or-flight response and are an essential component of compensation. Other major organs of this system include the kidneys and the brain. The endocrine system also includes several glands, such as the pancreas and the pituitary, thyroid, and adrenal glands.

Endocrine System Dysfunction

Dysfunctions of the endocrine system are primarily the result of organ or gland problems. Although trauma can cause injury to organs, endocrine dysfunctions typically are either present at birth or the result of illness. Endocrine disorders generally fall into one of two categories: too many hormones or not enough hormones.

Too Many Hormones. In some disease states, glands produce an excessive amount of hormones. Graves' disease, for example, is a condition in which the thyroid gland overproduces its hormone. Patients with this condition can suffer from difficulties such as inability to regulate temperature and fast heart rates.

Not Enough Hormones. More common are endocrine disorders where glands produce too few hormones. In Type 1 diabetes, the pancreas does not secrete enough of the hormone insulin. Insulin helps move glucose from our bloodstream into our body cells. Without enough insulin, our cells starve.

Adrenal Insufficiency. A number of conditions can affect the production of steroid hormones, such as cortisol and aldosterone, and impair adrenal performance. Although these medical conditions are relatively rare, several medications and other conditions can cause similar effects. Patients who have undergone an organ transplant take medications that suppress the immune system and can also suppress the normal function of the adrenal glands. Many patients also take prescribed steroids for conditions such as chronic respiratory illnesses. These patients can experience adrenal insufficiency if they stop taking their medication abruptly or if they are faced with physiologic stress such as trauma or severe illness. Although these situations are not common, they should be a consideration when assessing any patient who appears to be in shock.

For more information on endocrine disorders, see the chapter titled *Diabetic Emergencies and Altered Mental Status*.

The Digestive System

The digestive system consists of the esophagus, stomach, intestines, and a few associated organs. The digestive system allows food, water, and other nutrients to enter the body. It also controls the absorption of those substances into the bloodstream.

Digestive Dysfunction

Digestive disorders can seriously impact both hydration levels and nutrient transfer.

Gastrointestinal Bleeding. The digestive system is supported by a rich blood supply, which enables absorption of nutrients from the digestive tract into the bloodstream. Gastrointestinal (GI) bleeding can occur anywhere in the digestive tract from the esophagus to the anus. Digestive system bleeding can be slow and chronic or can present with hypovolemic shock from acute massive bleeding in the form of rectal bleeding or vomiting blood.

Vomiting and Diarrhea. Probably the most common digestive disorders are nausea, vomiting, and diarrhea. These are not diseases themselves but rather are symptoms of other disorders. Most commonly the combination of nausea, which may lead to vomiting, and diarrhea is caused by a viral or bacterial infection. When severe, the serious complications of vomiting and diarrhea include dehydration, malnutrition, and in some cases hypovolemic shock. Aside from primary digestive causes, nausea and vomiting can be signs of acute myocardial infarction (heart attack) and even certain strokes and brain injuries.

The Immune System

The immune system is responsible for fighting infection. It responds to specific body invaders by identifying them, marking them, and destroying them. The blood plays a major role in the immune system. Once a foreign body is identified, the body dispatches specialized cells and chemicals. White blood cells and antibodies are transported in the bloodstream to attack the invaders. (More information on this process can be found in the chapter titled *Allergic Reactions*.)

Officer Walker lost consciousness about three minutes into the ambulance transport. His collapsed lung had built up so much pressure that it dropped his blood pressure to a nonperfusing level. Luckily, though, this event occurred just as the ambulance was linking up with advanced life support. Because the EMTs recognized the shock state and because they were able to anticipate the worsening of the lung injury, their report to the oncoming paramedic led to an immediate decompression of Officer Walker's chest, a lifesaving step. Officer Walker regained consciousness in the recovery room after his emergency surgery. The team effort that saved his life started with his partner and carried through the EMTs, paramedics, nurses, and physicians. At each level, whether the responders knew it or not, an understanding of pathophysiology guided appropriate treatment.

This is a normal body response to infection or invasion by a foreign substance. An allergic reaction or anaphylactic reaction is an abnormally exaggerated version of this response that occurs as a result of a flaw in the immune system.

Hypersensitivity (Allergic Reaction)

An exaggerated immune response is referred to as ***hypersensitivity*** (also known as an allergic reaction). Hypersensitivity can occur in a response to certain foods, drugs, animals, or a variety of substances. In a hypersensitivity reaction, the immune system, in responding to these specific substances, releases chemical toxins that cause more of a reaction than necessary. The allergic reaction occurs when these chemicals affect more than just the designated invader.

hypersensitivity an exaggerated response by the immune system to a particular substance.

One of the chemicals released, called histamine, produces edema and, in some cases, a narrowing of the airways because of changes in blood vessel permeability. Other chemicals can cause dilation of the smooth muscles of blood vessels, resulting in a rapid drop in blood pressure and distributive shock. Hypersensitivity reactions range from minor and localized reactions to severe and life-threatening ones. Rapid identification and treatment is often lifesaving.

For more information on allergies and anaphylaxis, see the *Allergic Reactions* chapter.

Chapter Review

Key Facts and Concepts

- Pathophysiology allows us to understand how negative forces impact the normal function of the body.
- Pathophysiology helps us understand how common disorders cause changes in the body.
- Understanding how the body compensates for insults sheds light on the signs and symptoms we may see during assessment.
- Understanding what compensation looks like helps us rapidly identify potentially life-threatening problems.

Key Decisions

- Is the airway obstructed? Is it open? Will it stay open?
- Is air reaching the alveoli? Is breathing adequate?
- Is perfusion adequate in my patient? Is the patient in shock?
- Is anything interrupting the ventilation/perfusion match of this patient?

Chapter Glossary

aerobic (air-O-bik) ***metabolism*** the cellular process in which oxygen is used to metabolize glucose. Energy is produced in an efficient manner, with minimal waste products.

anaerobic (AN-air-o-bik) ***metabolism*** the cellular process in which glucose is metabolized into energy without oxygen. Energy is produced in an inefficient manner, with many waste products.

cardiac output the amount of blood ejected from the heart in one minute (heart rate · stroke volume).

chemoreceptors (ke-mo-re-cept-erz) chemical sensors in the brain and blood vessels that identify changing levels of oxygen and carbon dioxide.

dead air space air that occupies the space between the mouth and alveoli but that does not actually reach the area of gas exchange.

dehydration (de-hi-DRAY-shun) an abnormally low amount of water in the body.

diaphoresis (DI-uh-for-EE-sis) sweating; condition of cool, pale, and moist/sweaty skin.

edema (eh-DEE-muh) swelling associated with the movement of water into the interstitial space.

electrolyte (e-LEK-tro-lite) a substance that, when dissolved in water, separates into charged particles.

FiO_2 fraction of inspired oxygen; the concentration of oxygen in the air we breathe.

hydrostatic (HI-dro-STAT-ik) ***pressure*** the pressure within a blood vessel that tends to push water out of the vessel.

hypersensitivity an exaggerated response by the immune system to a particular substance.

hypoperfusion (HI-po-per-FEW-zhun) inability of the body to adequately circulate blood to the body's cells to supply them with oxygen and nutrients. A life-threatening condition. Also called *shock*. See also *perfusion*.

metabolism (meh-TAB-o-lizm) the cellular function of converting nutrients into energy.

minute volume the amount of air breathed in during each respiration multiplied by the number of breaths per minute.

patent (PAY-tent) open and clear; free from obstruction.

pathophysiology (path-o-fiz-e-OL-o-je) the study of how disease processes affect the function of the body.

perfusion (per-FEW-zhun) the supply of oxygen to and removal of wastes from the cells and tissues of the body as a result of the flow of blood through the capillaries.

plasma oncotic (PLAZ-ma on-KOT-ik) ***pressure*** the pull exerted by large proteins in the plasma portion of blood that tends to pull water from the body into the bloodstream.

shock See *hypoperfusion*.

stretch receptors sensors in blood vessels that identify internal pressure.

stroke volume the amount of blood ejected from the heart in one contraction.

systemic vascular resistance (SVR) the pressure in the peripheral blood vessels that the heart must overcome to pump blood into the system.

tidal volume the volume of air moved in one cycle of breathing.

V/Q match ventilation/perfusion match. This implies that the alveoli are supplied with enough air and that the air in the alveoli is matched with sufficient blood in the pulmonary capillaries to permit optimum exchange of oxygen and carbon dioxide.

Preparation for Your Examination and Practice

Short Answer

1. Define metabolism. Explain the necessary components of efficient metabolism.
2. Describe three types of respiratory dysfunction and how those dysfunctions affect the body.
3. Describe why it is important that blood vessels have the capability to dilate and constrict. How do these impact the cardiovascular system as a whole?
4. Define cardiac output. What are the key components of cardiac output?
5. Describe how the body might compensate for a challenge to the cardiopulmonary system. How might these compensations be seen in a patient?

Thinking and Linking

Pathophysiology, or the dysfunction of a particular system, can typically be identified through signs and symptoms. For the following situations, link each listed pathophysiology with its likely external manifestations to describe probable signs/symptoms, including changes in vital signs, that may result from the dysfunction.

PATHOPHYSIOLOGY	SIGN/SYMPTOM
Obstructed airway	
Bronchospasm (narrowed air passages)	
Vasoconstriction	
Heart rate too slow to maintain perfusion	

Critical Thinking Exercises

An understanding of cellular metabolism pathophysiology is important. The purpose of this exercise will be to consider some aspects of cellular metabolism.

1. When Officer Walker was shot, how did the chest injury impact his cellular metabolism? Why specifically did anaerobic metabolism become a problem?
2. Considering the requirements of normal cellular metabolism, discuss how each of the following systems and/or organs contributes to the delivery of those requirements:
   - Respiratory
   - Circulatory
   - Blood vessels
   - Blood

Pathophysiology to Practice

The following questions are designed to assist you in gathering relevant clinical information and making accurate decisions in the field.

1. We discussed that the heart plays a major role in compensation. Consider a patient with a traumatic injury to the heart. What impact on the patient's ability to compensate might an injury such as this have?
2. We discussed that the blood vessels play a major role in compensation. Consider a patient with an inability to control the diameter of the blood vessels (as in sepsis). What impact might an illness such as this have on the patient's ability to compensate?
3. Certain types of anemia decrease the amount of red blood cells in a patient's blood. What might be the impact of not having enough red blood cells? How might this condition affect that patient's ability to compensate for an illness or injury?

Street Scenes

It is 2000 hours. Your unit is dispatched to a run-down home for a man complaining of diarrhea. When you arrive, you notice a foul, fecal smell. You meet the patient, a 68-year-old man, in the living room. He complains of nausea and diarrhea over the past three days. He notes his bowel movements have been "very dark, almost black." He is awake, alert, and breathing at a rate of 24/min. His skin is slightly pale. You have a difficult time finding a radial pulse but feel a carotid pulse at 124.

Street Scene Questions

1. **What additional patient history should you obtain?**
2. **What does your primary assessment reveal about this patient's condition? How sick is he, and why?**
3. **Why might this patient not have a palpable radial pulse? How is this related to his heart and respiratory rates?**

You place the patient on high-concentration oxygen and continue your assessment while your partner readies the stretcher for transport. You locate a very weak radial pulse and obtain a blood pressure of 82/62. You notice no injuries but find his abdomen to be slightly tender in the left quadrants. You load the patient on the stretcher and prepare to transfer him to the ambulance.

Street Scene Questions

4. **Was a low blood pressure predictable based on your primary assessment?**
5. **What is the cause of this patient's low blood pressure?**
6. **Should you contact ALS (advanced life support, paramedic-level EMS) for this call, or simply transport the patient to the hospital yourself?**

When the patient stands to transfer from the chair to the stretcher, he becomes very dizzy and "feels like he is going to pass out." Once he lies down on the stretcher, he feels better.

En route to the hospital, you obtain a SAMPLE history. He states that his biggest problem tonight is the diarrhea, but his stomach hurts too. He has no allergies. He tells you he has a history of "drinking too much" and that he has had some "stomach problems because of it." He can't tell you what those problems are, but he "takes a pill for them." He hasn't been able to eat much over the past couple of days. In fact, he tells you he has been feeling weak for a few days and now the diarrhea has really made him feel bad.

You continue to transport him to the hospital. There he is diagnosed with a severe gastrointestinal bleed and prepared for surgery.

8 Life Span Development

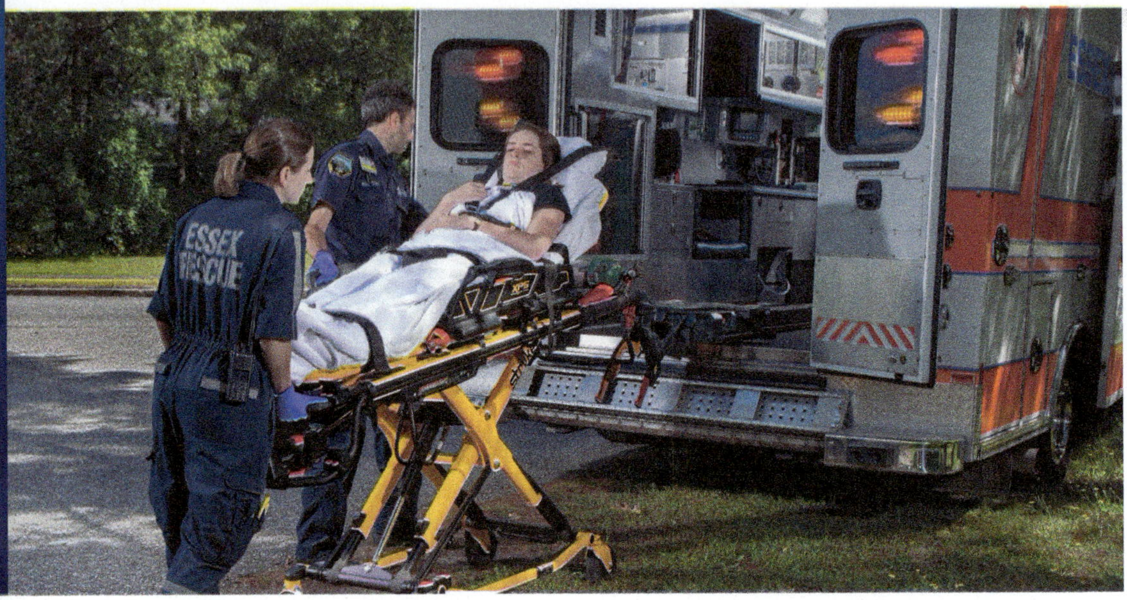

Related Chapters

The following chapters provide additional information related to topics discussed in this chapter:

6 Anatomy and Physiology

7 Principles of Pathophysiology

Standard

Life Span Development

Competency

Applies fundamental knowledge of life span development to patient assessment and management.

Core Concepts

- The physiologic (physical) characteristics of different age groups from infancy through late adulthood
- The psychosocial (mental and social) characteristics of different age groups from infancy through late adulthood

Outcomes

After reading this chapter, you should be able to:

8.1 Distinguish between the physiologic characteristics of people of different age groups. (pp. 186–196)

- Recall the physiologic characteristics of infants.
- Categorize infants' vital signs as normal or abnormal.

- Given descriptions of physical stimulation of an infant, explain the reflexes that should occur.
- Match infant age ranges with cognitive (mental) developmental milestones.
- Categorize toddlers' vital signs as normal or abnormal.
- Explain the increased susceptibility of toddlers to infectious diseases.
- Categorize a preschooler's vital signs as normal or abnormal.
- Categorize a school-age child's vital signs as normal or abnormal.
- Describe the physiologic changes that characterize adolescence.
- Differentiate between normal and abnormal adolescent vital signs.
- Compare the physiologic characteristics of early, middle, and late adulthood.
- Differentiate between normal and abnormal adult vital signs.

8.2 Compare the psychosocial characteristics of people. (pp. 186–196)

- Describe the cognitive (mental) and emotional characteristics expected in normally developing infants.
- Match toddler age ranges with cognitive (mental) developmental milestones.
- List the benefits to preschoolers of social interaction.
- Describe the psychosocial characteristics of school-age children.
- Describe the psychosocial characteristics of adolescents.
- Compare the psychosocial characteristics of early, middle, and late adulthood.

Key Terms

adolescence, *192*
bonding, *188*
early adulthood, *193*
infancy, *186*
late adulthood, *195*
middle adulthood, *194*
Moro reflex, *186*
palmar reflex, *186*
preschool age, *190*
rooting reflex, *187*
scaffolding, *188*
school age, *191*
sucking reflex, *187*
temperament, *188*
toddler phase, *188*
trust versus mistrust, *188*

Life Span Development looks at the physiologic (physical) and psychosocial (mental and social) changes that occur from birth to death. Although this chapter introduces you to typical changes that occur throughout the life span, we will follow one person, Jamie, as she develops through the following stages of life:

- Infancy
- Toddler phase
- Preschool age
- School age
- Adolescence
- Early adulthood
- Middle adulthood
- Late adulthood

Infancy (Birth to 1 Year)

infancy
stage of life from birth to 1 year of age.

If you have ever spent time around infants, you can attest to the phenomenal changes that occur during this first year of life. This is the period referred to as ***infancy***. The infant is a small bundle of joy, totally dependent on others, and grows to begin walking and developing a unique personality (Figure 8-1 and Figure 8-2).

CORE CONCEPT
The physiologic (physical) characteristics of different age groups from infancy through late adulthood

CORE CONCEPT
The psychosocial (mental and social) characteristics of different age groups from infancy through late adulthood

Physiologic Changes

As Jamie ages, her normal pulse rate and respiratory rate will decrease and her blood pressure will increase. Her vital signs are listed in Table 8-1. At birth, Jamie will weigh 6.6–7.7 pounds (3.0–3.5 kg). Her weight will likely double by 6 months and triple by 12 months. Her head will be equal to 25 percent of her total body weight.

While in her mother's uterus, Jamie's lungs did not function, and she had a different pattern of circulation before birth than after. The transition from fetal circulation to pulmonary circulation occurs quickly—usually within the first minutes or hours after birth.

Jamie's airway is shorter, narrower, less stable, and more easily obstructed than at any other stage in her life. She is primarily a "nose breather" until at least 4 weeks of age. Nasal congestion can cause difficulty breathing. She is also a diaphragm breather; thus, you may see more movement in her abdomen than the chest. Jamie will tire more easily when breathing difficulties occur because her accessory muscles are less mature and tire easily. She may be more susceptible to trauma, since her chest wall is less rigid and her lung tissue is more prone to trauma from pressure.

During pregnancy, certain antibodies that help protect from disease are passed to her from her mother. Jamie is also breast-fed, which provides her with antibodies to many of the diseases her mother has had. This helps protect Jamie until she can obtain her own antibodies, either from vaccination or exposure to diseases.

Moro reflex
a response to being startled in which the infant throws out both arms, spreads the fingers, then grabs with fingers and arms.

palmar reflex
a grasping reflex in which an infant grabs onto a finger placed in the infant's palm.

Jamie's nervous system includes four reflexes that will diminish over time:

- ***Moro reflex*** When you startle her, she throws her arms out, spreads her fingers, and grabs with her fingers and arms. These movements should be relatively equal on both sides.
- ***Palmar reflex*** When you place your finger in her palm, she grasps it. Within a couple of months, this merges with the ability to release an object from the hand.

FIGURE 8-1 A newborn infant.

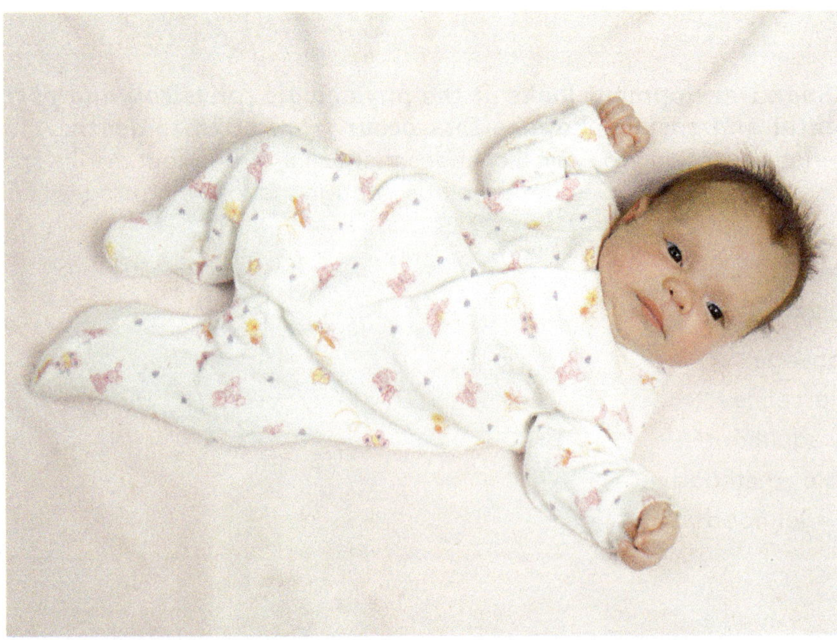

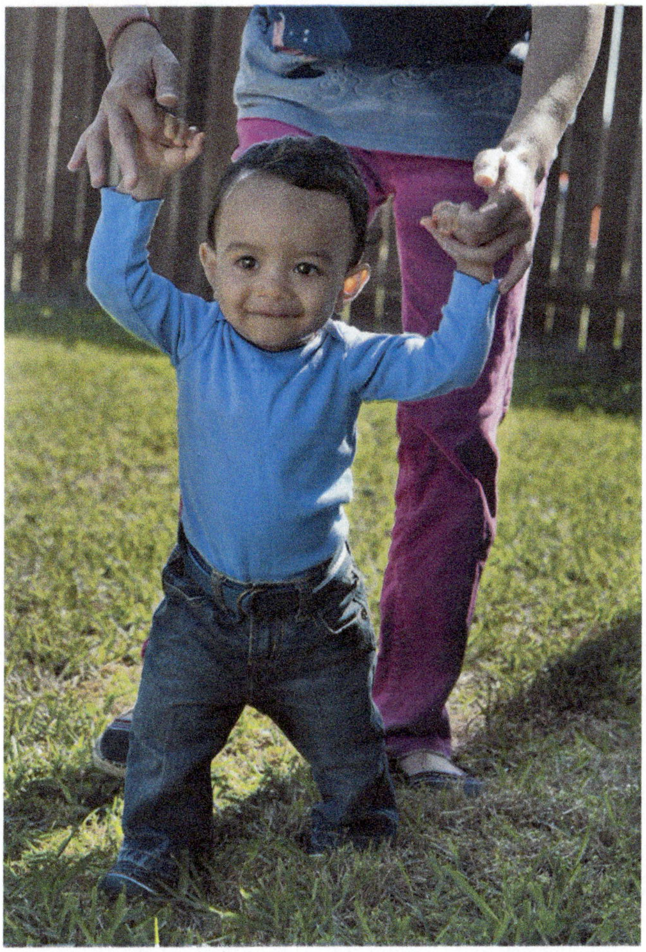

FIGURE 8-2 A year-old infant.

- ***Rooting reflex*** When you touch Jamie's cheek when she is hungry, she turns her head toward the side touched.
- ***Sucking reflex*** When you stroke Jamie's lips, she starts sucking. This reflex works in conjunction with the rooting reflex.

rooting reflex
a reflex response in which a hungry infant automatically turns toward the stimulus when the cheek or one side of the mouth is touched.

sucking reflex
a reflex in which stroking a hungry infant's lips causes the infant to start sucking.

Initially, Jamie will sleep from 16 to 18 hours in total throughout the day and night. This will soon change to about 4–6 hours during the day and 9–10 hours during the night. Although infants vary, usually by 2–4 months the infant will sleep through the night. Even though infants do sleep a lot, they are easy to awaken.

Jamie's extremities grow in length from a combination of growth plates (physis) located at both ends of the long bones (including the humerus, radius, femur, and so on.) As mentioned in the *Anatomy and Physiology* chapter, the bones at the top of the skull are not fused at birth. The "soft spot" where these bones meet is called a *fontanelle* (fawn-tawn-ELL). The posterior fontanelle usually closes by age 2 or 3 months, and the anterior one closes between 9 and 18 months. Looking at the anterior fontanelle, you can get a good idea of Jamie's state of hydration. Normally the fontanelle is level with, or slightly below, the surface of the skull. If the fontanelle is sunken, this indicates dehydration. If the fontanelle is bulging and the infant is not crying, you should suspect increased pressure inside the skull.

There are certain milestones during Jamie's first year. Some of these are listed in Table 8-2.

TABLE 8-1 Vital Signs: Infant

HEART RATE	RESPIRATORY VOLUME	RESPIRATORY RATE	SYSTOLIC BLOOD PRESSURE
100-170 for newborn 90-160 for infant up to 1 year	7-8 mL/kg at birth, increasing to 10-15 mL/kg at 1 year	30-60/minute (0-6 months) 24-30 (6-12 months)	50-70 mmHg for newborn About 90 mmHg up to 1 year

"Knowing how people change as they grow helps me clinically–and in dealing with all of my patients."

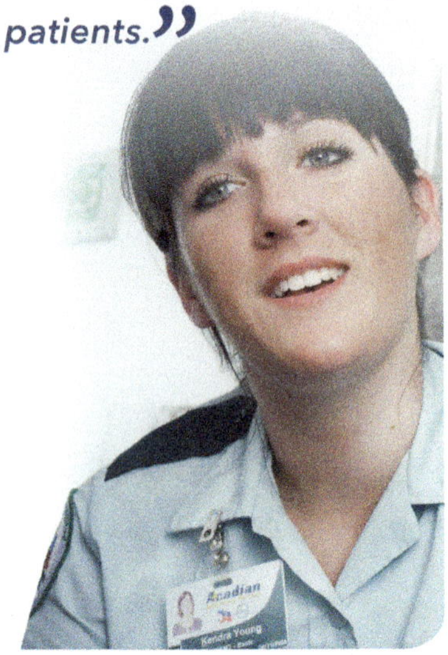

TABLE 8-2 Developmental Changes of the First 12 Months

AGE	CHARACTERISTICS
2 months	• Tracks objects with eyes • Recognizes familiar faces
3 months	• Moves objects to mouth with hands • Distinct facial expressions (smile, frown)
4 months	• Drools without swallowing • Begins to reach out to people
5 months	• Sleeps through the night without waking for feeding • Discriminates between family and strangers
5-7 months	• Begins to cut teeth
6 months	• Sits upright in high chair • Begins making one-syllable sounds
7 months	• Exhibits fear of strangers • Moods shift quickly (crying to laughing to crying)
8 months	• Begins responding to word *no* • Can sit alone • Can play peek-a-boo
9 months	• Responds to adult anger • Pulls self up to standing position • Explores objects by mouthing, sucking, chewing, and biting
10 months	• Pays attention to own name • Crawls well
11 months	• Attempts to walk without assistance • Begins to show frustration about restrictions
12 months	• Walks with help • Knows own name

bonding
formation of a close relationship through frequent association.

trust versus mistrust
concept developed from an orderly, predictable environment versus a disorderly, irregular environment.

scaffolding
building on what one already knows.

temperament
the infant's nature or personality, especially in terms of responding to the environment.

Psychosocial Changes

Jamie's primary means of communication is crying. Those close to Jamie will soon learn if she is crying because she is hungry, is tired, needs to be changed, or for some other reason.

Within the first six months, Jamie will bond with her caregivers and start displaying the following characteristics:

- ***Bonding*** This is her sense that her needs will be met. When she is hungry, she is fed. When she needs to be held, she is held.
- ***Trust versus mistrust*** Jamie likes an orderly, predictable environment. When her environment is disorderly and irregular, she develops anxiety and insecurity.
- ***Scaffolding*** She learns by building on what she already knows.
- ***Temperament*** This is her reaction to her environment.

Toddler Phase (12–36 Months)

toddler phase
stage of life from 12 to 36 months.

During the ***toddler phase*** physical, mental, and social development continue. Body systems continue to grow and refine themselves, and the toddler develops more individuality. This age group's curiosity has led to such affectionate terms as *curtain climbers* and *rug rats.*

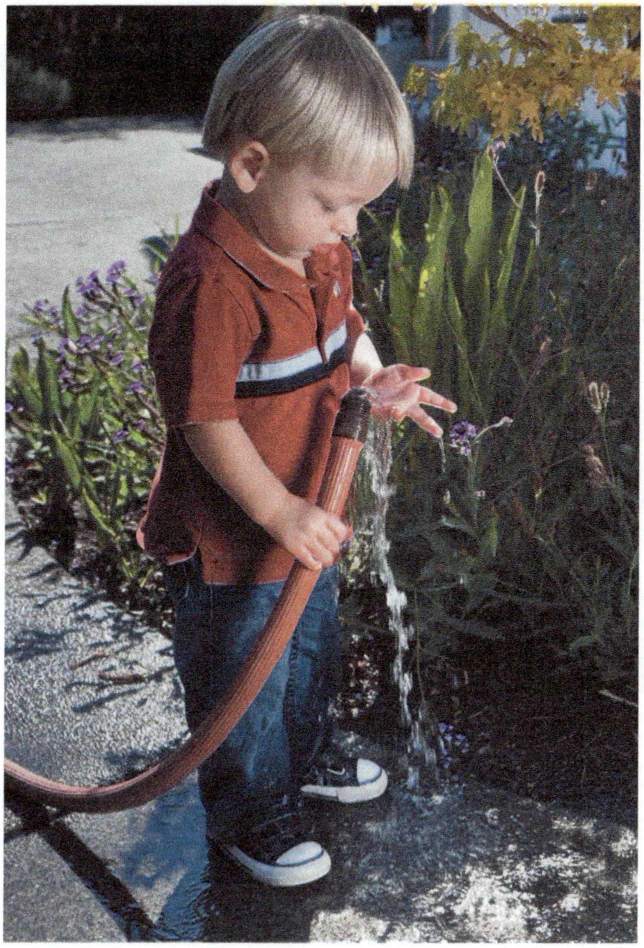

FIGURE 8-3 A toddler.

Their developing personality is sometimes referred to as the "terrible twos." Like all phases of childhood, these years can be a very rewarding time for both toddler and caregivers (Figure 8-3).

Physiologic Changes

Jamie's body temperature now ranges from 96.8°F to 99.5°F (36°C to 37.5°C). She will gain approximately 4.4 lb. (2.0 kg) per year. Her vital signs are listed in Table 8-3.

All of Jamie's body systems will continue to develop and improve in efficiency.

- **Pulmonary system.** Terminal airways branch and grow. Alveoli increase in number.
- **Nervous system.** Jamie's brain is now 90 percent of adult brain weight. Fine-motor skills develop.
- **Musculoskeletal system.** Muscle mass and bone density increase.
- **Immune system.** The toddler is more susceptible to illness. She develops immunity to pathogens as exposure occurs and through vaccination.
- **Teeth.** By 36 months of age, Jamie has all her primary teeth.

TABLE 8-3 Vital Signs: Toddler

HEART RATE	RESPIRATORY RATE	SYSTOLIC BLOOD PRESSURE
80-140/minute	24-40/minute	For ages 1 to 10 years: *Mean* systolic pressure is 90 + (age in years times 2), so mean systolic pressure for 2-year-olds is 94. This is an *average*, and individual blood pressures vary.

TABLE 8-4 Cognitive Developmental Changes from Infant to Preschooler

AGE	CHARACTERISTICS
12 months	• Begins to grasp that words "mean" something
18-24 months	• Begins to understand cause and effect • Develops separation anxiety, shown by clinging and crying when a parent leaves
24-36 months	• Begins developing "magical thinking" and engages in play-acting, such as playing house
3-4 years	• Masters the basics of language that will continue to be refined throughout childhood

Although Jamie is physiologically capable of being toilet-trained by 12–15 months of age, she is not psychologically ready until 18–30 months. It is important not to rush toilet training. She will let her parents know when she is ready. The average age for completion of toilet training is 28 months.

Psychosocial Changes

Cognitive development deals with the development of knowledge and thinking. Table 8-4 shows some of the cognitive development Jamie will experience.

Preschool Age (3–5 Years)

preschool age
stage of life from 3 to 5 years.

Preschool age is a time of continued physiologic and psychosocial development. This is often a time when preschoolers are put into social interaction situations such as day care or preschool (Figure 8-4).

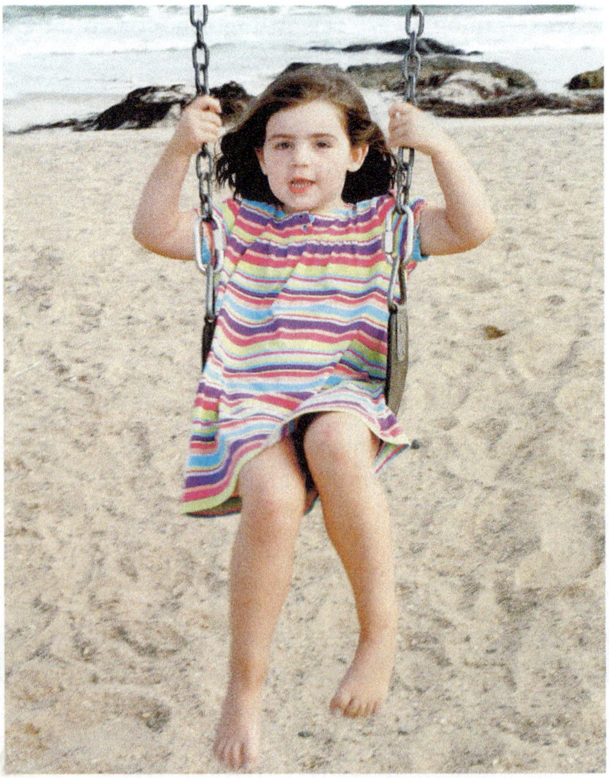

FIGURE 8-4 A preschooler.
(© Daniel Limmer)

TABLE 8-5 Vital Signs: Preschool Age

HEART RATE	RESPIRATORY RATE	SYSTOLIC BLOOD PRESSURE
70-120/minute	22-34/minute	For ages 1 to 10 years: *Mean* systolic pressure is 90 + (age in years times 2), so mean systolic pressure for 2-year-olds is 94. This is an *average*, and individual blood pressures vary.

Physiologic Changes

Jamie's body systems continue to develop and refine their various processes. Her vital signs are listed in Table 8-5.

Psychosocial Changes

Jamie attends a preschool, where she is involved with peer groups. Peer groups provide a source of information about other families and the outside world. Interactions with peers offer opportunities for learning skills, comparing herself to others, and feeling part of a group.

School Age (6–12 Years)

Whether attending a public or private school or being home-schooled, the stage of development referred to as ***school age*** opens vast opportunities for the child.

school age
stage of life from 6 to 12 years.

Physiologic Changes

Jamie's body temperature is between 96.8°F and 101.3°F (36°C and 36.5°C). She will gain 6.6 lb. (3 kg) and grow 2.4 inches (6 cm) per year (Figure 8-5). Her vital signs are listed in Table 8-6.

FIGURE 8-5 School-age children. *(Jacek Chabraszewski/Shutterstock)*

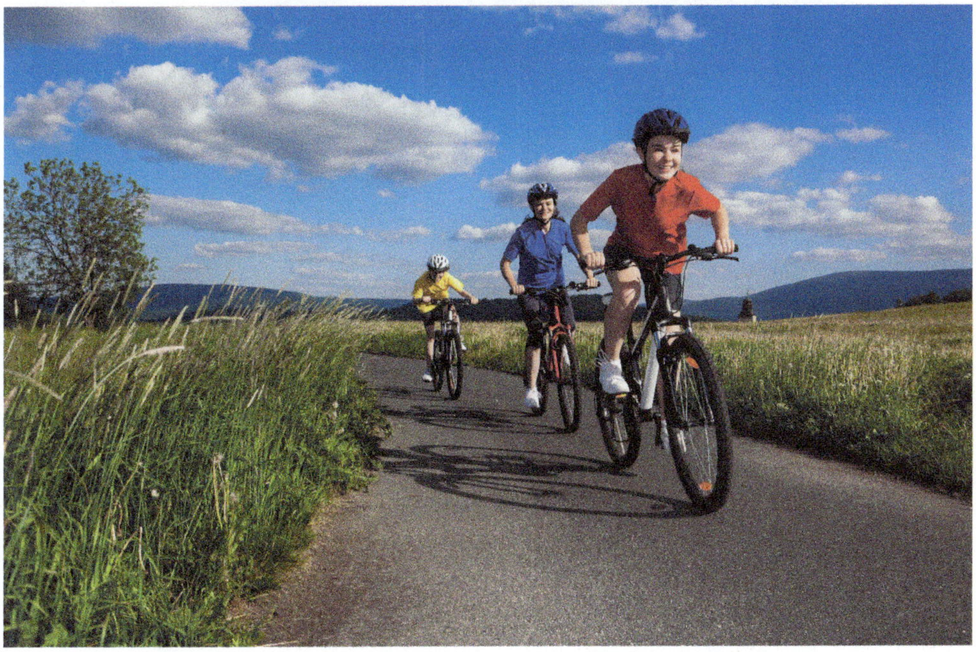

TABLE 8-6 Vital Signs: School Age

HEART RATE	RESPIRATORY RATE	SYSTOLIC BLOOD PRESSURE
65-120/minute	18-30/minute	For ages 1 to 10 years: Mean systolic pressure is 90 + (age in years times 2), so mean systolic pressure for 2-year-olds is 94. This is an average, and individual blood pressures vary.

One of the most obvious changes in Jamie during this time is the loss of her primary teeth. Replacement with permanent teeth begins.

Psychosocial Changes

This is a transition time for both Jamie and her parents. Her parents spend less time with her than they did at earlier ages and provide more general supervision. Jamie develops better decision-making skills and is allowed to make more decisions on her own.

Self-esteem develops and may be affected by popularity with peers, rejection, emotional support, and neglect. Negative self-esteem can be very damaging to further development.

As Jamie matures, moral development begins when she is rewarded for what her parents believe to be right and punished for what her parents believe to be wrong. With cognitive growth, moral reasoning appears, and the control of her behavior gradually shifts from external sources to internal self-control.

Adolescence (13–18 Years)

adolescence
stage of life from 13 to 18 years.

Although life span development is a continual process, dynamic physiologic and psychosocial changes occur during three major developmental ages: infancy, with the transition from fetal life to life in the world; ***adolescence***, with the transition from childhood to adulthood (Figure 8-6); and late adulthood, with its deterioration of systems.

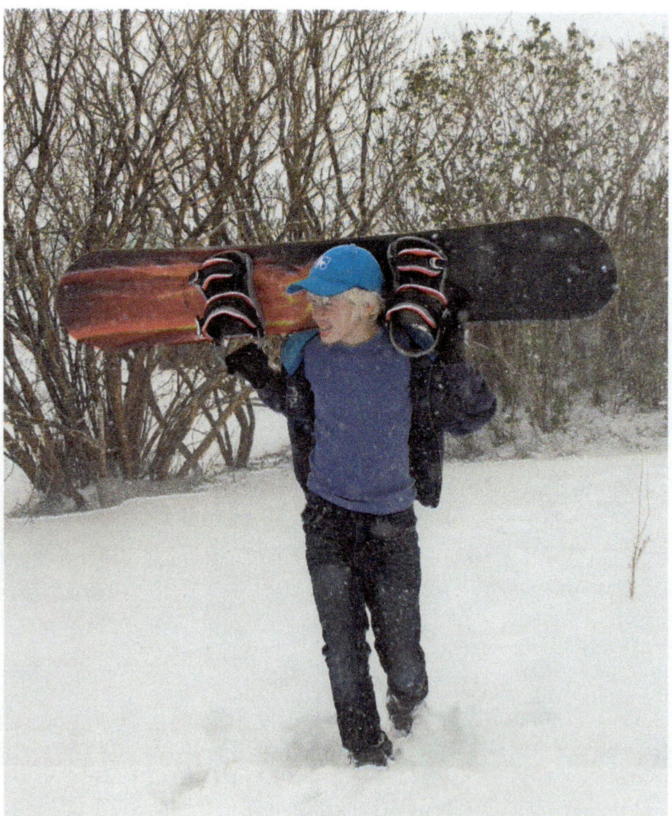

FIGURE 8-6 An adolescent.

TABLE 8-7 Vital Signs: Adolescence

HEART RATE	RESPIRATORY RATE	SYSTOLIC BLOOD PRESSURE
60-100/minute	12-20/minute	About 107-117

Physiologic Changes

During this stage, Jamie will usually experience a rapid two- to three-year growth spurt, beginning distally with enlargement of her feet and hands followed by enlargement of her arms and legs. Her chest and trunk enlarge in the final stage of growth. Girls are usually finished growing by the age of 16 and boys by the age of 18. In late adolescence, the average male is taller and stronger than the average female. Jamie's vital signs are listed in Table 8-7.

At this age, both males and females reach reproductive maturity. Secondary sexual development occurs, with noticeable development of the external sexual organs. In females, menstruation begins and breasts develop. The American Heart Association uses this development of sexual characteristics (puberty) as the point of transition when a patient is considered an adult (not a child) in its CPR guidelines.

Psychosocial Changes

Adolescence can be a time of serious family conflicts as the adolescent strives for independence and parents strive for continued control.

At this age, Jamie is trying to achieve more independence and develop her own identity. She becomes interested in sex and may find this embarrassing. She not only wants to be treated like an adult but also enjoys the comforts of childhood.

Body image is a great concern at this point in life. This is a time when eating disorders are common. It also is a time when self-destructive behaviors might begin, such as use of tobacco, alcohol, prescription or illicit drugs, cutting, and unsafe driving. Depression and suicide are alarmingly common in this age group.

As adolescents develop their capacity for logical, analytic, and abstract thinking, they begin to develop a personal code of ethics.

Early Adulthood (19–40 Years)

With great pomp and circumstance, the adolescent graduates from childhood to adulthood (Figure 8-7). Some say the best years are behind; some say the best years are ahead. But life is what you make of it, and ***early adulthood*** opens up great opportunities.

early adulthood
stage of life from 19 to 40 years.

Physiologic Changes

This is the period of life when Jamie will develop lifelong habits and routines. Her vital signs are listed in Table 8-8.

Peak physical condition occurs between 19 and 26 years of age, when all body systems are at optimal performance levels. At the end of this period, the body begins its slowing process.

Psychosocial Changes

The highest levels of job stress occur at this point in life, when Jamie is trying to establish her identity. Love develops, both romantic and affectionate. Childbirth is most common in this age group, with new families providing new challenges and stresses. Accidents are a leading cause of death in this age group.

TABLE 8-8 Vital Signs: Early Adulthood

HEART RATE	RESPIRATORY RATE	SYSTOLIC BLOOD PRESSURE
60-100/minute	12-20/minute	Less than 120

FIGURE 8-7 Young adults. *(Maridav/Shutterstock)*

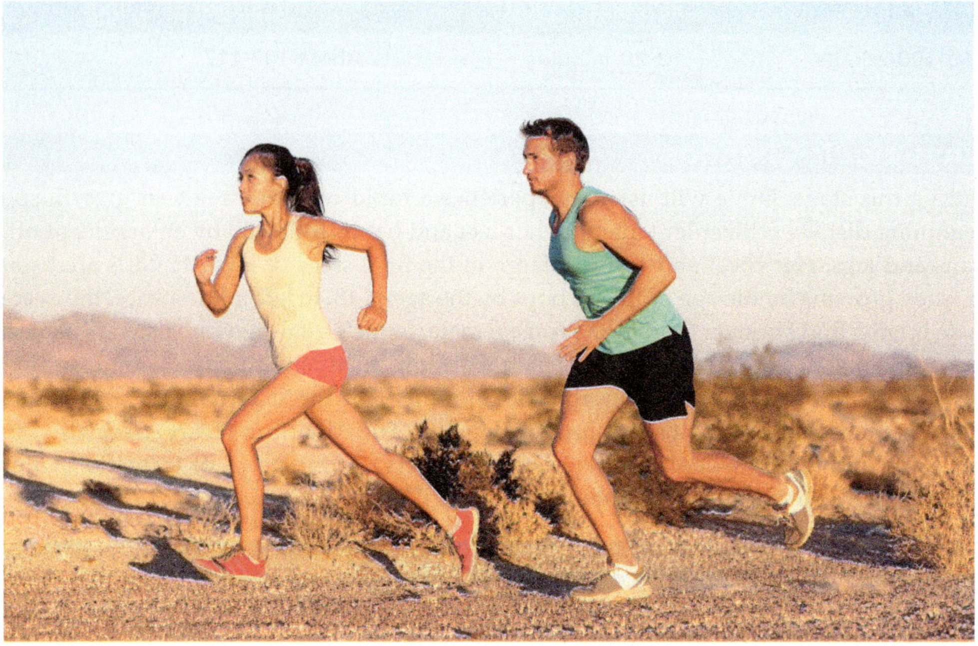

Middle Adulthood (41–60 Years)

middle adulthood stage of life from 41 to 60 years.

For most, ***middle adulthood*** includes a time of reflecting on how far they have come and where they want to go. This internal conflict is often called "midlife crisis."

Physiologic Changes

During this stage of development, Jamie has no significant changes in vital signs from early adulthood. She is starting to have some vision problems and is now wearing prescription glasses. Her cholesterol is a little high, and she is concerned about health problems. Cancer often develops in this age group, weight control becomes more difficult, and for women in the late 40s to early 50s, menopause commences. Heart disease is the major killer after the age of 40 in all age, sex, and racial groups (Figure 8-8).

FIGURE 8-8 Middle-aged adults. *(ViewStock/Getty Images)*

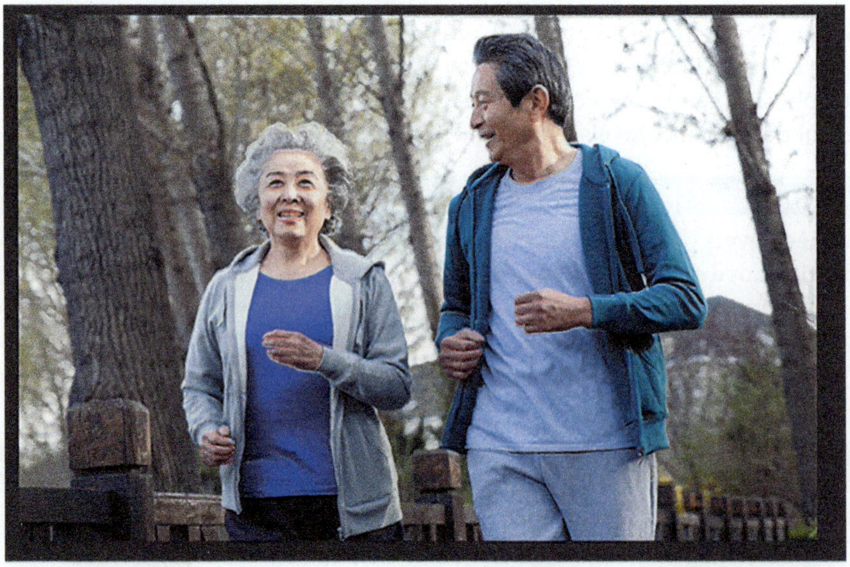

Psychosocial Changes

Jamie is becoming more task-oriented as she sees the time for accomplishing her lifetime goals diminish. Still, she tends to approach problems more as challenges than as threats. With her children starting lives of their own, she is experiencing empty-nest syndrome, the time after the last offspring has left home. This may also be a time of increased freedom and opportunity for self-fulfillment.

Jamie is concerned about her children as they start their new lives, and she is also concerned about caring for aging parents.

Late Adulthood (61 Years and Older)

Late adulthood is often referred to as the "twilight years." This stage of development brings about several physiologic and psychosocial changes, exceeded only by those seen during infancy or adolescence (Figure 8-9).

late adulthood stage of life from 61 years and older.

Physiologic Changes

Jamie's vital signs will depend on her physical and health condition. Her cardiovascular system becomes less efficient, and the volume of blood decreases. She is less tolerant of tachycardia (fast heart rate). Her respiratory system deteriorates and makes her more likely to develop respiratory disorders. Changes in the endocrine system result in decreased metabolism. Her sleep–wake cycle also is disrupted, causing her to have sleep problems. All other body systems are deteriorating as time progresses.

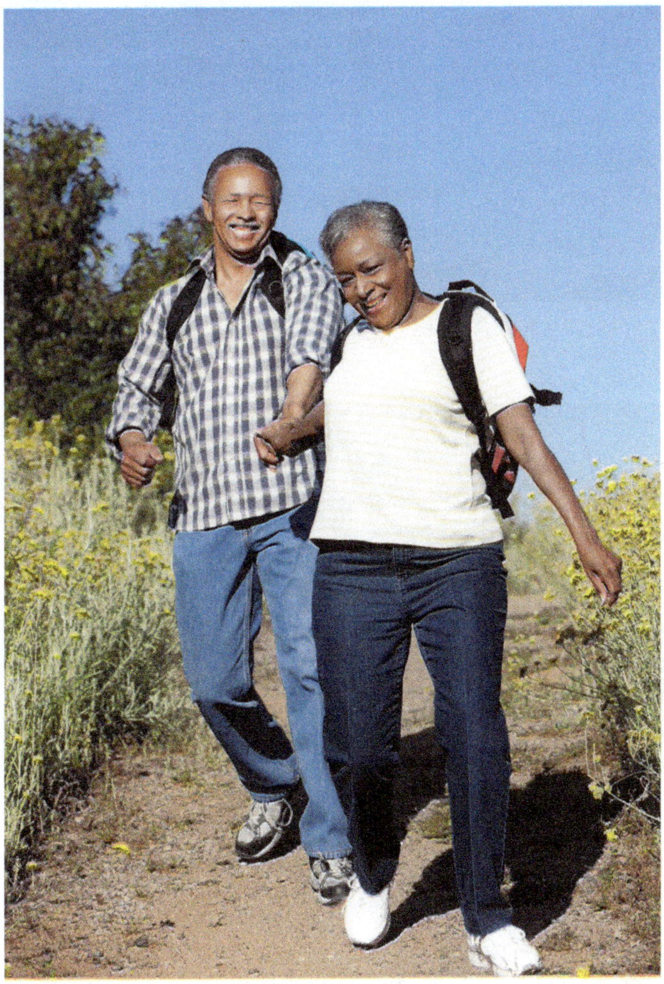

FIGURE 8-9 Older adults. *(Shutterstock)*

Psychosocial Changes

As Jamie ages, she will face many challenges. Motivation, personal interests, and the level of activities will enhance this later time of life. She faces the following challenges:

- **Living environment.** She wonders how long she can live independently and whether she will need to be in an assisted-living facility or perhaps a nursing home.
- **Self-worth.** Though she has slowed down a bit, she is concerned with producing quality work that benefits herself and others.
- **Financial burdens.** With limited income and increasing expenses, financial concerns weigh heavily on her decisions.
- **Death and dying.** She sees friends and relatives become ill and die. Concerns about her own health condition and mortality often come to mind.

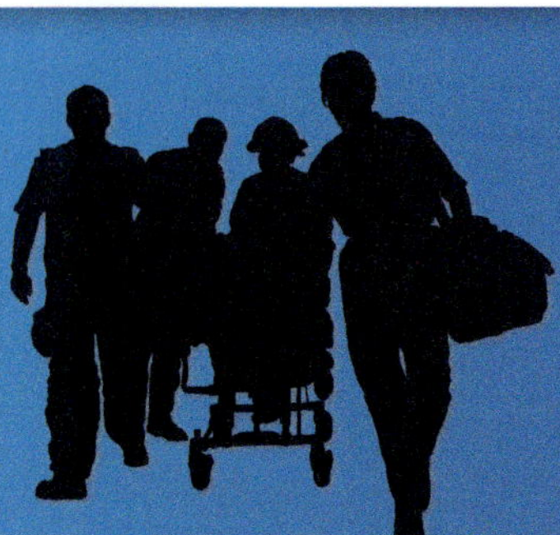

Think Like an EMT

Determining If Vital Signs Are Normal

Although you don't have to memorize vital signs (you can use a reference chart much of the time), you should have a general idea of whether vital signs are normal or abnormal for different age groups. For each of the vital signs in the following list, indicate whether you believe they are normal or abnormal. Note what the normal rate for each patient should be.

1. A 3-year-old boy who seems groggy and has a pulse of 60/minute
2. A 65-year-old man who feels like his heart is skipping beats and has a pulse of 130/minute
3. A 42-year-old man with a respiratory rate of 16 who fell off a curb and hurt his ankle
4. A 77-year-old woman with dizziness and a pulse of 56
5. A 3-month-old baby with a respiratory rate of 30

Point of View

"It is hard to believe I've been alive this long. Life has been good to me. It is my eighty-ninth birthday today. Things have changed a lot since I was born. I lost a sister to polio when she was little. People died right and left from the flu and pneumonia. Doctors then couldn't do anything like they do now. Somehow they keep me going."

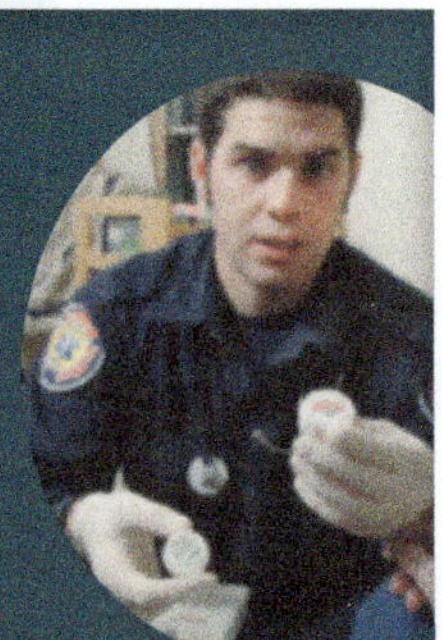

Chapter Review

Key Facts and Concepts

- Understanding the basic physiologic and psychosocial development for each age group will assist you in communicating with and assessing patients of various ages.
- Physiologic differences between the ages will also affect your care. Examples include differences in the respiratory systems of younger patients and the effect of preexisting medical conditions of older patients.
- Infants and young children have less developed and smaller respiratory structures, which can make respiratory conditions worse.
- Your ability to communicate with younger patients will depend on their stage of development. This can range from fear of strangers to separation anxiety from parents and embarrassment during adolescence. Older patients may have issues with denial or depression over medical conditions.

Key Decisions

How do I approach this patient most effectively based on developmental characteristics? Does the age of my patient pose any assessment or care challenges based on the physiologic development?

Chapter Glossary

adolescence stage of life from 13 to 18 years.

bonding the sense that needs will be met.

early adulthood stage of life from 19 to 40 years.

infancy stage of life from birth to 1 year of age.

late adulthood stage of life from 61 years and older.

middle adulthood stage of life from 41 to 60 years.

Moro reflex a response to being startled in which the infant throws out both arms, spreads the fingers, then grabs with fingers and arms.

palmar reflex a grasping reflex in which an infant grabs onto a finger placed in the infant's palm.

preschool age stage of life from 3 to 5 years.

rooting reflex a reflex response in which a hungry infant automatically turns toward the stimulus when the cheek or one side of the mouth is touched.

scaffolding building on what one already knows.

school age stage of life from 6 to 12 years.

sucking reflex a reflex in which stroking a hungry infant's lips causes the infant to start sucking.

temperament the infant's reaction to the infant's environment.

toddler phase stage of life from 12 to 36 months.

trust versus mistrust concept developed from an orderly, predictable environment versus a disorderly, irregular environment.

Preparation for Your Examination and Practice

Short Answer

1. For each of the following, decide which age group would most likely fit the description given:
   Decreased metabolism
   Toilet-trained
   Empty-nest syndrome
   Noticeable development of external sex organs
   Rooting reflex
   Self-destructive behaviors common
   Peak physical condition
   Twilight years
2. How would a child's response to EMS change from birth through adolescence?

Thinking and Linking

Thinking back to the Anatomy and Physiology *and* Principles of Pathophysiology *chapters, link information from those chapters to information in this chapter to answer the following questions:*

1. What is the difference between pediatric and geriatric bones? How would fractures be different between the two age groups?
2. How does heart rate change from birth through adulthood? Does the heart get stronger or weaker as a person enters late adulthood?
3. Does the respiratory system improve or decrease with age? Who is more likely to get a chronic respiratory condition, a child or geriatric patient?

Critical Thinking Exercises

Adolescent patients can offer special challenges to the EMT. The purpose of this exercise will be to consider how you might handle the challenge described here.

- You are called for a 16-year-old girl with abdominal pain. She is with friends at the park. She seems hesitant to answer any of your questions. What characteristic of adolescent development is most likely the cause of this? How could you overcome it?

Pathophysiology to Practice

The following questions are designed to assist you in gathering relevant clinical information and making accurate decisions in the field.

1. Your patient is a young child who has been thrown from a horse. Her vital signs seem mostly OK, but her heart rate is faster than normal. What does this cause you to suspect regarding her condition?
2. Elderly patients often take many medications. How will knowing what medications a patient takes help in your assessment and care of that patient?

Street Scenes

Your ambulance is called to an auto-versus-pedestrian collision. You arrive to find a child lying on the ground near the front of a mid-sized car. The child is crying and being held by his mother.

The driver meets you as you approach. She is crying and tells you she didn't see the child run out of the driveway into the path of her car until it was too late. She tells you she was fortunately going slowly–about 20-25 miles per hour.

You approach the scene and introduce yourself. The child appears to be 3 or 4 years old. He clings fiercely to his mother as you begin to talk. You see an abrasion on his right arm and another on the right side of his forehead.

Because of the mechanism of injury and abrasions on the patient's forehead, you decide you should provide spinal motion restriction precautions.

Street Scene Questions

1. How would you interpret the child's behavior of clinging to his mother? Do you believe it is a normal/good sign or a sign of serious injury?
2. Providing spinal motion restriction will mean restricting his movement. How do you anticipate the patient will respond to this?
3. Would involving the mother be helpful? How?

You continue to assess the child. You find his vital signs are pulse 102 strong and regular, respirations 28 and adequate, and blood pressure 96/58, and capillary refill time is less than 2 seconds. The boy's pupils react to light and appear to be of a normal size.

Street Scene Questions

4. Are these vital signs normal for this patient?
5. Do you need to memorize a list of vital sign ranges for various ages? If not, how would you know what is normal when on a call?
6. How should you explain your assessment and care to this child?

With the help of his mother and a stuffed animal from the ambulance, you are able to calm the child and immobilize him on a backboard. You splint his right arm. The child remains alert and is transported to the hospital uneventfully.

You later find that the child was very lucky and escaped serious injury. His only significant injury was a fracture of his arm–for which he was able to choose the color of his cast.

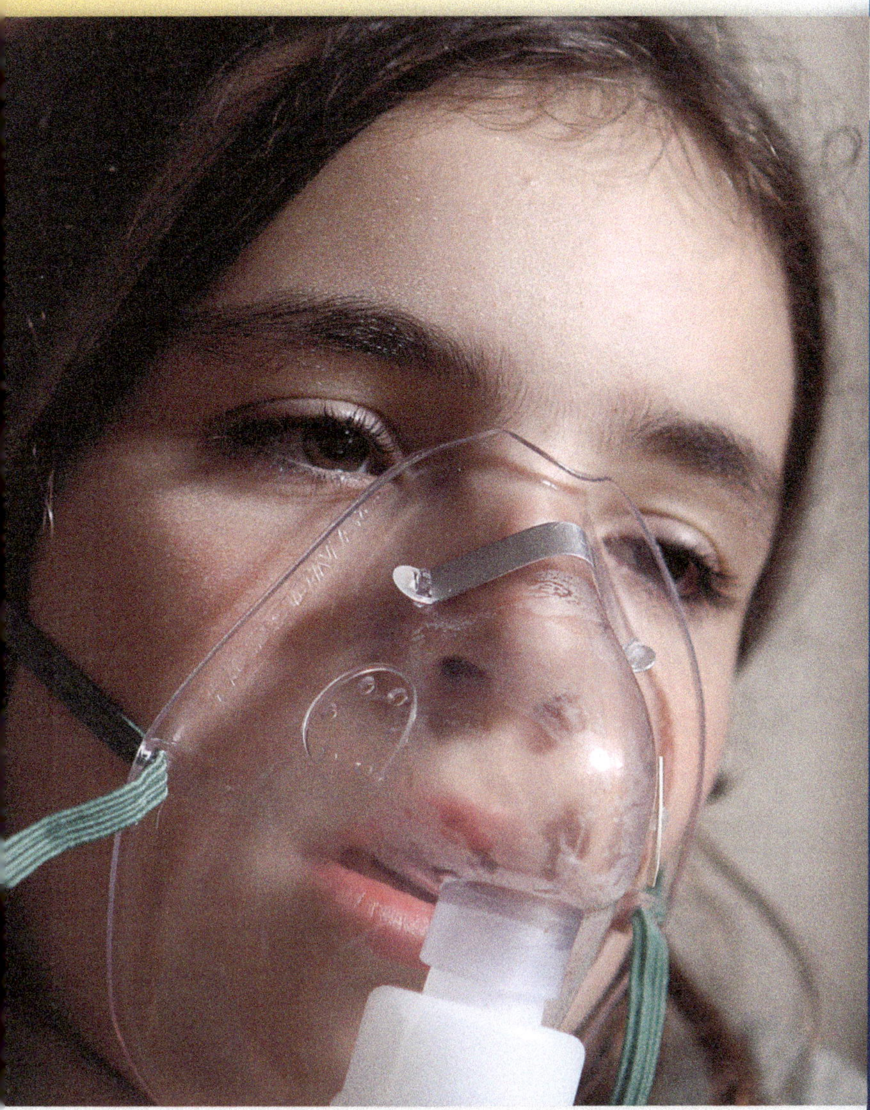

(© Daniel Limmer)

SECTION 2

Airway Management, Respiration, and Artificial Ventilation

CHAPTER 9
Airway Management

CHAPTER 10
Respiration and Artificial Ventilation

The *Airway Management, Respiration, and Artificial Ventilation* section contains two chapters that may be the most important chapters in this textbook. No patient will survive without an open airway or respiration.

Chapter 9 concerns a vital component of the primary assessment evaluation and maintenance of the airway. Airway physiology and pathophysiology are discussed, as are maneuvers for opening the airway, adjuncts for keeping the airway open, and various suctioning devices and techniques.

Chapter 10 discusses respiratory physiology and pathophysiology, adequate and inadequate breathing, positive pressure ventilation, and oxygen therapy. The chapter includes a final section on how you as an EMT—depending on your local protocols—may assist advanced providers with intubation of a patient, potentially while using certain blind intubation devices.

9 Airway Management

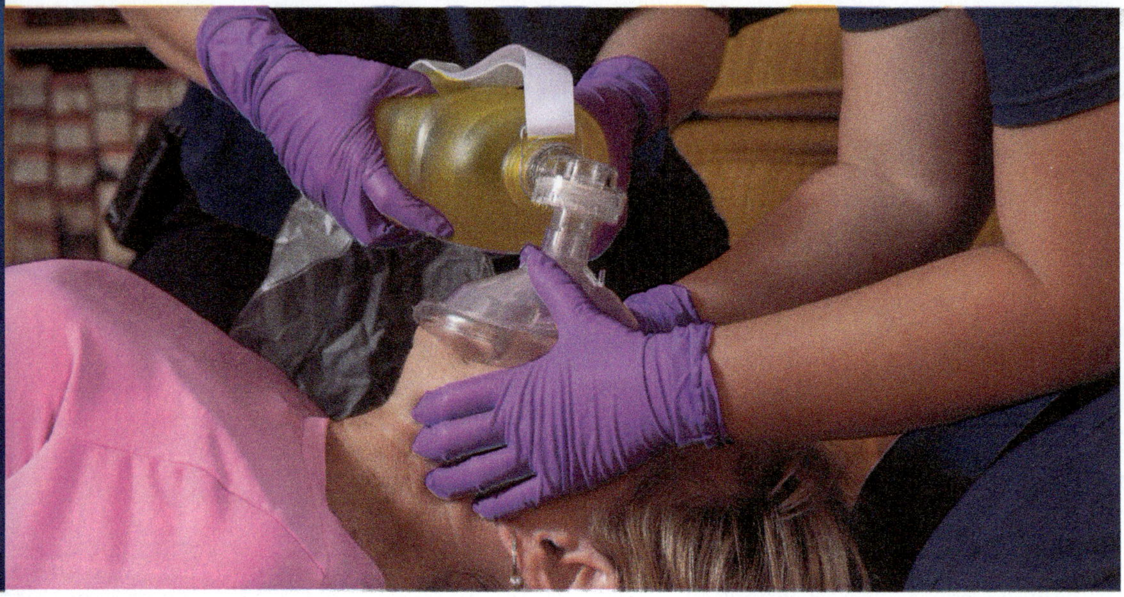

Related Chapters

The following chapters provide additional information related to topics discussed in this chapter:

Standard

Airway Management, Respiration, and Artificial Ventilation (Airway Management)

Competency

Applies knowledge (fundamental depth, foundational breadth) of general anatomy and physiology to patient assessment and management to ensure a patent airway, adequate mechanical ventilation, and respiration for patients of all ages.

Core Concepts

- Physiology of the airway
- Pathophysiology of the airway

- How to recognize an adequate or an inadequate airway
- How to open an airway
- How to use airway adjuncts
- Principles and techniques of suctioning

Outcomes

After reading this chapter, you should be able to:

9.1 Describe the structure and function of the normal airway. (pp. 203–206)

- Differentiate the structures of the upper airway from those of the lower airway.
- Match airway structures to their functions.

9.2 Explain concepts of airway pathophysiology. (pp. 206–210)

- List causes of obstruction of the upper and lower airway.
- List the steps to airway assessment in the primary assessment.
- Distinguish between signs that indicate absent breathing, inadequate airway, and adequate airway.
- List signs of inadequate airway that are more likely in children than in adults.
- Explain how to determine whether a patient's airway status may worsen.

9.3 Describe the use of manual maneuvers to open the airway. (pp. 210–216)

- Given a scenario, provide a rationale for selecting the type of manual maneuver that is best for the patient in the scenario.

9.4 Explain the use of adjunctive equipment to manage a patient's airway. (pp. 216–234)

- State the importance of having a suction device immediately available during airway management procedures.
- Given scenarios, identify adherence to general rules for using airway adjuncts.
- Describe how the features of an oropharyngeal airway allow it to provide an air passage in patients who cannot maintain their own airways.
- List the sequence of steps used in the insertion of an oropharyngeal airway.
- Identify instances when a nasopharyngeal airway offers benefits over an oropharyngeal airway.
- List the sequence of steps used in the insertion of a nasopharyngeal airway.
- Describe the minimum features required of suction units.
- Match the components and attachments of suction devices with their designed purposes.
- Suggest responses to complications encountered when suctioning a patient's airway.

- Recall the general rules that apply to all suctioning techniques.
- Describe decision-making considerations in choosing approaches to suctioning.

Key Terms

airway, *203*
bronchoconstriction, *207*
gag reflex, *217*
glottic opening, *203*
head-tilt, chin-lift maneuver, *213*
jaw-thrust maneuver, *213*
nasopharyngeal airway, *217*
oropharyngeal airway, *217*
patent airway, *203*
stridor, *207*
suctioning, *227*

The average person takes about 20,000 breaths per day. Those breaths deliver oxygen and remove carbon dioxide in an exchange vital to the well-being of the body cells. As we breathe, each of those breaths follows a distinct pathway of structures called the airway. These structures provide a channel for air that starts at the mouth and nose and ends at the gas-exchanging membranes of the alveoli. The airway includes the anatomy of the mouth and throat as well as the trachea and the thousands of small tubes that make up the lungs. In order for air to reach the alveoli, it must follow a clear and relatively unobstructed path, but maintaining an open and clear airway is anything but simple. In fact, EMS exists in large part because of the numerous and varied challenges that can affect airway patency. Physical obstructions such as foreign-body choking, secretions, and blood can all disrupt the flow of air. Structural problems, such as swelling, narrowing, or direct trauma, can also hinder air's movement. Regardless of the nature of the problem, when the path is blocked, bad outcomes occur. When air cannot reach the alveoli or be expelled normally, gas exchange cannot happen. Waste products build up and cellular metabolism fails. If not corrected, these problems will soon lead to death for the patient. As a primary goal, the EMT must assess, recognize, and immediately correct airway challenges. In fact, there are very few challenges that are more important.

In the *Anatomy and Physiology* chapter, you reviewed the anatomy and physiology of the respiratory system. In preparation for this chapter, you should study the following structures of the respiratory system and be able to label them on a blank diagram of the respiratory system: Figure 9-1, Figure 9-2, and Figure 9-3.

This chapter will also discuss a variety of topics you have previously covered in the CPR course you may have taken as a prerequisite to your EMT course. This information included providing rescue breathing, performing cardiopulmonary resuscitation (CPR), and treating airway obstructions in infants, children, and adults. We will discuss each of these topics, but for more detail you should review *Appendix A, Basic Cardiac Life Support Review,* in the back of this book.

FIGURE 9-1 The respiratory system.

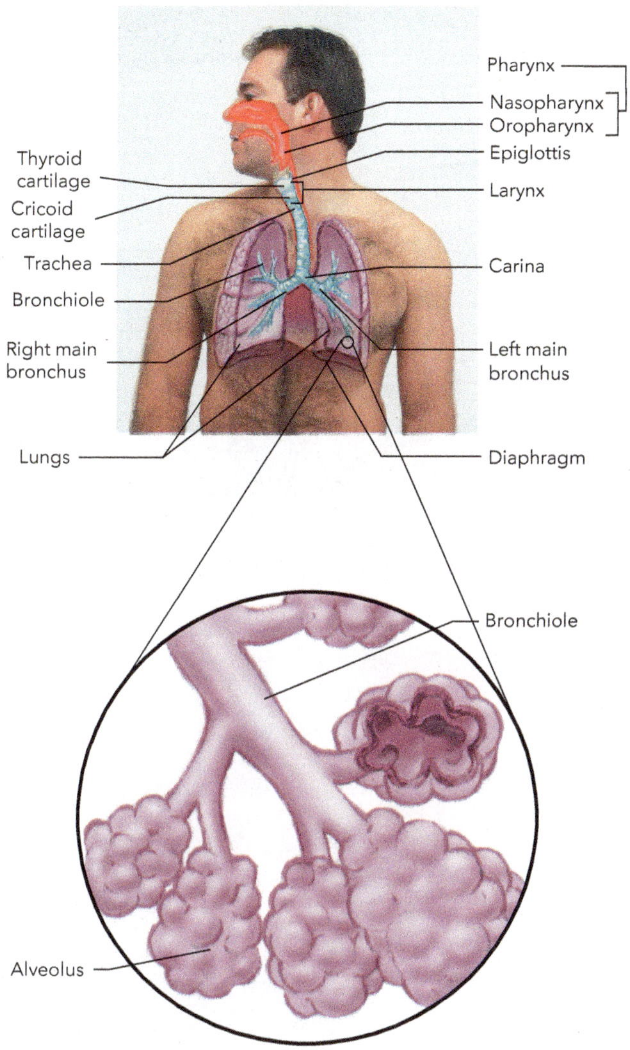

Airway Physiology

✱ CORE CONCEPT
Physiology of the airway

The movement of air into and out of the lungs requires an intact and open ***airway***, or ***patent airway***. That means that airflow is unobstructed and capable of moving freely along its path.

In the upper airway (Figure 9-2), air enters the body through the mouth and nose. The nose is specifically designed to accept air, and through a series of turns and curves, air is warmed and humidified as it proceeds through the nasal passages. The mouth is primarily designed to be the entrance to the digestive system, but it also is an entryway for air (especially in an emergency). Posterior and inferior to the mouth and nasal passages, air enters the throat, or *pharynx*. The pharynx is divided into three regions: the *oropharynx*, where the area of the mouth or oral cavity joins the pharynx; the *nasopharynx*, where the nasal passages empty into the pharynx; and finally, the *laryngopharynx*, the structures surrounding the entrance to the trachea.

The vocal cords are considered the glottic opening, and define the boundary between the upper and lower airway. The laryngopharynx, also known as the hypopharynx, is designed to provide structure to and protect the opening to the trachea. It also is the point of division between the upper airway and the lower airway. The entry point into the larynx, called the ***glottic opening***, is protected by a large leaflike structure called the *epiglottis*. This protective flap that sits above the glottic opening is designed to seal off the trachea during swallowing or in response to the gag reflex. The glottic opening is also protected by the vocal cords. These curtainlike fibers that line either side of the tracheal opening not only can close shut for protection but also vibrate with the passage of air to create the voice.

airway
the passageway by which air enters and leaves the body. The structures of the airway are the nose, mouth, pharynx, larynx, trachea, bronchi, and lungs.

patent airway
an airway (passage from nose or mouth to lungs) that is open and clear and will remain open and clear without interference to the passage of air into and out of the body.

glottic opening
the level of the vocal cords that defines the boundary between the upper and lower airways.

FIGURE 9-2 The upper airway.

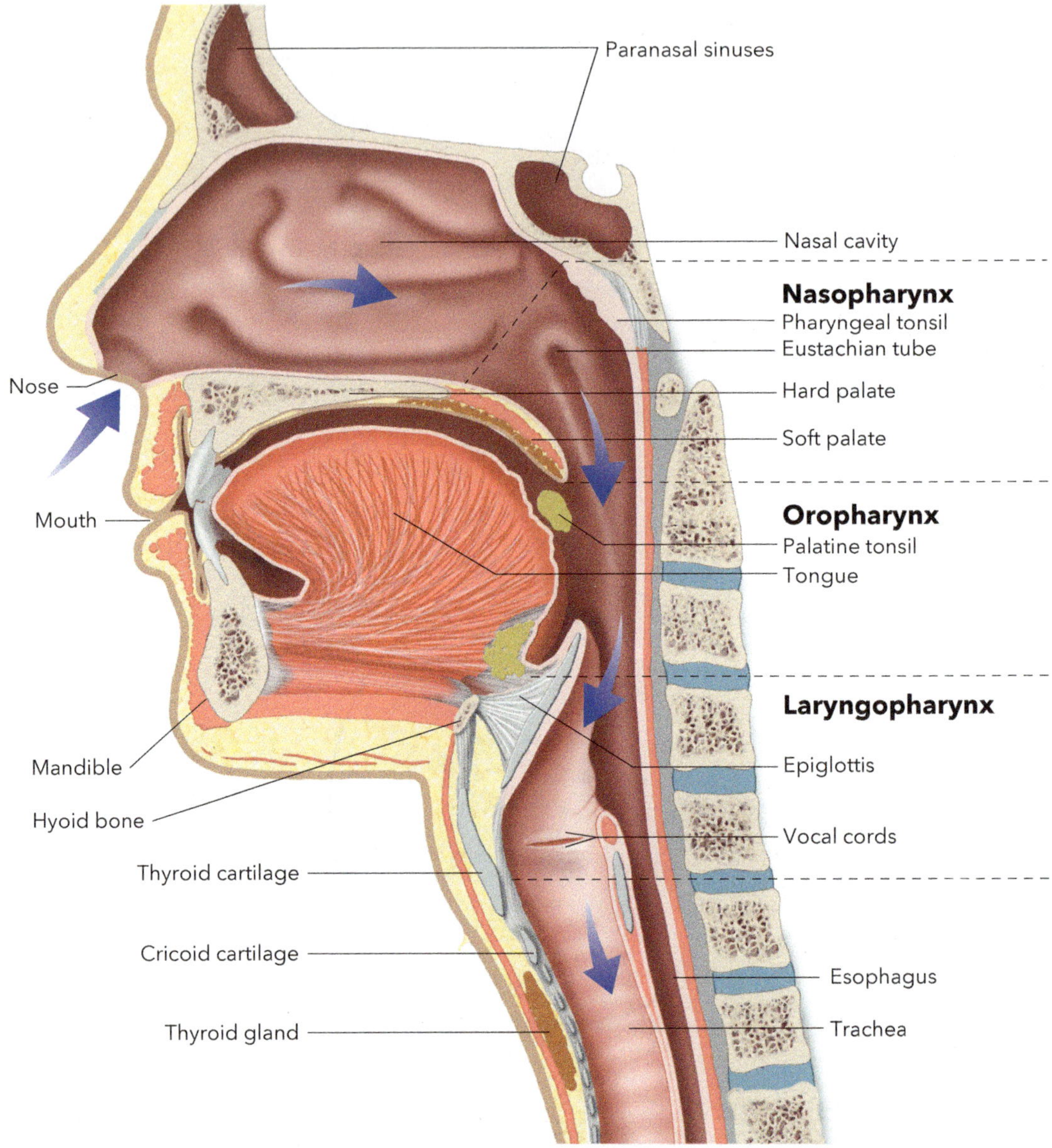

The larynx itself is supported and protected by cartilage (Figure 9-3). The shieldlike thyroid cartilage protects the front of the larynx and forms the Adam's apple. The cricoid ring, a complete circle of cartilage, forms the lower aspect of the larynx and provides structure to the superior trachea.

FIGURE 9-3 Larynx. *(Soleil Nordic/Shutterstock)*

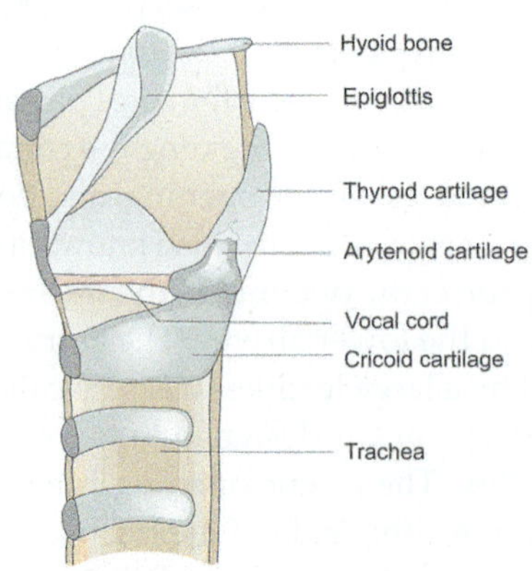

The lower airway (Figure 9-4) begins below the glottic opening and is composed of the trachea, bronchial passages, and the alveoli. From the glottic opening, air enters the trachea. The trachea is a tube protected by 16 rings of cartilage. These rings provide structure and prevent the trachea from collapsing. The top ring is the cricoid ring, which extends fully 360 degrees around. In the other rings, the cartilage extends only about three-fourths of the way around and is connected posteriorly by smooth muscle. The trachea branches at the *carina* and forms two mainstem bronchi. These large branches then further subdivide to form smaller and smaller air passages called bronchioles. All the air passages are supported by cartilage and are lined with smooth muscle. This smooth muscle allows the bronchioles to change their internal diameter in response to specific stimulation. The bronchioles end at the alveoli. Alveoli are tiny sacs that occur in grapelike bunches at the end of the airway. These alveoli are surrounded by pulmonary capillaries, and it is through their thin membranes that oxygen and carbon dioxide are diffused. (Gas exchange will be discussed in greater detail in the chapter titled *Respiration and Artificial Ventilation*.) It is important to remember that the bronchioles divide and travel in every direction. As a result, tiny bronchioles and the millions of alveoli to which they connect cover most anatomic regions of the chest from the collarbones to the diaphragm.

Pediatric Airway Physiology

The infant and child's neck muscles are immature, and the airway structures are shorter, narrower, and less rigid than an adult's. There are several other special characteristics about infants' and children's respiratory systems that you should know (Figure 9-5):

- The mouth and nose are smaller and more easily obstructed than in adults.
- The tongue takes up more space proportionately in the mouth than in adults.
- Newborns and infants typically breathe through their noses. Nasal obstruction can impair breathing.
- The trachea (windpipe) is softer and more flexible in infants and children.
- The trachea is narrower and is easily obstructed by swelling or foreign objects.
- The chest wall is softer, and infants and children tend to depend more on their diaphragms for breathing than do adults.

FIGURE 9-4 The lower airway. The bronchial tree. (*inset*) The alveolar sacs (clusters of individual alveoli).

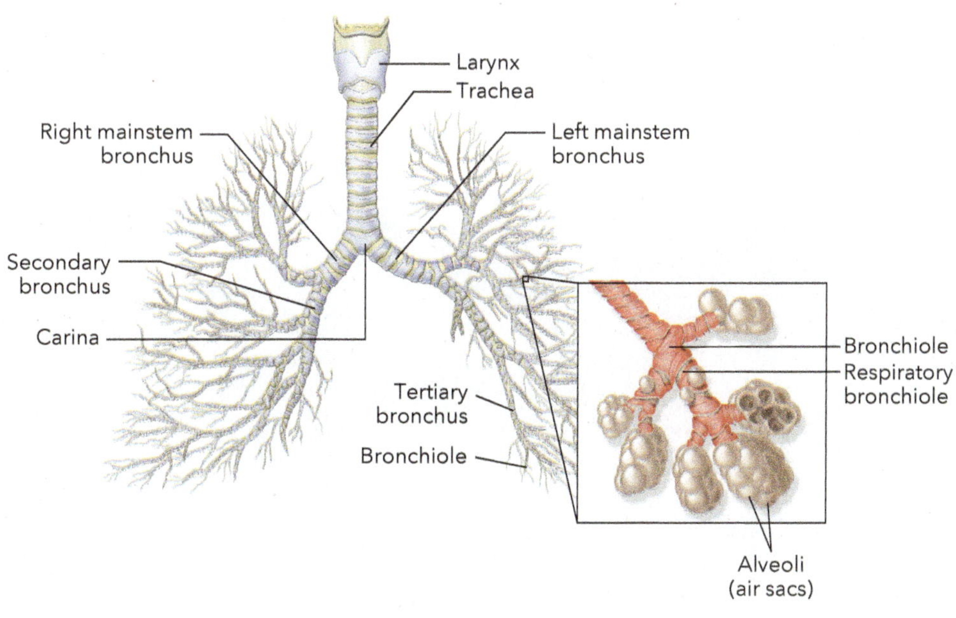

FIGURE 9-5 A comparison of child and adult respiratory passages.

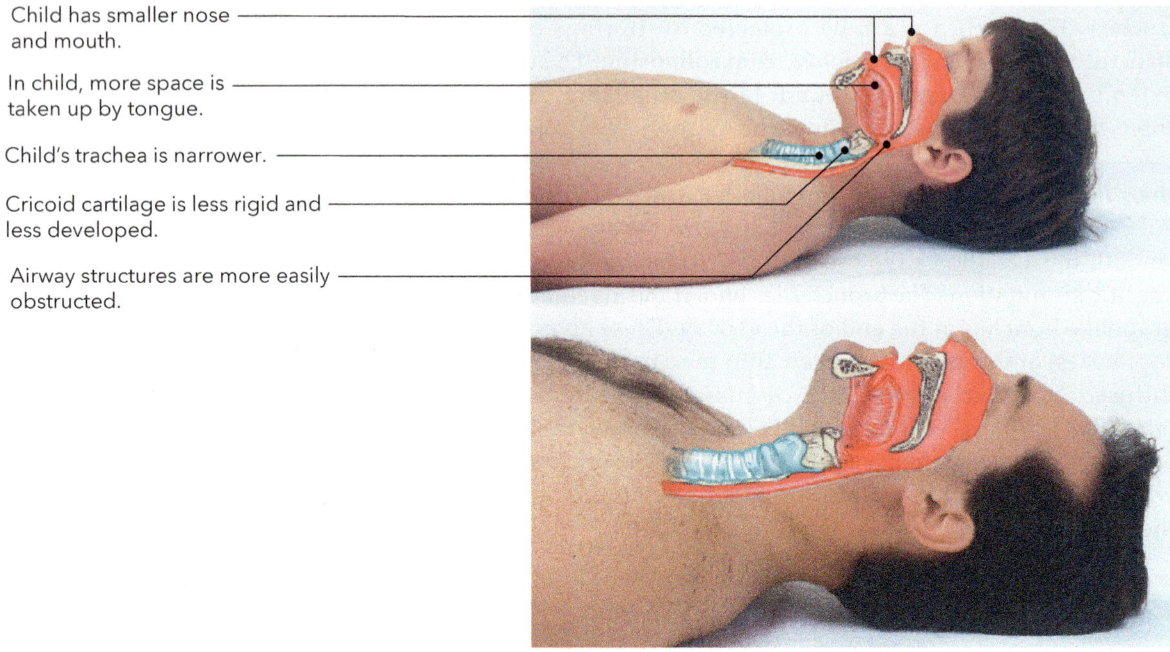

CORE CONCEPT
Pathophysiology of the airway

Airway Pathophysiology

For air to make the journey from the nose and mouth to the lungs, the pathway must be relatively unobstructed. A variety of obstructions can interfere with airflow. Foreign bodies such as food and small toys are common obstructions, as are fluids, including blood and vomit. The airway can even be obstructed by the patient. A patent airway requires control of more than 14 different muscle groups that support and keep open the channel of air. This is referred to as intact muscle tone. Conditions such as altered mental status and neurologic disorders can result in a loss of this muscle tone and lead to collapse of the airway. A common obstruction in a person with a decreased mental status is the tongue—or, more precisely, the epiglottis connected to the tongue. This obstruction occurs when a lack of muscle tone causes the tongue to relax and fall back. When it does, the epiglottis falls back and covers the entrance to the trachea. Often people consider this as the tongue obstructing the airway but, in reality, the epiglottis actually causes the obstruction. Patient position is often an associated factor in muscle tone–related airway obstruction. An unconscious or semiconscious patient lying flat (supine) is often at higher risk for the simple airway occlusion described above. This doesn't mean that the supine position is universally bad; it simply means that anytime a patient has an altered mental status, the airway must be carefully and continually monitored.

Point of View

"It happened so fast. I knew I was allergic to bees, but I never had a reaction that bad. It was like all of a sudden, I just couldn't breathe. I was fine just a few moments earlier, then my voice started to get real raspy and I could barely take a breath. I thought I was going to die. I remember the EMTs arriving, but not much more. I know they helped me with a dose of epinephrine, but by the time I regained consciousness, I was at the hospital. That medicine saved my life."

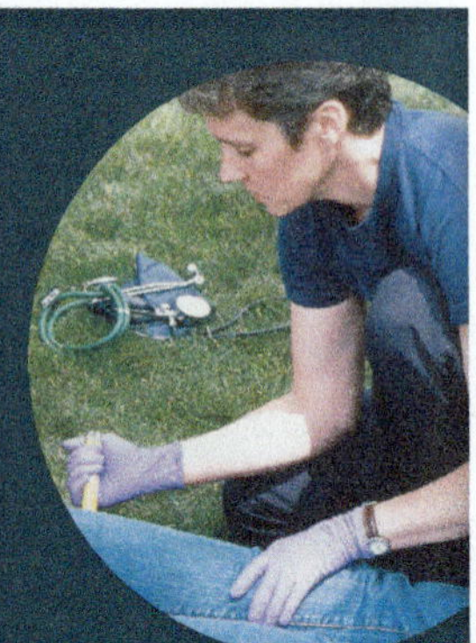

Airway obstruction can occur acutely, as in choking on a foreign body, or it can occur over time. Airway obstruction during a severe allergic reaction (anaphylaxis) from swollen airway tissues can rapidly lead to death if not treated immediately with epinephrine injection. Burns, blunt-force trauma, and certain infections can cause swelling of the tissues in and around the glottic opening. This can also impede the movement of air. Obstructions can also either completely or partially block the airway. As such, it is always important to evaluate the patency of an airway not just in the immediate sense but also in an ongoing sense. "Yes, the airway is open now, but will it stay open?"

In the lower airway, smooth muscle can constrict and decrease the internal diameter of the airway. Changing the internal diameter even slightly causes a significant increase in the resistance to airflow and can seriously impact the patient's ability to move air. This is commonly referred to as ***bronchoconstriction*** or bronchospasm, and is common in diseases such as asthma.

bronchoconstriction (BRON-ko-kun-STRIK-shun) the contraction of smooth muscle that lines the bronchial passages that results in a decreased internal diameter of the airway and increased resistance to airflow.

Sounds of a Partially Obstructed Airway

A partially obstructed airway can often be identified by the sounds of limited air movement. Understanding these sounds can help you better understand the pathophysiology of the obstruction.

- **Stridor.** Stridor is typically caused by severely restricted air movement in the upper airway. As air is forced by pressure through a partial obstruction, a high-pitched, sometimes almost whistling sound can be heard. Typically, stridor indicates a severely narrowed passage of air and suggests near obstruction. In stridor, the obstruction can be a foreign body, such as a toy, or it can be caused by swelling of the upper airway tissues, as in an infection.
- **Hoarseness.** Voice changes, such as stridor, often reflect a narrowing of the upper airway passages. Voice changes are often useful in assessing an ongoing airway issue. For example, in a person whose airway is swelling after a burn, you may note a normal voice to begin with, but a raspy voice as the swelling builds up around the vocal cords. The development of hoarseness is often an ominous sign.
- **Snoring.** Snoring is the sound of the soft tissue of the upper airway creating impedance (or partial obstruction) to the flow of air. Many persons normally snore while asleep, but snoring in the case of injury or illness can often indicate a decrease in mental status such that airway muscle tone is diminished. It is also an indication that the airway needs assistance to stay open.
- **Gurgling.** Gurgling is the sound of fluid obstructing the airway. As air is forced through the liquid, the gurgling sound is made. Common liquid obstructions include vomit, blood, and other airway secretions. Gurgling is a sign that immediate suctioning is necessary.

Patient Assessment

The Airway

There are really two questions you must consider when assessing a patient's airway: "Is the airway open?" and "Will the airway stay open?" (See Box 9-1.)

CORE CONCEPT

How to recognize an adequate or an inadequate airway

Is the Airway Open?

You can determine the presence of an airway in most patients by simply saying hello. The patient's ability to speak is an immediate indicator of moving air. At the same time, a person who is unable to speak, or one who speaks in an unusually raspy or hoarse voice, may be having difficulty moving air. ***Stridor*** is a high-pitched sound generated from partially obstructed airflow in the upper airway. This sound can be present on inhalation or exhalation (or both) and is an ominous sign of poor air movement. The sounds of breathing from the mouth and nose typically should be free of gurgling, gasping, wheezing, snoring, and stridor. You may also see patients use position to keep an airway open. When swelling obstructs airflow through the upper airway (typically due to infection),

stridor (STRI-dor) a high-pitched sound generated from partially obstructed airflow in the upper airway.

BOX 9-1 The Airway in the Primary Assessment–ABC

- Is the airway open?
- Is the patient able to speak?
- Look.
  - Visually inspect the airway to ensure it is free from foreign bodies and obvious trauma.
  - Look for visual clues of potential airway dangers such as facial burns, external neck trauma, and bleeding in and around the mouth and nose.
  - Look for visual signs of breathing such as the chest rising.
  - Look at the patient's position. Does the patient need to sit bolt upright to keep breathing?
- Listen.
  - Listen for the sound of breathing.
  - Listen for sounds of obstructed air movement such as stridor, snoring, gurgling, and gasping.
- Feel.
  - Feel for air movement at the mouth.
  - Feel the chest for rise and fall.
- Will the airway stay open?
  - Are there immediate correctable threats?
  - If no airway, then open it.
  - Consider how you might keep an unstable airway open.
  - Consider ALS for more definitive airway care.
- Are there potential threats that may develop later?
  - Reassess, reassess, reassess.
  - Assess for signs of impending collapse such as stridor or voice changes.
  - Consider conditions that may later threaten the airway (such as anaphylaxis).
  - Consider the patient's mental status. Can the patient maintain and protect the airway? Will that mental status likely change over time?

patients may present in the "sniffing position." You will notice a bolt-upright position with the head pitched forward as if attempting to smell something. In a person with a partially obstructed airway, this position can be critical to keeping air moving.

Often it is not immediately apparent whether an airway is open. In your CPR class, you may have learned about the Look-Listen-Feel method. If a person is unconscious, you may need to employ this method to ensure an airway is present. In this case, look at the chest to see whether it is rising and falling. The airway should also be visually inspected for foreign bodies, including objects and fluid. You should listen at the mouth for sounds of breathing while placing your hand on the patient's chest to feel for movement. You may also need to place your hand near the patient's mouth to feel for air flow. In these cases, you may detect subtle air movement that might not be apparent with visual observation alone.

Remember that you assess the airway as part of the primary assessment and that when you find a problem in the primary assessment, you must stop and fix that problem. In this case, if there is no airway present, stop and provide one. (We will discuss airway treatment later in this chapter.)

Will the Airway Stay Open?

The first part of this chapter discussed ensuring an open airway. That is certainly important, but of equal importance now will be ensuring that the airway stays open. Airway assessment is not just a moment in time, but rather a constant consideration, especially in a critical patient. In some cases you may need to immediately consider how to keep an airway open after establishing it. In a person with no ability to keep an airway open, you may manually open it with a head-tilt, chin lift. However, the moment you take your hands away, that airway will be lost. At this point you must consider additional steps. Similarly, if you identify a partially obstructed airway, you must ask yourself, "How long will it be until this airway is completely obstructed?" and "What are the necessary steps to take to prevent or resolve this problem?" Consider the following examples:

- You assess the airway of an unconscious victim of a fall off a ladder. She has no airway, so you apply the jaw thrust. The airway opens and she begins to breathe. However, when you take your hands away, the airway closes and she stops breathing. In this case the airway is open, but it will not stay open.
- You assess a child after multiple bee stings. He speaks to you with a hoarse voice but is breathing. You note stridor on inspiration. He has an airway, but his voice changes indicate that his airway is swelling and partially obstructing air movement. How long will he be able to move air? What steps must you take immediately to keep air moving?

Remember also that the ability to maintain an airway can change over time. As mental status decreases, so might the ability to protect an airway. Always reassess this capability and remember that just because your patient has an open airway now, there is no guarantee your patient will continue to have an open airway later.

Signs of an Inadequate Airway

Signs that would indicate no airway or a potentially inadequate airway include the following:

- There are no signs of breathing or air movement.
- There is evidence of foreign bodies in the airway, including blood, vomit, or objects such as broken teeth.
- No air can be felt or heard at the nose or mouth, or the amount of air exchanged is below normal.
- The patient is unable to speak or has great difficulty speaking.
- The patient's voice has an unusual hoarse or raspy quality.
- Chest movements are absent, minimal, or uneven. (Be aware, however, that patients can have chest movement even with an obstructed airway.)
- Movement associated with breathing is limited to the abdomen (abdominal breathing).
- Breath sounds are diminished or absent.
- Noises such as wheezing, stridor, snoring, gurgling, or gasping are heard during breathing.
- In children, there may be retractions (a pulling in of the muscles) above the clavicles and between and below the ribs.
- Nasal flaring (widening of the nostrils of the nose with respirations) may be present, especially in infants and children.

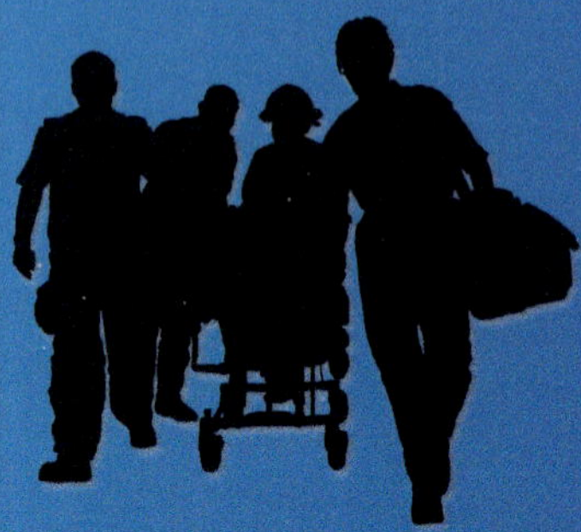

Think Like an EMT

Will the Airway Stay Open?

You have learned about the signs of an unstable airway. Use this information to consider whether the following patients have airways that will stay open.

1. A 16-year-old asthma patient who tells you he is tired and seems to be nodding off to sleep
2. A 72-year-old female who was recently diagnosed with pneumonia. Today she has called you because her breathing is much worse. She is breathing rapidly and has diminished lung sounds on the left side.
3. A 35-year-old male who tells you he is having trouble breathing. You notice he is drooling and is sitting bolt upright. When you attempt to lean him back on the stretcher, he coughs, gags, and repositions himself in a sniffing position.
4. A 16-month-old whose mother tells you the child has had a cold for two days and woke up with a cough tonight. The child is awake and alert but barking like a seal when coughing.

Opening the Airway

CORE CONCEPT
How to open an airway

Assessing the airway is one of the highest priorities of your assessment. When signs indicate an inadequate airway, a life-threatening condition exists. Prompt action must be taken to open and maintain the airway, as explained next.

For most patients, the airway can be assessed by simply assessing their speech. In a person with a diminished mental status, the procedures for airway evaluation, opening the airway, and artificial ventilation are best carried out with the patient lying supine (flat on the back). Scan 9-1 illustrates the technique for positioning a patient found lying on the floor or ground. Patients who are found in positions other than supine or on the ground should be moved to a supine position on the floor or stretcher for evaluation and treatment.

Any movement of a trauma (injured) patient before immobilization of the head and spine can produce serious injury to the spinal cord. If you suspect an injury that could have resulted in spinal trauma, protect the head and neck as you position the patient. Airway and breathing, however, have priority over protection of the spine and must be ensured as quickly as possible. If the trauma patient must be moved to open the airway or to provide ventilations, you will probably not have time to provide complete spinal precautions but, instead, will provide as much manual stabilization as possible.

Interpret the following as indications that head, neck, or spinal injury may have occurred, especially when the patient is unconscious and cannot tell you what happened or respond to assessment questions:

- Mechanism of injury is one that can cause head, neck, or spine injury. For example, a patient who is found on the ground near a ladder or stairs may have such injuries. Motor-vehicle collisions are another common cause of head, neck, and spine injuries.
- Any injury at or above the level of the shoulders indicates that head, neck, or spine injuries may also be present.
- Family or bystanders may tell you that an injury to the head, neck, or spine has occurred, or they may give you information that leads you to suspect it.

SCAN 9-1 Positioning the Patient for Basic Life Support

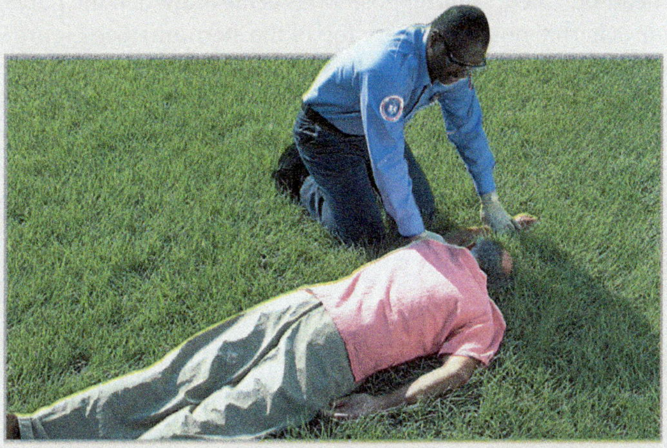

1. Straighten the legs and position the closer arm above the patient's head.

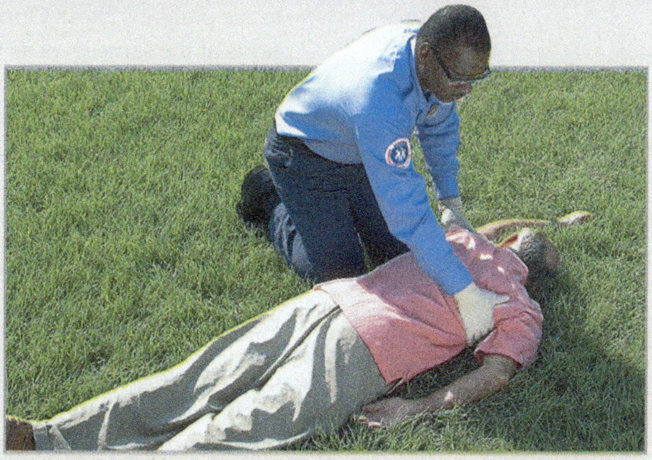

2. Grasp under the distant armpit.

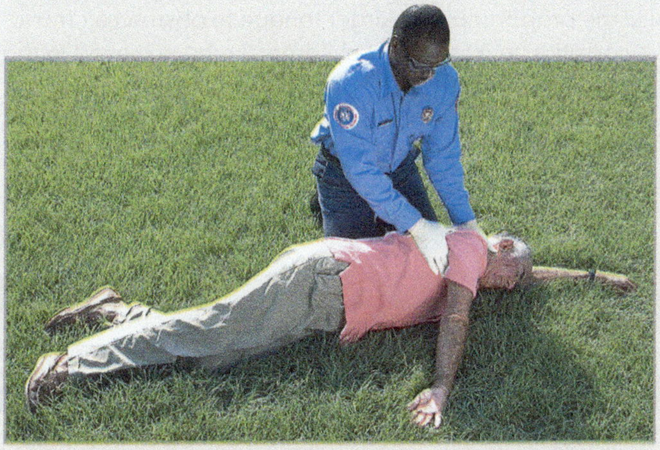

3. Cradle the head and neck and move the patient as a unit onto one side.

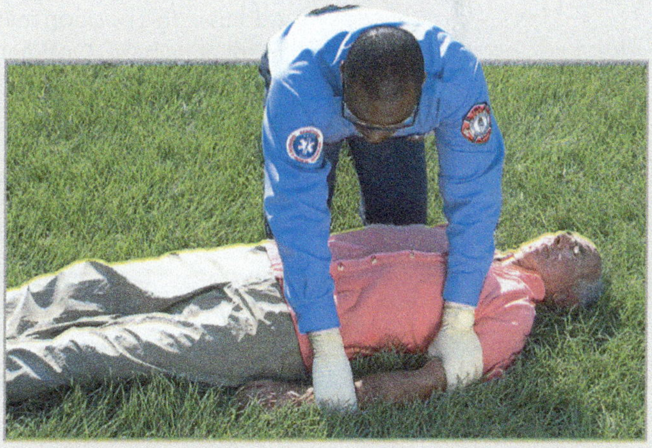

4. Move the patient onto the patient's back and reposition the extended arm.

NOTE: *This maneuver is used when the rescuer must act alone.*

Maintaining an Open Airway

Some patients will have an airway that is threatened but currently open. Often these patients are best managed simply by moving them to a proper position that facilitates continued air movement. In conscious patients, this frequently means allowing them to sit up and move themselves to their own preferred position. Conscious patients with a threatened airway will be very clear about the position they need to assume. In an unconscious or semiconscious patient with an intact airway, the head-elevated, sniffing position can often be helpful in maintaining a clear channel for air to follow.

Head-Elevated, Sniffing Position

In a supine patient, an optimal airway position can be achieved by creating a head-elevated, sniffing position. The slight elevation and anterior positioning of the head better aligns airway structures to allow for improved airway patency. In this position, the patient's head is moved in an anterior fashion to replicate the posture a person would take if that person were smelling flowers or sniffing an odor. In a supine patient, this position is typically achieved by placing about 1.5–2 inches (3–5 cm) of padding behind the patient's head. Not all patients will require padding, however. Different anatomy and different head size related to age can create unique positioning needs. It is important that you visualize and assess the requirements of each patient. Ideal positioning can be determined by assessing the position of the head relative to the patient's chest. Optimal head-elevated, sniffing position is achieved when the patient's ear is at the same level as the suprasternal notch (the very top of the sternum). See Figure 9-6. This is best visualized from a lateral viewpoint. Although this position is not absolutely necessary and may be contraindicated if the risk of spinal injury is present, it significantly enhances success when used in conjunction with other airway and breathing interventions.

Pediatric Note

Pediatric Airway Position

Children less than 4 years old often have a proportionately larger head with a larger occiput (the round posterior aspect of the skull). They also have a narrower, more flexible trachea. Laying a small child with altered mental status flat could result in flexion of the airway. This position would cause the head and neck to be flexed down toward the chest, and on the inside, the airway could be obstructed. (Exaggerated flexion of the airway causes the pliable trachea to bend unnaturally and block off the flow of air.) In addition, this position may cause the proportionately larger tongue to obstruct air movement at its base. Optimal airway position in infants and children can be achieved in the same manner as in adults, by aligning the patient's ear to the level of the suprasternal notch. Because of the proportionally larger head in pediatric anatomy, different areas may need to be padded to achieve this position. In small children, the head-elevated, sniffing position often requires padding to be placed behind the shoulders. In older or larger children, it may require padding behind the occiput, just as for adults.

Providing an Airway: Manual Airway Maneuvers

For any patient who does not have an intact airway, or for patients who lose their airway patency, you must intervene immediately. These patients require manual opening of the airway and may require ongoing interventions to support airway patency.

As stated previously, many airway problems are caused by lack of tone in the muscles that keep the airway open. As control over these muscles diminishes, muscles such as the tongue relax and allow the airway to be obstructed. Often position contributes to this problem. As the head flexes forward, the tongue may slide into the airway, causing the epiglottis to obstruct the airway. If the patient is unconscious, the tongue loses muscle tone, and muscles of the lower jaw relax. Since the tongue is attached to the lower jaw, the risk of airway obstruction is even greater during unconsciousness.

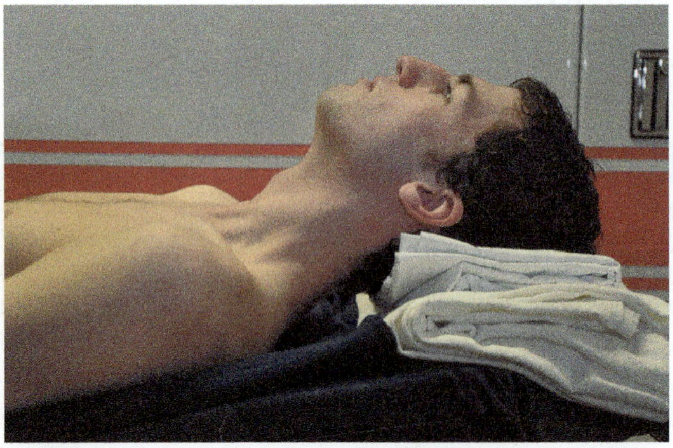

FIGURE 9-6 The head-elevated, sniffing position.
(© Edward T. Dickinson, MD)

FIGURE 9-7 Head-tilt, chin-lift maneuver, side view. *Inset* shows EMT's fingertips under the bony area at the center of the patient's lower jaw.

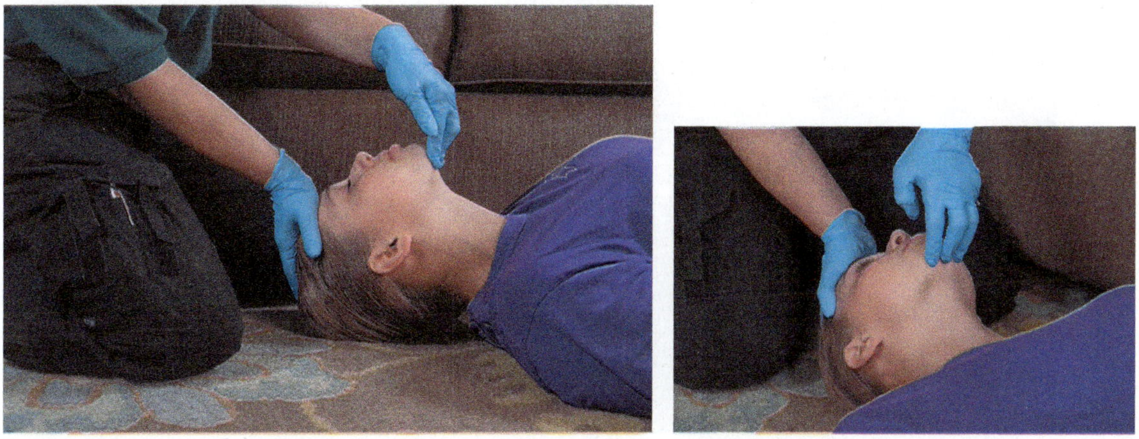

The basic procedures for opening the airway help to correct the position of the tongue and therefore move laryngeal tissues such as the epiglottis out of the way of the glottic opening.

Two procedures are commonly recommended for opening the airway: the head-tilt, chin-lift maneuver and the jaw-thrust maneuver, the latter being recommended when head, neck, or spine injury is suspected.

Head-Tilt, Chin-Lift Maneuver

NOTE: *If any indication of head, neck, or spine injury is present, do not use the head-tilt, chin-lift maneuver. (Use the jaw-thrust maneuver instead.) Remember that any unconscious and many conscious trauma patients should be suspected of having an injury to the head, neck, or spine.*

The ***head-tilt, chin-lift maneuver*** (Figure 9-7) uses head position to align the structures of the airway and provide for the free passage of air. The anterior movement of the jaw draws the tongue forward, away from the oral pharynx, and can usually resolve a simple obstruction.

To perform the head-tilt, chin-lift maneuver, follow these steps:

1. Once the patient is supine, place one hand on the forehead and place the fingertips of the other hand under the bony area at the center of the patient's lower jaw.
2. Tilt the head by applying gentle pressure to the patient's forehead.
3. Use your fingertips to lift the chin and to support the lower jaw. Move the jaw forward to a point where the lower teeth are almost touching the upper teeth. Do not compress the soft tissues under the lower jaw, which can obstruct the airway.
4. Do not allow the patient's mouth to be closed. To provide an adequate opening at the mouth, you may need to use the thumb of the hand supporting the chin to pull back the patient's lower lip. Do not insert your thumb into the patient's mouth (to avoid being bitten).

head-tilt, chin-lift maneuver a means of correcting blockage of the airway by the tongue by tilting the head back and lifting the chin. Used when no trauma or injury is suspected.

Jaw-Thrust Maneuver

NOTE: *The jaw-thrust maneuver is the only recommended airway procedure for unconscious patients with possible head, neck, or spine injury or unknown mechanism of injury.*

The ***jaw-thrust maneuver*** (Figure 9-8) is most commonly used to open the airway of an unconscious patient with suspected head, neck, or spine injury or unknown mechanism of injury.

NOTE: *The purpose of the jaw-thrust maneuver is to open the airway without moving the head or neck.*

Follow these steps:

1. Carefully keep the patient's head, neck, and spine aligned, moving the body as a unit as you place the patient in the supine position.

jaw-thrust maneuver a means of correcting blockage of the airway by moving the jaw forward without tilting the head or neck. Used when trauma or injury is suspected to open the airway without causing further injury to the spinal cord in the neck.

FIGURE 9-8 Jaw-thrust maneuver, side view. *Inset* shows EMT's finger position at angle of the jaw just below the ears.

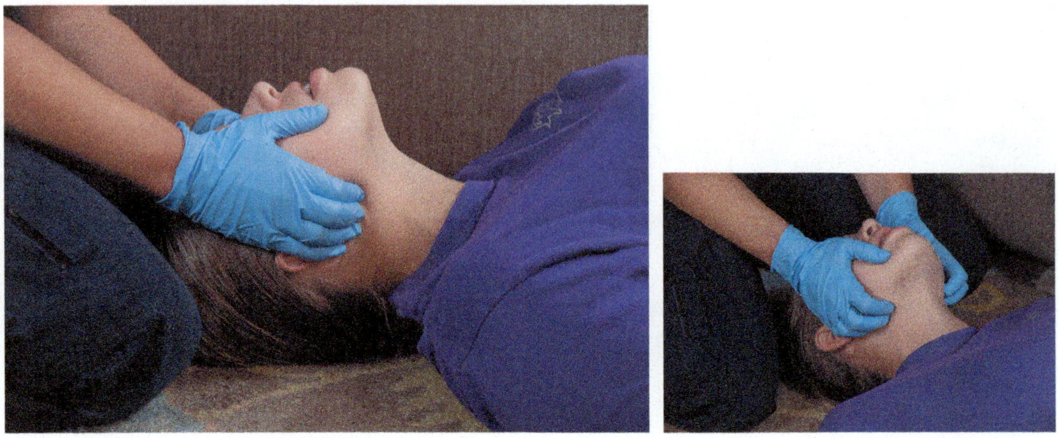

2. Kneel at the top of the patient's head. For long-term comfort, it may be helpful to rest your elbows on the same surface as the patient's head.
3. Carefully reach forward and gently place one hand on each side of the patient's lower jaw, at the angles of the jaw below the ears.
4. Using your index fingers, push the angles of the patient's lower jaw forward.
5. You may need to retract the patient's lower lip with your thumb to keep the mouth open.
6. Do not tilt or rotate the patient's head.

In addition to physically opening the airway with the head-tilt, chin-lift or the jaw-thrust maneuver, it is imperative that the airway also be cleared of any secretions, blood, or vomitus. The most effective way to clear the patient's airway is with a wide-bore, rigid-tip Yankauer suction device. *It is crucial to have a suction unit ready for immediate use when opening and maintaining the airway.* The equipment and techniques used for suctioning will be discussed later in this chapter.

Obstructed Airways

If an airway has been opened and it remains obstructed, you should consider the possibility of a foreign-body obstruction. If attempts to ventilate and reposition/reopen the airway fail, you must immediately move to foreign-body airway procedures. If possible, request advanced life support early, as ALS may offer additional foreign-body airway procedures. Although rapid transport may be necessary, never delay the initiation of foreign-body airway procedures in favor of transport.

Conscious Choking Adults and Children

The American Heart Association assigns choking to one of two categories—nonsevere or severe—depending on the extent to which the trachea is blocked. In severe choking, the trachea is fully blocked. No air is moving. These patients may still be conscious. They may be walking, grabbing, and fearful, but there will be no signs of air movement. These patients will not breathe, cough, or gasp. These patients require urgent intervention.

In nonsevere choking, the trachea is partially blocked but allows some air to be exchanged. These patients may speak (voice changes such as a hoarse or raspy voice can be an indication of nonsevere choking), cough, wheeze, or gasp. They may tell you they are choking. Stridor may be present. However, the key to identifying this category is the presence of at least some air movement. In general, these patients must be monitored carefully but be left alone to allow the body to do its best to clear the obstruction. Patients should be encouraged to cough and should be treated only if the obstruction becomes severe.

FIGURE 9-9 For a severe airway obstruction in an infant, alternate (A) back slaps with (B) chest thrusts.

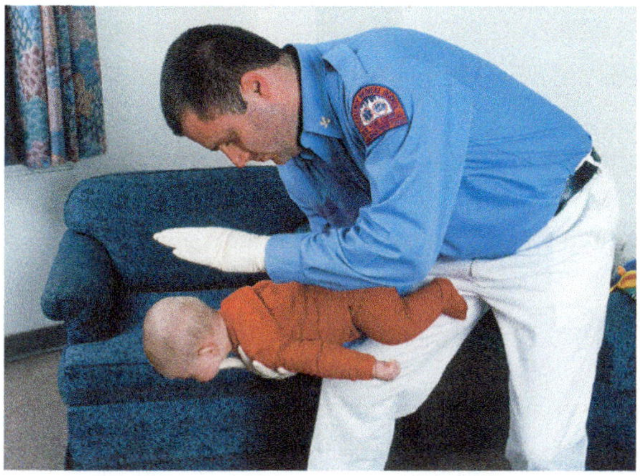
A

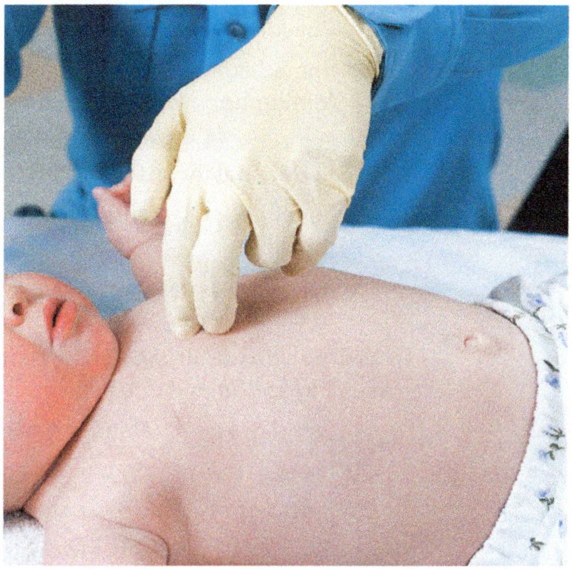
B

A conscious, severely choking adult patient would be treated with abdominal thrusts. To perform these, stand or kneel behind the patient. Place a fist over the patient's navel and then grab that fist with your other hand. Press your fist into the patient's abdomen with a quick, forceful upward thrust. Repeat this step until the obstruction is cleared or the patient becomes unconscious. If you cannot wrap both arms around the patient (as in a pregnant woman or an obese patient), move your hand placement over the patient's sternum.

Conscious Choking Infants

If a conscious infant (less than 1 year old) is choking severely, you must intervene immediately with back slaps and chest thrusts. To start, place the infant in a prone position along your forearm, with the head lower than the body (Figure 9-9A). Support the infant's head. With the heel of your other hand, deliver five back slaps forcefully between the infant's shoulder blades. If the obstruction is not resolved, cradle the infant between your two forearms and turn the infant over, taking care to support the head and neck. With the infant now lying supine, with the head lower than the body, place two fingers over the lower half of the patient's sternum, just below the nipple line, and deliver five rapid chest thrusts, compressing approximately one-half the anterior–posterior depth of the chest. (See Figure 9-9B.) Compress at a rate of one compression per second. Alternate back slaps and chest thrusts until the obstruction is cleared or the patient becomes unconscious.

Unconscious Choking

If the choking patient is unconscious, or if the patient becomes unconscious during other obstructed airway maneuvers, begin CPR. A more comprehensive discussion on both adult and pediatric CPR can be found in the chapter titled *Resuscitation*.

Patient Care

Care of the Patient with Severe Choking

Fundamental Principles of Care

Severe choking implies that the airway is completely blocked by a foreign body. It is indicated (and differentiated from nonsevere choking) by an inability to move air. Here the patient is not breathing, coughing, or speaking. This situation requires immediate intervention.

In patients with signs and symptoms indicating severe choking, take the following steps:

- Call for advanced life support assistance.
- Immediately assess for air movement. If no air movement is found, begin foreign-body airway maneuvers.
- For conscious adults and children (patients over the age of 1 year), initiate abdominal thrusts.
- For conscious infants (patients 1 year old or younger), initiate back slaps and chest thrusts.
- For any unconscious choking patient, or a patient who becomes unconscious due to choking, begin CPR.

For conscious adults and children (older than 1 year), follow these general guidelines for initiating abdominal thrusts:

- Stand or kneel behind the patient.
- Place a fist over the patient's navel and then grab that fist with your other hand.
- Press your fist into the patient's abdomen with a quick, forceful upward thrust.
- Repeat this step until the obstruction is cleared or the patient becomes unconscious.
- If you cannot wrap both arms around the patient (as in a pregnant woman or an obese patient) move your hand placement over the patient's sternum.

For conscious infants (1 year old or younger), initiate back slaps and chest thrusts. General guidelines for back blows and chest thrusts:

- Place the infant in a prone position along your forearm, with the head lower than the body.
- With the heel of your other hand, deliver five back slaps forcefully between the infant's shoulder blades.
- If the obstruction is not resolved, cradle the infant between your two forearms and turn it over.
- With the infant now lying supine and the head lower than the body, place two fingers over the lower half of the patient's sternum, just below the nipple line, and deliver five rapid chest thrusts, compressing approximately one-half the anterior-posterior depth of the chest.
- Compress at a rate of one compression per second.
- Alternate back slaps and chest thrusts until the obstruction is cleared or the patient becomes unconscious.

For any unconscious choking patient, or a patient who becomes unconscious due to choking, begin CPR.

Request ALS.

Airway Adjuncts

CORE CONCEPT
How to use airway adjuncts

If you determine that your patient does not have a patent airway, you must take action to secure it. The airway must be maintained throughout all care procedures.

The most common impediment to an open airway is a lack of airway muscle tone. When a patient becomes unconscious, the muscles relax. The tongue and tissues of the larynx will slide back into the pharynx and obstruct the airway. Even though a head-tilt, chin-lift maneuver or jaw-thrust maneuver will help open a patient's airway, the obstruction may resume once the maneuver is released. Sometimes even when the head-tilt, chin-lift maneuver or jaw-thrust maneuver is maintained, soft tissues and the tongue may continue to partially obstruct the airway.

Airway adjuncts—devices that aid in maintaining an open airway—may be used to initially assist in the opening of an airway, and may be continually used to help keep an airway open. There are several types of airway adjuncts.

The two most common airway adjuncts, whose main functions are to keep the tongue from blocking the airway, are the ***oropharyngeal airway*** (also known as the oral airway or OPA) and the ***nasopharyngeal airway*** (also known as the nasal airway or NPA). The structure and use of these airways can be understood by analyzing their names. *Oro* refers to the mouth; *naso*, the nose; and *pharyngeal*, the pharynx. Oropharyngeal airways are inserted into the mouth and help position the tongue properly. Nasopharyngeal airways are inserted through the nose and rest in the pharynx, also to help position the tongue properly.

oropharyngeal (OR-o-fah-RIN-jeul) ***airway***
a curved device inserted through the patient's mouth into the pharynx to help maintain an open airway.

nasopharyngeal (NAY-zo-fah-RIN-jeul) ***airway***
a flexible breathing tube inserted through the patient's nostril into the pharynx to help maintain an open airway.

gag reflex
vomiting or retching that results when something is placed in the back of the pharynx. This is tied to the swallow reflex.

Rules for Using Airway Adjuncts

Some general rules apply to the use of oropharyngeal and nasopharyngeal airways:

- Use an oropharyngeal airway only on patients who do not exhibit a ***gag reflex***. The gag reflex causes vomiting or retching when something is placed in the pharynx. When a patient is deeply unconscious, the gag reflex usually disappears, but it may reappear as the patient begins to regain consciousness. A patient with a gag reflex who cannot tolerate an oropharyngeal airway may be able to tolerate a nasopharyngeal airway.
- Open the patient's airway manually before using an adjunct device.
- When inserting the airway, take care not to push the patient's tongue into the pharynx.
- Have suction ready prior to inserting any airway.
- Do not continue inserting the airway if the patient begins to gag. Continue to maintain the airway manually, and do not use an adjunct device. If the patient remains unconscious for a prolonged time, you may later attempt to insert an airway to determine whether the gag reflex is still present.
- When an airway adjunct is in place, you must maintain the head-tilt, chin-lift maneuver or jaw-thrust maneuver and monitor the airway.
- After an airway adjunct is in place, continue to be ready to provide suction if fluid such as vomitus or blood obstructs the airway.
- If the patient regains consciousness or develops a gag reflex, remove the airway immediately.
- Use infection-control practices while maintaining the airway. Wear disposable gloves. In airway maintenance, there is a chance of a patient's body fluids coming in contact with your face and eyes. Wear a mask and goggles or other protective eyewear to prevent this contact.

Oropharyngeal Airway

Once a patient's airway is opened, an oropharyngeal airway can be inserted to help keep it open. An oropharyngeal airway is a curved device, usually made of plastic, that can be inserted into the patient's mouth. The oropharyngeal airway has a flange that will rest against the patient's lips. The rest of the device moves the tongue forward as it curves back to the pharynx.

There are standard sizes of oropharyngeal airways (Figure 9-10). Many manufacturers make a complete line, ranging from airways for infants to large adult sizes. An entire set should be carried to allow for quick, proper selection.

The airway adjunct cannot be used effectively unless you select the correct airway size for the patient. To determine the appropriate-sized oral airway, measure the device from the corner of the patient's mouth to the tip of the earlobe on the same side of the patient's face. An alternative method is to measure from the center of the patient's mouth to the angle of the lower jawbone. Do not use an airway device unless you have measured it against the patient and verified it as being the proper size. Remember that if an airway

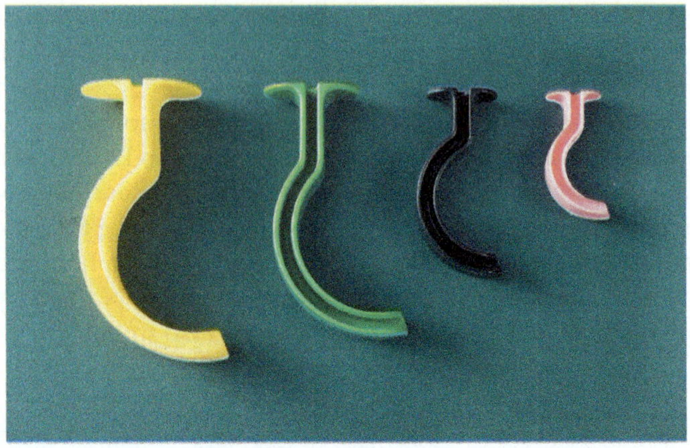

FIGURE 9-10 Oropharyngeal airways.

is too big, its distal tip will rest close to the esophagus and direct air into the stomach. If it is too small, it will not displace the tongue forward properly to open the airway. If the airway is not the correct size, do not use it on the patient.

To insert an oropharyngeal airway, follow these steps as shown in Scan 9-2:

1. Place the patient supine and use an appropriate manual method to open the airway. If no spinal injuries are suspected, use a head-tilt, chin-lift maneuver. If there are possible spinal injuries, use the jaw-thrust maneuver, moving the patient no more than is necessary to ensure an open airway. (The airway takes priority over the spine.)
2. Perform a crossed-finger technique to open the mouth—that is, cross the thumb and forefinger of one hand and place them on the upper and lower teeth at the corner of the patient's mouth. Spread your fingers apart to open the patient's jaws.
3. Position the airway device so its tip is pointing toward the roof of the patient's mouth.
4. Insert the device and slide it along the roof of the patient's mouth, past the soft tissue hanging down from the back (the uvula), or until you meet resistance against the soft palate. Be certain not to push the patient's tongue back into the pharynx. Any airway insertion is made easier by using a tongue blade (tongue depressor) or a rigid suction tip to assist in moving the tongue forward. In a few cases, you may have to use a tongue blade to hold the tongue in place. Watch what you are doing when inserting the airway. This procedure should not be performed by feel only.
5. Gently rotate the airway 180 degrees so the tip is pointing down into the patient's pharynx. This method prevents pushing the tongue back. Alternatively, insert the airway with the tip already pointing down toward the patient's pharynx, using a tongue depressor or rigid suction tip to press the tongue down and forward to avoid obstructing the airway. *This is the preferred method for airway insertion in an infant or child.* Some EMS systems allow an oropharyngeal airway to be inserted with the tip pointing to the side of the patient's mouth. The device is then rotated 90 degrees so its tip is pointing down the patient's pharynx. Use this approach only if it is part of the protocol of your EMS system

   NOTE: *Monitor the patient closely. If there is a gag reflex, remove the airway adjunct at once by following the anatomic curvature. You do not need to rotate the device when removing it.*
6. Position the patient. Place the nontrauma patient in a head-tilt position. If there are possible spine injuries, maintain cervical stabilization at all times during airway management.
7. Check to see that the flange of the airway is against the patient's lips. If the airway device is too long or too short, remove it and replace it with one that is the correct size.
8. Monitor the patient closely. If there is a gag reflex, remove the airway adjunct at once by following the anatomic curvature. You do not need to rotate the device when removing it.

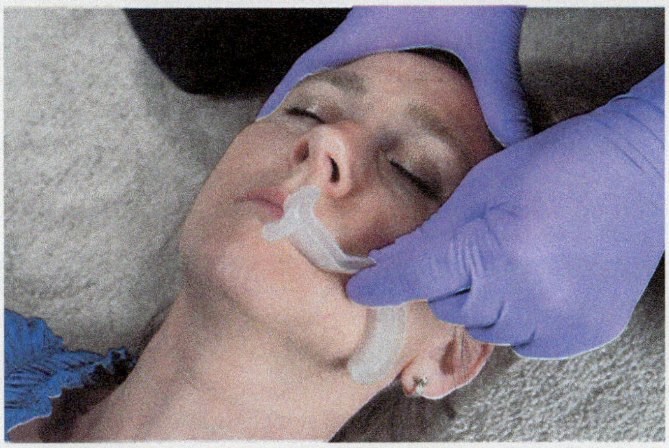

1. Ensure the oropharyngeal airway is the correct size by checking to make sure it either extends from the center of the mouth to the angle of the jaw or . . .

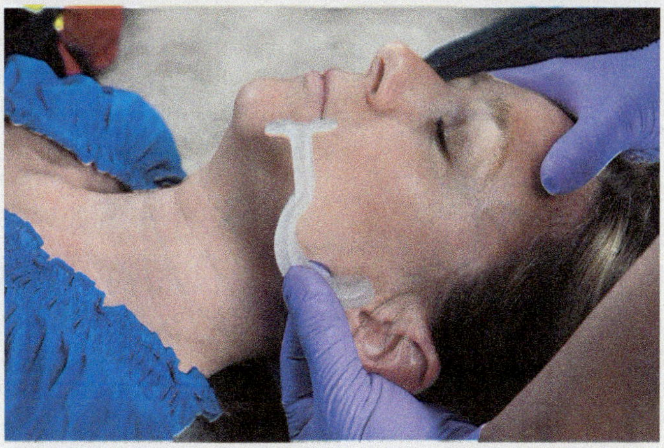

Measure from the corner of the patient's mouth to the tip of the earlobe.

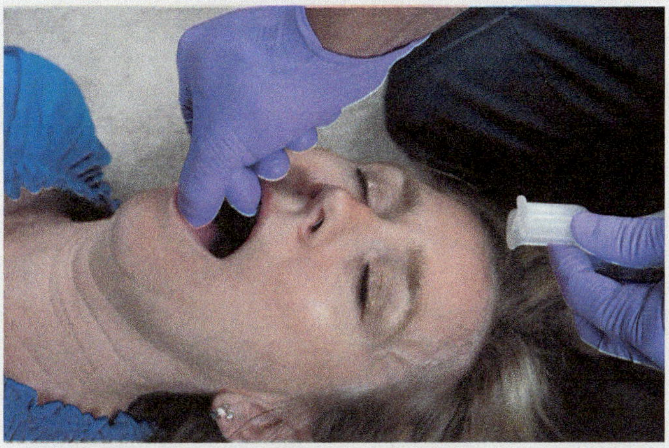

2. Use the crossed-fingers technique to open the patient's mouth.

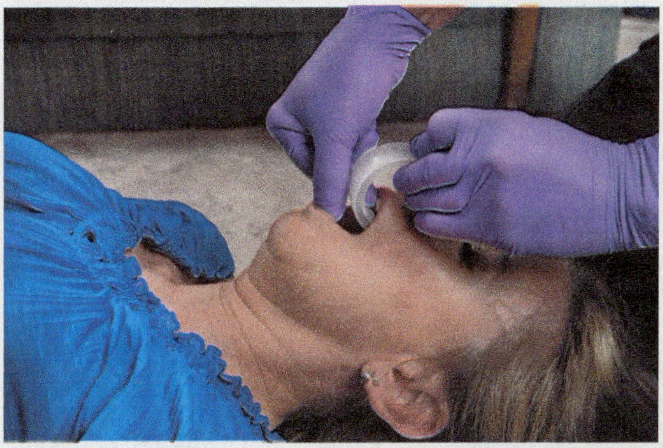

3. Insert the airway with the tip pointing to the roof of the patient's mouth.

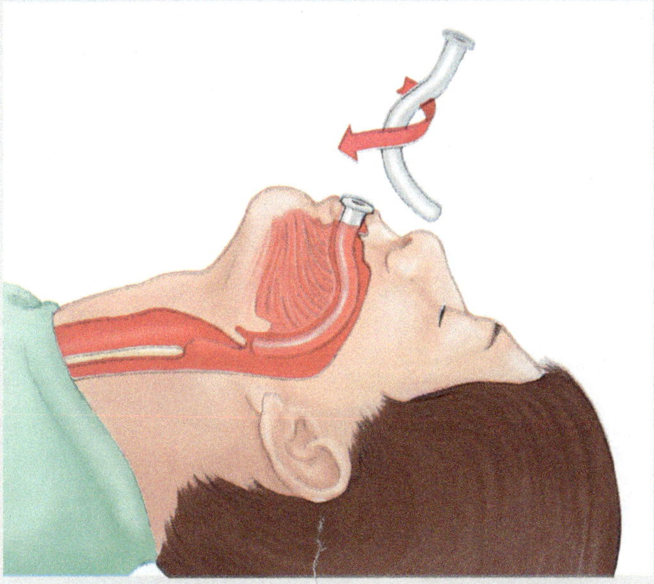

4. Rotate it 180 degrees into position. When the airway is properly positioned, the flange rests against the patient's mouth.

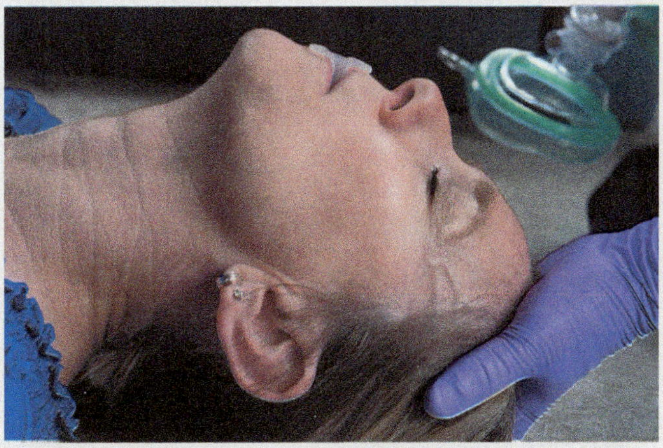

5. After proper insertion, the patient is ready for ventilation.

NOTE: *Monitor the patient closely. If there is a gag reflex, remove the airway adjunct at once by following the anatomic curvature. You do not need to rotate the device when removing it.*

Oropharyngeal Airways in Pediatric Patients

An oropharyngeal airway is inserted into a pediatric patient in essentially the same manner as with an adult (Scan 9-3). However, the larynx of an infant or a young child is more anterior and superior than that of an adult. As such, the oropharyngeal airway will be inserted straight in, without the need for rotation. A tongue depressor or rigid suction catheter is extremely useful during insertion to ensure that the tongue is not pushed backward by the advancing airway.

Nasopharyngeal Airway

The nasopharyngeal airway is a commonly used device because establishing it often does not stimulate the gag reflex. This allows the nasopharyngeal airway to be used in patients who have a reduced level of responsiveness but still have an intact gag reflex. Other benefits include the fact that it can be used when the teeth are clenched and when there are oral injuries.

You should carefully consider the use of a nasopharyngeal airway in a patient with signs of a basilar skull fracture. Although there is limited evidence, and the risk is likely very low, it is possible for adjuncts inserted into the nasal passageways to enter the brain cavity if the basilar skull is fractured. This risk should be considered a relative

SCAN 9-3 Inserting an Oropharyngeal Airway in a Child

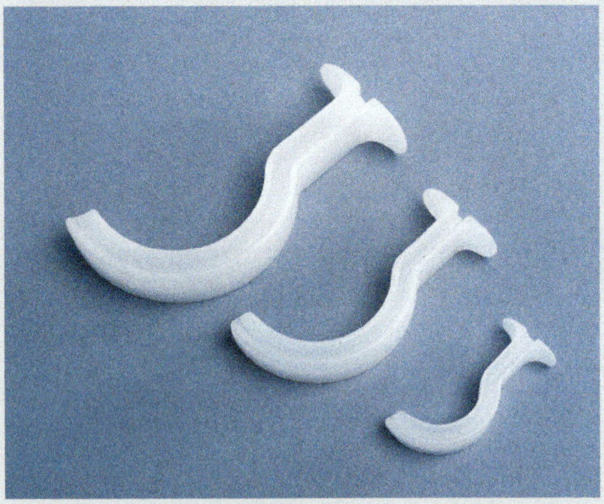

1. Oropharyngeal airways come in a variety of sizes.

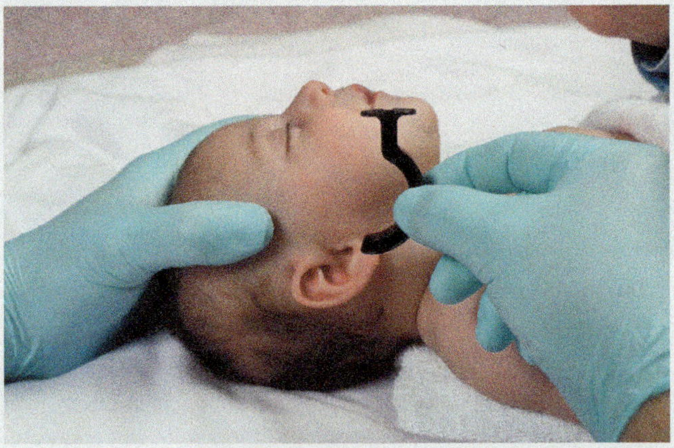

2. Size the airway by measuring from the corner of the mouth to the tip of the earlobe.

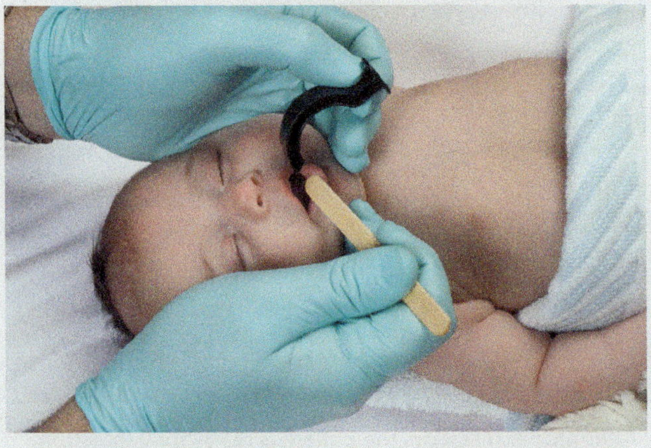

3. Use a tongue depressor to hold the tongue in position. Insert the airway with the tip pointing downward, toward the tongue and throat—the same position it will be in after insertion.

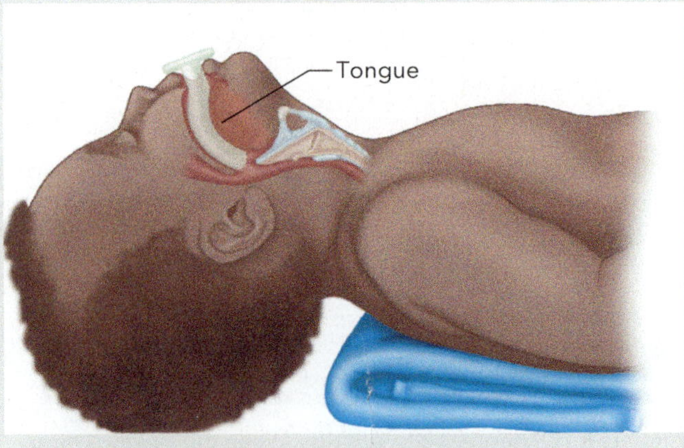

4. The oropharyngeal airway in position

contraindication, and the risks and benefits should be considered prior to insertion. Indicators of a basilar skull fracture would include severe facial trauma and/or cerebral spinal fluid leaking from the ears or nose. Nasopharyngeal airways may also be contraindicated in patients with epistaxis (nosebleed) or nasal trauma.

Use the soft, flexible nasal airway and not the rigid, clear plastic airway in the field. The soft ones are less likely to cause soft-tissue damage or bleeding. The typical sizes for adults are 34, 32, 30, and 28 French.

To insert a nasopharyngeal airway, follow these steps (see Scan 9-4):

1. Measure the nasopharyngeal airway from the patient's nostril to the tip of the earlobe or to the angle of the jaw. Choosing the correct length will ensure an appropriate diameter.
2. Lubricate the outside of the tube with a water-based lubricant before insertion. Do not use a petroleum jelly or any other type of non-water-based lubricant. Such substances can damage the tissue lining of the nasal cavity and the pharynx and increase the risk of infection.

SCAN 9-4 Inserting a Nasopharyngeal Airway

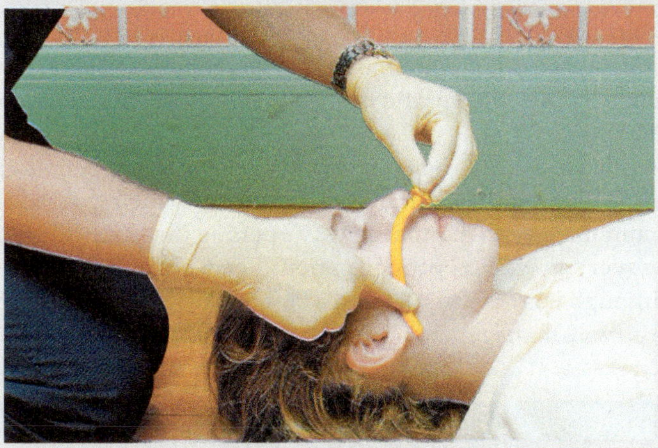

1. Measure the nasopharyngeal airway from the patient's nostril to the tip of the earlobe or to the angle of the jaw.

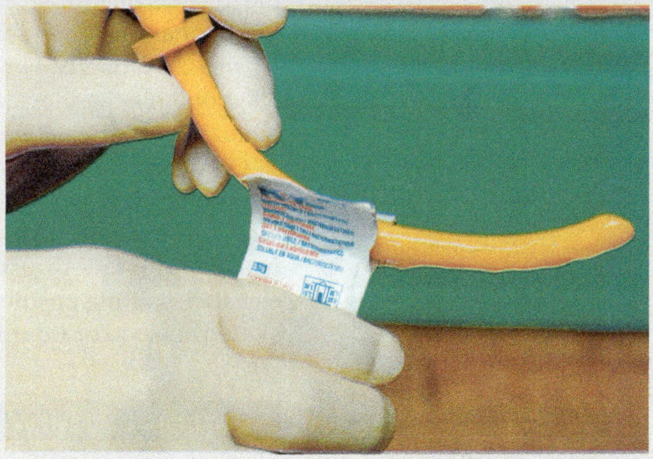

2. Apply a water-based lubricant before insertion.

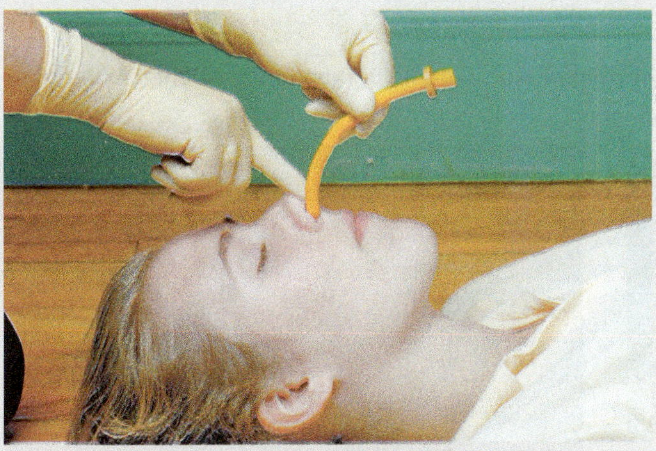

3. Gently push the tip of the nose upward and insert the airway. If the airway has a bevel, consider placing the beveled side toward the base of the nostril or toward the septum (wall that separates the nostrils).

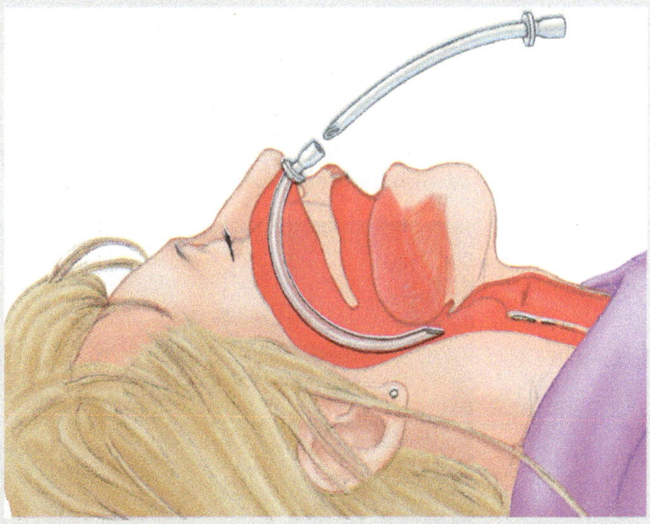

4. Advance the airway. Remember that the anatomy of the nasopharynx travels posteriorly and inferiorly, not upward. Gentle twisting of the nasopharyngeal airway on insertion can help navigate the folds of the nasal turbinates. Do not force the insertion. If significant resistance is met, withdraw and attempt insertion in the opposite nostril.

3. Gently push the tip of the nose upward and insert the airway. Keep the patient's head in neutral position. Most nasopharyngeal airways are designed to be placed in the right nostril. The bevel (angled portion at the tip) should point toward the base of the nostril or toward the septum (wall that separates the nostrils).
4. Insert the airway into the nostril. Gently advance the airway along the floor of the nasopharynx until the flange rests firmly against the patient's nostril. Never force a nasopharyngeal airway. Do not direct the nasal airway upward, or it will encounter the nasal turbinates and you will not be able to advance it. If you experience difficulty advancing the airway, pull the tube out and try the other nostril.

Pediatric Nasopharyngeal Airway

Nasopharyngeal airways can be used in pediatric patients (Figure 9-11A and Figure 9-11B). In very small patients (infants and small children), the diameter of the airway may limit its value as an adjunct. However, it can be considered in situations where other, more practical options have failed. Measuring and insertion procedures are the same as in adults.

Oropharyngeal and nasopharyngeal airways can be tremendous assets to the EMT when used properly. However, no device can replace the EMT. The proper use of these airways or any other device depends on the appropriate use, good judgment, and adequate monitoring of the patient by the EMT.

Oropharyngeal and nasopharyngeal airways help move soft tissue of the upper airway to provide clear passage for air. Although they can by themselves provide a patent airway, they are best used when combined with manual airway opening (head-tilt, chin-lift maneuver or jaw-thrust maneuver) as well as proper patient head positioning (head-elevated, sniffing position). Although it is easy to focus on a single tool or procedure, you should always consider all the airway management options that can benefit your patient.

Supraglottic Airways

Many systems now allow EMTs to insert supraglottic airways (Figure 9-12). Note that these devices are not universally allowed in all EMT scopes of practice. You should consult local protocol to determine availability in your area.

There are many types of supraglottic airways. These devices generally do not enter the trachea but rather isolate the glottic opening by occupying space in the larynx and hypopharynx.

FIGURE 9-11 (A) Using a nasopharyngeal airway with a pediatric patient. (B) Proper placement of a pediatric nasopharyngeal airway.

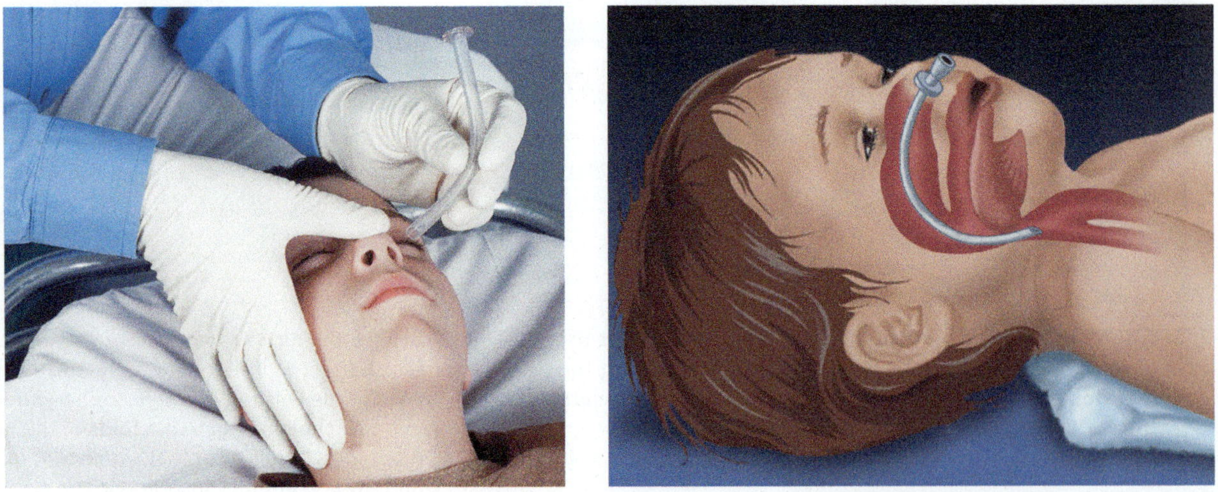

A

B

FIGURE 9-12 The King LT-D™ airway.

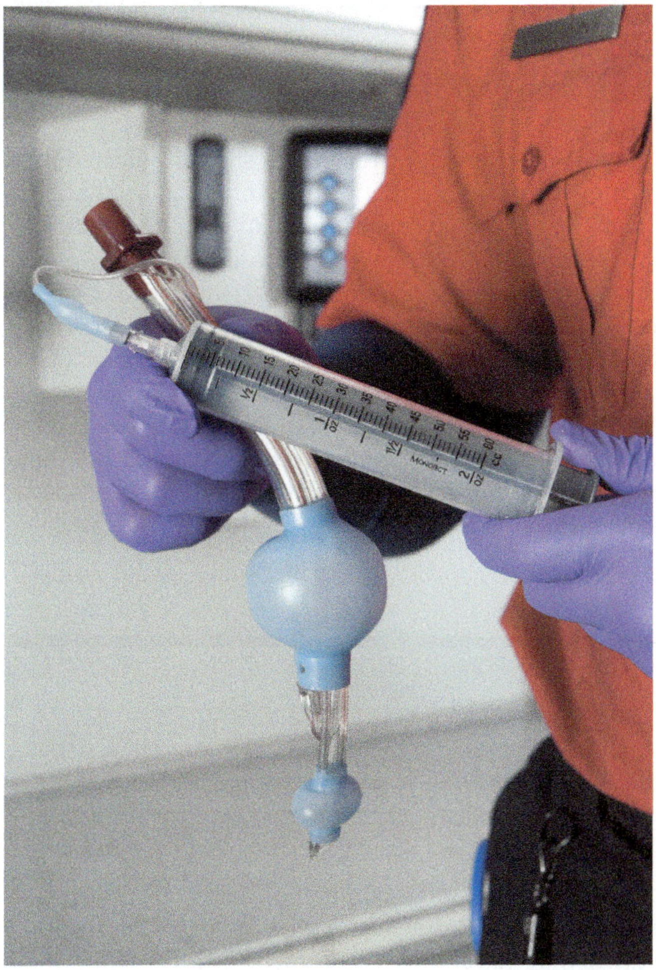

FIGURE 9-13 The laryngeal mask airway (LMA™).
(© Edward T. Dickinson, MD)

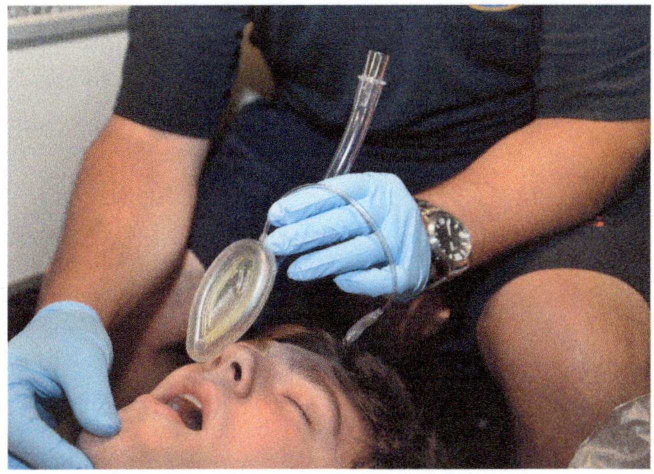

In most cases, insertion is a simple procedure that can be performed with the patient's head in a neutral position. There are a variety of different supraglottic airways available, and before using one, you should be thoroughly trained to the manufacturer's specific standards. However, some common features are discussed here.

Recognizing the Need for an Advanced Airway

Far too many practitioners think that an advanced airway is the answer to all airway problems. This simply is not true. Some patients will benefit from a supraglottic airway; others will not. If these devices are included in your scope of practice, it is essential to use your assessment to identify situations where their application will be of aid to the patient. In general, supraglottic airways are indicated when other basic airway-management measures have failed. If proper positioning, manual airway opening, and adjuncts cannot keep an airway open, a supraglottic airway may be of benefit. Also, supraglottic devices (such as the laryngeal mask airway in Figure 9-13) can help when an airway must be maintained over a relatively longer period, or as a bridge between simple maneuvers and endotracheal intubation. Prolonged transport times and some cardiac arrest events are examples of situations that may benefit from simple but reliable airway management over time. Supraglottic airways do not benefit patients who specifically need endotracheal intubation. Burn patients or anaphylactic patients who require intubation to protect against glottic swelling will not be helped by a supraglottic airway. Supraglottic airways cannot be used if the patient has a gag reflex.

Supraglottic Insertion Procedures

Although the specific insertion procedure for each supraglottic airway is beyond the scope of this text, there are common steps that should be discussed. As you prepare to insert a supraglottic airway, you must first prepare the patient, the EMS team, and the equipment you are about to use.

Preparing the Patient. Simple airway-maintenance procedures should be attempted first. If a patent airway can be achieved through patient positioning, manual airway opening (either head-tilt, chin-lift maneuver or jaw-thrust maneuver), and/or airway adjuncts, there is no urgent need for a supraglottic airway. These skills should always be attempted first. If a supraglottic airway is indicated, position the patient's head per manufacturer's recommendation. Most supraglottic airways suggest that the patient's head be positioned in the sniffing position discussed previously. Some devices suggest a neutral position prior to insertion. If possible, high-concentration oxygen should be administered to the patient prior to the insertion process. If using positive pressure ventilation, be sure the bag-valve-mask device is connected to flow concentration oxygen. Remember that the time it takes to insert the supraglottic airway is time that ventilations must cease. Preoxygenation diminishes the harmful effects of that brief period of time with no ventilation.

Pediatric Note

Supraglottic airways can be used in most pediatric patients. However, not all devices can be used in very young children and infants. Always consult manufacturer's recommendations and know how to select appropriate-sized devices for the pediatric patient.

To ensure an open airway to the level of the lungs, it is sometimes necessary to insert an endotracheal (through the trachea) tube. Endotracheal intubation is an advanced life support procedure in which EMTs may assist advanced-level providers. Furthermore, some EMS systems allow for the use of blind insertion airway devices. These devices and procedures will be discussed in the chapter titled *Respiration and Artificial Ventilation*.

Preparing the Team. Advanced airway insertion is a team activity and should begin with a brief "huddle" to discuss roles and responsibilities. Everyone on the scene should have a job and should know when and how to communicate. When multiple team members are present, specific duties should include suctioning, patient assessment, and equipment assistance.

Preparing the Device. Most supraglottic airways have sizing requirements. Some are sized by patient weight, others by the patient's height. Follow manufacturer's recommendations and be sure you have selected the appropriate device for the patient. Consider also any specific contraindications for its use before beginning. Some supraglottic airways require inflation of cuffs and balloons. If this is the case, syringes should be attached, and inflation must be checked prior to insertion. This check will specifically ensure that the appropriate equipment is available and that all balloons and cuffs are capable of being inflated properly before placement. Be sure suction is ready and confirm that mechanisms, such as end-tidal carbon dioxide detection, are available.

See procedures for insertion of a King airway (Scan 9-5) and an i-gel® device (Scan 9-6).

SCAN 9-5 Insertion of a King Airway

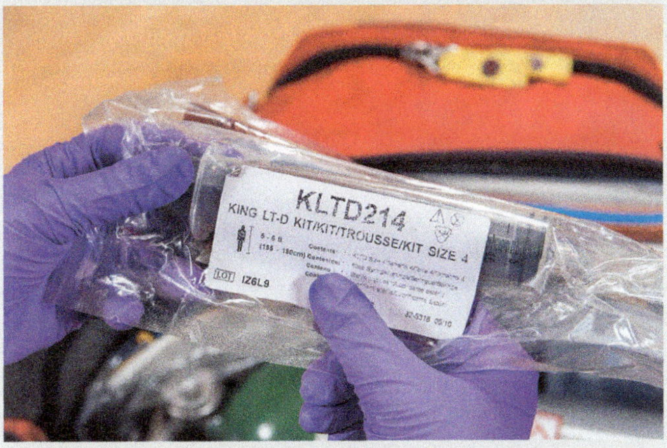

1. Select the appropriate-sized King airway based on patient height. Assemble equipment and test cuff patency. Remove all air from cuffs before insertion.

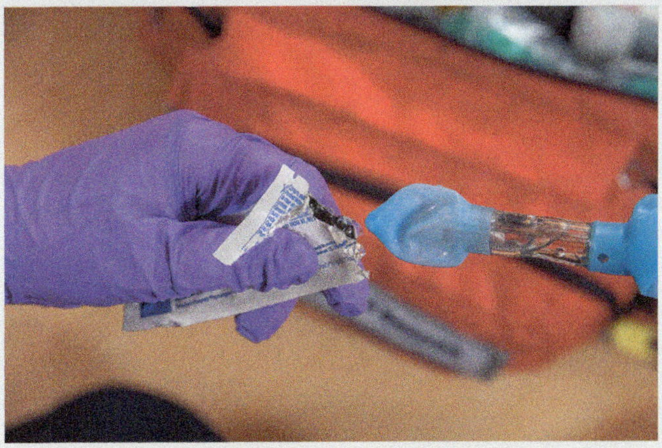

2. Apply water-based lubricant to distal tip of the device. Avoid applying lubricant to ventilation openings.

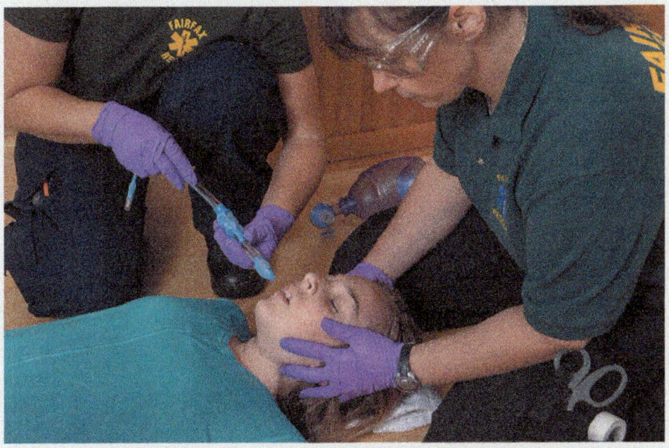

3. Preoxygenate the patient (if possible) and position the patient's head in the sniffing position.

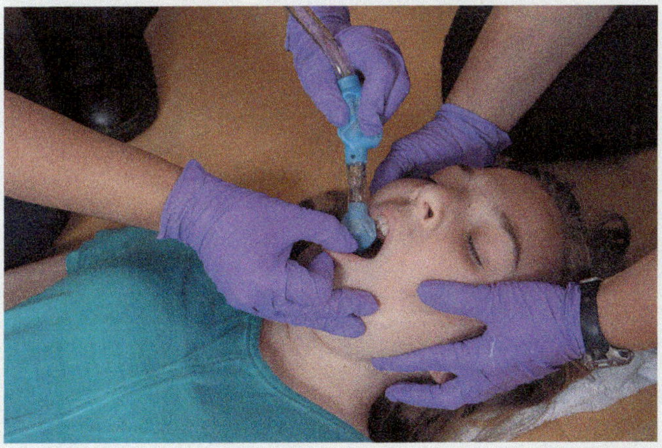

4. Perform a chin lift (unless contraindicated by spinal injury) and insert the device into the side of the mouth. The device should be rotated laterally. Advance just beyond the tongue.

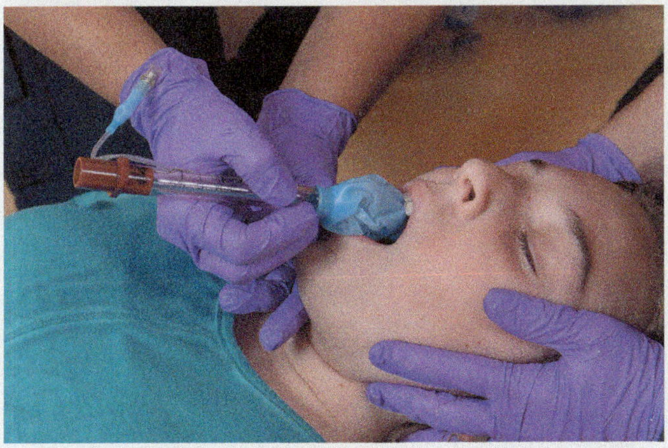

5. Continue to advance the device, turning it 45 degrees as it enters the hypopharynx. Do not force the device, and take care not to force the tongue backward.

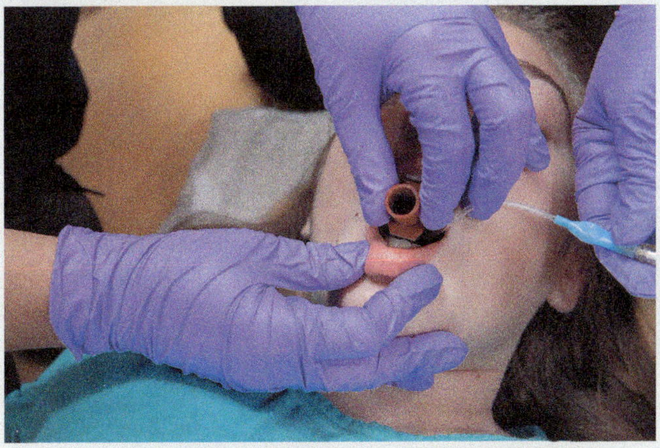

6. Advance until resistance is met, or the base of the connector aligns with the teeth.

(continued)

SCAN 9-5 Insertion of a King Airway *(continued)*

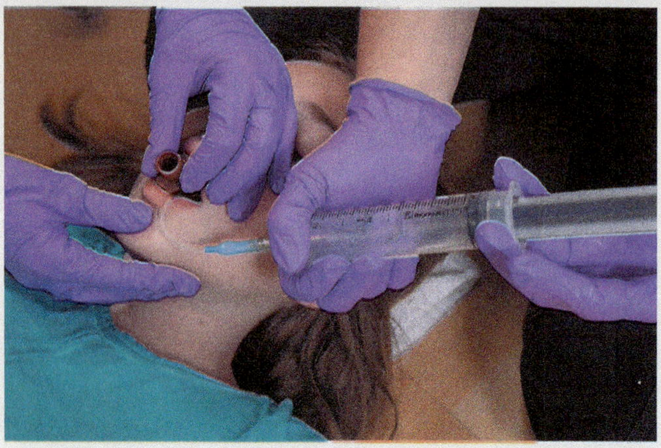

7. Inflate the cuffs to manufacturer-recommended volumes.

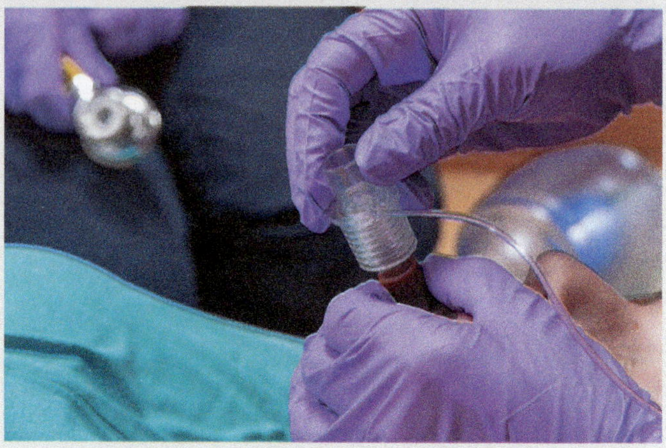

8. Attach bag-valve-mask device and attempt to ventilate. Look for appropriate chest rise.

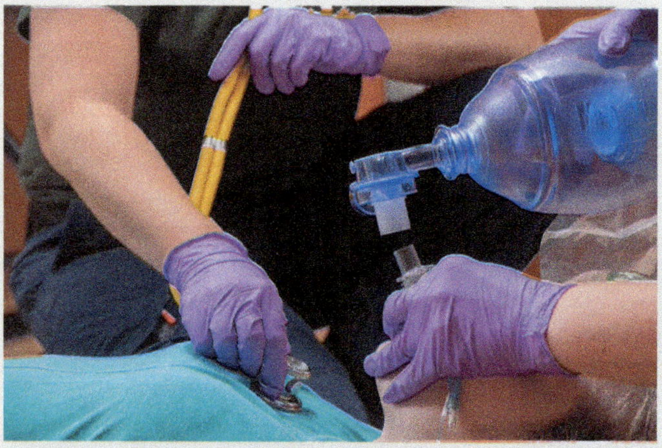

9. Confirm placement with end-tidal carbon dioxide detection; then secure the device. *(Manufacturer's instructions courtesy of King Systems* www.kingsystems.com*)*

SCAN 9-6 Insertion of an i-gel™ Airway

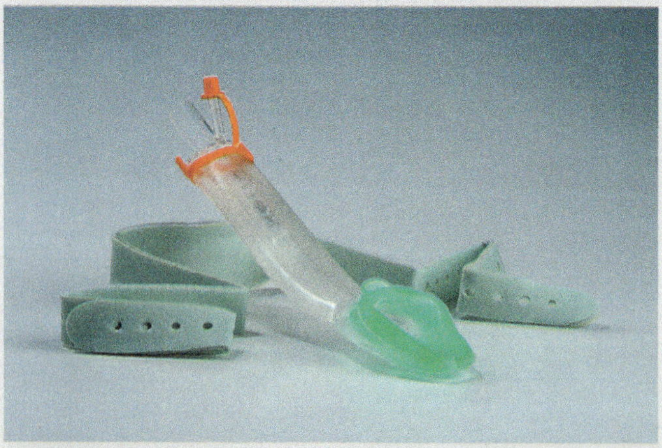

1. Select an appropriately sized i-gel device using the weight-based guidelines displayed on the airway and on the airway packaging.

2. Lubricate the front, back, and sides of the i-gel with a thin layer of water-based lubricant.

3. Place the patient in the head-elevated, sniffing position (unless contraindicated by spinal injury).

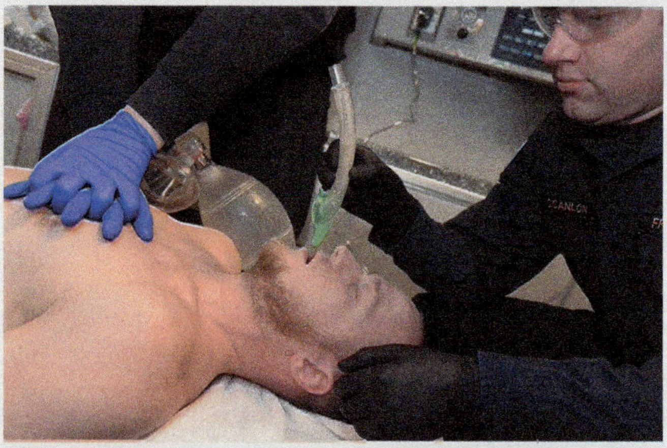

4. Position the i-gel so that it can be inserted anatomically in the direction of the hard palate. The open side of the distal cuff should be oriented toward the patient's tongue. Introduce the tip of the device into the mouth of the patient and insert in the direction of the hard palate. *(© Edward T. Dickinson, MD)*

SCAN 9-6 Insertion of an i-gel™ Airway *(continued)*

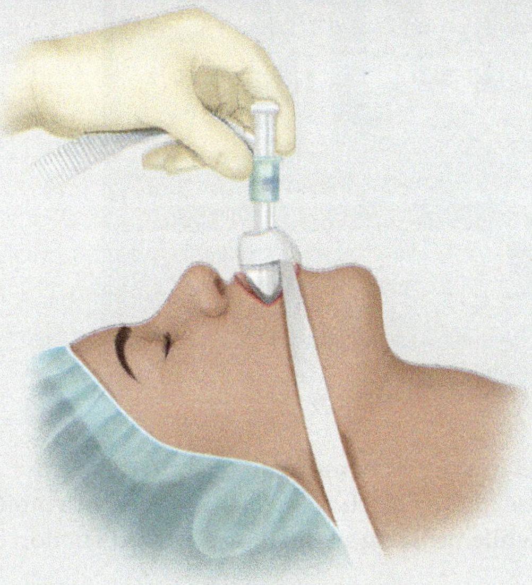

5. Insert the device until the patient's incisors are resting on the bite block. This will ensure that the tip of the airway is located at the upper esophageal opening and that the cuff is located against the laryngeal framework.
6. Secure the device. Slide the i-gel's strap underneath the patient's neck and attach to the hook ring. Take care not to overtighten the strap.

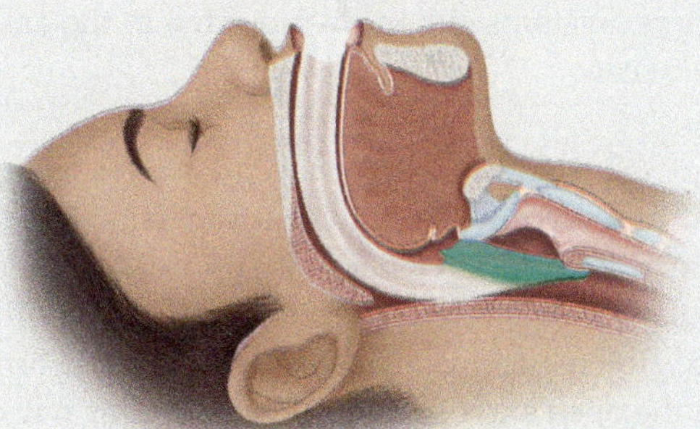

7. Attach a bag-valve-mask device and attempt to ventilate. Look for appropriate chest rise.
8. Confirm placement with end-tidal carbon dioxide detection; then secure the device.

Suctioning

The patient's airway must be kept clear of foreign materials, blood, vomitus, and other secretions. Materials that are allowed to remain in the airway may be forced into the trachea and eventually into the lungs. This will cause complications ranging from severe pneumonia to complete airway obstruction. ***Suctioning*** is the method of using a vacuum device to remove such materials. A patient needs to be suctioned immediately when fluids or secretions are present in the airway or whenever a gurgling sound is heard.

suctioning (SUK-shun-ing) use of a vacuum device to remove blood, vomitus, and other secretions or foreign materials from the airway.

Using Gravity to Clear an Airway

Very often, the best way to clear an airway is simply to use gravity. When large amounts of secretions or blood collect in the patient's mouth, it may be quite reasonable and often much faster than more technical alternatives to turn the patient to one side and allow liquids to drain from the mouth. This may not be possible in spine-injured patients, and a single responder may have difficulty moving a large patient alone. However, when possible, this method offers a simple, efficient step to take before suction devices are ready. It may also clear the obstruction altogether. When using this method, it is wise to turn the patient away from your body to avoid biohazards being splashed in your direction.

CORE CONCEPT
Principles and techniques of suctioning

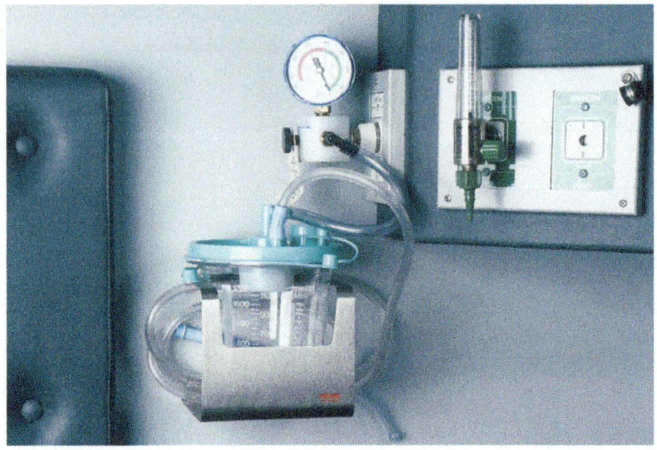

FIGURE 9-14 A mounted suction unit installed in the ambulance's patient compartment.

"Aspiration kills. Watch that airway constantly and suction, suction, suction."

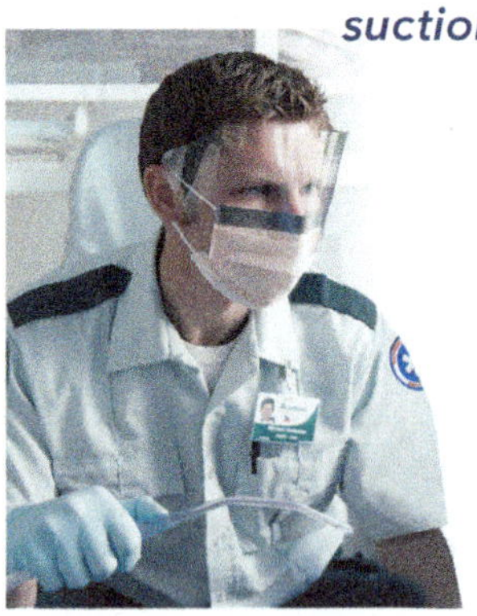

The lateral recumbent position and gravity may also enhance the capability of other suction devices. In cases of high-volume liquid obstruction, such as blood or vomitus, consider turning the patient to one side while utilizing manual or powered suction devices.

Suctioning Devices

Each suction unit consists of a suction source, a collection container for materials you suction, tubing, and suction tips or catheters. Systems either are mounted in the ambulance or are portable and may be brought to the scene.

Mounted Suction Systems

Many ambulances have a suction unit mounted in the patient compartment (Figure 9-14). These units are usually installed near the head of the stretcher so they are easily used. Mounted systems, often called onboard units, create a suctioning vacuum produced by the engine's manifold or an electrical power source. To be effective, suction devices must furnish an air intake of at least 30 liters per minute at the open end of a collection tube. This will occur if the system can generate a vacuum of no less than 300 mmHg when the collecting tube is clamped.

Portable Suction Units

There are many different types of portable suction units (Figure 9-15). They may be oxygen- or air-powered, electrically powered (by batteries or household current), or manually operated. The requirement for the amount of suction a portable unit must provide is identical to that of the fixed unit (30 liters per minute, 300 mmHg). It is important to have the ability to suction anywhere. Portable suction devices provide that ability.

FIGURE 9-15 (A) Battery-powered portable unit and (B) manually operated unit.

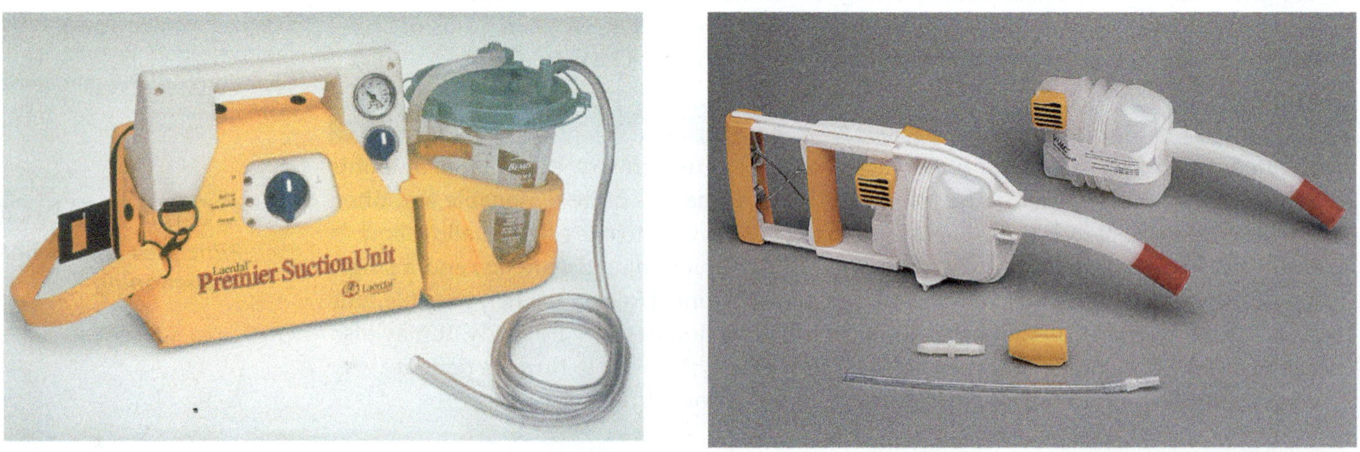

A

B

Tubing, Tips, and Catheters

For suctioning to be effective, the proper equipment must be used. Although a suction unit might be the most powerful available, it will do no good unless used with the proper attachments. Before operating a suction unit, you must have:

- Tubing
- Suction tips (Figure 9-16)
- Suction catheters
- Collection container
- Container of clean or sterile water

FIGURE 9-16 Suction catheter tips. (A) Rigid suction tip. (B) Cross-finger technique for rigid suction tip. (C) Detail showing air hole on side of suction device. (D) Soft suction catheter. *(© Daniel Limmer.)*

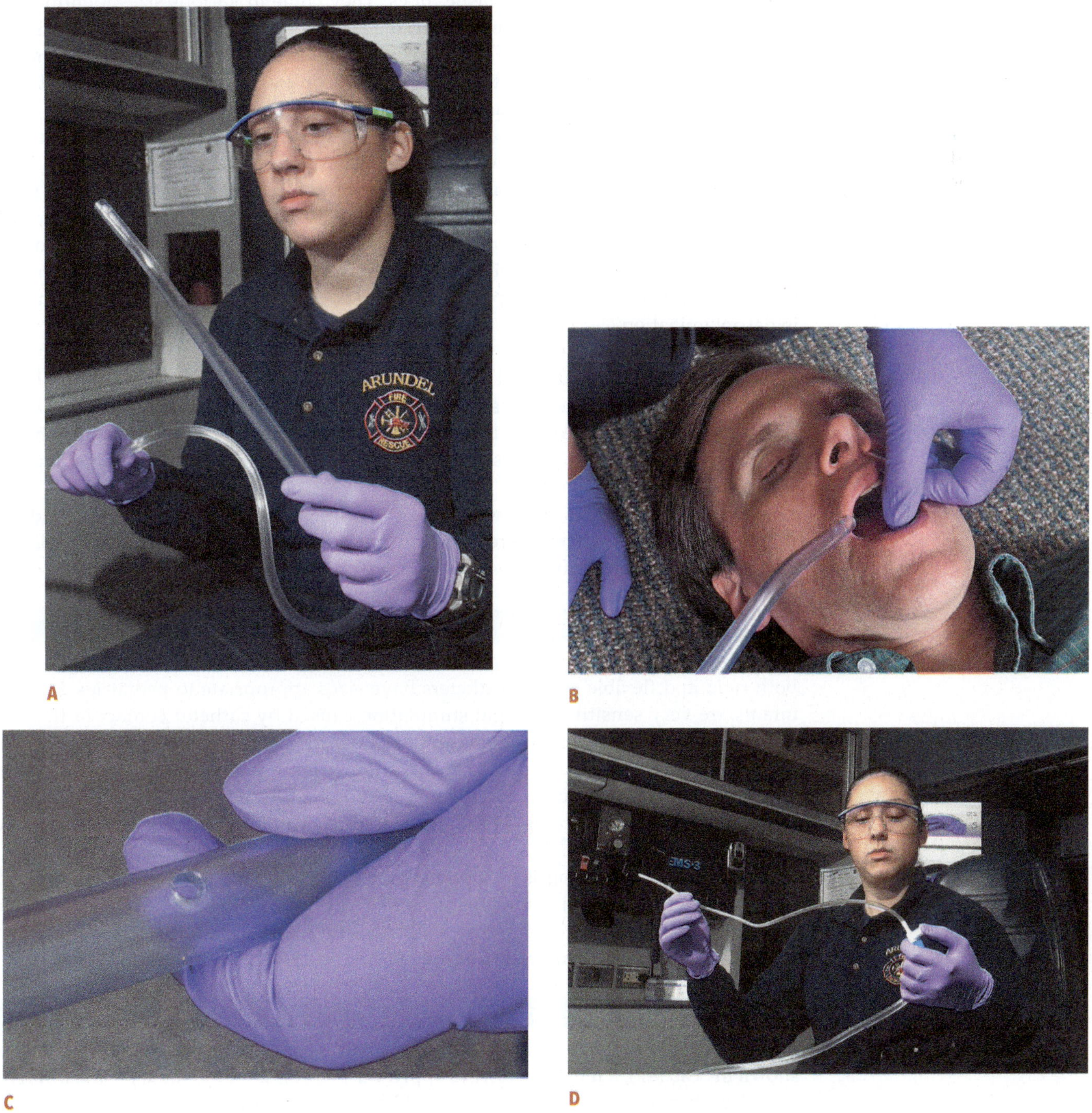

The *tubing* attached to a suction unit must be thick-walled, non-kinking, wide-bore tubing. This is because the tubing must not collapse due to the suction, must allow chunks of suctioned material to pass, and must not kink, which would reduce the suction. The tubing must be long enough to reach comfortably from suction unit to patient.

Currently the most popular type of *suction tip* is the rigid pharyngeal tip, also called Yankauer or tonsil-tip suction. (See Figure 9-16A.)

This rigid device allows you to suction the mouth and pharynx with excellent control over the distal end of the device. It also has a larger bore than flexible catheters. Most successfully used with an unresponsive patient, rigid-tip suction must be used with caution, especially if the patient is not completely unresponsive or may be regaining consciousness. When the tip is placed into the pharynx, the gag reflex may be activated, producing additional vomiting. It is also possible to stimulate the vagus nerve in the back of the pharynx, which can slow the heart rate. Therefore, be careful not to suction more than a few seconds at a time with a rigid tip, and never lose sight of the tip.

Suction catheters are flexible plastic tubes. They come in various sizes identified by a number "French." The larger the number, the larger the catheter. A 14 French catheter is larger than an 8 French catheter. These catheters are usually not large enough to suction vomitus or thick secretions, and they may kink. Flexible catheters are designed to be used in situations when a rigid tip cannot be used. For example, a soft catheter can be passed through a tube such as a nasopharyngeal or endotracheal tube or used for suctioning the nasopharynx. (A bulb suction device may also be used to suction nasal passages.)

Another important part of a suction device is the *collection container*. All units should have a nonbreakable container to collect the suctioned materials. These containers must be easily removed for disposal or decontamination. Remember to wear gloves, protective eyewear, and a mask not only while suctioning but also while cleaning the equipment. Most modern suction devices have disposable containers to eliminate the time and risks involved in decontamination.

Suction units also must have a *container of clean (preferably sterile) water* nearby. This water is used to clear matter that is partially blocking the tubing. When this partial blockage of the tube occurs, place the suction tip or catheter in the container of water. This will cause a stream of water to flow through the tip and tubing, usually dislodging the clog. When the tip or tubing becomes clogged with an item that will not dislodge, replace it with a new tip or tubing.

In the event of copious, thick secretions or vomiting, consider removing the rigid tip or catheter and using the large-bore, rigid suction tubing. After you are finished, place the standard tip back on for further suctioning.

Pediatric Suctioning

For the most part, suctioning in pediatrics is not very different than suctioning in adults. Both rigid and flexible suction catheters have sizes appropriate to pediatrics. However, infants are very sensitive to vagal stimulation caused by catheter contact in the hypopharynx. More so than adults, they can respond with a slowing of the heart rate. This is definitely not a contraindication to suctioning pediatric patients, but it does mean you should do your best to minimize necessary suctioning time and take care to avoid contact with the hypopharynx if possible. Careful assessment of the patient during suctioning should also occur.

Bulb syringe suctioning is a common procedure in infants and small children. This device can be very effective in clearing smaller airways. Bulb syringes are used to clear obstructed airways in the emergency childbirth setting and also to clear obstructing mucus from nasal passages in children with respiratory distress.

Techniques of Suctioning

Although there may be some variations in suction technique (a suggested technique is shown in Scan 9-7), a few rules always apply. *The first rule is always use appropriate infection-control practices while suctioning*. These practices include the use of protective eyewear, mask,

SCAN 9-7 Suctioning Techniques

If you are using a flexible catheter, measure it from the patient's earlobe to the corner of the mouth or from the center of the mouth to the angle of the jaw.

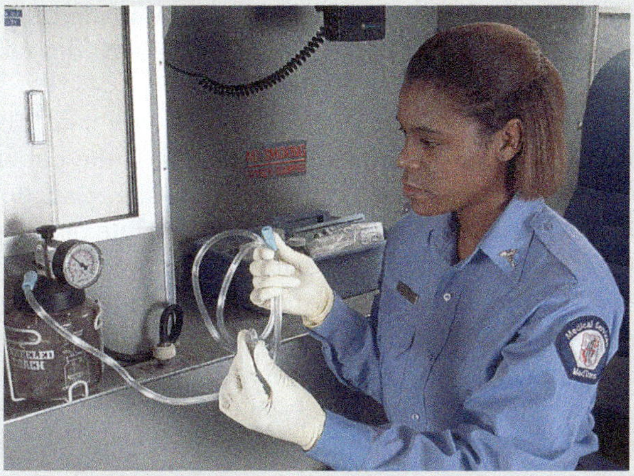

1. Turn the unit on, attach a catheter, and test for suction at the beginning of your shift.

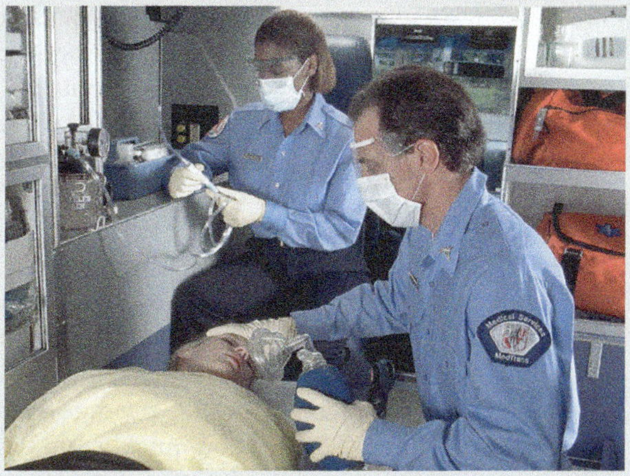

2. Position yourself at the patient's head and turn the patient's head or entire body to the side.

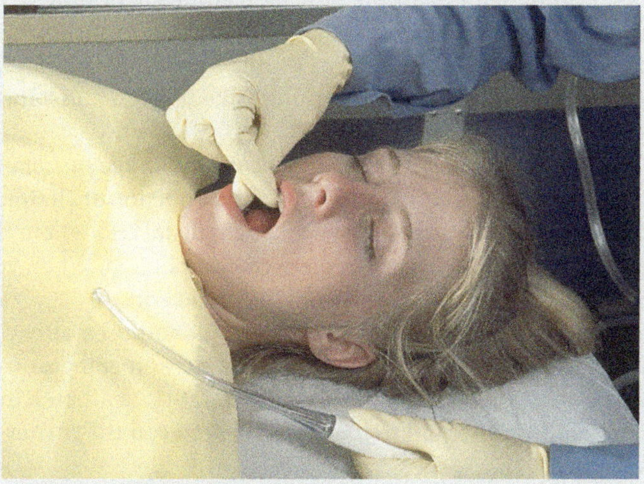

3. Open and clear the patient's mouth.

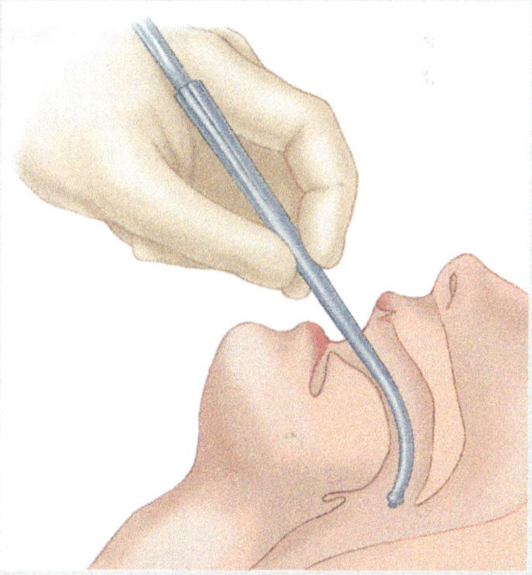

4. Place the convex side of the rigid tip against the roof of the mouth. Insert only as far as you can see or just to the base of the tongue.

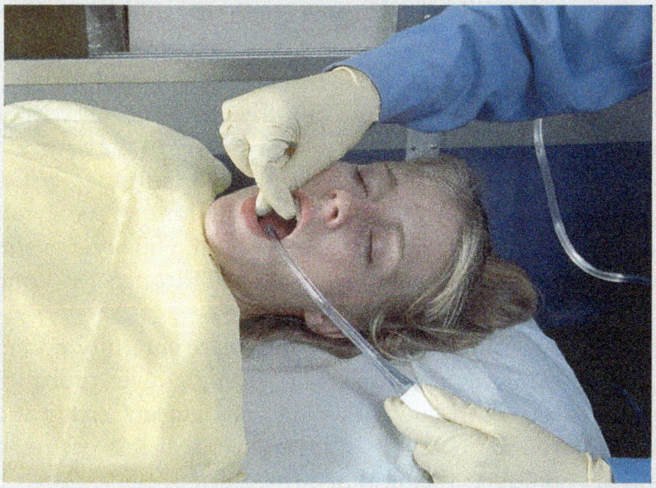

5. Apply suction only after the rigid tip is in place. Do not lose sight of the tip while suctioning. Suction while withdrawing the tip.

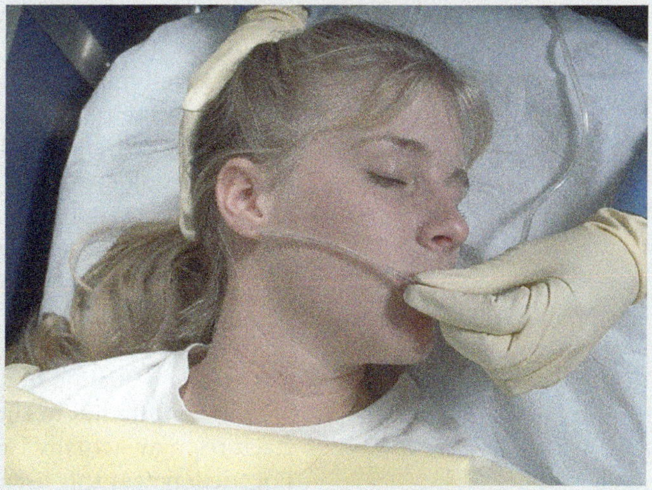

6. If you are using a flexible catheter, measure it from the patient's earlobe to the corner of the mouth or from the center of the mouth to the angle of the jaw.

and disposable gloves. Proper suctioning requires you to have your fingers around and sometimes inside the patient's mouth. Disposable gloves prevent contact between the EMT and the patient's bodily fluids. Protective eyewear and mask are also recommended, since these fluids might splatter, or the patient may gag or cough, sending droplets to your face, eyes, and mouth.

The second rule is to try limiting suctioning to no longer than 10 seconds at a time. This is because prolonged suctioning can cause hypoxia and vagal response. If the patient continues to vomit longer than 10 seconds, however, you still must continue to suction. Ventilating foreign matter into the lungs will also cause hypoxia and possible death. In short, suction quickly and efficiently for as short a time as possible.

Patients who need airway control and suctioning are often unconscious and may be in cardiac or respiratory arrest. Oxygen delivery to these patients is very important. During suctioning, the ventilations or other methods of oxygen delivery are discontinued to allow for the passage of the suction catheter. To prevent critical delays in oxygen delivery, suction quickly and efficiently until the airway is clear, then resume ventilations or oxygen delivery.

In a few cases, you will preoxygenate a patient before suctioning. This means that you will adequately ventilate the patient with supplemental oxygen before suctioning because oxygen levels will drop during suctioning—for example, during routine suctioning of an endotracheal tube. If you encounter a patient with vomitus or other materials in the airway, or if a patient vomits suddenly and unexpectedly, you should suction immediately, *without* preoxygenation. In these cases, preoxygenation would force foreign substances into the lungs, which can be fatal.

The third rule for suctioning is place the tip or catheter where you want to begin the suctioning, and suction on the way out. Most suction tips and catheters do not produce suction at all times. You have to start the suctioning. The tip or catheter will have an open, distal end where the suction is delivered. It will also have an opening, or port, in the proximal portion. When you put your finger over the proximal port, suctioning begins from the distal end.

It is not necessary to measure when using a rigid tip. Rather, you should be sure not to lose sight of the tip when inserting it. However, do measure the suction catheter in a manner similar to measuring for an oropharyngeal airway. The length of catheter that should be inserted into the patient's mouth is equal to the distance between the corner of the patient's mouth and earlobe.

Carefully bring the tip of the catheter to the area where suctioning is needed. Never jab or force the suction tip into the mouth or pharynx. Then place your finger over the proximal opening to begin the suctioning, and suction as you slowly withdraw the tip from the patient's mouth, moving the tip from side to side.

Suctioning is best delivered with the patient turned on the patient's side. This allows gravity to assist suction, as free secretions will flow from the mouth while suctioning is being delivered. Caution must be used in patients with suspected neck or spine injuries. In the patient requiring spinal precautions, suction the best you can without turning the patient. If all other methods have failed, as a last resort you may turn the patient's body as a unit, attempting to keep the neck and spine in line. It may also be beneficial to manually remove large particles prior to or during suctioning. As always, caution should be taken in placing your fingers in a patient's mouth. However, a shallow sweep will often help remove particles not able to be suctioned through the lumen of the suction device.

The rigid suction tip or flexible catheter should be moved into place carefully, and not forced. Rigid suction devices may cause tissue damage and bleeding. Never probe into wounds or attempt to suction away attached tissue with a suction device. Certain skull fractures may actually cause brain tissue to be visible in the pharynx. If this occurs, do not suction near this tissue; limit suctioning to the mouth.

Suction devices may also cause activation of the gag reflex and stimulate vomiting. In a patient who already has secretions that need to be suctioned, vomiting only makes things worse. If you advance a suction catheter or rigid suction tip and the patient begins to gag, withdraw the tip to a position that does not cause gagging, and begin suctioning.

Keeping an Airway Open: Definitive Care

At times, keeping an airway open will exceed the capabilities of the basic EMT. Medications and/or surgical procedures may be necessary to resolve the cause of airway obstruction. As an EMT, you should rapidly evaluate and treat airway problems, but also quickly recognize the need for more definitive care. In some systems, definitive care may be an advanced life support intercept. In other systems, definitive care might be the closest hospital. Either way, you must know your local system resources and recognize your capabilities and limitations.

Special Considerations

There are a number of special considerations in airway management:

- **Facial injuries.** Take extra care with the airway when patients have facial injuries (Figure 9-17). Because the blood supply to the face is so rich, blunt and penetrating injuries to the face frequently result in severe swelling or bleeding that may block or partially block the airway. Frequent suctioning may be required. Insertion of an airway adjunct or endotracheal tube may be necessary.

FIGURE 9-17 Severe facial injury may compromise airway management. (A) Severe laceration of the nose in an adult. (B) Child with injury to the jaw. *(Both: © David Effron, MD)*

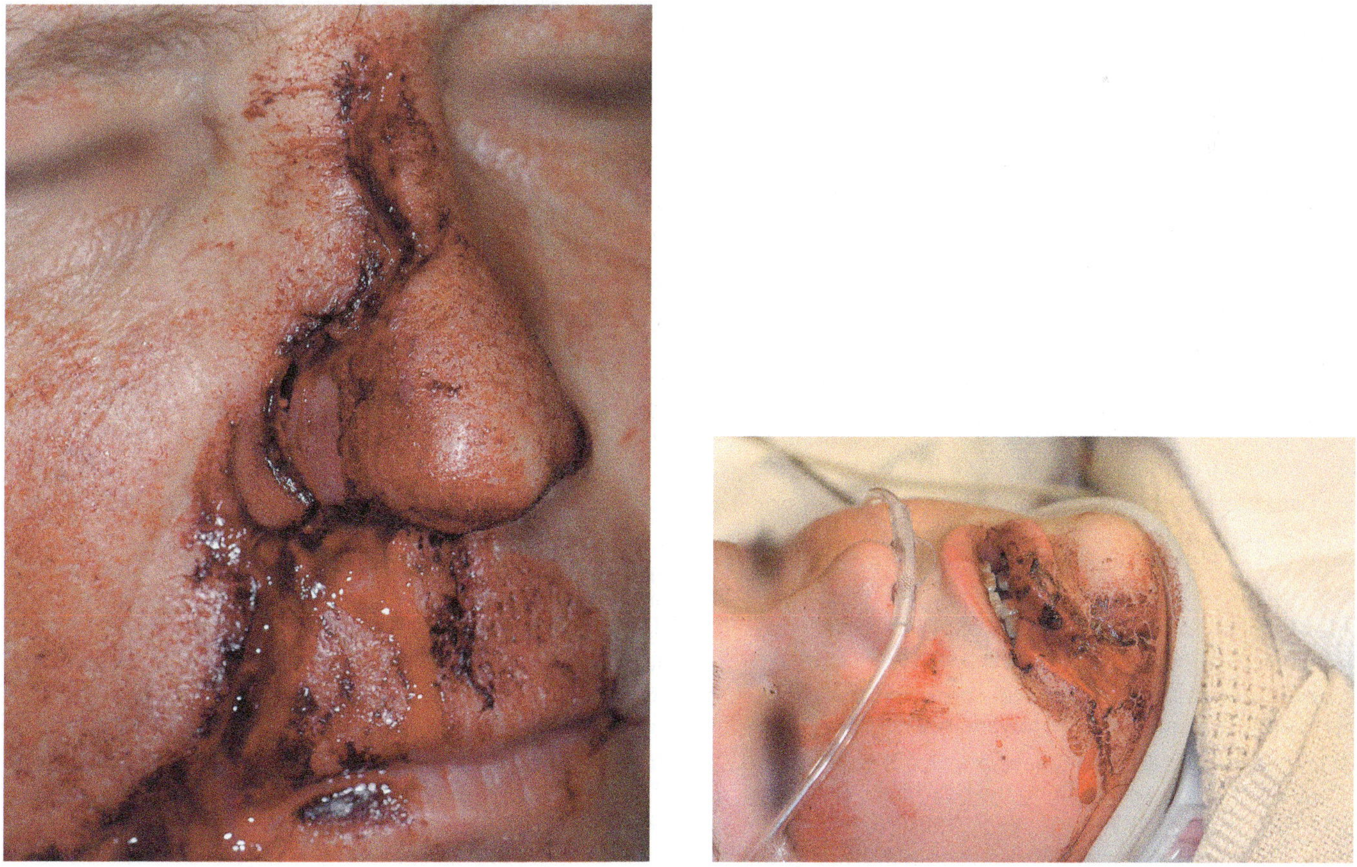

A B

- **Obstructions.** Many suction units are not adequate for removing solid objects such as teeth and large particles of food or other foreign objects. These must be removed using manual techniques for clearing airway obstructions, such as abdominal thrusts, chest thrusts, or finger sweeps, which you learned in your basic life support course and which are reviewed in Appendix A, *Basic Cardiac Life Support Review*, at the back of this book. You may need to log-roll the patient into a supine position to clear the oropharynx manually.
- **Dental appliances.** Dentures should ordinarily be left in place during airway procedures. Partial dentures may become dislodged during an emergency. Leave a partial denture in place if possible, but be prepared to remove it if it endangers the airway.

Chapter Review

Key Facts and Concepts

- The airway is the passageway by which air enters the body during respiration, or breathing.
- A patient cannot survive without an open airway.
- Airway adjuncts–the oropharyngeal and nasopharyngeal airways–can help keep the airway open.
- It may be necessary to suction the airway or to use manual techniques to remove fluids and solids from the airway before, during, or after artificial ventilation.

Key Decisions

- Is the airway open?
- Will the airway stay open?
- Do I need to suction the airway?
- Do I need an adjunct to keep the airway open?

Chapter Glossary

airway the passageway by which air enters and leaves the body. The structures of the airway are the nose, mouth, pharynx, larynx, trachea, bronchi, and lungs. *See also* patent airway.

bronchoconstriction (BRON-ko-kun-STRIK-shun) the contraction of smooth muscle that lines the bronchial passages that results in a decreased internal diameter of the airway and increased resistance to airflow.

gag reflex vomiting or retching that results when something is placed in the back of the pharynx. This is tied to the swallow reflex.

glottic opening the level of the vocal cords that defines the boundary between the upper and lower airways.

head-tilt, chin-lift maneuver a means of correcting blockage of the airway by the tongue by tilting the head back and lifting the chin. Used when no trauma, or injury, is suspected.

jaw-thrust maneuver a means of correcting blockage of the airway by moving the jaw forward without tilting the head or neck. Used when trauma or injury is suspected to open the airway without causing further injury to the spinal cord in the neck.

nasopharyngeal (NAY-zo-fah-RIN-jeul) ***airway*** a flexible breathing tube inserted through the patient's nostril into the pharynx to help maintain an open airway.

oropharyngeal (OR-o-fah-RIN-jeul) ***airway*** a curved device inserted through the patient's mouth into the pharynx to help maintain an open airway.

patent airway an airway (passage from nose or mouth to lungs) that is open and clear and will remain open and clear without interference to the passage of air into and out of the body.

stridor (STRI-dor) a high-pitched sound generated from partially obstructed airflow in the upper airway.

suctioning (SUK-shun-ing) use of a vacuum device to remove blood, vomitus, and other secretions or foreign materials from the airway.

Preparation for Your Examination and Practice

Short Answer

1. Name the main structures of the airway.
2. Explain why care for the airway is a vital part of emergency care.
3. Describe the signs of an inadequate airway.
4. Explain when the head-tilt, chin-lift maneuver should be used and when the jaw-thrust maneuver should be used to open the airway, and why each method should be used.
5. Explain how airway adjuncts and suctioning help in airway management.

Thinking and Linking

Think back to the Lifting and Moving Patients *chapter and link information from that chapter with information from this chapter as you consider the following questions:*

1. You are treating a patient with a spine injury who is immobilized on a backboard. He begins to vomit. In addition to suctioning, what do you do?
2. You are treating an unconscious patient with an unsecure airway. Thus far, you have had to maintain the airway using a head-tilt, chin-lift maneuver. You now prepare to move the patient and must negotiate a series of turns in a narrow hallway to get out of the house. What steps can you take to ensure the airway remains patent during extrication?

Critical Thinking Exercises

Airway assessment is a critical skill. The purpose of this exercise will be to consider how you might assess and manage patients with signs of an airway problem.

1. On arrival at the emergency scene, you find an adult female patient with gurgling sounds in the throat and inadequate breathing slowing to almost nothing. How do you proceed to protect the airway?
2. When evaluating a small child, you hear stridor. What does this sound tell you? What are your immediate concerns regarding this sound?
3. When assessing an unconscious patient, you note snoring respirations. Should you be concerned with this? If so, what steps can you take to correct this situation?

Pathophysiology to Practice

The following questions are designed to assist you in gathering relevant clinical information and making accurate decisions in the field.

1. Describe the signs of a partially obstructed airway.
2. Describe how an altered mental status might impact the airway of your patient.
3. Describe why trauma to the neck might be both an immediate and an ongoing threat to the airway.

Street Scenes

"Control to unit 144," your radio blurts out. You respond, "Go ahead, control." Dispatch tells you that you have a priority-one response to a man down, age unknown, found on the corner of Salina and Jefferson Street. Dispatch also notes that prearrival questioning indicates the patient is not breathing. Brian, your partner, drives, and while en route, you make sure that you have a plan. Brian will take the lead. When he pulls up to the scene, a frantic bystander is waving his arms. He points to a man lying on the ground who is not moving.

Street Scene Questions

1. **What is your first priority when starting to assess this patient?**
2. **What type of emergency care should you be prepared to give?**
3. **What equipment should you proceed into the scene with?**

As you approach, you observe a middle-aged man lying left lateral recumbent on the ground. The bystanders tell you they just found him and don't know how he got there. Your scene survey reveals no obvious trauma or bleeding. You address the patient in a loud voice, but he does not respond.

Street Scene Questions

4. **After ensuring the scene is safe, what are your immediate assessment priorities?**
5. **Describe the steps involved in assessing the airway of this unresponsive patient.**

Brian assists you in rolling the patient supine. Because you are unsure about the mechanism of injury, you maintain spinal precautions. You observe gurgling and snoring respirations. The patient has some chest rise, but there appears to be a substantial amount of vomit present in his airway.

Street Scene Questions

6. **What immediate actions must be taken to clear the airway?**
7. **Once the airway has been cleared, describe how you might open the airway.**

10 Respiration and Artificial Ventilation

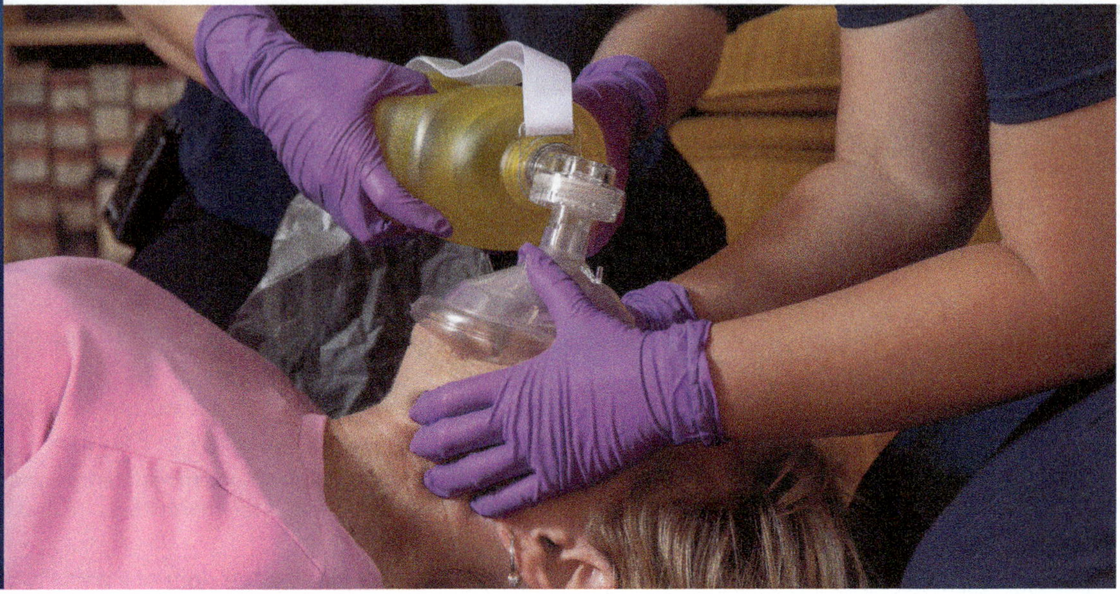

Related Chapters

The following chapters provide additional information related to topics discussed in this chapter:

Standard

Airway Management, Respiration, and Artificial Ventilation (Respiration, Artificial Ventilation)

Competency

Applies knowledge (fundamental depth, foundational breadth) of general anatomy and physiology to patient assessment and management to ensure a patent airway, adequate mechanical ventilation, and respiration for patients of all ages.

Core Concepts

- Physiology and pathophysiology of the respiratory system
- How to recognize adequate and inadequate breathing
- Principles and techniques of positive pressure ventilation
- Principles and techniques of oxygen administration

Outcomes

After reading this chapter, you should be able to:

10.1 Compare the physiology and pathophysiology of breathing. (pp. 239-241)

- Describe the mechanical process of breathing.
- Describe the physiology of respiration at the alveolar level.

10.2 Explain concepts of cardiopulmonary pathophysiology. (pp. 241-242)

- Explain how various conditions can interrupt the mechanical processes of breathing.
- Explain how various conditions can interrupt the process of gas exchange at the alveolar level.
- Explain how various impairments of circulation can interrupt the exchange of gases at the cellular level.

10.3 Summarize concepts of respiration. (pp. 243-248)

- List conditions necessary for adequate respiration.
- Recognize the consequences of inadequate breathing.
- Distinguish the pathophysiologies of respiratory distress and respiratory failure.

10.4 Describe the assessment of patients' breathing. (pp. 248-251)

- Describe the sequence of steps involved in assessing breathing.
- Evaluate breathing status based on assessment findings.
- Differentiate between patients who need only supplemental oxygen and those who need artificial ventilation with supplemental oxygen.

10.5 Summarize concepts of positive pressure ventilation. (pp. 251-264)

- Explain complications of positive pressure intervention.
- Describe the general approach to using artificial ventilation.
- Describe different techniques of artificial ventilation.
- Compare the approaches to artificial ventilation for patients with rapid breathing and those with slow breathing.
- Match the EMT's interventions with patients' respiratory statuses.
- Identify the equipment used with each technique of artificial ventilation.
- List the sequence of steps for using each technique of artificial ventilation.
- List modifications of artificial ventilation for stoma breathers.
- Describe the indications for using an automatic transport ventilator (ATV).

10.6 Explain concepts related to administering supplemental oxygen. (pp. 264-281)

- Describe the major issues to consider when making a decision to provide patients with supplemental oxygen.
- Compare the features of various portable and fixed oxygen cylinders used in EMS systems.
- Describe the EMT's obligations with respect to evaluating the supply of oxygen available.
- List the EMT's obligations with respect to safety related to oxygen use.

- Identify the equipment and supplies used in oxygen administration.
- Describe the purpose of each of the parts of an oxygen delivery system.
- List risks to patients who receive excessive amounts of supplemental oxygen.
- List the sequence of steps for preparing an oxygen delivery system for supplemental oxygen administration.
- Given a patient scenario, select the most appropriate approach to oxygen therapy.
- Describe considerations in responding to patients who have complications that can interfere with oxygen administration and artificial ventilation.
- Provide the rationales for modifying techniques of oxygenation and artificial ventilations in pediatric patients.

10.7 Explain the EMT's roles and responsibilities related to the use of advanced airway devices. (pp. 281-285)

- Recognize the types of devices used for advanced airway management.
- Identify what EMTs can do to assist in the advanced airway placement procedures.
- Describe considerations in ventilating a patient who has an advanced airway device in place.

Key Terms

alveolar ventilation, *239*
artificial ventilation, *251*
automatic transport ventilator (ATV), *264*
bag-valve mask (BVM), *259*
cellular respiration, *241*
cyanosis, *249*
diffusion, *241*
flowmeter, *268*
humidifier, *269*
hypoxia, *243*
nasal cannula, *276*
nonrebreather (NRB) mask, *275*
oxygen cylinder, *265*
partial rebreather mask, *277*
pocket face mask, *257*
positive pressure ventilation, *251*
pressure regulator, *268*
pulmonary respiration, *241*
respiration, *243*
respiratory arrest, *243*
respiratory distress, *243*
respiratory failure, *243*
stoma, *262*
tracheostomy mask, *278*
ventilation, *239*
Venturi mask, *277*

"Is the patient's airway open?" "Will it stay open?" In the chapter *Airway Management*, we discussed how you will use these questions as part of your primary assessment to immediately identify and manage problems associated with the movement of air in and out of the patient's lungs. But a clear pathway is not enough. To support life-sustaining oxygenation and ventilation, a patient requires a stimulus to breathe, proper regulation of that breathing, and the musculoskeletal function capable of moving air. Once you have secured the airway, you must turn your attention to the patient's ability to breathe. Two new questions must now be considered: "Is the patient breathing?" and if so, "Is breathing adequate?"

Breathing accomplishes two essential functions: It brings oxygen into the body and eliminates carbon dioxide. Although your body will tolerate the buildup of carbon dioxide longer than it will tolerate a lack of oxygen, both of these functions are absolutely necessary to support life. In the primary assessment, we will not only look at airway patency (whether the airway is open and clear), but also how well or how poorly air is being exchanged in the lungs. We will pair airway management with an assessment of breathing to ensure that both oxygenation and ventilation are occurring. If you determine that the patient's breathing is not meeting the body's needs, then you must take immediate corrective action. A thorough primary assessment combines a rapid evaluation of both airway *and* breathing, and identifies immediate life threats associated with the respiratory system.

In this chapter you will learn the skills necessary to identify and correct inadequate breathing. However, it is just as important to learn the decision-making process that will tell you when to employ those skills. You must learn not just *how to* but, equally important, *when to* assist a patient with breathing.

Physiology and Pathophysiology

Mechanics of Breathing

Air is moved into and out of the chest in a process called ***ventilation***. To move air, the diaphragm and the muscles of the chest are contracted and relaxed to change the pressure within the chest cavity. This changing pressure inflates and deflates the lungs. *Inhalation* is an active process. The muscles of the chest, including the intercostal muscles between the ribs, are engaged at the same time the diaphragm contracts in a downward motion. These movements increase the size of the chest cavity and create a negative pressure. This negative pressure pulls air in through the glottic opening and inflates the lungs. Conversely, *exhalation* is most commonly a passive process—that is, it occurs when the previously discussed muscles relax. As the size of the chest decreases, it creates a positive pressure and pushes air out. Because it is passive, exhalation typically takes slightly longer than inhalation. In certain disorders, like asthma and chronic obstructive pulmonary disease (COPD), narrowing of the airways can cause exhalation to become more of an active process. These patients are forced to engage accessory muscles to move air, and can often be identified by the unusual amount of effort and the prolonged timing of their exhalation (otherwise known as the expiratory phase of breathing).

ventilation
breathing in and out (inhalation and exhalation), or artificial provision of breaths.

CORE CONCEPT
Physiology and pathophysiology of the respiratory system

As we discussed in the chapter titled *Principles of Pathophysiology*, the amount of air moved in one breath (one cycle of inhalation and exhalation) is called *tidal volume*. A normal tidal volume is typically 5–7 mL per kg of body weight. The amount of air moved into and out of the lungs per minute is called *minute volume*. Minute volume is calculated by multiplying the tidal volume by the respiratory rate ($MV = TV \times RR$).

Ventilation (inhalation and exhalation) is ultimately designed to move air to and from the alveoli for gas exchange. However, not all the air we breathe reaches the alveoli. For example, an adult patient has an average tidal volume of roughly 500 mL. Of that 500 mL, only about 350 mL reaches the alveoli. The remainder occupies the trachea, bronchioles, and other non–gas-exchanging parts of the airway, known as *dead space* or *dead air space* (Figure 10-1). The alveoli are the only place where oxygen and carbon dioxide are exchanged with the bloodstream; therefore, the air in the dead space contributes nothing to oxygenating the body. The term ***alveolar ventilation*** refers to how much air actually reaches the alveoli.

alveolar ventilation
the amount of air that reaches the alveoli.

Alveolar ventilation is a very important concept to remember because some patients will go to extreme lengths to breathe without much air reaching the alveoli. Patients with severely narrowed and obstructed air passages will use great effort and display exaggerated chest wall movement, but the obstruction will prevent adequate alveolar ventilation. A less-than-thorough assessment might lead to a mistaken assumption that ventilation is adequate; however, a trained observer with a keen eye will quickly recognize the very real danger these patients face.

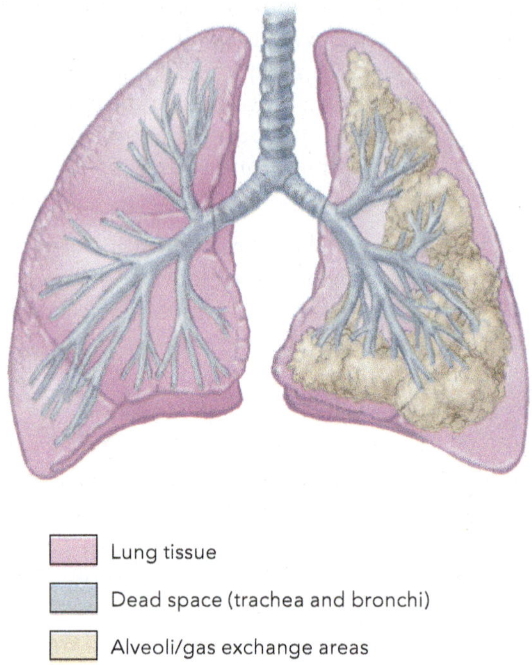

FIGURE 10-1 Dead air space; areas of the airway outside the alveoli/gas exchange areas.

Alveolar ventilation depends very much on tidal volume. Consider the following example:

An adult asthma patient has a normal tidal volume of 500 mL. Today, however, because his asthma attack has constricted his bronchiole tubes, he can move only 300 mL of tidal volume. If the air in the dead space remains constant at 150 mL, then only 150 mL of air reaches his alveoli per breath.

- Normal tidal volume: 500 mL × 16 breaths per minute = 8,000 mL
- Normal alveolar ventilation: 350 mL (500 − 150 dead air space) × 16 bpm = 5,600 mL
- Asthma attack tidal volume: 300 mL × 16 bpm = 4,800 mL
- Asthma attack alveolar ventilation: 150 mL (300 − 150 dead air space) × 16 bpm = 2,400 mL

Remember that alveolar ventilation can be altered through changes in rate as well as by changes in volume. A person breathing too slowly will have a decreased minute volume, so the amount of air reaching the alveoli per minute is decreased, just as it would be decreased by a reduction in tidal volume.

- Normal minute volume: 500 mL × 16 breaths per minute = 8,000 mL
- Slowed minute volume: 500 mL × 8 breaths per minute = 4,000 mL

Occasionally, very fast respiratory rates may decrease minute volume as well, not primarily because of rate but because the faster rate can affect the tidal volume. Fast breathing can, at times, limit the amount of time the lungs have to fill and therefore decrease tidal volume. Even though increasing the rate should increase minute volumes, exceptionally fast breathing will actually reduce minute volume and alveolar ventilation.

Physiology of Respiration

Alveoli form the ends of bronchiole tubes in the lungs. Bunches of these tiny air sacs are inflated and ventilated as air moves in and out of the most terminal reaches of the airway during breathing. Each alveolus is a bubble-like structure with air on the inside and pulmonary capillaries spanning its outside surface. This interface between air on the inside and circulating blood (in the pulmonary capillaries) on the outside creates the opportunity for life-sustaining gas exchange. Inhaled air fills the alveoli. The pulmonary capillaries bring circulating blood just to the other side of the microscopic alveolar-capillary membrane. These thin walls of the alveoli and the thin walls of the capillaries allow oxygen from the air in the alveoli to move into the blood to circulate throughout the body. The thin walls of the capillaries and alveoli also allow carbon dioxide to move from the blood into the alveoli to be expelled during exhalation.

The movement of gases from an area of high concentration to an area of low concentration is called ***diffusion***. The diffusion of oxygen and carbon dioxide that takes place between the *alveoli* and circulating blood is called ***pulmonary respiration***. Carbon dioxide is offloaded from the blood into alveoli, while oxygen from the air in the alveoli is loaded onto the hemoglobin and into the plasma of the blood, and transported to the cells. At the cells, through a similar but reversed process of diffusion, oxygen passes from the blood, across cell membranes, and into the cells, while carbon dioxide from the cells passes into the blood. The diffusion of oxygen and carbon dioxide that takes place between the *cells* and circulating blood is called ***cellular respiration*** (Figure 10-2).

diffusion
a process by which molecules move from an area of high concentration to an area of low concentration.

pulmonary respiration
the exchange of oxygen and carbon dioxide between the alveoli and circulating blood in the pulmonary capillaries.

cellular respiration
the exchange of oxygen and carbon dioxide between cells and circulating blood.

Remember: For this entire process to be working, the respiratory system must be appropriately matched up with a functioning cardiovascular system. The respiratory system must be moving air in and out of the alveoli, and the circulatory system must be transporting adequate amounts of blood between the cells and the alveoli. These two systems working in concert are often referred to as the *cardiopulmonary system* and also referred to as a ventilation–perfusion (V/Q) match, as was discussed in *Principles of Pathophysiology*. When either of these systems fails, the process of respiration is defeated.

Pathophysiology of the Cardiopulmonary System

Before proceeding, take a few minutes to review the concepts of pathophysiology of the cardiopulmonary system that were discussed in detail in *Principles of Pathophysiology*. Consider the following mechanical failures of the cardiopulmonary system that may occur:

- **Mechanics of breathing disrupted.** If the chest cannot create the necessary pressure changes, air cannot be moved in and out of the lungs. Breathing can be disrupted by a variety of causes, such as:
    - *A patient stabbed in the chest*. When the diaphragm moves downward, air is pulled into the chest cavity through the stab wound in addition to the normal drawing in of air through the glottic opening. Because of the air rushing into the chest through the stab wound, a negative pressure cannot be created to efficiently pull air into the lungs through the normal airway passages.
    - *A patient loses nervous control of respiration*. A patient may lose the ability to transmit messages through nerve tissue to innervate the muscles of respiration. This can occur in diseases such as myasthenia gravis and multiple sclerosis.
    - *A patient sustains painful chest wall injuries*. Pain and physical damage can both limit chest wall movement.
    - *A patient has airway problems such as bronchoconstriction*. If air cannot move, breathing cannot occur. Some diseases such as asthma and chronic obstructive pulmonary disease (COPD) can cause bronchial tubes to decrease in diameter and can limit the amount of air that can flow through them.
- **Gas exchange interrupted.** Sometimes the ability to diffuse oxygen and carbon dioxide is impaired. Consider the following examples:
    - *Low oxygen levels in the outside air, such as in confined-space rescue situations*. Here there simply is not enough oxygen in the air breathed in.
    - *Diffusion problems*. Some diseases, such as congestive heart failure and COPD, can limit the ability of alveoli to exchange oxygen and carbon dioxide. Here oxygenated air and blood reach the alveoli, but the alveoli themselves are not working.

- **Circulation issues.** There can be problems that prevent the blood from carrying enough oxygen to the body's cells, such as:
  - *Not enough blood*. If a person has lost a significant amount of blood, not enough blood can be circulated to the alveoli. If blood is not present at the interface with the alveoli, oxygen and carbon dioxide cannot be exchanged.
  - *Hemoglobin problems*. Occasionally respiration can be impaired if there is not enough hemoglobin, the oxygen-binding protein in the blood. For example, anemia is a disease that causes low amounts of hemoglobin in the blood. In other situations, as with a patient whose body pH becomes very acidotic, sufficient hemoglobin may be present but may have difficulty holding and transporting oxygen.

FIGURE 10-2 The processes of pulmonary and cellular respiration.

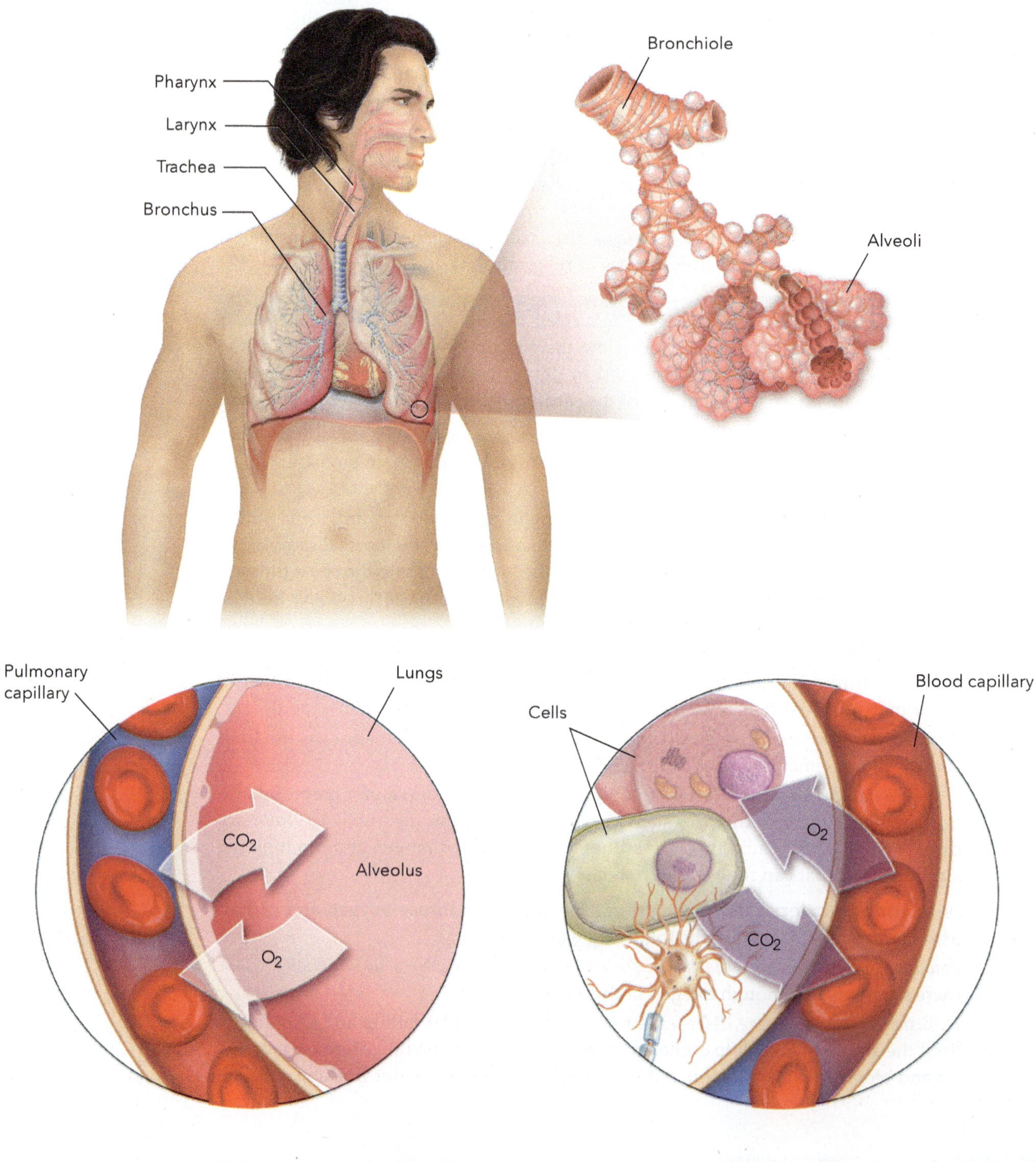

Respiration

As just discussed, *ventilation* is the term properly applied to the process of inhaling and exhaling, or breathing, whereas ***respiration*** refers to the exchange of gases between the alveoli and the blood (external respiration) and between the blood and the cells (internal respiration). However, in common speech, and in an overall sense, *respiration* means, simply, breathing in all its aspects.

respiration (RES-pir-AY-shun) the diffusion of oxygen and carbon dioxide between the alveoli and the blood (pulmonary respiration) and between the blood and the cells (cellular respiration). Also used to mean, simply, breathing.

Adequate and Inadequate Breathing

The brain and body cells need a steady supply of oxygen to accomplish the tasks of everyday living. Low levels of oxygen, or ***hypoxia***, will disrupt normal function. Although it is also important for carbon dioxide to be removed, the body will tolerate high levels of carbon dioxide (*hypercapnia*) for longer periods of time than it will tolerate hypoxia. As we evaluate breathing in a patient, we will assess severity based on how well the patient's cardiopulmonary system is accomplishing the goals of oxygenation and removal of carbon dioxide.

hypoxia (hi-POK-se-uh) an insufficiency of oxygen in the body's tissues.

CORE CONCEPT
How to recognize adequate and inadequate breathing

When the cardiopulmonary system fails, the body makes adjustments to compensate for hypoxia and/or a buildup of carbon dioxide. These adjustments are somewhat predictable and can help us recognize the severity of the patient's problem.

In most people, the urge to breathe is caused by the buildup of carbon dioxide. Special sensors in the cardiovascular system, called chemoreceptors, detect increasing levels of carbon dioxide as well as low levels of oxygen. When these sensors detect significant changes, especially a buildup of carbon dioxide, the respiratory system is stimulated to breathe more rapidly.

When a person's cardiopulmonary system cannot keep up with the body's current demands, carbon dioxide levels increase. In some situations hypoxia may also occur. The body typically responds with an increased respiratory rate to attempt to move more air in and out of the lungs. At this point, it is common for the patient to complain of the sensation of shortness of breath. The body will also typically respond by engaging the sympathetic (or fight-or-flight) nervous system. The sympathetic nervous system will increase heart rate in an attempt to move more blood (and transport more oxygen and carbon dioxide), and will constrict blood vessels, which also aids in the movement of blood.

In some cases the adjustments the body makes will keep up with added demands. For example, a patient will have a challenge, such as an asthma attack, and the patient's body will be compensating for that challenge. Increased respiratory rate, increased heart rate, and perhaps even position changes may be enough to meet the challenge and, at least minimally, the body's needs. The outward signs of these changes (e.g., vital signs, appearance, position) will indicate that the patient's system is working extra hard to meet the patient's needs. If these changes are effective, there will be signs that oxygen and carbon dioxide are being adequately exchanged. These signs include normal mental status, relatively normal skin color, and a pulse oximetry reading (measurement of blood oxygen saturation) that is within normal limits. These patients are classified as having ***respiratory distress***—that is, they have a challenge, but the compensatory mechanisms the body is providing are meeting their increased demands. They are, in fact, compensating.

respiratory distress increased work of breathing; a sensation of shortness of breath.

Unfortunately, some challenges are just too great for the body's compensatory mechanisms to overcome. In addition, most of the mechanisms of compensation, such as increased respiratory muscle use, come at a cost of increased oxygen demand. If the very nature of the problem is that there was not enough oxygen to begin with, the demand for oxygen will quickly overtake the limited supply. In these cases, compensation fails and the body's metabolic needs are not met. Hypoxia becomes profound, carbon dioxide builds to dangerous levels, and the muscles used for increased respiration begin to tire. This condition represents *inadequate breathing* and is called ***respiratory failure*** (Figure 10-3).

respiratory failure the inadequacy of breathing to the point where oxygen intake or the ventilation removal of carbon dioxide is not sufficient to support life.

Respiratory failure is especially important to recognize because it is often the precursor to the complete stoppage of breathing (***respiratory arrest***).

respiratory arrest when breathing completely stops.

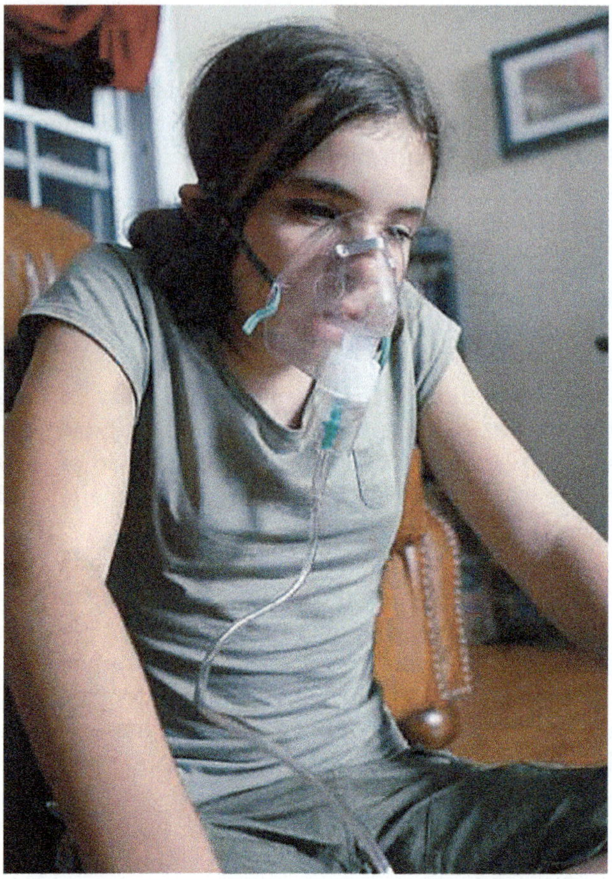

FIGURE 10-3 Respiratory distress usually involves accessory muscle use and increased work of breathing. Severe or prolonged respiratory distress can proceed to respiratory failure and inadequate breathing when the body can no longer work so hard to breathe. In this case, you will see a reduced level of responsiveness or an appearance of tiring, shallow ventilations, and other signs of inadequate breathing. *(© Daniel Limmer)*

As an EMT, you will use your primary assessment to evaluate patients and rapidly classify their respiratory status. In essence, you will be making the decision as to whether their breathing is adequate or inadequate.

Inadequate Breathing

When you note that a patient's breathing is absent, you will provide artificial ventilation. However, there is a time before respiration completely ceases when, although the patient may show some signs of breathing, these breathing efforts are not enough to support life. That is, the patient who continues to breathe in this manner will eventually develop respiratory arrest and die. This is deemed inadequate breathing. In inadequate breathing, either the *rate of breathing*, the *depth of breathing*, or both fall outside of normal ranges.

Recognizing inadequate breathing requires both keen assessment skills and prompt action (Table 10-1). Identifying this condition and providing ventilation to inadequately breathing patients may actually keep them alive and breathing in cases where they would have stopped breathing and died without your intervention (Figure 10-4).

Respiratory Distress to Respiratory Failure

Respiratory failure occurs when the mechanisms of respiratory compensation can no longer keep up with a respiratory challenge. To illustrate this process, let's review the progression of a patient having an asthma attack.

Patients with asthma have episodic attacks where their bronchiole tubes spasm and constrict. This leads to decreased airflow and decreased tidal volume. As minute volume and alveolar ventilation decrease, the body senses increased levels of carbon dioxide and slight hypoxia. The brain responds with an increased stimulus to breathe and activation of the sympathetic nervous system.

TABLE 10-1 Respiratory Conditions with Appropriate Interventions

CONDITION	SIGNS	EMT INTERVENTION	
ADEQUATE BREATHING Oxygenation and ventilation are sufficient to meet metabolic demands. Breathing may be challenged and the patient may be compensating (increased rate, accessory muscle use, etc.), but the effort is matching the patient's needs.	• Normal mental status • Rate and depth of breathing are adequate. • Air moving in and out of the chest • Skin color normal • Oxygen saturation normal	• Identify and treat respiratory challenge. • Consider supplemental oxygen (*nonrebreather mask* or *nasal cannula*).	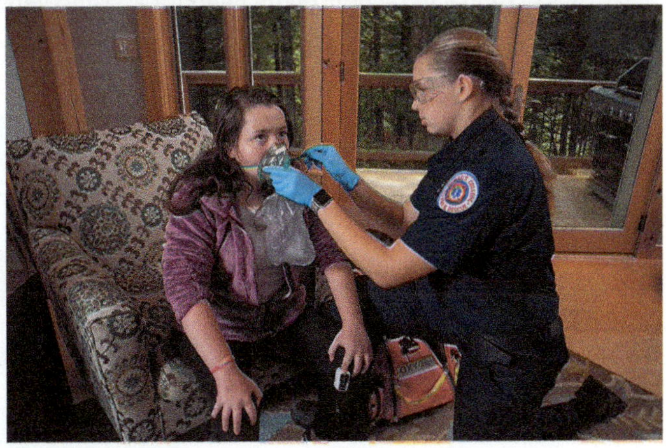
INADEQUATE BREATHING (RESPIRATORY FAILURE) Patient is breathing, but oxygenation and ventilation are insufficient to support life.	• Altered mental status • Patient has some breathing but not enough to live. • Rate and/or depth outside of normal limits • Shallow ventilations • Diminished or absent breath sounds • Noises such as crowing, stridor, snoring, gurgling, or gasping • Blue (cyanotic) or gray skin color • Decreased minute volume • Oxygen saturation low (< 95%)	Assisted ventilations (air forced into the lungs under pressure) with a *pocket face mask* or *bag-valve mask* **NOTE:** *A nonrebreather mask requires adequate breathing to pull oxygen into the lungs. It does not provide ventilation to a patient who is not breathing or who is breathing inadequately.*	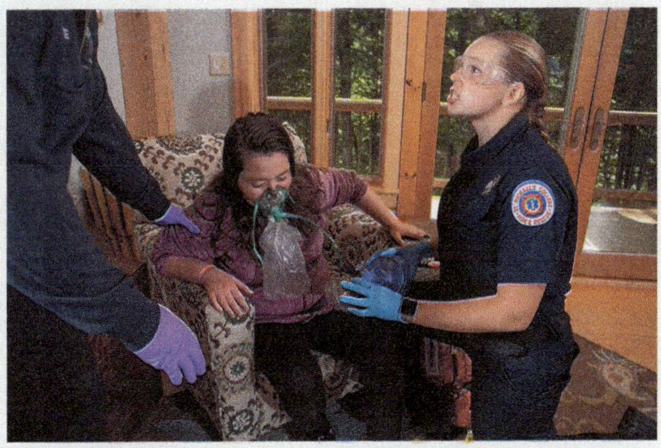
PATIENT IS NOT BREATHING AT ALL (RESPIRATORY ARREST)	• No chest or abdominal rise and fall • No evidence of air being moved from the mouth or nose • No breath sounds	Artificial ventilations with a *pocket face mask or bag-valve mask* at 10–12/minute for an adult or 12–20/minute for an infant or child **NOTE:** Do not *use oxygen-powered ventilation devices on infants or children.*	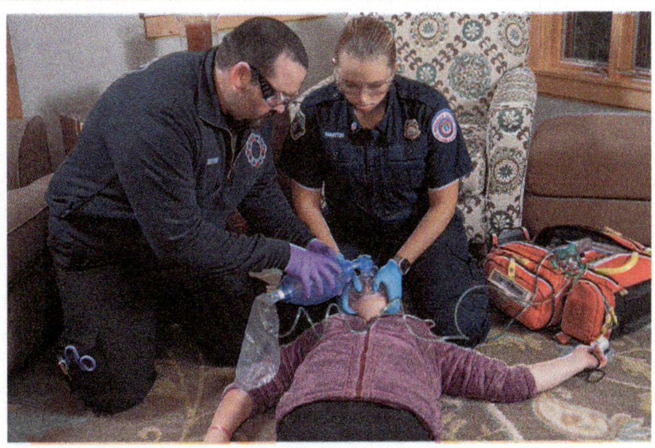

FIGURE 10-4 Along the continuum from normal, adequate breathing to no breathing at all, there are milestones where an EMT should apply a nonrebreather mask or nasal cannula, or switch to positive pressure ventilation with a pocket face mask or BVM for assisting the patient's own ventilations or providing artificial ventilation. It is essential to recognize the need for assisted ventilations, even before severe respiratory distress develops.

PATIENT'S CONDITION | **WHEN AND HOW TO INTERVENE**

Adequate breathing:
Speaks full sentences;
alert and calm

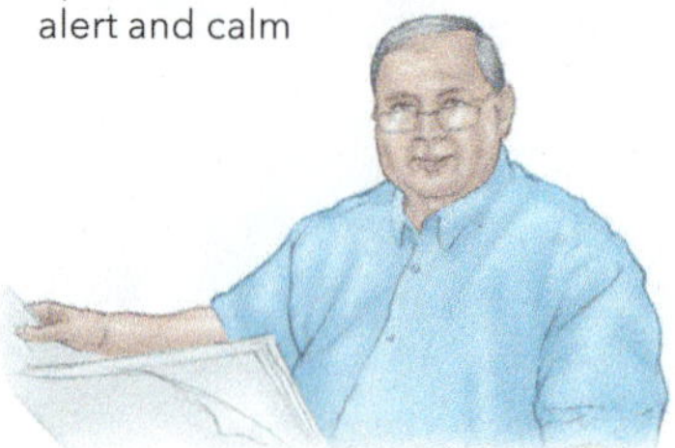

Nonrebreather mask or nasal cannula

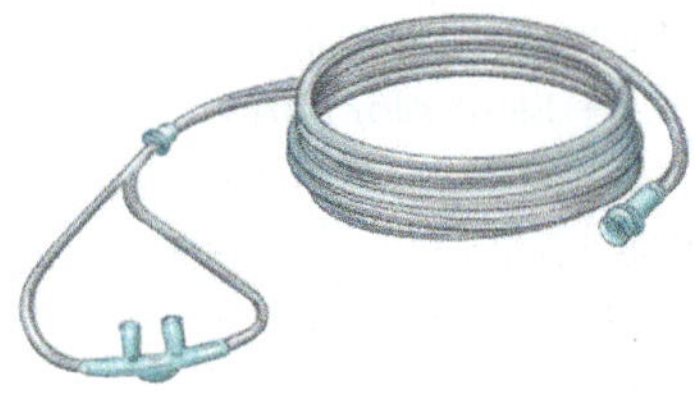

Increasing respiratory distress:
Visibly short of breath;
Speaking 3–4 word sentences;
Increasing anxiety

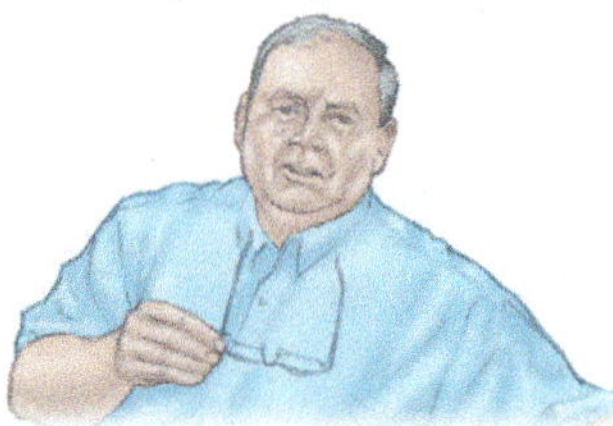

Nonrebreather mask

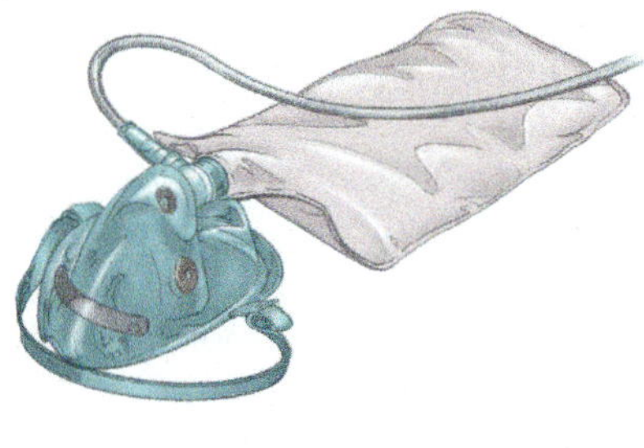

Key decision-making point:

Recognize inadequate breathing before respiratory arrest develops.

Assist ventilations before they stop altogether!

Severe respiratory distress:
Speaking only 1–2 word sentences;
Very diaphoretic (sweaty);
Severe anxiety

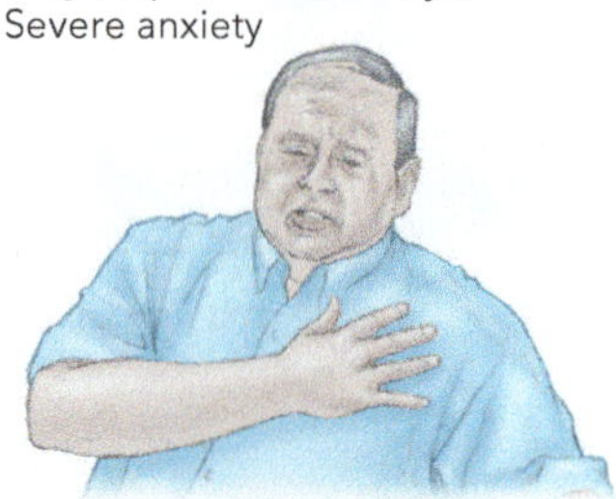

Assisted ventilations
Pocket face mask (PFM),
bag-valve mask (BVM)

Assist the patient's own ventilations, adjusting the rate for rapid or slow breathing

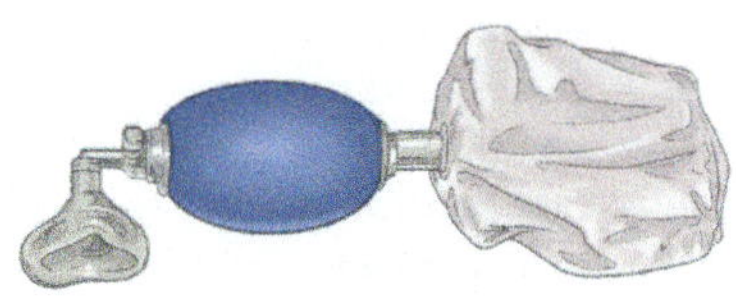

Continues to deteriorate:
Sleepy with head-bobbing;
Becomes unarousable

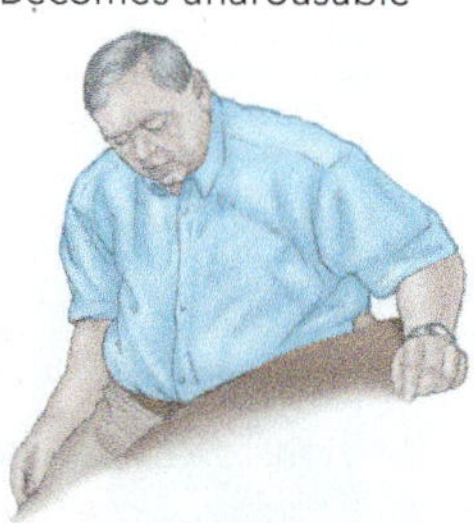

Respiratory arrest:
No breathing

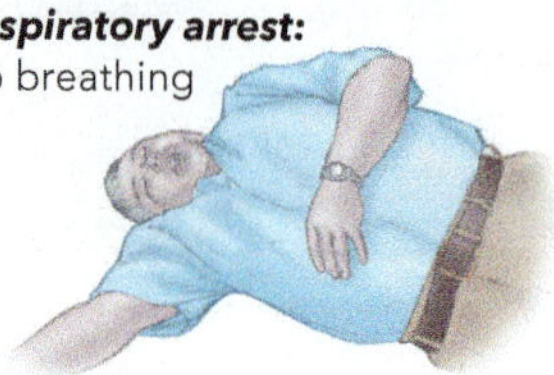

Artificial ventilation
Pocket face mask (PFM),
bag-valve mask (BVM)

Assisted ventilations at
10–12/minute for an adult or
20/minute for a child or infant

Inside the body, the respiratory system compensates. Respiratory rate and depth are increased in an attempt to increase alveolar ventilation. The heart pumps faster and harder in an attempt to move oxygen and carbon dioxide more quickly. Blood vessels constrict as the fight-or-flight response engages.

Outside the body, the patient may notice a sensation of shortness of breath. The person may complain, "I can't catch my breath." You may notice an increased respiratory rate and an increased work of breathing. It may simply look as if it is hard for the patient to breathe. You may hear wheezes, which are the sounds of the bronchoconstriction. You may also note the patient has slightly pale skin. However, since the patient's compensatory mechanisms are working, you should not see blue skin. Mental status is also normal, since adequate levels of oxygen are being supplied to the brain. At this point you would classify this patient as being in *respiratory distress*. The patient has a challenge, but needs are being met by compensatory mechanisms inside the body.

Unfortunately, the asthma attack continues. Inside the body, the patient's bronchiole tubes get narrower as they begin to swell in response to the attack. Tidal volume and alveolar ventilation decrease even more, and the brain now lacks sufficient oxygen. Carbon dioxide also has been building up and is beginning to interfere with normal function. As you reassess, you notice this patient is beginning to get anxious, maybe even a bit combative, as hypoxia increases and affects the brain. You notice it is harder to hear air moving when you auscultate the chest. The wheezes have become "tighter." Fingernails are now turning blue, and you notice a similar discoloration at the lips and around the eyes. *Respiratory failure* has begun. Compensation can no longer keep up with the body's needs.

As the attack continues, tidal volume and alveolar ventilation decrease even further. Hypoxia is now profound. The patient's body has become acidotic from retention of

Pediatric Note

The physiology and pathophysiology of pediatric breathing are very similar to those of breathing by adults. Pediatric patients too will have challenges, they will compensate, and they will experience adequate and inadequate breathing. Infants and children do, however, have some anatomic and physiologic differences that should be considered.

Compared to adults, children have a higher metabolic demand. In fact, they use oxygen twice as fast as adults do during metabolism. This translates to an aggressive need to maintain oxygenation, and significant complications when oxygenation is insufficient.

Children, in general, have a more pliable chest wall. When they are infants, their ribs flare outward at the bottom, flattening out the diaphragm. These anatomic differences mean that children rely more on respiratory rate during compensation than adults do. They also mean that significant accessory muscle use during breathing is less helpful than it is to compensating adults. Children simply use a lot more energy to achieve less-effective results during compensation.

NOTE: *Although pediatric patients are quite able to compensate during respiratory distress, the move from adequate to inadequate breathing can sometimes be subtle but rapid. Arrest can also occur abruptly. A critical assessment finding in pediatric patients with respiratory difficulty is the presence of a slow heart rate (bradycardia). Bradycardia in a pediatric patient with respiratory distress can be followed quickly by cardiac arrest from respiratory failure. The pediatric patient found to be in respiratory distress with associated bradycardia requires immediate artificial ventilation by pocket mask or bag-valve mask.*

Because of the high metabolic demands and the limitations associated with compensation, you must be attentive in your ongoing assessment and aggressive in preventing inadequate breathing. Treat respiratory conditions early and be aggressive with positive pressure ventilation when indicated.

too much carbon dioxide and from anaerobic metabolism (metabolism without enough oxygen present). The patient is growing tired. For a prolonged period now, the muscles of the chest have been working extra hard. These respiratory muscles demand oxygen that the patient's respiratory system cannot deliver. As a result, the respiratory muscles fatigue.

On the outside, mental status now is obviously severely impaired. The patient has become drowsy and can barely stay awake. The respiratory rate has slowed, and you note irregular breathing. Skin color is ashen with a definite bluish discoloration. The patient is now in profound respiratory failure. *Respiratory arrest* is imminent.

Patient Assessment

Assessing Breathing

As you assess breathing during the primary assessment, you should answer two important questions. The first question is "Is the patient breathing?" You can determine this simply by the patient's response to a simple "Hello." If the patient is unconscious, you may need to revert to BLS procedures and perform a look-listen-feel assessment. If the patient is not breathing, you must take immediate action to breathe for the patient. The second question you must answer is "If the patient is breathing, is it adequate?" Is the effort the patient is putting forth enough to support the patient's needs? If the answer is no, then you must intervene.

Signs of Adequate Breathing

To determine signs of adequate breathing, you should:

- *Look* for adequate and equal expansion of both sides of the chest when the patient inhales. If the patient has an obvious respiratory problem, expose and visually inspect the chest.
- *Listen* for air entering and leaving the nose, mouth, and chest. The sounds from the mouth and nose should be typically free of gurgling, gasping, crowing, wheezing, snoring, and stridor (harsh, high-pitched sound during inhalation). If the patient has an obvious respiratory problem or has a serious mechanism of injury, listen to both sides of the chest with a stethoscope. You should hear air moving in and out, and breath sounds (when auscultated or listened to with a stethoscope) should be present and equal on both sides of the chest.
- *Feel* for air moving out of the nose or mouth.
- Check for typical skin coloration. There should be no blue or gray colorations.
- Note the rate, rhythm, quality, and depth of breathing typical for a person at rest (Table 10-2).

Signs of Inadequate Breathing

Signs of inadequate breathing include the following:

- Altered mental status. The brain has no capacity to store oxygen. When metabolic needs are not met, brain functions fail. Signs of inadequate breathing include increasing anxiousness, confusion, lethargy, and loss of consciousness.

TABLE 10-2 Adequate Breathing

NORMAL RATES	QUALITY
Adult–12-20 per minute	Breath sounds–present and equal
Child–18-30 per minute	Chest expansion–adequate and equal
Infant–30-60 per minute	Minimum effort
RHYTHM	**DEPTH**
Regular	Adequate

- Chest movements are absent, minimal, or uneven.
- Slow pulse rate (bradycardia) in infants and children
- Movement associated with breathing is limited to the abdomen (abdominal breathing) or, especially in children, is exaggerated in alternating rise and fall of the chest and the abdomen (called *thoraco-abdominal breathing*). In these cases, the abdomen rises when the chest falls and vice versa. This paradoxical motion of the chest and abdomen can be an ominous sign of failing compensation.
- No air can be felt or heard at the nose or mouth, or the amount of air exchanged is below normal.
- Breath sounds are diminished or absent. Silent chest, especially in children, can be an ominous sign of poor alveolar ventilation.
- Noises such as wheezing, crowing, stridor, snoring, gurgling, or gasping are heard during breathing.
- Rate of breathing is too rapid or too slow.
- Breathing is very shallow, very deep, or appears labored.
- The patient's skin, lips, tongue, ear lobes, or nail beds are blue or gray. This condition is called ***cyanosis***, and the patient is said to be cyanotic.
- Inspirations are prolonged (indicating a possible upper airway obstruction) or expirations are prolonged (indicating a possible lower airway obstruction).
- Patient is unable to speak, or the patient cannot speak full sentences because of shortness of breath.
- In children, there may be retractions (a pulling in of the muscles) above the clavicles and between and below the ribs.
- Nasal flaring (widening of the nostrils of the nose with respirations) may be present, especially in infants and children.
- Low oxygen saturation reading (< 95%)
- Body position changes. As breathing becomes inadequate, many patients will rely on a bolt-upright or tripod position to assist with breathing. In particular, they will not be able to tolerate lying flat or perhaps even the semi-Fowler position.

cyanosis (SY-uh-NO-sis) a blue or gray color resulting from lack of oxygen in the body.

"If your patient's respirations aren't adequate to meet his body's needs, you have to be aggressive about helping him breathe."

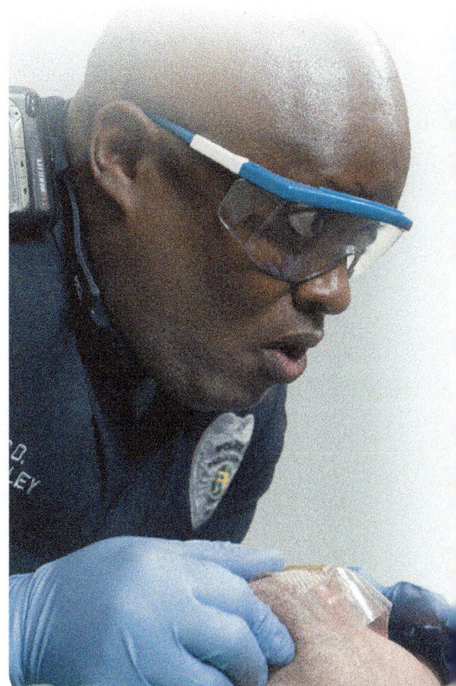

Respiratory Evaluation

NORMAL BREATHING *(ADEQUATE BREATHING)*	ADEQUATE BREATHING	INADEQUATE BREATHING	RESPIRATORY ARREST *(INADEQUATE BREATHING)*
Quiet, no unusual sounds	May have unusual sounds such as wheezing, stridor, or coughing.	Same as distress; beware absent sounds.	No sounds of breathing
Normal rate of breathing	Typically elevated rate of breathing; not excessively fast, though adequate minute volume	Often too fast or too slow Sometimes irregular or slowing Inadequate minute volume	None
Normal skin color	Sometimes normal or pale due to vasoconstriction	Pale or blue; sometimes mottled (blotchy)	Pale or blue
Normal mental status	Normal, sometimes agitated or anxious	Altered mental status	Typically unconscious or rapidly becoming unconscious

Occasionally respiratory arrest will be difficult to determine. Recall the steps of basic CPR. Look at the chest for rise and fall. Listen for the sounds of breathing. Feel for air movement. Although gasping breaths may occasionally be present, they should never be confused for normal breathing.

Hypoxia

As already noted, hypoxia is an insufficiency in the supply of oxygen to the body's tissues. There are several major causes of hypoxia. Consider the following scenarios:

- A patient is trapped in a fire. The air that the patient breathes contains smoke and reduced amounts of oxygen. Since the patient cannot breathe in enough oxygen, hypoxia develops.
- A patient has emphysema. This lung disease decreases the efficiency of the transfer of oxygen between the atmosphere and the body. Since the lungs cannot function properly, hypoxia develops.
- A patient overdoses on a drug that has a depressing effect on the respiratory system. The patient's respirations are only 5 per minute. In this case, the victim is not breathing frequently enough to support the body's oxygen needs. Hypoxia develops.
- A patient is losing blood. If bleeding leads to loss of hemoglobin, the patient's oxygen-carrying capacity is also lost. If oxygen cannot be transported to the cells, hypoxia occurs.

There are many causes of hypoxia in addition to the examples named, including occlusive problems such as stroke, myocardial infarction, and pulmonary embolism. The most important thing to know is how to recognize signs of hypoxia so that it can be treated. Hypoxia may be indicated by cyanosis (blue or gray color to the skin). In addition, when the brain suffers hypoxia, the patient's mental status may deteriorate. Restlessness or confusion may result.

As an EMT, your concern will be preventing hypoxia from developing or becoming worse and, when possible, reducing the level of hypoxia. This is done by addressing the cause of the problem and by administering supplemental oxygen.

Patient Care

Care of the Patient with Inadequate Breathing

Fundamental Principles of Care

When the patient's signs indicate inadequate breathing or no breathing (respiratory failure or respiratory arrest), a life-threatening condition exists, and prompt action must be taken. In *Airway Management*, we discussed the procedures for opening, clearing, and securing the airway. In some patients with respiratory failure, you may need to first address airway issues. You should review the *Airway Management* chapter for more information. The additional procedures to treat life-threatening respiratory problems are:

- Providing artificial ventilation to the nonbreathing patient and the patient with inadequate breathing
- Providing supplemental oxygen to the breathing patient who shows signs of hypoxia or distress

These procedures are discussed next and later in the chapter.

Decision Point

When Do I Intervene?

It can sometimes be difficult to determine when a patient needs your intervention. Often patients in respiratory failure will be breathing and conscious. It is important, however, to identify not just the presence of breathing but the adequacy of breathing. Even though the patient may still be breathing, if the signs of inadequate breathing are apparent, the patient absolutely needs your intervention. Keep in mind that what the patient is doing is not meeting the body's needs. If left unchecked, the patient's condition will progress to respiratory arrest. In general, it is better to be too aggressive than not aggressive enough. If the patient will allow you to intervene with a bag-valve mask, it generally means the patient needs it.

Positive Pressure Ventilation

If you determine that the patient is not breathing or that breathing is inadequate, you will need to provide artificial ventilation. *Ventilation* is the breathing of air or oxygen. ***Artificial ventilation***, also called ***positive pressure ventilation***, is the use of positive pressure to force air or oxygen into the lungs when a patient has stopped breathing or has inadequate breathing.

artificial ventilation
the use of positive pressure to force air or oxygen into the lungs when a patient has stopped breathing or has inadequate breathing. Also called *positive pressure ventilation.*

positive pressure ventilation
See artificial ventilation.

CORE CONCEPT
Principles and techniques of positive pressure ventilation

It is important to remember that when we use positive pressure, we use a force that is exactly the opposite of the force the body normally uses to draw air into the lungs. Under normal circumstances, the respiratory system creates a negative pressure within the chest cavity to pull in air. With artificial ventilations, we use positive pressure from outside to push air in. This change has some negative side effects that you must be conscious of and that you will need to limit by using proper technique.

The negative side effects of positive pressure ventilation are:

- **Decreasing cardiac output/dropping blood pressure.** Normally the heart uses the negative pressure of ventilation to assist the filling of its chambers with blood. When we use positive pressure to ventilate, we eliminate that negative pressure and filling assistance. Although the heart can typically compensate, the risk of causing a drop in blood pressure exists, especially when excessive positive pressures are used to ventilate. This risk from positive pressure can be minimized by using just enough volume to raise the chest.
- **Gastric distention.** Gastric distention is the filling of the stomach with air that occurs when air is pushed through the esophagus during positive pressure ventilation. The esophagus is the large expandable tube that leads from the hypopharynx to the stomach. Its opening is directly posterior to the smaller, nonexpandable opening of the trachea. When positive pressure is used to ventilate, air frequently is diverted into the esophagus and in turn inflates the stomach. Inflation of the stomach is referred to as gastric distention. Side effects of gastric distention include vomiting and restriction of the movement of the diaphragm. Gastric distention can be minimized by ventilating slowly with appropriate pressures; using airway adjuncts when ventilating; and establishing proper head position and airway-opening techniques.
- **Hyperventilation.** When we take over ventilations for a patient, it is important to pay attention to rate. There are any number of distractions and stressors that cause EMTs to ventilate too quickly, and you should know that there are negative consequences of this action. Hyperventilation causes too much carbon dioxide to be blown off. This causes a vasoconstriction (narrowing of the blood vessels) in the body and can limit blood flow to the brain. Always concentrate on maintaining proper ventilation rates while providing artificial ventilation.

Techniques of Artificial Ventilation

Various techniques are available to the EMT that can be used to provide artificial ventilation:

- Mouth-to-mask (preferably with high-concentration supplemental oxygen at 15 liters per minute)

- Two-rescuer bag–valve mask (BVM) (preferably with high-concentration supplemental oxygen at 15 liters per minute)
- One-rescuer bag–valve mask (preferably with high-concentration supplemental oxygen at 15 liters per minute)

NOTE: *Do not ventilate a patient who is vomiting or who has vomitus in the airway. Positive pressure ventilation will force the vomitus into the patient's lungs. Make sure the patient is not actively vomiting. Suction any vomitus from the airway before ventilating.*

No matter what method you use to ventilate the patient, you must ensure that the patient is being ventilated adequately. To determine the signs of *adequate* artificial ventilation, you should:

- Watch the chest rise and fall with each ventilation.
- Ensure that the rate of ventilation is sufficient—approximately 10–12 per minute in adults, 12–20 per minute in pediatric patients.

Inadequate artificial ventilation occurs when:

- The chest does not rise and fall with ventilations.
- Air escapes around the seal of the face mask or barrier device.
- The rate of ventilation is too fast or too slow.

Techniques used for artificial ventilation should also ensure adequate protection of the rescuer from the patient's body fluids, including saliva, blood, and vomit. For this reason, mouth-to-mouth ventilation is not recommended. A number of compact barrier devices are available for personal use (Figure 10-5).

NOTE: *The skill of assisting a patient's ventilations is difficult to master, as it requires careful watching for the chest rise and coordinating delivery of the pocket-mask or BVM ventilation.*

As noted earlier, ventilation will also be required on a patient who is breathing but doing so inadequately. This may be due to a very rapid but shallow rate or a very slow rate. In any case, keep in mind that it may be intimidating to ventilate (to use a pocket face mask or bag–valve mask on) a patient who is breathing and may even be aware of what you are doing. Follow these guidelines for ventilation of a breathing patient:

For a patient with rapid ventilations:

- Carefully assess the adequacy of respirations.
- Explain the procedure to the patient. Calm reassurance and a simple explanation such as "I'm going to help you breathe" are essential for the awake patient.
- Place the mask (pocket face mask or BVM) over the patient's mouth and nose.
- After sealing the mask on the patient's face, squeeze the bag with the patient's inhalation. Watch as the patient's chest begins to rise, and deliver the ventilation with the start of the patient's own inhalation. The goal will be to increase the volume of the breaths you deliver. Over the next several breaths, adjust the rate so you are ventilating fewer times per minute but with greater volume per breath (increasing the minute volume).

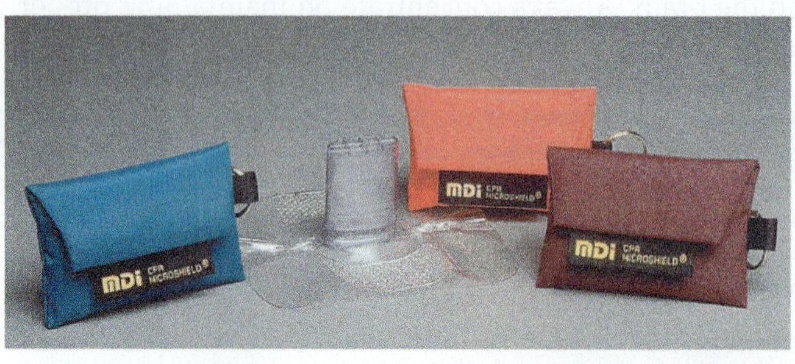

FIGURE 10-5 Examples of barrier devices.

For a patient with slow ventilations:

- Carefully assess the adequacy of respirations.
- Explain the procedure to the patient. Again, calm reassurance and a simple explanation such as "I'm going to help you breathe" are essential in the awake patient.
- Place the mask (pocket face mask or BVM) over the patient's mouth and nose.
- After sealing the mask on the patient's face, squeeze the bag every time the patient begins to inhale. If the rate is very slow, add ventilations in between the patient's own to obtain a rate of approximately 12 per minute (12–20 for children and infants) with adequate minute volume.

Face Mask Ventilation: Core Principles

There are two core principles essential to the delivery of effective face mask ventilations. These principles apply regardless of the technique used to administer the ventilation. Adequate face mask ventilations can only be achieved if the airway is open and the mask is properly sealed. Failure at either of these objectives will lead to failure of face mask ventilation.

Opening the Airway. The first essential concept of face mask ventilation is ensuring that the patient has an open and unobstructed airway before ventilations begin. This means that before a mask or barrier device is placed on the face, you should clear, suction, and position the airway. In the chapter on *Airway Management*, we discussed clearing and securing the airway. Those steps would be performed prior to positive pressure ventilation and are essential to the overall success of face mask ventilation. If necessary, review that chapter, before proceeding further.

The most important element of maintaining a patent airway during face mask ventilation (and the most common factor in failure) is simply maintaining the proper position of the patient's head. As discussed in *Airway Management*, the "head-elevated, sniffing position" is the optimal position for airway management. That same technique will be used with face mask ventilation to align airway structures, move the epiglottis off the glottic opening, and increase the likelihood of a patent airway. The head-elevated, sniffing position can be obtained with two basic sequential movements:

1. Flexion of the cervical spine—The first movement gently flexes the neck forward to create the basis of the sniffing position. (Visualize the movement of the neck necessary to smell a flower.) This is often accomplished by placing 2–5 cm of padding beneath the back of an adult's head. This flexion should move the head forward enough so that the hole of the ear aligns to the same level of the notch at the top of the sternum (otherwise known as the suprasternal notch). (See Figure 10-6A to C.) The outcome of your performance can be measured by physically visualizing where the head is positioned relative to the suprasternal notch.
2. Extension at the level of cervical vertebrae one and two (the atlanto-occipital joint)—While the neck remains in a flexed position, the head is now gently extended at the top of the neck. Imagine a person who is leaning forward and extending the head to smell a flower. This combination of a flexed neck and an extended head creates the sniffing position. Proper positioning can be checked by ensuring that the patient's face is parallel to the ceiling. Again, performance is measured by physically looking at the position of the head.

It is important to remember that anatomy can be vastly different from patient to patient. Some patients will need more padding; others will need none at all. The goal is to achieve the positional outcomes (ear at the level of the suprasternal notch and face parallel to the ceiling), not to apply a "one size fits all" approach. You should always visually assess your performance and adjust your technique based upon the unique characteristics of your patient.

Young pediatric patients can present specific anatomical challenges to obtaining the head-elevated, sniffing position. Children often have proportionally larger heads and particularly large occipital regions of the skull. (The occiput is the posterior portion of

FIGURE 10-6 Movements to achieve the head-elevated, sniffing position. (A) Neutral sniffing. (B) Flexion sniffing. (C) Sniffing.

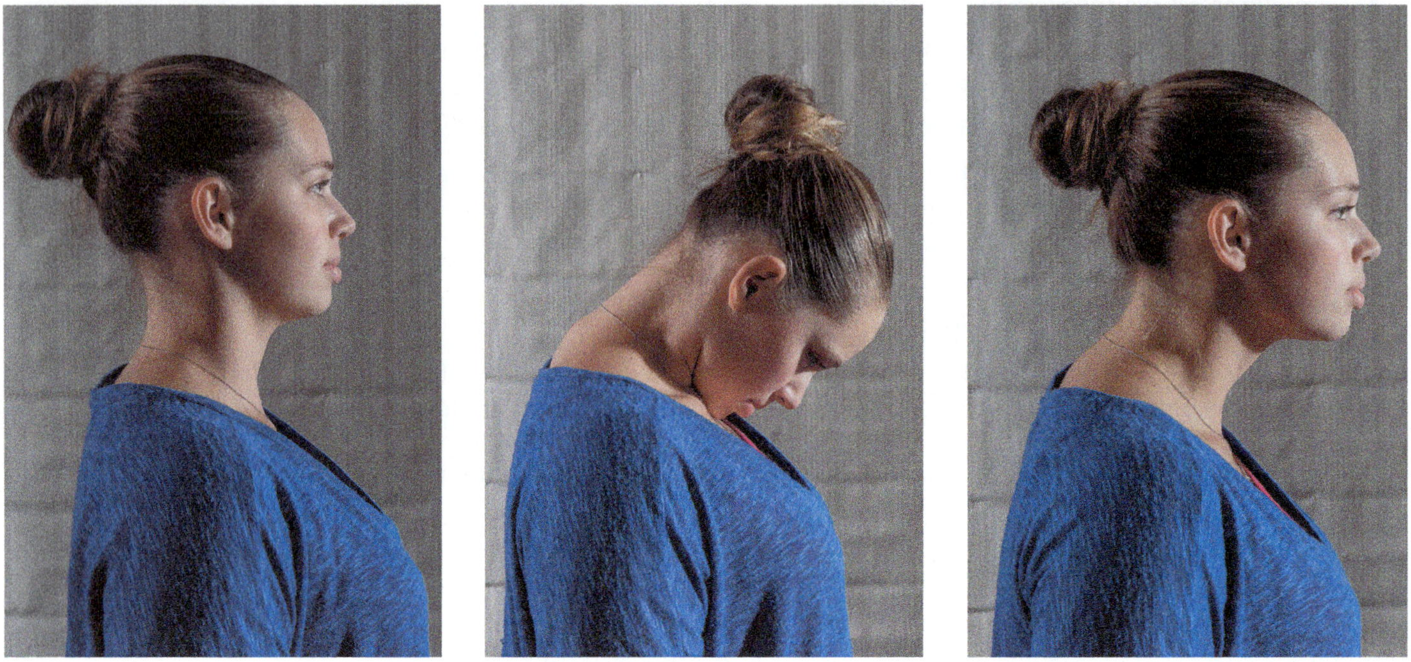

A B C

the skull.) Lying a young child flat can often cause hyperflexion of the neck and in some cases—especially in patients with altered mental status—can occlude the airway. Airway positioning must match the unique characteristics of every patient. In pediatrics, this means a wide range of interventions may be necessary to achieve optimal head-elevated, sniffing position. Typically, the youngest children (infants) will have the proportionally largest heads. In these patients, you may need to add padding beneath the shoulders to align the ear to the suprasternal notch (Figure 10-7). In preschool children, you may not need any padding, as the larger head may flex the neck just enough to achieve optimal positioning (Figure 10-8). School-age children may often require occipital padding, similar to adults. The key is to visualize each patient and adjust the amount and placement of padding according to the unique needs of the patient.

Patients who are morbidly obese (bariatric patients) frequently have airway patency problems during face mask ventilation. When supine, their large body mass can obstruct the airway and make the head-elevated, sniffing position fail. In a bariatric patient, if the traditional

FIGURE 10-7 Note the padding beneath the shoulders to achieve the head-elevated, sniffing position in a 3-year-old child.

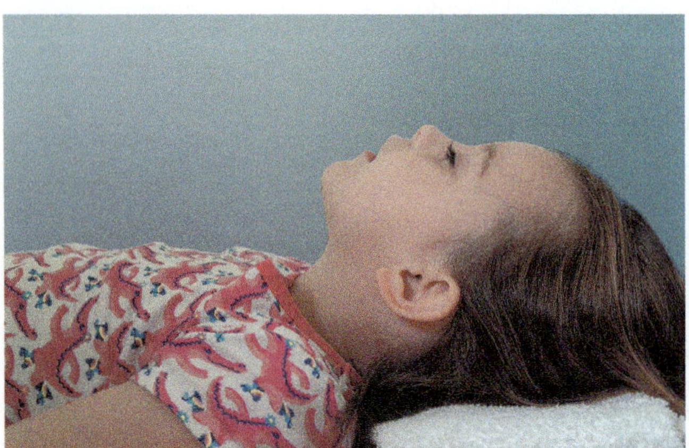

FIGURE 10-8 A 4-year-old child in head-elevated, sniffing position. Note the line from ear to chest showing proper alignment.

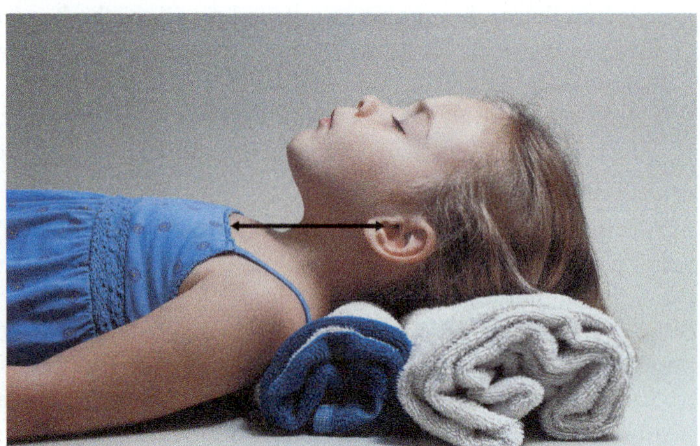

positioning fails, you should consider the "ramp" position (Figure 10-9). In the ramp position, the patient's torso is raised to a 45-degree angle and the head is allowed to plateau at the top of the ramp. It is important to note that the ramp position utilizes the same performance measures as the head-elevated, sniffing position. Even with the torso elevation, the patient's ear should align with the suprasternal notch and the face should be parallel to the ceiling.

Patients with spine injuries also present a unique challenge to the head-elevated, sniffing position. Experts disagree on the risk of exacerbating a spinal injury by moving a patient into the head-elevated, sniffing position, and there is a lack of applicable research. When considering face mask ventilation on a patient with a potential spine injury, it may be appropriate to attempt first to ventilate in a neutral position. If that position and airway adjuncts fail to maintain an open airway, you must then weigh the potential risks of exacerbating a spine injury against the risks of failure of ventilation. As always, follow local protocol.

Mask Seal

The second core principle of face mask ventilation is that the mask must be properly sealed to move air. A proper seal allows for the generation of positive pressure and is essential to moving air into the lungs. When the mask is improperly sealed, air escapes and pressure cannot be generated. Proper mask seal can be optimized by a number of initial considerations. First, ensure that you use the proper size mask for the patient. A properly sized mask should extend from the bridge of the patient's nose to the cleft of the chin and be wide enough to cover the entire mouth (Figure 10-10). Many face masks sizes

FIGURE 10-9 The ramp position. (A) The obese patient without a ramp. Note the angle of the line from ear to chest with improper alignment. (B) The obese patient with a ramp. Note the line indicating proper alignment. (C) Ramp and sniffing position for a patient with normal BMI. *((C) © Edward T. Dickinson, MD.)*

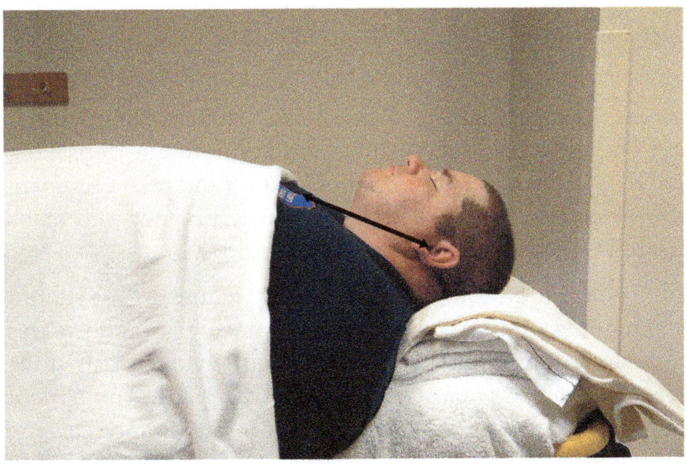

A

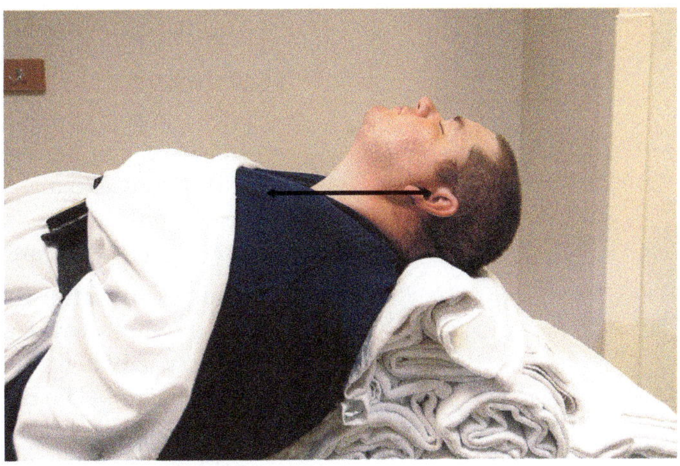

B

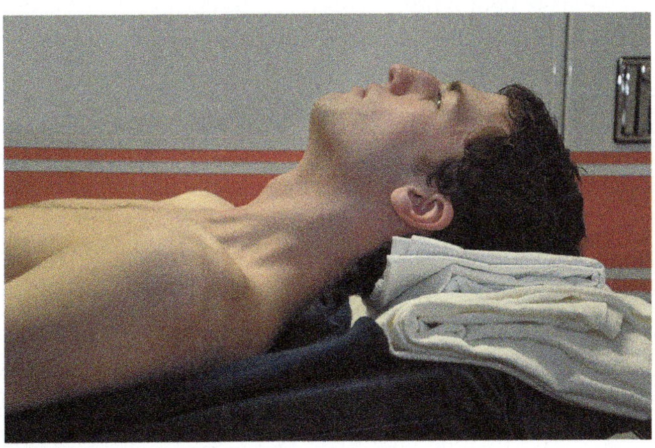

C

FIGURE 10-10 Mask sizing for face mask ventilation.

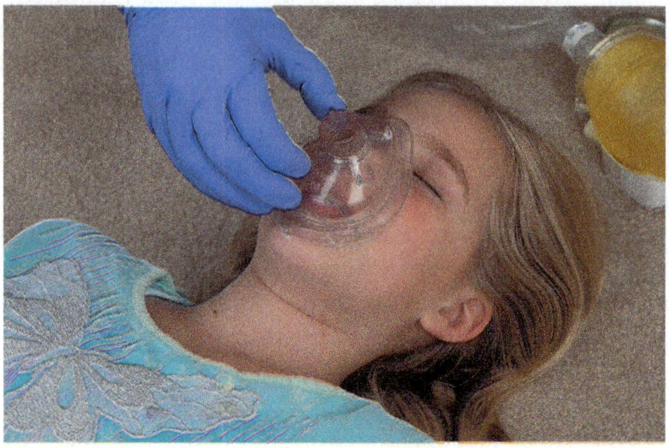

are available, from large adult to neonate. Make sure you select the correct one. Mask seal is also optimized by using two hands when creating a seal. Two-handed mask technique will be detailed later in this chapter.

Certain situations can cause difficulties in sealing a mask. Large, bushy beards can make air leaks likely. If this problem is causing ventilation failure, consider wetting the beard down with water or water-soluble lubricant.

Patients with dentures that have been removed can pose mask-seal issues. Removal of such appliances can change the size and structure of the jaw, making mask sizing awkward. If possible, leave dentures in place while providing positive pressure ventilation.

Optimizing Controllable Factors Prior to Positive Pressure Ventilation

Despite your best efforts to optimize the core concepts of face mask ventilation, difficulties can still arise. You should always be prepared for challenges and failure while deploying this skill. Because so many variables will be out of your control, you should take a moment before beginning to optimize the areas that you can change. Airway patency and mask seal are key, but there are other optimizing techniques you can consider.

- **Raise the patient's head.** It has long been held that airway management should be accomplished while the patient is supine. However, the supine position decreases the capacity of the lungs and allows the weight of the abdominal organs to restrict the movement of the diaphragm. In short, it is harder to breathe lying flat. Any patient with difficulty breathing will resist this position, so why are we insistent upon placing patients in just such a position when it is time to ventilate them ourselves? If protocol allows, consider elevating the torso to a 30-degree angle prior to providing face mask ventilations. This can often be as simple a step as slightly raising the head of the stretcher. The 30-degree angle increases lung capacity and maximizes the movement of the diaphragm.
- **Use an airway adjunct.** Unless there is a specific contraindication, such as gag reflex, an airway adjunct should always be inserted prior to providing face mask ventilation. An adjunct helps channel air to the trachea and minimizes the impact of sub-optimal position on airway patency. Proper head position must still be utilized, even if an adjunct has been placed, but the combination of position and an adjunct significantly reduces the risk of obstructed airway during ventilation.
- **Use a team.** Positive pressure ventilation is truly a team sport. There are simply too many considerations for one person to consider alone. Although it is true that certain situations dictate one-person ventilation, this should be considered extraordinary, and as a rule, this skill should be approached with multiple participants each focusing on specific ventilation-related tasks. For example, one person should focus solely on mask seal.

Both hands should be used to maintain mask contact with the face. At the same time, another person should focus on ventilation. This person should squeeze the bag, maintain the count, and visualize the chest wall for movement. These efforts should be coordinated in prior training or at least explained in a pre-skill huddle.

Mouth-to-Mask Ventilation

Mouth-to-mask ventilation is performed using a ***pocket face mask***. The pocket face mask is made of soft, collapsible material and can be carried in your pocket or bag (Figure 10-11). Many EMTs purchase their own pocket face masks for workplace or auto first aid kits.

pocket face mask
a device, usually with a one-way valve, to aid in artificial ventilation. A rescuer breathes through the valve when the mask is placed over the patient's face. It also acts as a barrier to prevent contact with a patient's breath or body fluids. It can be used with supplemental oxygen when fitted with an oxygen inlet.

Face masks have important infection-control features. Your ventilations (breaths) are delivered through a valve in the mask, so that you do not have direct contact with the patient's mouth. Most pocket masks have one-way valves that allow your ventilations to enter but prevent the patient's exhaled air from coming back through the valve and into contact with you (Figure 10-12).

Some pocket masks have oxygen inlets. When high-concentration oxygen is attached to the inlet, it delivers an oxygen concentration of approximately 50 percent. This is significantly better than the 16 percent oxygen concentration (in exhaled air) delivered by mouth-to-mask ventilations without supplemental oxygen.

Most pocket face masks are made of a clear plastic. This is important because you must be able to observe the patient's mouth and nose for vomiting or secretions that need to be suctioned. You also need to observe the color of the lips, an indicator of the patient's respiratory status. Some pocket face masks have a strap that goes around the patient's head. This is helpful during one-rescuer CPR, since it will hold the mask on the patient's face while you are performing chest compressions. However, it does not replace the need for proper hand placement on the mask.

To provide mouth-to-mask ventilation, follow the steps in Table 10-3:

FIGURE 10-11 Pocket face mask with a protective case that can be carried in a pocket or bag.

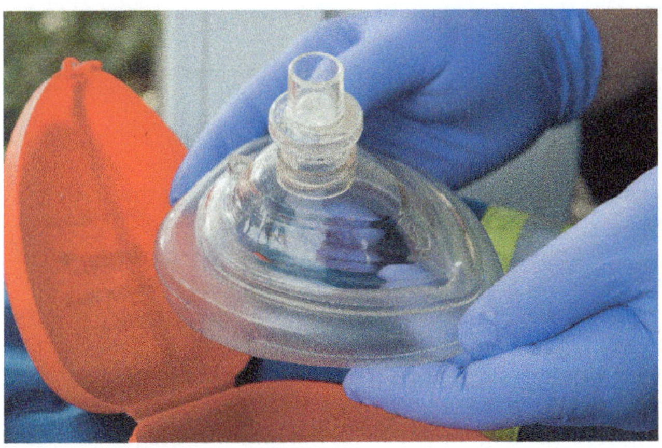

FIGURE 10-12 Use only a pocket mask with a one-way valve.

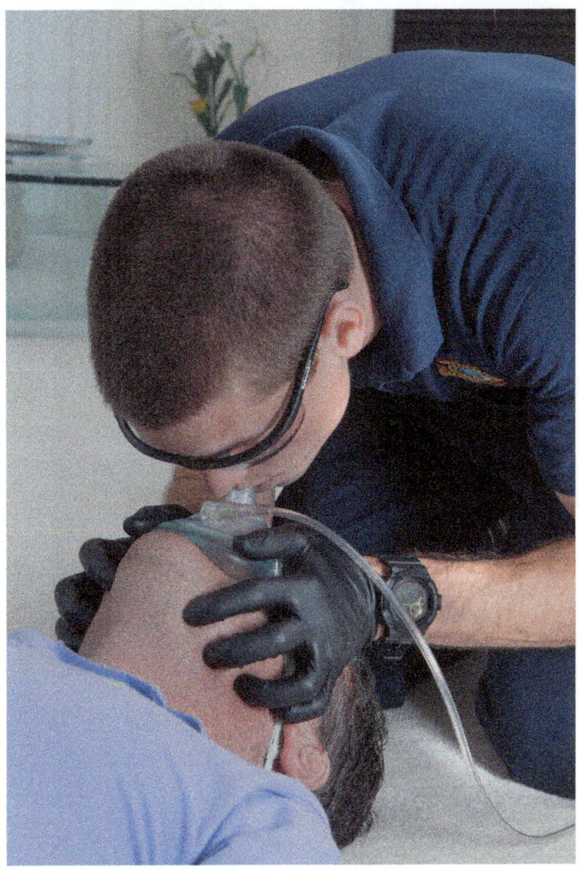

TABLE 10-3 Use of the Pocket Face Mask

PATIENT	USE OF THE POCKET FACE MASK
Patient *without* suspected spine injury–EMT at top of patient's head 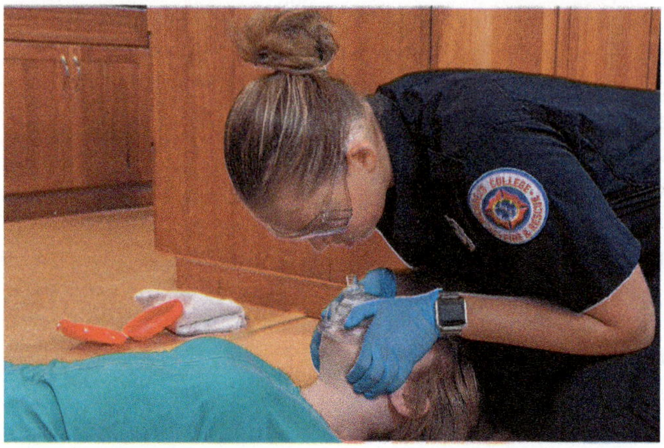	• Position yourself directly above (at the top of) the patient's head. • Place the patient in the head-elevated, sniffing position and insert an airway adjunct. • Apply the mask to the patient. Use the bridge of the patient's nose as a guide for correct position. • Place your thumbs over the top of the mask, your index fingers over the bottom of the mask, and the rest of your fingers under the patient's jaw. • Lift the jaw to the mask as you tilt the patient's head backward and place the remaining fingers under the angle of the jaw. • While lifting the jaw, squeeze the mask with your thumbs to achieve a seal between the mask and the patient's face. • Give breaths into the one-way valve of the mask. Watch for the chest to rise.
Patient *without* suspected spine injury–alternative position with EMT beside patient's head 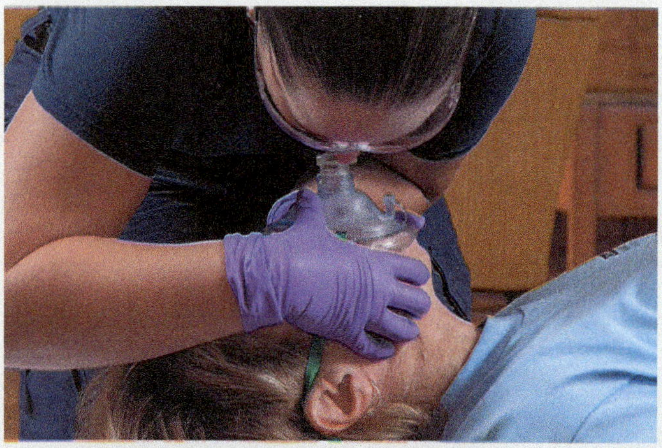	• Position yourself beside the patient's head. • Place the patient in the head-elevated, sniffing position and insert an airway adjunct. • Apply the mask to the patient. Use the bridge of the nose as a guide for correct position. • Seal the mask by placing your index finger and thumb of the hand closer to the top of the patient's head along the top border of the mask. • Place the thumb of the hand closer to the patient's feet on the lower margin of the mask. Place the remaining fingers of this hand along the bony margin of the jaw. • Lift the jaw while performing a head-tilt, chin-lift maneuver. • Compress the outer margins of the mask against the face to obtain a seal. • Give breaths into the one-way valve on the mask. Watch for the chest to rise.
Patient *with* suspected spine injury–EMT at top of patient's head 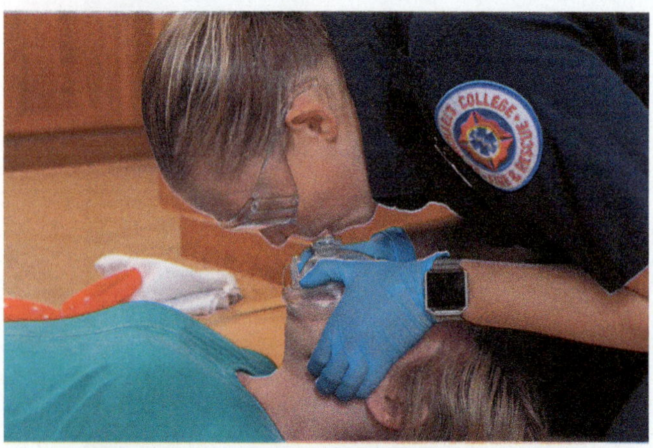	• Position yourself directly above (at the top of) the patient's head. • Place the patient in the head-elevated, sniffing position and insert an airway adjunct. • Apply the mask to the patient. Use the bridge of the patient's nose as a guide for correct position. • Place the thumb sides of your hands along the mask to hold it firmly on the face. • Use your remaining fingers to lift the angle of the jaw. ***Do not tilt the head backward***. • While lifting the jaw, squeeze the mask with your thumbs and fingers to achieve a seal. • Give breaths into the one-way valve on the mask. Watch for the chest to rise. NOTE: *Factors such as hand size, patient size, and dentures not in place may necessitate modifications in hand position and technique to achieve the necessary tight seal.*

Bag–Valve Mask

The ***bag-valve mask (BVM)*** is a handheld ventilation device. It may go by many names, including bag mask; bag–mask device; bag–valve–mask unit, system, device, or resuscitator; or simply BVM. The bag–valve–mask unit can be used to ventilate a nonbreathing patient and is also helpful to assist ventilations in the patient whose own respiratory attempts are not enough to support life, such as a patient with inadequate respirations or drug overdose. The BVM also provides an infection-control barrier between you and your patient. The use of the bag–valve mask in the field is often referred to as "bagging" the patient (Table 10-4).

bag-valve mask (BVM) a handheld device with a face mask and self-refilling bag that can be squeezed to provide artificial ventilations to a patient. It can deliver air from the atmosphere or oxygen from a supplemental oxygen supply system.

Bag–valve–mask units come in sizes for adults, children, and infants (Figure 10-13). Many different types of bag–valve–mask systems are available; however, all have the same basic parts. The bag must be a self-refilling shell that is easily cleaned and sterilized. (Some bag–valve–mask units are designed for single use and are then disposed of.) The system must have a non-jam valve that allows an oxygen inlet flow of 15 liters per minute. The valve should be nonrebreathing (preventing patients from rebreathing their own exhalations) and not subject to freezing in cold temperatures. Most systems have a standard 15/22 respiratory fitting to ensure a proper fit with other respiratory equipment, face masks, and endotracheal tubes.

The mechanical workings of a bag–valve–mask device are simple. Oxygen, flowing at 15 liters per minute, is attached to the BVM and enters the reservoir. When the bag is squeezed, the air inlet to the bag is closed, and the oxygen is delivered to the patient.

TABLE 10-4 Use of the Bag-Valve Mask

PATIENT	USE OF THE BAG-VALVE MASK
Patient *without* suspected spine injury 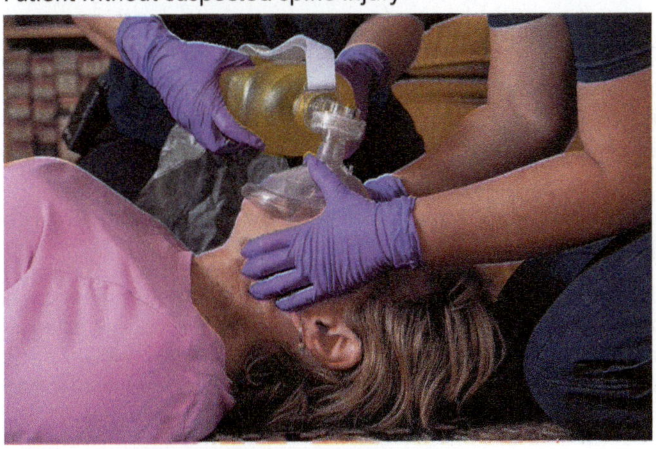	• Place the patient in the head-elevated, sniffing position and insert an airway adjunct. • Position your thumbs along the side of the mask. You will use your thumbs to press the mask downward onto the face. • Place the mask over the patient's face. Position the mask over the patient's nose and lower to the chin. (Large, round-style masks are centered first on the mouth.) Be sure that the mask is wide enough to cover the patient's mouth. • Use your index, middle, and ring fingers to bring the jaw up to the mask. • Connect the bag to the mask, and have an assistant squeeze the bag until the chest rises. • If the chest does not rise and fall, reevaluate the head position and mask seal. • If unable to ventilate, use another device (e.g., pocket face mask).
Patient *with* suspected spine injury 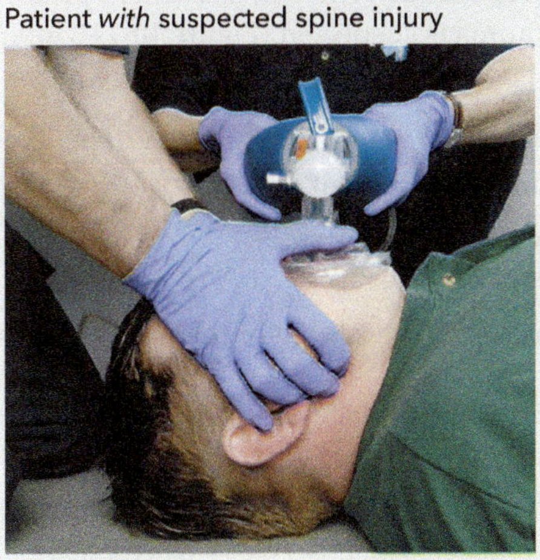	• Place the patient in the head-elevated, sniffing position or neutral position and insert an airway adjunct. • Have an assistant manually immobilize the head and neck. Immobilization of the head between your knees may be acceptable if no assistance is available. • Position your thumbs along the side of the mask. You will use your thumbs to press the mask downward onto the face. • Place the mask on the patient's face as previously described. • Use your index, middle, and ring fingers to bring the jaw up to the mask without tilting the head or neck. • Have an assistant squeeze the bag with two hands until the chest rises. • Continually evaluate ventilations.

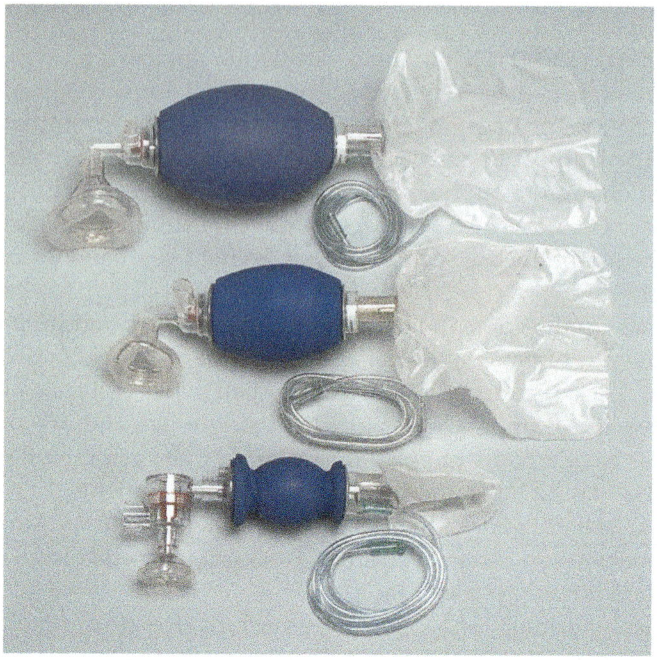

FIGURE 10-13 Adult, child, and infant bag-valve-mask units.

When the squeeze of the bag is released, a passive expiration by the patient will occur. While the patient exhales, oxygen enters the reservoir to be delivered to the patient the next time the bag is squeezed. BVM systems without a reservoir deliver approximately 50 percent oxygen. In contrast, systems with an oxygen reservoir provide nearly 100 percent oxygen. The bag itself will hold anywhere from 1,000 to 1,600 mL of air. This means that the bag–valve–mask system must be used properly and efficiently.

The most difficult part of delivering BVM artificial ventilations is obtaining an adequate mask seal so air does not leak out around the edges of the mask. It is difficult to maintain the seal with one hand while squeezing the bag with the other, and one-rescuer bag–valve–mask operation is often unsuccessful or inadequate for this reason. Therefore, it is strongly recommended that BVM artificial ventilation be performed by two rescuers. In two-rescuer BVM ventilation, one rescuer is assigned to squeeze the bag while the other rescuer uses two hands to maintain a mask seal.

NOTE: *Some older bag-valve masks have "pop-off" valves, designed to open after certain pressures are obtained. Studies have shown that pop-off valves may prevent adequate ventilations. BVM systems with pop-off valves should be replaced. A BVM system should also have a clear face mask so you can observe the lips for cyanosis and monitor the airway in case suctioning is needed.*

Two-Rescuer BVM Ventilation–No Trauma Suspected. When two rescuers perform bag–valve ventilation on a patient in whom no trauma is suspected (Figure 10-14), follow these steps:

1. Place the patient in the head-elevated, sniffing position and insert an airway adjunct.
2. Select the correct bag–valve mask size (adult, child, or infant).
3. Kneel at the patient's head. Position your thumbs along the side of the mask. You will use your thumbs to press the mask downward onto the face.
4. Place the apex, or top, of the triangular mask over the bridge of the patient's nose. Then lower the mask over the mouth and upper chin. If the mask has a large, round cuff surrounding a ventilation port, center the port over the patient's mouth. Ensure that the mask is wide enough to cover the patient's mouth.
5. Use your index, middle, and ring fingers to bring the patient's jaw up to the mask. *Maintain proper head position.*

FIGURE 10-14 Delivering two-rescuer BVM ventilation when no trauma is suspected in the patient. Note thumbs pressing the mask downward while fingers press jaw up.

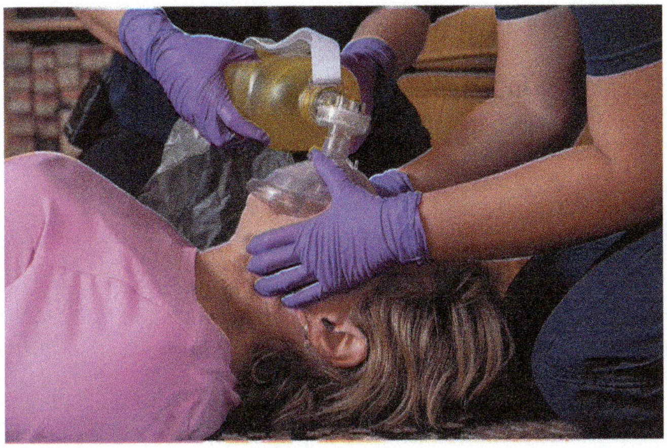

FIGURE 10-15 Delivering two-rescuer BVM ventilation while providing manual stabilization of the head and neck when trauma is suspected in the patient.

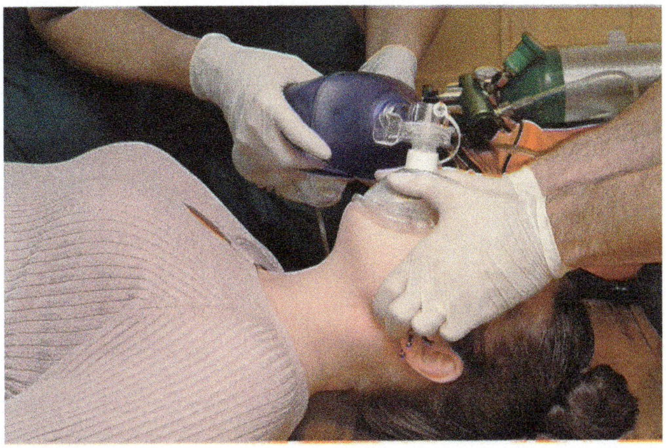

6. The second rescuer should connect the bag to the mask, if not already done. While you maintain the mask seal, the second rescuer should squeeze the bag gently until the patient's chest begins to rise. The second rescuer should squeeze the bag *once every 5–6 seconds for an adult, once every 3–5 seconds for a child or infant.*
7. The second rescuer should release pressure on the bag and let the patient exhale passively. While this occurs, the bag is refilling from the oxygen source.

Two-Rescuer BVM Ventilation–Spine Injury Suspected. When two rescuers perform bag–valve ventilation on a patient in whom trauma *is* suspected (Figure 10-15), follow these steps:

1. Place the patient in the head-elevated, sniffing position or neutral position and insert an airway adjunct.
2. Select the correct bag–valve mask size (adult, child, or infant).
3. Kneel at the patient's head. Position your thumbs along the side of the mask. You will use your thumbs to press the mask downward onto the face.
4. Use your index, middle, and ring fingers to bring the jaw upward, toward the mask, *without tilting the head or neck.*
5. Have the second rescuer gently squeeze the bag to ventilate the patient as previously described for the nonspine-injured patient.

One-Rescuer BVM Ventilation. As noted, use of a bag–valve mask by a single rescuer is the last choice of artificial ventilation procedure—behind use of a pocket face mask with supplemental oxygen; a two-rescuer bag–valve–mask procedure; and use of a flow-restricted, oxygen-powered ventilation device. You should provide ventilations with a one-rescuer bag–valve–mask procedure only when no other options are available.

When you perform bag–valve ventilation alone without assistance from a second rescuer, follow these steps:

1. Position yourself at the patient's head. Place the patient in the head-elevated, sniffing position and insert an airway adjunct.
2. Select the correct-sized mask for the patient. Position the mask on the patient's face as described previously for the two-rescuer BVM technique.
3. Form a "C" around the ventilation port with your thumb and index finger. Place your middle, ring, and little fingers along the bony prominence of the patient's jaw to hold the jaw to the mask.

4. With your other hand, gently *squeeze the bag once every 5–6 seconds. For infants and children, squeeze the bag once every 3–5 seconds.* The squeeze should cause the patient's chest to rise.
5. Release pressure on the bag and let the patient exhale passively. While this occurs, the bag is refilling from the oxygen source.

If the chest does not rise and fall during BVM ventilation, you should:

1. Reposition the head.
2. Check for escape of air around the mask, and reposition your fingers and the mask.
3. Check for airway obstruction or obstruction in the BVM system. Resuction the patient if necessary.
4. If none of these methods works, use an alternative method of artificial ventilation, such as a pocket mask or a flow-restricted, oxygen-powered ventilation device.

The BVM may also be used during CPR. In this situation, the bag is squeezed once each time a ventilation is to be delivered. In one-rescuer CPR, it is preferable to use a pocket mask with supplemental oxygen (Figure 10-16) rather than a BVM system. A single rescuer would take too much time picking up the BVM and obtaining a face seal each time a ventilation was to be delivered, in addition to the normal difficulty in maintaining a seal with the one-rescuer BVM technique.

NOTE: *Because proper decontamination of BVMs is often costly and time-consuming, many hospitals and EMS agencies use single-use, disposable BVMs. Bag-valve-mask devices designed for multiple uses should be completely disassembled and disinfected after each use.*

stoma
a permanent surgical opening in the neck through which the patient breathes.

Artificial Ventilation of a Stoma Breather. The BVM can be used to artificially ventilate a patient with a ***stoma***, a surgical opening in the neck through which the patient breathes. Patients with stomas who are found to be in severe respiratory distress or respiratory arrest frequently have thick secretions blocking the stoma. It is recommended that you suction the stoma often in conjunction with BVM-to-stoma ventilations.

As with other BVM uses, a two-rescuer technique is preferred over a one-rescuer technique. To provide artificial ventilation to a stoma breather using a BVM, follow these steps:

1. Clear any mucous plugs or secretions from the stoma.
2. Leave the head and neck in a neutral position, as it is unnecessary to position the airway prior to ventilations in a stoma breather.
3. Use a pediatric-sized mask to establish a seal around the stoma.
4. Ventilate at the appropriate rate for the patient's age.
5. If unable to artificially ventilate through the stoma, consider sealing the stoma and attempting artificial ventilation through the mouth and nose. (This may work if the

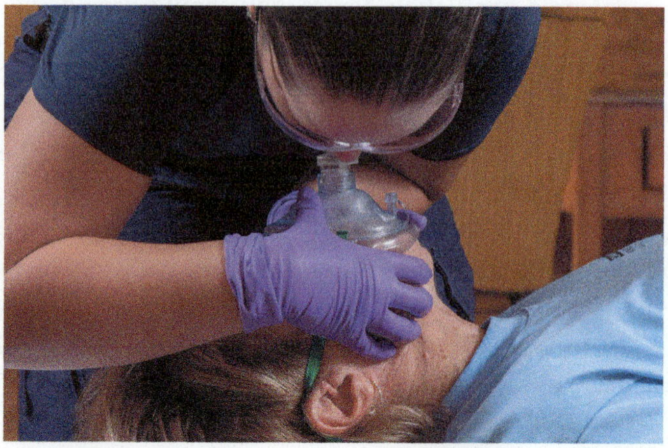

FIGURE 10-16 One-rescuer CPR using a pocket face mask with supplemental oxygen. The EMT is beside the patient. From this position, chest compressions can also be performed. The strap holds the pocket mask in place while the rescuer switches tasks.

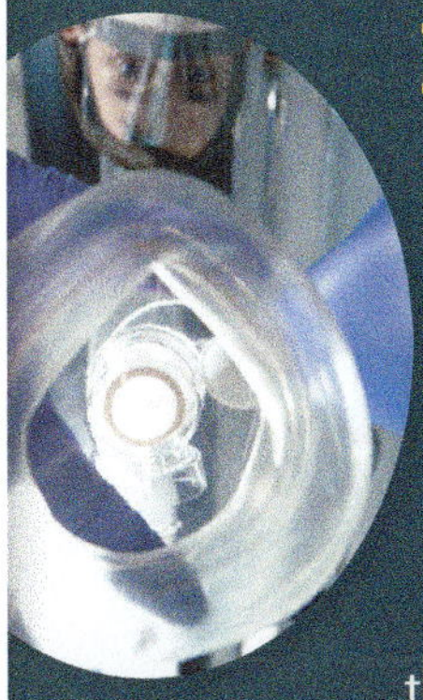

Point of View

"I still can't tell you why I didn't know it was coming on. I didn't feel right for a few days. Then it hit me. I couldn't move without feeling like I would suffocate. I just couldn't breathe. Couldn't catch my breath. I could tell it was serious when the EMTs came in. It showed in their faces.

"I think I must've started getting even worse because I remember feeling like I was losing it. I remember them trying to calm me down, but I really felt like I was going to have to be peeled off the ceiling of that ambulance.

"When they tried to put that big mask on my face, I felt like it was going to kill me, to take away all my air. I fought it. The EMTs kept calming me and putting that mask on my face. Somehow I calmed down a little, and they gave me air or oxygen or something. I made it to the hospital. The doctor told me that the EMTs may have saved my life.

"I appreciate that more than I can say–even if that mask felt pretty intimidating at the time."

trachea is still connected to the passageways of the mouth, nose, and pharynx. In some cases, however, the trachea has been permanently connected to the neck opening with no remaining connection to the mouth, nose, or pharynx.)

Ventilation Rates and Volume

Thus far we have discussed the core concepts and specific techniques of delivering positive pressure ventilations. These concepts and techniques are extremely important, but there are two more elements to positive pressure ventilation that must be considered. They are rate and volume.

Rate—Delivering positive pressure ventilation is a relatively infrequently used and relatively high-stress skill. It is very easy to let the pressure of the moment influence your ability to perform the skill properly. This is especially true when considering the rate of artificial ventilation. Far too often, ventilations are delivered too fast, and sometimes they are delivered too slowly. It is important to remember that improper rates can harm the patient. Ventilations delivered too slowly cause hypoventilation and can contribute to hypoxia and ventilation issues. Ventilations delivered too rapidly create an artificial hyperventilation and cause blood vessels to constrict. This vasoconstriction can decrease perfusion to the brain at a time when the brain is already likely hypoperfused. If possible, one person should focus only upon delivering proper ventilations while a second person focuses on maintaining the airway and mask seal. This focus allows concentration on proper ventilation rates. Adults should be ventilated 10–12 times per minute, or roughly once every 5–6 seconds. Pediatric patients should be ventilated 12–20 times per minute (infants typically require the higher rates within this range), or once every 3–5 seconds. Some systems have adopted external feedback devices that offer audible or visual indications when it is time to squeeze the bag. It may be reasonable to consider adoption of such feedback devices to prevent improper ventilation rates.

Volume—Just as the stress of the moment can impact rate, it is common to see patients being ventilated with excessive pressure and volume. Like hyperventilation, these excesses can also harm the patient. Ventilating too rapidly or with too much pressure is the most common cause of gastric distension, and as previously discussed, this inflation of the stomach limits the movement of the diaphragm and reduces the capacity of the lungs (especially in pediatric patients). To counter this excess, you should deliver ventilations slowly with gentle pressure. Consider using one hand or even two or three fingers to squeeze the bag. Ventilations should be delivered over 1 second. Excessive

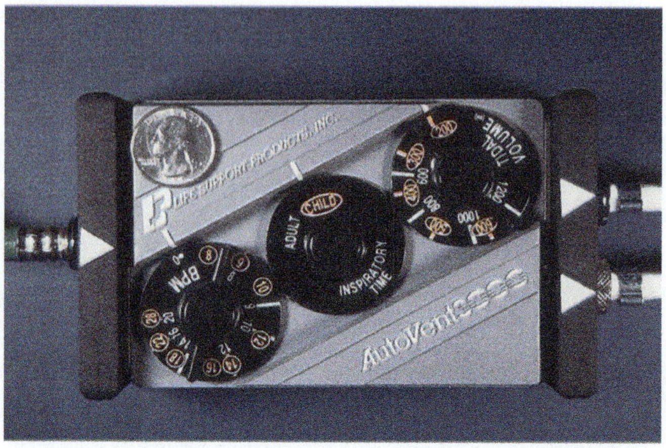

FIGURE 10-17 An automatic transport ventilator. The quarter is shown to provide a sense of scale. *(© Edward T. Dickinson, MD)*

volume (too much air) can cause pressure-related trauma to the lung tissue. Excessive volume also contributes to gastric distension. Volume-related issues can be minimized simply by ventilating only until the patient's chest begins to move. Remember that chest movement only occurs when most of lung fields are inflated. Even slight movement therefore indicates lung inflation. Do not ventilate to the full expansion of the chest. Again, keeping one person singularly focused on ventilation is a helpful strategy.

Automatic Transport Ventilator

automatic transport ventilator (ATV)
a device that provides positive pressure ventilations. It includes settings designed to adjust ventilation rate and volume, is portable, and is easily carried on an ambulance.

The ***automatic transport ventilator (ATV)*** (Figure 10-17) may be used in some EMS systems to provide positive pressure ventilations to a patient in respiratory arrest. The ATV has settings to adjust ventilation rate and volume. These ventilators are very portable and easily carried on ambulances. When prolonged ventilation is necessary, and when only one rescuer is available to ventilate a patient, the ATV may be beneficial. Caution must be used to be sure the respiratory rate is appropriate for the patient's size and condition. A proper mask seal is required for these devices to effectively deliver ventilation.

Oxygen Therapy

Importance of Supplemental Oxygen

Oxygen is a medication. When performed wisely, oxygen administration may be one of the most important and beneficial treatments an EMT can provide. The atmosphere provides approximately 21 percent oxygen. If a person does not have an illness or injury, that 21 percent is enough to support normal functioning. However, patients with whom EMTs come in contact are sick or injured, and often require supplemental oxygen.

CORE CONCEPT
Principles and techniques of oxygen administration

There are three major issues to consider in the supplemental oxygen decision process. Use these concepts to help guide your thinking.

- **Oxygen is a medication.** Like with any medication, a patient may be given too little or too much. All other medications are given based on need and therapeutic benefit. We must keep this in mind as a fundamental concept in oxygen delivery.
- **Oxygen can cause harm.** Current research indicates that oxygen can actually cause harm in reperfusion situations at the cellular level. In cases of heart attack and stroke, parts of the heart or brain are deprived of oxygen. As a result, toxic by-products of this anaerobic metabolism build up in the cells. When perfusion is restored to these areas, oxygen reacts with free radicals and other substances—causing significant damage at the cellular level—and may even send these toxins to other parts of the body as well. Although some cells will die as a result of the initial stroke or myocardial infarction, it is the surrounding cells that still have a chance to recover that are at greatest risk during reperfusion.
- **Oxygen should be administered based on your overall evaluation of the patient's presentation and possible underlying conditions.** Patients who have oxygen saturations below 94 percent and those who show signs of hypoxia or decompensation

(e.g., pale skin, altered mental status, cyanosis) should receive oxygen based on suspected hypoxia and in an effort to improve oxygen saturation. In a significant number of cases, a nasal cannula will be enough to raise saturation and benefit the patient with less potential for causing harm.

Always remember to *ventilate* rather than oxygenate patients in respiratory arrest. Consider the use of supplemental oxygen while using positive pressure to ventilate patients.

The 2015 American Heart Association guidelines deal with patients with acute coronary syndromes and stroke. Oxygen administration in trauma patients should be guided by a commonsense approach. If you had a patient with an isolated tibia and fibula fracture with no signs of shock or other injury, and an adequate oxygen saturation, oxygen would not be necessary. However, trauma patients showing signs of hypoperfusion, respiratory distress, or hypoxia should still receive high-concentration oxygen.

The decision to administer supplemental oxygen requires solid patient assessment and clinical judgment—both in the field and on your examinations for certification. Use this text, your instructor and Medical Director, and your protocols as additional sources to help you. As you progress through your class and discuss some of the clinical conditions for which you will be applying oxygen, it will become even more clear.

Oxygen Therapy Equipment

In the field, oxygen equipment must be safe, lightweight, portable, and dependable. Some field oxygen systems are very portable and can be brought almost anywhere. Other systems are installed inside the ambulance so oxygen can be delivered during transportation to the hospital.

Most oxygen-delivery systems (Figure 10-18) contain several items: oxygen cylinders, pressure regulators, and a delivery device (nonrebreather mask or cannula). When the patient is not breathing or is breathing inadequately, additional devices (such as a pocket mask or bag–valve mask) can be used to force oxygen into the patient's lungs.

Oxygen Cylinders

Outside a medical facility, the standard source of oxygen is the ***oxygen cylinder***, a seamless steel or lightweight-alloy cylinder filled with oxygen under pressure, equal to 2,000–2,200 pounds per square inch (psi) when the cylinders are full. Cylinders come in various sizes, identified by letters (Figure 10-19). The following cylinders are in common use in emergency care:

oxygen cylinder a cylinder filled with oxygen under pressure.

- *D cylinder* contains about 350 liters of oxygen.
- *E cylinder* contains about 625 liters of oxygen.
- *M cylinder* contains about 3,000 liters of oxygen.

FIGURE 10-18 An oxygen-delivery system.

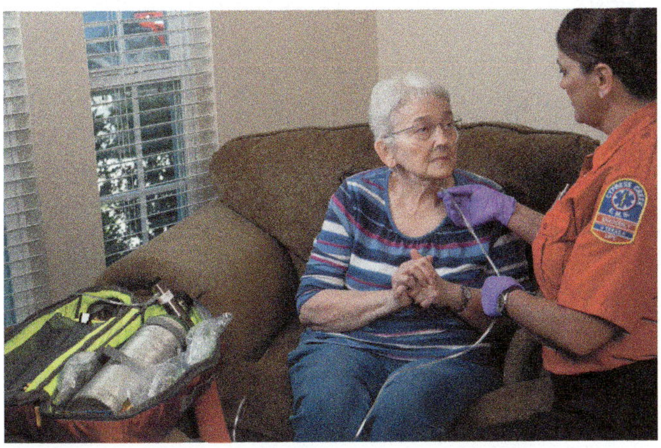

FIGURE 10-19 For safety, to prevent them from tipping over, oxygen cylinders must be placed in a horizontal position. If upright, they must be securely supported.

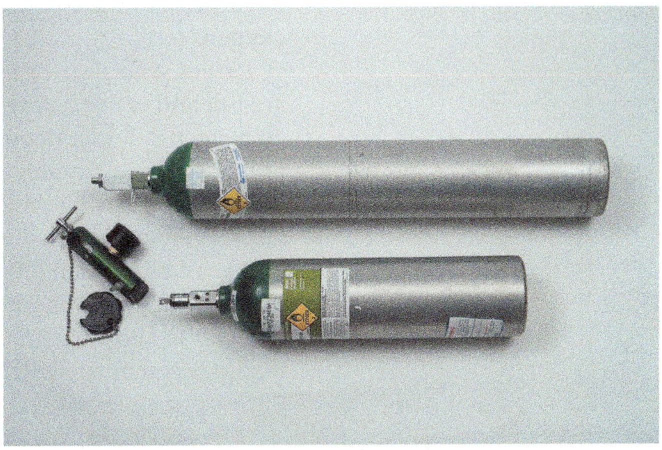

FIGURE 10-20 Larger cylinders are used for fixed systems on ambulances.

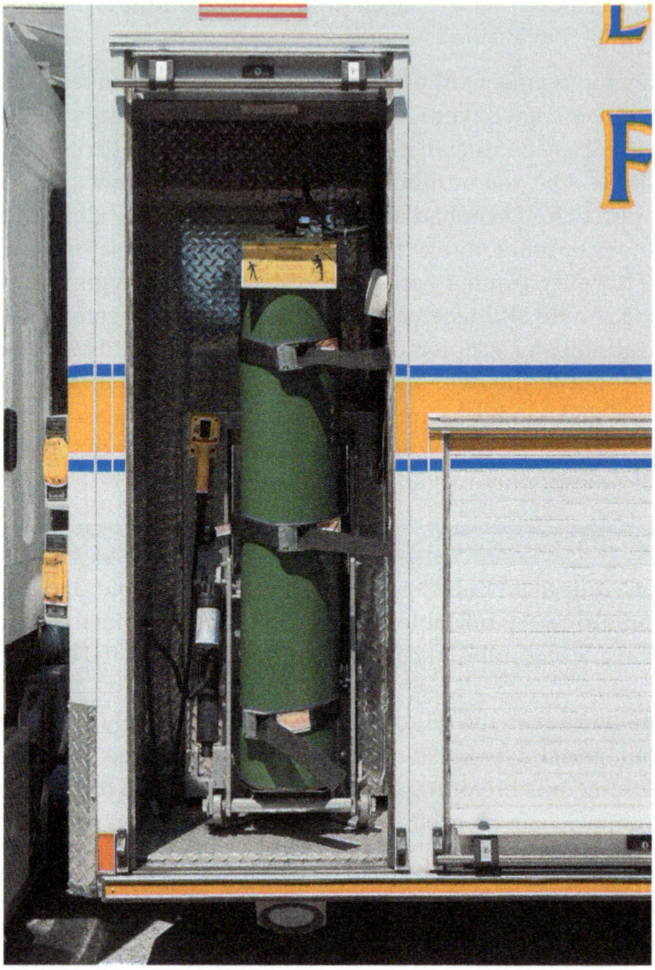

Fixed systems on ambulances (commonly called onboard oxygen) include the M cylinder and larger cylinders (Figure 10-20):

- *G cylinder* contains about 5,300 liters of oxygen.
- *H cylinder* contains about 6,900 liters of oxygen.

The United States Pharmacopoeia has assigned a color code to distinguish compressed gases. Green or green-and-white cylinders have been assigned to all grades of oxygen. Green is used in the United States. Europe is changing to white on the shoulder or top part of the tank. Unpainted stainless steel and aluminum cylinders are also used for oxygen. Regardless of the color, always check the label to be certain you are using medical-grade oxygen.

Part of your duty as an EMT is to make certain that the oxygen cylinders you will use are full and ready before they are needed to provide care. The length of time you can use an oxygen cylinder depends on the pressure in the cylinder and the flow rate. You cannot tell whether an oxygen cylinder is full, partially full, or empty just by lifting or moving the cylinder. The method of calculating cylinder duration is shown in Table 10-5.

Oxygen cylinders should never be allowed to empty below the safe residual, or the tank may be permanently damaged. The safe residual for an oxygen cylinder is when the pressure gauge reads 200 psi or above. Below this point, there is not enough oxygen in the cylinder to allow for proper delivery to the patient. Before the cylinder reaches the 200 psi reading, you must switch to a fresh cylinder.

TABLE 10-5 Oxygen Cylinders: Duration of Flow

Simple Formula

Gauge pressure in psi (pounds per square inch) minus the safe residual pressure (always 200 psi) times the constant (see following list) divided by the flow rate in liters per minute = duration of flow in minutes.

Cylinder Constants

D = 0.16	G = 2.41
E = 0.28	H = 3.14
M = 1.56	K = 3.14

Example

Determine the life of an M cylinder that has a pressure of 2,000 psi displayed on the pressure gauge and a flow rate of 10 liters per minute.

$$\frac{(2{,}000 - 200) \times 1.56}{10} = \frac{2{,}808}{10} = 280.8 \text{ minutes}$$

NOTE: *Some systems or services may require cylinder changes at specific psi levels. Always follow local guidelines.*

Safety is of prime importance when working with oxygen cylinders. You should:

- *Always* use pressure gauges, regulators, and tubing that are intended for use with oxygen.
- *Always* use nonferrous (made of plastic or of metals that do not contain iron) oxygen wrenches for changing gauges and regulators or for adjusting flow rates. Other types of metal tools may produce a spark should they strike against metal objects.
- *Always* ensure that valve seat inserts and gaskets are in good condition. This prevents dangerous leaks. Disposable gaskets on oxygen cylinders should be replaced each time a cylinder change is made.
- *Always* use medical-grade oxygen. Industrial oxygen contains impurities. The cylinder should be labeled *OXYGEN U.S.P.* The oxygen must not be more than 5 years old.
- *Always* open the valve of an oxygen cylinder fully, then close it half a turn to prevent someone else from thinking the valve is closed and trying to force it open. The valve does not have to be turned fully to be open for delivery.
- *Always* store reserve oxygen cylinders in a cool, ventilated room, properly secured in place.
- *Always* have oxygen cylinders hydrostatically tested every 5 years. The date a cylinder was last tested is stamped on the cylinder. Some cylinders can be tested every 10 years. A 10-year date may be followed by a five-pointed star.
- *Never* drop a cylinder or let it fall against any object. When transporting a patient with an oxygen cylinder, make sure the oxygen cylinder is placed in a carrying device or otherwise properly secured.
- *Never* leave an oxygen cylinder standing in an upright position without being secured.
- *Never* allow smoking around oxygen equipment in use. Clearly mark the area of use with signs that read *OXYGEN—NO SMOKING.*
- *Never* use oxygen equipment around an open flame.
- *Never* use grease, oil, or fat-based soaps on devices that will be attached to an oxygen supply cylinder. Take care not to handle these devices when your hands are greasy. Use greaseless tools when making connections.
- *Never* use adhesive tape to protect an oxygen tank outlet, or to mark or label any oxygen cylinders or oxygen delivery apparatus. The oxygen can react with the adhesive and debris, and cause a fire.
- *Never* try to move an oxygen cylinder by dragging it or rolling it on its side or bottom.

Pressure Regulators

pressure regulator
a device connected to an oxygen cylinder to reduce cylinder pressure so it is safe for delivery of oxygen to a patient.

The pressure in an oxygen cylinder (approximately 2,000 psi in a full tank, varying with surrounding temperature) is too high to be delivered to a patient. A ***pressure regulator*** must be connected to the cylinder to provide a safe working pressure of 30–70 psi.

On cylinders of the E size or smaller, the pressure regulator is secured to the cylinder valve assembly by a yoke assembly. The yoke is provided with pins that must mate with corresponding holes in the valve assembly. This is called a pin-index safety system. Since the pin position varies for different gases, this system prevents an oxygen-delivery system from being connected to a cylinder containing another gas.

NOTE: *You must maintain the regulator inlet filter. It has to be free of damage and clean to prevent contamination of and damage to the regulator.*

Cylinders larger than the E size have a valve assembly with a threaded outlet. The inside and outside diameters of the threaded outlets vary according to the gas in the cylinder. This prevents an oxygen regulator from being connected to a cylinder containing another gas. In other words, a nitrogen regulator cannot be connected to an oxygen cylinder, and vice versa.

Before connecting the pressure regulator to an oxygen supply cylinder, stand to the side of the main valve opening and open (crack) the cylinder valve slightly for just a second to clear dirt and dust out of the delivery port or threaded outlet.

Flowmeters

flowmeter
a valve that indicates the flow of oxygen in liters per minute.

A ***flowmeter***, which is connected to the pressure regulator, allows control of the flow of oxygen in liters per minute. Most services keep the flowmeter permanently attached to the pressure regulator. Low-pressure and high-pressure flowmeters are available.

Low-Pressure Flowmeters. Low-pressure flowmeters, specifically the pressure-compensated flowmeter and the constant flow selector valve (Figure 10-21A), are in general use in the field.

- **Pressure-compensated flowmeter.** This meter is gravity-dependent and must be in an upright position to deliver an accurate reading. The unit has an upright, calibrated glass tube in which there is a ball float. The float rises and falls according to the amount of gas passing through the tube. This type of flowmeter indicates the actual flow at all times, even though there may be a partial obstruction to gas flow (e.g., from a kinked

FIGURE 10-21 (A) Low-pressure flowmeters: (*left*) A pressure-compensated flowmeter; (*right*) a constant flow selector valve. (B) High-pressure flowmeter. High-pressure oxygen is delivered through hoses attached to a threaded connector.

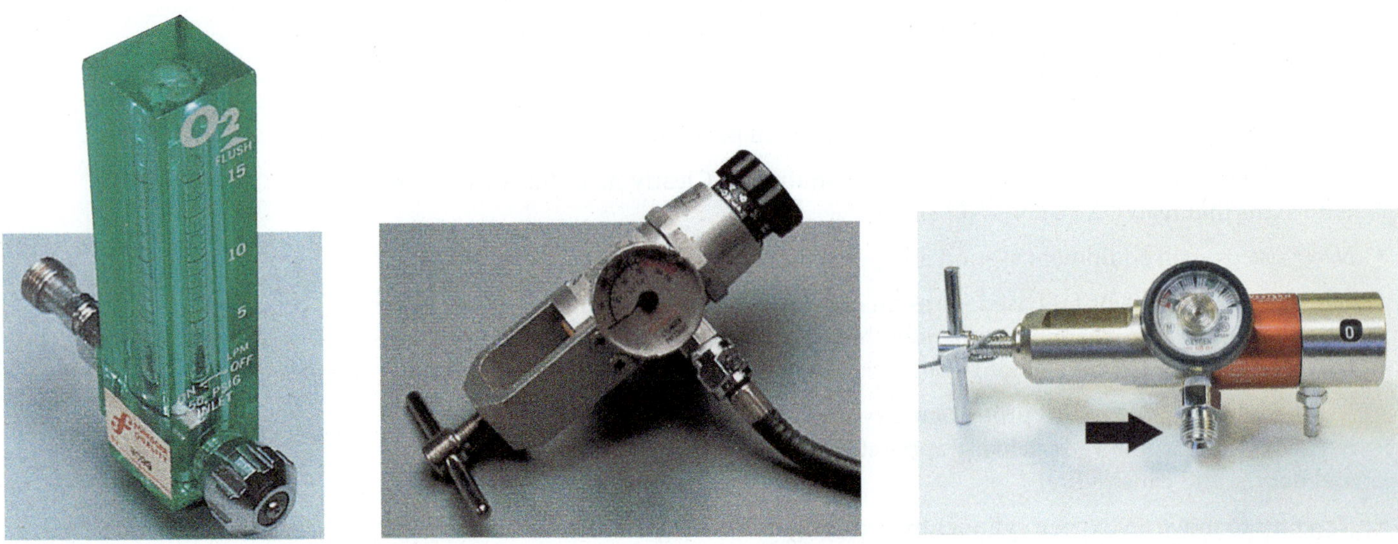

A

B

delivery tube). If the tubing collapses, the ball will drop to show the lower delivery rate. This unit is not practical for many portable delivery systems. Recommended use is for larger (M, G, and H) oxygen cylinders in the ambulance.

- **Constant flow selector valve.** This type of flowmeter, which is gaining in popularity, has no gauge and allows for the adjustment of flow in liters per minute in stepped increments (2, 4, 6, 8, and so on up to more than 15 liters per minute). It can be accurately used with the nasal cannula or nonrebreather mask and with any size oxygen cylinder. It is rugged and will operate at any angle.

When using this type of flowmeter, make certain that it is properly adjusted for the desired flow, and monitor it to make certain that it stays properly adjusted. All types of meters should be tested for accuracy as recommended by the manufacturer.

High-Pressure Flowmeters. The low-pressure flowmeters just listed will administer oxygen up to either 15 or 25 liters per minute. In some circumstances, however, oxygen is required at higher pressures. This may be necessary for oxygen-powered devices such as the Thumper™ CPR. There are several ways you will identify high-pressure connections. One is by observing a threaded connection on an oxygen regulator (Figure 10-21B). You may also see thick, green hose–type tubing connected to the high-pressure regulator.

Humidifiers

A ***humidifier*** can be connected to the flowmeter to provide moisture to the dry oxygen coming from the supply cylinder (Figure 10-22). Oxygen without humidification can dry out the mucous membranes of the patient's airway and lungs. In most short-term use, the dryness of the oxygen is not a problem; however, the patient is usually more comfortable when given humidified oxygen. This is particularly true if the patient has COPD or is a child.

humidifier a device connected to the flowmeter to add moisture to the dry oxygen coming from an oxygen cylinder.

A humidifier is usually no more than a nonbreakable jar of water attached to the flowmeter. Oxygen passes (bubbles) through the water to become humidified. As with all oxygen-delivery equipment, the humidifier must be kept clean. The water reservoir can become a breeding ground for algae, harmful bacteria, and dangerous fungal organisms. Always use fresh water in a clean reservoir for each shift. Sterile single-patient-use humidifiers are available and preferred.

In many EMS systems, humidifiers are no longer used, because they are not indicated for short transports and because of the infection risk. The devices may be beneficial on long transports and on certain pediatric patients with signs of inadequate breathing.

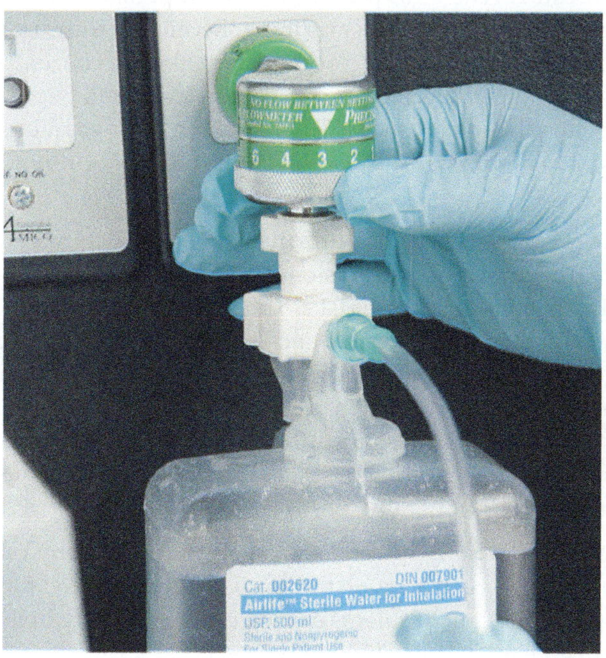

FIGURE 10-22 Humidifier in use on board an ambulance.

Hazards of Oxygen Therapy

Although the benefits of oxygen are often important, oxygen must be used carefully. The hazards of oxygen therapy may be grouped into two categories: nonmedical and medical.

Nonmedical hazards are extremely rare and can be avoided totally if oxygen and oxygen equipment are treated properly. Some of the most common hazards are:

- The oxygen used in emergency care is stored under pressure, usually 2,000–2,200 pounds per square inch (psi) or greater in a full cylinder. If the tank is punctured or a valve breaks off, the supply tank can become a missile. (Damaged tanks have been able to penetrate concrete walls.)
- Oxygen supports combustion, causing fire to burn more rapidly. It can saturate towels, sheets, and clothing, greatly increasing the risk of fire.
- Under pressure, oxygen and oil do not mix. When they come into contact, a severe reaction occurs that, for our purposes, can be termed an explosion. This is seldom a problem, but it can occur easily if you lubricate a delivery system or gauge with petroleum products or allow contact with a petroleum-based adhesive (e.g., adhesive tape).

Earlier in the chapter, we discussed how oxygen may be harmful in certain situations. The decision to administer oxygen and the amount given are based on a careful evaluation of the patient's condition and your skilled assessment. There are a few other situations to mention, and although they are extremely rare, they should be a part of your decision-making process.

- **Oxygen toxicity or air sac collapse.** These problems are caused in some patients whose lungs react unfavorably to the presence of oxygen, and also may result from too high a concentration of oxygen for too long a period of time. The body reacts to a sensed "overload" of oxygen with reduced lung activity and air sac collapse. This is extremely rare in the field.
- **Infant eye damage.** This condition may occur when premature infants are given too much oxygen over a long period of time (days). These infants may develop scar tissue on the retina of the eye. Oxygen by itself does not cause this condition, which is the result of many factors. Oxygen should never be withheld from any infant with signs of inadequate breathing.
- **Respiratory depression or respiratory arrest.** Over time, patients in the end stage of COPD may lose the normal ability to use the body's blood carbon dioxide levels as a stimulus to breathe. When this occurs, the COPD patient's body may use low blood oxygen as the factor that stimulates breathing. Because of this so-called hypoxic drive, EMTs have for years been trained to administer only low concentrations of oxygen to these patients for fear of increasing blood oxygen levels and wiping out their "drive to breathe." As with all patients, make decisions on oxygenation based on the patient's presented level of distress and pulse oximetry. Do not withhold oxygen from any patient in distress.
- **Exacerbation of underlying conditions.** As previously stated, oxygen has been demonstrated to contribute to reperfusion injury. Conditions such as myocardial infarction and stroke are subject to these risks. The risks of prolonged hyperoxia (very high levels of oxygen in the blood) are still unclear. In some animal models, hyperoxia has been linked with accelerated cell death and vasoconstriction. These risks have not been well demonstrated in human testing. However, if those risks are real, providing unnecessary oxygen is simply contributing to a problem. It is reasonable to assume that patients with reliable, normal oxygen saturations and no signs of hypoxia do not require additional oxygen therapy.

As an EMT, you will probably never see oxygen toxicity or any other adverse conditions that can result from oxygen administration. The time required for such conditions to develop is too long to cause any problems during emergency care in the field. The bottom line is: *Administer oxygen when clinically appropriate to do so!*

Administering Oxygen

Scan 10-1 and Scan 10-2 will take you step by step through the process of preparing the oxygen-delivery system, administering oxygen, and discontinuing the administration of oxygen. Do not attempt to learn on your own how to use oxygen-delivery systems. You should work with your instructor and follow your instructor's directions for the specific equipment you will be using.

SCAN 10-1 Preparing the Oxygen-Delivery System

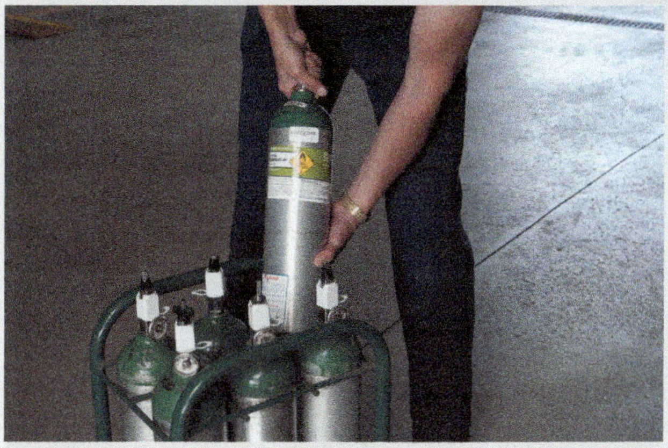

1. Select the correct cylinder. Check for the label *Oxygen U.S.P.*

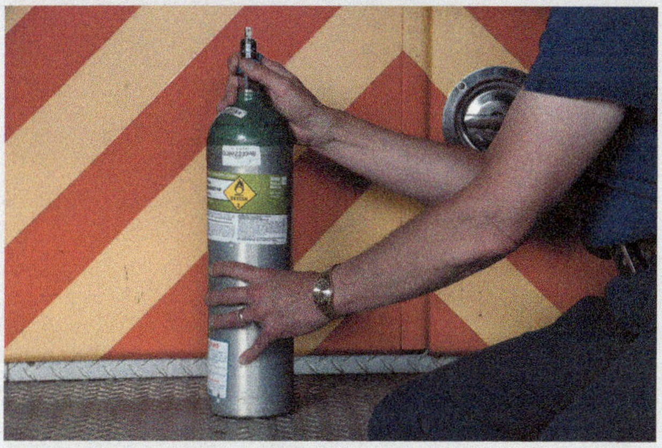

2. Place the cylinder in an upright position and stand to one side.

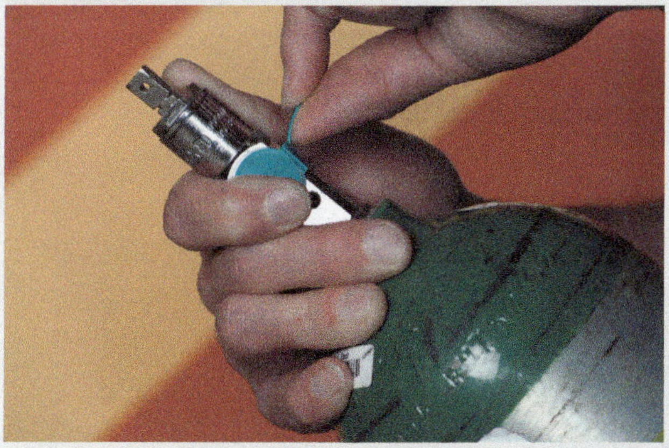

3. Remove the plastic wrapper or cap protecting the cylinder outlet.

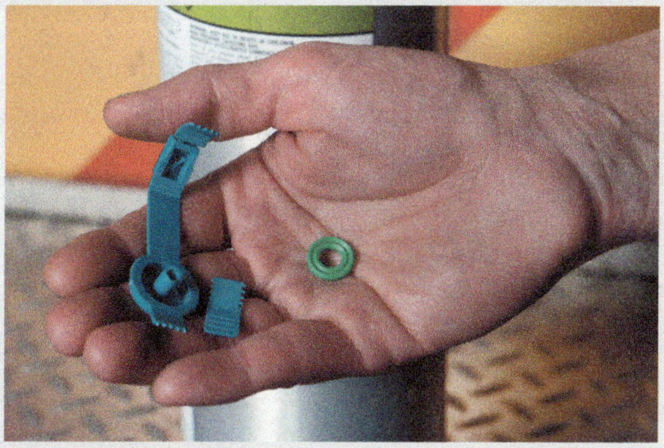

4. Keep the plastic washer.

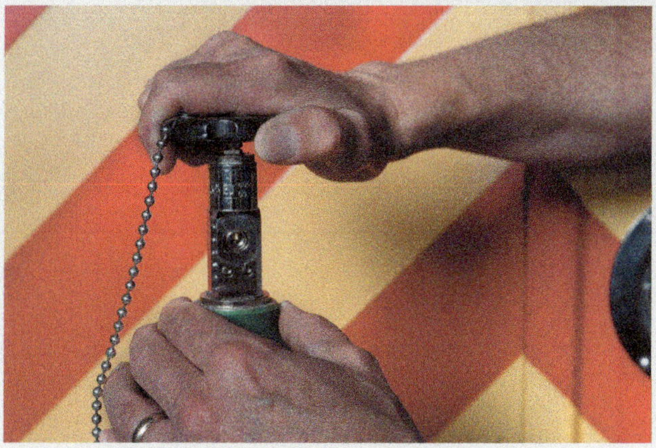

5. "Crack" the main valve for one second.

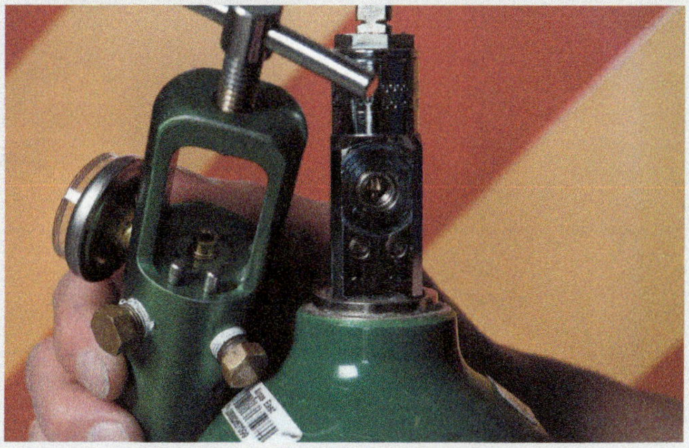

6. Select the correct pressure regulator and flowmeter.

(continued)

SCAN 10-1 Preparing the Oxygen-Delivery System *(continued)*

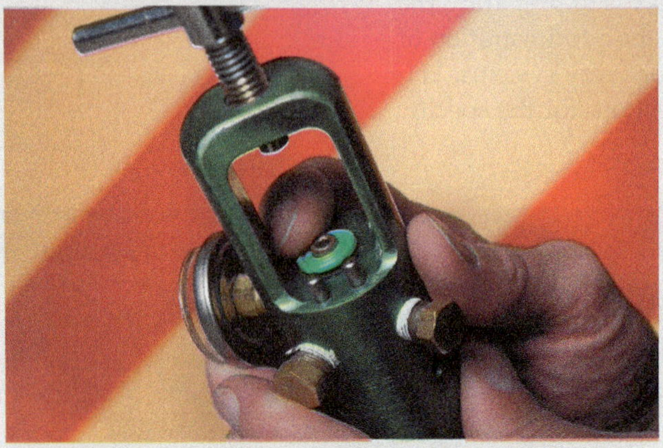

7. Place the cylinder valve gasket on the regulator oxygen port.

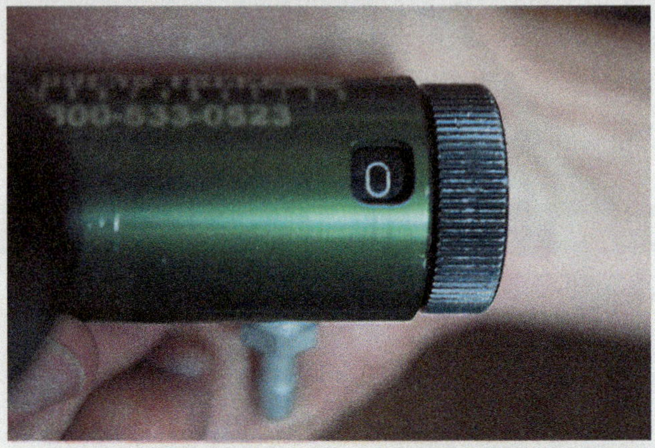

8. Make certain that the pressure regulator is closed.

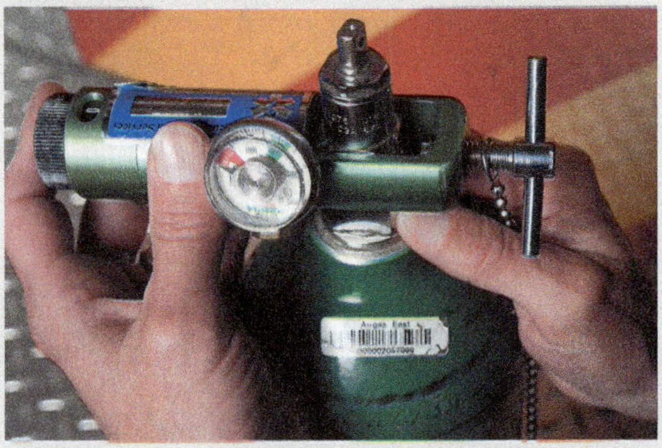

9. Align pins.

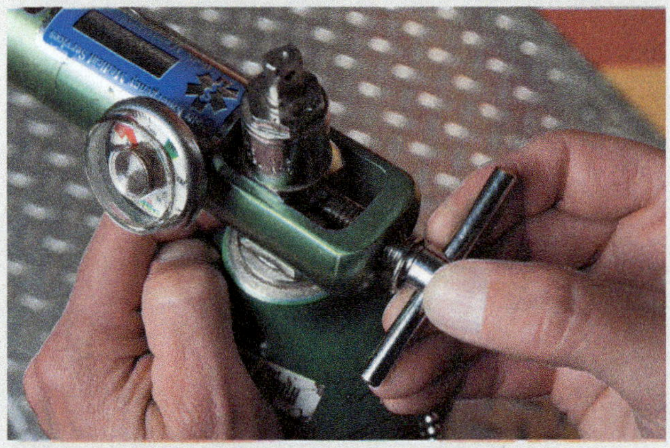

10. Tighten T-screw for pin yoke.

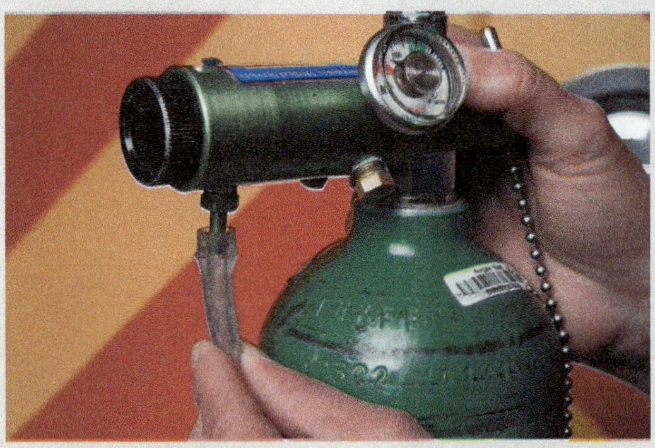

11. Attach tubing and delivery device.

SCAN 10-2 Administering Oxygen

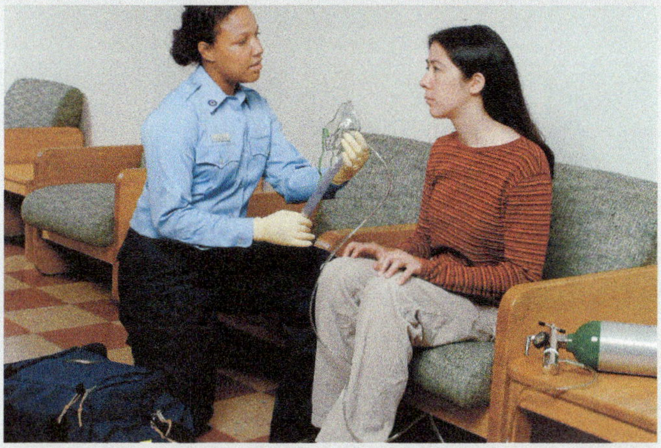

1. Explain to the patient the need for oxygen.

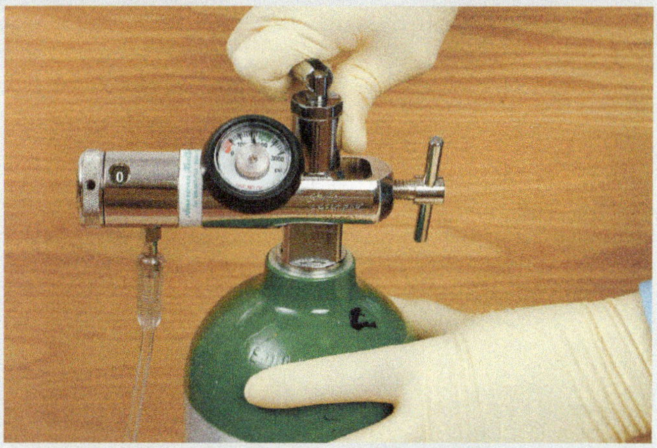

2. Open the main valve and adjust the flowmeter.

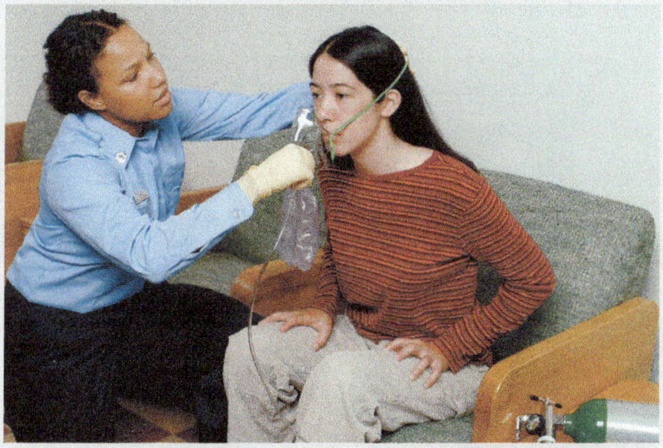

3. Place an oxygen-delivery device on the patient.

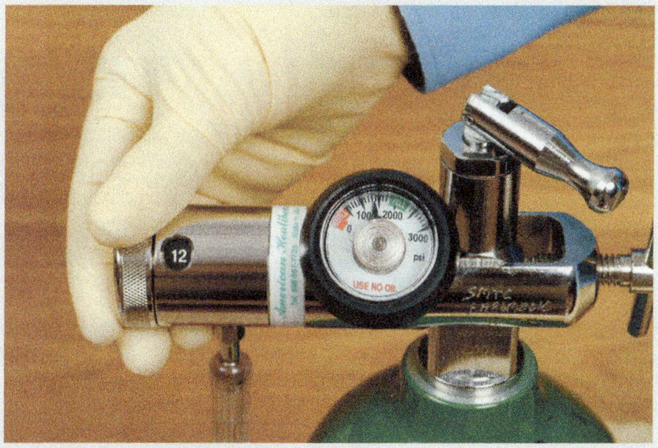

4. Adjust the flowmeter.

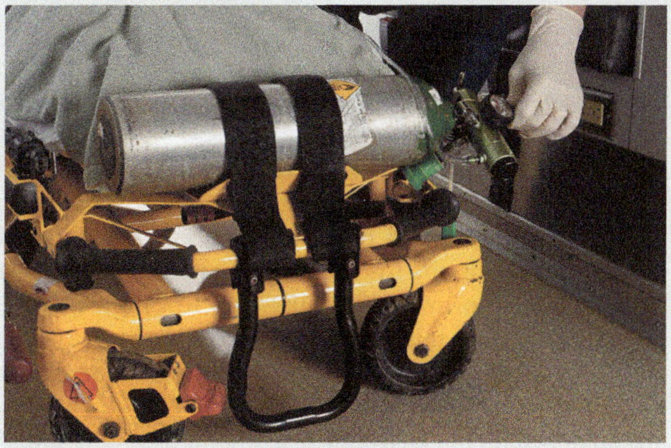

5. Secure the cylinder during transfer.

(continued)

SCAN 10-2 Administering Oxygen *(continued)*

Discontinuing Oxygen

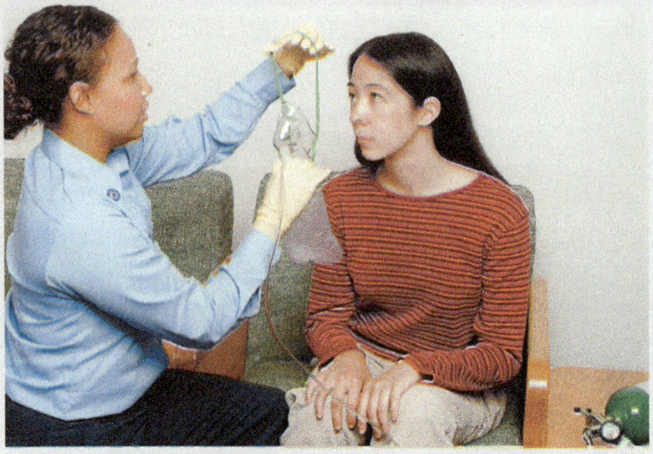

1. Remove the delivery device.

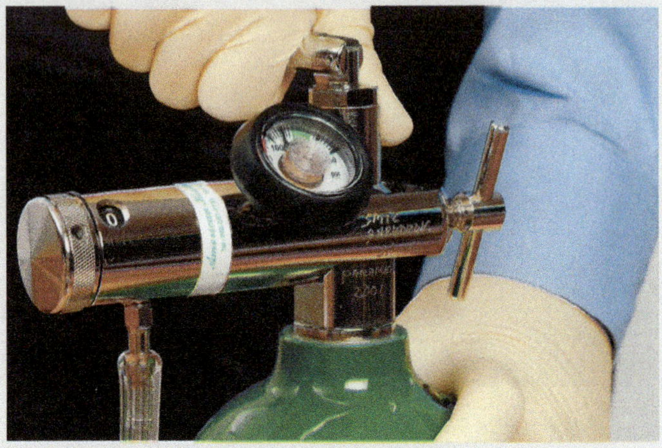

2. Close the main valve.

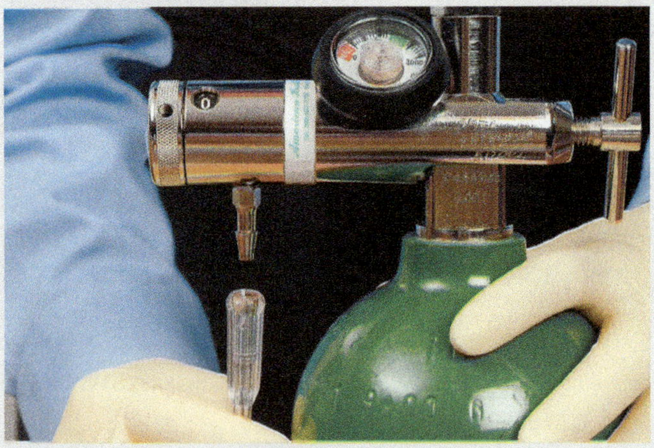

3. Remove the delivery tubing.

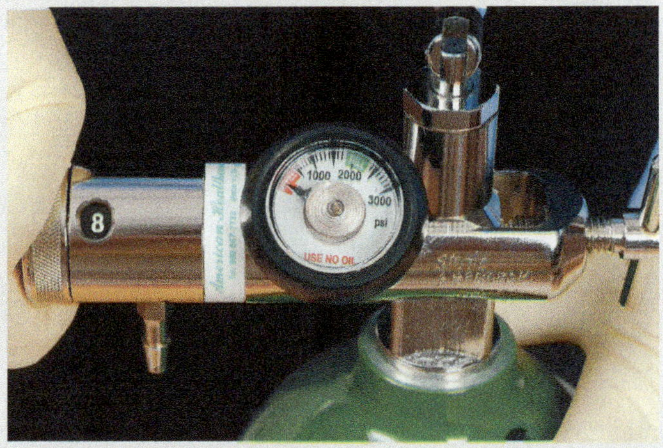

4. Bleed the flowmeter.

Supplemental Oxygen for Patients with Chest Pain? What is the Evidence?

Patients with chest pain traditionally have received high-concentration oxygen, but that teaching is now being questioned. There is little evidence of benefit or of harm from giving oxygen in the first few hours after an uncomplicated myocardial infarction (heart attack). This is primarily because very few high-quality studies have evaluated this question. Physiology tells us, though, that giving supplemental oxygen to healthy people may reduce the flow of blood through the coronary arteries, suggesting potential harm. The best treatment is not clear in patients with chest pain who are not short of breath or hypoxic, but in the face of no documented benefit and some potential harm, major organizations such as the American Heart Association and the International Liaison Committee on Resuscitation have recommended a selective approach to oxygen administration.

EMTs should administer supplemental oxygen to patients with chest pain who are short of breath or hypoxic, as determined by an oxygen saturation reading of less than 94 percent. Administer enough oxygen to relieve shortness of breath and bring the oxygen saturation to a normal level. For patients in mild distress, you may be able to do this with low-concentration oxygen through a nasal cannula. For patients in moderate to severe distress, you may need to give high-concentration oxygen via a nonrebreather mask. Local protocol may give more specific guidance on which patients to give oxygen to and how much to give them. As more research in this area is completed, these recommendations may change. This subject will be covered in more detail in the chapter titled *Cardiac Emergencies*.

Oxygen is administered to assist in the delivery of artificial ventilations to nonbreathing patients, as was discussed earlier in this chapter in the section titled *Techniques of Artificial Ventilation*. Oxygen is also very commonly administered to breathing patients for a variety of conditions. A number of oxygen-delivery devices and systems are used. Each has benefits and drawbacks. A device that is good for one patient may not be ideal for another. The goal is to use the oxygen-delivery device that is best for each patient.

For the patient who is breathing adequately and requires supplemental oxygen due to potential hypoxia, various oxygen-delivery devices are available. In general, however, the nonrebreather mask and the nasal cannula are the two devices most commonly used by the EMT to provide supplemental oxygen (Table 10-6).

Nonrebreather Mask

The ***nonrebreather (NRB) mask*** (Figure 10-23) is the EMT's best way to deliver high concentrations of oxygen to a breathing patient. This device must be placed properly on the patient's face to provide the necessary seal to ensure high-concentration delivery. The reservoir bag must be inflated before the mask is placed on the patient's face.

nonrebreather (NRB) mask a face mask-and-reservoir bag device that delivers high concentrations of oxygen. The patient's exhaled air escapes through a valve and is not rebreathed.

To inflate the reservoir bag, use your finger to cover the exhaust port or the connection between the mask and the reservoir. The reservoir must always contain enough oxygen so that it does not deflate by more than one-third during the patient's deepest inspiration. This can be maintained by the proper flow of oxygen (15 liters per minute). Air exhaled by the patient does not return to the reservoir (is not rebreathed). Instead, it escapes through a flutter valve in the face piece.

This mask will provide concentrations of oxygen ranging from 80 percent to 90 percent. The optimum flow rate is 12–15 liters per minute. New design features allow for one emergency port in the mask so the patient can still receive atmospheric air should the oxygen supply fail. This feature keeps the mask from being able to deliver 100 percent oxygen

TABLE 10-6 Oxygen-Delivery Devices

DEVICE	FLOW RATE	OXYGEN CONCENTRATION	APPROPRIATE USE
Nonrebreather mask	12-15 liters per minute	80-90 percent	Delivery system of choice for patients with signs of severe hypoxia and those short of breath, suffering severe injuries, or displaying an altered mental status
Nasal cannula	1-6 liters per minute	24-44 percent	Appropriate for patients with signs of hypoxia and those short of breath who need a small amount of supplemental oxygen or cannot tolerate a mask
Partial rebreather mask	9-10 liters per minute	40-60 percent	Usually not used in EMS. Some patients may use at home to treat ongoing respiratory diseases such as COPD.
Venturi mask	Varied, depending on device; up to 15 liters per minute	24-60 percent	A device used to deliver a specific concentration of oxygen. Device delivers 24-60 percent oxygen, depending on adapter tip and oxygen flow rate.
Tracheostomy mask	8-10 liters per minute	Can be set up to deliver varying oxygen percentages as required by the patient; desired percentage of oxygen may be recommended by the home care agency.	A device used to deliver ventilations/oxygen through a stoma or tracheostomy tube

FIGURE 10-23 Nonrebreather mask. In photo A, note the round disks–flutter valves that allow air exhaled by the patient to escape so it is not rebreathed. (Compare with Figure 10-25A, a partial rebreather that does not have the flutter valves.) B. nonrebreather mask.

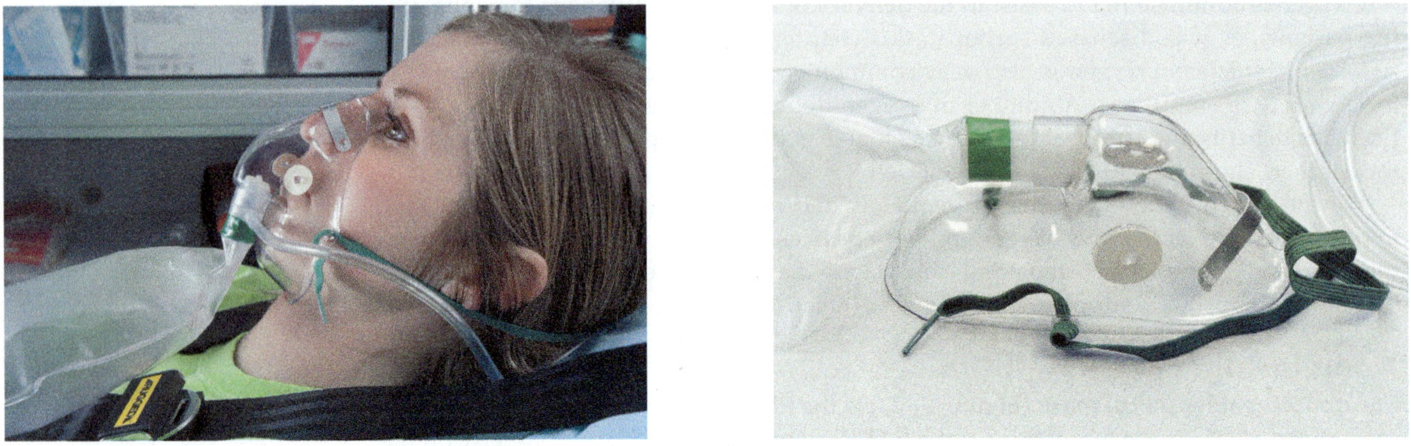

A

B

but is a necessary safety feature. The mask is excellent for use in patients with signs of hypoxia or who are short of breath or displaying an altered mental status.

Nonrebreather masks come in different sizes for adults, children, and infants.

Nasal Cannula

nasal cannula (NAY-zul KAN-yuh-luh)
a device that delivers low concentrations of oxygen through two prongs that rest in the patient's nostrils.

A ***nasal cannula*** (Figure 10-24) provides low concentrations of oxygen (between 24 percent and 44 percent). Oxygen is delivered to the patient by two prongs that rest in the patient's nostrils. The device is usually held to the patient's face by placing the tubing over the patient's ears and securing the slip-loop under the patient's chin.

The cannula is commonly used to help titrate oxygen saturation levels to 94 percent. Patients with signs of severe hypoxia may need a higher concentration than can be provided by a cannula. Some patients will not tolerate a mask-type delivery device, because they feel suffocated by the mask. For the patient who refuses to wear an oxygen face mask, the cannula still delivers a significant amount of oxygen. The cannula should be used when a patient will not tolerate a nonrebreather mask.

When a cannula is used, the liters per minute delivered should be no more than 4–6. At higher flow rates, the cannula begins to feel more uncomfortable, like a windstorm in the nose, and dries out the nasal mucous membranes.

FIGURE 10-24 Nasal cannula.

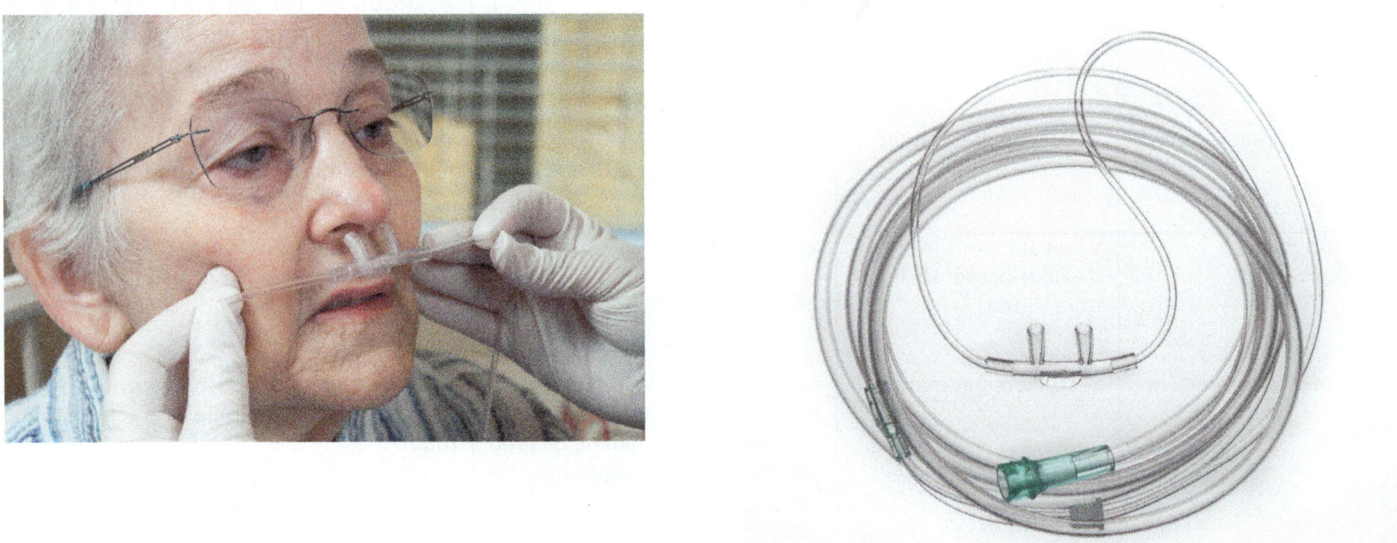

FIGURE 10-25 Partial rebreather mask. (Compare with Figure 10-23A. The partial rebreather mask does not have the flutter valves that a nonrebreather has, so the patient's exhaled air does not escape, and is partially rebreathed by the patient.)

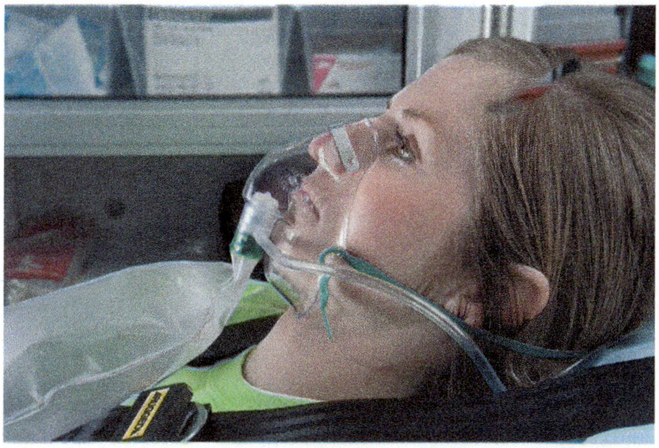

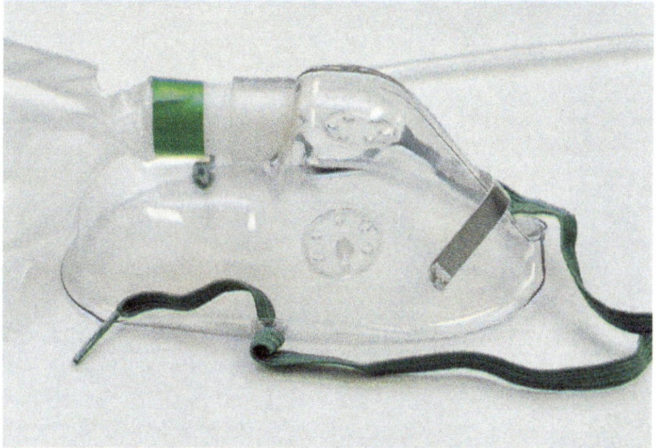

Partial Rebreather Mask

A ***partial rebreather mask*** (Figure 10-25) is very similar to a nonrebreather mask, with the exception that there is no one-way valve in the opening to the reservoir bag. This allows the patient to rebreathe about one-third of the exhaled air. This type of mask is used for some patients to preserve the carbon dioxide levels in their blood to stimulate breathing. Partial rebreather masks deliver 40 to 60 percent oxygen at 9–10 liters per minute. These masks are not typically used in EMS but may be encountered when caring for a patient who uses such a mask at home.

partial rebreather mask
a face mask and reservoir oxygen bag with no one-way valve to the reservoir bag, so some exhaled air mixes with the oxygen; used in some patients to help preserve carbon dioxide levels in the blood to stimulate breathing.

Venturi Mask

A ***Venturi mask*** (Figure 10-26) delivers specific concentrations of oxygen by mixing oxygen with inhaled air. The Venturi mask package may contain several tips. Each tip will provide a different concentration of oxygen when used at the flow rate designated on the tip. Some Venturi masks have a set percentage and flow rate, whereas others have an adjustable Venturi port. These devices are most commonly used on patients with COPD.

Venturi mask
a face mask-and-reservoir bag device that delivers specific concentrations of oxygen by mixing oxygen with inhaled air.

FIGURE 10-26 Venturi mask.

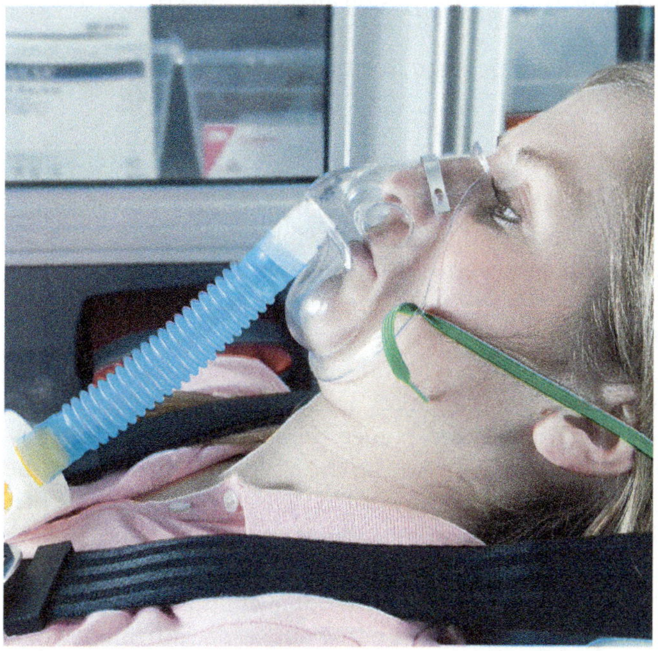

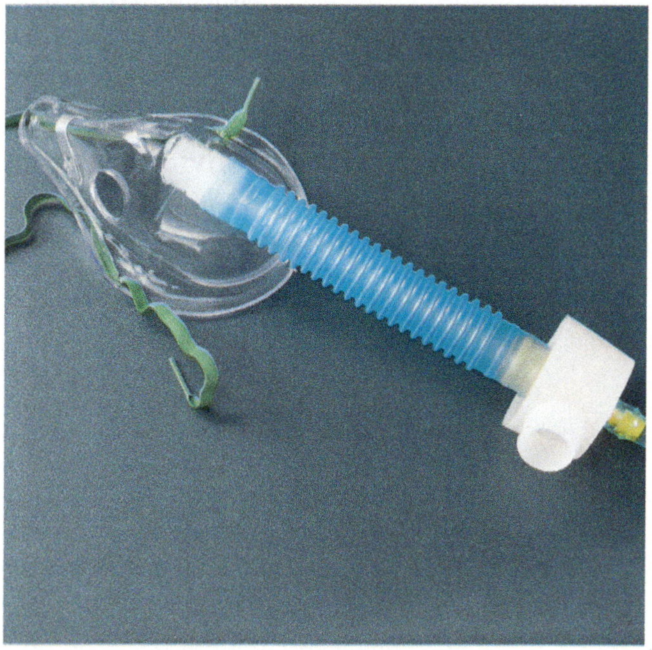

FIGURE 10-27 Tracheostomy mask.

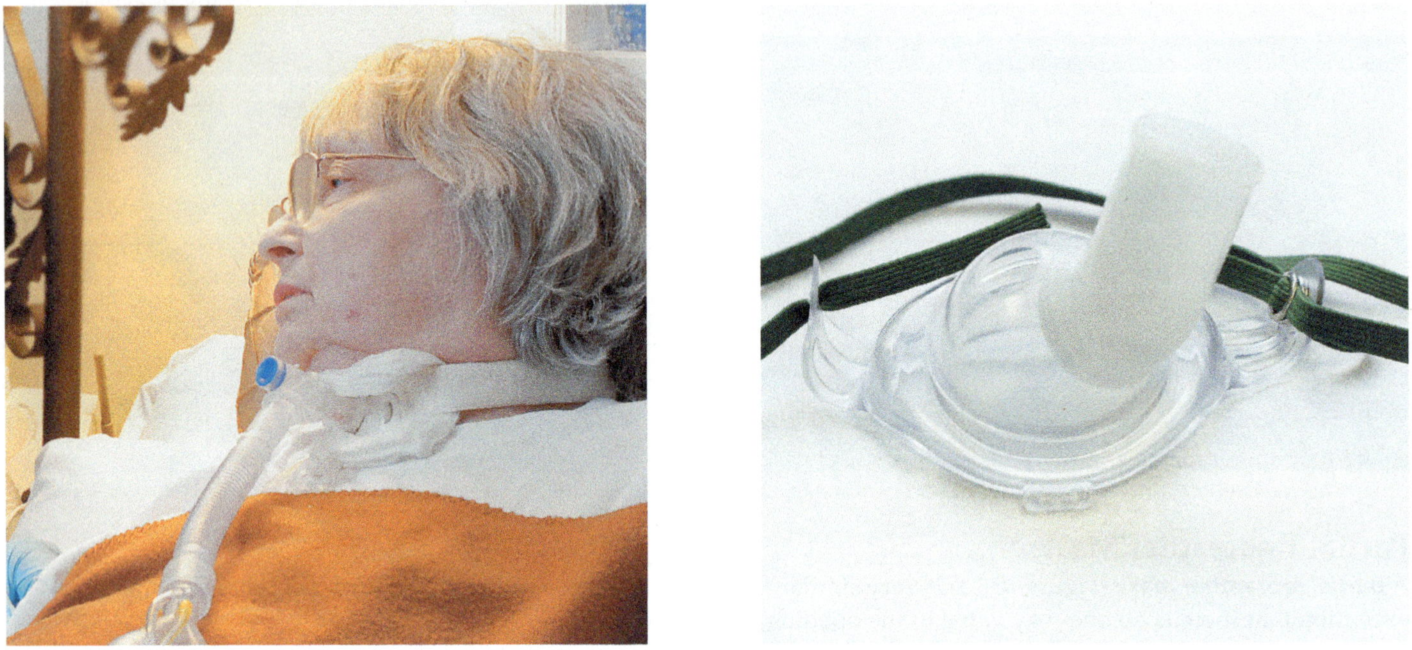

tracheostomy mask
a device designed to be placed over a stoma or tracheostomy tube to provide supplemental oxygen.

Tracheostomy Mask

A ***tracheostomy mask*** (Figure 10-27) is designed to be placed over a stoma or tracheostomy tube to provide supplemental oxygen. It is typically a small, cuplike mask that fits over the tracheostomy opening and is held in place by an elastic strap placed around the neck. These masks are connected to 8–10 liters per minute of oxygen via supply tubing.

CPAP

Continuous positive airway pressure, or CPAP, has been shown to offer benefits as an oxygen-delivery device. Although the primary benefit of CPAP is pressure and not necessarily oxygen, there are several situations emerging in which CPAP is used as an oxygen-delivery device. For example, CPAP is increasingly being used to preoxygenate patients prior to placement of an advanced airway. Although this would not necessarily be in the EMT's scope of practice, it is reasonable to envision an EMT being part of a larger advanced life support team.

The use and application of CPAP will be discussed in more detail in the chapter *Respiratory Emergencies.*

Providing Pediatric Patients Supplemental Oxygen

As in adults, high-concentration oxygen should be administered to children in respiratory distress, those with inadequate respirations, and those in possible shock. Hypoxia is the underlying reason for many of the most serious medical problems with children. Inadequate oxygen will have immediate effects on the heart rate and the brain, as shown by a slowed heart rate and an altered mental status.

However, infants and young children are often afraid of an oxygen mask. For these patients who will not tolerate a mask or nasal cannula, try a "blow-by" technique. In this technique you hold, or have a parent hold, the oxygen tubing or the pediatric nonrebreather mask 2 inches (5 cm) from the patient's face so the oxygen will pass over the face and be inhaled (Figure 10-28). Some departments use blow-by oxygen devices that resemble stuffed animals. These commercially made products may be less threatening to a child than traditional oxygen devices. Follow the manufacturer's recommendations regarding liter flow per minute when using these devices. Some children respond well when oxygen tubing is pushed through the bottom of a paper cup, especially if the cup is

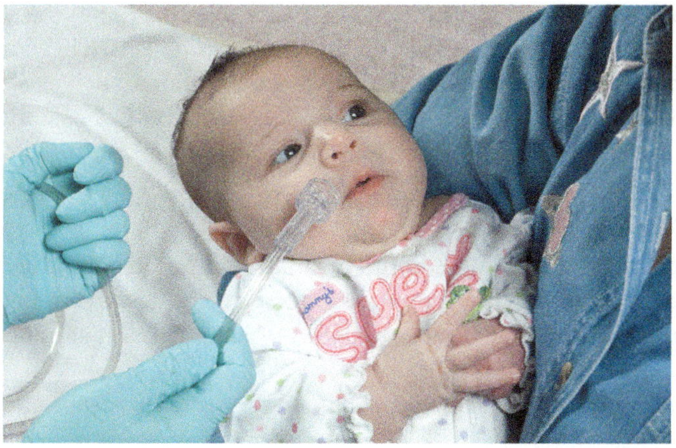

FIGURE 10-28 You can deliver oxygen to an infant using the blow-by method.

colorful or has a picture drawn inside it. Hand the cup to the child or ask a parent to hold it. Infants and young children instinctively explore new things by bringing them up to their mouths, so when they handle and explore the cup, they will breathe in the oxygen. Do not use a Styrofoam cup. Styrofoam may flake, and the child could inhale the particles.

Remember that a nonrebreather mask will always provide more efficient oxygen delivery, and many children tolerate it well. Use blow-by only if more efficient administration methods fail.

Special Considerations

There are a number of special considerations in airway management:

- **Facial injuries.** Take extra care with the airway if a patient has facial injuries. Because the blood supply to the face is so rich, blunt injuries to the face frequently result in severe swelling or bleeding that may block or partially block the airway. Frequent suctioning may be required. In addition, insertion of an airway adjunct or endotracheal tube may be necessary.

Think Like an EMT

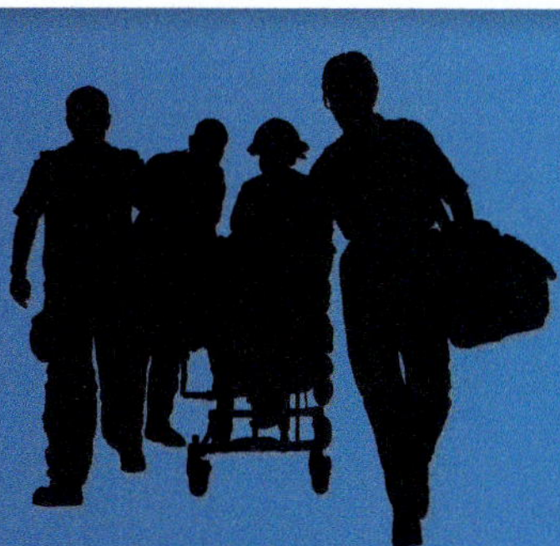

Oxygen or Ventilation?

You have learned several methods to administer supplemental oxygen and to provide ventilations to a patient. The decision on whether to provide supplemental oxygen (e.g., nonrebreather mask or cannula) or to ventilate (e.g., BVM) is one of the most important decisions you will make.

For each of the following patients, decide whether you would administer oxygen or ventilate the patient.

1. A patient who was found on the floor by a relative. He has no pulse or respirations.
2. A 14-year-old patient who has a broken femur. She is alert; pulse 110, strong and regular; respirations 28, rapid, and deep.
3. A 64-year-old male with chest pain. He is alert; pulse 56; respirations 18 and normal.
4. A 78-year-old patient with COPD. He has had increasing difficulty breathing over the past few days. He responds verbally but is not oriented. His pulse is 124; respirations 36 and shallow.

- **Obstructions.** Many suction units are not adequate for removing solid objects such as teeth and large particles of food or other foreign objects. These must be removed using manual techniques for clearing airway obstructions, such as abdominal thrusts, chest thrusts, or finger sweeps, which you learned in your basic life support course and which are reviewed in *Appendix A, Basic Cardiac Life Support Review,* at the back of this book. You may need to log roll the patient into a supine position to clear the oropharynx manually.
- **Dental appliances.** Dentures should ordinarily be left in place during airway procedures. Partial dentures may become dislodged during an emergency. Leave a partial denture in place if possible, but be prepared to remove it if it endangers the airway.

Pediatric Note

There are several special considerations that you must take into account when assessing and managing breathing in an infant or child. (Review Figure 9-5 comparing adult and child airways in the *Airway Management* chapter.)

Anatomic Considerations

- In infants and children, the tongue takes up more space proportionally in the mouth than in adults. Always consider using an airway adjunct when performing artificial ventilation.
- The trachea (windpipe) is softer and more flexible in infants and children. Furthermore, small children often have a proportionally larger head, which makes it more difficult to maintain a patent airway. Often padding is necessary behind their shoulders to provide a proper airway position. Always consider this when performing artificial ventilation.
- The chest wall is softer, and infants and children tend to depend more on their diaphragms for breathing. Gastric distention can severely impair the movement of the diaphragm and therefore seriously decrease tidal volumes in children.
- A child's metabolism consumes oxygen at a higher rate than adults do. Although they compensate well, hypoxia will often occur more rapidly, and decompensation can be swift.

Management Considerations

- When ventilating, avoid excessive pressure and volume. Use only enough to make the chest rise.
- Use properly sized face masks when providing ventilations, to ensure a good mask seal.
- Flow-restricted, oxygen-powered ventilation devices are contraindicated (should not be used) in infants and children, unless you have a pediatric unit and have been properly trained in its use.
- Use pediatric-sized nonrebreather masks and nasal cannulas when administering supplemental oxygen.
- Infants and children are prone to gastric distention during ventilations, which may impair adequate ventilations.

Assisting with Advanced Airway Devices

You may be called to assist an advanced EMT or paramedic with an advanced airway device. There are two basic types of devices, each with different procedures for use:

1. **Devices that require direct visualization of the glottic opening (endotracheal intubation).** A device called a laryngoscope is used to visualize the airway while the tube is guided into the trachea.
2. **Devices that are inserted blindly, meaning without having to look into the airway to insert the device.** These devices include the King LT-D™ airway, iGel®, and laryngeal mask airway (LMA™).

In most states, the decision to use the advanced device and insertion of the device are limited to advanced-level providers. (Always refer to your local protocol.) The EMT may be called on to assist in patient preparation for insertion of the device. The most important thing an EMT can do to further the success of the insertion and benefit to the patient is to assure a patent airway and quality ventilations prior to insertion of the device. Fortunately this is something EMTs should be doing all the time.

NOTE: *Be especially careful not to disturb the endotracheal tube. Movement of the patient to a backboard, down stairs, and into the ambulance can easily cause displacement of the tube. If the tube comes out of the trachea, the patient receives no oxygen and will certainly die.*

Preparing the Patient for Intubation

Before the paramedic inserts the endotracheal tube, you may be asked to give the patient extra oxygen. This is referred to as hyperoxygenation, and it can easily be accomplished by ventilating with a bag–valve–mask device that is connected to oxygen and includes a reservoir. To do this, ventilate at a normal rate. Do not administer more than 20 breaths per minute for more than 2–3 minutes or administer breaths more forcefully during this time. Increasing the force of ventilations (bag squeeze) will force air into the stomach and cause vomiting. Occasionally, a high-flow nasal cannula (administering supplemental oxygen at a rate as high as 15 liters per minute) may be used to support preoxygenation and passive oxygenation during placement of the advanced airway. Although EMTs would not traditionally use a nasal cannula at this high flow rate, this specific preoxygenation scenario may warrant it. CPAP is also commonly used to prepare conscious and breathing patients for intubation.

The paramedic will then position the patient's head in the head-elevated, sniffing position. The paramedic will remove the oral airway and pass the endotracheal tube (Figure 10-29) through the mouth, into the throat, past the vocal cords, and into the trachea. This procedure requires using a laryngoscope to move the tongue out of the way and provide a view of the vocal cords. The tube may also be passed through the nose. This does not require visualization of the airway.

To maneuver the tube past the vocal cords correctly, the paramedic will need to see them. You may be asked to help by gently pressing on the throat to push the vocal cords into the paramedic's view. You will do this by pressing your thumb and index finger just to either side of the throat over either the thyroid cartilage (Adam's apple) or the cricoid cartilage, the ring-shaped cartilage just below the thyroid cartilage, and gently directing the throat upward toward the patient's right (Figure 10-30). This motion of Bringing Up and to the Right Position is referred to as the BURP maneuver.

Once the tube is properly placed, the cuff is inflated with air from a 10-cc syringe. While holding the tube, the paramedic ensures proper tube placement by using at least two methods, including auscultation of both lungs and the epigastrium and using a capnometry

FIGURE 10-29 (A) The endotracheal tube and (B) endotracheal tube with stylet in place.

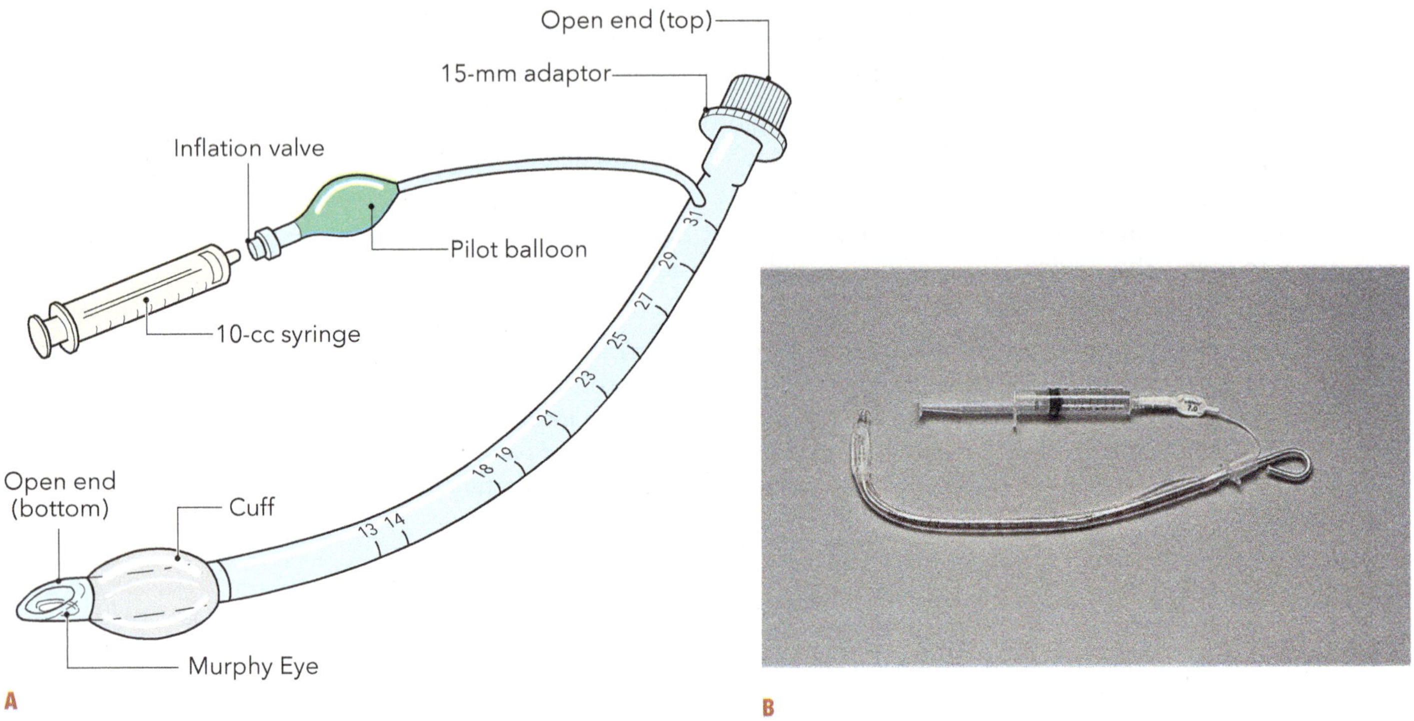

FIGURE 10-30 In the BURP maneuver, press your thumb and index finger on either side of the throat over the cricoid cartilage and gently direct the throat upward and toward the patient's right. *(© Edward T. Dickinson, MD)*

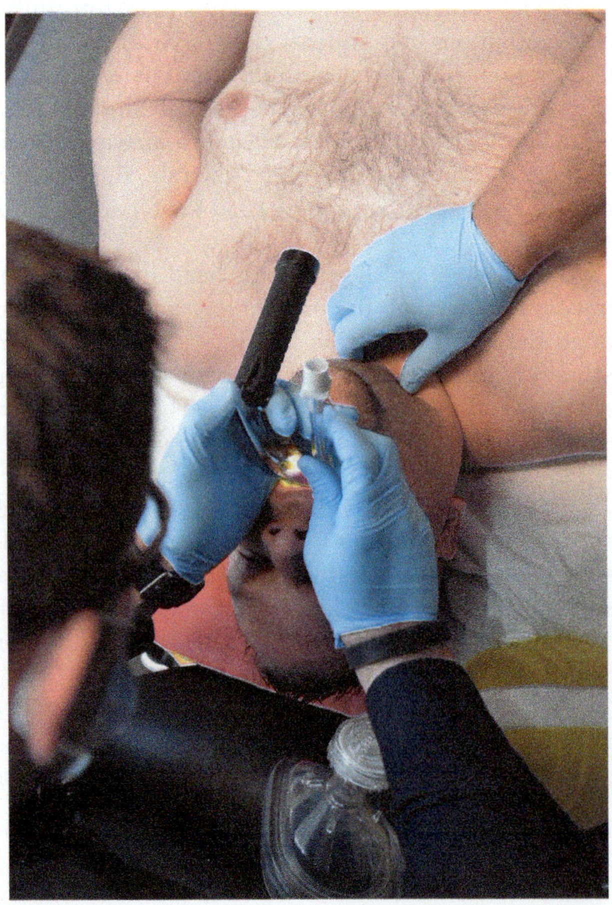

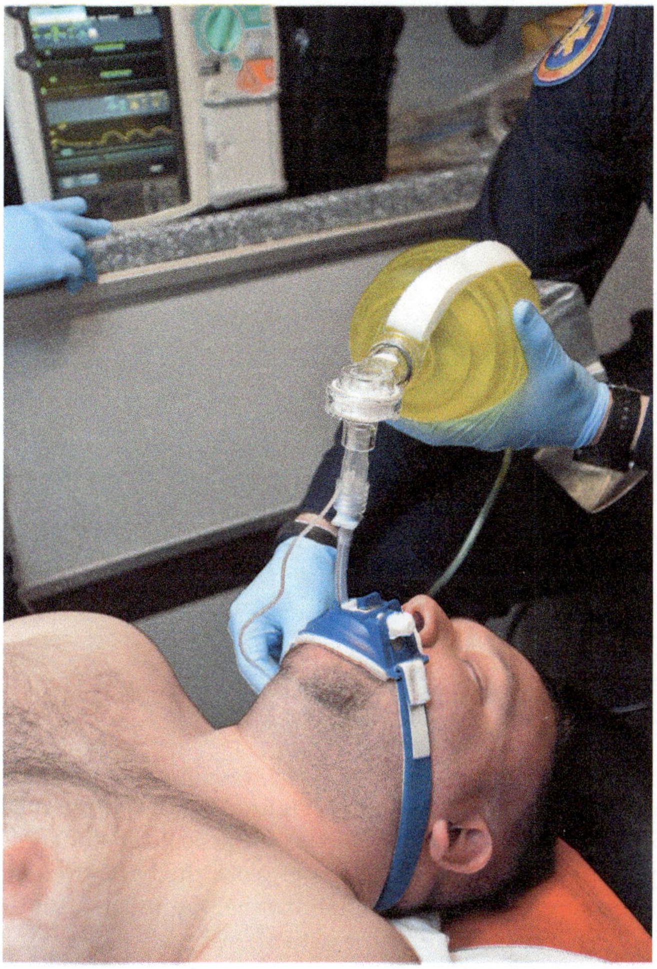

FIGURE 10-31 An end-tidal CO_2 detector can confirm proper placement of the endotracheal tube. *(© Edward T. Dickinson, MD)*

or an end-tidal CO_2 detector device (Figure 10-31). If the tube has been correctly placed, there will be sounds of air entering the lungs but no sounds of air in the epigastrium. Air sounds in the epigastrium indicate that the tube has been incorrectly placed in the esophagus instead of the trachea, so air is entering the stomach instead of the lungs. The tube position must be corrected immediately by removing the tube, reoxygenating the patient, and repeating the process of intubation.

The correctly positioned tube is anchored in place with a commercially made tube restraint. The entire procedure of intubation—including the last ventilation, passing the tube, and the next ventilation—should take less than 30 seconds.

You might be asked to assist the advanced providers by monitoring the lung and epigastric sounds throughout the call. Most systems now use continuous end-tidal carbon dioxide detection when an endotracheal tube is in place as one method of monitoring tube placement.

If the tube is pushed in too far, it will most likely enter the right mainstem bronchus, preventing oxygen from entering the patient's left lung. (You can identify this by noting breath sounds on the right side with no sounds over the left or the epigastrium.)

If the tube is pulled out, it can easily slip into the esophagus and send all the ventilations directly to the stomach (indicated by breath sounds over the epigastrium), denying the patient oxygen. Tube displacement is a fatal complication if it goes unnoticed.

Ventilating the Intubated Patient

When you are asked to ventilate an intubated, or "tubed," patient, keep in mind that even very little movement can displace the tube. Look at the gradations on the side of the tube. In the typical adult male, for example, the 22-cm mark will be at the teeth when the tube is properly placed. If the tube moves, report this to the paramedic immediately.

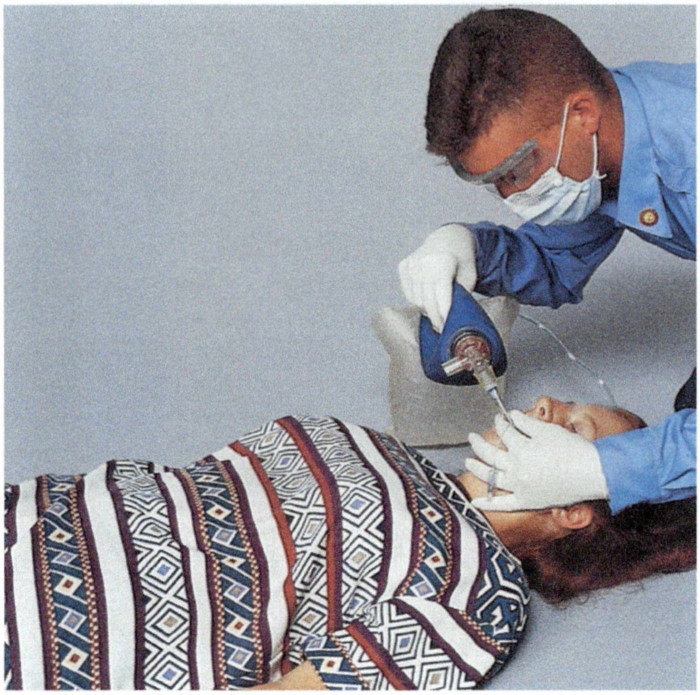

FIGURE 10-32 Make sure the endotracheal tube does not move. Hold it with two fingers against the patient's teeth.

Ventilate about 10 times per minute, or every 6 seconds. Hold the tube against the patient's teeth with two fingers of one hand (Figure 10-32). Use the other hand to work the bag–valve–mask unit. (A patient with an endotracheal tube offers less resistance to ventilations, so you may not need two hands to work the bag.) If you are ventilating a breathing patient, be sure to provide ventilations that are timed with the patient's own respiratory effort as much as possible, so the patient can take full breaths. It is also possible to help the patient increase the patient's respiratory rate, if needed, by interposing extra ventilations. Remember these cautions:

- Pay close attention to what the ventilations feel like. Report any change in resistance. Increased resistance when ventilating with the bag–valve mask is one of the first signs of air escaping through a hole in the lungs and filling the space around the lungs, which is an extremely serious problem. A change in resistance can also indicate that the tube has slipped into the esophagus.
- When the patient is defibrillated, carefully remove the bag from the tube. If you do not, the weight of the unsupported bag may accidentally displace the tube.
- Watch for any change in the patient's mental status. A patient who becomes more alert may need to be restrained from pulling out the tube. In addition, an oral airway generally is used as a bite block (a device that prevents the patient from biting the endotracheal tube). If the patient's gag reflex returns along with increased consciousness, you may need to pull the bite block out a bit.

Finally, during a cardiac arrest in the absence of an IV line for administering medications, you may be asked to stop ventilating and remove the BVM. The paramedic may then inject a medication such as epinephrine down the endotracheal tube.

Assisting with a Trauma Intubation

Occasionally you will be asked to assist in the endotracheal intubation of a patient with a suspected cervical spine injury. Since using the sniffing position, which involves elevating the neck, risks worsening cervical spine injury, some modifications are necessary. Your role will change as well. You may be required to provide manual in-line stabilization during the whole procedure.

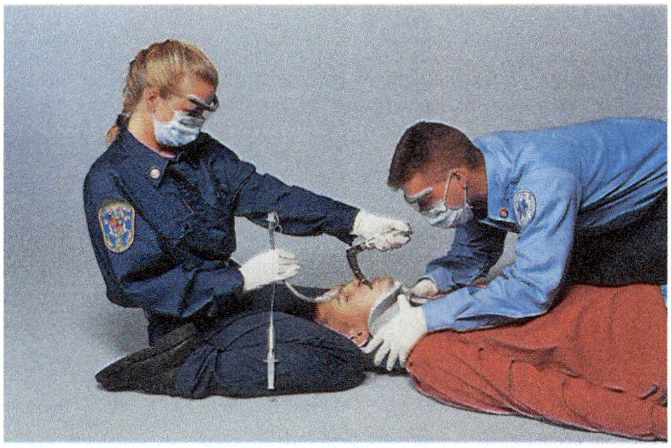

FIGURE 10-33 To assist in the intubation of a patient with suspected cervical spine injury, maintain manual stabilization throughout the procedure.

To accomplish this, the paramedic will hold manual stabilization while you apply a cervical collar. In some EMS systems, the patient may be intubated without a cervical collar in place but with attention to manual stabilization during and after intubation. Since the paramedic must stay at the patient's head, it will be necessary for you to stabilize the head and neck from the patient's side (Figure 10-33). Once you are in position, the paramedic will lean back and use the laryngoscope, which will bring the vocal cords into view. The patient can then be tubed.

After intubation, you will hold the tube against the teeth until placement is confirmed with both an esophageal detector device and auscultation of both lungs and the epigastrium. Then the tube is anchored. At that time, you can change your position to a more comfortable one. However, until the patient is immobilized on a long backboard, it will be necessary to assign another EMS worker to maintain manual stabilization while you ventilate the patient. Never assume that a collar provides adequate immobilization by itself. Manual stabilization must be used in addition to a collar until the head is taped in place on the backboard.

Chapter Review

Key Facts and Concepts

- Respiratory failure is the result of inadequate breathing, breathing that is insufficient to support life.
- A patient in respiratory failure or respiratory arrest must receive artificial ventilations.
- Oxygen can be delivered to the nonbreathing patient as a supplement to artificial ventilation.
- Oxygen can also be administered as therapy to the breathing patient whose breathing is inadequate or who is cyanotic, cool and clammy, short of breath, suffering chest pain, suffering severe injuries, or displaying an altered mental status.

Key Decisions

- Is the patient breathing? Is the patient breathing adequately (ventilating *and* oxygenating)? Does the patient need supplemental oxygen?
- Is there a need to initiate artificial ventilation?
- Are my artificial ventilations adequate (proper rate and volume)?

Chapter Glossary

alveolar ventilation the amount of air that reaches the alveoli.

artificial ventilation forcing air or oxygen into the lungs when a patient has stopped breathing or has inadequate breathing. Also called *positive pressure ventilation*.

automatic transport ventilator (ATV) a device that provides positive pressure ventilations. It includes settings designed to adjust ventilation rate and volume, is portable, and is easily carried on an ambulance.

bag-valve mask (BVM) a handheld device with a face mask and self-refilling bag that can be squeezed to provide artificial ventilations to a patient. It can deliver air from the atmosphere or oxygen from a supplemental oxygen-supply system.

cellular respiration the exchange of oxygen and carbon dioxide between cells and circulating blood.

cyanosis (SY-uh-NO-sis) a blue or gray color resulting from lack of oxygen in the body.

diffusion a process by which molecules move from an area of high concentration to an area of low concentration.

flowmeter a valve that indicates the flow of oxygen in liters per minute.

humidifier a device connected to the flowmeter to add moisture to the dry oxygen coming from an oxygen cylinder.

hypoxia (hi-POK-se-uh) an insufficiency of oxygen in the body's tissues.

nasal cannula (NAY-zul KAN-yuh-luh) a device that delivers low concentrations of oxygen through two prongs that rest in the patient's nostrils.

nonrebreather (NRB) mask a face mask-and-reservoir bag device that delivers high concentrations of oxygen. The patient's exhaled air escapes through a valve and is not rebreathed.

oxygen cylinder a cylinder filled with oxygen under pressure.

partial rebreather mask a face mask and reservoir oxygen bag with no one-way valve to the reservoir bag, so some exhaled air mixes with the oxygen; used in some patients to help preserve carbon dioxide levels in the blood to stimulate breathing.

pocket face mask a device, usually with a one-way valve, to aid in artificial ventilation. A rescuer breathes through the valve when the mask is placed over the patient's face. It also acts as a barrier to prevent contact with a patient's breath or body fluids. It can be used with supplemental oxygen when fitted with an oxygen inlet.

positive pressure ventilation *See* artificial ventilation.

pressure regulator a device connected to an oxygen cylinder to reduce cylinder pressure so it is safe for delivery of oxygen to a patient.

pulmonary respiration the exchange of oxygen and carbon dioxide between the alveoli and circulating blood in the pulmonary capillaries.

respiration (RES-pir-AY-shun) the diffusion of oxygen and carbon dioxide between the alveoli and the blood (pulmonary respiration) and between the blood and the cells (cellular respiration). Also used to mean, simply, breathing.

respiratory arrest when breathing completely stops.

respiratory distress increased work of breathing; a sensation of shortness of breath.

respiratory failure the reduction of breathing to the point where oxygen intake is not sufficient to support life.

stoma a permanent surgical opening in the neck through which the patient breathes.

tracheostomy mask a device designed to be placed over a stoma or tracheostomy tube to provide supplemental oxygen.

ventilation breathing in and out (inhalation and exhalation), or artificial provision of breaths.

Venturi mask a face mask-and-reservoir bag device that delivers specific concentrations of oxygen by mixing oxygen with inhaled air.

Preparation for Your Examination and Practice

Short Answer

1. Describe the signs of respiratory distress.
2. Describe the signs of respiratory failure.
3. Name and briefly describe the techniques of artificial ventilation (mouth-to-mask or BVM).
4. For BVM ventilation, describe recommended variations in technique for one or two rescuers and for a patient with trauma suspected or trauma not suspected.
5. Describe how positive pressure ventilation moves air differently from how the body normally moves air.
6. Name patient problems that would benefit from administration of oxygen, and explain how to decide what oxygen-delivery device (nonrebreather mask, nasal cannula, or other) should be used for a particular patient.

Thinking and Linking

Think back to the Airway Management *chapter and link information from that chapter with information from this chapter to describe how the process of moving air in and out of the chest might be interfered with by the following dysfunctions:*

1. Penetrating trauma to the chest
2. A spinal injury that paralyzes the diaphragm
3. Bronchoconstriction that narrows the air passages
4. A rib fracture
5. A brain injury to the respiratory control center in the medulla

Critical Thinking Exercises

Careful assessment is needed to decide whether a patient needs artificial ventilation. The purpose of this exercise will be to apply this skill in the following situations.

1. On arrival at the emergency scene, you find an adult female patient who is semi-conscious. Her respiratory rate is 7 per minute. She appears pale and slightly blue around her lips. What immediate actions are necessary? Is this patient in respiratory failure, and if so, what signs and symptoms indicate this? Does this patient require artificial ventilations?
2. On arrival at the emergency scene, you find an adult male patient sitting bolt upright in a chair. He looks at you as you come into the room, but he is unable to speak more than two words at a time. He seems to have a prolonged expiratory phase; you hear wheezes, and his respiratory rate is 36. What immediate actions are necessary? Is this patient in respiratory failure, and if so, what signs and symptoms indicate this? Does this patient require artificial ventilations?
3. On arrival at the scene of a motor-vehicle crash, you find an adult female patient pacing outside her damaged vehicle. She appears to be breathing very rapidly but acknowledges you as you approach. Her color seems normal, and her respiratory rate is 48. What immediate actions are necessary? Is this patient in respiratory failure, and if so, what signs and symptoms indicate this? Does this patient require artificial ventilations?

Pathophysiology to Practice

The following questions are designed to assist you in gathering relevant clinical information and making accurate decisions in the field.

1. Describe the elements you would assess to determine whether a patient was breathing adequately.
2. You are assessing a breathing patient. Describe what findings might indicate the need to initiate artificial ventilations despite the fact the patient continues to breathe.
3. Describe how you would determine that you have delivered enough air (volume) when ventilating using a bag-valve mask.

Street Scenes

"Dispatch to unit 401, respond to 244 Lisbon Street for a patient with shortness of breath." En route, you make a preliminary plan with your partners, Danielle and Jim. You discuss what equipment the team will bring in and briefly review the immediate life threats associated with shortness of breath. Going into the apartment building, you bring in the stretcher, jump kit, oxygen, portable suction, and BVM unit.

As you approach the apartment, you notice that the hall smells of cigarette smoke. The odor is worse as you enter the unit. Your patient is found sitting at the kitchen table. He is a tall, thin, 70-year-old man. He appears anxious and is obviously having trouble breathing.

Street Scene Questions

1. **What is your first priority when starting to assess this patient?**
2. **Assuming his airway is patent, what are the essential elements in assessing this patient's breathing?**
3. **What type of emergency care should you be prepared to give?**

As you assess the patient, you note he is breathing rapidly with an audible wheeze. He seems very tired. He can speak only one or two words at a time, and you notice that his fingernails are blue. You also notice that his respiratory rate slows down and becomes slightly irregular from time to time.

Street Scene Questions

4. **Is this patient's breathing adequate? Why or why not?**
5. **Does this patient require artificial ventilation?**

The team decides that this patient is in respiratory failure, is tiring out, and needs immediate ventilation. You connect the BVM to high-concentration oxygen and begin to ventilate the patient. At first the patient is uncooperative and you find it difficult to time your ventilations with his. However, after a few breaths, your timing begins to work. About every fourth patient breath, you administer a breath to help increase tidal volume. The patient becomes more and more comfortable with this.

Jim continues the assessment while Danielle requests advanced life support (ALS) backup and prepares for rapid transport.

You continue ventilating as the team loads the patient and initiates transport.

3 SECTION

Patient Assessment

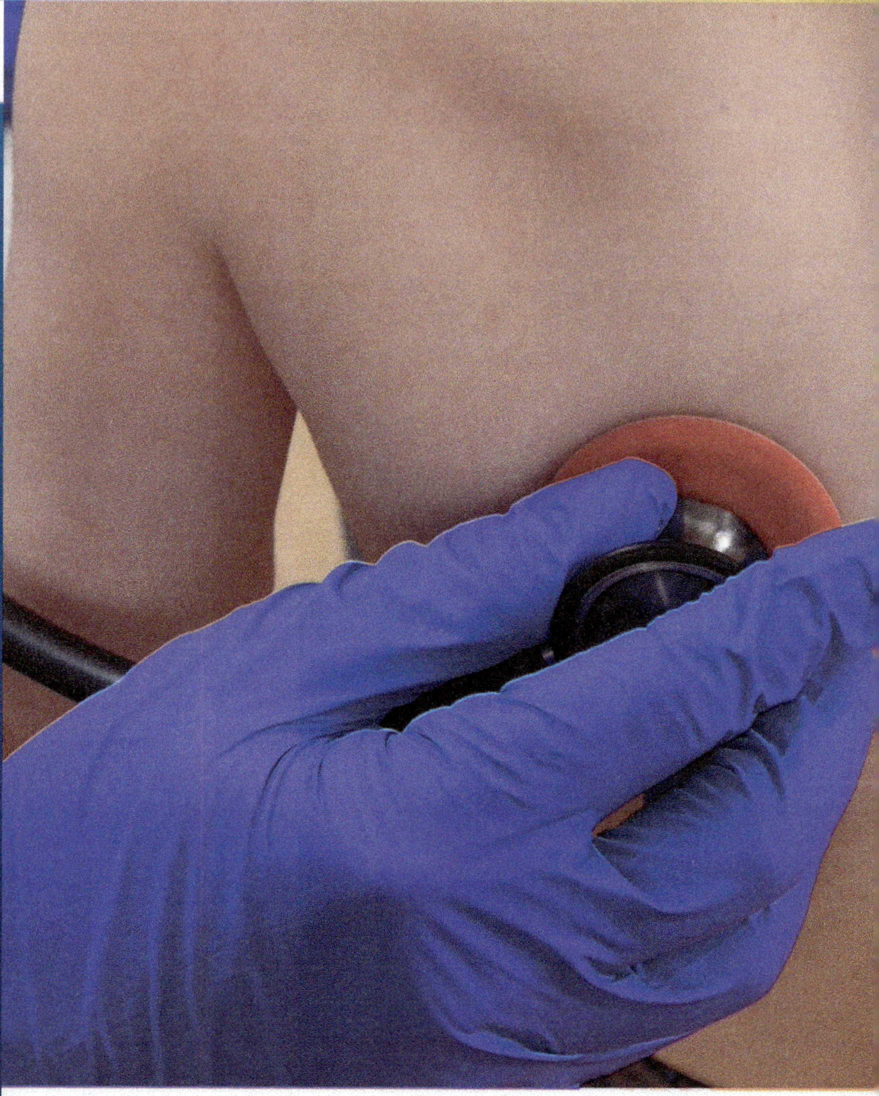

The elements of patient assessment are presented in this section. Before you reach a patient, you will perform a *scene size-up* to determine scene safety and evaluate the nature of the call, number of patients, and need for additional resources. When the scene is safe, your first task is to find and immediately care for any life threats as you perform the *primary assessment*.

Next you will perform the *secondary assessment*, during which you will obtain a patient history and perform a more detailed assessment. You will also measure vital signs and make use of appropriate monitoring devices. This section will detail the assessment of patients in a variety of situations, including medical and trauma emergencies. En route to the hospital, you will perform frequent and careful *reassessment*. Throughout the patient assessment, you will be working toward forming your EMT field diagnosis of the patient's condition, making use of critical thinking and decision-making skills. Finally, you will use the important skills of communication and documentation in assessment and throughout your patient care.

11

Scene Size-Up

Related Chapters

The following chapters provide additional information related to topics discussed in this chapter:

Standard

Assessment (Scene Size-Up)

Competency

Applies scene information and patient assessment findings (scene size-up, primary and secondary assessment, patient history, and reassessment) to guide emergency management.

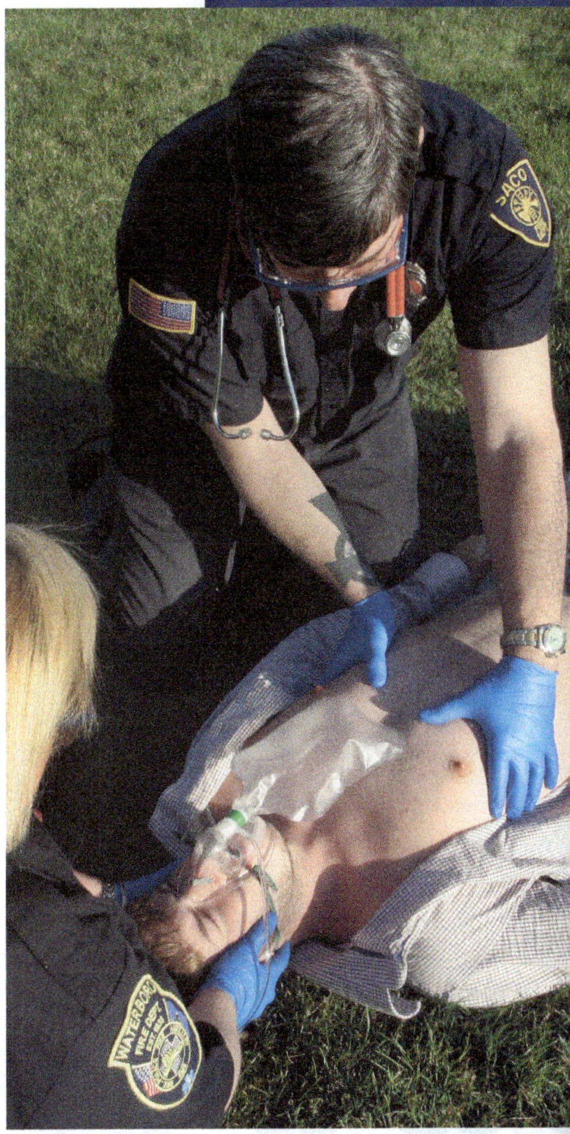

(© Daniel Limmer)

Core Concepts

- Identifying hazards at a scene
- Determining if a scene is safe to enter
- Mechanisms of injury and how they relate to patient condition
- Determining what additional assistance may be needed at a scene

Outcomes

After reading this chapter, you should be able to:

11.1 Analyze each of the components of scene size-up. (pp. 290–309)

- Recognize potential hazards at a scene.
- Explain the rationale for the priority of determining scene safety.
- Identify any modifications required to your personal protective equipment based on specific characteristics of a scene.
- Relate observations about the mechanism of injury to suspicions for patterns of patient injuries.
- Identify sources of information to advise you about the nature of a medical patient's illness.
- Given a scenario, determine the need for additional resources.

Key Terms

blunt-force trauma, *306*
danger zone, *294*
index of suspicion, *307*
mechanism of injury, *299*
nature of the illness, *307*
penetrating trauma, *306*
scene size-up, *290*

Scene Size-Up

scene size-up
steps taken when approaching the scene of an emergency call: checking scene safety, taking Standard Precautions, noting the mechanism of injury or nature of the patient's illness, determining the number of patients, and deciding what, if any, additional resources to call for.

CORE CONCEPT
Identifying hazards at a scene

Scene size-up is the first part of the patient assessment process. It begins as you approach the scene, surveying it to determine if there are any threats to your own safety or to the safety of your patients or bystanders, to determine the nature of the call, and to decide whether you will need additional help. (See *Visual Guide: Scene Size-Up*.)

However, scene size-up is not confined to the first part of the assessment process. These considerations should continue throughout the call, since emergencies are dynamic, always-changing events. You may find, for example, that patients, family members, or bystanders who were not a problem initially become increasingly hostile later in the call, or that vehicles or structures that seemed stable suddenly shift and pose a danger.

After your initial scene size-up, you will become more directly involved in patient assessment and care. However, it is a good idea to remember the key size-up elements throughout the call, to prevent dangerous surprises later.

You can obtain important information from just a brief survey of the scene. For example, you might see a downed electrical wire at the scene of a vehicle collision, a potentially deadly situation for you as the EMT, your patient, and bystanders. Further observations of the scene are likely to reveal more important information about the mechanism of injury. For example, damage to the steering wheel or windshield would be a strong indicator of potential chest, head, or neck injury caused by driver impact with those surfaces. A deployed airbag would cause you to assess for injuries that airbags might cause, especially to an infant or child front-seat passenger (Figure 11-1).

FIGURE 11-1 Clues such as (A) exterior damage, (B) a deployed air bag, or (C) a damaged windshield may lead you to suspect certain types of injuries. *(Photos A and B: © Daniel Limmer)*

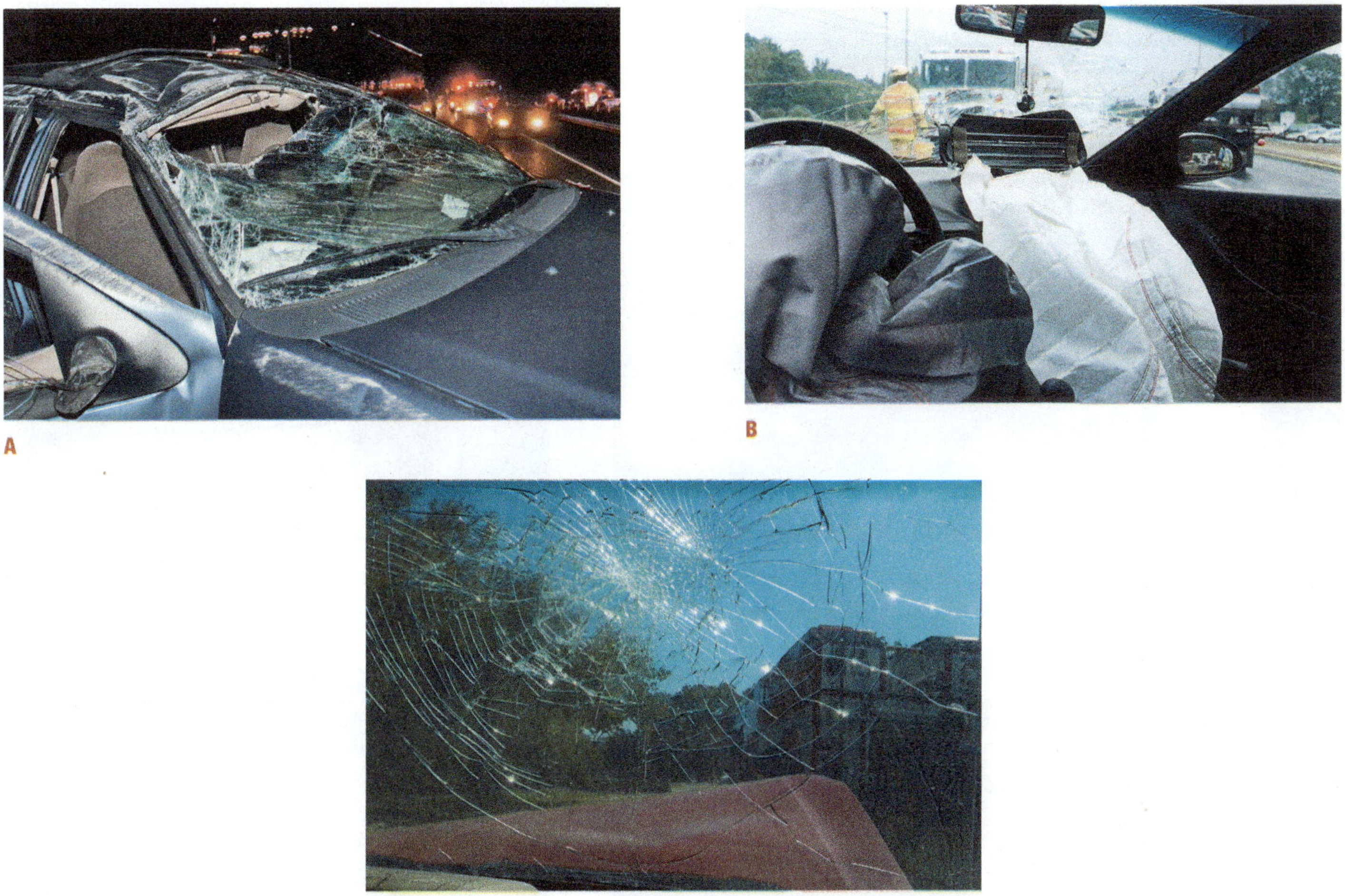

A B C

Just as important as your observations will be the actions you take to obtain needed assistance and prevent further injury. For example, if there were two patients at a collision, you would request that a second ambulance be dispatched to the scene—more, if you discovered that there were additional passengers. If there were also a downed wire at that scene, posing a danger of electrocution and fire, you would notify the fire department as well as the power company and the police department. In addition, you would take steps to keep bystanders clear of traffic, the collision, and the patients.

Scene Safety

The only predictable thing about emergencies is that they are often unpredictable and can pose many dangers if you are not careful.

CORE CONCEPT
Determining if a scene is safe to enter

Before you arrive on-scene, the dispatcher may relay important information to you. A well-trained emergency medical dispatcher (EMD) uses a set of questions to determine information that may affect you directly. For example, if the caller tells the EMD of particular hazards, you could immediately call for additional specialized assistance. You will learn more about the questions an EMD asks in the *EMS Operations* chapter.

Often you will arrive at a scene where there are police, firefighters, and even other ambulances already present. In a situation such as this, do not assume that the scene is safe or that others have taken care of any hazards. Always perform your own size-up, no matter who arrives first. Scan for scene hazards, infection-control concerns, mechanisms of

11 Scene Size-Up

EXAMINE THE SCENE, MINIMIZE DANGERS, PLAN AHEAD

Identify hazards

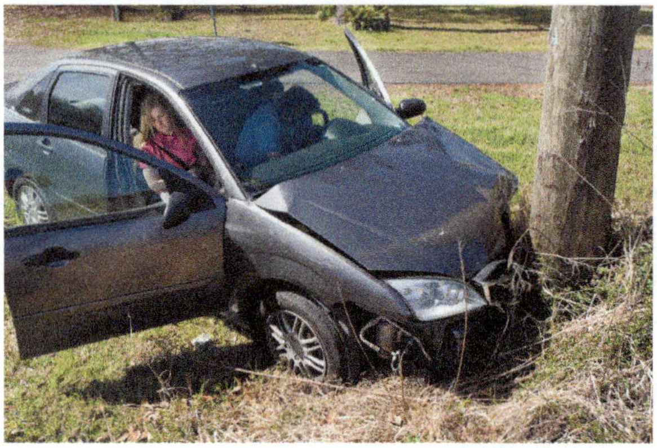

Examine for mechanism of injury or nature of illness (medical patient).

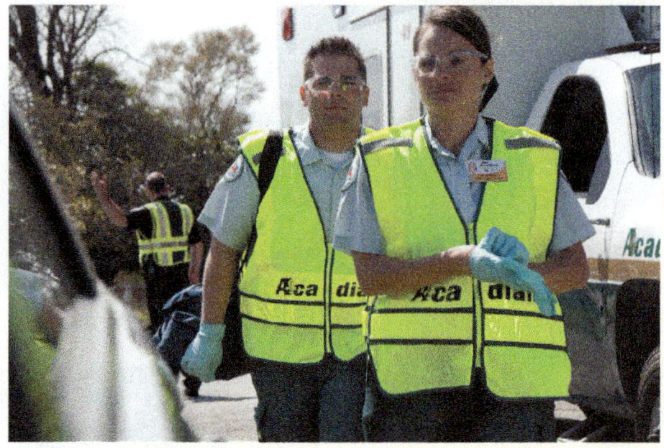

Take appropriate Standard Precautions.

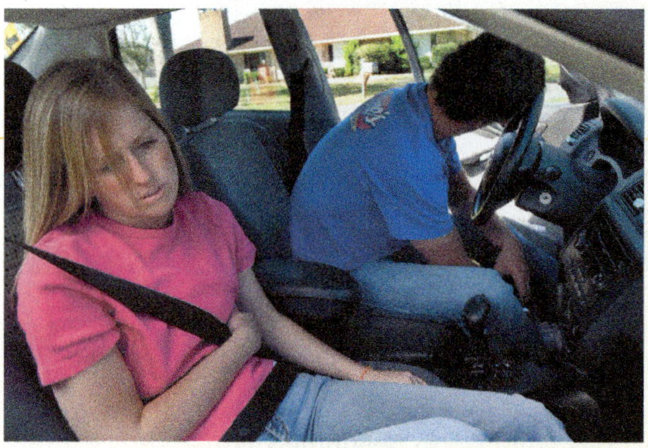

Determine number of patients.

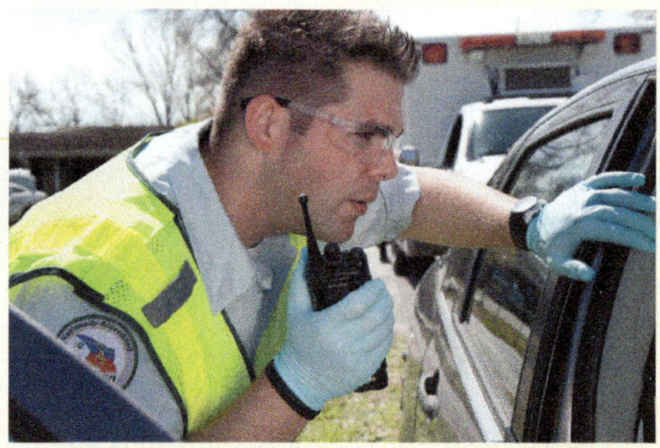

Radio for additional resources early.

"Call for help right away. If you wait, it will be too late."

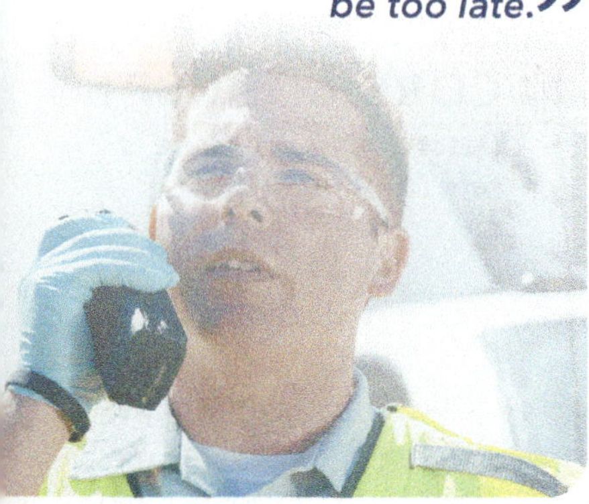

injury, and number of patients. The scene size-up begins even before the ambulance comes to a stop. Observe the scene while you approach and again before you exit the vehicle.

The following are scene size-up considerations you should keep in mind when you approach a crash or hazardous material emergency:

As you near the collision scene:

- Look and listen for other emergency service units approaching from side streets.
- Look for signs of a collision-related power outage, such as darkened areas, which suggest that wires are down at the collision scene.
- Observe traffic flow. If there is no opposing traffic, suspect a blockade at the collision scene.
- Look for smoke in the direction of the collision scene—a sign that fire has resulted from the collision.

When you are within sight of the scene (Figure 11-2):

- Look for clues indicating escaped hazardous materials, such as placards, a damaged truck, escaping liquids, fumes, or vapor clouds. If you see anything suspicious, stop the ambulance immediately and consult your hazardous materials reference book or hazardous materials team, if one is available. (See more information under Establishing the Danger Zone.)
- Look for collision victims on or near the road. A person may have been thrown from a vehicle as it careened out of control, or an injured person may have walked away from the wreckage and collapsed on or near the roadway.
- Look for smoke not seen at a distance.
- Look for broken utility poles and downed wires. At night, direct the beam of a spotlight or flashlight on poles and wire spans as you approach the scene. Keep in mind that wires may be down several hundred feet from the crash vehicles.
- Be alert for persons walking along the side of the road toward the collision scene. Curious onlookers are often oblivious to vehicles approaching from behind.
- Watch for the signals of police officers and other emergency service personnel. They may have information about hazards or the location of injured persons.

FIGURE 11-2 Your first sighting of the scene will give you many clues about the type and extent of injuries you may encounter. (A) Hurricane. (B) Fire. (C) Train wreck. (D) Suicide scene; note that suicide with toxic gas can create a grave danger for rescue workers. *((A) Terray Sylvester/REUTERS/Newscom; (B) CHINE NOUVELLE/SIPA/Newscom; (C) Alex Milan Tracy/Sipa USA/Newscom)*

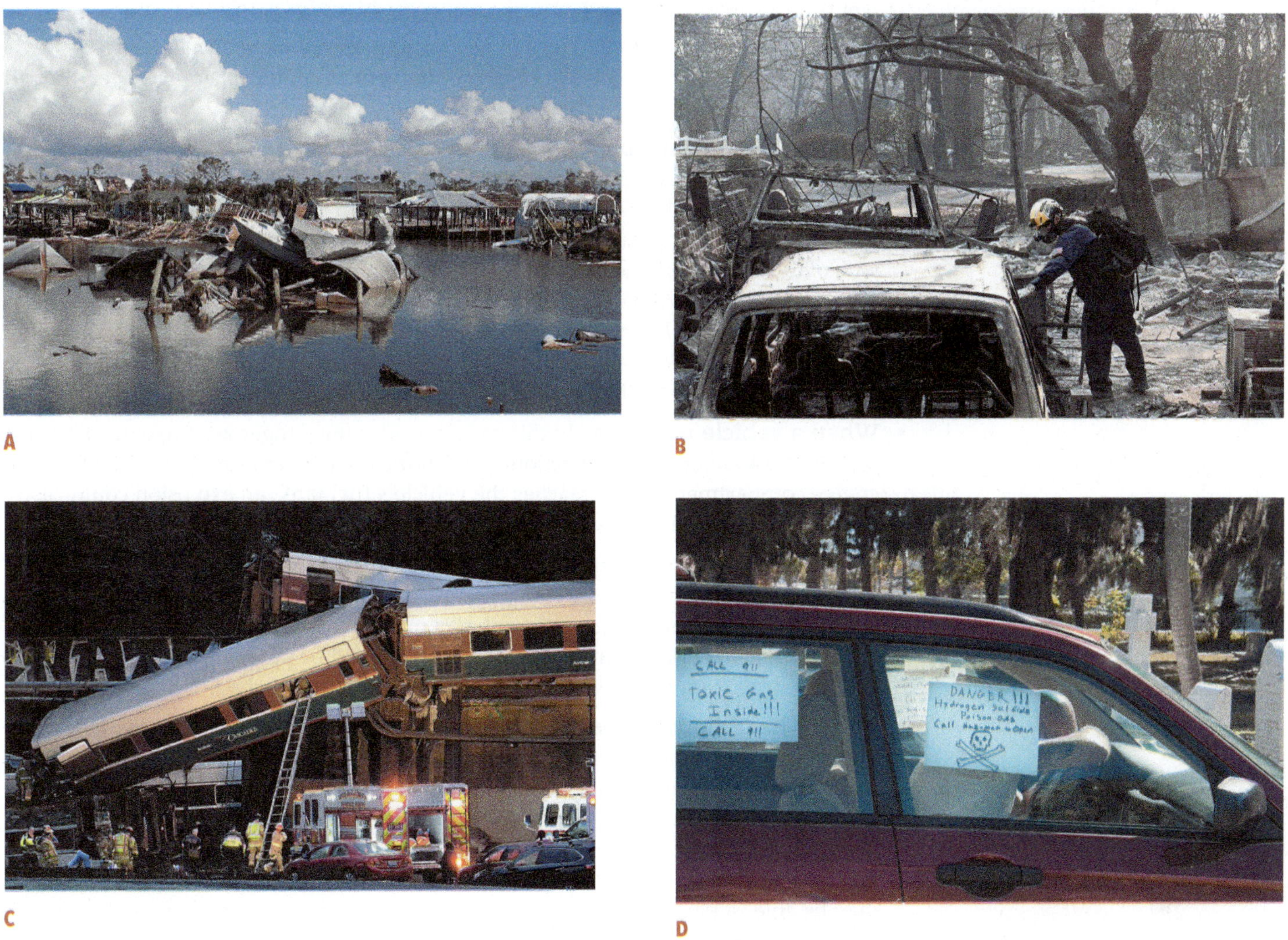
A
B
C
D
TOXIC Gas Inside!!!
CALL 911
DANGER!!!
Poison Gas

As you reach the scene:

- If personnel are at the scene and using the incident command/management system, follow the instructions of the person in charge. This may involve the positioning of the ambulance, wearing protective equipment and apparel, determining where to find the patients, or being aware of specific hazards. The Incident Commander (the responder responsible for the overall coordination of activities at the scene) may be able to provide you with lifesaving information regarding unstable conditions such as the stability of a building and the possibility of structural collapse.

  Don appropriate protective apparel, including head protection, a bunker coat (or similar clothing that will protect you from sharp edges), and an ANSI-approved reflective vest that goes over your coat. You should have extrication gloves easily available in a pocket. When temperature and weather are significant factors, be sure to protect yourself with clothing that will keep you dry and at the appropriate temperature.

  Sniff for odors such as gasoline or diesel fuel. Pay attention to any unusual odor that may signal a hazardous material release.

Establishing the Danger Zone

danger zone
the area around the wreckage of a vehicle collision or other incident within which special safety precautions should be taken.

A ***danger zone*** exists around the wreckage of every vehicle collision, within which special safety precautions must be taken. The size of the zone depends on the nature and severity of collision-produced hazards (Scan 11-1). An ambulance should never be parked within the danger zone. Follow these guidelines in establishing the danger zone:

- **When there are no apparent hazards.** In this case, consider the danger zone to extend at least 50 feet (15.2 meters) in all directions from the wreckage. The ambulance will be away from broken glass and other debris, and it will not impede emergency service personnel who must work in or around the wreckage. When using highway flares to protect the scene, make sure that the person igniting them has been trained in the proper technique.
- **When fuel has been spilled.** In this case, consider the danger zone to extend a minimum of 100 feet (30.4 meters) in all directions from the wreckage and fuel. In addition to parking outside the danger zone, park upwind, if possible. (Note the direction of the wind by observing flags, smoke, and so on.) Thus, the ambulance will be out of the path of dense smoke if the fuel ignites. If fuel is flowing away from the wreckage, park uphill as well as upwind. If parking uphill is not possible, position the ambulance as far from the flowing fuel as possible. Avoid gutters, ditches, and gullies that can carry fuel to the ambulance. Do not use flares in areas where fuel has been spilled. Use orange traffic cones during daylight and reflective triangles at night.
- **When a vehicle is on fire.** In this case, consider the danger zone to extend at least 100 feet (30.4 meters) in all directions, even if the fire appears small and limited to the engine compartment. If fire reaches the vehicle's fuel tank, an explosion could easily damage an ambulance parked closer.
- **When wires are down.** In this case, consider the danger zone as the area in which people or vehicles might be in contact with energized wires if the wires pivot around their points of attachment. Even though you may have to carry equipment and stretchers for a considerable distance, the ambulance should be parked at least one full span of wires away from the poles to which broken wires are attached.
- **When a hazardous material is involved.** In this case, check the *Emergency Response Guidebook (ERG)*—published by the U.S. Department of Transportation, Transport Canada, and the Secretariat of Communications and Transportation of Mexico—for suggestions as to where to park, or ask the Incident Commander to request advice from an agency such as CHEMTREC (Chemical Transportation Emergency Center, Washington, D.C.; 24-hour hotline 800-424-9300 or 703-527-3887). In some cases, you may be able to park 50 feet (15.2 meters) from the wreckage, as when no hazardous

SCAN 11-1 Establishing the Danger Zone

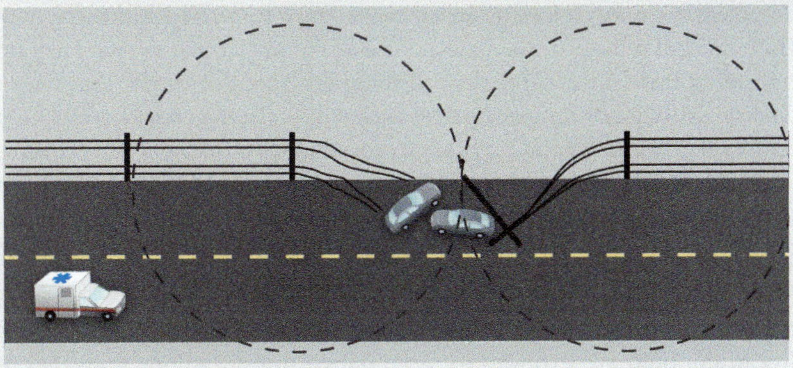

Downed Lines
In incidents involving downed electrical wires and damaged utility poles, the danger zone should extend beyond each intact pole for a full span and to the sides for the distance that the severed wires can reach. Stay out of the danger zone until the utility company has deactivated the wires, or until trained rescuers have moved and anchored them.

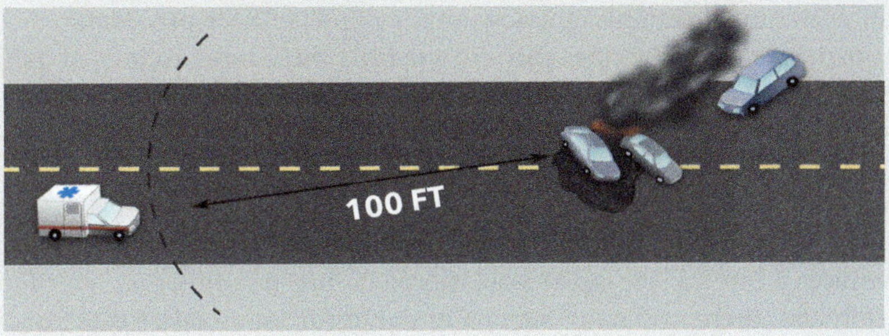

Vehicle on Fire
If no other hazards are involved, such as dangerous chemicals or explosives, the ambulance should park no closer than 100 feet (about 30 meters) from a burning vehicle. Park upwind.

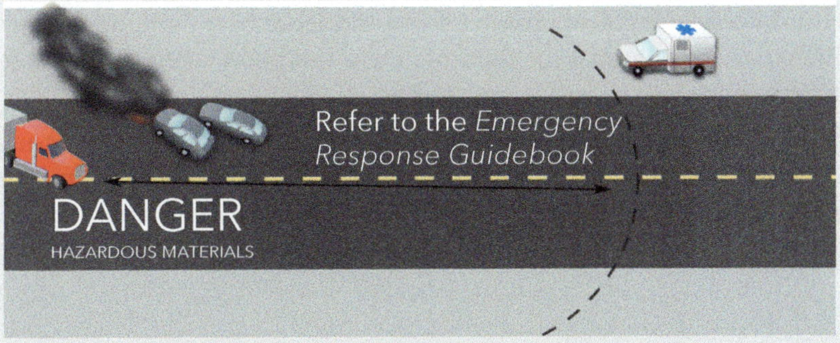

Hazardous Material Threatened by Fire
When hazardous materials are either involved in or threatened by fire, the size of the danger zone is dictated by the nature of the material. Use binoculars to read the placard on the truck and refer to the *Emergency Response Guidebook* for a safe distance to establish your command post. Park upwind.

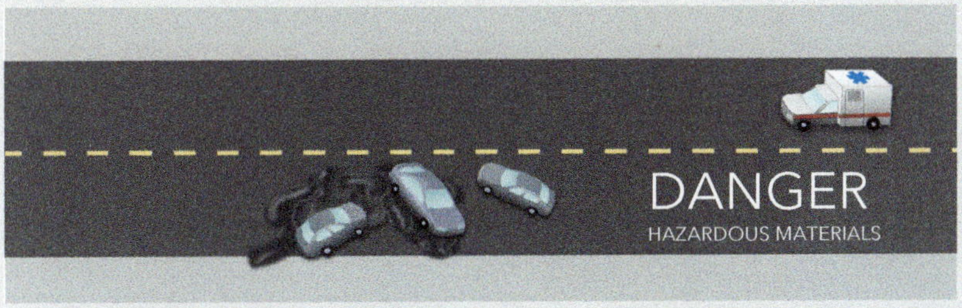

Spilled Fuel
The ambulance should be parked upwind from flowing fuel. If this is not possible, the vehicle should be parked as far from the fuel flow as possible, avoiding gutters, ditches, and gullies that may carry the spill to the parking site. Remember, your ambulance's catalytic converter is an ignition source over 1000 degrees Fahrenheit (538 degrees Celsius).

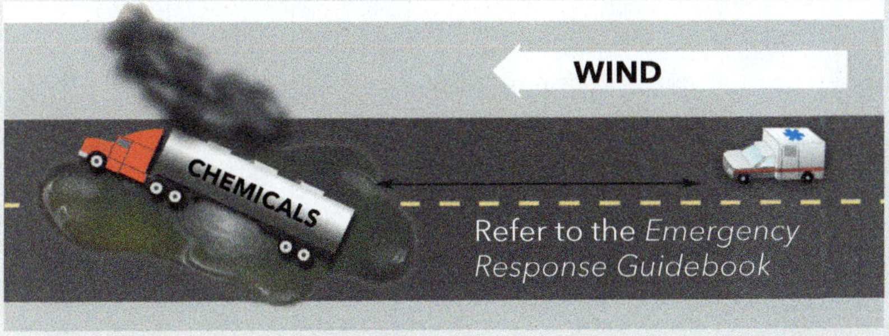

Hazardous Materials
Leaking containers of dangerous chemicals may produce a health as well as a fire hazard. When chemicals have been spilled, whether fumes are evident or not, the ambulance should be parked upwind. if the hazardous material is known, seek advice from experts such as CHEMTREC through the Incident Commander.

material has been spilled or released. In other cases, you may be warned to park 2000 feet (609.6 meters) or more from the wreckage, as when there is the possibility that certain high explosives may detonate. In all cases, park upwind from the wreckage when you discover that a hazardous material is present at a collision site. Park uphill if a liquid is flowing but on the same level if there are gases or fumes that may rise. Park behind some artificial or natural barrier if possible. (In the chapters *EMS Operations* and *Highway Safety and Vehicle Extrication*, you will learn more about parking the ambulance. In *Hazardous Materials, Multiple-Casualty Incidents, and Incident Management*, you will learn more about hazardous materials.)

Crime Scenes and Acts of Violence

Another significant danger faced by the EMT is violence. Crime risks vary, but it is certain that EMTs working in the field are exposed to more dangerous situations than they were even a few years ago. Shootings at elementary and secondary schools, colleges, and shopping malls, as well as terrorist incidents, are now on the minds of EMS providers.

Although a majority of calls go by uneventfully, the EMT must be conscious of dangers from many sources, including other human beings (Figure 11-3). EMTs often envision violence as occurring at bar fights or on the street, but domestic violence (violence in the home) is also a cause for concern.

Protection from violence is as important as protection from the dangers at a vehicle collision. As an EMT, you should never enter a violent situation to provide care. Safety at a violent scene requires a careful size-up as you approach. Just as a downed wire signals danger at a collision site, there are many signals of danger from violence that you may observe as you approach the scene, such as:

- **Fighting or loud voices.** If you approach a scene and see or hear fighting, threatening words or actions, or the potential for fighting, there is a good chance that the scene will be a danger to you.
- **Weapons visible or in use.** Any time you observe a weapon, you must use an extreme amount of caution. The weapon may actually be in the hands of an attacker (a grave danger) or simply in sight. Weapons include knives, guns, and martial arts weapons as well as any other items that may be used as weapons.

FIGURE 11-3 Crowds are a potential source of violence. *(Mark Ide/Science Source)*

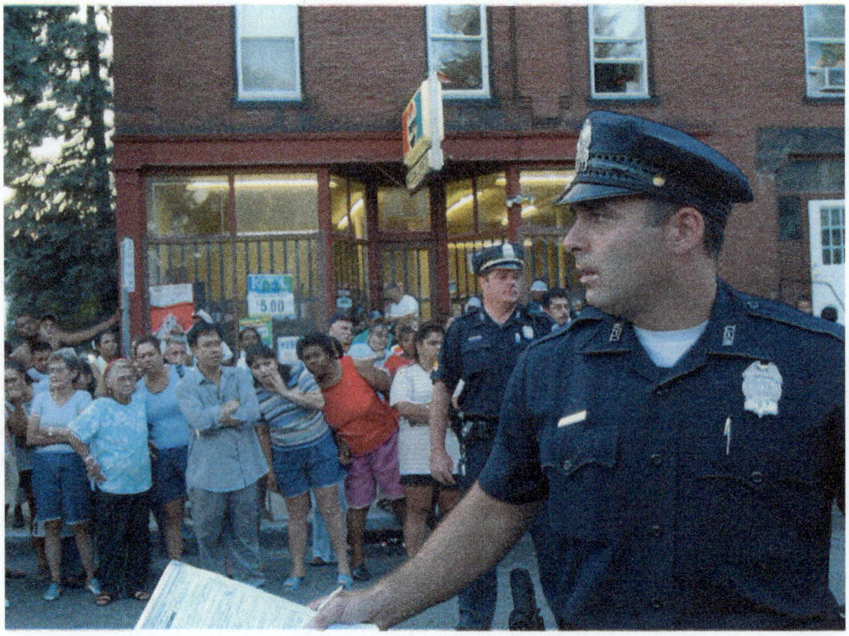

- **Signs of alcohol or other drug use.** When alcohol or other drugs are in use, a certain unpredictability exists at any scene. It will not take long for you to observe unusual behavior from a person under the influence of one of these substances. This behavior may result in violence toward emergency personnel at the scene. In addition, there are hazards associated with the drug culture, such as street violence and the presence of contaminated needles.
- **Unusual silence.** Emergencies are usually active events. A call that is "too quiet" should raise your suspicions. Although there may be a good reason for the silence, extra care should be taken.
- **Knowledge of prior violence.** If you or a member of your crew has been to a particular location for calls involving violence in the past, extra caution must be used on subsequent calls to the same location. Neighbors may sometimes volunteer information about previous incidents.

Whether the call is residential or in the street, observe the scene for the signs of danger listed previously and any others you may find (Figure 11-4). This brief danger assessment may be all that is required to prevent harm to you or your crew during the call.

If you observe signs of danger, there are actions that you must take to protect yourself. You learned about these actions in the chapter *Well-Being of the EMT*. The specific actions you should take depend on many factors, including your training, the type of danger, and the help available to you.

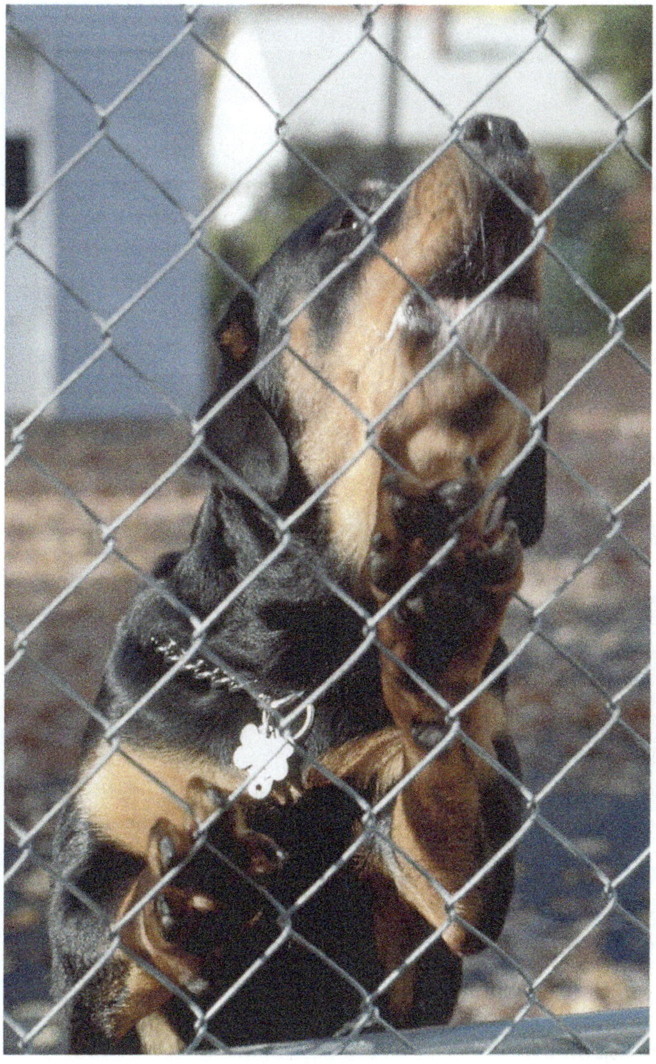

FIGURE 11-4 Whether the call is to a residence or to the street, a variety of hazards may be present.

Point of View

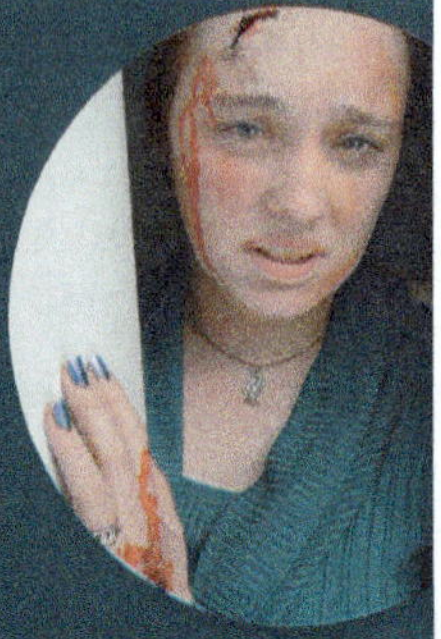

"I am still a relatively new EMT. Everyone always said you never know what you will find when you respond to a call. Well, I found out about this pretty early in my EMS career.

"My crew and I were sent to a 'fall' at a residence in a decent part of town. We pulled up to the house. Everything looked calm—but sometimes you just can't tell from the outside. We went to the door. We stood to the sides of the door like we were trained. We knocked. The woman came to the door, and she looked like she had been through a war. I started to move like I was going into the house, but she pushed the door closed a bit more and kind of peeked out. My first thought was to say, 'Come on. Let us in. We need to take care of you.' She put her weight behind the door and wouldn't let us in. Then it hit me. She didn't fall. Whatever had happened, she was trying to protect us.

"I asked her to step outside so we could talk but she refused. I motioned for my other crew members to get back to the rig and mouthed, 'Call for help.'

"I felt so helpless. I didn't want her to go back inside, but I was already on borrowed time and should be retreating. 'Come out here. Please!' I urged in a forced whisper. She looked behind her and then shut the door in my face.

"I moved rapidly to the rig, watching my back. We drove out of sight. Two police cruisers came by pretty quickly. I filled them in on what I had seen. They went to the scene. About five minutes later, the dispatcher radioed us to go back in. They had a man in handcuffs. The woman was crying. I'm still not sure whether she was crying because she was hurt or because he was arrested. The look in her eyes was so vacant.

"Always, always, always size up the scene. I always wonder what would've happened if I wasn't cautious going to that call."

There may be a time you will be able to safely rescue a patient from a burning vehicle before the engine compartment burns, or a situation where you are able to place a victim of violence in the ambulance and quickly leave the scene, but there will be other times you will have to make a difficult choice. You might determine that it is too risky to help a patient and that you must retreat from the scene, even if it has negative consequences for the patient. These situations present difficult choices.

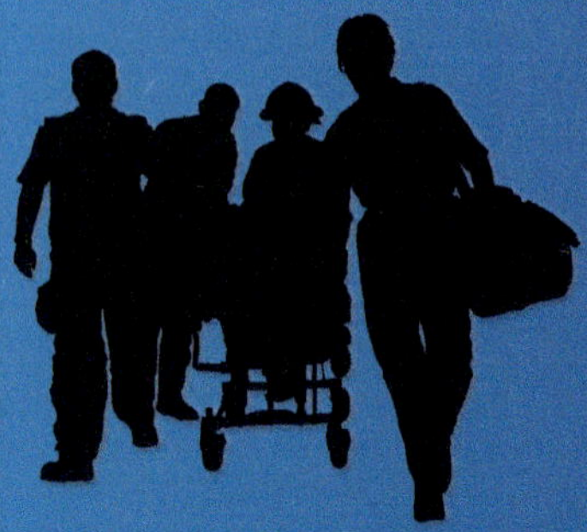

Think Like an EMT

Should I or Shouldn't I?

In each of the following situations, list some things you might consider when deciding whether to stay and help the patient or to retreat to a safe location.

1. A patient is inside a car that is on fire.
2. You are having lunch at a food truck when you hear shots ring out. Three men flee the scene and one man is down on the ground, bleeding.
3. While in the supermarket shopping for your crew's dinner, you hear screaming and someone shrieks, "OH MY GOD! SHE'S BEEN STABBED!"
4. You are in a city park and a child falls from a swing, striking his head on a rock. There is significant bleeding. You have no protective gloves.

Standard Precautions

As you perform your initial size-up of the scene, there are many important points to consider. One very important aspect of personal protection—and one that you will need long after you have addressed any physical dangers—is Standard Precautions, also called body substance isolation (BSI).

You learned about Standard Precautions and personal protective equipment (PPE) in the chapter *Well-Being of the EMT*. Body substances include blood, saliva, and any other body fluids or contents. All body substances can carry viruses and bacteria. Your patient's body substances can enter your body through cuts or other openings in your skin. They can also easily enter your body through your eyes, nose, and mouth. You are especially at risk of being infected by a patient's body substances when the patient is bleeding, coughing, or sneezing, or whenever you make direct contact with the patient, as in mouth-to-mouth ventilation. Infection is a two-way street, of course. You can also infect the patient.

For example, at a vehicle collision that is likely to have caused severe injuries with bleeding, all personnel should wear protective gloves and eyewear. Since this potential hazard can be spotted before there is any contact with the patient, everyone should be wearing gloves before beginning patient care. If a patient requires suctioning or spits up blood, this would be another indication for protective eyewear and a mask. Whenever a patient is suspected of having tuberculosis or another disease spread through the air, wear an N-95 or high-efficiency particulate air (HEPA) respirator to filter out airborne particles the patient exhales or expels.

A key element of Standard Precautions is always to have personal protective equipment readily available, either on your person or as the first items you encounter when opening a response kit. Remember that taking proper Standard Precautions early in the call and evaluating the need for such precautions throughout the call will prevent needless exposure later on.

Nature of the Call

After you have ensured scene safety and taken the appropriate Standard Precautions, it is important to determine the nature of the call by identifying the mechanism of injury or the nature of the patient's illness.

Mechanism of Injury

The ***mechanism of injury*** is what causes an injury (e.g., a rapid deceleration causes the knees to strike the dash of a car; a fall on ice causes a twisting force to the ankle) (Scan 11-2).

mechanism of injury
a force or forces that may have caused injury.

Certain injuries are considered common to particular situations. Injuries to bones and joints are usually associated with falls and vehicle collisions; burns are common to fires and explosions; penetrating soft-tissue injuries can be associated with gunshot wounds; and so on.

CORE CONCEPT

Mechanisms of injury and how they relate to patient condition

Even if you cannot determine the exact injury the patient has sustained, knowing the mechanism of injury may allow you to predict various injury patterns. For example, in many situations you will examine and possibly restrict movement of the patient's spine because of the mechanism of injury and your assessment. Knowing that the patient has fallen should suggest that you also check for an injured arm or leg.

Motor-Vehicle Collisions. Identifying the mechanism of injury is important when dealing with motor-vehicle collisions. Vehicles are safer than ever, with supplemental restraint systems (airbags, side impact curtains, and others) that can prevent serious injury—but these can cause some injuries themselves. Consider the following when an airbag has deployed:

- The airbag may have a nontoxic powder that will be found on the patient and in the car. If you arrive very quickly after the crash, you may see this powder in the air and mistake it for smoke.

SCAN 11-2 Mechanism of Injury and Affected Areas of the Body

MECHANISM OF INJURY

The force that produced the injury, its intensity and direction.

TYPES OF FORCE

- Direct
- Twisting
- Forced Flexion or Hyperextension
- Indirect

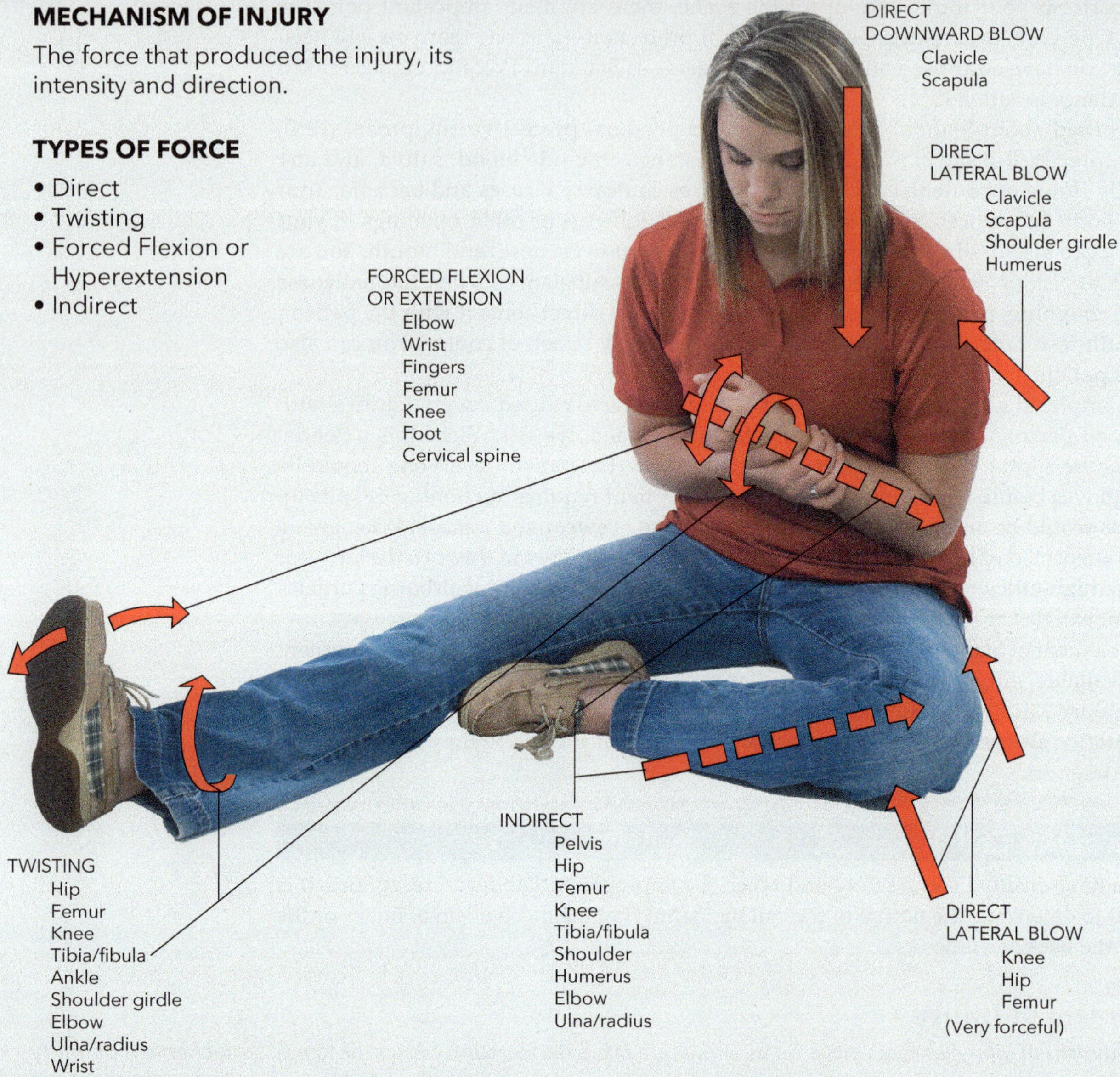

- The airbag itself may occasionally cause injuries. These may range from abrasions that occur during deployment to fractures of extremities that may have been in the path of the bag during deployment. (See Figure 11-5.)
- Airbags often cause damage to the windshield during deployment. Do not mistake this for damage done by the patient's striking the windshield.
- Air bags may deploy and turn objects in their path into projectiles. This is also relevant in the ambulance. Do not install or place items where they are in the path of airbag deployment.

While airbags and more efficient passenger restraint systems have dramatically reduced injuries in collisions, there are times when people don't use restraint systems (seat belt and shoulder harness) or they wear them improperly. It should also be noted that airbags only deploy once. If there are additional collisions in a crash after the airbag has deployed, the patient will not be protected. Some older vehicles may not have airbags or other modern safety systems.

In collisions where safety systems are not in place, or when multiple collisions occur, you may see telltale patterns of damage in the vehicle which relate to injuries on the patient. For example, a collapsed or bent steering column suggests that the driver has

FIGURE 11-5 (A) Facial impact of airbag in a child. (B) Fractured hand from airbag. *(Both: © Edward T. Dickinson, MD.)*

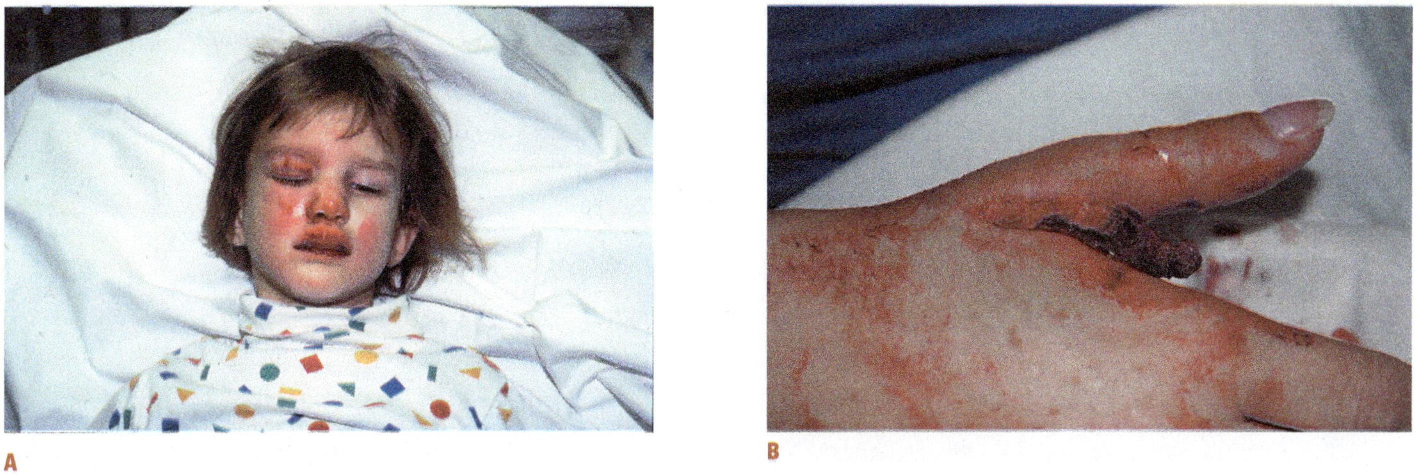

suffered a chest-wall injury with possible rib or even lung or heart damage. A shattered, blood-spattered windshield points to the likelihood of a forehead or scalp laceration and possibly a severe blow to the head that may have caused a head or spinal injury.

The law of inertia—that a body in motion will remain in motion unless acted upon by an outside force (e.g., being stopped by striking something)—explains why there are actually three collisions involved in each motor-vehicle crash. The first collision is the vehicle's striking an object. The second collision is when the patient's body strikes the interior of the vehicle. The third collision occurs when the organs of the patient strike surfaces within the body (Figure 11-6).

FIGURE 11-6 There are three collisions in a motor-vehicle crash: (A) a vehicle collision, when the vehicle strikes an object; (B) a body collision, when the person's body strikes the interior of the vehicle; and (C) an organ collision, when the person's organs strike interior surfaces of the body.

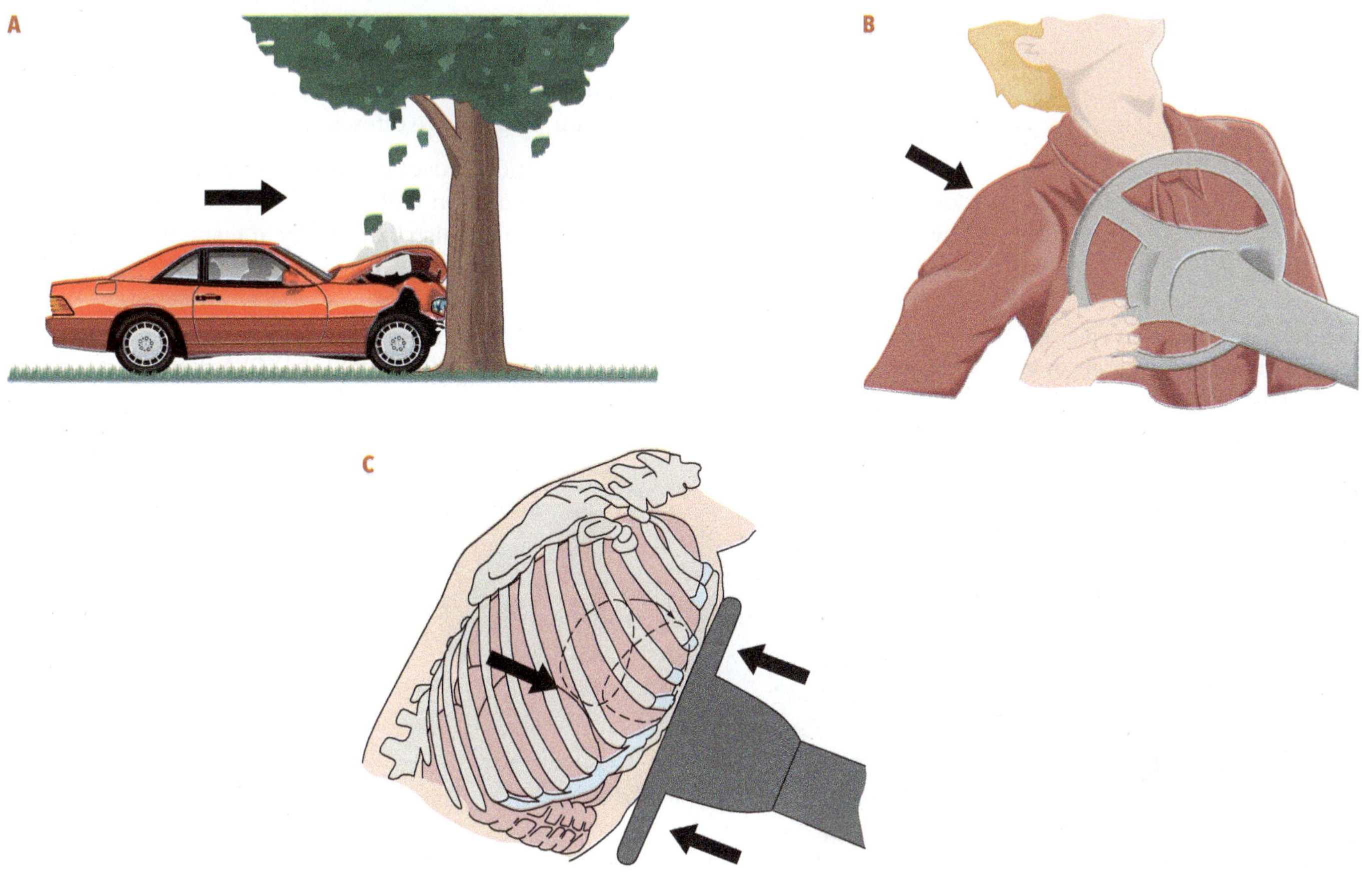

FIGURE 11-7 (A) A head-on impact. (B) Seatbelt neck and chest abrasions in a child. *((A) Kevin Link/Science Source; (B) © David Effron, MD)*

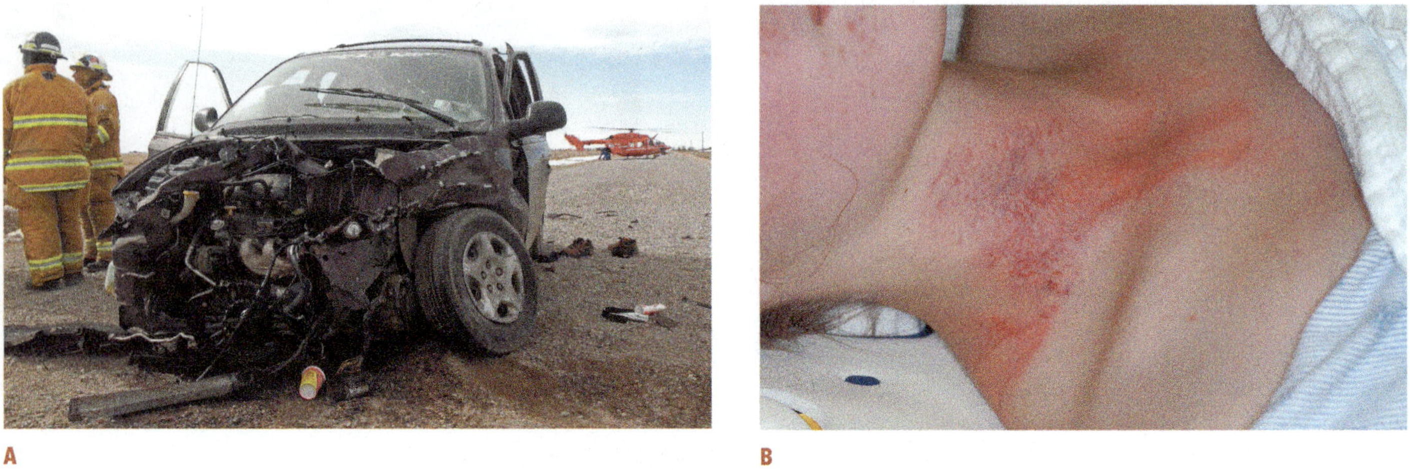

Identifying the type of motor-vehicle collision also provides important information on potential injury patterns:

- **Head-on collisions.** These have a great potential for injury to all parts of the body. Two types of injury patterns are likely: the up-and-over pattern and the down-and-under pattern. In the first pattern, the patient follows a pathway up and over the steering wheel, commonly striking the head on the windshield (especially when not wearing a seat belt), causing head and neck injuries. In addition, the patient may strike the chest and abdomen on the steering wheel, causing chest injuries or breathing problems and internal organ injuries. In the second pattern, the patient's body follows a pathway down and under the steering wheel, typically striking the knees on the dash, causing knee, leg, and hip injuries (Figure 11-7 and Figure 11-8).

  Airbags are designed to deploy in front-end impacts. Airbags have a significant role in the prevention of serious injury—and may actually cause some injuries, albeit minor, themselves. If an airbag has deployed, be sure to move the deflated bag so you can fully examine the steering wheel. Remember that airbags deploy only once. If there were subsequent impacts, an airbag would have offered no protection to the patient.
- **Rear-end collisions.** These are common causes of neck and head injuries. The law of inertia states not only that a body in motion will remain in motion unless acted on by an outside force (as discussed earlier) but also that a body at rest will remain at rest unless acted on by an outside force (such as being pushed or jerked). This explains why

FIGURE 11-8 In a head-on collision, an unrestrained person is likely to travel in (A) an up-and-over pathway causing head, neck, chest, and abdominal injuries or in (B) a down-and-under pathway causing hip, knee, and leg injuries. (C) A deploying airbag can also cause injuries.

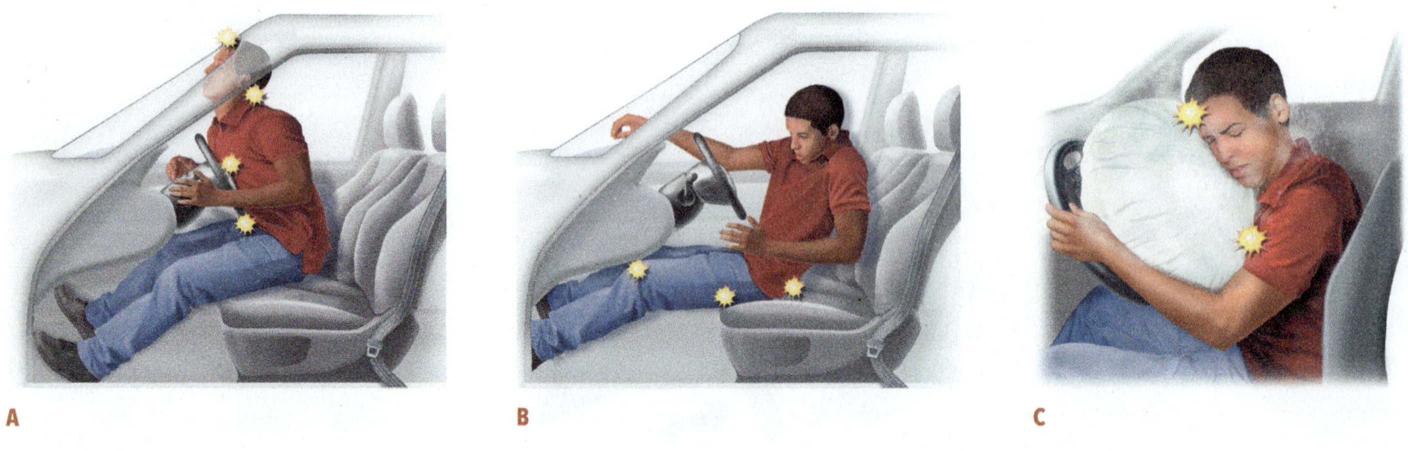

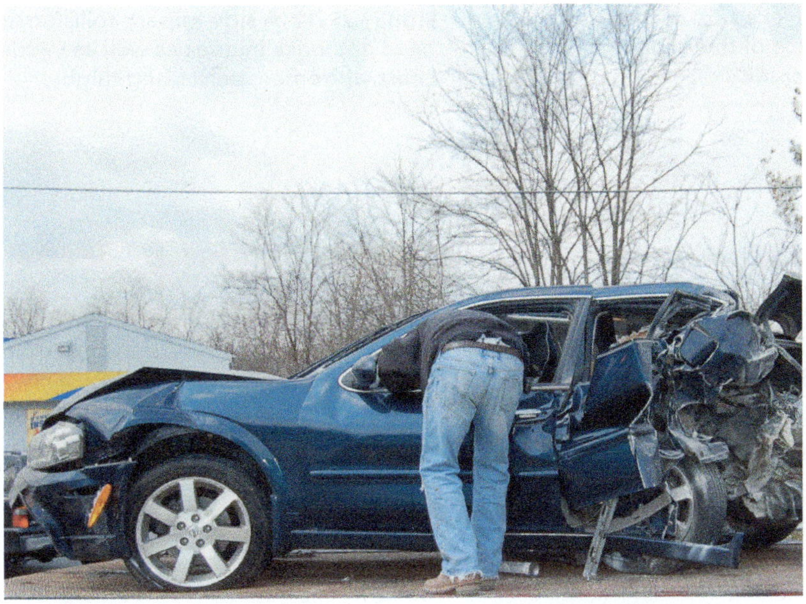

FIGURE 11-9 Rear impact.
(© Edward T. Dickinson, MD)

neck injuries are common in a rear-end collision—the head remains still as the body is pushed violently forward by the seat back, jerking the neck backward (if a headrest was not properly placed) and then forward (Figure 11-9 and Figure 11-10).

- **Side-impact collisions (broadside or "T-bone").** These collisions have other injury patterns. The head tends to remain still as the body is pushed laterally, causing injuries to the neck. The head, chest, abdomen, pelvis, and thighs may be struck directly, causing skeletal and internal injuries (Figure 11-11 and Figure 11-12). Many vehicles are now equipped with side-impact or side-curtain airbags, which are designed to protect occupants from side-impact collisions.
- **Rollover collisions.** These can be the most serious, because of the potential for multiple impacts. Rollover collisions frequently cause ejection of anyone who is not wearing a seat belt. Expect any type of serious injury pattern (Figure 11-13 and Figure 11-14).
- **Rotational impact collisions.** These involve cars that are struck and that then spin. The initial impact often causes subsequent impacts. (The spinning vehicle strikes another vehicle or a tree.) As in a rollover collision, this can cause multiple injury patterns.

FIGURE 11-10 In a rear-end collision, the unrestrained person's head is jerked violently (A) backward then (B) forward, causing neck, head, and chest injuries.

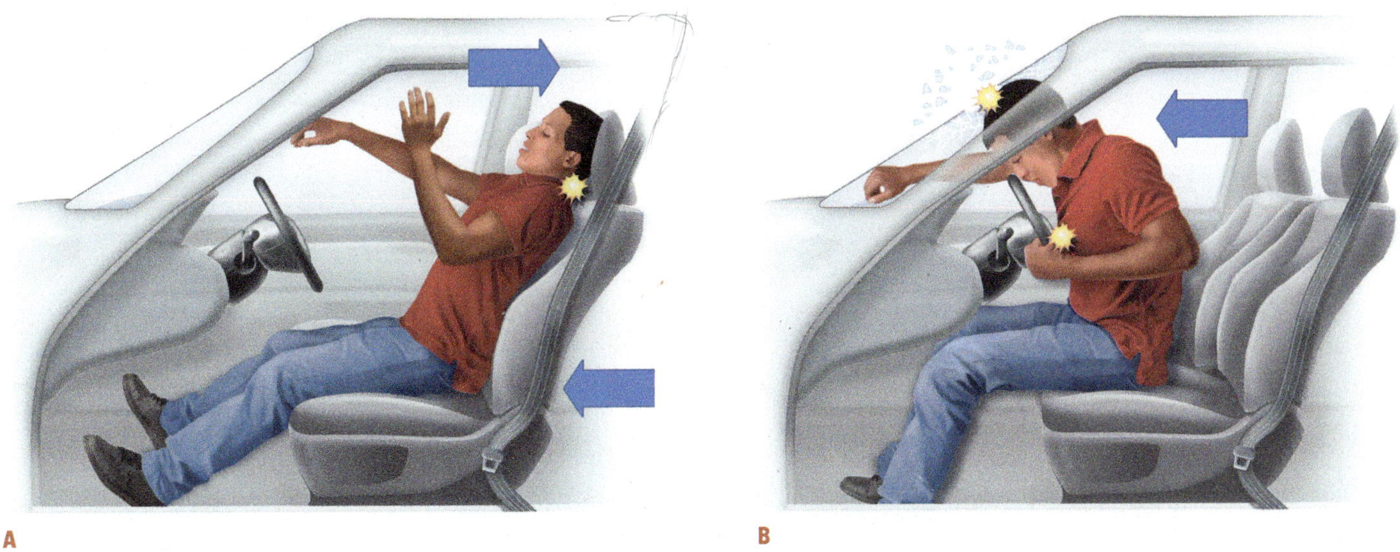

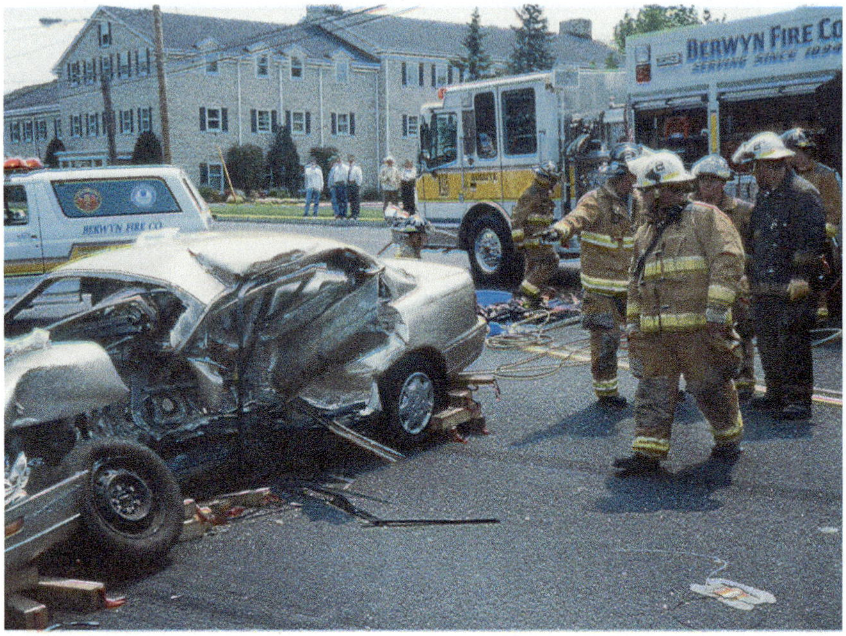

FIGURE 11-11 Side impact sustained to the driver's side of the car. In this crash, the driver would experience the force of the impact directly. Multiple injuries are likely. *(© Edward T. Dickinson, MD)*

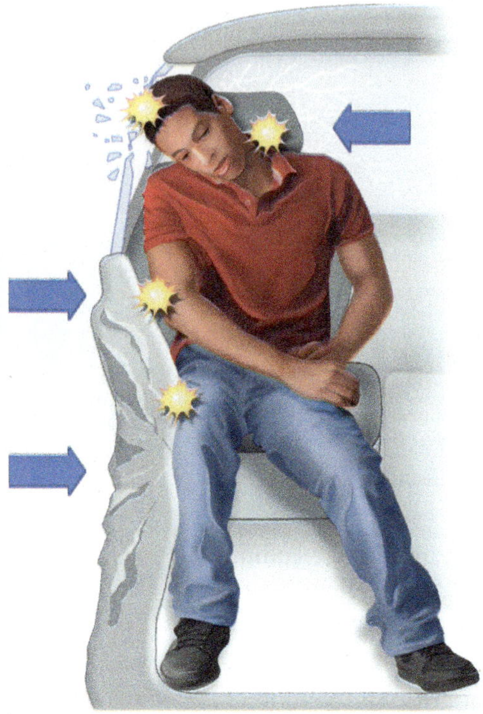

FIGURE 11-12 A side-impact collision may cause head and neck injuries as well as injuries to the chest, abdomen, pelvis, and thighs.

An important aspect of mechanism-of-injury determination is to find out where the patient was sitting in the vehicle, if lap and shoulder belts were used, and whether airbags deployed. Note any deformities in the steering wheel, dash, pedals, or other structures within the vehicle.

You will often be able to observe important clues regarding mechanism of injury before you even exit the ambulance. At a head-on collision, for instance, you can anticipate up-and-over or down-and-under injury patterns for a driver who remains in the car and multiple injury patterns for a driver who is thrown from the car. For either patient, anticipate external injuries (from the collision of the body with auto interiors and pavement)

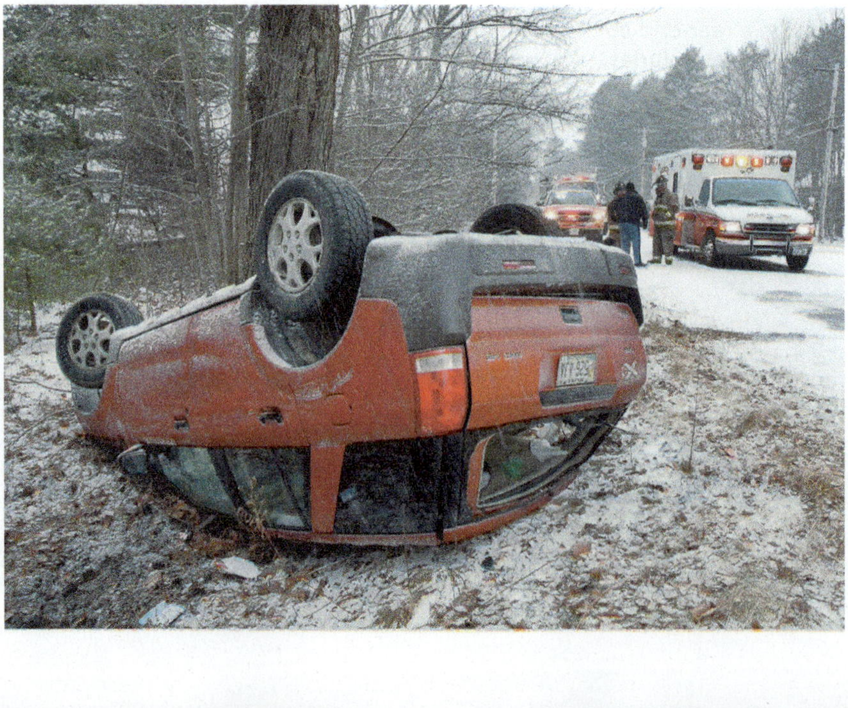

FIGURE 11-13 Rollover collision. *(© Daniel Limmer)*

FIGURE 11-14 In a rollover collision, the unrestrained person will suffer multiple impacts and possibly multiple injuries.

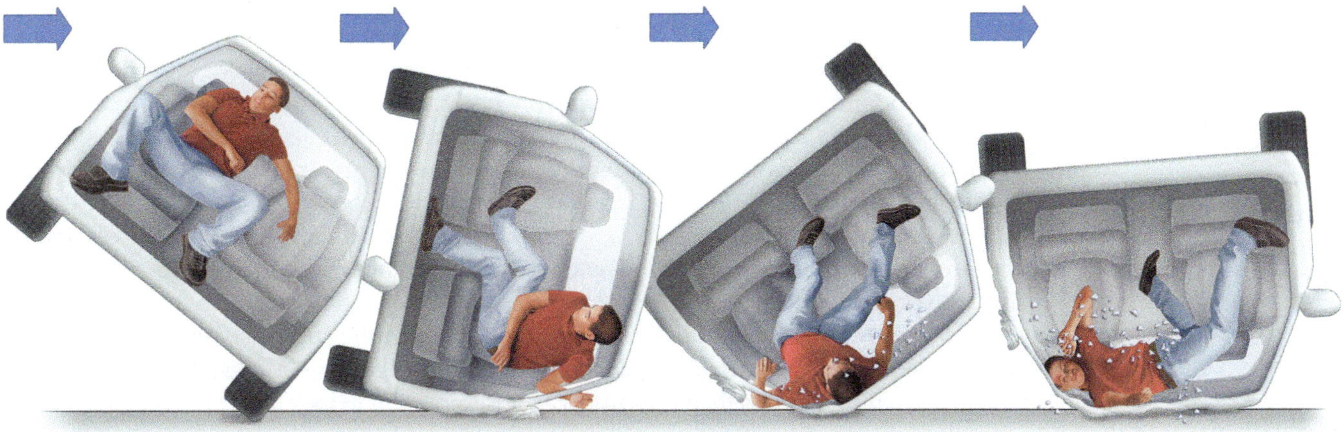

and internal injuries (from collision of organs with the interior of the body as well as from external blunt-force or penetrating trauma). When a patient appears to have been the driver of a vehicle, look for damage to the windshield, steering wheel, dash, and pedals when you are able to do a close-up inspection. You should also observe for damage to other interior surfaces, which might indicate there were additional passengers who might be patients.

Injuries involving motorcycles and all-terrain vehicles also have the potential to be serious. These vehicles offer the operator and passengers little protection in the event of a collision. Determine whether the patient was wearing a helmet that offered some protection from head injury. Also attempt to determine whether the patient was ejected. In some cases, the operator will be thrown from the bike, and will strike and severely injure hips, thighs, or legs.

Falls. Falls are another cause of injury where the extent and pattern of damage may be determined by the characteristics of the fall (Figure 11-15). Important factors to consider are the height from which the patient fell, the surface the patient fell onto, the part of the patient that hit the surface, and anything that interrupted the fall.

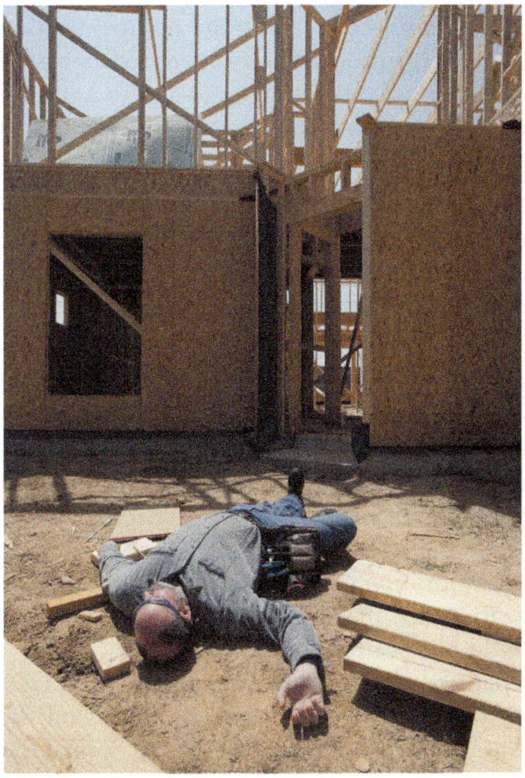

FIGURE 11-15 The characteristics of a fall may provide valuable clues to a patient's injuries.

In falls, injury to the part of the body that comes in contact with the ground or another hard surface is only the beginning of the trauma experienced by the patient. The force is also transmitted to adjoining parts of the body. For example, think of a person who dives into a shallow body of water and strikes the head. Although the head will be injured, the force travels on to the cervical and thoracic spine, very possibly resulting in severe spinal cord injury and paralysis. Similarly, when a patient jumps from a height and lands squarely on one or both feet, there is trauma to the feet but also to the ankles, legs, and even the pelvis. Always assess along the path of the energy. It is likely that you will find additional injuries.

The general guideline from the U.S. Department of Health and Human Services and the Centers for Disease Control and Prevention is that a fall of greater than 20 feet (6 meters) for an adult or greater than 10 feet (3 meters) for a child under age 15—or more than 2–3 times the child's height—is considered to be a severe fall for which transport to a trauma center is recommended. This is a reasonable guideline, but it doesn't guarantee a resulting injury (or rule out injury if the fall is less than this distance). It is important to look at all factors at the scene in combination with the patient's complaint, vital signs, and your physical examination findings. When in doubt, assign the patient a high priority for rapid packaging and prompt transport.

penetrating trauma
injury caused by an object that passes through the skin or other body tissues.

Penetrating Trauma. ***Penetrating trauma***, or injury caused by an object that passes through the skin or other body tissue, also has characteristics that may help in determining the extent of injury. These wounds are classified by the velocity, or speed, of the item that caused the injury. Low-velocity items are those that are propelled by hand, such as knives. Low-velocity injuries are usually limited to the area that was penetrated. Remember that there can be multiple wounds, and the blade may have been moved inside the patient, so there can be damage to multiple vital organs.

Medium-velocity wounds are usually caused by handguns. Some forcefully propelled items, such as an arrow launched from a compound bow or a ballistic knife, will also cause greater velocities than the same items propelled by hand.

Bullets propelled by a high-powered or assault-type rifle travel at a high velocity. Medium- and high-velocity injuries can cause damage almost anywhere in the body. Bullets cause damage in two ways (Figure 11-16):

- **Damage directly from the projectile.** The bullet itself will damage anything in its path. The damage depends on the size of the bullet, its path, and whether it fragments (breaks up into smaller projectiles), with the fragments taking different paths. The path of the bullet once it is inside the body is unpredictable, since it may be deflected by bone or other tissue onto a totally different course as it tumbles through the body. There is often damage to organs and tissues that are not in a straight line between the entrance and exit wounds.
- **Pressure-related damage, or cavitation.** This means that the energy of the bullet as it enters the body creates a pressure wave that causes a cavity considerably greater than the size of the bullet. This cavity is temporary, but it may damage items in its path.

blunt-force trauma
injury caused by a blow that does not penetrate the skin or other body tissues.

Blunt-Force Trauma. ***Blunt-force trauma*** is injury caused by a blow that strikes the body but does not penetrate the skin or other body tissues (e.g., when one is struck by a baseball bat or thrown against a steering wheel). The energy from a blunt-force blow will travel through the body, often causing serious injury to and even rupture of internal organs and vessels. The resulting compromise of body functions, hemorrhage, or spillage of organ contents into the body cavity may have more severe consequences for the patient than a penetrating injury. Yet signs of blunt-force trauma are often subtle and easy to overlook. The skin may appear reddened at the site of the blow, but in the prehospital setting, the bluish coloration characteristic of a bruise may not have had time to appear. Your main clue that such an injury may exist will often be the presence of a mechanism of injury that could have caused this kind of injury.

Identifying the mechanism of injury will help you, as an EMT, to determine what injuries are possible and to treat these injuries accordingly, even if signs and symptoms are not present. Never assume, based on the mechanism of injury, that there are no injuries. Even very minor collisions may cause injuries.

FIGURE 11-16 Bullets cause damage in two ways: from the bullet itself (A and C) and from cavitation, which is the temporary cavity caused by the pressure wave that is absorbed by the tissue (B).

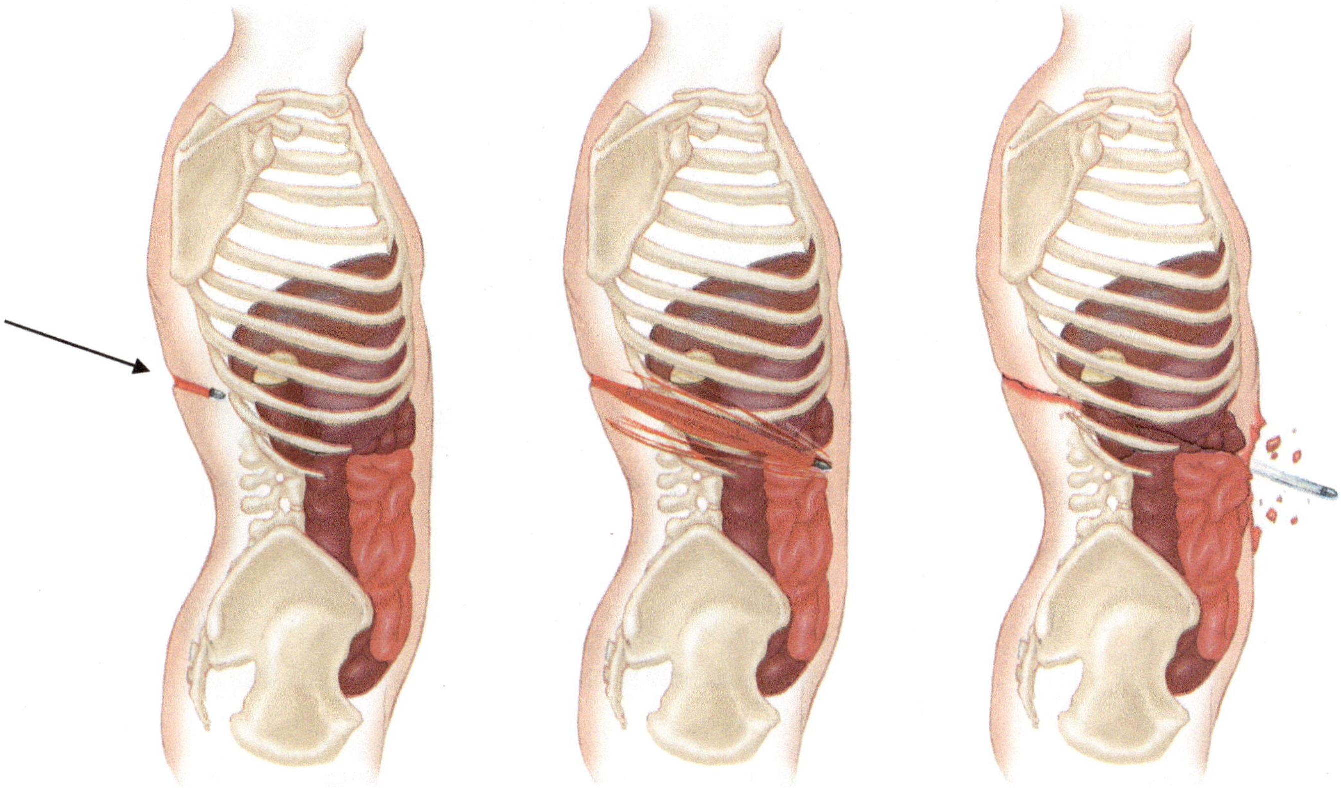

Maintain a high ***index of suspicion***—a keen awareness that there may be injuries—based on the mechanism of injury.

index of suspicion awareness that there may be injuries.

Nature of the Illness

Identifying the ***nature of the illness*** for a medical patient serves the same purpose as identifying the mechanism of injury for a trauma patient: finding out what is or what may be wrong with the patient. To begin identifying the nature of a patient's illness during the scene size-up, you must scan the entire scene. Information may be obtained from many sources:

nature of the illness what is medically wrong with a patient.

- **The patient.** When conscious and oriented, patients will be a prime source of information about their condition throughout the assessment process.
- **Family members or bystanders.** These people can also provide important information, especially for the unconscious patient. Even when patients are conscious and able to tell you about their condition, always consider the information from others who are present. Patients who are disoriented or confused may provide information that is either partially true or even untrue. Use information from all sources to piece the patient assessment puzzle together.
- **The scene.** While you are sizing up the scene for safety, make note of other factors that may be clues to the patient's condition. You may observe medications, which you will make a mental note to examine later. You may be struck by dangerous or unsanitary living conditions for this particular patient. This is important to note and mention to the emergency department personnel later.

Number of Patients and Adequacy of Resources

CORE CONCEPT
Determining what additional assistance may be needed at a scene

The final part of the scene size-up is determining if you have sufficient resources to handle the call. If, for example, you noted at a two-car collision that there were at least two patients—one driver still in the car and the other thrown to the pavement—you would immediately request an additional ambulance. As you approach the scene, you should

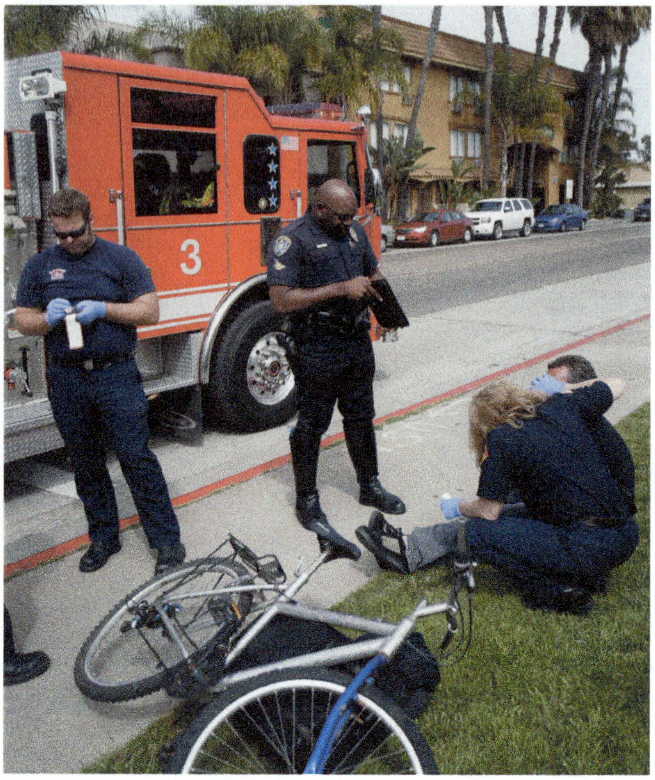

FIGURE 11-17 Actively look for any additional patients, such as pedestrians or cyclists. *(Kevin Link/ Science Source)*

actively look for clues that there may be additional patients—other passengers or pedestrians involved in the collision (Figure 11-17)—and if so, you should immediately call for additional ambulances.

Sometimes you may discover a need for additional resources even in a situation that, at first, would not seem to require them. For example, you may not feel that a single-patient medical call could tax your resources, but consider the following scenarios where you may find yourself needing extra help:

- Your ambulance is called to respond to an elderly woman with chest pain. You are greeted at the door by her husband, who does not look well. He denies any complaints but is sweaty and holding his chest. Your first patient tells you that her husband has a heart condition.
- A single patient experiences back pain. This is usually not a reason for additional assistance, but this patient is in a third-floor apartment (with no elevator) and weighs 425 pounds (193 kilograms).
- Your ambulance is called for a patient with "general weakness." Upon the arrival of yourself and your partner, two more persons in the same family develop the same flulike symptoms. You appropriately suspect carbon monoxide poisoning, since they admit that they have been having furnace problems.

In each of these situations, what appeared to be a routine one-patient call actually turned out to be more. An important part of scene size-up is to recognize these situations and call for help immediately. As the call progresses and you get more involved in patient care, it is less likely that you will remember to call for the additional help. It may also be too late when the help arrives if you do not call immediately.

Your response can range from simply calling for another ambulance to care for the ill husband in the first situation, or extra personnel to help move the 425-pound (193-kg) man in the second, to activating a multiple-casualty incident for the family with carbon monoxide poisoning. (You will learn about multiple-casualty incidents in *Hazardous Materials, Multiple-Casualty Incidents, and Incident Management*.) Try to anticipate the maximum numbers of patients and radio for help accordingly. Follow local protocols.

Think Like an EMT

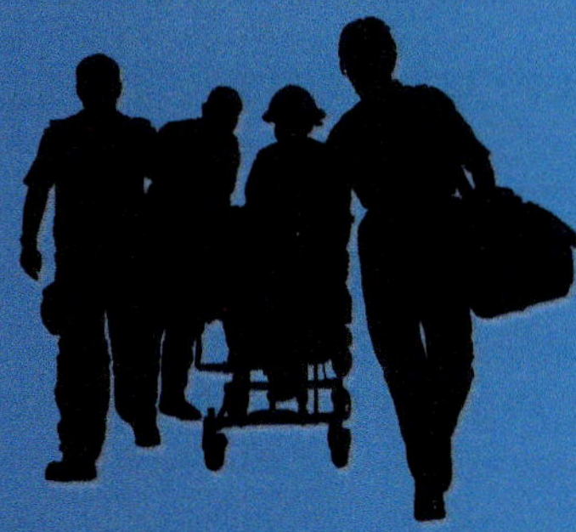

Determining Areas of Concern at the Scene

The scene size-up is a vital part of any call. For each of the following scenes, determine a few areas of concern you would want to check before proceeding to the patient. Remember each of the components of the scene size-up. You shouldn't try to think of every possibility, only the most likely ones. Practice the critical thinking process of evaluating a scene–something you will do on every call.

1. An 18-wheeler with an enclosed trailer slid off the road into a ditch in an ice storm. The vehicle is in the ditch, leaning to the right.
2. A van and a passenger car collided on an interstate highway.
3. You arrive at an office building and see people running out the front and side doors in a panic. One person appears bloody and is running toward your ambulance.
4. You respond to a residence with the fire department and arrive on scene first. A resident meets you at the end of the driveway and tells you there is a strong smell of natural gas in the house.
5. You respond to a construction site for a fall.

Chapter Review

Key Facts and Concepts

- Scene size-up is the first part of the patient assessment process.
- It is important during scene size-up to determine what, if any, threats there may be to your own safety and to the safety of others at the scene, then to take appropriate Standard Precautions.
- Next, it is important to determine the nature of the call by identifying the mechanism of injury or the nature of the patient's illness.
- Finally, you must take into account the number of patients and other factors at the scene to determine if you will need additional help.

Key Decisions

- Is it safe to approach the scene?
- What precautions should my crew and I take to protect ourselves at the scene?
- What personal protective equipment should I put on, and what should I have available?
- Can I safely access or help a patient, or is it too dangerous?
- What does the scene suggest about the mechanism of injury?
- What is the nature of illness?
- How many patients are present, and what additional assistance should I call for?

Chapter Glossary

blunt-force trauma injury caused by a blow that does not penetrate the skin or other body tissues.

danger zone the area around the wreckage of a vehicle collision or other incident within which special safety precautions should be taken.

index of suspicion awareness that there may be injuries.

mechanism of injury a force or forces that may have caused injury.

nature of the illness what is medically wrong with a patient.

penetrating trauma injury caused by an object that passes through the skin or other body tissues.

scene size-up steps taken when approaching the scene of an emergency call: checking scene safety, taking Standard Precautions, noting the mechanism of injury or nature of the patient's illness, determining the number of patients, and deciding what, if any, additional resources to call for.

Preparation for Your Examination and Practice

Short Answer

1. For each of the following dangers, describe actions that must be taken to remain safe at a collision scene.
   - Leaking gasoline
   - Toxic or hazardous material spill
   - Vehicle on fire
   - Downed power lines
2. List several indicators of violence or potential violence at an emergency scene.
3. Describe several situations where it is appropriate to wear disposable gloves. Describe situations where you would also wear protective eyewear and mask. Describe situations where you would wear an N-95 or HEPA respirator.
4. Describe common mechanism-of-injury patterns.
5. List sources of information about the nature of a patient's illness.
6. List several medical and trauma situations where you may require additional assistance.

Thinking and Linking

Use the information you learned in earlier chapters to answer the following questions:

1. You respond to a head-on collision of two automobiles late at night. There are no apparent fluids leaking, no smoke involved, no wires down, and no abnormal smells. What PPE should you put on as you exit the ambulance? What PPE should you have available close by, in case it is needed?
2. A patient has stab wounds to the lower anterior ribs and lower posterior ribs. What organs are most at risk of injury from the different wounds?
3. As you are assessing an alert passenger in a car that was hit from behind, you suddenly smell smoke. What technique should you use to remove the patient from the vehicle?
4. You responded to a call with possible domestic violence. Because the scene did not appear to be safe, you did not go into the house, but retreated and called for police assistance. Another EMT says that you committed abandonment when you did that. What is your response?

Critical Thinking Exercises

You can and should start planning your scene size-up en route, on the basis of dispatch information. The purpose of this exercise will be to apply this skill in the following situation.

You are called to the scene of a shooting at a fast-food restaurant. En route, you plan your scene size-up strategy. What actions do you anticipate taking on arrival?

Pathophysiology to Practice

The following questions are designed to assist you in gathering relevant clinical information and making accurate decisions in the field.

1. A patient has stab wounds to the anterior lower ribs and the lower posterior ribs. What organs are most at risk of injury from the wounds located:
   - In the lower left lateral ribs?
   - In the lower right lateral ribs?
   - In the lower posterior ribs on either side?
2. Would any of your answers change if you discovered that the patient was in the fetal position, in a defensive posture, when stabbed?

Street Scenes

It is the middle of the night, and you are hoping to get a few hours of sleep. You are just getting relaxed when the monitor activates. "Ambulances Bravo 5 and Delta 2 with heavy rescue to the Avenue A off-ramp for Interstate 55 to the report of a two-vehicle crash."

You are the first EMS responder to arrive, and as you approach the scene, you see both vehicles: one a passenger vehicle, the other a truck with a placard. As you do a scene size-up, you try to get the "big picture." You are concerned about where to stage your ambulance because of traffic, safety of crews, possible gasoline leaking, and not knowing what the placard on the truck identifies. You notify the dispatcher that you are on the scene and request that the Highway Patrol be notified for traffic-control assistance. You find a location upwind about 100 yards (about 91.5 meters) from the scene. You place warning markers to alert traffic and to mark the staging area for other responding units. You are putting on your turnout gear with helmet, goggles, and gloves, including a reflective vest, when heavy rescue arrives. You talk with the captain, who tells you that the heavy rescue crew will stabilize the vehicles and handle the battery disconnects and gasoline leaks. You point out the placard that needs to be checked out.

Street Scene Questions

1. What other scene size-up issues are left to consider?
2. Is this scene now safe, or do other precautions need to be taken?
3. What Standard Precautions should be considered?

The crew from heavy rescue approaches the scene, stabilizes the vehicles, and motions you forward. The Highway Patrol has closed off traffic, and the captain from heavy rescue tells you that there is no hazardous material concern. On scene, you determine that the drivers were the only occupants of the vehicles. You check one patient and, at the same time, your partner checks the other. Your patient has significant facial cuts and bruises, and complains of leg pain. You realize that the extrication gloves you are wearing will not provide the proper Standard Precautions, so you put proper disposable gloves on immediately. After you try unsuccessfully to open the driver's-side door next to your patient, you realize that heavy rescue is required. The captain has already alerted the rescue crew, and they are almost ready to use pry tools. You learn that your partner's patient is conscious and alert with no specific complaints.

Street Scene Questions

4. When the second ambulance arrives, where should it be located in relation to the collision scene?
5. What precautions should you take to protect the patients from any further harm while they are being extricated from the vehicles?
6. How should you plan to make sure that you can safely get the patient from the scene to the ambulance?

As heavy rescue finishes getting their tools ready, you set a protective cloth over your patient. You explain what is being done and stay close for reassurance. While this is going on, the second ambulance arrives and parks close to the second collision vehicle, and the crew takes over patient care. Your ambulance is relatively far away, so you ask your partner to bring it closer to prevent having to carry your patient a long distance. This makes packaging the patient for transport safer and easier. The remainder of the call is uneventful, with both patients transported safely to the hospital emergency department.

12 Primary Assessment

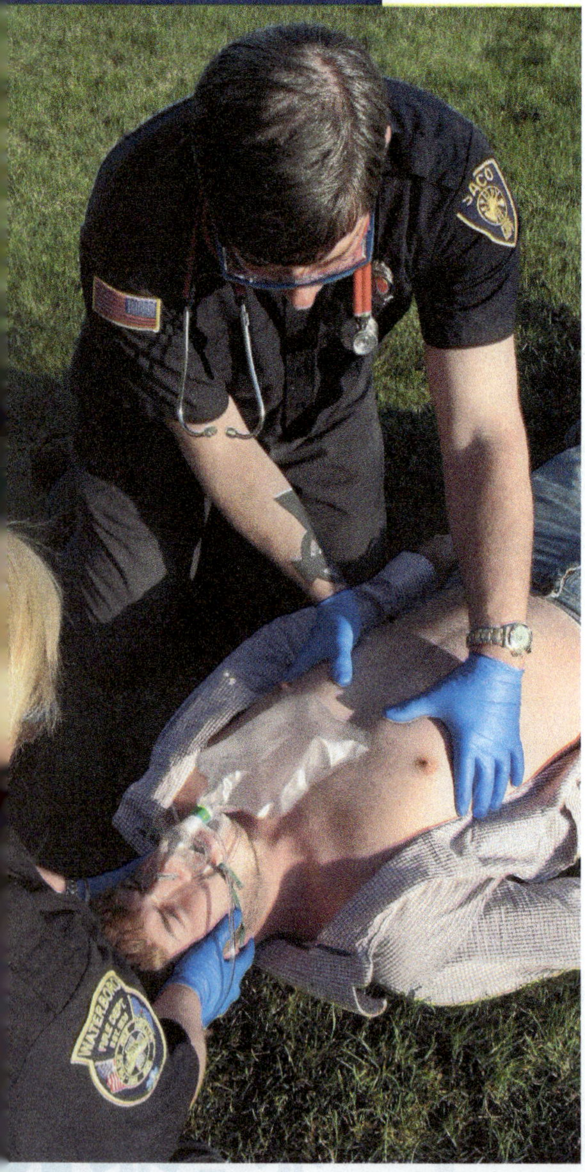

(© Daniel Limmer)

Related Chapters

The following chapters provide additional information related to topics discussed in this chapter:

Standard

Assessment (Primary Assessment)

Competency

Applies scene information and patient assessment findings (scene size-up, primary and secondary assessments, patient history, and reassessment) to guide emergency management.

Core Concepts

- Deciding on the approach to the primary assessment
- Manual stabilization of the head and neck when necessary
- The general impression
- Assessment of mental status using the AVPU scale

- Identifying and treating problems with the airway, breathing, and circulation
- Making a priority decision

Outcomes

After reading this chapter, you should be able to:

12.1 Summarize the general approach to primary assessment. (pp. 314–321)

- Describe the components of the primary assessment.
- Describe why the steps of primary assessment are ongoing.
- Given a scenario, determine the sequence of the primary assessment steps.
- Describe the actions to be taken upon finding specific problems during the primary assessment.
- Compare the approaches to stable, potentially unstable, and unstable patients.
- Describe the concept of manual stabilization of the head and neck.

12.2 Summarize the specific components of the primary assessment. (pp. 321–329)

- Given a description of mental status, categorize a patient's status using the Alert/Verbal/Painful/Unresponsive (AVPU) approach.
- Given a description of primary assessment findings, categorize the patient as stable, potentially stable, or unstable.

12.3 Explain the concept of clinical judgment applied to the primary assessment. (pp. 330–334)

- Explain the evolution of clinical judgment from novice to expert EMTs.
- Explain how observations can modify the EMT's interpretation of the chief complaint.
- Analyze a primary assessment.

Key Terms

A-B-Cs, *322*
AVPU, *321*
chief complaint, *321*
general impression, *318*
interventions, *315*
manual stabilization, *318*
mental status, *321*
primary assessment, *314*
priority, *327*
spinal motion restriction, *318*

The primary assessment is a key part of patient care. Not only is it the first time you physically reach your patient, it is the time when you will be called to identify and take immediate action for problems that can kill your patient. You may be called to suction a patient's airway or to perform CPR. You may also be called on to identify subtle signs of shock early so that the patient can quickly be taken to appropriate care. While you are doing these critical interventions, you will also be getting a solid idea of your patient's overall condition. Is it serious or not? This impression will help you make decisions as you continue your assessment.

If the primary assessment could be boiled down to one sentence, it would be this: Quickly and efficiently identify and treat any threats to your patient's life.

CORE CONCEPT

Deciding on the approach to the primary assessment

primary assessment
the first element in a patient assessment; steps taken for the purpose of discovering and dealing with any life-threatening problems. The six parts of primary assessment are: (1) forming a general impression, (2) assessing mental status, (3) assessing airway, (4) assessing breathing, (5) assessing circulation, and (6) determining the priority of the patient for treatment and transport to the hospital.

The Primary Assessment

The ***primary assessment*** is the portion of the patient assessment during which you will focus exclusively on life threats—specifically those that interfere with airway, breathing, and circulation. This chapter deals with this vital part of the assessment process. You may also hear the primary assessment referred to as the *primary survey* or *initial assessment*. It is always the first element in the total assessment of the patient.

Approach to the Primary Assessment

As an EMT, you will see many different patients with varied medical and traumatic conditions. The primary assessment can—and should—vary depending on several factors that include the patient's condition, how many EMTs are on the scene, and other priorities you determine as you assess your patient.

Although it may seem easiest to assume that you will assess each patient in A-B-C order (airway, breathing, circulation), this is not necessarily the case for all patients. In your CPR course, you were taught a C-A-B (circulation [compressions], airway, breathing) approach to the first steps in your assessment of a patient who appears lifeless and has no pulse. In short, you will perform your primary assessment in the way your patient needs it most.

Consider the following patient conditions and situations:

- You are called to a responsive patient who dropped a concrete block on his foot and is in considerable pain.
- You are eating in a restaurant and observe a man with what appears to be a complete airway obstruction.
- You arrive at the side of a patient who had passed out and is now moaning. She has vomited.
- You are called for a "man down" and see a person on the ground who does not appear to be moving or breathing.
- You are called for an industrial accident and find a woman who looks pale, sweaty, and about to pass out. She has blood spurting from her thigh.

In the responsive patient who dropped a block on his foot, you will perform a primary assessment, but little action will be required. The other patients will require you to perform many vital actions. The man who is choking needs to have his airway cleared as a first priority. The woman who passed out is in immediate need of suction. The "man down" will likely need CPR. For this patient, compressions and defibrillation are your first priorities. The woman with spurting blood is essentially bleeding to death. In this case you must immediately take action to stop the bleeding.

Remember that you will not be alone on an ambulance. Professional rescuers (EMTs are included in this category) will often work in a team environment in which multiple tasks may be accomplished immediately and simultaneously. In this case, there is no need to wonder whether you should open the airway first or stop the bleeding first, because both may be done at the same time. It is also possible that a friend, family member, or even the patient may be able to help control bleeding while you do other important tasks.

Decision Making in the Primary Assessment

The mnemonic *A-B-C* can help you remember the things you have to do in the primary assessment but not the exact order in which you must perform them. To determine exactly what you will do and in what sequence during the primary assessment, there are certain general considerations you will take into account.

- Any vomit in the airway that enters the lungs is very serious and often fatal. The stomach contents contain solids that may obstruct the airway, as well as strong acids that can cause irritation within the airway. Some patients are saved by defibrillation but later die because of aspiration pneumonia or pneumonitis. *It is a vital component of the primary assessment to suction the airway as soon as needed and before ventilating.*

- Exsanguinating (very severe, life-threatening) bleeding must be stopped immediately. Damage to major vessels, especially arteries, can cause death extremely rapidly from bleeding. *Life-threatening bleeding must be controlled immediately.*
- Breathing and circulation are obviously vital for life. You must make sure your patient is breathing and breathing adequately to support life. *In cases where there appears to be no breathing or only very occasional, ineffective breaths (agonal breathing), you should check for a pulse and begin CPR if necessary.*
- If immediate interventions such as bleeding control or CPR are not required, you will shift into an important but less urgent mode in which you will administer oxygen appropriate for the patient's condition and evaluate for shock.

Again, the order in which these interventions are performed depends on the patient's specific condition and the number and priority of the urgent conditions just listed that you are presented with. Remember: Multiple EMTs can accomplish multiple priorities simultaneously.

Performing the Primary Assessment

Keep in mind that the first steps of the primary assessment will depend on your initial impression of the patient. As already noted, if the patient shows signs of life, you will begin to work through the A-B-Cs in an order dictated by your patient's priorities. If the patient appears lifeless—that is, not moving and apparently not breathing—you will take a different course of action and shift toward resuscitation, beginning with chest compressions and preparation of the defibrillator if the patient is pulseless. (Review Figure 12-1.)

The primary assessment is generally considered to have six parts (See Visual Guide to Primary Assessment):

- Forming a general impression
- Assessing the patient's mental status (and manually stabilizing the patient's head and neck, when appropriate)
- Assessing the patient's airway
- Assessing the patient's breathing
- Assessing the patient's circulation
- Determining the patient's priority

CORE CONCEPT

Stabilization and protection of the trauma patient's head and neck when appropriate

NOTE: *If, during the primary assessment, you discover any life-threatening condition, you must immediately perform the appropriate* ***interventions*** *(actions to correct those problems).*

interventions actions taken to correct or manage a patient's problems.

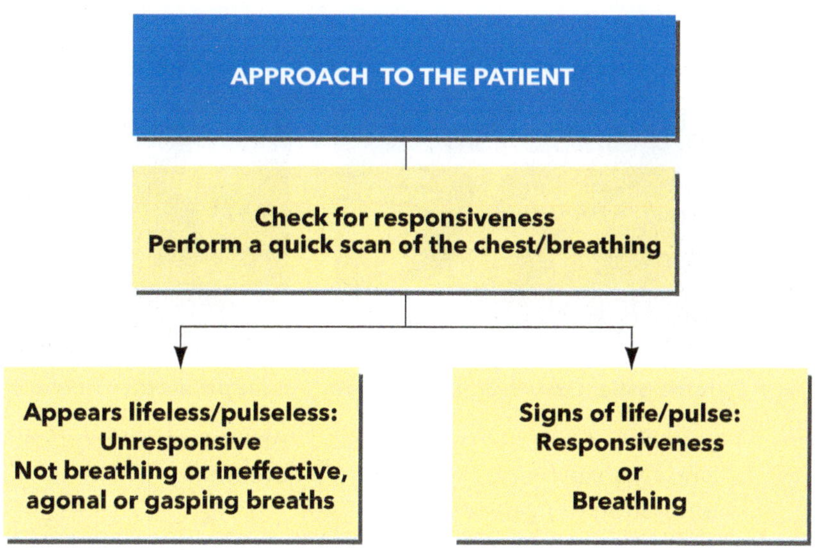

FIGURE 12-1 First approach to the patient: determining if the patient appears lifeless or if the patient has signs of life.

12 Primary Assessment

Identify and Treat Life Threats

GENERAL IMPRESSION: *Chief Complaint and AVPU*

Key Decision:

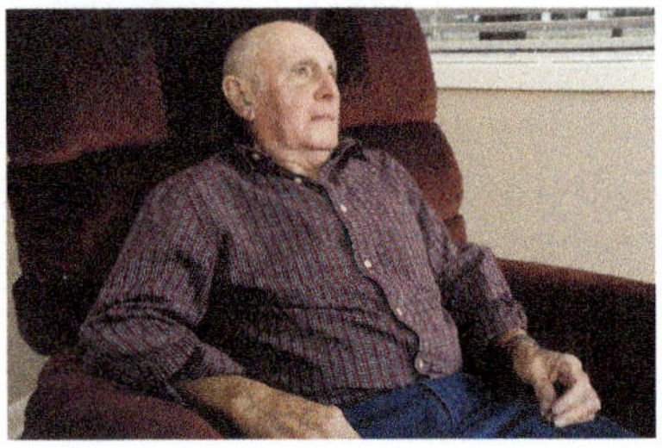

How does the patient look?

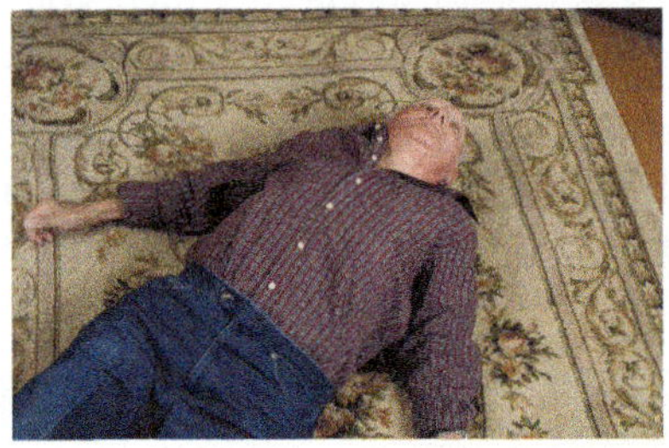

If the patient is apparently lifeless (no breathing or agonal breathing), go directly to a pulse check and the C-A-B approach.

You may perform **airway**, **breathing**, and **circulation** in any order.

This is dependent on the patient's presentation and emergent needs. Multiple parts of the primary assessment can be performed simultaneously when more than one EMT is present.

AIRWAY

Key Decision:

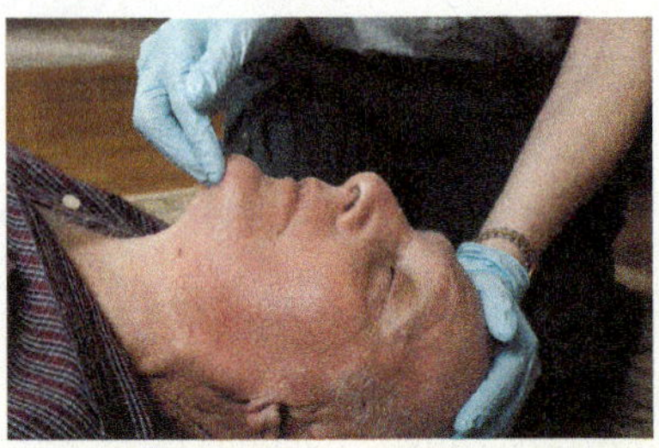

Open the airway.

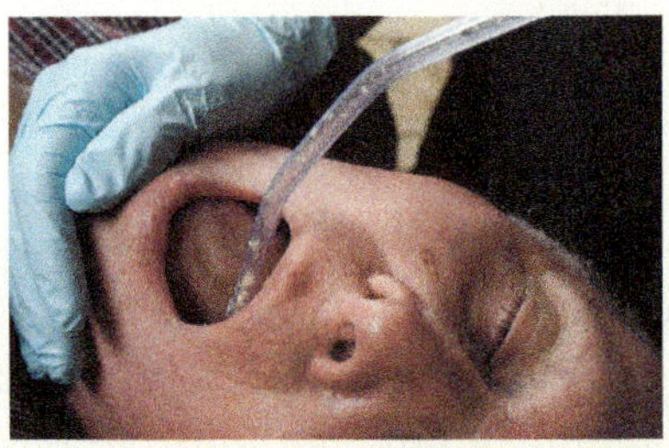

Suction if necessary.

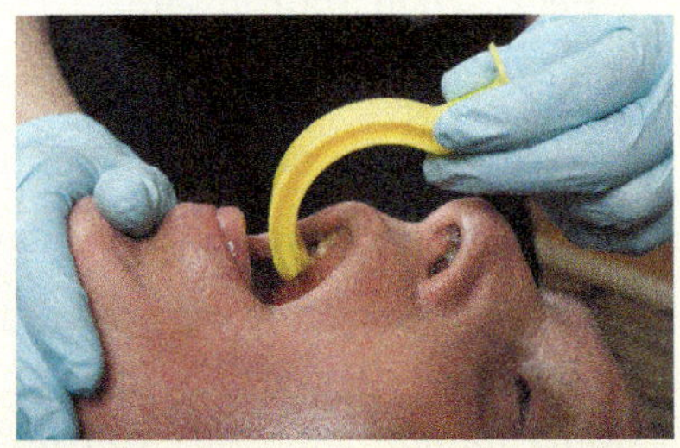

Place an oral or nasal airway if indicated.

BREATHING

Key Decision:

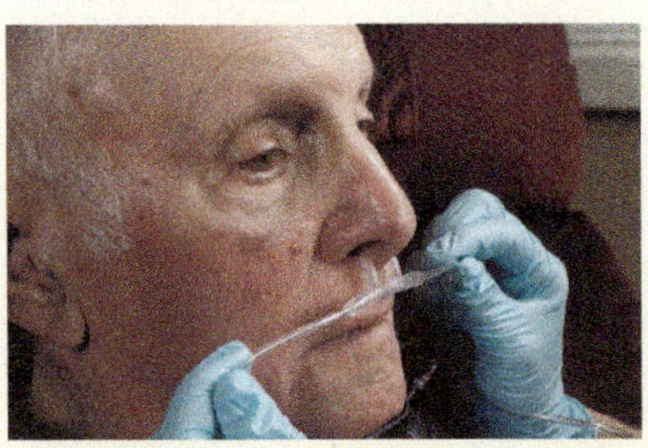

Is the patient breathing?

Oxygen saturation readings below 94%

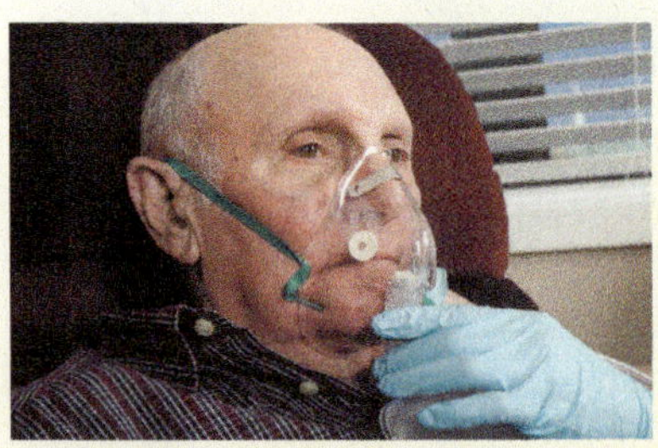

Is the patient breathing adequately?

Significant respiratory distress and hypoxia (very low oxygen saturation or cyanosis)

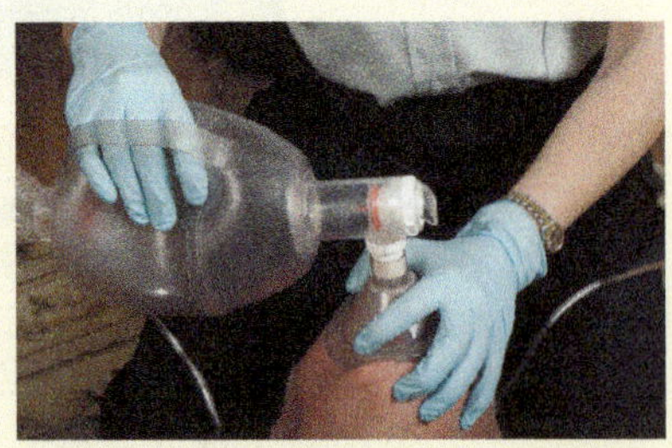

Is the patient hypoxic?

Absent or inadequate breathing

CIRCULATION

Key Decision:

Does the patient have a pulse?
Does the patient have signs of shock?
Does the patient have life-threatening bleeding?

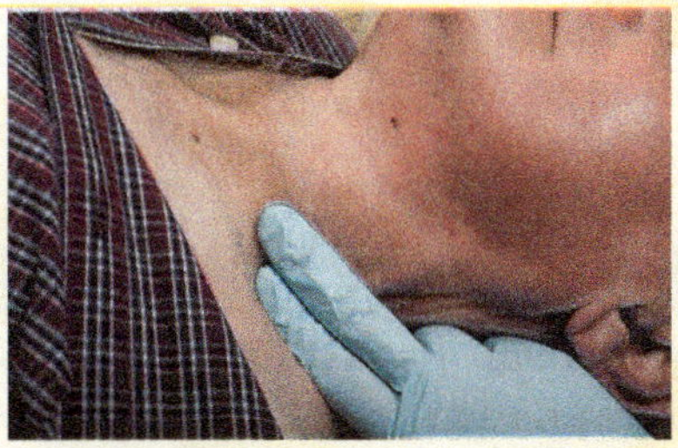

Unresponsive

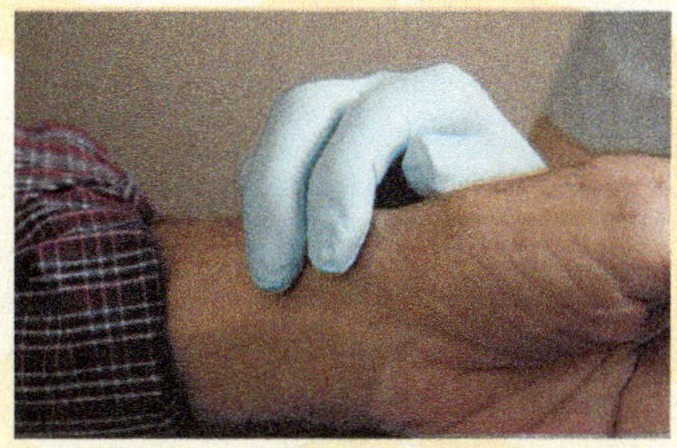

Responsive

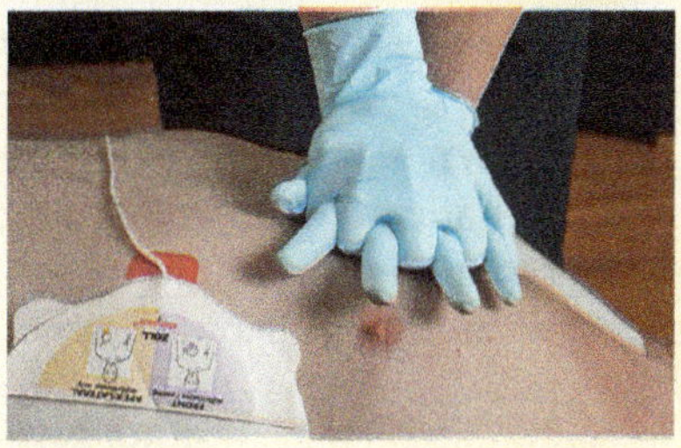

If pulseless, perform CPR and apply defibrillator.

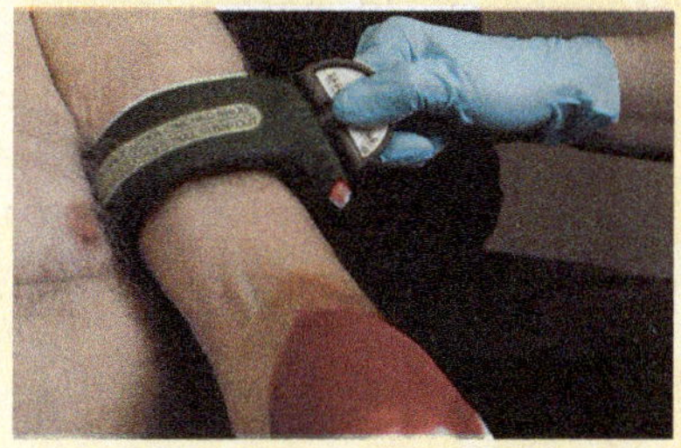

Control life-threatening bleeding. Treat for shock.

PRIORITY DETERMINATION

Key Decision:

How do I handle this patient from this point on?

Stable: slower pace, more detailed secondary examination

Potentially unstable: expedite transport, fewer assessments and interventions on scene

Unstable: rapid transport, only lifesaving assessment and interventions on scene

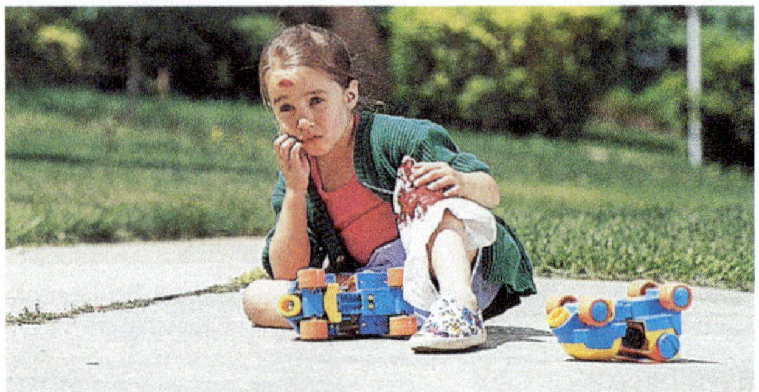

FIGURE 12-2 Forming a general impression includes your immediate assessment of the environment and the patient's chief complaint and appearance.

Form a General Impression

general impression impression of the patient's condition that is formed on first approaching the patient, based on the patient's environment, chief complaint, and appearance.

CORE CONCEPT
The general impression

Forming a ***general impression*** helps you to determine how serious the patient's condition is and to set priorities for care and transport. It is based on your immediate assessment of the environment and the patient's chief complaint and appearance (Figure 12-2).

The environment can provide a great deal of information about the patient. It frequently offers clues—to the EMT who looks for them—about the patient's condition and history. One of the most important things the environment can sometimes tell you is what happened. Is there an overturned ladder, indicating that the patient may have fallen? Has the patient been exposed to a cold outdoor environment for a long time? Or is there no apparent mechanism of injury, leading you to presume that the patient has a medical problem rather than trauma (an injury)? Although the EMT cannot rely completely on the patient's environment to rule out trauma, when combined with the chief complaint (e.g., the patient complaining of symptoms that sound more like a medical problem than an injury), environmental clues become extremely useful.

Beginning Spinal Motion Restriction

spinal motion restriction a procedure for limiting movement of the head, neck, and spine when spinal injury is possible or likely

manual stabilization using one's hands to prevent movement of a patient's head and neck until a cervical collar can be applied.

Spinal motion restriction (SMR) is a procedure in which you restrict movement of the head, neck, and spine when spinal injury is possible or likely. In this early part of your patient assessment, your primary concern will be to treat the patient's life-threatening conditions while not aggravating a potential spine injury.

You should apply this initial spinal motion restriction to the head and neck on first contact with any patient you suspect may have an injury to the spine based on mechanism of injury, history, or signs and symptoms. You will continue it throughout the call unless a physical examination determines it is not necessary.

When you apply the initial SMR, your object is to hold the patient's head still in a neutral, in-line position. This is called ***manual stabilization*** of the head and neck (Figure 12-3).

FIGURE 12-3 Manual stabilization of the head and neck. (A) When your patient is sitting up, position yourself just behind the patient and hold the patient's head by spreading your fingers over the sides of the head and placing your thumbs behind the ears. (B) When your patient is supine, kneel behind the patient and spread your fingers and thumbs around the sides of the patient's head to hold it steady.

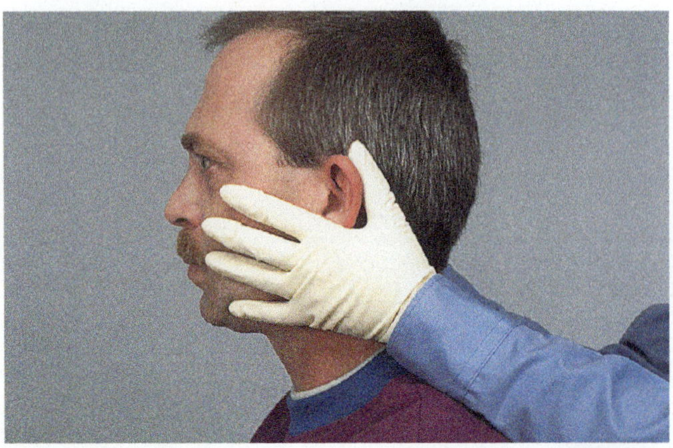

A

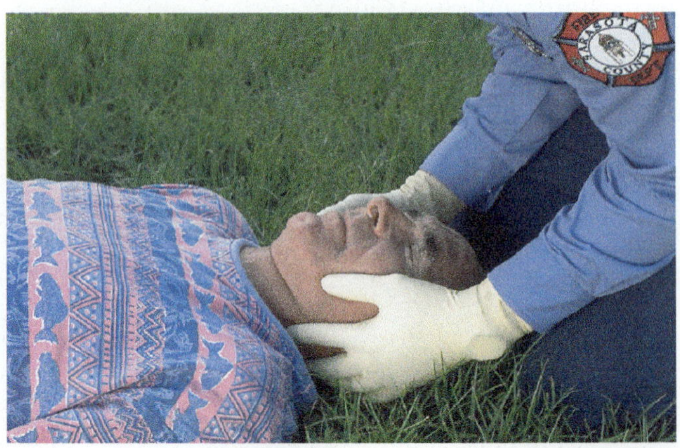

B

The head should be facing forward and not be turned to either side or tilted forward or backward. You must be careful not to pull or twist the patient's head but rather to hold it still and to remind the patient not to try to move it.

If your patient is in another position (for example, crumpled on one side) or is being moved by other EMS personnel, adapt the technique to the best of your ability to hold the head in a steady position in line with the spine. When the patient is finally moved to a supine position, more traditional manual stabilization may be performed.

There are times when you are at a scene alone, when there are multiple patients, or when the patient has serious injuries that require your attention (and your hands). You may find you need to ventilate a patient, and you are having trouble doing so while maintaining motion restriction of the head and neck. In these cases, spinal motion restriction is not the highest priority.

If you are alone and are treating a patient who needs airway maintenance, ventilation, or bleeding control, you should perform those tasks and minimize motion of the head and neck as best you can. Likewise, the American Heart Association acknowledges that it can be difficult to ventilate a patient using the jaw-thrust technique. If you are unable to ventilate while maintaining motion restriction, some movement of the spine may be necessary to ventilate effectively.

Remember that there may be more than one way to restrict motion of the spine during the primary and secondary assessments. Patients who are experiencing neck pain often self-splint and naturally restrict movement. You may instruct a responsive patient not to move the head and neck. This may be done by instructing the patient to maintain the nose on the same imaginary line as the umbilicus (belly button) at the center of the body until manual stabilization may be initiated, and a cervical collar is placed.

EMS systems have specific guidelines for when to use and when not to use manual stabilization and spinal motion restriction. If this is the case in the system where you work, you should familiarize yourself with the local protocols and follow them.

The "Look Test"

At this point, experienced providers often get a feeling about the patient's condition. This feeling comes from environmental observations as well as from the brief but valuable information obtained by that first look at the patient as you approach. Some call this the "look test." You will develop more of this instinctual approach to assessment as you gain experience.

The chapter *The Principles of Pathophysiology* explains many of the things listed here as clinical topics. This chapter will discuss how and why the following clinical topics play a part in your assessment. For now, we will tell you some of the things experienced EMTs use to identify patients who may be critical, such as:

- **Patients who appear lifeless.** Patients who appear to be lifeless—who have no movement or apparent evidence of breathing, or have only gasping breathing—will be resuscitated by beginning CPR compressions and preparing your defibrillator as soon as possible if they are found to be pulseless.
- **Patients who have an obvious altered mental status.** An altered mental status can indicate many underlying conditions, from hypoxia to shock to diabetes to overdose to seizure. During the primary assessment, your concern is not the cause of the altered mental status; it is the impact it will have on your patient and your assessment and care decisions. In this case:
  - Your primary assessment will be more aggressive because of a higher potential for life-threatening problems, including vomitus or secretions in the airway and the need for ventilation.
  - Your subsequent assessments will likely be done more quickly, to expedite transport.
- **Patients who appear unusually anxious and those who appear pale and sweaty.** These signs are indicators of possible shock. Recognizing these signs at the earliest possible moment will help you to identify this potentially serious condition early. In this case:
  - Recognizing anxiety, pallor, and sweatiness early will prompt you to look for other signs of shock as you complete your primary assessment, including observation of rapid pulse and respiratory rates.

- Identification of shock will help you make the decision to classify the patient as unstable or potentially unstable and will expedite your assessment and care.
- Recognizing potential shock early in the call will help you perform appropriate assessments later. In cases of suspected trauma, you will match this information with the mechanism of injury, the patient's complaint, and assessment findings. In the medical patient, identifying shock may help you identify a body system to examine later (e.g., the gastrointestinal tract for indications of GI bleeding or the cardiac system for signs and symptoms of a heart attack).

- **Obvious trauma to the head, chest, abdomen, or pelvis.** Experienced EMTs identify serious trauma to these areas as injuries that can cause airway problems, profound shock, or death.
  - Head injuries are serious because the brain is housed within the skull. Also, because the head bleeds a lot when injured, the airway may require significant attention and care.
  - The integrity of the chest is vital for breathing. When the chest is injured, normal adequate breathing may be disrupted by rib injury, collapsed lungs, and bleeding from the major blood vessels within the mediastinum.
  - The abdomen not only contains a rich blood supply, but it also contains many organs that may be injured during trauma.
  - Injury to the pelvis can cause severe—and even fatal—bleeding.
- **Specific positions indicate distress.** The tripod position (Figure 12-4) indicates significant difficulty breathing, whereas Levine's sign (Figure 12-5) indicates significant chest pain or discomfort. Seeing either of these signs tells two things: The level of chest discomfort or respiratory distress is severe, and the patient's complaints (cardiac and respiratory) are among the most serious medical complaints, indicating a high priority.

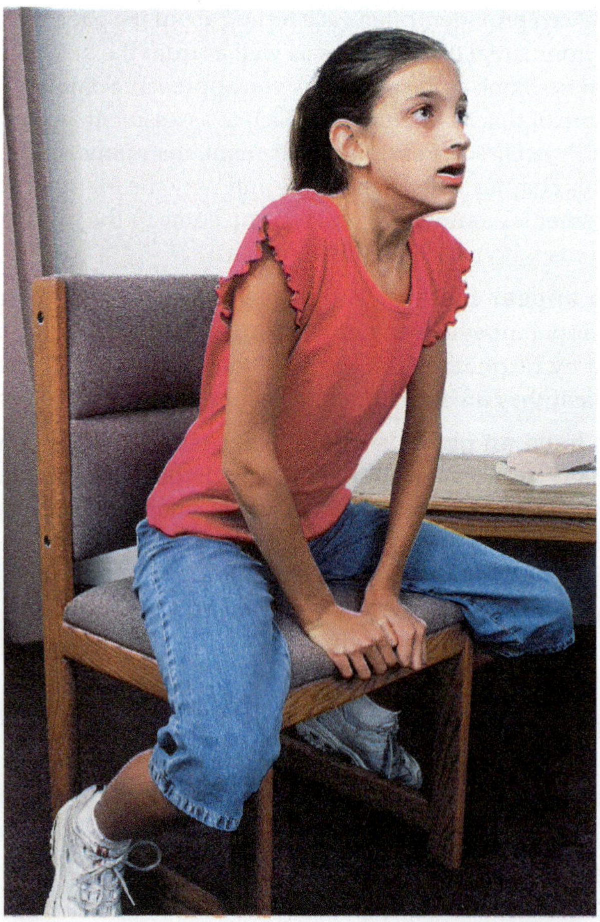

FIGURE 12-4 In cases of severe difficulty breathing, patients may assume the tripod position–sitting upright, leaning forward, and supporting themselves with arms locked in front of them.

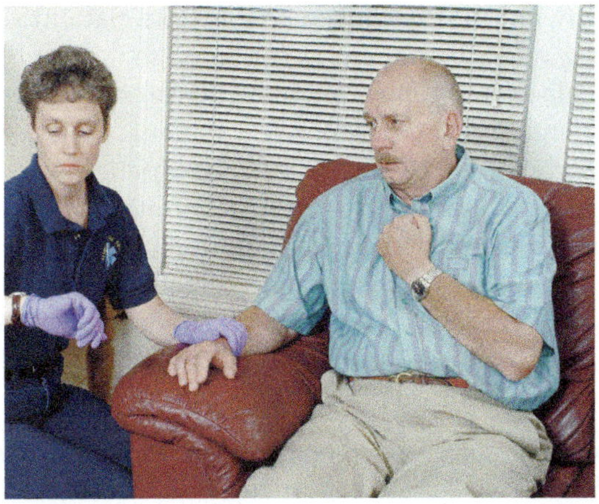

FIGURE 12-5 The classic sign of chest pain is Levine's sign, a fist clenched over the chest.

The clinical clues just listed are not all-inclusive. There are many indications—some very subtle—that something is wrong with a patient. Something as seemingly simple as a patient's saying "I feel weak" or "I'm not myself" may indicate a serious problem. You should also remember that these signs are only part of the information you will gather. You will find unstable patients who present with none of these signs and patients with very minor complaints who look serious.

Most important, remember that the presence of any of these signs usually indicates a serious condition, but absence of these signs does not guarantee that the patient is stable.

The Chief Complaint

The ***chief complaint*** is the reason EMS was called, usually in the patient's own words. It may be as specific as abdominal pain or as vague as "not feeling good." In any case, it is the patient's description of why you were called. This may be different than the patient's actual problem. A patient may complain of left shoulder or jaw pain when the actual problem is a myocardial infarction. The chief complaint gives you a place to start with your history and physical examination.

chief complaint
in emergency medicine, the reason EMS was called, usually in the patient's own words.

You form a general impression by looking, listening, and smelling. You look for the patient's age and sex—which are usually easy to determine once the patient is in sight. You look at the patient's position to see if it indicates an injury, pain, or difficulty in breathing. You listen for sounds such as moaning, snoring, or gurgling respirations. You sniff the air to detect any smells such as hazardous fumes, urine, feces, vomitus, or decay.

Something that is more difficult to describe than your direct observations—but just as important—is the feeling or sense you get when you arrive at the scene or encounter the patient. You may become anxious when you see a patient who exhibits no outward signs of illness or injury yet "just doesn't look right" to you. Or you may feel reassured when you are dispatched to a "sick baby" but see that the infant is alert and smiling. After you gain some practice assessing and managing patients, you may develop a sixth sense that clues you in to the severity of a patient's condition. This is part of what is called *clinical judgment*, judgment based on experience in observing and treating patients. Some people find it easier than others to cultivate this ability, but even those who have excellent clinical judgment do not depend on it alone. A systematic approach to finding threats to life is the best way to make sure they are not missed.

Assess Mental Status

Determining the patient's ***mental status***, or level of responsiveness, will usually be easy, since most patients are alert and responsive; that is, they are awake and will talk and answer questions sensibly. Some, even if not awake, will still respond to verbal stimuli, such as talking or shouting. At a lower level of responsiveness, the patient will respond only to painful stimuli, such as pinching a toe or ear, or squeezing the trapezius muscle between the neck and the shoulder. The lowest and most serious status is unresponsiveness, when the patient will not respond even to a painful stimulus. An easy way to keep these levels of responsiveness in mind is by remembering the letters ***AVPU***, for *alert*, *verbal response*, *painful response*, and *unresponsive*.

mental status
level of responsiveness.

AVPU
a memory aid for classifying a patient's level of responsiveness or mental status. The letters stand for **A**lert, **V**erbal response, **P**ainful response, **U**nresponsive.

CORE CONCEPT
Assessment of mental status using the AVPU scale

A patient may be awake but confused. An awake patient's mental status can be described by specifying what the patient is "oriented to." Most EMS systems document orientation to person, place, and time. Patients who can speak clearly can almost always tell you their name (orientation to person). A few patients are oriented to person but cannot tell you where they are (orientation to place). Some patients are oriented to person and place but cannot tell you the time, day, or date (orientation to time). A few EMS systems include additional questions to determine orientation.

A depressed mental status may indicate a life-threatening problem such as insufficient oxygen reaching the brain or shock. If the level of responsiveness is lower than alert, provide oxygen based on the patient's oxygen saturation and level of distress and consider the patient a high transport priority.

Assess the A-B-Cs

A-B-Cs airway, breathing, and circulation.

You will always check the ***A-B-Cs***—airway, breathing, and circulation—as you look for life-threatening problems. Remember as you perform the primary assessment that there are two purposes: to identify and correct life threats with airway, breathing, and circulation, and to gather information (e.g., indications of severity/priority, and signs of illness or injury) that will help you later in your assessment.

You were introduced to the initial decision-making scheme earlier in the chapter. Figure 12-6 shows an expanded view of the primary assessment. Remember that you will use these components in the order that is most appropriate for your patient's condition (Scan 12-1 and Scan 12-2).

CORE CONCEPT
Identifying and treating problems with the airway, breathing, and circulation

Airway

If the patient is alert and talking clearly or crying loudly, you know that the airway is open. If the airway is not open or is endangered (the patient is not alert, is supine, or is breathing noisily), take measures to open the airway, such as the jaw-thrust or head-tilt, chin-lift maneuver; suctioning; or insertion of an oropharyngeal or nasopharyngeal airway. If the airway is blocked, perform clearance procedures.

Breathing

Once an open airway is ensured, assess the patient's breathing. There are four general situations that call for assistance with breathing, listed here from most to least severe:

- **If the patient is in respiratory arrest with a pulse,** perform rescue breathing.
- **If the patient is not alert and the patient's breathing is inadequate (with an insufficient minute volume because of decreased rate or depth, or both),** provide positive pressure ventilations with oxygen.

Point of View

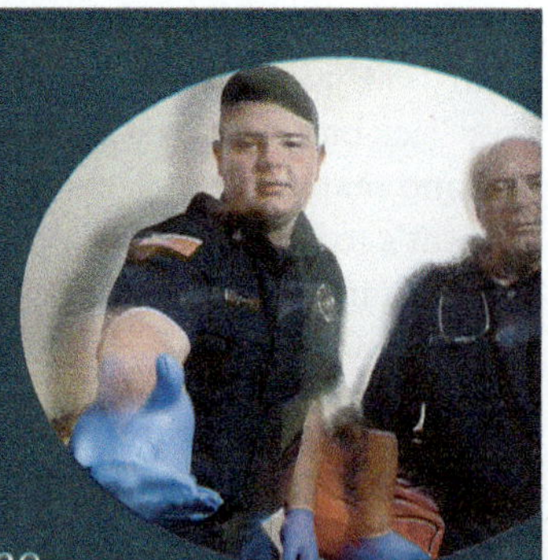

"I thought I'd just lie down for a nap. I wasn't feeling that well. Most everything from then on is really a blur. I remember my wife trying to wake me up. I can't even tell you how much time had passed.

"The next thing I knew, here were these two big guys standing over me in dark clothes. I had a hard time focusing on them . . . or even hearing them. I know this sounds silly, but it was like everyone on Earth was walking through air and I was walking through Jell-O. It took me extra time to do everything–extra time to hear or think or do something simple like move my arms. They'd ask me a question, and I couldn't even think about the right answer, and they moved on to the next question. It felt like all I was doing was mumbling.

"All I can say is that it was one of the scariest things I have ever experienced. Turns out my blood sugar was off. I'm glad EMS was there to help, that's for sure, although my recollection of it is still fuzzy."

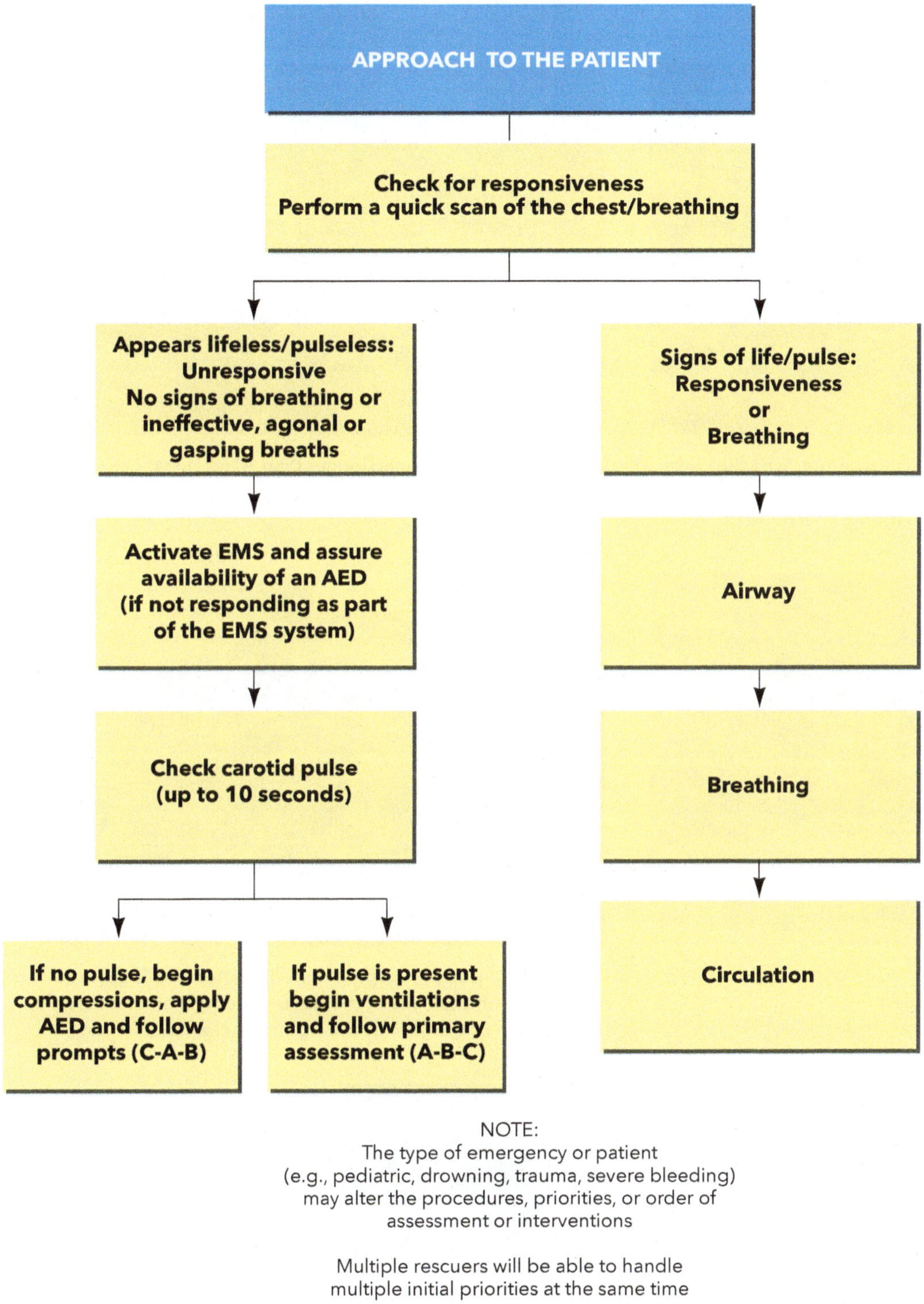

FIGURE 12-6 The approach to the patient: two pathways.

- **If the patient has some level of alertness and the patient's breathing is inadequate,** assist the patient's ventilations with 100 percent oxygen. Synchronize your ventilations with the patient's own respirations so they are working together, not against each other.
- **If the patient's breathing is adequate but there are signs or symptoms suggesting respiratory distress or hypoxia,** provide oxygen based on the patient's need as determined by the pulse oximetry reading, your examination, and the patient's complaint and level of distress.

Part of the primary assessment includes correcting certain conditions you may find. Injuries to the chest can reduce the rate and depth of breathing and significantly impact the functioning of the lungs. An example of a condition you will look for is an injury that penetrates the chest, leaving an open wound. You will identify these injuries by observing

"The most important things we can do for our patients are in the A-B-Cs."

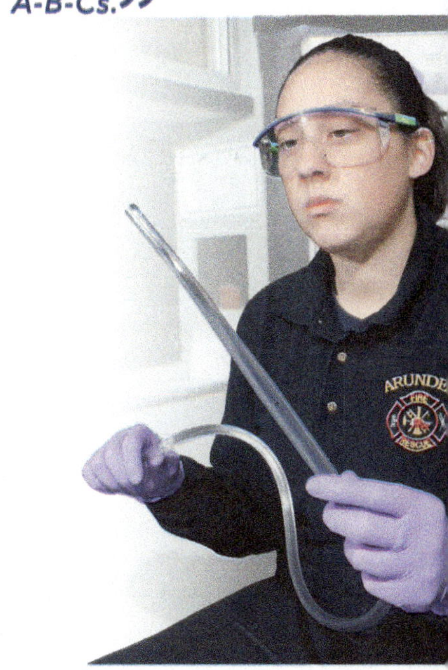

(© Daniel Limmer)

SCAN 12-1 Primary Assessment–Patient is Apparently Lifeless

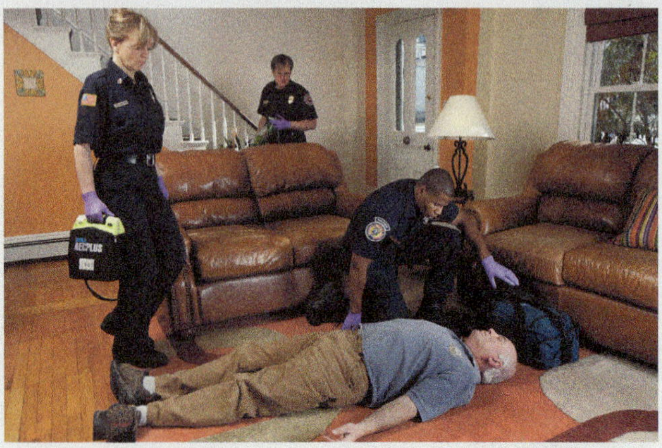

1. Look for signs of life, including movement. Scan the chest for signs of breathing. If no sign of life such as breathing (or only gasping breathing) is found, check the pulse.

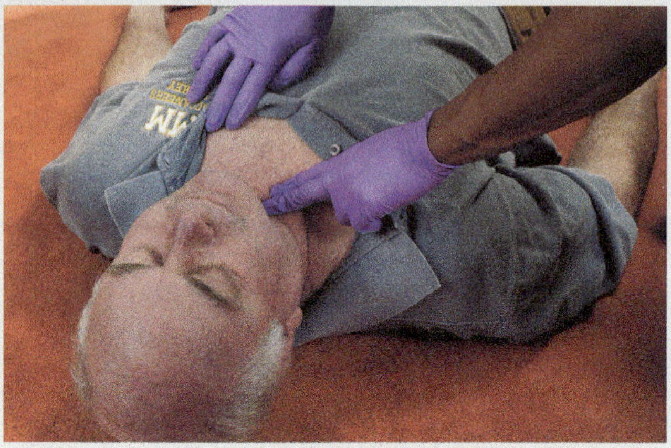

2. Check the pulse for no longer than 10 seconds.

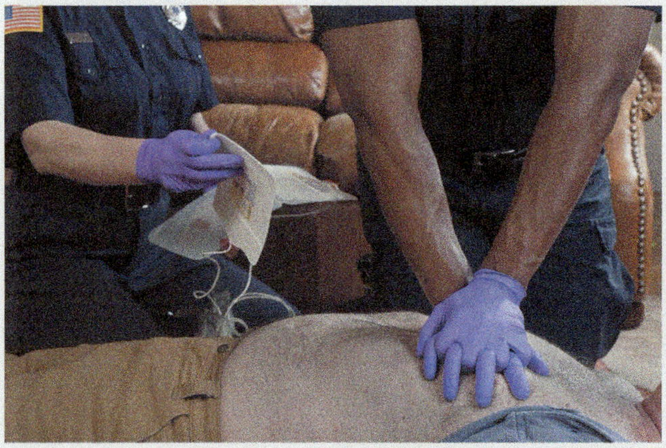

3. If no pulse is detectable, begin CPR compressions while the defibrillator is being readied.

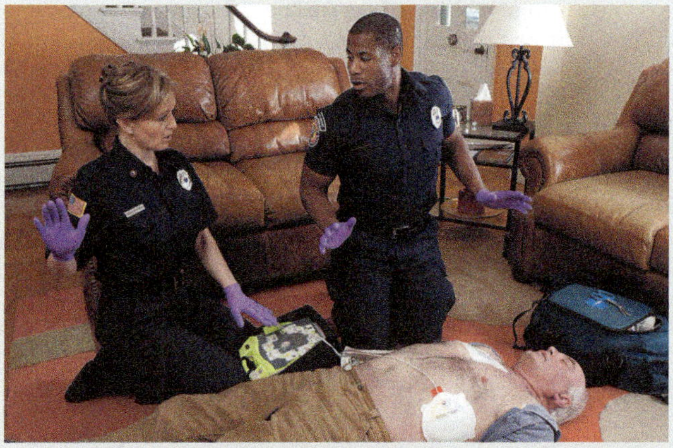

4. Clear the patient. Apply the defibrillator and follow the voice prompts. (Use of the defibrillator will be discussed in depth in the *Cardiac Emergencies* chapter.)

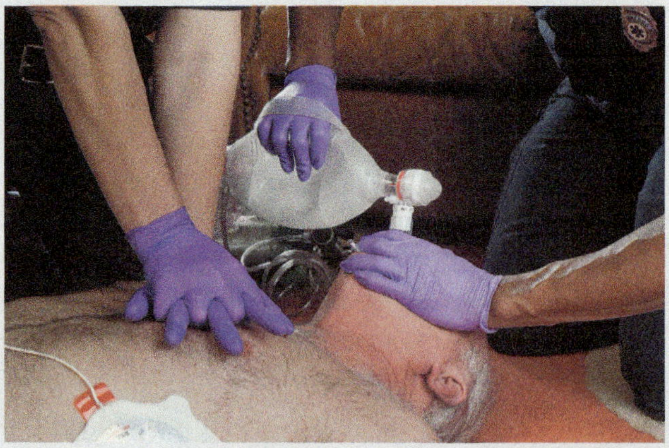

5. Continue resuscitation. Multiple rescuers can handle multiple assessment tasks simultaneously.

SCAN 12-2 Primary Assessment–Patient With A Pulse

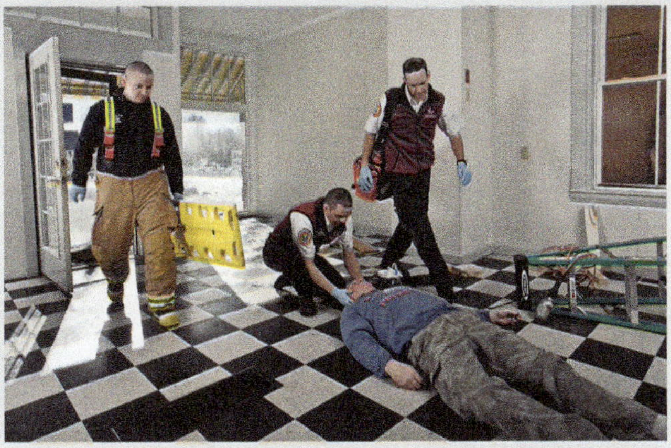

1. Develop a general impression and obtain a chief complaint if possible. Take spinal precautions if trauma is suspected.

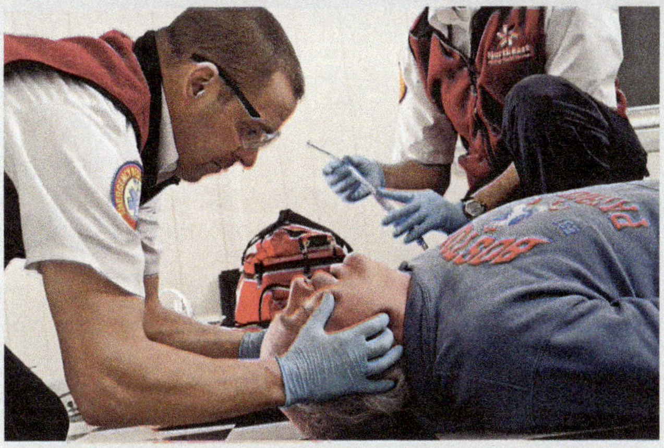

2. Open the airway. Provide manual stabilization of the head and neck if indicated.

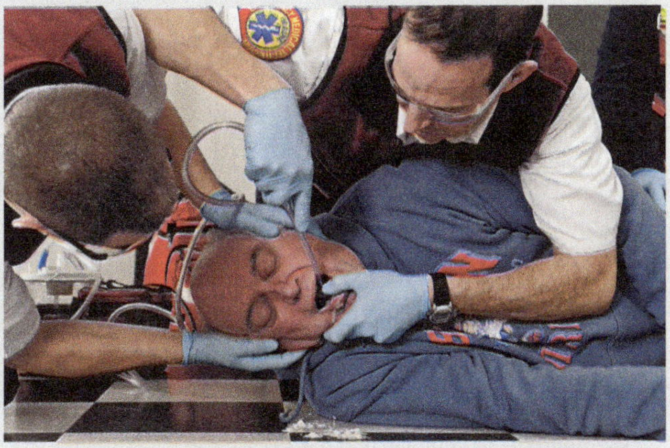

3. Suction if necessary. Note that spinal motion restriction is maintained.

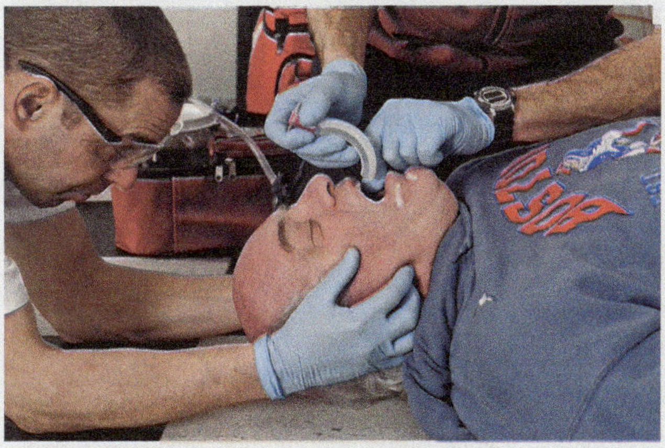

4. Insert an oral or nasal airway if required to maintain a patent airway.

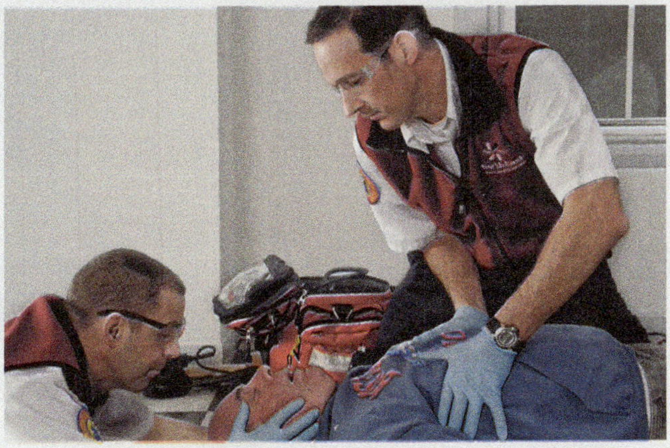

5. Evaluate breathing for rate and depth.

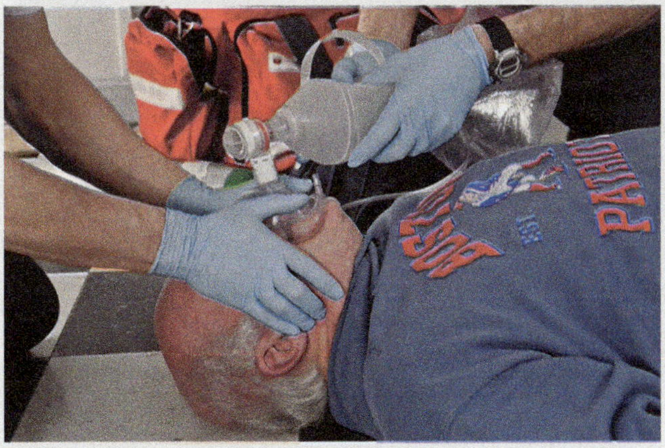

6. Apply positive pressure ventilation to patients who are not breathing or are breathing inadequately.

(continued)

SCAN 12-2 Primary Assessment–Patient With A Pulse *(continued)*

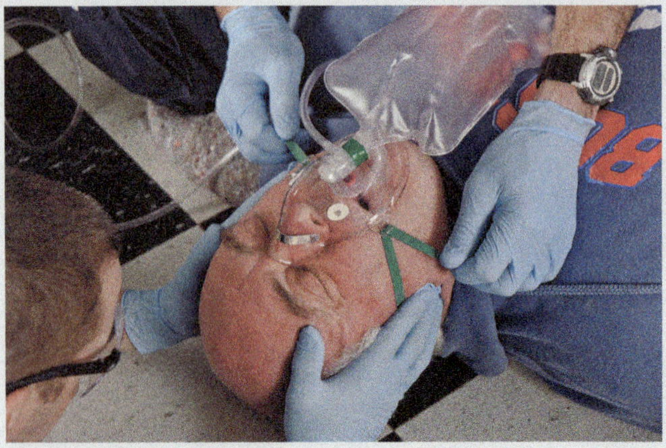

7. Provide oxygen based on pulse oximetry reading, patient complaint, and patient condition.

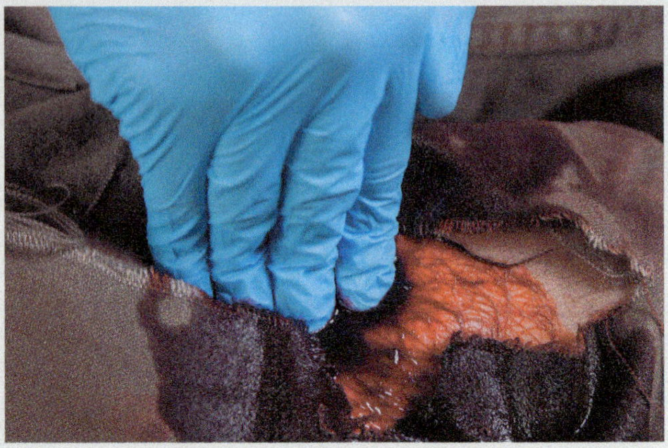

8. Identify bleeding and apply direct pressure as quickly as possible.

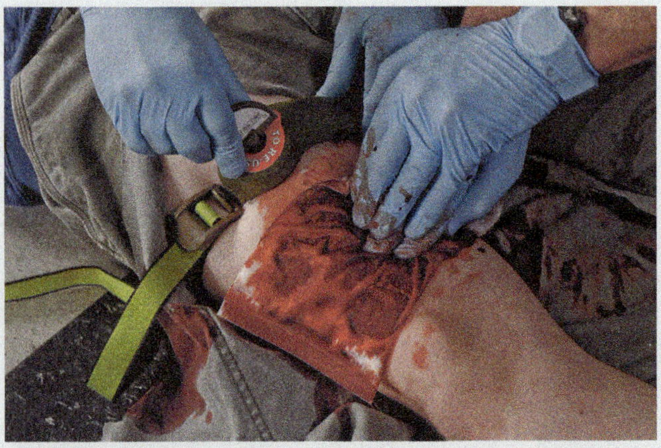

9. Apply a tourniquet and control life-threatening bleeding.

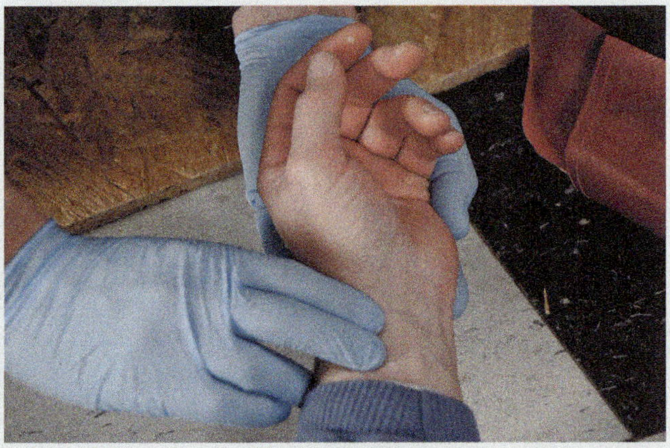

10. Evaluate circulation. Check the pulse.

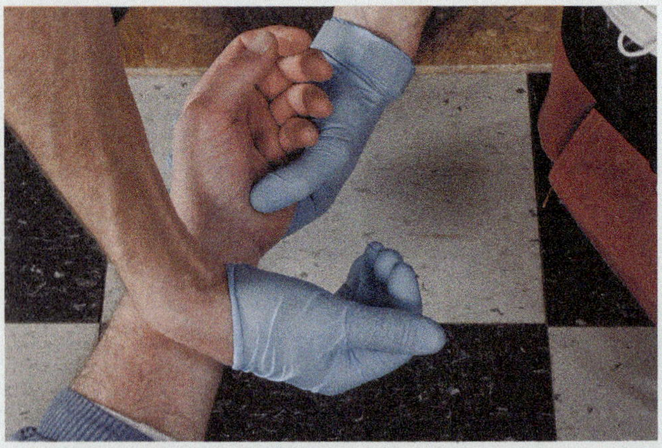

11. Evaluate circulation. Check skin color, temperature, and condition.

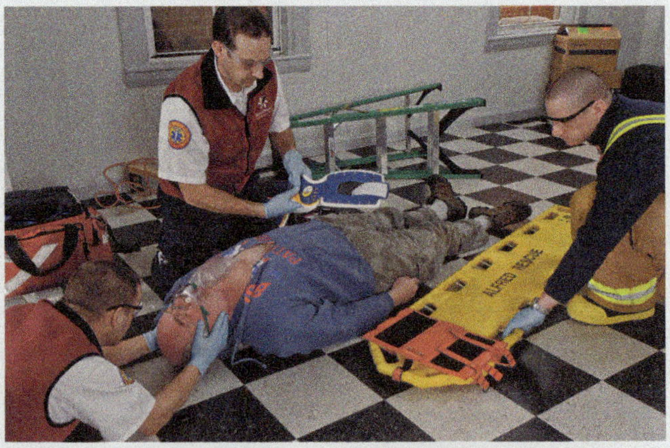

12. Make a status/transport priority decision and request ALS or other assistance as necessary.

and palpating the chest cavity. Although you won't be taught how to care for these chest injuries until later in the book, for now remember that it will be important to look for these life-threatening conditions in the primary assessment.

Circulation

Once any breathing problems are corrected, assess the patient's circulation. Begin by taking the patient's pulse. If the patient was lifeless on your initial approach, you will have begun CPR at that point. Keep in mind, however, that cardiac arrest is not the only possible life-threatening circulation problem. Shock and severe blood loss are also life-threatening.

To evaluate circulation, assess pulse, skin, and bleeding. If the patient is light-skinned, you can check the pulse and skin at the same time. As you take the radial pulse, note whether the skin at the wrist is warm, pink, and dry—indicating good circulation—or pale and clammy (cool and moist), suggesting shock, which is a serious condition. If your patient is dark-skinned, you can check the color of the lips or nail beds, which should be pink.

You don't have to take the pulse for a full 30 seconds and obtain an exact rate. During the primary assessment, there are only three possible results of the pulse check that you will be looking for:

1. Within normal limits
2. Unusually slow
3. Unusually fast

Anything other than normal is concerning and may indicate a serious condition. You will get used to different pulse rates as you practice. This will allow you to identify these three types of pulse rates easily—especially in combination with other things (e.g., a very rapid pulse in the presence of trauma, or a very slow pulse in a patient who has chest pain, both indicating an unstable, high-priority patient).

Also check for and control severe bleeding. If even one large vessel or several smaller ones are bleeding, a patient can lose enough blood in just a minute or two to die. Quick control of severe external bleeding can be lifesaving. Transport decisions should take into account the potential for shock resulting from inadequate circulation and blood loss. Although the bleeding-control step is mentioned here, it may be performed in the earliest parts of the primary assessment. Remember that the order in which you provide care in is determined by choosing to address the condition that would be likely to kill the patient first.

Keep in mind that to perform a primary assessment, you must touch your patient. Even when you encounter an alert patient, you should still feel for a pulse, as well as for skin temperature and condition. These may help you identify shock early—a potentially lifesaving assessment.

Determine Priority

Any life-threatening airway, breathing, or circulation problem must be treated as soon as it is discovered. Once life threats are under control, you will decide on the patient's ***priority*** for immediate transport versus further on-scene assessment and care.

priority
the decision regarding the need for immediate transport of the patient versus further assessment and care at the scene.

A useful approach to decision making is to classify a patient as stable, potentially unstable, or unstable. Although there are few hard-and-fast rules for how to determine stability, several principles will help you.

CORE CONCEPT
Making a priority decision

- **To be stable, a patient needs to have vital signs that are in the normal range or just slightly abnormal.** If they are abnormal, they must be small deviations from normal or easily explained by factors other than injury and illness (e.g., sweating on a hot day or slightly increased pulse because of fever). Stable vital signs are not the only requirement for a stable classification, but they are necessary.
- **A threat to the airway, breathing, or circulation, either actual or imminent, rules out stable.** This puts a patient in either the unstable or potentially unstable category, depending on the severity of the patient's condition.
- **There are many times when it is not crystal clear what a patient's problem is, so there will be many possible diagnoses, some more serious than others.** When a

patient does not have any immediate threats to life but you believe the patient may deteriorate because of the nature of the problem, you should consider the potentially unstable category for the patient. This means you will not delay transport, but it does not necessarily mean you will use lights and siren to transport the patient to the hospital.

- **A patient's priority can change.** For example, an unconscious diabetic patient with low blood sugar would initially be unstable because of the threat to the airway. If the patient became awake enough to swallow oral glucose, then became alert and oriented, it would be appropriate to change this patient's priority to stable.

Although most patients do not need immediate transport, a few do. Therefore, you must be able to determine which patients fall into which category. *If any life-threatening problem cannot be controlled or threatens to recur, or if the patient has a depressed level of responsiveness, the patient has an immediate priority for transport to the hospital, with assessment and care continuing en route.*

A number of findings indicate a high priority for transport (Table 12-1) (i.e., the patient is categorized as unstable or potentially unstable). These are conditions for which there usually is little or no treatment that can be given in the field that will make a difference in how well the patient does. You will learn more about these conditions in later chapters.

Primary assessment steps and interventions are summarized in Table 12-2.

TABLE 12-1 High-Priority Conditions

• Poor general impression
• Unresponsive
• Responsive, but not following commands
• Difficulty breathing
• Shock
• Complicated childbirth
• Chest pain consistent with cardiac problems
• Uncontrolled bleeding
• Severe pain anywhere

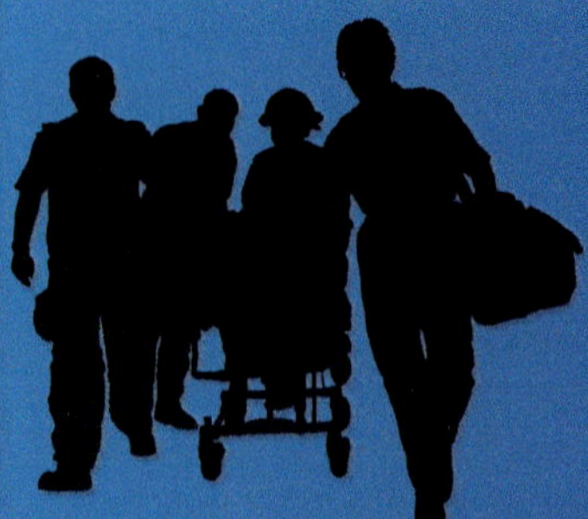

Think Like an EMT

Determining Priority

At the end of the primary assessment, you will make a priority determination. This determination is a key decision that will affect the rest of your assessment and care. Patients deemed a high priority will receive a streamlined assessment process leading to prompt transport. Patients who are not a high priority will receive their assessment and care at a slower (although not slow) pace. Determine whether each patient described here should be classified as a high or low priority at the end of the primary assessment.

1. A responsive patient who is having difficulty breathing and is unable to lie flat on the ambulance cot
2. A man who passed out at a wedding and is still unresponsive
3. A responsive child who got her foot caught in bike spokes and may have broken the foot
4. A responsive patient who describes severe pain in his abdomen
5. A patient who only moans (doesn't respond with words or actions) and appears to have ingested alcohol

TABLE 12-2 Primary Assessment Steps and Interventions

MEDICAL PATIENT		TRAUMA PATIENT	
RESPONSIVE	**UNRESPONSIVE**	**RESPONSIVE**	**UNRESPONSIVE**
1. *General impression:* Form general impression of patient's condition.	**1.** *General impression:* Form general impression of patient's condition.	**1.** *General impression:* Form general impression of patient's condition. Evaluate mechanism of injury. **Intervention:** Manual stabilization of head and neck if you suspect spinal injury.	**1.** *General impression:* Form general impression of patient's condition. Evaluate mechanism of injury. **Intervention:** Manual stabilization of head and neck if you suspect spinal injury.
2. *Mental status:* AVPU (alert)	**2.** *Mental status:* AVPU (responsive to only verbal or painful stimulus, or not responsive) **Intervention:** Recognize that hypoxia or shock may be a cause of altered mental status. Administer oxygen, as appropriate, during your treatment in breathing (#4 below).	**2.** *Mental status:* AVPU (alert)	**2.** *Mental status:* AVPU (responsive to only verbal or painful stimulus, or not responsive) **Intervention:** Oxygen administration. For patients with shock, hypoxia, or severe injuries, you will administer high-concentration oxygen.
3. *Airway* is open.	**3.** *Airway* is compromised. **Interventions:** Open airway with head-tilt, chin-lift maneuver; consider oro- or nasopharyngeal airway; suction as needed. For foreign-body obstruction, use abdominal thrusts or other blockage-clearing technique.	**3.** *Airway* is open.	**3.** *Airway* is compromised. **Interventions:** Open airway with jaw-thrust maneuver; consider oro- or nasopharyngeal airway; suction as needed. For foreign-body obstruction, use abdominal thrusts or other blockage-clearing technique.
4. *Breathing:* Look for rise and fall of chest, and listen and feel for rate and depth of breathing. Look for work of breathing (use of accessory muscles, retractions). Assess oxygen saturation. **Interventions:** Administer oxygen based on the patient's oxygen saturation reading, complaint, and level of distress. If breathing becomes inadequate, provide positive pressure ventilations and high-concentration oxygen.	**4.** *Breathing:* Look for rise and fall of chest, and listen and feel for rate and depth of breathing. Look for work of breathing (use of accessory muscles, retractions). Assess oxygen saturation. **Interventions:** Administer oxygen based on the patient's oxygen saturation reading, complaint, and level of distress. Position patient on side. If breathing is inadequate, provide positive pressure ventilations with oxygen. If respiratory arrest develops, perform rescue breathing.	**4.** *Breathing:* Look for rise and fall of chest, and listen and feel for rate and depth of breathing. Look for work of breathing (use of accessory muscles, retractions). **Interventions:** Patients with minor or isolated injuries usually do not require oxygen. Administer oxygen based on the patient's oxygen saturation reading, complaint, and level of distress. If respiratory failure develops, provide positive pressure ventilations and high-concentration oxygen.	**4.** *Breathing:* Look for rise and fall of chest, and listen and feel for rate and depth of breathing. Look for work of breathing (use of accessory muscles, retractions). Expose and palpate the chest for signs of trauma that will affect breathing. **Interventions:** Administer oxygen based on the patient's oxygen saturation reading, complaint, and level of distress. If breathing becomes inadequate, provide positive pressure ventilations with oxygen. If respiratory arrest develops, perform rescue breathing.
5. *Circulation:* Pulse; bleeding; skin color, temperature, condition **Interventions:** Control bleeding. Treat for shock. If cardiac arrest occurs, perform CPR.	**5.** *Circulation:* Pulse; bleeding; skin color, temperature, condition **Interventions:** Control bleeding. Treat for shock. If cardiac arrest occurs, perform CPR.	**5.** *Circulation:* Pulse; bleeding; skin color, temperature, condition **Interventions:** Control bleeding. Treat for shock. If cardiac arrest occurs, perform CPR.	**5.** *Circulation:* Pulse; bleeding; skin color, temperature, condition **Interventions:** Control bleeding. Treat for shock. If cardiac arrest occurs, perform CPR.
6. *Priority:* A responsive patient's priority depends on chief complaint, status of A-B-Cs, and other factors.	**6.** *Priority:* An unresponsive patient is automatically a high priority for immediate transport.	**6.** *Priority:* A responsive patient's priority depends on chief complaint, status of A-B-Cs, and other factors.	**6.** *Priority:* An unresponsive patient is automatically a high priority for immediate transport.

Patient Characteristics and Primary Assessment

Patient assessment takes different forms, depending on the following patient characteristics:

- Whether the patient has a medical problem or trauma (injury)
- Whether the patient has an altered mental status
- Whether the patient is an adult, a child, or an infant

How can the steps of primary assessment be applied to such varied types of patients? The following scenarios—plus some final paragraphs—will help to show you.

Mr. Schmidt—*A Responsive Adult Medical Patient*

One afternoon, you are dispatched to "an elderly man whose stomach hurts." Mrs. Schmidt greets you at the door and leads you to her husband.

General Impression

As you approach the sofa where Mr. Schmidt is sitting, you see that he is an older male who appears ill and in pain. You see nothing around him to suggest that he has been injured. All of this suggests a medical problem rather than an injury.

Mental Status, Airway, and Breathing

You introduce yourself by saying "Hello, Mr. Schmidt. I'm Gerry Jones. I'm an emergency medical technician from the Fairfield Ambulance Service. How can I help you?" "My stomach hurts," he replies. As you ask questions, you note that Mr. Schmidt is alert and answering clearly. The fact that he is speaking in a normal way indicates that his airway is open. You can hear that his breathing is not labored. You look at his chest and note that his breathing is normal in rate and depth. You place the pulse oximetry probe on his finger and see that he is at 98 percent. There is no need to administer oxygen at this time.

Circulation

"I'm going to check your pulse," you explain as you reach for his wrist. You quickly assess Mr. Schmidt's circulation by palpating his radial pulse, observing his skin, and looking for bleeding. Although you do not stop to count exactly how fast his pulse is, you can tell that it is normal in rate and strength, and regular in rhythm. The skin at his wrist is pink, warm, and dry. No blood is evident anywhere around him.

Priority

With the information you have gathered in just a few seconds, you conclude that Mr. Schmidt has no problems that are likely to kill him in the next few minutes. Therefore, you decide he is probably stable. No immediate lifesaving measures are required, and neither is immediate transport to the hospital. You are able, instead, to move ahead with the next steps of your assessment as Mr. Schmidt continues to rest on the sofa. Note that categorizing a patient as stable does not mean you can sit back and have a leisurely conversation with the patient on the way to the hospital. There are many causes of abdominal pain; most of them are not life-threatening, but there is the possibility the patient will deteriorate. You will need to keep a close eye on him. You will learn more about this in the discussion of reassessment in the *Secondary Assessment* chapter.

Mrs. Malone—*An Unresponsive Adult Medical Patient*

Your dispatcher sends you to an "unconscious" woman. Her daughter says she cannot wake her mother, Mrs. Malone, and leads you to the bedroom.

General Impression

An older woman in nightclothes is lying on her back in bed. Her eyes are closed, and she is not moving.

Mental Status

You say loudly, "Mrs. Malone, can you hear me?" In response to your question, she moans a little, so you know she responds to a verbal stimulus. In your report you will describe both the stimulus (verbal) and the response (moaning). If Mrs. Malone had not responded to verbal stimulus, you would have scanned her chest for indications of breathing. If she didn't appear to be breathing, you would check the pulse, move her to the floor, and begin compressions if necessary. If the patient is breathing, you should continue the primary assessment by inflicting a painful stimulus to try to get a response from her.

Airway and Breathing

Because she is lying on her back, Mrs. Malone's airway is threatened by her tongue. Since patients with depressed responsiveness are always at risk for airway problems, you know that you need to be aggressive about opening and maintaining her airway. Even though you haven't heard any sounds indicating partial airway obstruction (such as snoring or gurgling), your partner (having ruled out trauma) removes the pillow, tilts her head back, and lifts her chin.

Next you evaluate her breathing by bringing your ear next to her mouth and looking for movement of her chest and abdomen as you listen and feel for the movement of air with your ear. You determine the depth of Mrs. Malone's respirations and whether her breathing rate is slow or fast. If you found that her breathing was inadequate, you would ventilate Mrs. Malone with 100 percent oxygen.

Her respirations are in the normal range and appear to be deep, but you give Mrs. Malone high-concentration oxygen by nonrebreather mask anyway, because her oxygen saturation is low and her level of responsiveness is depressed. You put in a nasopharyngeal airway and move Mrs. Malone onto her side to help protect her airway.

Circulation

Mrs. Malone's pulse is strong, regular, and in the normal range for rate. You look for blood but find none. The skin at her wrist is cool and dry. Because Mrs. Malone is dark-skinned, you assess for skin color at her lips and nail beds, which are pale. Although the pulse and bleeding check are normal, the pallor and coolness of her skin are abnormal. This reinforces your decision to administer oxygen by nonrebreather mask.

Priority

The priority of this patient is high, because her mental status is depressed, her airway is at risk, and her skin indicates a circulation problem. You arrange immediate transport to the hospital for this unstable patient, and plan to continue assessment and care en route.

■ Clara Diller—*A Responsive Child Trauma Patient*

You respond to the scene where, the dispatcher says, a child has fallen.

General Impression

As you get out of the ambulance, you see a girl who is about 5 years old sitting on the sidewalk. She is crying and holding a bloody cloth on her knee. The mechanism of injury is apparent: A pair of skates indicates that she has probably taken a tumble while skating.

Mental Status, Airway, and Breathing

When you reach the patient, you kneel next to her and introduce yourself. You ask what happened. She confirms your suspicion that she fell down while trying out her new skates. When you ask her, she tells you her name is Clara Diller and that her head and knee hurt. Since she is crying and answers your question easily, you determine that her mental status is alert and her airway is clear.

It doesn't appear that Clara hit her head. The fall seems to have affected only her knee, so you don't need to use any spinal motion restriction techniques.

Circulation

You feel Clara's radial pulse. It is slightly rapid but strong and regular. You look around her and see no blood except on the cloth and on her knee. Since it is hard to tell how much bleeding may be under the cloth, you tell Clara you want to look at her knee. You see a 2-inch (5-cm) laceration which is oozing some blood, so you put the cloth back on and ask the neighbor who takes care of Clara to apply a little pressure to it. When you felt Clara's radial pulse, you noted that her skin was warm, pink, and dry. You also assess her capillary refill by pressing on the end of her fingernail. The color in the nail bed returns to pink in less than 2 seconds, so all indications are that Clara's circulation is good.

Pediatric Note

Because Clara is a child, several other factors were different in her case than they were for your adult patients, Mr. Schmidt and Mrs. Malone.

Since children are often shy or distrustful of strangers or adults, you made a special effort to gain Clara's trust by kneeling to her level as you talked with her. You had the time to do this because the injuries didn't appear severe, and Clara seemed stable. Responsive children need to have some trust in the EMT. This may take a minute or two, but the general impression will guide you in determining how long to spend developing a rapport with the child.

Infants and children breathe faster than adults, and their hearts beat faster, which you kept in mind when you evaluated Clara's breathing and circulation. Anxiety about the fall and your arrival alone are enough to slightly raise her pulse.

A special part of checking circulation in infants and children is capillary refill. Nail beds are typically pink in healthy, normal people. When the end of the fingernail is gently pressed, it turns white. When the pressure is released, the nail bed turns pink again very quickly, usually in less than 2 seconds. In children, this may help you to evaluate the circulation of blood. In an infant or small child with small nail beds, press the back of the hand or top of the foot instead. Count "one-one thousand, two-one thousand" or say "capillary refill." If the nail or skin regains its pink color in the time it takes to say one of these, it is probably normal. Abnormal responses include prolonged or absent capillary refill (taking too long to turn pink again, or not turning pink again at all). These usually indicate problems with circulation.

Capillary refill may be used on adults, but in some cases may be unreliable. In some adults, especially in the elderly, it is normal for capillary refill to take longer than 2 seconds. Even in infants and young children, capillary refill can be affected by factors such as the weather. Cold temperatures will prolong capillary refill. In other words, it should be used as one factor to consider in determining the priority of the young patient, but not the only one.

An infant has an airway that is different from an adult's, so opening an infant's or child's airway means moving the head to a neutral position–not tilting it back, the way an adult's airway is opened. The mental status of unresponsive infants is typically checked by talking to the infant and flicking the feet.

Priority

Based on the information you have gathered, you determine that Clara's priority for immediate transport is low. She has no significant mechanism of injury and no immediately life-threatening problems. There is no evidence that she was struck by a car or hit any object other than the sidewalk. You categorize her as stable.

■ **Brian Sawyer**–*An Unresponsive Adult Trauma Patient*

At the scene of a motor-vehicle collision, you go to the aid of a young man who has been thrown from his car.

General Impression

The young man appears to be approximately 25 years old. His eyes are closed, and he is not moving. As you approach, you can hear snoring respirations. The mechanism of injury, the collision and the fact that he is quite a distance from his vehicle are obvious. A police officer tells you that the patient's name is Brian Sawyer.

Mental Status and Airway

Your partner moves to stabilize Brian's head, and the two of you position him on his back. Your partner attends to Brian's airway as you begin to check his mental status. He doesn't respond to your calling his name, and he is unresponsive to a pinch of the trapezius muscle in his shoulder.

Your partner has started to treat the airway problem you both heard, snoring respirations that mean partial obstruction of the airway. Your partner manually stabilizes Brian's head at the same time that he does a jaw thrust, which relieves the snoring sound. You listen closely and hear no other noises from his airway. If you heard gurgling or saw fluid in Brian's airway, you would suction him promptly.

Breathing and Circulation

To evaluate breathing, you look, listen, and feel. Brian has respirations that appear somewhat elevated but of adequate depth. Because he is unresponsive but has adequate respirations, you decide to give Brian high-concentration oxygen by nonrebreather mask as soon as you finish checking his circulation. You start to assess circulation by feeling the radial pulse. It is rapid and weak. There is no blood on or near the patient that you can see. His skin is pale, cool, and sweaty. You select an oropharyngeal airway and insert it, then apply a nonrebreather mask with 15 liters per minute of high-concentration oxygen.

Priority

The priority you assign Brian is high. He is unresponsive to pain, and his rapid, weak pulse; pale, rapid respirations; and clammy skin are signs of shock. You will spend as little time on the scene as possible with this unstable patient. You plan to monitor his airway, place a cervical collar on him, maintain spinal motion restriction, and get him to an appropriate facility quickly. Since you and your partner will both be needed to care for this patient en route to the hospital, you radio for additional personnel to drive the ambulance.

Comparing the Primary Assessments

The four patients—Mr. Schmidt, Mrs. Malone, Clara Diller, and Brian Sawyer—were very different in their characteristics. Notably:

- Mr. Schmidt and Mrs. Malone were medical patients, whereas Clara Diller and Brian Sawyer had suffered trauma.
- Both Mr. Schmidt and Clara Diller were responsive, and neither was a priority for immediate transport. However, both Mrs. Malone and Brian Sawyer had altered mental statuses and airway and circulation problems that made them high priorities for immediate transport to the hospital.
- Clara Diller was a child, whereas the other three patients were adults.

There were a few obvious differences in the primary assessments of these patients. For example, both Clara Diller and Brian Sawyer, as trauma patients, required consideration of c-spine stabilization and possible immobilization of the head and spine. In contrast, Mr. Schmidt and Mrs. Malone, as medical patients with no evidence of any mechanism of injury, did not. For all four patients, the purpose of the primary assessment was to discover and correct any life-threatening problems. Mrs. Malone and Brian Sawyer had more problems to correct (mainly airway problems), so there were more actions to take. Therefore, the primary assessment of these two patients took a little longer than the primary assessment of Mr. Schmidt and Clara Diller.

In spite of these differences, the main thing to note is that the primary assessment steps were the same for all of them: forming a general impression; assessing mental status; checking airway, breathing, and circulation (and correcting any immediately life-threatening problems as soon as they were found); and making a priority decision regarding immediate transport versus continued on-scene assessment and care.

These steps of the primary assessment must be followed for every patient, no matter whether that patient has a medical condition or trauma; is responsive or unresponsive; is an infant, child, or adult—and no matter how mild or serious that patient's condition may seem to be. If these steps are not followed consistently, it is very possible to overlook and neglect to manage a life-threatening problem.

To consider how the steps of the primary assessment are applied to responsive and unresponsive medical and trauma patients, review Table 12-2. For a summary of how the steps of the primary assessment are applied to adults, children, and infants, see Table 12-3.

TABLE 12-3 Primary Assessment of Adults, Children, and Infants

	ADULTS	CHILDREN 1-5 YEARS	INFANTS TO 1 YEAR
Mental Status	AVPU: Is patient alert? Responsive to verbal stimulus? Responsive to painful stimulus? Unresponsive? If alert, is patient oriented to person, place, and time?	As for adults	If not alert, shout as a verbal stimulus, flick feet as a painful stimulus. (Crying would be infant's expected response.)
Airway	Trauma: jaw-thrust maneuver. Medical: head-tilt, chin-lift maneuver. Both: Consider oro- or nasopharyngeal airway, suctioning.	As for adults; see the *Airway Management* chapter and Appendix A, BCLS Review for special child airway techniques. If performing head-tilt, chin-lift maneuver, do so without hyperextending (stretching) the neck.	As for children; see the *Airway Management* chapter and BCLS Review for special infant airway techniques.
Breathing	If respiratory arrest, perform rescue breathing. If depressed mental status and inadequate breathing, give positive pressure ventilations with 100 percent oxygen. Administer oxygen based on the patient's oxygen saturation reading, complaint, and level of distress	As for adults, but normal rates for children are faster than for adults. (See the chapter *Vital Signs and Monitoring Devices* for normal child respiration rates.) If oxygen is necessary, a parent may have to hold oxygen mask to reduce the child's fear of mask.	As for children, but normal rates for infants are faster than for children and adults. (See the chapter *Vital Signs and Monitoring Devices* for normal infant respiration rates.)
Circulation	Assess skin, radial pulse, and bleeding. If patient is in cardiac arrest, perform CPR. See the chapter *Bleeding and Shock* on how to treat for bleeding and shock.	Assess skin, radial pulse, bleeding, and capillary refill. See the *Vital Signs and Monitoring Devices* chapter for normal child pulse rates (faster than for adults). If patient is in cardiac arrest, perform CPR. See BCLS Review for child techniques. See the *Bleeding and Shock* chapter.	Assess skin, brachial pulse, bleeding, and capillary refill. See the *Vital Signs and Monitoring Devices* chapter for normal infant pulse rates (faster than for children and adults). If patient is in cardiac arrest, perform CPR. See BCLS Review for special infant techniques. See the *Bleeding and Shock* chapter.

Chapter Review

Key Facts and Concepts

- The primary assessment is a systematic approach to quickly finding and treating immediate threats to life.
- The general impression, although somewhat subjective, can provide extremely useful information regarding the urgency of a patient's condition.
- The determination of mental status follows the AVPU approach.
- Evaluating airway, breathing, and circulation quickly but thoroughly will reveal immediate threats to life that must be treated before the EMT proceeds further with assessment.
- Your approach to a patient will vary depending on how the patient presents. The American Heart Association recommends a C-A-B approach for patients who appear lifeless and apparently are not breathing or have only agonal respirations. This begins with a pulse check and chest compressions if there is no pulse.
- If your patient shows signs of life (e.g., moving, moaning, talking) and is breathing, you will take a traditional A-B-C approach.
- Remember that the mnemonic *A-B-C* is a guide to interventions that may be taken. You will choose your interventions based on the patient's immediate needs. They may be done in any order that fits the patient's needs.
- The patient's priority describes how urgent the patient's need to be transported is and how to conduct the rest of your assessment.

Key Decisions

- Is this patient medical or trauma; responsive or unresponsive; adult, child, or infant?
- Does this patient have any signs of life?
- Does this patient require a C-A-B approach (likely in cardiac arrest)? Does the patient therefore require chest compressions and defibrillation as the first priority?
- Do I need to stop and suction the airway, insert an artificial airway, administer oxygen, or ventilate the patient?
- Is the patient's condition stable enough to allow further assessment and treatment at the scene?

Chapter Glossary

A-B-Cs airway, breathing, and circulation.

AVPU a memory aid for classifying a patient's level of responsiveness or mental status. The letters stand for alert, verbal response, painful response, unresponsive.

chief complaint in emergency medicine, the reason EMS was called, usually in the patient's own words.

general impression impression of the patient's condition that is formed on first approaching the patient, based on the patient's environment, chief complaint, and appearance.

interventions actions taken to correct or manage a patient's problems.

manual stabilization using one's hands to prevent movement of a patient's head and neck until a cervical collar can be applied.

mental status level of responsiveness.

primary assessment the first element in a patient assessment; steps taken for the purpose of discovering and dealing with any life-threatening problems. The six parts of primary assessment are: (1) forming a general impression, (2) assessing mental status, (3) assessing airway, (4) assessing breathing, (5) assessing circulation, and (6) determining the priority of the patient for treatment and transport to the hospital.

priority the decision regarding the need for immediate transport of the patient versus further assessment and care at the scene.

spinal motion restriction a procedure for limiting movement of the head, neck, and spine when spinal injury is possible or likely.

Preparation for Your Examination and Practice

Short Answer

1. List factors you will take into account in forming a general impression of a patient.
2. Explain how to assess a patient's mental status with regard to the AVPU levels of responsiveness.
3. Explain how to assess airway, breathing, and circulation during the primary assessment. Explain the interventions you will take for possible problems with airway, breathing, and circulation.
4. Explain the C-A-B approach to the primary assessment, and explain the circumstances in which the C-A-B approach would be appropriate.

5. Explain the A-B-C approach to the primary assessment, and explain the circumstances in which the A-B-C approach would be appropriate.
6. Explain what is meant by this statement in the chapter: "The order in which these interventions [airway, breathing, circulation] are performed depends on the patient's specific condition and the number and priority of urgent conditions . . . that you are presented with."
7. Explain what is meant by this statement in the chapter: "Multiple EMTs can accomplish multiple priorities simultaneously."
8. Explain what is meant by the term *priority decision*.
9. Explain what special interventions are required in the following situations:
   - If a patient has suffered trauma
   - If a patient is unresponsive

Thinking and Linking

Think back to the Respiration and Artificial Ventilation *chapter and link information from that chapter (regarding oxygen administration and artificial ventilation) with information from this chapter as you consider the following situation:*

- Your patient, injured in a car crash, is breathing at 6 breaths per minute. Would you administer oxygen by nonrebreather mask or provide artificial ventilations? Describe the technique you would use.

Critical Thinking Exercises

Determining a patient's priority status is a critical skill within the primary assessment. For each of the following patients, state whether the patient's priority is stable, potentially unstable, or unstable, and explain your reasoning:

1. A 26-year-old male found unresponsive on the ground outside a bar who is now waking up after you attempted to insert a nasopharyngeal airway
2. A 60-year-old female complaining only of weakness who appears pale and sweaty, is alert, and has no problem with the A-B-Cs, but just "looks" to you as though she is very sick
3. A 6-month-old infant who vomited but appears happy and is reacting appropriately to the people and things around her now
4. A patient who tells you that she has severe difficulty breathing
5. A patient who has ingested too much alcohol and is vomiting
6. A patient who is doubled over, screaming, because of abdominal pain

For each of the following patients, determine which portion of the primary assessment would be performed first (C-A-B approach or A-B-C approach) and explain your reasoning:

1. A patient who is unresponsive with arterial bleeding coming from his neck
2. A patient with a broken ankle and no other apparent injury
3. A patient who is not moving and does not appear to be breathing

Pathophysiology to Practice

The following questions are designed to assist you in gathering relevant clinical information and making accurate decisions in the field.

1. Describe how administration of oxygen to an unresponsive patient might lead you to change a patient's priority.
2. An older adult patient with Alzheimer's disease is acting abnormally, according to his family. He is alert and oriented to name but not place or time. His family says this is his normal mental status. What priority should you assign him and why?
3. A middle-aged male is lying on the street after he was hit by a car. He appears unresponsive as you approach. You notice that he is bleeding from a laceration on his forearm and making gurgling sounds from his airway. If you are alone, what factors do you consider in deciding what to do first? Why?

Street Scenes

Your patient is a 78-year-old unconscious male who was shaving with his electric razor when he fell to the floor. You hear snoring respirations as you initiate manual spinal motion restriction precautions and determine that the patient responds to painful stimuli. You then perform a jaw-thrust maneuver, continue to assess the airway and breathing, and confirm that the patient has snoring respirations. With the help of your partner, you insert an oropharyngeal airway, reassess breathing, and observe labored respirations and cyanosis around the lips. After you give the patient high-concentration oxygen by nonrebreather mask, you assess his circulation. In a minute or so, the patient regains consciousness, and his skin color improves. He tells you his name is Danya and explains that he had suddenly felt lightheaded, sat down, and must have passed out. Later, during transport, you keep the patient on oxygen, take another set of vital signs, and gather a patient history.

Street Scene Questions

1. What should be done immediately on contact with an unconscious patient who has fallen?
2. What are some considerations when opening the airway of an unconscious patient?
3. Using the AVPU scale, what is the level of responsiveness of a patient who responds to your calling out the patient's name?

When you return to quarters, you hope to get a short break, but it's just minutes before you receive a call for a 7-year-old patient reported to be unresponsive at the Mount Hope Elementary School. On arrival, you are directed to the athletic field, where the coach and school nurse tell you that Joey Sullivan had a seizure for the second time this month. His eyes are closed, he is not moving, and his skin color appears normal. Your partner gets down next to the patient to assess his mental status. "Hey, Joey!" she calls out. He does not respond. She pinches a fingernail firmly. There is still no response. "Unresponsive to pain," she says to you. When she tilts Joey's head back, there is a good deal of saliva visible in his mouth. Suctioning removes it without difficulty, and you administer oxygen to the patient by nonrebreather mask. You turn Joey onto his side and get a complete set of vital signs as your partner gets the stretcher. By the time you place Joey on the stretcher, he is becoming more responsive. Because of his improving mental status, you downgrade his priority and transport him to the hospital.

Street Scene Questions

4. Would knowing the cause of Joey's seizures change how you performed his primary assessment?
5. For Joey, what is the best position to prevent airway problems from occurring?
6. How did Joey's priority change during this call?

13 Vital Signs and Monitoring Devices

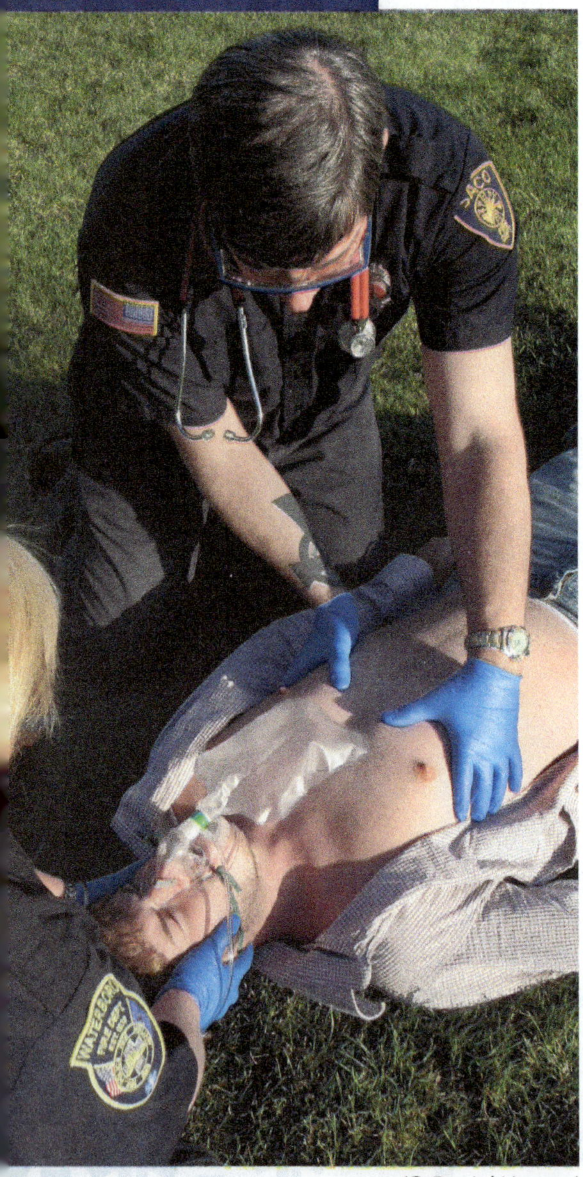

(© Daniel Limmer)

Related Chapters

The following chapters provide additional information related to topics discussed in this chapter:

Standard

Assessment (Monitoring Devices)

Competency

Applies scene information and patient assessment findings (scene size-up, primary and secondary assessments, patient history, and reassessment) to guide emergency management.

Core Concepts

- How to obtain vital signs, including pulse, respirations, blood pressure, skin, temperature, and pupils
- How to document vital signs on a prehospital care report
- How to use various monitoring devices

Outcomes

After reading this chapter, you should be able to:

13.1 Explain the contribution of vital signs to the patient assessment process. (pp. 340–359)

- Describe the physiologic processes indicated by each vital sign.
- Explain causes of abnormal vital signs.
- Describe modifications of assessing circulation in children.
- Compare vital signs of infants and children with those of adults.
- Describe the techniques for assessing each of the vital signs.
- Integrate vital signs with other assessment findings to refine the patient's priority.
- Recognize characteristics that can lead to difficulty or false readings when obtaining vital signs.
- Compare auscultation, palpation, and automatic blood pressure monitor approaches to obtaining a blood pressure.

13.2 Explain the contribution of information from monitoring devices to patient assessment. (pp. 359–365)

- Identify patients for whom the use of a monitoring device will provide useful information.
- Outline the steps of using various monitoring devices.
- Interpret findings of pulse oximetry.
- Recognize blood glucose level normal ranges.
- Identify situations that can lead to difficulty or false readings when using a monitoring device.

Key Terms

auscultation, *352*
blood pressure, *350*
blood pressure monitor, *352*
brachial artery, *352*
brachial pulse, *344*
bradycardia, *341*
carotid pulse, *344*
constrict, *349*
diastolic blood pressure, *350*
dilate, *349*
oxygen saturation (SpO_2), *359*
palpation, *352*
pulse, *340*
pulse oximeter, *359*
pulse quality, *344*
pulse rate, *340*
pupil, *349*
radial pulse, *344*
reactivity, *349*
respiration, *345*
respiratory quality, *346*
respiratory rate, *345*
respiratory rhythm, *347*
sphygmomanometer, *352*
systolic blood pressure, *350*
tachycardia, *341*
vital signs, *340*

Following the primary assessment and control of any immediate life threats, you will begin a more thorough assessment of your patient. An essential element of this assessment will be measuring vital signs. Vital signs are measurable things such as pulse, blood pressure, and respirations. Because they reflect the patient's condition—and changes in the patient's condition—you will take them early and repeat them often.

Gathering the Vital Signs

When you begin to assess a patient, some things are obvious or easy to discover. For example, the most important part of patient assessment is the chief complaint, the reason the patient called for EMS. Usually the patient will describe the complaint. Other parts of assessment that are usually apparent as soon as you see and talk to the patient are age, sex, and general alertness. However, not all parts of your assessment are so obvious or so easy to find out. The vital signs, for example, are major components of assessment that will take a few minutes to complete.

Vital signs are gathered on virtually every EMS patient. Occasionally a patient will be so seriously injured or ill that you are not able to get this information because you are too busy treating immediate threats to life. This is the exception, however. The vast majority of patients you will encounter as an EMT should have an assessment that includes vital signs measurement. If you do not get this information, you may remain unaware of important conditions or trends in patient conditions that require you to provide particular treatments in the field or that prompt transport to a hospital.

Where do vital signs fit into the sequence of patient assessment? After the primary assessment to find and treat immediate life threats (which was the subject of the *Primary Assessment* chapter), you will conduct a more thorough assessment that includes a secondary assessment (which will be the subject of *Secondary Assessment* chapter). Vital signs will be obtained during this part of the assessment process.

Vital Signs

vital signs
outward signs of what is going on inside the body, including respiration; pulse; skin color, temperature, and condition (plus capillary refill in infants and children); pupils; and blood pressure.

Vital signs are outward signs of what is going on inside the body. They include pulse; respiration; skin color, temperature, and condition (plus capillary refill in infants and children); pupils; and blood pressure. Although oxygen saturation is not considered to be a vital sign, many EMS providers include it with their consideration of the vital signs. (See Visual Guide: Vital Signs Evaluation.)

CORE CONCEPT

How to obtain vital signs, including pulse, respirations, blood pressure, skin temperature, and appearance of pupils

Evaluation of these indicators can provide you, as an EMT, with valuable information. The first measurements you obtain are called the baseline vital signs. You can gain even more valuable information when you repeat the vital signs and compare them with the baseline measurements. This allows you and other members of the patient's health care team to see trends in the patient's condition and to respond appropriately.

Another sign that gives important information about a patient's condition is mental status. Although it is not considered one of the vital signs, you should assess the patient's mental status whenever you take the vital signs. The *Primary Assessment* described how to evaluate mental status.

NOTE: *It is essential that you record all vital signs as you obtain them, along with the time at which you took them.*

Pulse

pulse
the rhythmic beats felt as the heart pumps blood through the arteries.

The pumping action of the heart is normally rhythmic, causing blood to move through the arteries in waves—not smoothly and continuously, at the same pressure, like water flowing through a pipe. A fingertip held over an artery where it lies close to the body's surface and crosses over a bone can easily feel the characteristic "beats" as the surging blood causes the artery to expand. What you feel is called the ***pulse***. When taking a patient's pulse, you are concerned with two factors: rate and quality (Figure 13-1).

Pulse Rate

pulse rate
the number of pulse beats per minute.

The ***pulse rate*** is the number of beats per minute. The number you get will allow you to decide if the patient's pulse rate is normal, rapid, or slow (Table 13-1).

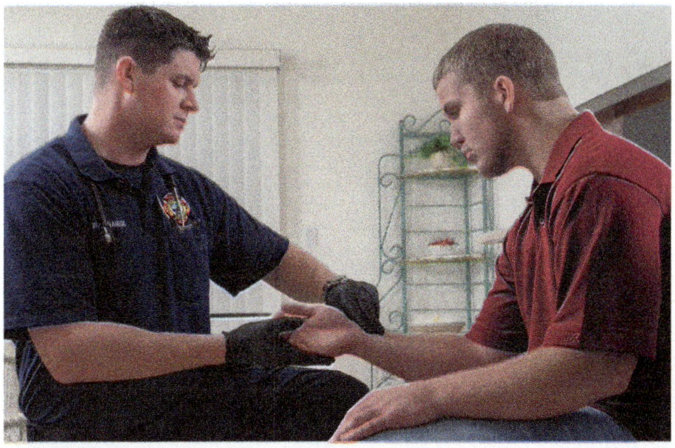

FIGURE 13-1 Assess pulse rate and quality. Count for 30 seconds and multiply by 2 to obtain the beats per minute.

Pulse rates vary among individuals. Factors such as age, physical condition, degree of exercise just completed, medications or other substances being taken, blood loss, stress, and body temperature all have an influence on the rate. The normal rate for an adult at rest is between 60 and 100 beats per minute. Any pulse rate above 100 beats per minute is rapid, whereas a rate below 60 beats per minute is slow. A rapid pulse is called ***tachycardia***. In contrast, a slow pulse is called ***bradycardia***. Athletes, because of their conditioning, may have a normal at-rest pulse rate between 40 and 50 beats per minute. This is slow but does not indicate poor health. However, the same pulse rate in a nonathletic or elderly person may indicate a serious condition. You should be concerned about the typical adult whose pulse rate stays above 100 or below 60 beats per minute.

In an emergency, it is not unusual for the pulse rate to fluctuate temporarily between 100 and 140 beats per minute. If the pulse rate is higher than 150, or if you take a patient's pulse several times during care on scene and find a pulse rate staying above 120 beats or below 50 beats per minute, consider this a sign that something may be seriously wrong with the patient, and transport as soon as possible.

tachycardia
(TAK-uh-KAR-de-uh)
a rapid pulse; any resting pulse rate above 100 beats per minute in an adult.

bradycardia
(BRAY-duh-KAR-de-uh)
a slow pulse; any pulse rate below 60 beats per minute.

TABLE 13-1 Pulse

NORMAL PULSE RATES (BEATS PER MINUTE AT REST)	
Adult	60-100
Adolescent 11-18 years	60-100
School age 6-10 years	65-120 (awake; slightly lower when asleep)
Preschoolers	70-120 (awake; slightly lower when asleep)
Toddler 1-3 years	80-140 (awake; slightly lower when asleep)
Infant 0-12 months	90-160 (awake; slightly lower when asleep)
Newborn	100-170 (awake; slightly lower when asleep)
PULSE QUALITY	**SIGNIFICANCE/POSSIBLE CAUSES**
Rapid, regular, and full	Exertion, fright, fever, high blood pressure, first stage of blood loss
Rapid, regular, and thready Irregular	Shock, later stages of blood loss Abnormal electrical activity in the heart
Slow	Head injury, drugs, some poisons, some heart problems, lack of oxygen in children
No pulse	Cardiac arrest (clinical death) **NOTE:** If a patient is awake and talking to you but has no carotid pulses, ask if the patient has a ventricular assist device.

13 Obtaining Vital Signs

THE SIX VITAL SIGNS

Pulse

Presence
Strength
Regularity

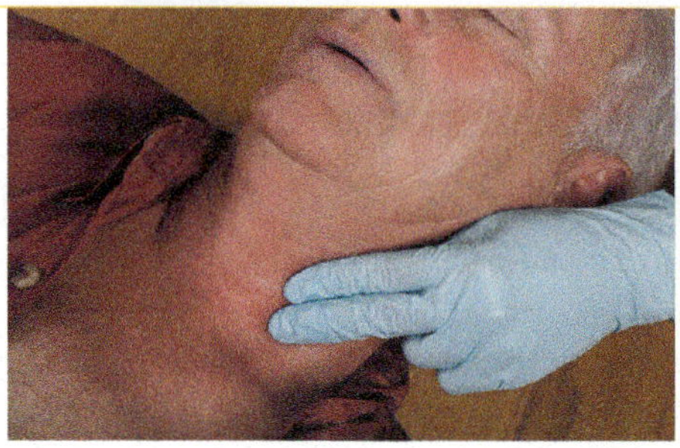

Unresponsive patient

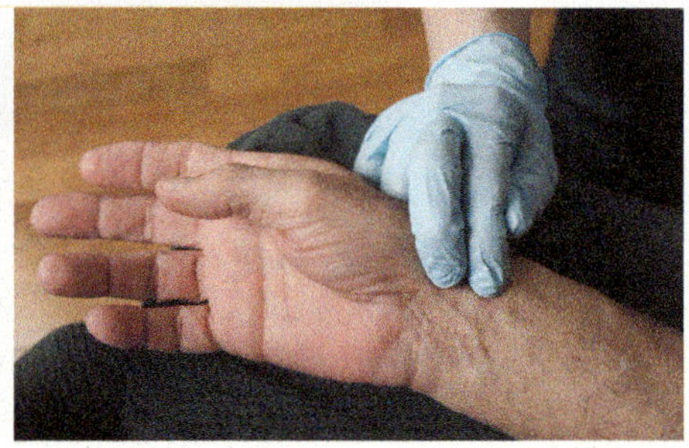

Responsive patient

Blood Pressure

Systolic
Diastolic
Palpation–systolic only

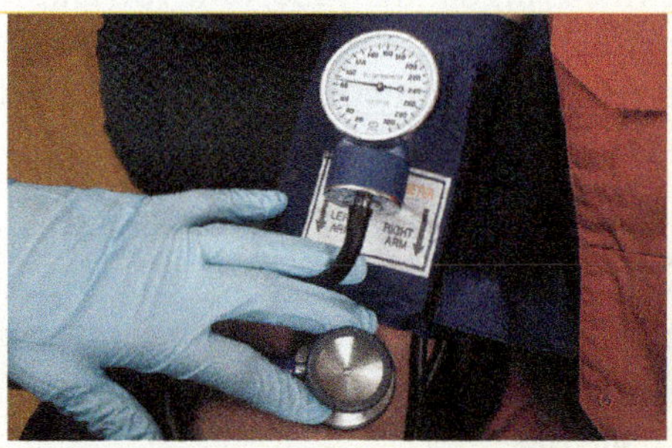

Auscultation

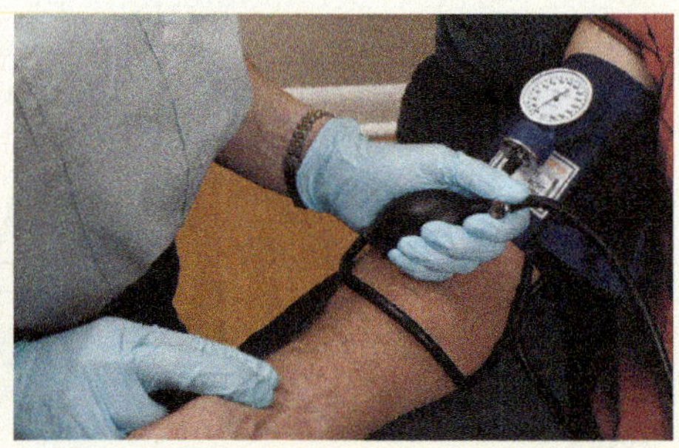

Palpation

Skin

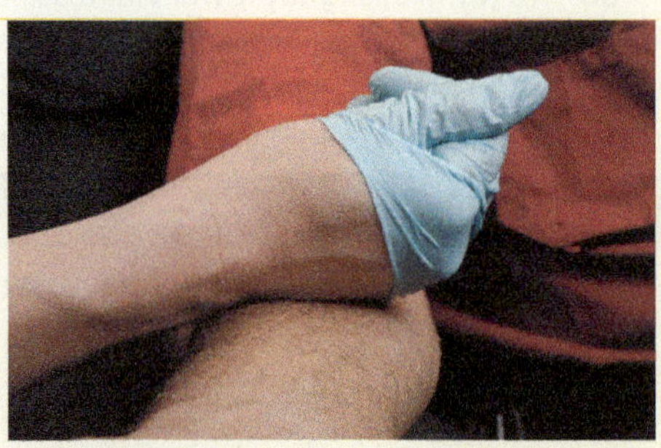

Color, temperature, and condition

Respirations

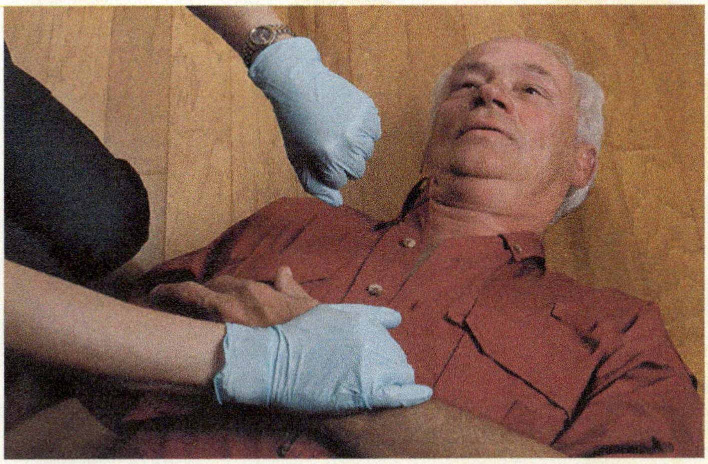

Rate and depth

Pupils

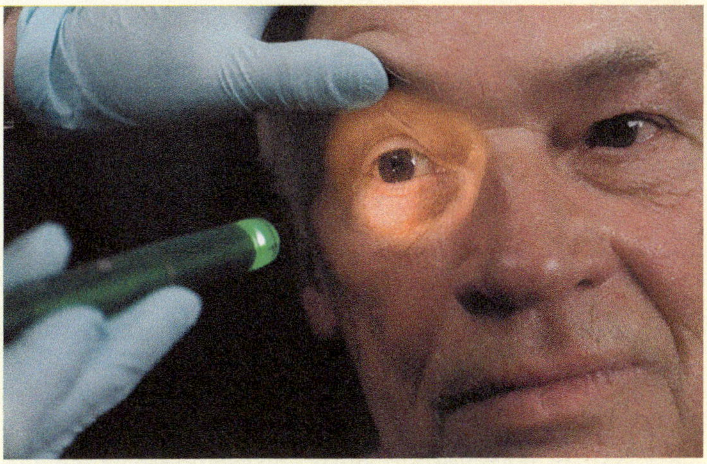

Size and reactivity

Pulse Oximetry

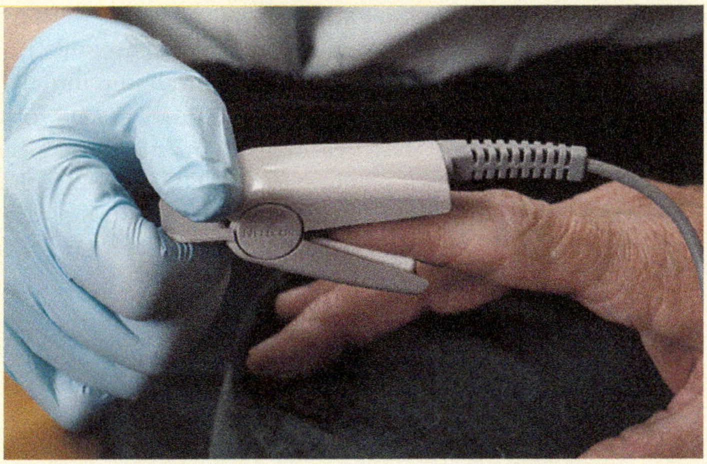

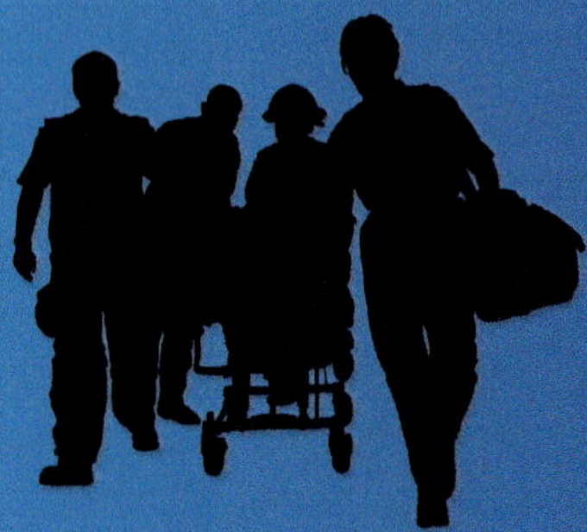

Think Like an EMT

Solving Assessment Problems

An accurate set of vital signs is an important foundation for critical decision making. For each of the common EMS situations that follow, describe how you would solve the problem you are faced with. In some cases, you may think of more than one potential solution.

1. You are trying to count the respiratory rate of a very talkative middle-aged male. Every time you think you're beginning to get an accurate count, he starts talking again.
2. You are about to put a blood pressure cuff on a 40-year-old male when he says that you can't put the cuff on that arm. He is a kidney dialysis patient and says he has a shunt in that arm. Because of the small room he is in, you can't get over to his other side.
3. The patient is an unconscious 32-year-old female who was thrown from a car when it flipped over. When you attempt to check the pulse at the patient's wrist, you search and search but can't find it.

Pediatric Note

A high pulse in an infant or child is not as great a concern as a low pulse. A low pulse may indicate imminent cardiac arrest.

Pulse Quality

pulse quality the rhythm (regular or irregular) and force (strong or weak) of the pulse.

Two factors determine ***pulse quality***: rhythm and force. *Pulse rhythm* reflects regularity. A pulse is said to be regular when intervals between beats are constant. When the intervals are not constant, the pulse is irregular. You should report and document irregular pulse rhythms.

Pulse force refers to the pressure of the pulse wave as it expands the artery. Normally the pulse should feel as if a strong wave has passed under your fingertips. This is a strong or full pulse. When the pulse feels weak and thin, the patient has a thready pulse. Many disorders can be related to variations in pulse rate, rhythm, and force (Table 13-1).

radial (RAY-de-ul) ***pulse*** the pulse felt at the wrist.

brachial (BRAY-key-al) ***pulse*** the pulse felt in the upper arm.

carotid (kah-ROT-id) ***pulse*** the pulse felt along the large carotid artery on either side of the neck.

Pulse rate and quality can be determined at a number of points throughout the body. During the determination of vital signs, you should initially find a ***radial pulse*** in patients 1 year of age and older. This is the wrist pulse, named for the radial artery found on the lateral (thumb) side of the forearm. In an infant who is 1 year old or younger, you should find the ***brachial pulse*** in the upper arm (Figure 13-2) rather than the radial pulse. If you cannot measure the pulse on one arm, try the pulse of the other arm. When you cannot measure the radial or brachial pulse, use the ***carotid pulse***, felt along the large carotid artery on either side of the neck. Be careful when palpating a carotid pulse in a patient. Excessive pressure on the carotid artery can result in slowing of the heart, especially in older patients. If you have difficulty finding the carotid pulse on one side, try the other side, but *do not assess the carotid pulses on both sides at the same time.*

To measure a radial pulse, find the pulse site by placing your first three fingers on the thumb side of the patient's wrist just above the wrist crease (toward the shoulder). Do not

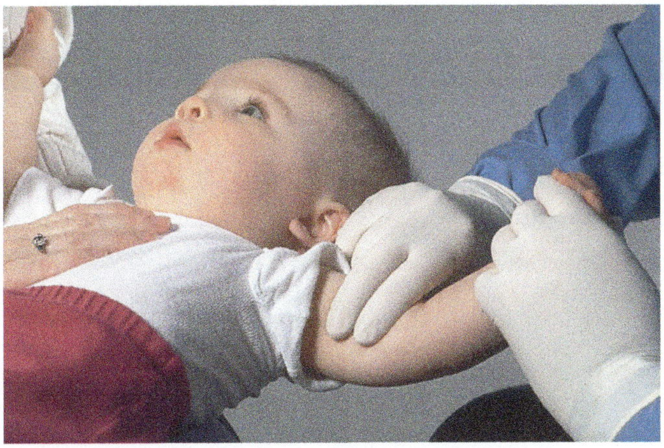

FIGURE 13-2 Palpating a brachial pulse in an infant. *(© Daniel Limmer)*

use your thumb. It has its own pulse that may cause you to measure your own pulse rate. Slide your fingertips toward the thumb side of the patient's wrist, keeping one finger over the crease. Apply moderate pressure to feel the pulse beats. If the patient has a weak pulse, you may need to apply greater pressure. But take care—if you press too hard, you may press the artery shut. Remember: If you experience difficulty, try the patient's other arm.

Count the pulsations for 30 seconds and multiply by 2 to determine the beats per minute. While you are counting, judge the rhythm and force. Record the information: for example, "Pulse 72, regular and full," and the time of determination.

If the pulse rate, rhythm, or force is not normal, continue with your count and observations for a full 60 seconds.

There is a situation where you may not be able to feel a pulse, but the patient is awake and talking to you. This is when he has a ventricular assist device, a pump implanted in the chest that helps the heart move blood through the circulatory system. Because many of these devices propel blood continuously and not in waves the way the heart does, there is no change in the pressure in the arteries. This means there is no pulse and no way to measure blood pressure.

CORE CONCEPT
How to document vital signs on a prehospital care report

Respiration

The act of breathing is called ***respiration***. A single breath is considered to be the complete process of breathing in (called *inhalation* or *inspiration*) followed by breathing out (called *exhalation* or *expiration*). For the determination of vital signs, you are concerned with two factors: rate and quality (Figure 13-3).

respiration (res-puh-RAY-shun) the act of breathing in and breathing out.

Respiratory Rate

The ***respiratory rate*** is the number of breaths a patient takes in one minute (Table 13-2). The rate of respiration is classified as *normal*, *rapid*, or *slow*. The normal respiration rate for an adult at rest is between 12 and 20 breaths per minute. Keep in mind that age, sex, size,

respiratory (RES-puh-ruh-tor-e) ***rate*** the number of breaths taken in one minute.

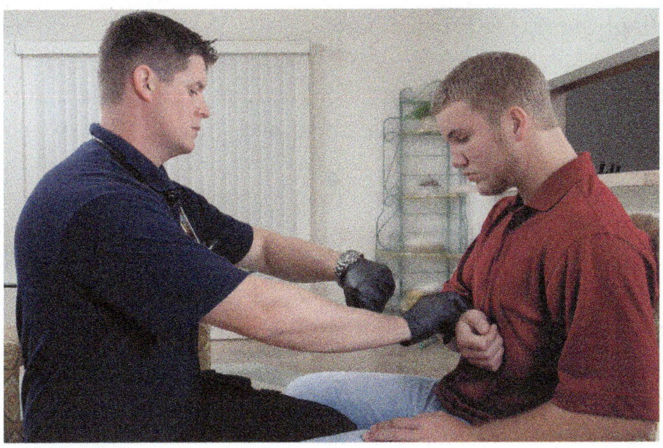

FIGURE 13-3 Assess respiration rate and quality. Count for 30 seconds and multiply by 2.

TABLE 13-2 Respirations

NORMAL RESPIRATORY RATES (BREATHS PER MINUTE, AT REST)	
Adult	12-20 Above 24: serious Below 10: serious
Adolescent (13-18 years)	12-20
School age (6-12 years)	18-30
Preschooler (3-5 years)	22-34
Toddler (1-3 years)	24-40
Infant	30-60 (0-6 months), 24-30 (6-12 months)
Newborn	30-60 (over 60 considered tachypnea)
RESPIRATORY SOUNDS	**POSSIBLE CAUSES/INTERVENTIONS**
Snoring	Airway blocked/open patient's airway; prompt transport
Wheezing	Medical problem such as asthma/assist patient in taking prescribed medications; prompt transport
Gurgling	Fluids in airway/suction airway; prompt transport
Crowing (harsh sound when inhaling)	Medical problem that cannot be treated on the scene/prompt transport

physical conditioning, and emotional state can all influence breathing rates. For example, fear and other emotions experienced during an emergency can cause an increase in respiratory rate. Unusually fast or slow respiratory rates may require you to act by administering oxygen or providing ventilations to the patient in respiratory failure.

Respiratory Quality

respiratory (RES-puh-ruh-tor-e) ***quality*** the normal or abnormal (shallow, labored, or noisy) character of breathing.

Respiratory quality, the quality of a patient's breathing, may fall into any of four categories: *normal, shallow, labored,* or *noisy*. Normal breathing means that the chest or abdomen moves an average depth with each breath and the patient is not using the accessory muscles (look for pronounced movement of the shoulder, neck, or abdominal muscles) to breathe. How can you tell if breathing is normal? Normal depth of respiration is something you can learn to judge by watching healthy people breathe when at rest.

Shallow breathing occurs when there is only slight movement of the chest or abdomen. This is especially serious in the unconscious patient. It is important to look not only at the chest but also at the abdomen when assessing respiration. Many resting people breathe more with their diaphragm (the muscle between the chest and the abdomen) than with their chest muscles.

Labored breathing can be recognized by signs such as an increase in the work of breathing (the patient has to work hard to move air in and out), the use of accessory muscles, nasal flaring (widening of the nostrils on inhalation), and retractions (pulling in) above the collarbones or between the ribs, especially in infants and children. You may also hear stridor (a harsh, high-pitched sound on inspiration), grunting on expiration (especially in infants), or gasping.

Noisy breathing is obstructed breathing (when something is blocking the flow of air). Sounds to be concerned about (Table 13-2) include snoring, wheezing, gurgling, and crowing. A patient with snoring respirations needs to have the airway opened. Wheezing may respond to prescribed medication that the patient has and that you may be able to assist the patient in taking. Gurgling sounds usually mean that you need to suction the patient's airway. Crowing (a noisy, harsh sound when breathing in) may not respond to any treatment you give. The patient who is crowing needs prompt transport—as do all patients with difficulty breathing.

Respiratory Rhythm

Respiratory rhythm is not important in most of the conscious patients you will see. This is because the regularity of an awake patient's breathing is affected by the patient's speech, mood, and activity, among other things. If you observe irregular respirations in an unconscious patient, however, you should report and document it.

respiratory (RES-puh-ruh-tor-e) ***rhythm***
the regular or irregular spacing of breaths.

Start counting respirations as soon as you have determined the pulse rate. Many individuals change their breathing rate if they know someone is watching them breathe. For this reason, do not move your hand from the patient's wrist or tell the patient you are counting the respiratory rate. Immediately after you have counted pulse beats, begin to watch the patient's chest and abdomen for breathing movements. Count the number of breaths taken by the patient during 30 seconds and multiply by 2 to obtain the breaths per minute. While counting, note the rate, quality, and rhythm of respiration. Record your results; for example, "Respirations are 16, normal, and regular." Then record the time of your assessment.

Skin

The color, temperature, and condition of the skin can provide valuable information about your patient's circulation. There are many blood vessels in the skin. Since the skin is not as important to survival as some of the other organs (such as the heart and brain), the blood vessels of the skin will receive less blood when a patient has lost a significant amount of blood or the ability to adequately circulate blood. Constriction (growing smaller) of the blood vessels causes the skin to become pale. For this reason, the skin can provide clues to blood loss as well as a variety of other conditions.

The best places to assess skin color in adults are the nail beds, the inside of the cheek, and the inside of the lower eyelids. Tiny blood vessels called capillaries are very close to the surface of the skin in all of these places, so changes in the blood are quickly reflected at these sites. They are also more accurate indicators than other sites in adults with dark complexions. In infants and children, the best places to look are the palms of the hands and the soles of the feet. In patients with dark skin, you can check the lips and nail beds.

Ordinarily the color you see (Table 13-3) in any of these places is pink. Abnormal colors include pale, cyanotic (blue–gray), flushed (red), and jaundiced (yellow). Pale skin frequently indicates poor circulation of blood. A common cause of this in the field is loss of blood. Cyanotic skin is usually a result of not enough oxygen getting to the red blood cells. Flushed skin may be caused by exposure to heat. Jaundice is a yellowish tint

TABLE 13-3 Skin Color

SKIN COLOR	SIGNIFICANCE/POSSIBLE CAUSES
Pink	Normal in light-skinned patients; normal at inner eyelids, lips, and nail beds of dark-skinned patients
Pale	Constricted blood vessels, possibly resulting from blood loss, shock, hypotension, emotional distress
Cyanotic (blue-gray)	Lack of oxygen in blood cells and tissues resulting from inadequate breathing or heart function
Flushed (red)	Exposure to heat, emotional excitement
Jaundiced (yellow)	Abnormalities of the liver
Mottled (blotchy)	Occasionally in patients with shock

TABLE 13-4 Skin Temperature and Condition

SKIN TEMPERATURE/CONDITION	SIGNIFICANCE/POSSIBLE CAUSES
Cool, clammy	Sign of shock, anxiety
Cold, moist	Body is losing heat.
Cold, dry	Exposure to cold
Hot, dry	High fever, heat exposure
Hot, moist	High fever, heat exposure
"Goose pimples" accompanied by shivering, chattering teeth, blue lips, and pale skin	Chills, communicable disease, exposure to cold, pain, or fear

to the skin from liver abnormalities. An uncommon skin coloration is mottling, a blotchy appearance that sometimes occurs in patients, especially children and the elderly, who are in shock.

To determine skin temperature (Table 13-4), feel the patient's skin with the back of your hand. A good place to do this is the patient's forehead (Figure 13-4). Note if the skin feels normal (warm), hot, cool, or cold. If the patient's skin seems cold, then further assess by placing the back of your hand on the abdomen beneath the clothing. At the same time, notice the patient's condition—is the skin dry (normal), moist, or clammy (both cool and moist)? Look for "goose pimples," which are often associated with chills. Many patient problems are exhibited by changes in skin temperature and condition. Continue to be alert for major temperature differences on various parts of the body. For example, you may note that the patient's trunk is warm but the left arm feels cold. Such a finding can reveal a problem with circulation.

Pediatric Note

In infants and children under 6 years of age, you should also evaluate capillary refill. Press on the nail bed–or the top of the hand or foot–and watch how long it takes for the normal pink color to return after you release it. Normally this takes no more than 2 seconds. If it takes longer, the patient's blood is probably not circulating well. Abnormal responses include prolonged and absent capillary refill. This sign is not reliable in infants or children who have been exposed to cold temperatures.

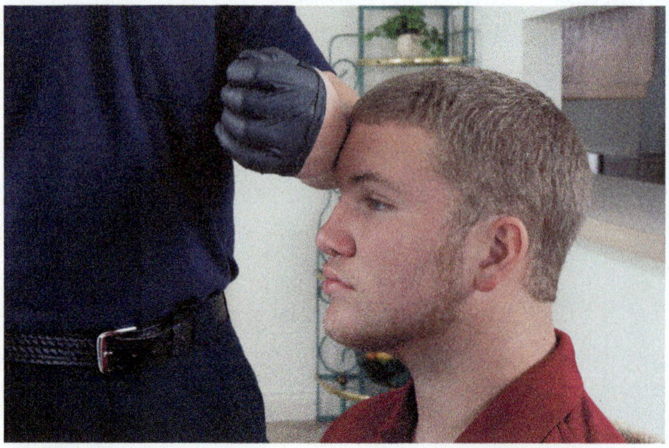

FIGURE 13-4 Determining skin temperature.

Pupils

The ***pupil*** is the black center of the eye. One of the things that cause it to change size is the amount of light entering the eye. When the environment is dim, the pupil will ***dilate*** (get larger) to allow more light into the eye. When there is a lot of light, the pupil will ***constrict*** (get smaller). Therefore, you will check a patient's pupils by shining a light into them (Figure 13-5 and Figure 13-6). When you check pupils, you should look for three things: size, equality, and ***reactivity*** (reacting to light by changing size). Under ordinary conditions, pupils are neither large nor small, but midpoint. Dilated pupils are extremely large. In fact, it is usually difficult to tell what color eyes the patient has if the pupils are dilated. Both pupils are normally the same size, and when a light shines into them, they react by constricting. The rate at which they constrict should be equal. Nonreactive (fixed) pupils do not constrict in response to a bright light.

pupil
the black center of the eye.

dilate (DI-late)
get larger.

constrict (kon-STRIKT)
get smaller.

reactivity (re-ak-TIV-uh-te)
in the pupils of the eyes, reacting to light by changing size.

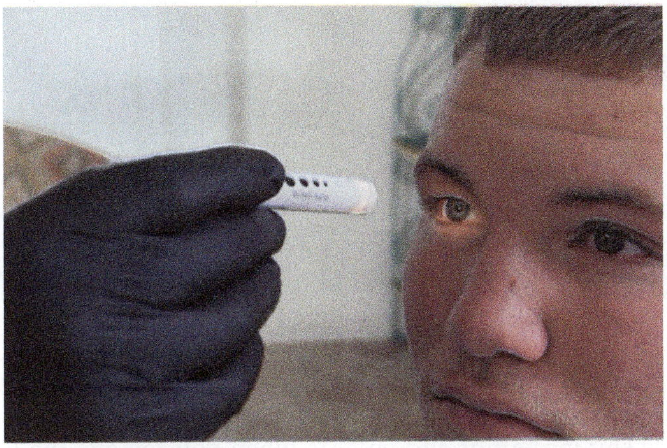

FIGURE 13-5 Examining the pupils.

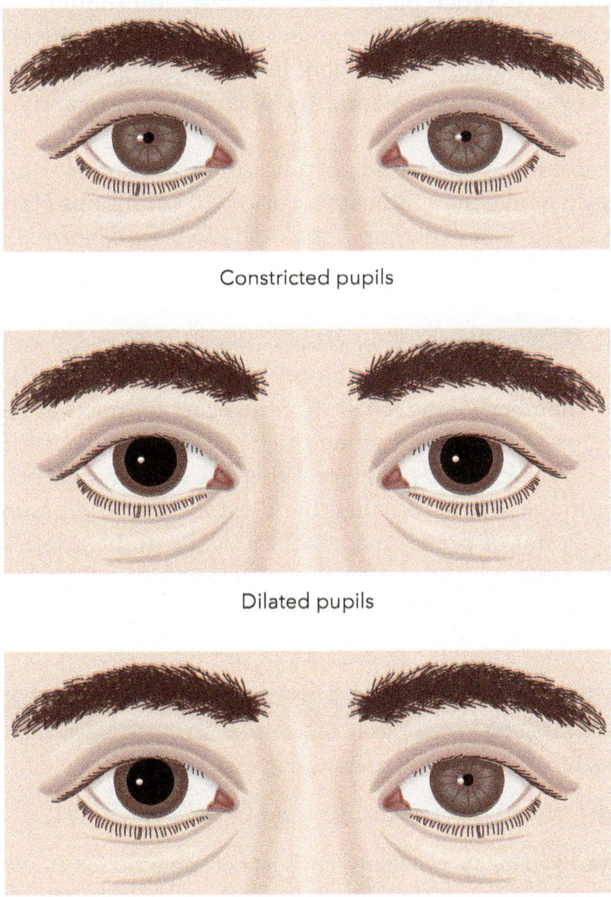

Constricted pupils

Dilated pupils

Unequal pupils

FIGURE 13-6 (A) Constricted, (B) dilated, and (C) unequal pupils.

FIGURE 13-7 Unequal pupils can be a sign of the influence of a topical drug (one placed directly on the eye, such as an eye drop) or of head or eye injury. *(© Edward T. Dickinson, MD)*

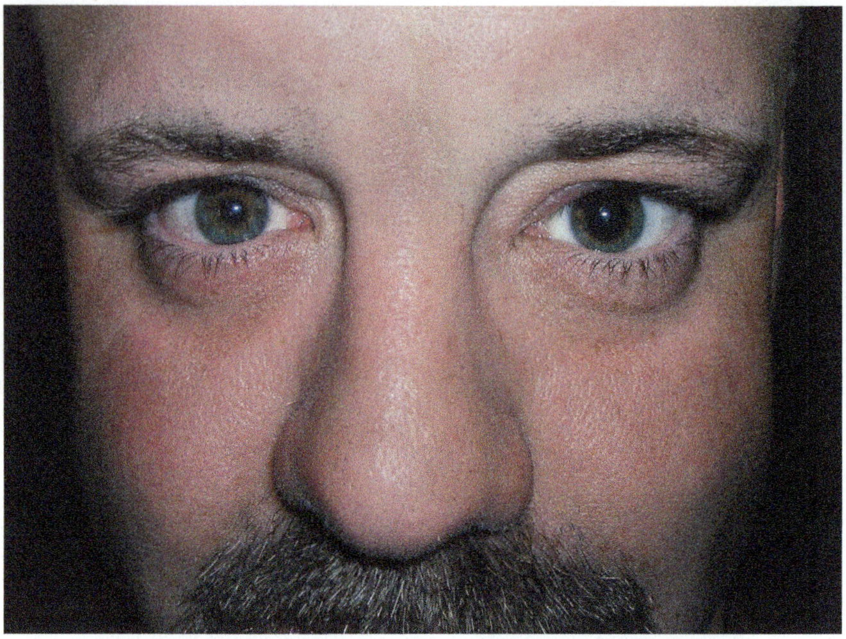

To check the patient's pupils, first note their size before you shine any light into them. Next, cover one eye as you shine a penlight into the other eye. The pupil should constrict when the light is shining into it and enlarge when you remove the light. Repeat this process with the other eye. When performing this test, you should cover the eye you are not examining, because light entering one eye usually affects the size of the pupils in both eyes. When you are examining a patient in direct sunlight or very bright conditions, initially cover both eyes. After a few seconds, uncover one eye and evaluate it. Cover it again and repeat with the other eye.

Pupils that are dilated, constricted to pinpoint size, unequal in size or reactivity (Figure 13-7), or nonreactive may indicate a variety of conditions (Table 13-5), including drug influence, head injury, or eye injury. Any deviations from normal should be reported and documented.

blood pressure
the force of blood against the walls of the blood vessels.

systolic (sis-TOL-ik) ***blood pressure***
the pressure created when the heart contracts and forces blood out into the arteries.

diastolic (di-as-TOL-ik) ***blood pressure***
the pressure remaining in the arteries when the left ventricle of the heart is relaxed and refilling.

Blood Pressure

The force of blood against the walls of the blood vessels is called ***blood pressure***. Each time the ventricle (lower chamber) of the left side of the heart contracts, it forces blood out into the circulation. The pressure created when the heart contracts and forces blood into the arteries is called the ***systolic blood pressure***. When the left ventricle relaxes and refills, the pressure remaining in the arteries is called the ***diastolic blood pressure***. These two pressures indicate the amount of pressure against the walls of the arteries, and together are known as the blood pressure. When you take a patient's blood pressure, you report the systolic pressure first and the diastolic second—for example, as "120 over 80," or "120/80."

TABLE 13-5 Pupils

PUPIL APPEARANCE	SIGNIFICANCE/POSSIBLE CAUSES
Dilated (larger than normal)	Fright, blood loss, drugs, prescription eye drops
Constricted (smaller than normal)	Drugs (narcotics), prescription eye drops
Unequal	Stroke, head injury, eye injury, artificial eye, prescription eye drops
Lack of reactivity	Drugs, lack of oxygen to brain

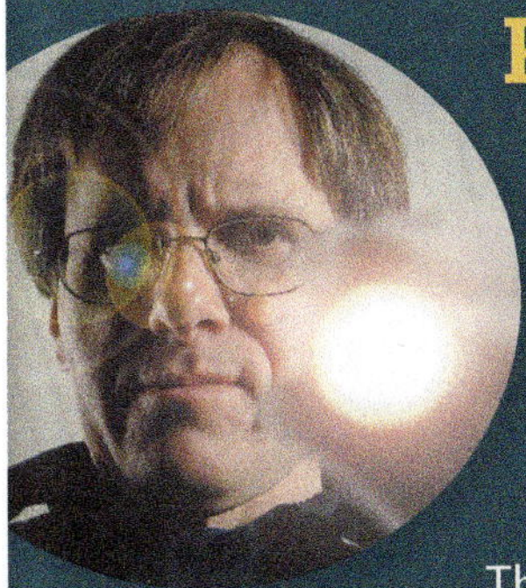

Point of View

"I have to tell you, people are glad when the ambulance shows up, but it is intimidating as hell. Pardon my language and everything, but I remember when I hit my head and passed out. It was like the cavalry came into my kitchen.

"My sister-in-law is an EMT. She talks about medical things like other people talk about going shopping. Really easy, like something you do every day. But when the EMTs came to my house, I was a little intimidated. They started doing this and checking that. It was hard enough to focus after just getting my bell rung. I couldn't even start to answer their questions, and to make things worse, they kept shining a flashlight in my eyes.

"On the way to the hospital, it got better. Actually, I think my head got clearer and it turns out they were worried about me. Something about 'altered mental status.' Maybe that means I was kind of nuts. We had a nice talk, and they told me it was good news that my pupils looked OK (Aha! That's why they were shining that light in my eyes) and also good news that I was talking with them now.

"I just finally felt like I had some control over what was going on."

One blood pressure reading in isolation may not be very meaningful. You will need to take several readings over a period of time while care is provided at the scene and during transport. Changes in blood pressure can be very significant. The patient's blood pressure may be normal in the early stages of some very serious problems, only to change rapidly in a matter of minutes.

Pulse and respiratory rates vary among individuals, but blood pressure is a little different (Table 13-6). A normal blood pressure is a systolic pressure of no more than 120 millimeters of mercury (mmHg) and a diastolic pressure of no more than 80 mmHg. *Millimeters of mercury* refers to the units on the blood pressure gauge. If an adult has a systolic pressure of 140 mmHg or greater or a diastolic pressure of 90 mmHg or greater, the person has hypertension (high blood pressure). Readings between these limits (121–139 mmHg systolic and 81–89 mmHg diastolic) indicate a condition sometimes called

TABLE 13-6 Blood Pressure

BLOOD PRESSURE NORMAL RANGES	SYSTOLIC
Adult	Less than or equal to 120
Adolescent	About 107–117
Ages 1 to 10 years	Mean systolic pressure is 90 + (age in years times 2) Example: mean systolic pressure for 2-year-olds is 90 + 4. This formula is an average, and individual blood pressures vary.
Infant	About 90
At day 10	90
At birth	50–70
BLOOD PRESSURE	**SIGNIFICANCE/POSSIBLE CAUSES**
High blood pressure	Medical condition, exertion, fright, emotional distress, or excitement
Low blood pressure	Athlete or other person with normally low blood pressure; blood loss; late sign of shock
No blood pressure	Patient with a ventricular assist device in the chest

FIGURE 13-8 Positioning blood pressure cuff.

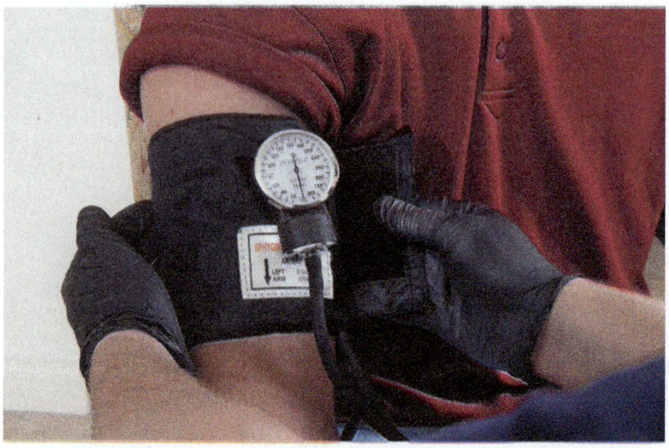

prehypertension. This means the patient is at risk of developing some of the complications of hypertension, such as heart disease, stroke, or kidney disease.

One of the most important factors that determine the normal range of vital signs is age. Infants and children have faster pulse and respiratory rates and lower blood pressures than adults. Compare the ranges for infants and children with those for adults as displayed in the tables in this chapter.

Serious low blood pressure is generally considered to exist when the systolic pressure falls below 90 mmHg. Many individuals under stress (such as that caused by having the ambulance come to their home) will exhibit a temporary rise in blood pressure. More than one reading will be necessary to decide if a high or low reading is only temporary. If the blood pressure drops, your patient may be developing shock. (However, other signs are usually more important early indicators of shock.) Report any major changes in blood pressure to emergency department personnel without delay.

sphygmomanometer (SFIG-mo-mah-NOM-uh-ter) the cuff and gauge used to measure blood pressure.

To measure blood pressure with a ***sphygmomanometer*** (the cuff and gauge), first place the stethoscope around your neck. Position yourself at the patient's side and place the blood pressure cuff on the patient's arm (Figure 13-8). The cuff should cover two-thirds of the upper arm, elbow to shoulder. Be certain that there are no suspected or obvious injuries to this arm. There are several patient populations where the use of a blood pressure cuff must be avoided on one arm due to pre-existing conditions. When determining a blood pressure in patients who have had a breast removed (mastectomy) or those who have an arm dialysis graft or fistula (see chapters titled *Hematologic and Renal Emergencies* and *Emergencies for Patients with Special Challenges*), the arm opposite the surgical procedure should be utilized. Similarly, a blood pressure cuff should not be placed directly on top of an IV catheter site. There should be no clothing under the cuff. If you can expose the arm sufficiently by rolling the sleeve up, do so, but make sure that this roll of clothing does not become a constricting band.

brachial (BRAY-key-al) ***artery*** the major artery of the arm.

auscultation (os-kul-TAY-shun) listening. A stethoscope is used to auscultate for characteristic sounds.

palpation touching or feeling. A pulse or blood pressure may be palpated with the fingertips.

blood pressure monitor a machine that automatically inflates a blood pressure cuff and measures blood pressure.

Wrap the cuff around the patient's upper arm so the lower edge of the cuff is about 1 inch (2.5 cm) above the crease of the elbow. The center of the bladder must be placed over the ***brachial artery***, the major artery of the arm. The marker on the cuff (if provided) should indicate where you place the cuff in relation to the artery. However, many cuffs do not have markers in the correct location. Tubes entering the bladder are not always in the right location either. According to the American Heart Association, the only accurate method is to find the bladder center. Apply the cuff so it is secure but not overly tight. You are now ready to begin your determination of the patient's blood pressure.

Three common techniques are used to measure blood pressure with a sphygmomanometer: (1) ***auscultation***, when a stethoscope is used to listen for characteristic sounds (Figure 13-9); (2) ***palpation***, when the radial pulse or brachial pulse is palpated (felt) with the fingertips (Figure 13-10); and (3) ***blood pressure monitor***, when a machine controls inflation of the cuff and detects changes in blood flow in the artery (Figure 13-11 and Figure 13-12). Palpation is not as accurate as auscultation, since only an approximate systolic pressure can be determined. Palpation is used when there is too much noise

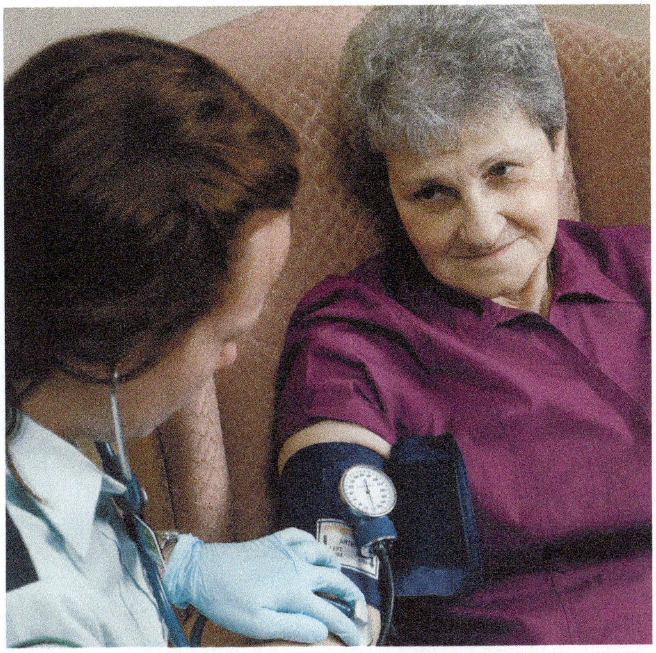

FIGURE 13-9 Measuring blood pressure by auscultation. Correct blood pressure cuff size is crucial for accuracy.

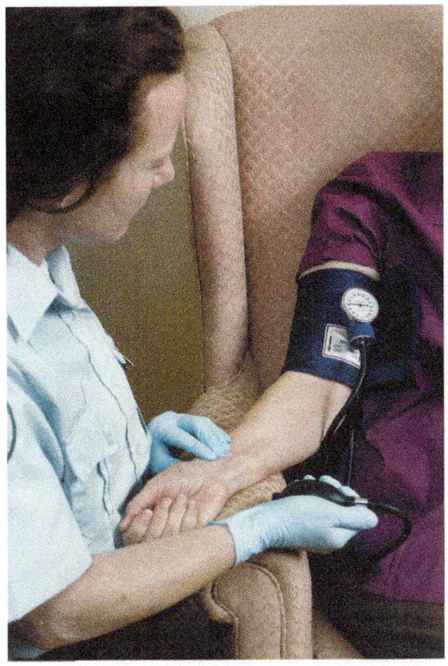

FIGURE 13-10 Measuring blood pressure by palpation.

around a patient to allow the use of the stethoscope. Blood pressure monitors are improving in quality, and many emergency departments and EMS agencies use them.

Determining Blood Pressure by Auscultation

1. **Prepare.** The patient should be seated or lying down. If the patient has not been injured, support the patient's arm at the level of the heart.
2. **Position the cuff and the stethoscope.** Place the cuff snugly around the upper arm so the bottom of the cuff is just above the elbow. With your fingertips, palpate the brachial artery at the crease of the elbow (Figure 13-13). Place the earpieces of the stethoscope in your ears. (The earpieces should be pointing forward in the direction of your ear canals.) Position the diaphragm of the stethoscope directly over the brachial

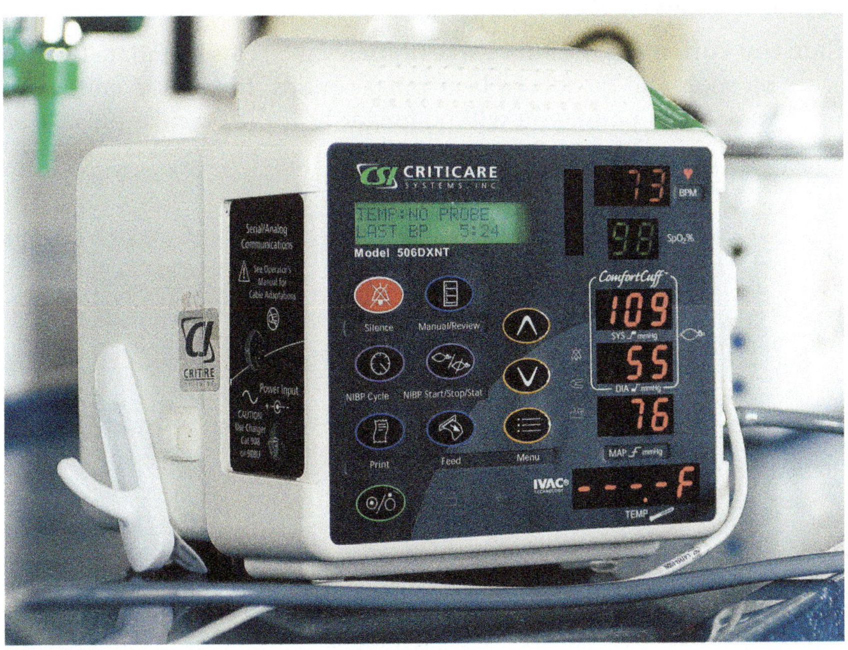

FIGURE 13-11 An automatic blood pressure monitor.

FIGURE 13-12 (A and B) Automated blood pressure cuff as part of an ECG monitor. (C and D) Stand-alone automated blood pressure cuff.

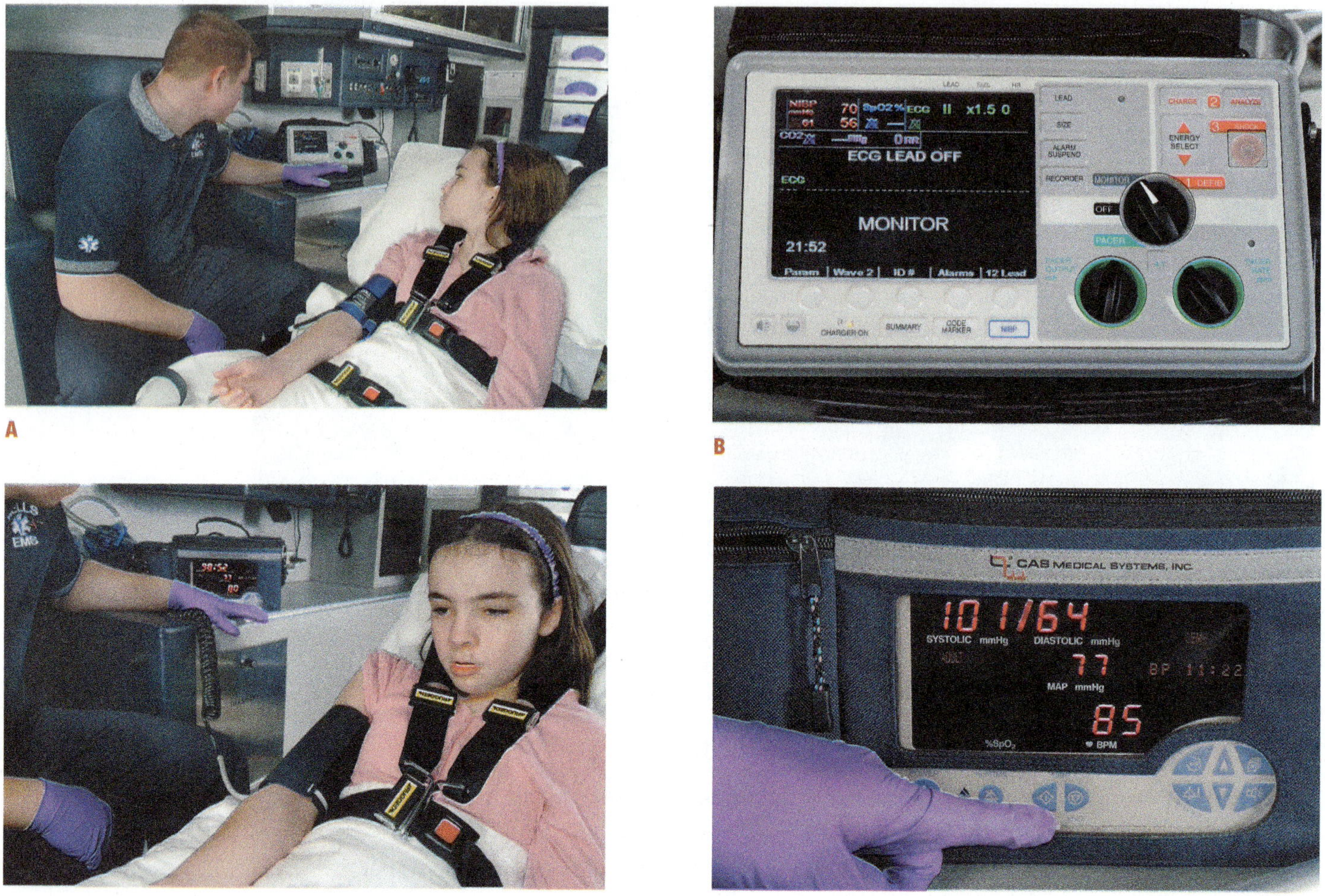

A B C D

pulse, or over the medial anterior elbow (front of the elbow) if no brachial pulse can be found. Do not place the head of the stethoscope underneath the cuff, since this will give you false readings.

3. **Inflate the cuff.** With the bulb valve (thumb valve) closed, inflate the cuff. As you do so, you soon will be able to hear pulse sounds. Inflate the cuff, watching the gauge. At a certain point, you will no longer hear the brachial pulse. Continue to

FIGURE 13-13 When measuring blood pressure by auscultation, locate the brachial artery by palpation before placing the stethoscope.

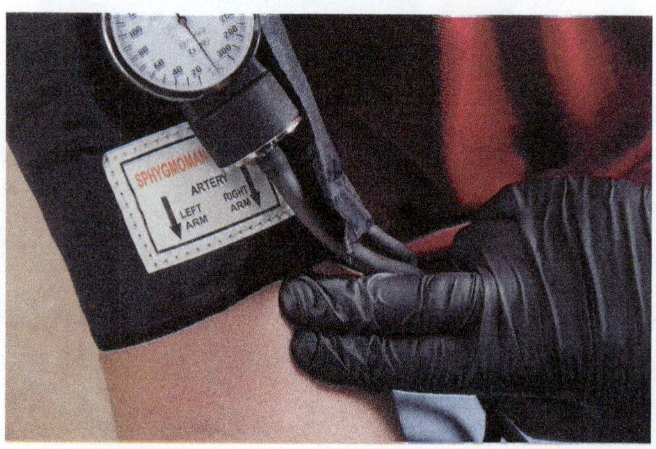

inflate the cuff until the gauge reads 30 mm higher than the point where the pulse sound disappeared.

4. **Obtain the systolic pressure.** Slowly release air from the cuff by opening the bulb valve, allowing the pressure to fall smoothly at the rate of approximately 5–10 mm per second. Listen for the start of clicking or tapping sounds. When you hear the first of these sounds, note the reading on the gauge. This is the systolic pressure.
5. **Obtain the diastolic pressure.** Continue to deflate the cuff, listening for the point at which these distinctive sounds fade. When the sounds turn to dull, muffled thuds, the reading on the gauge is the diastolic pressure. Sometimes you will not be able to hear a change in these sounds. When this happens, the point at which the sounds disappear is the diastolic pressure.
6. **Record measurements.** After obtaining the diastolic pressure, let the cuff deflate rapidly. Record the measurements and the time—for example, "Blood pressure is 140/90 at 1:10 p.m." Blood pressure is reported in even numbers. If a reading falls between two lines on the gauge, use the higher number.

If you are not certain of a reading, repeat the procedure. You should use the other arm or wait 1 minute before reinflating the cuff. Otherwise, you will tend to obtain an erroneously high reading. If you are still not sure of the reading, try again or get some help. Never make up vital signs!

NOTE: *Some patients who have high systolic blood pressures will have the pulse sounds disappear as you deflate the cuff but reappear as you continue with deflation. When this happens, false readings may be obtained. If you determine a high diastolic reading, wait 1-2 minutes and take another reading. As you inflate the cuff, feel for the disappearance in the radial pulse to ensure that you are not measuring a false diastolic pressure. Listen as you deflate the cuff down into the normal range. The diastolic pressure is the reading at which the last clear sound takes place.*

When the heartbeat is irregular, the interval between heartbeats can vary a great deal. You may obtain an artificially low blood pressure reading if you pass the systolic or diastolic pressure between two widely separated beats, especially if you deflate the cuff quickly. If the patient's heartbeat is irregular, you should deflate the cuff a little more slowly and listen even more carefully to obtain an accurate reading.

Determining Blood Pressure by Palpation

1. **Position the cuff and find the radial pulse.** Apply the cuff as described for auscultation. Then find the radial pulse on the arm to which the cuff has been applied. If a radial pulse cannot be palpated, find the brachial pulse.
2. **Inflate the cuff.** Make certain that the adjustable valve is closed on the bulb and inflate the cuff to a point where you can no longer feel the radial pulse. Note this point on the gauge and continue to inflate the cuff 30 mmHg beyond this point.
3. **Obtain and record the systolic pressure.** Slowly deflate the cuff, noting the reading at which the radial pulse returns. This reading is the patient's systolic pressure. Record your findings as, for example, "Blood pressure 140 by palpation" or "140/P" and the time of the determination. (You cannot determine a diastolic reading by palpation.)

Determining Blood Pressure by Blood Pressure Monitor

CORE CONCEPTS
How to use various monitoring devices

1. **Position the cuff.** Apply the cuff as described for auscultation.
2. **Inflate the cuff.** Press the button that tells the monitor to begin inflating the cuff.
3. **Obtain and record the blood pressure.** After the monitor has finished deflating the cuff, it will indicate the patient's blood pressure on a screen. If it cannot get a blood pressure, it will tell you. Some monitors will give not only the systolic and diastolic pressures but also the mean arterial pressure (MAP). As this is not typically used in prehospital care, do not let it distract you from the numbers you are seeking.

Pediatric Note

Obtain a blood pressure on every patient who is more than 3 years old. Blood pressures are difficult to obtain with any accuracy on infants and children younger than 3, and have little bearing on the patient's field management. You can get more useful information about the condition of an infant or very young child by observing for conditions such as a sick appearance, respiratory distress, or unconsciousness. See Scan 13-1 regarding vital signs on a child. Follow your local protocols.

Unless medical direction advises otherwise, the first blood pressure you get should be with the auscultation method. Although the quality of blood pressure monitors has been improving, these machines still make errors and occasionally fail. This may be more likely to happen in the prehospital environment. The blood pressure obtained by auscultation is the standard against which other blood pressures will be compared. If a reading from the blood pressure monitor is very different from the auscultated blood pressure, recheck the blood pressure yourself by auscultation or palpation.

Many blood pressure monitors have timers you can set to take the blood pressure every 5 minutes, every 15 minutes, or at some other interval determined by the operator. This can provide a useful reminder to the EMT when it is time to check the rest of the vital signs again.

It is important that the EMT follow the manufacturer's directions and local medical direction in using an automated blood pressure monitor or any other device used in patient assessment.

Vital signs are usually taken more than once. How frequently they should be repeated depends on the patient's condition and your interventions. Stable patients need repeat vital signs at least every 15 minutes. Unstable patients need repeat vital signs at least every 5 minutes. Also repeat vital signs after every medical intervention. Record every reading of the vital signs (Figure 13-14), because if you don't write them down, you probably won't remember them.

Temperature

The human body continuously generates and loses heat but manages to maintain a temperature within a narrow range that allows chemical reactions and other activities to take place inside the body. For most patients an EMT encounters, the temperature will not be important, although for some it may be. This includes cases where the patient may be hypothermic or hyperthermic (with a below-normal or above-normal temperature, often from a change in the environment), febrile (feverish), or suffering from a generalized infection (septic).

One very important use for temperature is in screening for influenza. Many EMS systems now record patient data electronically, which has allowed health departments to evaluate EMS data during flu season to see if there has been an outbreak of the disease in a particular area. By looking for patients with signs and symptoms consistent with influenza, including fever, public health specialists may be able to detect outbreaks earlier than ever before.

You learned earlier in this chapter about skin color, temperature, and condition. In this section, we are dealing not with the surface temperature of the skin but with the body's core temperature, or the closest we can get to measuring it. The core temperature reflects the level of heat inside the trunk, where the heart, lungs, and digestive organs function. Since it is usually not practical to place a thermometer inside someone's heart or stomach, we measure the closest substitute available. Traditionally this is either an oral or rectal temperature, but it is also possible to get an axillary temperature in the armpit (axilla).

SCAN 13-1 Taking Vital Signs on a Child

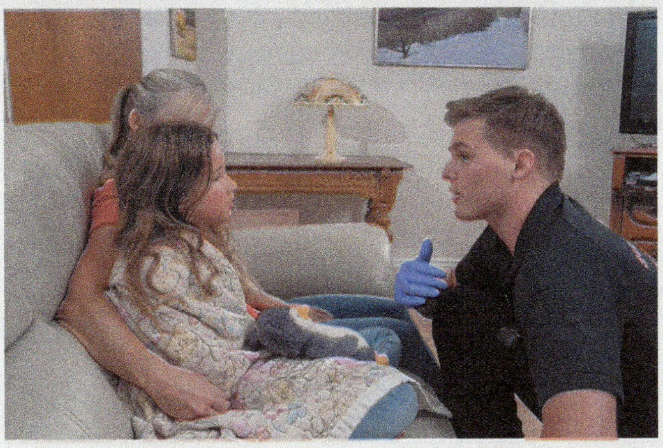

1. EMT talks to child. Get down at the patient's level. Explain what you will be doing, using terms the child will understand.

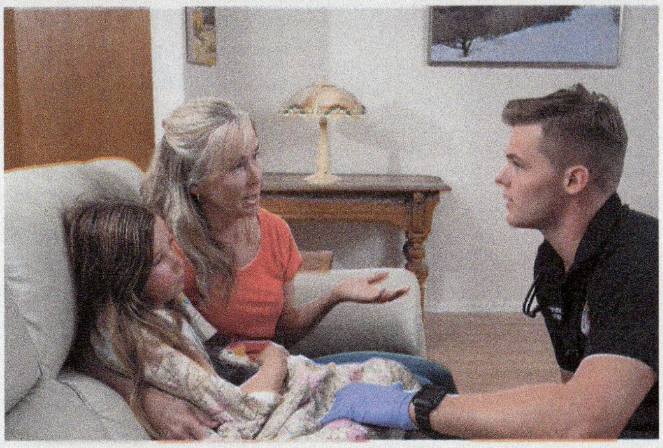

2. EMT talks to the parent. Parents may be present, and can assist with vital signs by helping keep the child calm. Parents can also report changes in mental status and in many cases provide the best patient history.

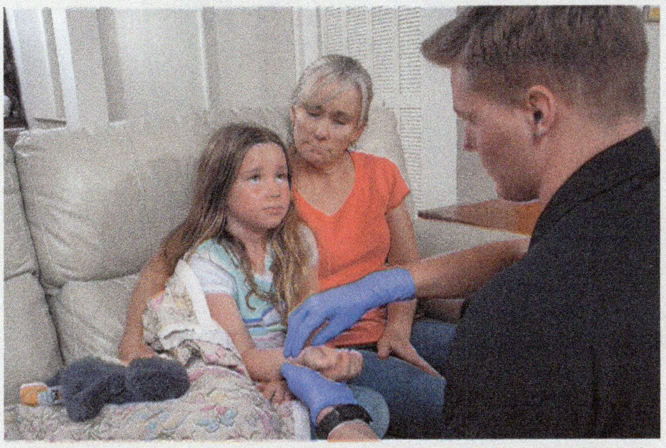

3. EMT takes a radial pulse. Comfort the child and take "easy" vital signs (pulse and respiration) first to help reduce anxiety.

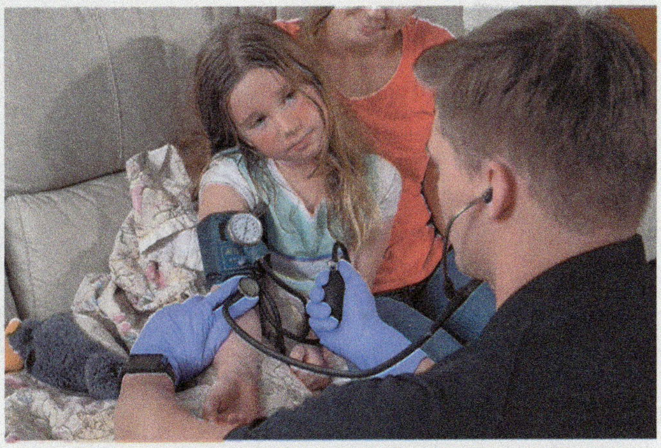

4. EMT takes BP. Make sure blood pressure cuff is properly sized. In infants and younger pediatric patients, blood pressure readings may not be accurate, and circulatory status can be reliably obtained by other means.

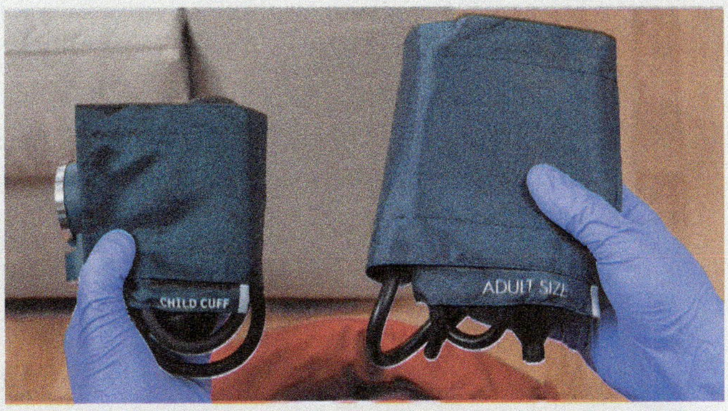

5. Two sizes of pediatric BP cuffs. Use of properly sized cuffs will provide accurate readings.

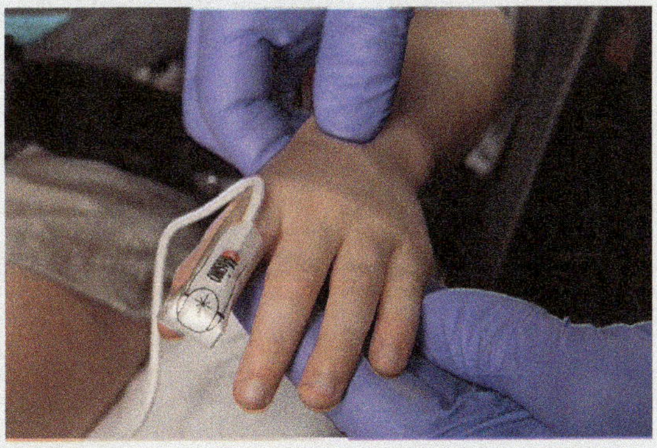

6. Pediatric pulse oximeter. Use properly sized devices for pediatric patients.

FIGURE 13-14 The prehospital care report (run sheet) provides spaces for recording vital signs.

Time	Pulse	Respirations	Blood Pressure
1410	88 str, reg	28	132/84
Pupils	**Skin Color**	**Skin Temperature**	**Skin Condition**
Equal ☑ Unequal ☐	Normal ☐	Cold ☐	Moist ☑
Reactive (L) (R)	Pale ☑	Cool ☑	Dry ☐
Nonreactive L R	Cyanotic ☐	Warm ☐	
Dilated ☐	Flushed ☐	Hot ☐	
Normal Size ☑	Jaundiced ☐		
Constricted ☐			

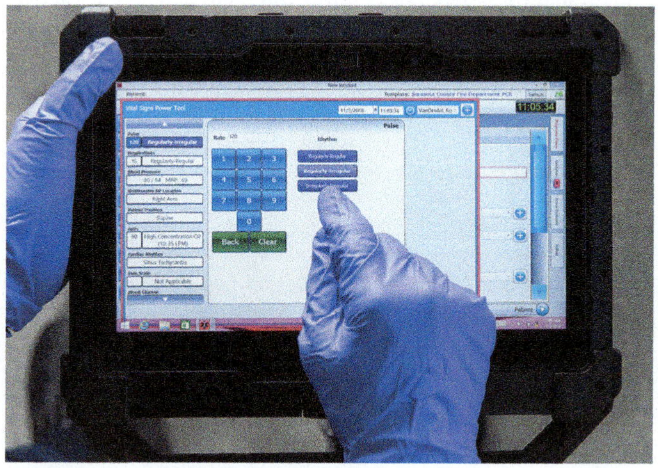

Although glass thermometers are usually accurate, the conditions EMTs encounter in the field make them undesirable. Putting a piece of glass into the patient's mouth, then traveling over bumpy roads in the back of a moving ambulance, risks injuring the patient from broken glass. A quicker way to get an oral temperature is to use an electronic thermometer (Figure 13-15), which usually provides a reading in just a few seconds. This is also safer and more hygienic, since these machines usually employ metal probes with disposable plastic covers. To get a temperature with an electronic thermometer, put a new plastic cover over the probe, insert it under the patient's tongue, and follow the

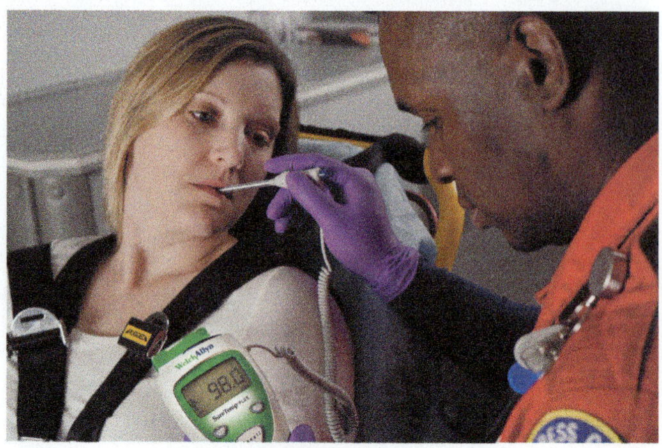

FIGURE 13-15 An electronic thermometer is safer, more hygienic, and quicker to produce a reading than a glass thermometer.

manufacturer's instructions. When an oral temperature is not practical, you can sometimes get an axillary temperature. Rectal temperatures are not usually practical or necessary in the field.

Tympanic thermometers that measure the temperature in the ear are commercially available and frequently used, but are not accurate enough for EMS use. Numerous evaluations of these devices have consistently found that the margin of error is quite wide. Many patients are misclassified as having abnormally high or low temperatures by tympanic devices. Forehead thermometers, strips placed on the forehead, are also not accurate enough for EMTs to use.

A normal temperature is not necessarily 98.6°F (37°C). A person's normal temperature depends on the time of day, activity level, age, where the temperature is measured, and simple genetics—some people just have a higher or lower normal temperature than other people. Temperature rises and falls at different times of the day and night and usually rises with increased physical activity. Older people tend to have lower temperatures than younger people. A rectal temperature is often about 1 degree Fahrenheit higher than an oral temperature, and an axillary temperature is frequently about a degree lower. Most people have a typical temperature somewhere near 98.6°F (37°C), but many healthy people walk around with temperatures that are not "normal" by these traditional measures. In general, a healthy, normal person will have a temperature greater than 96.8°F (36°C) and less than 101.3°F (38.5°C).

"Vital signs are important. Trends in vital signs tell the story."

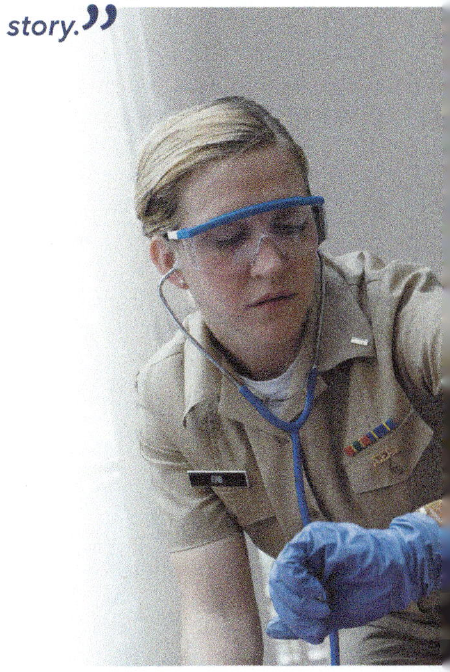

Monitoring Devices

Oxygen Saturation

EMTs and other health care providers commonly measure the level of oxygen circulating through a patient's blood vessels. A measurement of oxygen saturation is not a vital sign, but many EMS providers incorporate it into their gathering of vital signs. Your EMS system may have specific guidance on when to perform this measurement.

The device that measures oxygen saturation of the blood, called a ***pulse oximeter*** (Figure 13-16), sends different colors of light into the tissue at the end of a finger or on an earlobe and measures the amount of light that returns. The machine then determines the proportion of oxygen in the blood and displays the ***oxygen saturation (SpO_2)*** percentage.

pulse oximeter
an electronic device for determining the amount of oxygen carried in the blood, known as the oxygen saturation or SpO_2.

oxygen saturation (SpO_2)
the ratio of the amount of oxygen present in the blood to the amount that could be carried, expressed as a percentage.

FIGURE 13-16 A pulse oximeter with sensor applied to the patient's finger.

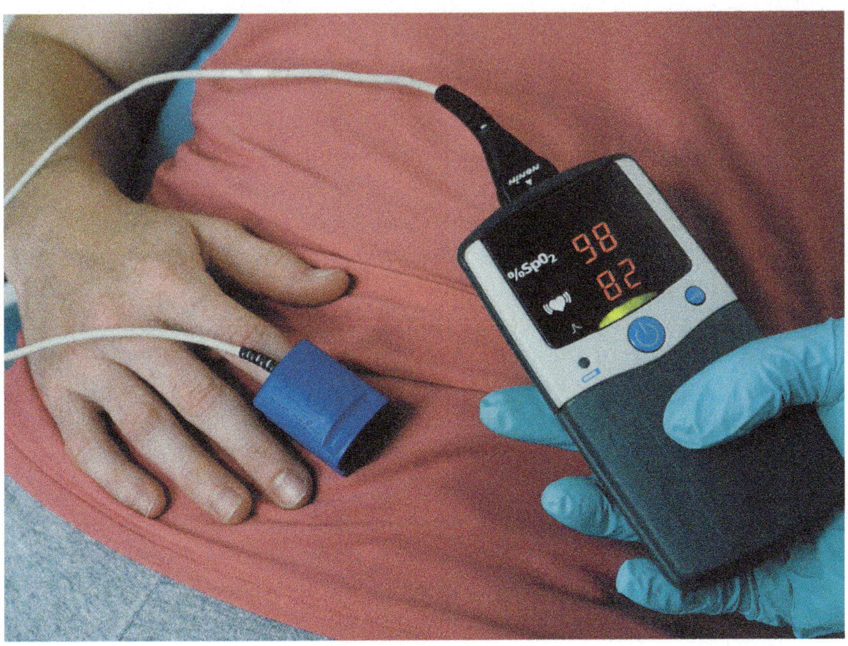

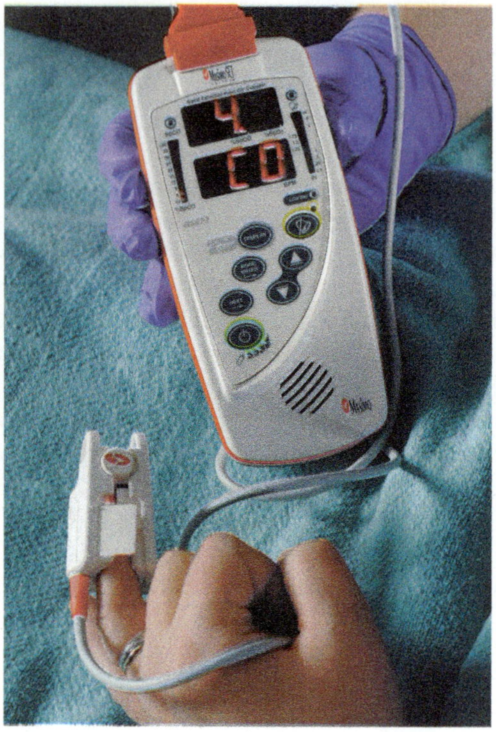

FIGURE 13-17 A CO-oximeter detects carbon monoxide as well as oxygen levels in the blood.

A different kind of oximeter uses different wavelengths of light that allow it to measure carbon monoxide (CO) as well as oxygen. For this reason, it is sometimes called a CO-oximeter (Figure 13-17). Future versions of this device will very likely be more accurate, less expensive, and easier to use than early models. Interpreting CO-oximeter readings in a particular clinical situation can be challenging, so if you use a CO-oximeter, be sure to follow your local protocols regarding its application and interpretation.

When to Use a Pulse Oximeter

If your service has a pulse oximeter, you should have a protocol governing when to use it. Generally, this will include many patients, including those complaining of respiratory problems or otherwise at risk for hypoxia. When used properly, the device can help you to assess the effectiveness of artificial respirations, oxygen therapy, and bronchodilator (inhaler) therapy.

Interpreting Pulse Oximeter Readings

The oxygen saturation, or SpO_2, is typically 96 percent to 100 percent in a normal healthy person. A value of nearly 96 percent may sound good, but that is not really the case. A reading of 91 percent to 95 percent indicates mild hypoxia, 86 percent to 90 percent indicates significant or moderate hypoxia, and 85 percent or less indicates severe hypoxia. The American Heart Association does not recommend oxygen administration for some types of patients unless the pulse oximetry is below 94 percent.

Oxygen administration requires clinical judgment along with the pulse oximetry reading. If the patient has any of the following conditions, administer high-concentration oxygen by nonrebreather mask (or bag–valve mask, if the patient's respiratory rate and depth are inadequate): exposure to carbon monoxide; moderate to severe hypoxia (saturation less than 90 percent); or severe respiratory distress, especially when combined with low saturation readings or peripheral perfusion so poor that you cannot get a reliable pulse oximeter reading. On the other hand, if the patient is in mild respiratory distress or has an oxygen saturation reading between 91 percent and 95 percent, you can administer low-concentration oxygen by nasal cannula. In all situations where you administer oxygen, you should reassess the patient periodically to determine whether to continue or to change the amount of oxygen you are administering. A patient who has improved significantly on high-concentration oxygen may not need it any longer and may be fine with low-concentration oxygen later.

NOTE: *Oxygen is a drug, and in some cases may actually cause harm. Your oxygenation decisions should be based on your assessment, the patient complaint, the level of distress, your protocols, and pulse oximetry readings.*

Cautions: The following cautions apply to interpreting pulse oximetry readings:

- The oximeter is inaccurate with patients in shock and hypothermic patients (those whose body temperatures have been lowered by exposure to cold), because not enough blood is flowing through the capillaries for the device to get an accurate reading.
- The oximeter will produce falsely high readings in patients with carbon monoxide and certain other uncommon types of poisoning. This is because carbon monoxide binds with hemoglobin in the blood, producing the red color read by the device. Because cigarettes produce carbon monoxide, chronic smokers may have 10 percent to 15 percent of their hemoglobin bound to carbon monoxide. This means their oxygen saturation readings will be higher than the actual oxygen saturation.
- Excessive movement of the patient can cause inaccurate readings, as can nail polish, if the device is attached to a finger. Carry acetone wipes to quickly remove the nail polish from a patient's fingernail before attaching the oximeter. Anemia and hypovolemia are other potential causes of falsely high oxygen saturation readings.
- The accuracy of the pulse oximeter should be checked regularly, following the manufacturer's recommendations. The batteries used to power the device must be in good condition, and the probe needs to be kept clean to get accurate readings.
- Pulse oximetry is also useful when evaluating the effect of an intervention you have instituted (when you hope the SpO_2 goes up or remains high) and alerting you to a deterioration in the patient's oxygen saturation (when the SpO_2 starts going down). When evaluating the effect of an intervention you have performed, remember not to rely solely on the oximeter for indications of the patient's condition. Treat the patient, not the device.

Determining Oxygen Saturation

1. Connect the sensor lead to the monitor and clip it onto a fingertip (toe or distal foot in an infant).
2. Turn the device on. After a few seconds, the device should display the SpO_2 and heart rate. Make sure the heart rate displayed on the monitor screen is the same as the patient's pulse rate (which you palpated already). If the heart rate shown on the pulse oximeter does not match the pulse rate that you have determined, it is likely that the oxygen saturation will not be an accurate reading either.
3. If you get a poor signal or "trouble" indicator, try repositioning the sensor on the finger or moving it to a different finger.
4. Once you get an accurate reading, check the oximeter reading every 5 minutes. A convenient time to do this is when you check the patient's vital signs.

Blood Glucose Meters

One of the many advances in managing diabetes has been the development of portable, reliable blood glucose meters. The portability, low cost, and accuracy of blood glucose meters have made it practical to carry them on the ambulance. They are easy to use, and since they are routinely used by patients (Figure 13-18), many EMS systems allow EMTs to use blood glucose meters that are carried on the ambulance. Your protocols will tell you whether you are allowed to carry and use a blood glucose meter.

People with diabetes now routinely test the level of glucose in their blood at least once a day, and sometimes as often as five or six times a day. By determining the amount of

FIGURE 13-18 Many EMS systems allow EMTs to use blood glucose meters that are carried on the ambulance.

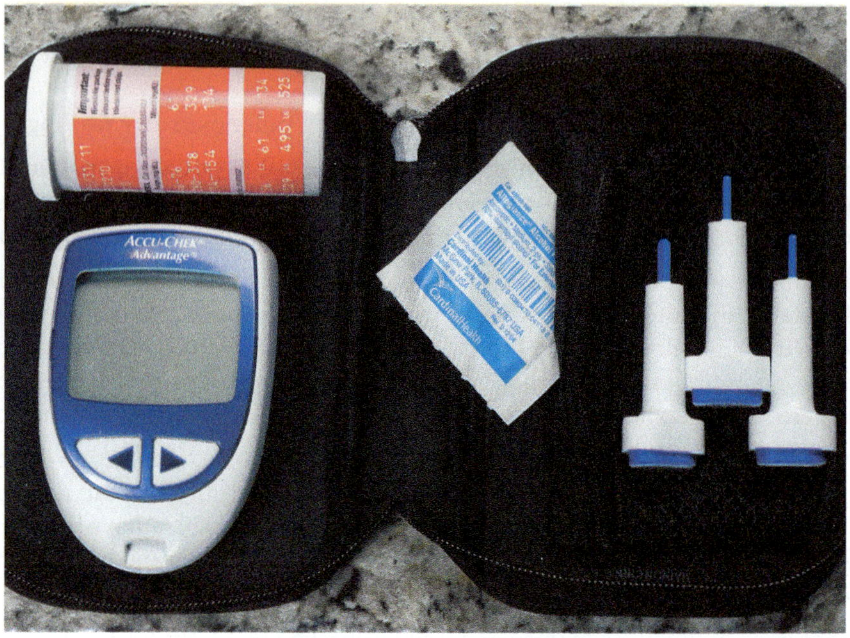

glucose in their blood, they can determine very precisely how much insulin they should take and how much and how often they should eat. Keeping blood glucose levels as close to normal as possible leads to significantly fewer diabetes-related complications (heart disease, blindness, and kidney failure, to name a few), so people with diabetes have a strong motivation to keep their blood glucose level within the normal range.

A blood glucose meter is used by placing a drop of the patient's blood on a test strip. The blood is traditionally obtained by pricking a finger, although some blood glucose meters allow patients to obtain the blood from other areas, such as the forearm. The blood glucose meter evaluates the change in chemical composition of the material on the strip and displays a number that correlates to the glucose concentration in the person's blood. In the United States, this number usually shows the amount of glucose in milligrams per deciliter (100 mL) of blood (expressed as mg/dL), also called milligrams percent. Outside of the United States, the meter may use a different system of measuring glucose to report results.

Using a Blood Glucose Meter

NOTE: *EMTs must have permission from medical direction or local protocol to perform blood glucose monitoring using a blood glucose meter.*

If the patient has a blood glucose meter, the patient or a family member can use it to determine the patient's blood glucose level. Generally, EMTs should not use a patient's blood glucose meter. There are many different types of these devices on the market, each with its own instructions for use, which may be very different from device to device. In addition, there is no way for the EMT to know whether the test strips have been stored properly or when the device was last calibrated. These facts are very important if the reading is to be accurate.

If you have blood glucose meters on the ambulance, they must be calibrated and stored according to the manufacturer's recommendations. Take Standard Precautions. When using a blood glucose meter (Scan 13-2), you will follow these steps:

1. Prepare the device, including a test strip and lancet.
2. Use an alcohol prep to cleanse the patient's finger.
3. After allowing the alcohol to dry, use the lancet to perform a finger stick on the patient. Wipe away the first drop of blood that appears. Squeeze the patient's finger if necessary

SCAN 13-2 Using a Blood Glucose Meter

NOTE: *EMTs must have permission from medical direction or by local protocol to perform blood glucose monitoring using a blood glucose meter.*

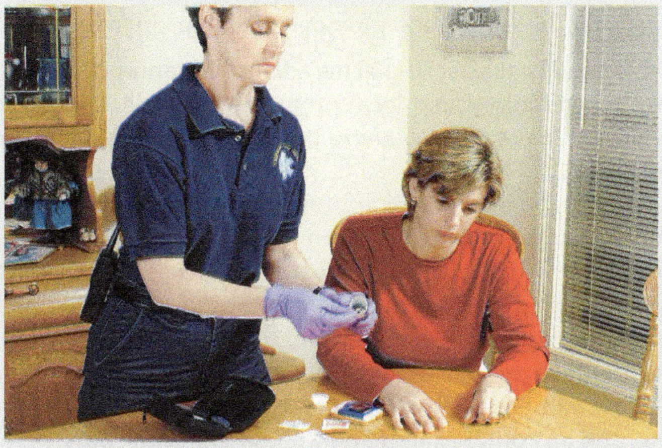

1. Prepare the blood glucose meter, including a test strip and a lancet.

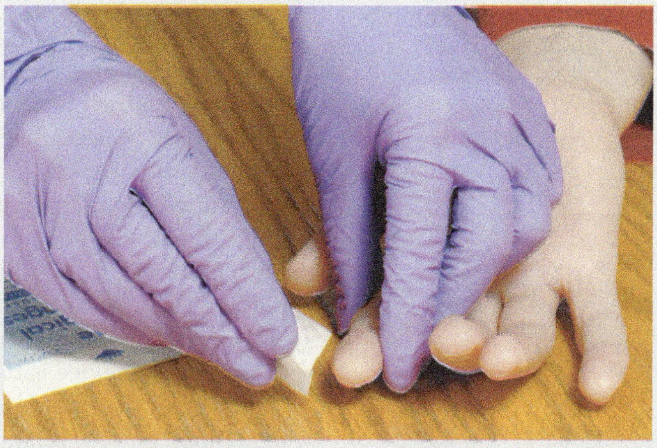

2. Cleanse the skin with an alcohol preparation. Allow the alcohol to dry before performing the finger stick.

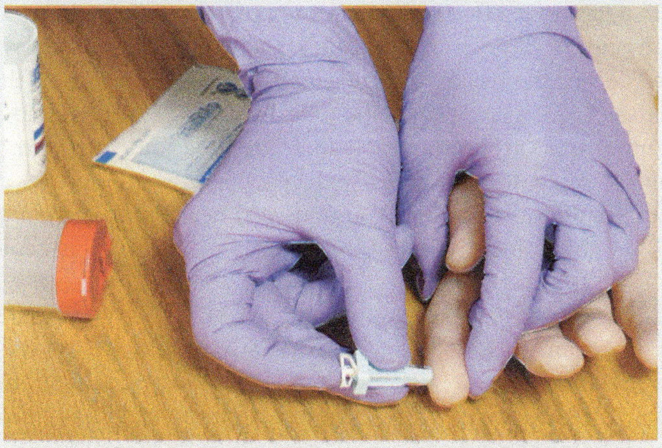

3. Use the lancet to perform a finger stick. Wipe away the first drop of blood that appears. Squeeze the finger if necessary to get a second drop of blood.

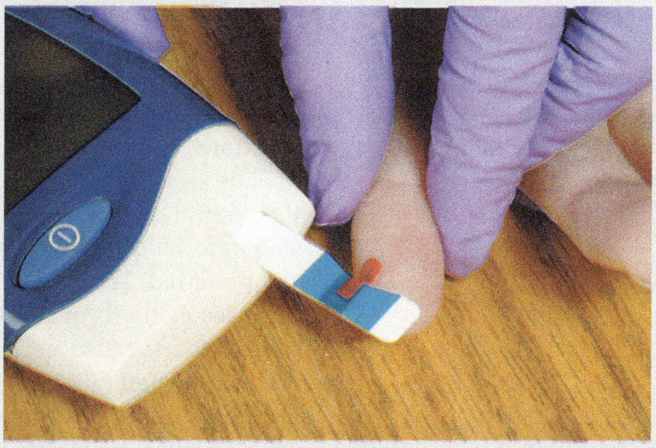

4. Apply the blood to the test strip. This may be done by holding the strip next to the finger to draw the blood into the strip.

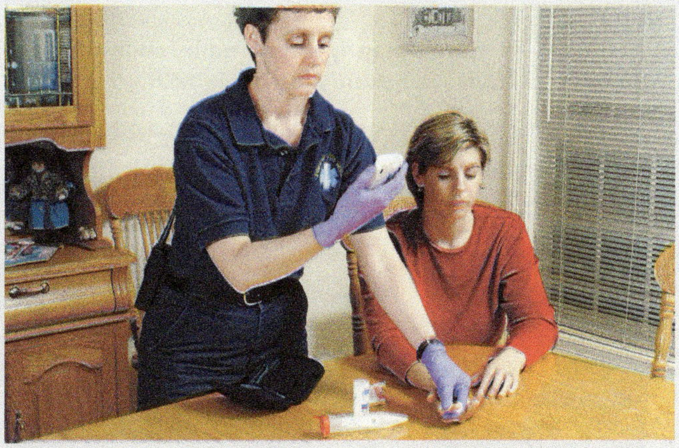

5. Read the blood glucose level displayed on the blood glucose meter. (It may take 10 or 15 seconds for the device to provide a reading.) Assess the puncture site and apply direct pressure or a bandage to the site if bleeding continues.

to get a second drop of blood. Holding the patient's hand lower than the heart and warming the hand may increase blood flow.

4. Apply the blood to the test strip. This is often done by holding the strip up to the finger and drawing the blood into the strip.
5. The blood glucose meter analyzes the sample and provides a reading, often in seconds.

A normal blood glucose level is usually at least 70–100 mg/dL (milligrams per deciliter) depending on the manufacturer's instructions and local protocols. You will learn in the chapter titled *Diabetic Emergencies and Altered Mental Status* how to interpret this information and apply it to the patient's care.

Although many people use blood glucose meters appropriately and accurately, it is quite common to get an inaccurate reading, especially when the device is not used properly. It is critical, for any health care provider who is using a blood glucose meter to test a patient's blood, to have the proper training in use of the device and be thoroughly familiar with its care and maintenance. Calibration and testing on a regularly scheduled basis are essential if the device is to give accurate results.

Remember that the blood glucose monitor (meter) is just one tool in your patient assessment. Blood glucose monitoring, and any other examination, should never be done before performing a thorough primary assessment. Some areas recommend that the blood glucose measurements be done while en route to the hospital.

Capnography

Pulse oximetry measures the amount of oxygen in the bloodstream but does not tell you what happens once the oxygen reaches the tissues. Capnography is a testing method that tells us indirectly how well the tissues are using oxygen (and performing other physiologic functions) by measuring the amount of carbon dioxide exhaled, called end-tidal carbon dioxide, or $ETCO_2$. Capnography shows a number and a "graph" on a screen (Figure 13-19) that indicates how much CO_2 the patient is exhaling. You may also hear of capnometry, a similar technique that provides just the number without the graph. Capnography is generally preferred. The normal level of $ETCO_2$ is 35–45 mmHg.

These methods of assessment are typically used by advanced EMTs and paramedics, but EMTs may also use them in certain EMS systems. Patients who may be assessed with these methods include those who have an advanced airway, who are being ventilated (including those receiving CPR), who are in respiratory distress, who have been sedated, who have certain metabolic conditions, or who are very sick or at risk of deteriorating.

There are two ways in which capnography can be applied. A patient who is breathing spontaneously has a special nasal cannula (Figure 13-20) applied that allows for a small

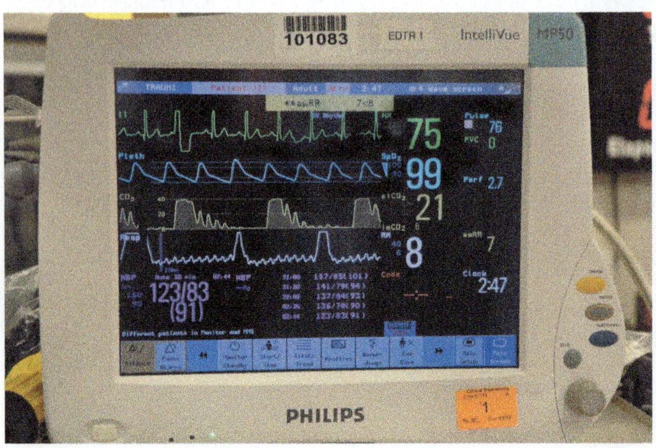

FIGURE 13-19 Capnography graph. *(© Edward T. Dickinson, MD)*

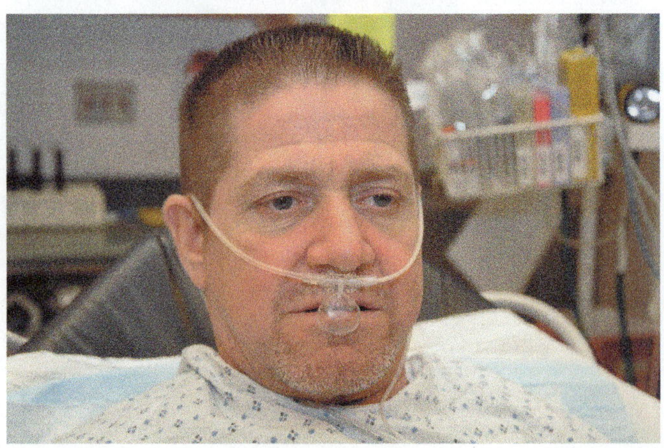

FIGURE 13-20 Capnography measured by special device on nasal cannula. *(© Edward T. Dickinson, MD)*

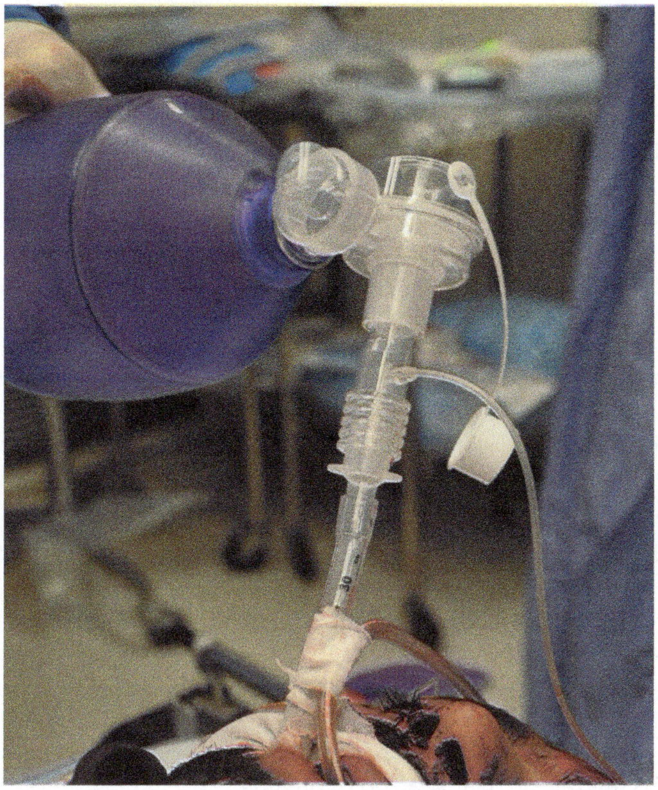

FIGURE 13-21 Capnography device on plastic "collar" between bag-valve and mask. *(© Edward T. Dickinson, MD)*

amount of exhaled air to go down a separate small tube to the monitor, where it is analyzed and the result is displayed on the screen. In the ventilated patient, on the other hand, there is a plastic "collar" (Figure 13-21) that fits between the bag–valve and the mask (or advanced airway). It, too, has a small tube that carries exhaled CO_2 to the monitor.

Capnography can be very helpful in certain circumstances. For example, if you are doing CPR, a sudden substantial increase in end-tidal CO_2 frequently indicates the return of spontaneous circulation and is an indication that you should stop compressions to check for a pulse. End-tidal CO_2 can assist in determining the presence or absence of certain conditions, or can suggest certain interventions. If you use capnography in your EMS system, you will receive additional training in how and when to use it.

Chapter Review

Key Facts and Concepts

- You can gain a great deal of information about a patient's condition by taking a complete set of baseline vital signs, including pulse, respirations, skin, pupils, and blood pressure.
- The EMT must become familiar with the normal ranges for pulse, respirations, and blood pressure in adults and children.
- Trends in the patient's condition will become apparent only when vital signs are repeated, an important step in continuing assessment.
- How often you repeat the vital signs will depend on the patient's condition: at least every 15 minutes for stable patients and at least every 5 minutes for unstable patients.

Key Decisions

- Do I have time to obtain vital signs, or is the patient so unstable that I should get the patient en route to the hospital?
- When should I apply a pulse oximeter to a patient with difficulty breathing? Without difficulty breathing?
- Are abnormal vital signs a result of an illness or injury, or are they the result of some other factor?
- Under what circumstances might it be appropriate to check vital signs on a stable patient every 5 minutes?

Chapter Glossary

auscultation (os-kul-TAY-shun) listening. A stethoscope is used to auscultate for characteristic sounds.

blood pressure the force of blood against the walls of the blood vessels.

blood pressure monitor a machine that automatically inflates a blood pressure cuff and measures blood pressure.

brachial (BRAY-key-al) ***artery*** the major artery of the arm.

brachial (BRAY-key-al) ***pulse*** the pulse felt in the upper arm.

bradycardia (BRAY-duh-KAR-de-uh) a slow pulse; any pulse rate below 60 beats per minute.

carotid (kah-ROT-id) ***pulse*** the pulse felt along the large carotid artery on either side of the neck.

constrict (kon-STRIKT) get smaller.

diastolic (di-as-TOL-ik) ***blood pressure*** the pressure remaining in the arteries when the left ventricle of the heart is relaxed and refilling.

dilate (DI-late) get larger.

oxygen saturation (SpO_2) the ratio of the amount of oxygen present in the blood to the amount that could be carried, expressed as a percentage.

palpation touching or feeling. A pulse or blood pressure may be palpated with the fingertips.

pulse the rhythmic beats felt as the heart pumps blood through the arteries.

pulse oximeter an electronic device for determining the amount of oxygen carried in the blood, known as the oxygen saturation or SpO_2.

pulse quality the rhythm (regular or irregular) and force (strong or weak) of the pulse.

pulse rate the number of pulse beats per minute.

pupil the black center of the eye.

radial (RAY-de-ul) ***pulse*** the pulse felt at the wrist.

reactivity (re-ak-TIV-uh-te) in the pupils of the eyes, reacting to light by changing size.

respiration (res-puh-RAY-shun) the act of breathing in and breathing out.

respiratory (RES-puh-ruh-tor-e) ***quality*** the normal or abnormal (shallow, labored, or noisy) character of breathing.

respiratory (RES-puh-ruh-tor-e) ***rate*** the number of breaths taken in one minute.

respiratory (RES-puh-ruh-tor-e) ***rhythm*** the regular or irregular spacing of breaths.

sphygmomanometer (SFIG-mo-mah-NOM-uh-ter) the cuff and gauge used to measure blood pressure.

systolic (sis-TOL-ik) ***blood pressure*** the pressure created when the heart contracts and forces blood out into the arteries.

tachycardia (TAK-uh-KAR-de-uh) a rapid pulse; any pulse rate above 100 beats per minute, for an adult.

vital signs outward signs of what is going on inside the body, including respiration; pulse; skin color, temperature, and condition (plus capillary refill in infants and children); pupils; and blood pressure.

Preparation for Your Examination and Practice

Short Answer

1. Name the vital signs.
2. Explain why vital signs should be taken more than once.

Thinking and Linking

Think back to the Respiration and Artificial Ventilation *chapter, and link information from that chapter (regarding oxygen administration and artificial ventilation) with information from this chapter (regarding oxygen saturation) as you consider the following situations:*

1. You are assessing a patient who complains of "feeling dizzy." On primary assessment, her breathing appears to be adequate, but when you apply the pulse oximeter during vital signs measurement, you note that her blood oxygen saturation reading is 92 percent. You know that a normal reading would be at least 96 percent. What intervention should you take to improve this patient's oxygen saturation? What technique and equipment would you use?
2. At the scene of a motor-vehicle collision, you are caring for a patient with multiple injuries. Because his breathing was obviously inadequate (shallow and rapid), you initiated artificial ventilation with a bag-valve-mask unit. However, a subsequent reading on this pulse oximeter shows his blood oxygen saturation level—even with assisted ventilations—is only 90 percent. What can you do to attempt to improve his oxygen saturation level?

Critical Thinking Exercises

Vital signs assessments are a critical part of patient assessment. The purpose of this exercise will be to consider how you might deal with the following challenges to obtaining accurate vital signs.

1. How much time should the EMT spend looking for a pulse when the radial pulse is absent or extremely weak?
2. How should you react when the blood pressure monitor gives a reading that is extremely different from previous readings you got?
3. How can you get an accurate pulse oximeter reading on a patient with thick artificial nails?

Pathophysiology to Practice

The following questions are designed to assist you in gathering relevant clinical information and making accurate decisions in the field.

1. Sometimes a patient's heart will have an electrical problem and beat more than 200 times a minute. Why is the pulse so weak in such a patient?
2. When someone has lost a significant amount of blood, the adrenal glands secrete epinephrine (adrenaline), which causes pale, sweaty skin. What effect does epinephrine have on blood vessels, leading to this condition?
3. Why is chronically high diastolic pressure strongly associated with heart disease?

Street Scenes

You are just sitting down to relax when the dispatcher calls to notify you of a 73-year-old female patient with abdominal pain at 19 Oakwood Lane. Before getting to the scene, you and your partner agree that you will do the patient interview and he will assess vital signs. When you arrive, you find the patient sitting at her kitchen table. She tells you her name is Ms. Socorro Alvarez. She says she has stomach pain, "But I don't need to go to the hospital."

As you look at this patient, you find that you aren't confident that this is a good decision. You start to think A-B-Cs and realize that her airway is obviously open and clear, but her breathing seems a little rapid.

Street Scene Questions

1. **What is your primary concern for this patient?**
2. **What vital signs should be taken even if a no-transport decision is being considered?**
3. **Ideally, what should the patient history include?**

You mention to Ms. Alvarez that since she called EMS, she must be concerned. Then you ask her permission to assess her vital signs and ask her a few questions. She consents. "Tell me about the abdominal pain you had today," you begin. She explains that the pain was pretty bad and worse than the pain she had yesterday. "It is a sharp pain," she says. "It got much worse when I had a bowel movement." She tells you that her stools are black and tarry, she hasn't eaten today, and she was cleaning the kitchen when this last "attack" came on.

After your partner takes the patient's vital signs, he tells you that her pulse is 110 and thready, respirations are 28, and blood pressure is 100/70. You ask the patient if she knows her usual blood pressure, and she tells you 150/90. The pulse oximeter is unable to get a reliable reading.

Street Scene Questions

4. **What other patient history information should be obtained?**
5. **Should you take another set of vital signs?**
6. **How might you get the patient to rethink her decision not to be transported?**

You ask the patient if she is taking any medication. When she hands you two bottles from the kitchen table, you notice that her skin is pale and clammy. You write down the names of the medications and ask if she has any allergies. She tells you she is allergic to penicillin. You tell the patient that you think she really needs to go to the hospital and be seen by a doctor. You explain that her pulse is high and some of the other information she has provided needs to be evaluated. Your partner takes another set of vital signs and reports that the pulse is now 120 and thready. The other vital signs have not changed. Finally, after a bit more talk, the patient gives consent for transport.

You load the patient onto a stretcher and provide oxygen. The transport to the hospital is less than 10 minutes and uneventful. En route, your partner gives the radio report and you obtain another set of vital signs. After you transfer patient care to the emergency department personnel and are doing your paperwork, you notice a great deal of activity around her. After a while, a woman approaches and tells you that she is Ms. Alvarez's daughter. "The doctor told me that Mama is bleeding internally," she says, "and that she needed immediate medical attention. Thank you."

14 Principles of Assessment

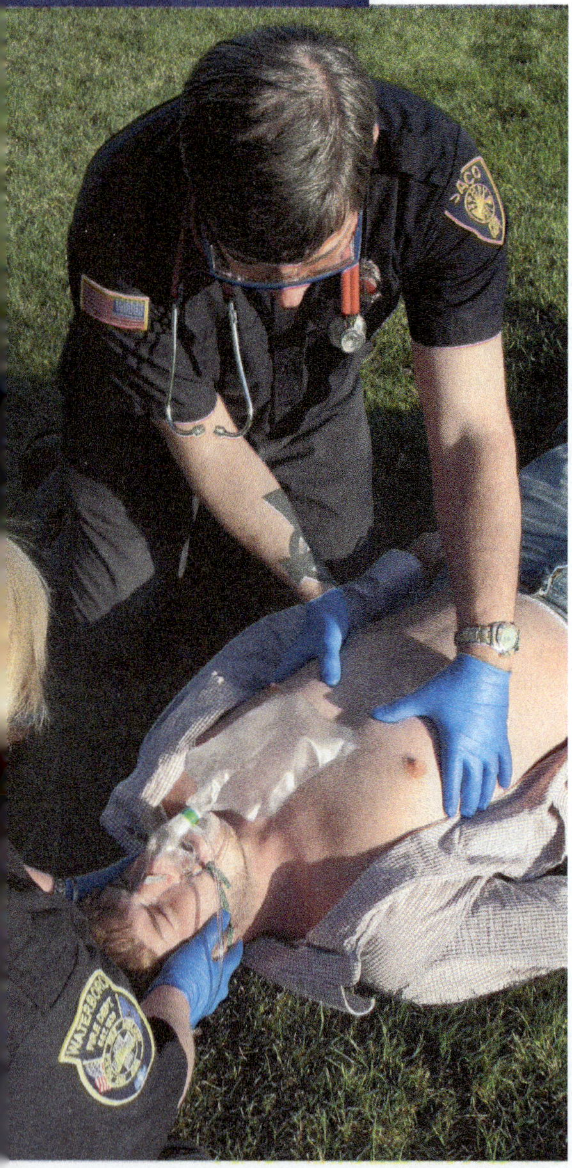
(© Daniel Limmer)

Related Chapters

The following chapters provide additional information related to topics discussed in this chapter:

Standards

Assessment (Secondary Assessment; Reassessment)

Clinical Behavior/Judgment (Decision Making)

Competencies

Applies scene information and patient assessment findings (scene size-up, primary and secondary assessments, patient history, and reassessment) to guide emergency management.

Initiates basic interventions based on assessment findings intended to mitigate the emergency and provide limited symptom relief while providing access to definitive care.

Core Concepts

- How examinations are conducted
- History-taking techniques
- Physical examination techniques
- Body system examinations
- Critical thinking concepts for the EMT

Outcomes

After reading this chapter, you should be able to:

14.1 Explain techniques that are useful in obtaining the patient history. (pp. 370–377)

- Distinguish between circumstances when collecting a complete history is better facilitated by open-ended or closed-ended questions.
- Apply the OPQRST mnemonic to gain additional information about a complaint.
- Apply the SAMPLE mnemonic to organize information gathering.

14.2 Describe the general techniques of physical examination. (pp. 377–391)

- Compare the type of information that can be obtained through each general technique of physical examination.
- Provide the information you anticipate getting from different body systems when deciding to use a general technique of physical examination.

14.3 Analyze your approach to decision making in EMS scenarios. (pp. 391–398)

- Compare EMTs' process of diagnosis with that of emergency physicians.
- Explain the impact of experience on diagnostic processes.
- Given a short description of an EMT setting, recognize common cognitive biases.

14.4 Evaluate your approach to decision making in EMS scenarios. (pp. 398–400)

- Compare the features of experienced physicians' thinking with EMTs' thinking.
- Evaluate your approach to thinking like an EMT.

Key Terms

chief complaint, *372*

closed-ended question, *371*

crepitation, *390*

diagnosis, *391*

differential diagnosis, *393*

history of the present illness/injury (HPI), *372*

jugular vein distention (JVD), *384*

open-ended question, *371*

past medical history (PMH), *370*

OPQRST, *372*

SAMPLE, *373*

You are called to a patient with a complaint of altered mental status. The patient's family say she doesn't seem to be acting right. She is lethargic and only responds occasionally.

You will first conduct an initial assessment as described in the chapter *Primary Assessment*. But what happens next? How will you determine what the patient's condition is—an important part of determining what treatment you will provide? As you are probably aware, you have many options for a patient with altered mental status, including administering glucose (for diabetic conditions), administering naloxone for opioid overdose, providing oxygen (administered prudently for hypoxia), performing a stroke scale to determine if the patient is having a stroke—and more.

Your secondary assessment is very important. This is where you will search for the findings that will guide you to the best treatment decisions for your patient. While many worry about what treatment to provide for a patient, the fact is that your treatments are decided by application of a protocol. The most important thing you can do is a thorough assessment to reach the correct conclusion or preliminary diagnosis.

Principles of Assessment

CORE CONCEPT
How examinations are conducted

This section will teach you techniques of assessment that will help form your secondary assessment process. You will learn about history taking, which is asking questions about patients' current problem and past medical conditions, and methods of physical examination. You will learn how to do this for both adult and pediatric patients.

The Patient History

past medical history (PMH) information gathered regarding the patient's health problems in the past.

A number of techniques are used in assessment. These techniques are sometimes collectively referred to as the history and physical examination. This section will discuss techniques involved in taking the history and conducting the physical exam. Remember that the history has two different components: history of the present illness (HPI) and the patient's ***past medical history (PMH)***.

History-Taking Techniques

CORE CONCEPT
History-taking techniques

The history is obtained by talking to the patient. If you are unable to talk to the patient, you will try to obtain the history, as best as you can, from family members, bystanders, medications present, and other things you observe at the scene (e.g., a home oxygen cylinder).

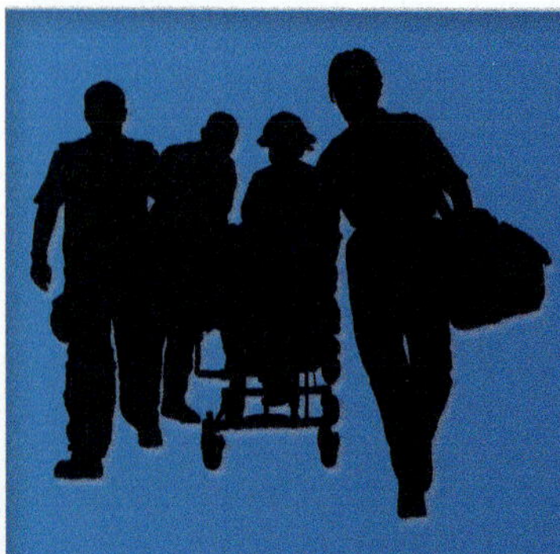

Think Like an EMT

Critical Thinking and Decision Making

A successful secondary assessment relies on solid clinical judgment and critical thinking. How do you decide which exams to do when? How do you know when your patient is critical or not? These are important decisions based on information you get from your patient.

You won't have to master critical thinking and decision making at this point in your course, but the need to develop these skills must be acknowledged here. You will get much more practice during your course.

The hallmark of successful EMTs is the ability to adapt their assessments to the patients, to be thorough, and to make good decisions as they go along.

To obtain a history, it is helpful to develop a rapport with the patient. This is done by getting to the same physical level as the patient (when safe and appropriate), demonstrating empathy for the patient's problem or condition, and listening carefully. Few things are more frustrating to a patient than being asked a question, answering it, and hearing the same question again because the EMT didn't remember the answer.

Generally it is best to begin with an ***open-ended question***. This means a question to which the patient can't give just a "yes" or "no" answer. Imagine that you are beginning your history on a patient who called because of a headache. Which would get you started better and provide the most information?

open-ended question a question requiring more than just a "yes" or "no" answer.

What can you tell me about your headache?
Or
Do you have a headache?

By asking, "What can you tell me about your headache?" you have asked a broad question. Patients can answer as they choose, but they must answer in some detail. If a patient replies, "Well, it hurts," you can keep going with, "Can you tell me more about the headache?" or "Can you describe the pain to me?"

It is unlikely that any patient will predict all the things you will need to know about the headache and give you all of that information in the first answer, so you will continue with additional questions as necessary. For example, you may ask, "How long have you had the headache?" and "Does the pain radiate anywhere?" The more chances you give patients to tell you things in their own words, the better the information you will obtain.

There are exceptions, however, to the rule of asking open-ended questions. You may see a patient who looks pale and very sick, and looks ready to pass out. In this case, ask questions quickly, including ***closed-ended questions***, questions that can be answered "yes" or "no." When you sense this is a serious emergency, you must take control of the situation. "Do you feel like you are going to pass out?" is a closed-ended question but one that must be answered immediately.

closed-ended question a question requiring only a "yes" or "no" answer.

Additional techniques of communication are discussed in the chapter titled *Communication and Documentation*.

You will use history taking to obtain a picture of what is going wrong with the patient. Remember that the questions you ask will help you fill in this picture. Sometimes problems will be very obvious, such as with a person who was just shot, but other times problems will be more challenging to identify. With these patients, you will use history taking to assemble and recognize patterns that point to known disorders. For example, if a 50-year-old male told you he has chest pain, it would be very important to understand how that pain came about. He might tell you that the pain came on suddenly while he was sitting on the couch and that the pain was associated with respiratory distress and sweating. When you learn more about cardiac emergencies, you will recognize these findings as a pattern that would point to a myocardial infarction. On the other hand, if he told you that his pain began after an earlier car crash in which he struck his chest on the steering wheel, the pattern of a traumatic injury would emerge. As you can imagine, these scenarios require very different treatment plans. Structured and purposeful history taking allows you to identify these patterns and make good decisions on your patients' behalf. As you proceed further in your course, you will learn more about specific disorders and pathophysiologies. As you fill in more and more information, you will be better prepared to recognize patterns and tailor your history taking to arrive at a functional diagnosis.

Remember that diagnosing is often a complicated process. Patients frequently have multiple, mixed problems, and not every situation will be identifiable to you. This ambiguity is allowable and is frequently embraced by paramedics and physicians. Creating a treatment plan does not always require a clear and definite diagnosis. In emergency medicine, we often seek to identify not "what is wrong with the patient," but rather "what does this patient need?" We provide for that need while a more complicated diagnosis is sought. As you develop your patient assessment skills, you will hone your technique to match these desired outcomes.

Ideally, you will create a structure and plan for your assessment that is consistent and reproducible. Consistency is crucial not only to developing a thorough approach, but also to performing this approach under stress. Although you may tailor questions to look for specific patterns, there are key elements that every patient history should consider.

A patient history usually starts with simply asking patients what is wrong. What are they complaining of and how did the problem come about? These elements are referred to as the ***chief complaint*** and the ***history of the present illness/injury (HPI)***.

chief complaint
the patient's statement that describes the symptom or concern associated with the primary problem the patient is having.

history of the present illness/injury (HPI)
the events and or mechanism leading up to the patient's current problem.

OPQRST
a memory aid in which the letters stand for questions asked to get a description of the present illness: onset, provocation, quality, region/radiation, severity, time.

TABLE 14-1 OPQRST

O	Onset
P	Provocation
Q	Quality
R	Radiation, region
S	Severity
T	Time

OPQRST (see Table 14-1) is a memory aid used to develop information pertaining to the chief complaint and history of the present illness/injury. The letters stand for categories of questions asked to gather information: onset, provocation, quality, region/radiation, severity, and time.

Here are some examples of OPQRST questions:

- **Onset.** What were you doing when the pain or problem began?
- **Provocation.** Does anything seem to trigger the pain or problem? Does anything make it feel better?
- **Quality.** Can you describe the pain or problem for me?
- **Region; radiation.** Where is the pain? Will you please point toward it? Does it seem to shoot or spread anywhere?
- **Severity.** How bad is the pain or problem? If zero is no pain or problem and ten is the worst you can imagine, what number would you say your pain or problem is right now?
- **Time.** When did the pain or problem start? Has it changed at all since it started? Consider whether the patient's complaint had a sudden or gradual onset. (For example, pneumonia generally has a gradual onset, while an asthma attack has a more rapid onset.)

Remember to begin with open-ended questions. Allow patients to answer in their own words. Listen carefully to their answers. In the case of abdominal pain, there are additional questions you will likely want to ask once you get the patient's own description and answers. These will vary from patient to patient, and you will tailor these questions to help you identify specific patterns. Examples include:

- Does the pain feel better or worse when you eat food? (This may indicate an ulcer or digestive issue.)
- Does the pain radiate to your shoulder? (Pain from some abdominal organs tends to radiate to the shoulder. The patient may not be aware that shoulder pain is related to the present condition.)
- I see that you have your legs drawn up. Does that make you feel better?

Once you discuss the chief complaint and history of the present illness/injury, it may be appropriate to expand on how the problem came about and if it matches problems they have had in the past. Questions from OPQRST such as those about onset and time may be followed by requests for more detailed information such as, "What were you doing when the problem started?" or "Were you feeling ok, prior to the onset?" Overall, you are seeking to develop a clear picture of the events and circumstances that led the patient to call EMS. Occasionally it may be appropriate simply to ask why the patient called the ambulance. (Beware, however, not to allow the tone of this question to become judgmental in terms of whether or not they should have called an ambulance.) Do not forget to consider prior trauma in seemingly medical problems or medical problems in seemingly traumatic events. Consider the following:

- A child has awakened with shortness of breath. Although this complaint seems medical, it would change entirely if you found out that the child had been in a car crash the previous day.

- A woman complains of chest pain after a minor car crash. Although it would be easy to associate the chest pain with the trauma of the crash, this complaint would change entirely if the patient disclosed that the chest pain started prior to the crash and that she was driving herself to the hospital.

The patient's medical history is very important, and should be discussed. Although many conditions appear independent of prior history, a large number of problems are related to previous medical conditions. Consider asking patients if they have ever been hospitalized, and if so, for what? Are there any prior medical conditions? For example, if the patient has chest pain today, but has, in the past, had three heart attacks, there is a high likelihood that the problem of today is related to the past medical condition. Past medical history can be extremely relevant in patients who are unconscious or unable to communicate. A history of diabetes in an unconscious patient is an extremely important finding. A history of asthma in a patient with respiratory distress will likely point you to an appropriate treatment plan. Past medical history can also complicate unrelated, current problems. For example, patients with a history of asthma are at a higher risk of dying from severe allergic reactions. Patients with a history of chronic lung disease decompensate faster from chest injuries. Although past medical history may not be the most important finding, it can shed much light onto a patient's current problem.

Once you have inquired about past medical history, you should also ask about current medications. Patient medications can help you understand past medical history and can sometimes identify conditions not previously discussed. Consider the following exchange:

EMT: "Sir, do you have any past medical history or problems?"

Patient: "No."

EMT: "Do you take any medications?"

Patient: "Yes, I take insulin."

Although the patient failed to disclose he had diabetes, the fact that he takes insulin would strongly indicate this and would be a point for further questioning by the EMT. Daily medications can also affect unrelated conditions. For example, beta-blocker medications taken to treat high blood pressure can limit increases in heart rate and affect the body's compensation efforts. Certain medications also make patients more susceptible to heat or cold injuries.

Additional questions to consider would pertain to patient allergies and last oral intake. Depending upon the nature of the problem, allergies or recent meals may be relevant. For example, patients with gallbladder problems can develop abdominal pain after eating fatty meals. Patients experiencing a new-onset skin rash may be developing a severe allergic reaction. Knowing prior allergies is very important.

It is also appropriate to ask patients about their recent travel history. With the appearance of diseases such as Ebola and respiratory viruses that originate in other parts of the world, determining if the patient has been out of the country recently or exposed to someone who has been out of the country has become increasingly important.

The mnemonic ***SAMPLE*** (Table 14-2) is a memory aid that can be used like a checklist for patient assessment. Although experienced providers learn to ask questions based on the patient presentation, pattern recognition, and differential diagnosis, the SAMPLE mnemonic is an excellent way to ensure the most meaningful components of the patient have been addressed.

Here are some examples of SAMPLE history questions:

- **Signs and symptoms.** What's wrong? (This is a reminder to get the history of the present illness.)
- **Allergies.** Are you allergic to medications or foods, or do you have environmental allergies? Do you have a medical identification tag describing your allergies?

SAMPLE
a memory aid in which the letters stand for elements of the past medical history: signs and symptoms, allergies, medications, pertinent past history, last oral intake, and events leading to the injury or illness.

TABLE 14-2 SAMPLE History

S	Signs and symptoms
A	Allergies
M	Medications
P	Pertinent past medical history
L	Last oral intake
E	Events

"The history provides most of the information you'll need for the medical patient. Get the right information."

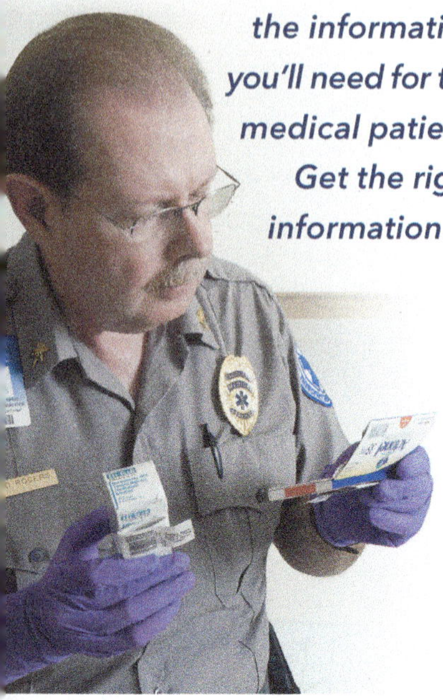

- **Medications.** What medications are you currently taking or are you supposed to be taking (prescription, over-the-counter, or recreational)? Are you on birth control pills (for females of childbearing age)? Do you have a medical identification tag with the names of medications on it? Do you take any herbal supplements or vitamins or minerals?
- **Pertinent past history.** Have you been experiencing any medical problems? Have you been feeling ill? Have you recently had any surgery or injuries? Have you been seeing a doctor? What is your doctor's name?
- **Last oral intake.** When did you last eat or drink? What did you eat or drink? (Food or liquids can cause symptoms or aggravate a medical condition. Also, if a patient will need to go to surgery, the hospital staff must know when the patient last had anything to eat or drink, since stomach contents can be vomited while a patient is under anesthesia, which is a very dangerous occurrence.)
- **Events leading to the injury or illness.** What sequence of events led to today's problem (e.g., the patient passed out, then got into a car crash versus got into a car crash, then passed out)?

Experienced EMTs know that a good history question gives you two more good additional history questions. The ultimate goal is to get the most relevant information to help direct your care.

History taking helps develop a picture, but remember that it is only one element of the secondary assessment. Findings here must be confirmed, developed, and cross-checked with the other elements of the secondary assessment. In many ways, patient assessment is similar to the scientific method used in laboratories every day. In a lab, a hypothesis (or suspected outcome) is proposed. Scientists then test this hypothesis to prove whether it is true. In patient assessment, we develop and test possibilities. Like scientists developing a hypothesis, we use the chief complaint and the history of the present illness to see patterns and identify likely problems, pathologies, or diagnoses. In EMS, as in science, we will use further assessment to test our ideas and to turn those possibilities into probabilities. For example, when a mother tells you her daughter developed difficulty breathing after playing outside, you might suspect a severe allergic reaction. You might ask the mother about possible exposures (such as a bee sting). You might further ask if there was a history of allergy to bee stings. If the answers led you in this direction, you might look to identify a pattern. You will soon learn that severe allergic reactions, otherwise known as anaphylaxis, develop quickly and are commonly associated with wheezing and gastrointestinal distress. This knowledge might lead your patient history questioning toward asking whether these conditions or symptoms are present. If so, the possibility then becomes a probability. Now you must test your hypothesis.

From a general perspective, preschoolers can usually be interviewed if you take your time and keep your language simple. School-age children will be able to describe more clearly how they feel and what happened. They will talk with you honestly but may feel that the injury or illness is a punishment for something they did. They must be reassured and told it is all right to feel sick or hurt or to cry. Before telling the child something or asking a question, take a second to think about how the child might interpret what you are about to say. This may help you to minimize the child's confusion or anxiety. Do not use sarcasm or teasing. Often preschoolers do not understand that you are joking. Even older children may feel powerless to answer back or defend themselves.

Include parents, teachers, and/or care providers in your interview. Since they are often the most valuable source of information for your assessment, do not exclude them. Seeing that familiar adults are being included gains the child's confidence if you follow up by talking directly to the child. If the parents are injured, the child needs to know that someone is caring for the child as well.

All patients have some degree of fear at the emergency scene. Infants and children are usually more fearful than adults because they lack experience with illness and injury. In addition to this, children are easily frightened by the unknown. Since so many details of the emergency scene are unknowns, it is easy to see why emergencies can be scary for children. The elements associated with the emergency (pain, noise, bright lights, cold) can set off a panic reaction in infants.

Pediatric Note

Most of the components of the pediatric assessment are the same as you would perform on an adult. There are, however, subtle but important differences with pediatric patients (Figure 14-1). Very young children (infants) may simply not be able to use words, and toddlers and preschoolers may be reluctant to communicate because of stranger and separation anxiety. It is important to adjust your expectations to the developmental stage of your patient. The chapter *Life Span Development* discusses these developmental stages and should be reviewed for a better understanding of pediatric history taking.

FIGURE 14-1 Engaging on the same level as the patient and focusing closely on what the patient says are two ways of ensuring that you will obtain good information.

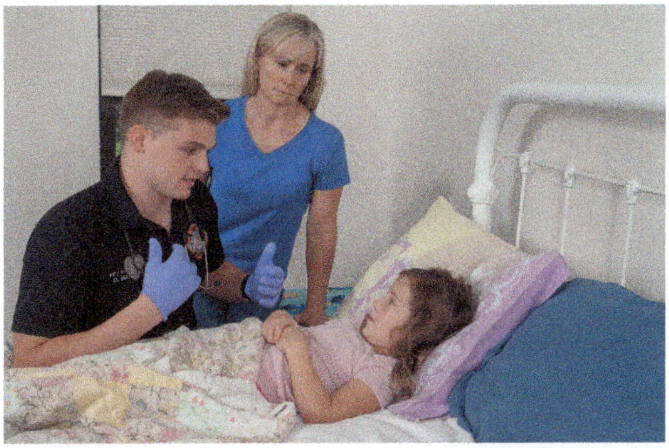

A When possible, take more time and explain. Get down to the patient's level. This has the advantage of making you (a stranger) less physically intimidating to the child.

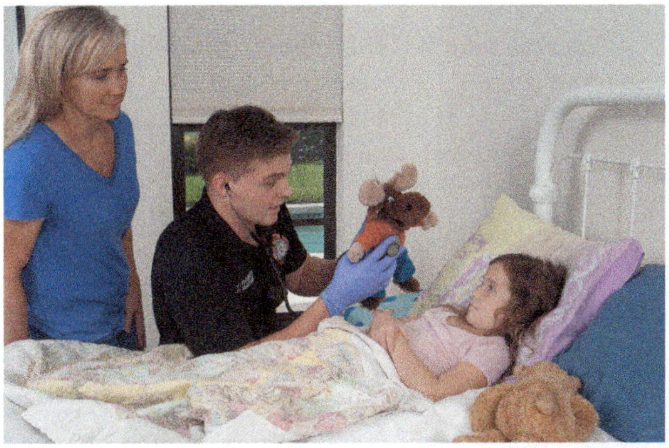

B Many EMS agencies have toys or special pediatric devices to occupy or distract a child during assessment, care, and transport.

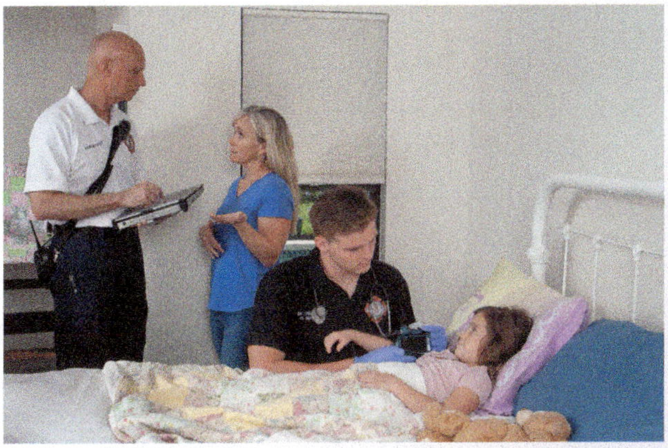

C A child may not be able to answer history questions; in these cases, a parent can be a valuable source of information. Make sure to tell the child what will happen. For example, tell the child that the blood pressure cuff will pinch a little. Honesty builds trust.

D Use terms the pediatric patient will understand. For example, a child patient may not understand if you ask if the pain "radiates" anywhere.

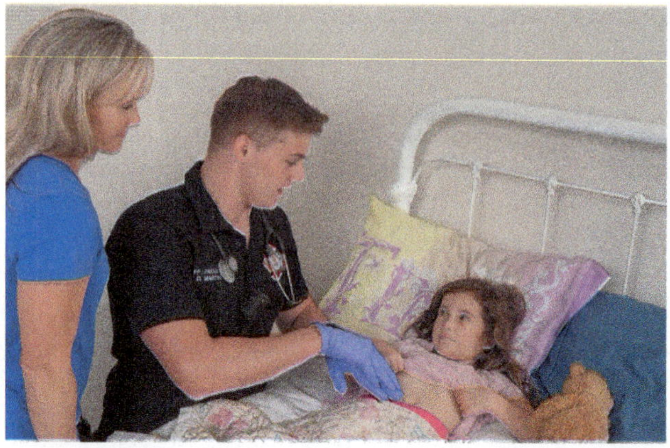

E Consider the patient's development level and need for modesty, which are different than for an adult.

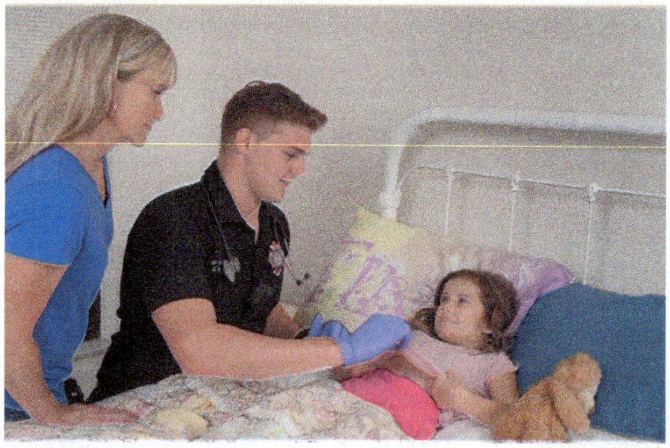

At an emergency, if children do not understand you, or if they believe that you do not understand them, their fear will increase. To communicate, children must remain calm. Putting children at ease is a very important part of the care you must provide. Some children, when stressed, will act like a younger child. This is called *regression*.

Any problems faced by the child will be intensified if the parents are not at the scene. Children find security through their parents when facing new problems or emergencies. Asking for mom or dad may be the child's first priority, even above that of having your help.

When dealing with pediatric patients, you should:

1. Identify yourself simply by saying, "Hi, I'm Pat. What's your name?"
2. Let the child know that the parents have been called or will be called.
3. Determine if there are life-threatening problems, and immediately treat them. If there are none, continue at a relaxed pace. Fearful children cannot tolerate a rapidly paced assessment and confusing questions from a stranger.
4. Let children have any nearby toy that they may want.
5. Kneel or sit at the child's eye level. Ensure that bright light is not directly behind you and shining into the child's eyes.
6. *Smile.* This is a familiar sign from adults that reassures children.
7. Touch the child or hold the child's hand or foot. A child who does not wish to be touched will let you know. Smile and provide comfort through your conversation.
8. Explain equipment before use and explain each step as you do it, using simple, concrete language.
9. Let the child see your face, and make eye contact without staring at the child. Speak directly to the child; use words the child can understand. Be sure the child can hear you.

10. Stop occasionally to find out if the child understands. Never assume the child understood you, but find out by asking questions (if the child is old enough to respond).
11. *Never lie to the child.* When something may hurt, be honest but reassuring, telling the child you will be there to help.

The Physical Examination

The physical examination, like the patient history, is a vital element of the secondary assessment. Performed before, during, or after patient history, it too helps develop a clinical picture and can identify problems not recognized in the primary assessment. Commonly, physical examination and patient history are used together to create and confirm probabilities developed from assembling patterns. For example, in the previous scenario, the patient history raised the probability of a severe allergic reaction. Physical examination can help confirm this suspicion. Patient history has led you to form a hypothesis. You must now test your hypothesis. You will soon learn that severe allergic reactions commonly cause swelling, rash, and low blood pressure. Here a physical examination can help prove or disprove the probability. Observation, inspection, and auscultation will look for the signs commonly associated with severe allergy. If they are present, your probability just became even more probable.

Physical Examination Techniques

CORE CONCEPT
Physical examination techniques

There are three techniques you will use in your physical examination. These are observe, auscultate, and palpate. The technique or techniques you use will depend on the patient's complaint. Using the severe allergic reaction example from earlier, you may observe the patient's skin for the formation of a rash; you may listen to the lungs for abnormal sounds such as wheezing; and you may palpate her hands and feet to identify swelling. The techniques you choose will depend on your patient's complaint and presentation.

- **Observe.** Observation is looking at the patient for an overall sense of patient condition as well as evaluating the chief complaint (Figure 14-2A). It may seem like a very simple technique, but the results are very important. You may use observation in many ways. A patient may have a chief complaint of a shoulder injury. You can observe the area for deformity and compare it visually with the uninjured shoulder. In another example, a patient may tell you that nothing is wrong, or that there is only mild distress. Your observations may note a pained expression, difficulty moving, or another example that the situation is more serious than the patient believes or is saying.
- **Auscultate.** Auscultation is listening for signs of an abnormal condition (Figure 14-2B). In most cases, auscultation is done with a stethoscope, although some sounds (e.g., wheezing) can sometimes be heard without the stethoscope.
- **Palpate.** Some situations and conditions will require palpation (Figure 14-2C). This involves feeling an area for deformities or other abnormal findings. You will palpate the abdomen of a patient who complains of pain there. You will also palpate as part of a full-body examination of a trauma patient (discussed later in this chapter).

FIGURE 14-2 (A) Observe the patient for an overall sense of the patient's condition. (B) Auscultate (listen) for abnormal sounds within the body. (C) Palpate (feel) for deformities and other abnormal findings.

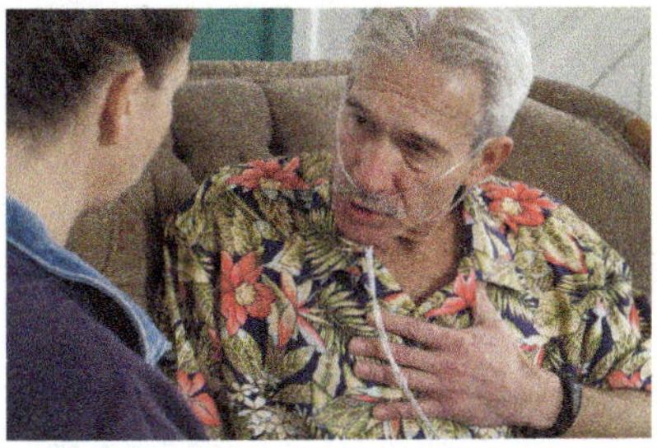

A

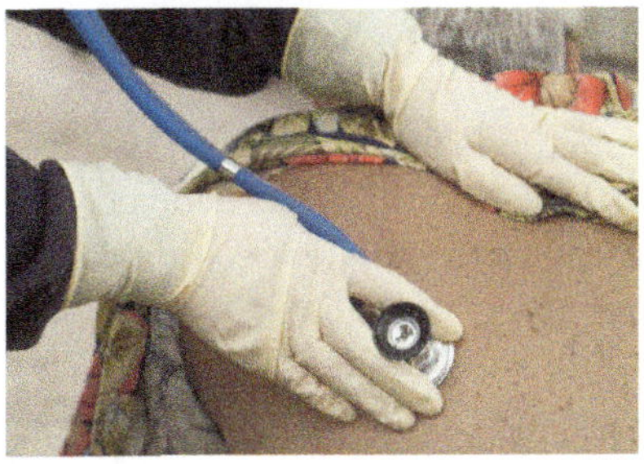

B

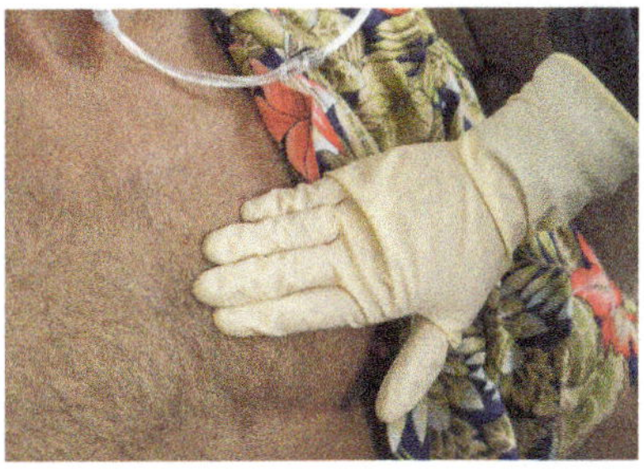

C

Pediatric Physical Exam

Young pediatric patients are often frightened by physical examination. Aggressive examination techniques often lead to crying and significant agitation. Although agitated and crying children can still be assessed, an upset state can impact clinical conditions such as respiratory distress, and certainly changes assessment findings. When possible, you should approach frightened children slowly and start from the least invasive parts of their body to the most invasive. In adults, we normally perform the physical examination in head-to-toe order; on alert infants and small children, this is reversed. Starting with the toes or trunk and working your way toward the head will let the child get used to you and your touch before you attempt to touch around the head and face. Playing with the infants' feet often puts them at ease.

Do not use any equipment on the child without first explaining what you will do with it. Many children fear the medical items that are familiar to the EMT, thinking they will cause pain. Always tell the child what you are going to do as you take vital signs and perform a physical exam. Do not try to explain the entire procedure at once. Instead, explain each step as you do it. Use simple language and remember that children tend to take things literally. If you tell a young child "I'm going to take your pulse," the child may think you are going to take something away. Instead, say, "I'm going to hold your wrist for a minute." If the child is older, explain why. Unless there are possible injuries that indicate the child should not be moved, a young child should be held on a parent's lap during a physical exam. Many EMS teams carry clean stuffed animals (such as teddy bears) that can be given to a child during the physical exam. The toys can provide comfort to the child and allow you to explain the examination by using the toy as a model. Point to an area on the toy to show the child where you must touch and where you will bandage when you need to provide emergency care. This type of one-to-one communication also helps build parent and bystander confidence, letting them know that a professional, compassionate EMT is caring for the child. (If you use a toy, allow the child to keep it.)

Never lie to the child about something that hurts. Tell children when part of the examination may hurt. If they ask if they are sick or hurt, be honest, but be sure to add that you are there to help and will not leave. Let the child know that other people also will be helping.

Most very young children will suffer no embarrassment when you remove or reposition clothing during the exam. Nonetheless, protect the child from the stares of onlookers. Many children around the ages of five to eight go through a stage of intense modesty. You may have to keep explaining why you must remove certain articles of clothing. Many parents, teachers, and day care personnel teach children that strangers should not remove their clothing or touch them. The children that you examine may not understand your intentions and may resist. Some children may become upset because they feel you are taking something away from them. Take your time and do not rush children into accepting all that is happening. Remember that children rapidly lose body heat, so if you expose them, quickly cover them with a blanket.

The assessment of an infant or child is done to look for the same signs of injury and illness and to prove or disprove the same probabilities as in the case of the adult patient. See Scan 15-7, The Pediatric Physical Examination.

Body System Examinations

CORE CONCEPT
Body system examinations

Under older methods of training, EMTs were taught to assess using a set series of steps for every patient. EMS education has evolved over the years, the most notable change involving expanded assessment knowledge and procedures.

Many students would finish class and ask, "But how will I know what to say to patients in the back of the ambulance?" This is because rote or generic assessment steps that are applied to every patient really don't work. The principle behind body system exams is to give you a series of different yet relevant exams and exam techniques based on the patient's complaint and the parts of the body or body systems this complaint is likely to involve. These body system examinations will fit into your overall secondary examination of the patient.

One of the reasons that body system exams are now taught to EMTs is that you have learned—and will continue to learn—pathophysiology (the study of how disease processes affect body functions), which provides a deeper understanding of the conditions you will be assessing.

You will need to choose which body system or systems to examine for each patient. For some patients, you may choose one; for others, several systems will be examined. This is part of the decision-making process mentioned earlier in the chapter.

There are many techniques of body system assessment. The following sections will present complete and relevant techniques. Your instructor may teach you additional methods of assessing different body systems.

The sections that follow also list history questions. These will be questions that are specific to each condition and are not designed to elicit a complete history.

Additional assessment concepts will be presented in the chapters that cover specific types of emergencies.

The SAMPLE and OPQRST mnemonics listed earlier can be used to remember what to ask and to focus questions relevant to each of the body systems.

As you read the following information, you may want to refer to the *Visual Guide, Medical Body System Exams.*

Respiratory System

Emergencies involving the respiratory system are a frequent source of EMS calls because dysfunction in this system results in shortness of breath or trouble with normal breathing. Between asthma, pneumonia, and chronic lung conditions, respiratory complaints are found in the young and old. Assessing the respiratory system is done by a variety of techniques.

NOTE: *The most important determination you can make when assessing the respiratory system is whether the patient is breathing adequately. You must constantly be alert for respiratory failure. If at any point respiratory failure is observed, you will discontinue your assessment and ventilate the patient immediately.*

Respiratory Assessment—History

Obtain a history of existing respiratory conditions and the medications taken for each. Determine if those medications have been taken as prescribed. Determine if signs and symptoms of this episode match those of previous episodes.

- Determine the onset. Many respiratory conditions can be differentiated by how abruptly or slowly they came on. Asking a simple question such as "How long have you had this shortness of breath?" can significantly help in making a diagnosis.
- Dyspnea on exertion—Is it increasingly difficult for patients to catch their breath after they have exerted themselves (e.g., climbing a flight of stairs)? Do not ask patients to exert themselves to determine this.
- Weight gain—Does the patient report recent, rapid weight gain or that the patient's clothes fit more tightly? This may indicate fluid buildup (heart failure).
- Orthopnea—Does the patient have difficulty breathing when lying down? This occurs in several respiratory conditions, including heart failure.
- Does the patient sleep on pillows? Has the patient required more pillows recently?
- Does the patient have a cough? Has the cough been productive? If so, what does the patient cough up?
- Has the patient had any respiratory conditions recently (e.g., flu, bronchitis, or cold)?
- Does the patient have a chronic illness that affects the respiratory system (e.g., asthma or emphysema/COPD)?

VISUAL GUIDE

14 Medical Body System Exams

Where you perform the exam depends on *patient priority* and *status*: unstable patient–in the ambulance; stable patient–on scene

Perform a history

The body system exam(s) you choose are based on the information you obtain in the history.

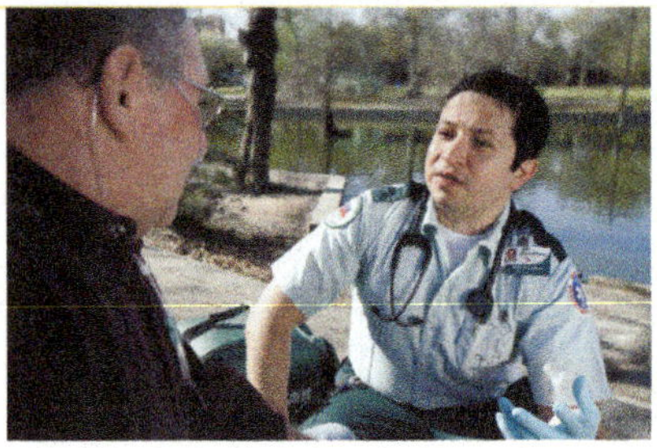

Body Systems Exam:

Respiratory

Work of breathing and position
Lung sounds
Pedal and sacral edema
Pulse oximetry

Respiratory Specific History

Dyspnea on exertion
Orthopnea
Weight gain

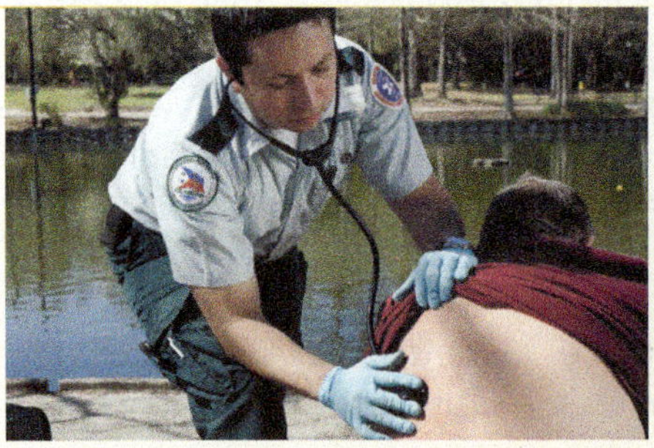

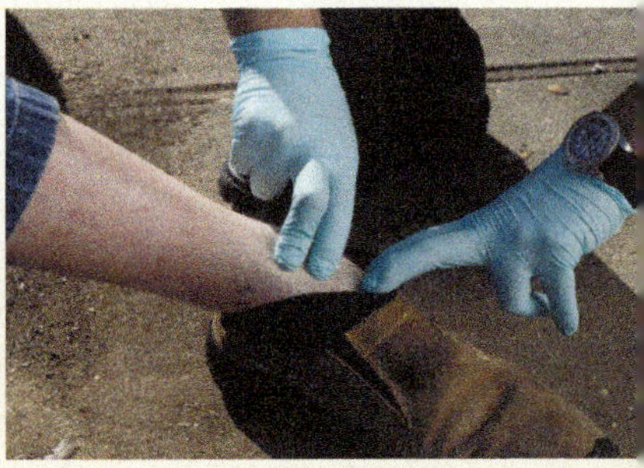

Body Systems Exam:

Cardiovascular

Check pulse (presence/rate/regularity)
Skin color/temperature/condition
Blood pressure
Orthostatic blood pressure changes
Jugular vein distention (JVD)
Many components of the respiratory exam also apply to the cardiovascular system.

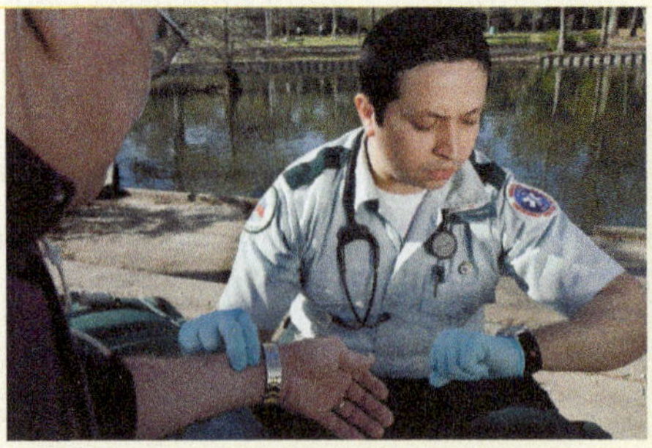

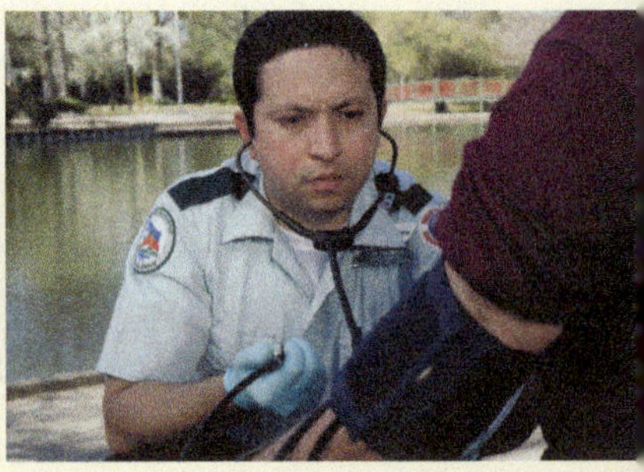

Body Systems Exam:

Neurologic

Cincinnati Prehospital Stroke Scale (or other approved scale)
Pupils
Monitoring mental status changes over time

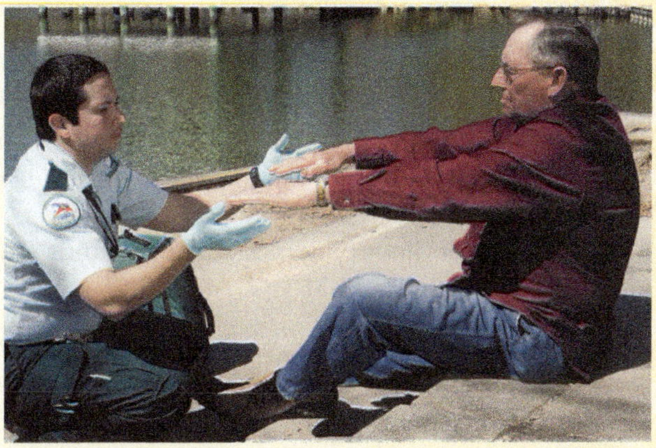

Body Systems Exam:

Endocrine

Blood glucose monitoring
Skin color/temperature/conditions
Breath odors
Excessive hunger, thirst, or urination
Pupils
Monitoring mental status changes over time

Diabetic Specific History
Oral intake
Medication history/use
Recent illness

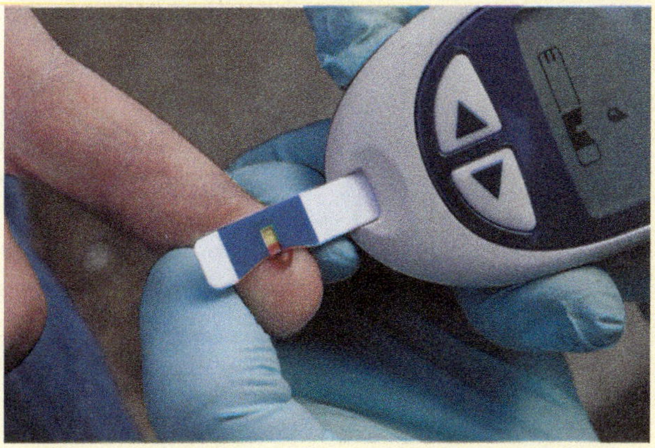

Body Systems Exam:

GI/GU

Palpation of abdominal quadrants

GI/GU Specific History
Input/output amount and frequency
Question or observe for bright red or digested blood in vomit, stool, or urine
Menstrual history and pregnancy where appropriate

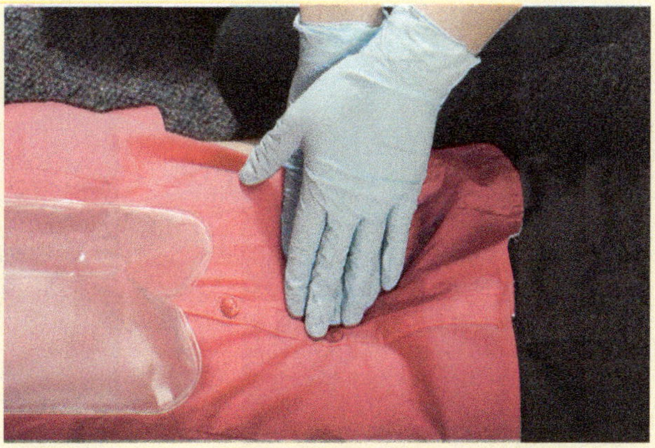

Respiratory Assessment—Physical Examination

Some of the most important parts of the respiratory assessment are performed before ever touching the patient. During your size-up and primary assessment, you made observations about your patient. These included two important assessments that apply to the respiratory system:

- Mental status—altered mental status may be caused by decreased oxygen delivery to the brain.
- Level of respiratory distress and work of breathing—since you have been observing your patient for some time, you likely have already noticed the level of distress the patient is in. Specifically note accessory muscle use and of the effort put forth to breathe.

Now, as part of the secondary assessment, make these evaluations:

- Observe chest wall motion—the chest wall should expand significantly and equally. Any alteration to this indicates an underlying problem such as trauma to the chest wall or pneumothorax.
- Auscultate lung sounds—you will listen for the presence and absence of lung sounds. You may also hear abnormal sounds, including wheezes (indicating airway narrowing) and popping or crackling sounds (rhonchi and rales, indicating fluid in the airway) (Figure 14-3).
- Use pulse oximetry—measure the oxygen saturation of the blood (Figure 14-4).
- Observe edema—edema may be heard in the lungs. It may also be observed in other parts of the body. Check the ankles for dependent edema (Figure 14-5). This will appear as puffy, swollen ankles. In patients who are bedridden, edema may be observed in the abdomen and flanks.
- Fever—does the patient have a fever? This may indicate an infectious process such as pneumonia.

Cardiovascular System

Assessment of the cardiovascular system involves two major parts of the body: the heart and the blood vessels. It also involves two major patient presentations: the cardiac patient and the patient in shock or with a vascular problem. Assessment of the cardiovascular system applies to the patient with acute coronary syndrome as well as to the trauma patient in shock.

The respiratory system is so closely aligned with the cardiovascular system that history questions and assessments for the respiratory system are commonly used during the

FIGURE 14-3 Auscultate to listen for the presence and absence of lung sounds.

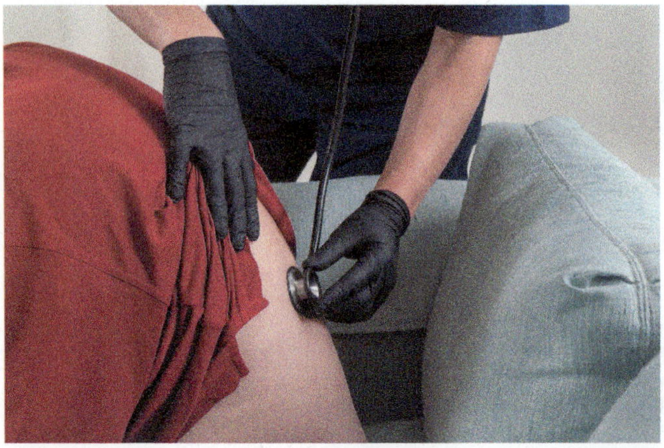

FIGURE 14-4 Use pulse oximetry to measure oxygen saturation of the blood.

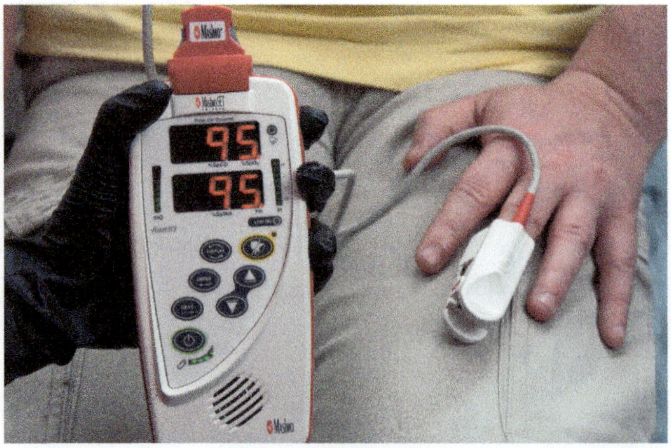

FIGURE 14-5 Check for edema (swelling).

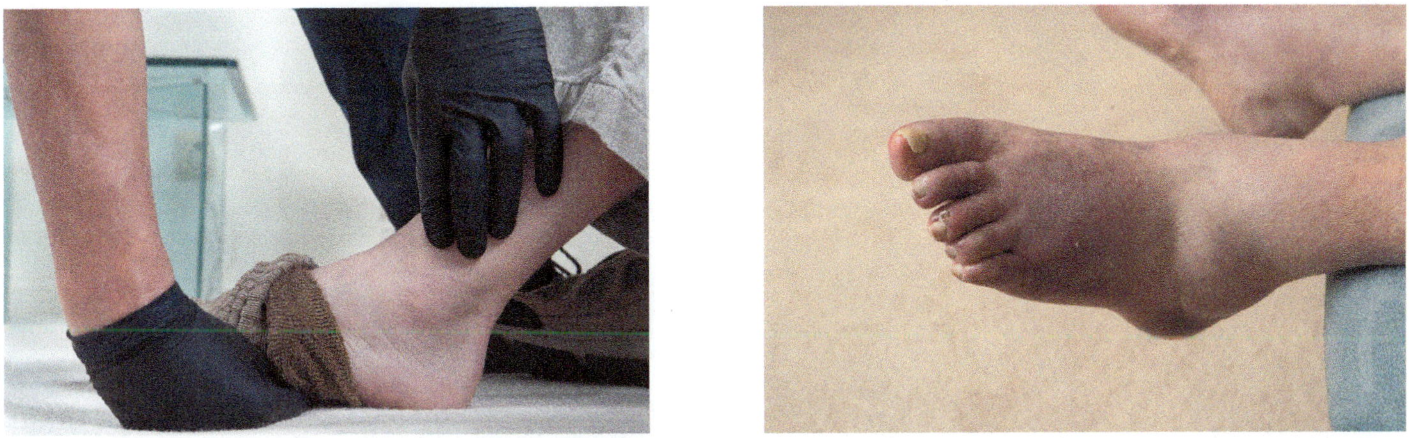

A B

cardiovascular examination and vice versa. Use them as appropriate. You will use the assessment techniques and history questions that apply to the patient you are treating.

Cardiovascular Assessment—History

The following are elements of a cardiovascular system history:

- Obtain a history of existing cardiac conditions and the medications taken for each. Determine if the medications have been taken as prescribed.
- Determine if signs and symptoms of this episode match previous episodes. (This question is valid for any medical condition.)
- Obtain a description of any chest discomfort using the OPQRST mnemonic.
- Determine specific characteristics of the discomfort—does the discomfort change with position, breathing or movement?

Cardiovascular Assessment—Physical Examination

A variety of conditions may cause chest discomfort. These range from heart attack to broken ribs to pneumonia. Use the techniques in this section that pertain to the history and presentation of your patient.

- Look for signs that the condition may be severe—including skin color, temperature, and condition (Figure 14-6). Pale, cool and/or moist skin indicates a more serious condition. (This may also be done in the primary assessment.) Note the mental status. Altered mental status can indicate poor perfusion to the brain.

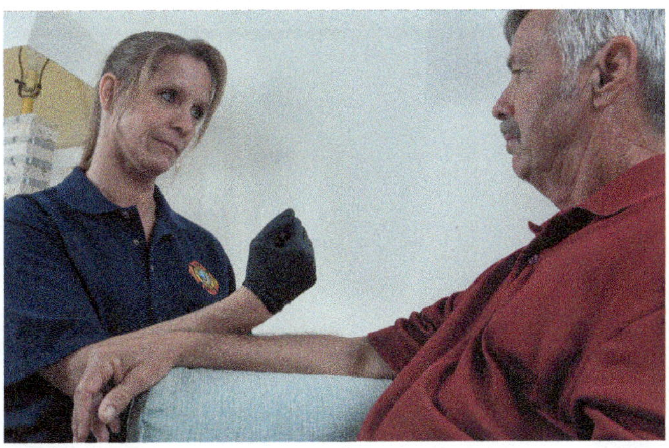

FIGURE 14-6 Check skin color, temperature, and condition.

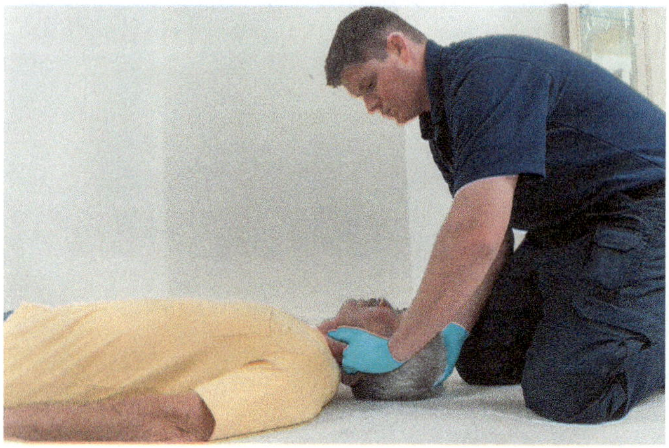

FIGURE 14-7 Check for the presence of a carotid pulse.

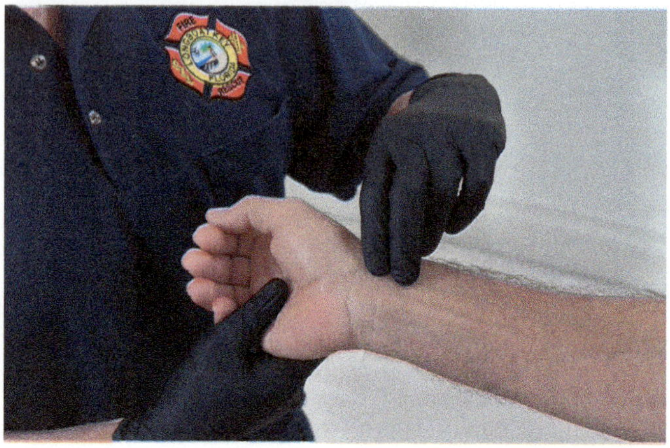

FIGURE 14-8 Check for presence and strength of a radial pulse.

- Obtain a pulse (Figure 14-7)—be alert for unusually high or low rates and pulses that are irregular. Also determine whether a radial pulse is present and if it is strong or weak (Figure 14-8). An absent or weak radial pulse may indicate poor perfusion.
- Obtain a blood pressure (Figure 14-9)—the blood pressure may be normal, hypertensive, or hypotensive. During transport, consider taking a blood pressure on both arms. Determine if there is a significant difference between the two (greater than 20 mmHg). This may indicate aortic aneurysm.
- Note the pulse pressure—a narrow or narrowing pulse pressure (the difference between the systolic and diastolic pulse pressures) may indicate shock.
- Look for ***jugular vein distention (JVD)*** (Figure 14-10)—JVD may indicate heart failure or other obstructive conditions within the chest.
- Palpate the chest—is the chest tender to palpation in one specific area? This may indicate trauma.
- Observe posture and breathing—is the patient guarding the patient's chest? This may indicate injury. Shallow breathing may also indicate chest trauma because deep breaths cause pain.

jugular (JUG-yuh-ler) ***vein distention (JVD)*** bulging of the neck veins.

Nervous System

There are two main elements to the nervous system examination. The first has to do with mental status. Mental status is an important indicator of the functioning of the brain. Decreases in oxygen and low perfusion will cause altered mental status. There are,

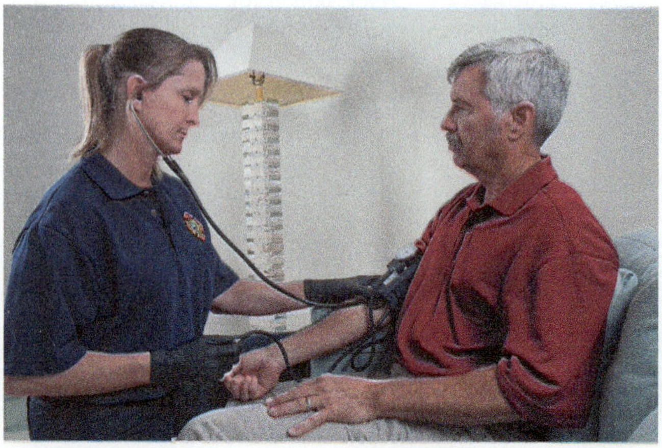

FIGURE 14-9 Obtain a blood pressure reading.

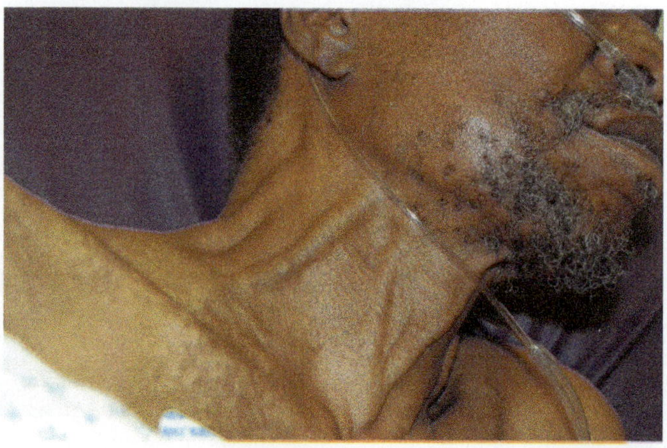

FIGURE 14-10 Look for jugular vein distention (JVD). *(© Edward T. Dickinson, MD)*

however, many causes of altered mental status, including stroke, tumors, and dementia. (Hypoglycemia will be discussed in the section on the endocrine system.)

The second major component of the nervous system exam is examination of the body for signs of dysfunction. You may find changes in stroke patients (facial asymmetry, slurred speech), as well as in motor-vehicle collisions where trauma causes damage to the spine (weakness or inability to move extremities).

Neurologic Assessment—History

Depending on the patient's current mental status, you may need to get some or all of the following information from a relative or bystander.

- Determine the patient's mental status—you will determine the patient's mental status in regard to the ability to know person, place, time, and purpose (Figure 14-11).
- Determine the patient's normal state of mental functioning—some patients may not have normal functioning to begin with (e.g., patients with dementia or Alzheimer's disease). In these cases you should determine any changes from the patient's baseline.
- Obtain a history of neurologic conditions—the patient may have had previous strokes or transient ischemic attacks (TIAs). You may also encounter patients with neurologic conditions such as amyotrophic lateral sclerosis (Lou Gehrig's disease) or Guillain-Barré syndrome.
- Note the patient's speech—you will note slurring during conversation with the patient. There are other speech problems and patterns that indicate brain dysfunction, including inability to speak at all and speaking inappropriate words.

Neurologic Assessment—Physical Examination

Following are elements of the neurologic physical examination:

- Perform a stroke scale (Figure 14-12)—use the Cincinnati Prehospital Stroke Scale (CPSS) or another system-approved scale.
- Check peripheral sensation and movement—you should check each extremity for movement (e.g., "Wiggle your fingers for me") and sensation. These should be equal. Unequal or absent findings may indicate spinal injury.
- Gently palpate the spine for tenderness or deformity (Figure 14-13).
- Check extremity strength—have the patient squeeze your fingers with the patient's hands (grip strength [Figure 14-14]) and have the patient raise and lower a foot against the force of your hands. The findings should be equal bilaterally. Inequality or lack of movement may indicate spinal injury.

FIGURE 14-11 Talk to the patient to determine the patient's mental status.

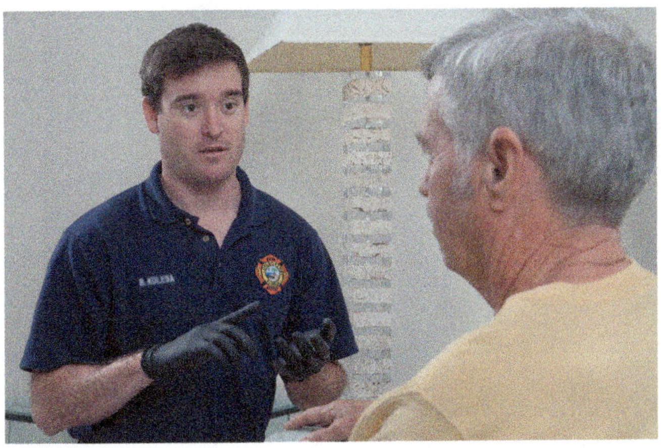

FIGURE 14-12 Observe for signs of stroke, such as arm drift, facial asymmetry, and speech difficulty.

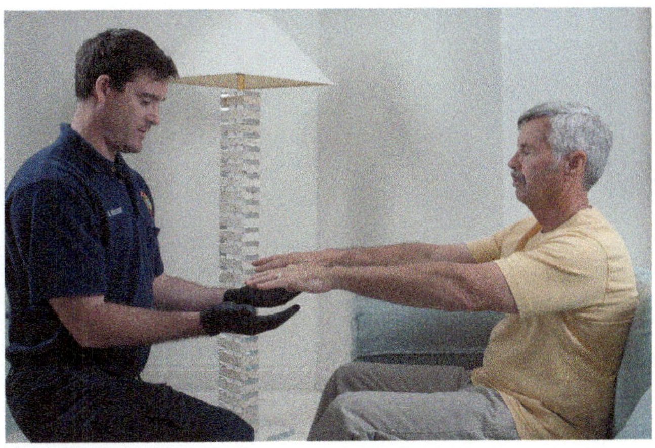

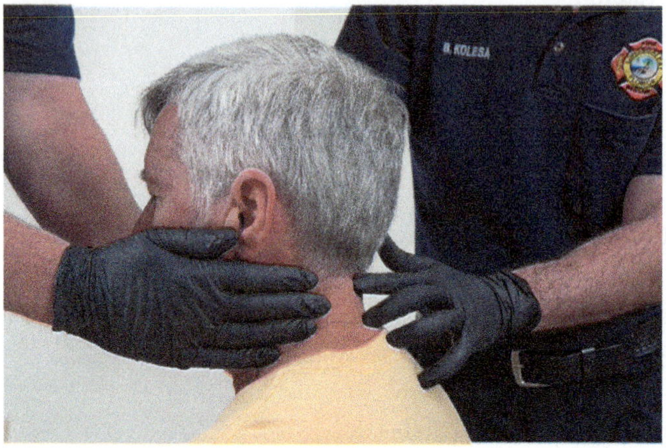

FIGURE 14-13 Palpate the spine for tenderness or deformity.

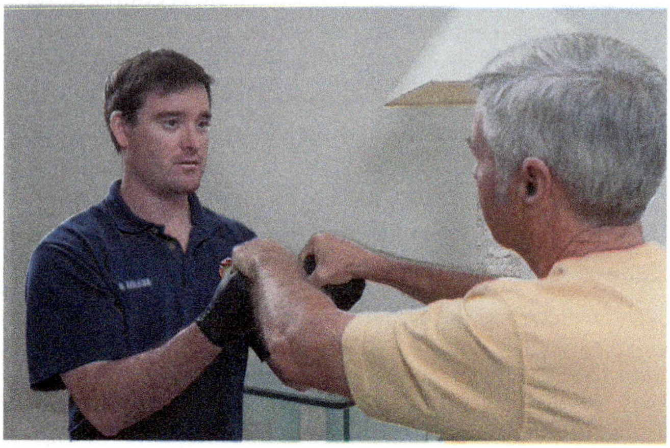

FIGURE 14-14 Check the patient's grip strength.

- Check the patient's pupils for equality and reactivity (Figure 14-15).
- If the patient is walking, examine the patient's gate. Can the patient keep on balance? Is the patient capable of walking the way the patient normally does? Take care not to allow patients to stand if they are already dizzy or have balance issues. Fall risk would be high in these patients.

Endocrine System

The endocrine system is composed of glands that produce and secrete hormones. These can affect everything from growth to heart rate. The most common endocrine emergency is with a diabetic patient. This section will focus primarily on the diabetic emergency.

Some components of the history won't be available from the patient with an altered mental status. This can be obtained from family members or bystanders.

Endocrine Assessment—History

Following are elements of the endocrine system history:

- Obtain a history of endocrine conditions. The patient may have a history of diabetes mellitus or thyroid disease.
- Determine whether the patient takes medications and when they were last taken. Was this a normal dose? Has the patient changed the dose recently?
- Determine whether the patient has eaten. Determine the quantity of food and when it was ingested. Is this the same as or different than usual?
- Have patients been exerting themselves at an unusual level? If so, more or less exertion?

FIGURE 14-15 Check the pupils for equality and reactivity.

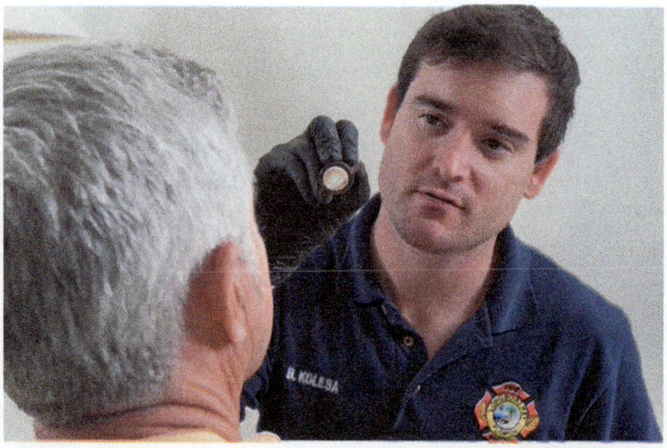

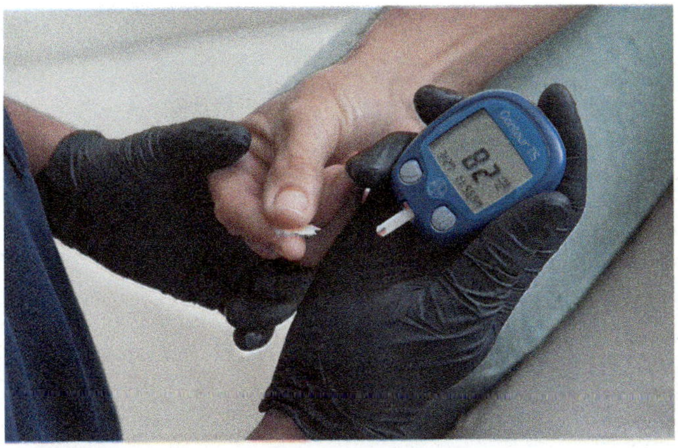

FIGURE 14-16 Obtain a blood glucose reading if protocols permit.

- Is the patient currently sick? Illness can change the patient's metabolism and calorie needs. Patients may also change medication levels if they are ill.
- Has the patient taken a blood glucose reading recently? Does the patient generally keep blood glucose under control, or does it fluctuate?
- Ask if the patient has an insulin pump. These may malfunction or be programmed incorrectly, causing increased insulin to be released in to the body.

Endocrine Assessment—Physical Examination

Following are elements of the endocrine system physical examination:

- Evaluate the patient's mental status. Hypoglycemia with altered mental status is generally treated by EMTs except in patients unable to control their own airways.
- Observe the patient's skin—cool, moist skin may occur in hypoglycemia.
- Obtain a blood glucose level (if allowed to do so by protocol) (Figure 14-16). The normal blood glucose range is 70–100 mg/dL (3.8–5.5 mmol/L).
- Look for an insulin pump. This may be providing too much insulin, causing hypoglycemia.
- Look for medical jewelry that identifies the patient as a diabetic.

Gastrointestinal System

The gastrointestinal system is spread throughout the body, although we largely think of abdominal organs when we think of this system. If you trace the path of food from when we ingest it to when we excrete it, we are looking at the entire gastrointestinal system.

When assessing the gastrointestinal system, we generally look at what has gone in, what has come out, and what it looks like when it comes out.

Remember that there may be trauma to the gastrointestinal system anywhere from the mouth progressing distally to the anus. This may be caused by many different events, including motor-vehicle collisions, falls, violence, and sexual assault.

Gastrointestinal Assessment—History

When taking a history for the gastrointestinal system, small details are important. Be sure to ask detailed questions—even when the questions may not be pleasant.

- Pain or discomfort—does the patient complain of any pain? Get a full and accurate description using the OPQRST mnemonic. Does the pain begin or get better after eating?
- Oral intake—part of the SAMPLE history, oral intake is important. You should determine a recent intake history of both solids and liquids. Determine if this has varied from the norm.
- Does the patient have a history of any gastrointestinal issues? Does the patient take any medications?

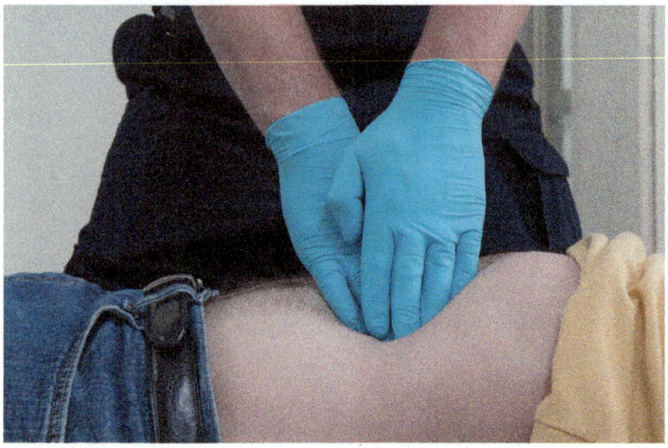

FIGURE 14-17 Palpate the abdominal quadrants.

- Vomiting—has the patient vomited? How much and how frequently? What did the vomit look like? (Of particular note are material that appears like coffee grounds and dark or bright red blood visible in the vomit.)
- Bowel movements—has the patient had bowel movements recently? If so, how frequently? How does this compare with normal? What did the stool look like? Dark, tarry stools may indicate digested blood. Bright red blood may be observed in the stool or on toilet tissue.

Gastrointestinal Assessment—Physical Examination

Following are elements of the gastrointestinal system physical examination:

- Observe the patient's position—a patient with abdominal complaints may take a fetal (knees to chest) position for comfort or may guard the abdomen to prevent others from touching it.
- Assess the abdomen—inspect then palpate the abdominal quadrants (Figure 14-17). Palpate the area or areas of pain last. Some are instructed to auscultate the abdomen for bowel sounds. If you do this, do it before palpation.
- Inspect other parts of the gastrointestinal system as appropriate.
- If there is vomitus or feces available, inspect it. Note the volume and color of the material. Be particularly observant for signs of gastrointestinal bleeding.

Immune System

The immune system can cause a number of physical problems, but the most relevant for EMS is the allergic reaction. Assessment deals with identifying signs and symptoms of an allergic reaction and determining whether the reaction is severe (anaphylaxis) or not. This is a case where the physical examination has more relevance in the medical patient, since allergic reactions cause signs such as hives on the skin and wheezing.

Immune System—Patient History

Following are elements of the immune system history:

- Does the patient have any allergies, or has the patient had a reaction to a substance or sting in the past?
- Has the patient been exposed to a known allergen or to a substance known to commonly cause allergic reactions (such as a new antibiotic medication or an insect sting)?
- If the patient has allergies, what are typical reactions like? Have previous reactions been severe and caused EMS response or hospitalization?
- Does the patient have a history of asthma?

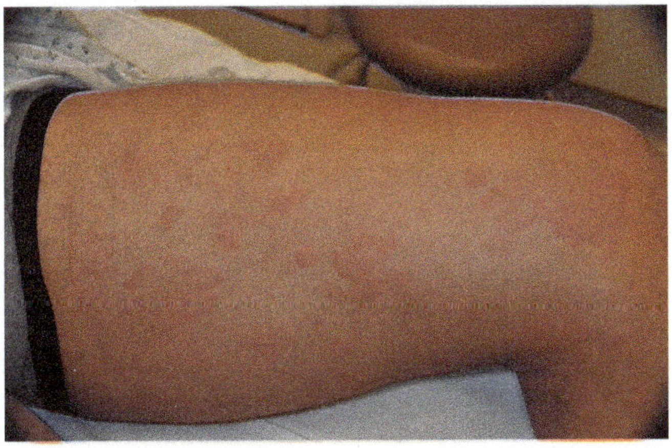

FIGURE 14-18 Inspect the skin for hives. *(© Edward T. Dickinson, MD)*

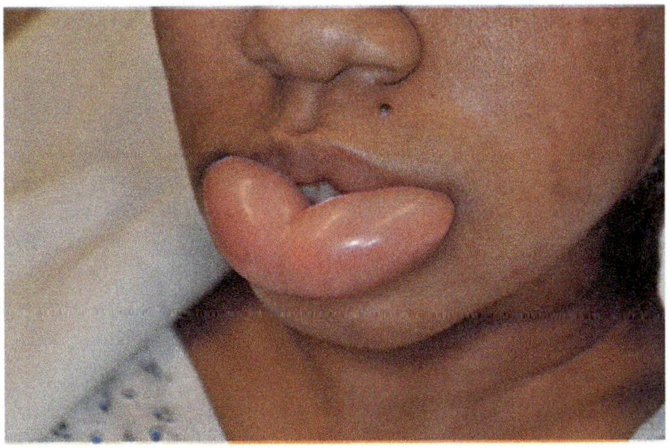

FIGURE 14-19 Inspect the face, lips, and mouth for swelling. *(© Edward T. Dickinson, MD)*

- Does the patient feel tightness in the chest or throat, difficulty breathing, or swelling around the face or mouth and tongue?
- Does the patient have GI distress (abdominal pain or cramping or diarrhea)?
- Does the patient have itchiness or a rash?
- Does the patient have medications for allergic reactions, such as an epinephrine auto-injector?

Immune System—Physical Examination

Following are elements of the immune system physical examination:

- Inspect the point of contact with the allergen. Do you see a stinger (bee sting) or evidence of allergic reaction such as systemic swelling or swelling in the mouth or airway?
- Inspect the patient's skin for a widespread rash or hives (Figure 14-18).
- Inspect the face, lips, and mouth for swelling (Figure 14-19).
- Listen to the patient speak. is the patient's voice hoarse or raspy? Do you hear stridor?
- Listen to the patient's lungs to ensure adequate breathing. Note if wheezes are present.

Musculoskeletal System

In the *Anatomy and Physiology* chapter, you learned that there are hundreds of bones in various shapes throughout the body. The musculoskeletal examination assesses these bones for injury.

While there are a few medical musculoskeletal system diseases, they are very rare. The musculoskeletal system is most commonly injured by trauma. This is the setting in which most musculoskeletal examinations will be performed as part of a complete trauma examination (discussed in the chapter *Secondary Assessment*).

Musculoskeletal Assessment—History

Since musculoskeletal assessment is usually performed during traumatic incidents, the history is usually taken after the physical assessment. This history usually provides less information than the physical assessment, but there are times it will be helpful:

- Ask if the patient has had prior injuries in the area you suspect injury.
- Ask if the patient takes blood-thinning medications, or medications that may delay clotting. This may help predict bleeding that can be severe and difficult to control.

FIGURE 14-20 Inspect for signs of musculoskeletal injury such as deformity. *(© Edward T. Dickinson, MD)*

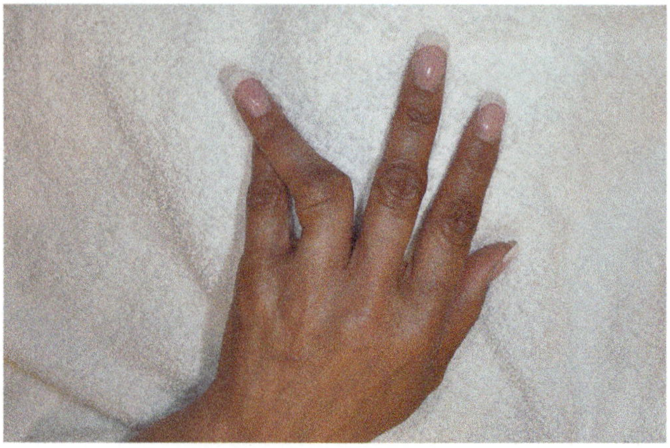

FIGURE 14-21 Look for bruising. *(© Edward T. Dickinson, MD)*

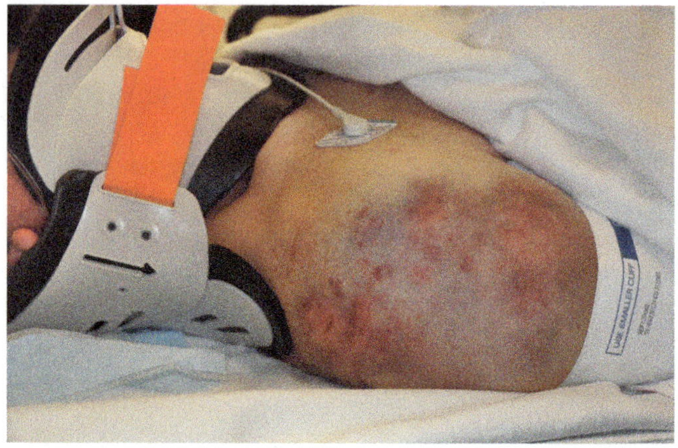

- Ask if the patient has any underlying diseases or conditions that might make fractures more common (osteoporosis, certain cancers and chemotherapy, diseases of the spine, etc.)
- Use the history to determine if a medical problem (e.g., loss of consciousness) caused the traumatic injury.

Musculoskeletal Assessment—Physical Examination

Following are elements of the musculoskeletal system physical examination:

- Inspect the patient for signs of musculoskeletal injury such as deformity (Figure 14-20), swelling, or bruising (Figure 14-21).
- Palpate areas in which you suspect injury (Figure 14-22). Palpate gently if deformities are obvious. Palpation should never cause injury.
- Compare sides of the body and note any asymmetry (Figure 14-23).
- Be alert for ***crepitation*** (the feeling of bone ends rubbing together) as you palpate.
- In a head-to-toe assessment, you will palpate all major body areas and extremities. This is often done when there are multiple injuries or the patient is unresponsive and unable to tell you where the injury is.

crepitation (krep-uh-TAY-shun) the grating sound or feeling of broken bones rubbing together.

FIGURE 14-22 Palpate areas where you suspect injury. Palpate gently so as not to cause unnecessary pain or further injury.

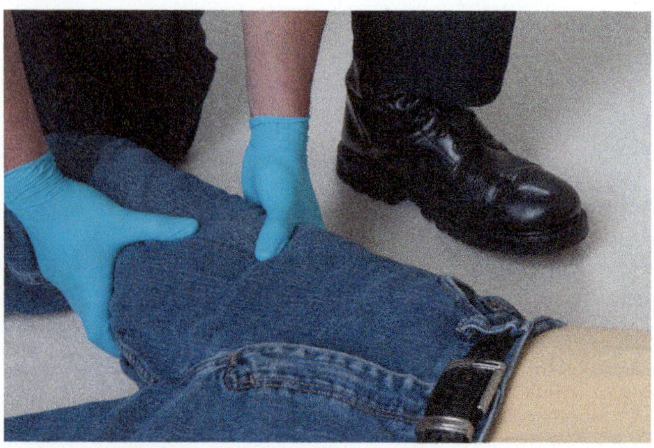

FIGURE 14-23 Compare sides of the body for any asymmetry (here, a right shoulder dislocation). *(© Edward T. Dickinson, MD)*

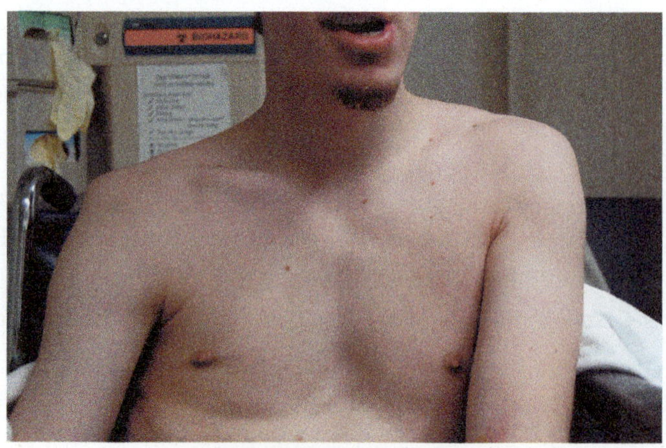

Pediatric Note

In traumatic accidents, children often have fears and concerns that differ from adults, as far as body image, disfigurement, and understanding of what is going to happen (Figure 14-24). Being aware of the child's perspective can help you be more effective at the scene. Children also have physical differences that are crucial to keep in mind when treating pediatric patients.

FIGURE 14-24

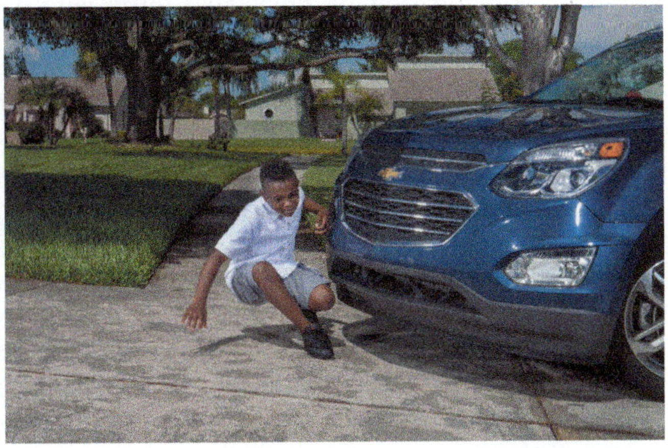

A Child involved in collision with a car. Note that the area of impact from a vehicle may be higher on a child than on an adult.

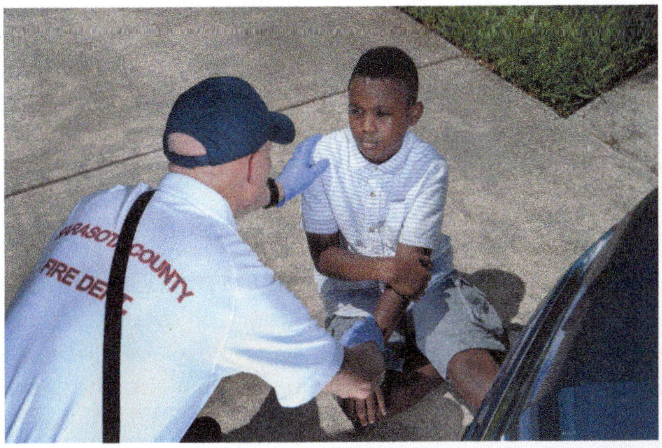

B EMT talking to and examining the child at his level. A friendly voice and direct eye contact can help to calm a frightened child.

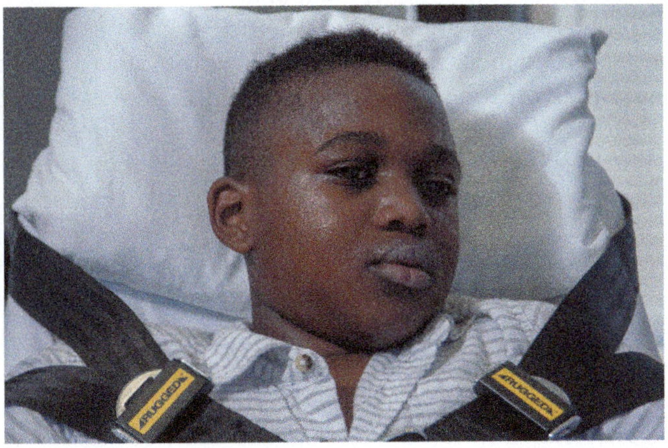

C Children may have different injury patterns than adults because of their head size, growth and development, and activities (e.g., when struck by a car as a pedestrian or bicyclist). Early stages of shock in children may be more difficult to detect, leading to what seems to be a sudden appearance of compensation. Be alert for tachycardia and changes in mental status.

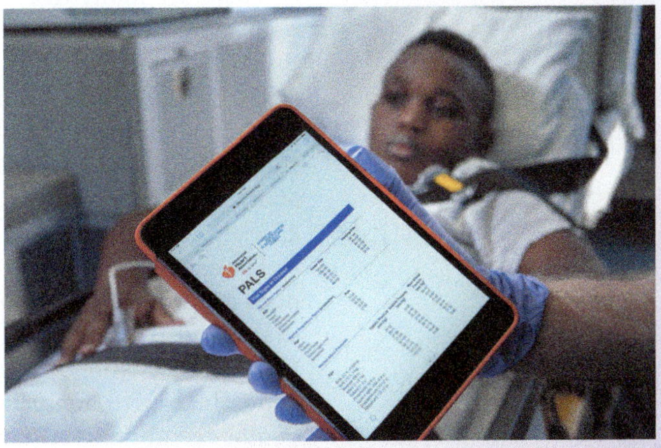

D Vital signs for pediatric patients are different than those for adults. Use references rather than memory to be sure of the normal range for various age groups.

Critical Thinking and Decision Making

Diagnosis is critical in medical care. For years, however, EMTs have heard "EMTs don't diagnose." In reality, there are conditions that EMTs have to diagnose, such as cardiac arrest. There are also conditions that EMTs don't diagnose, such as tetanus. However, paramedics and

diagnosis
a description or label for a patient's condition that assists a clinician in further evaluation and treatment.

emergency physicians don't typically make the diagnosis of tetanus either. What's the difference between the diagnosis an EMT makes and the diagnosis other health care providers make?

Cardiac arrest is at one end of a spectrum of diagnoses that stretches all the way from minor conditions such as a cut finger to liver lacerations, lung cancer, and beyond. EMTs learn enough to diagnose a few things, although the EMT's conclusion may be a very generalized diagnosis. For example, an EMT may say that a patient has abdominal pain of unknown cause. Although this sounds vague, it is the same diagnosis emergency physicians may use when, after both laboratory and radiologic testing, the cause of a patient's abdominal pain still cannot be determined. Of course, the emergency physician has the training, experience, and resources to rule out (exclude) and diagnose many more causes of abdominal pain than an EMT does. For that reason, the emergency physician's diagnosis is more specific than the EMT's diagnosis. Nonetheless, there are some similarities between how EMTs function in the field and how emergency physicians function in the emergency department. Obviously, as an EMT with only about 200 hours of training, you are not expected to have the same depth of knowledge or expertise in diagnosis and emergency care as a physician with thousands of hours of classroom and clinical training.

EMT Diagnosis and Critical Thinking

CORE CONCEPT
Critical thinking concepts for the EMT

An EMT's diagnosis is a description or label for a patient's condition, based on the patient's history, physical exam, and vital signs, that assists the EMT in further evaluation and treatment. It may be referred to by other names: field diagnosis, presumptive diagnosis, or working diagnosis. No matter the name, they all refer to how EMTs come to a conclusion, after assessing a patient, about the nature of the patient's condition (or sometimes what it is not). The process of reaching a diagnosis involves a great deal of simultaneous activity, both physical and intellectual. It is sometimes difficult to determine in the field how much information to get and when to get it. The process that assists the EMT in doing this is called critical thinking.

"My skills make me a good EMT. My thinking and decision making make me a great EMT."

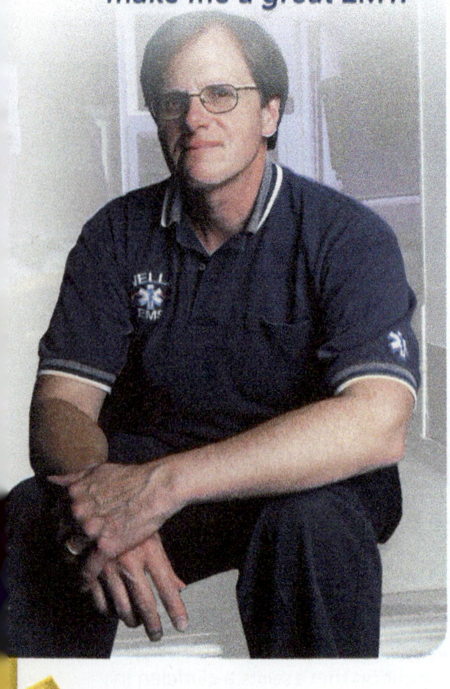

There are many descriptions of critical thinking. It is an analytical process that can help someone think through a problem in an organized and efficient manner. It is also thinking that is reflective, reasonable, and focused on deciding what to do in a particular situation. Some people describe it as an attitude of inquiry that involves the use of facts, principles, theories, and other pieces of information. All of these descriptions contain some truth. However, this section is going to focus primarily on critical thinking as an analytical process that can help someone think through a problem in an organized and efficient manner.

For example, suppose an EMT is assessing a patient with abdominal pain. The EMT does a primary assessment, gathers the patient history, performs a pertinent physical exam, and institutes treatment and transport. After completing all of these steps, the EMT still is unsure of what is causing the patient's condition. The patient might have an abdominal aortic aneurysm, pancreatitis, gallstones, a duodenal ulcer, or any of a variety of other conditions. Although a physician may be able to diagnose many of these specific conditions, that ability usually requires a significant amount of training, experience, clinical skill, laboratory tests, imaging, and perhaps even consultation with a specialist. How would a clinician determine what was wrong with this patient?

How a Clinician Reaches a Diagnosis

Different clinicians have different levels of training and experience, time, technology, and other resources. Despite all of these differences, they all have to reach some kind of conclusion about what is wrong with the patient and what kind of treatment to administer. All clinicians begin with the same basic approach: Gather information, consider possibilities, and reach a conclusion. The way they implement these steps, however, varies significantly.

The Traditional Approach to Diagnosis in Medicine

The first step in the traditional approach to diagnosis is assessing the patient (Figure 14-25). Next the clinician draws up a list of conditions or diagnoses that could be causing the

FIGURE 14-25 The traditional approach to reaching a diagnosis includes interviewing the patient in the controlled environment of a clinic or office.

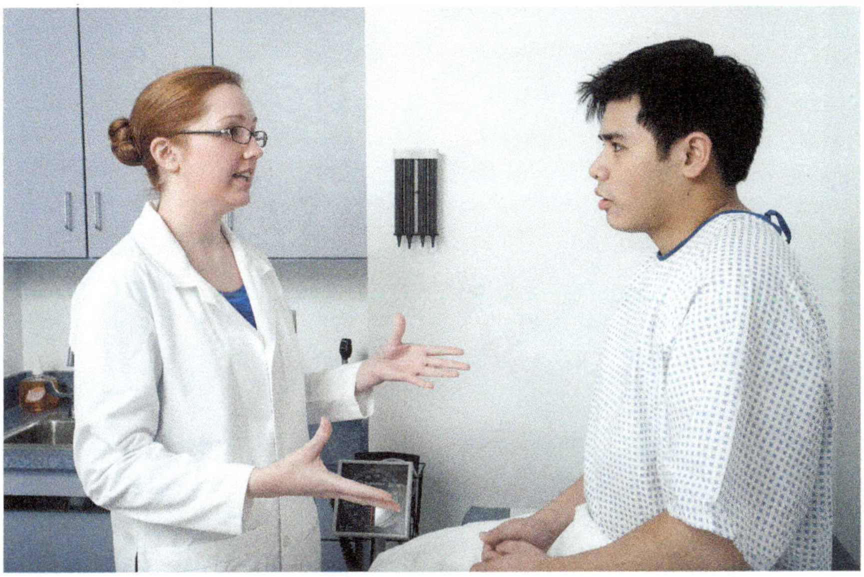

patient's condition. This list is called a ***differential diagnosis*** or just "the differential." To determine which of the potential diagnoses is correct, the patient receives further evaluation and perhaps some tests to rule in or rule out the diagnoses on the list. Once the results of the assessment and tests are known, the clinician considers those results and excludes conditions that are unlikely to be correct. In the end, this results in a diagnosis (or in some cases, a few possible diagnoses). Sometimes, as a result of the additional assessment, the list becomes longer before it can be narrowed down (Figure 14-26).

differential diagnosis a list of potential diagnoses compiled early in the assessment of the patient.

The Emergency Medicine Approach to Diagnosis

The emergency physician often does not have the time or the resources to use the traditional approach to reach a diagnosis. Instead, because of the unique circumstances and environment of the emergency department, the goals are to rule out life-threatening conditions, to narrow the range of possible diagnoses, and to institute urgent treatment. Part of the treatment may often be referral to the patient's own physician or a specialist to conduct further evaluation once the emergency physician determines that the patient's condition does not require admission to the hospital.

The first step in the emergency department, therefore, is to quickly rule out or identify and treat immediate life threats. Once that is done, the physician gathers information from

TRADITIONAL APPROACH TO DIAGNOSIS IN MEDICINE

Patient assessment (history, physical exam, vital signs, tests)

List of possible causes/diagnoses (differential diagnosis)

↓

Further evaluation

↓

Consider results of evaluation

↓

Narrow the list (may have to consider additional possibilities before reaching a diagnosis)

FIGURE 14-26 The traditional approach to diagnosis in medicine.

FIGURE 14-27 The emergency physician assesses patients in the busy, hectic atmosphere of an emergency department. *(© Edward T. Dickinson, MD)*

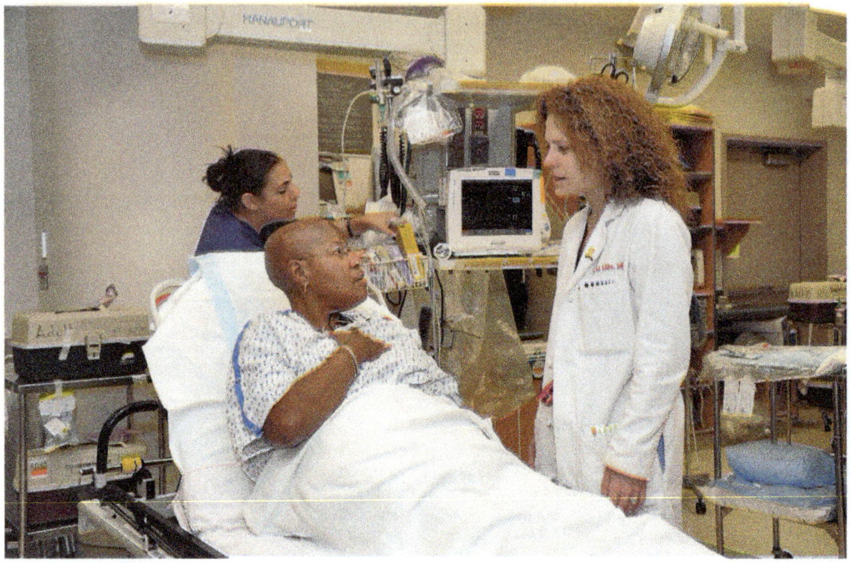

the patient, family, and friends and performs a physical exam (Figure 14-27). The focus of much of the questioning and assessment is to rule out the worst-case scenarios (i.e., the conditions that may threaten the patient's life or quality of life later on). The emergency physician looks for red flags, which are signs or symptoms that suggest the possibility of a particular problem that is very serious. For example, sudden onset of tearing pain in the abdomen that radiates to the back is a red flag that suggests an abdominal aortic aneurysm.

The information obtained from the secondary assessment guides the clinician in formulating a differential diagnosis, leading the clinician to ask further questions and order particular tests. However, not every test is available to the physician in the ED. A patient with a four-week-old knee injury will probably have to wait to get an MRI (magnetic resonance imaging) to see what is going on inside the joint. The emergency physician is therefore working with less information than the physician in an office environment. Once additional information is available from the laboratory and other tests, the physician considers it and comes to a diagnosis and disposition. The diagnosis may be very specific, such as appendicitis, or it may be as general as abdominal pain of unknown cause (Figure 14-28).

FIGURE 14-28 The emergency medicine approach to reaching a diagnosis.

EMERGENCY MEDICINE APPROACH TO DIAGNOSIS

Primary assessment to find and treat immediate threats to life

Patient assessment (history, physical exam, vital signs, tests) with special attention to looking for red flags

Consider the most serious conditions associated with the patient's presentation and rule them in or out (rule out the worst-case scenario)

List of possible causes/diagnoses (differential diagnosis)

↓

Further evaluation in light of time and resources available in the ED

↓

Consider results of evaluation

↓

Narrow the list (may have to re-state the chief complaint as the diagnosis)

All of this occurs in the busy, hectic environment of the emergency department, where the physician may be caring for four or five (or more) patients simultaneously and is frequently being interrupted with additional information or questions.

The EMS Approach to Diagnosis

The EMT has a lot in common with the emergency physician. The EMT has limited resources available, has few treatment options (although those options are very important), and knows time is of the essence. Unlike the emergency physician, however, the EMT usually cannot care for four or five patients simultaneously. Since the EMT has to go to the patient, the EMT is unavailable for other patients until that first patient has been delivered to another clinician. This puts pressure on the EMT to be very efficient; the sooner duties with one patient are complete, the sooner the EMT can get to the next. The EMT also works in an uncontrolled environment (Figure 14-29). For example, the emergency physician does not usually have to worry about being bitten by a patient's dog. However, emergency physicians do occasionally encounter violent patients in the ED, just as the EMT does in the field.

The tools the EMT has available in the field differ too. Although the amount of technology used in the field has increased tremendously over the past 10–20 years, EMTs have nowhere near the resources available in an ED. An EMT can merely evaluate a patient's vital signs and oxygen level of the blood, whereas the emergency physician can order multiple blood tests and imaging studies such as X-rays, ultrasounds, and CT (computed tomography) scans. The EMT's education focuses narrowly on certain conditions that have high statistical morbidity (illness) or mortality (death), whereas the emergency physician completes at least three years of postgraduate training after four years of medical school. Most important, much of that education is spent seeing thousands of patients and learning assessment and management skills under supervision.

All of this means that although the EMT will follow many of the same steps the emergency physician does in reaching a diagnosis, most of the EMT's diagnostic steps will be abbreviated or limited. The EMT's primary assessment finds and treats the patient's immediate life threats. Secondary assessment—consisting of the patient's history, physical exam, vital signs, and a few tests—comes next, with special attention devoted to looking for red flags. Simultaneously, the EMT begins treatment that may be beneficial and is not harmful. The most common example of this is administering oxygen.

The EMT then considers the most serious conditions associated with the patient's presentation that can be treated in the field and quickly rules them in or out, so important treatment can be administered as quickly as possible. If the patient has no life-threatening conditions and no red flags, the EMT creates a mental list of possible causes or diagnoses

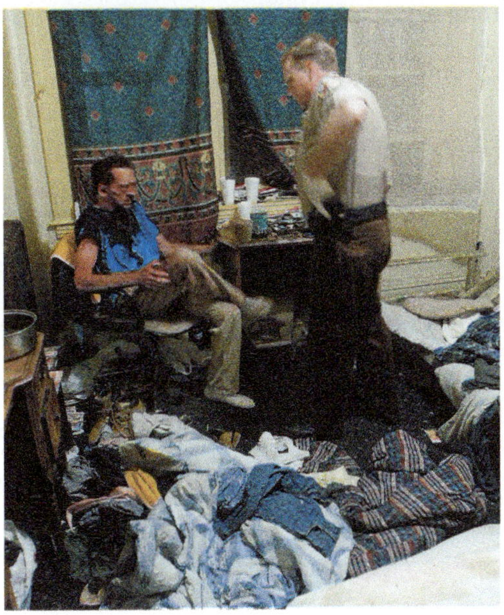

FIGURE 14-29 The EMT assesses a patient in the uncontrolled environment of the field. *(Mark Ide/Science Source)*

FIGURE 14-30 The EMS approach to reaching a diagnosis.

EMS APPROACH TO DIAGNOSIS

Primary assessment to find and treat immediate threats to life

Patient assessment (history, physical exam, vital signs, tests) with special attention to looking for red flags
Simultaneously, the EMT begins treatment that may be beneficial and is not harmful, e.g., oxygen

Consider the most serious conditions associated with the patient's presentation that can be treated in the field and rule them in or out

List of possible causes/diagnoses (differential diagnosis) if time allows

↓

Further evaluation in light of limited time available and restricted resources present in the field

↓

Consider results of evaluation

↓

Narrow the list (may have to restate the chief complaint as the diagnosis)

(a differential diagnosis). This list will often be short; e.g., in a patient with abdominal pain, the differential may be abdominal aortic aneurysm, gastrointestinal bleeding, dehydration, and all other causes of abdominal pain.

Next, depending on the situation, there may be further evaluation limited by the time and resources available in the field. This further evaluation may take place while en route to the hospital. After considering the results of any additional evaluation, the EMT may be able to narrow the list of possible diagnoses. In many cases, this may simply be a restatement of the chief complaint (e.g., abdominal pain) as the diagnosis (Figure 14-30).

Although these three approaches to diagnosis—traditional, emergency medicine, and EMS—have a lot in common, some differences clearly exist (Table 14-3).

TABLE 14-3 Approaches to Reaching a Diagnosis

	TRADITIONAL APPROACH	EMERGENCY MEDICINE APPROACH	EMS APPROACH
Goal	Reach definitive diagnosis and institute treatment	Rule out life-threatening conditions, narrow range of possible diagnoses, and institute urgent treatment	Rule out life-threatening conditions, narrow range of possible diagnoses, institute treatment when supported by protocols, as well as treatments important to patient survival and comfort Transport for more extensive assessment and treatment
Pace	Leisurely	Efficient	Urgent; dependent on patient condition and priority
Thoroughness	Very thorough	Focused	Limited in the field
Assessment tools and tests	Wide range of tests patient can be sent for	Limited to pertinent tests that are available at the time of the patient's presentation	Tools pertinent to finding some conditions, such as BP cuff, stroke scales, blood glucose monitor, and pulse oximeter
Extent of patient rapport	Significant	Limited	Limited with short transport times, greater with long transport times
Range of possible diagnoses	Extensive	Moderate	Limited

Approach to Diagnosis in Medicine—Shortcuts and Biases

Very experienced physicians do not always use the traditional approach of drawing up an extensive list and narrowing it down. Instead, they have learned shortcuts (also called heuristics) that speed up the process of reaching a diagnosis. These shortcuts, based on pattern recognition, help make physicians better, more efficient clinicians. The expert clinician can quickly recognize certain features of a patient's presentation that significantly narrow the diagnostic possibilities. The experienced physician can also quickly determine what further evaluation is necessary to rule in or rule out certain possibilities. As a result, highly experienced physicians can reach difficult diagnoses or conclusions more quickly than newer physicians, who need more time to consider the possibilities.

Shortcuts to diagnosis have limitations, of course. Experienced clinicians understand this and keep in mind avoidable traps so their conclusions are as accurate as possible.

As you gain experience in the medical field, you can start to develop shortcuts like experienced physicians do. In doing so, however, you will need to understand the advantages and shortcomings of shortcuts, or heuristics. Here are some of the more common heuristics and their biases:

- **Representativeness.** Representativeness means that when you encounter a patient with a certain group of signs and symptoms that resemble a particular condition, you assume the patient has that condition. Representativeness is at the heart of pattern recognition and is an important heuristic. What is its disadvantage? Patients don't always present with the typical signs and symptoms of a condition. As a result, when a patient doesn't fit the classic pattern, it is easy for the health care provider to mistakenly conclude the patient doesn't have that condition. For example, older patients with myocardial infarctions sometimes deny chest pain and complain instead of shortness of breath or weakness as their chief complaint.

  To avoid this trap, remain aware of its possibility. Remind yourself that patients don't read the textbooks and can present with uncommon or atypical signs or symptoms.

  A way to summarize representativeness is to think of the saying "If it looks like a duck and quacks like a duck, it must be a duck—except when it isn't."

- **Availability.** Availability is the urge to think of things because they are more easily recalled, often because of a recent exposure. For example, if an EMT has a patient with chest pain who is diagnosed with a dissecting thoracic aneurysm, the next time there is a patient with chest pain, the EMT is more likely to think of dissecting thoracic aneurysm as a possibility, even though the condition is much less common than angina and myocardial infarctions. Because of recent exposure to this condition, the EMT may overestimate its frequency.

  You can reduce your chances of falling into this trap by asking yourself just how common the particular condition that you're considering is, and whether you're considering it mainly because it matches information that is easily available. One way to think of the problem of availability is the EMT's tendency to say "You have the same thing my last patient had!"

- **Overconfidence.** Being an EMT requires a significant degree of confidence. Without it, the EMT is unable to function in a chaotic environment. Overconfidence, however, can work against the EMT. Thinking you know more than you really do can lead to many problems. A good way to avoid this tendency is to be aware of the limits of your knowledge and ability. Be careful in your assessment. Surveys consistently show that people think they know more than they actually do.

  When faced with a clinical situation, try to be as objective as possible when evaluating how much evidence has been gathered and whether it has been gathered in a logical and thorough fashion. Try to keep your ego out of this self-evaluation as much as possible. You can summarize the problem of overconfidence as "Of course I know what to do. I'm an EMT!"

- **Confirmation bias.** Clinicians commit confirmation bias by looking primarily for evidence that supports the diagnosis they already have in mind. By doing so, they may very well overlook evidence that refutes or reduces the probability of that diagnosis. This commonly occurs when the patient's presentation includes a lot of information and the clinician feels it's easier to go with one diagnosis rather than look for others.

  To avoid this pitfall, look for data that refutes the diagnosis you have in mind or reduces the likelihood of it. In other words, look for contrary data and consider competing hypotheses. The tendency to look only for information that supports what you already think is reflected in the saying "It must be right; I thought of it!"

- **Illusory correlation.** Human beings are able to draw conclusions about how the world works because they are able to see how one thing causes another. However, this human tendency can be misleading sometimes. Very often, one event may appear to cause another when, in fact, the two events are either coincidental or both caused by the same thing, leading to illusory correlation. For example, some believe that fluoridated water causes cancer. It is true that cities that have fluoridated their water have a higher rate of cancer than rural areas. Therefore, it would be very easy to conclude that one caused the other. However, when you look more closely at the data, you discover that cities are more likely than rural areas to fluoridate their water. Cities have higher rates of cancer than rural areas in general. Furthermore, cities that fluoridate have the same incidence of cancer as cities that do not fluoridate. Therefore, the appearance of cause and effect in this case is an illusion.

  To avoid this illusion, be skeptical about instances where one thing appears to cause another. Consider how the appearance of two things together may be just coincidence or, alternatively, consider that they may both have the same cause. An easy way to remember illusory correlation is to think of this example: "Most ice cream is eaten during the summer. Most drownings occur in the summer. Therefore, ice cream causes drowning."

- **Anchoring and adjustment.** In this situation, an EMT considers a particular condition to be likely, and later thinking is anchored to that hypothesis. The EMT may adjust in time, but sometimes not as much as necessary, because of the starting point. For example, an EMT may initially think that an unconscious intoxicated person is unconscious because "She's just drunk." When information appears that the patient may have sustained head trauma, the EMT may cling to the hypothesis that the patient's real problem is just intoxication.

  To avoid this, be careful not to jump to conclusions and determine a diagnosis on the basis of just a few signs or symptoms. Do a thorough assessment. The tendency to cling to your first conclusion is exemplified in the saying "You get only one chance to make a first impression."

- **Search satisfying.** It can be very satisfying to finally determine what is causing a patient's problem. However, once that happens, it is easy to stop looking for other causes of potential problems. This is called "search satisfying." The problem with search satisfying is that you can miss a secondary diagnosis (many EMS patients have more than one problem) or just be mistaken about the primary diagnosis. If you don't look for other problems, you will probably not detect them.

  A good way to prevent this problem is to keep an open mind about other possibilities and to evaluate each diagnosis before accepting it. This principle is well stated in the saying "Don't count your chickens before they hatch."

How an EMT Can Learn to Think Like an Experienced Physician

The following list features attitudes and understandings you can develop to help you think like an expert.

- **Learn to love ambiguity.** Ambiguity is at the core of EMS. Working in EMS means you are going out into unknown situations armed with limited education and experience (compared with physicians and many other clinicians) and equipped with limited tools and treatments. You are expected to make decisions, including some life-or-death decisions, in a very short period of time before you transport the patient to definitive care. You will not be able to gather the same amount of information that staff in a hospital does, and you have a limited range of treatments to provide your patients. No matter how conscientious and knowledgeable you are, you will run into situations where you just can't find a definitive answer to the question of why a patient is sick. That is the nature of EMS. By accepting that uncertainty as a natural part of what you do, you will actually become a better provider, able to understand the limitations of your knowledge and how this affects your patient care.

- **Understand the limitations of technology and people.** No one is perfect. Every human being makes errors. Some people go about procedures in ways you would never think of doing. Once you accept this, you will find it easier to work in the everyday world, where things don't always go as you planned. When you get information from someone else, whether a crew member, patient, or bystander, consider the source. How accurate and reliable do you judge the source to be? Is there a potential source of bias that might affect the way that person reports information? Is there a limited skill level or lack of familiarity with EMS that should make you consider how to process information from someone else?

  Similarly, no piece of equipment is perfect. Every mechanical or electronic device is subject to failure, whether from low batteries, inappropriate use, or excessive wear. When you get a reading from a device that doesn't make sense for the clinical picture in front of you, don't accept it as necessarily correct. If possible, have the device repeat the reading. Consider how the unexpected result could affect your management of the patient. In the end, you may need to make a decision regarding whether to accept an anomalous reading or go with your clinical judgment. Whether you made the correct decision is often not clear until later.
- **Realize that no one strategy works for everything.** No matter how experienced and skilled you become, you will encounter situations that don't work well for your particular approach to EMS calls. In such cases, it is important to be flexible and able to use more than just a single tactic. Times such as these are when experts think like new clinicians. They have to formulate a longer list than usual of differential diagnoses and rule them in or out.
- **Form a strong foundation of knowledge.** Expert clinicians may use different approaches to thinking through problems, but one thing they all have in common is a strong foundation of knowledge. They are extremely familiar with the signs and symptoms of conditions they are expected to encounter. They are also very aware of conditions that can mimic those diseases. They keep up to date with new information on associated conditions that sometimes accompany those diseases. They have both the tools (the thinking processes) and the supplies (the knowledge to apply those tools).
- **Organize the data in your head.** Create what experts call elaborated knowledge. Once you can list the signs and symptoms of a disease, work in the other direction. Take signs and symptoms and consider what other diseases they may be associated with. This actually creates new connections in your brain and provides practice for what you actually will do in the field. Reflect on how the presence or severity of a particular sign or symptom changes the probability of a particular disease or condition. At first, concentrate on a few diseases that have similar chief complaints. Study them until you know the signs and symptoms of each, and work from the signs and symptoms back to the problem.
- **Change the way you think.** Once you have mastered the presentations of several conditions, compare and contrast them. Determine what features the conditions have in common and what features set them apart from each other. Rephrase the symptoms a patient provides so they match more closely the way a disease is described.

For instance, if a young male patient complains of 9/10 pain in the middle of his stomach that hit him like a thunderbolt, characterize this as the sudden onset of severe pain in the center of the abdomen.

- **Learn from others.** Your EMT class is only part of your education. Take advantage of the exposure you get to expert clinicians, and ask them to think out loud when they are solving problems. This will familiarize you with the ways an expert looks for information, processes it, and uses it to reach a diagnosis.
- **Reflect on what you have learned.** An essential part of being an expert clinician is learning from your experiences. Contrary to popular belief, people don't only learn from their mistakes. People learn even more from their successes. When someone succeeds in a venture, this reinforces the behavior that led to the success and leads to good habits. After a patient contact, especially a challenging one, evaluate your behavior. What did you do well? What can you do better? What did you learn that you didn't know before? What knowledge do you need to be more accurate and efficient in the future?

Keep in mind that once you have reached a possible diagnosis, your work is not necessarily over. You should continue looking for data that will help to rule in or rule out the conditions you are considering. All patients may have more than one thing wrong with them, so don't stop looking for causes too early. Your conclusion may also be wrong, so it is good to continue thinking about what may be wrong with a patient.

These steps can be used not only when reaching a diagnosis, but also with many other problems. Being aware of how you think gives you a powerful tool for improving your information-gathering and thought processes. Keep in mind that when you are faced with an unfamiliar situation, you should go back to the basics. Do your assessment and follow the general principles outlined in your EMT course.

Reaching a diagnosis is a process you can learn. However, be careful not to expect too much of yourself at the beginning—the process of thinking critically is developed through study, practice, and reflection. It will take time to develop this skill. In the meantime, don't let anyone force you to go further than your level of competence. Know the boundaries of your knowledge, skill, and judgment. Overconfidence can be dangerous. Strive to learn more by study and observation of more experienced providers. Most important, don't let attempts to reach a diagnosis delay patient care that is safe and appropriate.

Point of View

"Probably the best lesson I learned about critical thinking was to listen. You can't figure out what is going on without the facts. Sometimes it's the little pieces of information you could easily overlook. Other times it is the thought between the words that doesn't come out but you know it is there. Sure, you'll assess and take vitals. But trust me. You'll never find what you need to know unless you listen."

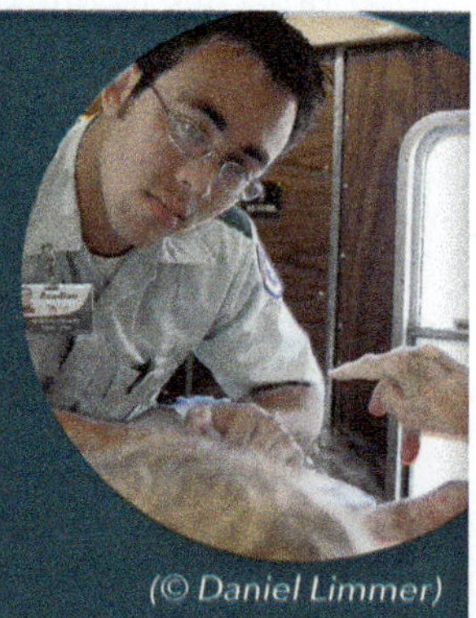

(© Daniel Limmer)

Chapter Review

Critical Thinking and Decision Making

Key Facts and Concepts

- EMTs make diagnoses in the field, although they may not be as extensive or detailed as physicians' diagnoses.
- The traditional approach to reaching a diagnosis is to assess the patient, draw up a list of differential diagnoses, assess further to rule in or rule out different conditions, and narrow the list until you reach a conclusion.
- Highly experienced physicians don't always use the traditional approach. They use heuristics (shortcuts) in combination with their experience and training, which speeds up the process of reaching a diagnosis.
- Potential pitfalls of heuristics include representativeness, anchoring and adjustment, overconfidence, confirmation bias, illusory correlation, and search satisfying.
- Learn to think more critically by accepting the ambiguity of EMS working conditions, understanding limitations of people and technology, forming a strong foundation of knowledge, and organizing the data in your mind.
- When considering the cause of a patient's condition, don't let your search for a cause delay your treatment of the patient.

Key Decisions

- Have I addressed life threats before beginning the assessment and diagnostic process?
- Does this patient have an obvious problem, or do I need to think more critically?
- Are there other potential causes besides the obvious one for this patient's condition?
- Have I considered other reasonable possibilities?
- What other information should I get to confirm or refute the working diagnosis?
- How specific does my field diagnosis have to be to determine the right treatment?
- What is best for the patient?

Chapter Glossary

chief complaint the patient's statement that describes the symptom or concern associated with the primary problem the patient is having.

closed-ended question a question requiring only a "yes" or "no" answer.

crepitation (krep-uh-TAY-shun) the grating sound or feeling of broken bones rubbing together.

diagnosis a description or label for a patient's condition that assists a clinician in further evaluation and treatment.

differential diagnosis a list of potential diagnoses compiled early in the assessment of the patient.

history of the present illness (HPI) information gathered regarding the symptoms and nature of the patient's current concern.

jugular (JUG-yuh-ler) ***vein distention (JVD)*** bulging of the neck veins.

open-ended question a question requiring more than just a "yes" or "no" answer.

OPQRST a memory aid in which the letters stand for questions asked to get a description of the present illness: **o**nset, **p**rovocation, **q**uality, **r**adiation, **s**everity, **t**ime.

past medical history (PMH) information gathered regarding the patient's health problems in the past.

SAMPLE a memory aid in which the letters stand for elements of the past medical history: **s**igns and symptoms, **a**llergies, **m**edications, **p**ertinent past history, **l**ast oral intake, and **e**vents leading to the injury or illness.

Preparation for Your Examination and Practice

Short Answer

1. How would you describe critical thinking?
2. What are the differences in the way an emergency physician reaches a diagnosis compared with the way an EMT reaches a diagnosis?
3. What are "search satisfying" and "confirmation bias"?
4. What questions would you ask to get a history of the present illness from a patient with a chief complaint of chest pain?

Thinking and Linking

Consider what you have studied so far about pathophysiology and patient assessment and link what you have already learned with the information presented in this chapter as you answer the following questions.

1. Why are patients who are *pale and sweaty* considered more serious than patients who aren't? How will seeing pale and sweaty patients affect your critical thinking and decision making?
2. Why are patients who are *anxious and restless* considered more serious than patients who aren't? How will seeing anxious and restless patients affect your critical thinking and decision making?
3. Why are patients with an *altered mental status* considered more serious than patients who aren't? How will seeing a patient with altered mental status affect your critical thinking and decision making?

Critical Thinking Exercises

For the following patients, determine how the critical thinking process will interact with the patient assessment process you learned in the previous chapters. First determine your priorities. Then describe what information you may want to obtain for diagnosis where appropriate.

1. A 52-year-old man complains of chest pain while sitting at his desk at work. He appears alert and oriented. He tells you he thinks it may "just be stress."
2. You are called to a 67-year-old man who was reportedly "acting unusually" when he became unresponsive. His wife said he complained of an odd feeling in his arm, and his speech was slurred before he became unresponsive.
3. An 18-year-old snowboarder took a fall and thinks he may have broken his ankle.
4. A 41-year-old woman has difficulty breathing and a little pain when she breathes in deeply. She is alert but a little anxious.

Street Scenes

You are called to a patient with an altered mental status at an assisted-living facility. The staff tells you that Mr. Ronson is normally very active and vibrant, "like the mayor of this place." But today he just isn't himself. He just sits in the chair and doesn't talk. "It is so unlike him," they say.

You arrive at the patient's side and introduce yourself. The patient turns his head toward you and acknowledges you with a grunting noise. His color appears OK. He is breathing deeply and regularly. His radial pulse is strong at about 60 beats per minute and regular. You quickly check his pulse oximetry reading, and it is 96 percent. You place him on 2 liters of oxygen via nasal cannula.

The attendant gives you a list of medications taken by the patient. They tell you he is diabetic and has had two heart attacks and one stroke. He also has high blood pressure and high cholesterol.

Street Scene Questions

1. **Assuming that your primary assessment is completed, what would be your next assessment steps?**
2. **What body systems may be contributing to this altered mental status?**
3. **How do the medications impact your history taking and decision making?**

You further find that Mr. Ronson lives alone. He was fine when he went to bed last night and was laughing and joking with the staff. His vital signs are pulse 58, strong and regular; respirations 22 and adequate; blood pressure 164/92; pupils equal and reactive; skin warm and slightly moist.

His medications all seem to match the conditions the staff reported. He has taken the meds with assistance from the staff. He has no known allergies and last ate yesterday afternoon. No one saw Mr. Ronson after he went to bed last night, so the events leading up to the current situation are unclear. He does appear able to follow your directions but not able to answer questions.

Street Scene Questions

4. **What assessments would you perform on this patient and why?**
5. **What is your transport priority for the patient?**
6. **At what point would you call for an ALS intercept?**

Mr. Ronson is able to perform a Cincinnati Prehospital Stroke Scale, and does not show signs of stroke. Checking his blood glucose levels, you find a level of 32 mg/dL, which is significantly below normal. Because of his mental status, you are concerned about his ability to swallow, so you notify ALS and request an intercept. Fortunately, they are close and respond before you leave the scene. They begin an IV and administer dextrose. Mr. Ronson was joking again before he reached the hospital.

The medics commend you for figuring out what was wrong and for the initial report when they got to the scene.

Secondary Assessment

15

Related Chapters

The following chapters provide additional information related to topics discussed in this chapter:

Standards

Assessment (Secondary Assessment; Reassessment)

Clinical Behavior/Judgment (Decision Making)

Competencies

Applies scene information and patient assessment findings (scene size-up, primary and secondary assessments, patient history, and reassessment) to guide emergency management.

Initiates basic interventions based on assessment findings intended to mitigate the emergency and provide limited symptom relief while providing access to definitive care.

Core Concepts

- Components of the secondary assessment
- Secondary assessment of the responsive medical patient
- Secondary assessment of the unresponsive medical patient
- Secondary assessment of the trauma patient with minor injury
- Secondary assessment of the trauma patient with serious injury or multisystem trauma
- Detailed physical exam

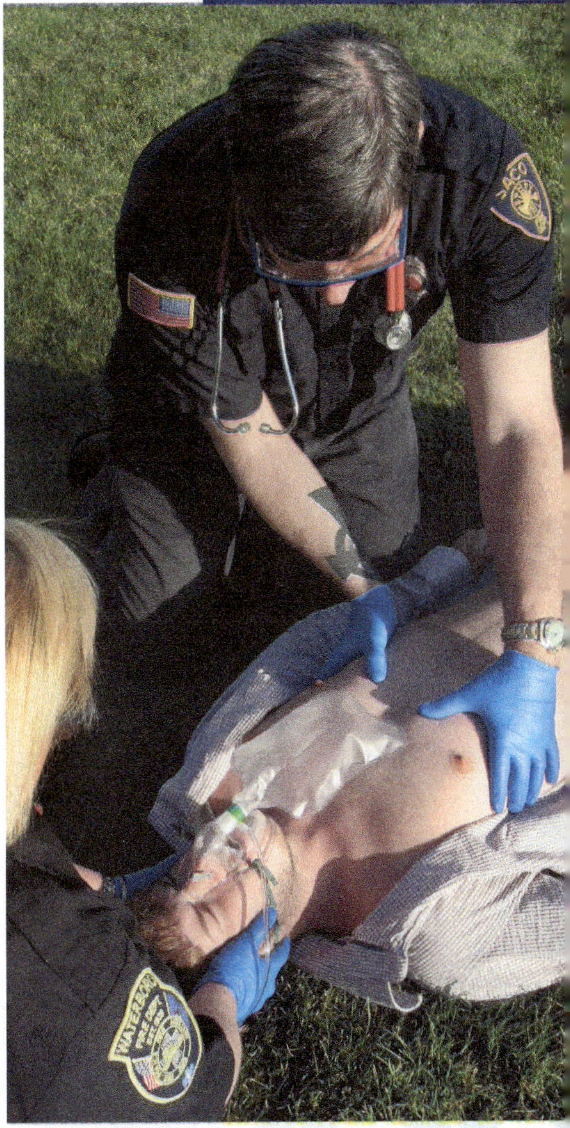

(© Daniel Limmer)

Outcomes

15.1 Describe the integration of the secondary assessment into the overall patient care process. (pp. 404–407)

- State the purpose of the secondary assessment.
- List the components of secondary assessment.
- Describe modifications to the approach to secondary assessment based on patients' situational factors.

15.2 Describe secondary assessment of medical patients. (pp. 407–419)

- Compare approaches you would take to responsive and unresponsive patients.

15.3 Describe secondary assessment of trauma patient with serious or multisystem injuries. (pp. 420–428)

- Adapt secondary assessment techniques based on the suspected body system involved.

15.4 Analyze your approach to decision making in EMS scenarios. (pp. 428–450)

- Compare the secondary assessment approaches to trauma patients with minor injuries and those with serious or multisystem injuries.

Key Terms

detailed physical exam, *448*
distention (dis-TEN-shun), *438*
history of the present illness or injury (HPI), *406*
medical patient, *405*
paradoxical motion, *438*
past medical history (PMH), *406*
priapism, *439*
rapid trauma assessment, *428*
reassessment, *407*
sign, *406*
stoma, *438*
symptom, *407*
tracheostomy, *438*
trauma patient, *405*

"Her breathing is not right," says the mother of your 7-year-old patient. "She has been this way since she came back in the house a few minutes ago and she is getting worse." Before coming into the home, you completed a scene survey, and now, as mom explains what is going on, you quickly work through a primary assessment. The young girl is breathing adequately at this point, but she is wheezing and working hard to breathe. That voice in your head is telling you she is in trouble. You have to make a plan. You have to do something . . . but what?

EMS is a collection of moments just like this. Sometimes these moments are big, critical, or complex, and sometimes they are small and simple, but every day, EMS practitioners of all levels are faced with decisions that affect the well-being of their patients. So far you have learned the initial elements of patient assessment. You have learned about safety and situational awareness in the context of a scene survey. You have also learned to identify and treat immediate life threats in the context of the primary assessment, but these elements are most commonly snap decisions made from quick observations. Sometimes patient care decisions require more thought and more information.

The secondary assessment addresses the need for a more thorough review and looks specifically at problems not dealt with in the primary phases. Here you will seek more information and use a more thorough examination to develop an understanding of the immediate patient needs. You will confirm initial findings and look to determine the root cause of outward signs and symptoms. In many cases, you will use this information to diagnose and treat a specific problem within your scope of practice.

Sometimes the moments of EMS require snap decision making and immediate action, but more often, quality patient care comes from gathering information and informed thinking. This is the heart of the secondary assessment. Make no mistake: Even though the secondary assessment is completed after the primary assessment, its findings can be just as time-sensitive and just as critical as those found in earlier elements of patient assessment. As in the scenario described above, patient care plans are frequently developed under stress and in suboptimal conditions. This is why a structured patient assessment is so important. The sequence of identifying the need for immediate action and then processing additional information as it becomes available allows the overstressed brain to find clarity in chaos. It allows us to act when action is most necessary, but also to think and develop plans when time allows. In this chapter, you will discuss this process of assessment and reassessment and close the loop on the assessment cycle. Think-act-reassess. That is a recipe for success in these moments.

The Secondary Assessment

The primary assessment could be described as a time of reaction. Here you observe and react to specific findings. Key assessments are designed to rapidly identify life threats, and immediate action is taken. In the secondary assessment, you will use history taking and physical examination to gather information, make plans, and diagnose. Your interventions will now be linked to critical thinking and will be specifically targeted to address an underlying pathophysiology. In this portion of the assessment, you literally find out what is wrong with the patient and treat accordingly.

The secondary assessment is performed after the scene size-up and the primary assessment. There are important reasons for this. You must be sure you are functioning at a safe scene and that you have all the resources you need. You must also be sure the patient has no immediate life threats that require prompt intervention. For example, it would be dangerous to start a lengthy secondary examination on a patient who is breathing inadequately and requires ventilation. With critical patients, the secondary assessment is frequently conducted in the ambulance after transport has been initiated. In some cases, critical interventions may take priority and supersede the need to conduct much of a secondary assessment at all. Conversely, you may find there is no need to rush with a stable patient, and some or all of your secondary assessment may be performed on scene.

Another reason it is good to get into the habit of making sure you complete the scene size-up and primary assessment before beginning the secondary assessment is that many practical skills examinations deduct points or consider it a failure to begin any part of the secondary assessment before the size-up or primary assessment. This is designed to mimic the importance of that order in the field.

Components of the Secondary Assessment

The secondary assessment can be performed on any patient. Typically, patients are categorized into three main types based on the nature of their underlying complaint:

- ***Medical patient***—a patient with one or more medical diseases or conditions
- ***Trauma patient***—a patient suffering from one or more physical injuries
- **Unknown patient**—a patient with a problem of an undetermined nature

medical patient
a patient with one or more medical diseases or conditions.

trauma patient
a patient suffering from one or more physical injuries.

CORE CONCEPT
Components of the secondary assessment

When performing a secondary assessment, you will generally complete three basic components: physical examination, patient history, and vital signs. Although we will present them in this order, there is not necessarily a need to maintain a "first, second, third" linear approach. In fact, high-performing teams will often combine elements in a single coordinated effort.

- **Physical examination.** This part of the secondary assessment, as the name implies, is where you will use your senses to examine the patient. You may feel for injuries, listen for abnormal breathing sounds, and look for swelling. It is important to use your senses to their fullest to get the most relevant information.
- **Patient history.** The history is obtained by asking questions. Most commonly, questions will be answered by the patient, but answers may also come from family or even bystanders. These answers to your questions will provide you with vital information about your patient. You will use questions to confirm suspicions, seek additional information, and differentiate possible problems from probable problems. You will ask about the patient's current condition or complaint—the ***history of the present illness or injury (HPI)***—and you will ask whether the patient has had any prior medical problems and if the patient takes any medications—the ***past medical history (PMH)***.
- **Vital signs.** You will take vital signs such as pulse, respirations, blood pressure, and pulse oximetry (measuring oxygen saturation of the blood), and you will assess the skin (color, temperature, and condition) and the pupils of the eyes. This set of vital signs will present an immediate picture of patient stability (is the patient's blood pressure too low or the patient's heart rate too fast or slow?) and also establishes a baseline for comparison of future measurements. (Have your interventions improved the patient's status? Is the patient decompensating?) Vital signs were covered in the chapter *Vital Signs and Monitoring Devices*.

history of the present illness or injury (HPI)
information gathered regarding the symptoms and nature of the patient's current concern.

past medical history (PMH)
information gathered regarding the patient's health problems in the past.

The order in which you perform these three components of the secondary assessment depends on many factors. Some of these are as follows:

- With many medical patients, you will perform the history first because the history provides the most relevant information for a medical patient. You will then perform a physical examination based on what you find in the history.
- In trauma patients, the hands-on physical examination often provides the most information. You may initially ask patients if they hurt anywhere, but then you will do a hands-on assessment to be sure. In some patients, you will examine the entire body (called a head-to-toe examination), and in other patients, those with minor injuries, you might just palpate one area (such as a possibly broken wrist).
- Patients who are unresponsive obviously can't answer your questions. In this case you must get the information from family and bystanders when you can. The physical examination will also be a primary source of information here.
- Seriously injured or ill patients will require you to do all of the same things, but you may do them in a slightly different order or at a different pace. For example, a serious trauma patient will get a primary assessment and a very quick secondary assessment (sometimes called a rapid physical examination) to check for major injuries before transport. The same goes for some medical patients (e.g., those with heart attack and stroke) because they must be transported promptly to the hospital for lifesaving interventions.

From the history and physical examination, you will gather signs and symptoms that result from the patient's condition and that give clues to what that condition may be.

It is important to know the difference between a sign and a symptom.

- A ***sign*** is something you can see. It may be an extremity deformed from trauma or ankles swollen from fluid accumulation after a heart attack.

sign
something regarding the patient's condition that you can see.

- A ***symptom*** is something the patient tells you. An example might be abdominal pain or difficulty breathing. You usually aren't able to see it, but it is something the patient feels and tells you about.

symptom
something regarding the patient's condition that the patient tells you.

Patient assessment is a dynamic process. You may be called to six patients in a row and not perform patient assessment the same way for any two of them—and all the different ways you performed the assessment may be correct. This is because the way the assessment is best performed will depend on the type of patient, on whether the patient is stable, and on how many EMTs you have on scene. Keep in mind, for example, that one EMT may be taking a history from the patient while another talks to a family member or bystander to get additional information. It is common for one EMT to obtain vital signs while another takes a history from the patient.

Always remember that your assessment doesn't stop with the secondary assessment. You will continually assess the patient in a process called ***reassessment***, discussed in the chapter *Reassessment*.

reassessment
a procedure for detecting changes in a patient's condition. It involves four steps: repeating the primary assessment, repeating and recording vital signs, repeating the physical exam, and checking interventions.

Secondary Assessment of the Medical Patient

The goals of patient assessment are the same regardless of the type of illness or injury. A secondary assessment on any patient is designed to paint a clinical picture, recognize patterns, and identify any immediate medical needs. Although the goals are the same, the approach may vary depending on the nature of the problem and the communication abilities of the patient. Assessing a medical patient typically means that you will focus more attention on history and less on physical examination. In a trauma patient, that ratio is reversed. Here, injuries typically require immediate examination and patient history will play a smaller role. You will still complete a physical examination on medical patients and a history on trauma patients, but the circumstances will dictate their relative priorities.

Because the history is so important for the medical patient assessment, you will use different approaches for the responsive and the unresponsive medical patient. This is because the patient who is responsive can answer history questions, while the patient who is unresponsive (or has a significantly diminished mental status) cannot. Therefore, this section is broken into two parts, discussing the secondary assessment of the responsive medical patient and that of the unresponsive medical patient.

As previously stated, the secondary assessment has three parts: patient history, physical exam, and baseline vital signs. The goals are the same, but the sequence of these parts, as well as the order in which you might ask patient history questions, differ for the responsive medical patient and for the unresponsive medical patient (Table 15-1).

Responsive Medical Patient

CORE CONCEPT
Secondary assessment of the responsive medical patient

As you learned in the chapter *Primary Assessment*, it makes a great deal of difference in the assessment process whether the patient is responsive or unresponsive. This is especially true of the medical patient. In trauma patients, there are often many external signs of trauma or injury, but this is not true of a patient with a medical condition. The most important source of information about a medical patient's condition is what the patient can tell you. This is why, when the patient is awake and responsive, obtaining the patient's history comes first (Scan 15-1).

A good example of the kind of patient you will see often is one who is awake and has a medical problem with no immediately life-threatening problems. After you finish the primary assessment for this patient, perform a secondary assessment. This will tell you what you need to know to administer the proper treatment. You will sometimes encounter medical patients who are a high priority for transport because of the serious nature of their conditions.

Obtain a Patient History

The interview you do with a responsive medical patient is similar to the interview a physician conducts before a physical examination. It is a conversational information-gathering effort.

TABLE 15-1 Assessment of the Responsive and Unresponsive Medical Patient

RESPONSIVE MEDICAL PATIENT	UNRESPONSIVE MEDICAL PATIENT
1. Gather the chief complaint and the history of the present illness using a body system approach. Use mnemonics such as OPQRST to help get detailed information from the patient: **O**nset **P**rovocation **Q**uality **R**adiation **S**everity **T**ime	**1.** Conduct a rapid physical exam. Focus on body systems and areas related to the suspected condition (if known): Head Neck Chest Abdomen Pelvis Extremities Posterior
2. Gather a past medical history from the patient. Use SAMPLE to ensure a comprehensive history: **S**igns and **s**ymptoms **A**llergies **M**edications **P**ertinent past history **L**ast oral intake **E**vents leading to the illness	**2.** Obtain baseline vital signs: Respirations Pulse Skin Pupils Blood pressure Oxygen saturation
3. Conduct a physical exam (focusing on the area the patient complains about and the related body systems).	**3.** Gather the history of the present illness (OPQRST) from family or bystanders: **O**nset **P**rovocation **Q**uality **R**adiation **S**everity **T**ime
4. Obtain baseline vital signs: Respirations Pulse Skin Pupils Blood pressure Oxygen saturation	**4.** Gather a past medical history (SAMPLE) from bystanders or family: **S**igns and **s**ymptoms **A**llergies **M**edications **P**ertinent past history **L**ast oral intake **E**vents leading to the illness

NOTE: This table shows the general order of steps. You may alter this order in accordance with the situation and the number of EMTs available, and when the patient's condition warrants immediate action due to immediate life threats.

Not only will you gain needed information from the interview, but you will also reduce the patient's fear and promote cooperation.

Although relatives and bystanders may serve as sources of information, the most important source is the patient. Do not interview relatives and bystanders before you interview the patient unless the patient is unresponsive or unable to communicate. You may gain information from bystanders and medical identification devices later, while you are conducting the physical examination.

You will ask history questions based on the body system or systems you believe are responsible for the patient's condition based on the patient's chief complaint and your observations. The reason you should also use your observations is that patients may be distracted by one complaint and not be aware of or forget to tell you of another. An example is a patient who complains of general weakness where you note the patient guarding the abdomen.

Try to ask open-ended questions, that is, questions that the patient answers with responses other than "yes" or "no." For example, do not ask, "Is your chest pain dull and

SCAN 15-1 Examination of the Responsive Medical Patient

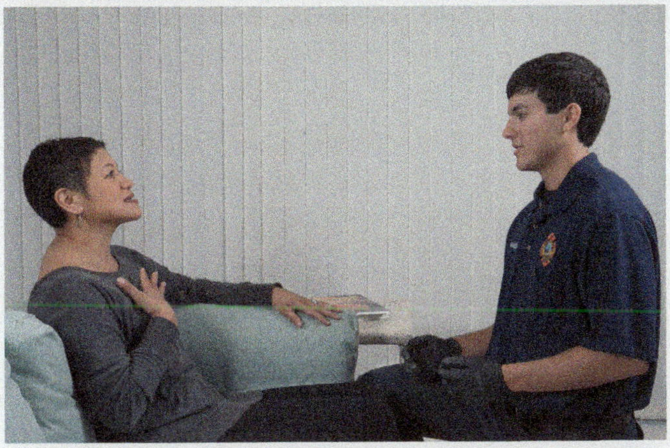

1. **CHIEF COMPLAINT AND HISTORY OF PRESENT ILLNESS.** Ask questions based on the body system or systems affected. You will determine the systems to examine based on the patient's complaint and your observations. Use the OPQRST questions when necessary to get a description of the patient's complaints:
   Onset
   Provocation
   Quality
   Radiation
   Severity
   Time

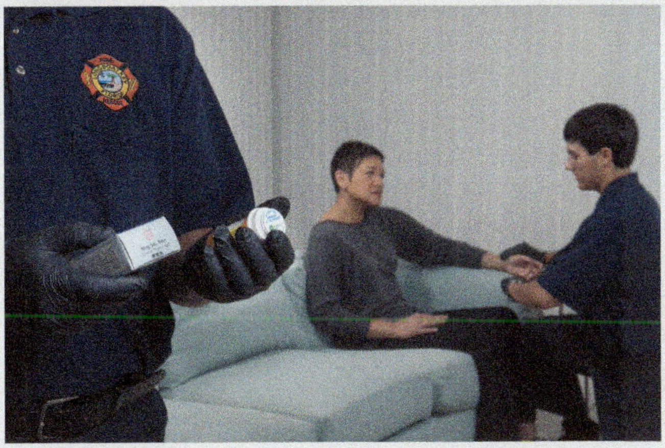

2. **PAST MEDICAL HISTORY.** Ask the SAMPLE questions:
   Signs and symptoms
   Allergies
   Medications
   Pertinent past history
   Last oral intake
   Events leading to the illness

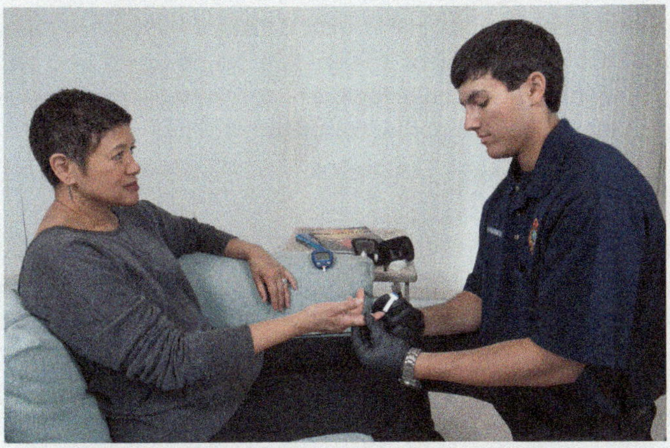

3. **PERFORM A PHYSICAL EXAMINATION OF THE RELEVANT BODY SYSTEMS.** Perform an assessment of the relevant body parts or systems:
   Respiratory
   Cardiovascular
   Neurologic
   Endocrine
   Gastrointestinal
   Reproductive
   Genitourinary

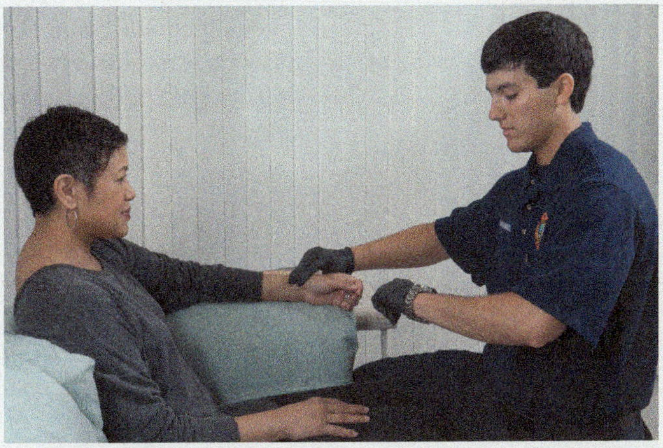

4. **VITAL SIGNS.** Assess the patient's baseline vital signs:
   Respiration
   Pulse
   Skin color, temperature, condition (and capillary refill in infants and children)
   Pupils
   Blood pressure
   Oxygen saturation (if appropriate for the patient's chief complaint)

(continued)

SCAN 15-1 Examination of the Responsive Medical Patient *(continued)*

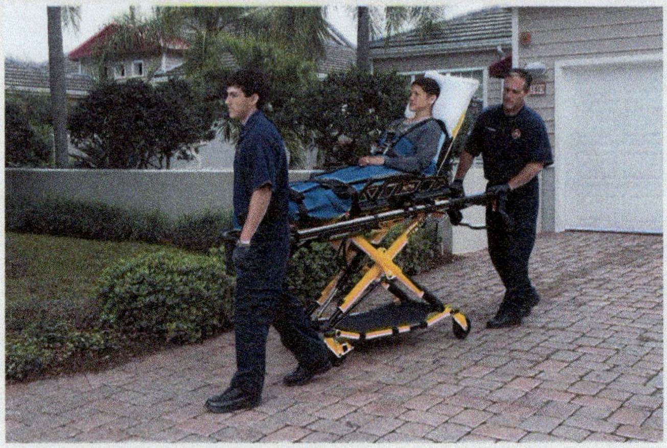

5. INTERVENTIONS AND TRANSPORT. Perform interventions as needed and transport the patient. Contact on-line medical direction as needed.

crushing?" Ask instead, "How would you describe your pain?" In this way, you will avoid giving the patient the impression that you want a particular answer. If the patient seems to be unable to describe the pain, you can try giving several choices: "Is your pain dull, or sharp, or burning?"

Find out the patient's age; then get the rest of the past medical history and the name of the patient's personal physician. Use the SAMPLE mnemonic, as defined in Table 14-1, and the list of the SAMPLE questions provided earlier in the chapter *Principles of Assessment*.

Tailoring the Physical Exam for Specific Chief Complaints

If you obtain the history of the present illness and the past medical history as they have been described up until now, you will obtain a great deal of information. Many times, however, you can gain additional important information by tailoring the history to the patient's chief complaint. This means asking questions pertinent to that complaint.

Perform a Physical Exam

With responsive medical patients, the EMT's physical exam is usually brief. You will gather most of the important assessment information in this type of patient from the history and vital signs. Table 15-2 lists some of the physical exam steps you should take when evaluating patients with certain chief complaints. For example, if your patient has difficulty breathing, you should listen to the patient's chest with a stethoscope for the presence and equality of breath sounds. If you have received additional education on recognizing specific types of breath sounds, you should attempt to do so. For a patient who is at risk for hypoxia, such as this one, you should also check oxygen saturation. If your patient has a complaint that does not fit into any of the categories you learned in your EMT course, you should focus the exam on the body part that the patient has a complaint about. For example, if the patient complains of thigh pain, you will inspect and palpate the patient's thigh.

Obtain Baseline Vital Signs

A complete set of baseline vital signs taken during the secondary assessment is essential to the assessment of a medical patient. Later assessments of the vital signs will be compared against this baseline set of vital signs to determine trends in the patient's condition. If you are using an automatic blood pressure device, you should also take a manual blood pressure to verify the accuracy of the device, and again at any point the device reports a significant change in blood pressure.

TABLE 15-2 Secondary Assessment: Specific Medical Complaints

TYPE OF COMPLAINT	ADDITIONAL HISTORY	PHYSICAL EXAM
Shortness of breath	Cough Fever or chills Dyspnea on exertion Weight gain (indicates fluid) Has a prescribed bronchodilator?	Lung sounds (presence and equality) Wheezing Work of breathing and position Pulse oximetry (oxygen saturation) Pedal or sacral edema
Chest pain or discomfort	Has prescribed nitroglycerin? Taking aspirin?	Skin color, temperature, and condition Blood pressure Pulse (including strength and regularity) Lung sounds (presence and equality) Jugular vein distention Ankle edema Oxygen saturation
Mental status changes or neurologic complaints	Headache Seizure	FAST (Face-Arm-Speech-Time) Face: Does one side of the patient's face droop? (Ask the patient to smile.) Arms: Can the patient hold both arms in front of the patient? Speech: Is the patient's speech clear and understandable? Time: Time is critical. If the patient exhibits any of these signs (even if they go away), call 9-1-1.
Allergic (involves components of the cardiovascular and respiratory systems)	Time of exposure Time of symptom onset	Stinger Rash/hives (urticaria) Lung sounds (presence and equality) Face and neck edema Oxygen saturation
Abdominal pain	Fever Nausea and vomiting Diarrhea or constipation Blood in vomit or feces; may be bright red (fresh) or dark (digested) Menstrual history	Inspect and palpate all four quadrants of the abdomen.
Altered mental status with a diabetic history	Oral intake Medication history History of recent illness Excessive hunger, thirst, urination	Blood glucose monitoring Skin color, temperature, and condition Mental status Unusual breath odors

Administer Interventions and Transport the Patient

In later chapters you will learn when to provide treatment for specific medical conditions. Remember that a decision for prompt transportation of critical patients or those with specific complaints (e.g., chest pain or suspected stroke) is part of a treatment plan. The only treatment you have learned about so far that might be appropriate for a responsive patient is oxygen.

Unresponsive Medical Patient

CORE CONCEPT

Secondary assessment of the unresponsive medical patient

The sequence of assessment for an unresponsive medical patient differs from the sequence of assessment for a responsive medical patient. If the patient were responsive, the first step of your secondary assessment would be talking with the patient to obtain the history of the present illness and the past medical history, followed by the physical exam and baseline vital signs.

For an unresponsive patient, the process is reversed. (Review Table 15-1 and see Scan 15-2.) You will begin the rapid physical examination based on any information you gather at the scene, then complete a set of baseline vital signs. After these procedures, you will gather as much of the patient's history as you can. Since you cannot obtain a history from an unresponsive patient, you should attempt to get relevant information from any

Think Like an EMT

Challenges in History Gathering

Obtaining a history is a key part of the assessment of the medical patient. However, some patients are easier to get a history from than others. Consider what you might say and do to improve your history gathering in the following circumstances:

1. A 79-year-old female keeps talking, saying a lot about things that have nothing to do with the problem you are there for.
2. A 16-year-old female is surrounded by her family. She has abdominal pain that you suspect may be from a pregnancy, but you have not yet asked her if she might be pregnant.
3. A 32-year-old male with diabetes has not eaten lately, according to his family. He is alternately combative and quiet. When you ask him questions, he gives you a vacant stare and says nothing.
4. A 22-year-old male college student, his roommate tells you, has been acting strangely the past few weeks. The patient is now sitting on his bed with his knees drawn up against his chest, rocking back and forth, saying things that don't make sense to you.

Pediatric Note

When gathering a history from a child, be sure to kneel or find another way to get on the same level with the child. Put questions in simple language the child can understand. Note that much of the history for a child and all of the information for an infant will need to be gathered from the parents, guardian, or other adult caretaker.

Point of View

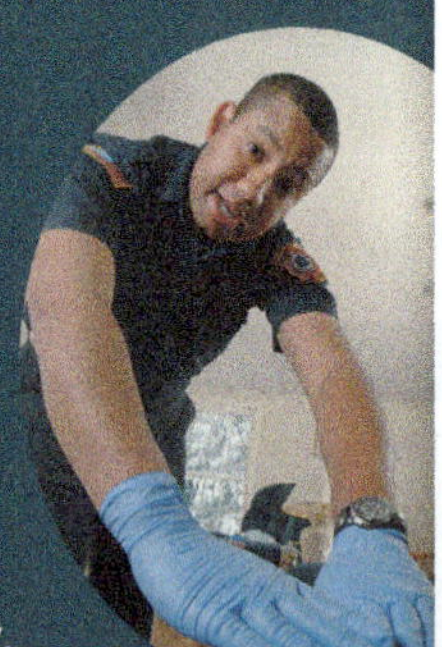

"At first I thought it might be a stomach bug. You know how your belly gets kind of achy? But then it got worse. The pain was strong. And came in waves. I curled up in a ball and asked my husband to call the ambulance. I knew something was really wrong.

"By the time the ambulance got to the house, I had vomited. But it still was painful. And it still wasn't the flu. I could tell.

"The EMT was very nice. He asked where it hurt and then pushed on my belly. He was pretty gentle, but it hurt anyhow. He also asked me questions. Everything from if I thought I had a fever to if I was pregnant to when I ate last . . . even when I pooped last. He sure was thorough.

"Well, I can look back at it now and laugh . . . now that they took out my appendix and I'm walking around again. But it sure wasn't funny then."

relatives or bystanders who may be present (e.g., "He said he was having indigestion, and then he passed out!").

Another difference between the secondary assessment for the responsive and for the unresponsive patient is the nature of the physical exam. For a responsive patient, you will be able to focus your exam on just the part of the body the patient mentions in the patient's complaint. Since an unresponsive patient cannot tell you where the problem is, and bystanders can provide only limited information, you will need to do a rapid assessment of the entire body.

SCAN 15-2 Examination of the Unresponsive Medical Patient

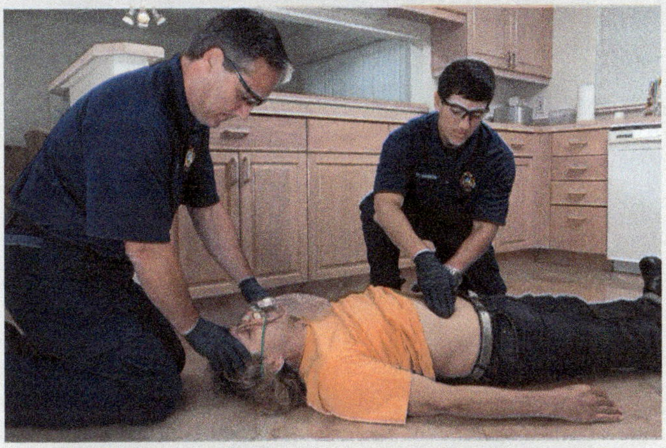

1. **RAPID PHYSICAL EXAM.** Perform a rapid assessment of the entire body:
   - Head
   - Neck
   - Chest
   - Abdomen
   - Pelvis
   - Extremities
   - Posterior

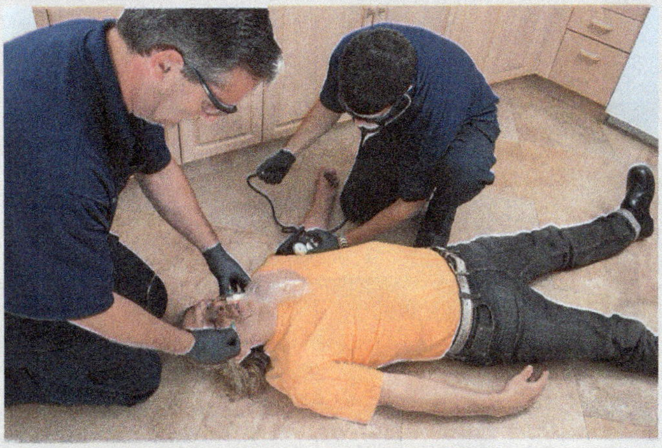

2. **VITAL SIGNS.** Assess the patient's baseline vital signs:
   - Respiration
   - Pulse
   - Skin color, temperature, condition (and capillary refill in infants and children)
   - Pupils
   - Blood pressure
   - Oxygen saturation

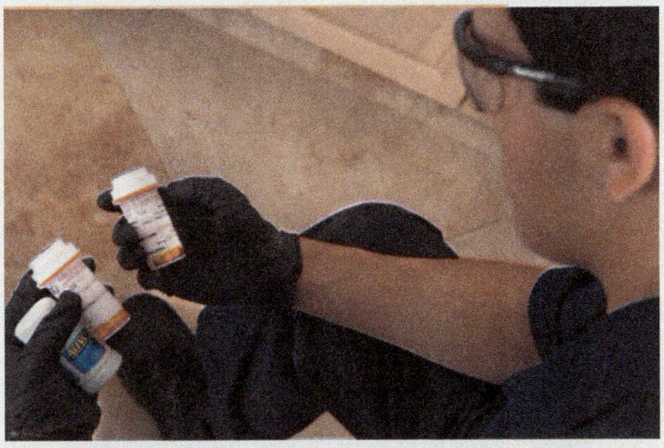

3. **MEDICAL HISTORY.** Interview family and bystanders for information about the present illness (OPQRST) and also the SAMPLE history:
   - Signs and symptoms
   - Allergies
   - Medications
   - Pertinent past history
   - Last oral intake
   - Events leading to the illness

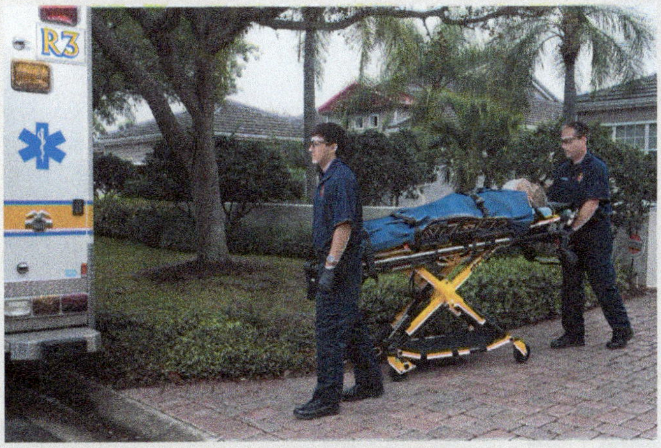

4. **INTERVENTIONS AND TRANSPORT.** Perform interventions as needed and transport the patient. Contact on-line medical direction as needed.

15 Medical Patient Assessment

Develop a General Impression

Observe and approach the patient.

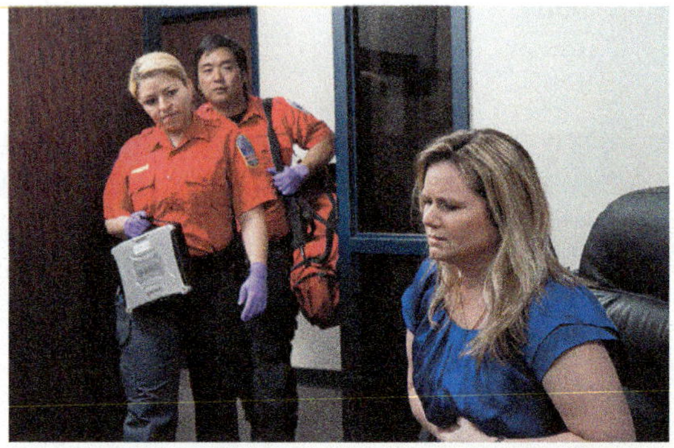

PRIMARY ASSESSMENT

Responsive

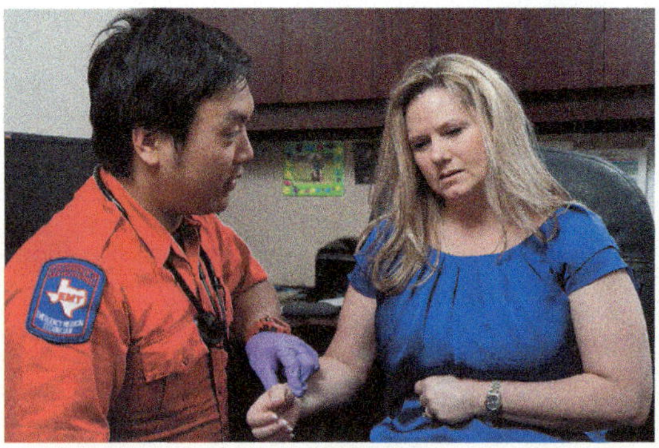

Ensure adequate breathing.
Check pulse and skin for signs of shock.

Unresponsive

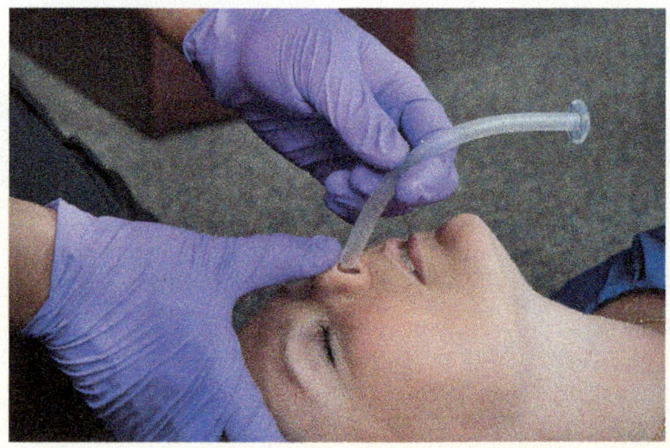

Immediate ABCs
Suction
Airway adjuncts

Ventilation if necessary
Circulation

Supplemental Oxygen Indicated

NOTE: *Upon approach, if patient appears lifeless and is not breathing, begin with circulation and a pulse check as part of C-A-B.*

Determine Priority

SECONDARY ASSESSMENT

Responsive

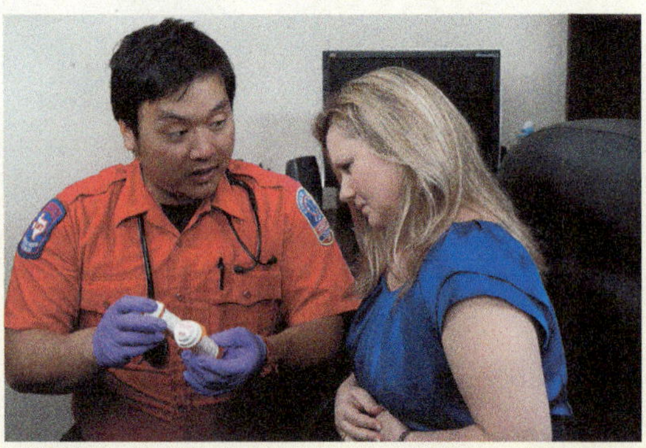

History first
Body systems exams as appropriate

Unresponsive

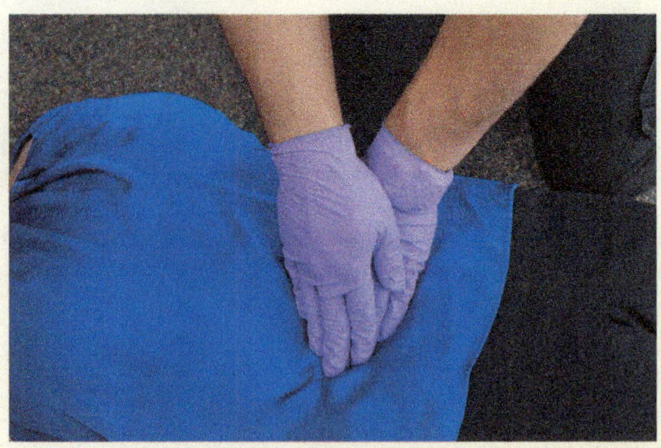

Body systems exams first
History
Expedited pace

Vital Signs

Interventions (en route for serious or unstable patients)

Transport

Timing, priority, and destination based on patient's condition

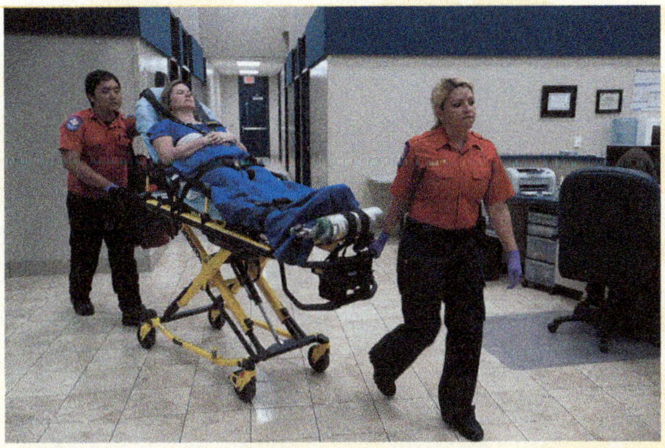

Reassessment

About every 5 minutes for unstable patients
About every 15 minutes for stable patients
Repeat primary assessment.
Reassess chief complaint.
Check interventions.
Repeat vital signs.

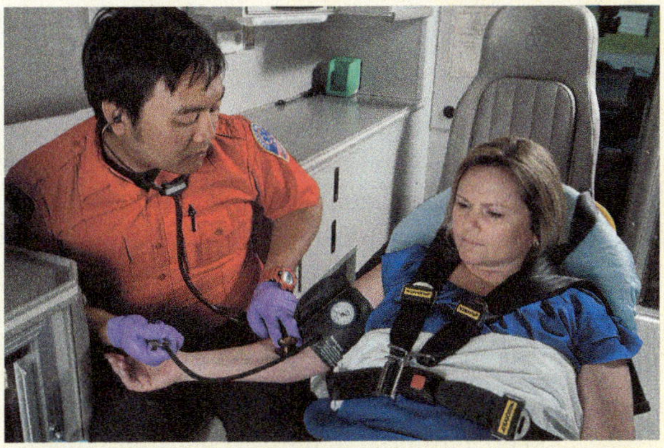

Notify the Hospital

Provide a concise report.
Notify any specialized teams:
Cardiac (suspected myocardial infarction/chest pain), Stroke

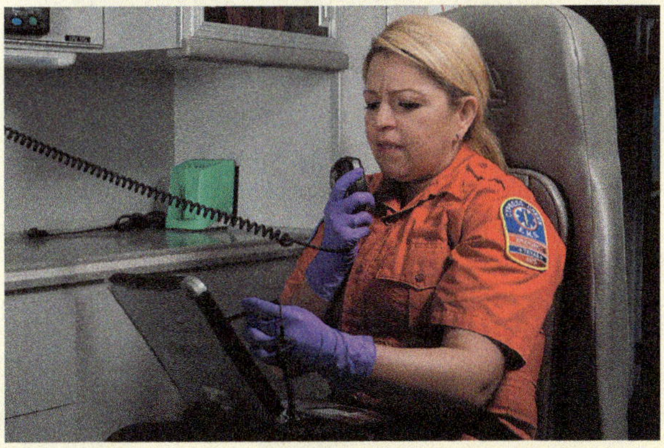

Throughout the Call

Provide comfort and reassurance.
Be alert for changes in the patient's condition.

Finally, since the patient is unresponsive, the patient will automatically be a high priority for transport and will likely require airway maintenance throughout the call. This means that all of the exam components you perform will be done quickly but accurately while integrating steps to transport.

Perform a Rapid Physical Exam

The physical exam of an unresponsive medical patient will be similar to the head-to-toe physical exam for a trauma patient. You will rapidly assess the patient's head, neck, chest, abdomen, pelvis, extremities, and posterior. As you assess each area, you will look for signs of injury. Other things to look for in the medical patient include:

- **Neck.** Jugular vein distention, medical identification devices.
- **Chest.** Presence and equality of breath sounds.
- **Abdomen.** Distention, firmness, or rigidity.
- **Pelvis.** Incontinence of urine or feces.
- **Extremities.** Pulse, motor function, sensation, oxygen saturation, medical identification devices.

Check for Medical ID Devices. Medical identification devices can provide important information. One of the most commonly used medical identification devices is the Medic Alert emblem shown in Figure 15-1. More than one million people wear a medical identification device in the form of a necklace or a wrist or ankle bracelet. One side of the device might have a Star of Life emblem. The patient's medical problem is engraved on the reverse side, along with a telephone number to call for additional information.

When you are performing the physical exam, look for necklaces and bracelets or wallet cards. Never assume you know the form of every medical identification device. The occasional patient may even wear medical ID information as a tattoo. Check any necklace or bracelet carefully, taking care when moving the patient or any of the patient's extremities. You should alert the emergency department staff when you arrive that the patient is wearing or carrying medical identification, and tell them what condition it relates to (diabetes or a heart condition, for example).

Check Pupils. It is easy to forget to check the pupils of a patient who is unresponsive. Try to keep in mind that *the most important time to check the pupils is when the patient's eyes are closed!*

Obtain Baseline Vital Signs

Assess the patient's pulse, respirations, skin, pupils, and blood pressure, and note any abnormalities. Determine the patient's oxygen saturation (Figure 15-2). Be sure to record your observations so later vital sign assessments can be compared with these baseline observations. If you have an automated blood pressure monitoring device, use it after you have obtained a manual blood pressure or in accordance with local protocol. This will allow you to be confident that the machine reading is correct.

FIGURE 15-1 Look for medical identification devices, which commonly display the Medic Alert emblem.

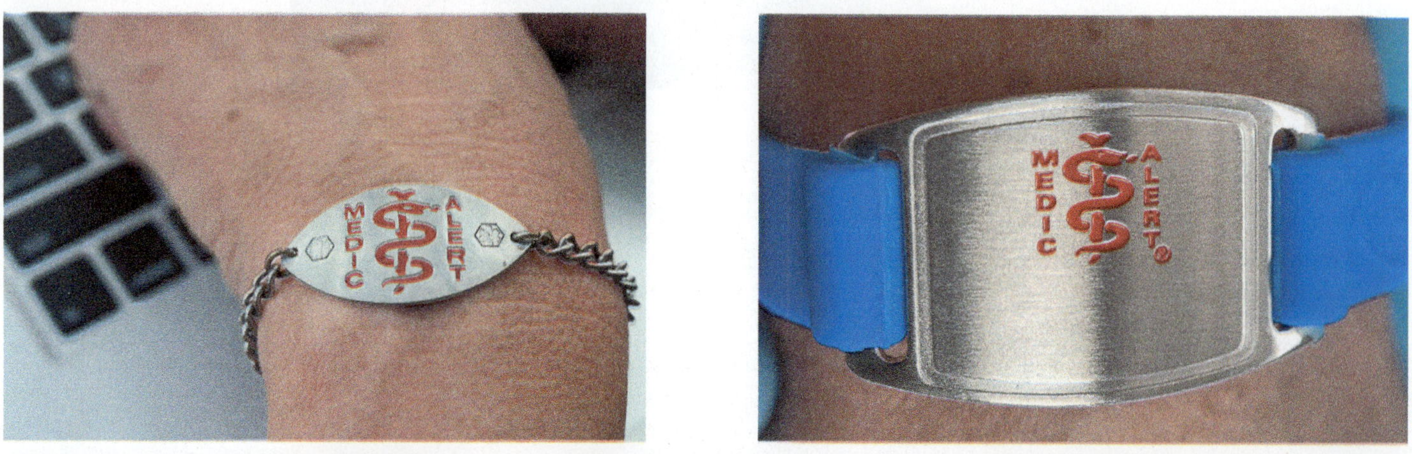

FIGURE 15-2 Use pulse oximetry to check oxygen saturation levels.

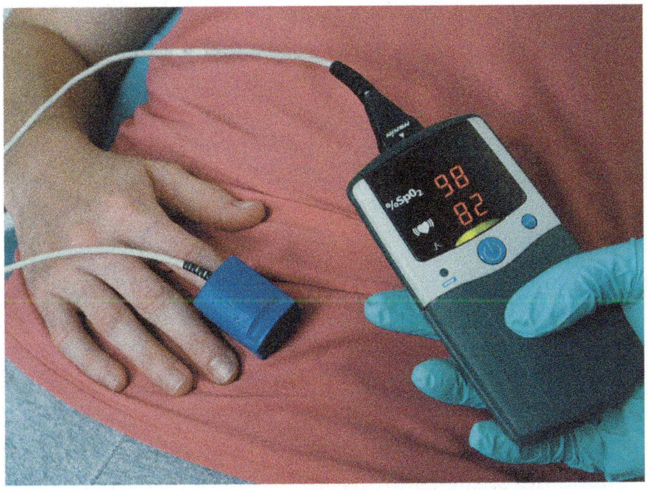

FIGURE 15-3 Obtain a past medical history. If the patient is unable to respond or to respond clearly, obtain as much information as possible from others who may know or have observed the patient. *(Mark Ide/Science Source)*

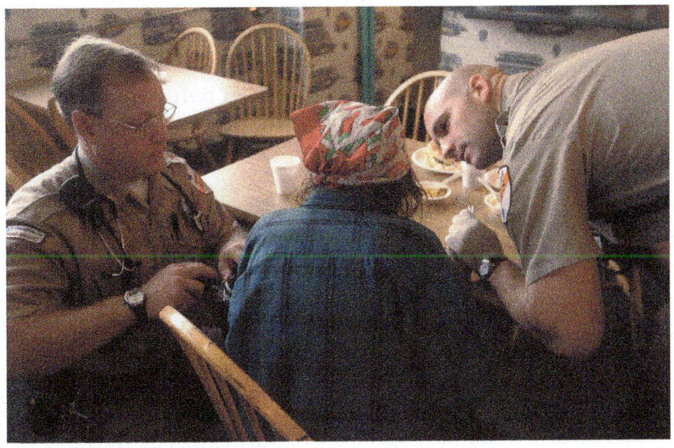

Consider a Request for ALS Personnel

In accordance with local protocols, and if advanced life support personnel are available, consider at this time if the additional services paramedics can provide would benefit your patient.

If you are serving in a rural area or other location where you do not have the option of requesting advanced life support, and if you are very distant from a hospital, there may be a closer local clinic or other health facility that has an arrangement to provide advanced care. Consider whether it is worth a delay to stop at such a facility for the special care that may help stabilize your patient before you continue transport to the hospital.

If arrangements such as these exist where you work as an EMT, you must be familiar with the types of patients this facility can help. The arrangements should be in writing, to reduce confusion and prevent loss of precious time with critical patients.

Obtain a Patient History

Since an unresponsive patient or one with an impaired mental status (Figure 15-3) cannot talk or respond competently, you will have to interview bystanders, if any, to get as much information as possible. When interviewing bystanders, determine if any are relatives or friends of the patient. They usually have more information to provide about past problems than other bystanders would have. Learn which of the bystanders saw what happened. When questioning bystanders, you should ask:

- **What is the patient's name?** If the patient is obviously a minor, ask if the parent or guardian is present or if the parent or guardian has been contacted.
- **What happened?** You may be told that the patient fell off a ladder, appeared to faint, fell to the ground and began seizing, was hit on the head by a falling object, or other possible clues.
- **Did you see anything else?** For example, was the patient clutching the chest or head before falling?
- **Did the patient complain of anything before this happened?** You may learn of chest pain, nausea, concern about odors where the patient was working, or other clues to the problem.
- **Does the patient have any known illnesses or problems?** This may provide you with information about heart problems, alcohol abuse, allergies, or other problems that could cause a change in the patient's condition.
- **Is the patient taking any medications?** Be sure to use the word *medications* or *medicines*. If you say "drugs" or some other term, bystanders may not answer you, thinking that you are asking questions as part of a criminal investigation. In rare cases you may

feel that the bystanders are holding back information because the patient was abusing drugs. Remind them that you are an EMT and you need all the information they can give you so proper care can begin.

Remember that multiple crew members can perform parts of the history while the physical exam is being performed. If someone witnessed the patient become unresponsive, that person may have very valuable information, such as any complaints the patient had before becoming unresponsive and the patient's medical history. Although the patient can't confirm this information, it may be very valuable in your assessment and care.

Administer Interventions and Transport the Patient

There is not usually much information gained from the secondary assessment of an unresponsive medical patient that will change treatment in the field. The most important thing to look for is a mechanism of injury or signs that would make you suspect a spine injury. Either of these would mean that you need to immobilize the patient's spine. Most of the time, the information you gather in your assessment of unresponsive medical patients will be particularly helpful to the staff in the emergency department. Emergency physicians and nurses depend on EMTs to evaluate the scene carefully and to gather as much useful information as possible that they cannot get in the hospital.

Mid-Chapter Review

Secondary Assessment of the Medical Patient

Key Facts and Concepts

- The secondary assessment of the medical patient takes two forms, depending on whether the patient is responsive.
- You assess the responsive patient by obtaining a patient history, then performing a physical exam of affected parts of the body before getting baseline vital signs.
- Since unresponsive medical patients cannot communicate, it is appropriate to start the assessment with a rapid physical exam. Baseline vital signs come next; then you interview family, friends, and bystanders to get any history that can be obtained.
- You might not change any field treatment as a result of the information gathered here, but the results of the assessment may be very important to the emergency department staff.

Key Decisions

- Is the patient responsive enough to provide a history?
- If a patient cannot provide a history, can someone present at the scene do so?
- What kind of secondary assessment does the patient's chief complaint suggest?

Preparation for Your Examination and Practice

Short Answer

1. Explain how and why the secondary assessment for a medical patient differs from the secondary assessment for a trauma patient.
2. Explain how and why the secondary assessment for a responsive medical patient differs from the secondary assessment for an unresponsive medical patient.

Thinking and Linking

Think back to the Scene Size-Up *chapter and link information from that chapter with information from this chapter as you consider the following situation.*

- You are at the home of an elderly man whose wife called 911 because her husband was complaining of chest pain. While assessing your patient, the wife begins to complain of shortness of breath. Now you have two patients. What should you do?

Critical Thinking Exercises

Getting a history from a medical patient can require a good deal of skill. The purpose of this exercise will be to consider how you might obtain a history in the following situations.

1. You are trying to get information from the very upset son of an unresponsive man. He is the only available family member. He is so upset that he is having difficulty talking to you. How can you quickly get him to calm down and give you his father's medical history?
2. You are interviewing a very pleasant older man. Unfortunately, your assessment is taking a long time, because he does not answer your questions, and instead starts talking about other things. He lives alone and appears to be lonely. How should you handle this?

Pathophysiology to Practice

The following question is designed to assist you in gathering relevant clinical information and making accurate decisions in the field.

- A patient has a history as a three-pack-a-day smoker. How is this likely to affect the patient's blood pressure? Why?

Street Scenes

Just as you are about to sit down to eat lunch, your ambulance is dispatched to a local health club for a 50-year-old female having an asthma attack. Upon arrival, you find the scene to be safe. Taking Standard Precautions, you are directed to the women's locker room, where you find your patient sitting on a workout bench.

"Hello. How can we help you today?" you ask. Your general impression is of an alert middle-aged woman in moderate respiratory distress.

"Oh, I'm having an asthma attack," she says. You can see her airway is open, but her breathing is rapid and moderately labored. You observe no bleeding, find her skin to be normal, and determine her radial pulse to be slightly rapid but strong and regular.

Street Scene Questions

1. **What priority is this patient?**
2. **What are the next steps in the management of this patient?**

Satisfied there are no life threats for which you have to provide immediate intervention, you determine this patient's priority to be medium in severity with the potential to get worse.

"What's your name?" you ask. She replies that her name is Grace.

"What were you doing when the difficulty breathing started?" you ask. It turns out she had been exercising on the treadmill. You note that she is speaking in complete sentences and does not have to stop every few words to catch her breath. You ask Juan, your partner, to begin administering oxygen by way of a nonrebreather mask. While Juan is doing that, you continue your examination.

Street Scene Questions

3. **What part of the secondary assessment should follow next?**
4. **What signs or symptoms would you look for to determine if the patient was getting better or worse?**

"What do you think caused your shortness of breath?" you ask. She replies that she's had a mild case of asthma for about 10 years and that it is exercise-induced. You ask how long she has been having trouble breathing with this episode. "About ten minutes," she replies.

You know that many asthmatics carry their own medication for asthma, so you ask what medications she is taking. "I have an inhaler, but I left it at home. I think it's called Al Butterball or something like that." You suggest the name "albuterol," and she nods her head.

You ask if she is allergic to anything, and she shakes her head no. While you listen to lung sounds, Juan obtains baseline vitals. You note that the lung sounds are equal but noisy, like a whistling sound. Juan informs you that her pulse is 120 and regular; skin is warm and dry; respirations are 24 and slightly labored; and her blood pressure is 130/70. Her oxygen saturation is 96 percent.

Grace accepts your offer to transport her to the emergency department, so you put her on the stretcher in her position of comfort, sitting up. During the short trip to the hospital, you use the radio to inform the emergency department of your patient's condition and treatment, take another set of vital signs, and reassess the patient. She appears to be a little better, but her breathing is still slightly labored and a little noisy. She does not have any signs suggesting that she is getting worse, things such as retractions above the clavicles and between the ribs, the ability to speak only a few words at a time, or cyanosis, particularly of the lips and nail beds. After you transfer Grace to the care of the emergency department staff, you return to service.

Secondary Assessment of the Trauma Patient

For assessment of the trauma patient, remember that *trauma* means "injury." Injuries can range from slight to severe, from a cut finger to a massive wound. (Refer to the *Visual Guide, Trauma Patient Assessment*.) Often you will not be able to see the injury or how serious it is, especially if it is internal. Even when you can't see the wound, you will still be required to make important decisions such as priority for leaving the scene (expedited or routine) and the proper amount of care to perform on the scene versus in the ambulance en route.

Generally, there is a combination of factors that will help you determine how serious or potentially serious the patient is. These include:

- The location of the injury or injuries on the patient
- The patient's mental status
- The patient's airway status
- Vital signs
- The mechanism of injury
- The patient's age or the presence of preexisting conditions

There are many terms to describe a seriously injured patient. These patients may be called simply "serious" or "critical." Others may use the term "high-priority patient." In any case, there are some patients you will want to transport rapidly, spending minimal time on the scene, while others will have minor injuries and no need for rapid transport. These less serious patients will receive more care on scene because they are not a high priority for transport. This section will describe the assessment and on-scene strategies for both patient types.

Of course, in the real world, there will be patients who seem to fall somewhere in the middle, between these two categories. You might not be sure they are high-priority for transport. In this case, use the material in this section to make the best decision possible, and remember that you can upgrade or downgrade the priority based on additional information as you develop it. Generally, if you aren't sure, err on the side of caution and transport as high-priority until proven otherwise.

The procedures for a trauma patient who does not have significant injury are discussed in the following section. The procedures for a patient who does have a significant or serious injury will be discussed later in the subsequent section. Table 15-3 lists and contrasts the procedures for these two categories of trauma patient.

Trauma Patient with Minor Injury/Low Priority

CORE CONCEPT

Secondary assessment of the trauma patient with minor injury

In this case, the patient is likely oriented and complaining of an isolated injury or minor injuries. Your size-up and primary assessment have provided quite a bit of information about your patient already. You checked the patient's circulation during the primary assessment, and there were no signs of shock. The mechanism of injury didn't seem significant. Instead of examining the patient from head to toe, you focus your assessment on just the areas that are clearly injured, or that the patient tells you are painful, or that you suspect may be injured because of the mechanism of injury. The assessment will include a history of the present illness, a physical exam, a set of baseline vital signs, and a past medical history.

Determine the Chief Complaint

Remember that the chief complaint is what the patient tells you is the matter. For example, one patient may tell you she has cut her finger. Another may complain of pain after twisting an ankle.

Obtain a Patient History

Although history taking will likely be less extensive in a trauma patient compared with that for a medical patient, understanding the clinical picture and how the patient's past medical history relates to the current problem are no less important. It will be important to immediately inquire about the *history of the present illness/injury (HPI)*, as it will define how the

TABLE 15-3 Secondary Assessment–Trauma Patient

NOT SERIOUSLY INJURED	MORE SERIOUSLY INJURED
AFTER SCENE SIZE-UP AND PRIMARY ASSESSMENT:	***AFTER SCENE SIZE-UP AND PRIMARY ASSESSMENT:***
1. Determine the chief complaint and elicit information about how the patient was injured (history of the present illness).	1. Determine the chief complaint and rapidly elicit information about how the patient was injured (history of the present illness).
2. Perform the physical exam based on the chief complaint and mechanism of injury.	2. Continue spinal precautions (if indicated).
3. Assess baseline vital signs.	3. Consider requesting advanced life support personnel.
4. Obtain a past medical history.	4. Perform rapid trauma assessment.
	5. Assess baseline vital signs.
	6. Obtain a patient history.

current injury occurred. Presumably, you have already addressed this in your scene size-up by examining the mechanism of injury, but it will be worthwhile to discuss it further with the patient. Gather information on how the injury occurred in addition to relevant details. For example, if the patient was in a motor-vehicle collision, find out where the patient was in the vehicle, whether the patient was wearing lap and shoulder belts, and the speeds of the vehicles involved. If the patient was on a bicycle or motorcycle, ask whether the patient was wearing a helmet when the incident occurred. If the patient was stabbed or shot, find out the size and type of knife or type of gun and ammunition (only if it is possible to do so safely). A much more important question in shootings is "How many shots did you hear?" (This is more important than ammunition and such details because it tells you whether you need to worry about one hole or, potentially, lots of holes.)

In general, what you should try to find out in the history of the present illness for a trauma patient is:

- The nature of the force involved (blunt, such as from hitting the steering wheel; penetrating, such as from a knife or a saw; crushing, such as from something heavy falling on the patient).
- The direction and strength of the force.
- Equipment used to protect the patient.
- Actions taken to prevent or minimize injury.
- Areas of pain and injuries resulting from the incident.

If the patient is unable to provide this information because of an altered mental status, use the procedures described later in this chapter on how to assess a patient with a significant mechanism of injury.

Do not forget the other elements of a patient history when assessing a trauma patient. Examine the chief complaint with OPQRST and review past medical history, medications, allergies, and last oral intake. Each of these questions can be relevant to even minor traumatic injuries. For example, a small head bruise is far more meaningful if it is determined that the patient takes blood thinners, for the risk of intracerebral hemorrhage is much higher.

"Trauma assessment is a hands-on process."

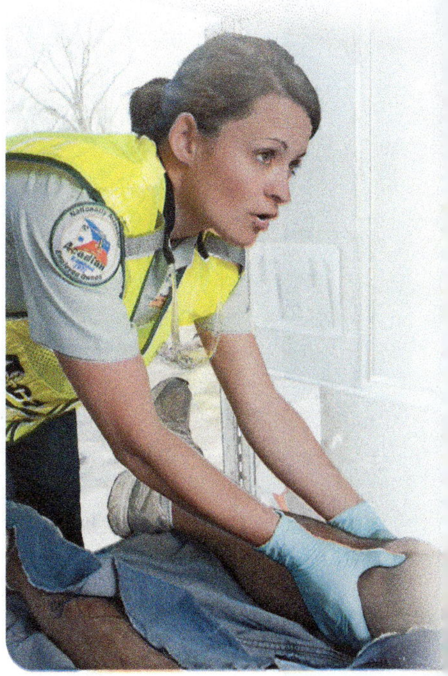

Perform a Physical Exam

Your decision on which areas of a patient's body to assess will depend partly on what you can see (e.g., the cut on the patient's finger) and what the patient tells you (the chief complaint, perhaps "My ankle hurts"). But you will not rely on just these obvious signs and symptoms. You will also pay attention to potential injuries the mechanism of injury causes you to suspect. For example, if the patient with the painful ankle suffered the injury by falling down a flight of steps, you should suspect that the patient may have more than just an ankle injury—including a head injury that could be more serious.

15 Trauma Patient Assessment

Rapidly Identify and Correct Life Threats

Size up the Scene

Provide c-spine stabilization based on severity of injury or mechanism and/or complaint of pain.

Primary Assessment

Massive hemorrhage
Airway
Breathing
Circulation

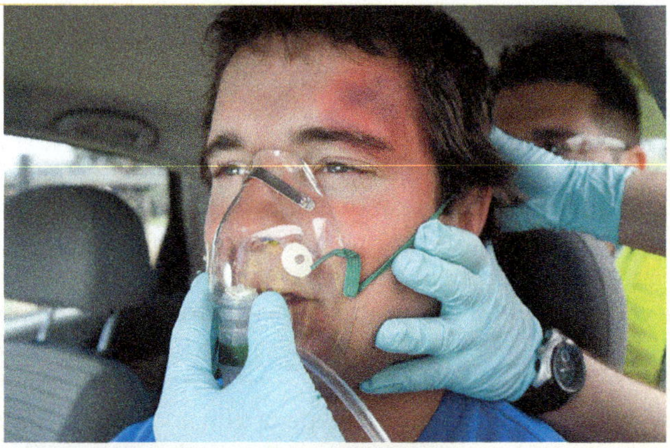

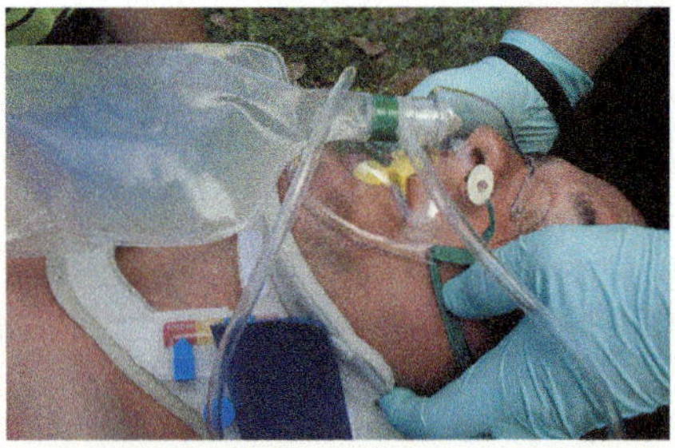

Maintain the airway.

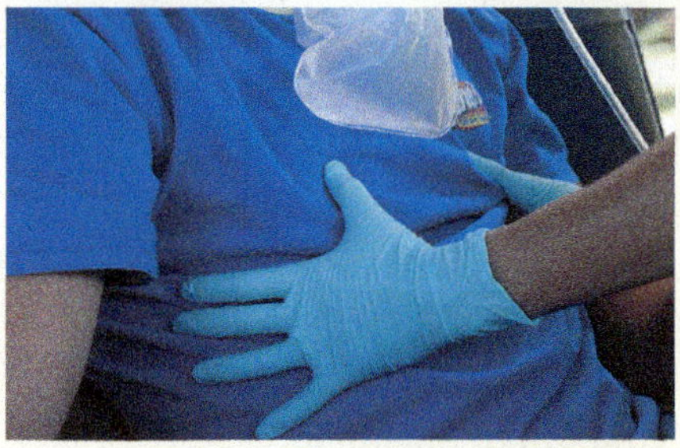

Assess for injuries that could affect breathing. Apply oxygen or ventilate as needed.

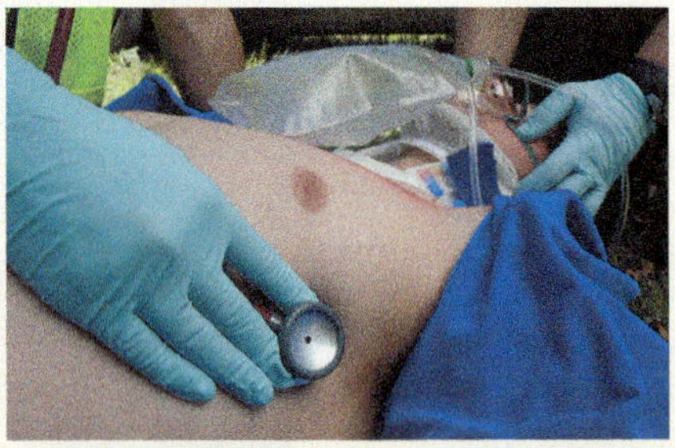

Listen for and compare lung sounds bilaterally.

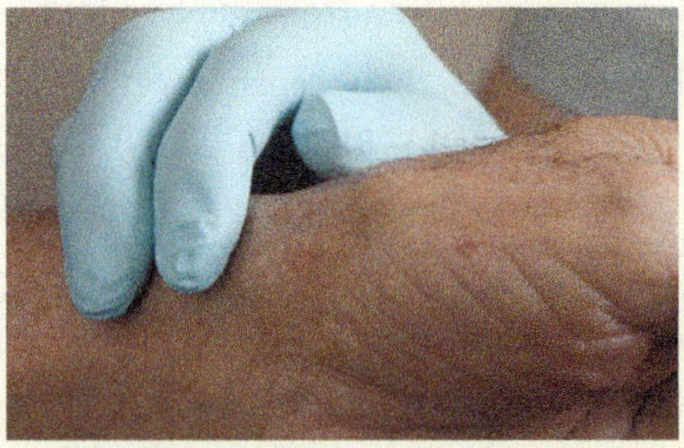

Check for signs of shock.

Priority Determination

Does my patient have serious injury requiring prompt transport from the scene?

OR

Does the patient have minor and/or isolated non-life-threatening injury?

On-Scene Examination

Serious or multiple injuries:

Rapid head-to-toe exam:
head, neck, chest, abdomen, pelvis, extremities, posterior

Minor or isolated injury:

Slower, focused exam

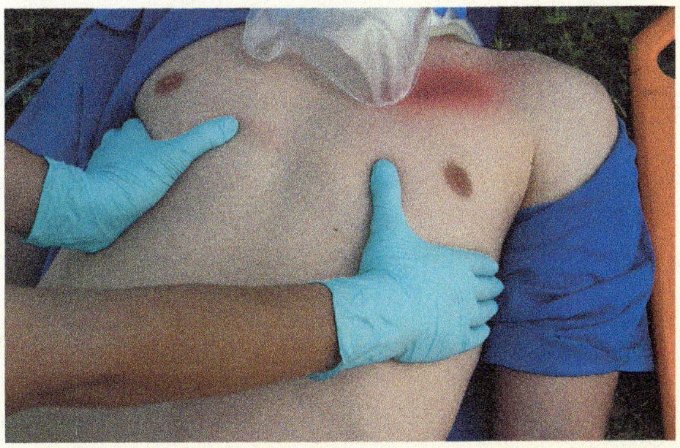

Transport

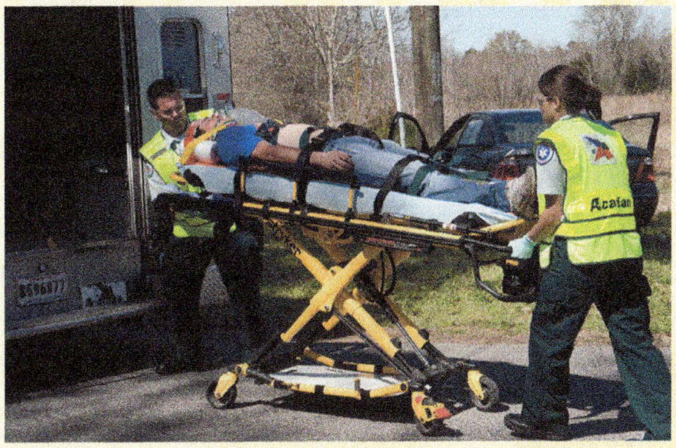

Perform Detailed Assessment and Reassessments En Route

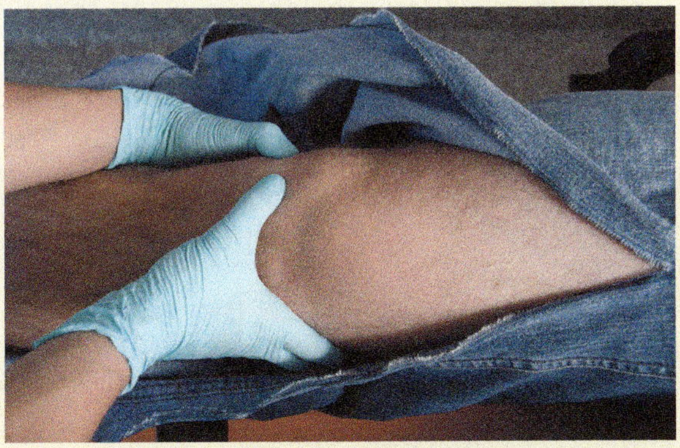

Notify Receiving Hospital

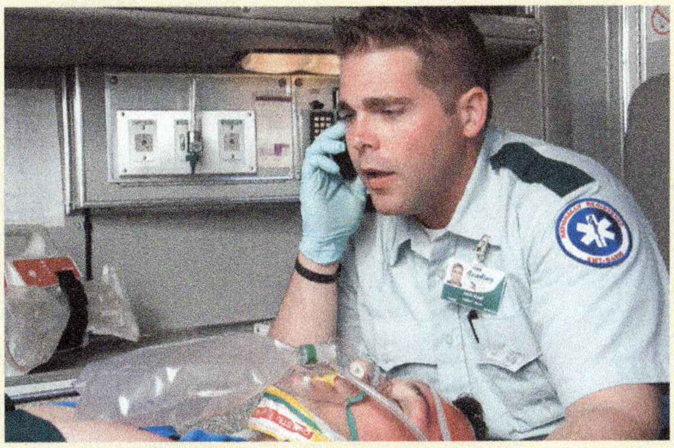

As already discussed for the medical patient, there are three techniques of physical examination that an EMT must master: observation, palpation, and auscultation. When you *observe*, you look for abnormalities in symmetry (e.g., differing chest expansion on one side as compared with on the other), color (e.g., pale, flushed, black and blue, blisters), shape (e.g., swelling, deformity, lacerations, punctures, penetrations), and movement (e.g., strength and equality of hand grip strength, ability to raise an arm). When you *palpate*, you press on possibly injured or affected areas to determine abnormalities in shape, temperature (e.g., hot, cool), texture (e.g., smooth, wet, abraded), and sensation (e.g., tenderness, ability to detect touch). *Auscultation* means listening; in the context of emergency care, it usually refers to listening with a stethoscope. You will listen to a patient's chest for abnormalities such as decreased or absent breath sounds, typically comparing one side of the chest to the other.

There are many signs of trauma an EMT may detect on physical exam. Which irregularities you search for will depend on the circumstances of the patient and the situation.

One aid some EMTs use to remember the types of injuries to look for is the acronym *DCAP-BTLS*, which stands for 'deformities, contusions, abrasions, punctures and penetrations, burns, tenderness, lacerations, and swelling.' It may not be practical (and it would be very time-consuming) to look at every body part and recite the DCAP-BTLS mnemonic during your examination, but it is good way to keep in mind that there are many types of possible injuries.

Deformities are just what they sound like: parts of the body that no longer have the normal shape. Common examples are broken or fractured bones that push up the skin over the bone ends. *Contusions* is the medical term for bruises. *Abrasions*, or scrapes, are some of the most common injuries you will see. *Punctures and penetrations* are holes in the body, frequently the result of gunshot wounds and stab wounds. When they are small, they are easy to overlook. *Burns* may be reddened, blistered, or charred-looking areas. *Tenderness* means that an area hurts when pressure is applied to it, as when it is palpated. Pain (which is present even without any pressure) and tenderness frequently, but not always, go together. *Lacerations* are cuts—open wounds that sometimes cause significant blood loss. *Swelling* is a very common result of injured capillaries bleeding under the skin.

Wounds, tenderness, and deformities is a method of classification that is simpler to remember than DCAP-BTLS but that covers a similar range of signs and symptoms you should watch for in the patient with trauma or suspected trauma. Wounds, tenderness, and deformities are the categories that will be summarized later in Table 15-5 and that will be referred to throughout the physical examination portions of this section.

Point of View

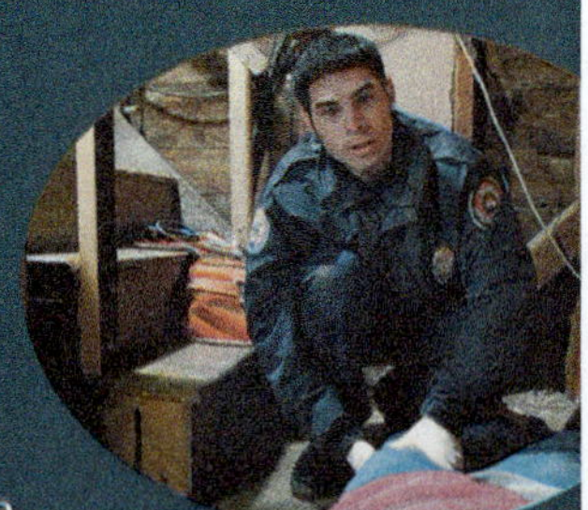

"I was putting some boxes up in the loft in our barn. I must've missed a step. I fell down the first few stairs and felt a 'crack' in my leg. I heard it, but man, I really felt it snap. If that wasn't proof enough, it hurt more than anything I ever felt before. It was broken!

"The EMTs came. They were great, but I gotta tell you, even when they said they'd be careful, they made horrible pain even worse. When the one EMT examined my leg, I thought I was going to jump out of my skin. Any little movement was just so painful.

"They put a splint on and took me to the hospital. I won't even tell you how much the bumps hurt on the ride to the hospital. I don't want to be a complainer, but, well, it hurts to break your leg. Let me tell you."

To find these signs and symptoms, you will need to expose the patient. This means removing or cutting away clothing so you can see and palpate the area or areas of the body you are assessing. Compare normal with injured areas to determine if an abnormality exists. Be sure to tell the patient what you are doing and offer reassurance as necessary. Protect the patient's privacy, and take steps to prevent unnecessarily long exposure to cold.

Obtain Baseline Vital Signs

As in a medical patient, early vital signs provide an immediate snapshot of stability and a baseline for future assessment.

Spinal Motion Restriction–Applying a Cervical Collar

Most EMS systems will apply a cervical collar to any patient who requires spinal precautions. Assessing the need for spinal precautions will be discussed in the chapter *Trauma to the Head, Neck, and Spine*, but it may be reasonable to begin these precautions early in the assessment process.

Several types of cervical-spine immobilization devices are on the market. It is important that you select one that is rigid (stiff, not easily movable) and the right size. The traditional soft collar that you occasionally see someone wearing on the street has no role in immobilizing a prehospital patient's cervical spine.

The wrong-size immobilization device may actually harm the patient by making breathing more difficult or obstructing the airway. Whatever device is used must not obstruct the airway. If the proper-sized collar is not available, it is better to place a rolled towel around the neck (to remind the patient not to move the head) and tape the patient's head to the backboard.

The techniques for selecting the right-sized cervical collar and for applying a cervical collar are presented in Scan 15-3. As you study the scan and practice applying a cervical collar, consider the following:

- Make certain that you have completed the primary assessment and that you have cared for all life-threatening problems before you apply the collar.
- Use the mechanism of injury, level of responsiveness, location of injuries, and any spinal protocols that apply to determine the need for cervical immobilization. Apply a rigid cervical collar whenever any of these factors leads you to believe that spine injury is a possibility.
- Assess the patient's neck prior to placing the collar. Once the collar is in place, you will not be able to inspect or palpate the back of the neck.
- Reassure the patient. Having a cervical collar applied around your neck can be a constricting and frightening experience. Explain the procedure to the patient.
- Make sure the collar is the right size for the patient. The proper-sized rigid collar depends more on the length of the patient's neck than on the width. A large patient may not be able to wear a large collar. A small patient with a long neck may need your largest collar. The front height of the collar should fit between the point of the chin and the chest at the suprasternal (jugular) notch—the *U*-shaped dip where the clavicle and sternum meet. Once in place, the collar should rest on the clavicles and support the lower jaw. It should not stretch the neck (too high), it should not support the chin (too short), and it should not constrict the neck (too tight).
- Remove the patient's necklaces and large earrings before applying the collar.
- Keep the patient's hair out of the way.
- Keep the patient's head in the in-line anatomical position (a neutral position with head facing front, not tilted forward or back or turned to either side) when applying manual stabilization and the collar.

SCAN 15-3 Applying a Cervical Collar

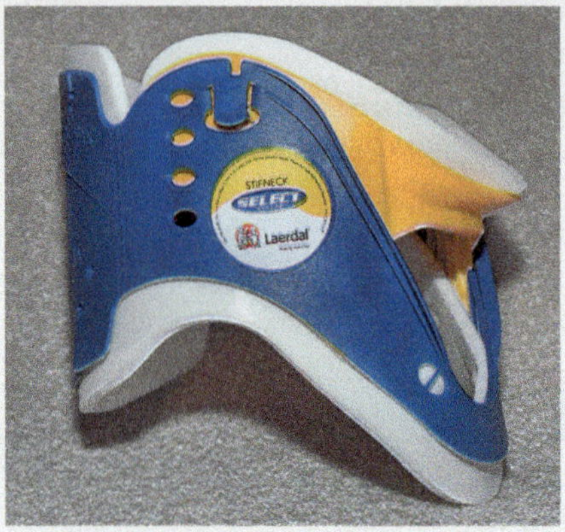

STIFNECK® SELECT™ *(© Edward T. Dickinson, MD)*

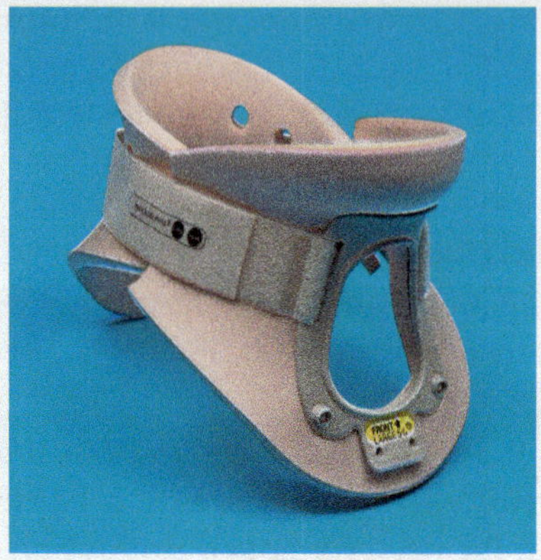

WIZLOC Cervical Collar.

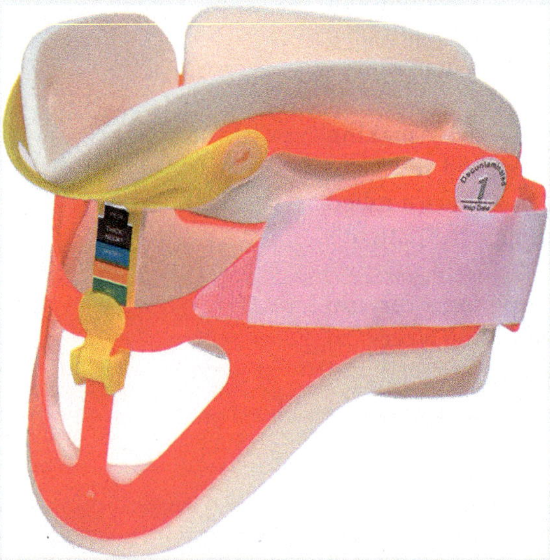

Philadelphia Cervical Collar™ Patriot Adult and Pediatric.

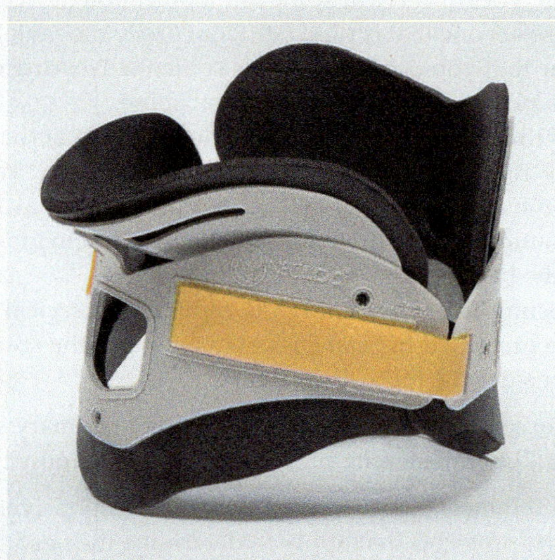

NEC-LOC™ rigid extrication collar, opened. Rigid cervical collars are applied to protect the cervical spine. Do not apply a soft collar.

SIZING A CERVICAL COLLAR

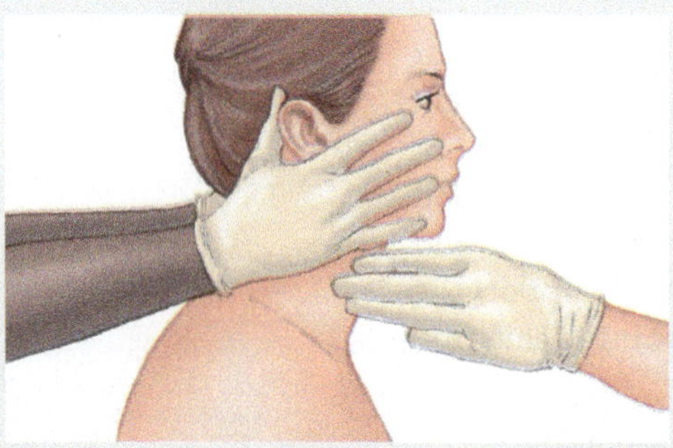

1. Measure the patient's neck.

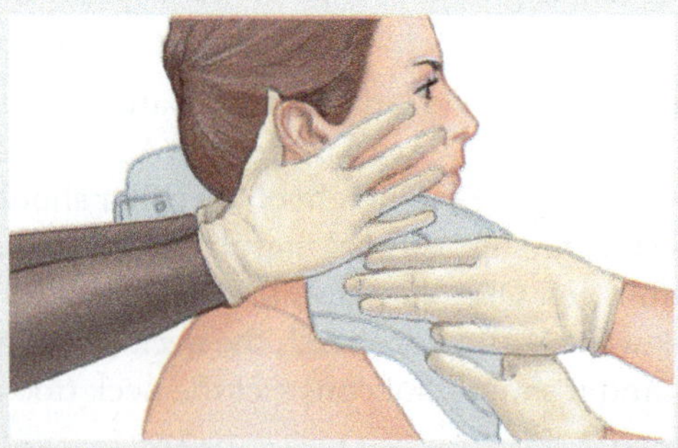

2. Measure the collar. The chin piece should not lift the patient's chin and hyperextend the neck. Make sure the collar is not too small or tight, which would make the collar act as a constricting band.

SCAN 15-3 Applying a Cervical Collar *(continued)*

APPLYING AN ADJUSTABLE COLLAR TO A SEATED PATIENT

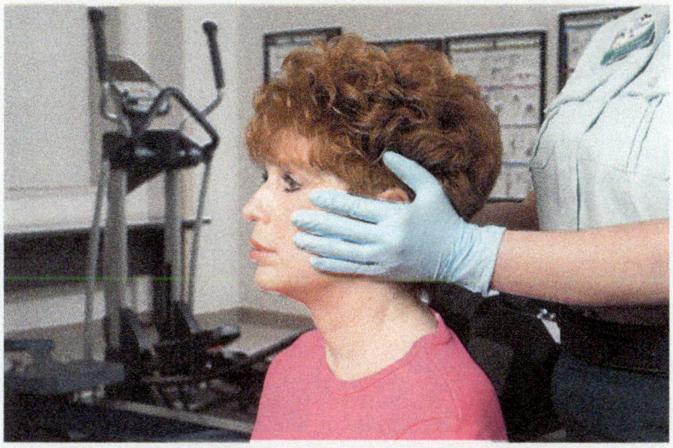

1. Stabilize the head and neck from the rear.

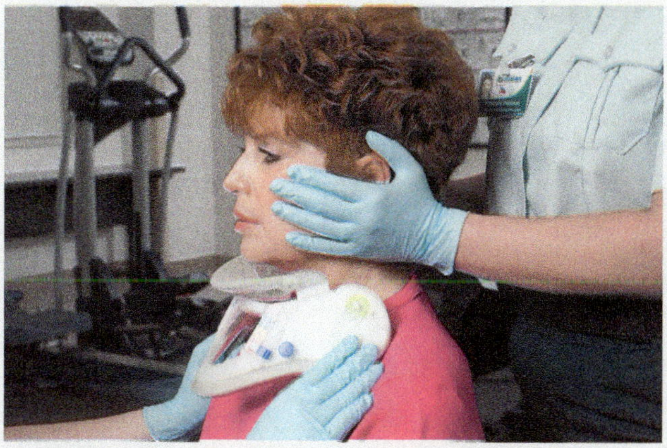

2. Properly angle the collar for placement.

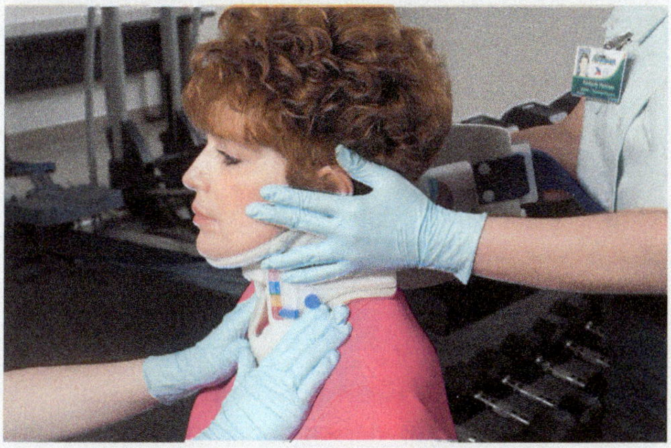

3. Position the collar.

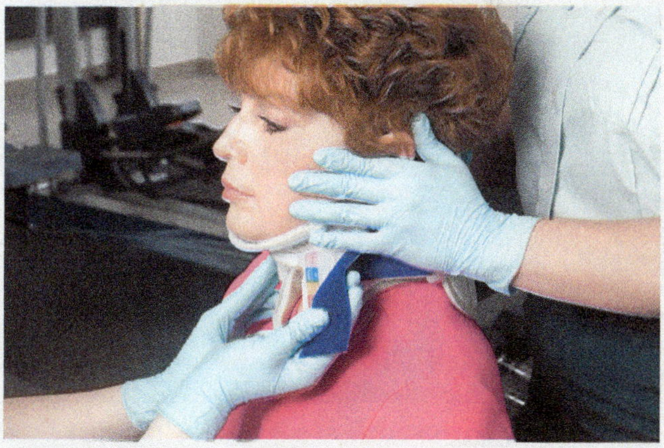

4. Begin to secure the collar.

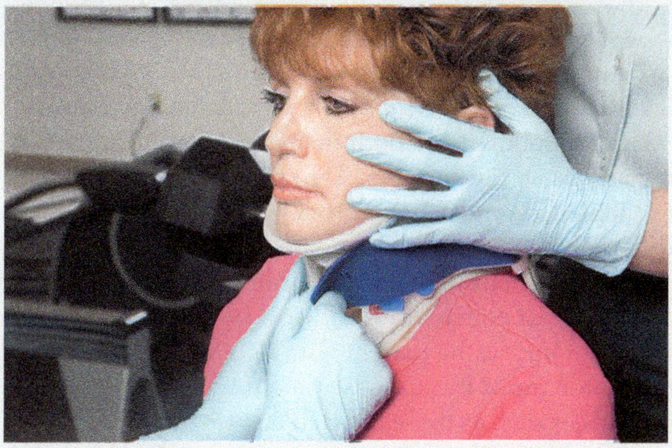

5. Complete securing the collar.

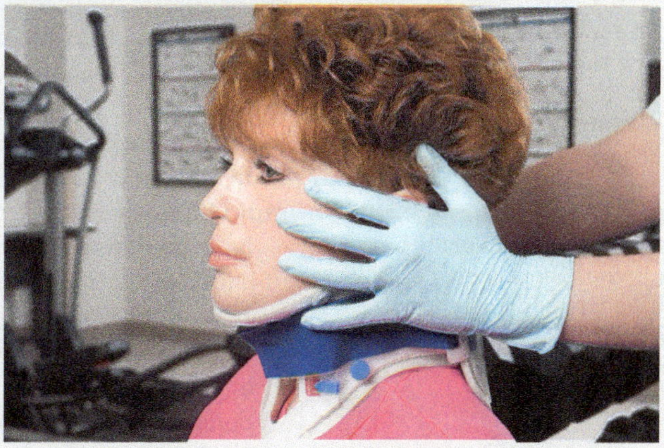

6. Maintain manual stabilization of the head and neck.

(continued)

SCAN 15-3 Applying a Cervical Collar *(continued)*

APPLYING AN ADJUSTABLE COLLAR TO A SUPINE PATIENT

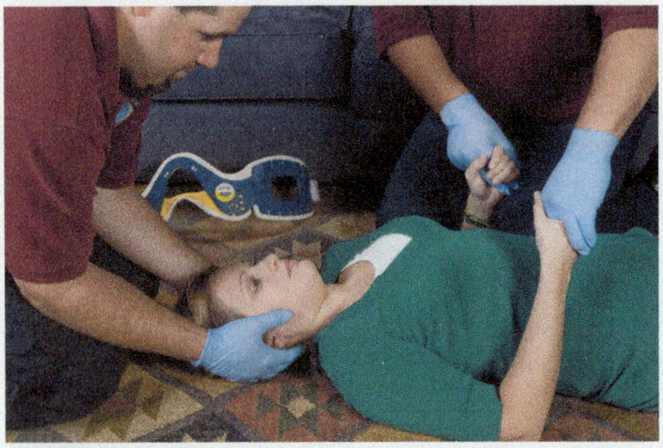

1. Kneel at the patient's head, and stabilize the head and neck.

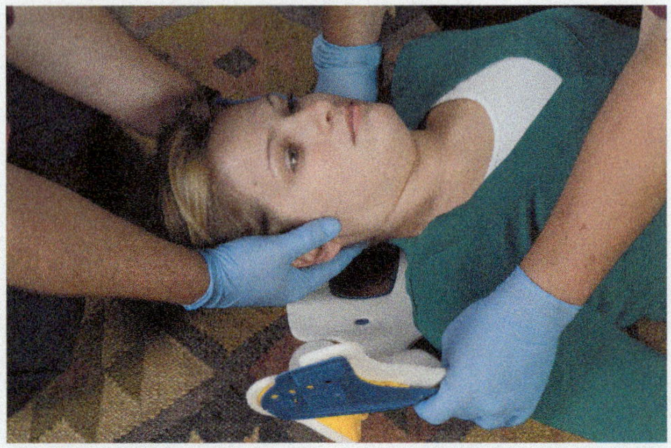

2. Set the collar in place.

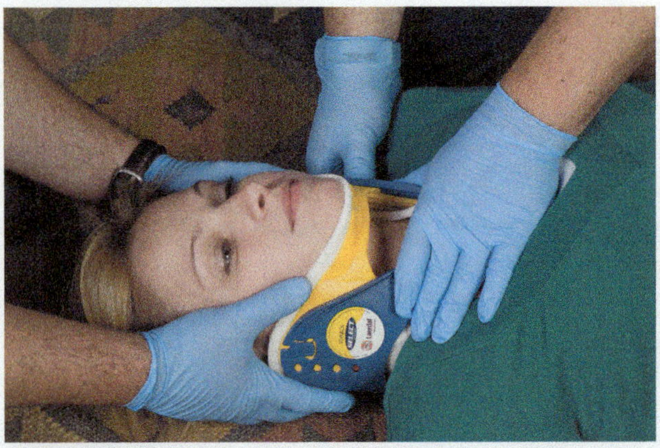

3. Secure the collar.

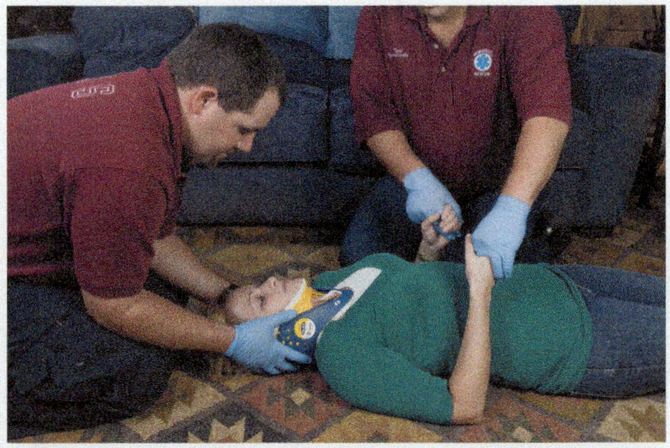

4. Continue to manually stabilize the head and neck.

CORE CONCEPT

Secondary assessment of the trauma patient with serious injury or multisystem trauma

rapid trauma assessment a rapid assessment of the head, neck, chest, abdomen, pelvis, extremities, and posterior of the body to detect signs and symptoms of injury.

Trauma Patient with Serious Injury or Multisystem Trauma/High Priority

When you have a patient you have determined is unstable or is potentially unstable because of problems found in the primary assessment or because of a significant mechanism of injury (Figure 15-4), you will do all of the following: Continue manual stabilization of the head and neck, consider requesting advanced life support (ALS) personnel, and perform a ***rapid trauma assessment***. (Review Table 15-3 and see Scan 15-4.)

Note that there are several additional steps for the patient with a significant mechanism of injury compared with the steps for the patient with no significant mechanism of injury (e.g., manual stabilization and ALS request consideration). Also note that instead of a physical exam focused just on the area of injury, the patient with a significant mechanism of injury receives a complete, head-to-toe rapid trauma assessment.

Some patients who undergo experiences such as those listed in Box 15-1 will escape without serious injury, but many more will not be so lucky. For this reason, you should consider the mechanism of injury as one part of your determination of your patient's condition.

Although the mechanism of injury can provide a lot of information about the kinds of injuries a patient may have, there is still the possibility that patients will have hidden injuries. These injuries are considered to be hidden because patients may have no signs or symptoms initially but nevertheless have serious conditions that may become apparent only later.

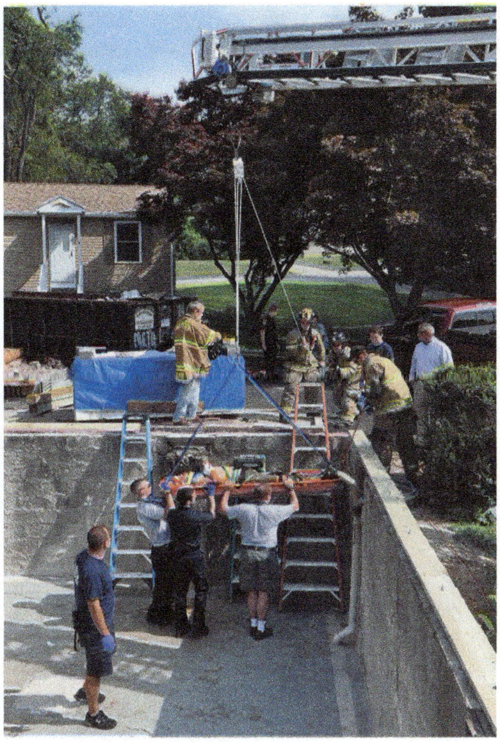

FIGURE 15-4 Mechanism of injury, such as for this worker who fell into a cement foundation, may help you predict injuries and is one factor in determining patient stability and making transport decisions. *(© Edward T. Dickinson, MD)*

BOX 15-1 Field Triage: Significant Mechanisms of Injury

Guidelines for Field Triage of Injured Patients

Transport to a hospital that provides trauma care if any of the following are identified:

- Falls
  - Adults: fall > 20 feet (6.1 meters) (one story = 10 feet [3 meters])
  - Children aged < 15 years: fall > 10 feet (3 meters) or 2-3 times child's height
- High-risk auto crash
  - Intrusion: >12 inches (30 cm) to the occupant site or >18 inches (46 cm) to any site
  - Ejection (partial or complete) from automobile
  - Death in same passenger compartment
  - Vehicle telemetry data consistent with high risk of injury
  - Auto versus pedestrian/bicyclist thrown, run over, or with significant (> 20 mph/32 kph) impact or motorcycle crash > 20 mph (32 kph)

Source: Adapted from Centers for Disease Control and Prevention, Guidelines for Field Triage of Injured Patients, Recommendations of the National Expert Panel on Field Triage, Morbidity and Mortality Weekly Report (MMWR), January 23, 2009, Vol. 58, No. RR-1.

Pediatric Note

Infants and children are more fragile than adults. This means that a child may sustain the same injury as an adult, but from less force. For this reason, there are additional mechanisms of injury that the EMT needs to consider significant when children and infants are concerned. (Review Box 15-1.)

Remember that, because of children's smaller stature, injuries that would affect an adult's knee or thigh might affect a child's abdomen, chest, neck, or skull.

(Text continues on p. 433.)

SCAN 15-4 Physical Examination of the Trauma Patient

Reassess the mechanism of injury and actual injury. If the mechanism of injury is not significant (e.g., patient has a cut finger), focus the physical exam on only the injured part. If the mechanism of injury is significant:

- Continue spinal precautions.
- Consider requesting ALS personnel.
- Reconsider transport decision.
- Reassess mental status.
- Perform a rapid trauma assessment.

HISTORY OF THE PRESENT ILLNESS

Rapidly determine what happened to the patient to cause injury.

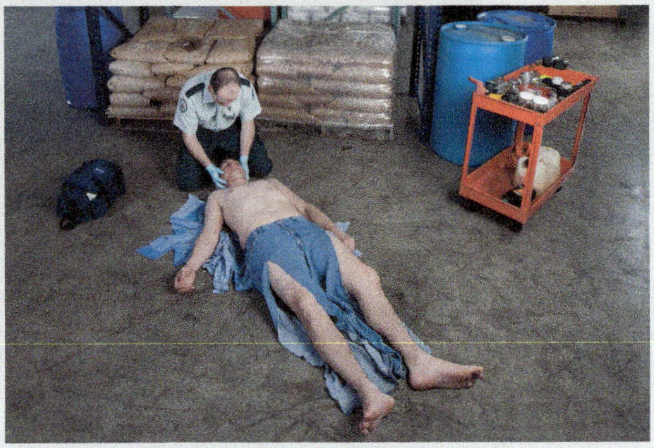

RAPID TRAUMA ASSESSMENT

Rapidly assess each part of the body.

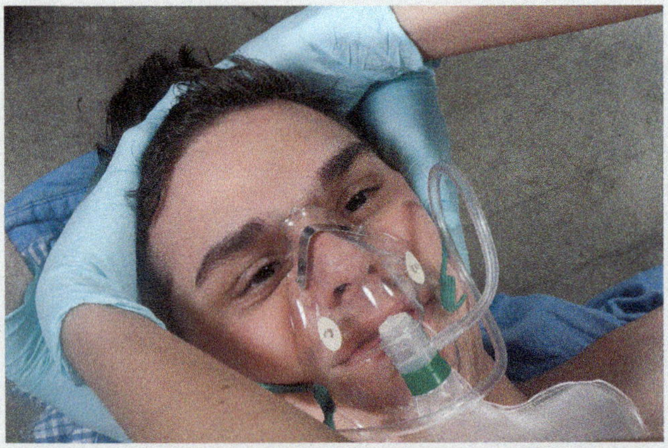

HEAD: Check for wounds, tenderness, and deformities plus crepitation.

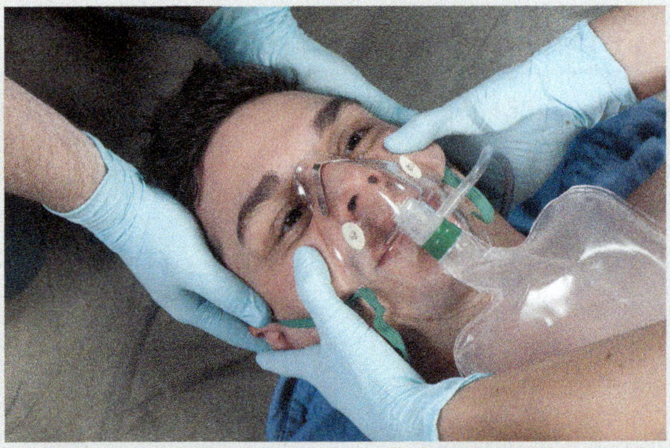

FACE: Check for wounds, tenderness, and deformities.

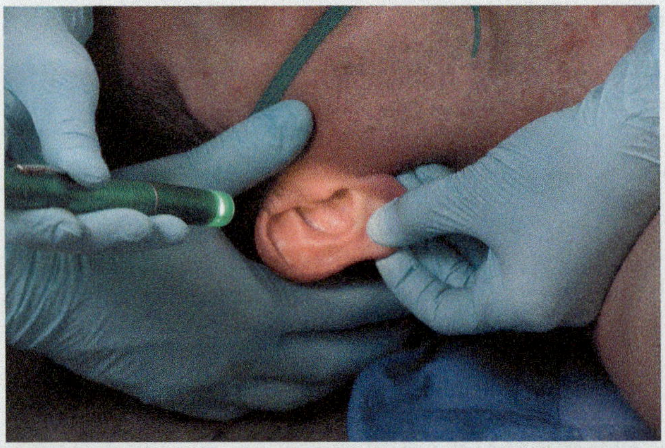

EARS: Check for wounds, tenderness, and deformities, plus drainage of blood or clear fluid.

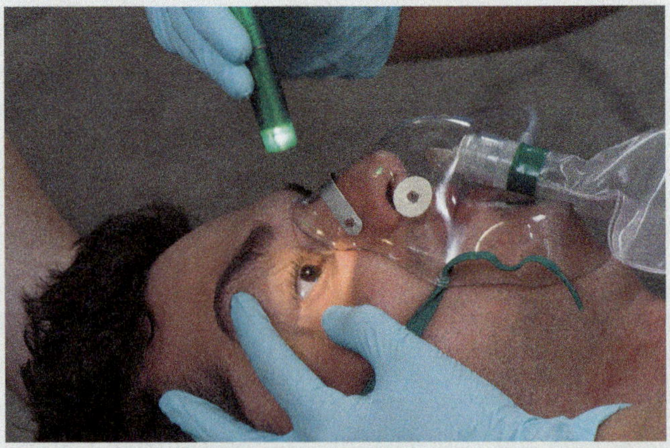

EYES: Check for wounds, tenderness, and deformities, plus discoloration, unequal pupils, foreign bodies, and blood in the anterior chamber.

SCAN 15-4 Physical Examination of the Trauma Patient *(continued)*

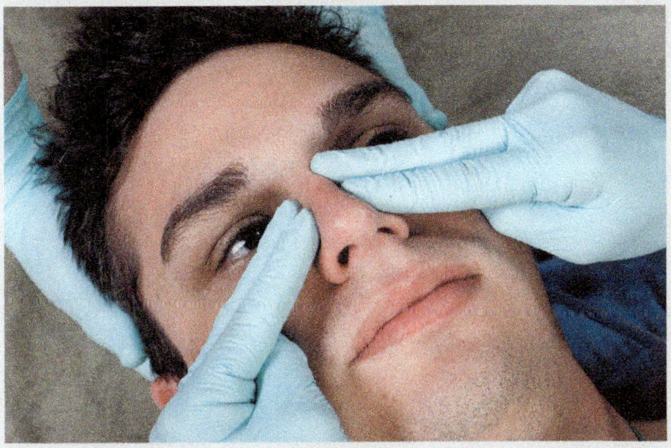

NOSE: Check for wounds, tenderness, and deformities, plus drainage of blood or clear fluid.

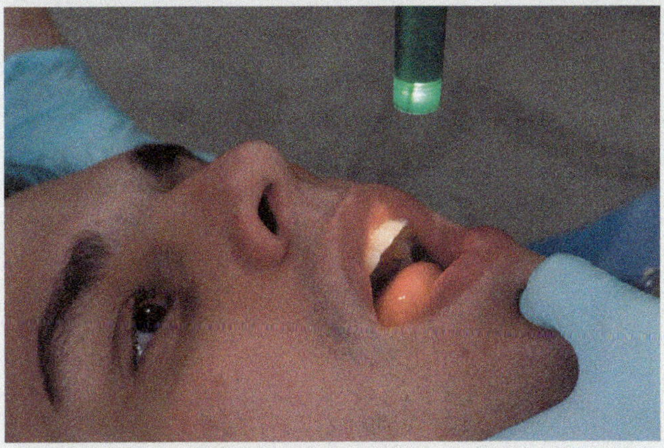

MOUTH: Check for wounds, tenderness, and deformities, plus loose or broken teeth; objects that could cause obstruction, swelling, or laceration of the tongue; unusual breath odor; or discoloration.

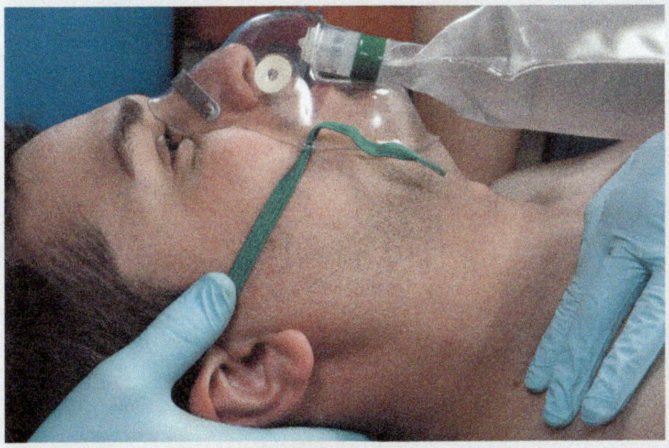

NECK: Check for wounds, tenderness, and deformities, plus jugular vein distention and crepitation.

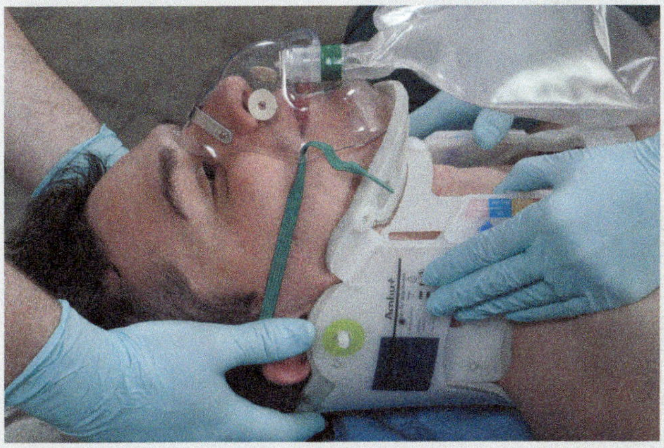

APPLICATION OF COLLAR: Once the neck has been examined, apply the cervical collar.

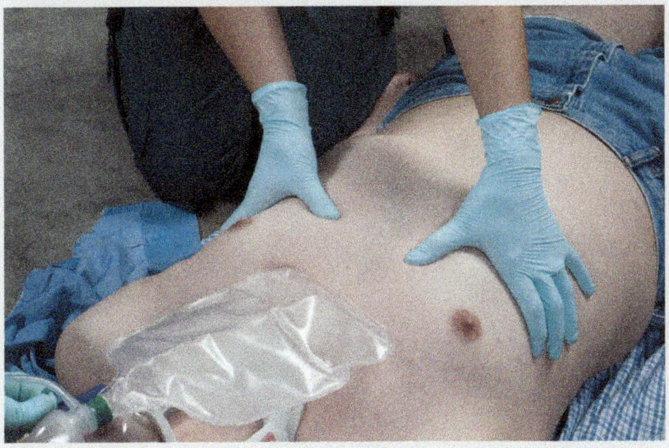

CHEST: Inspect and palpate for wounds, tenderness, and deformities, plus crepitation and paradoxical motion.

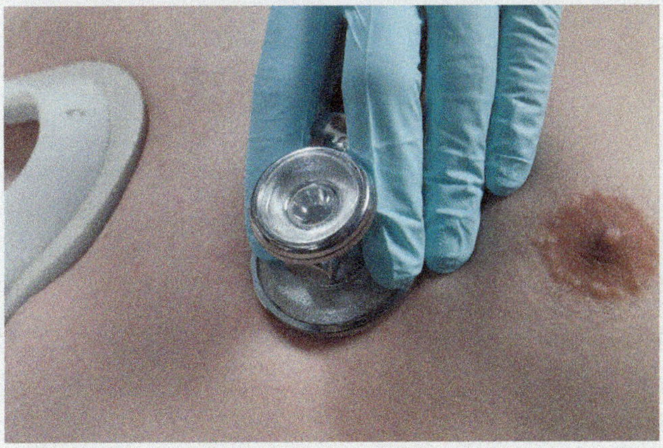

CHEST: Auscultate for breath sounds (presence, absence, and equality).

(continued)

SCAN 15-4 Physical Examination of the Trauma Patient *(continued)*

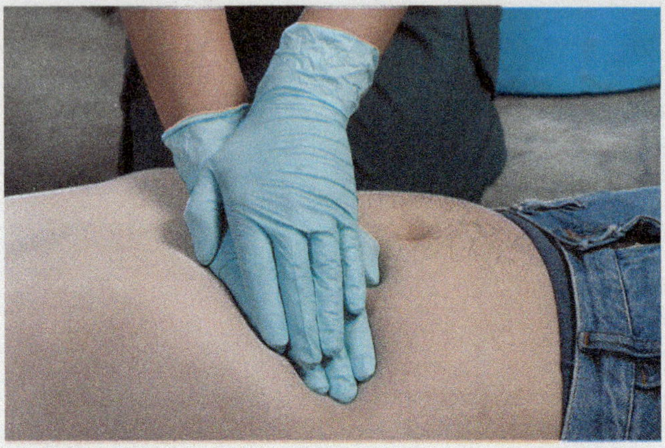

ABDOMEN: Check for wounds, tenderness, and deformities, plus firm, soft, and distended areas.

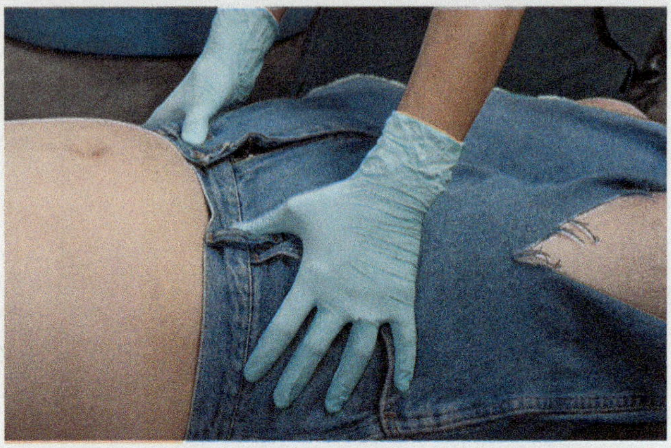

PELVIS: Check for wounds, tenderness, and deformities using gentle compression for tenderness and gentle motion.

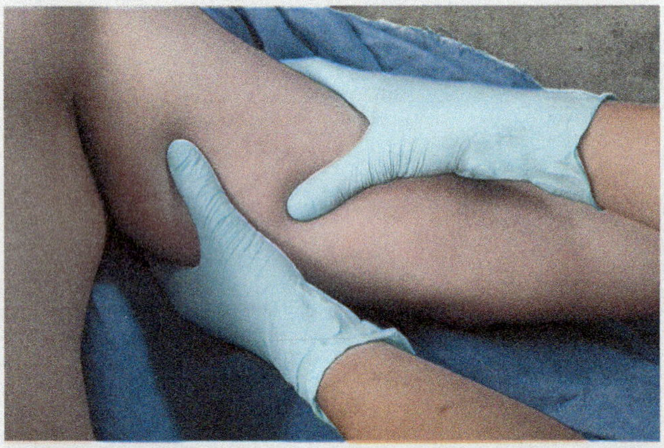

UPPER EXTREMITIES: Check for wounds, tenderness, and deformities.

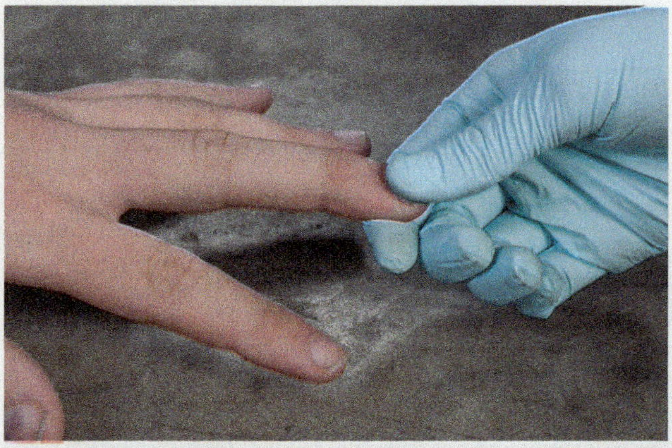

UPPER EXTREMITIES: Check for circulation, sensation, and motor function.

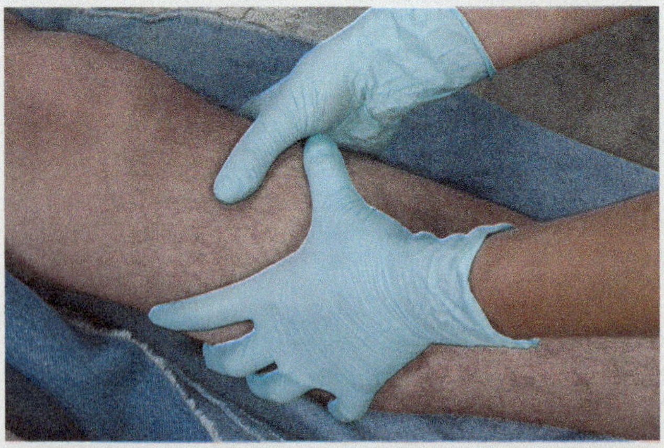

LOWER EXTREMITIES: Check for wounds, tenderness, and deformities.

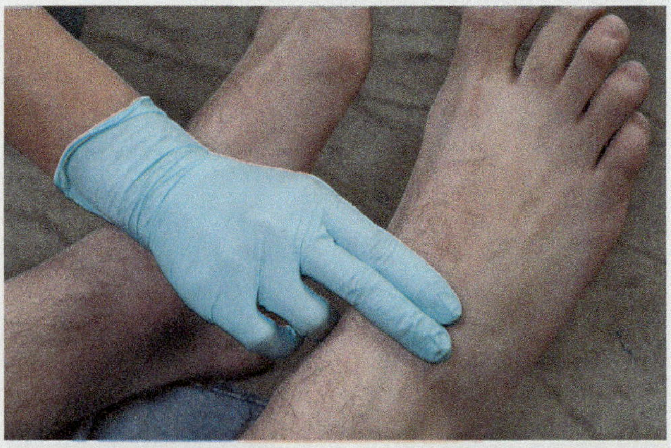

LOWER EXTREMITIES: Check for circulation, sensation, and motor function.

SCAN 15-4 Physical Examination of the Trauma Patient *(continued)*

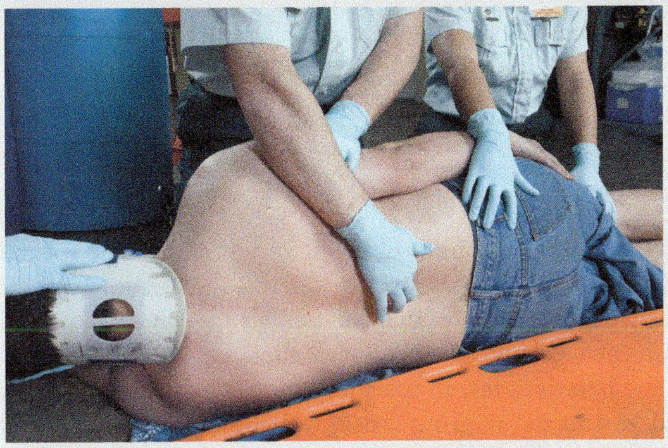

POSTERIOR: Check for wounds, tenderness, and deformities. (To examine posterior, roll patient using spinal precautions.)

VITAL SIGNS

Assess the patient's baseline vital signs:

- Respiration
- Pulse
- Skin color, temperature, condition (capillary refill in infants and children)
- Pupils
- Blood pressure
- Oxygen saturation (if directed by local protocol)

OBTAIN A PATIENT HISTORY IF POSSIBLE

Interview patient or (if patient is unresponsive) family and bystanders to get as much information as possible about the patient's problem. Use SAMPLE:

Signs and symptoms.
Allergies.
Medications.
Pertinent past history.
Last oral intake.
Events leading to problem.

INTERVENTIONS AND TRANSPORT

Contact on-line medical direction, and perform interventions as needed.
Package and transport the patient.

Seat belt injuries are a good example. There is no doubt that, when properly used, seat belts save lives by preventing drivers and passengers from hitting hard objects inside a vehicle and by preventing them from being ejected. But seat belts can also cause injuries. When patients are in high-velocity collisions, the force of being thrown forward against buckled seat belts will occasionally cause injury to the bowel and other abdominal organs. Similarly, patients with seat belt marks on the upper chest and side of the neck may have sustained trauma to the major arteries in the neck that supply the brain. These injuries may not become apparent for several hours or even days. It is important to realize that even people who were wearing seat belts may have sustained serious injuries.

Airbags save lives; however, they do not provide total protection from injury (Figure 15-5). Airbags prevent occupants from going through the windshield or hitting hard objects inside the vehicle. However, they protect occupants only once, even if the vehicle sustains collisions with several other vehicles or objects. They are most effective

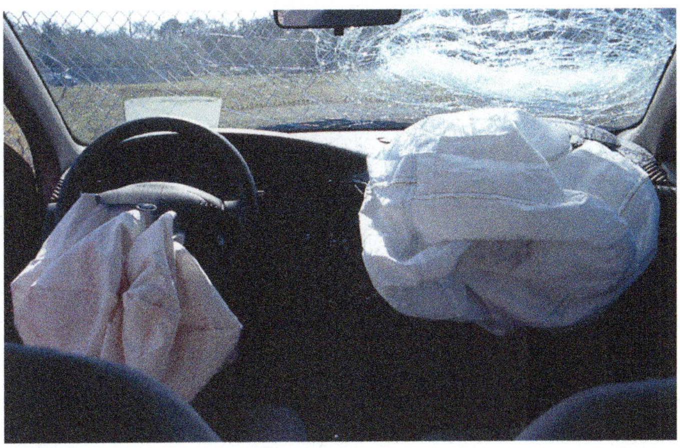

FIGURE 15-5 An airbag can prevent injuries. However, once deployed, it can also conceal important information about the patient's mechanism of injury. When you see a deployed airbag, remember to "lift and look."

TABLE 15-4 Significant Injuries and Signs of Significant Injuries

Unresponsive or altered mental status
Penetrating wound of the head, neck, chest, or abdomen (e.g., stab and gunshot wounds)
Airway that is not patent
Respiratory compromise
Pallor, tachycardia, and other signs of shock

when used in combination with seat belts. In a few instances, especially with a small driver or passenger (particularly a child), or when the front seat is pulled far forward or when a seat belt is not in place to keep the person from being thrown forward, the expanding airbag may cause injury. Also, the driver may sustain an arm injury because of improper positioning of hands on the steering wheel, or may sustain a chest injury from hitting the steering wheel after the bag deflates. When inspecting a vehicle in which an airbag has deployed, you should look at the steering wheel. Whenever you see a bent or broken steering wheel, you should treat the patient like every other patient who has a significant mechanism of injury. A good way to find this kind of damage is to remember to "lift and look" under the airbag after the patient has been removed from the vehicle.

Side-impact airbags, sometimes called side-curtain airbags, are becoming more common. They offer great potential to protect vehicle occupants from side-impact collisions but may also cause injuries discussed earlier with seat belts and airbags.

You should not use mechanism of injury alone as a tool for determining patient priority and assessment strategies. Study in this area is still needed to indicate more clearly which patients will benefit from expedited assessment, treatment, and transport. Although you will note the method of injury (MOI) for potential use by hospital staff, you will do a rapid trauma assessment for the patient with a significant injury regardless of whether the patient has a significant MOI. The overall patient picture depends on many factors. Table 15-4 lists some examples of significant injuries and signs of significant injuries.

Continue Spinal Precautions

During the primary assessment, it may be appropriate to manually stabilize the patient's head to prevent cervical-spine injury. Follow local protocols on spinal precautions.

Consider a Request for Advanced Life Support Personnel

Some areas of the country, particularly urban and suburban areas, have advanced life support (ALS) personnel—paramedics who respond with EMTs when they are transporting patients who might benefit from the additional interventions paramedics can provide. If this is the case where you practice as an EMT, you should familiarize yourself with your local protocols. Rural EMTs do not always have this option, but they may have other means by which to improve the patient's care before arrival at a hospital.

In some areas that are very distant from hospitals, local clinics arrange to provide advanced care to certain kinds of patients. For example, if an ambulance is an hour away from the closest hospital, but a local clinic is only 10 minutes away, the ambulance may be able to stop there with a patient in cardiac arrest. There are limits, though, on what can be done at health care centers such as these. Many of them would not be able to provide additional care that is worth a delay in transport for awake trauma patients.

If arrangements such as these exist where you work as an EMT, you must be familiar with the types of patients your clinic can help. The arrangements should be memorialized in writing to reduce confusion and prevent loss of precious time with critical patients. In any case, the patient with serious trauma must ultimately, if at all possible, be transported to a trauma center.

Perform a Rapid Trauma Assessment

A patient to whom you have assigned a high priority needs a quickly performed physical exam, known as the rapid trauma assessment. This requires only a few moments and should be performed at the scene, before loading the patient into the ambulance, even though the

TABLE 15-5 Physical Exam/Trauma Assessment

BODY PART	WOUNDS, TENDERNESS, AND DEFORMITIES	PLUS
Head	Wounds, tenderness, and deformities	Crepitation, ear drainage, skull depression
Neck	Wounds, tenderness, and deformities	Jugular vein distention, crepitation
Chest	Wounds, tenderness, and deformities	Paradoxical motion, crepitation, breath sounds (present, absent, equal)
Abdomen	Wounds, tenderness, and deformities	Firmness, softness, distention
Pelvis	Wounds, tenderness, and deformities	Pain, tenderness, motion
Extremities	Wounds, tenderness, and deformities	Distal circulation, sensation, motor function
Posterior	Wounds, tenderness, and deformities	

patient is a high priority for transport. The care that you provide en route will be based on the results of this rapid assessment, and you will obtain valuable information to relay to the hospital staff so that they can be prepared for your patient.

During the rapid trauma assessment, you will be able to detect injuries that may later threaten life or limb. You may also find life-threatening injuries that you did not find during the primary assessment. When dealing with a responsive patient, you should ask the patient before and during the trauma assessment about any symptoms.

To perform the rapid trauma assessment, you will use your sense of sight to inspect and your sense of touch to palpate different areas of the body. You may also use your sense of hearing to detect abnormal sounds, not just from the airway but also from other areas, such as the sound of crepitation (broken bones rubbing against each other). You may use your sense of smell as well to detect odors such as gasoline, urine, feces, or vomitus. You will evaluate the patient from head to toe, in the sequence described next.

The signs and symptoms you will assess in each area are summarized in Table 15-5. Remember, however, that this is a quick evaluation, so you will not spend a lot of time on any one area.

Rapid Assessment of the Head. Gently palpate the cranium for wounds, tenderness, and deformities, as well as the sound or feel of broken bones rubbing against each other, known as crepitation. Run your gloved fingers through the patient's hair and palpate gently. A good way to check the back of the head in a supine patient is to start with your fingers at the top of the neck and carefully slide them upward toward the top of the patient's head. If there is blood on your gloves, there is an open wound. However, if you do not see any blood on the floor or ground, then you do not need to apply a dressing to the wound right away.

Inspect and palpate the face for wounds, tenderness, and deformities by looking at and then gently palpating the cheekbones, forehead, and lower jaw. The bones in the face are fragile and may break when subjected to significant forces.

Inspect and palpate the ears, searching for wounds, tenderness, and deformities, as well as drainage of blood or other fluids. If these are found, they are important pieces of information to pass on to the emergency department staff because they may be indications of injury to the skull (Figure 15-6). Also gently bend each ear forward to look for any bruising. Although it is typically a sign that develops later, a bruise behind the patient's ear is called Battle's sign and is another important sign of skull injury to tell hospital staff about.

Next assess the eyes, inspecting for the usual wounds, tenderness, and deformities, as well as discoloration, unequal pupils, foreign bodies, and blood in the anterior chamber (front) of the eye. Blood in the anterior chamber is not common; however, when present, it is a sign that the eye sustained significant force and is bleeding inside (Figure 15-7).

Inspect and palpate the nose for injuries or signs of injury. Look not only for wounds, tenderness, and deformities but also for drainage and bleeding.

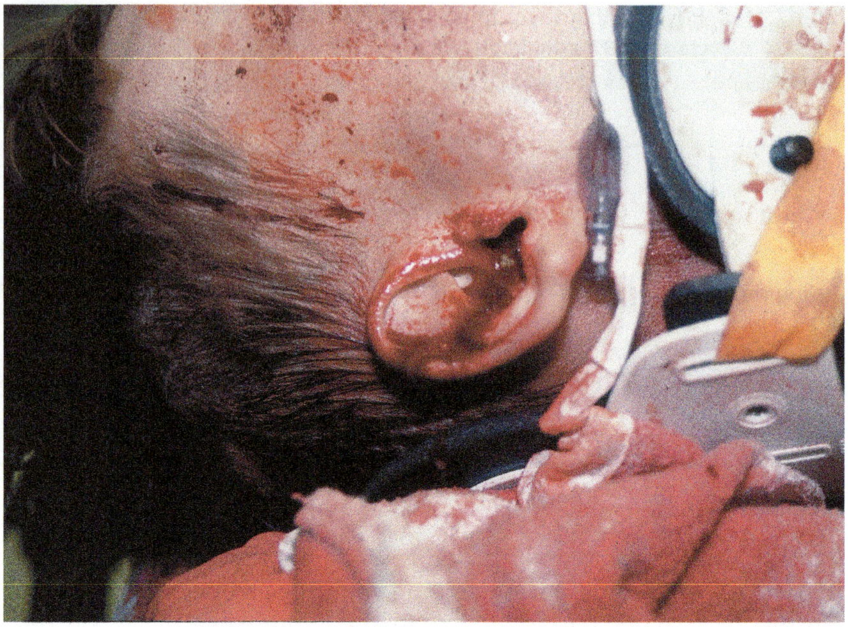

FIGURE 15-6 Blood and cerebrospinal fluid draining from the ear of a trauma patient. *(© Edward T. Dickinson, MD)*

FIGURE 15-7 Blood in the anterior chamber of the eye is a sign that the eye has sustained considerable force. *(Photo: © Edward T. Dickinson, MD)*

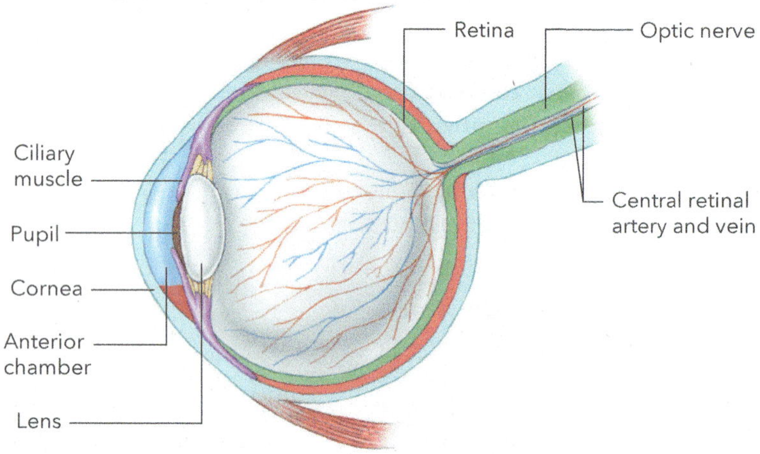

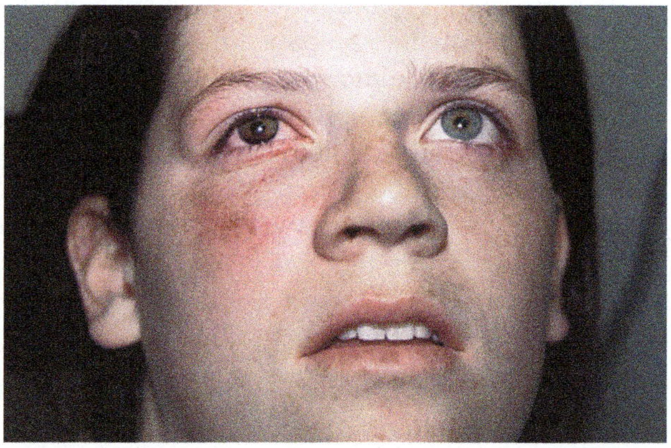

When assessing the ears and nose, you may find blood or clear fluid draining from them. Blood may be from a laceration of that area, or it may be coming from inside the skull. Clear fluid may be just from a runny nose or it may be cerebrospinal fluid (CSF). You should prevent an ear or nose that is draining blood or clear fluid from getting any dirtier than it is at that point. CSF surrounds the brain and spinal cord, and if it is leaking out, then bacteria can get into the brain. Similarly, a wound from inside the skull that is leaking blood can also provide a route for bacteria to get in. Figure 15-8A summarizes signs of brain injury. Figure 15-8B is a photo of a patient with Battle's sign (a late sign of head injury), and Figure 15-8C is a CT scan of that same patient.

Open the patient's mouth and look for wounds, tenderness, and deformities; loose or broken teeth; other objects that could cause obstruction; swelling or lacerations of the tongue; unusual breath odor; and discoloration. A foreign body such as a broken tooth is a potential source of airway obstruction and must be removed as soon as possible from the patient's mouth. The most common unusual breath odor is from alcoholic beverages. Other conditions besides alcohol, though, can cause similar odors.

FIGURE 15-8 (A) Battle's sign and other signs of brain injury. (B) A patient with Battle's sign. (C) CT scan of that same patient. *(Photos B and C: © Edward T. Dickinson, MD)*

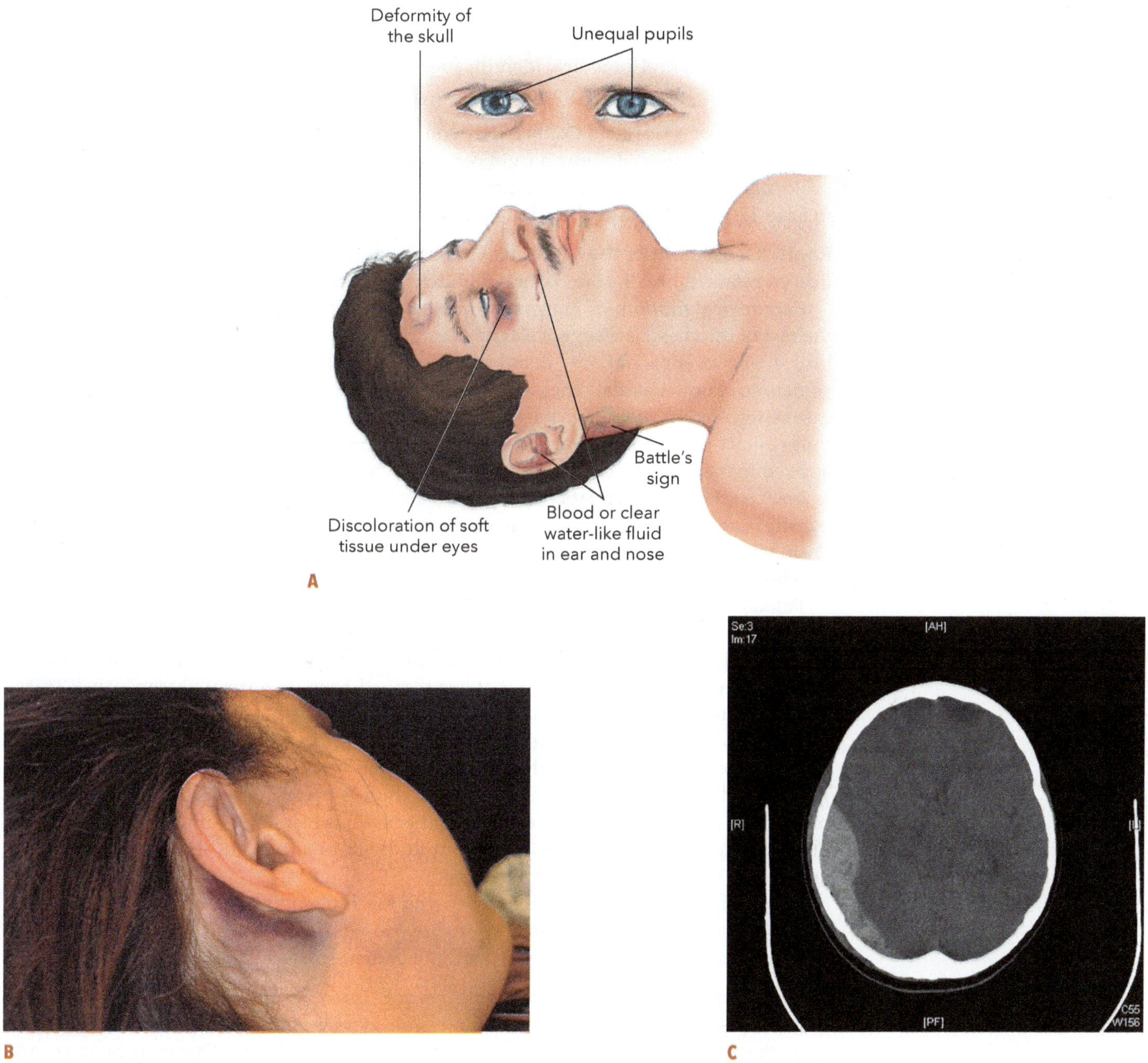

Rapid Assessment of the Neck. Assess the neck for wounds, tenderness, deformities, and jugular vein distention (JVD). (Review Figure 14-9.) JVD is present when you can see the patient's neck veins bulging. The neck veins are usually not visible when the patient is sitting up. If they are bulging when the patient is upright, it means that blood is backing up in the veins because the heart is not pumping effectively. This could be the result of a tension pneumothorax (air trapped in the chest) or cardiac tamponade (blood filling the sac around the heart). However, it is normal to see bulging of the neck veins when the patient is lying in a horizontal position or with the head down. Flat neck veins in a patient who is lying down may be a sign of blood loss, showing that there is not enough blood to fill them. When you see *flat* neck veins in a *flat* patient, think "blood loss." To summarize, *either* neck veins that are bulging when the patient is sitting up *or* neck veins that are flat when the patient is flat are abnormal and should be noted during the exam.

stoma (STO-ma)
a permanent surgical opening in the neck through which the patient breathes.

tracheostomy (tray-ke-OS-to-me)
a surgical incision held open by a metal or plastic tube.

paradoxical (pair-uh-DOCK-si-kal) ***motion***
movement of a part of the chest in the opposite direction to the rest of the chest during respiration.

distention (dis-TEN-shun)
a condition of being stretched, inflated, or larger than normal.

Another thing you might find when assessing the patient's anterior neck is a surgical opening. A ***stoma*** is a permanent surgical opening in the neck through which the patient breathes. A ***tracheostomy*** is a surgical incision held open by a metal or plastic tube. If the patient requires artificial ventilation, you may need to provide it through the stoma, as described in the chapter *Respiration and Artificial Ventilation.*

You may also find a medical identification medallion on a necklace when assessing the neck. Note the information on the necklace if you find one.

Application of a Cervical Collar. After you assess the patient's head and neck, it may be appropriate to size and apply a rigid cervical spine immobilization collar if indicated by protocols. Use the principles and methods that were described earlier in this chapter and in Scan 15-3 and in the chapter *Trauma to the Head, Neck, and Spine.*

Rapid Assessment of the Chest. Next assess the chest for wounds, tenderness, deformities, crepitation, breath sounds, and paradoxical motion.

Paradoxical motion, or movement of part of the chest in the opposite direction from the rest of the chest, is a sign of a serious injury. It usually occurs when several ribs have broken at two ends and are "floating" free of the rest of the rib cage. (This condition is sometimes known as flail chest.) The opposite motion of the broken section is obvious during respiration, moving inward when the lungs expand with air and outward when the lungs empty (Figure 15-9). Paradoxical motion also indicates that a great deal of force was applied to the patient's chest; in other words, there was a significant mechanism of injury.

You can check for crepitation and paradoxical motion of the chest at the same time. Start by palpating the patient's clavicles (collarbones). Next, gently feel the sternum (breastbone). Position your hands on the sides of the chest and feel for equal expansion of both sides of the chest. During this process, you may feel broken bones or floating paradoxical segments.

Palpate the entire rib cage for deformities. Use your hands to apply gentle pressure to the sides of the rib cage. If there is an injured rib and the patient is able to respond, the patient will tell you that it hurts. Occasionally you may detect a crackling or crunching sensation under the skin from air that has escaped from its normal passageways. This is called subcutaneous emphysema.

Listen for breath sounds (Scan 15-5) just under the clavicles in the mid-clavicular line and at the bases of the lungs in the mid-axillary line. Notice whether the breath sounds are present and equal. A patient who has breath sounds that are absent or very hard to hear on one side may have a collapsed lung or other serious respiratory injury. There are many other characteristics of breath sounds, but in the trauma patient, presence and equality are the two things to look for at this time.

It is important to remember that when you reach the point of examining the patient's chest in the rapid trauma assessment, you need to expose the chest if you have not already done so. However, keep the weather and the patient's privacy in mind when doing this.

Rapid Assessment of the Abdomen. When you assess the abdomen for wounds, tenderness, and deformities, also check for firmness, softness, and distention. The term ***distention*** is another way of saying the abdomen appears larger than normal. One of its causes can be internal bleeding. Whether the abdomen is abnormally distended or not may be a very difficult judgment to make, so do not spend a lot of time on it. You may also see a colostomy or ileostomy when you inspect the abdomen. This is a surgical opening in the abdominal wall with a bag in place to collect excretions from the digestive system. If you see such a bag, leave it in place and be careful not to cut it if you cut clothing away.

Palpate the abdomen by gently pressing down once on each abdominal quadrant. (Picture the abdomen divided into four segments—upper left, upper right, lower left, and lower right—and press on each quadrant in turn.) If the patient tells you there is pain in a specific area of the abdomen, palpate that site last. When practical, make sure your hands are warm. Press in on the abdomen with the palm side of your fingers, depressing the surface about 1 inch (2.5 cm). Many EMTs prefer to use two hands, one on top of the other at the fingertips. Normally the abdomen is soft. Firmness of the abdomen can be a sign of injury to the organs in the abdomen and of internal bleeding.

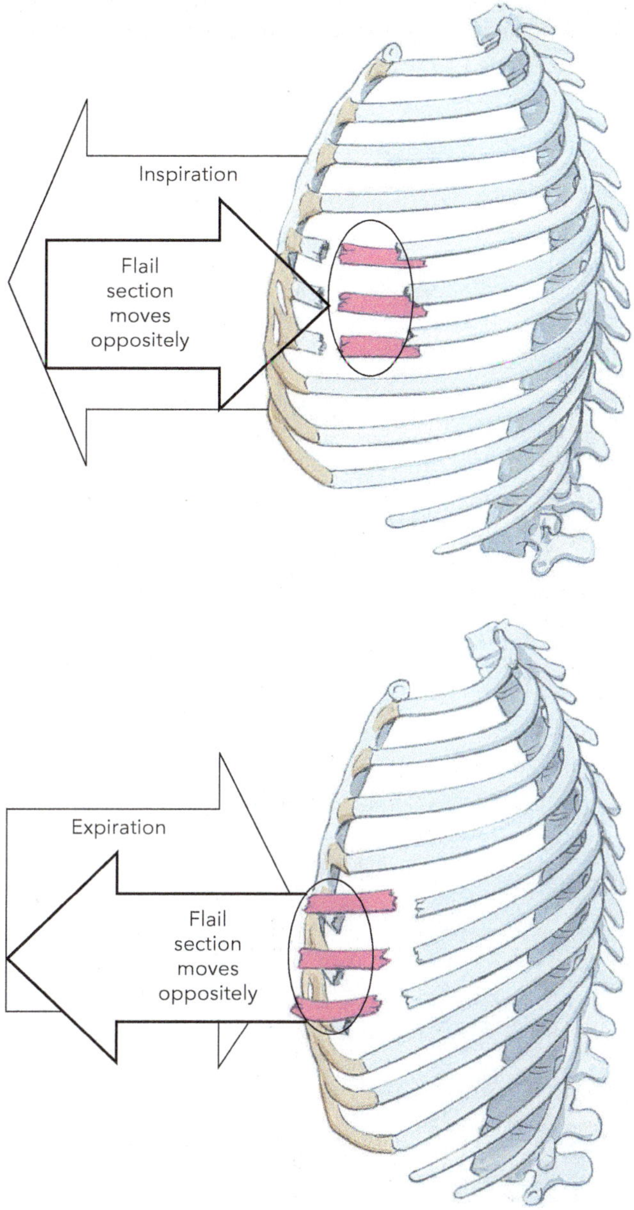

FIGURE 15-9 Paradoxical motion.

Another finding you may occasionally come across when palpating a patient's abdomen is a pulsating mass. This may be an enlarged aorta. If you do feel such pulsations, do not press any farther into the abdomen. Doing so could cause further injury to a weakened blood vessel.

Rapid Assessment of the Pelvis. Next assess the pelvis for wounds, tenderness, and deformities. You may observe bleeding or ***priapism***, a persistent erection of the penis that can result from spinal cord injury or certain medical problems. If the patient is awake, palpate the pelvis gently, stopping as soon as the patient identifies pain in the pelvis. Consider the complaint of pain as reason enough to treat the patient for an injury to the pelvis. Continuing to palpate or compress the painful pelvis of a conscious patient will not give you any more useful information, but it can produce excruciating pain and, if done too strenuously, may injure the patient.

priapism (PRY-ah-pizm) persistent erection of the penis that may result from spinal injury and some medical problems.

An unconscious patient, however, cannot tell you if the pelvic area hurts. Therefore, you will gently compress the pelvis of the unconscious patient to detect tenderness (if there is enough responsiveness to pain to cause the patient to flinch or groan) and motion of the bones (indicating instability or broken bones). These signs will help you determine whether you need to treat the unconscious patient for a pelvic injury.

SCAN 15-5 Assessing Breath Sounds

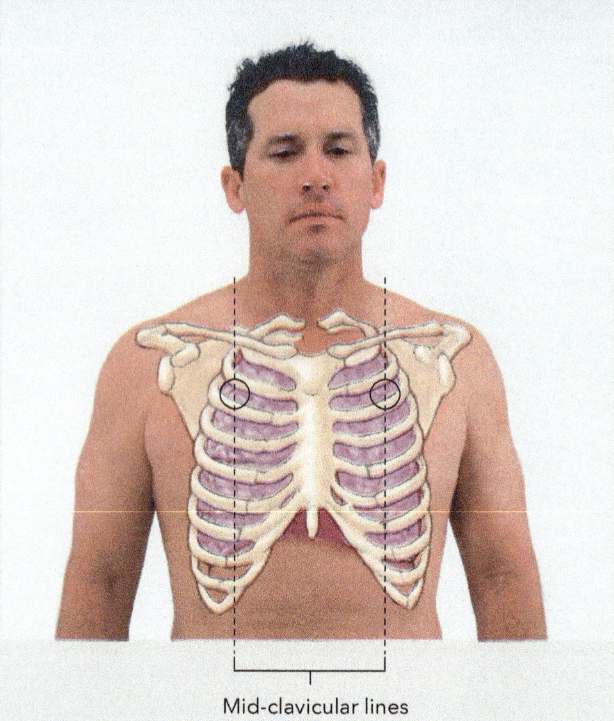

Listen at the mid-clavicular lines.

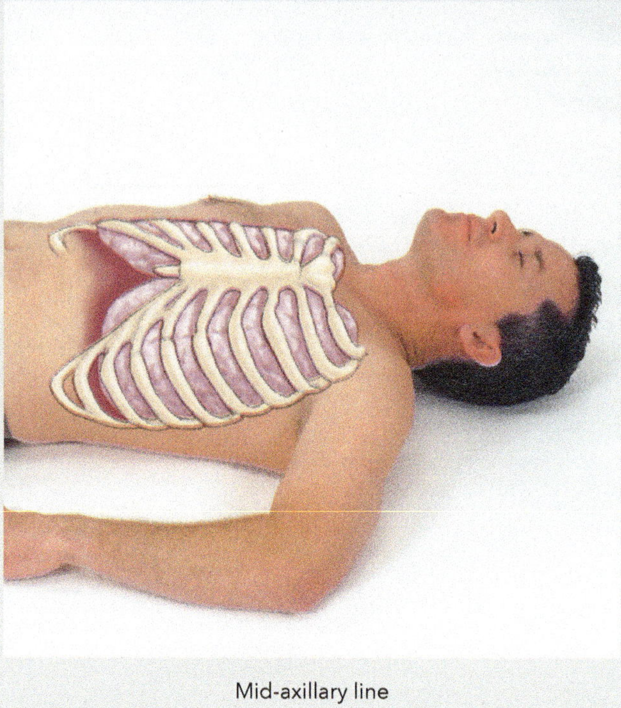

Listen at the mid-axillary lines.

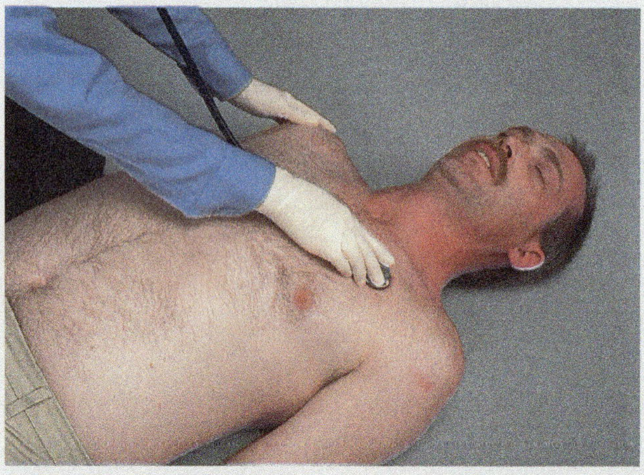

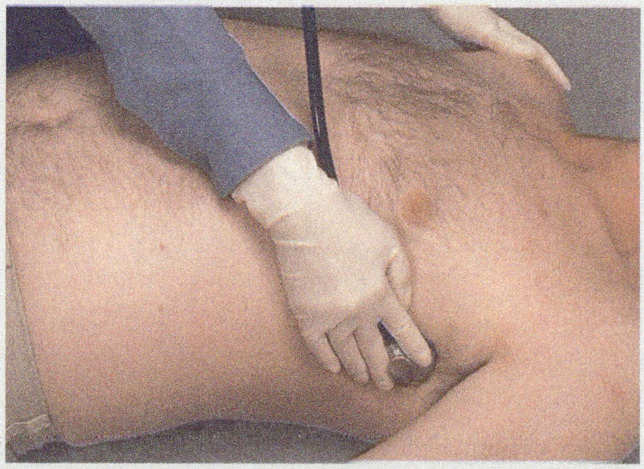

Listen at the mid-clavicular and the mid-axillary lines on both sides of the chest. Is air entry present? Absent? Equal on both sides?

Rapid Assessment of the Extremities. Quickly assess all four extremities for wounds, tenderness, and deformities, as well as distal circulation, sensation, and motor function—that is, whether a pulse is present, the patient has feeling in the hands and feet, and the patient can move the hands and feet (Scan 15-6). In a conscious patient, you will touch the patient's hand or foot and ask whether the patient can feel your touch. If you are not sure whether the patient is telling you the truth, you can ask where on the hand or foot you are touching the patient. You can also test movement in the extremities of conscious patients by asking them to squeeze your fingers and to move their feet against your hands.

If you find a deformity, diminished function, or other indication of injury to an extremity in a patient who is a high priority for transport, you will not splint the extremity at the scene but will treat it en route.

SCAN 15-6 Assessing Distal Function

Assess all four extremities for distal circulation, sensation, and motor function. Diminished function may be a sign of injury that has compromised circulation, motor function, or nerve function. Distal function should be checked both before and after any interventions such as splinting, bandaging, and immobilization and at intervals during transport to be sure such interventions are not interfering with distal function. If distal function has become compromised, adjust your interventions as necessary.

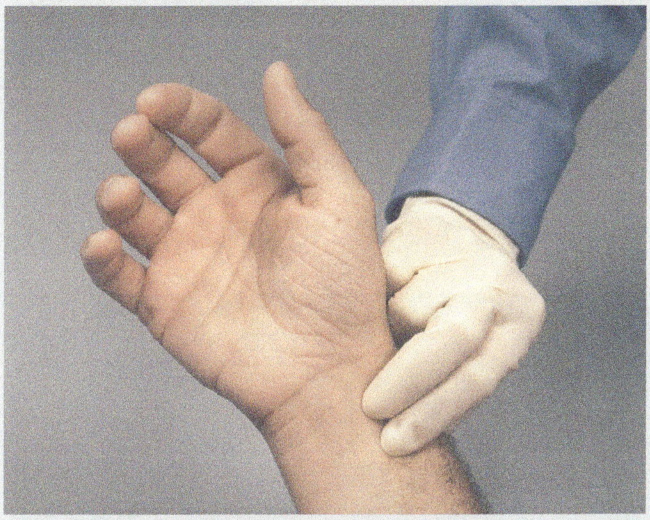

1. Assess distal circulation in the upper extremities by feeling for radial pulses.

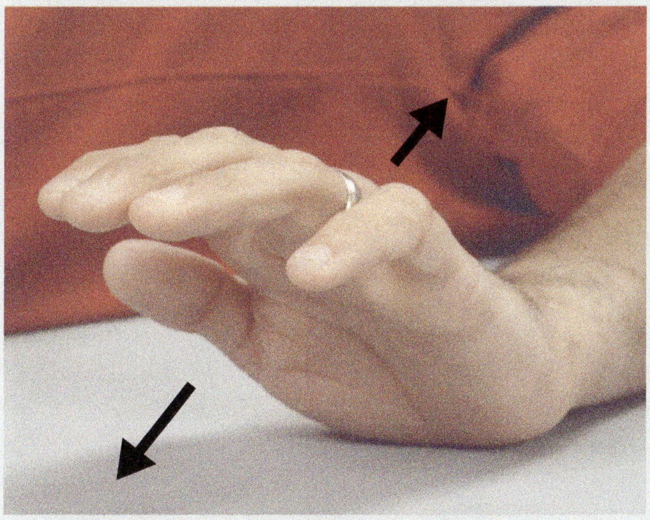

2. Assess distal motor function by checking the patient's ability to move both hands.

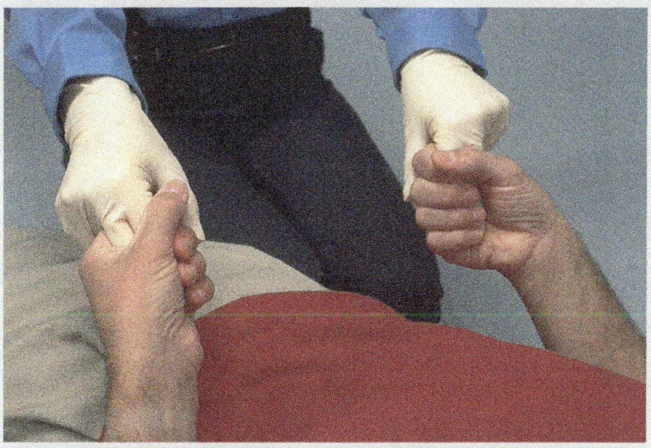

3. Assess strength in the hands by asking the patient to squeeze your fingers.

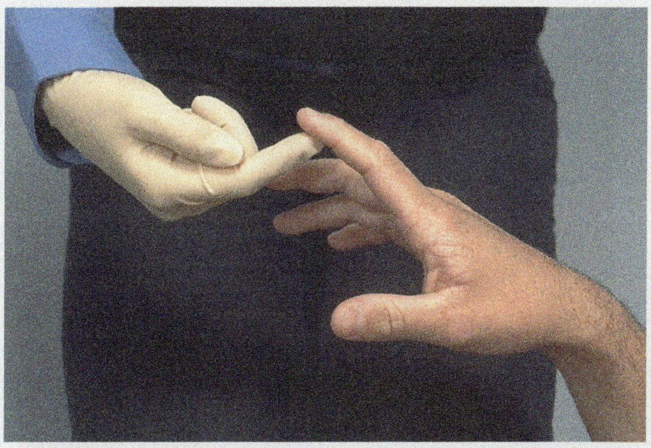

4. Assess distal sensation to the upper extremities by asking the patient "Which finger am I touching?" (Be sure the patient cannot see which finger.)

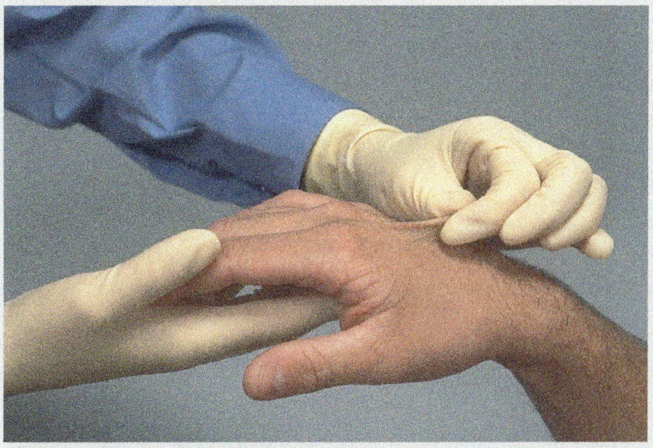

If the patient is unresponsive, check distal sensation in the upper extremities by pinching the back of the hand. Watch and listen for a response.

(continued)

SCAN 15-6 Assessing Distal Function *(continued)*

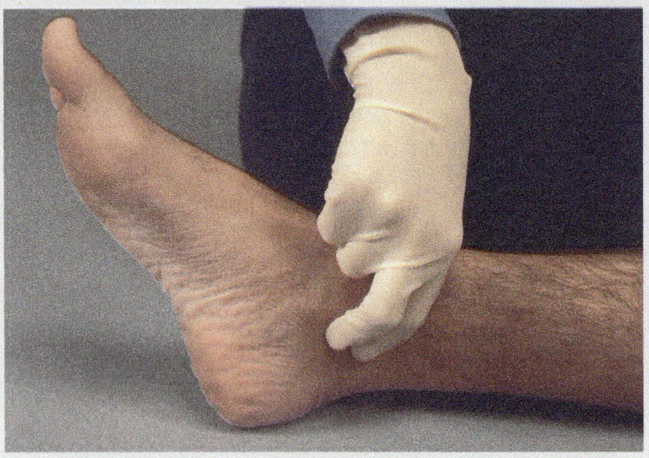

5. Check distal circulation in the lower extremities by feeling the posterior tibial pulse just behind the medial malleolus of the ankle, or . . .

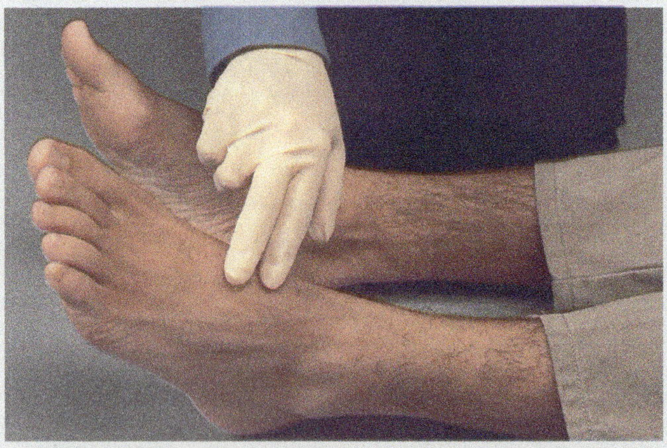

. . . feel the dorsalis pedis pulse at the top of the foot.

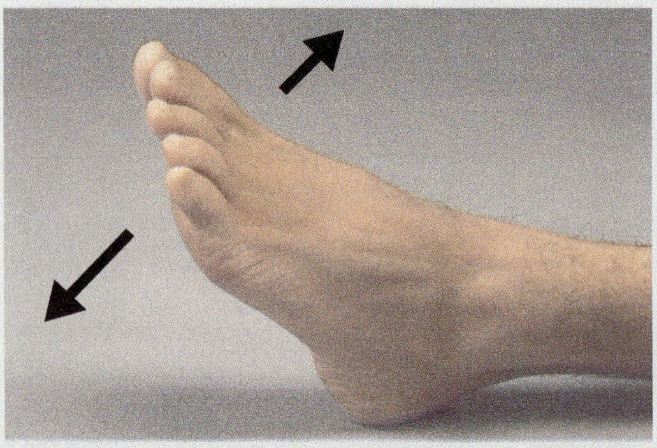

6. Assess distal motor function by checking the patient's ability to move the feet.

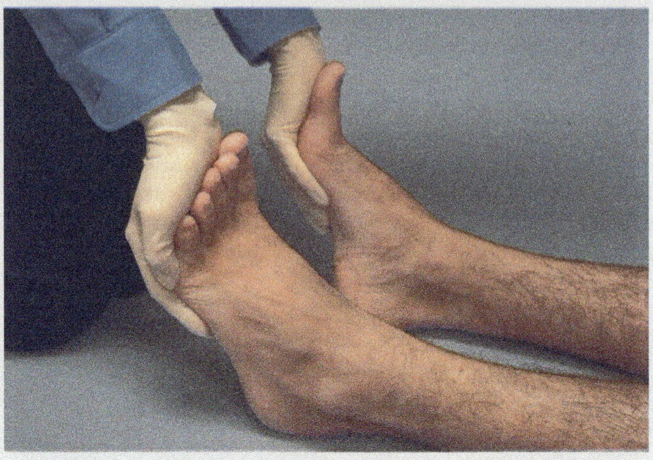

7. Assess strength in the feet and legs by asking the patient to push against your hands.

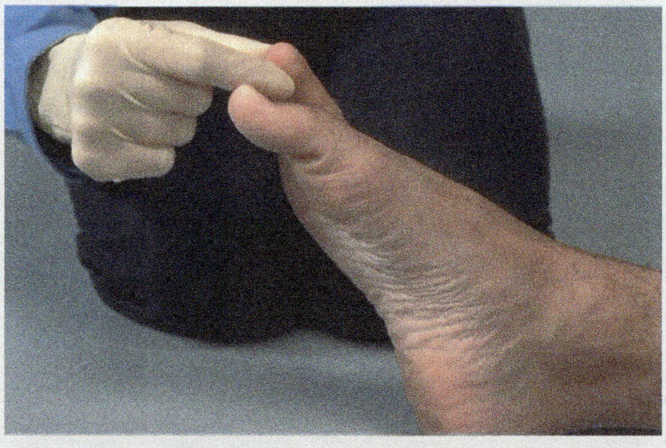

8. Assess distal sensation in the lower extremities by asking the patient "Which toe am I touching?" (Be sure the patient cannot see which toe.)

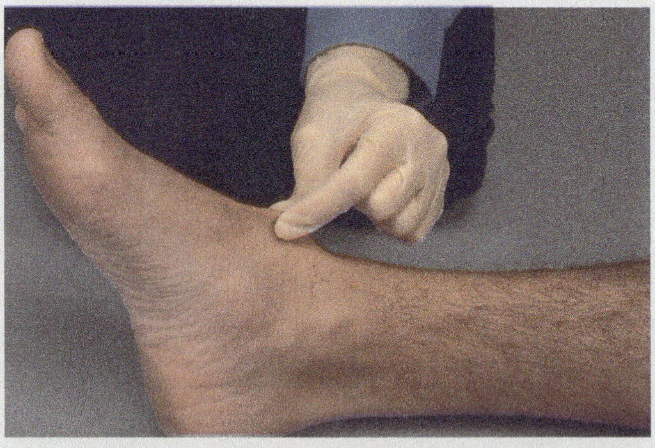

If the patient is unresponsive, check distal sensation in the lower extremities by pinching the top of the foot. Watch and listen for a response.

Rapid Assessment of the Posterior Body. Roll the patient onto the patient's side as a unit (you will learn how to do a log-roll maneuver in the chapter *Trauma to the Head, Neck, and Spine*) and assess the posterior body, inspecting and palpating for wounds, tenderness, and deformities in the area of the spine and to the sides of the spine, the buttocks, and the posterior extremities. This may be a good opportunity to slide in an extrication device, such as a backboard or soft sleeve, to enable movement of the patient. Follow local protocols.

One method of stabilizing an injured pelvis is forming a pelvic wrap from a folded sheet or using a commercially available pelvic sling. (You will learn about how to apply a pelvic wrap in the chapter *Musculoskeletal Trauma*.) Become familiar with how local medical direction wishes you to manage these patients.

Obtain Baseline Vital Signs and Past Medical History. Quickly obtain a set of baseline vital signs, as discussed in the chapter *Vital Signs and Monitoring Devices*. If using a pulse oximeter as part of your assessment, apply it now (or earlier if your local protocol suggests doing so). If the patient is unresponsive, you will not be able to get a past medical history from the patient. If there is a friend or family member nearby, that person may be able to give you information about the patient's medical history.

Some General Principles

Several important principles to remember when examining a patient, which are mentioned throughout the chapter, are summarized in the following list:

- Tell the patient what you are going to do. In particular, let the patient know when there may be pain or discomfort. Stress the importance of the examination, and work to build the patient's confidence. Ask the patient if he or she understands what you are doing, and explain your actions again if needed.
- Expose any injured area before examining it. By exposing areas, you can see such things as bruises and puncture wounds. Let the patient know when you must lift, rearrange, or remove any article of clothing. Do all you can to ensure the patient's privacy.
- Try to maintain eye contact. Do not turn away while you are talking or while the patient is answering your questions.
- Apply your spinal protocols. Many serious trauma patients will receive spinal motion restriction because of the seriousness of their injuries or an altered mental status that prevents a full spinal examination. Others, because of the type of injury or lack of apparent spinal trauma, may not require motion restriction. Be sure you know your spinal protocols before you encounter a trauma patient.

Think Like an EMT

Rapid Trauma or Focused Exam?

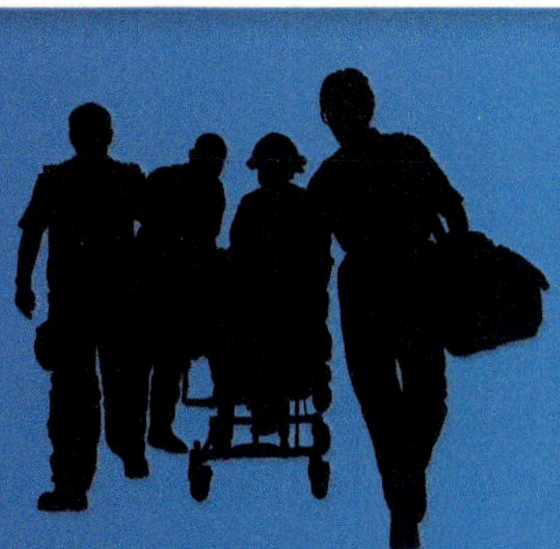

For each of the following patients, determine if you should perform a head-to-toe rapid trauma assessment or, instead, a physical exam focused on a specific area or injury.

1. Your patient was found unresponsive after being ejected from a vehicle in a rollover collision.
2. Your patient tripped and believes he broke his wrist. He complains of no other injuries.
3. Your patient complains of only minor neck pain after a frontal impact accident in which there was considerable damage and airbag deployment.
4. Your patient fell about six feet (1.8 meters) from a tree and believes he broke his ankle. Bystanders tell you he briefly lost consciousness.

- During the physical exam, you may stop or alter the assessment process to provide care that is necessary and appropriate for the priority of the patient. For a patient who is not a priority for rapid transport, you may pause to bandage a bleeding wound, even if the bleeding is not life-threatening, or to splint an injured extremity.
- During the rapid trauma assessment, apply a cervical collar if spine injury is suspected. For a patient who is a priority for rapid transport, treatments such as controlling non-life-threatening bleeding or splinting an injured extremity may take place en route to the hospital if time and the patient's condition permit.

Pediatric Examination

Head. Do not apply pressure to an infant's fontanelles ("soft spots"). The skin over the anterior fontanelle is normally level with the top of the skull or slightly sunken. It may bulge naturally when the infant cries or be abnormally sunken if the infant is dehydrated. Meningitis and head trauma cause the fontanelle to bulge due to increased intracranial pressure. Collisions involving infants and children can often produce head injuries (Figure 15-10 and Scan 15-7).

Nose and Ears. Look for blood and clear fluids coming from the nose and ears. Suspect skull fractures if either type of fluid is present. Children are nose breathers, so mucus or blood clot obstructions will make it hard for them to breathe.

Neck. Children are vulnerable to spinal cord injuries because of their proportionately larger and heavier heads. The neck offers less support because muscles and bone structures are less developed. In medical emergencies, the neck may be sore, stiff, or swollen. Young children may have significant spinal cord injuries even with no injury to the spinal bones because children's bones are often incompletely calcified and, therefore, difficult to fracture. However, traumatic force that did not fracture the child's spinal bones may have been transferred to the spinal cord, resulting in spinal cord injury. Therefore, do not allow the absence of bony abnormality to the neck or spine lead you to conclude that there is no spinal cord injury.

FIGURE 15-10 There are special areas to consider during pediatric assessment.

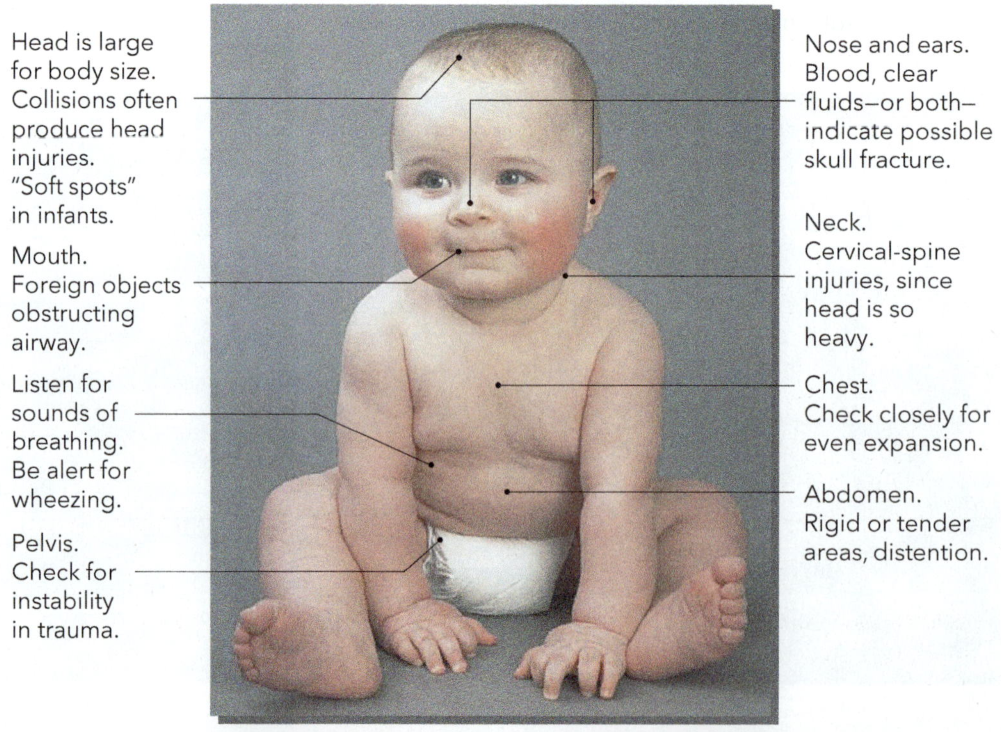

SCAN 15-7 The Pediatric Physical Examination

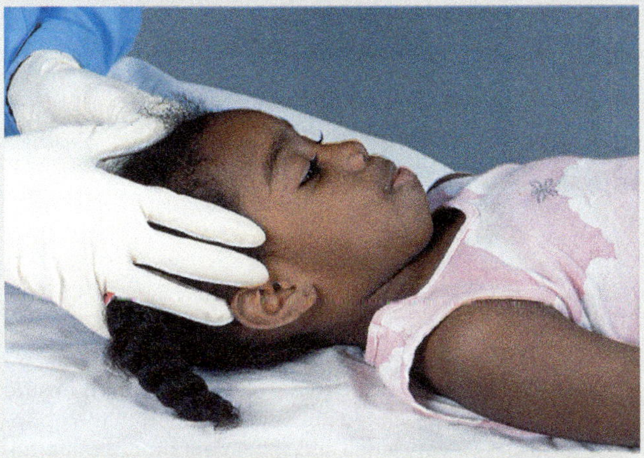

1. Examine the head. Look for bruising, or for blood or clear fluid draining from the nose or ears. Palpate gently for soft or spongy areas, skull irregularities, or crepitus (feeling of grinding bone fragments). Check the fontanelles in infants.

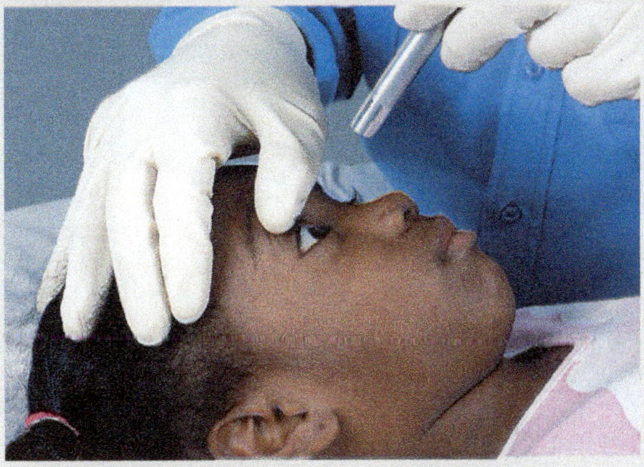

2. Check the eyes. The pupils should be equal in size and reactive to light.

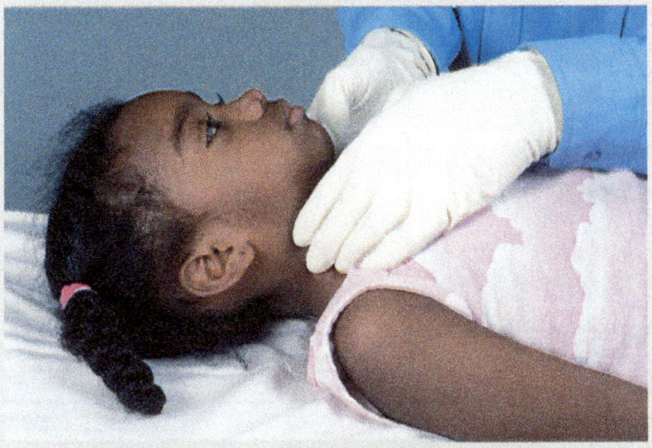

3. Examine the neck. Check for the position of the trachea, swollen neck veins, stiffness, tenderness, or crepitus.

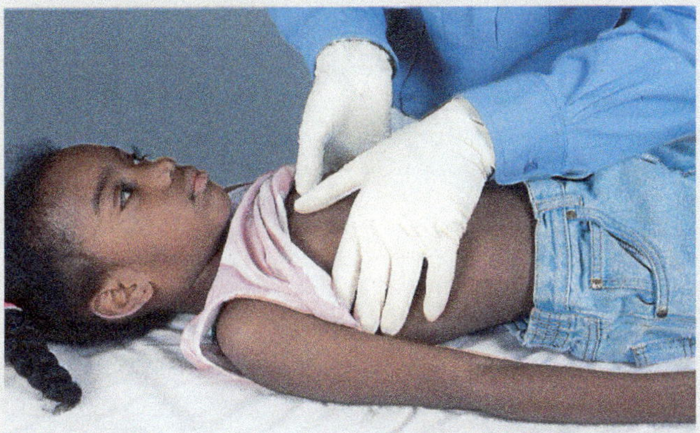

4. Examine the chest. Check for bruising, equal chest rise and fall, and crepitus. Watch for signs of breathing difficulty.

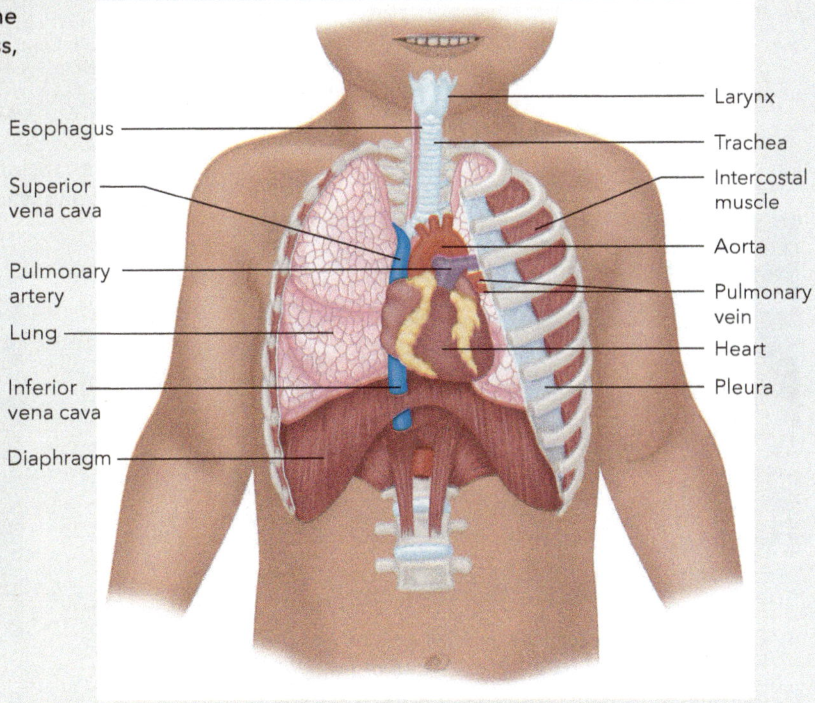

While examining the chest, be aware of the contents of the thorax.

(continued)

SCAN 15-7 The Pediatric Physical Examination *(continued)*

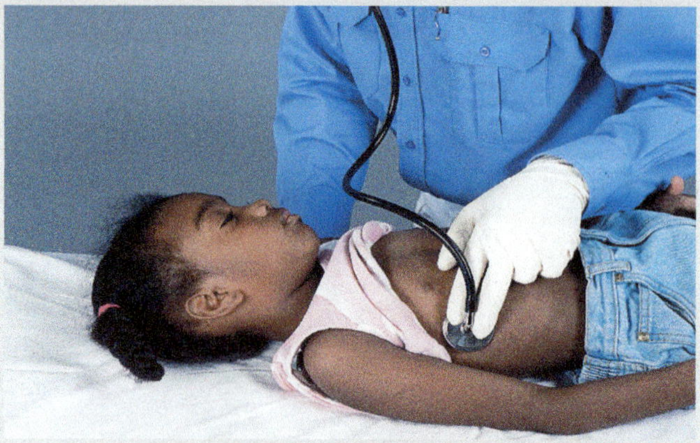

5. Auscultate for breath sounds over all lung fields.

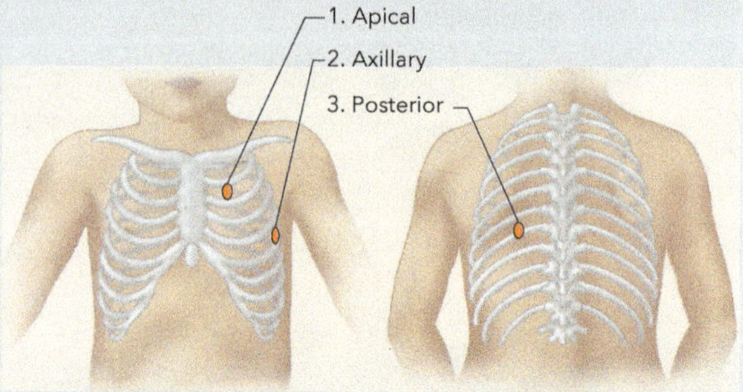

Auscultation sites. In infants, the lateral lung fields are best evaluated from the mid-axillary position to ensure that sounds appreciated are not referred from the opposite lung. The very small and thin infant thorax can artificially transmit sounds from one side of the chest to the other when auscultated from the front or back.

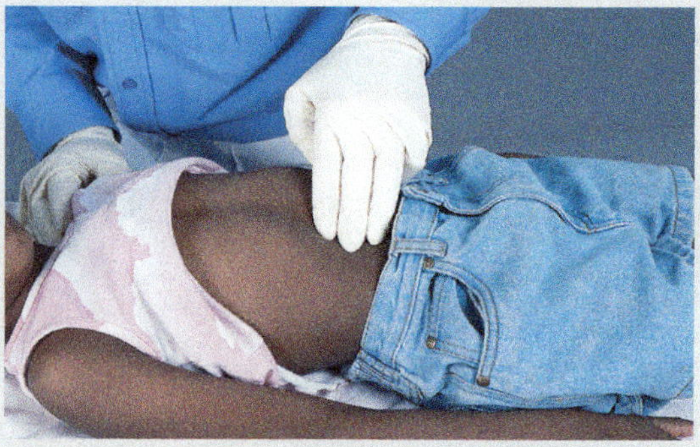

6. Examine the abdomen. Check for bruising, tenderness, or guarding. Look for swelling that may indicate swallowed air.

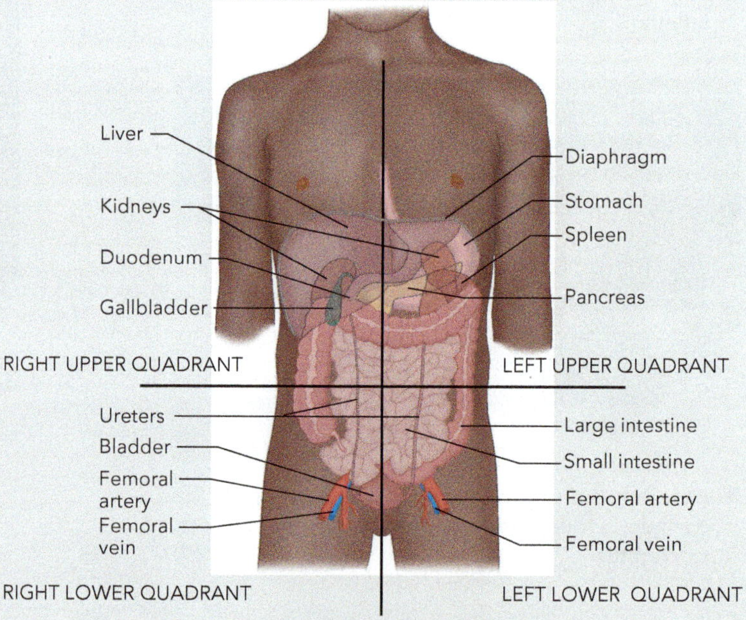

Divide the abdomen into quadrants and examine each one while remembering which organs are located in each quadrant.

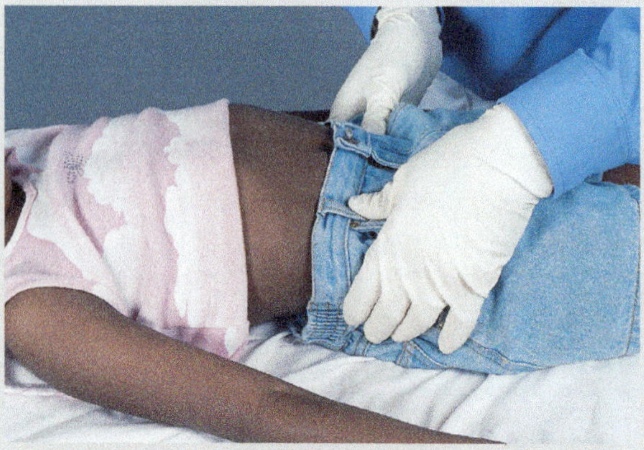

7. Examine the pelvis for tenderness, swelling, bruising, or crepitus. If the patient complains of pain, injury, or other problems in the genital area, assess for bruising, swelling, or tenderness in that area.

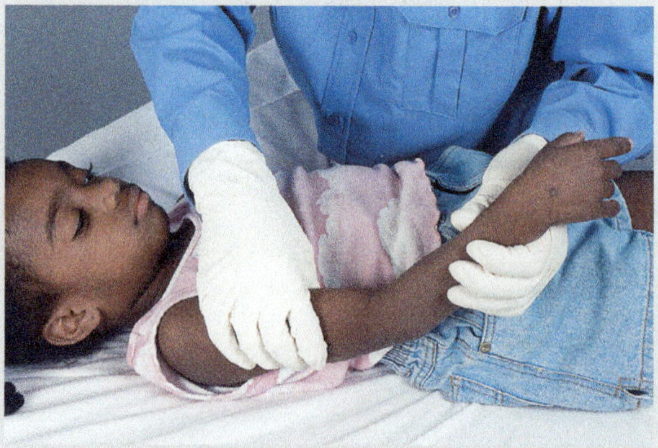

8. Examine the extremities. Evaluate pulses, sensation, and warmth. Look for unequal movement.

SCAN 15-7 The Pediatric Physical Examination *(continued)*

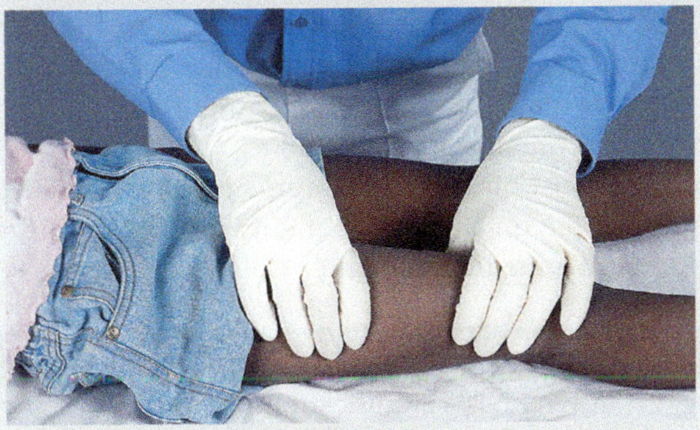

9. If you have immobilized an extremity, check the patient's capillary refill, peripheral pulses, and sensory status (if age-appropriate) and compare them with the other arm or leg.

NOTE: *You may choose a toe-to-head approach in lieu of the head-to-toe approach shown in this scan, depending on the patient's age, the level of apprehension the patient exhibits, and the severity of the patient's condition.*

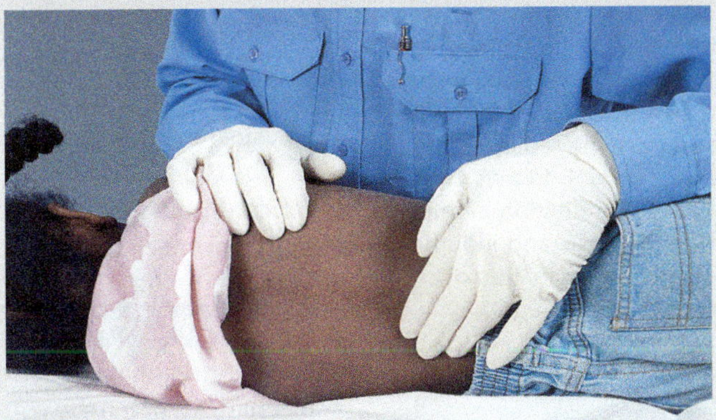

10. Examine the back. Assess for tenderness, bruising, and crepitus. If the child requires immobilization, the back can be checked while the child is being log-rolled onto the spine board.

Airway. Keep the infant's head in the neutral position and the child's head in the neutral-plus or sniffing position (chin thrust forward to maintain an open airway). If there is no suspicion of spinal injury, place a flat, folded towel under the patient's shoulders to get the appropriate airway alignment. Children's airways are more pliable and smaller than adults'. Hyperextension or hyperflexion may close off the airway. For medical respiratory problems, the child will probably want to sit up.

Chest. Listen closely for even air entry and the sounds of breathing on both sides of the chest. Be alert for wheezes and other noises. Check for symmetry, bruising, paradoxical movement, and retraction of the sternum or the muscles between the ribs. Remember that a child's soft ribs may not break, but there may be underlying injuries to the organs within the chest.

Abdomen. Note any rigid or tender areas and distention. Because a child's abdominal organs (especially the spleen and liver) are large in relation to the size of the abdominal cavity, and because there is little protection offered by the still-undeveloped abdominal muscles, these organs are more susceptible to trauma than an adult's. Because most children 8 years of age or younger are abdominal breathers, any injury that impedes the movement of the diaphragm can compromise a young child's breathing.

Pelvis. In the event of trauma, check for stability of the pelvic girdle.

Extremities. Perform an assessment with capillary refill and distal pulse, including a neurologic component for motor function with a sensation check. With an infant or young child, you do not have to press on a nail bed. You can quickly check capillary refill by squeezing a hand or foot, forearm, or lower leg. Check for painful, swollen, and deformed injury sites. (The bones of an infant or child are more pliable, so they bend, splinter, and buckle before they fracture.)

CORE CONCEPT
Detailed physical exam

Detailed Physical Exam

The primary assessment and the rapid trauma assessment are done quickly because of the necessity of getting the seriously injured or ill patient into the ambulance and to the hospital without delay. En route to the hospital, you may have time to do a more complete patient

detailed physical exam an assessment of the head, neck, chest, abdomen, pelvis, extremities, and posterior of the body to detect signs and symptoms of injury. It differs from the rapid trauma assessment only in that it also includes examination of the face, ears, eyes, nose, and mouth during the examination of the head.

assessment known as the ***detailed physical exam***. If you are not on a transporting unit and the ambulance has not arrived, you may do the detailed physical exam at the scene.

The purpose of the detailed physical exam is to gather additional information about the patient's injuries and conditions. Some of this information may help you to determine the proper treatment for the patient, and some of the information you gather in the detailed physical exam will assist the emergency department staff.

The detailed physical exam is performed most often on the trauma patient with a significant injury or mechanism of injury, less often on a trauma patient with no significant injury or mechanism of injury, and seldom on a medical patient.

Trauma Patient with a Significant Injury

For a trauma patient who is not responsive, or who has a significant injury or an unknown mechanism of injury, you will have assessed almost the entire body during the rapid trauma assessment—but very quickly. For this patient, a detailed physical exam may reveal signs or symptoms of injury that you missed or that have changed since the rapid trauma assessment.

Before Beginning the Detailed Physical Exam

It is important to remember that you should perform the detailed physical exam only after you have performed all critical interventions. The best way to ensure this is to repeat your primary assessment before you begin the detailed physical exam. To do this, reassess your general impression of the patient, focusing on the patient's mental status, plus airway, breathing, and circulation.

If you are treating a severely injured patient, you may be too busy to begin or complete the detailed physical exam at all. This is not a failure on your part. Your responsibility is to give the patient the best care possible under the difficult conditions found in the field. If you do not do a complete assessment, but you keep a critical patient's airway, breathing, and circulation intact, you have helped the patient far more than if you had done the complete assessment. *Performing a detailed physical exam is always a lower priority than addressing life-threatening problems.* Box 15-2 shows the place of the detailed physical exam among the priorities and sequence of assessment.

Performing the Detailed Physical Exam

If you have not already exposed the patient, you need to do so now. Since you are now in the enclosed ambulance, it is much easier to protect the patient's privacy and protect the patient from exposure to the environment.

The detailed physical exam will look a lot like the rapid trauma assessment that you did during the secondary assessment. You will look for the familiar signs of wounds, tenderness, and deformity.

The detailed physical exam is similar to the rapid trauma assessment—with some important differences:

- The exam usually takes place in the ambulance, en route. Noise and motion may interfere with some procedures.

BOX 15-2 Detailed Physical Exam in the Sequence of Assessment Priorities

1. Scene size-up
2. Primary assessment and critical interventions for immediately life-threatening problems
3. Patient history, rapid physical exam, vital signs, plus interventions as needed
4. Repeat primary assessment for immediately life-threatening problems. Provide critical interventions as needed.
5. Detailed physical exam (time and critical-care needs permitting)
6. Reassessment for life-threatening problems, plus reassessment of vital signs. Provide critical interventions as needed.

- If spinal precautions have been taken or if splinting devices are in place, you must work around them—for example, by examining the neck through openings in the rigid collar, and examining only as much of the posterior as you can reach.

There are only a few differences in the rest of the exam compared with what you did in the rapid trauma assessment. These differences result from either the different environment (the back of the ambulance) or the treatment you have already given to the patient (e.g., cervical collar).

When you assess the neck, you may be limited by the cervical collar that you placed on the patient during the secondary assessment (rapid trauma assessment). You will not be able to inspect or palpate the back of the neck, but you will be able to assess for wounds, tenderness, deformities, jugular vein distention (JVD), and crepitation through the openings in the collar. You should make sure the collars you use have these openings. Remember that some degree of JVD may be a normal finding in a supine patient but is always an abnormal finding in a seated patient.

Reassessing the chest can be a challenge in a moving ambulance. You can reassess for anything you can palpate, such as crepitation or flail chest. However, because of road noise, breath sounds may be difficult to hear. Just keep in mind that you are auscultating for the presence and equality of breath sounds in your trauma patient, not the different kinds of abnormal sounds that are more common in medical patients. If you are unable to hear breath sounds because of road noise, it is generally better to continue transporting the patient to the hospital. It makes little sense to stop the ambulance and delay transport unless you can do something to treat an abnormality you find. Reassess the abdomen and pelvis as in the rapid assessment.

Any deformities or other indications of a musculoskeletal injury to an extremity found during the rapid trauma assessment will most likely have been temporarily immobilized by securing the patient to the stretcher or long spine board. It is unlikely that taking time to splint such injuries would have been appropriate at the scene, when rapid transport was a priority. En route to the hospital, if the patient's other injuries are not keeping you too busy, it may be a good time to apply a splint to an injured extremity after you perform the detailed physical exam. You will learn splinting techniques in the chapter *Musculoskeletal Trauma*.

When it comes to reassessing the posterior body, it would most likely be inappropriate to roll the patient while the ambulance was in motion. Unless there is a significant change or new finding, your primary concern at this point is to evaluate as much of the posterior body as you can reach for other injuries that may have been missed earlier. Simply reassess the flanks (sides) and as much of the spinal area as you can touch without moving the patient.

Although the rest of the detailed physical exam is essentially the same as the rapid trauma assessment, you have more time, so you can be more thorough. This is especially true with long transports in rural or wilderness areas.

Your next priority is to make sure that the emergency department is ready for your patient by using the ambulance radio or cellular phone to notify the emergency department of the patient's condition. Depending on how far you are from the hospital and what your local protocols say, you may do this step before the detailed physical exam. If you have not yet notified the hospital, you should do it now. You will learn more about what to say to hospital personnel and how to say it in the chapter *Communication and Documentation*.

Trauma Patient Who Is Not Seriously Injured

When caring for a trauma patient who is responsive and has no significant injury or mechanism of injury, you will have focused your assessment on just the areas the patient tells you hurt, plus those areas that you suspect may be injured based on the mechanism of injury.

This kind of patient received all the assessment they needed while still at the scene. The patient does not generally need a detailed physical exam. It is important to keep a high index of suspicion, though. When in doubt, do a detailed physical exam. Be aware of the responsive trauma patient's fear and need for emotional support.

You should perform a detailed physical exam on a trauma patient who has a significant injury (or mechanism of injury) and on any patient who has an unclear or unknown mechanism of injury. However, the detailed physical exam typically takes a different form in trauma patients than in medical patients. This is because there are usually few signs an EMT can find in the physical exam of a medical patient that are significant or about which an EMT can or should do anything. Most of the assessment information on medical patients comes from the history and vital signs.

Occasionally you may come across a patient who could be either medical or trauma—or both. For example, imagine you have responded to an elderly man who is found alone and unconscious, slumped over the steering wheel of his car. The car is off the road and there is no damage to it. Did the patient lose consciousness first, then drive his car off the road, or did he drive off the road and get knocked out from a blow to the head? The safest and best thing to do for a patient such as this is generally to treat them as a trauma patient who gets a rapid trauma assessment and, if there is time, a detailed physical exam—but whenever possible, also get a history from any witnesses you can find.

Chapter Review

Secondary Assessment of the Trauma Patient

Key Facts and Concepts

- The patient without a significant mechanism of injury receives a history of the present illness and physical exam focused on areas that the patient complains about and areas that you think may be injured based on the mechanism of injury.
- Next, gather a set of baseline vital signs and a patient history.
- For the patient with a significant injury or MOI, provide spinal precautions, consider whether to call advanced life support personnel (if available), get a brief patient history, and perform a rapid trauma assessment.
- In the rapid trauma assessment, look for wounds, tenderness, and deformities, plus certain additional signs appropriate to the part being assessed (as summarized in Table 15-5). Systematically examine the head, neck, chest, abdomen, pelvis, extremities, and posterior body.
- After assessing the neck, it may be appropriate to apply a cervical collar. After completing the physical assessment, provide spine motion restrictions and get a baseline set of vital signs and a past medical history.
- After you have performed the appropriate critical interventions and begun transport, the patient may receive a detailed physical exam en route to the hospital.
- The detailed physical exam is very similar to the rapid trauma assessment, but there is time to be more thorough in the assessment. The detailed physical exam does not take place before transport unless transport is delayed.
- The detailed physical exam is most appropriate for the trauma patient who is unresponsive or has a significant injury or unknown MOI.
- A responsive trauma patient with no significant injury or MOI will seldom require a detailed physical exam.

Key Decisions

- Does this patient have an injury or mechanism of injury severe enough to suggest a rapid trauma assessment is appropriate?
- Should we apply a cervical collar to this patient?
- How should the task of assessment be divided when there are two EMTs at the scene?

Chapter Glossary

detailed physical exam an assessment of the head, neck, chest, abdomen, pelvis, extremities, and posterior of the body to detect signs and symptoms of injury. It differs from the rapid trauma assessment only in that it also includes examination of the face, ears, eyes, nose, and mouth during the examination of the head.

distention (dis-TEN-shun) a condition of being stretched, inflated, or larger than normal.

history of the present illness (HPI) information gathered regarding the symptoms and nature of the patient's current concern.

medical patient a patient with one or more medical diseases or conditions.

paradoxical (pair-uh-DOCK-si-kal) ***motion*** movement of a part of the chest in the opposite direction to the rest of the chest during respiration.

past medical history (PMH) information gathered regarding the patient's health problems in the past.

priapism (PRY-ah-pizm) persistent erection of the penis that may result from spinal injury and some medical problems.

rapid trauma assessment a rapid assessment of the head, neck, chest, abdomen, pelvis, extremities, and posterior of the body to detect signs and symptoms of injury.

reassessment a procedure for detecting changes in a patient's condition. It involves four steps: repeating the primary assessment, repeating and recording vital signs, repeating the physical exam, and checking interventions.

sign evidence of the patient's condition that you can see.

stoma (STO-ma) a permanent surgical opening in the neck through which the patient breathes.

symptom something regarding the patient's condition that the patient tells you.

tracheostomy (tray-ke-OS-to-me) a surgical incision held open by a metal or plastic tube.

trauma patient a patient suffering from one or more physical injuries.

Preparation for Your Examination and Practice

Short Answer

1. Should rapid trauma assessment be performed on all patients regardless of mechanism of injury?
2. What are the steps for rapid trauma assessment?
3. When do you provide a detailed physical examination on a patient who has experienced trauma?

Thinking and Linking

Think back to the Scene Size-Up *chapter and link information from that chapter with information from this chapter as you consider the following situation:*

1. You approach a scene and observe a pretty spectacular crash–a lot of damage to the vehicle. You think this could mean significant injury to your patient. Think of what you may find in the secondary assessment that would validate or disprove that observation.
2. List the steps of the rapid trauma assessment, and describe the kind of patient for whom the rapid trauma assessment is appropriate.
3. List the areas covered in the detailed physical exam. What do you look and feel for as you assess each of these areas?
4. You have been dispatched to the scene of a car that struck a light pole. You have gained access to the front seat and are beginning your assessment of a female adolescent who appears to be seriously injured. From the corner of your eye, you suddenly notice that the transformer is starting to spark. What should you do?

Critical Thinking Exercises

Trauma can take many forms and vary from minor to critical. The purpose of this exercise will be to consider how you might deal with the following situations.

1. You are assessing a patient who fell three stories. He is unresponsive and bleeding into his airway. The driver of the ambulance is positioning the vehicle and bringing equipment to you. How do you balance the patient's need for airway control (he requires frequent suctioning) with your need to assess his injuries?
2. As an EMT, how would you balance the need for appropriate on-scene assessment and treatment with the need for speed in getting the patient to the hospital in each of the following situations?
   - You arrive at a residence to find a patient who explains that he has accidentally cut his finger with a kitchen knife. The cut is bleeding profusely.
   - You arrive at a schoolyard to find a girl who bystanders say was shot by a rival gang member. She is lying in a pool of blood but is able to speak to you.
   - You are called to respond to a man who has been found unconscious on a sidewalk next to an apartment building in the middle of the night. There were no witnesses to explain what may have happened to him.

Pathophysiology to Practice

The following question is designed to assist you in gathering relevant clinical information and making accurate decisions in the field.

- A patient with a chest injury may have a lung collapse. Why are the breath sounds on the injured side typically decreased or absent when the chest cavity is filled with air, which usually transmits sounds very well?

Street Scenes

It's Saturday night and you've been assigned to one of the ambulances that covers downtown, where there is usually some kind of excitement going on. As you sit in quarters, you're listening to the scanner. The police seem to be busy with a variety of calls—disturbances, domestics, and larcenies, to name a few. Then you hear on the police frequency: "Dispatch, we need an ambulance ASAP. We have a stabbing here." You don't wait for your pager to activate before you're in the ambulance bay with your partner. The pager follows shortly: "Delta 55, respond to 1512 Broadway, outside, for a stabbing. Police on the scene, and scene is secure."

Your response takes only a few minutes. When you arrive, you see a male in his twenties lying on the sidewalk. "What happened?" you ask him.

"Some punks punched me in the face and threw me into the street when they stole my wallet."

At this point, you tell the patient not to move his head. The patient continues, "When I tried to fight them off, they stabbed me in the chest."

The patient's airway is open, but he is out of breath and his breathing is rapid and shallow. You check the chest and see the entrance wound. You listen for breath sounds. There is silence on the side of the wound. You put on an occlusive dressing and administer oxygen by nonrebreather mask. You then rapidly check for external bleeding.

Street Scene Questions

1. What is the priority of this patient?
2. What should be done next?
3. When should vital signs be taken?

You and your partner agree that this patient needs to be rapidly transported to the trauma center. Your partner gets a cervical collar and the stretcher. You perform a rapid physical exam from head to toe. The patient has abrasions on the left cheek, the left wrist is swollen with pain on movement, and there is tenderness in both lower abdominal quadrants. Your partner takes a set of vital signs. You decide to do the patient history in the ambulance. You transfer the patient to the stretcher. During the move, you check the patient's back for any wound, bleeding, or tenderness.

Once the patient is loaded in the ambulance, your partner starts toward the hospital with red lights and siren. The patient is still conscious, but he is having trouble talking in complete sentences. He reports a lot of discomfort. You think there may be pressure building up in his chest because of an injury to the lung.

Street Scene Questions

4. What should you do next?
5. What should be done for the detailed physical exam, if there is time before reaching the trauma center?

You are confident that you need to treat the patient's worsening difficulty breathing. You lift the corner of the occlusive dressing and hear some air escape. The patient starts to breathe easier almost immediately. You take another set of vital signs. Then you secure the bandage over the chest wound again. You turn your attention to the detailed exam, starting at the head, then moving to the chest and abdomen, and finally ending with all four extremities and as much of the back as you can reach. With each location, you check for wounds, tenderness, and deformities.

The remainder of the transport is uneventful. You transfer the patient to the hospital with an updated prehospital care report that includes the latest set of vital signs.

Reassessment

16

Related Chapters

The following chapters provide additional information related to topics discussed in this chapter:

11 Scene Size-Up
12 Primary Assessment
13 Vital Signs and Monitoring Devices
17 Communication and Documentation

Standards

Assessment (Secondary Assessment; Reassessment)
Clinical Behavior/Judgment (Decision Making)

Competencies

Applies scene information and patient assessment findings (scene size-up, primary and secondary assessments, patient history, and reassessment) to guide emergency management.

Initiates basic interventions based on assessment findings intended to mitigate the emergency and provide limited symptom relief while providing access to definitive care.

Core Concepts

- Observing trends during reassessment
- Reassessment for stable and for unstable patients

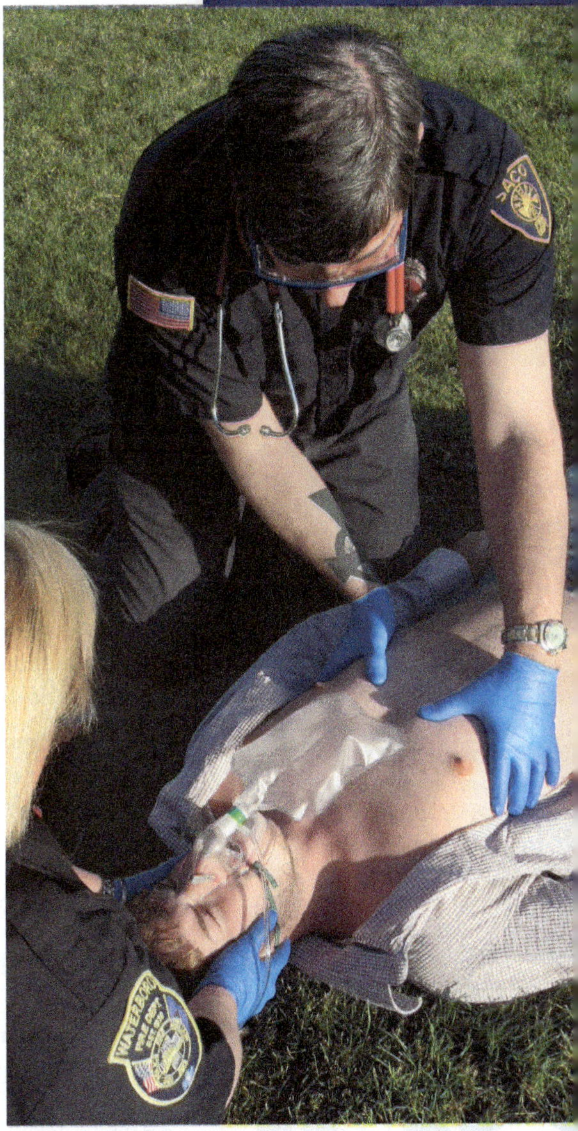

(© Daniel Limmer)

Outcomes

After reading this chapter, you should be able to:

16.1 Analyze the components in your approach to re-evaluating patients in EMS scenarios. (pp. 454–459)

- Evaluate patient status based on trending assessment findings.
- Compare the approaches to reassessing stable and unstable patients.

Key Terms

reassessment, *454* trending, *457*

"Never let your guard down. Assess, reassess, and then assess again. You aren't done until you get to the hospital."

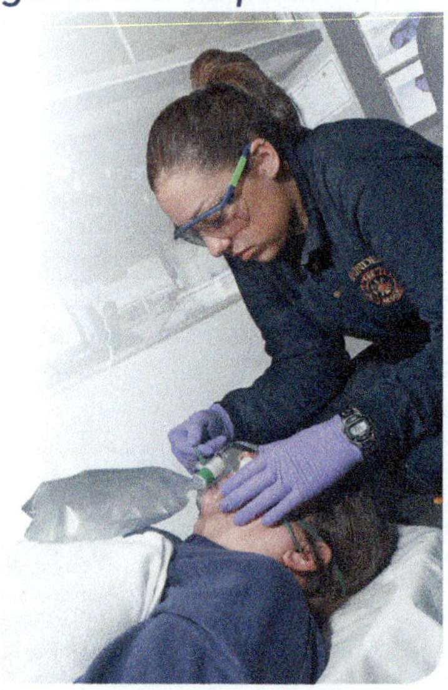

Reassessment

It is important to observe and reobserve your patient, not only to determine the patient's condition at first sight, but also to detect any changes. The patient may exhibit an obvious change, such as loss of consciousness, or more subtle differences, such as restlessness, anxiety, or sweating. These may indicate a change in circulation. Some patients may take a turn for the worse before they reach the hospital, although this is uncommon. In some cases, you may see patient improvement, possibly in response to interventions you perform. You will be able to detect these changes by performing a series of steps called ***reassessment***.

reassessment
a procedure for detecting changes in a patient's condition. It involves four steps: repeating the primary assessment, repeating and recording vital signs, repeating the physical exam, and checking interventions.

You will perform reassessment on every patient after you have finished performing interventions and, often, after you have done the detailed physical exam. Sometimes you may skip doing a detailed physical exam because you are too busy taking care of life-threatening problems, or you have a medical or noncritical trauma patient for whom the detailed physical exam would not yield useful information. *Reassessment, however, must never be skipped except when lifesaving interventions prevent you from doing it*. Even in the latter situation, one partner can often perform the reassessment while the other continues lifesaving care.

Throughout the assessment procedures that take place on the way to the hospital, remember to explain to a conscious patient what you are doing, to talk in a reassuring tone, and to consider the patient's feelings, such as anxiety or embarrassment.

Components of Reassessment

During the reassessment, you will repeat key elements of assessment procedures you have already performed. For example, you will repeat the primary assessment (to check for life-threatening problems), reassess vital signs, repeat the physical exam related to the patient's specific complaint or injuries, and check any interventions you have performed. (See Scan 16-1.)

Pediatric Note

Remember to maintain eye contact with a conscious child, stay on the child's level as much as possible, and explain what you are doing in a quiet and reassuring voice.

SCAN 16-1 Reassessment

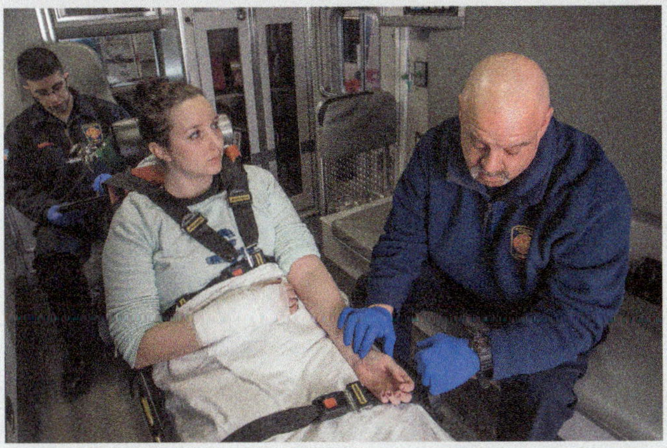

1. Repeat the primary assessment.

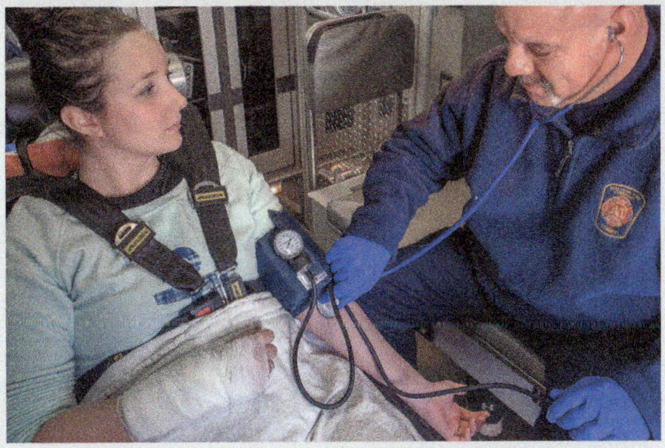

2. Reassess and record vital signs.

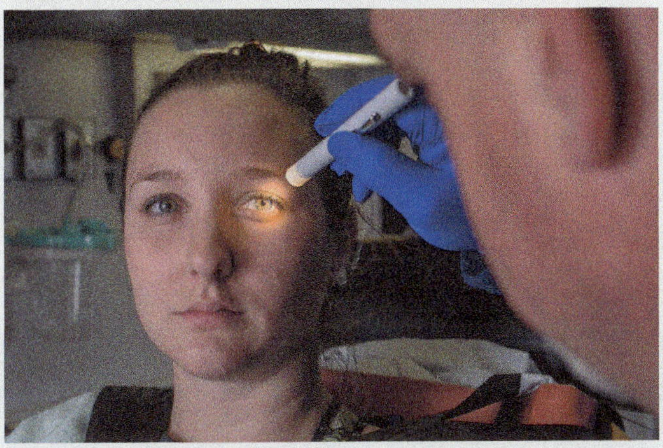

3. Repeat pertinent parts of the secondary assessment.

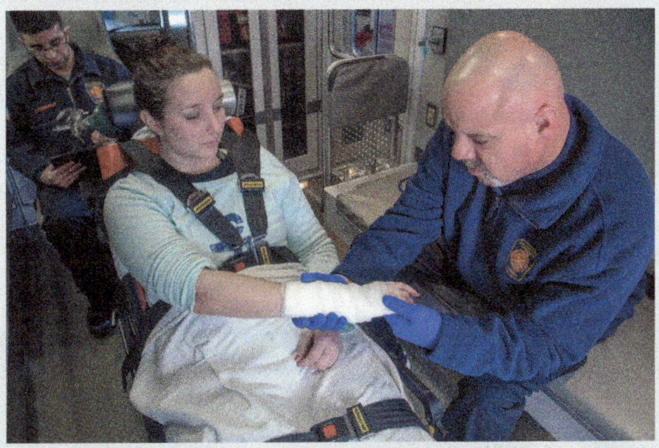

4. Check interventions.

Repeat the Primary Assessment

Begin reassessment by repeating the primary assessment to recheck for life-threatening problems:

- Reassess mental status.
- Maintain an open airway.
- Monitor breathing for rate and quality.
- Reassess the pulse for rate and quality.
- Monitor skin color and temperature.
- Reestablish patient priorities.

Remember, life-threatening problems that were not present or that were brought under control during the primary assessment may develop or redevelop before the patient reaches the hospital. For example, the mental status of the patient who was responsive and alert may begin to deteriorate, which is a significant trend and a worrisome sign. The airway that was open may become occluded, patients who were breathing adequately on their own may now require respiratory support, and other signs—such as a rapid pulse, cool skin, and pallor—may indicate the onset of shock. Life threats must be continually watched, and managed immediately when discovered.

Pediatric Note

The mental status of an unresponsive child or infant can be checked by speaking loudly (verbal stimulus) or flicking the feet (painful stimulus). Crying would be an expected response from a child with an adequate mental status.

Reassess and Record Vital Signs

During the secondary assessment, you took and recorded a set of baseline vital signs: pulse, respiration, skin, pupils, and blood pressure. During reassessment, you will reassess and record the vital signs, comparing the results with the earlier baseline measurements and any other vital sign measurements you may have taken (for example, during the detailed physical exam, if you conducted one). Reevaluate oxygen saturation if you previously assessed it.

It is especially important to record each vital sign measurement as soon as you obtain it. In this way, you will not need to worry about remembering the different numbers you get for pulse rate, blood pressure, respiratory rate, and oxygen saturation. When you have more than one set of vital signs, it becomes even easier to forget them if you have not written them down. Another reason to document your reassessment is so you can see trends in the patient's condition, which we will discuss later in this chapter.

Point of View

"Do you know what I hate? I hate when a medical person does a test and doesn't tell you what the result is.

"The EMTs were polite and knew what they were doing, but I really wish they would have told me what my blood pressure was. And my pulse. They take it, write it down, talk about it, but they don't tell me what it is.

"I take mine at home and write it down so my doctor can see how I am doing between appointments. I've had high blood pressure for years. I was going to ask, but they were so busy. I didn't want to bother them."

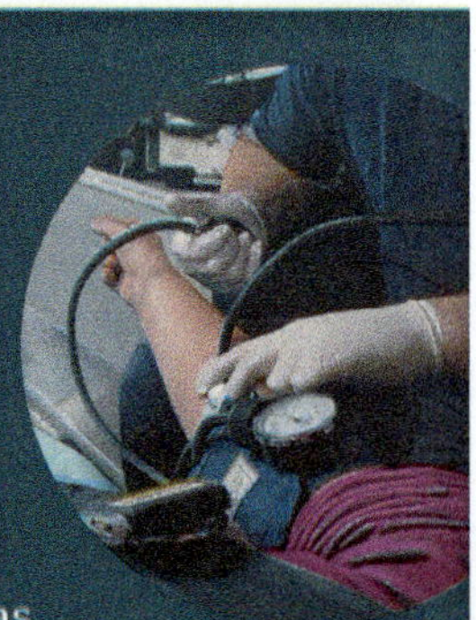

Repeat Pertinent Parts of the History and Physical Exam

A patient's chief complaint may change over time, especially with regard to its severity. Ask the patient about changes in symptoms, especially ones that you anticipate because of treatments you have administered. At the same time, be careful not to suggest particular answers to the patient.

You may also find changes as you repeat the physical exam. For example, a chest injury may become apparent as muscles get tired and you see paradoxical motion that was not present or noticeable when you first assessed the patient. (Paradoxical motion is present when a part of the chest goes in as the patient inhales and goes out as the patient exhales, opposite to the motion of the rest of the chest.) The abdomen may become distended, a sign that you are especially likely to see if you have a long transport. As you learn more about specific injuries and illnesses in later chapters, you will learn more signs to look for in your reassessment.

Check Interventions

Whenever you check the interventions that you have performed for a patient, try to take a fresh look at the patient. Attempt to be as observant as if you had never seen the patient before. This may help you to evaluate the adequacy of your interventions more objectively and to adjust them as necessary. Always do the following:

- Ensure adequacy of oxygen delivery and artificial ventilation.
- Ensure the management of any bleeding is effective.
- Ensure adequacy of other interventions.

Situations change. The fact that you put the patient on oxygen initially does not prevent the tank from running out later, or the tubing from becoming kinked or disconnected. A good habit to develop is to check the entire path of the oxygen from the tank to the patient. This means looking at the regulator on the tank and confirming that it has sufficient oxygen, and that the flowmeter is set to the proper flow. Make sure that the tube is firmly connected to the regulator. Follow the tubing and make sure there are no kinks that would prevent the flow of oxygen. Look at the mask or cannula. Make sure the tubing is connected to it and that it is the proper device. Confirm that it is properly positioned on the patient's face and, if it is a nonrebreather mask, that the nonrebreather bag does not completely deflate when the patient inhales. Increase the flow rate if it does. With practice, this sequence of steps will take just a few seconds.

Wounds that have stopped bleeding can start bleeding again, so it is important to check them as part of reassessment. Check any bandage you have applied and make sure it is dry, with no blood seeping through. When an unbandaged wound is in a location where you cannot see it, gently palpate it with gloved hands and check your gloves for blood.

Also be sure to check other interventions, such as cervical collars, stretcher straps, and splints. Any of these can slip and need adjustment.

CORE CONCEPT
Observing trends during reassessment

Observing Trends

Because reassessment is a means of determining ***trending*** (changes over time) in the patient's condition, you will need to repeat the reassessment steps frequently. Be sure to record your findings and compare them with earlier findings. It is important to notice and document any changes or trends. In later chapters, you will learn about specific trends to look for in patients' vital signs. For example, when you reach the chapter *Bleeding and Shock*, you will learn about trends in the pulse rate and blood pressure as signs of shock.

trending
changes in a patient's condition over time, such as slowing respirations or rising pulse rate, that may show improvement.

Based on your findings, you may need to institute new treatments or adjust treatments you have already started. Your findings, in particular any trends you have noted, will also be important information for the hospital staff, and will let them know if the patient's condition is improving or deteriorating.

CORE CONCEPT
Reassessment for stable and for unstable patients

Reassessment for Stable and Unstable Patients

The patient's condition, as well as the length of time you spend with the patient, will determine just how often you will conduct the reassessment. The more serious the patient's condition, the more often you will do it. Remember that with an unstable patient, you will likely be in a constant state of reassessment and care. Some guidelines suggest reassessing your patient at these intervals:

- Every 15 minutes for a stable patient, such as a patient who is alert, has vital signs in the normal range, and has no serious injury
- Every 5 minutes for an unstable or potentially unstable patient, such as a patient who has an altered mental status; difficulty with airway, breathing, or circulation, including severe blood loss; or vital signs indicating instability or potential instability

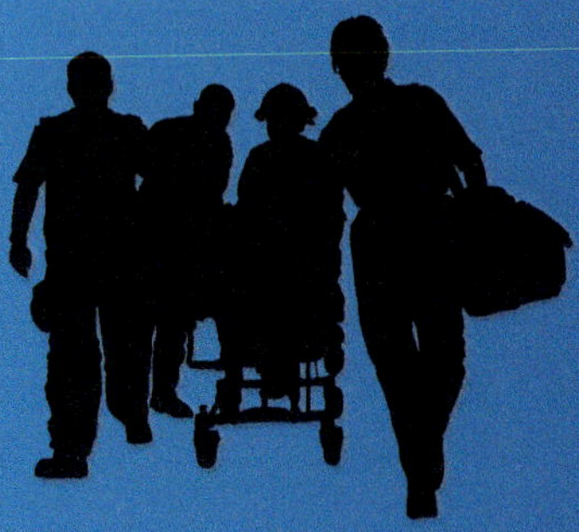

Think Like an EMT

Trending Vital Signs

Observing a trend in vital signs—trending—is more valuable than getting an individual set of vital signs. Observing trends is essential for making accurate decisions regarding transport destination and whether ALS may be necessary. Look at the following sets of vital signs for three patients and determine the trend for each patient.

1. A 32-year-old male fell about 15 feet (4.5 meters) from a roof and has multiple injuries. His vital signs have been:

TIME	PULSE	BLOOD PRESSURE	RESPIRATORY RATE	SKIN
2140	88	120/90	20, shallow	Pale but dry
2155	98	100/80	22, shallow	Pale but dry
2200	110	90/60	24, full	Pale but dry

How would you describe the trend of his vital signs: deteriorating, essentially unchanged, returning to normal, or not possible to determine?

2. A 64-year-old female fell to the floor and is complaining of hip pain. Her vital signs have been:

TIME	PULSE	BLOOD PRESSURE	RESPIRATORY RATE	SKIN
1330	108	160/90	24, shallow	Pale but dry
1345	112	150/90	20, shallow	Pale but dry
1350	96	140/80	20, full	Pale but dry

How would you describe the trend of her vital signs: deteriorating, essentially unchanged, returning to normal, or not possible to determine?

3. A 19-year-old female injured her left ankle and lower leg in a soccer game. Her vital signs have been:

TIME	PULSE	BLOOD PRESSURE	RESPIRATORY RATE	SKIN
1922	108	126/96	20, shallow	Pale and sweaty
1930	116	110/80	22, shallow	Pale and sweaty
1935	124	90/70	22, full	Pale and sweaty

How would you describe the trend of her vital signs: deteriorating, essentially unchanged, returning to normal, or not possible to determine?

Whenever you believe there may have been a change in the patient's condition, repeat at least the primary assessment. In this way, you will detect signs of life-threatening conditions as soon as possible. When in doubt, repeat reassessment every 5 minutes or as frequently as possible (Figure 16-1).

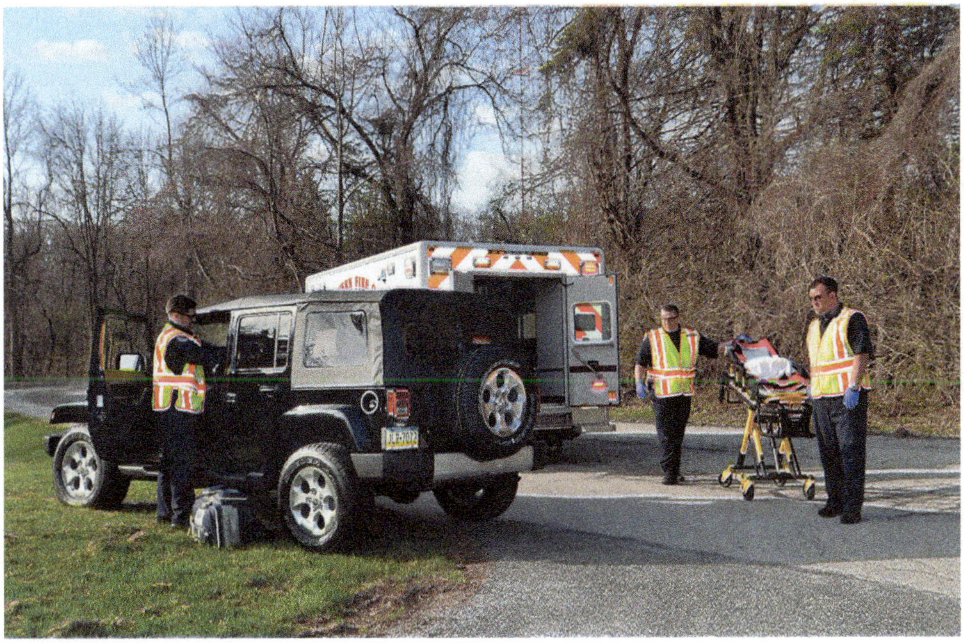

FIGURE 16-1 In rural EMS, long transport distances and times may dictate many reassessments—at least every 15 minutes for a stable patient, at least every 5 minutes for an unstable patient.
(© Edward T. Dickinson, MD)

Chapter Review

Key Facts and Concepts

- Reassessment is the last step in your patient assessment.
- You should generally reassess a stable patient at least every 15 minutes and an unstable patient at least every 5 minutes.
- Elements of reassessment include repeating the primary assessment, repeating and recording vital signs, repeating pertinent parts of the history and physical exam, and checking any treatments or interventions you performed for the patient.
- Treatments you need to check include oxygen, bleeding, spinal motion restriction, and splints.

Key Decisions

- Has the patient's condition changed in any way that indicates the need for new interventions? Is the airway clear? Is breathing adequate? Is circulation intact?
- Are the interventions I performed functioning as they should?
- Do I need to adjust any of the interventions I initially applied?

Chapter Glossary

reassessment a procedure for detecting changes in a patient's condition. It involves four steps: repeating the primary assessment, repeating and recording vital signs, repeating the physical exam, and checking interventions.

trending changes in a patient's condition over time, such as slowing respirations or rising pulse rate, that may show improvement.

Preparation for Your Examination and Practice

Short Answer

1. Name the four steps of reassessment, and list what assessments you will make during each step.
2. Explain the value of recording, or documenting, your assessment findings, and explain the meaning of the term *trending*.

Thinking and Linking

Think back to the Principles of Pathophysiology *chapter and link information from that chapter with information from this chapter as you consider the following situation.*

- You are transporting an 80-year-old man with general weakness that, according to his description, has been coming and going all morning. His initial vital signs were pulse 84, blood pressure 130/80, respirations 18 and full, SpO_2 98 percent. En route, he tells you that he's having one of his "weak spells" and that he's also dizzy. You check his vital signs again and find the following: pulse 180, blood pressure 90/70, respirations 22 and full, SpO_2 95 percent. How would an extremely rapid pulse cause such a change in vital signs and his chief complaint?

Critical Thinking Exercises

The reassessment must be conducted with the same care and attention to needed interventions as in the primary and secondary assessments. The purpose of this exercise will be to consider how you might manage certain situations you might discover during reassessment.

- What do you need to do if your reassessment turns up one of these findings?
  1. Gurgling respirations
  2. Bag on nonrebreather mask collapses completely when the patient inhales
  3. Snoring respirations

Pathophysiology to Practice

The following question is designed to assist you in gathering relevant clinical information and making accurate decisions in the field.

- Your patient is having an asthma attack. Her breathing rate is normal at 12 breaths per minute, but her blood oxygen level (SpO_2) is too low. Why?

Street Scenes

You receive a call for an elderly woman with a possible stroke. After taking the appropriate Standard Precautions, you ensure scene safety and enter the house. An older man, identifying himself as the patient's husband, meets you at the door. As he leads you to the kitchen, he explains that he came home after being out for a while and found his wife unable to stand up. When you reach the kitchen, you find Althea Stokes sitting in a chair.

Your general impression is of an older woman who appears awake but is slumped onto her left side. As you introduce yourself, you notice the patient's eyes are open and she appears awake, but her speech is slow and slurred. She does not appear to be in pain. A small amount of saliva is drooling onto her blouse. Her airway is open (at least for the moment); breathing appears normal and unlabored; there is no sign of bleeding; and her radial pulse is strong, slightly rapid, and very irregular. You assign Mrs. Stokes a medium priority as a medical patient. In your basic-life-support system, calling for advanced life support is not an option.

Street Scene Questions

1. **How does the patient's mental status affect the way you maintain the patient's airway?**
2. **What questions should you ask the patient and her husband?**

You wipe the saliva away from the patient's mouth and consider how to maintain her airway. If she loses consciousness, you should be prepared to suction. In the meantime, you make a mental note to keep an eye on further potential threats to her airway.

Since the patient is having difficulty speaking, you get most of the history from Mr. Stokes. His 82-year-old wife is usually alert and very active, he informs you. She was fine when he left about four hours ago, but when he came home, she was slumped over in the chair and couldn't seem to move her left arm and leg. When you ask Mrs. Stokes if she is having any pain or difficulty breathing, she slowly responds with slurred speech, "No, I'm not." As your partner gathers vital signs, you look at the patient more carefully. The right side of her face seems to be drooping, especially her cheek and upper eyelid. When you ask her to hold her arms out in front of her, she picks up her right arm but can barely move her left one. When you ask her to smile, only the left side of her face moves. Her pupils are equal and reactive to light. Her vital signs are pulse 92 and irregular, blood pressure 180/96, respirations 20 and unlabored, and her pulse oximetry reads 96 percent.

According to Mr. Stokes, the only medical problem his wife has is high blood pressure, for which she takes just one medication, Vasotec. She has no allergies to medications. She is a patient of Dr. Newman and has not been hospitalized recently.

You take special care to put Mrs. Stokes on her left side on the stretcher, so she is still able to move her right arm and saliva will not obstruct her airway.

Street Scene Question

3. **How should you perform a reassessment on this patient?**

En route, you contact the receiving hospital and report on the patient's condition and treatment. You repeat her vital signs and this time get a pulse of 88 and irregular, blood pressure of 170 by palpation, and respirations of 22 and unlabored. Her pulse oximetry has not changed. When you ask the patient how she feels now, she replies in a clear voice, "Why, much better, young man." Surprised at this sudden improvement, you proceed to assess her again. She can now hold both arms up in front of her with her eyes closed. When she smiles, there is no longer any sign of a deficit. Cheered up by this turn of events, you confirm that her husband's version of events is accurate. You also learn that Mrs. Stokes has led an interesting life, having been a history teacher for 40 years.

About five minutes after this improvement, you notice that the patient seems to be having trouble speaking again. When you ask her to hold her arms out in front of her, she is able to pick both of them up, but her left arm drifts off and falls down. Her smile barely shows her teeth. When you ask her to repeat the phrase "You can't teach an old dog new tricks," she can get only the first few words out, and only with great difficulty. Concerned about these changes in the patient's condition, you call the hospital again and advise them of the developments.

When you arrive at the emergency department a few minutes later, Mrs. Stokes's condition has not changed again. The nurse undresses her, and the emergency physician assesses her as you prepare the ambulance for the next call and complete your patient care report. Just as you are finishing the report, the doctor comes out of the patient's room. "Well, I'm glad you brought this patient here," he says. "We can offer Mrs. Stokes the opportunity to participate in a research project evaluating a new experimental treatment for stroke."

"Do you think she's really having a stroke?" you ask. "Her condition kept changing, getting better and then getting worse again."

Knowing that understanding the manifestations of a disease in a patient is an important part of quality improvement, the doctor tells you, "We often see changes in the condition of stroke patients in the first few hours of the episode. It can make assessment a real challenge. I'm glad you were able to detect the changes and let us know about them."

With a new appreciation for the value of a reassessment, you return to your service area, ready for another call.

17

Communication and Documentation

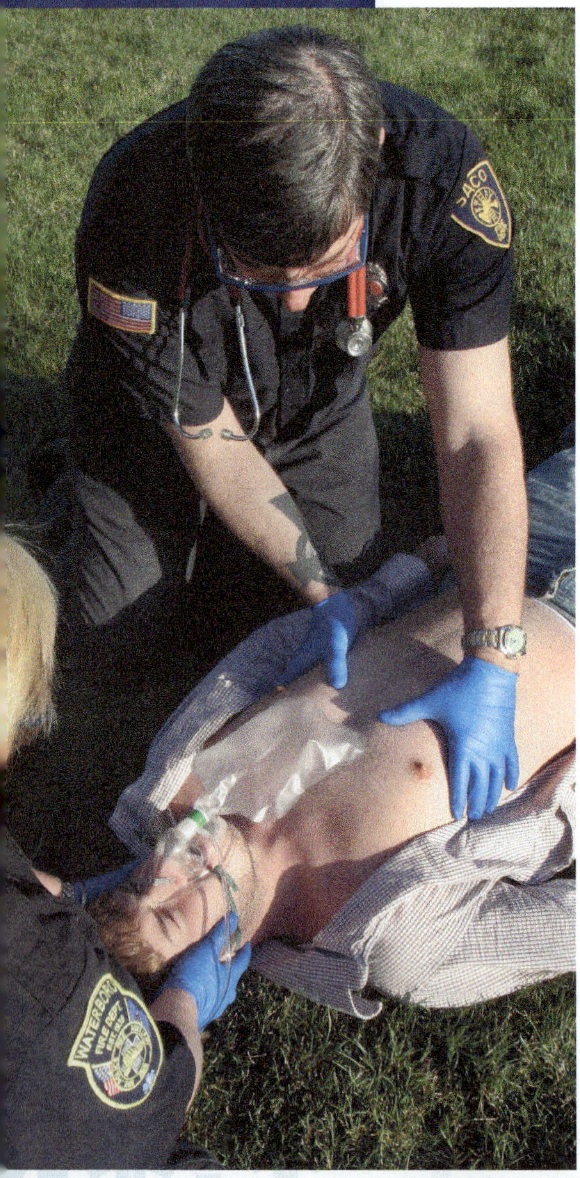
(© Daniel Limmer)

Related Chapters

The following chapters provide additional information related to topics discussed in this chapter:

4 Medical, Legal, and Ethical Issues
12 Primary Assessment
13 Vital Signs and Monitoring Devices
15 Secondary Assessment
18 General Pharmacology
39 Hazardous Materials, Multiple-Casualty Incidents, and Incident Management

Standard

Preparatory (Documentation; EMS System Communication)

Competency

Uses fundamental knowledge of the EMS system, safety/well-being of the EMT, and medical/legal and ethical issues in the provision of emergency care.

Core Concepts

- Radio procedures used at various stages of the EMS call
- Delivery and format of a radio report to the hospital
- Delivery and format of a verbal hand-off report to the hospital
- Communication skills used when interacting with other members of the health care team
- Communication skills used when interacting with the patient
- Components of and procedures for the written prehospital care report
- Legal aspects and benefits of documentation
- Documentation concerns in patient refusal

Outcomes

After reading this chapter, you should be able to:

17.1 Compare public safety radio communications systems to best practices. (pp. 464–469)

- Describe the features of communication system components.
- Describe the impact of each component of a communication system on the delivery of patient care.
- Assess portrayals of radio communication for compliance with basic principles of radio communication.
- Assess portrayals of radio medical reports for the correct use of each of the components of a radio medical report.

17.2 Evaluate the various types of interpersonal communications EMTs have with others. (pp. 469–474)

- Compare the verbal patient report when transferring patient care to hospital personnel to the radio patient report given en route.
- Explain professional ways to overcome a communication problem.
- Describe the importance of communicating with all health care providers involved in patient care at the scene.
- Describe the general guidelines for engaging in therapeutic communication.
- Describe modification of approaches to patients with communication challenges.
- Given a portrayal of an episode of therapeutic communication, identify what went well and what did not go well.

17.3 Generate a written prehospital care report from a portrayal of patient care. (pp. 474–490)

- Describe each of the functions of a prehospital care report.
- Identify the purposes of the National Highway Transportation Safety Administration (NHTSA) data elements.
- Identify the Patient Information and Administrative Information elements of the NHTSA minimum data set.
- Identify the minimum NHTSA data required to communicate effectively through the narrative of a prehospital report.
- Explain the importance of each of the required elements of the narrative portion of a written prehospital care report.
- Explain how to ensure your written prehospital care report complies with confidentiality requirements.
- Explain the documentation required when a patient refuses emergency prehospital care and transportation.
- Give examples of how the quality and completeness of your written prehospital care reports can serve you and others, in the near and far future.
- Explain the consequences of falsification of prehospital care report information.
- Describe the proper correction of errors and late entries in prehospital care reports.
- Explain modifications to the EMT's documentation in special situations.

Key Terms

base station, *464*
cell phone, *465*
drop report (or transfer report), *476*
mobile radio, *464*
portable radio, *464*
repeater, *465*
telemetry, *465*
watt, *464*

You will learn about several types of communication in this chapter: radio communication, the verbal report at the hospital, interpersonal communication, and documentation. As the term implies, radio communication is conducted by radio. Technology has allowed cell phones and other equipment to be used in areas where radio transmissions were previously the only choice. The verbal report is your chance to convey information about your patient directly to the hospital personnel who will be taking over the patient's care. Interpersonal communications are important in dealing with other EMTs, the patient, family and bystanders, medical direction, and other members of the EMS system.

Documentation is an important part of the patient care process and lasts long after the call. The report you write will become a part of the patient's permanent hospital record. As records of your agency, your reports and those written by other EMTs become a valuable source for research on trends in emergency medical care and a guide for continuing education and quality improvement. Your report may also be used as evidence in a legal case. Documentation has short-term benefits as well. Noting vital signs and a patient's history will help you remember important facts about the patient during the course of the call.

Communications Systems and Radio Communication

Radio equipment is often taken for granted, since it is now so common (Figure 17-1). However, the development of radio links between dispatchers, mobile units, and hospitals has been one of the key contributors to improvement in EMS over the years. Imagine if you had to call the dispatcher by phone every few minutes to see if there was a call! Without radio transmissions from ambulances, hospitals would be unable to prepare for the arrival of patients as they do now.

Communications Systems

There are a number of components to any radio or communications system: base stations, mobile radios, portable radios, repeaters, cell phones, telemetry, and other devices.

- ***Base station*** setup with two-way radios that are at a fixed site, such as a hospital or dispatch center.
- ***Mobile radios*** are two-way radios that are used or affixed in a vehicle. Most are actually mounted inside the vehicle. These devices have lower transmitting power than base stations. The unit used to measure output power of radios is the ***watt***. The output of a mobile radio is generally 20–50 watts, with a range of 10–15 miles (about 16–24 km).
- ***Portable radios*** are handheld two-way radios with an output of 1–5 watts. This type of radio is important because it will allow you to be in touch with the dispatcher, medical direction, and other members of the EMS system while you are away from the ambulance.

base station
setup with two-way radios at a fixed site, such as a hospital or dispatch center.

mobile radio
a two-way radio that is used or affixed in a vehicle.

watt
the unit of measurement of the output power of a radio.

portable radio
a handheld two-way radio.

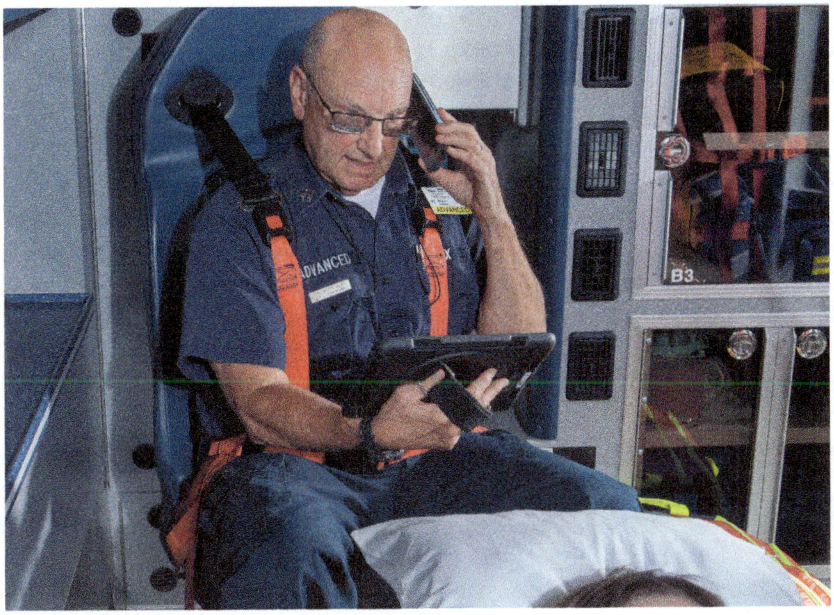

FIGURE 17-1 Communication from the ambulance can be by radio or cell phone.

- ***Repeaters*** are devices that are used when transmissions must be carried over a long distance. Repeaters may be in ambulances or placed in various areas around an EMS system. The repeater picks up signals from lower-power units, such as mobile and portable radios, and retransmits them at a higher power. The retransmission is done on another frequency (Figure 17-2).
- ***Cell phones*** are phones that transmit through the air to a cell tower. In many areas where the distances or expense are too great to set up a conventional EMS radio system, cell phones allow EMS communications through an already established commercial system.
- ***Telemetry*** is the process of sending and receiving data wirelessly. In EMS, this may be an electrocardiogram (ECG), vital signs, or other patient-related data. Some systems allow EMTs to acquire and transmit ECGs to the hospital.

repeater
a device that picks up signals from lower-power radio units, such as mobile and portable radios, and retransmits them at a higher power. It allows low-power radio signals to be transmitted over longer distances.

cell phone
a phone that transmits through the air instead of over wires, so the phone can be transported and used over a wide area.

telemetry
the process of sending and receiving data wirelessly.

FIGURE 17-2 Example of an EMS communication system using repeaters.

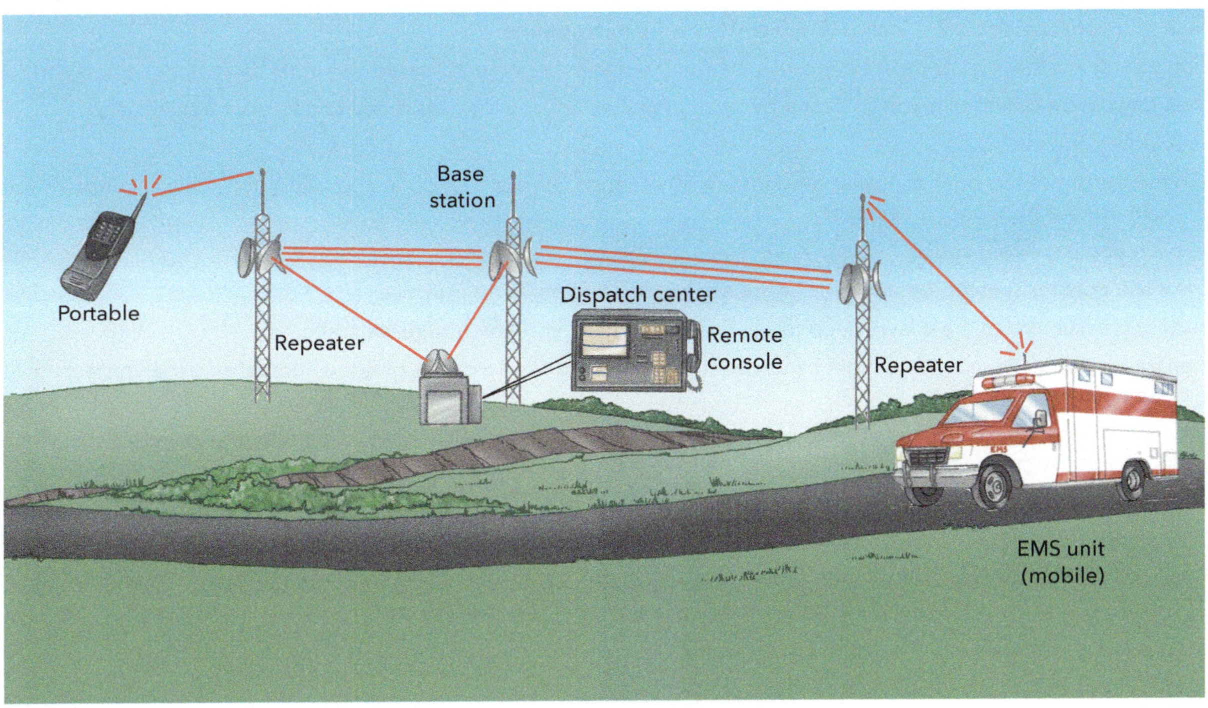

New technology is developing almost constantly. Computers and tablets are being used to record information at the patient's side. This information may be wirelessly transmitted to dispatch and to the hospital. These same devices permit transmission of some standard messages, such as ambulance identification or arrival at the scene, by punching a key. The messages are transmitted in a condensed form that helps keep busy frequencies less crowded.

Since radios are so important to EMS today, many systems have backup radios. This means that in the event of power failure or malfunction, another option is available. For example, if the base station fails, there may be a backup radio or alternative power supply available. If the mobile radio in your ambulance malfunctions, portable radios or phones may be used in its place.

Note that radio systems require preventive maintenance and repair, just like the ambulance and your other EMS equipment. Radio equipment must be treated with care on a daily basis and not mishandled.

Radio Communication

EMS is just one of many public services that use radio communication. To maintain order on the airwaves, the Federal Communications Commission (FCC) assigns and licenses radio frequencies. This prevents two or more agencies from trying to use the same frequency and interfering with each other's communications. There are also strict rules about interfering with emergency radio traffic and prohibiting profanities and offensive language.

Some general rules for radio transmissions should always be followed. These rules prevent delays and allow all persons to use the frequencies. Although there may be some minor variations within your EMS system, always keep in mind the principles shown in Box 17-1.

BOX 17-1 Principles of Radio Communication

Follow These Principles when Using the EMS Radio System:

- Make sure that your radio is on and the volume is adjusted properly.
- Reduce background noise by closing the vehicle window when possible.
- Listen to the frequency and ensure that it is clear before beginning a transmission.
- Press the "press to talk" (PTT) button on the radio, then wait one second before speaking. This prevents cutting off the first few words of your transmission.
- Speak with your lips about 2-3 inches (5-7.5 cm) from the microphone.
- When calling another unit or base station, use their unit number or name, followed by yours. "Dispatcher, this is Ambulance 2."
- If the unit you are calling tells you to "Stand by," wait until they tell you they are ready to take your transmission.
- Speak slowly and clearly.
- Keep the transmissions brief. If it takes longer than 30 seconds, stop at that point and pause for a few seconds so emergency traffic can use the frequency if necessary.
- Use plain English. Avoid codes.
- Do not use phrases such as "be advised." These are implied and serve no purpose.
- Courtesy is assumed, so there is no need to say "Please," "Thank you," or "You're welcome."
- When transmitting a number that might be unclear (15 may sound like 16 or 50), give the number and then repeat the individual digits. Say "Fifteen, one-five."
- Anything said over the radio can be heard by the public on a scanner. Do not use the patient's name over the radio. For the same reason, do not use profanities or statements that tend to slander any person. Use objective, impartial statements.
- Use "we" instead of "I." As an EMT, you will rarely be acting alone.
- "Affirmative" and "Negative" are preferred over "Yes" and "No" because the latter are difficult to hear.
- Give assessment information about your patient but avoid offering a field diagnosis of the patient's problem. For example, say "Patient complains of abdominal pain" rather than "Patient probably has appendicitis."
- Avoid slang or abbreviations that are not authorized.
- Use EMS frequencies only for authorized EMS communication.

Radio Transmissions throughout the Call

CORE CONCEPT
Radio procedures used at various stages of the EMS call

The initial call for help received by the emergency medical dispatcher (EMD) most often comes via telephone but may also be radioed from another agency, such as the police. After proper information is obtained, the EMD dispatches the units. The following is a sample flow of information between the dispatcher and units in the field. You are the EMT on ambulance number 6:

Dispatcher: Ambulance 6. . . .

You: Ambulance 6. Go ahead.

Dispatcher: Ambulance 6, respond to 1243 Magnolia Boulevard—that's one-two-four-three Magnolia Boulevard—for an assault. The police are en route. Stand by at the corner of Magnolia and Third until the police report the scene secure.

You: Ambulance 6 received that. Will stand by at Magnolia and Third.

Without prompt and efficient dispatch and receipt of information, the ambulance could easily be sent to the wrong location. In this situation, the dispatcher also relayed important safety information. Since the call was for an assault, the dispatcher "staged" the ambulance, or ordered it to stand by, until the scene was safe.

You respond to the assigned location, reporting your arrival to the dispatcher:

You: Dispatcher, Ambulance 6 is arriving at the staging area.

Dispatcher: Message received, Ambulance 6. I will advise you when the scene is secure.

Most scenes are safe. However, in this case the dispatcher has decided, from the nature of the call and other information obtained, that it is not. Police arrive at the scene and separate the parties involved in the assault. The police radio the dispatcher and advise that the scene is secure. The next transmission is to your ambulance:

Dispatcher: Ambulance 6, the police report that the scene is secure. Respond in.

You: Message received by Ambulance 6. (You drive two blocks to the scene and report to the dispatcher.)

You: Dispatcher, Ambulance 6 is at the scene.

Dispatcher: Ambulance 6 at the scene at 1310 hours.

The dispatcher records all the times according to the 24-hour clock: the time of the original call, the time the ambulance was dispatched, the time when the ambulance reached the staging area, and finally the time when the ambulance arrived at the scene. Should this case go to court, the records of the dispatch center, your care report, and the dispatch audiotape of the call may be subpoenaed. Unless there is a need for medical direction or assistance from the scene, the next call will be when you are en route to the hospital:

You: Dispatcher, Ambulance 6 is en route to Mercy Hospital with one patient.

Dispatcher: Ambulance 6 en route to Mercy Hospital at 1323 hours.

You will call the hospital via radio or phone to advise staff there of the status of your patient and the estimated time of arrival (ETA). When arriving at the hospital, you again advise the dispatcher:

You: Ambulance 6 is arriving at Mercy Hospital.

Dispatcher: Ambulance 6 at Mercy at 1334 hours.

You will note that the dispatcher gives the time after most transmissions. This will allow you to record times if they are required on your patient care record. The dispatcher also usually briefly repeat the message to ensure acknowledgment of the right unit.

After turning the patient over to the hospital staff and preparing the ambulance for the next run, you will advise the dispatcher that you are leaving the hospital. You may also find it part of your local procedure to advise the dispatcher when you are back in your district or area and when you are back in quarters. Many transmissions are made between the mobile radio within the ambulance and the dispatcher at a base station. In some EMS systems, simple standard communications such as being enroute, arriving on the scene, and arriving at the hospital are transmitted by pushing a button on a mobile data terminal (MDT) mounted in the ambulance, rather than by a verbal radio transmission. MDT use reduces congestion on busy radio frequencies.

Remember, when you have one available, bring your portable radio with you whenever you leave the ambulance. You may need to call for assistance during scene size-up if hazards or multiple patients are found, and the portable radio allows you to do that without running back to the ambulance to make the call on the fixed unit.

Radio Medical Reports

CORE CONCEPT
Delivery and format of a radio report to the hospital

"Your report to the hospital should be clear and concise. They should know exactly what to expect."

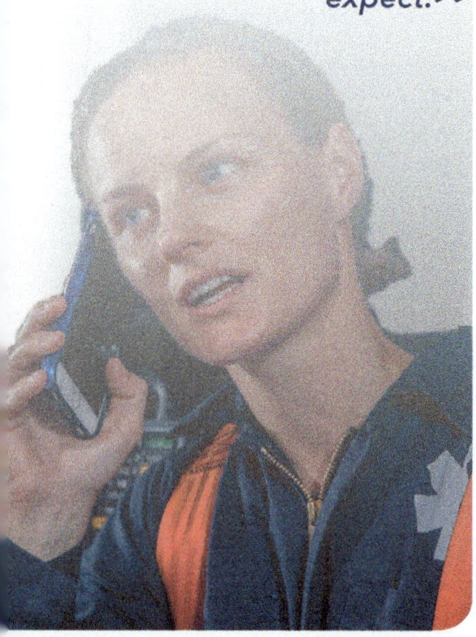

Reports must be made to medical personnel as part of almost every call. These reports may be by radio, verbally (in person), in writing, or in all three ways. The radio report is specifically structured to present pertinent facts about the patient without providing more detail than necessary. Too much detail ties up the radio frequency and takes up the time of hospital personnel.

In an effort to protect patient privacy, some hospitals encourage EMTs to use a cell phone en route to the emergency department rather than the radio. Follow your local protocols.

Experienced EMTs try to "paint a picture" of the patient in words. This requires knowledge of radio procedure and practice. If you have a critical patient, your radio report should make that clear. This can be done by describing the chief complaint, injuries, vital signs, treatments, and mechanism of injury. Even with critical patients, you must keep a clear, steady tone to your voice. Resist the urge to talk fast or appear excited, as it will prevent effective communication.

Keep in mind that the purpose of a radio or phone report is to give the hospital staff sufficient information to determine where the patient should go (e.g., major trauma room) and to have the appropriate personnel there when the patient arrives. In general, you do not need to provide details like the patient's medications or allergies, because this information will not change either of the items above. Giving this information will only prolong the time needed for the report. Of course, exceptions to these principles include reporting an overdose or an allergic reaction.

A medical radio report has 12 parts. The following example, broken into its individual parts, shows a report you might make to the hospital:

1. **Unit identification and level of provider**
   "Memorial Hospital, this is Community BLS Ambulance 6 en route to your location . . . "
2. **Estimated time of arrival**
   ". . . with a 15-minute ETA."
3. **Patient's age and sex**
   "We are transporting a 68-year-old male patient . . ."
4. **Chief complaint**
   ". . . who complains of diffuse pain in his abdomen."
5. **Brief, pertinent history of the present illness**
   "The pain is sharp, started two hours ago, is rated 3/10 in severity, and is accompanied by slight nausea."
6. **Major past illnesses**
   "The patient has a history of high blood pressure."
7. **Mental status**
   "He is alert and oriented, never lost consciousness."
8. **Baseline vital signs**
   "His vital signs are pulse 88 regular and full, respirations 20 and unlabored, skin normal, and blood pressure 134 over 88; oxygen saturation is 98 percent."

9. **Pertinent findings of the physical exam**
"Our exam revealed tenderness in both upper abdominal quadrants. They did not appear rigid."

10. **Emergency medical care given**
"For care, we have placed him in a position of comfort."

11. **Response to emergency medical care**
"The level of pain has not changed during our care. Mental status has remained unchanged. Vital signs are basically unchanged."

12. **Contact medical direction if required or if you have questions.**
"Does medical direction have any orders?"

After giving this information, you will continue with reassessment of the patient en route to the hospital. During that time, additional vital signs will be taken, there may be changes in the patient's condition, or you may discover new information about the patient, particularly on long transports. In some systems you should radio this additional information to the hospital in a follow-up radio call while en route. (Follow local protocols.)

When you contact medical direction, you may be given orders. EMTs have an increasing number of medications and skills they may use to help patients. The on-line physician may order you to assist in administering the patient's own medication, order the administration of a medication you carry on the ambulance, or give other orders. In any case, the communication between you and medical direction must be clear and concise to avoid misinterpretations that can inadvertently harm the patient. For example, a patient may have a medication called nitroglycerin for chest pain. This medication, as you will learn in *General Pharmacology*, is one that you may assist the patient in taking. (Follow local protocols.) The medication should be given only if the patient's blood pressure is above a certain level. If there is a misunderstanding between you and the physician, and this medication is ordered improperly, harm may come to the patient.

To avoid misunderstanding and miscommunication, use the following guidelines when communicating with medical direction:

- Give the information to medical direction clearly and accurately. Speak slowly and clearly. The physician's orders will be based on what you report.
- After receiving an order for a medication or procedure, repeat the order word for word. You may also ask to do a procedure or give a medication and be denied by medical direction. Repeat this also.
- If an order is unclear, ask the physician to repeat it. After you have a clear understanding of the order, repeat it back to the physician.
- If an order appears to be inappropriate, question the physician. There may have been a misunderstanding, and your questioning may prevent the inappropriate administration of a medication. If the physician verifies the order, the physician may explain the order to you.

The Verbal Report

At the hospital, you will give a written report on your patient to hospital personnel, as explained later in the chapter. However, since it will take some time to complete your prehospital care report, the first information you give to hospital personnel will be your verbal report.

As you transfer your patient to the care of the hospital staff, introduce the patient by name. Then summarize the same kind of information you gave over the radio, pointing out any information that is updated or different from your last radio report. Include the following in your verbal report:

CORE CONCEPT
Delivery and format of a verbal hand-off report to the hospital

- Chief complaint
- History that was not given previously
- Additional treatment given en route
- Additional vital signs taken en route

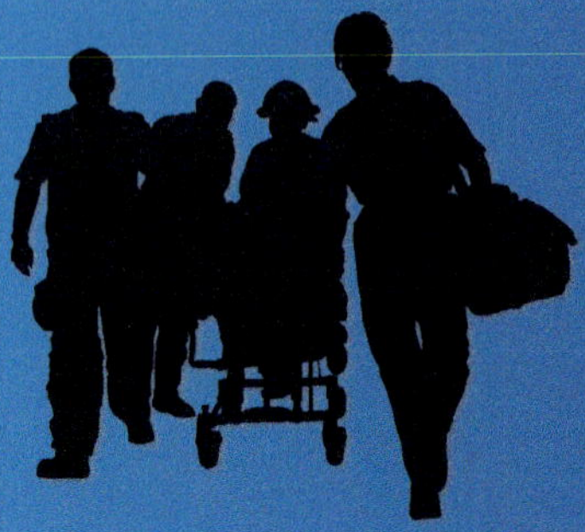

Think Like an EMT

Communication Challenges

Communication may take various forms in EMS: written, face-to-face verbal, or by radio or phone. Make your decisions based on the form of communication that would be best in the following scenarios.

1. You are en route to a call of unknown nature for an older adult patient. Emergency medical responders arrived at the scene about five minutes ago, and you are still ten minutes from the scene. Dispatch has not called you on the radio with an update on the patient's condition. What are some of the reasons this might be the case? How should you proceed?
2. A 17-year-old male patient drank a large amount of alcohol and then passed out, according to his friends, who called 911. When you arrive, you find the patient initially unresponsive to painful stimuli and then, a few minutes later, able to slur some words when you ask him questions. A few minutes after that, he withdraws when you apply a painful stimulus. How should you describe his mental status to the hospital while you are en route?
3. You are at the scene of a two-car motor-vehicle collision and would like to give the local hospital some warning that you will be transporting a severely injured patient in a few minutes. Unfortunately, when you try to call the hospital on the radio, they are unable to understand what you are saying. How should you proceed?
4. You have just arrived at the scene of a 34-year-old man with diabetes who is "out of it," according to what the caller told Dispatch. One of his friends, trying to be helpful, tells you that he thinks the patient is "conscious but unresponsive." Confused as to what this might mean, you proceed to the patient and find him sitting in a chair, staring straight ahead, not saying anything. When you ask him a question, he doesn't answer and doesn't even look at you. When you pinch his arm, he looks down at his arm but doesn't respond in any other way. How can you describe this patient's mental status in a way that will give the hospital an accurate impression of what is going on? *Hint*: Describe what you observe instead of trying to attach labels to this patient.

Interpersonal Communication

CORE CONCEPT

Communication skills used when interacting with other members of the health care team

Team Communication

As an EMT, you are part of a team of health care professionals. For example, at the scene, you may need to communicate with first responders (trained emergency medical responders or others who have reached the scene and provided care before your arrival) or with advanced providers (advanced EMTs or paramedics) (Figure 17-3). The most recent CPR guidelines talk about a "pit crew" approach. This requires excellent communication for all members of the team to work together for maximum efficiency.

On many medical calls, a home health care aide or family member may be at the scene and be able to provide you with valuable information about the patient and the present emergency (Figure 17-4). You will need to speak candidly and respectfully with these members of the health care team to gather important information about the patient and complete any necessary and appropriate transfer of care.

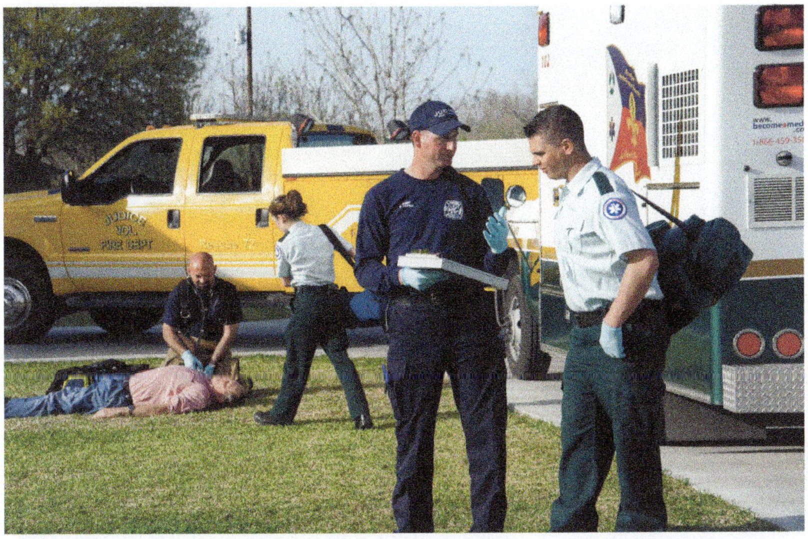

FIGURE 17-3 You may need to communicate with emergency medical responders or advanced EMS personnel at the scene.

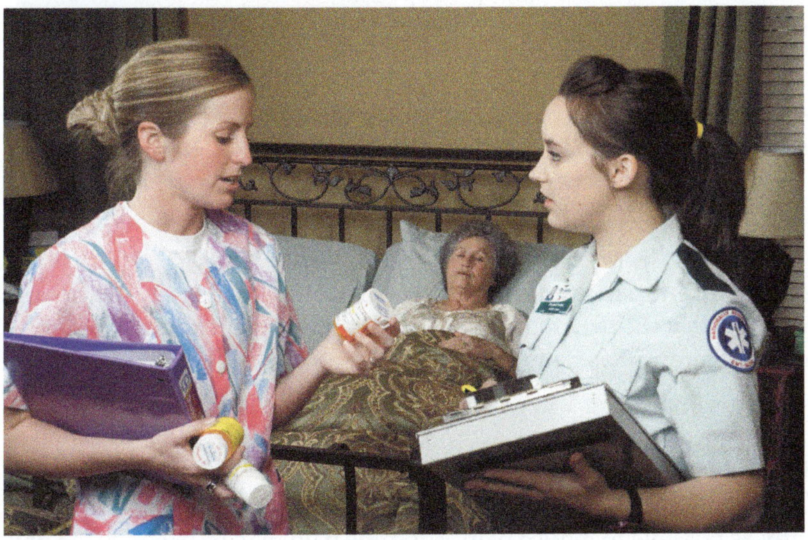

FIGURE 17-4 You may need to communicate with a home health aide or family member about the patient's condition and present emergency.

Therapeutic Communication

Although communication between two or more human beings is a skill learned over the years, many people still do not communicate as well as they could. Communicating with patients and others who are in crisis is even more difficult (Figure 17-5). Although interpersonal communication could be presented as a course in itself, the following guidelines will help when dealing with patients, families, friends, and bystanders:

CORE CONCEPT

Communication skills used when interacting with the patient

- **Use eye contact.** Make frequent eye contact with your patient. It shows that you are interested in your patient and that you are attentive. Failure to make eye contact signals that you feel uneasy around the patient. (If your patient is avoiding eye contact, consider that in some cultures eye contact is considered rude. You may want to match your behavior to the patient's in this situation.)
- **Be aware of your position and body language.** Your positioning with respect to the patient is important. If you are higher than the patient, you may appear intimidating. If possible, position yourself at or below the patient's eye level (Figure 17-6). This will be less threatening to the patient. Body language is also important. Standing with your arms crossed or not directly facing the patient (a closed stance) sends a signal to the patient that you are not interested. Use a more open stance (arms down, facing the patient), when it can be done safely, to communicate a warmer attitude.

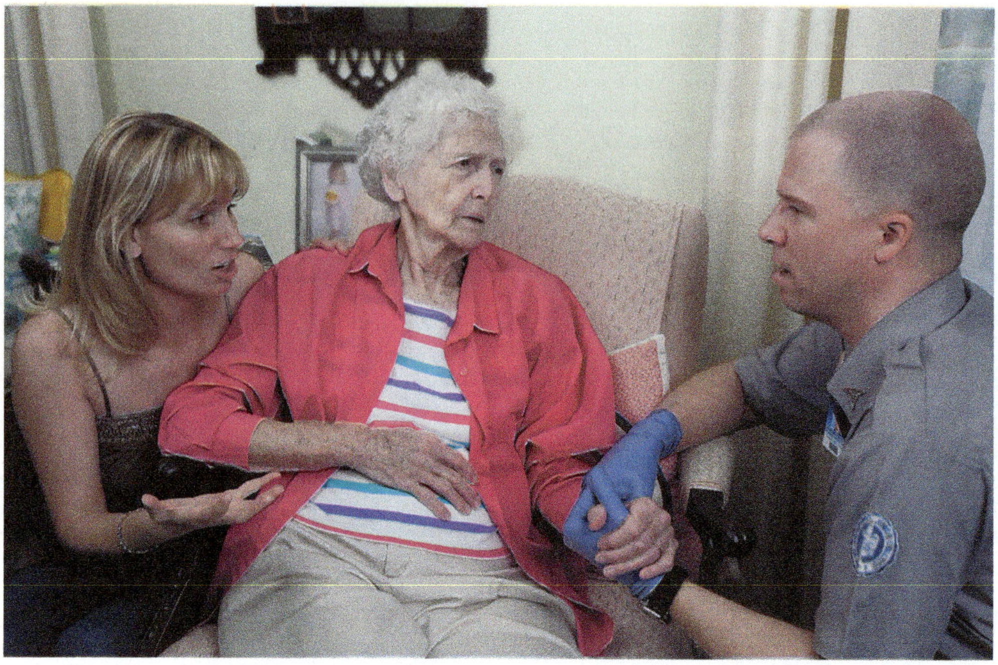

FIGURE 17-5 Communicating with patients and others who are in crisis requires skill and tact.

A closed or more serious stance may sometimes be beneficial, however, when you need to calm or direct bystanders at the scene. Standing above a patient may convey authority and can be done to gain control when necessary.

Watch the patient's body language to see how your communication is going. If the patient uses a closed stance, your communication efforts may not be working.

- **Use language the patient can understand.** Speak slowly and clearly. Do not use medical or other terms that the patient will not understand. Explain procedures before they are performed, to prevent anxiety.
- **Be honest.** Honesty is important. You will frequently be asked questions that you will not have the answer to: "Is my leg broken?" "Am I having a heart attack?" At other times you will know the answer to the question, but it is not pleasant: "Will it hurt when you put that splint on?" If the answer is "Yes," tell the truth. Explain that you will do it as gently as possible to reduce pain, but some pain may be experienced. It is much worse to lie to patients and have them find out that you were not being truthful. This will erode the patient's confidence in you as well as in other EMTs and medical personnel the patient may meet later on.

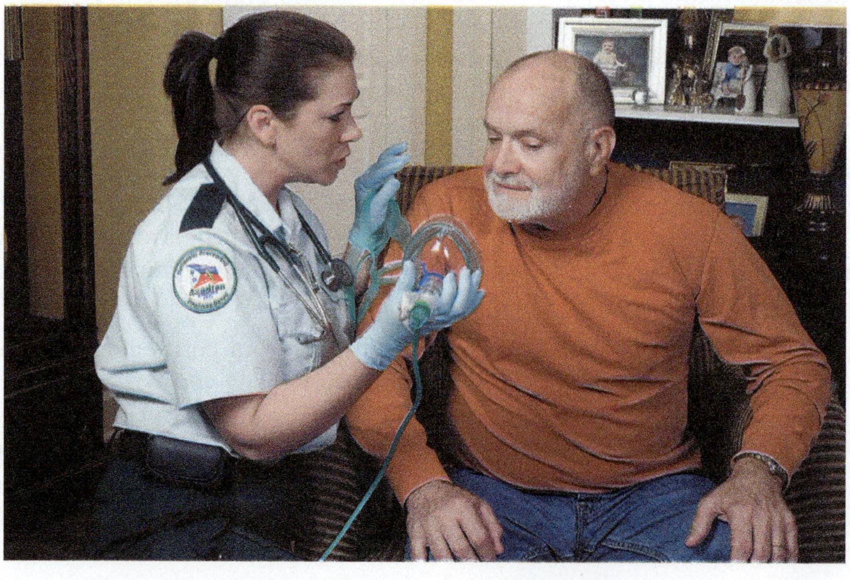

FIGURE 17-6 Position yourself at or below the patient's eye level to be less intimidating and to aid communication.

- **Use the patient's proper name.** Especially with senior citizens and other adults, do not assume familiarity. As a general rule, call patients as they introduce themselves to you. If a person many years older than you introduces himself as William Harris, it might be best to call him Mr. Harris as a sign of respect. Immediately calling him "Bill" when he clearly stated his name was "William" would be disrespectful. If, after you call him "Mr. Harris," he says "Please call me Bill," you have shown respect and can then use the less formal name. If in doubt, ask what the patient would like to be called.
- **Listen.** If you ask the patient a question, get an answer, then have to ask the same question again, it will show the patient that you were not listening. If you are not listening, the patient will feel that you are not interested or that you just don't care. If you ask a question, wait for the answer. Then write it down so you will not forget.

If a person has a mental disability or is hard of hearing, speak slowly and clearly. Do not talk down to the patient. Patients with a hearing disability may read lips. In any case, seeing your lips may help the patient understand what you are saying. Therefore, be sure that a deaf or hearing-impaired person can see your mouth when you talk. Remember that a person who is blind or who has a visual deficit can usually hear, so do not give in to the temptation to speak loudly or unnaturally. For the visually impaired person, you will want to take extra effort to explain anything that is happening that the patient cannot see.

You may also find people who do not speak the same language that you do. In this case, use an interpreter, a manual, or a phone app that provides translations. Phone companies often provide this service. Family members are not always familiar with medical terminology, so you should be cautious in using it. It is sometimes possible to get a professional translating service through the phone company or hospital. You may also find that your communications center or medical direction has someone available who speaks the patient's language.

Older adults are a rapidly growing segment of the population who often need EMS care. These older patients may have medical problems simply because of their age. They may also be more prone to falls and serious injury from trauma due to the condition of their bones and body systems.

Many older patients are well oriented and physically able. Others, however, may have problems with hearing, sight, or orientation that have come on with age. These patients may seem confused or may simply find it difficult to communicate. In spite of their sensory limitations, of course, these patients still have needs and feelings. They deserve patience, kindness, and understanding—along with proper emergency care (Figure 17-7).

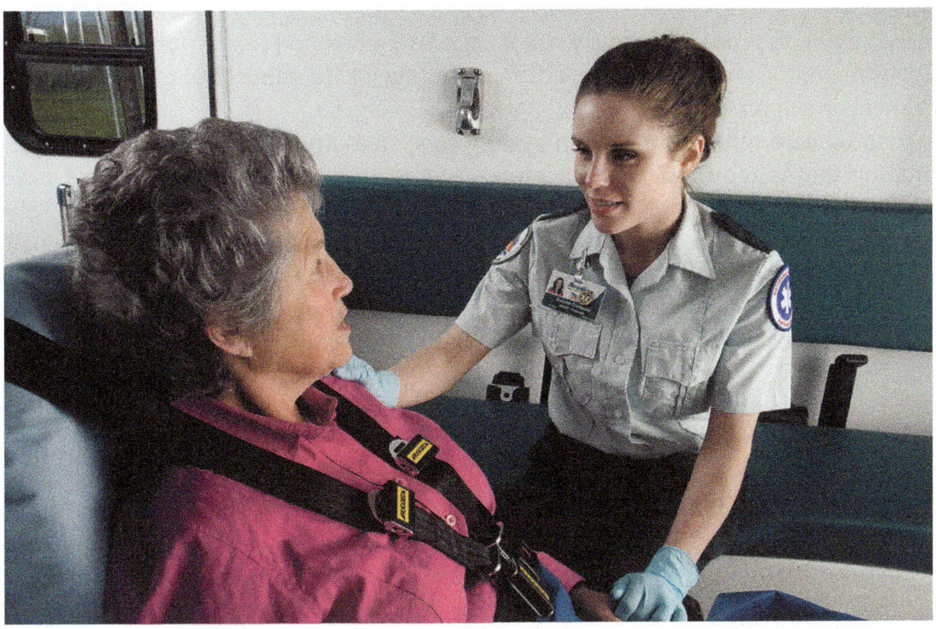

FIGURE 17-7 Be considerate of the older adult patient.

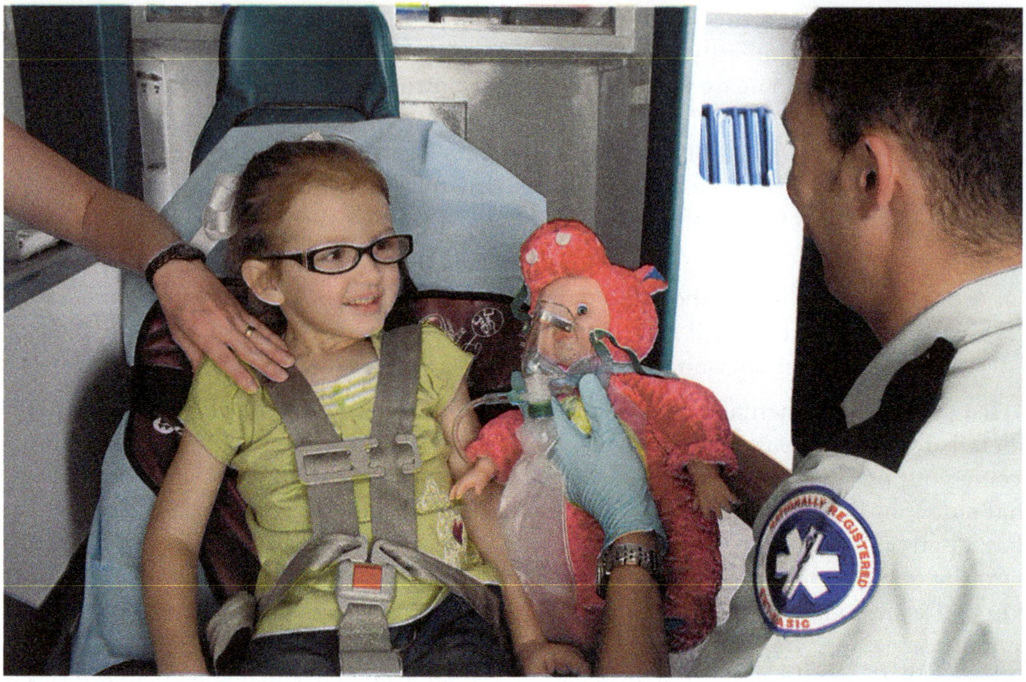

FIGURE 17-8 Stay at a child's eye level or lower.

Since children sometimes can be difficult to assess and communicate with, it is often best to involve the parents of the child when communicating. Two rules of communication with children are critically important:

- Always come down to the child's level (Figure 17-8). Never stand above a child, as you will literally tower over the child and appear very intimidating. Crouching down reduces the size difference and greatly improves communication. If the child is not critically ill, you might even take the time to sit on the floor and get slightly below the child in the beginning.
- Children often sense lies even more quickly than adults do. It is important to tell the truth to children. Remember, you may be the first contact from the EMS system that the child has ever had. Work to make it positive.

Prehospital Care Report

CORE CONCEPT
Components and procedures for the written prehospital care report

The record that you produce during a call is called a prehospital care report or, informally, a PCR. Your region or service may use a different name for the same kind of document, such as trip sheet or run report.

Prehospital care reports vary from system to system and state to state. Although the information that is required to complete each is relatively similar, the method used to record the data may be somewhat different.

Many prehospital care reports are now done by direct data entry (Figure 17-9). This can take several forms. Laptops, tablets, and pen-based computers (Figure 17-10) are commonly used. They allow the EMT to enter information about a call directly into the device. Receiving hospitals have data connections that allow for transfer of information. Many of these devices are Web-based. With this method, the EMT also has the option of signing on to a secure website, using computers at the hospital and at the station to enter the data. Depending on the hospital, the EMT may need to use a printer at a receiving hospital to print out a hard copy of the report for the emergency department staff.

Written reports are those that have narrative portions, areas to record vital signs in written-number form, and fields to complete (Figure 17-11). These are used in some areas and will also serve as a backup should computer entry be unavailable. The term *written* is used in this chapter to describe both computer-based and handwritten reports.

FIGURE 17-9 (A) Printout of an electronic prehospital care report. (B) As an electronic report appears on the computer screen. *(© Courtesy of ImageTrend, Inc.)*

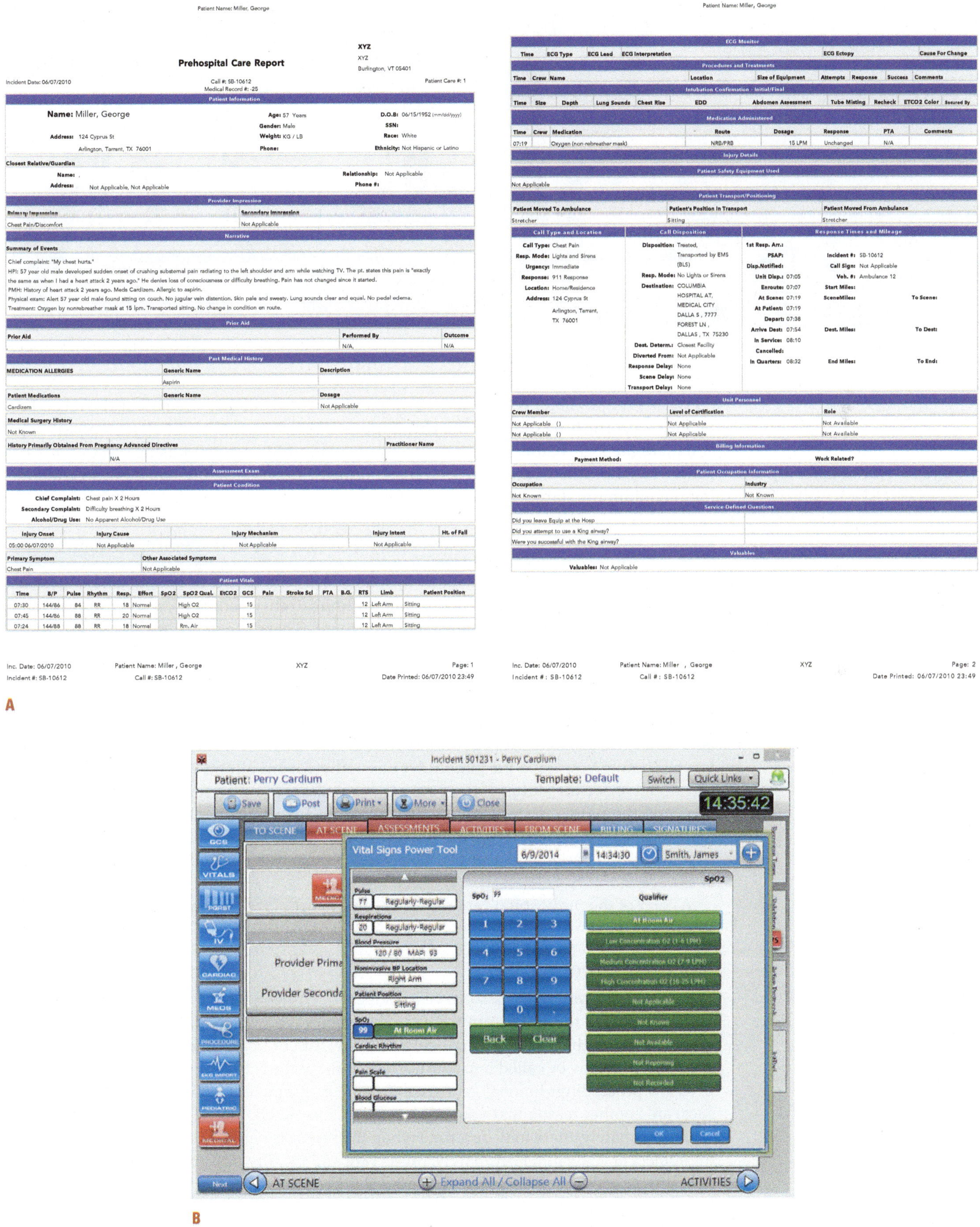

FIGURE 17-10 Direct data devices as documentation tools: (A) a laptop pen-based computer and (B) a pen-based computer with PCR form on the screen.

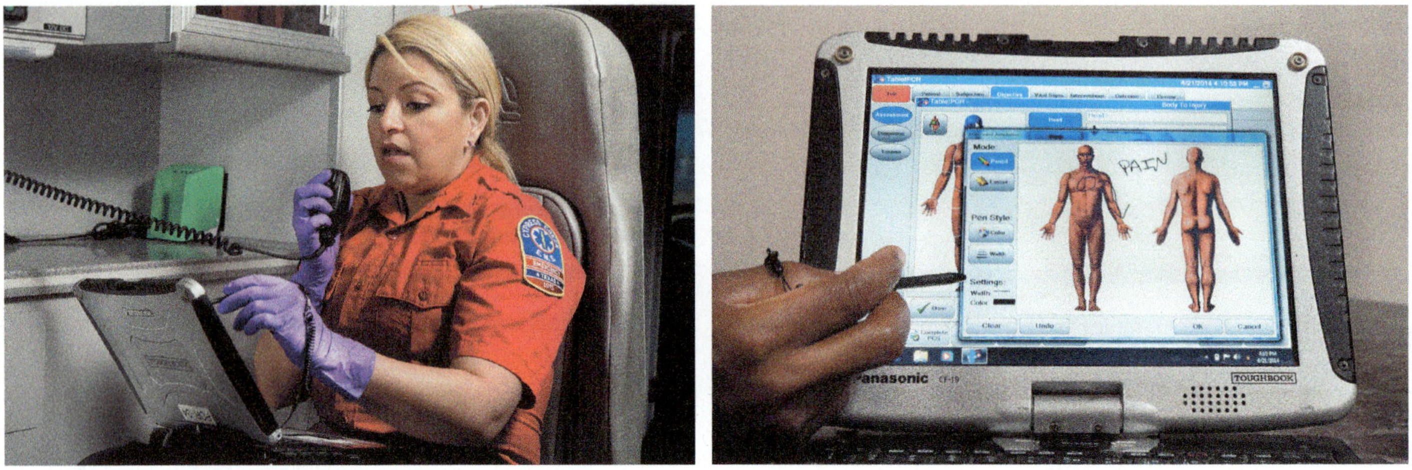

A B

drop report (or transfer report) an abbreviated form of the PCR that an EMS crew can leave at the hospital when there is not enough time to complete the PCR before leaving.

Whenever possible, you should complete the PCR while you are still at the receiving facility with fresh memory of the call (Figure 17-12). Since it is not always possible to complete the PCR before a crew has to leave, many EMS agencies using electronic data collection employ a ***drop report (or transfer report)***. This is an abbreviated report containing the minimum data set, described later.

Functions of the Prehospital Care Report

The prehospital care report has many functions. It is the record of patient care, serves as a legal document, provides information for administrative functions, aids education and research, and contributes to quality improvement. These functions are discussed in the following paragraphs.

Patient Care Record

The prehospital care report conveys important information about the patient to members of the EMS system and beyond. Although you provide a verbal report to the hospital staff before you leave the patient, your written record allows emergency department personnel to see the status of the patient when you arrived on scene, the care you gave, and how the patient's status may have changed during your care. An example of this would be the emergency department staff looking back at your original set of vital signs to compare the patient's current condition with the patient's condition when first found at the scene.

A copy of the prehospital care report becomes part of the patient's permanent hospital record.

Legal Document

The prehospital care report also serves as a legal document, which may be called for at any legal proceeding resulting from the call. The person who wrote the report will ordinarily go to court with the form. If the patient was the victim or perpetrator of a crime, the report and the writer may be called into court to testify about the call during criminal proceedings. Civil law proceedings for negligence in injuries (e.g., if a patient falls in a shopping mall and sues) are another reason that your report may be examined.

Unfortunately, there may be a time when the report is being examined because you are the subject of a lawsuit. Fortunately, this is rare and usually preventable. In a case such as this, the report in which you documented the circumstances and the care you gave will be very important.

FIGURE 17-11 Example of a prehospital care report with fill-in boxes and a narrative space. Paper PCR form with blanks.

STATE EMS

PRESS DOWN, YOU ARE MAKING THREE COPIES.

RUN REPORT #	Mo. Day Year	M T W Th F S Sun	SERVICE NAME	SERVICE NO.	VEHICLE NO.	ALS ☐ Performed ☐ Back-up called	SERVICE RUN NO.
746118							

NAME | BILLING INFORMATION

STREET OR R.F.D.

CITY/TOWN | STATE | ZIP

AGE/DATE OF BIRTH | ☐ Male ☐ Female | PHONE

INCIDENT LOCATION: | ADDRESS | CITY/TOWN

TRANSPORTED TO: | TREATING/FAMILY PHYSICIAN | CREW LICENSE NUMBERS

TRANSPORTATION/COMMUNICATIONS PROBLEMS

☐ Medical
☐ Cardiac
☐ Poisoning/OD
☐ Respiratory
☐ Behavioral
☐ Diabetic
☐ Seizure
☐ CVA
☐ OB/Gyn
☐ Other______

☐ Trauma
☐ Multi-Systems Trauma
☐ Head
☐ Spinal
☐ Burn
☐ Soft Tissue Injury
☐ Fractures
☐ Other______

☐ Code 99

R	L	LUNG SOUNDS
☐	☐	CLEAR
☐	☐	ABSENT
☐	☐	DECREASED
☐	☐	RALES
☐	☐	WHEEZE
☐	☐	STRIDOR

TYPE OF RUN
☐ Emergency Transport
☐ Routine Transfer
☐ Emergency Transfer
☐ No Transport
☐ Refused Transport

TIME	CODE		ODOMETER
		Call Received	
		Enroute	
		At Scene	
		From Scene	
		At Destination	
		In Service	

☐ MEDICATIONS ☐ ALLERGIES

CHIEF COMPLAINT:

TIME	PULSE	RESP	BP	PUPILLARY RESPONSE	SKIN	VERBAL RESPONSE	MOTOR RESPONSE	EYE-OPENING RESPONSE	CAPILLARY REFILL
			/			5 4 3 2 1	6 5 4 3 2 1	4 3 2 1	☐ Normal ☐ None ☐ Delayed
			/			5 4 3 2 1	6 5 4 3 2 1	4 3 2 1	☐ Normal ☐ None ☐ Delayed
			/			5 4 3 2 1	6 5 4 3 2 1	4 3 2 1	☐ Normal ☐ None ☐ Delayed

☐ MVA ☐ Concern AOB/ETOH SEAT BELTS: ☐ Used ☐ Not Used ☐ N/A ☐ Helmet Used

MUTUAL AID: Assisted/Assisted by Service # ______ Time Called: ______

PATIENT'S SUSPECTED PROBLEM: 746118

☐	Cleared Airway	☐	Extrication
☐	Artificial Respiration/BVM	☐	Cervical Immobilization
☐	Oropharyngeal Airway	☐	KED/Short Board
☐	Nasopharyngeal Airway	☐	Long Board
☐	CPR-Time:	☐	Restraints
☐	Bystander CPR	☐	Traction Splinting
☐	AED	☐	General Splinting
☐	Suction	☐	Cold Application
☐	Oxygen-LPMin __ ☐ Nasal ☐ Mask	☐	MAST Inflated
☐	Pulse Oximetry	☐	
☐	Autovent	☐	

☐ Medication Administered | ☐ Defib Lic.# ____ | MEDICAL CONTROL ☐ Written Order/Protocol ☐ Verbal Order/Protocol

☐ Monitor | ☐ Chest Decomp | IV ☐ SUC LIC.# ____ Total Attempts ___

☐ Pacing | ☐ Caricothyrotomy | ☐ UNSUC LIC.# ____ ___

EOA ☐ SUC LIC.# ____ Total Attempts ___ ☐ UNSUC LIC.# ____ ___

ET ☐ SUC LIC.# ____ Total Attempts ___ ☐ UNSUC LIC.# ____ ___

LIC #	EKG RHYTHM	TIME	MEDS/DEFIB/C-VERT	DOSE W/S	ROUTE

NAME OF E.D. TREATING PHYSICIAN ______ SIGNATURE OF CREW MEMBER IN CHARGE ______ COPY 1 HOSPITAL

FIGURE 17-12 (A) Example of a prehospital care report. A PCR report. (B) An EMT completes her prehospital care report, using a computer in the receiving hospital ED.

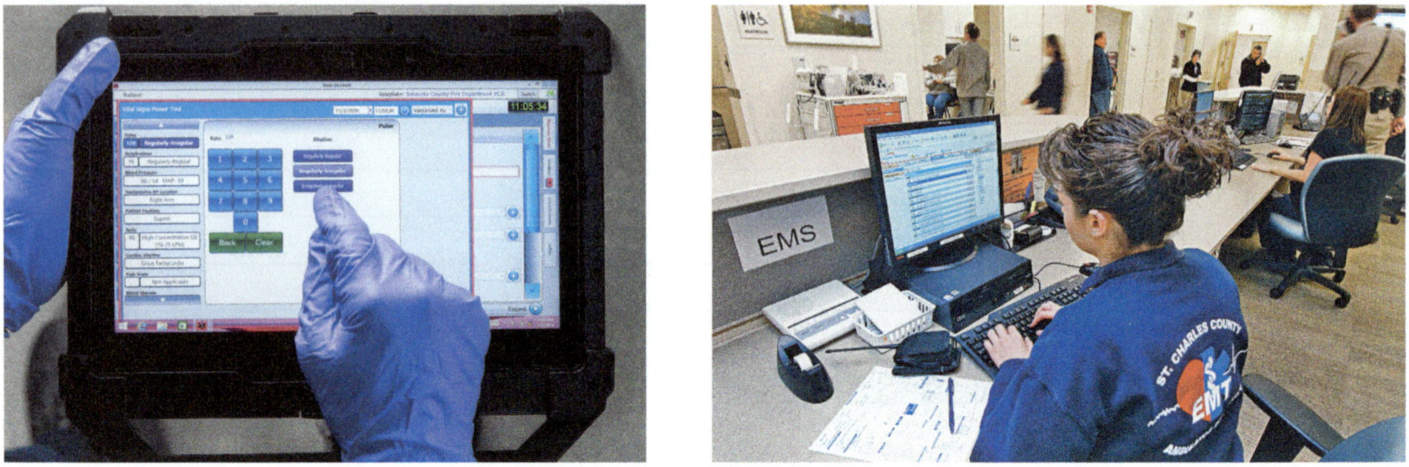

A

B

Administrative Data

Depending on the service you belong to, you may have to obtain insurance and billing information from the patient or patient's family. This may be recorded on your prehospital care report, on a separate form, or on both.

Education and Research

Your report may be examined later as part of a research project. Analysis of statistics compiled from prehospital care reports can reveal patterns and trends in EMS management and care. For example, analysts may see instances in which response time could be improved, or different ways of scheduling and deploying units to prepare for busy areas and times. Statistics also may justify a request for additional resources.

Prehospital care reports can help management keep track of each EMT's experience and skills. Extra practice may be scheduled during continuing education sessions for skills that the reports reveal are underused, for instance. When an unusual or uncommon type of call takes place, the prehospital care report may be used as a demonstration of how to document such a case after it is stripped of data that might identify the patient.

Quality Improvement

Most organizations have a quality improvement (QI)—also known as a quality assurance (QA) or continuous quality improvement (CQI)—system in place by which calls are routinely reviewed for conformity to current medical and organizational standards. Examination of prehospital care reports is one major way of conducting this review. At times, QI evaluations reveal excellent care by an EMT team that deserves special recognition and a "pat on the back."

Completion of the Prehospital Care Report

Because of all the purposes the prehospital report serves, it is essential that it be completed as soon as possible after the call, ideally before you leave the hospital. Timely completion of the report will ensure that it is readily available to the hospital providers as they make important patient-care decisions. You also want to complete the report while the events of the call are fresh in your mind, to ensure accuracy. Your EMS agency will likely have specific policies about how quickly the prehospital reports must be completed.

Elements of the Prehospital Care Report

Data Elements

Each individual box in the prehospital care report is called a *data element*. Although some elements may seem insignificant, each is actually an important part of the report and of the description of the patient and patient responses. These elements are necessary for research as well as for documenting the call.

BOX 17-2 NHTSA Minimum Data Set

Patient Information

This information is gathered at the time of the EMT's initial contact with a patient on arrival at the scene, following all interventions, and on arrival at the medical facility:

- Chief complaint
- Level of responsiveness (AVPU)–mental status
- Systolic blood pressure for patients greater than 3 years old
- Skin perfusion (capillary refill) for patients less than 6 years old
- Skin color and temperature
- Pulse rate
- Respiratory rate and effort

Administrative Information (Run Data)

- Time of incident report
- Time unit notified
- Time of arrival at patient
- Time unit left scene
- Time of arrival at destination
- Time of transfer of care

To aid in evaluation and research across states and regions, the National Highway Traffic Safety Administration (NHTSA) has developed a data set of more than four hundred elements. There is a standardized definition of what each element means, so regions and states can consolidate and compare their data. There is also a minimum data set containing a much smaller number of elements that all prehospital care reports should have nationwide. The NHTSA data set has been adopted by many states, which are in the process of implementing it. The minimum data set is summarized in Box 17-2.

The prehospital care report can be broken down into two sections: run data and patient information. The format for data varies, depending on whether it is a paper report or an electronic report, as well as on the specific information required by your service. Formats you may encounter include check boxes, short answers, and narrative sections for longer answers. Review Figure 17-9 (an electronic report) and Figure 17-11 (a paper report) as you read about the following report elements.

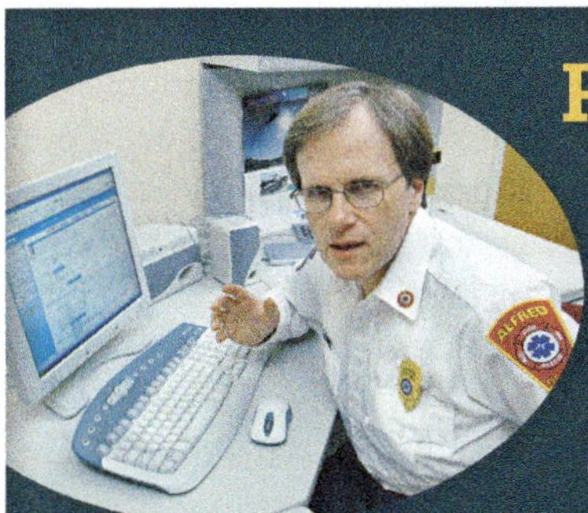

Point of View

"I remember the day I found out the right way to do documentation.

"I turned in a run report one evening. When I came in to work the next day, the chief called me in. He wasn't happy. And looking back, he had reason not to be. It wasn't my best work. I had listened to my partner. He has been around for 25 years. He told me to just put down a couple of sentences and the vitals, said it was a 'no-brainer.'

"Now I know that if I got sued, it would've looked bad. But the thing that really got me is when the chief told me it looked like I was doing a poor job. I know I took good care of that patient. And I even helped contact her family on the cell phone so someone would be at the hospital for her.

"I don't want a bad report to go to the QI committee–or to court–but most important, I am proud of what I do. The chief made me realize my reports should reflect that pride. And believe me, now they do."

Run Data

Spaces for run data, which may be provided at the beginning or end of the report form, include the agency name, date, times, call number, unit personnel and levels of certification, and other basic information as mandated by your service. Times recorded must be accurate and synchronous (by clocks or computers that show the same time). Be sure to use the time as given by the dispatcher when noting times on your report. There may be a difference of several minutes between the time displayed on your watch and the dispatch center's official time. Computer-aided dispatch systems that synchronize with computerized patient care reports use the same times. This time difference may seem insignificant, but is actually very important in such areas as determining how long a patient has been in cardiac arrest, trends in patient condition, or measurement of system efficiency in response times.

Patient Information

This section contains information about the patient. Specifically, it typically includes:

- Patient's name, address, and phone number
- Patient's sex, age, and date of birth
- Patient's weight
- Patient's race and/or ethnicity
- Billing and insurance information (in many jurisdictions).

Information Gathered During the Call

Following the run data and basic patient information, prehospital care reports provide areas for information about the entire call. This information may include:

- Your general impression of the patient
- A narrative summary of events throughout the call, including the chief complaint, history of the present illness, past medical history, physical exam, and care
- Specific sections to detail prior aid, past medical history, physical exam results, vital signs, ECG results, procedures and treatments, medications administered, and other information about the call as required by your service
- Transport information.

Narrative Sections

The narrative section or sections of a prehospital care report are less structured than the fill-in or check-box sections. They provide space to write information about the patient that cannot fit into fill-in blanks or check boxes. In a paper report, the space provided for narratives is still somewhat limited. In an electronic report, however, the space for the narrative will typically expand as needed. Even though the electronic space is expandable and you want to include all important information, you should still strive to write clearly and concisely as a courtesy to those who will need to read your report.

Experienced EMTs consider a good prehospital care report one that "paints a picture" of their patient. The report, as mentioned previously, is read by many people and is a vital part of the patient's record. When hospital personnel or your quality improvement team read your report, it should tell the patient's story fully and appropriately.

Remember, you were involved throughout the call and are familiar with the patient, the patient's chief complaint, and the care you gave. The people who read your report will have no prior knowledge of the call or the patient. It is imperative that you provide complete, accurate, and pertinent information about your patient and present the information in a logical order.

NOTE: *The simple fact that there is no pain or complaint of difficulty does not mean that the patient should not be treated. If the patient's medical condition or mechanism of injury so indicates, treat the patient despite the absence of pain or other symptoms and document accordingly.*

The following guidelines will help you prepare narrative portions of your prehospital care reports.

- **Include both objective and pertinent subjective information.** Objective statements are those that are observable, measurable, or verifiable, such as, "The patient has a swollen, deformed extremity." This is backed up by your visual observation. An objective statement might also be "The patient's blood pressure was 110/80," based on a measurement you took.

  Subjective information is information from an individual point of view. It may be provided by the patient as a symptom. ("I feel dizzy.") It also may be provided by the EMT, such as your general impression of the patient. ("Patient appears to have difficulty breathing.") Avoid subjective statements that are merely opinions, are beyond your level of training or scope of practice ("I do not believe that the leg is broken" or "Patient is probably having a heart attack"), or are irrelevant. ("Patient's daughter was rude.")

  Prehospital care reports are designed to be factual documents. Use objective statements whenever possible and only pertinent subjective statements. If you record something you did not observe yourself, put it in quotation marks (e.g., "A bystander stated that 'The patient passed out at the wheel before crashing' "). Placing a statement in quotation marks and identifying the source lets readers of the report know where the information came from.

  The chief complaint is another piece of information that is sometimes given in quotation marks. Patients who are conscious and oriented will usually tell you why they or someone else called you. ("My chest hurts.") If the patient is not conscious or oriented, the person who called EMS may provide the chief complaint. ("She said he 'felt faint and then passed out.' ") Since the chief complaint is in someone else's words, it should be placed in quotation marks.

  In documenting your assessment procedures, remember to document important observations about the scene, such as suicide notes, weapons, and any other facts that would be important for patient care but not available to the emergency department personnel.

- **Include pertinent negatives.** These are examination findings that are negative (things that are not true) but are important to note. For example, if a patient has chest pain, you will ask if the patient has difficulty breathing. If the patient says nothing, that statement is an important piece of negative information. On your prehospital care report, you would note, "The patient said nothing when asked about difficulty breathing." Negative information often applies to trauma patients. For example, if the mechanism of injury indicates that there may be an injury to the arm but the patient says there is no pain, you would note, "The patient denies pain in right arm." Documenting pertinent negatives lets other medical professionals know that you thought to examine these areas and that the findings were negative. Not documenting them might leave the reader wondering if this area was explored at all.

- **Avoid radio codes and nonstandard abbreviations.** Codes you may use on the radio may not be familiar to hospital personnel, so do not use them in written documentation. Abbreviations, when used properly, make writing efficient and accurate. However, using nonstandard abbreviations will cause confusion and possibly lead to errors in patient care.

- **Write legibly and use correct spelling.** A prehospital care report will have absolutely no value if it cannot be read, so take the time to make your handwriting readable. Unclear writing, misread by others, may cause errors that could harm the patient. In addition, your QI team will be unable to read the report for review, and it will have no value for research or training. Spelling is also important. If you cannot properly spell a word, look it up (many ambulances and emergency departments have medical dictionaries) or use another word. If you are typing your narrative, be sure the word that your spell checker suggests is the word you want to use.

- **Use medical terminology correctly.** Be sure that any medical terms you employ are used correctly. If you are not sure of the meaning of a term, look it up in a medical dictionary or use everyday language to describe the condition instead. Careless use of medical terms could make your report unclear or cause a misunderstanding that might result in harm to the patient.
- **If it's not written down, you didn't do it.** This is a statement that you will most likely hear from your instructor and experienced EMTs in the field. It explains an important concept of EMS documentation. Make sure that you document all your interventions thoroughly. If you did not document them, it will appear as if they were never performed when the call is later reviewed.

The prehospital care report's most important function is to present an accurate representation of the patient's condition throughout the call, the patient's history and vital signs, treatments performed, and changes or lack of changes in the patient's condition following treatments.

Special Documentation Issues

CORE CONCEPT
Legal aspects and benefits of documentation

Legal Issues

There are several legal issues pertaining to prehospital care reports and other documents you may be asked to complete. These include issues of confidentiality, patient refusals, falsification, and error correction.

Confidentiality

The prehospital care report itself and the information it contains are strictly confidential. The information must not be discussed with or distributed to unauthorized persons. The Health Insurance Portability and Accountability Act (HIPAA) requires ambulance services that are covered by the law to take certain steps to safeguard patient confidentiality (Figure 17-13). This typically includes placing completed PCRs into a locked box. HIPAA, state, and local regulations will indicate to whom the information may be distributed. Obviously, the receiving hospital must receive patient care information so it can treat the patient properly. Most reports have a copy that will be left at the hospital. Confidentiality issues were discussed in the *Medical, Legal, and Ethical Issues* chapter.

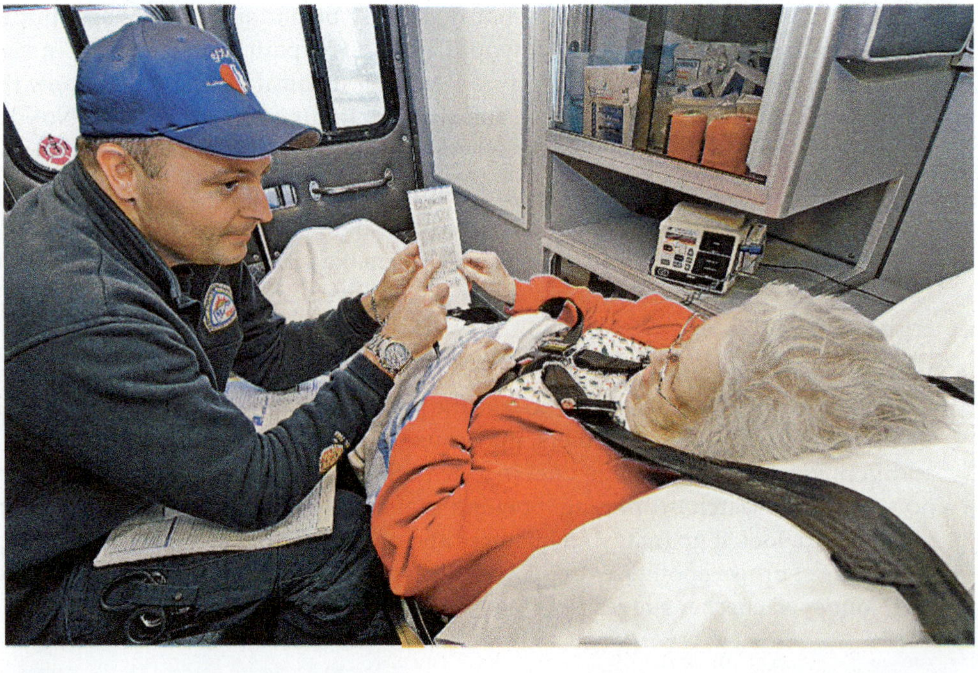

FIGURE 17-13 An EMT explains a HIPAA privacy information leaflet to a patient.

Patient Refusals

The *Medical, Legal, and Ethical Issues* chapter also discussed the issue of liability when patients refuse treatment. It is one of the foremost causes of liability for EMTs and their EMS systems. The chapter presented several suggestions on what to do when a patient refuses care or transportation.

CORE CONCEPT
Documentation concerns in patient refusal

Document all actions you take to persuade the patient to go to the hospital. In addition, you will have to make notes on the patient's capacity, or the ability to make an informed, rational decision regarding medical needs. If the patient is not capable of making this determination for any reason—including age, intoxication (alcohol and/or other drugs), mental competency, or the patient's medical condition—you must document any actions you take to protect the patient. The patient must be informed of the potential consequences of not going to the hospital or of refusing your care.

The fact that a patient refuses transport to a hospital does not mean that you should not perform an assessment. If the patient greets you with a statement such as "I don't know why my daughter called, because I'm not going anywhere," you may still be able to persuade the patient to get "checked out." Perform as much of a secondary assessment as possible, including vital signs. Document all of your findings and emergency care given on the prehospital care report. This information will be important to give to medical direction when you talk to them. Be sure to consult medical direction, according to your local protocols, whenever there is a patient refusal.

Most EMS agencies have a refusal-of-care form to use in the event that you have done your best to persuade the patient to accept care or transport and the patient still refuses. This form may be either part of the prehospital care report or a separate document. You should make sure the patient reads and signs this form (Figure 17-14). It is rare that a patient will refuse to sign the form. If so, be sure to document this as well and note the names of witnesses to the refusal. If possible, when a patient refuses to sign a refusal

Think Like an EMT

Choosing How and What to Document

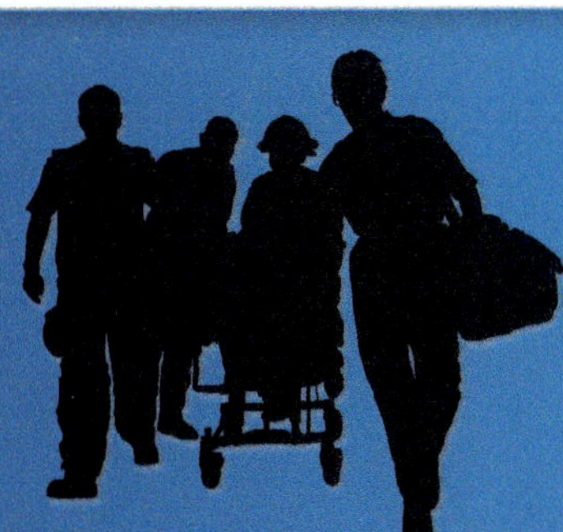

Documentation is an important and challenging duty for the EMT. The documentation you produce may be looked at years later in criminal and civil cases–as well as be reviewed by your QI committee. You will need to make decisions about how and what you document, as you will see in the following scenarios.

1. After the police secure the scene, you treat a man and woman who apparently had a dispute. Neither sustained any life-threatening injuries, so you have time to gather more information at the scene. Even though you and your partner evaluate them in different rooms, they are still angry and trading insults. The boyfriend claims she is a two-timing slut who has syphilis and chlamydia. The girlfriend claims he is an alcoholic and a drug addict. How much of this should you document on the PCR? How should you phrase any information you obtained in this way?
2. Three years after documenting a call, you receive a notice to appear for a deposition regarding it. So much time has passed that you don't remember the call. Should you review the PCR before you go? Why or why not?
3. When you treat a 3-year-old girl for an arm injury, you suspect she has been abused. How do the privacy rules of HIPAA affect what you may and what you should do with regard to reporting this situation to the authorities?

FIGURE 17-14 Example of a refusal information sheet.

GUIDELINES

REFUSAL INFORMATION SHEET

PLEASE READ AND KEEP THIS FORM!

This form has been given to you because you have refused treatment and/or transport by Emergency Medical Services (EMS). Your health and safety are our primary concern, so even though you have decided not to accept our advice, please remember the following:

1) The evaluation and/or treatment provided to you by the EMS providers is not a substitute for medical evaluation and treatment by a doctor. We advise you to get medical evaluation and treatment.

2) Your condition may not seem as bad to you as it actually is. Without treatment, your condition or problem could become worse. If you are planning to get medical treatment, a decision to refuse treatment or transport by EMS may result in a delay which could make your condition or problem worse.

3) Medical evaluation and/or treatment may be obtained by calling your doctor, if you have one, or by going to any hospital Emergency Department in this area, all of which are staffed 24 hours a day by Emergency Physicians. You may be seen at these Emergency Departments without an appointment.

4) If you change your mind or your condition becomes worse and you decide to accept treatment and transport by Emergency Medical Services, please do not hesitate to call us back. We will do our best to help you.

5) DON'T WAIT! When medical treatment is needed, it is usually better to get it right away.

I have received a copy of this information sheet.

PATIENT SIGNATURE: ______________________ DATE: ______

WITNESS SIGNATURE: ______________________ DATE: ______

AGENCY INCIDENT #: ______________ AGENCY CODE: ______

NAME OF PERSON FILLING OUT FORM: ____________________

G 11A

FIGURE 17-15 Document a patient refusal of care thoroughly in the narrative portion of the prehospital care report.

The 49 year old female patient, according to her daughter, "passed out" suddenly. She was in that condition for about 3-5 minutes. The daughter stated that the patient "came to" gradually. Upon our arrival she was fully conscious and oriented. The daughter denies observing any seizure activity. She states that the patient passed out in a chair and did not fall or injure herself as a result of the incident. The patient denies any problems such as chest pain or difficulty breathing. She denies allergies. Her last oral intake was about 2 hours ago (sandwich and coffee). The patient denies any past medical history or current medications.

Vital signs noted above show no abnormalities between two sets taken at a 15 minute interval. The patient refuses transportation to the hospital and has signed the refusal form attached to this report. Her daughter is present with her at her residence and witnessed the refusal. The patient appears to have capacity and be oriented. She was advised to call back at any time should she need our assistance or transportation to the hospital of her choice. She was also advised that her failure to go to the hospital may result in a return or worsening of the previous symptoms which, depending on the underlying cause, could result in a serious medical problem or even death.

The patient's daughter will stay with her for several hours and then provide follow-up calls throughout the evening to make sure the patient is all right. The patient was encouraged to contact her family physician for follow-up care as soon as possible. Since the patient did not have one, a sticker listing our phone number was placed on her phone. We contacted medical direction about the situation and spoke to Dr. Baker at Mercy Hospital. She had no further suggestions.

form, get the witnesses to sign a statement confirming that the patient has refused care or transport.

You should also include information about the patient refusal in the narrative section of the prehospital care report. Figure 17-15 shows a handwritten sample documentation of a patient refusal that might go into the narrative portion of the prehospital care report.

You will note that the narrative shown in Figure 17-15 contains many points of information, including pertinent negatives. The report states that the patient "denies" chest pain or difficulty in breathing. Statements from the patient's daughter are noted as to the source: "according to her daughter . . . " and "The daughter denies seeing any seizure activity."

Before you leave patients who have refused care or transport, be sure to make and document alternative care suggestions, such as encouraging them to seek care from a doctor. Try to be sure that a responsible family member or friend remains with the patient. Make sure that the responsible person also understands that the patient should seek care. Never convey the impression that you are annoyed about being called to the scene "for nothing." Make certain patients understand that if the condition worsens, or even if they change their minds, EMS should be called, and you or another EMT team will gladly come back.

Falsification

Prehospital care reports document the information obtained and the care rendered during the call. False entries or misrepresentations on a report are usually intended to cover up serious flaws in assessment or in care. However, falsification may actually make the problem look worse when it is uncovered.

Two types of errors may be committed during a call: of omission and commission. Errors of omission are those in which an important part of the assessment or care was left out. An example is oxygen. If a patient is experiencing shortness of breath, oxygen is an appropriate treatment. If it is overlooked for any reason, never write that oxygen was administered when it was not.

Occasionally, because of events during transport to a hospital, an EMT may be able to get only one set of vital signs. Never be tempted to write down an extra set of vital signs when they were not taken. Document only the vital signs that were taken. If there is a reason you have taken only one set, document the reason (e.g., "The patient became combative and disoriented en route, preventing a second set of vital signs").

Errors of commission are actions performed on the patient that are wrong or improper. An example of this is incorrect administration of medication. There are certain medications that you will be able to administer or assist the patient in self-administering. This is a great responsibility. If a medication was administered when it was not indicated, it is important to tell medical direction and document the incident on the prehospital care report. Failure to document exactly what happened may have a further negative effect on the patient's care. The hospital may think that the patient's condition is due to some other cause. In other situations, the hospital may re-administer the medication, not realizing that it had already been given.

Document the situation surrounding any error of omission or commission and explain exactly what happened. Document what was done to correct the situation, including advising medical direction and verbally notifying hospital personnel.

Falsification or misrepresentation on a prehospital care report leads to poor patient care because the facts were not documented, and hospital personnel may be misled about the patient's condition and the care received. Falsification or misrepresentation may also lead to the suspension or revocation of your certification or license as an EMT.

You will avoid falsifications if you follow this principle: Write everything important that did happen and nothing that didn't.

Correction of Errors

Prehospital care reports are not always written in ideal circumstances. You may even find yourself being dispatched to another call before you finish writing up your last one. In situations such as this, you may inadvertently write incorrect information on the report.

Any time there is incorrect information on the report, it must be corrected.

If your system uses an electronic PCR without paper copies, log in and get access to the PCR. You may need an administrator at your service to unlock it for you. Correct the data and add an addendum that explains the change you made and why.

FIGURE 17-16 Cross out an error with a single line and initial the change, as in this handwritten example.

COMMENTS PATIENT COMPLAINS OF PAIN IN HIS ~~RIGHT~~ DL LEFT SHOULDER THAT RADIATES TO THE LEFT ARM.

If your system uses paper reports and the form is still intact (all copies attached and not yet distributed), or if you are correcting the paper copy of a computer-generated form, draw a single horizontal line through the error, initial it, then write the correct information beside it (Figure 17-16). Do not completely cross out the error or obliterate it. This may appear to be an attempt to cover up a mistake in patient care. Follow your agency's guidelines for changing information in the computerized run report program. Changes are usually logged with the date and time of the change and the name of the EMT who made the change. It is important that changes are identified and the report is marked as amended. You may need to send copies of the amended report to those who received copies previously.

If the error is discovered at a later date, after the report has been submitted, draw a single line through the error, mark the area with your initials and the date, and add the correct information to the end of the report or in a separate note. This should be done in a different-colored ink when possible, so the change will be obvious. Copies of the report may have already been distributed to other agencies, your quality improvement committee, insurance companies, or attorneys. A corrected copy may need to be sent. Make sure that you place the date on the changes, so the most recent copy is identifiable. If information has been omitted and you wish to add it, be sure also to date this information and place your initials by the added information.

Whether you need to submit a copy of the revised form to the receiving hospital will probably depend on the seriousness of your change. Follow your agency's procedures for correction of errors.

Special Situations

Multiple-Casualty Incidents

An incident in which there are many patients or injuries—such as a multiple-vehicle collision, a major fire, or a plane crash—causes many logistical problems for an EMS system. Documentation of information for individual patients may be difficult. Patients in a multiple-casualty incident (MCI) will probably be moved from one treatment area to another at the scene, then receive transport to a hospital. Patients may be transported to several different hospitals. It is very important to keep information with patients from an MCI scene as they move through the system. This is often done through the use of a triage tag (Figure 17-17). This tag is affixed to the patient and used to record the patient's chief complaint and injuries, vital signs, and treatments given. Later in the emergency, the tag will be used to complete a traditional prehospital care report.

When completing a prehospital care report for a patient involved in a multiple-casualty incident, it will not be possible to provide the detail that you would normally provide for a single-patient call. This is an understandable consequence of the MCI. Your region or agency may have requirements for what information must be completed on the report during an MCI.

FIGURE 17-17 During a multiple-casualty incident, triage tags are used to document information for each patient. (B) EMT with triage tag. *(Photo B: © Steve Salengo)*

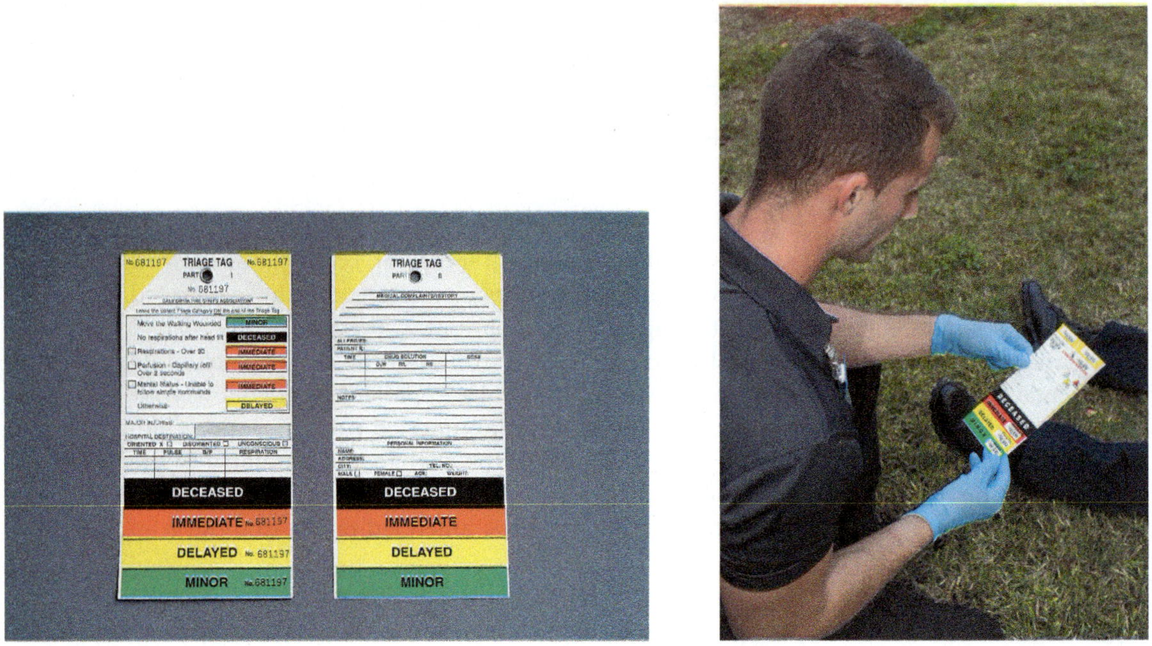

A B

Special Situation Reports

Many states use a supplemental form for advanced life support (ALS) calls or additional documentation for calls that were complex or involved (Figure 17-18).

Your activities as an EMT may also take you to some unusual situations that will require documentation on a form other than a prehospital care report. Such forms are usually specific to a local agency rather than mandated statewide (Figure 17-19). Some examples of situations that might require this kind of special report include:

- Exposure to infectious disease
- Injury to yourself or another EMT
- Hazardous or unsafe scenes to which other crews should be alerted
- Referrals to social service agencies for elderly or other patients in need of home care
- Mandatory reports for child or elder abuse.

This list is not all-inclusive. If there is any situation that requires extra documentation, the special report form may be the place to note it. It is important to remain accurate and objective when filling out this type of report, especially in an unusual or emotional situation. Follow local guidelines for the documentation of confidential information in these reports and for distribution of copies to appropriate agencies or persons.

FIGURE 17-18 Example of a supplemental form. *(New York State Department of Health)*

USE BALL POINT PEN ONLY.

M D Y
DATE   RUN NO.

CONTINUATION FORM for the Prehospital Care Report

Press Down Firmly. You're Making 4 Copies.

AGENCY CODE   VEH. ID

Name   Agency Name   Enter PCR ID# (Top Center of PCR)

ADDITIONAL HISTORY & PHYSICAL EXAM FINDINGS   Weight in Kilograms

R BREATH SOUNDS L	NECK VEINS	EDEMA	ABDOMEN
☐ Normal ☐ ☐ Decreased ☐ ☐ Absent ☐ ☐ Rales ☐ ☐ Rhonchi ☐ ☐ Wheezes ☐	☐ Normal ☐ Distended **TRACHEAL SHIFT** R ☐ L ☐	☐ Pedal ☐ Sacral ☐ Ascites ☐ Other	☐ Normal ☐ Tender ☐ Rigid ☐ Distended ☐ Other

SERIAL VITAL SIGNS, EKG, RHYTHMS, MEDICATIONS AND TREATMENT

TIME	RESP.	PULSE	B.P.	LEVEL OF CONSCIOUSNESS	EKG RHYTHMS	DEFIBRILLATION CARDIOVERSION	MEDICATIONS	DOSE	ROUTE
	Rate: ☐ Regular ☐ Shallow ☐ Labored	Rate: ☐ Regular ☐ Irregular		☐ Alert ☐ Voice ☐ Pain ☐ Unresp.	☐ NSR ☐ Brady ☐ Asystole ☐ IVR ☐ V. Fib. ☐ V. Tach. ☐ PVC ☐ SVT ☐ Other		☐ Epinephrine ☐ Dopamine ☐ Naloxone ☐ Atropine ☐ Sodium Bicarb. ☐ Bretylium ☐ Dextrose ☐ Isoproterenol ☐ Nitroglycerin ☐ Lidocaine ☐ Lasix ☐ Other		☐ IV ☐ ET ☐ IM ☐ SL ☐ SQ ☐ PO ☐ Nebulizer
	Rate: ☐ Regular ☐ Shallow ☐ Labored	Rate: ☐ Regular ☐ Irregular		☐ Alert ☐ Voice ☐ Pain ☐ Unresp.	☐ NSR ☐ Brady ☐ Asystole ☐ IVR ☐ V. Fib. ☐ V. Tach. ☐ PVC ☐ SVT ☐ Other		☐ Epinephrine ☐ Dopamine ☐ Naloxone ☐ Atropine ☐ Sodium Bicarb. ☐ Bretylium ☐ Dextrose ☐ Isoproterenol ☐ Nitroglycerin ☐ Lidocaine ☐ Lasix ☐ Other		☐ IV ☐ ET ☐ IM ☐ SL ☐ SQ ☐ PO ☐ Nebulizer
	Rate: ☐ Regular ☐ Shallow ☐ Labored	Rate: ☐ Regular ☐ Irregular		☐ Alert ☐ Voice ☐ Pain ☐ Unresp.	☐ NSR ☐ Brady ☐ Asystole ☐ IVR ☐ V. Fib. ☐ V. Tach. ☐ PVC ☐ SVT ☐ Other		☐ Epinephrine ☐ Dopamine ☐ Naloxone ☐ Atropine ☐ Sodium Bicarb. ☐ Bretylium ☐ Dextrose ☐ Isoproterenol ☐ Nitroglycerin ☐ Lidocaine ☐ Lasix ☐ Other		☐ IV ☐ ET ☐ IM ☐ SL ☐ SQ ☐ PO ☐ Nebulizer
	Rate: ☐ Regular ☐ Shallow ☐ Labored	Rate: ☐ Regular ☐ Irregular		☐ Alert ☐ Voice ☐ Pain ☐ Unresp.	☐ NSR ☐ Brady ☐ Asystole ☐ IVR ☐ V. Fib. ☐ V. Tach. ☐ PVC ☐ SVT ☐ Other		☐ Epinephrine ☐ Dopamine ☐ Naloxone ☐ Atropine ☐ Sodium Bicarb. ☐ Bretylium ☐ Dextrose ☐ Isoproterenol ☐ Nitroglycerin ☐ Lidocaine ☐ Lasix ☐ Other		☐ IV ☐ ET ☐ IM ☐ SL ☐ SQ ☐ PO ☐ Nebulizer
	Rate: ☐ Regular ☐ Shallow ☐ Labored	Rate: ☐ Regular ☐ Irregular		☐ Alert ☐ Voice ☐ Pain ☐ Unresp.	☐ NSR ☐ Brady ☐ Asystole ☐ IVR ☐ V. Fib. ☐ V. Tach. ☐ PVC ☐ SVT ☐ Other		☐ Epinephrine ☐ Dopamine ☐ Naloxone ☐ Atropine ☐ Sodium Bicarb. ☐ Bretylium ☐ Dextrose ☐ Isoproterenol ☐ Nitroglycerin ☐ Lidocaine ☐ Lasix ☐ Other		☐ IV ☐ ET ☐ IM ☐ SL ☐ SQ ☐ PO ☐ Nebulizer
	Rate: ☐ Regular ☐ Shallow ☐ Labored	Rate: ☐ Regular ☐ Irregular		☐ Alert ☐ Voice ☐ Pain ☐ Unresp.	☐ NSR ☐ Brady ☐ Asystole ☐ IVR ☐ V. Fib. ☐ V. Tach. ☐ PVC ☐ SVT ☐ Other		☐ Epinephrine ☐ Dopamine ☐ Naloxone ☐ Atropine ☐ Sodium Bicarb. ☐ Bretylium ☐ Dextrose ☐ Isoproterenol ☐ Nitroglycerin ☐ Lidocaine ☐ Lasix ☐ Other		☐ IV ☐ ET ☐ IM ☐ SL ☐ SQ ☐ PO ☐ Nebulizer
	Rate: ☐ Regular ☐ Shallow ☐ Labored	Rate: ☐ Regular ☐ Irregular		☐ Alert ☐ Voice ☐ Pain ☐ Unresp.	☐ NSR ☐ Brady ☐ Asystole ☐ IVR ☐ V. Fib. ☐ V. Tach. ☐ PVC ☐ SVT ☐ Other		☐ Epinephrine ☐ Dopamine ☐ Naloxone ☐ Atropine ☐ Sodium Bicarb. ☐ Bretylium ☐ Dextrose ☐ Isoproterenol ☐ Nitroglycerin ☐ Lidocaine ☐ Lasix ☐ Other		☐ IV ☐ ET ☐ IM ☐ SL ☐ SQ ☐ PO ☐ Nebulizer

COMMENTS:

MEDICAL FACILITY CONTACTED

CREW			
ADDITIONAL NAME—CREW ☐ EMS-FR ☐ EMT ☐ AEMT #	ADDITIONAL NAME—CREW ☐ EMS-FR ☐ EMT ☐ AEMT #	ADDITIONAL NAME—CREW ☐ EMS-FR ☐ EMT ☐ AEMT #	ADDITIONAL NAME—CREW ☐ EMS-FR ☐ EMT ☐ AEMT #

EMS 100A (11/86) provided by NYS-EMS PROGRAM

AGENCY COPY/**WHITE**   HOSPITAL PATIENT RECORD COPY/**PINK**   RESEARCH COPY/**BLUE**   EXTRA SERVICE COPY/**GREEN**

PAGE ______ OF ______

FIGURE 17-19 Example of a special incident report.

Special Incident Report

Department of Emergency Medical Services

Date of Incident: ______ **Time:** ______ **REMO #:** ______

Town Run #: ______ **Reported by:** ______ **Zone:** ______

Type of Incident: ☐ MCI ☐ Rescue ☐ Personnel Matter ☐ Injury ☐ Accident with an EMS vehicle
☐ Infectious Disease Exposure ☐ Scene Conflict ☐ Other ______

Total # of Patients: ☐ #P-1: ____ ☐ #P-2: ____ ☐ #P-3: ____ ☐ #P-0: ____
Elapsed Scene Time: *(First unit arrival to last unit to hospital)* ______
Total Time of Incident: ______

Describe the Incident Below:
Attach any additional documentation such as news clippings and the pre-hospital care report.
Attach additional sheets if necessary.

Signature: ______ **Date:** ______

Office Use Only
This incident relates to: ☐ Day Operation: TOT ______ ☐ Night Operation: TOT: ______ ☐ Administration: TOT: ______

Disposition: ______

Date: ______

Notifications/Copies: ☐ Director ☐ Deputy Director ☐ Supervisors
☐ Deputy Supervisors ☐ Senior Medics ☐ Zone Coordinator(s)
☐ Other ______ Zone: ☐ 2 ☐ 3 ☐ 4

Chapter Review

Key Facts and Concepts

- When calling in patient information, include these elements:
  - Unit identification and level of provider
  - Estimated time of arrival
  - Patient's age and sex
  - Chief complaint
  - Brief, pertinent history of the present illness
  - Major past illnesses
  - Mental status
  - Baseline vital signs
  - Pertinent findings of the physical exam
  - Emergency medical care given
  - Response to emergency medical care
  - Contact made with medical direction if required or if you have questions
- When completing the prehospital care report, or PCR, include the following:
  - Patient's name, address, date of birth, age, sex
  - Billing and insurance information (in many jurisdictions)
  - Nature of the call
  - Mechanism of injury
  - Location where the patient was found
  - Treatment administered before arrival of the EMT (by bystanders, emergency medical responders, or others)
  - History of the present illness, including signs and symptoms
  - Past medical history
  - Baseline and subsequent vital signs
  - Secondary assessment
  - Care administered and the effect that the care had on the patient (e.g., improved; no change)
  - Changes in condition throughout the call
- A PCR may be a legal document in a court proceeding.
- The PCR should be completed as soon as possible after the completion of the call.
- Data from PCRs may help determine future treatments, trends, research, and quality improvement.
- Your report should "paint a picture" of your patient and the condition, accurately describing your contact with the patient throughout the call.

Key Decisions

- What radio procedure should I follow at this (or any) stage of the call?
- What elements should I include in the medical radio report?
- What information about this patient must I include in the care report?
- What steps must I take to avoid legal issues during communication and documentation for this call?

Chapter Glossary

base station a two-way radio at a fixed site such as a hospital or dispatch center.

cell phone a phone that transmits through the air instead of over wires, so the phone can be transported and used over a wide area.

drop report (or transfer report) an abbreviated form of the PCR that an EMS crew can leave at the hospital when there is not enough time to complete the PCR before leaving.

mobile radio a two-way radio that is used or affixed in a vehicle.

portable radio a handheld two-way radio.

repeater a device that picks up signals from lower-power radio units, such as mobile and portable radios, and retransmits them at a higher power. It allows low-power radio signals to be transmitted over longer distances.

telemetry the process of sending and receiving data wirelessly.

watt the unit of measurement of the output power of a radio.

Preparation for Your Examination and Practice

Short Answer

1. List the steps of a medical radio report, and describe the communication that may be necessary during each part.
2. List several guidelines for effective interpersonal communication with patients.
3. Explain what is meant by "objective" and "subjective" information in the narrative portion of the prehospital care report. Explain what is meant by "a pertinent negative."
4. Explain how spelling and the use of codes, abbreviations, and medical terms relate to writing a clear and accurate narrative report.
5. List some important steps to take and information to include when documenting a patient refusal.

Thinking and Linking

Think back to the Vital Signs and Monitoring Devices *chapter and link information from that chapter with information from this chapter as you consider the following situation:*

- Five minutes before arrival at the hospital, you obtain a pulse of 108 on your critically injured patient. As you are writing up your prehospital care report, your partner tells you that just as you arrived at the hospital, he was taking the patient's pulse and got a rate of 59. You are stunned. How could the patient's pulse have dropped from 108 to 59? Then common sense kicks in. "You forgot to multiply by two," you tell him. "The pulse must have been 118." How did you figure out that the rate of 59 had not been multiplied by two? What is the reason for multiplying by two?

Critical Thinking Exercises

It is important to be able to organize your radio and written reports correctly. The purpose of this exercise will be to consider how you might organize the information provided.

1. The following information, describing a patient, is in random order. Organize the information and present a medical radio report as if you were radioing the hospital.
   - Chest pain radiating to the shoulder
   - 56 years old
   - Oxygen applied at 15 liters per minute via nonrebreather
   - Alert and oriented
   - Female
   - Came on 20 minutes ago while mowing the lawn
   - History of high blood pressure and diabetes
   - ETA 20 minutes
   - Pulse 86, respirations 22, skin cool and moist, blood pressure 110/66, SpO_2 96 percent
   - Oxygen relieved the pain slightly
   - Denies difficulty breathing
   - You are requesting orders from medical direction
   - You are on Community BLS Ambulance 4
   - Lung sounds equal on both sides
   - Placed in a position of comfort
2. Write a narrative report for the same call. What did you include in the narrative that you did not include in the radio report? Why?

Street Scenes

You and your partner have just finished a call involving a motor-vehicle crash with two vehicles. It was the first call of the day, just after you had checked out the ambulance but before you had time for breakfast. It is now 9:30 a.m. and you are sitting at a desk in the emergency department, doing the prehospital care report. Although the patient didn't seem to be hurt badly, he had been complaining of lower-back pain. Based on the patient complaint and the patient assessment, you decided to do a full immobilization.

Street Scene Question

1. **What information is important to include in the prehospital care report?**

Although your partner is hurrying you, you write a very complete and thorough prehospital care report. You detail the patient's pulses, motor function, and sensation in all extremities before and after immobilization, including the fact that you observed the patient had difficulty moving his left foot and that he said it felt numb. The patient also told you that he was wearing only a lap-style seat belt at the time of the crash and that he had a considerable amount of pain. He had not moved from the vehicle prior to the arrival of EMS.

Street Scene Questions

2. **What is the importance of doing an accurate and thorough prehospital care report?**
3. **Should you have your partner read and comment on the prehospital care report before considering it complete?**
4. **What are the ramifications of having a prehospital care report in the hospital record that is different from the original copy on file with your EMS agency?**

After writing your prehospital care report, your partner reviews it, and you leave a copy at the hospital for inclusion with the hospital chart. You manage to make it to breakfast, and you put this call behind you.

A few months later, the director of your ambulance service stops you and asks if you remember this call. You think for a moment but have only a vague recollection. The director informs you that the patient has started a lawsuit and claims that he sustained damage as the result of prehospital care. She says that the prehospital care report was reviewed by the ambulance service's lawyer, who believes that it provides a very good defense, and the case will probably be dismissed. The director lets you read a copy of the prehospital care report. As you read it, you start to remember the call. You had forgotten about the patient's complaint of pain and other symptoms.

As she walks away, the director tells you that the good documentation you provided will make all the difference in how this case gets decided. This is very different from a case she had a few years ago when an EMT changed the service's copy of the PCR after leaving a copy at the hospital. In that case, the lawyer for the plaintiff noticed the discrepancies and made things very difficult for the ambulance service.

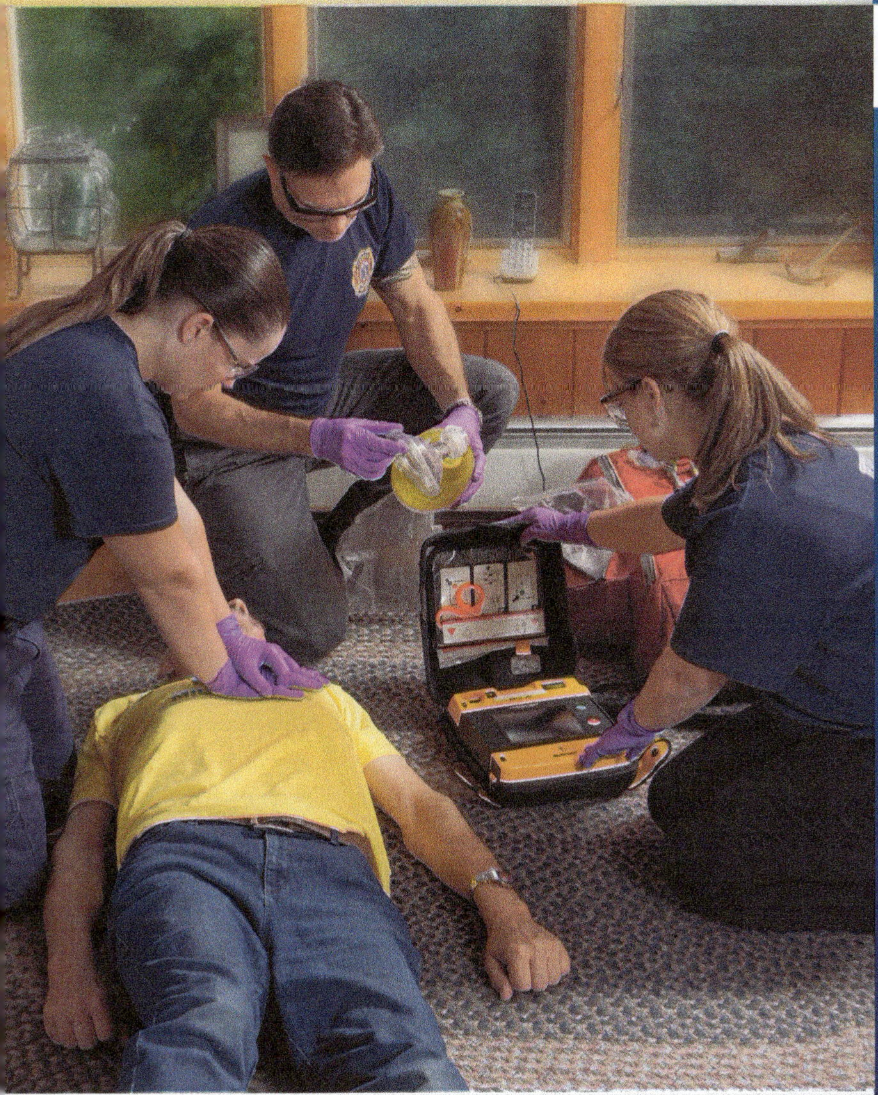

SECTION 4

Medical Emergencies

Medical emergencies are usually caused by a disease or malfunction within the body. This section begins with a chapter on pharmacology (Chapter 18), or the study of drugs and medicines, focusing on the drugs EMTs are permitted to administer or help administer.

The remaining chapters focus on types of medical emergencies that commonly prompt emergency calls to EMS, including breathing difficulty (Chapter 19); chest pain and discomfort (Chapter 20); resuscitation (Chapter 21); diabetic emergencies and conditions that may present with altered mental status, including seizures and stroke (Chapter 22); allergic reactions (Chapter 23); infectious diseases and sepsis (Chapter 24); poisoning and overdose (Chapter 25); abdominal pain and discomfort (Chapter 26); behavioral and psychiatric emergencies, including suicide attempts (Chapter 27); and hematology and nephrology (emergencies resulting from blood and kidney/renal disorders) (Chapter 28).

18 General Pharmacology

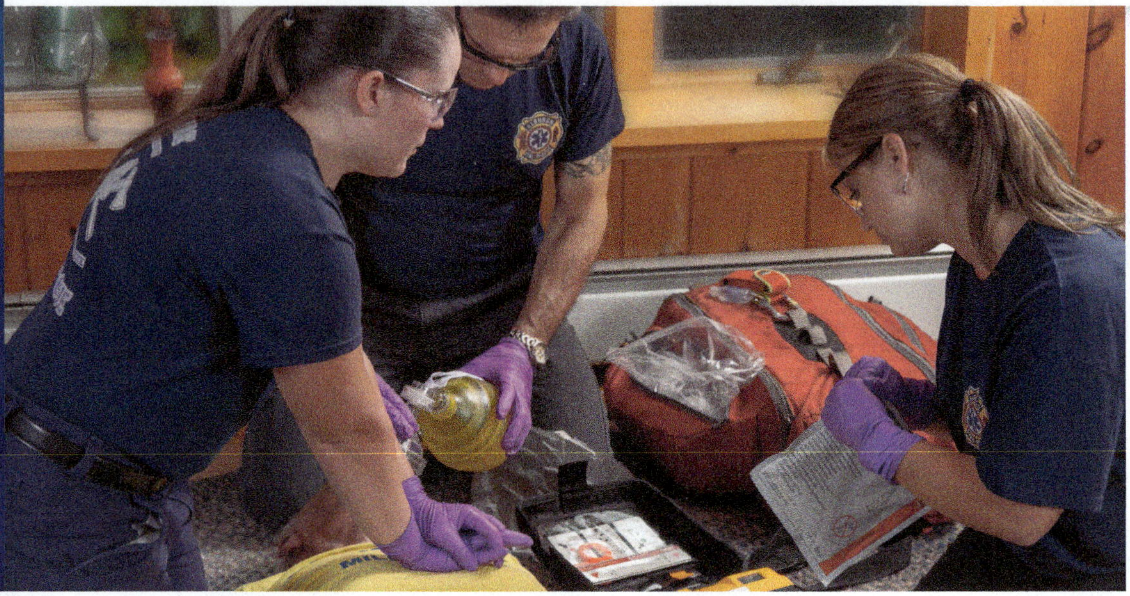

Related Chapters

The following chapters provide additional information related to topics discussed in this chapter:

10 Respiration and Artificial Ventilation

19 Respiratory Emergencies

20 Cardiac Emergencies

22 Diabetic Emergencies and Altered Mental Status

23 Allergic Reactions

25 Poisoning and Overdose Emergencies

Standards

Pharmacology (Content Areas: Principles of Pharmacology; Medication Administration; Emergency Medications)

Competency

Applies fundamental knowledge of the medications that the EMT may assist with/administer to a patient during an emergency

Core Concepts

- Which medications may be carried by the EMT
- Which medications the EMT may help administer to patients
- What to consider when administering any medication

- The role of medical direction in medication administration
- How the EMT may assist with IV therapy

Outcomes

After reading this chapter, you should be able to:

18.1 Describe medications EMTs may carry on the ambulance and administer. (pp. 496–499)

- Describe the actions of specific medications carried on the ambulance (e.g., aspirin, oral glucose, oxygen, naloxone).
- Identify the reason an EMT would administer a medication carried on the ambulance.
- Identify the routes by which medications carried on the ambulance are administered to the patient by the EMT.
- Identify generic and trade names of all medications carried on the ambulance and those prescribed to patients with which EMTs may assist.

18.2 Describe patients' own prescription medications which EMTs may assist patients in taking. (pp. 499–503)

- Describe the actions of bronchodilators, nitroglycerin, epinephrine auto-injectors, and force protection medication.
- Describe the role of medical direction in assisting with administration of patients' prescribed medications.
- Relate the actions of albuterol and epinephrine to the correction of the pathophysiology of anaphylaxis and asthma.

18.3 Explain general concepts of pharmacology. (pp. 503–510)

- Distinguish between chemical, generic, and trade names of drugs.
- Assess patient and context to determine the indications and contraindications for a medication before you give it.
- Anticipate desired effects, known side effects, and untoward effects of drugs before you give them.
- Recognize the occurrence of desired effects, untoward effects, and side effects in a patient.
- Describe the importance of clinical judgment in administering medications.
- Compare the two types of medical authorization under which an EMT can administer medications.
- Describe the importance of checking expiration dates and following the Five Rights of medication administration.
- Describe each of the routes of drug administration.
- Describe how pharmacodynamics affect judgments about medication administration.
- Identify the steps of reassessment and documentation required after administering a medication.
- Describe common categories of medications and herbal remedies that you will find used by patients in the field.

18.4 Explain the EMT's role in assisting with intravenous (IV) therapy. (pp. 510–514)

- Identify the parts of the equipment and supplies required for IV therapy.
- Outline the steps of preparing the IV fluid and intravenous tubing.
- Recognize other tasks EMTs can assist with, if asked, when assisting with IV therapy.
- Describe how to troubleshoot an IV that is not running, running too slowly, or running too quickly.

Key Terms

aspirin, *497*
atomizer, *506*
contraindications, *504*
enteral, *504*
epinephrine, *501*
indications, *504*
inhaler, *499*
naloxone, *499*
nitroglycerin, *501*
oral glucose, *497*
oxygen, *498*
parenteral, *504*
pharmacodynamics, *507*
pharmacology, *496*
side effect, *504*
untoward effects, *504*

AS AN EMT, *you will be trusted with the task of administering medications in emergency situations.* This important responsibility requires you to use critical decision-making skills and pay attention to detail. Although in many cases these medications may be lifesaving, there is the potential to do significant harm to the patient when they are administered incorrectly.

The study of drugs—their sources, characteristics, and effects—is called ***pharmacology***. This chapter introduces the terminology, basic principles, and rules about pharmacology. We will discuss medications EMTs carry on the ambulance and review prescribed medications you may assist the patient in taking with approval from medical direction. You will learn the forms of medications your patients may be taking as well as the names for common types of medications and why they are used.

Although you will learn many facts and terms regarding medications, remember that nothing replaces good judgment and proper decision making. As always, the most important tool you carry is your brain.

NOTE: *Although EMS personnel use the terms medications and drugs interchangeably, the public often associates the word drugs with illegal or abused substances. When dealing with the public, therefore, use the term medicines or medications.*

Medications EMTs Can Administer

pharmacology
(FARM-uh-KOL-uh-je)
the study of drugs, their sources, their characteristics, and their effects.

You will be able to administer or assist with at least these seven medications in the field: aspirin, oral glucose, oxygen, prescribed bronchodilator inhalers, nitroglycerin, epinephrine auto-injectors, and naloxone. Some systems permit EMTs to administer certain additional drugs. The information that follows is a brief introduction to each of these drugs.

Your local system may allow additions to this medication list. It is beyond the scope of this text to include all the possibilities. However, if your system uses medications that are not covered here, be sure to obtain the appropriate information and education for those medications before administering them to a patient. In any case, you will need to be aware of whether you need on-line medical direction to administer a medication or you can administer it off-line under conditions described in a protocol or standing orders.

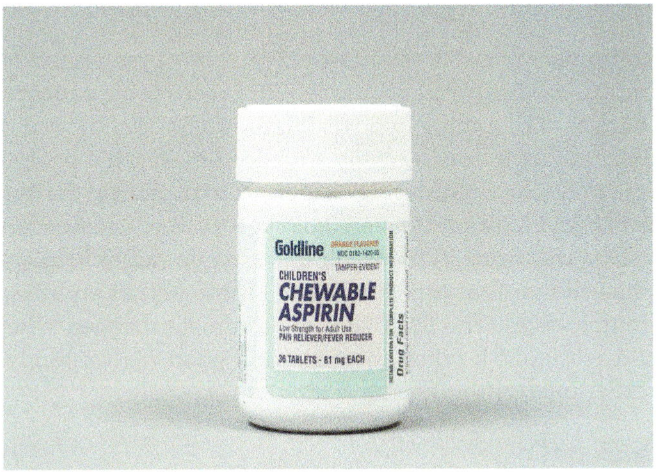

FIGURE 18-1 Aspirin is administered to patients with chest pain of a suspected cardiac origin.

Aspirin

CORE CONCEPT
Which medications may be carried by the EMT

You may have taken a simple ***aspirin*** to relieve a headache or treat a fever. In the world of EMS, however, aspirin has a much more important role. As an EMT, you will administer aspirin to patients with chest pain of a suspected cardiac origin (Figure 18-1). In the event a heart attack is occurring, aspirin reduces the blood's ability to clot and works to prevent the clot formation that causes damage to the heart. Studies have demonstrated that the administration of aspirin to patients having a heart attack (myocardial infarction) can significantly reduce their chance of death. It is an exceptionally important medication under these circumstances. Fortunately, it is also very simple to administer. As many ambulances do not carry drinking water, most services will carry chewable low-dose aspirin, and the patient will simply be asked to chew and swallow the appropriate dose. There are very few reasons not to administer aspirin to a patient having chest pain of a suspected cardiac origin. However, some patients do have allergies, and others have gastrointestinal bleeding that can be made worse by the administration of aspirin. Always follow your local protocols for administration guidelines.

aspirin
a medication used to reduce the clotting ability of blood to prevent and treat clots associated with myocardial infarction.

Oral Glucose

Glucose is a kind of sugar. ***Oral glucose*** is a form of glucose that can be taken by mouth as a treatment for a conscious patient (who is able to swallow) with an altered mental status and a history of diabetes. Too much diabetic medication (such as insulin or oral drugs) coupled with too little food (especially too few carbohydrates) will lead to low blood sugar. The brain is very sensitive to low levels of sugar, and this is commonly a cause of altered mental status. Oral glucose usually comes as a tube of gel (Figure 18-2) that you can apply to a tongue depressor and place between the patient's cheek and gum or under the tongue. This allows the patient to swallow the glucose, so it can be absorbed easily into the digestive tract and bloodstream, which carries it to the brain. This action may begin to reverse the patient's potentially life-threatening condition. The procedure for administering oral glucose will be found in the chapter titled *Diabetic Emergencies and Altered Mental Status*.

oral glucose (GLU-kos)
a form of glucose (a kind of sugar) given by mouth to treat an awake patient (who is able to swallow) with an altered mental status and a history of diabetes.

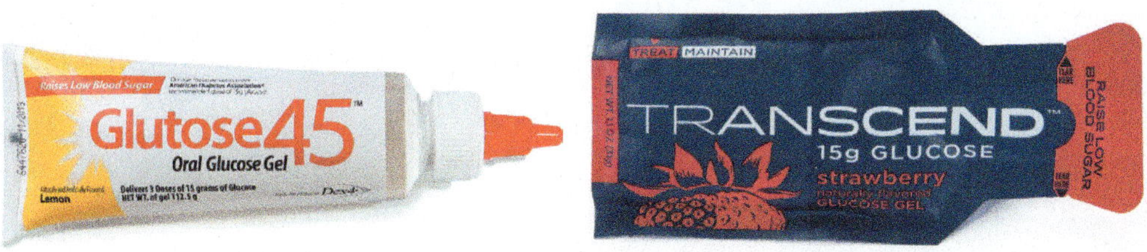

A B

FIGURE 18-2 Oral glucose may help a patient with diabetes. (A) Oral glucose tube. (B) Alternate brand of glucose.

oxygen
a gas commonly found in the atmosphere. Pure oxygen is used as a medication to treat any patient whose medical or traumatic condition may cause the patient to be hypoxic, or low in oxygen.

Oxygen

Oxygen is a gas commonly found in the atmosphere. Pure oxygen is used as a medication to treat any patient whose medical or traumatic condition causes the patient to be hypoxic (low in oxygen) or in danger of becoming hypoxic (Figure 18-3). Throughout this text, you have learned—and will continue to learn—many situations in which a patient should be given oxygen. Specific methods of administering oxygen are explained in the *Resuscitation* chapter.

Until a few years ago, EMTs administered oxygen to all patients except those with very minor problems. This was done in the belief that oxygen might help and could not hurt. Recent research has shown that this is not true. Too much of anything can be harmful under certain circumstances. The EMT should administer oxygen when there is a good reason and should withhold it when there is not a good reason to give it. It should be treated like any other medication you have at your disposal.

Activated Charcoal

NOTE: *Some systems allow the administration of activated charcoal. Therefore, although it is not one of the most commonly carried medications, we discuss it here briefly. Always consult local protocol to confirm which medications you are allowed to carry and administer.*

Activated charcoal is a powder prepared from charred wood, usually premixed with water to form a slurry for use in the field (Figure 18-4). It is used to treat only certain poisonings or overdoses when a substance is swallowed and is in the patient's digestive tract for a prolonged period of time. Activated charcoal will adsorb some poisons (bind them to the surfaces of the charcoal) and help prevent them from being absorbed by the body. The procedure for administering activated charcoal will be found in the *Poisoning and Overdose Emergencies* chapter.

FIGURE 18-3 Oxygen is a commonly used, but powerful, medication.

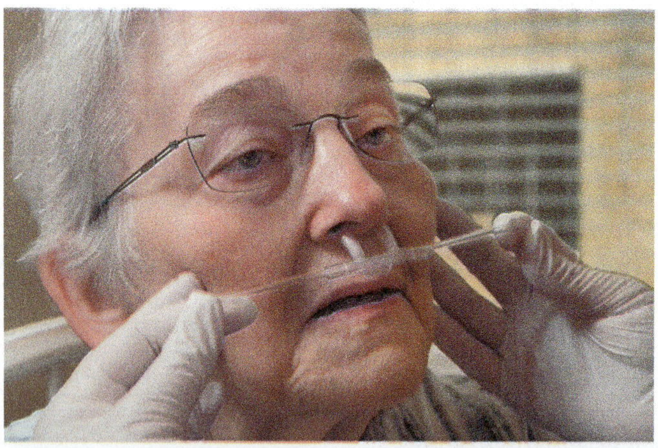

FIGURE 18-4 Activated charcoal is only occasionally used in poisoning cases.

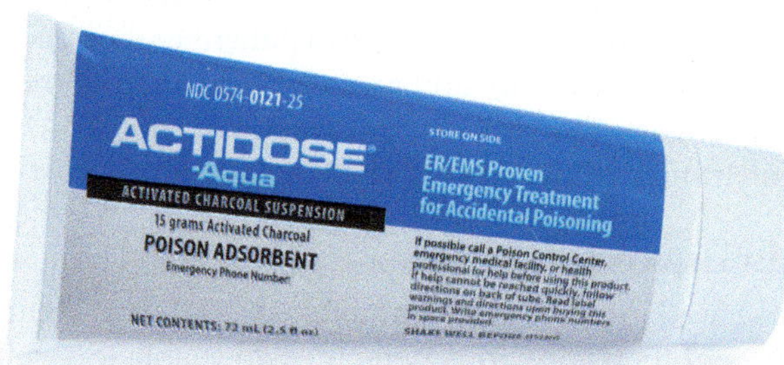

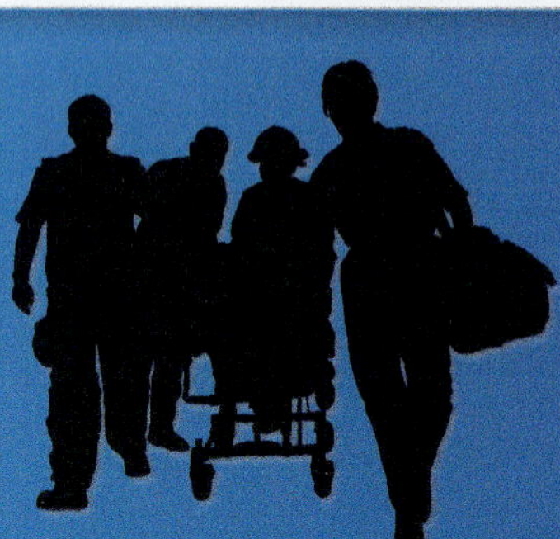

Think Like an EMT

We Are Really Close to the Hospital. Should I Give Aspirin?

You are treating a 68-year-old woman complaining of sudden-onset "tightness" in her chest and nausea. You have done a thorough patient assessment and administered high-concentration oxygen. Local protocols allow the administration of aspirin, but you are only 5 minutes away from the hospital. Should you give the patient the medication?

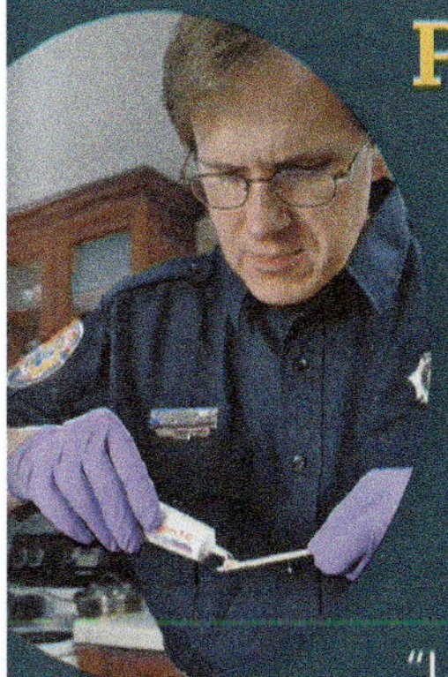

Point of View

"I woke up and checked my blood sugar. It was a little higher than I expected. I ate a light breakfast and took a few extra units of insulin, as my endocrinologist explained for me to do.

"The next thing I know, my husband was looking very concerned. Then the ambulance showed up. I remember the EMTs being there, but I couldn't make out what they were saying. I remember wanting so much to talk to them, but the words weren't coming out right.

"I saw the sugar. They put it in my mouth on the tongue blade. I am not sure how long it took. I was pretty out of it. But suddenly the world was again in focus—like someone adjusted the camera lens and everything was clear.

"I saw the EMTs smiling at me. My husband still had a worried look. But I was OK. I could think and talk and function again. I must have taken too much insulin or read the meter wrong. Thank goodness for the EMTs—and for that sugar."

Naloxone

When someone takes too much of a narcotic, the person can lose consciousness; become unable to protect the airway; and, most important of all, go into respiratory failure with slow, shallow breathing. Narcotics, especially in large or high concentration doses, slow the respiratory drive and can even cause respiratory arrest. ***Naloxone***, trade name Narcan®, one of the few antidotes in medicine, can reverse the effects of a narcotic very quickly (Figure 18-5). Although it is usually injected, naloxone is also effective when administered as a fine spray into the nose. The mucous membranes in the nose can absorb very fine droplets of certain medications and feed them into the circulatory system, allowing them to exert an effect in other parts of the body. If you give naloxone to someone who is unconscious and in respiratory failure but who has not had a narcotic, it will have no effect. If the mucous membranes are damaged or blocked in a patient who has taken a narcotic, intranasal administration will not work and you will need to use your airway management skills. More details on the use of atomized naloxone will be found in the chapter *Poisoning and Overdose Emergencies*.

naloxone
an antidote for narcotic overdoses.

EMTs Assisting with Prescribed Medications

CORE CONCEPT
Which medications the EMT may help administer to patients

Bronchodilator Inhalers

Patients can carry various medications to help them through a period of difficulty breathing. Most often, patients with diseases such as asthma, emphysema, or chronic bronchitis carry a bronchodilator, a medication designed to enlarge constricted bronchial tubes, making breathing easier. Many of these medications can be carried in an ***inhaler***, which contains an aerosol form of a medication the patient can spray directly into the airway (Figure 18-6). Examples of these medications include albuterol (Ventolin® HFA, Proventil®, Volmax®) and levalbuterol (Xopenex®).

inhaler
a spray device with a mouthpiece that contains an aerosol form of a medication that a patient can spray into the airway.

Since many bronchodilators also have an effect on the heart, an increased heart rate and patient jitteriness are common side effects of treatment.

Be sure to determine that the inhaler is actually the patient's and not that of a family member or bystander. You may need to have permission from medical direction to help a patient self-administer a prescribed inhaler. This permission from medical direction may come by phone or radio, or there may be a standing medical order that permits you to assist a patient with this kind of medication. *Always comply with the protocols of your EMS system.* More details on the use of a prescribed inhaler will be found in the chapter titled *Respiratory Emergencies*.

FIGURE 18-5 Naloxone, trade name Narcan®, one of the few antidotes in medicine, can reverse the effects of a narcotic very quickly. (A) Narcan® with syringe and atomizer at left, prefilled syringe and atomizer at right. (B) Narcan® being administered to patient. (C) Close-up of Narcan® inhaler. *(Photos B and C: Edward T. Dickinson, MD)*

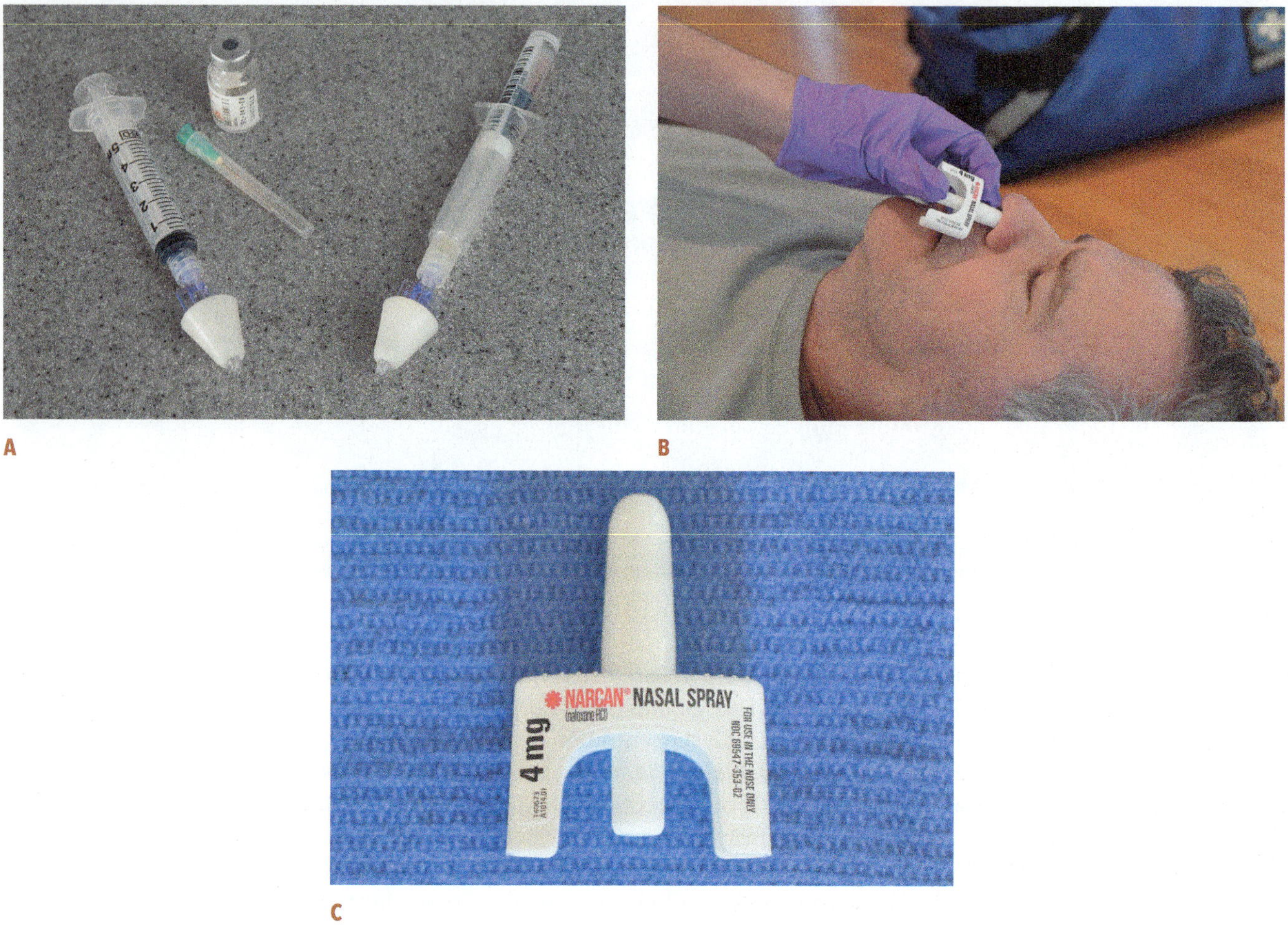

FIGURE 18-6 (A) A prescribed inhaler may help a patient who has respiratory problems. (B) A spacer attached to the inhaler helps the patient by allowing the medication to be released into the spacer, where it remains airborne for a time so the patient can inhale it without feeling rushed—as might be the case if inhaling it directly, without the spacer. (C) EMT assisting with spacer.

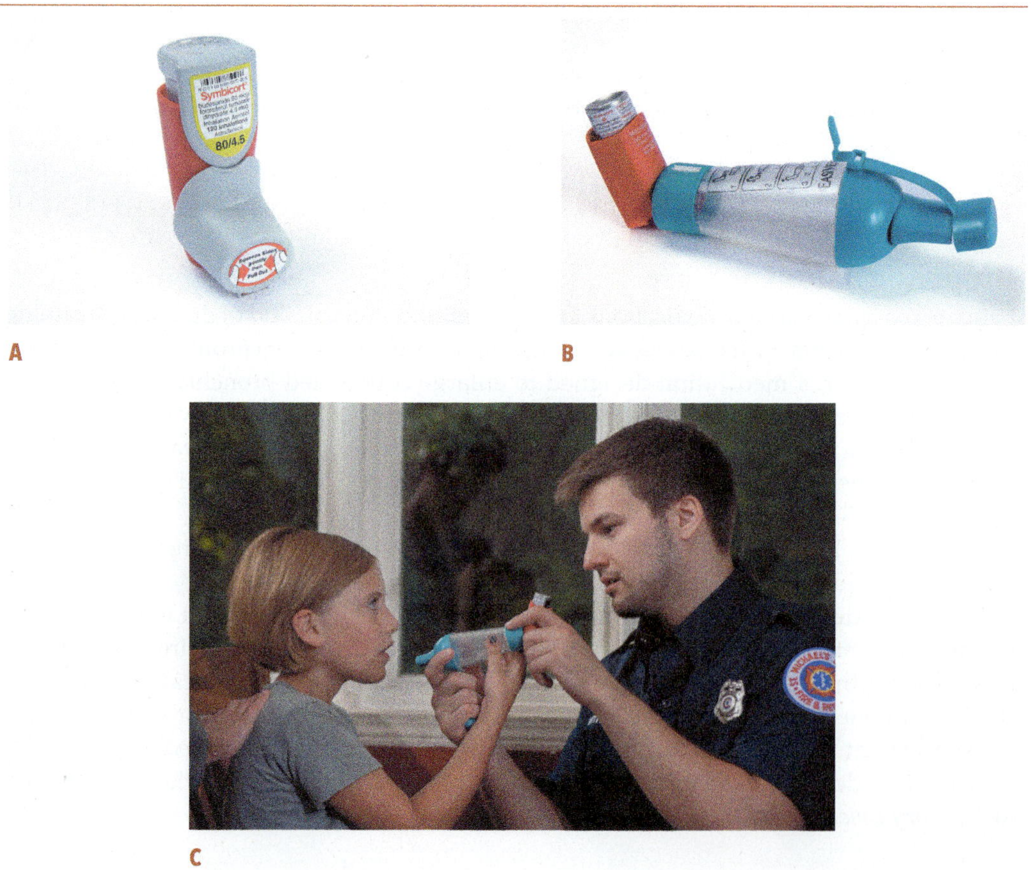

Nitroglycerin

Many patients with problems such as recurrent chest pain or a history of heart attack carry ***nitroglycerin*** pills or spray. Nitroglycerin pills are dissolved sublingually (under the tongue); the spray is administered on or under the tongue and is allowed to absorb (i.e., is not swallowed immediately). Patients should avoid swallowing nitroglycerin in any form because doing so would lead to its being neutralized in the stomach. Nitroglycerin (Figure 18-7) is a drug that helps to dilate the coronary vessels, which supply the heart muscle with blood. It is often called just "nitro." A common trade name is Nitrostat®.

nitroglycerin (NYE-tro-GLIS-uh-rin) a drug that helps to dilate the coronary vessels that supply the heart muscle with blood.

This drug is taken by the patient who has chest pain believed to be cardiac in origin. It is not uncommon for EMTs to treat patients who have already taken a nitroglycerin pill or who are carrying a bottle of nitroglycerin tablets and have not thought to try one. (Many patients are instructed by their physician to take up to three nitroglycerin pills for their chest pain and, if the chest pain persists, to call EMS.)

Be sure to determine that the nitroglycerin is actually the patient's and not that of a family member or bystander. Also determine whether the patient has recently taken anything to treat erectile dysfunction, such as sildenafil (Viagra®), vardenafil (Levitra®), tadalafil (Cialis®), or similar medication. If so, the patient should not take nitroglycerin, because of the possibility of a serious negative interaction with these drugs.

You may need to obtain permission from medical direction by phone or radio, or there may be a standing medical order that permits you to assist a patient with nitroglycerin administration. *Always comply with the protocols of your EMS system.* More information on assisting a patient in taking nitroglycerin will be found in the *Cardiac Emergencies* chapter.

Since nitroglycerin causes a dilation of blood vessels, a drop in the patient's blood pressure is always a potential side effect of administration. If this should occur, you should lay the patient flat and contact medical direction again for advice.

Epinephrine Auto-Injectors

When a patient is highly allergic to something such as shellfish, penicillin, or a bee sting, exposure to it may lead to a very severe reaction that may cause life-threatening changes in the airway and circulation (anaphylaxis). The reaction can be reversed by administering **epinephrine**, a medication that will help to constrict the blood vessels and relax airway passages.

epinephrine (ep-uh-NEF-rin) a drug that helps to constrict the blood vessels and relax passages of the airway. It may be used to counter a severe allergic reaction.

Because severe allergic reactions may reach a life-threatening stage in a very short time, epinephrine must be administered quickly. Many patients who are prone to severe allergic reactions carry an epinephrine auto-injector (Figure 18-8). This is a syringe with a spring-loaded needle that will release and inject epinephrine into the muscle when the auto-injector is pushed against the thigh. There are several different varieties of auto-injector on the market. Epi-Pen® is the trade name of a commonly carried epinephrine auto-injector.

FIGURE 18-7 Nitroglycerin is often prescribed for chest pain. Forms of nitroglycerin include (A) tablets and (B) a spray.

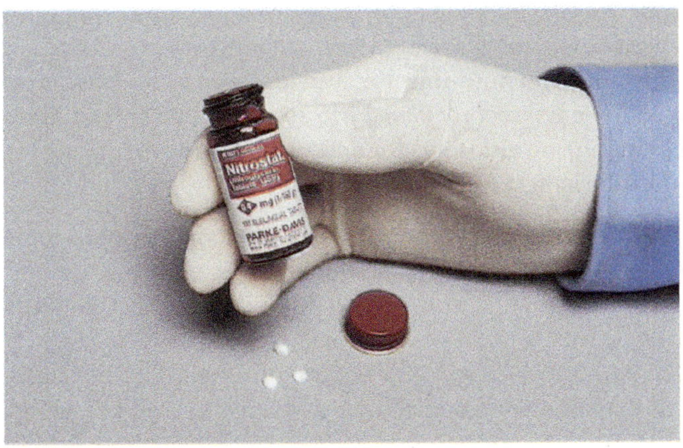

A

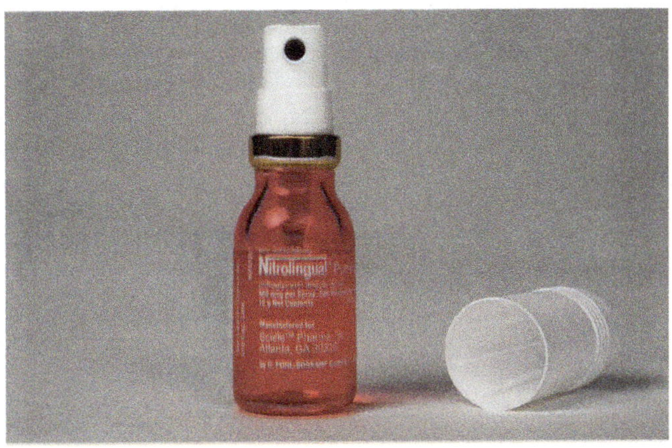

B

FIGURE 18-8 An epinephrine auto-injector can reverse a severe allergic reaction. (A) Adult and pediatric Epipens®. (B) Generic epinephrine auto-injector. (C) Epinephrine auto-injectors.

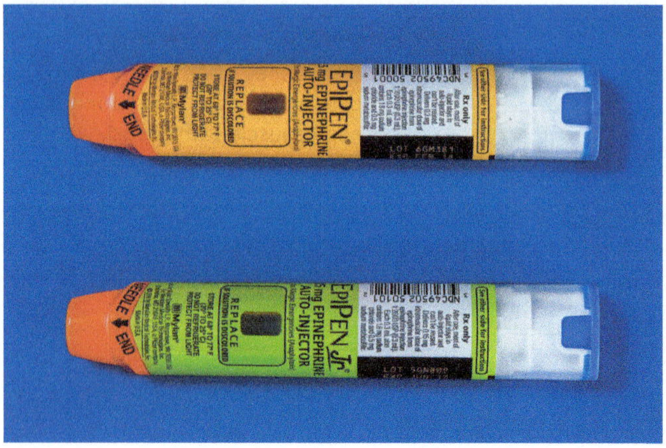

A

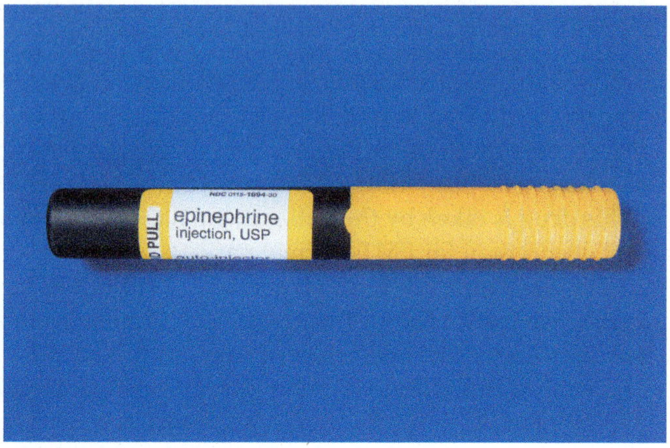

B

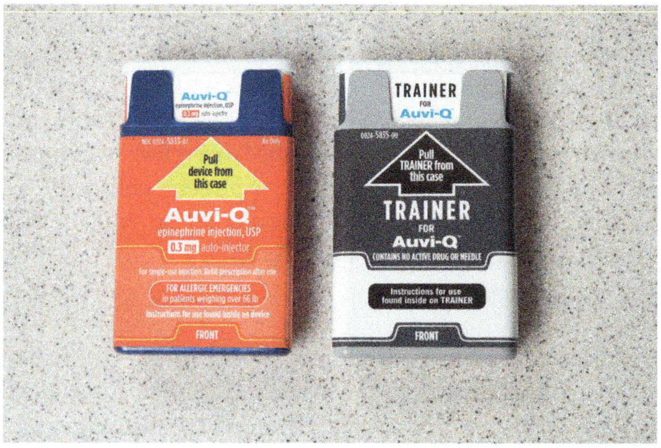

C

Adrenaclick® is a similar device. Auvi-Q® is the trade name of an epinephrine auto-injector that gives voice instructions for its use. If you need to assist a patient with the use of an epinephrine auto-injector, be sure to determine that the auto-injector is actually the patient's and not that of someone else.

Since epinephrine has a potent effect on the heart and vascular system, increased heart rate and blood pressure commonly occur after its administration to the patient.

You may need to seek permission from medical direction, or there may be a standing order permitting you to assist a patient who has an epinephrine auto-injector. In some systems, EMTs carry and are trained to use epinephrine auto-injectors to treat patients with anaphylaxis. Because of the significant expense associated with an auto-injector, EMTs in some areas carry epinephrine that is not in an auto-injector, and are trained to draw it up and administer it. *Always comply with the protocols of your EMS system.* More information on assisting a patient in using an epinephrine auto-injector and preparing epinephrine for administration without an auto-injector is in the chapter *Allergic Reactions.*

How Medications for Asthma and Anaphylaxis Work. Medications are valuable tools to help patients in the most serious of medical emergencies. Some medications are carried by EMTs, whereas others belong to the patients. You may be allowed to assist patients with taking their medications.

The following chart discusses the pathophysiology of two common emergency presentations, asthma and anaphylaxis, and explains how medications available to the EMT work.

CONDITION	PATHOPHYSIOLOGY	ACTION OF MEDICATIONS
Asthma	Small airways become reactive and constrict. Air does not move in and out easily, and exhaling is more difficult. This results in air trapping. On auscultation of a full respiratory cycle, you will notice that the expiratory phase is prolonged. "Triggers" such as exercise, allergens, respiratory viruses, and even aspirin and nonsteroidal anti-inflammatory drugs (NSAIDs) cause this reaction.	Albuterol is a medication very commonly used during asthma attacks. It is available in an inhaler and in a small-volume nebulizer (SVN). Albuterol must actually enter the smaller airways; it acts on contact. Albuterol acts on the $beta_2$ receptors of the sympathetic nervous system, which results in dilation of the airways. The fact that albuterol acts primarily on the β-specific receptors means there will be limited cardiac side effects (such as rapid heart rate).
Anaphylaxis	Anaphylaxis is a life-threatening response of the immune system. Anaphylaxis affects major systems such as the circulatory and respiratory systems and, if untreated, can cause death. Anaphylaxis begins when the body overreacts to an antigen. Common causes of anaphylaxis are bee stings, peanut butter, and medication allergies. The allergic reaction (begun when an antigen meets antibodies within the body) causes the body to release a variety of substances, including histamine, which cause vasodilatation and shock as well as bronchoconstriction. These substances also alter vascular permeability, allowing fluid to enter and swell the airways, lips, tongue, and throat.	The epinephrine auto-injector carried by patients and on many ambulances provides immediate and significant benefit to those suffering from anaphylaxis. Epinephrine causes vasoconstriction (which reverses shock) by acting on the alpha receptors of the sympathetic nervous system. It reduces vascular permeability and the edema found in the face and airways. Epinephrine also causes bronchodilation to open constricted bronchioles through the beta receptors in the sympathetic nervous system.

Force Protection Medications

Many systems also carry "force protection medications" such as atropine in auto-injector form to treat responders in the event of a chemical weapons attack. Typically, you would administer these medications to yourself and your partner if you found yourself exposed to certain weapons of mass destruction, such as nerve gas. Local protocols will determine which of these medications (if any) are carried. Follow local guidelines for administration.

General Information about Medications

Drug Names

Every drug or medication is listed in a comprehensive government publication called the *U.S. Pharmacopoeia* (USP). Each drug is listed by its generic name (a general name that is not the brand name of any manufacturer). However, each drug actually has at least three names: the chemical name, the generic name, and one or more trade (brand) names given the drug by various manufacturers. As mentioned earlier, Epi-Pen® is the trade name of an epinephrine auto-injector. Chemical names and technical formulas are used only by scientists or manufacturers. For example, the chemical names for epinephrine are 1,2-Benzenediol, 4-[(1R)-1-hydroxy-2-(methylamino)ethyl]-, or (-)-3, 4-Dihydroxy-α-[2(methylamino)ethyl] benzyl alcohol, but the chemical formula for epinephrine is $C_9H_{13}NO_3$, You can tell the difference between trade (brand) names and generic names by the way they appear in print. A trade name, e.g., Ventolin® HFA, is capitalized. A generic name is not—e.g., albuterol, the generic name for Ventolin® HFA.

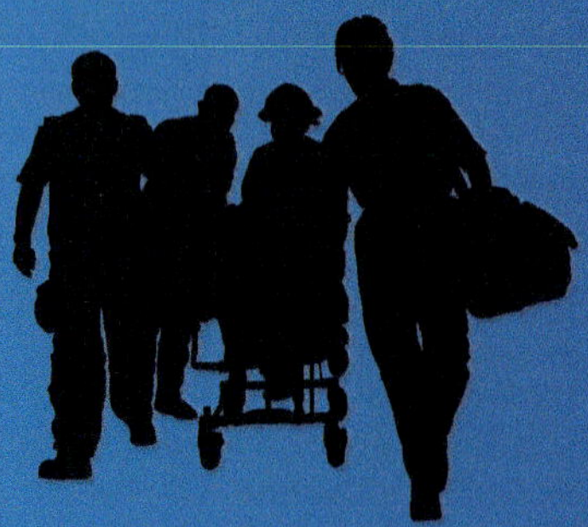

Think Like an EMT

ALS Is on the Way. Should I Assist the Patient with Her Inhaler?

You are treating a 21-year-old asthma patient. She has been having an "asthma attack" for about 20 minutes. The patient complains of severe shortness of breath, and your assessment confirms her difficulties. You have completed a thorough patient assessment, administered high-concentration oxygen, and called for ALS. The patient has a prescribed albuterol inhaler that you are allowed to assist her with based on your protocols. However, you note that ALS is only 5-8 minutes away. Should you assist with the medication, or simply wait for the paramedics to arrive?

What You Need to Know When Giving a Medication

indications
specific signs or circumstances under which it is appropriate to administer a drug to a patient.

contraindications (KON-truh-in-duh-KAY-shunz)
specific signs or circumstances under which it is not appropriate and may be harmful to administer a drug to a patient.

side effect
any action of a drug other than the desired action.

untoward (un-TORD) ***effect***
an effect of a medication in addition to its desired effect that may be potentially harmful to the patient.

CORE CONCEPT
What to consider when administering any medication

parenteral (pair-EN-tur-al)
referring to a route of medication administration that does not use the gastrointestinal tract, such as with an intravenous medication.

enteral (EN-tur-al)
referring to a route of medication administration that uses the gastrointestinal tract, such as swallowing a pill.

Every drug has an ***indication*** or indications—that is, specific signs, symptoms, or circumstances under which it is appropriate to administer the drug to a patient. For example, nitroglycerin is indicated when a patient has chest pain or squeezing, dull pressure. Each drug also has ***contraindications***, or specific signs, symptoms, or circumstances under which it is not appropriate and may be harmful to administer the drug to the patient. For example, nitroglycerin is contraindicated (should not be given) if the patient has low blood pressure because nitroglycerin, in dilating the blood vessels, causes a slight drop in the systolic blood pressure. As noted earlier, nitroglycerin is also contraindicated if the patient has recently taken Viagra or a similar medication, because of possible serious negative interactions.

A ***side effect*** is any action of a drug other than the desired action. Some side effects are predictable, such as the drop in blood pressure from nitroglycerin. If you were not aware of the side effect of a drop in blood pressure and gave the drug to a patient who started out with low blood pressure, the results could be devastating. The patient's blood pressure might "bottom out," which is definitely not a desirable effect for a cardiac patient. Often medications have unintended effects; that is, effects that occur in addition to the specific reason the drug was administered. Occasionally these effects can be classified as ***untoward effects***, or effects that are not only unexpected, but also potentially harmful to the patient.

Medications come in many different forms. A few examples are:

- Compressed powders or tablets, such as nitroglycerin pills
- Liquids for use outside the digestive tract, such as in an injection. This route is called the ***parenteral*** route and refers to bypassing the GI tract. An example of this type of medication would be epinephrine from an auto-injector.
- Liquids to be taken orally (such as a cough syrup). This route uses the digestive tract to reach the bloodstream and is known as an ***enteral*** route.
- Liquid that is vaporized, such as a fixed-dose nebulizer
- Gels, such as the paste in a tube of oral glucose
- Suspensions, such as the thick slurry of activated charcoal in water
- Fine powder for inhalation, such as that in a prescribed inhaler
- Gases for inhalation, such as oxygen
- Sublingual (under-the-tongue) sprays, such as a nitroglycerin spray

Medication Safety and Clinical Judgment

Administering or assisting with medications is a serious responsibility since if medications are given incorrectly, they can cause serious harm to the patient. As an EMT, you need to use good judgment and carefully consider any medication you administer.

The back of an ambulance is a dynamic place. There are many distractions and many decisions you will have to make. However, when it comes time to make decisions about medications, you need to focus. Medication administration should be undertaken only after a thorough patient assessment. You must be aware of all the factors that go into safe medication administration. You must understand not only how this medication would impact any patient in general but also how it will impact your current patient under the current, specific circumstances.

Know the medication. If you are unsure about it, look it up. Never guess. Medical direction may be required for permission, but it may also be contacted for assistance. Ask questions. An EMT must multitask routinely, but when it comes to medication administration, you need to be singular of focus. This is the time to think only about the task at hand.

Once the medication is administered, you cannot take it back. Focus, clear thinking, and good judgment—all will help ensure a proper and safe treatment.

Medication Authorization

CORE CONCEPT
The role of medical direction in medication administration

As an EMT, you will be authorized to administer medications by your medical director. This medical director may be service-level, regional-level, or even state-level. The authorization to administer medications can come in two different manners:

1. **Off-line medical direction.** In this case, you will not actually speak to a physician to ask permission. Off-line medical direction uses "standing orders"—that is, orders written down in the form of protocols. Providers learn these protocols and administer medications guided by the specific circumstances and conditions previously outlined in their rules and regulations.
2. **On-line medical direction.** In this case, you will need to speak directly to a physician (or designee) to obtain verbal permission to administer a medication. Verbal confirmation is required. As an EMT, you should always be diligent to ensure you have heard and correctly understand the instructions. A useful technique to employ is the "echo technique." In this technique, you will listen to the order and repeat the order back. The physician then should give you a verbal confirmation that what you have heard is correct. Use of this process significantly reduces medication errors. If at any time you are confused or have a question, speak up. Asking for clarification while on-line always is appropriate.

The Five Rights

Before administering a medication to any patient, confirm the order and write it down. ***Ensure that the medication is within its expiration date.*** Then check the "five rights" by asking yourself the following questions as you select the medication:

1. **Do I have the right patient?** Does this medication belong to the patient? Is this the same patient for whom medical direction approved a medication order?
2. **Is it the right time to administer this medication?** Have I made the right decision to administer the medication based on what I am seeing? Is it appropriate under these circumstances to give this particular medication?
3. **Is this the right medication?** Did I pick up the right bottle? Am I sure this is the correct medication?
4. **Is this the right dose?** Have I double-checked? Am I sure I am giving the correct amount?
5. **Am I giving this medication by the right route of administration?**

NOTE: *Once you have administered a medication, be sure to document it fully and in a timely manner.*

Routes of Administration

The route by which the drug is administered affects the rate at which the medication enters the bloodstream and arrives at its target organ to achieve its desired effect. EMTs use the following routes of administration:

- **Oral, or swallowed** This route is very safe and has few complications associated with administration. However, since the medication must be digested to take effect, it also takes longer for the medication to become effective. Oral medications are typically given in pill or capsule form; however, liquids can also be an option. Patients simply swallow the medication. In EMS, most oral medications are given in chewable pill form (such as aspirin), since water for swallowing pills is often not available.
- **Sublingual, or dissolved under the tongue** This route also accesses the body through the mouth; however, in this case, the medication is typically placed under the tongue and allowed to dissolve. As it dissolves, the medication is absorbed by the vascular soft tissue of the mouth. This route is faster than swallowing pills, but absorption sometimes is difficult if circulation is poor (as in shock). More information on assisting a patient with sublingual nitroglycerin can be found in the chapter *Cardiac Emergencies*.
- **Inhaled, or breathed into the lungs, usually as tiny aerosol particles (such as from an inhaler) or as a gas (such as oxygen)** Inhaled medications are breathed in through the respiratory system, and the medication is absorbed into the bloodstream through the alveoli. This is typically a simple process of putting a mask on your patient (as with oxygen). However, inhaled medications can be delivered via inhalers or nebulizers as well. More details on the use of a prescribed inhaler will be found in the chapter *Respiratory Emergencies*.
- **Intranasal, or sprayed into the nostrils** To use the intranasal route, you spray very fine droplets of medication into one or both nostrils with an ***atomizer***. If the capillaries in the mucous membranes are intact and not blocked, certain medications can be absorbed into the circulatory system and have an effect very similar in strength and speed to an injection of the same medication. The intranasal route works only with certain medications. You use it by attaching a special device (an atomizer) to the end of the medication-filled syringe. Pushing firmly on the plunger forces the liquid out of the atomizer in very small droplets.

atomizer
a device attached to the end of a syringe that atomizes medication (turns it into very fine droplets).

- **Intravenous, or injected into a vein** The intravenous route is beyond the scope of the EMT level. However, you should know that this is a fast and precise way to administer medications into the body by directly accessing the bloodstream through a vein.
- **Intramuscular, or injected into a muscle (parenteral)** The intramuscular route injects medication directly into the muscle. There, blood vessels can rapidly absorb the medication and transfer it to other parts of the body. This method of administration is very fast and allows for the effects of medication to occur rapidly. It can, however, be affected by poor circulation (as in shock), and it also has a much higher complication rate than do the oral and sublingual routes. This route typically uses a needle, as in an auto-injector, to deliver the medication. When you break the integrity of the skin's defenses with the needle, infections can occur. More information on assisting a patient in using an auto-injector can be found in the *Allergic Reactions* chapter.
- **Subcutaneous, or injected under the skin** Subcutaneous injections are very similar to intramuscular injections except that they deliver medications into the layers of the skin rather than into the muscle. This results in a slightly slower absorption than with intramuscular injections.
- **Intraosseous, or injected into the bone marrow cavity** New technology (the "IO gun" or "IO drill") allows rapid placement of a rigid needle into the bone marrow cavities of long bones such as the tibia. This technology, with compelling research that shows medications and fluids injected into the marrow reach the central circulation as fast as those given IV, has made the IO route popular among ALS providers and emergency physicians in emergencies such as cardiac arrests.

- **Endotracheal, or sprayed directly into a tube inserted into the trachea** This route is used in some ALS systems. Endotracheal medications are administered through a tube inserted into the trachea to be absorbed by the tissue of the lungs. Recent evidence has questioned the effectiveness of this route, however, because lung tissue has very unpredictable absorption rates. Yet you may find this route still used as a last resort.

Pharmacodynamic Considerations

Pharmacodynamics is the study of the effects of medications on the body. It is important to consider pharmacodynamics any time you administer a medication. You should ask questions such as "What effect will this medication have, and how will it affect my patient specifically?" Remember that patient-specific factors can change how a medication will work. For example, a smaller, lighter patient, such as a pediatric patient, will require less medication to achieve the desired effect. Often, geriatric patients will have difficulty eliminating medications, and therefore will feel the effects of medications longer. Consider age- and weight-related dose changes (Figure 18-9), and always understand how the medication will affect your specific patient before administering it.

pharmacodynamics (FARM-uh-KO-die-nam-ICS) the study of the effects of medications on the body.

Reassessment and Documentation

After administering any medication, you must reassess your patient. Essentially, you should begin your patient assessment again and look for any changes—improvements, deteriorations, or unintended effects—that the medication might have caused. Reassessment should occur immediately and be frequently repeated, especially with medications that take time to be effective.

It is also important to clearly document the medications you have administered. Good documentation must include the name of the medication (spelling counts), the dose of the medication, the route by which you administered it (be specific, as in "injected into the right upper thigh"), the time of administration, and any effects you noted. Remember that the hospital will continue to give the patient medications and must know what has already been administered to carry out a safe treatment plan.

"The more you know medications, the more you know your patient."

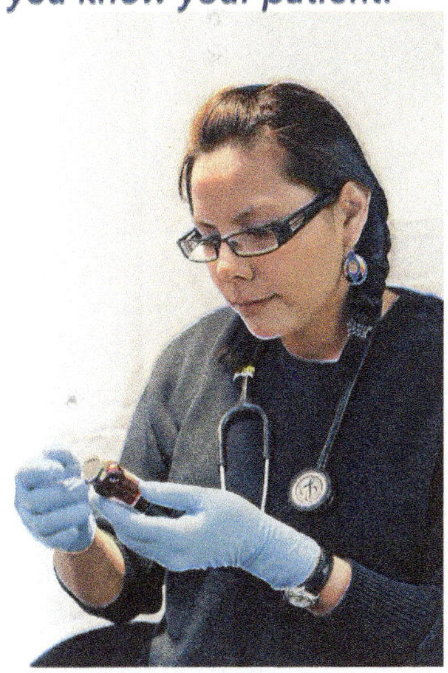

(Kevin Link/Science Source)

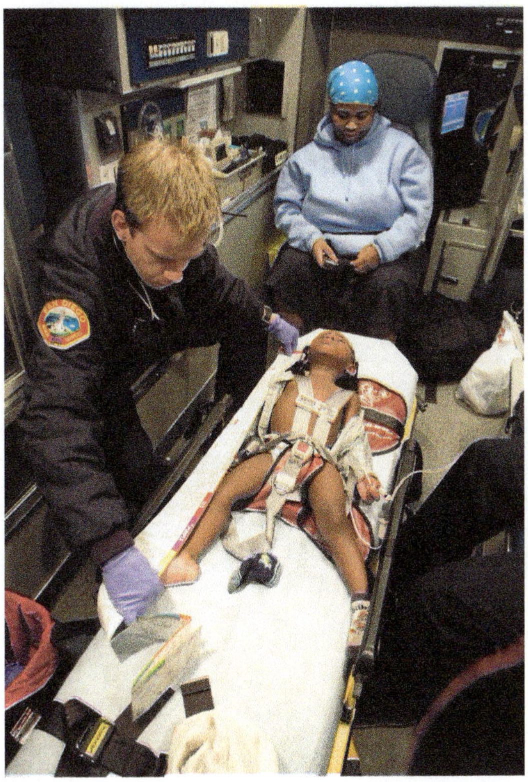

FIGURE 18-9 EMT using a Broselow™ tape, a length-based measurement tool that helps to estimate correct dosages for pediatric medications, sizing of medical devices such as an endotracheal tube, and determining the amount of energy used for manual defibrillation by ALS providers. *(© Daniel Limmer)*

Medications Patients Often Take

It would be impossible to learn and carry around in your head all the types of medications you might discover your patients are taking. However, the medications a patient is taking may be a clue to a preexisting medical condition or, if improperly used, a cause of the patient's current problem. For example, a patient who is taking antihypertensives and antidiabetics might also be taking or misusing other medications that can contribute to an altered mental status—perhaps phenytoin (Dilantin®) to control seizures, codeine for pain, or propranolol (Inderal®) for a heart rhythm disorder. Some medications that may be prescribed to a patient for daily use in managing a respiratory condition (one example would be beclomethasone, another would be Advair® [Figure 18-10]) should not be used to reverse an acute attack or to alleviate breathing difficulty.

It is a good idea to have a resource from which you can get additional information about a patient's medications en route to the hospital. Most EMTs carry with them, or have easily available access to, a pocket guide that contains useful information such as commonly used drug abbreviations. These pocket guides usually list the most commonly prescribed medications along with the general category of that medication, to help you understand what the medication may be used for. A version of this guide is available that can be downloaded to a smartphone. This is often more comprehensive than the paper version and more easily updated. Several programs are available, some of them at very little or no cost. However, remember that your main purpose in finding out what medications the patient is taking is not to make a field diagnosis but to report this information to medical direction and hospital personnel.

Table 18-1 lists the eight most common categories of medications you will find in the field that are relevant to patient care, with a few examples of medications in each category. Table 18-2 lists some common herbal agents patients sometimes take. A sizable number of people use these preparations, but they do not always think of them as medications that they should tell you about when you ask them what medications they take. Some of these agents have powerful effects, both intended and unintended, and should be recorded on the prehospital care report. Many also have interactions with prescription or over-the-counter medications. There are many other drugs and drug categories in addition to those listed in the tables.

FIGURE 18-10 (A) Advair® is a medication that may be prescribed to a patient for daily management of a respiratory disease. It should not be used for emergency treatment of an acute attack or breathing difficulty. (B) Breo® system.

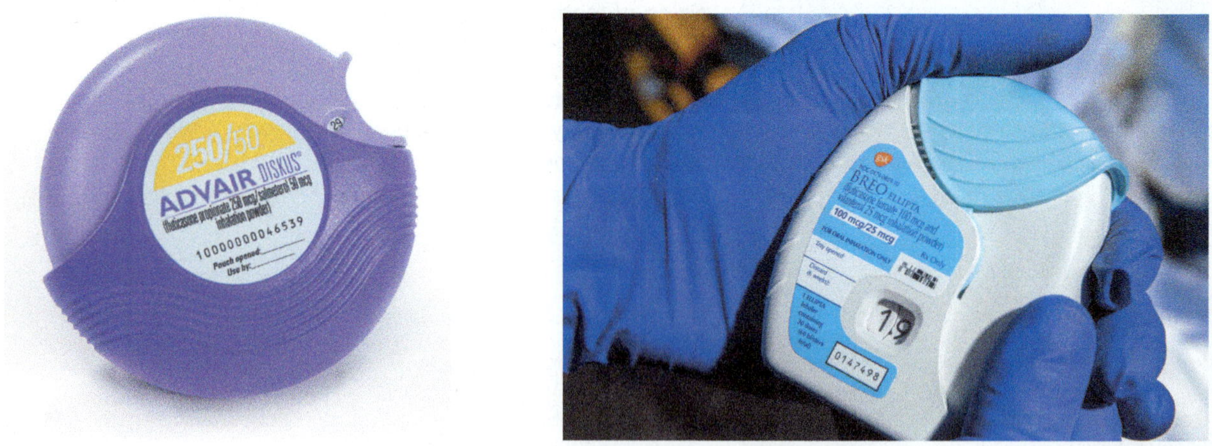

A B

TABLE 18-1 Medications Patients Often Take

ANALGESICS: DRUGS PRESCRIBED FOR PAIN RELIEF	
• acetaminophen (Anacin-3, Panadol, Tempra, Tylenol*) • aspirin (Ecotrin, Emprin) • codeine • ibuprofen (Actiprofen, Advil, Excedrin IS, Motrin, Novoprofen, Nuprin) • indomethacin (Indocin)	• morphine (Astramorph PF, Duramorph, MS Contin, Roxanol) • nalbuphine (Nubain) • naproxen (Naprosyn, Aleve) • oxycodone (OxyContin) • propoxyphene (Darvon)
ANTIDYSRHYTHMICS: DRUGS PRESCRIBED FOR HEART RHYTHM DISORDERS	
• carvedilol (Coreg) • digoxin (Lanoxin) • disopyramide (Norpace) • metoprolol (Lopressor, Toprol XL)	• propranolol (Inderal) • procainamide (Procan SR, Pronestyl) • verapamil (Calan, Calan SR, Isoptin, Isoptin SR, Verelan)
ANTICONVULSANTS: DRUGS PRESCRIBED FOR PREVENTION AND CONTROL OF SEIZURES	
• carbamazepine (Epitol, Tegretol) • ethosuximide (Zarontin) • gabapentin (Neurontin) • lamotrigine (Lamictal) • levetiracetam (Keppra)	• phenobarbital (Solfoton) • phenytoin (Dilantin) • primidone (Mysoline) • topiramate (Topamax) • valproic acid (Depakene)
ANTIHYPERTENSIVES: DRUGS PRESCRIBED TO REDUCE HIGH BLOOD PRESSURE	
• amlodipine (Norvasc) • captopril (Capoten) • clonidine (Catapres) • hydrochlorothiazide (HydroDiuril, Oretic)	• hydralazine (Apresoline, Hydralazine HCL) • methyldopa (Aldomet) • nifedipine (Adalat, Adalat CC, Procardia) • prazosin (Minipress)
BRONCHODILATORS: DRUGS THAT RELAX THE SMOOTH MUSCLES OF THE BRONCHIAL TUBES. THESE MEDICATIONS PROVIDE RELIEF OF BRONCHIAL ASTHMA AND ALLERGIES AFFECTING THE RESPIRATORY SYSTEM	
• albuterol (Proventil, Ventolin HFA, Volmax) • albuterol/ipratropium (Combivent, DuoNeb) • ipratropium (Atrovent) • levalbuterol (Xopenex)	• metaproterenol (Alupent, Metaproterenol sulfate, Metaprel) • montelukast (Singulair) • salmeterol (Serevent) • zafirlukast (Accolate)
ANTIDIABETIC AGENTS: DRUGS PRESCRIBED TO DIABETIC PATIENTS TO CONTROL HYPERGLYCEMIA (HIGH BLOOD SUGAR)	
• glimepiride (Amaryl) • glipizide (Glucotrol) • glyburide (DiaBeta, Glynase PresTab, Micronase)	• insulin (Humulin, Novolin, NPH, Humalog) • metformin (Glucophage) • rosiglitazone maleate (Avandia)
ANTIDEPRESSANT AGENTS: DRUGS PRESCRIBED TO HELP REGULATE THE EMOTIONAL ACTIVITY OF THE PATIENT TO MINIMIZE THE PEAKS AND VALLEYS IN THEIR PSYCHOLOGICAL AND EMOTIONAL STATES	
• amitriptyline (Elavil) • amoxapine (Asendin) • bupropion (Wellbutrin) • citalopram (Celexa) • clomipramine (Anafranil) • escitalopram (Lexapro) • fluoxetine (Prozac) • imipramine (Tofranil)	• nefazodone (Serzone) • nortriptyline (Aventyl, Pamelor) • paroxetine (Paxil) • protriptyline (Vivactil) • sertraline (Zoloft) • trimipramine (Surmontil) • venlafaxine (Effexor)
BLOOD THINNERS	
PRESCRIBED ANTI-COAGULANT AGENTS	PRESCRIBED ANTI-PLATELET AGENTS
• apaxiban (Eliquis) • dabigatran etexilate (Pradaxa) • injected low-molecular-weight heparin (Lovenox) • rivaroxaban (Xarelto) • ticagrelor (Plavix) • warfarin (Coumadin)	• aspirin • clipidogrel (Plavix) • ticagrelor (Brilinta)

NOTE: Generic names are lowercase. Trade names (®) are capitalized.

TABLE 18-2 Herbal Agents and What They Are Sometimes Used For

HERBAL AGENT	SOMETIMES USED FOR
Gingko or gingko biloba	Dementia, poor circulation to the legs, ringing in the ears
St. John's wort	Depression
Echinacea	Prevention and treatment of the common cold
Garlic	High cholesterol
Ginger root	Nausea and vomiting
Saw palmetto	Swollen prostate
Hawthorn leaf or flower	Heart failure
Evening primrose oil	Premenstrual syndrome
Feverfew leaf	Migraine prevention
Kava kava	Anxiety
Valerian root	Insomnia

After any medication is given to a patient, it is important that you reassess the patient to see what effects the drug has had. Obtain another set of vital signs and compare them with the vital signs that you took before administering the medication. Ongoing patient assessment should include an evaluation of the changes in the patient's condition and vital signs after administration of medication. Be sure to document the patient's response to each drug intervention—for example, "The patient's respiratory distress decreased after five minutes of high-concentration oxygen by nonrebreather mask."

CORE CONCEPT
How the EMT may assist with IV therapy

Assisting with IV Therapy

Setting Up an IV Fluid Administration Set

IV therapy is an advanced life support procedure. In this procedure, an intravenous (IV) catheter is inserted into a vein so blood, fluids, or medications can be administered directly into the patient's circulation. A blood transfusion is almost always given at the hospital, whereas infusions of other fluids and many medications can be done in the field.

There are two ways fluids and medications may be administered into the vein. One of these is through a heparin or saline lock (Figure 18-11). In this case, a catheter is placed into the vein. A small cap or lock is placed over the end of the catheter that protrudes from the skin. This lock contains a port through which you can administer medication. There is no

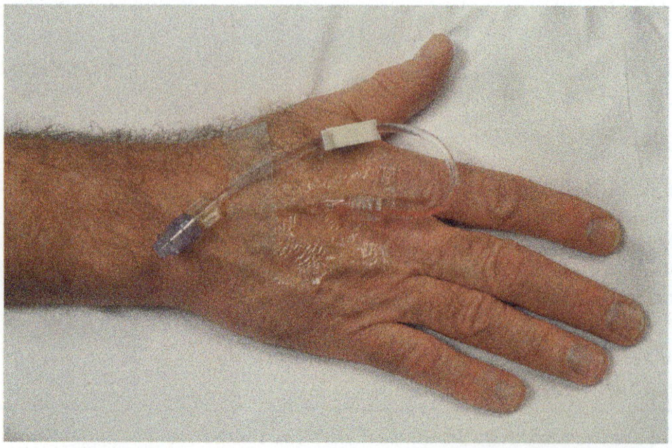

FIGURE 18-11 A saline or heparin lock can be used when fluid is not likely to be administered but medication administration or IV access may be needed later on. *(© Edward T. Dickinson, MD)*

IV bag attached to a saline lock. It is used in cases where fluid isn't likely to be administered but the administration of medications and/or the need for IV access later on is likely.

The second way fluids can be administered is though the traditional IV bag, which hangs above the patient and constantly flows fluids and medications into the patient.

The bag of fluid that feeds the IV is usually a clear plastic bag that collapses as it empties. The administration set is the clear plastic tubing that connects the fluid bag to the needle, or catheter. There are three important parts to this tubing:

1. The *drip chamber* is near the fluid bag. There are two basic types: the micro drip (also sometimes called mini drip) and the macro drip. The micro drip chamber is used when minimal flow of fluid is needed (with children, for example). Sixty small drops from the tiny metal barrel in the drip chamber equal 1 cubic centimeter (cc), or 1 milliliter (mL). The macro drip is used when a higher flow of fluid is needed (for a multitrauma patient in shock, for example). There is no little barrel in the drip chamber of the macro drip, and just 10–15 large drops equal 1 cc, or 1 mL.
2. The *flow regulator* is located below the drip chamber. It is a device that can be pushed up or down to start, stop, or control the rate of flow.
3. The *drug or needle port* is below the flow regulator. The paramedic can inject medication into this opening.

An extension set includes an extra length of tubing, which can make it easier to carry or disrobe the patient without accidentally pulling out the IV.

In most cases, a paramedic or AEMT will insert the IV into the patient's vein. However, you may be enlisted to help set up the IV administration set. If so, you will need to take the following steps:

1. Take out and inspect the fluid bag (Figure 18-12). The bags come in a protective wrapping to keep them clean. If you are setting up the IV, you must remove the wrapper, then inspect the bag to be sure it contains the fluid that has been ordered. Check the expiration date to make sure the fluid is usable, and look to see that the fluid is clear and free of particles. Squeeze the bag to check for leaks. Occasionally the fluid comes in a bottle. If so, be sure it is free of cracks. If anything is wrong, report the problem and inspect another bag or bottle.
2. Select the proper administration set. Uncoil the tubing, and do not let the ends touch the ground or any other surface (Figure 18-13).
3. Connect the extension set to the administration set, if an extension set is to be used.
4. Make sure the flow regulator is closed. To do this, roll the stopcock away from the fluid bag.

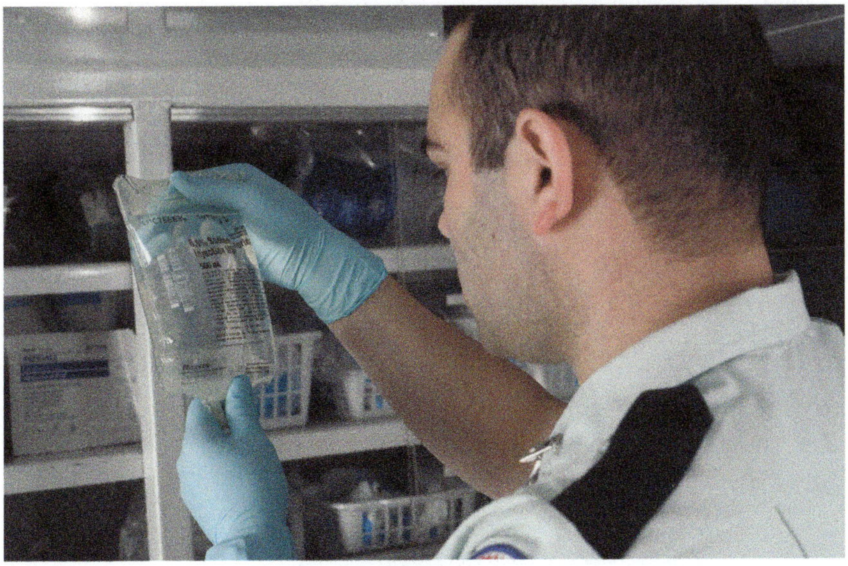

FIGURE 18-12 Inspect the IV bag to be sure it contains the solution that was ordered, it is clear, it does not leak, and it has not expired.

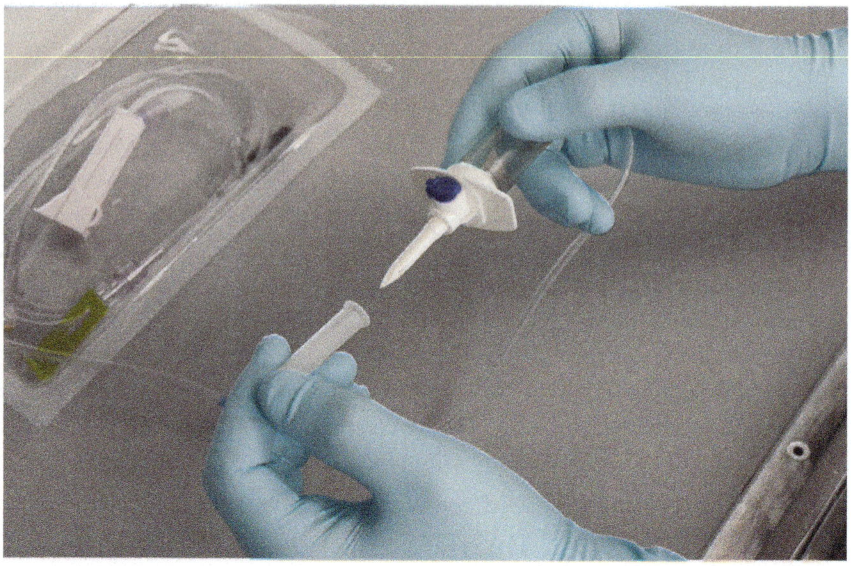

FIGURE 18-13 Setting up the IV administration set includes removing the protective coverings from the port of the fluid bag and the spiked end of the tubing.

5. Remove the protective covering from the port of the fluid bag and the protective covering from the spiked end of the tubing. Insert the spiked end of the tubing into the fluid bag with a quick twist (Figure 18-14). Do this carefully. Maintain sterility. If these parts touch the ground or any other surfaces, they must not be used. Introducing germs or dirt directly into a patient's bloodstream can be extremely serious and possibly fatal.
6. Hold the fluid bag higher than the drip chamber. Squeeze the drip chamber a time or two to start the flow. Fill the chamber to the marker line (approximately one-third full).
7. Open the flow regulator and allow the fluid to flush all the air from the tubing (Figure 18-15). You may need to loosen the cap at the lower end to get the fluid to flow. Maintain the sterility of the tubing end and replace the cap when you are finished. Most sets can be flushed without removing the cap. Be sure that all air bubbles have been flushed from the tubing to avoid introducing a dangerous air embolism into the patient's vein.
8. Turn off the flow (Figure 18-16).

Make certain that the setup stays clean until the paramedic removes the needle and connects the IV tubing to the catheter inside the patient's vein. Occasionally, the paramedic will draw blood from the vein to obtain samples before inserting the IV. You may

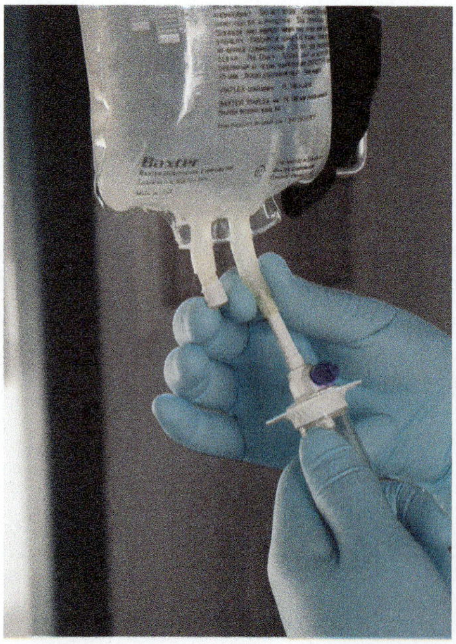

FIGURE 18-14 Insert the spiked end of the tubing into the fluid bag.

FIGURE 18-15 Open the flow regulator.

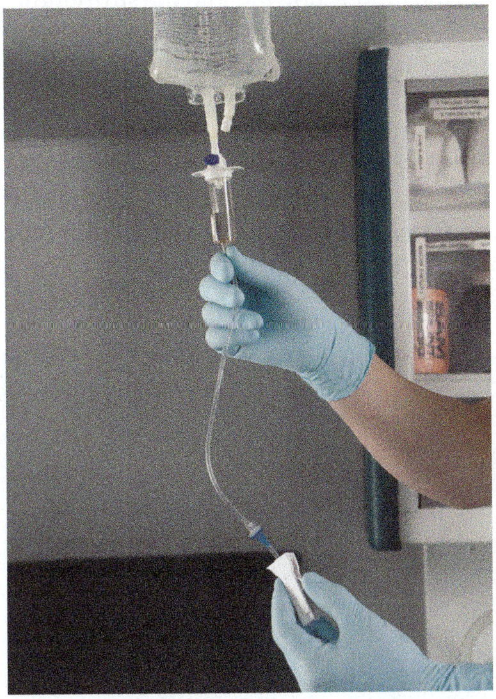

FIGURE 18-16 Turn off the flow.

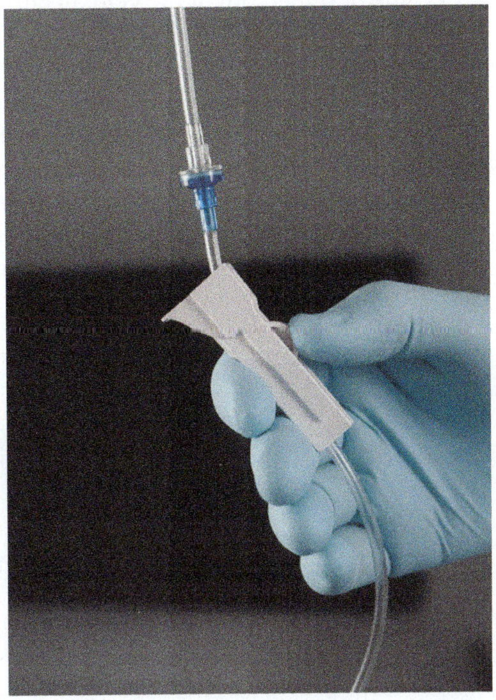

be asked to assist by placing the blood in sample tubes and labeling the tubes with the patient's name and any other information that your hospital requires. Remember that these tubes are potential carriers of pathogens. Be sure to take Standard Precautions. Carry the blood tubes to a safe place where they will not be in danger of breaking.

Do not be surprised if you are asked to hold up the patient's arm for a few minutes during a cardiac arrest. During cardiac arrest, medications can be more effective if the arm is temporarily raised after a drug is injected into the IV.

Maintaining an IV

An IV must continue to flow at the proper rate once it has been inserted into the patient's vein. However, a number of things may interrupt the flow. If you are charged with maintaining an IV, be sure to check for and correct the following problems:

- The constricting band used to raise the vein for insertion of the needle may have been mistakenly left on the patient's arm, perhaps covered by a sleeve.
- The flow regulator may be closed.
- The clamp may be closed on the tubing.
- The tubing may kink.
- The tubing may get caught under the patient or equipment.

The position of the IV or of the patient's arm also may need to be adjusted. Some IVs flow only when the patient's arm or IV site is in a certain position. Adjusting or even splinting the arm may be helpful as long as the splint is not too tight. Since the IV flow usually depends on gravity, be sure that the bag is held well above the IV site and the patient's heart.

Insufficient flow can cause blood to clot in the catheter. This can be prevented by adjusting the flow to an adequate "keep the vein open," or KVO, rate. Although the KVO rate varies, it is usually about 30 drops per minute for a micro drip and 10 drops per minute for a macro drip set. If the drip chamber is overfilled, clamp the tubing, invert the drip chamber, and pump some fluid back into the bag.

An IV with a flow rate that is too fast is called a "runaway IV." It can rapidly overload the patient with fluid and cause serious problems, especially in an infant or child. The IV will need to be adjusted to the proper rate.

An infiltrated IV is one where the needle has either punctured the vein and exited the other side or pulled out of the vein. In either case, the fluid is flowing into the surrounding tissues instead of into the vein. An unnoticed infiltrated IV can be very dangerous. Certain high-concentration medications (such as 50 percent dextrose) can cause the death of the surrounding tissue. In addition to complaining of pain, the patient will show swelling at the site (noticeable in all but some obese patients). The person in charge of maintaining the IV must stop the flow and discontinue the IV according to local protocol. If you are not authorized to do this, report the problem immediately to the paramedic or medical direction.

If you learn how to help advanced life support personnel start an IV, set up an administration set, label blood tubes, and maintain an IV, valuable time can be saved at the scene and during transport.

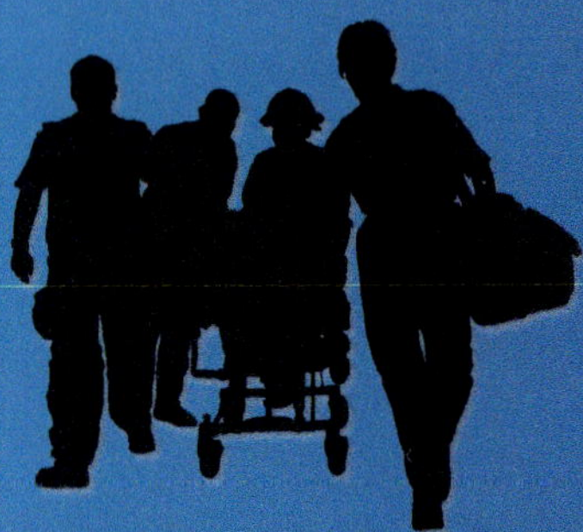

Think Like an EMT

How or Whether to Assist with Medications

Your decisions on how to assist patients with their medications—or whether to assist them at all—are a critical part of your practice as an EMT. The following questions will test your knowledge and decision making in this vital area.

1. You are treating a patient who has chest pain. He tells you his wife has nitroglycerin. He asks if he should take her pills. What should you tell him?
2. You are treating a patient who is diabetic. She appears very sleepy, and responds only to loud verbal stimulus by briefly opening her eyes. The patient's sister says, "Give her some sugar!" Should you? Why or why not?
3. Your COPD patient is breathing 48 times per minute shallowly. His wife believes his "lung problems" have been acting up. Would the patient's inhaler help him?

Chapter Review

Key Facts and Concepts

- Aspirin, oral glucose, and oxygen are medications that the EMT may administer to a patient under specific conditions that are carried on the ambulance.
- The EMT may assist the patient in taking prescribed inhalers, nitroglycerin, and epinephrine in auto-injectors.
- You may be able to administer intranasal naloxone, or may encounter patients who have received it from a layperson.
- You may need to have permission from medical direction to administer or assist the patient with a medication. Follow local protocols.
- There is a wide variety of medications that a patient may be taking. You will try to find out what medications a patient is taking when you take the SAMPLE history (signs and symptoms, allergies, medications, pertinent past history, last oral intake, and events leading to the injury or illness). These drugs may be identified by a variety of generic and trade names. Your main purpose in finding out what medications the patient is taking is to report this information to your medical director or hospital personnel.
- When administering a medication, first check the expiration date. Keep the five rights in mind: right patient, right medication, right dose, right route, and right time. Fully document all medication administration as soon as possible.

Key Decisions

- Should I administer aspirin?
- Should I assist the patient with prescribed medication?
- What medications is my patient taking, and what information about the patient's current condition can I obtain based on those medications?
- How do the patient's medications potentially affect the current condition?

Chapter Glossary

aspirin a medication used to reduce the clotting ability of blood to prevent and treat clots associated with myocardial infarction.

atomizer a device attached to the end of a syringe that atomizes medication (turns it into very fine droplets).

contraindications (KON-truh-in-duh-KAY-shunz) specific signs or circumstances under which it is not appropriate and may be harmful to administer a drug to a patient.

enteral (EN-tur-al) referring to a route of medication administration that uses the gastrointestinal tract, such as swallowing a pill.

epinephrine (ep-uh-NEF-rin) a drug that helps to constrict the blood vessels and relax passages of the airway. It may be used to counter a severe allergic reaction.

indications specific signs or circumstances under which it is appropriate to administer a drug to a patient.

inhaler a spray device with a mouthpiece that contains an aerosol form of a medication that a patient can spray into the airway.

naloxone an antidote for narcotic overdoses.

nitroglycerin (NYE-tro-GLIS-uh-rin) a drug that helps to dilate the coronary vessels that supply the heart muscle with blood.

oral glucose (GLU-kos) a form of glucose (a kind of sugar) given by mouth to treat an awake patient (who is able to swallow) with an altered mental status and a history of diabetes.

oxygen a gas commonly found in the atmosphere. Pure oxygen is used as a drug to treat any patient whose medical or traumatic condition may cause hypoxia, or low oxygen.

parenteral (pair-EN-tur-al) referring to a route of medication administration that does not use the gastrointestinal tract, such as an intravenous medication.

pharmacodynamics (FARM-uh-KO-die-nam-ICS) the study of the effects of medications on the body.

pharmacology (FARM-uh-KOL-uh-je) the study of drugs, their sources, their characteristics, and their effects.

side effect any action of a drug other than the desired action.

untoward (un-TORD) ***effect*** an effect of a medication in addition to its desired effect that may be potentially harmful to the patient.

Preparation for Your Examination and Practice

Short Answer

1. Name the drugs that are commonly carried on the ambulance and may be administered by the EMT under certain circumstances.
2. Name the drugs that the EMT may assist the patient in taking if they have been prescribed and if administration has been approved by medical direction.
3. Medications may take the form of tablets. Name several other forms in which medications may appear.
4. Describe the difference between on-line medical direction and off-line medical direction. Provide examples of each.
5. Name several routes by which medications may be administered.

Thinking and Linking

Medication administration is a key intervention the EMT may perform during patient assessment and transport. Think back to the chapter Secondary Assessment, *especially the sections on assessment of the trauma patient and medical patient and reassessment, as you answer the following question.*

- List the "five rights" of medication administration, and discuss why each is important. What would the potential risk to the patient be if each were not checked prior to administration?

Critical Thinking Exercises

Administering medications to the patient is a serious responsibility. How would you act in the following situation?

- A patient is complaining of chest pain. "Here's some nitroglycerin," says a family member. "Give him that." What do you do?

Pathophysiology to Practice

The following question is designed to assist you in gathering relevant clinical information and making accurate decisions in the field.

- In this chapter, we have discussed the need to reassess the patient after the administration of any medication. What elements would you reassess? What findings might be significant?

Street Scenes

It is winter and cold, so you are not too surprised when the dispatcher tells you to respond to the mall for a 62-year-old male patient with chest pain. During winter, many cardiac patients walk for exercise in the mall, and this is not the first cardiac call you have had there. When you arrive, you find the patient sitting in a chair. You introduce yourself and your partner, ask the patient his name, and then say, "Well, Mr. Edwards, why was EMS called?"

"I was doing my usual morning walk," he explains, "when I started to get chest pain. I thought it might go away but it didn't. I got concerned and asked the security guard to call 911."

As your partner takes a set of vital signs, you ask the patient, "On a scale of zero to ten, with ten being the worst pain you've ever had, how would you rate the chest pain you're having now?" He tells you that it is a seven. You ask him to describe the pain and to point to where it is located. He says that it feels like a dull pain and points to the center of his chest. He also says the pain does not radiate. The patient seems pale, and his skin is dry. After a bit more questioning, he tells you the last time this happened, he took nitro for relief.

Street Scene Questions

1. What additional patient history should you obtain?
2. Should you let the patient take nitroglycerin? Why or why not?
3. Are vital signs important if nitroglycerin is going to be taken by the patient?

You ask Mr. Edwards if he has nitroglycerin with him now. He says his wife has it, but she went to a store in another part of the mall and should be back shortly. You then ask about other medications, and the patient tells you he is on propranolol and a diuretic. Next you ask if he has ever had a heart attack. The patient tells you that he had one about a year and a half ago with an angioplasty. Vital signs are pulse 90, blood pressure 120/90, and respirations of 24 and labored. When his wife shows up, she attempts to administer a pill, but you ask her to wait.

Street Scene Questions

4. What information do you want to know about the nitroglycerin?
5. How should the nitroglycerin be administered?
6. When should vital signs be taken again?

At your request, the patient's wife gives you the nitroglycerin bottle so you can check the expiration date. At the same time, you check to make sure that it is the patient's specific prescription. It all checks. According to standing orders in your system, if a patient has these signs and symptoms, including a systolic blood pressure over 100, you may give a nitro dose without having radio contact with medical direction. You tell the patient that you are going to put the pill under his tongue and he should let it dissolve. You specifically tell Mr. Edwards not to swallow.

About a minute after you give Mr. Edwards the pill, he complains of a slight headache. You tell him this is a possible side effect of taking nitro and not to be concerned. After another minute goes by, you ask the patient to rate the chest pain on a scale of zero to ten again. "About a two," he replies. "In fact, the pain is almost gone," he tells you. Your partner takes another set of vital signs, since a patient's blood pressure can drop when taking nitro, but there is no change. You package the patient for transport and move to the ambulance, making sure you keep the AED close by. You give Mrs. Edwards a short update and explain to her that you will take the nitroglycerin bottle with the patient. The transport to the hospital is uneventful, and you take another set of vital signs en route.

19

Respiratory Emergencies

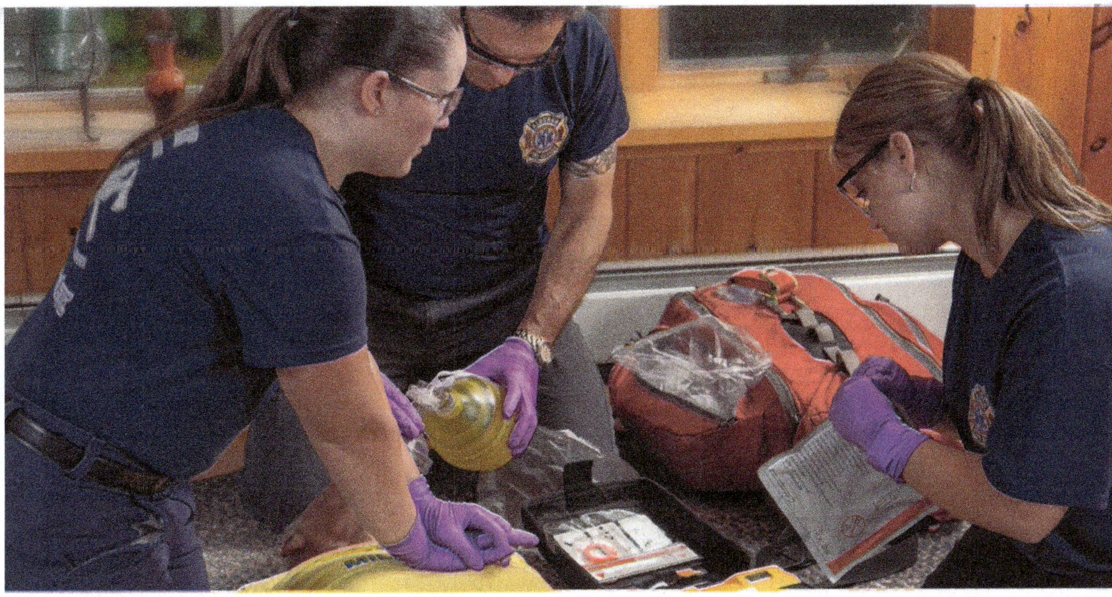

Related Chapters

The following chapters provide additional information related to topics discussed in this chapter:

- **3** Lifting and Moving Patients
- **6** Anatomy and Physiology
- **7** Principles of Pathophysiology
- **9** Airway Management
- **10** Respiration and Artificial Ventilation
- **12** Primary Assessment
- **13** Vital Signs and Monitoring Devices
- **15** Secondary Assessment
- **20** Cardiac Emergencies

Standard

Medicine (Content Areas: Respiratory)

Competency

Applies fundamental knowledge to provide basic emergency care and transportation based on assessment findings for an acutely ill patient.

Core Concepts

- How to identify adequate breathing
- How to identify inadequate breathing

- How to identify and treat a patient with breathing difficulty
- Use of continuous positive airway pressure (CPAP) to relieve difficulty breathing
- Use of a prescribed inhaler and how to assist a patient with one
- Use of a prescribed small-volume nebulizer and how to assist a patient with one

Outcomes

After reading this chapter, you should be able to:

19.1 Explain a patient's breathing status. (pp. 520–522)

- Summarize the coordinated processes required of the cardiopulmonary system to maintain perfusion.
- Outline the assessment procedure for determining the adequacy of respiration.
- Describe the mechanics of inspiration and expiration.

19.2 Distinguish between descriptions of a patient who is breathing adequately and one who is not. (pp. 522–526)

- Discern adequate from inadequate respiratory rate.
- Discern adequate from inadequate respiratory rhythm.
- Discern adequate from inadequate breathing quality.
- Relate the differences in pediatric anatomy and physiology to the differences observed in inadequate breathing in children compared with adults.

19.3 Select the most appropriate intervention sequence for a description of a patient with inadequate breathing. (pp. 526–528)

- Recommend the prioritized treatment for a patient with inadequate breathing.
- Describe the considerations in choosing the means of providing artificial ventilation to a patient.
- Contrast the characteristics of inadequate artificial ventilation with those of adequate artificial ventilation.
- Describe differences in the respiratory interventions for children versus those for adults.

19.4 Outline the assessment process for a patient complaining of difficulty breathing. (pp. 528–534)

- Recognize the different ways patients may describe a chief complaint that tells you they are having difficulty breathing.
- Describe immediate observations that give an early means of differentiating between adequate and inadequate breathing in a patient complaining of difficulty breathing
- Describe the adaptation of the *OPQRST* mnemonic to a patient with a chief complaint of difficulty breathing.
- Recall symptoms that a patient with shortness of breath may complain of.
- Describe specific observations that EMTs should look for in the assessment of a patient with difficulty breathing.

- Describe the auscultation of the lungs in a patient with difficulty breathing.
- Describe the characteristics of abnormal breath sounds.
- Describe the underlying problem that produces each of the abnormal breath sounds.
- Recognize how vital signs may be altered in a patient with a chief complaint of difficulty breathing.
- Describe how the pulse oximeter should be integrated in assessment of a patient complaining of difficulty breathing.

19.5 Propose a treatment plan for a representation of a patient with breathing difficulty. Describe the components of the general approach to caring for a patient with difficulty breathing. (pp. 534–538)

- Select the best oxygen administration modality for a patient complaining of difficulty breathing.
- Describe how continuous positive airway pressure (CPAP) works.
- List the indications for treating a patient with CPAP.
- List the contraindications for treating a patient with CPAP.
- Describe the procedure for treating a patient with CPAP.
- Describe how different complications of CPAP can be recognized.

19.6 Recommend a diagnosis-based treatment plan for a patient with difficulty breathing. (pp. 538–546)

- Describe the features of chronic obstructive pulmonary disease (COPD).
- Describe the features of asthma.
- Describe the features of pulmonary edema.
- Describe the features of pneumonia.
- Describe the features of spontaneous pneumothorax.
- Describe the features of pulmonary embolism.
- Describe the features of epiglottitis.
- Describe the features of croup.
- Describe the features of bronchiolitis.
- Describe the features of cystic fibrosis.
- Describe the features of viral respiratory infections.

19.7 Identify common medications used for patients with difficulty breathing. (pp. 546–551)

- Differentiate between the types of inhaled medications EMTs may give to a patient with difficulty breathing and those they may not give.
- List the indications for assisting a patient with a metered-dose inhaler.
- List the contraindications of treating a patient with a metered-dose inhaler.
- Provide the instructions a patient needs to use the inhaler.
- Recall the rights of medication administration.
- List the side effects of the inhaled medications EMTs assist with.
- Describe the steps in assisting a patient with using a prescribed inhaler.
- Compare the use of a small-volume nebulizer with that of a metered-dose inhaler.

Key Terms

bronchoconstriction, *546*
continuous positive airway pressure (CPAP), *535*
exhalation, *521*
expiration, *521*
inhalation, *521*
inspiration, *521*

Breathing is how we stay alive. The movement of oxygen and carbon dioxide in and out of the cells is critical to almost every human function, but we live in a world where challenges to that capability are all around us. Degenerative conditions, like chronic obstructive pulmonary disease and heart failure, threaten the very structures where gas exchange takes place. Chronic and episodic conditions, like asthma or respiratory infections, suddenly obstruct the exchange of air in the lungs. Trauma can also impact the anatomy and control mechanisms necessary to the function of breathing. All these conditions (and many more) are among the reasons that EMTs exist. In bringing emergency medical care to the field, we have been selected to intervene, to assess, and to treat patients with serious challenges to their cardiopulmonary systems. Our job is to see that patient needs are met. Because breathing adequately is essential to staying alive, we must recognize the situations where the cardiopulmonary system is failing and act swiftly to rectify the problem.

In the chapters *Anatomy and Physiology* and *Principles of Pathophysiology*, you learned about the value of oxygenation, ventilation, and perfusion. In the chapters *Airway Management*, *Respiration and Artificial Ventilation*, and *Primary Assessment*, you learned to use your primary assessment to recognize and treat inadequate breathing. In this chapter, we will tie this information together with a more comprehensive view of specific respiratory challenges and discuss the effective interventions used to treat them. It may be appropriate to review those prior chapters before you begin.

Respiration

Respiratory Anatomy and Physiology

In the chapter *Anatomy and Physiology*, you learned about the anatomy of the respiratory system. You learned that the lungs and heart occupied the space within the closed container of the chest cavity and that the lower border of this cavity was formed by the diaphragm. You also learned that air flowed from the mouth and nose, through the trachea, and to the alveoli of the lungs, where gas exchange takes place. But, to truly understand the respiratory system, you also must consider the physiology of how air is moved.

The Pressures of the Respiratory System

To move air, the respiratory system changes pressure within the chest cavity. Negative pressure is used to move air in and positive pressure is used to move air out. These changes in pressure are generated by contraction and relaxation of the respiratory system muscles.

It can be helpful to think of the respiratory system like a syringe used to draw up a medication. Like a syringe pointed upwards, the respiratory system has a small opening at the top it uses to introduce air. This is called the glottic opening, and it is at the very top of the trachea, seated in the hypopharynx. (See Figure 9-3.) A syringe also has a cavity that is filled when medication is drawn in. In the case of the respiratory system, this cavity would be the chest itself and, more specifically, the lungs. As air is introduced, the lungs are filled, and the chest cavity is expanded. The bottom border of the syringe would be the plunger, which moves up and down to change the size of the syringe cavity. By depressing the plunger, or moving it upward, the cavity becomes smaller, and pressure within the syringe increases. By withdrawing the plunger, or moving it downward, the cavity of the syringe becomes larger and pressure within decreases. Decreasing pressure would then draw the medication in through the small hole at the top of the syringe.

The physiology of the respiratory system uses a similar process. To initiate **inspiration** (a breath in), the thin, umbrella-shaped muscle of the diaphragm contracts and physically moves lower toward the abdomen. At the same time the muscles between the ribs, the intercostal muscles, expand the chest wall. The net effect of these movements is to increase the size of the chest cavity and decrease the pressure within the lungs. This negative pressure pulls air into the glottic opening, and the lungs inflate. During **expiration** (a breath out), the process is reversed. The diaphragm and intercostal muscles relax, and the size of the chest cavity decreases. Internal pressure increases. With increased pressure, air is pushed out of the glottic opening, and the lungs empty. This process is illustrated in Figure 19-1.

Because inhalation requires contraction of muscles and forcible movement of the diaphragm, it is often referred to as an "active" process. Exhalation is conversely referred to as a "passive" process because, in most cases, pressure change occurs due to simple relaxation.

- **Inspiration.** The active process that uses the contraction of several muscles to increase the size of the chest cavity is called ***inspiration***. In this process, the intercostal (rib) muscles and the diaphragm contract. The diaphragm lowers and the ribs move upward and outward. The expanding size of the chest cavity then causes air to flow into the lungs. Another term for inspiration is ***inhalation***.
- **Expiration.** A passive process, ***expiration*** involves the relaxation of the rib muscles and diaphragm. The ribs move downward and inward, while the diaphragm rises. This movement causes the chest cavity to decrease in size and causes air to flow out of the lungs. Another term for expiration is ***exhalation***.

Review in the *Anatomy and Physiology* chapter how oxygen and carbon dioxide are exchanged through the alveoli and capillaries of the lungs and through the capillaries and cells throughout the body. The exchange of oxygen and carbon dioxide, both in the lungs and in the body's cells, is critical to support life. There are many things that can go wrong within the body that will alter this vital exchange. Primarily these are problems with the respiratory system or the circulatory system, as were described in the chapter *Principles of Pathophysiology*. This chapter will further discuss the respiratory system as well as problems with breathing, and their effects on the body. Problems with the circulatory system will be discussed in greater detail in the *Cardiac Emergencies* chapter.

inspiration (IN-spuh-RAY-shun) an active process in which the intercostal (rib) muscles and the diaphragm contract, expanding the size of the chest cavity and causing air to flow into the lungs.

inhalation (IN-huh-LAY-shun) another term for inspiration.

expiration (EK-spuh-RAY-shun) a passive process in which the intercostal (rib) muscles and the diaphragm relax, causing the chest cavity to decrease in size and forcing air from the lungs.

exhalation (EX-huh-LAY-shun) another term for expiration.

FIGURE 19-1 The process of respiration.

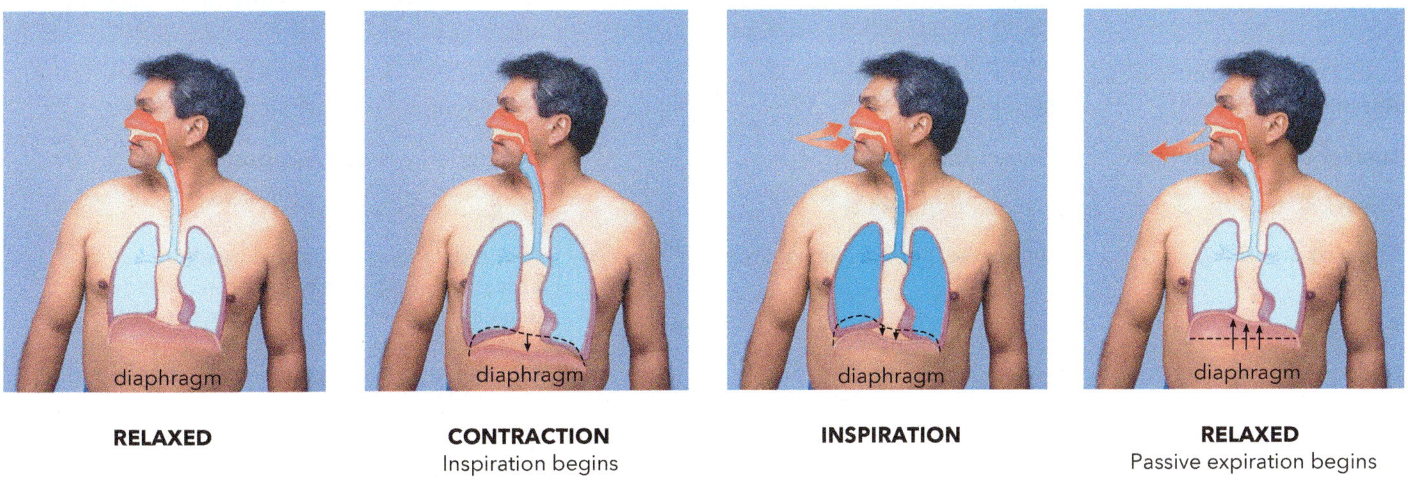

Pediatric Note

In very young children, particularly neonates and infants, the structure of the rib cage flares outward at the bottom. In adults, the structure curves inward. This outward flare in infants causes the diaphragm to be comparatively much flatter, and therefore less able to move, than an adult's diaphragm. The chest walls of young children are also more flexible than those of adults. As a result, it is often harder for young children to generate the negative pressure to control breathing. Under normal circumstances, these differences do not pose a problem, but when a respiratory challenge occurs, the pediatric respiratory system has a more difficult time compensating. Adults use more muscles of the chest and try to take stronger and deeper breaths, but young children are limited to increasing the respiratory rate to aid breathing. This strategy can be effective, but it also uses a great deal more energy than the compensation efforts of an adult.

CORE CONCEPT

How to identify adequate breathing

Adequate Breathing

Control of breathing occurs in our brain. Changing levels of carbon dioxide and oxygen, and the pH of our blood and cerebrospinal fluid signal the medulla oblongata to stimulate breathing. Impulses travel through the nervous system to the muscles of breathing to constantly adapt the rate and volume of breathing constantly to meet the needs of the body. Times of higher oxygen demand, such as during heavy exercise, stimulate rapid breathing, while periods of lower demand, such as while sleeping, slow the rate. Adequate breathing is a constant balancing act that matches supply with demand.

As you learned in the *Respiration and Artificial Ventilation* chapter, breathing may be classified as adequate or inadequate. Simply stated, adequate breathing is breathing that is sufficient to support life. Inadequate breathing fails to meet the demands of metabolism. Your ability to assess the adequacy of a patient's breathing is vital to the patient's survival (Table 19-1).

Adequate breathing demonstrates certain findings that are considered "normal." When breathing adequately, patients will generally have a normal mental status and be moving air when breathing. They will be able to speak relatively normally without having to catch their breath. Their color will be normal and their oxygen saturation level will typically be

TABLE 19-1 Adequate and Inadequate Breathing

	ADEQUATE BREATHING	INADEQUATE BREATHING
Rate	Adult: 12-20/minute; school-age child: 18-30/minute; infant (0-6 months): 30-60/minute	Above or below normal rates for the patient's age group
Rhythm	Regular	May be irregular
Quality of Breath Sounds	Present and equal	Diminished, unequal, or absent
Chest Expansion	Adequate and equal	Inadequate or unequal
Effort of Breathing	Unlabored, normal respiratory effort	Labored: increased respiratory effort; use of accessory muscles (may be pronounced in infants and children and involve nasal flaring, seesaw breathing, grunting, and retractions between the ribs and above the clavicles and sternum)
Depth	Adequate	Too shallow

in the normal range. An assessment of adequate breathing is determined by observing all of these findings as well as rate, rhythm, and quality of breathing:

- **Rate.** Rates of breathing that are considered normal vary by age. For an adult, a normal rate is 12–20 breaths per minute. For a school-age child, it is 18–30 breaths per minute. For an infant, it is 30–60 breaths per minute. Remember that breathing rates are very situational and you must always consider the context in which you are measuring them. For example, an infant might have a significantly higher rate when crying than another infant who is sleeping. Extremes of rate (higher or lower) are only meaningful if they affect the other expectations of adequate breathing. An infant who has a fast respiratory rate when crying is likely fine if mental status, color, and oxygen saturation are all within normal range. On the other hand, a fast respiratory rate combined with an altered mental status, cyanosis, or low oxygen saturation would be a cause for concern and be considered inadequate breathing that required immediate intervention. Extremes of rate should still be considered a significant finding even when adequate breathing is present, because they can point to the presence of a physiologic challenge and compensation for that challenge.
- **Rhythm.** Normal breathing rhythm will usually be regular. Breaths will be taken at regular intervals and will last for about the same length of time. Remember that talking and other factors can make normal breathing slightly irregular.
- **Quality.** Breath sounds, when auscultated with a stethoscope, will normally be present and equal when the lungs are compared with each other. When observing the chest cavity, both sides should move equally and adequately to indicate a proper air exchange. The depth of the respirations must be adequate.

"Respiratory assessment means not just making sure air is moving in and out but judging how well it's moving in and out."

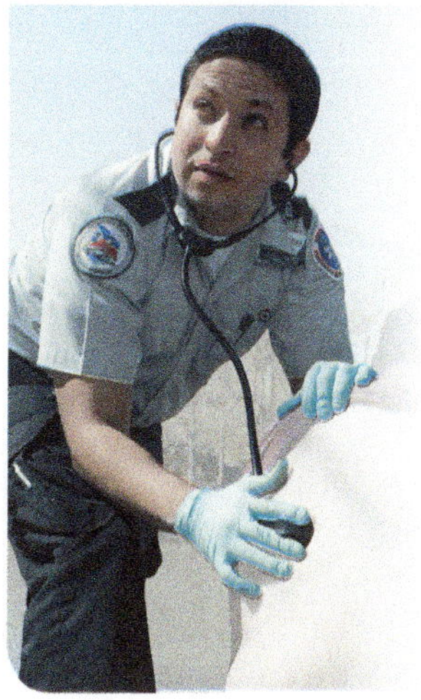

It should be noted that a patient can have a respiratory challenge, like an asthma attack, and still be breathing adequately. The body has an amazing ability to compensate for even the worst challenges, and although signs of respiratory distress may be present, the patient's metabolic needs may still be met. Increases in respiratory rate and depth as well as accessory muscle use and positioning can all be used to respond to a challenge and compensate for its effects. It is very common to encounter a patient who is short of breath and working hard to breathe, but who still is breathing adequately. Our goal in such patients is to support their compensatory efforts (by administering oxygen, for example), identify the respiratory challenge, and offer treatment (such as a metered-dose inhaler) if possible. Most importantly, we want to keep such patients breathing adequately and prevent decompensation to inadequate breathing. Of course, patients in respiratory distress are always at risk to decompensate and should be monitored carefully.

Inadequate Breathing

Inadequate breathing is breathing that is not sufficient to support life. If left untreated, this condition will surely lead to death. One of your most important tasks as an EMT is to identify and treat patients with inadequate breathing. The primary assessment, initiated at first contact with the patient, will be your first opportunity to identify the presence of inadequate breathing. Remember that breathing is a dynamic process; it constantly needs to be reassessed. What started as adequate can quickly progress to inadequate. (See Table 19-1.) Assessment and treatment of breathing should begin early in the call and continue throughout your time with the patient.

CORE CONCEPT
How to identify inadequate breathing

Patient Assessment

Inadequate Breathing

Among the first organs affected by hypoxia is the brain. The brain is constantly working and requires a reliable supply of oxygen and nutrients to continue functioning. It also has no capacity to store oxygen or nutrients. Therefore, when its supply is interrupted, brain function will be impaired. Inadequate breathing is very often first demonstrated by mental status changes. Sometimes these changes can be subtle. The patient may become anxious or develop a "feeling of impending doom," but as hypoxia develops these changes become more dramatic. Confusion, combativeness, lethargy (dull, tired, and disinterested affect), and somnolence (sleepiness) all precede an unconscious state if hypoxia is not corrected. Somnolence will also occur as levels of carbon dioxide rise. The skin too will show evidence of hypoxia. Deoxygenated red blood cells make the blood appear blue or purple and will cause certain areas of the skin to become gray or bluish in appearance. This condition is called cyanosis and will first appear around the eyes and in the fingernail beds. Cyanosis is a profound warning that severe hypoxia is present. You may also see other systems of the body engage to attempt to compensate for inadequate breathing. A rapid heart rate, rapid breathing, and sweaty skin are all signs of the "fight or flight" response mounted by the brain and central nervous system in response to a respiratory challenge. Inadequate breathing is also characterized by the following findings:

- **Fast respiratory rate.** Respiratory rate usually increases in response to a respiratory challenge. Patients with difficulty breathing typically increase their breathing rate as the challenge becomes worse. Although a fast rate alone does not identify inadequate breathing, it is certainly a clue that compensation is occurring, and identifies the need for a more detailed assessment.
- **Slowing or irregular respirations.** When compensation fails or when a respiratory challenge overwhelms the body's ability to compensate, breathing can often become irregular and slow before it stops altogether. Slowing rates and irregular breathing, in the context of other signs of inadequate breathing (especially altered mental status), are dangerous findings that point to an inadequate state.
- **Inability to speak.** The ability or inability to speak normally correlates well to the patient's level of respiratory distress. An inability to speak in normal sentences, of more than only one or two words before having to take a breath is an important indicator of a severe problem. Inability to speak should be considered a key warning sign, particularly in the presence of other indicators of inadequate breathing.
- **Silent chest.** In severe respiratory problems (most commonly in severe asthma), air movement can become so diminished that no lung sounds can be heard upon auscultation with a stethoscope. The patient may still be attempting to breathe, and the chest wall may be moving, but narrowed airways simply do not allow for air movement in the lungs. Silent chest is a particularly ominous finding in children.
- **Low oxygen saturation despite supplemental oxygen.** A reliable finding of low oxygen saturation is an indication of hypoxia and a sign that breathing is not meeting the oxygenation needs of the body. Sometimes this can be treated and improved with supplemental oxygen. However, when supplemental oxygen fails to improve the hypoxia, and when low saturation is found in the context of other signs of inadequate breathing, it should be considered a dangerous finding.
- **Agonal respirations.** Agonal respirations (also called dying respirations) are sporadic, irregular breaths that are usually seen just before respiratory arrest. They are shallow and gasping with only a few breaths per minute. This breathing pattern is clearly a sign of inadequate breathing.
- **Rhythm.** The rhythm of breathing is not an absolute indicator of adequate or inadequate breathing. A patient who is talking or is aware of having the patient's respirations observed may have slight irregularities, even though breathing is adequate. The rhythm of inadequate breathing may be irregular, but a patient could have a regular rate, even when breathing is inadequate.
- **Quality.** When breathing is inadequate, breath sounds may be diminished or absent. The depth of respirations (tidal volume) will be inadequate or shallow. Chest expansion may be inadequate or unequal, and respiratory effort is increased. You may note the use of accessory muscles (e.g., muscles of the neck and abdomen) in breathing. Breathing may also be labored. Since oxygenation of the body's tissues is reduced, the skin may be pale or cyanotic (blue) and feel cool and clammy to the touch. If you can get an oxygen saturation level, it will usually be low.

In patients with diminished responsiveness, sounds such as snoring and gurgling also indicate a serious airway problem that requires immediate intervention.

Decision Points

- Is the patient breathing?
- Is the patient breathing adequately?
- Do I have an intervention to help this patient?
- Will this patient benefit from ALS?

Pediatric Note

Respiratory problems can be very serious in infants and children. Although children rarely have heart attacks or other problems of adulthood, respiratory conditions are a leading killer of infants and children. With this in mind, you must begin respiratory treatment of infants and children with a thorough and accurate assessment and prompt, proper care.

The structure of infants and children's airways differs somewhat from that of adults:

- **Airway.** All airway structures are smaller in an infant or child than in an adult, and therefore are more easily obstructed.
- **Tongue.** Infants and children's tongues are proportionally larger and therefore take up more space in the mouth than an adult's tongue.
- **Trachea.** The trachea is smaller, softer, and more flexible in infants and children, which may lead to obstruction from swelling or trauma more easily than in adults. The cricoid cartilage is less developed and less rigid.
- **Diaphragm.** Infants and children depend more heavily on the diaphragm for respiration, since the chest wall is softer. This is why infants and small children in respiratory distress exhibit "seesaw breathing," in which the movement of the diaphragm causes the chest and abdomen to move in opposite directions.

Be aware that some signs of inadequate breathing are unique to or more prominent in infants and children. Be on the lookout for these signs:

- Nasal flaring (widening of the nostrils)
- Grunting
- Seesaw breathing (As the child breathes in, the diaphragm descends, causing the abdomen to lift and the chest to sink. The reverse happens as the diaphragm relaxes during exhalation).
- Retractions (pulling in of the muscles) between the ribs (intercostal), above the clavicles (supraclavicular), and above the sternum (suprasternal)

Progression of Inadequate Breathing to Cardiac Arrest in Infants and Children

Perhaps the most startling feature in the spectrum of respiratory distress and respiratory failure in pediatrics is when cardiac arrest suddenly occurs. Respiratory failure is the leading cause of cardiac arrest in children. Infants and children tend to compensate well for respiratory challenges, but when those mechanisms fail, they tend to do so abruptly. When the respiratory failure occurs, the pediatric heart often slows and then stops. A slow heart rate (bradycardia) is never normal in an infant or child in respiratory distress. It is a sign of severe hypoxia and heralds imminent cardiac arrest. These patients should receive immediate ventilation with high-flow oxygen with an appropriately sized bag-valve-mask (BVM) device.

Patient Care

Care of the Patient with Inadequate Breathing

Fundamental Principles of Care

There is a wide range of function between adequate respirations and complete stoppage of breathing (respiratory arrest). You must pay careful attention to the patient's breathing throughout the call. It is not enough to simply make sure a patient is breathing. The patient must be breathing adequately! If at any time you find that a patient is not breathing adequately, the treatment of this condition is your first patient care priority (Table 19-2).

TABLE 19-2 Appropriate EMT Interventions for Respiratory Conditions

CONDITION	SIGNS	EMT INTERVENTION	
Adequate Breathing Patient is breathing adequately but needs supplemental oxygen due to a medical or traumatic condition.	• Normal mental status • Rate and depth of breathing adequate • Air moves freely in and out of the chest. • Skin color normal • Pulse oximetry within normal range	Consider supplemental oxygen to maintain normal pulse oximetry. Treat the underlying problem. (Assist with patient inhaler or nebulizer; consider CPAP.)	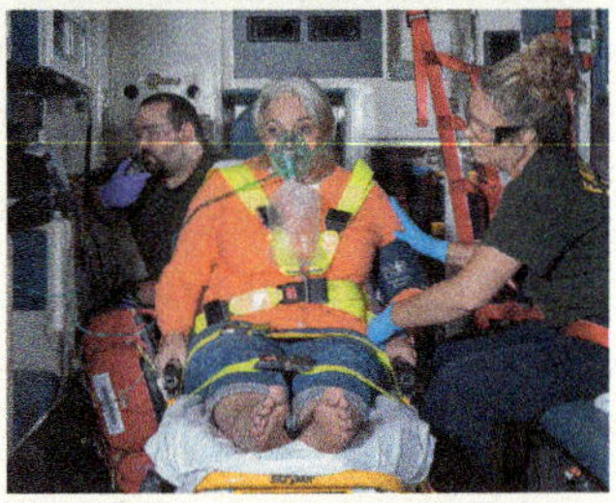
Inadequate Breathing Patient is moving some air in and out, but it is slow or shallow and not enough to live.	• Altered mental status • Patient has some breathing but not enough to live. • Rate and/or depth outside of normal limits • Shallow ventilations • Diminished or absent breath sounds • Noises such as crowing, stridor, snoring, gurgling, or gasping • Blue (cyanosis) or gray skin color • Decreased minute volume • Low pulse oximetry despite supplemental oxygen	Assisted ventilations (positive pressure ventilations) with a pocket face mask or bag-valve mask. See chapter text about adjusting rates for rapid or slow breathing. **NOTE:** *A nonrebreather mask requires adequate breathing to pull oxygen into the lungs. It does not provide ventilation to a patient who is not breathing or who is breathing inadequately.*	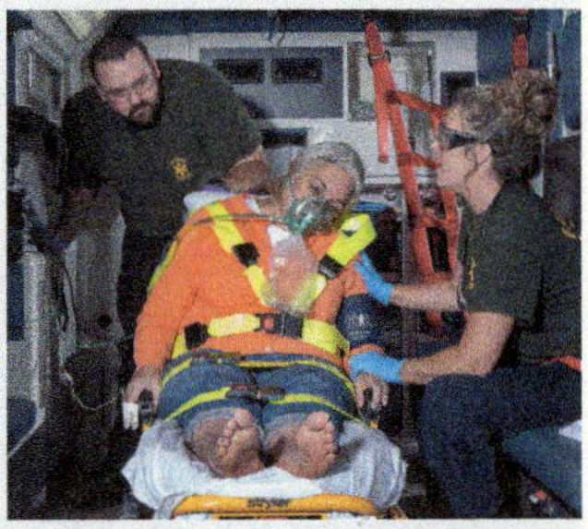

TABLE 19-2 Appropriate EMT Interventions for Respiratory Conditions (*Continued*)

CONDITION	SIGNS	EMT INTERVENTION	
No Breathing at All	• No chest rise • No evidence of air being moved from the mouth or nose • No breath sounds	Assisted ventilations with a pocket face mask; bag-valve mask at 10-12/minute for an adult and 12-20/minute for an infant or child **NOTE:** *Do not use oxygen-powered ventilation devices on infants or children.*	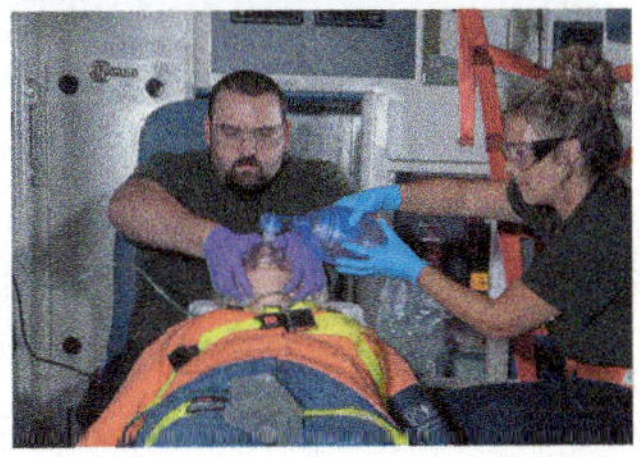

When you determine, by the signs that were discussed under the previous Patient Assessment feature, that a patient's breathing is inadequate, you will provide assisted ventilation with supplemental oxygen. Consider the following methods:

- Pocket face mask with supplemental oxygen
- Two-rescuer bag-valve mask with supplemental oxygen
- One-rescuer bag-valve mask with supplemental oxygen

The means of providing artificial ventilation were discussed in the chapter *Respiration and Artificial Ventilation*. Make sure that you are properly trained with the device that you are using for ventilation. If supplemental oxygen is not immediately available, begin artificial ventilation without supplemental oxygen, and attach the oxygen supply to the mask as soon as it is available.

If you are uncertain about whether a patient's breathing is inadequate and requires artificial ventilation, provide artificial ventilation. In the rare circumstance when a patient with inadequate breathing is conscious enough to fight artificial ventilation, transport immediately and consult medical direction.

Adequate and Inadequate Artificial Ventilation

Like breathing, artificial ventilation can be adequate or inadequate. When you are performing artificial ventilation adequately, the chest will rise and fall with each artificial ventilation. The adequate rate for artificial ventilation is 10–12 breaths per minute for adults, and 12–20 per minute for infants and children. Do not hyperventilate the patient. Hyperventilating leads to elimination of more carbon dioxide, which changes the blood chemistry and can result in constriction of the blood vessels in the brain, leading to decreased perfusion of the brain.

When you provide artificial ventilation without chest compressions (in a patient with a pulse), monitor the pulse carefully. With adequate artificial ventilation, the pulse rate should return to normal or near normal. Since the pulse in adults will usually increase when there is a lack of oxygen, a pulse that remains the same or increases may indicate inadequate artificial ventilation. Naturally, if the pulse disappears, this indicates that the patient is in cardiac arrest and needs chest compressions (CPR).

Pediatric Note

Although pediatric patients differ from adults in many ways, few differences are more important in emergency care than those within the respiratory system.

When adult patients experience a decrease in oxygen in the bloodstream (hypoxia), their pulse increases. In infants and children with respiratory difficulties, you may observe a slight increase in pulse early, but soon the pulse will drop significantly. As mentioned earlier, a low (bradycardic) pulse in infants and small children in the setting of a respiratory emergency means trouble.

If you observe a pulse below the expected rates for infants and children, evaluate your ventilations or oxygen therapy thoroughly. In ventilations, make sure that you have an open airway and that the chest rises slightly with each breath. Nothing is more important for infants and children than adequate airway care. In any situation, make sure that the oxygen tank has not run out and that the tubing has not kinked or slipped off the delivery device or oxygen cylinder.

For any patient—adult, child, or infant—if the chest does not rise and fall with each artificial ventilation or the pulse does not return to normal, check that you are maintaining an open airway via the head-elevated, sniffing position. Suction fluids and foreign matter from the airway as necessary, or perform abdominal thrusts and finger sweeps as needed to clear large airway obstructions. (Deliver alternating series of back blows and chest thrusts to clear airway obstructions in infants. Do not perform blind finger sweeps in infants or children; remove only visible objects.) Insert an oropharyngeal or nasopharyngeal airway as needed to maintain a patent airway. If you are using supplemental oxygen, check that all connections are secure and that the tubing has not kinked.

In infants and children, it is especially important to distinguish between an upper airway obstruction and a lower airway disease if there appears to be a blockage of the airway. If the airway is blocked by the tongue, blood, secretions, or debris, suction the airway and consider inserting an oropharyngeal or nasopharyngeal adjunct to help maintain an open airway.

Infants and children are also subject to respiratory infections (e.g., croup) that may result in swelling of the airway passages. In such cases, probing or placing anything in the patient's mouth or pharynx may set off spasms in the vocal cords.

Refrain from placing anything in the patient's mouth, administer oxygen, provide ventilations as needed, and transport as quickly as possible if you see any signs of a serious respiratory problem, such as:

- Wheezing, stridor, or grunting
- Increased breathing effort
- Flared nostrils or retracted muscles of breathing
- Rapid breathing
- Pale or cyanotic lips or mouth.

CORE CONCEPT

How to identify and treat a patient with breathing difficulty

Breathing Difficulty

Breathing difficulty, or "shortness of breath," is a frequent chief complaint that describes a patient's feeling of labored or difficult breathing. Although there are objective signs associated with breathing difficulty (as the following text will show), the difficulty as the patient reports it to you is a subjective perception of the patient. The amount of distress the patient feels may or may not reflect the actual severity of the condition. The adequacy of breathing may be more or less than the patient feels it is. Therefore, do not rely entirely on the patient's report to decide the seriousness of the condition. Perform an assessment to help you make that determination.

Patient Assessment

Breathing Difficulty

The most important element of the assessment of a patient with breathing difficulty is the primary assessment. Here you will begin by differentiating immediately whether breathing is adequate or inadequate. The primary assessment will also identify any necessary immediate interventions. If your patient is breathing inadequately and positive pressure ventilations are indicated, your assessment may have to stop there. Lifesaving interventions will always take priority. However, in most cases, teamwork will enable you to move on to the secondary assessment once airway and breathing have been controlled.

The secondary assessment for patients with respiratory emergencies involves obtaining an appropriate patient history and an assessment of the respiratory system. If time permits, a more detailed physical examination may also be appropriate. The *OPQRST* memory aid can be adapted to address the chief complaint of difficulty breathing, and can be very useful. Consider the following interview questions:

O—Onset. When did your difficulty breathing begin? Did it come on slow/fast? (In some cases of chronic respiratory illness, it may also be appropriate to ask if there was a specific time when the difficulty breathing became significantly worse).

P—Provocation. What were you doing when this came on? Does anything make the shortness of breath worse? Have you been short of breath when exerting yourself?

Q—Quality. Do you have a cough, and if so, are you bringing anything up with it?

R—Radiation. Do you have pain or discomfort anywhere else in your body? Does it seem to spread to any other part of your body?

S—Severity. On a scale of one to ten, how bad is your breathing trouble? (Ten is worst, one best.)

T—Time. How long have you had this feeling?

Associated symptoms. Do you have any pain or discomfort? Do you have any other symptoms, like fever or chills? Have you noticed any weight gain in the past few days?

Alternatively, consider using the *SAMPLE* mnemonic to complete a thorough patient history. In addition to inquiring about the **S**igns and **s**ymptoms of respiratory complaint, ask about **A**llergies. Ask if they have taken any prescribed **M**edications or done anything else to help relieve their condition. What medications do they take every day? Remember that these medications can help identify existing medical conditions. **P**ast medical history is also important (especially if they have had breathing problems in the past). Ask patients about their **L**ast oral intake. Another good question to ask is about **E**vents, such as whether the patient has recently traveled to an area of the world that is experiencing an infectious respiratory outbreak or has had close contact with someone who has recently traveled to such an area. A complete patient history allows you to assemble a problem list and consider a differential diagnosis. This may affect the treatment you provide and the treatment provided later at the hospital.

After assessing the adequacy of respirations, you should gather vital signs and perform a physical exam focused on the respiratory system. This includes the following (see also Figure 19-2):

Observing

- Altered mental status, including restlessness, anxiety, or depressed level of consciousness
- Unusual anatomy (barrel chest)
- The patient's position, including:
  - Tripod position (patient leaning forward with hands on knees or another surface)
  - Sitting with feet dangling, leaning forward.
- Work of breathing, including:
  - Retractions
  - Use of accessory muscles to breathe

FIGURE 19-2 Signs and symptoms of breathing difficulty. *(© Ray Kemp/911 Imaging)*

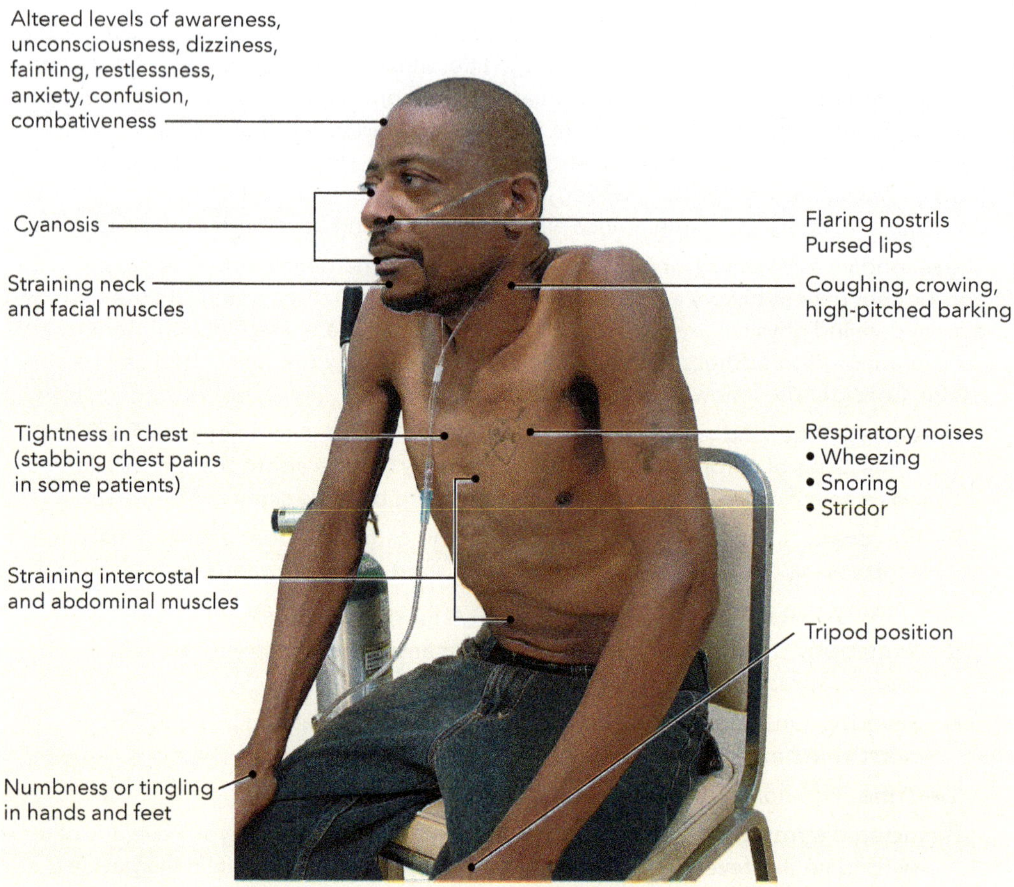

    - Flared nostrils
    - Pursed lips
    - The number of words the patient can say without stopping, described as one-word dyspnea, two-word dyspnea, and so on.
- Pale, cyanotic, or flushed skin
- Pedal edema, swelling around the calves, ankles, and feet
- Sacral edema, swelling around the low back in bedridden patients
- Noisy breathing, which may be described as:
    - Audible wheezing (heard without stethoscope)
    - Gurgling
    - Snoring
    - Stridor (harsh, high-pitched sound during breathing, usually due to upper airway obstruction)
    - Coughing
- Oxygen saturation, or SpO_2, reading of less than 95 percent on the pulse oximeter.

Auscultating

- Lung sounds on both sides during inspiration and expiration

Evaluating vital sign changes, which may include:

- Increased pulse rate
- Decreased pulse rate (especially in infants and children)

- Changes in the breathing rate (above or below normal levels)
- Changes in breathing rhythm
- Hypertension or hypotension.

Special Considerations Regarding Pulse Oximeter Readings

The *Vital Signs and Monitoring Devices* chapter discussed use of the pulse oximeter to determine the oxygen saturation of the patient's blood and identify hypoxic patients (patients with less-than-adequate oxygenation). Although the other signs and symptoms listed previously are certainly enough to identify hypoxia, the pulse oximeter will allow you to obtain a precise numerical reading.

If you have a pulse oximeter immediately available, place the sensor on the patient's finger before applying oxygen. This will give you a "room air" reading and give you the patient's saturation before you apply oxygen. When you apply oxygen to the patient, the reading should improve. Document both readings on the report. *Never delay the necessary administration of oxygen to obtain a reading. If the pulse oximeter is not immediately available, apply oxygen immediately and apply the pulse oximeter when it becomes available.*

Special Considerations Regarding Auscultation of Lung Sounds

When you auscultate the patient's lungs with a stethoscope, you may hear breath sounds that are normal or diminished in volume. You may also hear abnormal sounds such as wheezing, rhonchi, and crackles. Although there is no single universally agreed-on system for describing these sounds, some of the more common descriptions appear in the following list.

- *Wheezes* are high-pitched sounds that will seem almost musical in nature. The sound is created by air moving through narrowed air passages in the lungs. It can be heard in a variety of diseases but is common in asthma and sometimes in chronic obstructive lung diseases such as emphysema and chronic bronchitis. Wheezing is most commonly heard during expiration.
- *Crackles* are (as the name indicates) a fine crackling or bubbling sound heard on inspiration in the lower airway. The sound is caused by fluid in the alveoli or by the opening of closed alveoli. Some people refer to crackles as *rales*.
- *Rhonchi* are lower-pitched sounds that resemble snoring or rattling. They are caused by secretions in larger airways, as might be seen with pneumonia or bronchitis, or when materials are aspirated (breathed) into the lungs. The difference between crackles and rhonchi is not always obvious and is somewhat subjective. However, rhonchi generally are louder than crackles.
- *Stridor* is a high-pitched sound that is heard on inspiration. It is an upper airway sound indicating partial obstruction of the trachea or larynx. Stridor is usually audible without a stethoscope.

Listen for these lung sounds on both sides over the patient's chest (upper and lower), at the mid-axillary line, and over the patient's back (upper and lower) (Figure 19-3). Listening to the lungs in several areas may help to localize the patient's problem since some sounds may be present in the lower lobes (e.g., crackles from acute pulmonary edema), whereas others may be present throughout the lungs (e.g., wheezes from an asthma attack). You may also observe changes over time when listening to lung sounds. An asthmatic patient who has used an inhaler may feel that breathing is easier, and the wheezes may diminish. Wheezing can also become coarser and easier to hear as the medication takes effect and airways begin to open up. Be careful, however. Sometimes the wheezes will also disappear when a patient's condition worsens and breathing becomes inadequate. This is because the patient is not moving enough air in and out of the lungs anymore to create the wheezing.

Although lung sounds can be useful, they are only a rough indicator of what is going on inside the patient's chest. Only movement or vibrations that are strong enough to be transmitted through the tissue of the chest are audible with your stethoscope. Remember that your patient's overall status is more important than the lung sounds.

FIGURE 19-3 Auscultate for breath sounds on the upper and lower chest, the upper and lower back, and at the mid-axillary line.

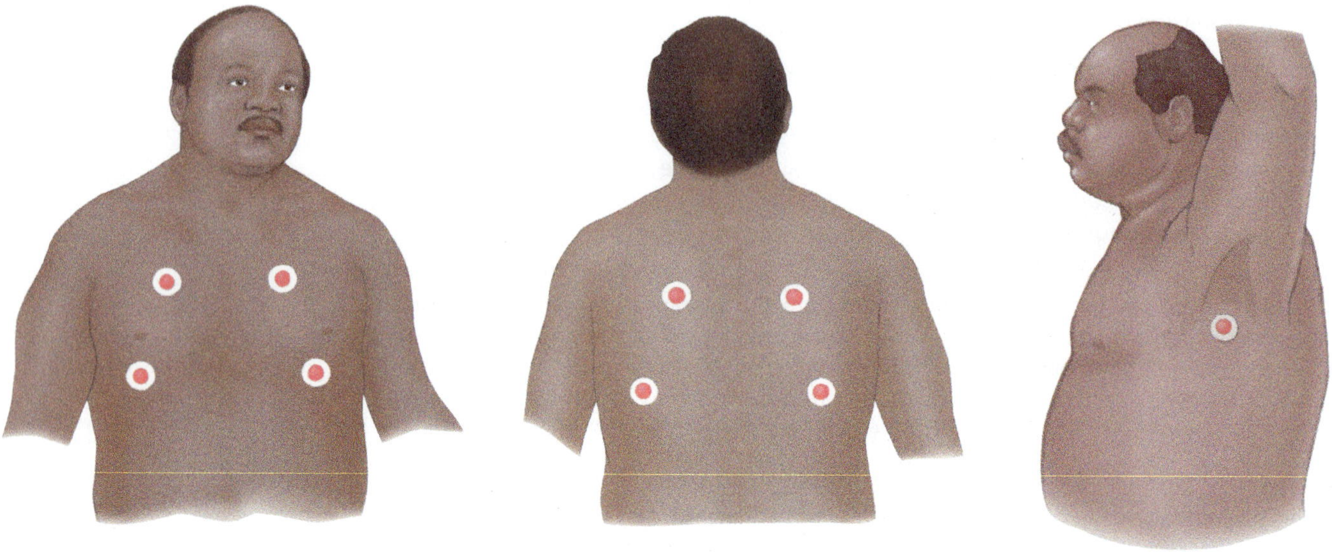

It is important to remember that a patient with breathing difficulty may have either adequate or inadequate breathing. You may encounter two patients, at different times, who tell you that they are having difficulty breathing ("I can't catch my breath" or a similar complaint). One patient may be having minor difficulty due to a preexisting respiratory condition but still have adequate breathing. This condition is not life-threatening. The other patient, who has offered exactly the same complaint, may be having a problem, such as an allergic reaction, and severe difficulty breathing. Your examination of this patient may reveal inadequate breathing that is life-threatening and requires immediate artificial ventilation.

Difficulty breathing may have many causes, ranging from ongoing medical conditions to illnesses such as pneumonia and other infections to cardiac problems that cause disturbances in the respiratory system.

Pediatric Respiratory Distress

Respiratory disorders are a great concern in infants and children. For the pediatric patient, it is important to distinguish whether the probable cause of the breathing difficulty is an upper airway problem or a lower airway problem. The care that you would give for an upper airway obstruction is not indicated for a lower airway disorder. Also, because respiratory problems can have such serious consequences in infants and children, it is critical to be alert for early signs of respiratory failure.

Recognizing respiratory distress or respiratory failure is an important goal in the assessment of a pediatric patient with difficulty breathing. Gather information quickly from the parents and do a rapid assessment of the child. Unless there are clear indications of foreign body airway obstruction, do not put a tongue depressor in the child's mouth to examine the airway. This may cause local injury or spasms that can totally obstruct the upper airway.

Recognize the following signs of early respiratory distress that are specific to infants and children (Figure 19-4):

- Nasal flaring
- Retraction of the muscles above, below, and between the sternum and ribs
- Stridor (high-pitched, harsh sound)

FIGURE 19-4 (A) Signs of respiratory distress in children. (B) Tripod breathing. (C) Altered mental status. (D) Retractions.

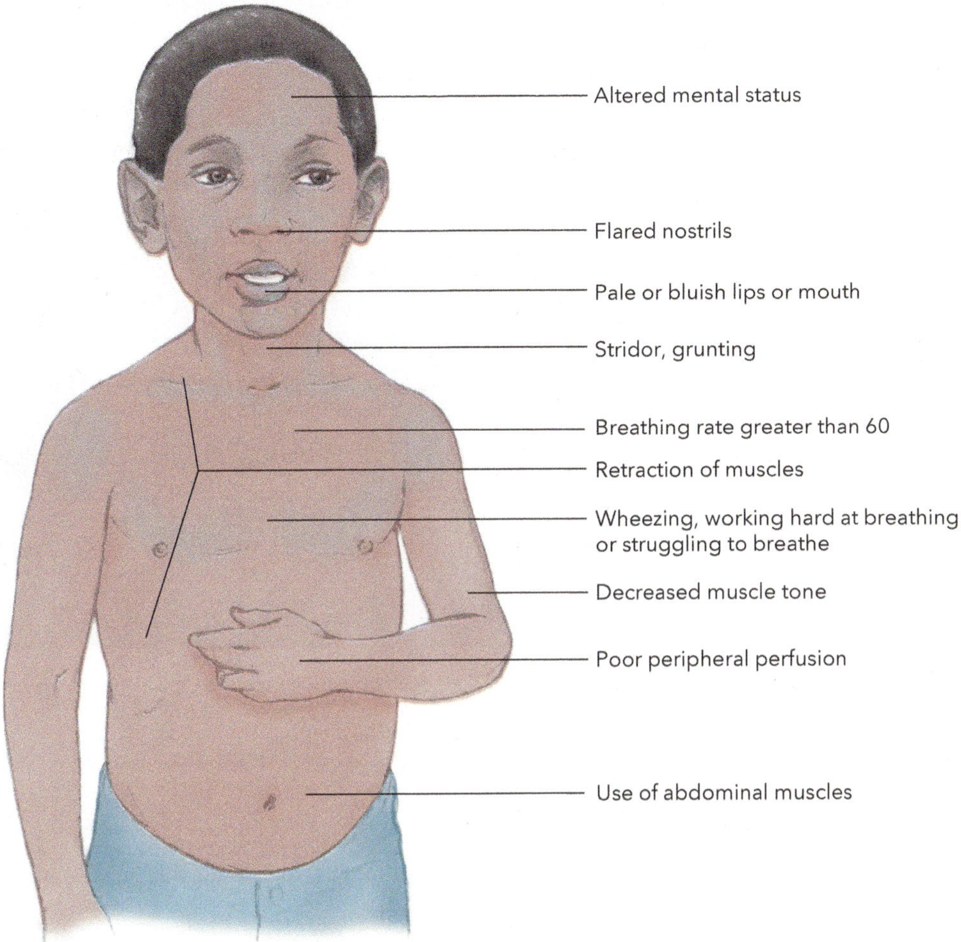

A

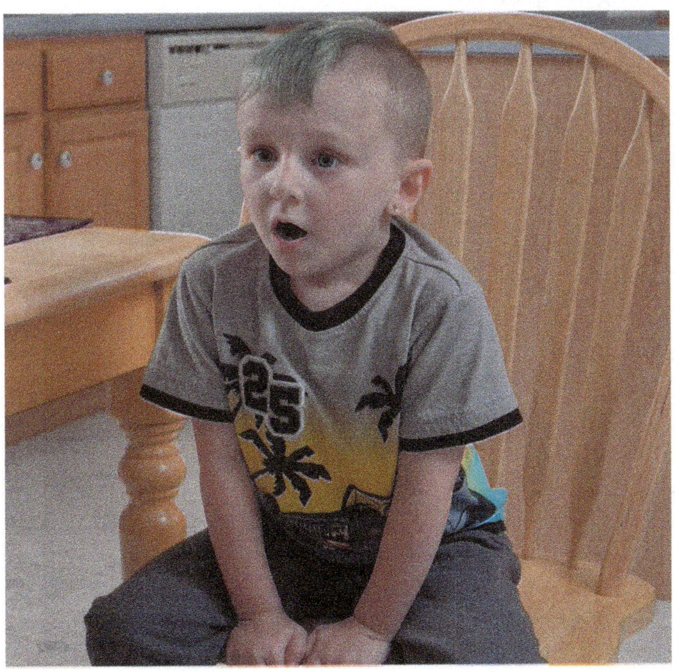

B

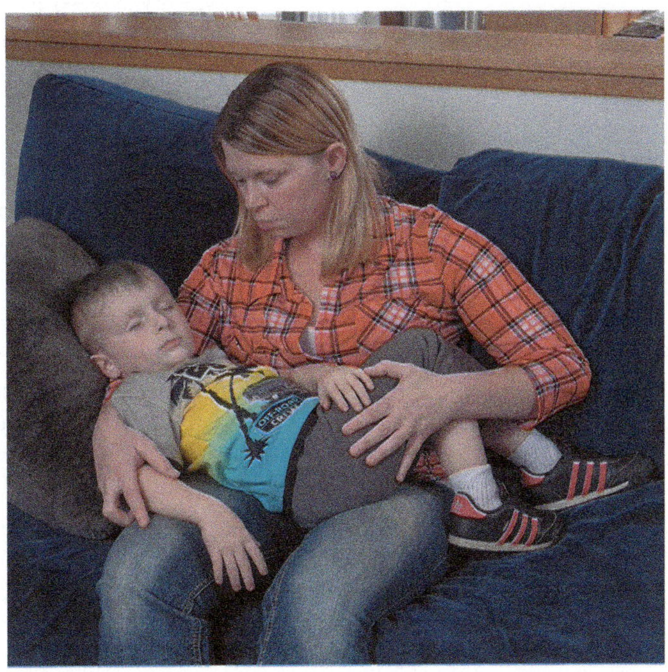

C

(continued)

FIGURE 19-4 *(Continued)*

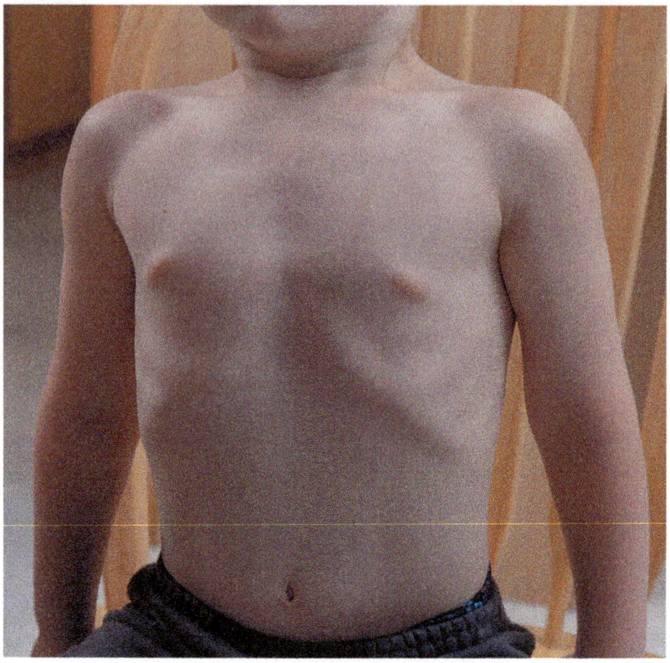

D

- Grunting
- Decreased muscle tone
- Decreased mental status
- Poor peripheral perfusion (capillary refill greater than 2 seconds)
- Decreased heart rate (a late sign)

Decision Points

- Is the pediatric patient breathing adequately?
- Is the pediatric patient breathing inadequately?

Patient Care

Care of the Patient with Breathing Difficulty

Fundamental Principles of Care

A patient with a respiratory condition requires an immediate evaluation to rapidly identify and treat respiratory failure. If respiratory failure is not found, treatment will focus on preventing hypoxia and correcting the root cause of the respiratory problem.

When a patient is suffering from breathing difficulty, provide the following care:

- **Assessment.** Assess the airway and breathing during the primary assessment and frequently throughout the call. Assist respiration with artificial ventilations and oxygen whenever the patient has or develops inadequate breathing.
- **Oxygen.** Provide supplemental oxygen when hypoxia is suspected or when signs of hypoxia are present. If a hypoxic patient is breathing adequately but is in significant respiratory distress, consider a nonrebreather mask at 15 liters per minute or a nasal cannula at 6 liters per minute to achieve and maintain a pulse oximetry of 95 percent. If the patient has inadequate breathing, provide supplemental oxygen while performing artificial ventilation.
- **Positioning.** If the patient is experiencing breathing difficulty but is breathing adequately, place the patient in a position of comfort. Most patients with breathing difficulty feel they can breathe better sitting up.

- **Prescribed inhaler.** If the patient has a prescribed inhaler or nebulizer, you may be able to assist the patient in taking this medication. This would be done after consultation with medical direction, often during transportation to the hospital. (More information on prescribed inhalers and nebulizers will be provided later in this chapter.)
- **Continuous positive airway pressure (CPAP).** CPAP can be used to treat specific conditions like acute pulmonary edema, and can provide beneficial second-line support in conditions that cause bronchoconstriction. The indications for CPAP can vary from system to system, so consult local protocol before use.

Continuous Positive Airway Pressure (CPAP)

CORE CONCEPT

Use of continuous positive airway pressure (CPAP) to relieve difficulty breathing

Many EMS systems have adopted ***continuous positive airway pressure***, or ***CPAP***, into the EMT scope of practice. Although the application of CPAP will be discussed here, it is important for you to check your local protocols to identify whether this intervention is in your scope of practice.

CPAP is a unique combination of noninvasive positive pressure and supplemental oxygen. Most CPAP systems combine high-flow oxygen and air to create a degree of positive pressure at a mask worn by the patient. While the positive pressure generated by CPAP is not enough for artificial respirations and *should never be used in situations where artificial ventilation would be indicated*, the positive pressure it generates can be therapeutic in specific problems, such as acute pulmonary edema and drowning, where expanding collapsed alveoli is essential.

continuous positive airway pressure (CPAP) a form of noninvasive positive pressure ventilation (NPPV) consisting of a mask and a means of blowing oxygen or air into the mask to prevent airway collapse or to help alleviate difficulty breathing.

Many and varied CPAP devices are available, and it is beyond the scope of this text to describe how each device generates pressure. You should always be familiar with the CPAP system you are using and always follow manufacturer's instructions for use. However, most CPAP systems do have common elements that are worthy of a brief overview here:

- Flow generation: The effects of CPAP are created by generating high levels of air flow at the CPAP mask. In some cases, air flow can be as high as 70 liters per minute. While this may seem very high compared with supplemental oxygen delivery devices like a nonrebreather mask, the air flow from a CPAP mask would best be compared to a gentle breeze. Most devices use either a combination of air and high-flow oxygen or simply air to generate this flow. Some are powered by a mechanical device called a Down's flow generator, while others use a simple Venturi system. The amount of oxygen delivered through a CPAP device depends on how much oxygen is used in the generation of flow. Some devices use high-flow oxygen and can be adjusted to offer high concentration flow. Others use room air and therefore offer only room-air levels of oxygen to the patient. You must know your system to understand how much oxygen can be administered through it. No matter the method of flow generation, it is the flow that allows the vital pressure of CPAP to be created.
- Positive end expiratory pressure (PEEP): By inhaling and exhaling against the flow of air created by CPAP, patients increase the pressure within their respiratory system. This pressure is referred to and measured as positive end expiratory pressure, or PEEP. PEEP is the pressure within the respiratory system at the end of an exhalation, and it is that increase in pressure that is most helpful when treating respiratory distress. Increased pressure in the respiratory system helps keep small airways and alveoli from collapsing and can prevent fluid from entering the alveoli in pulmonary edema. The "C" in CPAP stands for "continuous," so most systems have a popoff valve (either adjustable or fixed) designed to regulate otherwise-changing pressures between inhalation and exhalation (Figure 19-5). If the device you are using has a PEEP adjustment, you must set an initial PEEP level and be prepared to adjust this level throughout treatment. Most CPAP systems are designed to provide 7–15 centimeters of water PEEP.
- Mask seal: Similar to positive pressure ventilation, a mask seal must be created and maintained to deliver the effects of CPAP efficiently. Most systems utilize a face mask similar to those used in conjunction with a bag–mask device. Commonly, there is also a harness that covers the patient's head, used to keep the CPAP mask in place.

FIGURE 19-5 (A) Adjustable CPAP PEEP valve with variable flow generator. (B) EMT adjusting flow.

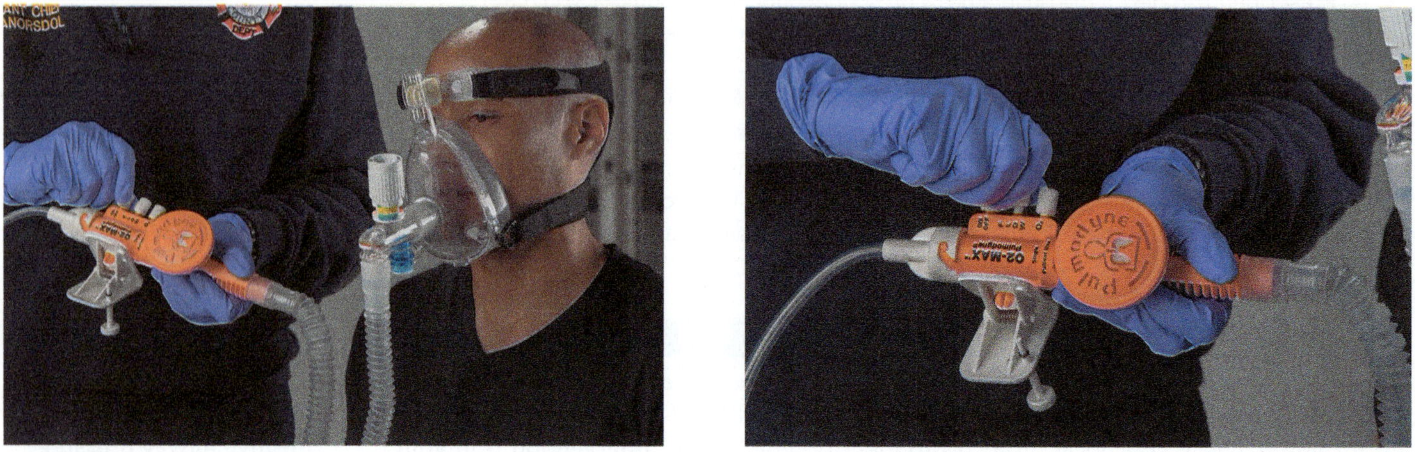

A

B

While mask seal is not as essential here as it is in positive pressure ventilation, you should monitor to prevent air leaks and therefore maximize CPAP's therapeutic effects.

Prehospital indications for CPAP use are still evolving. Common indications include:

- **Pulmonary edema and drowning.** In this situation, fluid leaks from the pulmonary capillaries into the tissue around the alveoli. This fluid can collapse small airways and, in severe cases, leak into the alveoli itself. When this happens, gas exchange is impaired. The pressure generated by CPAP prevents the movement of this fluid and pneumatically splints the small airways open.
- **Asthma and COPD.** In asthma and COPD, small airways are constricted and collapse under the increased pressure used to exhale. Alveoli are also at risk of closing at the end of exhalation. The pressures generated by CPAP help splint open these collapsed airways and often make it easier for patients to breathe. CPAP can also provide valuable supplemental oxygen.
- **Respiratory failure.** In some systems, CPAP is used as an intermediary step between supplemental oxygen and artificial ventilation. As compensation begins to fail, some patients will experience fatigue of the respiratory muscles. It is this fatigue that causes slowing rates and, in some cases, respiratory arrest. CPAP, by splinting open airways and providing supplemental oxygen, can sometimes make breathing easier and buy time for therapies to take effect. These are very dangerous situations, however, as a patient must be breathing for CPAP to work. Constant reassessment is necessary.

Contraindications for CPAP generally fall into two classes: anatomic–physiologic and pathologic. Anatomic–physiologic contraindications include mental status so depressed that the patient cannot protect the airway or follow instructions; lack of a normal, spontaneous respiratory rate (CPAP increases the volume of air the patient breathes but does not increase the patient's respiratory rate); inability to sit up; hypotension, generally considered to be less than 90 mmHg; and inability to get and maintain a good mask seal.

Pathologic contraindications include nausea and vomiting; chest trauma, particularly when a pneumothorax is possible; shock; upper gastrointestinal bleeding or recent gastric surgery; and any condition that would prevent a good mask seal, such as congenital facial malformations, facial trauma, or burns.

There are other conditions in which, even though CPAP may not be contraindicated, the EMT nevertheless needs to exercise caution: claustrophobia or inability to tolerate the mask and seal; history of inability to use CPAP; secretions so copious that they need to be suctioned; and a history of pulmonary fibrosis.

Although CPAP is frequently effective in relieving patients' difficulty breathing, the EMT needs to be aware of some side effects. Since CPAP works by maintaining a positive pressure throughout the respiratory cycle, less blood is able to return to the heart through the veins. Ordinarily, when inspiration occurs, the pressure in the thoracic cavity decreases enough that it promotes the return of blood to the heart. When CPAP is being used, the pressure in the lungs causes less blood to return to the heart, so the cardiac output decreases, frequently resulting in a drop in blood pressure. In some patients, the drop may be enough to make the patient hypotensive. For this reason, the patient needs to have a systolic blood pressure of at least 90 mmHg in order to consider use of CPAP.

When the lungs are subject to continuous positive pressure, there is a risk that the pressure may cause a weak area to rupture, leading to lung collapse (pneumothorax). This risk is increased in patients with chronic respiratory conditions such as COPD and asthma. However, COPD patients with difficulty breathing are commonly treated with BiPAP (bilevel positive airway pressure) in the emergency department. This is similar to CPAP but somewhat more complex.

Patients who are vomiting (or nauseated, putting them at risk of vomiting) have an increased risk of aspiration because positive pressure can push air into the stomach, resulting in gastric distention. This can lead to vomiting and blowing of the vomitus into the airway and lungs.

A less dangerous side effect, though one very uncomfortable for the patient, is drying of the corneas of the eyes. Even a small leak at the top of the mask can lead to a high volume of air blowing directly into the eyes, especially if transport time is long.

To apply CPAP (Scan 19-1), explain to the patient that you are applying a mask that is going to flow air. The mask may feel strange, but should help the patient feel better within a couple of minutes. If the patient has never had CPAP before, it may help to allow the patient to hold the mask initially. Once the patient gets used to it and starts to feel some improvement, you can attach the straps that will hold the mask in place. Start with a low level of PEEP. Many systems start between 5 and 7 centimeters of water (cm H_2O) and then adjust to a therapeutic level.

Patients with pulmonary edema commonly achieve benefit at or around 10 centimeters H_2O. Some CPAP systems also allow for the adjustment of oxygen concentration. Although it may be tempting to provide high concentrations, remember that the therapeutic effects of CPAP most commonly are derived from pressure, not oxygen. In Venturi-driven CPAP systems, it is common for pressure to drop as oxygen concentrations are increased. While supplemental oxygen may be necessary, maintaining flow and pressure is frequently more important. Use the information provided to you by the pulse oximeter to help titrate the concentration of oxygen being administered. Always keep the true goal of CPAP in mind.

Reassess the patient's mental status, vital signs, and level of dyspnea frequently. If the patient's mental status or respiratory condition deteriorates, remove the CPAP and begin ventilating the patient with a bag mask.

Follow your local protocols as to when to apply CPAP, how much PEEP to start with, how frequently to increase it, and how high to go.

SCAN 19-1 CPAP

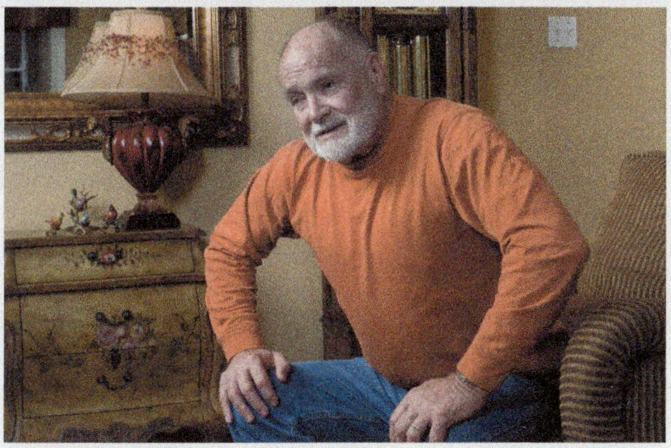

1. Assess to be sure that the patient meets the criteria for CPAP.

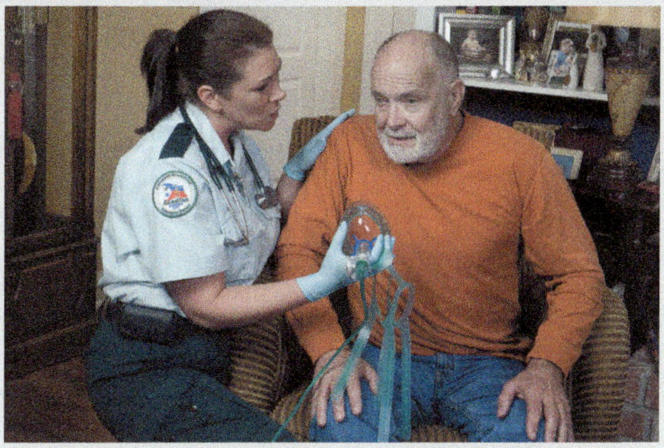

2. Explain the device to the patient. The mask and snug seal may initially cause the patient to feel smothered and anxious.

(continued)

SCAN 19-1 CPAP *(continued)*

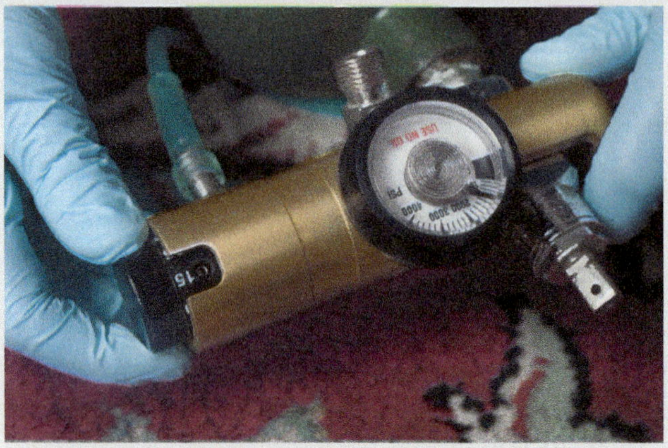

3. Start flow to the mask and adjust PEEP and oxygen settings per protocol.

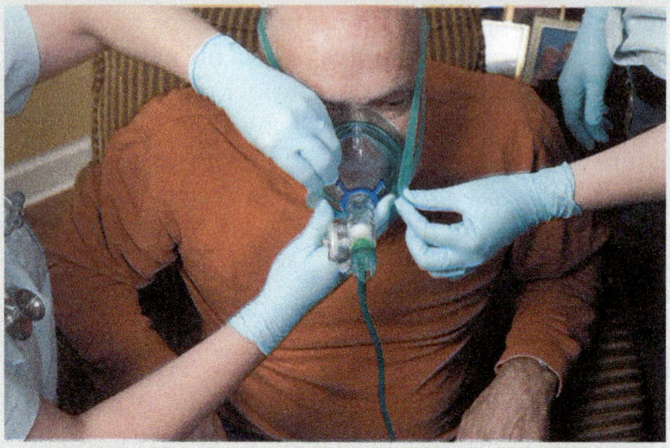

4. Apply the mask to the patient's face. Continue to calm and reassure the patient.

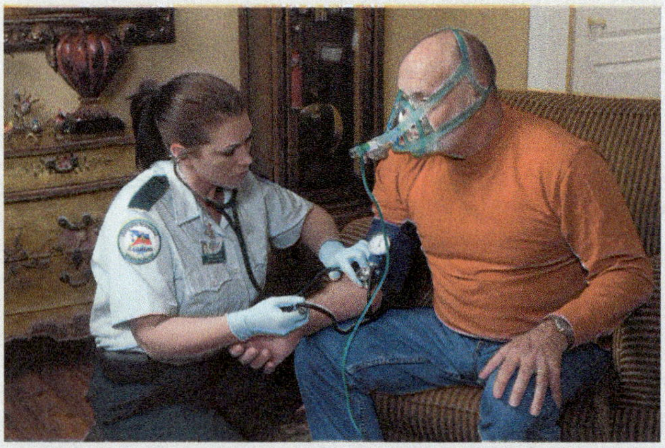

5. Reassess and monitor the patient.

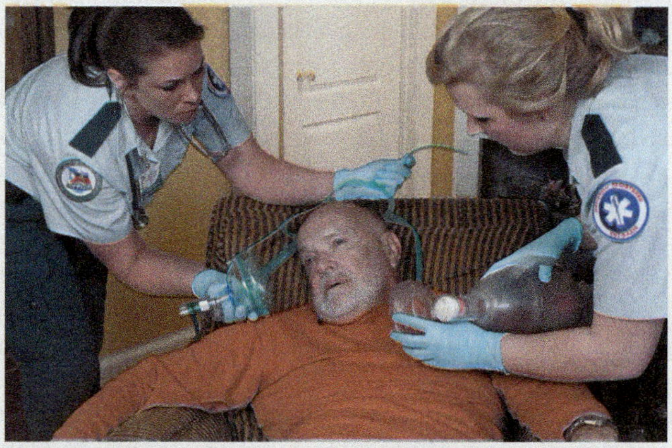

6. Discontinue CPAP and ventilate the patient if breathing becomes inadequate.

Respiratory Conditions

Although treatment in the field is very similar for different respiratory diseases, the EMT may find it useful to understand some of the more common causes of respiratory distress, along with the signs and symptoms associated with them.

Chronic Obstructive Pulmonary Disease (COPD)

Emphysema—as well as chronic bronchitis, and many undetermined respiratory illnesses that cause the patient problems like those seen in emphysema—are all classified as chronic obstructive pulmonary disease (COPD).

COPD is most commonly a problem of middle-aged or older patients (Figure 19-6). This is because these disorders ordinarily take time to develop as tissues in the respiratory tract react to irritants. Cigarette smoking causes the overwhelming majority of cases of COPD. Occasionally, other irritants such as chemicals, air pollutants, or repeated infections cause this condition.

Chronic bronchitis and emphysema are compared in Figure 19-7. In chronic bronchitis, the bronchiole lining is inflamed and excess mucus is formed. The cells in the bronchioles that normally clear away accumulations of mucus are not able to do so. The sweeping apparatus on these cells, the cilia, has been damaged or destroyed.

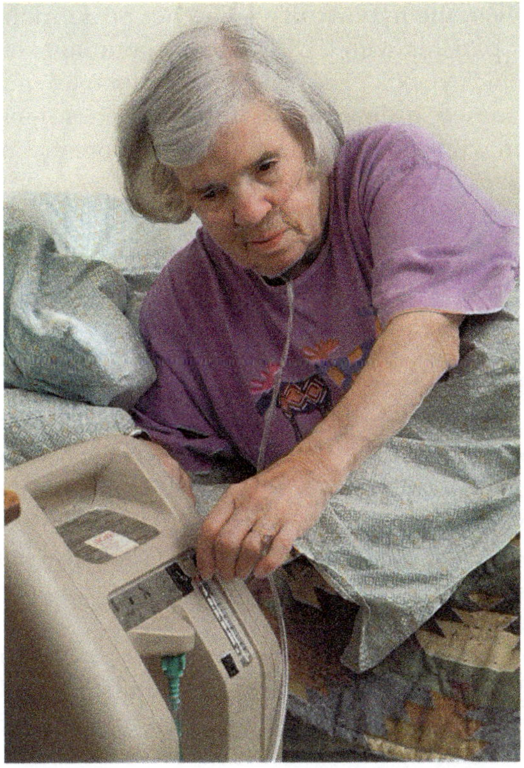

FIGURE 19-6 A patient with chronic obstructive pulmonary disease (COPD) on home oxygen. *(© Michal Heron)*

In emphysema, the walls of the alveoli break down, greatly reducing the surface area for respiratory exchange. The lungs begin to lose elasticity. These factors combine to allow stale air laden with carbon dioxide to be trapped in the lungs, reducing the effectiveness of normal breathing efforts.

Many COPD patients will exhibit characteristics of both emphysema and chronic bronchitis. Usually the reason a COPD patient calls the ambulance is that a recent upper respiratory infection has caused an acute worsening of chronic disease. This may cause the patient to experience a fever and cough up green or dark sputum.

A small number of COPD patients develop a hypoxic drive to trigger respirations. In patients without COPD, the brain stem determines when to breathe based on increased levels of carbon dioxide in the blood. Since COPD patients develop a tolerance to their body's high levels of carbon dioxide, the brain learns to rely, instead, on low oxygen levels as the trigger to breathe. The higher oxygen levels that result from oxygen administration may, in rare cases, signal the COPD patient to reduce or even to stop breathing (leading to respiratory arrest).

FIGURE 19-7 Chronic bronchitis and emphysema are chronic obstructive pulmonary diseases.

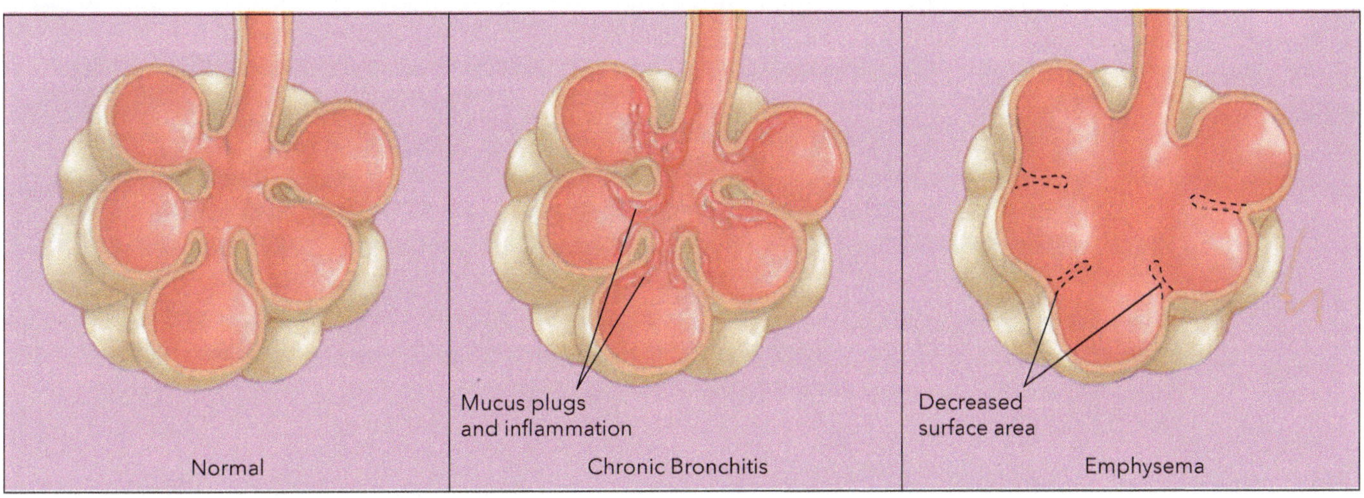

In most cases, however, the hypoxic drive will not be a problem in the prehospital setting. (Indeed, many patients with COPD are on continuous home oxygen by nasal cannula because of chronic hypoxia.) The patient's need for oxygen will outweigh any risk involved with administration. If the patient is hypoxic or has signs of hypoxia, a higher concentration of oxygen will be required in spite of the potential problems. If oxygen is indicated to treat the COPD patient, do not withhold it.

Constantly monitor the patient. If the patient's breathing becomes inadequate or stops, be prepared to assist respirations through artificial ventilation; then contact medical direction.

Asthma

Seen in young and old patients alike, asthma is a chronic disease that has episodic exacerbations, or flare-ups. It is a disease that seems to affect the patient at irregular intervals. This is far different from chronic bronchitis and emphysema, both of which continuously afflict the patient. Asthma also differs from chronic bronchitis and emphysema in that it does not produce a hypoxic drive. An asthma attack or flare can be life-threatening. Between episodes, the asthmatic patient can lead a normal life. Many use steroid inhalers for their chronic condition to reduce inflammation in the airways, with albuterol administered only for a "rescue" during a flare.

Attacks can be precipitated by insect stings, air pollutants, infection, strenuous exercise, or emotional stress. When an asthma attack occurs, the small bronchioles that lead to the air sacs of the lungs become narrowed because of contractions of the muscles that make up the airway. To complicate matters, there is an overproduction of thick mucus. The combined effects of the contractions and the mucus cause the small passages to practically close down, severely restricting air flow.

The air flow is mainly restricted in one direction. When the patient inhales, the expanding lungs exert an outward pull, increasing the diameter of the airway and allowing air to flow into the lungs. During exhalation, however, the opposite occurs and the stale air becomes trapped in the lungs. This requires the patient to exhale the air forcefully, producing the characteristic wheezing sounds associated with asthma.

There is no known way to prevent asthma, but episodes of distress can often be prevented by use of appropriate medications and careful attention to avoiding items that trigger attacks.

Point of View

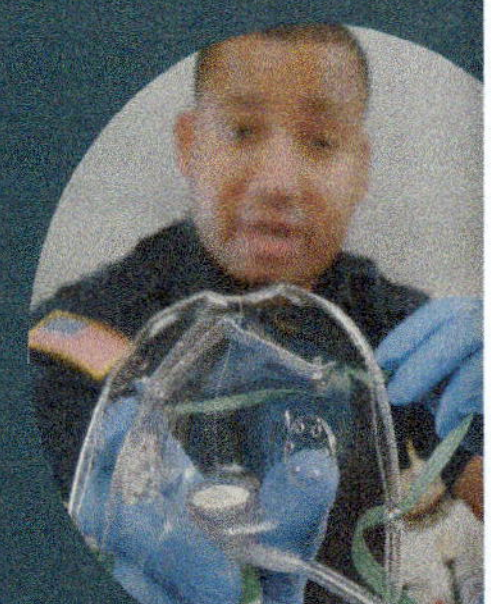

"I couldn't breathe. I mean, I really couldn't breathe. I felt like I couldn't get air in and out, and I was pretty sure I was going to die.

"I tell you this because I feel bad about how I yelled at the EMT. I can't remember everything, but I seem to remember being downright nasty. You see, I have asthma but have never had an attack like that before.

"My husband called the EMTs, and they came to the house pretty quickly. But my breathing was getting worse and worse and, well, like I said, I wasn't sure I'd live through this one. It makes you crazy.

"When the EMT tried to put that mask on my face, I felt like I was being smothered. Even though I know it's supposed to help, I couldn't stop myself from lashing out at the EMT. I pushed his hand away and yelled. I can't imagine what it must've looked like or what was going through his mind while I was yelling at him.

"He finally got me to put the mask on. He was very patient and calm. The oxygen did help me, but it wasn't easy. By the time we got to the hospital, I felt a little better. And I apologized to him. He told me not to worry about it. But I do.

"I really hope this never happens again."

Pulmonary Edema

Patients with heart failure, formerly referred to as congestive heart failure or CHF, may experience difficulty breathing because of fluid that accumulates in the lungs, preventing them from breathing adequately. The abnormal accumulation of fluid in or around the alveoli of the lungs is known as pulmonary edema. It typically occurs because the left side of the heart has been damaged, often by a myocardial infarction (heart attack) or chronic hypertension. Since the left side of the heart receives blood from the lungs, the inability to pump blood out results in pressure building up and going back to the lungs. Since there is only one layer of cells lining the alveoli and one layer of cells covering the adjoining capillaries, when pressure builds up, it is relatively easy for fluid to cross this thin barrier and accumulate in the tissue around the alveoli and—in severe cases—in the alveoli themselves. If the weight of the fluid collapses the alveoli and if fluid occupies the lower airways, it is difficult for gas exchange to occur. This challenge causes the sensation of shortness of breath and often results in hypoxia.

Patients with heart failure often have both left-sided heart failure and right-sided heart failure. Since the right side of the heart receives its blood from the systemic circulation (everything besides the lungs), pressure backs up into the systemic circulation. This becomes visible as edema in the lower parts of the body, typically the lower legs. In bedridden patients, the legs are not the lowest part of the body. Instead, fluid accumulates in the sacral area of the lower back. Sometimes the patient with heart failure will also have jugular vein distention (JVD) (Figure 19-8), and accumulation of fluid in the abdominal cavity.

When the patient lies down at night to sleep, the fluid in the body moves back into the circulation. This means it can easily overload the system and leak into the lungs, leading at first to mild dyspnea that can be relieved by sleeping propped up on one pillow, then two pillows or even three pillows. At some point the amount of fluid becomes too much, and the patient awakens acutely short of breath with the feeling of drowning.

The most common diagnostic indication of acute pulmonary edema is a prior history of heart failure. A patient who can speak will likely tell you of a history of similar problems associated with heart failure. The patient often describes feeling a little worse each night for the past several days. There may also have been a weight gain of several pounds in just a few days, perhaps accompanied by the need for a larger belt. Respiratory distress associated with acute pulmonary edema typically comes on abruptly, and patients commonly describe a sudden onset of difficulty breathing. Other signs and symptoms include anxiety, pale and sweaty skin, tachycardia, hypertension, respirations that are rapid and labored, and low oxygen saturation. In severe cases, you may hear a gurgling sound from the lungs, even without a stethoscope, each time the patient breathes. When you auscultate the lungs, you will usually hear crackles or sometimes wheezes. In severe cases the patient may cough up frothy sputum, which is usually white but sometimes tinged pink.

Treatment includes high-concentration oxygen by mask, unless breathing is inadequate and you need to ventilate the patient. If at all possible, keep the patient's legs in a

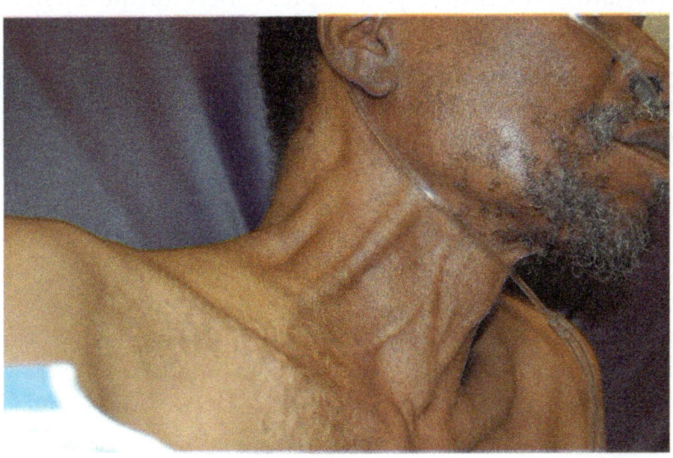

FIGURE 19-8 Jugular vein distention (JVD) in a patient with heart failure. *(© Edward T. Dickinson, MD)*

dependent position (hanging down). Bringing the legs up may push more fluid into the already overloaded circulatory system and make matters worse. As noted earlier, CPAP may be very useful in these patients, since it increases the pressure in the alveoli and prevents fluid from shifting. It also can splint open the small airways.

Although most cases of pulmonary edema you see will be the result of heart failure or MI, there are some noncardiac causes. Some people, for example, when exposed to the low atmospheric pressure of high altitudes, may develop pulmonary edema. In this case, the heart is fine. The most important treatment for these patients is to bring them back to normal altitude and atmospheric pressure. You should administer high-concentration oxygen until this can be accomplished. Pulmonary edema can also present in drowning patients and in patients who have inhaled toxins and drugs (like inhaled or smoked opioids).

Although traditionally called *congestive heart failure*, this condition is now usually just called *heart failure*, to reflect the reality that many patients don't develop the congestion (with blood) of the body's organs. This condition, whatever it is called, is quite common and is fortunately much more treatable than it used to be. Many patients who would not have survived more than a year or two just a decade ago are now living active lives, thanks to strict diet modification (low-sodium), modern pharmacology, and sometimes use of advanced electronic pacemakers that make the heart beat more efficiently.

Pneumonia

Pneumonia is an infection of one or both lungs caused by bacteria, viruses, or fungi. It results from the inhalation of certain microbes that then grow in the lungs and cause inflammation. People with COPD or other respiratory diseases are more likely to get pneumonia. People with chronic health problems are also at higher risk.

Some of the most common signs and symptoms of pneumonia include coughing (mucus can be greenish, yellow, or occasionally bloody), fever, chest pain, and severe chills. Most, but not all, patients complain of shortness of breath, either with or without exertion; chest pain that is sharp and pleuritic (worsens on inhalation); headache; pale, sweaty skin; fatigue; and confusion, especially in the elderly. Sometimes an older person will have only a few other signs or symptoms besides confusion. When you auscultate the chest, you may hear crackles on one side in just one region.

Prehospital care consists of supportive treatment that you would administer to any patient with difficulty breathing. If the patient is hypoxic, administer supplemental oxygen. In some EMS systems, EMTs apply CPAP to these patients. In some cases, pneumonia can be severe enough to cause inadequate breathing, and will require artificial respirations. If the pneumonia is thought to be bacterial, the patient will receive antibiotics at the emergency department. The cause of the pneumonia, the severity of the patient's condition, and the patient's state of general health will determine whether the patient needs to be admitted to the hospital.

Immunization with a vaccine that prevents the most common types of bacterial pneumonia is an important and effective part of prevention for the elderly and those with chronic health conditions.

Spontaneous Pneumothorax

When a lung collapses without injury or any other obvious cause, it is called a spontaneous pneumothorax. This is usually the result of rupture of a bleb, a small section of the lung that is weak. Once the bleb ruptures, the lung collapses and air leaks into the thorax. Certain conditions and activities place patients at higher risk of a spontaneous pneumothorax. Patients with COPD and a history of smoking are at highest risk. Tall, thin people are also more likely to have a weak spot that can rupture with just a cough.

The patient with a collapsed lung typically has sharp, pleuritic chest pain and shortness of breath, although these may be mild when the pneumothorax is small. When the area involved is larger, the patient will often tire easily, be tachycardic, breathe fast, have a low oxygen saturation, and exhibit cyanosis.

In the patient with a classic spontaneous pneumothorax, auscultation will reveal breath sounds that are decreased or absent on the side with the injured lung. The breath sound exam is not always reliable, however, as some patients with a pneumothorax may have perfectly normal breath sounds. As the pneumothorax worsens, patients can develop JVD and hypotension. These findings indicate a life-threatening problem.

If a pneumothorax is suspected, and the patient has significant respiratory distress, contact ALS immediately. Administer oxygen and treat the patient like anyone else who is short of breath. As mentioned earlier, CPAP is contraindicated in patients with a suspected pneumothorax. Most patients with a pneumothorax will need to have a small catheter or a larger plastic chest tube inserted between the ribs, then into the pleural space around the collapsed lung. The catheter will help remove the air, allowing the lung to re-expand.

Pulmonary Embolism

Blood usually travels through the vessels in the lung, eventually getting to the capillaries, where oxygen and carbon dioxide are exchanged. When something that is not blood—such as a blood clot, air, or fat—tries to go through these blood vessels, it gets stuck and blocks an artery in the lungs. This is a dangerous condition known as a pulmonary embolism.

The most common example of a pulmonary embolism is a blood clot that starts in a vein, often a vein in the leg or in the pelvis. This dangerous type of clot is called a deep vein thrombosis (DVT). The common reasons a DVT occurs include lying down or sitting in one position for an extended period, having active cancer, or having a limb immobilized in a cast. All these conditions can result in pooling of the blood in the veins that makes it more likely to clot and form a thrombus.

Other things can block the pulmonary arteries, though not as often as a blood clot. A significant amount of air introduced into a vein can cause great harm and even death. If fat gets into the circulation—for example, from the marrow of a fractured bone—the same results can occur.

The signs and symptoms of a pulmonary embolism are extremely variable, making this life-threatening condition difficult to detect. The classic presentation is sudden onset of sharp, pleuritic chest pain (worsens with breathing in and out); shortness of breath; anxiety; a cough (sometimes with bloody sputum); tachycardia; and tachypnea. Unfortunately, few patients with a pulmonary embolism present in this way. The patient may also complain of feeling light-headed or dizzy, with pain and swelling in one or both legs. If the clot is large, the patient may be hypotensive or go into cardiac arrest.

Administer oxygen and treat the patient like anyone else who is short of breath. Keep a high index of suspicion for pulmonary embolism in patients with recent immobilizations and those with a previous history of DVT.

Pulmonary embolus can sometimes be prevented by avoiding long periods of inactivity, refraining from smoking, taking appropriate medication when there is a high risk of forming clots, and getting care for DVT before it leads to a pulmonary embolism.

Epiglottitis

When an infection inflames the area around and above the epiglottis, the tissue swells. If it swells enough, it can actually occlude, or close off, the airway. Epiglottitis used to be a disease of children, but it is now much less common in children than in adults in the United States. This is primarily the result of childhood vaccination against *Haemophilus influenzae* type B, the bacterium that used to cause most cases of epiglottitis in children. Currently, pediatric cases of epiglottitis are usually limited to children who have not been fully vaccinated.

The typical adult with epiglottitis is a male in his forties who may have had a recent cold. Symptoms include sore throat and painful or difficult swallowing. In severe cases, the patient may be in the tripod position, to increase the glottic opening as much as possible. Other signs may include a sick appearance, muffled voice, fever, and drooling because of the pain and difficulty in swallowing. An alarming sign is stridor. This indicates the airway already has a significant degree of obstruction.

In contrast to the slower onset of symptoms in adults with epiglottitis, children who have this disease often experience a sudden onset. Although children between 2 and 7 years of age used to be the most likely to experience epiglottitis, it can now appear in a child of any age. The presentation of a still child leaning forward in the tripod position, drooling, and appearing to be in distress should alert the EMT to the possibility of this disease.

Treatment for epiglottitis includes doing as much as possible to make the patient calm and comfortable. This means you should *not* inspect the throat. Administer high-concentration oxygen if you can do it without alarming the patient. Transport as soon as possible to an emergency department capable of dealing with this type of patient. Be sure to advise the staff when you expect to arrive, so that the proper personnel can be there. Because of the possibility of sudden closure of the airway, use of lights and siren is justified for a patient in this condition unless you are very close to the hospital. If untreated, up to 10 percent of children with this disease may die. Adults can tolerate the swelling better, because their airways are larger in caliber, but there is still a risk of losing the airway.

Most cases of childhood epiglottitis can be prevented by administration of the *Haemophilus influenzae* type B vaccine. Adult epiglottitis can result from infection by many different microbes, so there is no reliable way to prevent it in adults.

Croup

Croup is caused by a group of viral illnesses that result in inflammation of the larynx, trachea, and bronchi. It is typically an illness of children 6 months to about 4 years of age, and it often occurs at night. Tissues in the airway (particularly the upper airway) become swollen and restrict the passage of air. This problem sometimes follows a cold or other respiratory infection.

The classic presentation of croup is the development of a loud, barking cough and hoarse voice, usually occurring just after bedtime. Associated breathing difficulty typically resolves when the child moves to an upright position (like when being held by a parent). However, croup can be severe and cause inadequate breathing, indicated by signs of hypoxia (cyanosis, altered mental status, etc.) and signs of significant breathing difficulty, like inspiratory stridor. If signs of inadequate breathing are present, initiate artificial respirations and transport immediately. If the patient is in respiratory distress but is breathing adequately, call advanced life support (ALS) and initiate gentle transport. Consider supplemental oxygen if the patient is hypoxic. Allow the patient to remain in a position of comfort.

Bronchiolitis

Bronchiolitis is a condition in which small airways become inflamed because of viral infection. Although a wide array of viruses can cause bronchiolitis, the most common cause is the respiratory syncytial virus, or RSV. RSV typically affects children younger than 5 years and is the most common cause of hospitalization for infants. RSV is typically seasonal and peaks throughout the fall and early winter. As bronchiolitis is caused by a virus, it is commonly associated with other cold-like symptoms such as a runny nose, fever, and general illness. Symptoms typically progress over a few days and worsen to include respiratory distress. It is also common for multiple children in the house to be sick with similar symptoms.

Bronchiolitis can cause significant respiratory distress and progress to inadequate breathing. Artificial ventilation may be necessary. If the patient is hypoxic or shows signs of hypoxia, treat with supplemental oxygen. Consider using a bulb syringe to suction the nose if it is obstructed by mucus. Clearing the nose of an infant can significantly improve minute ventilation.

Cystic Fibrosis

A genetic disease that appears in childhood, cystic fibrosis (CF) causes thick, sticky mucus that accumulates in the lungs and digestive system. The mucus can cause life-threatening lung infections and serious problems with digestion. Signs and symptoms may include:

- Coughing with large amounts of mucus from the lungs
- Fatigue

- Frequent occurrences of pneumonia, characterized by fever, more coughing than usual, worse shortness of breath than usual, more sputum than usual, and loss of appetite
- Abdominal pain and distention
- Coughing up blood
- Nausea
- Weight loss

If you encounter a patient with CF, the patient or the patient's parent will be able to tell you about how the disease affects the patient. Historically, CF was a disease of childhood, and patients died young. Thanks to advances in pulmonary care, today half of CF patients in the United States are 18 years of age or older. Patients or parents will be very familiar with the disease and what usually works for them. Use their knowledge to your advantage.

Viral Respiratory Infections

Like bronchiolitis in children, viral respiratory infections are common in adults. In fact, the Centers for Disease Control and Prevention state that upper respiratory infections (such as the common cold) affect more than 17 billion people each year. There are many presentations of respiratory infections, but they often start with a sore or scratchy throat with sneezing, a runny nose, and a feeling of fatigue. There may be a fever and chills. The infection can spread into the lungs, causing shortness of breath, especially in those who have chronic health conditions. The cough can be persistent and may produce sputum that is yellow or greenish. Symptoms usually persist for 1–2 weeks. Influenza, otherwise known as the flu, is a particularly dangerous viral infection, killing between 12,000 and 56,000 people each year. The danger of influenza is specifically associated with its ease of transmission from one person to another. The average person who contracts the flu will transmit it to between 3 and 5 other people.

Although similar to the common cold, influenza symptoms are typically more intense and last longer. Influenza is also more commonly associated with fever, headaches, and body aches than is the common cold. Patients with influenza can experience respiratory distress as well.

Because the signs and symptoms of respiratory infections are so similar, and because infections often resemble the symptoms of many other diseases, it may be impossible for an EMT to diagnose a specific problem or condition. When faced with unclear symptoms, you should provide supportive care and administer oxygen if the patient is hypoxic or if signs of hypoxia are present.

Remember that viral infections are very contagious. These diseases are spread by inhalation of and contact with respiratory droplets, so you must protect yourself from infection. If you suspect your patient has a respiratory infection, you should don eye protection, gloves, and a protective surgical mask before making contact. Although the most common respiratory viruses, such as influenza and even measles, are stopped by a simple surgical mask, emerging and novel respiratory illnesses may in the future require a higher level of filtration. All EMTs should be properly fitted for an N-95 mask and use it as needed.

Unlike bacterial respiratory infections where antibiotics are used to treat and cure the infection, viral respiratory infections are treated with supportive care such as supplemental oxygen for hypoxia and bronchodilators for wheezing. Even antiviral medications that are used to treat influenza only shorten the course of the infection; they do not cure the infection.

Good hygiene can help prevent viral respiratory infections. Before touching your hand to your nose or eyes, be sure it is clean. If you have shaken hands with someone who is carrying the virus, it can be transmitted to you and introduced into your system through the mucous membranes of the nose and eyes. Alcohol-based hand sanitizer can be very helpful. Avoiding the spray of a sick person who is sneezing or coughing will also reduce your risk of contracting a viral respiratory infection.

EMTs should also be good practitioners of infection control. Vaccinations, such as those that protect against influenza, measles, and mumps, are important steps to take not only to keep yourself safe, but also to prevent the spread of disease. If you do get sick, stay home and prevent spreading your illness to patients who may not be as capable of compensating for infection. Use cough etiquette; cough or sneeze into your elbow or a tissue rather than your hand. Remember that the control of infection is a burden that we must all share.

The Prescribed Inhaler

CORE CONCEPT

Use of a prescribed inhaler and how to assist a patient with one

A patient with asthma, COPD, or similar chronic illness may have an inhaler prescribed by a physician. You will need to get permission from medical direction to help the patient use the inhaler. This may be accomplished by phone/radio or by standing order, depending on your local protocols. Keep in mind that a patient may have overused the inhaler prior to your arrival, so it is important to determine exactly when and how many times the inhaler has been used. Be sure to give this information to medical direction.

The metered-dose inhaler gets its name from the fact that each activation of the inhaler provides a metered, or exactly measured, dose of medication. Most patients simply refer to the device as their "inhaler" or "puffer." The inhaler is prescribed for patients with respiratory problems that cause ***bronchoconstriction*** (constriction, or blockage, of the bronchi that lead from the trachea to the lungs) or other types of lung obstructions. The inhalers contain a drug that dilates, or enlarges, the air passages, making breathing easier. These drugs are in the form of a fine powder. The timing of the activation of the inhaler in relation to a deep breath is very important to prevent the fine powder from coming to rest on the moist inner surface of the mouth. The medication will work only if it comes in contact with lung tissue directly. Studies have shown that inhalers can be very beneficial—but only when used properly.

bronchoconstriction constriction, or blockage, of the bronchi that lead from the trachea to the lungs.

Spacer devices (Figure 19-9) make the exact timing necessary to use an inhaler less critical. The inhaler is activated into the spacer device. The medication stays airborne inside the chamber and can then be inhaled directly into the lungs.

When patients use an inhaler, they often are excited or nervous because they are short of breath. Many do not use their inhalers properly. Some people have never had proper instruction in use of their inhalers. Make sure to calm the patient the best you can and coach the patient to use the inhaler properly, as follows:

1. As with any medication, ensure that you have the right patient, the right time, the right medication, the right dose, and the right route. Check the expiration date. Make sure the inhaler is at room temperature or warmer. Shake the inhaler vigorously several times. If the metered-dose inhaler is new or has not been used for several days or weeks, you should first prime the inhaler by depressing it at least once before use with the patient. Some metered-dose inhalers require more than one activation to prime properly. If proper use is unclear, refer to the medication instructions on the packaging or contact medical control.
2. Make sure that the patient is alert enough to use the inhaler properly. Use a spacer device if the patient has one available. If a spacer is used, ensure that the inhaler is seated properly in the holder on the spacer.

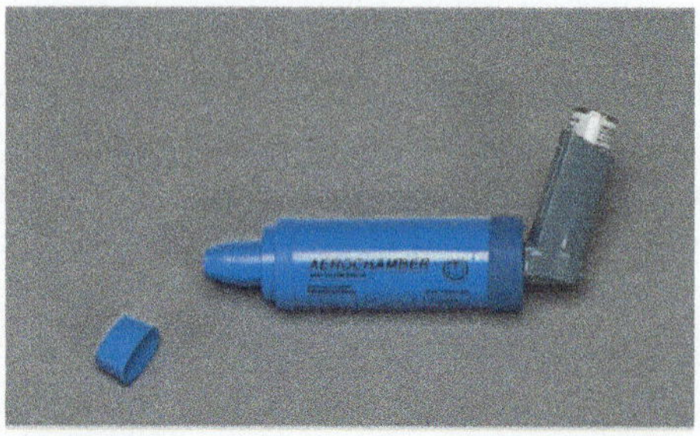

FIGURE 19-9 A spacer between the inhaler and patient makes the timing during inhaler use less critical.

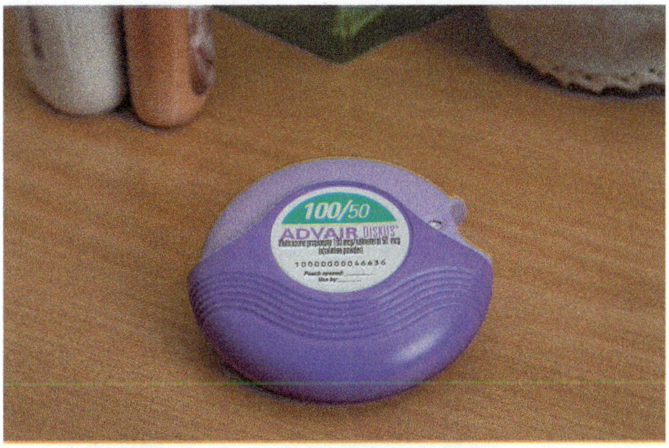

FIGURE 19-10 The Advair® inhaler.

3. Make sure the patient first exhales deeply.
4. Instruct patients to insert the mouthpiece into their mouth, past their teeth, and above their tongue. They should hold the inhaler upright and press down once on the top of the canister to activate the spray as they inhale slowly and deeply. If using a spacer, a whistling sound would indicate that the patient inhaled too rapidly.
5. After patients inhale, instruct them to hold their breath for 5–10 seconds or as long as possible (if 5 seconds is too long), so the medication can be absorbed. This may be difficult with patients who are anxious or severely short of breath, but unless the medication is held in the lungs, it will have minimal or no value. After holding their breath, they may breathe out slowly.
6. If medical control has ordered more than one puff of medication, you should wait 15–30 seconds between administrations.

Your role will involve more coaching than it will actually administering the medication. The proper sequence for administration of a prescribed inhaler is shown in Scan 19-2. Inhalers are described in detail in Scan 19-3. Follow local protocols and consult medical direction, if required, before assisting a patient with an inhaler.

NOTE: *There are many types of drugs used in prescribed inhalers. The so-called rescue inhalers act immediately in an emergency to reverse airway constriction. Fast-acting emergency inhalers include inhalers that contain albuterol (Ventolin ®HFA, Proventil®, Volmax®) or levalbuterol (Xopenex®), and combination inhalers contain albuterol and ipratropium (Combivent®). Other inhalers are not for use in emergencies; rather, they are used daily to help reduce inflammation and prevent attacks. These medications (e.g., beclomethasone, Flovent®, or Advair®–Figure 19-10) should not be used to reverse an acute attack, nor should they be used in the event of breathing difficulty or airway constriction.).*

The Small-Volume Nebulizer

CORE CONCEPT
Use of a prescribed small-volume nebulizer and how to assist a patient with one

The medications used in metered-dose inhalers can also be administered by a small-volume nebulizer (SVN). Nebulizing a medication involves running oxygen or air through a liquid medication. The patient breathes the vapors created. Small-volume nebulizers are used in hospitals and ambulances; they are also prescribed to patients. Patients with chronic respiratory conditions such as asthma, emphysema, or chronic bronchitis may have these devices in their homes.

Unlike the inhaler, which is used in only one breath, a nebulizer produces a continuous flow of aerosolized medication that can be taken in during multiple breaths over several minutes, giving the patient a greater exposure to the medication.

Some states have begun to allow EMTs to carry and administer nebulized medications such as albuterol, whereas other states may allow EMTs to assist with a home nebulizer when allowed by medical direction. Scan 19-4 demonstrates the use of an oxygen-powered nebulizer similar to those carried on ambulances. Follow your local protocols regarding the use of nebulized medications.

SCAN 19-2 Prescribed Inhaler–Patient Assessment and Management

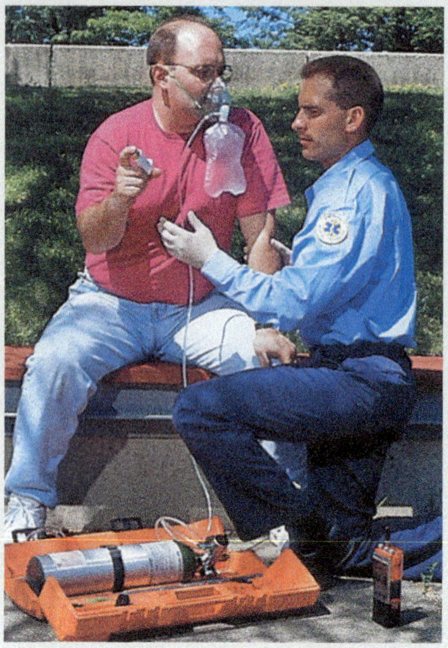

1. The patient has the indications for use of an inhaler: signs and symptoms of breathing difficulty and an inhaler prescribed by a physician.

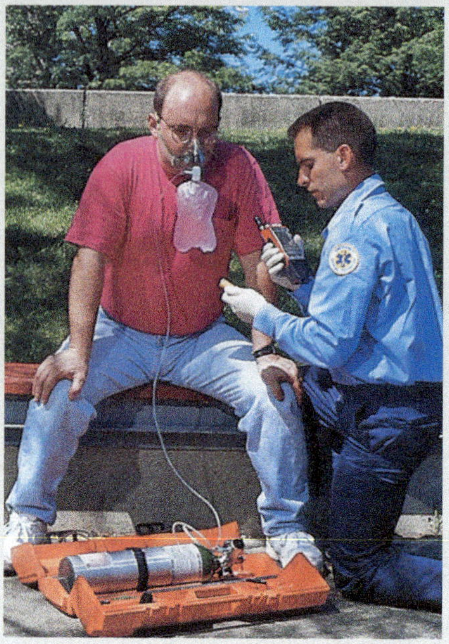

2. Contact medical direction and obtain an order to assist the patient with the prescribed inhaler. (Follow local protocols.)

3. Verify the expiration date of the inhaler.

4. Ensure the five "rights":
   - Right patient
   - Right time
   - Right medication
   - Right dose
   - Right route

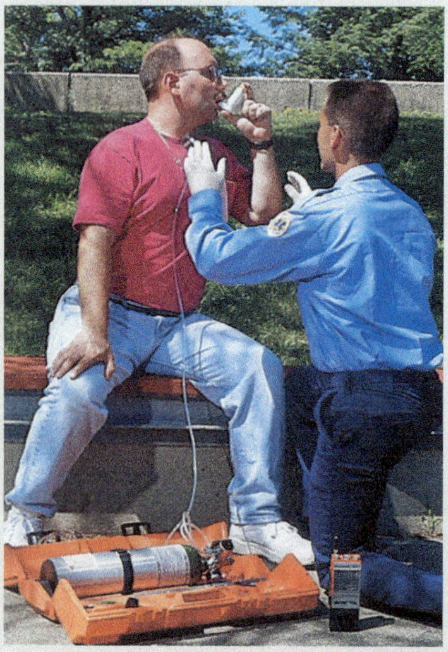

5. Shake and prime the inhaler, make sure the inhaler is at room temperature or warmer, and make sure the patient is alert.
   Coach the patient in the use of an inhaler. Tell the patient to exhale deeply, press the inhaler to activate the spray, inhale, and hold the breath so that medication can be absorbed.

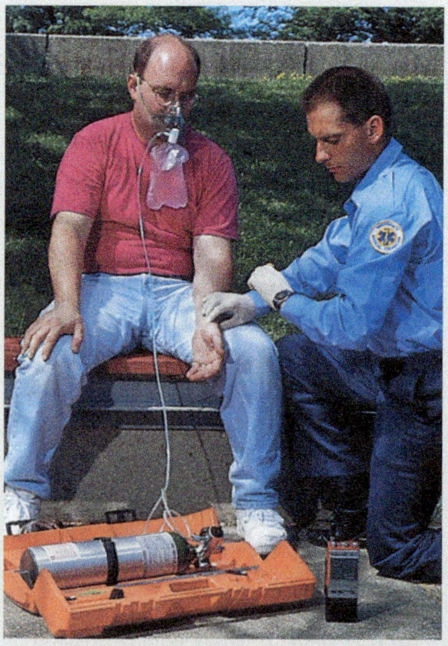

6. After use of the inhaler, reassess the patient: Take vital signs, perform a focused exam, and determine if breathing is adequate.

7. Document the time of administration, the medication given, the dose given, and route of administration (inhaled).

SCAN 19-3 Prescribed Inhaler

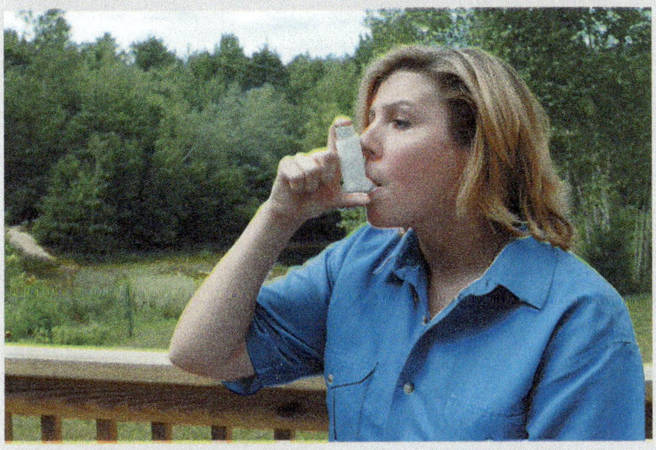

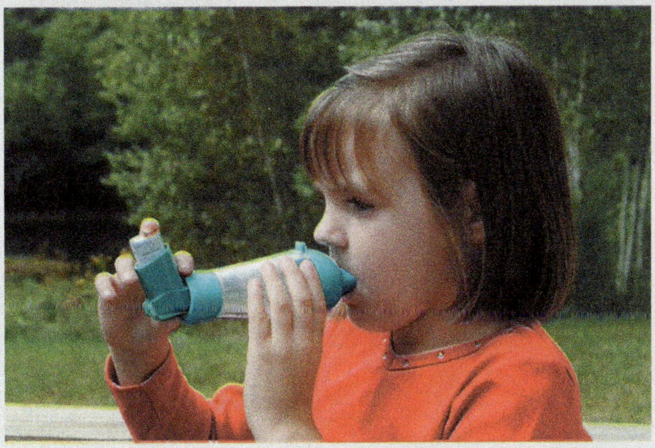

MEDICATION NAME

1. Generic: albuterol, metaproterenol, ipratropium
2. Trade: Proventil®, Ventolin®HFA, Alupent®, Metaprel®, Combivent®

INDICATIONS

Meets all the following criteria:

1. Patient exhibits signs and symptoms of respiratory emergency.
2. Patient has physician-prescribed handheld inhaler.
3. Medical direction gives specific authorization to use.

CONTRAINDICATIONS

1. Patient is unable to use the device (e.g., not alert).
2. Inhaler is not prescribed for the patient.
3. No permission has been given by medical direction.
4. The patient has already taken the maximum prescribed dose prior to the EMT's arrival.

MEDICATION FORM

Handheld metered-dose inhaler

DOSAGE

Number of inhalations based on medical direction's order or physician's order

ADMINISTRATION

1. Obtain an order from medical direction, either on-line or off-line.
2. Check the expiration date of the inhaler.
3. Ensure the right patient, right time, right medication, right dose, and right route, and that the patient is alert enough to use the inhaler.
4. Check whether the patient has already taken any doses.
5. Ensure the inhaler is at room temperature or warmer.
6. Shake the inhaler vigorously several times and prime if necessary.
7. Have the patient exhale deeply.
8. Instruct patients to insert the mouthpiece of the inhaler into their mouth, past their teeth, and above their tongue.
9. Have patients depress the handheld inhaler as they begin to inhale slowly and deeply.
10. Instruct patients to hold their breath for 5-10 seconds, or as long as possible, so the medication can be absorbed.
11. Resume supplemental oxygen therapy if indicated.
12. Wait 15-30 seconds and repeat the second dose if so ordered by medical direction.
13. If patients have a spacer device for use with the inhaler (device for attachment between inhaler and patient to allow for more effective use of medication), it should be used.
14. Document medication administration.

ACTIONS

Beta-agonist bronchodilator dilates bronchioles, reducing airway resistance.

SIDE EFFECTS

1. Increased pulse rate
2. Tremors
3. Nervousness

REASSESSMENT STRATEGIES

1. Gather vital signs.
2. Perform a focused reassessment of the chest and respiratory function.
3. Observe for deterioration of the patient; if breathing becomes inadequate, provide artificial respirations.

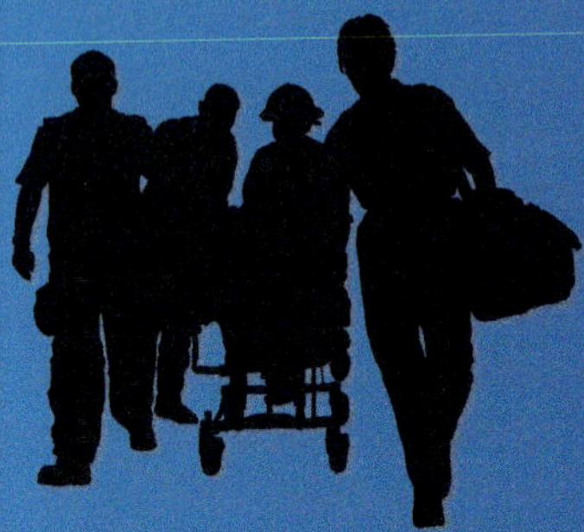

Think Like an EMT

Administering a Prescribed Inhaler

As an EMT, you may be allowed to assist a patient in using a prescribed inhaler. Certain inhalers deliver a medication that relaxes narrowed airways and provides tremendous benefit to the patient when they are used properly.

For each of the following situations, decide whether you should assist the patient with the inhaler.

1. You are called to a 14-year-old patient who complains of difficulty breathing. He tells you he has a history of asthma. The patient's pulse is 104, strong and regular; respirations 28 with audible wheezes; blood pressure 130/84; skin warm and dry. The patient's parents are present. The inhaler is prescribed to the patient.
2. You are called to a 67-year-old patient who complains of difficulty breathing. The patient tells you she has a history of breathing problems but does not know specifically which ones. Her vital signs are pulse 122, strong and regular; respirations 28 with audible wheezes; blood pressure 104/64; skin cool and dry. The patient's daughter presents an inhaler, saying, "This is mine, but it's what I use when I'm wheezing."
3. You are called to a 24-year-old female who was exercising when she developed difficulty breathing. She has a history of asthma. You find her looking tired and weak. Her vital signs are pulse 142, respirations 42 and shallow, blood pressure 96/56, skin cool and moist. You do not hear any wheezes. A friend ran and got the patient's inhaler from her car.

Small Volume Nebulizer (SVN) Medications

There are typically three types of medications administered prehospitally through small-volume nebulizers. They are:

- Albuterol: Albuterol is a medication that dilates the bronchial passageways by engaging beta receptors associated with the sympathetic nervous system. It is relatively fast-acting and is generally the first line of therapy in a bronchoconstricted patient.
- Ipratropium bromide: Ipratropium bromide is a bronchodilator that accomplishes its goal by blocking bronchoconstriction associated with the parasympathetic nervous system. It is an anticholinergic medication. Ipratropium has a slower onset compared with albuterol, and also lasts longer.
- DuoNeb™: DuoNeb™ is a formulation that combines both albuterol and ipratropium bromide. It therefore provides bronchodilation through beta stimulation and by blocking parasympathetic bronchoconstriction. This mix of medication is often used as a first-line agent to treat bronchoconstriction.

The side effects and precautions with nebulized medications are the same as those noted in Scan 19-3 for prescribed inhalers. Patients may experience an increased pulse rate, tremors, nervousness, or a "jittery" feeling. Patients who are not breathing adequately will not benefit from a nebulizer since they are not breathing deeply enough to get the medication into their lungs.

Local protocol will determine the dose, rate, and interval of medications administered through a small-volume nebulizer.

SCAN 19-4 Small-Volume Nebulizer (SVN)–Patient Assessment and Management

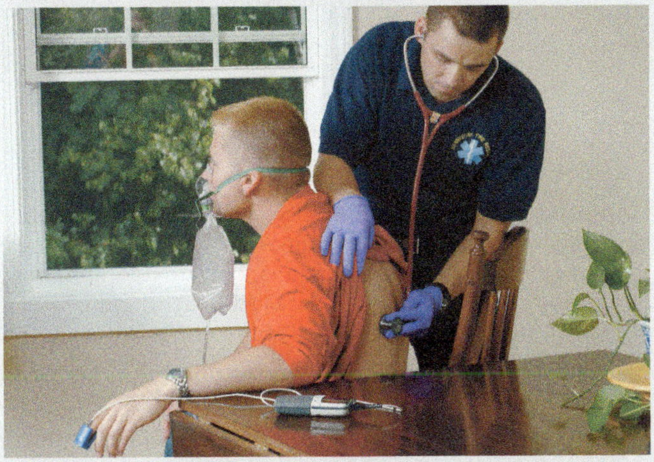

1. Identify the patient as a candidate for nebulized medication per protocol (e.g., history of asthma with respiratory distress). Administer oxygen and assess vital signs. Be sure the patient is not allergic to the medication.

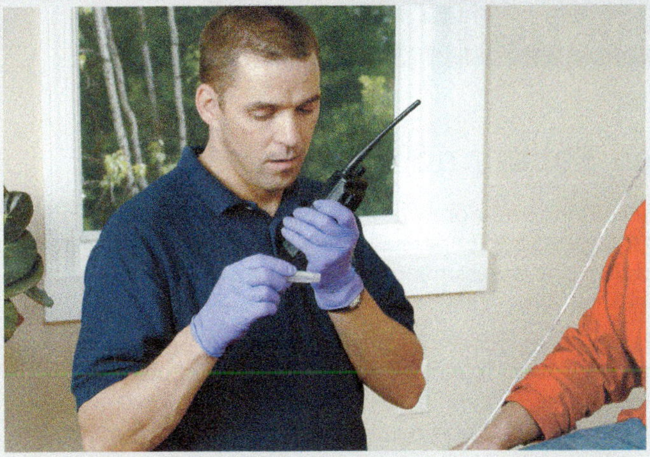

2. Obtain permission from medical direction to administer or assist with the medication.

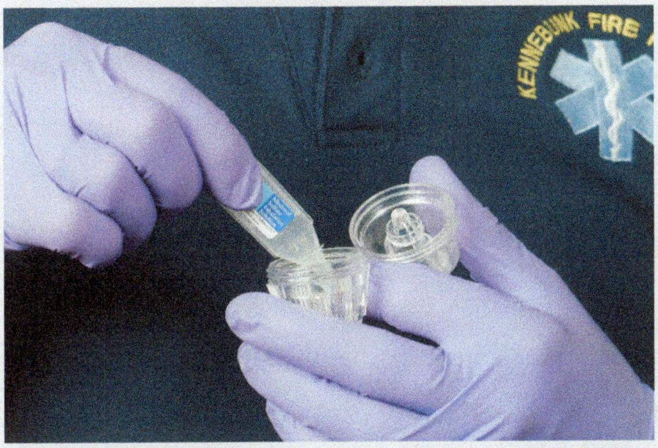

3. Verify the expiration date of the medication. Ensure the five rights (right patient, right time, right medication, right dose, right route). Prepare the nebulizer. Put the liquid medication in the chamber. Attach the oxygen tubing and set the oxygen flow for 6–8 liters per minute (or according to manufacturer's recommendations).

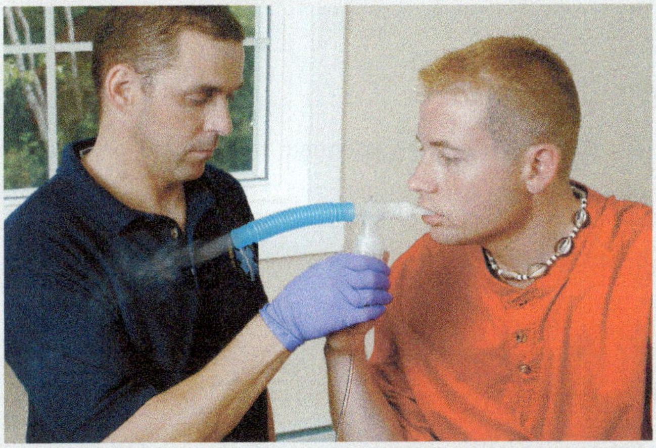

4. Have the patient seal the lips around the mouthpiece and breathe deeply and then hold the breath for 2–3 seconds, if possible. Continue until the medication is gone from the chamber.

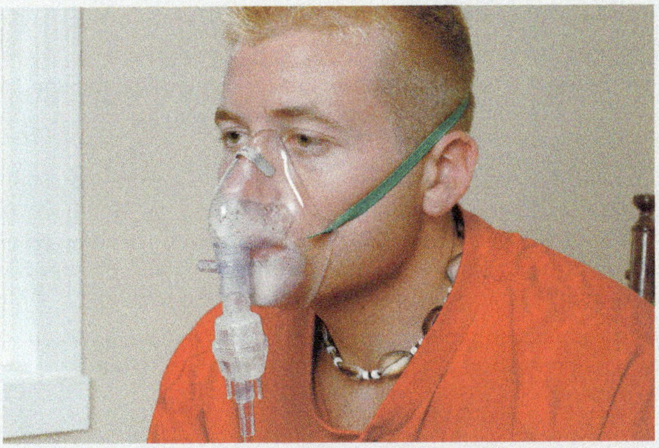

5. Or use an alternative device—a mask delivers the medication.

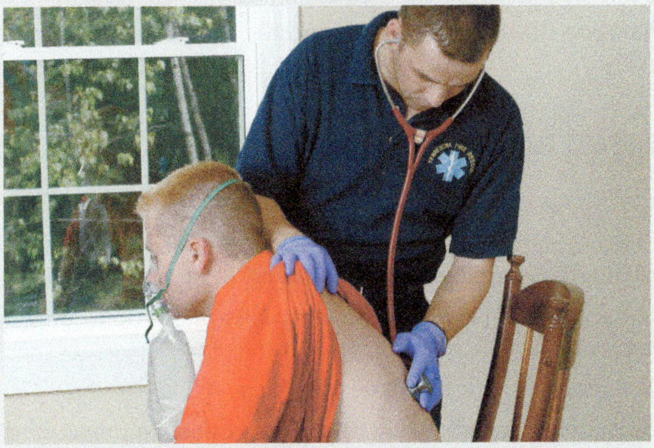

6. After use of the nebulizer, reassess the patient's level of distress and vital signs. Additional doses may be authorized by medical direction if the patient continues to be in distress and the patient is not having adverse effects from the medication.

7. Document the time of administration, the medication given, the dose given, and route of administration (inhaled) for each dose given.

Chapter Review

Key Facts and Concepts

- Respiratory emergencies are common complaints for EMTs. It is important to understand the anatomy, physiology, pathophysiology, assessment, and care for patients experiencing these emergencies.
- Patients with respiratory complaints (which are closely related to cardiac complaints) may exhibit inadequate breathing. Rapid respirations indicate serious conditions, including hypoxia, cardiac and respiratory problems, and shock.
- Very slow and shallow respirations are often the endpoint of a serious condition and are a precursor to death.
- The history usually provides significant information about the patient's condition. In addition to determining a pertinent past history and medications, determine the patient's signs and symptoms with a detailed description including OPQRST and events leading up to the episode.
- Important physical examination points include checking the patient's work of breathing, inspecting accessory muscle use, gathering pulse oximetry readings, assuring adequate and equal lung sounds bilaterally, examining for excess fluid (lungs, ankles, and abdomen), and gathering vital signs.
- Several medications are available that may help correct a patient's difficulty in breathing.

Key Decisions

- Is the patient's breathing adequate, inadequate, or absent?
- What are the appropriate oxygenation or ventilation therapies?
- Should I assist a patient with or administer any medications?
- Do I have protocols and medications that may help this patient?
- Does the patient have a presentation and condition that may fit these protocols?
- Are there any contraindications or risks to using medications in my protocols?

Chapter Glossary

bronchoconstriction constriction, or blockage, of the bronchi that lead from the trachea to the lungs.

continuous positive airway pressure (CPAP) a form of noninvasive positive pressure ventilation (NPPV) consisting of a mask and a means of blowing oxygen or air into the mask to prevent airway collapse or to help alleviate difficulty breathing.

exhalation (EX-huh-LAY-shun) another term for expiration.

expiration (EK-spuh-RAY-shun) a passive process in which the intercostal (rib) muscles and the diaphragm relax, causing the chest cavity to decrease in size and force air from the lungs.

inhalation (IN-huh-LAY-shun) another term for inspiration.

inspiration (IN-spuh-RAY-shun) an active process in which the intercostal (rib) muscles and the diaphragm contract, expanding the size of the chest cavity and causing air to flow into the lungs.

Preparation for Your Examination and Practice

Short Answer

1. What would you expect a patient's respiratory rate to do when the patient gets hypoxic? Why?
2. What would you expect a patient's pulse rate to do when the patient gets hypoxic? Why?
3. List the signs of inadequate breathing.
4. Would you expect to assist with the patient's prescribed inhaler when the patient is experiencing heart failure? Why or why not?
5. List some differences between adult and infant/child respiratory systems.
6. List the signs and symptoms of breathing difficulty.

Thinking and Linking

Think back to the chapters Lifting and Moving Patients, Airway Management, *and* Respiration and Artificial Ventilation, *and link information from those chapters with information from this chapter as you consider the patients listed.*

Assume that each patient is on the second floor of the house and that your wheeled stretcher will not go beyond the front door. For each, decide in which position and via which device you would transport the patient down a flight of stairs. You will consider both the patient's comfort and clinical needs in the decision.

Once you choose the transportation device, explain how you will also safely transport a "D" cylinder of oxygen down the stairs with the patient.

1. A 15-year-old patient having an asthma attack
2. A 77-year-old man in minor distress who reports he has a slight fever and believes his phlegm has changed color
3. A 44-year-old woman who overdosed on sleeping pills and is not breathing
4. An 82-year-old woman who is barely responsive, appears sleepy, and has slow, shallow breaths
5. A 69-year-old man with difficulty breathing and severely swollen ankles who has to sleep propped up by two pillows, and whose wife states he has been diagnosed with heart failure

Critical Thinking Exercises

Being able to determine whether breathing is not adequate is a critical skill. For each of the following patients, state whether the patient's breathing seems adequate or inadequate—and explain your reasoning.

1. A 45-year-old male patient experiences severe difficulty in breathing. His respirations are 36 per minute and very shallow. He has minimal chest expansion and can barely speak.
2. A 65-year-old female tells you that she has trouble breathing. Her respirations are 20 per minute and slightly labored. Her respirations are regular, and there appears to be good chest expansion.
3. A 3-year-old patient recently had a respiratory infection. Her parents called because she is having difficulty breathing. You observe retractions of the muscles between the ribs and above the collarbones, as well as nasal flaring. The child seems drowsy. Respirations are 40 per minute.

Pathophysiology to Practice

The following questions are designed to assist you in gathering relevant clinical information and making accurate decisions in the field.

1. Is it possible for a patient to have fluid in the lungs without having swollen ankles? Why or why not?
2. Would you expect a longer inspiratory cycle or expiratory cycle in an asthma patient? Explain your answer.
3. Can a patient experience respiratory distress and a pulse oximetry reading of 98 percent? Why or why not?

For each of the following patients, decide which condition is most likely. Although minimal information is presented for each patient, your knowledge of the conditions will guide you to the correct choice and help hone your decision making and intuition in the field.

A. COPD

B. Heart failure

C. Asthma

1. 10-year-old patient
2. 82-year-old patient who recently finds she can't sleep lying down
3. 76-year-old patient who reports difficulty breathing with fever and increased mucus production
4. A patient who has had a prior heart attack with difficulty breathing and who reports gaining five pounds (2.27 kg) in the past 2–3 days
5. A very skinny elderly man who is constantly on a nasal cannula at 2 liters per minute at home
6. A 35-year-old man who has difficulty breathing while playing racquetball

Street Scenes

Your pager is activated, and the only information the dispatcher provides is "A female patient with difficulty breathing." The dispatcher also advises you that the ALS response unit is unavailable. On arrival, you find Mrs. Carmela Bartolone in a lawn chair with her husband and neighbor standing next to her, trying to get her to slow her breathing. You ask some quick medical questions and realize that the neighbor saw what happened, the husband has the medical history, and the patient can't talk in full sentences because of severe dyspnea.

Street Scene Questions

1. **What is the first thing you should do for this patient?**
2. **What questions should you ask the husband? The neighbor?**

After you perform a primary assessment, you decide to get patient information from the husband. He states that Mrs. Bartolone has emphysema from many years of smoking two packs of cigarettes a day. He says this same type of attack happened once before, about six months ago. At that time, she was taken to the hospital and needed to be intubated and placed on a ventilator. She is on a number of medications, which he needs to get from inside the house. He reports no known allergies or other medical history.

From what you can gather, Carmela Bartolone spends many of her days housebound on a home oxygen unit. On this particular spring day, she felt that she should work in her flower garden. As she started to pull weeds, she failed to realize how much her rate of breathing was picking up. She soon found herself unable to catch her breath, and was unable to get back to the house. The neighbor who saw Carmela's breathing problem asked if she needed anything. Carmela's response was "Get help!"

Street Scene Questions

3. What is the significance of the medical history provided by the husband?
4. How much oxygen should the patient receive?

The fact that Mrs. Bartolone had to be put on a ventilator 6 months ago makes you realize that this patient is at risk of deteriorating very quickly. As you evaluate her breathing again, you note her respiration rate is still rapid. Your partner counts it at 36. You notice the patient's lips are bluish, her nostrils are flaring, and she is pushing herself up in the chair to make it easier to breathe. Your partner informs you that the patient is using the muscles of the chest and stomach to help her breathe. Mrs. Bartolone is becoming less restless because she is getting drowsy, a sign that action is needed. Your partner recommends that you assist ventilations with a bag-valve mask, and you concur. As you start to hook up the oxygen reservoir, the husband returns with Carmela's inhalers and tells you she gets only 2 liters per minute on her home unit. He also tells you that the doctor stressed she should not get more than that.

Street Scene Questions

5. Is the patient a good candidate for use of an inhaler?
6. Should this patient be considered a high priority, with lights and siren, for transport to the hospital?

You and your partner agree that this patient needs ventilations assisted with high-concentration oxygen and transport without delay. Her normal 2 liters per minute of oxygen are not enough to oxygenate her in this condition. You transport the patient while assisting ventilations. You would like to help her use her inhaler, but your protocol requires the patient to be alert. (She is drowsy.) In addition, you know you are doing the patient a lot of good by ventilating her with high-concentration oxygen.

While en route, your partner notifies the hospital by radio of the patient's condition, treatment being provided, and an ETA of ten minutes. You are able to ventilate the patient well by yourself, but that also means you are unable to get repeat vital signs. Keeping your priorities in mind, you continue ventilating Mrs. Bartolone and estimate her pulse rate by checking it quickly and frequently between ventilations. The patient seems more alert as you arrive at the emergency department. There you provide a prehospital care report to the waiting physician, which includes the patient history you obtained from the husband. As you start to leave the patient area, the doctor thanks you for being aggressive in assisting ventilations.

Cardiac Emergencies

20

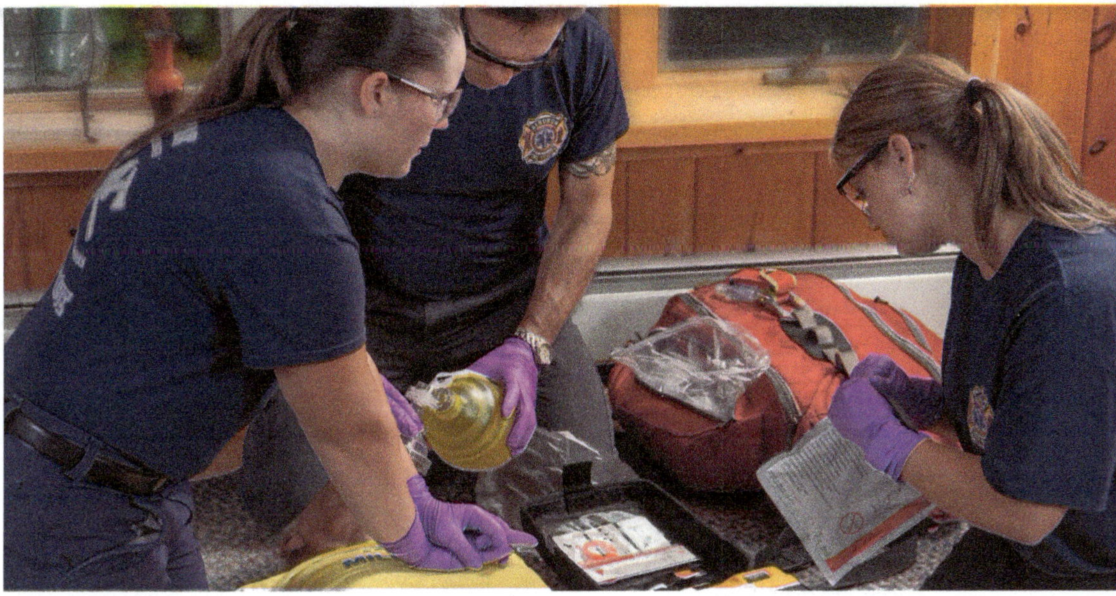

Related Chapters

The following chapters provide additional information related to topics discussed in this chapter:

3 Lifting and Moving Patients
6 Anatomy and Physiology
10 Respiration and Artificial Ventilation
12 Primary Assessment
13 Vital Signs and Monitoring Devices
15 Secondary Assessment
22 Diabetic Emergencies and Altered Mental Status
26 Abdominal Emergencies
Appendix A Basic Cardiac Life Support Review

Standard

Medicine (Cardiovascular)

Competency

Applies fundamental knowledge to provide basic emergency care and transportation based on assessment findings for an acutely ill patient.

Core Concepts

- Aspects of acute coronary syndrome (ACS)
- Conditions that may lead to a cardiac emergency

Outcomes

After reading this chapter, you should be able to:

20.1 Explain the anatomy and physiology of the cardiovascular system. (pp. 557–558)

- Describe the flow of blood through the heart's chambers.
- Describe the flow of blood from the heart, to the body, and back to the heart.

20.2 Explain the concept of acute coronary syndrome (ACS). (pp. 558–559)

- Recognize the signs and symptoms of acute coronary syndrome.
- Describe the concept of cardiac compromise.

20.3 Outline management when presented with a portrayal of a patient presenting with signs and symptoms of acute coronary syndrome. (pp. 559–569)

- Evaluate the patient's signs and symptoms against those for ACS.
- Describe the role of positioning for a patient with ACS.
- Describe the practice for administering oxygen to a patient with suspected ACS.
- Describe the pharmacology of medications that EMTs can administer to patients with suspected ACS.
- Describe the EMT's responsibilities with respect to administering aspirin to a patient with suspected ACS.
- Describe the EMT's responsibilities with respect to administering nitroglycerin to a patient with suspected ACS.
- Identify criteria for immediate transport of a patient with ACS signs and symptoms.
- Explain the teamwork required to carry out interventions while transporting an ACS patient to the hospital.
- Explain the advantage of prehospital 12-lead electrocardiograms (ECGs).

20.4 Illustrate how the underlying pathophysiology of the various causes of cardiac conditions poses threats to the patient. (pp. 570–577)

- Describe the relationship between coronary artery disease, angina pectoris, and acute myocardial infarction (AMI).
- Describe the concept of a dysrhythmia.
- Relate the pathophysiology of heart failure to its presenting signs and symptoms.
- Describe the concept of an aneurysm.
- Identify conditions that interfere with the mechanical work of the heart.

Key Terms

acute coronary syndrome (ACS), *558*

acute myocardial infarction (AMI), *572*

aneurysm, *576*

angina pectoris, *570*

bradycardia, *559*

cardiac compromise, *558*

cardiovascular system, *557*

coronary artery disease (CAD), *570*

dyspnea, *559*

dysrhythmia, *572*

embolism, *572*

heart failure (HF); also called *congestive heart failure (CHF)*, *574*

nitroglycerin, *570*

occlusion, *572*

pedal edema, *574*

pulmonary edema, *575*

tachycardia, *559*

thrombus, *572*

Cardiovascular disease kills more than half a million people in the United States each year. It is, in fact, the leading cause of death. In the coming year, it is projected that roughly 700,000 people will have a heart attack and about 15% of those people will die from the event. The survivors will join the ranks of the more than 85 million people living in the United States with the effects of cardiovascular disease.

As you can imagine, EMS frequently encounters those 85 million patients with cardiovascular disease. Whether it be at the start of symptoms of their first heart attack, or when living with a failing heart is just too difficult, or even as the patients collapse in cardiac arrest, EMS plays a critical role. Patients with cardiovascular disease pose a wide range of challenges in the prehospital world and present with emergent situations that range from relatively simple to utterly critical. As an EMT, you will serve as the entry point into the health care system for a great many of these patients, so you must be prepared to recognize and treat these everyday challenges.

This chapter will begin the discussion on the assessment and treatment of cardiovascular disease. The chapter titled *Resuscitation* will continue with the very specific topic of resuscitation. Before we start, it may be appropriate to review anatomy, physiology, and pathophysiology of the cardiovascular system in *Anatomy and Physiology* and *Principles of Pathophysiology*.

Cardiac Anatomy and Physiology

The ***cardiovascular system*** is made up of the heart, the blood vessels, and blood. The system is tasked with perfusing the cells of the body. It carries out this task continually, without pause, and the body relies upon the constant supply of oxygenated blood to fuel metabolism and to power literally every function from digestion to conscious thought. In the chapter *Anatomy and Physiology*, key cardiovascular structures and functions were outlined, including:

cardiovascular system the heart and the blood vessels.

- Composition of the blood (red and white blood cells, platelets, and plasma)
- Flow of blood through the chambers of the heart (the atria and ventricles)
- Flow of blood through the arteries, veins, arterioles, venules, and capillaries, and the names and positions of major blood vessels
- Circulation of blood between the heart and the lungs, and between the heart and the rest of the body.

It is important to recall these concepts and functions as we begin to explore how the cardiovascular system can be disrupted.

The key central component of the cardiovascular system is the heart. Fundamentally, the heart is a very simple organ tasked with only one job: to pump blood. But the manner in which it accomplishes this task is quite complex. As described in *Principles of Pathophysiology*, the heart combines the generation and distribution of its own electrical charge with the mechanical response by its cells to create the rhythmic and unceasing pumping action that delivers blood to the body. In the cardiac conduction system, an electrical charge is created, and this energy is passed from cell to cell along a specialized pathway. As energy

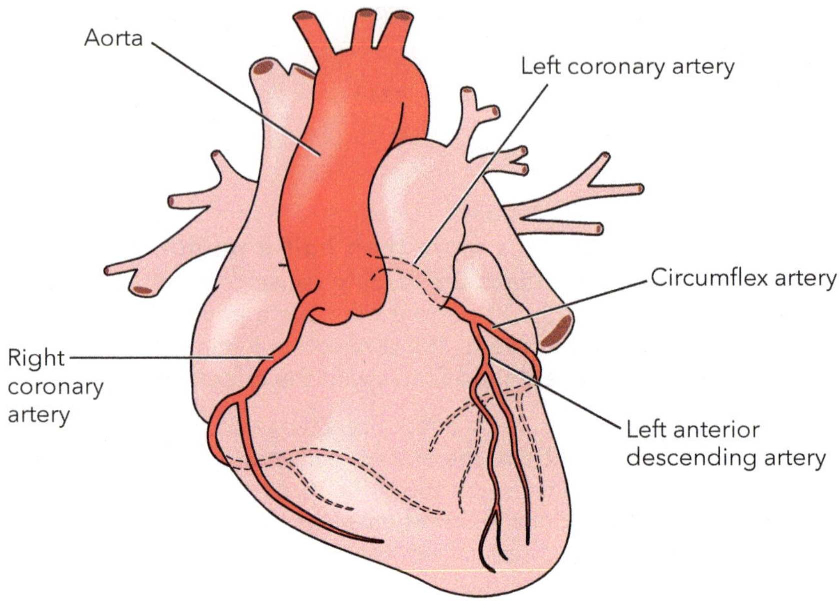

FIGURE 20-1 The coronary arteries. *(Blamb/Shutterstock.)*

is distributed along this pathway, it spreads to all the cells of the heart and, if conditions are correct, this energy stimulates a mechanical contraction of those cells that creates the mechanical squeeze used to push blood. This cycle repeats itself tens of thousands of times each day, and perfusion is achieved.

Remember that the heart is a muscle, and to perform this nonstop action, it requires a constant supply of oxygen and nutrients. The heart is the first organ perfused by oxygenated blood leaving the heart. It receives its supply of blood via the coronary arteries that branch off the very base of the aorta and spread throughout the heart muscle. (See Figure 20-1.) The heart has no reserve of oxygen, so any interruption in its supply of oxygenated blood results in significant problems. The hard-working cells of the heart rapidly become hypoxic and will quickly die if left without perfusion.

Acute Coronary Syndrome

acute coronary syndrome (ACS)
a blanket term used to represent any symptoms related to lack of oxygen (ischemia) in the heart muscle. Also called *cardiac compromise*.

cardiac compromise
see acute coronary syndrome.

CORE CONCEPT
Aspects of acute coronary syndrome (ACS)

Acute coronary syndrome (ACS), sometimes called ***cardiac compromise***, is a blanket term that refers to any time when the blood supply to the cells of the heart is blocked or disrupted, resulting in symptoms for the patient. This can occur abruptly, as when a clot suddenly develops in a coronary artery, causing a heart attack, or it can occur over time, as when a coronary artery is narrowed due to a buildup of plaque. In both cases, the outcome is the same: Cells of the heart muscle go without the oxygenated blood they desperately need. If the situation is not corrected, those cells will die.

ACS indicates that the cells of the heart are going without adequate oxygenated blood. This hypoxic condition is commonly referred to as *ischemia*. When ischemia occurs, the affected cells do not have enough oxygenated blood to conduct metabolism, and when metabolism fails, the functioning of those cells is impaired. As the hypoxic state worsens, cells become damaged and eventually die. Some body cells, like those of bone and skin, can endure long periods of ischemia, but cells that are constantly working, such as the heart and brain cells, die quickly without an adequate supply of blood. Although dead cells cannot be revived, most damage and ischemic states can be corrected by restoring perfusion. This concept will be a key outcome in treating acute coronary syndrome. But, to treat acute coronary syndrome, we must first recognize it.

Different types of cells respond differently to ischemic conditions like ACS. The first sign of ischemia in brain tissue is the failed function of those cells. Ischemic conditions like stroke are often identified by an inability of the patient to carry out simple functions like movement or speech.

Chest discomfort is a finding that many patients with acute coronary syndrome will experience. As heart cells become ischemic, pain receptors are engaged, causing an uncomfortable feeling. However, the discomfort of ischemic heart cells is not always felt as pain. Some will describe the sensation as "pressure" or "squeezing." They might use words like "discomfort" or "aching." The discomfort is also not limited to the chest. ACS discomfort is occasionally localized or can radiate (the sensation of pain centered in one area but extending to another) to the jaw, neck, either arm, and the upper abdomen (also known as the epigastrium). Some patients do not experience pain at all. Indeed, some patients only report profound generalized weakness as their symptom. ACS without pain is a relatively common finding in older adult, female, and/or diabetic patients.

There are several other findings that are commonly associated with ischemia in the heart. Shortness of breath, otherwise known as ***dyspnea***, is very common. This finding is especially common in older patients and women. Nausea and/or vomiting is also a common finding associated with acute coronary syndrome. Fainting or near fainting, otherwise known as *syncope*, can also be present when heart cells become ischemic. Some patients will simply report vague symptoms such as fatigue or dyspnea on exertion as their primary complaint.

dyspnea (DISP-ne-ah) shortness of breath; labored or difficult breathing.

There are also specific signs you will see in some of these patients, including the sudden onset of sweating and an abnormal pulse or blood pressure. Many patients who have sudden onset of sweating think they are coming down with the flu, but this may result from the denial that is common in these patients. They refuse to acknowledge, at least consciously, that they may be having heart problems. The pulse may be abnormally slow (slower than 60 beats per minute, called ***bradycardia***) or abnormally fast (faster than 100 beats per minute, ***tachycardia***), and can be irregular. Some patients complain of palpitations, which are irregular or rapid heartbeats they feel as a fluttering sensation in the chest. A few patients are hypotensive (systolic blood pressure less than 90), whereas others are hypertensive (systolic greater than 140 or diastolic greater than 90).

bradycardia (bray-di-KAR-de-ah) slow heart rate, usually less than 60 beats per minute.

tachycardia (tak-e-KAR-de-ah) fast heart rate, more than 100 beats per minute.

A patient with ACS is often anxious. In some patients this takes the form of a feeling of impending doom, which the patient may express to you or others. Occasionally, you will see a patient whose anxiety displays itself through irritability and a short temper.

As you can see, recognizing acute coronary syndrome can be complicated. A wide net needs to be cast to capture all the potential patients.

Since the signs and symptoms of an ACS can vary so greatly, it is much safer for the EMT to treat all patients with the pattern of symptoms described above as though they were having a heart problem. In the past, it was common practice to try and suggest that ACS was not occurring by asking patients questions about elements of their history. It was assumed that certain answers would "rule out" the possibility of ACS. While it is true that some historical findings can make ACS a less likely diagnosis, research has clearly shown that it is far safer to assume ACS if any part of the historical pattern matches findings associated with ACS. Some common cardiovascular disorders will be discussed later in this chapter to assist you in recognizing and treating the symptoms associated with such disorders. Definitive diagnosis and care will be provided at the hospital.

Management of Acute Coronary Syndrome

The management of a patient with ACS is detailed in the following text and in Scan 20-1.

Patient Assessment

Acute Coronary Syndrome

After performing your primary assessment, perform a history and physical exam. Explore the chief complaint and the present illness by asking the OPQRST questions. (Inquire about **o**nset, **p**rovocation, **q**uality, **r**adiation, **s**everity, and **t**ime.) Also get a past medical history (allergies, medications the patient may be taking, pertinent past history, last oral intake, and events leading to the present emergency). Then take baseline vital signs.

The following signs and symptoms are often associated with ACS:

- Pain, pressure, or discomfort in the chest, jaw, neck, arms, or upper abdomen
- Difficulty breathing
- Palpitations
- Sudden onset of sweating and nausea or vomiting
- Syncope
- Anxiety (feeling of impending doom, irritability)
- Unusual generalized weakness (especially common in older women)
- Abnormal pulse (rapid, slow, or irregular)
- Abnormal blood pressure

Physical Examination

Although there are few physical findings that point directly to acute coronary syndrome, you should when possible conduct a systems exam and complete a thorough physical evaluation. Certain findings indicate the discomfort common with ACS. These include:

- Grabbing or clutching the center of the chest (also known as Levine's sign)
- Sweating
- Pale or gray skin
- Anxiousness or restlessness associated with a "feeling of impending doom."

Other findings indicate a past medical history of cardiac problems. Although this past history does not necessarily indicate ACS is occurring today, it does increase the likelihood. These findings include:

- Acute pulmonary edema (Note that this can be an acute-onset problem directly linked to ACS.)
- Swollen ankles and feet
- Medic alert jewelry indicating cardiac problems.

12-lead ECG

In many states, EMTs are acquiring 12-lead ECGs to speed the process of recognizing electrocardial findings associated with acute myocardial infarction. Although interpretation of 12-lead ECG is outside the scope of practice for an EMT, the placement of chest leads and acquisition of a printed tracing have been adopted by many states. In addition, the ability of an EMT to electronically transmit an ECG to the destination hospital significantly speeds the diagnostic process and is an excellent example of how teamwork leads to improved outcomes.

Preparing a Patient for an ECG

To acquire a 12-lead ECG, a series of sticky electrodes are placed on the patient's chest. These electrodes are designed to sense electrical activity of the heart and are connected via wire to a cardiac monitor. Electrical activity sensed by the electrodes is measured by the monitor and displayed on the monitor's screen. Most monitors also enable you to print an electronic tracing of the measured electrical activity. This printed or electronically submitted tracing is referred to as a 12-lead electrocardiogram, or ECG.

To obtain an accurate 12-lead ECG, the monitor leads must be placed directly on the chest and should have secure contact with the skin. Clothing and jewelry must be removed from the area of placement and the skin should be gently wiped with a towel or soft cloth to remove sweat and dead skin cells prior to placement of the lead. If the patient has significant chest hair, a safety razor should be used to clear the area where the electrode will be placed. Once the leads have been properly placed, the EMT typically will press a button on the cardiac monitor to begin the analysis and print the tracing. There may also be additional steps to transmit findings to the destination hospital.

NOTE: *The function and use of a 12-lead monitor is specific to the particular monitor defibrillator. Different devices have different steps for acquisition of 12-lead ECG. The discussion here is designed to provide an overview of the process, not to offer specific instructions. Prior to using any cardiac monitor to obtain an ECG, refer to state and local protocols and follow manufacturer's recommendations for specific operating procedures.*

12-lead ECG Placement

To obtain a 12-lead ECG, electrodes must be placed in very specific positions on the patient's body. Accuracy and reliability of the electronic tracing are dependent on proper placement, so care should be taken to achieve optimal placement. It may be reasonable to utilize a schematic or checklist to recall the anatomic location for each lead.

It is important to note that although the 12-lead ECG provides 12 separate "electrical views" of the heart, it is actually obtained by physically applying only 10 ECG leads to the patient. Each lead is specifically labeled to identify the position in which it should placed. Almost all ECG leads are also color coded to identify proper positioning, but there can be some variability in the precise colors used. When in doubt, always default to using the imprinted lead name ("V1", etc.) rather than the lead color to determine proper placement.

After properly preparing the patient, place the ECG leads in the following locations:

Step 1–Place the limb leads.

Most monitors begin the process of obtaining a 12-lead ECG by attaching electrodes to the patient's arms and legs. Classically, the lead identified by a white color is placed on the patient's right arm or shoulder and the lead identified by a black color is placed on the patient's left arm or shoulder. Some systems suggest placing these electrodes on the patient's wrists, but in general, placement higher up the arm will prevent movement and shaking of the extremity from interfering with the ECG analysis. The American Heart Association simply recommends that all limb leads on arms be placed below the joint of the shoulder and limb leads on legs be placed below the inguinal fold (or roughly the joint of the hip). As always, follow local protocols (Figure 20-2).

Once the arm leads have been placed, electrodes will be placed on the legs. Most commonly, a red lead is placed on the patient's left leg. This electrode is commonly placed on the patient's ankle but can also be placed further up the leg, as described above. Most monitors also require placement of a green grounding lead. This lead is placed on the patient's right leg (Figure 20-3).

Step 2–Place the V1 and V2 leads. The leads that are placed on the chest are referred to as "chest leads" and designated V1 through V6. Each of these leads has a specific geographic placement site on the chest. They are typically placed in a specific order, as placement of one relates to placement of the next lead. This sequence typically starts with placement of V1 and V2.

Lead V1 is placed at the level of the 4th intercostal space (the space between the 4th and 5th rib) just to the patient's right of the sternum. The 4th intercostal space can be

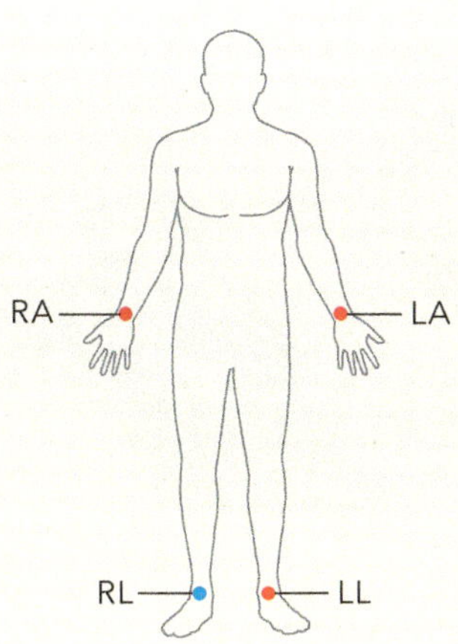

FIGURE 20-2 Placement of arm and leg leads.

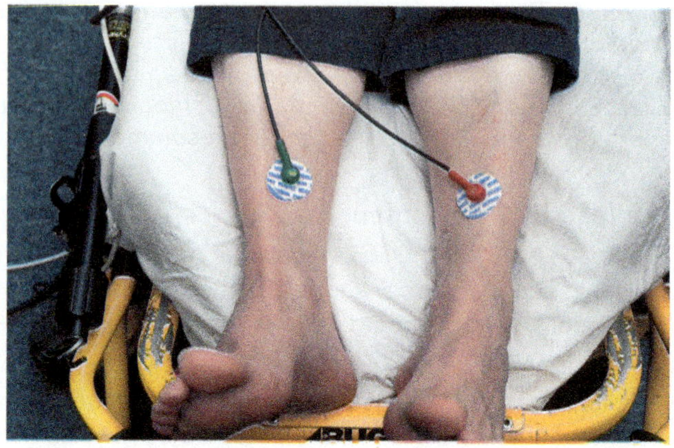

FIGURE 20-3 Placement of leg leads.

found by gently palpating the ribs and counting down from the collar bone (remember that the clavicle covers the 1st intercostal space) or by identifying the horizontal joint in the sternum below the suprasternal notch. This joint is called the angle of Louis and sits adjacent to the 2nd intercostal space. Palpating and visualizing this joint can offer a quick reference on intercostal placement. V1 is first placed at the 4th intercostal space just to the patient's right of the sternum, then V2 can be placed at the same intercostal level just to the patient's left of the sternum.

Step Three–Place V4 and V3. Next you must place lead V4. V4 is placed in the 5th intercostal space at the mid-clavicular line. Once you have placed V2, simply drop down one intercostal space. The midclavicular line can be found by visualizing the patient's clavicle, which extends from the suprasternal notch to the acromion joint of the shoulder. The midclavicular line is the midway point between the suprasternal notch and the acromion joint. In most patients, this line would correspond to an area just lateral to the patient's nipple.

There are often questions about where to place V4 if a patient has large breasts. Although a breast can be moved to place a lead directly on the chest wall, very often this movement causes the lead to be moved out of proper geographic placement. Most expert agree that it is better to simply place a chest lead on top of breast tissue (in proper placement) than to attempt to move the breast.

V4 is then placed in the 5th intercostal space at the midclavicular line. V3 can then be placed halfway between V2 and V4 (Figure 20-4).

Step Four–Place V5 and V6. Once lead V4 has been placed, attaching V5 and V6 is relatively simple. V5 and V6 are also placed in the 5th intercostal space. V5 is placed on the anterior axillary line and V6 is placed on the axillary line. Recall from the chapter *Anatomy and Physiology* that the axillary line is the imaginary line that would divide the body into front and back halves. The anterior axillary line then is the line that would be drawn halfway

FIGURE 20-4 Placement of V4 and V3.

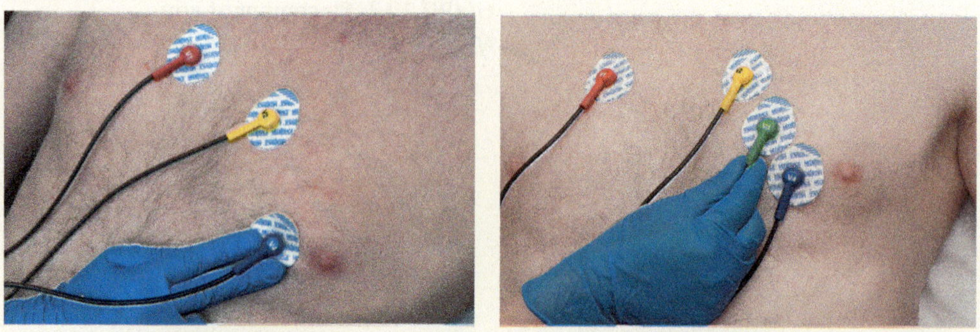

Placement of Lead V4 **Placement of Lead V3**

from the axillary line to the front of the body. It divides the front half in half again. V6 would be attached at the axillary line and V5 would be attached at the anterior axillary line. Some providers find it useful to attach V6 at the easier-to-identify axillary line and then simply attach V5 halfway between V6 and V4 (Figure 20-5). As always, follow local protocol.

Once all the leads have been placed, you will then obtain a 12-lead ECG. This is most commonly completed by turning on the monitor defibrillator and pressing a designated "12-lead" or "Acquire" button. It is helpful to ask the patient to hold still for the few seconds it takes to acquire the ECG. Typically, acquisition is demonstrated by the printing of an ECG tracing or an audible indication that acquisition is complete. Again, these details will be reviewed in a training specific to your monitor defibrillator.

ECG leads are generally left on the patient in the prehospital setting, as serial acquisitions may be indicated.

FIGURE 20-5 Placement of V5 and V6.

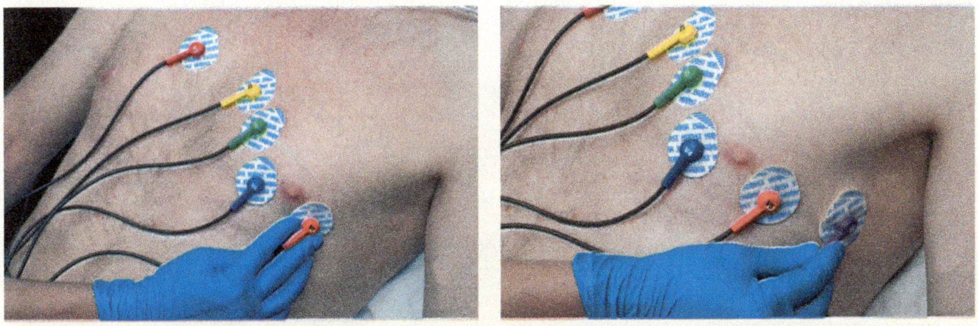

Placement of Lead V5

Placement of Lead V6

SCAN 20-1 Managing Acute Coronary Syndrome

First Take Standard Precautions.

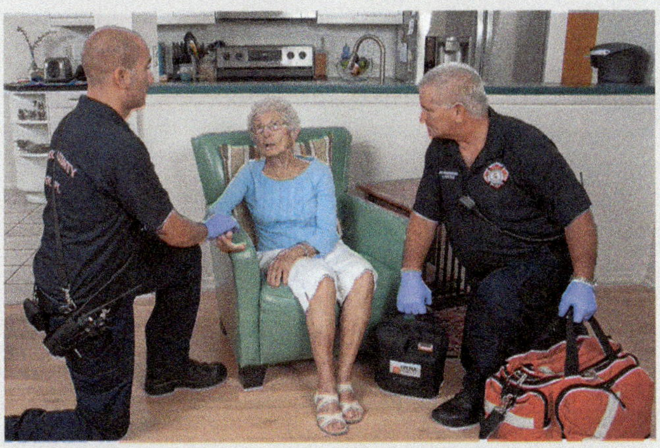

1. Perform the primary assessment.

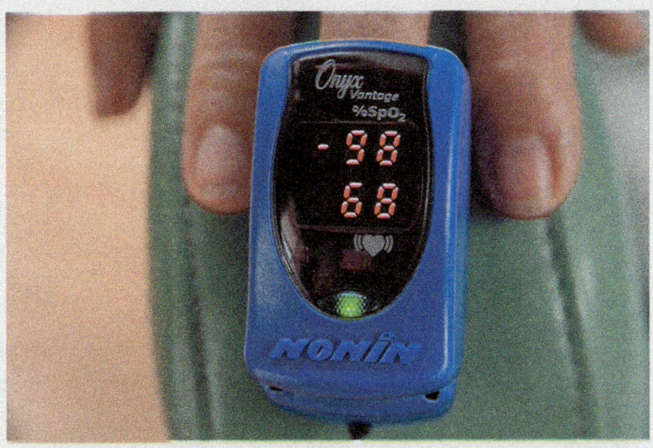

2. Determine oxygen saturation. Provide supplemental oxygen if the patient is hypoxic or shows signs of hypoxia. Oxygen should be considered in acute coronary syndrome patient with dyspnea as well. Adjust to raise the oxygen saturation to at least 94 percent. Perform the history and physical exam for a medical patient. Document the findings.

(continued)

SCAN 20-1 Managing Acute Coronary Syndrome *(continued)*

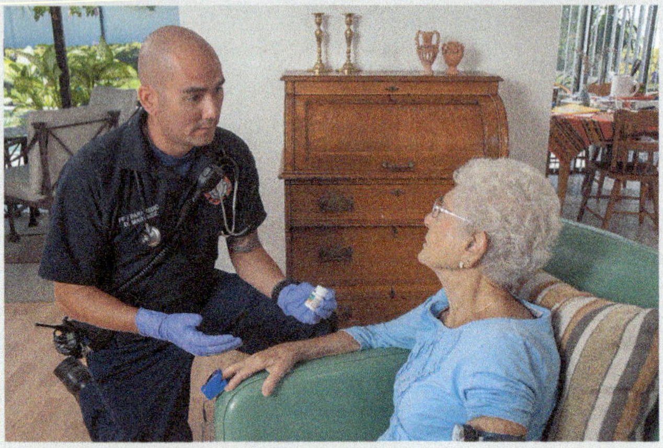

3. Ask if the patient is allergic to aspirin and if the patient has taken any aspirin recently.

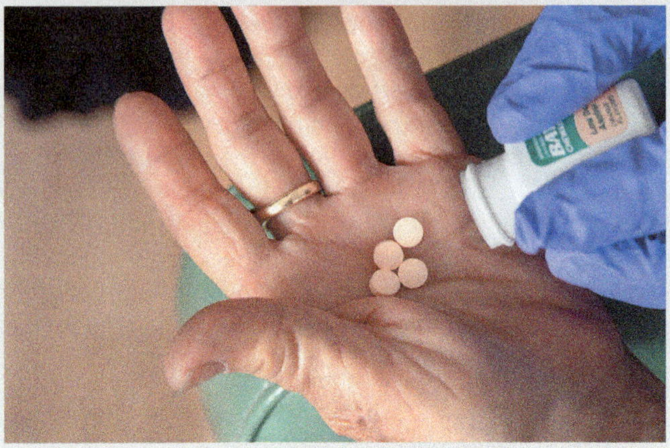

4. Administer chewable aspirin, if appropriate.

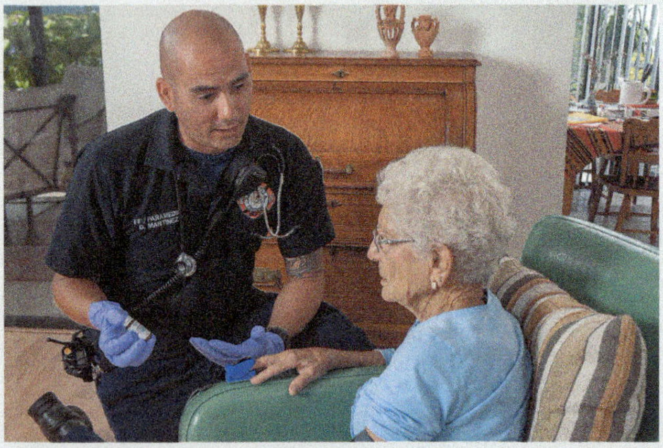

5. If the patient meets nitroglycerin criteria and has prescribed nitroglycerin, ask the patient about the last dose taken.

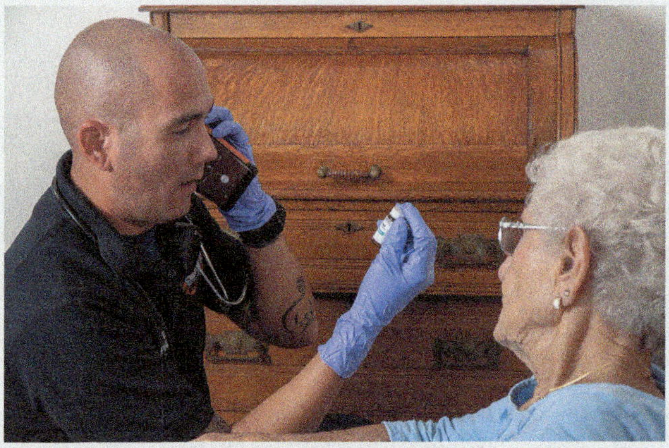

6. Check the expiration date of the medication. Then follow the five rights: right patient, right time, right drug, right dose, and right route. Follow local protocols and consult medical direction before assisting the patient with taking medication.

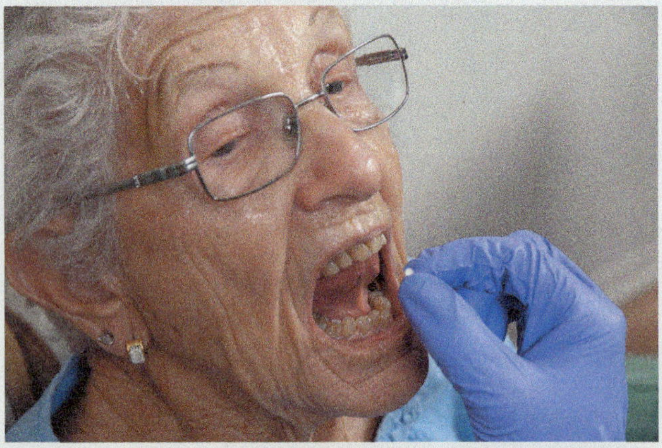

7A. Ask the patient to open the mouth and lift the tongue. Place a nitroglycerin tablet under the tongue, or . . .

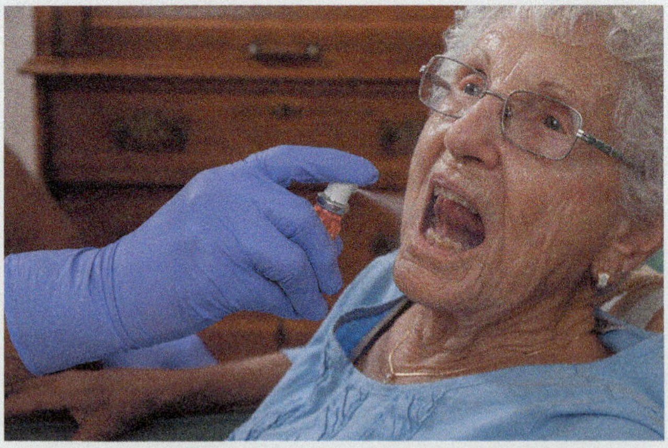

7B. If the nitroglycerin is in spray form, spray the medication under the tongue according to label directions. With either method of delivery, have the patient close the mouth and hold the nitroglycerin under the tongue, where the medication will be absorbed quickly. The patient should *not* swallow until the medication is absorbed.

SCAN 20-1 Managing Acute Coronary Syndrome *(continued)*

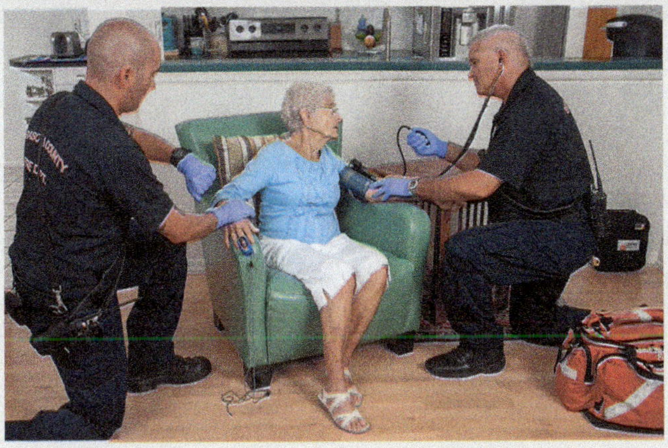

8. Reassess the patient. Document both medication administration and reassessment findings.

Patient Care

Care of the Patient with Acute Coronary Syndrome

Fundamental Principles of Care

When patients present with acute coronary syndrome, a fundamental principle is to assume the worst possible scenario and treat them as though they are having a cardiac event. Excellent care of the ACS patient is achieved through teamwork at all levels. EMTs begin early recognition and fundamental care such as aspirin and nitroglycerin and then continue care by working with advanced providers to deliver the patient to an appropriate facility. It is the combination of efforts at each level and integrated management that offer the patient the best outcome.

Follow these steps for the emergency care of a patient with suspected ACS:

- Place the patient in a position of comfort, typically sitting up. This is especially true of patients with difficulty breathing. Patients who are hypotensive (systolic blood pressure less than 90) will usually feel better lying down. Occasionally, you will see a patient who has both difficulty breathing and hypotension. In this case, it may be very difficult to find a good position. The best way to determine the proper position is to ask the patient what position will relieve the breathing difficulty without causing weakness or light-headedness.
- Determine if oxygen should be administered to the patient. Oxygen should be administered to patients who are hypoxic (saturations less than 94 percent) and those who are in respiratory distress. The goal is to get the patient's oxygen saturation to a minimum of 94 percent.

There has been a dramatic shift in oxygen-administration theory. In the past, everyone with chest pain or discomfort was given oxygen by nonrebreather mask. You may hear people talk about this or even see protocols that still mention high-concentration oxygen. Laboratory and animal studies suggest that administering more oxygen than necessary may lead to the production of certain chemical entities that can be harmful, so current recommendations are to administer only enough oxygen to bring the patient's oxygen saturation level up to 94 percent. See Table 10-1 Respiratory Conditions with Appropriate Interventions in the chapter called *Respiration and Artificial Ventilation* and consider the following as you decide on oxygen therapy for your ACS patient:

- Patients who are in respiratory failure, who are experiencing agonal breaths, and who are apneic will receive high-concentration oxygen via ventilations with a BVM or pocket face mask.
- Patients who have low oxygen saturations or otherwise appear critical should receive high-concentration oxygen with the intent to bring the oxygen saturation

above 94 percent and relieve discomfort and anxiety. This may be done by a mask or nasal cannula.

- Patients who complain of chest pain or discomfort but who are alert and otherwise not in significant distress and who have an oxygen saturation of at least 94 percent should not receive oxygen. These patients should be monitored carefully in the event distress develops or oxygen saturation levels decline. If either occurs, administer oxygen as described above.
- Transport immediately if the patient has any one of the following:
  - No history of cardiac problems
  - History of cardiac problems but does not have nitroglycerin
  - Systolic blood pressure below 90–100 (Use the minimum systolic number in this range that is designated by your EMS system.)
- If you are trained, equipped, and authorized to do so, obtain a 12-lead electrocardiogram. Follow local protocol with regard to whether you should transmit it to a hospital or physician for interpretation. Determining whether the patient has an ST-elevation myocardial infarction (STEMI) may be extremely important in deciding the most beneficial kind of treatment for the patient and where you will transport the patient.

  In areas with more than one hospital, there may be one or two facilities with special treatment available for cardiac patients. Almost all hospitals can administer an intravenous drug to dissolve the clot that is causing insufficient oxygenation of the heart. A more effective way to unclog the coronary artery is to insert a catheter with a balloon at the tip into the arterial system and thread it into the coronary arteries. When the balloon reaches the narrow section of the artery, it is inflated, compressing the obstructive material against the side of the blood vessel and opening up circulation to the heart muscle again. This is called *percutaneous coronary intervention (PCI)* and is often better than the fibrinolytic or "clot buster drug" approach when it is done early (within a few hours of onset of symptoms). Only hospitals with special facilities and available staff can do this, however. If your EMS system has the ability to transport patients to a hospital with this capability, there will be a local protocol that you should follow describing when, where, and how you should transport patients with certain signs and symptoms.
- If you are allowed to do so by your local protocol, administer up to 325 mg of aspirin by mouth (Scan 20-2). Aspirin given for acute coronary syndrome should be chewed, not swallowed.

  Do NOT administer aspirin if:
  - The patient is at risk for aspiration or cannot swallow.
  - The patient has taken a full dose (325 mg) of aspirin within the last 6 hours.
  - The patient has an aspirin allergy.
  - The patient has a history of recent gastrointestinal bleeding. Contact medical control for guidance in these situations.
  - The patient is already taking a prescribed blood thinner. (Some systems may allow aspirin administration with some blood thinners. Follow local protocol and, if in doubt, contact medical control prior to administration of aspirin.)
- If you are allowed by local protocol, assist the patient in taking nitroglycerin (Scan 20-3) if *all* of the following conditions are met:
  - Patient complains of chest discomfort or pain. (Consider also discomfort in other areas commonly associated with ACS. If in doubt, contact medical control.)
  - Patient has a history of cardiac problems.
  - Patient's physician has prescribed nitroglycerin (NTG).
  - Patient has the nitroglycerin at hand.
  - Systolic blood pressure meets your protocol criteria (usually greater than 90–100 systolic).

- Patient has not taken Viagra®, Levitra®, Cialis®, or a similar drug for erectile dysfunction within 48–72 hours. (Use the time within this range that is designated by your EMS system.)
- Medical direction authorizes administration of the medication.

• After giving one dose of the nitroglycerin, give a repeat dose in 5 minutes if *all* of the following conditions are met:
  - Patient experiences no relief or only partial relief.
  - Systolic blood pressure remains greater than 90–100 systolic.
  - Medical direction authorizes another dose of the medication.

• Administer a maximum of three doses of nitroglycerin, reassessing vital signs and chest pain after each dose. If the blood pressure falls below 90–100 systolic, treat the patient for shock (hypoperfusion). Transport promptly.

SCAN 20-2 Aspirin

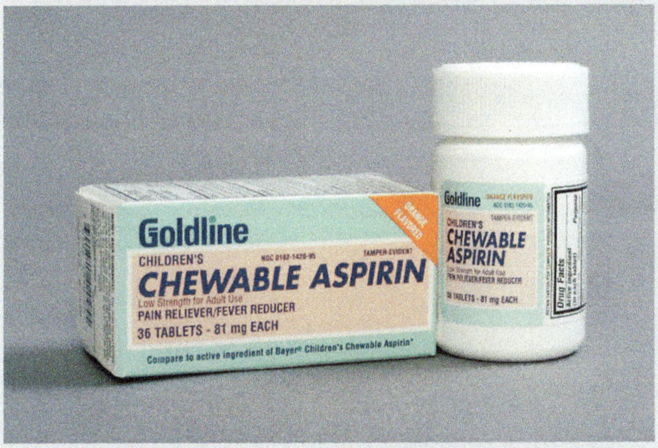

MEDICATION NAME

1. Generic: aspirin
2. Trade: many available

INDICATIONS

All of the following conditions must be met:

1. Patient complains of chest discomfort or pain or discomfort in an area commonly associated with acute coronary syndrome.
2. Patient is not allergic to aspirin.
3. Patient is not already taking any medications to prevent clotting.
4. Patient has no other contraindications to aspirin.
5. Patient is able to swallow without endangering the airway.
6. Medical direction authorizes administration of the medication.

CONTRAINDICATIONS

1. Patient is unable to swallow without endangering the airway.
2. Patient is allergic or sensitive to aspirin.
3. Patient has gastrointestinal ulcer or recent bleeding.
4. Patient has a known bleeding disorder.
5. Medical direction may decide if the benefit of giving aspirin to a patient who has one of the following conditions outweighs the risk:
   a. Already taking a blood-thinning medication to prevent clotting (including aspirin)
   b. Pregnancy
   c. Recent surgery

MEDICATION FORM

Tablet; many EMS systems use baby aspirin, usually supplied as 81 mg chewable tablets.

DOSAGE

162–325 mg (two to four 81 mg tablets of chewable baby aspirin). Aspirin does not usually need to be administered more than once in the early treatment of cardiac problems.

ADMINISTRATION

1. Gather a history and perform a physical exam appropriate for a cardiac patient.
2. Contact medical direction if no standing orders.
3. Check the expiration date. Ensure the right medication, right patient, right time, right dose, and right route.
4. Ensure the patient is alert.
5. Ask the patient to chew the tablets.
6. Document medication administration, route, and time.
7. Perform reassessment.

ACTIONS

1. Prevents blood from clotting as quickly, leading to increased survival after myocardial infarction.
2. When administered to cardiac patients, aspirin is not being used to relieve pain.

(continued)

SCAN 20-2 Aspirin *(continued)*

SIDE EFFECTS

1. Nausea
2. Vomiting
3. Heartburn
4. If patient is allergic, bronchospasm and wheezing
5. Bleeding

REASSESSMENT STRATEGIES

1. Perform reassessment.
2. Evaluate the patient for new onset of difficulty breathing from bronchospasm.
3. Any bleeding resulting from the aspirin is very unlikely to occur before the patient arrives at a hospital.
4. Record the assessments.

NOTE: *Transportation of a patient with a heart condition must be carried out in a thoughtful, calm, and careful fashion. A rough ride with sudden starts, stops, and turns, and siren wailing, is likely to increase the patient's fear and apprehension, placing additional stress on the heart. Speed is important, as the patient must reach the hospital quickly. However, the judicious use of siren or horn must be balanced against the possibility of worsening the patient's condition.*

SCAN 20-3 Nitroglycerin

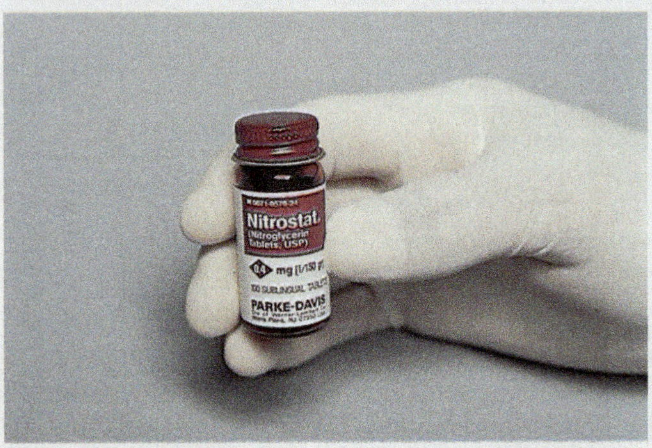

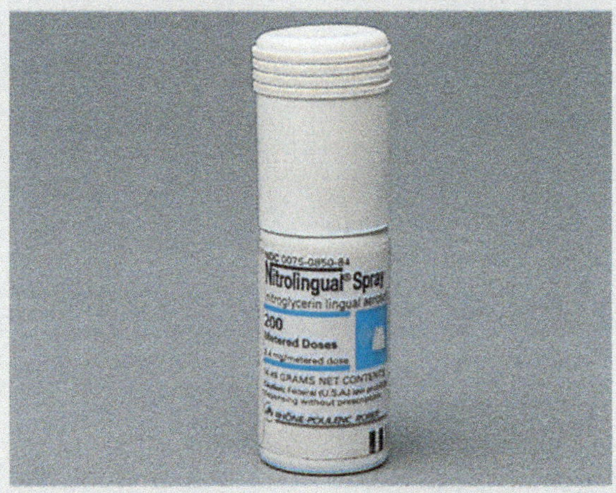

MEDICATION NAME

1. Generic: nitroglycerin
2. Trade: Nitrostat®, Nitrolingual®

INDICATIONS

All the following conditions must be met:

1. Patient complains of chest discomfort or pain or discomfort in an area commonly associated with acute coronary syndrome.
2. Patient has a history of cardiac problems.
3. Patient's physician has prescribed nitroglycerin (NTG).
4. Systolic blood pressure is greater than 90 systolic.
5. Medical direction authorizes administration of the medication.

CONTRAINDICATIONS

1. Patient has hypotension or a systolic blood pressure below 90.
2. Patient has a head injury.
3. Patient is an infant or child.
4. Patient has already taken the maximum prescribed dose.
5. Patient has recently taken Viagra®, Cialis®, Levitra®, or another drug for erectile dysfunction.

MEDICATION FORM

Tablet or sublingual (under the tongue) spray

DOSAGE

One dose. Repeat in 5 minutes, if less than complete relief, if systolic blood pressure remains above 90, and if authorized by medical direction, up to a maximum of three doses.

ADMINISTRATION

1. Perform a focused assessment for the cardiac patient.
2. Take the patient's blood pressure. (Systolic pressure must be above 90–100. Use the number designated by your EMS system.)
3. Contact medical direction, if no standing orders.

SCAN 20-3 Nitroglycerin *(continued)*

4. Check the expiration date. Then ensure the right patient, right time, right medication, right dose, and right route.
5. Ensure the patient is alert.
6. Question the patient on the last dose taken and effects. Ensure understanding of the route of administration.
7. Ask the patient to lift the tongue to the roof of the mouth. Place the tablet or spray dose under the tongue (while wearing gloves) or have the patient place the tablet or spray under the tongue.
8. Have the patient keep the mouth closed with the tablet under the tongue (without swallowing) until dissolved and absorbed.
9. Recheck the patient's blood pressure within 2 minutes.
10. Document medication administration, route, and time.
11. Reassess the patient.

ACTIONS

1. Relaxes blood vessels.
2. Decreases workload of heart.

SIDE EFFECTS

1. Hypotension (Lowers blood pressure.)
2. Headache
3. Pulse rate changes

REASSESSMENT STRATEGIES

1. Monitor blood pressure.
2. Ask patient about effect on pain relief.
3. Seek medical direction before readministering.
4. Record assessments.

Pediatric Note

Children usually have very healthy hearts, so it is rare for an EMT to see a pediatric patient with a cardiac problem. Most such problems are congenital (the child is born with them), so they are discovered before the newborn leaves the nursery. You may see a child who has had cardiac surgery or has learned to live with the problem through changes in lifestyle or medication. In cases such as these, parents are frequently very well informed and can be of great assistance.

Think Like an EMT

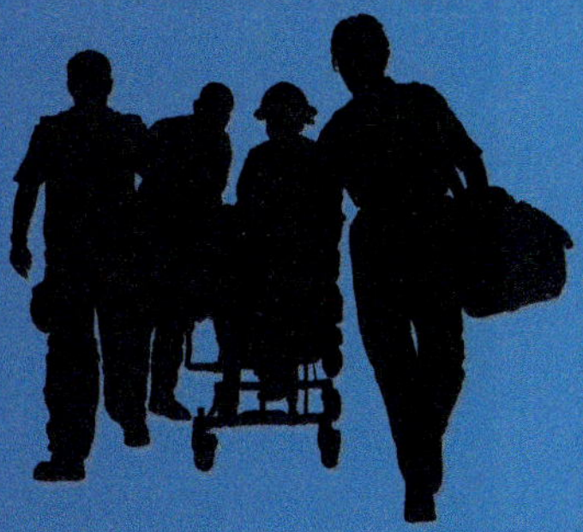

Meeting Sublingual Nitroglycerin Criteria

You are treating a patient with chest pain. For each scenario provided, decide whether this patient meets the general criteria for sublingual nitroglycerin administration. Each of the patients has nitroglycerin prescribed by his cardiologist.

1. You are treating an 84-year-old patient with chest pain. His wife tells you that he began having a sensation in his chest he thought was indigestion about two hours ago. The patient is very pale and sweaty and appears sleepy. His pulse is 104 and slightly irregular, respirations 28 and adequate, and blood pressure 94/66.
2. You are treating a 68-year-old male patient who has a history of angina pectoris. He tells you that he began having chest discomfort just after eating dinner. The discomfort is in the center of his chest and is described as a heavy feeling. It feels like the last time he had a heart problem. His vital signs are pulse 92, strong and regular; respirations 20 and adequate; blood pressure 138/92; and skin warm and moist.
3. You are treating a 49-year-old male patient complaining of pain in his "stomach." He states the pain is below his diaphragm and radiates to the left side. He has taken one nitroglycerin spray without relief. The patient states this pain is not like his one heart attack. His vital signs are pulse 68, strong and regular; respirations 18 and adequate; blood pressure 112/68; and skin warm and dry.

"Heart attack calls require teamwork from the scene to the hospital. I work with ALS and notify the hospital early to give the patient the best chance of full recovery."

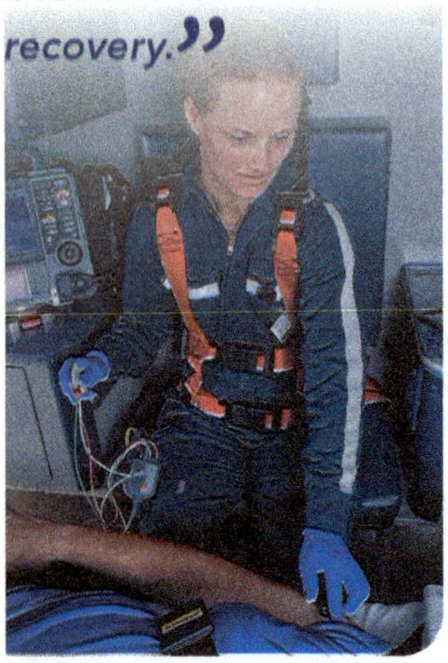

Cardiovascular Disorders

Heart problems can be caused by a number of disorders that affect the condition and function of the blood vessels and the heart. The majority of cardiovascular emergencies are caused, directly or indirectly, by changes in the inner walls of arteries. These arteries can be part of the systemic (total body), pulmonary (lung), or coronary (heart) circulatory systems. Problems with the heart's electrical and mechanical functions also cause cardiovascular emergencies.

Coronary Artery Disease

As we discussed in the Acute Coronary Syndrome section, the heart muscle is perfused by the coronary arteries. These arteries descend from the aorta and reach all areas of the heart. Vital oxygenated blood is delivered to the cells of the heart via these vessels, and as long as they keep blood flowing, perfusion of the heart is maintained.

When the coronary arteries are narrowed or blocked, blood flow is reduced, thereby reducing the amount of oxygen delivered to the heart. Conditions that narrow or block the arteries of the heart are commonly called ***coronary artery disease (CAD)***. Coronary artery disease is a serious health problem that results in hundreds of thousands of deaths yearly in the United States.

CORE CONCEPT
Conditions that may lead to a cardiac emergency

coronary artery disease (CAD)
diseases that affect the arteries of the heart.

CAD is often the result of the buildup of fatty deposits on the inner and middle walls of arteries. This buildup causes a narrowing of the inner vessel diameter, restricting the flow of blood. Fats and other particles combine to form this deposit, known as plaque. As time passes, calcium can be deposited at the site of the plaque, causing the area to harden.

Some factors that put a person at risk of developing CAD, such as heredity (a close relative who has CAD) and age, cannot be changed. However, there are many risk factors that can be modified to reduce the risk of coronary artery disease. These include hypertension (high blood pressure), obesity, lack of exercise, elevated blood levels of cholesterol and triglycerides, and cigarette smoking.

Many patients have more than one of these risk factors. Fortunately, the damage caused by the second group of risk factors may be reversed or slowed by changing behavior. Smokers can return to the risk level of a nonsmoker soon after quitting. Medication and weight loss can lower high blood pressure. Improved diet and exercise can help the other controllable factors.

Coronary artery disease is not typically an emergency by itself. Millions of people live with this disease each year. However, it is the progression of this disease, the narrowing of blood vessels over time, that frequently leads to specific disorders that we would consider an emergency.

Angina Pectoris

angina pectoris (AN-ji-nah [or an-JI-nah] PEK-to-ris)
signs of acute coronary syndrome (usually chest pain) occurring when blood supply to the heart is reduced and a portion of the heart muscle is not receiving enough oxygen.

Angina pectoris means, literally, a pain in the chest. In this condition, coronary artery disease has narrowed the arteries that supply the heart. During times of exertion or stress, the heart works harder. The portion of the myocardium supplied by the narrowed artery becomes starved for oxygen. When the myocardium is deprived of oxygen, chest discomfort (angina pectoris) is the most frequent result (Figure 20-6). This discomfort is sometimes called an angina attack. It is important to remember that chest pain is not the only symptom associated with the ischemia of angina pectoris. While pain or discomfort is common, the ischemia caused by a narrowed coronary artery can also cause shortness of breath, nausea, sweating, and syncope.

Since the symptoms of angina pectoris come on with increased stress or exertion, they will frequently diminish when the patient stops the exertion. As the oxygen demand of the heart returns to normal, the symptoms subside. Seldom does this attack last longer than 5 minutes once the patient returns to rest.

nitroglycerin
a medication that dilates the blood vessels.

Possession of nitroglycerin is a good indication that the patient has a history of this condition. ***Nitroglycerin*** is a prescribed medication that dilates the blood vessels. Although

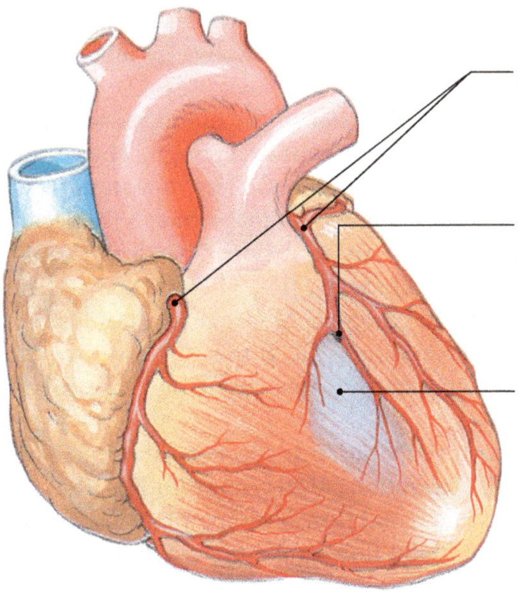

FIGURE 20-6 Angina pectoris, or chest pain, results when a coronary artery is partially blocked, depriving an area of the myocardium of oxygen during exertion.

nitroglycerin will dilate arteries, including the coronary arteries, it predominantly dilates veins. This results in more blood staying in the veins of the body, so there is less blood coming back to the heart. With less blood to pump out, the heart does not have to work as hard. Nitroglycerin is available in tablets that are placed under the patient's tongue to dissolve, as well as sprays and patches. The patches have adhesive that keeps them on the skin, gradually releasing nitroglycerin throughout the day.

Most angina patients are advised by their doctors to take nitroglycerin for chest pain. Patients are usually told to rest and are allowed to take three nitroglycerin doses over a 10-minute period. If there is no relief of symptoms after that time, they are instructed to call for help.

Usually angina is very predictable. Exertion causes symptoms, and rest makes those symptoms go away. However, as vessels get more and more narrow, this condition can occur more frequently and with less specific provocation. It becomes increasingly difficult to differentiate this problem from the symptoms associated with a myocardial infarction.

Assessing and Treating Angina Pectoris

The most difficult task in treating a patient with angina pectoris is to differentiate the symptoms from acute myocardial infarction. In most cases, we simply cannot. Patients with angina pectoris will potentially complain of any and all acute coronary syndrome symptoms, including discomfort, dyspnea, nausea, and syncope. The one potentially differentiating factor, however, is the subsiding of symptoms. By definition, the symptoms associated with angina pectoris resolve with rest. In some cases, the original dispatch complaint of chest pain (for example) will have subsided prior to or shortly after the arrival of EMS. Complete resolution of symptoms would suggest angina pectoris. Symptoms of myocardial infarction do not typically resolve on their own.

Even so, a patient who complains of any of the symptoms of ACS should be assumed to be having a myocardial infarction until proven otherwise. Treat the symptomatic angina pectoris patient in the same manner as described in the acute coronary syndrome section. Consider oxygen, administer nitroglycerin and aspirin, obtain a 12-lead ECG, and transport. If all symptoms have resolved, contact medical control. It may be appropriate to transport the patient for a more detailed evaluation.

Acute Myocardial Infarction

The narrowing of the coronary arteries sets the stage for several other cardiac conditions. As plaque accumulates and hardens, it can create weak areas of the vessel and make rupture

occlusion (uh-KLU-zhun) blockage, as of an artery, by fatty deposits.

thrombus (THROM-bus) a clot formed of blood and plaque attached to the inner wall of an artery or vein.

embolism (EM-bo-lizm) blockage of a vessel by a clot or foreign material brought to the site by the blood current.

acute myocardial infarction (AMI) (ah-KUTE MY-o-KARD-e-ul in-FARK-shun) the condition in which a portion of the myocardium dies as a result of an occlusion; often called a heart attack by laypersons.

dysrhythmia (dis-RITH-me-ah) a disturbance in heart rate and rhythm.

possible. This condition, known as an aneurysm, will be discussed in more detail later in this chapter. The narrowing of the vessel also sets the stage for blood flow to be blocked by an ***occlusion***.

As plaque accumulates, the inner diameter of the blood vessel narrows. In addition, the inner lining of that vessel can become hard and rough. The rough surface formed inside the artery can facilitate formation of blood clots, which narrow the artery even more. The clot and debris from the plaque form a ***thrombus***. A thrombus can reach a size where it blocks blood flow and causes an occlusion. The clot may also break loose to become an ***embolism*** and move to occlude the flow of blood somewhere downstream in a smaller artery. In cases of partial or complete blockage, the tissues beyond the point of blockage will be starved of oxygen and may die. If this blockage involves a large area of the heart (as in a heart attack) or the brain (causing one kind of stroke), the results may be quickly fatal.

The blocking of a coronary artery by the formation of a thrombus or by an embolism is known as an ***acute myocardial infarction (AMI)*** (Figure 20-7). Often called a *heart attack* by laypersons, an AMI results when blood flow is interrupted and myocardial cells begin to die. Rarely, the interruption of blood flow to the myocardium may be due to the rupturing of a coronary artery (aneurysm).

The occlusion of blood in an acute myocardial infarction can cause two very dangerous categories of problems: ischemia and dysrhythmias. Ischemia that leads to injury of cells and cell death can disturb the electrical function of the heart. As cells die, the very precise distribution and route of electrical current that normally causes the rhythmic contractions of the heart can be disrupted and cause new and sometimes deadly patterns of conduction. A ***dysrhythmia*** occurs when electricity is distributed abnormally through the heart, causing harmful changes to rate, rhythm, and pumping ability. As discussed previously, patients with an occluded coronary artery can develop tachycardia, bradycardia, and even deadly dysrhythmias like ventricular fibrillation. If a patient dies from a myocardial infarction, it is likely because of a dysrhythmia.

A myocardial infarction can also cause mechanical problems within the heart itself. As cells die from hypoxia, the function of those cells is lost. If the blockage affects enough cells, the pumping action of the heart can be affected. Although this is a rare situation compared with electrical problems, mechanical failure must be considered. Occasionally myocardial infarction can affect areas of the heart, such as the muscles that close the valves. Multiple heart attacks can also result in a cumulative effect that simply diminishes function to an unsafe level. Either way, these conditions can result in acute inability of the heart to function properly mechanically. This very deadly condition is called *cardiogenic shock* and typically results in a dramatic drop in blood pressure.

FIGURE 20-7 (A) Cross-section of a myocardial infarction and (B) a heart with normal and infarcted tissue at lower left area. *(Photo B: Biophoto Associates/Science Source)*

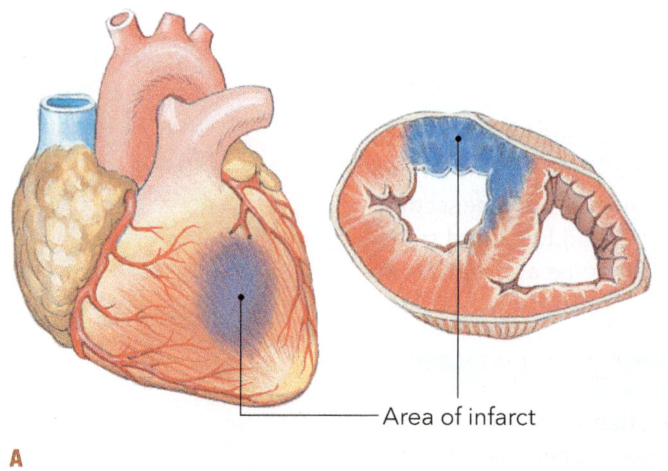

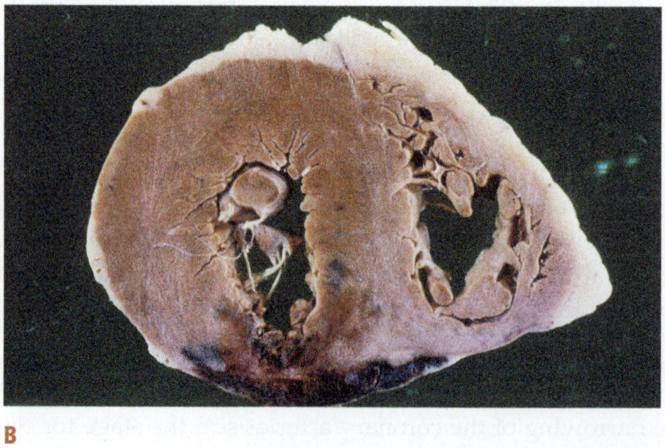

More than 700,000 cases of AMI occur in the United States each year, and cardiovascular disease causes hundreds of thousands of deaths annually. A major portion of these deaths are cases of *sudden death*, a cardiac arrest that occurs within 2 hours of the onset of symptoms. In most cases, sudden death occurs outside of hospitals. The patient may have no prior symptoms of coronary artery disease. Nearly 25 percent of these individuals have no previous history of cardiac problems.

The treatment of AMI has changed radically in recent years. Previously, patients were admitted to coronary care units, where they were observed and, when emergencies occurred, treated with varying degrees of success. Now some patients receive treatment with medications called *fibrinolytics* to dissolve the clot that is blocking the coronary artery. To be most effective, these medications must be administered early. With each hour that passes before they are administered, they become less likely to dissolve the clot. An even more effective way to unclog the coronary artery is to insert a catheter into the blocked artery with a balloon that can be inflated to reopen circulation to the heart (a procedure known as *balloon angioplasty*), or to insert a tiny stent (pipe) within the artery to restore blood flow. Patients with myocardial infarctions must reach the hospital quickly. The expression that "time is muscle" reminds emergency providers that the sooner patients with AMI reach the hospital and undergo these types of procedures to restore blood flow to the heart, the greater their chance to survive the AMI with less permanent damage to the heart muscle.

A patient who leaves the hospital after an AMI will usually be told to take aspirin every day to prevent another episode. The patient will also probably be told to take a medication known as a *beta blocker*. Beta blockers are a group of medications that slow the heart and make it beat less strongly. This would not usually be considered a good thing, but in post-AMI patients, it results in a decrease in the work the heart has to do. This actually benefits the heart and leads to longer and better lives for these patients.

Assessment and Treatment of a Myocardial Infarction

Conduct a primary and secondary assessment on a suspected acute myocardial infarction patient as described in the Acute Coronary Syndrome section. Take care in the primary assessment to ensure that the patient has a pulse and is breathing. (Some AMI patients will present in cardiac arrest.) Use the secondary assessment to identify signs and symptoms associated with ischemia and an occluded coronary vessel.

A myocardial infarction will exhibit the pattern of symptoms described in the ACS section. Chest, jaw, neck, arm, and epigastrium discomfort are common. Dyspnea is the most common finding in AMI patients over the age of 60. Nausea and/or vomiting, syncope, and sweating are also common. Remember that not every patient having an acute MI will experience discomfort. Some patients will only complain of fatigue or dyspnea on exertion. About one in ten patients will experience cardiac arrest as the first symptom of acute myocardial infarction. Care of these patients will be discussed in detail in the chapter *Resuscitation*.

The most important treatment for a suspected myocardial infarction is transport. Whether the patient will receive fibrinolytics or angioplasty, these interventions both occur in the hospital setting. When the pattern of ACS is recognized, the first step you should take is to initiate transport.

Most EMS systems now have a mechanism for activating a system of care designed to treat patients with acute myocardial infarction. These systems recognize the time-sensitive nature of a heart attack and are designed to initiate definitive care as soon as possible. Some hospitals are designated as cardiac centers specifically equipped to manage these patients. Your system may have specific protocols identifying criteria for immediate transport of suspected AMI patients to these facilities. Even in settings where cardiac systems of care are not present, rapid transport of a suspected AMI patient is still a priority.

A 12-lead ECG is an important element of the care of a suspected AMI patient. A 12-lead ECG can identify specific electrical patterns associated with acute myocardial infarction and allow for the specific "ruling in" of a heart attack. This positive identification allows therapies to be more aggressive and gives the opportunity for definitive AMI patients to take precedence over others. As previously stated, many systems have integrated 12-lead ECG acquisition into the EMT scope of practice. If protocols allow, you should acquire and transmit an ECG as soon as possible for a suspected AMI patient.

If an AMI is suspected, contact ALS. Most advanced providers can interpret 12-lead ECG and will have more options for treating dangerous dysrhythmias.

Be prepared for cardiac arrest. Although this is relatively uncommon, even in a confirmed AMI patient, it can occur. It may be reasonable to bring an automated external defibrillator (AED) into the patient's house and keep it close by during care.

A suspected AMI patient should also receive aspirin and nitroglycerin as detailed in previous sections. (Review Scan 20-2 and Scan 20-3.)

Take steps to keep the AMI patient calm. This may mean choosing to defer a lights-and-siren transport. Always weigh benefits and risks based upon your particular circumstance. Suspected AMI patients should not be allowed to walk, because increased demand on the heart can make the ischemia worse.

Transport the patient immediately, taking into account the most appropriate destination. Always follow local protocols.

Heart Failure and Acute Pulmonary Edema

heart failure (HF)
the failure of the heart to pump blood with normal efficiency; also known as *congestive heart failure (CHF)*.

Heart failure (also known as ***congestive heart failure*** *or* ***CHF)*** is a progressive condition in which the heart is unable to pump blood with normal efficiency. Although there are several subtypes of heart failure, typically the condition implies that one or both ventricles can no longer fill properly or pump an adequate amount of blood to meet the demands of the cardiovascular system. Heart failure is not the same as cardiac arrest. In cardiac arrest, the heart literally is unable to pump blood. In heart failure, pumping of the heart continues; it is just inefficient compared with the needs of the cardiovascular system. The inefficient pumping associated with heart failure leads to several unwelcome consequences. Inefficient pumping means that the heart's ability to perfuse body tissues is impaired. Heart failure patients may struggle to accomplish even simple exercise-related tasks. Walking to the mailbox may be an impossible chore without a break halfway. Inadequate pumping can also leave very limited ability to compensate for a challenge. A person with heart failure may simply not be able to increase the heart rate to counter blood loss. And finally, inefficient pumping can cause fluid to back up and at times cause dangerous breathing problems.

When a ventricle fails to eject an appropriate proportion of the blood that has filled it, pressure builds up in the blood vessels that feed that ventricle. For example, if the right ventricle fails to pump efficiently, pressure builds up in the right atrium and in the superior and inferior vena cava. This pressure backup can be visibly seen in right-sided failure; these patients frequently have jugular venous distention (JVD) resulting from the pressure of the vena cava backing up the jugular veins. In high-pressure states, the body will attempt to even that pressure off by leaching fluid from the capillaries. In right-sided failure, this fluid can often be seen as swelling and fluid buildup in the abdomen, resulting from high pressure and fluid leakage in the capillaries around the liver; and swelling in the ankles and feet, otherwise known as ***pedal edema***, resulting from fluid leaking from capillaries in the extremities. A more dangerous fluid shift occurs when the left ventricle pumps inefficiently.

pedal edema
accumulation of fluid in the feet or ankles.

When the left ventricle fails, pressure builds in the left atria and then in the pulmonary vein. Pressure in the pulmonary vein causes the capillaries surrounding the alveoli in the lungs to leak. Fluid creeps across the one-celled membrane of the capillaries and occupies space around and eventually in the alveoli itself. Fluid around the alveoli can cause the tiny air sacs to collapse. When fluid leaches into the alveoli, it occupies space where gas exchange used to occur. This impairs the body's ability to diffuse oxygen and carbon dioxide. Fluid shifting into the lungs is referred to as ***pulmonary edema*** and can be a life-threatening problem for the patient. Evidence of this shift is often first seen as respiratory distress in the patient; it can also be identified by the presence of crackles on auscultation of the lungs.

pulmonary edema accumulation of fluid in the lungs.

Both right-sided and left-sided heart failure can be chronic conditions. You may see the signs and symptoms of either one every day. Left-sided heart failure complications, particularly pulmonary edema, typically occur in a more acute fashion—that is, they develop abruptly, typically after a significant increase in cardiac workload. For example, a patient with chronic left-sided failure might develop pulmonary edema after attempting to climb a flight of stairs. The additional exercise demand on the heart increases pressure just enough to initiate the pulmonary edema. Pulmonary edema is also occasionally associated with the development of a new myocardial infarction or with the onset of a dysrhythmia.

Assessment and Treatment of Heart Failure

Heart failure in and of itself is not necessarily an emergency. Thousands of people live each day with varying degrees of pumping inefficiency. Although their lifestyles may have required significant changes, the presence of failure does not necessarily imply an emergent issue. Heart failure is most commonly identified in the secondary assessment. Most heart failure patients will describe a history of heart failure (also called congestive heart failure) when questioned about existing medical conditions. Patients with chronic heart failure also take specific medications designed to control pressure and fluid levels. Beta blockers like metoprolol, ACE inhibitors like captopril, and diuretics like Lasix® (sometimes described as a "water pill") all point to a history of heart failure. Signs of fluid buildup also help identify chronic heart failure patients. Pedal edema, swelling in the abdomen or buttocks, and JVD all are associated with inefficient pumping. Many patients with heart failure are trained to weigh themselves at home to constantly assess their fluid status. A weight gain of more than a few pounds is usually considered significant.

If failure develops acutely, as it often does with pulmonary edema, you will likely see evidence of fluid in the lungs. Difficulty breathing, crackles, and even coughing up of pink, frothy sputum may be found. Patients with pulmonary edema also very commonly have a history of chronic heart failure and may also have pedal edema, have JVD, and take heart failure medications.

To assess a patient with heart failure properly, start with a primary assessment. Patients with pulmonary edema often decompensate to inadequate breathing and require positive pressure ventilation. If possible, use OPQRST and SAMPLE to obtain a thorough patient history. Use a detailed system assessment of the cardiovascular system to identify signs of inefficient pumping like crackles, JVD, or pedal edema.

Assess and reassess vital signs. The presence of pulmonary edema can occur with both fast and slow dysrhythmias, and can be associated with either very high or very low blood pressures.

The treatment of heart failure is typically limited to treatment of an acute presentation like pulmonary edema. If pulmonary edema is present, contact ALS immediately. Patients with pulmonary edema need immediate treatment and often decompensate rapidly.

If protocols allow, consider the application of CPAP to treat pulmonary edema. (See the *Respiratory Emergencies* chapter for more specific details on treating this disorder.) CPAP can be especially effective in treating pulmonary edema because its resultant increased airway pressures help open up wet alveoli and improve oxygen exchange in the lungs. Some EMS systems allow EMTs to administer nitroglycerin to treat acute pulmonary edema. Nitroglycerin in this case is used to dilate blood vessels and take workload off the heart. Consult your local protocols to determine if this is possible in your area.

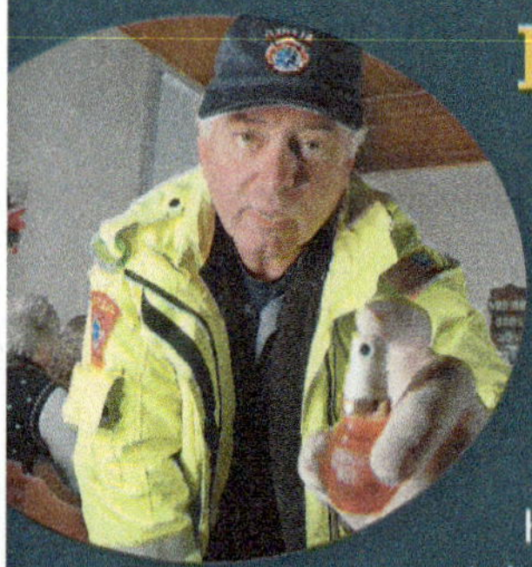

Point of View

"I couldn't believe I was having chest pain. How cruel was it that I'd prayed I wouldn't have another heart attack–and where do I get chest pain again? Church. Not only did my chest hurt, but I was so embarrassed.

"I was so embarrassed and worried that I forgot I had the nitro spray with me. The EMTs came and checked me over and asked me if I'd ever had pain like this before. That was when I remembered. I never had to use it before. They put a spray under my tongue before they wheeled me out of church because it was quite a distance to the ambulance. It actually helped.

"When we got to the ambulance, I told them that my pain felt better. When they found out that I still had some pain, they checked me again and then gave me another spray. I have to say I relaxed a bit when the pain went away.

"When you have chest pain, you think you are going to die. It is a great feeling suddenly realizing that the pain is gone. You really think you have a chance of living. Wow."

Aneurysm

aneurysm (AN-u-rizm) the dilation, or ballooning, of a weakened section of the wall of an artery.

Aneurysm is a cardiovascular disorder that stems from weakened sections in the arterial walls. This weakening can be congenital but can also be associated with the buildup of plaque described earlier. An aneurysm can occur in any artery, but it commonly affects arteries in the chest, abdomen, or brain. In an aneurysm, a weakened area of the artery expands and dilates outward under the pressure of normal blood flow. Occasionally, blood breaks through the inner lining of the artery and works its way into the middle layers of the vessel. This further weakens and dilates the artery. When a weakened section of an artery bursts, there can be rapid, life-threatening internal bleeding (Figure 20-8). Tissues beyond the rupture can be damaged because the oxygenated blood they need is escaping and not reaching them. If a major artery ruptures, death from shock can occur very quickly. The two most common sites of aneurysms that you will encounter in emergency situations are the aorta (see the *Abdominal Emergencies* chapter) and the brain. (See the information on stroke and other causes of altered mental status in the *Diabetic Emergencies and Altered Mental Status* chapter.) When an artery in the brain ruptures, a severe form of stroke occurs. The severity depends on the site of the stroke and the amount of blood loss.

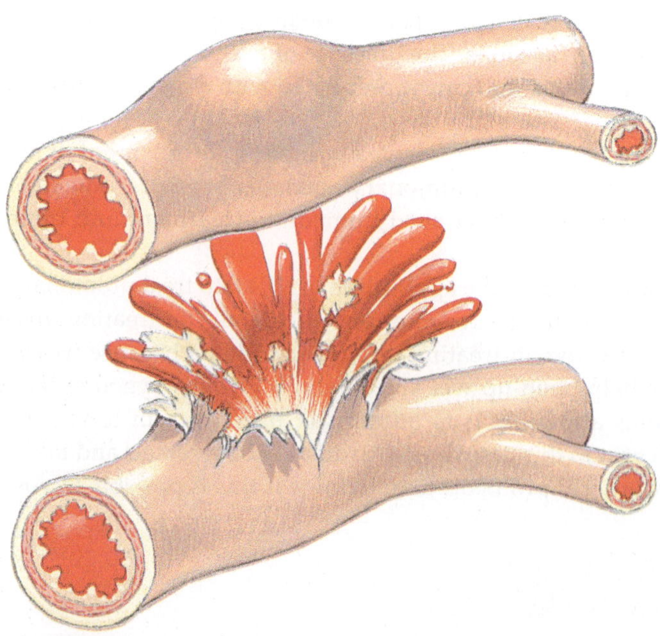

FIGURE 20-8 A weakened area in the wall of an artery will tend to balloon out, forming a saclike aneurysm, which may eventually burst.

Pediatric Note

Most pediatric cardiac disorders are congenital in nature. That means they are present at birth. The difficulty of identifying other cardiac conditions lies in the fact that often they have just appeared and are new, instead of being a known, ongoing issue. There are several pediatric cardiac conditions that cause sudden cardiac arrest. Assessment and care of cardiac arrest will be discussed in detail in the *Resuscitation* chapter.

Some pediatric patients manage ongoing cardiac disorders ranging from birth defects to acquired diseases. These conditions are very rare and too diverse to discuss in detail in this text. However, when managing any pediatric patient with an unknown or unclear chronic condition, you should:

- Consult with caregivers to establish a baseline for the child.
- Discuss with caregivers why EMS has been called. How is the current situation different than the expected baseline?
- Manage primary assessment issues like respiratory failure and cardiac arrest in the same way you would with other patients.
- Consult medical control if you are unclear about assessment or treatment priorities.
- Transport the patient to a facility capable of managing the patient's ongoing condition. (Always follow local protocol.)

Chapter Review

Key Facts and Concepts

- Patients with acute coronary syndrome (ACS) can have many different presentations. Some complain of pressure or pain in the chest with difficulty breathing and a history of heart problems. Others may have just mild discomfort that they ignore for several hours or that goes away and returns. Some patients having heart attacks have no chest discomfort at all.
- Use a thorough secondary assessment to identify the signs and symptoms associated with the pattern of acute coronary syndrome.
- Because of the many possible presentations and the potentially severe complications of acute coronary syndrome, it is important to have a high index of suspicion and to treat patients with these symptoms aggressively. The treatment will not hurt them and may help them.
- Patients with suspected ACS who are hypoxic or short of breath need oxygen and prompt, safe transportation to definitive care. You may be able to assist patients who have their own nitroglycerin in taking it, thereby relieving pain and anxiety.
- Definitive treatment for an acute myocardial infarction occurs at the hospital. Treat suspected AMI as a time-sensitive disorder. Consider appropriate transportation destinations, activate systems of care, and obtain early 12-lead ECG, if possible.
- Aspirin and nitroglycerin are first-line medications associated with the treatment of acute coronary syndrome.
- Heart failure is a chronic condition that can have life-threatening acute presentations. Recognize the signs and symptoms of acute pulmonary edema and treat aggressively.

Key Decisions

- Is the pattern of signs and symptoms associated with acute coronary syndrome present?
- Is oxygen indicated in this patient with acute coronary syndrome?
- Is this patient with possible acute coronary syndrome (ACS) a candidate for aspirin or nitroglycerin?
- What is the best hospital destination for this patient with possible ACS?
- Do I need to activate the cardiac system of care?

Chapter Glossary

acute coronary syndrome (ACS) a blanket term used to represent any symptoms related to lack of oxygen (ischemia) in the heart muscle. Also called *cardiac compromise*.

acute myocardial infarction (AMI) (ah-KUTE MY-o-KARD-e-ul in-FARK-shun) the condition in which a portion of the myocardium dies as a result of occlusion; often called a heart attack by laypersons.

aneurysm (AN-u-rizm) the dilation, or ballooning, of a weakened section of the wall of an artery.

angina pectoris (AN-ji-nah [or an-JI-nah] PEK-to-ris) pain in the chest occurring when blood supply to the heart is reduced and a portion of the heart muscle is not receiving enough oxygen.

bradycardia (bray-di-KAR-de-ah) when the heart rate is slow, usually less than 60 beats per minute.

cardiac compromise see acute coronary syndrome.

cardiovascular system the heart and the blood vessels.

coronary artery disease (CAD) diseases that affect the arteries of the heart.

dyspnea (DISP-ne-ah) shortness of breath; labored or difficult breathing.

dysrhythmia (dis-RITH-me-ah) a disturbance in heart rate and rhythm.

embolism (EM-bo-lizm) blockage of a vessel by a clot or foreign material brought to the site by the blood current.

heart failure (HF) the failure of the heart to pump efficiently, leading to excessive blood or fluids in the lungs, the body, or both; formerly known as *congestive heart failure (CHF)*.

nitroglycerin a medication that dilates the blood vessels.

occlusion (uh-KLU-zhun) blockage, as of an artery, by fatty deposits.

pedal edema accumulation of fluid in the feet or ankles.

pulmonary edema accumulation of fluid in the lungs.

tachycardia (tak-e-KAR-de-ah) when the heart rate is fast, more than 100 beats per minute.

thrombus (THROM-bus) a clot formed of blood and plaque attached to the inner wall of an artery or vein.

Preparation for Your Examination and Practice

Short Answer

1. What position is best for a patient with:
   a. Difficulty breathing and a blood pressure of 100/70?
   b. Chest pain and a blood pressure of 180/90?
2. List two contraindications for the administration of aspirin.
3. List two contraindications for the administration of nitroglycerin to a patient with acute coronary syndrome.
4. List three signs or symptoms associated with acute pulmonary edema.

Thinking and Linking

Think back to the chapter Lifting and Moving Patients *and link information from that chapter with information from this chapter as you consider the following situation:*

1. Your patient is experiencing difficulty breathing, chest pressure, and a blood pressure of 160/100. What is the best way to transfer her down a flight of stairs?

Think back to the chapter Medical, Legal, and Ethical Issues *and link information from that chapter with information from this chapter as you consider the following situation:*

2. Your patient complains of crushing pain to the center of the chest, radiating to the left shoulder. His vital signs are within normal limits. He is alert. You tell him that he needs to go the hospital, but he says he doesn't want to go. You explain that he has signs and symptoms of a heart attack and that if he doesn't go to the hospital, he could die. He says, "I understand that but I'm not going to the hospital. Period." What should you do now?

Critical Thinking Exercises

Survival of a heart attack is clearly linked to early intervention. Whether it be "clot busting" medications or balloon angioplasty, obtaining definitive care early is the best way to reduce mortality in this disorder.

1. What role does obtaining a prehospital 12-lead ECG play in your local system of care?
2. Is there an appropriate situation when by-passing the closest hospital for another hospital may be in the best interest of the patient suffering an apparent acute MI?

Pathophysiology to Practice

The following questions are designed to assist you in gathering relevant clinical information and making accurate decisions in the field.

1. A 66-year-old male patient is complaining of excruciating central chest pain radiating to his back. He tells you his doctor said he has a "bubble" on a blood vessel in his chest. His pulse is 64 and regular, blood pressure 126/82, respirations 16 and unlabored. What medical condition is the patient most likely describing? What are the risks and benefits of administering aspirin and nitroglycerin in this situation?
2. You are treating an elderly male patient with heart failure who is complaining of severe difficulty breathing that has worsened over the past few hours. He takes numerous medications but admits that he ran out of his "water pill" a few days ago. Since then, he has noticed that his weight has increased by several pounds and his belt has been getting tighter. He has also awakened short of breath and needs to sleep propped up on two pillows. How are these signs and symptoms related to the patient's HF?

Street Scenes

Mary is an active 70-year-old who lives by herself in an apartment. She just returned home from shopping and is sitting down, eating lunch, when she feels some chest discomfort that she believes is indigestion. She thinks it will go away, but it doesn't. She stops eating and goes into the living room to sit on the couch, which makes her feel out of breath. She thinks about calling her doctor but doesn't want to be a bother. Unfortunately, the discomfort is now turning into pain, and she feels numbness in her left arm. So, she finally calls her doctor and asks what to do. After hearing the symptoms, her doctor calls 911 to have an ambulance take her to the hospital. Almost two hours have passed since Mary started having signs and symptoms.

You are having a late lunch, which you have only half finished, when a tone comes over your radio. "Ambulance 32, respond to a 70-year-old female experiencing chest pain at 45 Packard Road, apartment 2-D, a third-party call from a physician's office."

When you arrive on scene, your partner says he knows a stair chair will be needed to get the patient from the second floor. He gets the stair chair, and you get the first-in bag.

Street Scene Question

1. **What type of emergency equipment needs to be taken to the side of every potential cardiac patient?**

You proceed to the patient's apartment. As you enter, you notice the patient sitting on the couch, looking pale and anxious. You ask her why EMS was called. She responds by telling you about her discomfort and her trouble breathing. She also mentions that the pain has become worse. You ask the patient when the pain started and what she was doing when it started. You ask her to describe the pain and to rate the severity on a scale of zero to ten (with ten being the worst pain she can imagine). She answers, "Three in the beginning, but now it is eight." Your partner comes through the door with the AED, and you give him a quick overview. You both agree that the ALS unit needs to be requested. You radio the dispatcher, who gives you an ETA of five minutes.

Street Scene Questions

2. **What described symptoms suggest acute coronary syndrome?**
3. **What assessment information do you need to obtain next?**

Your partner gets a set of vital signs, including a room air oxygen saturation of 89 percent, so you place the patient on a nonrebreather mask at 15 liters per minute. You get further history, with the most significant additional information being high blood pressure, for which she takes medication and has been compliant.

Street Scene Question

4. **What are your immediate treatment priorities?**

The oxygen improves the patient's saturation to 95 percent. You decide to switch the patient to a nasal cannula and are able to maintain the normal saturation. You move the patient to the stair chair and then move her to the ambulance. Shortly after loading, you note that Mary has become confused. She looks very pale. Your partner reassesses vital signs while you repeat the primary assessment. Mary is breathing adequately, but her blood pressure has dropped. You lay her flat and begin transport. A 12-lead ECG is obtained, transmitted to the hospital, and turned over to the paramedics when they intercept your ambulance halfway to the cardiac care center. They identify an inferior wall acute myocardial infarction. Transport is continued.

At the hospital, you turn over care to the cardiac care team. You and the paramedic offer a patient handoff verbal report and Mary is whisked off to the catheterization lab. The door to catheterization time was significantly reduced by your report and early 12-lead ECG. You find out later that Mary is expected to make a full recovery.

21 Resuscitation

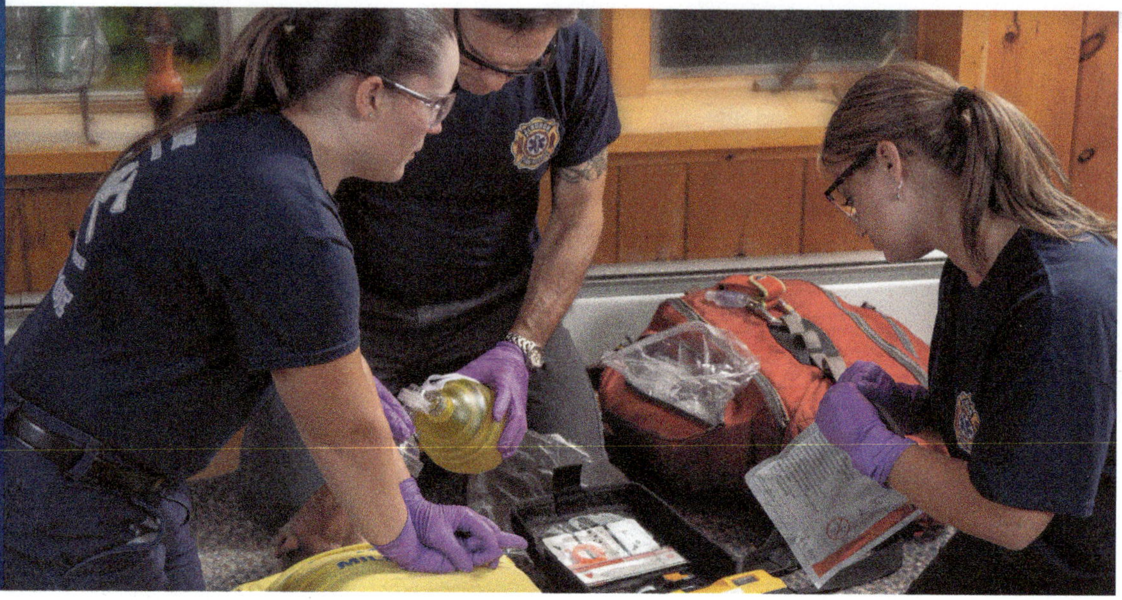

Related Chapters

The following chapters provide additional information related to topics discussed in this chapter:

- **3** Lifting and Moving Patients
- **6** Anatomy and Physiology
- **10** Respiration and Artificial Ventilation
- **12** Primary Assessment
- **13** Vital Signs and Monitoring Devices
- **15** Secondary Assessment
- **20** Cardiac Emergencies
- **22** Diabetic Emergencies and Altered Mental Status
- **26** Abdominal Emergencies
- Appendix A Basic Cardiac Life Support Review

Standard

Medicine (Cardiovascular)

Competency

Applies fundamental knowledge to provide basic emergency care and transportation based on assessment findings for an acutely ill patient.

Core Concepts

- Cardiac arrest and the chain of survival
- Management of a cardiac arrest patient
- Use of an automated external defibrillator (AED)
- Special considerations in AED use
- Use of mechanical cardiopulmonary resuscitation (CPR) devices

Outcomes

After reading this chapter, you should be able to:

21.1 Explain the pathophysiology of cardiac arrest. (pp. 583-589)

- Describe conditions that may trigger cardiac arrest.
- Identify key signs of cardiac arrest.

21.2 Summarize the importance of EMS systems' use of the chain of survival as a means of improving outcomes from cardiac arrest. (pp. 589-612)

- Explain the features of each component of the chain of survival.
- Explain how each component of the chain of survival is intended to improve cardiac arrest outcomes.
- Describe the treatment sequence by which EMTs manage a patient in cardiac arrest.
- Identify circumstances when a mechanical CPR device is advantageous.
- Compare the two types of mechanical CPR devices an EMT may use.
- Describe types and operation of automated external defibrillators (AEDs).
- Explain the integration of CPR and AED use in a patient in cardiac arrest.
- Explain how roles change during the transition of patient care.
- Describe the EMT's approach to different patient responses to treatment, including regaining a pulse and going back into cardiac arrest.
- Describe modifications to cardiac arrest management for pediatric patients.

21.3 Summarize the EMT's obligations with respect to terminating resuscitative efforts before arriving at the hospital. (p. 612)

- Identify the circumstances of the cardiac arrest that must be present prior to an individual EMT's stopping resuscitative efforts.
- Identify the criteria that must be reported to medical direction when requesting an order to cease resuscitative efforts.

21.4 Identify special circumstances in resuscitation that the EMT may encounter. (pp. 612-616)

- Explain the teamwork required to carry out interventions in coordination with others or while transporting a patient with ACS to the hospital.
- Describe the significance to cardiac arrest management of cardiac implants and surgeries.

Key Terms

agonal breathing, *585*
apnea, *587*
asphyxial cardiac arrest, *585*
asystole, *584*
cardiac arrest, *583*
cardiopulmonary resuscitation (CPR), *591*
chain of survival, *583*
commotio cordis, *585*
compression fraction, *593*
defibrillation, *583*
dysrhythmia, *584*
pulseless electrical activity (PEA), *584*
return of spontaneous circulation (ROSC), *599*
sudden cardiac arrest, *585*
ventricular fibrillation (VF), *584*
ventricular tachycardia (V-tach), *584*

"He's not breathing!" is the first thing you hear as you enter the house. What you thought would be a routine shortness of breath call clearly has taken a turn for the worse. The patient's wife is frantic. She waves you to the back bedroom and pleads with you to hurry. In the bedroom you find him. The patient is prone on the floor. His skin is blue, and he is not moving. "Hello, sir," you say as you gently shake his shoulder. No response. As you observe his chest, you see no breathing. You feel no pulse. As if reading your mind, your partner, Grace, speaks up to say, "You better get us some help. I'm starting compressions."

In this moment, the patient in front of you is staring death in the face. Unresponsive, pulseless, and not breathing indicate that he is in ***cardiac arrest***. This means that his heart is not pumping and blood is not flowing in the cardiovascular system. With every ticking second, his brain becomes more and more hypoperfused. Oxygen is not being exchanged, and metabolism has ceased. Cells throughout his body are injured because of the growing hypoxia. Without a rapid reversal, the damage will become permanent, and the patient will die. In fact, few patients survive this moment. Nationwide, the survival of out-of-hospital cardiac arrest is less than 15 percent. However, you can offer him a chance. For all the highly technical advances in medicine, the two interventions this patient needs to survive this event are ultimately provided within the EMT scope of practice. Quality chest compressions and early defibrillation are the only chance and really the only interventions ever proven to alter outcomes. That's right; despite all the paramedics, nurses, and doctors and all the medicines, procedures, and tests, research continues to show that the only reliable and reproducible solutions are the compressions and defibrillation you will deploy right then and there.

Now of course, teamwork is still important. The best outcome for this or any patient in cardiac arrest will come when the chain of survival is engaged. ***Chain of survival*** is a term used by the American Heart Association to describe the key elements of emergency cardiac care. It is discussed in a later section of this chapter, but in brief, its components include:

- Recognition and activation of the emergency response system (and prevention strategies, especially for children)
- Immediate high-quality CPR
- Rapid ***defibrillation***
- Basic and advanced emergency medical services
- Advanced life support and postarrest care.

Cardiac arrest survival is optimized by weaving each element of care together. More patients survive when dispatchers augment the capabilities of bystanders; when team leaders orchestrate integrated basic and advanced life support (BLS and ALS) interventions; and when on-scene cardiac arrest care transitions smoothly to postarrest care and appropriate transport. Furthermore, we now understand that the quality of interventions and attention to detail matter greatly. Not only must responders work together, they must work together well and perform each task at a high level. This underscores the need for team leadership and defines a clear need for pre-event training.

High-performance cardiac arrest management combines each of these elements beneath an umbrella of quality. First defined by Dr. Mickey Eisenberg in Seattle, high-performance CPR is an integrated process that begins with systems planning; incorporates regimented training rich with performance feedback; utilizes incident command in cardiac arrest situations; and focuses with laser beam precision on the application of key interventions such as chest compressions and defibrillation. High-performance cardiac arrest management also carefully analyzes team performance and the quality of interventions in an ongoing effort to constantly improve.

It is difficult to argue with the success of high-performance cardiac arrest management. In communities that have adopted Dr. Eisenberg's strategies, survival in witnessed cardiac arrest has peaked at higher than 50 percent. Although that high rate of survival may not be possible in every community, it is reasonable to expect that integrating key strategies will demonstrate outcome improvements.

This chapter will focus on treating the cardiac arrest patient. We will discuss the EMT's role in overall system improvement but focus most of our time on actual cardiac arrest care. The lessons of high-performance cardiac arrest management will be integrated throughout our approach, and it is our intent that care discussed in this chapter will reflect national best practices. As always, consider your own local scope of practice and protocols before responding.

The Pathophysiology of Cardiac Arrest

In the chapter *Anatomy and Physiology*, you learned about the structure and function of the heart. Before beginning this chapter, you should review:

- Flow of blood through the chambers of the heart (the atria and ventricles)
- The cardiac conductive system (the electrical impulses and specialized muscles that cause the heart to contract)
- Flow of blood through the arteries, veins, arterioles, venules, and capillaries
- Circulation of blood between the heart and the lungs and between the heart and the rest of the body
- Shock (hypoperfusion).

The heart is a simple organ. In fact, it has only one job: to pump blood. To achieve this goal, however, an elaborate combination of electrical and mechanical functions must work together with precise timing and coordinated effort. As you recall from the chapter *Anatomy and Physiology*, the heart creates its own electrical stimulation and sends that depolarization along a predetermined path, the cardiac conduction pathway. This electrical stimulation is intended to cause the surrounding muscle to contract in a specific sequence to get the top-down, atrial-first-then-ventricular pumping action that pushes blood into the vessels and ultimately out to the rest of the body. The chapters *Anatomy and Physiology* and *Principles of Pathophysiology* also explained that the pumping muscle of the heart requires a reliable and uninterrupted supply of oxygenated blood to sustain function and that without that oxygenated blood, function could fail. Finally, in the chapter *Cardiac Emergencies*, you learned that blockages in the coronary vessels, commonly associated with acute coronary syndrome, could cause areas of the heart to become ischemic and could lead to both electrical and mechanical dysfunction. If these elements are not clear, take a moment to review the pertinent sections.

cardiac arrest
a state in which the heart is no longer pumping blood.

chain of survival
a metaphor that describes the key elements of cardiac arrest management. Each link in the chain describes a different but interconnected intervention; when combined, these interventions offer optimal care.

defibrillation
delivery of an electrical shock to stop the fibrillation of heart muscles and restore a normal heart rhythm.

Mechanical Failure of the Heart

The heart can stop pumping effectively due to mechanical problems. By far the most common mechanical reason that the heart ceases to function correctly is loss of normal heart muscle (myocardial) structure. This can result from myocardial infarction, where large areas of the heart muscle die because of lack of blood flow. It might be caused by conditions like chronic hypertension, which causes the heart muscle to become abnormally thick, reducing pumping efficiency. Profound mechanical dysfunction can also result from loss of normal heart valve function. For example, a narrowing (stenosis) of the aortic valve can block normal outflow of blood from the left ventricle. In addition, mechanical failure can be caused by direct trauma to the chest or heart. Blunt and penetrating injuries can damage chambers of the heart or cause conditions like *pericardial tamponade*. In cardiac tamponade, blood (or other fluids) occupy the space between the heart and the pericardial sac. If the pressure increases enough, this blood in the pericardial sac can restrict movement and filling of the ventricles.

Any of these conditions can cause the pumping action of the heart to fail. If impairment of normal heart mechanics is substantial enough, the heart's pumping efficiency may not be able to generate a pulse or maintain adequate systemic blood pressure. The eventual effect would be cardiac arrest.

Many of these mechanical conditions can occur even when normal electrical function of the heart is maintained. This is important to remember when we discuss electrical dysfunctions and defibrillation. Although most cardiac arrest is associated with an electrical problem, and defibrillators are specifically geared to identify electrical dysfunction, not every cardiac arrest case is caused by an electrical problem. When paramedics using a cardiac monitor during a cardiac arrest see an organized electrical rhythm that is referred to as ***pulseless electrical activity (PEA)***, this most commonly indicates a mechanical failure with intact organized electrical function.

pulseless electrical activity (PEA)
a condition in which the heart's electrical rhythm remains relatively normal, yet the mechanical pumping activity fails to follow the electrical activity, causing cardiac arrest.

Electrical Dysfunction of the Heart

Although mechanical dysfunction can be the root cause of cardiac arrest, electrical issues are far more common. Under normal circumstances, individual heart cells move tiny charged electrolyte particles, called *ions*, in and out of the cells to generate an electrical charge. This charge cascades from one cell to another to create the electrical movement called conduction of electrical impulses. Heart muscle cells are unique in that they can generate their own electrical impulses, but normal electrical conduction of the heart flows through a specialized cardiac conduction pathway. This pathway sequentially stimulates the muscles of the atria to contract, followed by stimulating the muscles of the ventricles to contract. A microscopic component of the cell called the sodium potassium pump must be engaged to carry ions to their designated starting points. The sodium potassium pump requires energy to complete its task and so relies on a constant supply of oxygenated blood. When this supply of oxygen is interrupted (as during a myocardial infarction), ions cannot be moved normally, and the electrical distribution system fails. Without proper electrical stimulus, the mechanical aspects do not function, and blood is not pumped.

If the electrical system fails completely and no electricity is created, a condition called ***asystole*** occurs. On a cardiac monitor, this would be recognized as a flat line, demonstrating an absence of energy.

More often, disruption of the heart's normal electrical function leads to a ***dysrhythmia***. In the chapter *Cardiac Emergencies*, you learned that ischemia can lead to unusually slow or unusually fast rhythms. If the electrical disruption is severe enough, it can also lead to dysrhythmias that cause cardiac arrest. Specifically, ***ventricular tachycardia (V-tach)*** and ***ventricular fibrillation (VF)*** occur when electrical dysfunction causes chaotic and inappropriate electrical distribution through the heart. These dysrhythmias are commonly caused by hypoxic cells responding electrically in an uncoordinated way. In both dysrhythmias, there is electrical and mechanical response, but pumping fails because the responses are chaotic and/or uncoordinated. In ventricular tachycardia, both ventricles pump so rapidly that they have no time to fill, and so there is no or inadequate blood to pump. In ventricular fibrillation, chaotic mechanical response to chaotic electrical activity leads to a quivering motion of the heart that fails to pump any blood. Dysrhythmias like ventricular tachycardia and ventricular fibrillation lead to sudden cardiac arrest (described next). They appear abruptly, are difficult to predict, and result in sudden collapse of the patient.

asystole (ay-SIS-to-le)
a condition in which the heart has ceased generating electrical impulses. Commonly called *flatline*.

dysrhythmia (dis-RITH-me-ah)
a disturbance in heart rate and rhythm.

ventricular tachycardia (V-tach) (ven-TRIK-u-ler tak-i-KAR-de-uh)
a condition in which the heartbeat is quite rapid; if rapid enough, ventricular tachycardia will not allow the heart's chambers to fill with enough blood between beats to produce blood flow sufficient to meet the body's needs.

ventricular fibrillation (VF) (ven-TRIK-u-ler fib-ri-LAY-shun)
a condition in which the heart's electrical impulses are disorganized, preventing the heart muscle from contracting normally.

The good news is that the electrical dysfunction of VF and V-tach is often correctable if treated rapidly. As you will learn in coming sections, automated external defibrillators are used to identify and fix these uncoordinated patterns of cardiac electrical activity and provide EMTs with the best opportunity to reverse these deadly dysrhythmias.

Sudden vs. Asphyxial Cardiac Arrest

Cardiac arrest is often described by the manner in which the heart stops pumping, either *sudden* or *asphyxial*. ***Sudden cardiac arrest*** typically refers to an abrupt onset of a dysrhythmia like ventricular fibrillation or tachycardia. Sudden dysrhythmias account for more than 85 percent of all arrest situations, and most of these dysrhythmias (roughly 89 percent) are caused by acute coronary syndrome. Other possible causes of sudden cardiac arrest are congenital heart conditions, illnesses, and toxins. Even sudden blunt trauma to the anterior chest, such as being struck by a baseball or diving chest first onto hard ground, can lead to sudden cardiac arrest dysrhythmias. This mechanism of cardiac arrest is known as ***commotio cordis***. In sudden cardiac arrest, the most concerning problem is the failure of the heart pump. Oxygen levels in the blood tend to be relatively normal at the beginning of the cardiac arrest period.

sudden cardiac arrest
a cardiac arrest occurring due to the abrupt onset of a dysrhythmia.

commotio cordis (com-mo-shee-o cord -iss)
a cardiac arrest caused by acute blunt force trauma to the anterior chest.

Asphyxial cardiac arrest implies that the heart has stopped pumping due to issues related to systemic hypoxia. Conditions like respiratory problems and shock, which lead to low oxygen levels in the blood, cause this type of cardiac arrest. Systemic hypoxia leads to reduced perfusion of cardiac muscle cells. Without proper oxygenation, the always-hungry myocardium becomes ischemic and prone to life-threatening dysrhythmias. Asphyxial cardiac arrest is typically found in patients with serious illnesses and injuries. Increased acidity in the blood from metabolic or respiratory failure is also a common contributor to asphyxial cardiac arrests. Examples of patients with asphyxial cardiac arrest are patients with cardiac arrest due to severe asthma and patients in arrest after decompensating from shock. Asphyxial cardiac arrest tends to appear with more warning than does sudden cardiac arrest. Both sudden and asphyxial cardiac arrest are treated similarly, but it is important to remember that patients with asphyxial cardiac arrest generally have very low oxygen levels and elevated carbon dioxide levels in their blood. Quality ventilations are important for these patients during CPR.

asphyxial cardiac arrest
(aus-fix-ial)
a cardiac arrest caused by systemic hypoxia, typically due to a respiratory disorder or shock.

Agonal Respirations

When the heart stops suddenly, oxygenated blood is present not only in the circulatory system but also in the brain and the muscles that control respiration—in particular, the intercostal muscles and the diaphragm. Since there is still some oxygen in the medulla, it is able to send occasional impulses through the nervous system to stimulate the respiratory muscles. ***Agonal breathing*** (gasping respirations) occurs as a primal reflex to the cardiac arrest state. Often when the heart stops beating, the central nervous system signals the respiratory system to literally gasp for life. As the patient inhales, the pressure in the thorax decreases. This encourages more blood to return to the heart. When the patient exhales, the pressure in the thorax increases, promoting movement of blood into the coronary arteries. Since the heart valves push blood one way, this also increases blood flow to the aorta, carotid arteries, and the brain. This small amount of oxygen may actually allow the medulla to continue to send out impulses to the respiratory muscles again, leading to a cycle in which the body attempts to resuscitate itself.

agonal breathing
irregular, gasping breaths that precede apnea and death.

Unfortunately, when agonal breathing does occur, it cannot go on forever. The amount of oxygen delivered to the medulla decreases with time, leading to fewer breaths and a downward spiral ending in death, unless someone intervenes to improve perfusion (through CPR) and to restart the heart's electrical rhythm (through defibrillation). The word *agonal* refers to something that occurs just before death (the same word root as *agony*), so these respirations are traditionally referred to as *agonal respirations*. It is important to note that agonal respirations do not occur in all cardiac arrests.

When someone suddenly goes into cardiac arrest and collapses, up to half the time the patient may exhibit these irregular, gasping breaths that do not look normal and can be confusing. Agonal respirations are the body's attempts to prevent death, but they will only last a few moments, usually less. They are usually less frequent than normal respirations and more sudden and dramatic, not smooth and natural like normal breaths; sometimes they are very brief and weak. Patients who exhibit agonal respirations have a high probability of survival when resuscitative measures (CPR and defibrillation) are provided, probably because agonal respirations are more often associated with shockable rhythms, and they are an indication of the presence of oxygen in key areas such as the heart and brain.

When you encounter a patient with agonal respirations, do not let these respirations confuse you. If you don't feel a pulse (or if you are not sure you feel a pulse), perform chest compressions. Patients who have just gone into cardiac arrest have the greatest chance of survival with immediate high-quality chest compressions and rapid defibrillation.

Likewise, if you are compressing the chest when the patient suddenly takes a spontaneous, gasping breath, or even displays movement such as opening eyes or moving limbs, check the patient. Unless you are sure you feel a pulse, resume compressions. Take this as a good sign, however. You are providing enough oxygen to the brain, heart, and muscles for some impulses to get through to the respiratory and other muscles.

The Effects of Cardiac Arrest

When the heart fails to pump, blood stops moving, and cells are robbed of essential oxygen and nutrients. Organs that require a constant supply of oxygen, like the heart and brain, are damaged immediately, while organs like skin and bone can withstand an interrupted supply longer. As the systemic hypoxia builds, more cells die and more organs fail. If uncorrected, the organism itself (the person) dies. This process occurs not over the course of hours but within minutes. The chance of survival literally shrinks with each passing second.

Although the absolute timing is not clear, a pattern certainly exists that demonstrates cardiac arrest is most survivable in the immediate few minutes after its onset. Statistically, adult patients who suffer sudden cardiac arrest from ventricular fibrillation or ventricular tachycardia have a better survival rate than those with asphyxial cardiac arrest, largely because rapid defibrillation can correct the dysrhythmia. Conversely, the longer that defibrillation is delayed from the time of cardiac arrest, the lower the chance of survival. The likelihood of survival decreases exponentially as each minute passes and as systemic hypoxia and its metabolic consequences increase. The goal must be to intervene as early as possible and to stop this process in a time frame where organs are still salvageable, and survival is most possible.

Pediatric Cardiac Arrest

Most adult cardiac arrests are sudden and are caused by acute coronary syndrome. Most pediatric cardiac arrests are very different. In infants and children, only about 20 percent of cardiac arrests are caused by sudden dysrhythmias, and very few are caused by blockages of the coronary arteries. In children, cardiac arrests are generally asphyxial in nature. They occur due to prolonged systemic hypoxia as would be caused by choking, shock, or a respiratory problem. Unlike cardiac arrest in adults, which is typically an unexpected and sudden event, in children cardiac arrest is generally a predictable outcome after steady decompensation.

Patient Assessment

Beware! Cardiac arrest causes tunnel vision. Walking into a life-threatening, time-sensitive situation with many interventions to consider can be a stressful event. Situations like these cause our own sympathetic nervous systems to engage in a fight-or-flight response. Part of that natural response is for our body to focus on what it selects as the most immediate threat (in this case, the patient). This can cause what is referred to as *perceptual narrowing*, or tunnel vision. Many providers enter a cardiac arrest situation and focus solely on the patient. However, situational awareness is also important. Before engaging the patient, take a deep breath. Look left and look right. See the whole scene. Make sure what might have killed the patient is not about to kill you or your team. Use that situational awareness to gather scene clues that may help identify an underlying condition or problem that led to the cardiac arrest. Remember that situational awareness, combined with solid team coordination, is necessary to orchestrate the multiple interventions needed to serve the patient best.

Because cardiac arrest care is extremely time-sensitive, it is important to recognize rapidly when the condition has occurred. The primary assessment is uniquely geared toward rapid recognition of cardiac arrest, but it is only useful if applied consistently. The primary assessment quickly identifies the three key features of a cardiac arrest patient:

1. **Unresponsiveness:** Cardiac arrest causes rapid loss of consciousness, so first check for any level of response. This is most commonly done by announcing yourself or calling out the patient's name as you approach the patient. Some patients with diminished levels of consciousness may require a gentle nudge or jostle to respond. If no response is present, be highly suspicious of a cardiac arrest state.
2. ***Apnea*** (absence of breathing): Normal breathing ceases in cardiac arrest states. Use the primary assessment to assess immediately for air movement. Look at the chest and abdomen for predictable rise and fall. If the patient is not breathing, cardiac arrest is likely. In some systems, the combination of apnea and unresponsiveness is enough to assume cardiac arrest and may be indication enough to begin chest compressions. An apneic, unresponsive patient has a high probability of being in cardiac arrest. Watch for agonal breathing. These breaths occur during cardiac arrest and should not be confused with normal breathing. Agonal breaths are typically shallow and irregular, and occur only a few times per minute—or they may not occur at all. Agonal breaths are much slower than normal breaths. Agonal breaths are an indication of cardiac arrest.
3. **Absence of pulse:** In a cardiac arrest state, the pumping heart has failed, and no pulse will be palpable. If indicated, check the carotid pulse for no more than 10 seconds. If no pulse is found, immediately begin chest compressions. Central pulses such as the carotid pulse are more reliable for identifying cardiac arrest than are peripheral pulses (such as the radial pulse). Low blood pressure states can cause peripheral pulses to be lost even though the heart is still pumping.

apnea (Ap-ne-ah) the absence of breathing.

If cardiac arrest is identified, primary assessment stops and chest compressions should be started immediately. In a noncardiac arrest patient, apnea signals the need for airway management and positive pressure ventilations.

Although the steps of the primary assessment are essential, the approach to a cardiac arrest patient is largely established by the view from the door. Both responsiveness and breathing are assessed as you make first contact. Other visual clues, like severe cyanosis or unnatural positioning, may help identify the cardiac arrest state.

Pediatric Note

Pediatric cardiac arrest is recognized by the same key features that identify adult cardiac arrest: responsiveness, breathing, and pulse. In infants and small children, the carotid pulse may be difficult to assess. In these patients, you can palpate a brachial or femoral pulse instead (Figure 21-1).

The indication to start chest compressions must also be slightly adjusted for the pediatric patient. A heart rate less than 60 beats per minute in an infant should be considered nonperfusing and should indicate chest compressions. For older children, use patient assessment to drive the decision to start chest compressions. For example, a 2-year-old who is unconscious and hypotensive with a heart rate of 58 should have ventilations started immediately, and compressions should be begun if the heart rate does not promptly respond to ventilations. On the other hand, an alert 8-year-old with a normal blood pressure and a heart rate of 60 likely does not need immediate intervention.

FIGURE 21-1 To assess the pulse of an infant or small child, check the (A) brachial pulse or (B) femoral pulse in an infant.
(© Daniel Limmer)

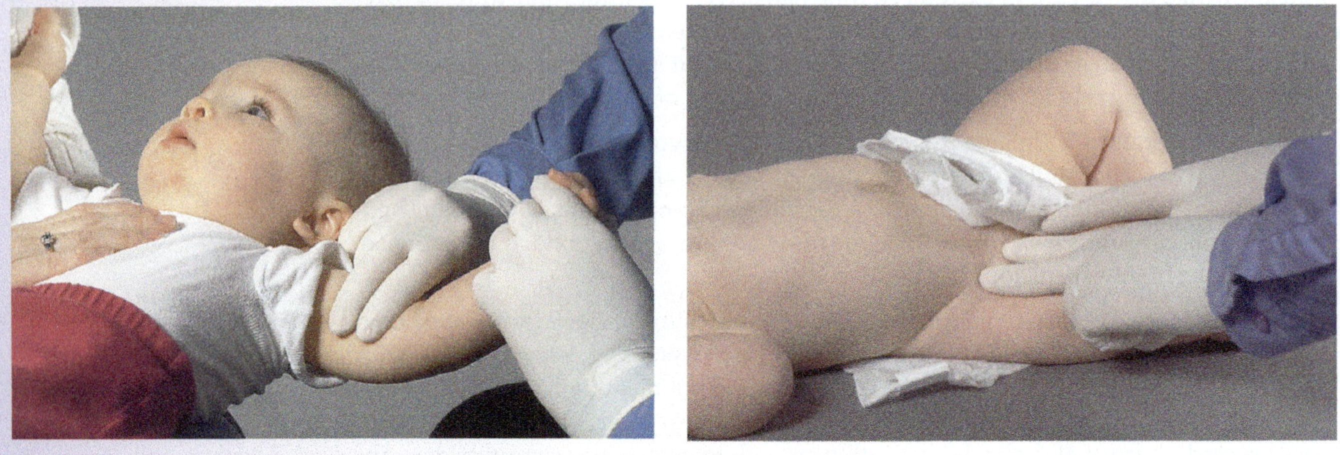

A B

Sudden Unexpected Infant Death Syndrome (SUIDS)

In 2016, there were about 3,600 sudden unexpected infant deaths (SUIDS) in the United States. These deaths occur among infants less than 1 year old and have no immediately obvious cause.

The three commonly reported types of SUIDS are the following:

- Sudden infant death syndrome (SIDS)
- Unknown cause
- Accidental suffocation and strangulation in bed

In 2016, there were about 1,500 deaths due to SIDS, 1,200 deaths due to unknown causes, and about 900 deaths due to accidental suffocation and strangulation in bed. Many possible causes for SUIDS have been investigated but are not well understood. The problem is not caused by external methods of suffocation or by vomiting or choking. The problem may be related to nerve cell development in the brain or the tissue chemistry of the respiratory system or the heart. Some relationships have been drawn to family history of SIDS and respiratory problems, but there is still no accepted reason these babies die.

When asleep, the typical SUIDS patient will show periods of cardiac slowdown and temporary cessation of breathing known as sleep apnea. Eventually the infant will stop breathing and will not start again on its own. Unless the infant is reached in time, the episode will be fatal. The baby's condition is most commonly discovered in the early morning when the parents go to wake the baby.

It is not up to you, as an EMT, to diagnose SUIDS. All you or the parents will know is that the baby is in respiratory or cardiac arrest. You will treat the baby as you would any patient in this condition:

1. Unless there is rigor mortis (stiffening of the body after death) or lividity, a condition in which cardiac arrest causes small capillaries to break down and cause bruising in the lower (dependent) areas of the body, you should provide resuscitation.
2. Be certain that the parents receive emotional support and that they understand that everything possible is being done for the child at the scene and during transport.

CORE CONCEPT
Cardiac arrest and the chain of survival

Parents who lose a child to SUIDS often suffer intense feelings of guilt from the moment they find the child. Whether or not the parents express such guilt, remind them that SUIDS occurs to apparently healthy babies who are receiving the best of parental care. Do not speak with a suspicious tone or ask inappropriate questions. Do not be embarrassed to express your sorrow for their loss. If you are questioning whether you should resuscitate

Think Like an EMT

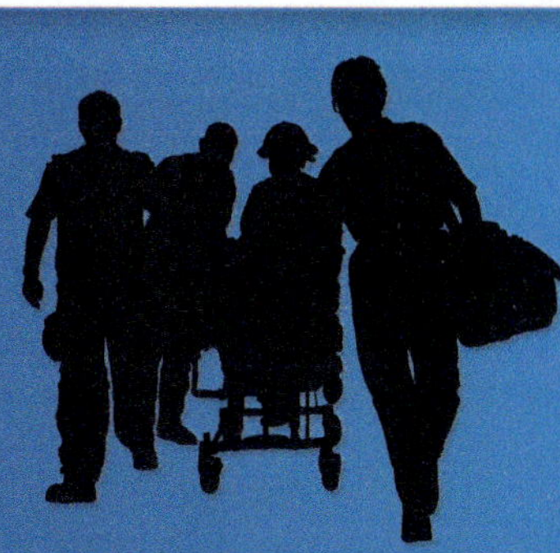

Is My Patient Really in Cardiac Arrest?

Given the previously discussed criteria, decide which of the following patients require immediate chest compressions.

1. A 77-year-old female has a severe exacerbation of COPD. She has been working hard to breathe all evening and has been struggling since you arrived. Approximately 2 minutes ago, she stopped responding to you. She is now breathing slowly at 8 breaths per minute (down from approximately 40 per minute). She is cyanotic but has a carotid pulse of 130.
2. A 1-month-old female is found in her crib. She is not breathing and not responsive. Your assessment also notes rigor in her extremities and dependent lividity on her back.
3. An 8-month-old female has had severe respiratory distress due to bronchiolitis for 24 hours. You've noticed over the past 30 seconds that her breathing has slowed and now has stopped. She is cyanotic and not moving. You get no response when you shake her gently. Your partner cannot feel a brachial pulse.

the baby or not, always resuscitate. It is better to resuscitate when it isn't necessary than to fail to resuscitate when it is.

Improving Cardiac Arrest Survival

One of the mantras of Seattle's Resuscitation Academy is "It takes a system to save a victim." This mantra represents the idea that survival in cardiac arrest is not the result of a single intervention or a medication, but rather the sum total of many different but coordinated functions dedicated to offer that patient the best chance for life. In EMS, it is easy to get hyperfocused on a specific step such as chest compressions or defibrillation, but it is truly more important to see the value of a systems-based approach. High-performing systems incorporate bystander CPR; the distribution of public access to automatic external defibrillators; dispatcher training and prearrival instructions; response procedures; and quality measured resuscitation steps to build a systems approach to survival. Each element is held in equal value and resources are dedicated to all. Although you may be just starting your EMS career and therefore not yet participating in system-level planning, it is never too early to understand this big picture.

Chain of Survival

The American Heart Association has summarized the most important factors that affect survival of cardiac arrest patients in its chain-of-survival concept. The chain has five elements: (1) recognition and activation of the emergency response system, (2) immediate high-quality CPR, (3) rapid defibrillation, (4) basic and advanced emergency medical services, and (5) advanced life support and postarrest care. These steps reflect the systems approach to survival outlined above. An EMS system where each of these links is strong is much more likely to resuscitate a cardiac arrest patient than a system with weaknesses anywhere along the chain.

An underlying theme of the chain of survival is teamwork. Although many of the actions you should take to resuscitate someone are described as though you are alone or working with very little help, you will usually have at least one other person, if not more, to work with you. It is essential that you and your teammates work together in a coordinated fashion to maximize the chance of your patient's survival. The need for teamwork also extends to others beyond the first ambulance crew at the scene, including bystanders, ALS teams, emergency medical responders, public safety officers, emergency department physicians and staff, and cardiac catheterization lab staff. High-quality resuscitation efforts involve a choreographed approach. Resuscitation teams should work together like a race car pit crew to deliver high-quality interventions and to maximize survival. High-quality teams develop and practice resuscitation strategies before the call. They utilize incident command procedures and practice efficient communication skills. During CPR, providers position themselves for maximum efficiency and minimum interruption of chest compressions. In high-performance resuscitation, different scopes of practice and certification work hand in hand to optimize team performance. As an EMT, you could be a team leader with a paramedic reporting to you. You might also be a team member delivering chest compressions or managing an airway.

High-performance resuscitation requires many interventions to be accomplished at once. There must be coordination for these combined activities to work in the patient's favor. Having clear expectations that everyone is aware of goes a long way toward achieving that goal. This will allow simple things such as primary assessment to be more efficient, as one person checks the pulse and another gets equipment ready and positioned properly. It also facilitates complex activities such as getting the patient to the cardiac catheterization lab at the right time, so the appropriate people are present and prepared. Often this team coordination is a planned and practiced event. But even in situations where teams are thrown together at the time of the response, quality leadership and communication will improve outcomes.

Link One: Recognition and Activation of the Emergency Response System

When cardiac arrest occurs, a race against the clock begins. As discussed previously, the likelihood of survival decreases as every second passes. To optimize survival, resuscitation must begin immediately after primary assessment. As EMTs, we typically think of driving fast and getting compressions started immediately, but to optimize survival, efforts must begin even before that.

The challenge in most EMS systems is that our response times are relatively fixed. On average it takes 8–10 minutes (and in many cases much more time) for an ambulance to arrive at the side of a patient. Without efforts starting before our arrival, our interventions begin in most cases outside of that narrow window of cardiac arrest survivability. From a systems approach, that means we need to train citizens, family members, and bystanders to recognize cardiac arrest, and to activate and begin resuscitation prior to the arrival of EMS. Key points within this link include teaching those who witness someone collapse or find someone unresponsive to call emergency medical services quickly. Of equal importance is the training of emergency medical dispatchers to recognize potential cardiac arrest situations and help bystanders to initiate chest compressions. This is commonly referred to as dispatcher-aided CPR or pre-arrival instructions. It does not matter whose hands are providing those chest compressions. Bystanders initiating resuscitation efforts alone or prodded by a dispatcher offer a key mechanism to stop that ticking clock and expand the window of survival.

Point of View

"Vern collapsed and I didn't know what to do. It was so sudden. I called 911. The minutes till they arrived seemed like forever. One of the EMTs came to me and explained what was going on. The CPR and the shocks were so forceful! I may never totally understand it, but I have Vern back with me now and I owe it all to them."

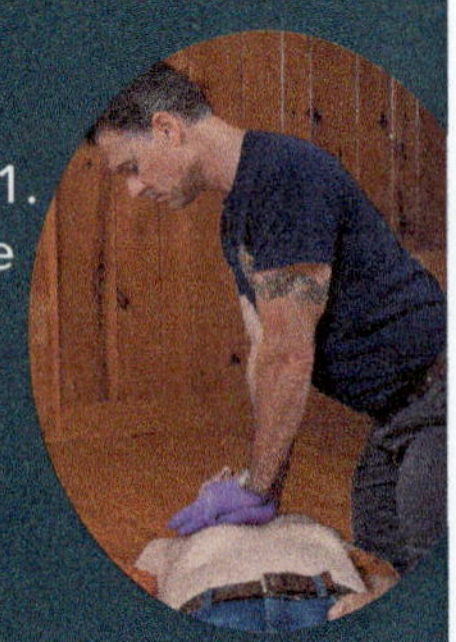

EMTs play a vital role in this link. Many services offer public CPR training, and many collaborate with dispatch to enhance services. Even simple public service messages regarding recognition of cardiac arrest help enhance these capabilities. Although we tend to dismiss these nonclinical interventions, they are no less important and sometimes more important than the more commonly practiced steps of resuscitation.

Link Two: Immediate High-Quality CPR

In cardiac arrest, the cardiovascular system comes to a standstill, and cells starve for oxygenated blood. With every passing minute, vulnerable organs and organ systems are damaged and die. ***Cardiopulmonary resuscitation (CPR)*** counteracts this process. Chest compressions, when completed effectively, mimic the effects of the heart and move blood through the cardiovascular system. The provider of those chest compressions becomes an external pump for the body. With attention to detail, quality compressions can replace roughly 20 percent to 25 percent of cardiovascular function. Although certainly less than normal, this limited blood flow may be enough to support the very low metabolic usage of a patient in cardiac arrest, getting blood flow to the brain and to the muscle of the heart itself. These pressures are commonly referred to as *cerebral* and *coronary perfusion pressures;* in animal models, they are accurate predictors of successful resuscitation. In other words, if our efforts can sustain even diminished blood pressure and flow to the brain and the heart, the chance of survival increases.

cardiopulmonary resuscitation (CPR) actions taken to revive a person by keeping the person's heart and lungs working.

All CPR is not alike. To reach acceptable cerebral and coronary perfusion pressures, we must pay attention to the details of our resuscitative efforts. The following are key elements of quality CPR:

- **Hand placement:** For all patients, the point of compression should be the lower third of the patient's sternum. For adults, the rescuer should place the heel of one hand on the center of the victim's chest (which is the lower half of the sternum) and the heel of the other hand on top of the first so that the hands are overlapped and parallel. For a child, the hand position remains the same, but the second, overlapping hand may not be necessary to compress to a proper depth. For an infant, a lone provider should use the two-finger chest compression technique. Here, two fingers are placed over the lower half of the infant's sternum. The two-thumb encircling hands technique (Figure 21-2) is recommended when CPR is provided by two rescuers. Encircle the infant's chest with both hands; spread your fingers around the thorax, and place your thumbs together over the lower half of the sternum.

FIGURE 21-2 (A) Two-finger technique for infant chest compressions. (B) Two-thumb encircling technique for infant chest compressions.

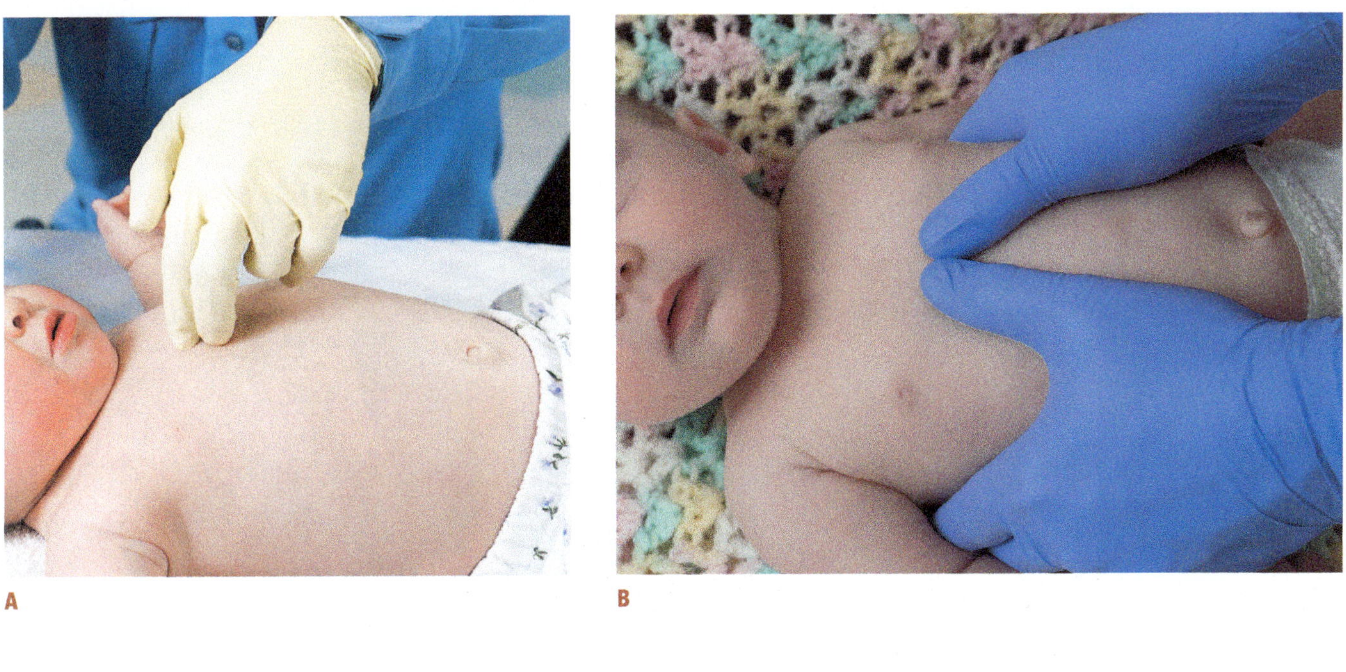

A

B

- **Compression depth:** Chest compressions facilitate the movement of blood in the cardiovascular system in two ways. First, the compression itself increases pressure within the chest and essentially squeezes blood out of the heart and lungs. To complete this function, the depth of compression must be sufficient. Secondly, the full recoil of the chest creates a negative pressure inside the chest that draws blood back into the heart, priming the pump for the next squeeze. To accomplish this, the compressor must allow the chest to completely recoil without leaning on the chest following compression. For adults, rescuers should compress to a depth of at least 2 inches (5 cm) and then allow an equal amount of time for the chest to recoil. For infants and children (until puberty), rescuers should compress at least one-third the anterior–posterior diameter of the chest. This equates to approximately 1.5 inches (3.8 cm) in infants and 2 inches (5 cm) in children. The quality of compressions is improved by good CPR form. If two hands are used, hands should overlap with interlocked fingers. Elbows should be locked, and the weight of the shoulders should drive the compression. The pivot point should be at the waist, not the elbows. (See Figure 21-3.) Remember that even after 1 minute of chest compressions, rescuers commonly fatigue, decreasing the quality and depth of compressions. For this reason, no rescuer should compress for longer than 2 minutes, if avoidable, and a team leader should offer continuous feedback on performance. Many cardiac monitor defibrillators offer feedback on rate and depth of compression. When available, these devices should be used to ensure quality. When possible, compressions should be performed with the patient laying supine on a firm surface to facilitate proper chest wall movement. Soft, cushiony surfaces give way when compressed, limiting the pressure changes and movement of blood.
- **Compression rate:** When performing CPR, consider how the heart works. It creates pressure in the cardiovascular system not with one pump but through the many contractions per minute it generates. It does not pause. In fact, if the heart did pause, even for a matter of seconds, a healthy person would immediately feel the effects. When doing CPR, we must mirror the habits of a healthy heart. Remember that adequate cerebral and coronary perfusion pressures are generated through a consistent and appropriate rate of compressions. Remember also that every pause in compressions drops those pressures to an inadequate level, and a series of compressions must be used to regain them. High-performance CPR pays specific attention to sustaining an appropriate rate. For infants, children, and adults, the chest should be compressed at a rate of 100–120 compressions per minute. Again, quality should be ensured either by a team leader or via an external feedback device. Compressing too slowly does not generate adequate cerebral and coronary perfusion pressure. Compressing too rapidly does not allow the heart adequate time to fill with blood.

FIGURE 21-3 Proper CPR form.

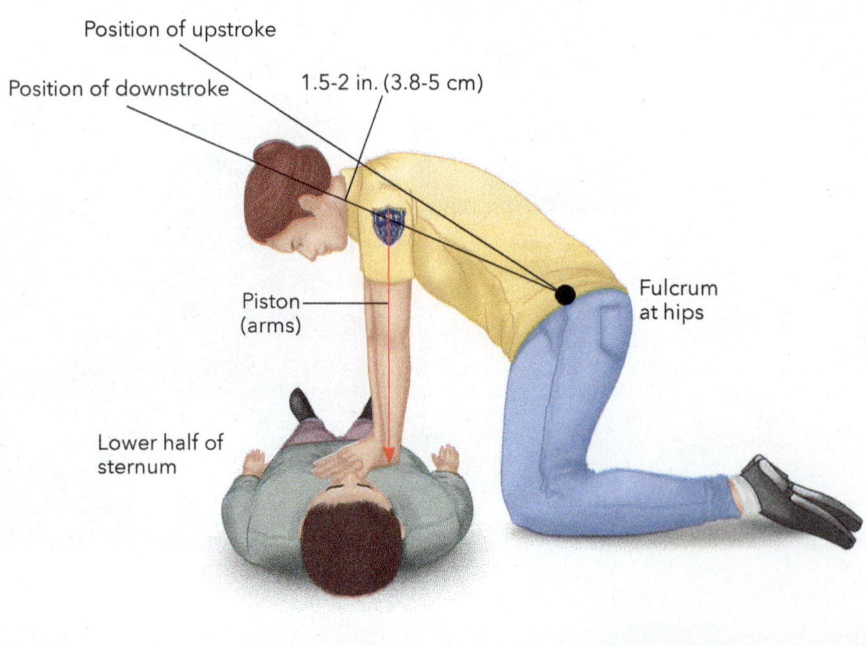

- **Minimizing pauses in compressions:** High-quality CPR also means minimizing pauses in compressions. As just described, any pause in chest compressions drops cerebral and coronary perfusion pressure. This means that during the pause, the brain and heart are not receiving oxygenated blood. Research has shown a clear link between the length and number of pauses and patient survival. Even counting pauses by the second, the more we pause, the less likely it is that resuscitation will be successful. To that end, many systems use a term called ***compression fraction*** to measure the quality of CPR. Compression fraction measures the amount of time chest compressions were performed compared with the total amount of time rescuers were on scene. High-performance systems aim for compression fractions above 90 percent and take active steps to avoid pausing chest compressions. These steps include:
    - Initiating chest compressions immediately upon arrival. Unless there is an immediate danger or an inability to perform the actual skill, chest compressions should start where the patient lies.
    - Clearing rescuers during the automated external defibrillator analysis phase and not delaying shocks for additional clearing. (Defibrillation steps will be discussed in greater detail later in this chapter.)
    - Preplanning and practicing compressor change-out to avoid unnecessary delays of chest compressions.
    - Minimizing the urgency of transport in the initial phases of the resuscitation. If chest compressions and defibrillation are ongoing, the team should stay in place to complete these vital steps. Transport should occur only after the initial interventions have been performed and only if those interventions are unsuccessful.
    - Training as a team, including ALS providers, in realistic situations to identify errors and improve performance.
    - Training with the tools of resuscitation, especially mechanical CPR devices, to prevent unnecessary delays associated with unfamiliar use.

compression fraction
the amount of time chest compressions are being performed compared with the total time of patient contact.

- **Rescue breathing:** In most cases, chest compressions are paired with rescue breathing. In cardiopulmonary resuscitation, *cardio-* refers to chest compressions and *-pulmonary* refers to the lungs. American Heart Association guidelines suggest that compressions should be started immediately upon recognition of the cardiac arrest, but then ventilations should be integrated at a ratio of 2 ventilations to 30 compressions. In pediatric patients, if two rescuers are present, this ratio can be adjusted to 2:15. Scan 21-1 describes high-performance CPR.

SCAN 21-1 High-Performance CPR

First Take Standard Precautions.

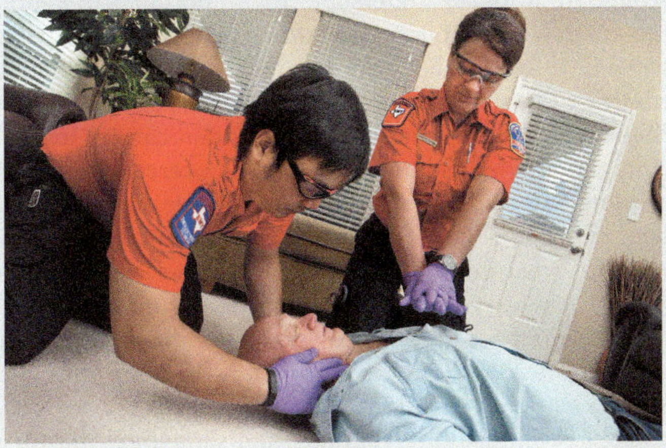

1. EMT 1 checks pulse while EMT 2 hovers, hands ready to start CPR.

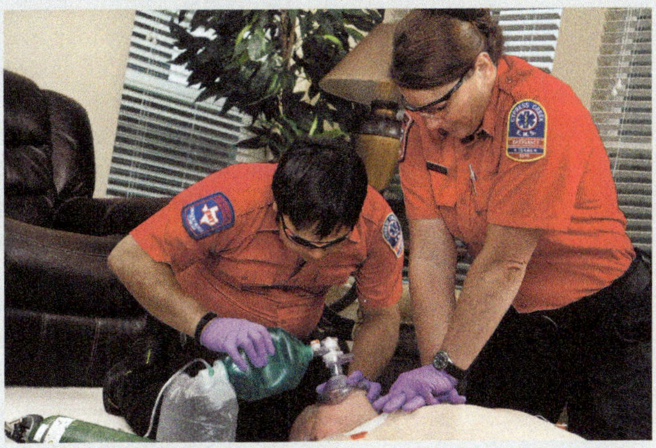

2. EMT 1 provides bag-valve-mask ventilation while EMT 2 performs chest compressions.

(continued)

SCAN 21-1 High-Performance CPR *(continued)*

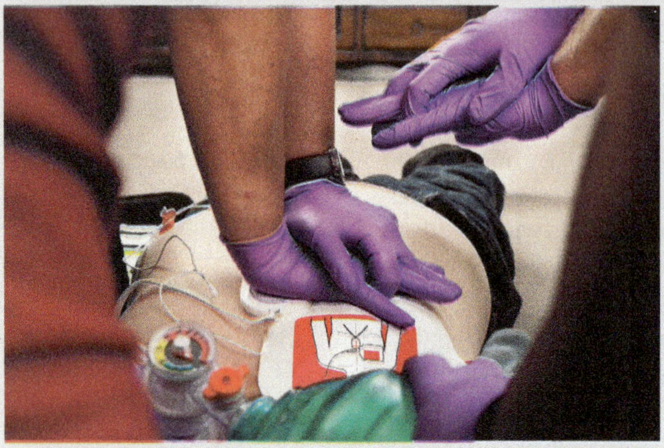

3. EMT 1 continues bag-valve-mask ventilation. EMT 2 continues CPR as EMT 3 hovers, hands ready to spell EMT 2 with chest compressions.

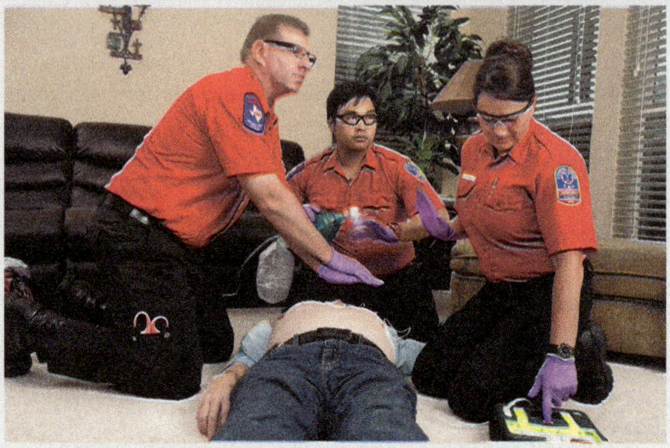

4. Once the AED is applied, EMTs suspend ventilation and chest compressions while AED analyzes the rhythm. Providers should clear the patient in this phase, in preparation for the shock to be delivered.

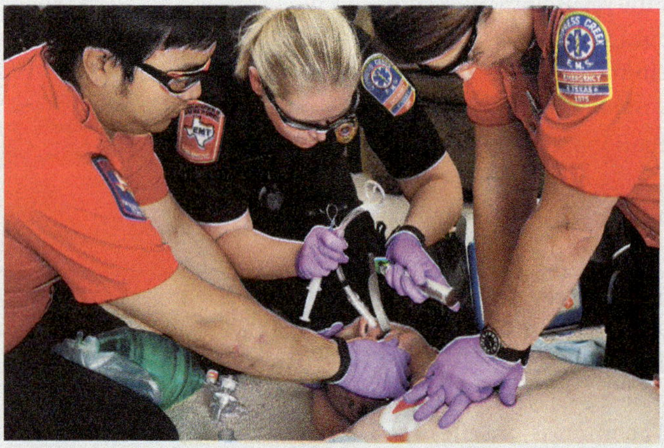

5. Advanced life support (ALS) arrives and establishes an airway.

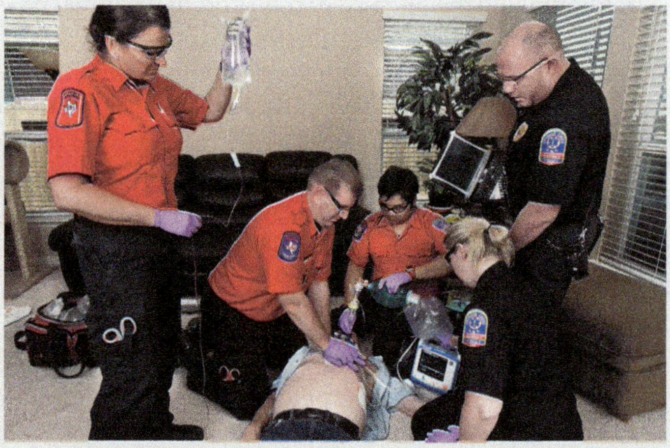

6. ALS and EMTs work as a team.

As an EMT, you will generally deliver CPR that follows the standards of the American Heart Association. Research is ongoing to better understand the importance of ventilation in CPR. Rapidly evolving research has led to local variations in how the ventilation component of CPR is done in some EMS system. For example, we know that ventilations should always play a role in pediatric CPR, since the most common cause of cardiac arrest is hypoxia. The need for ventilations in adults suffering from sudden cardiac arrest is less clear. Some systems have integrated what is referred to as cardiocerebral resuscitation and removed the need for immediate ventilations. Their arguments suggest that in sudden cardiac arrest, the patient is not hypoxic, and the most important need is chest compressions to support circulation. Breathing interrupts compressions and therefore could disrupt that most vital goal. In these systems, rescuers provide continuous chest compressions (most commonly for the first 5 minutes) and delay providing ventilations. Some systems apply a nonrebreather mask to allow for passive oxygenation caused by changing pressures in the chest. The evidence is still unclear. It is true that systems that utilize cardiocerebral resuscitation have similar survival rates (and sometimes improved survival rates) compared with those for traditional systems, but there is not yet enough evidence to make a conclusive decision on which method is better. Other systems have integrated what are referred to as "asynchronous ventilations," which means they deliver

FIGURE 21-4 Mechanical CPR device–the Physio Control LUCAS™ device. (A) LUCAS™ device on patient. (B) Close-up of controls.

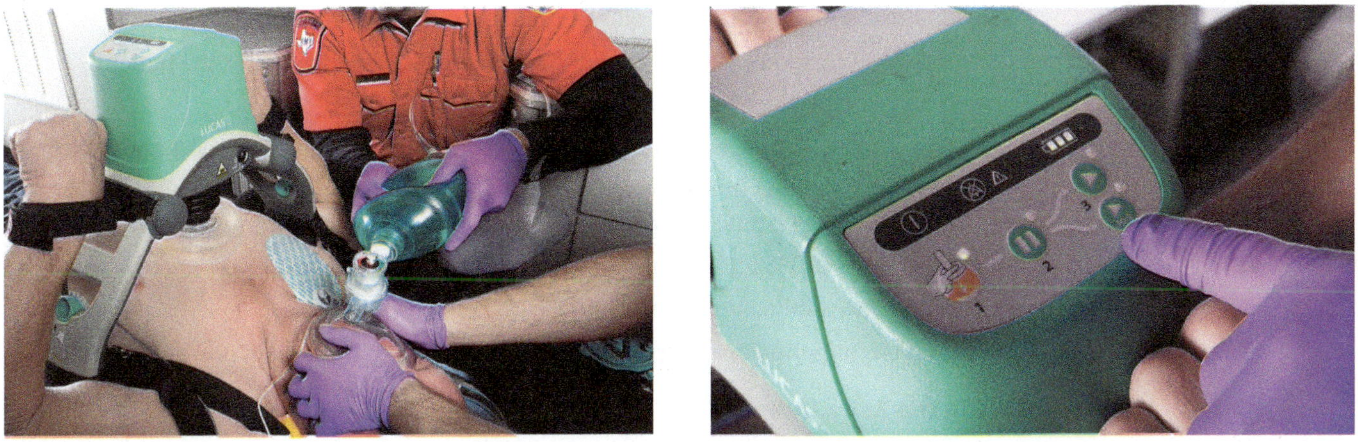

A B

relatively low-volume ventilations without interrupting compressions. Most commonly, an asynchronous ventilation approach would deliver a gentle ventilation every 10 compressions without a specific pause for a breath. What we know for sure is that the science of CPR is rapidly evolving. Always follow your local protocols, but be aware that what you are taught today about CPR may change in the future.

Mechanical CPR Devices. Some EMS systems utilize mechanical CPR devices. Machines like the Physio Control LUCAS™ (Figure 21-4) or the Zoll AutoPulse™ (Figure 21-5) deliver chest compressions at a preprogrammed rate. These devices commonly use a battery or a compressed gas, like oxygen, to power compressions. The advantages of a mechanical CPR device include consistency of rate and depth and the fact that the machine never tires. These devices can provide great assistance in situations where human resources are scarce. Disadvantages of these mechanical devices include a significant training curve and potential delays in chest compressions while the device is being set up. Research as to the effectiveness of these devices as compared with that of manual chest compressions is still inconclusive. It is reasonable to believe that they are not less effective than human-delivered compressions, but little evidence supports their necessarily being better. More research is needed. In the meantime, follow local protocols.

The following text shows how the devices would be worked into a typical cardiac arrest situation.

FIGURE 21-5 (A) The Zoll AutoPulse™ device on a patient. (B) The control panel.

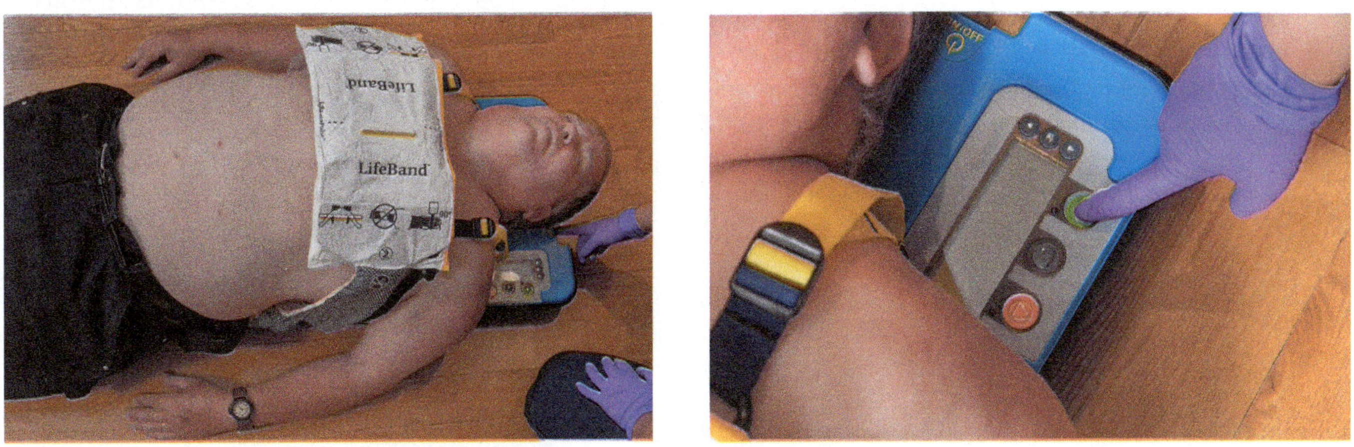

A B

Using the LUCAS™ CPR Device.

- Take Standard Precautions.
- Ensure CPR is in progress and effective.
- Stop CPR just long enough to put the LUCAS™ base plate under the patient.
- Attach the LUCAS™ upper part and restart CPR.
- Position the suction cup so the lower edge is just above the lower end of the sternum.
- With the machine in the "Adjust" mode, position the pressure pad so it touches the chest without putting any pressure on it.
- Push the "ACTIVE (Continuous)" or "ACTIVE (30:2)" button to start compressions.
- Apply the stabilization strap before moving the patient.
- Upon termination of arrest or return of spontaneous circulation, power down the unit.

Using the Zoll AutoPulse™.

- Take Standard Precautions.
- Ensure CPR is in progress and effective.
- Align the patient on the AutoPulse™ platform.
- Close the Lifeband™ chest band over the patient's chest.
- Press Start. (AutoPulse™ is designed to do the compressions automatically.)
- Provide bag–mask ventilation at a rate of 2 ventilations for every 30 compressions. Each ventilation should be given over 1 second to provide visible chest rise.
- If an advanced airway is in place (ETT, LMA, or Combitube), there are no longer cycles of compressions to ventilations. The compression rate is a continuous 100 per minute, and the ventilation rate is 8–10 per minute.
- After 2 minutes of CPR, reassess for shockable rhythm.

Link Three: Rapid Defibrillation

CORE CONCEPT
Use of mechanical cardiopulmonary resuscitation (CPR) devices

Chest compressions maintain a minimal amount of cardiovascular pressure and can preserve vital organs in a cardiac arrest state. They are essential to a successful resuscitation, but they rarely can save a patient alone. To achieve a successful resuscitation, the heart must begin pumping again. To make this happen, the life-threatening dysrhythmia must be corrected. An automated external defibrillator (AED) is used to address this problem.

An AED (Figure 21-6) is really two devices in one. First, it is a sensor. It uses electrodes connected to the patient's chest to sense and recognize specific cardiac dysrhythmias. AEDs are designed to recognize ventricular fibrillation and ventricular tachycardia, and they are very good at doing just that. In fact, an average AED has an accuracy greater than 95 percent in detecting and differentiating those rhythms. That means that it very rarely will miss a dysrhythmia it has been programmed to detect, and the odds of its mistaking an interpretation (for example, confusing a nonarrest rhythm for one that requires defibrillation) are

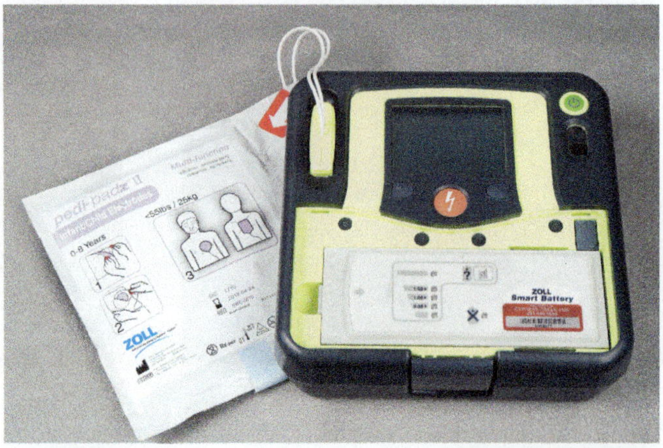

FIGURE 21-6 AED (shown with pediatric pads).

astronomically low. The second role of an AED is defibrillation. When it finds ventricular fibrillation or ventricular tachycardia, it will offer the ability to transfer energy from its battery and discharge that energy out through the electrodes and into the patient. This is very important because this energy is used to stop life-threatening dysrhythmias.

In the chapter *Cardiac Emergencies*, you learned that dysrhythmias occur when the electrical conduction of the heart is disturbed. Normally, heart cells generate their own energy and transfer that energy from cell to cell to stimulate mechanical contraction. A dysrhythmia occurs when this precise conduction is disturbed. In the *Cardiac Emergencies* chapter, you also learned that dysrhythmias in the ventricles, like ventricular fibrillation or ventricular tachycardia, are life-threatening because they cause a failure of those large sections of the heart to pump. Defibrillation interrupts dysrhythmias by introducing an external electrical charge. Energy is transferred from one AED electrode to the other and therefore passes the energy through the heart. When this electricity travels through the heart, it depolarizes the heart cells it touches. Depolarization briefly interrupts the heart cells' own electrical function and resets them. The goal of defibrillation therefore is to introduce external energy to enough heart cells to cause a global resetting of electrical function in the organ itself. The dysrhythmia represents incorrect electrical function. Defibrillation briefly pauses that function and requires conduction to then restart. If the intervention works properly, that restart will cause normal electrical function in the heart to resume. In many ways, defibrillation is like restarting your computer when an error occurs. By pressing the "Off" button, you interrupt the problem that has occurred, and the global reset hopefully restores normal function. Unfortunately, defibrillation doesn't always work.

Two rhythms other than ventricular fibrillation and ventricular tachycardia can cause cardiac arrest. *Asystole*, the absence of electrical activity, can cause the heart to stop pumping. *Pulseless electrical activity* (PEA), which is normal electrical activity without a mechanical response, can cause a similar failure. Unfortunately, defibrillation cannot be used in these dysrhythmias. In asystole, there is no electrical distribution to reset, and PEA is not caused by an electrical problem, so defibrillation is equally useless. In these cases, an AED will fail to identify its main targets of ventricular fibrillation and ventricular tachycardia, and will simply offer a "No shock advised" message. The patient will still be in cardiac arrest, just not a candidate for defibrillation. Luckily, nonshockable dysrhythmias are found in less than 15 percent of cardiac arrest patients (although they are found at a higher rate in pediatric patients). When defibrillation is not indicated, your efforts must focus on quality chest compressions in the hope that increased blood flow to the heart muscle might create a shockable situation at the next analysis. (The sequence of resuscitation will be discussed in detail later in the chapter.)

Defibrillation can be delivered through an AED, as described above, but it can also be delivered manually. Paramedics and physicians frequently use cardiac monitor/defibrillators to visually identify a dysrhythmia and choose to deliver a shock. This is referred to as *manual defibrillation*. For most EMTs, however, defibrillation will come from an AED. Don't worry, though; AEDs are, in most cases, just as efficient.

Defibrillation is also classified by the type of shock delivered. A *monophasic* defibrillator sends a single shock (this is what *monophasic* means) from the negative pad to the positive pad. A *biphasic* defibrillator sends the shock first in one direction then the other.

When considering the global approach to a cardiac arrest, access to defibrillation is an extremely high priority. In fact, the vast majority of saves come from the combination of early, quality CPR and rapid defibrillation. With the chain of survival in mind, it should be your goal to deliver a defibrillator to any cardiac arrest patient as soon as possible. Although we typically associate defibrillators with emergency medical services, remember that public-access AEDs are an equally important component in this link. AEDs now are distributed in malls, airports, schools, and many other public places (Figure 21-7). These public-access devices offer a vital opportunity to decrease the time it takes for defibrillation to reach a patient. EMS services should support and promote the distribution of AEDs in their communities as a core factor in improving cardiac arrest survival. In addition to true public-access defibrillators, AEDs are distributed to police departments, fire departments, and other municipal services. These devices also enhance the systemwide response capability and should be supported and fostered by EMS.

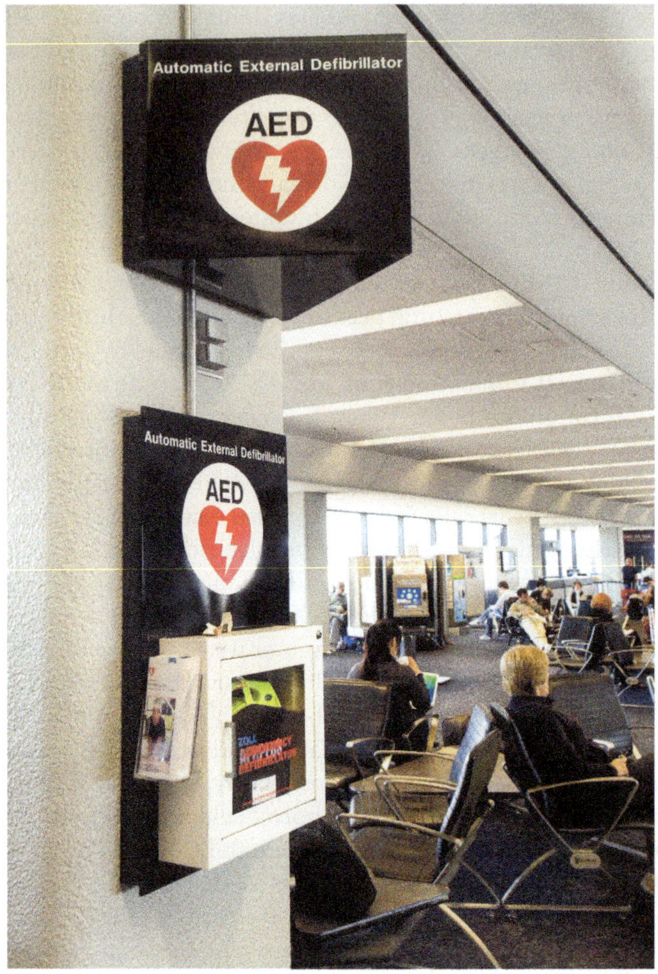

FIGURE 21-7 Public-access defibrillator.

CORE CONCEPT
Use of an automated external defibrillator (AED)

Keep in mind the ticking clock. For every second that passes without defibrillation, survival odds decrease. We will soon discuss the sequence of interventions in cardiac arrest, but for now, keep in mind that every patient in cardiac arrest requires an AED as soon as possible.

Link Four: Basic and Advanced Life Support

Emergency medical services (EMS) supplies the basic and advanced life support link in the chain of survival. So far, we have discussed early activation, quality CPR, and rapid defibrillation, and hopefully by now you can see how EMS integrates with the role of bystanders, dispatchers, and other first responders. Although we tend to focus on our own resuscitation efforts, it is important to remember the importance of the larger, systemwide approach.

Basic life support, in the form of quality compressions and rapid defibrillation, is truly the key to cardiac arrest survival. This care begins with bystanders, and is enhanced by first responders, but truly lives with EMTs. As the saying goes, "EMTs own CPR," and it is absolutely true that, for a cardiac arrest patient, few other interventions matter. To that end, EMTs should take pride that the care they deliver is the most meaningful care, and should develop capabilities to provide those interventions with the highest quality.

But quality cardiac arrest care is a team effort. Team leaders foster teamwork and ensure quality, EMTs manage basic life support, and AEMTs and paramedics provide advanced procedures and medications. Although the most important focus should be on the delivery of compressions and defibrillation, the best outcomes occur when each level works as part of the larger team.

High-performing teams practice their roles in cardiac arrest. Many teams have predetermined roles for each provider and communicate those expectations prior to beginning the resuscitation. Some departments utilize checklists in which the team leader can fill positions as resources become available. The "triangle of life" (see Figure 21-8) is a

FIGURE 21-8 Predetermined cardiac arrest roles–the "triangle of life." *(Adapted from Austin/ Travis County Medical Director.)*

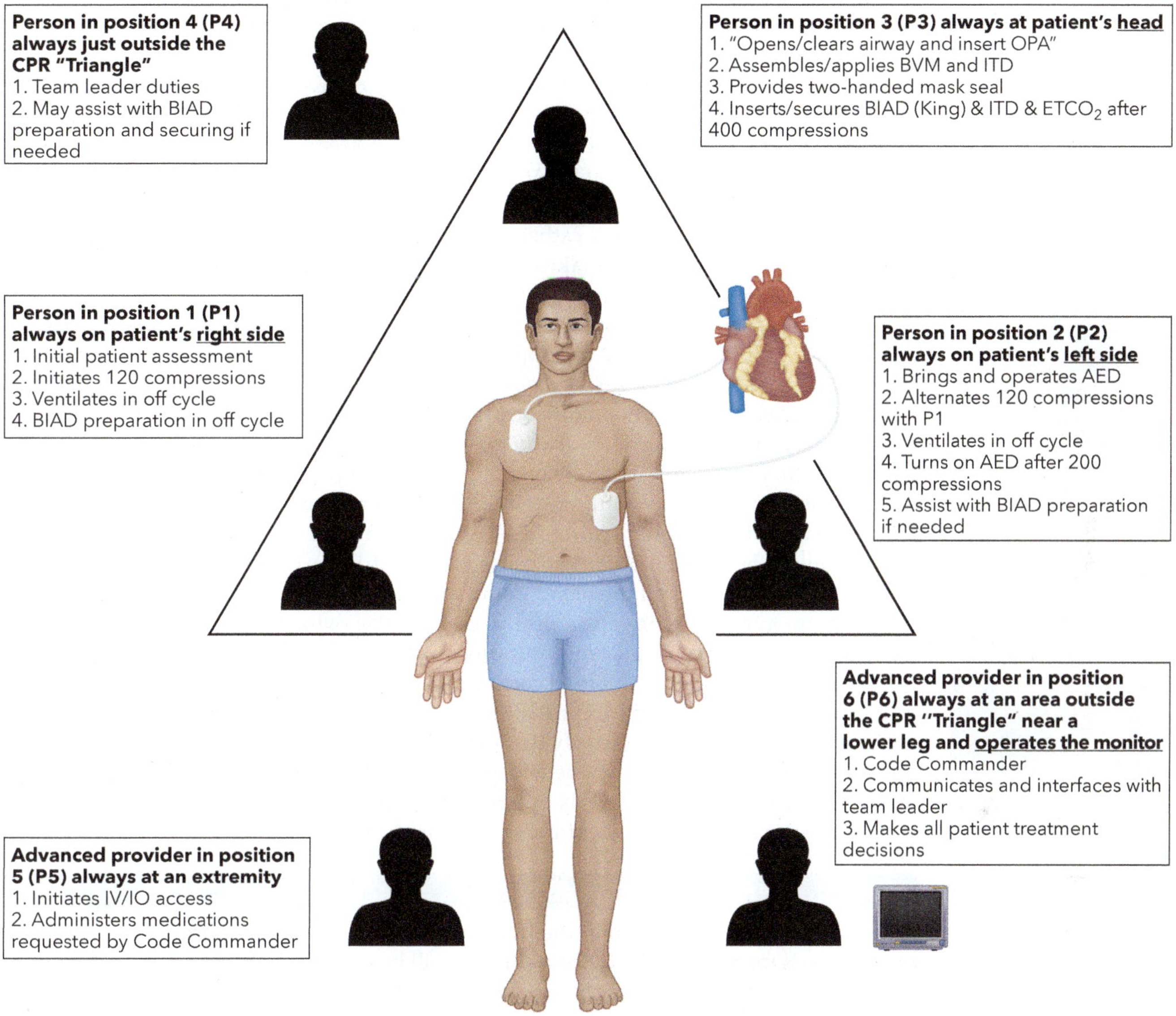

commonly used term; the triangle represents the first three providers attending the patient. On either side of the patient, one provider delivers compressions and the other attaches the AED. At the head of the patient, the third provider manages the airway and delivers ventilations. As additional providers enter the scene, the team leader may add advanced life support outside the triangle to obtain venous access and deliver medication, or rotate another provider in to perform chest compressions or assist with bag–mask ventilation.

Not every response situation can be preplanned. However, it is important to remember that organization and attention to detail contribute to overall survival.

Link Five: Advanced Life Support and Postarrest Care

Integrated postarrest care means coordinating numerous different means of assessment and interventions that, together, maximize the patient's chance of neurologically intact survival. Perhaps the most important step is to first recognize that a ***return of spontaneous circulation (ROSC)*** has occurred. ROSC occurs when the heart begins to beat on its own again. Most commonly, this is recognized by a patient's starting to breathe. Spontaneous breathing can be identified by visualizing regular, predictable movement of the chest. Less commonly, the patient may regain partial or complete mental status. Sometimes this is indicated by verbalizations, but it can also be demonstrated by purposeful movements. There have been numerous case reports of patients regaining some measure of consciousness

return of spontaneous circulation (ROSC) the heart beating again after successful resuscitation.

"The first time I did CPR, I was nervous—very nervous. But it really does come down to just doing it—and doing it right. Pump hard. Pump fast. Don't stop."

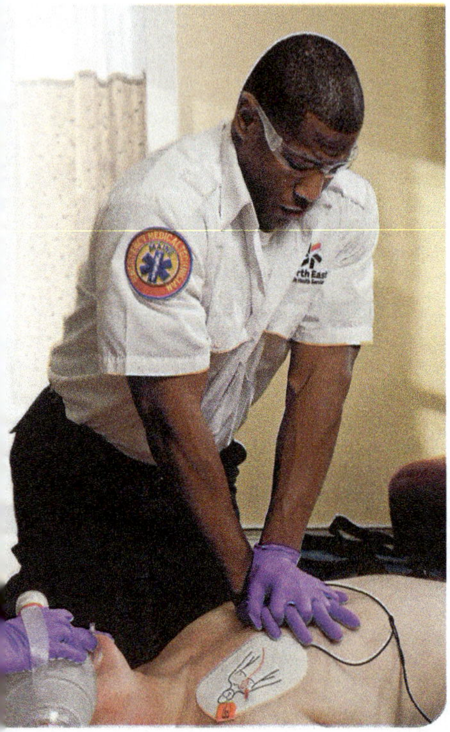
(© Daniel Limmer)

CORE CONCEPT
Management of a cardiac arrest patient

because of quality CPR. The return of a pulse is, of course, an indicator of circulation, but beware; pulse checks are notoriously unreliable. Even experienced health care providers are prone to thinking a pulse is present when it is not. Always err on the side of continuing resuscitation if in doubt.

If ROSC can be confirmed, care must shift from a cardiac arrest mode to a postarrest model. Remember that you may have resolved the most immediate life threat, but the underlying cause of the original arrest is likely still present. For most adult patients, this cause is acute coronary syndrome. As such, a key postarrest priority will be to initiate immediate transport to an appropriate receiving hospital. Some systems direct postarrest patients to hospitals with cardiac catheterization capabilities. Always follow local protocol.

Advanced life support care takes a higher priority in postarrest care. Management of the airway, blood pressure, and carefully controlled ventilation are key concerns. If ALS is not on scene, now is the time to seek them out. Advanced airway procedures and medications may be necessary to support the resuscitated patient. When managing the airway prior to ALS arrival, keep in mind the urgent need to keep air moving. Even brief hypoxia increases the likelihood of rearrest and death. Be aggressive in clearing potential obstructions, and ensure proper airway positioning. As patients regain consciousness, be aware that they can begin to choke on adjuncts used during resuscitation. Have suction ready. If the patient is not breathing, deliver positive pressure ventilations at a normal rate (10–12 breaths/minute for adults and 12–20 breaths/minute for children). Take care not to hyperventilate. Hyperventilation can cause vasoconstriction of cerebral blood vessels, and postarrest patients need all the blood going to their brain that they can get. If the patient is breathing, guard the airway carefully. Use a pulse oximeter to titrate supplemental oxygen to reach at least 95 percent saturation, but if the pulse oximeter is not available or is inaccurate, err on the side of high concentrations of oxygen.

In many systems, it may be important to obtain a 12-lead ECG on postarrest patients. In this case, the ECG may help identify that patient whose arrest was caused by a myocardial infarction. As an EMT, you may be allowed to complete that skill yourself and transmit the results; you may facilitate this by arranging for advanced life support intercept; or you may assist the ALS provider in obtaining the 12-lead ECG.

Management of Cardiac Arrest

EMTs own CPR! Remember that the interventions you can provide are exactly what the patient needs for a successful outcome. There will be no one on this scene more important than you. That said, resuscitation success is maximized by an application of the chain of survival. As we discuss the steps of resuscitation, it is important to keep this team approach in mind.

The rest of this chapter will emphasize the actual steps you must take to provide resuscitation. Specific emphasis will be given to the role of defibrillation and high-performance CPR. Managing a patient in cardiac arrest means you need to be able to:

- Perform one-rescuer and team-based CPR.
- Administer defibrillation with an AED.
- Take Standard Precautions to protect yourself (and patients).
- Use an automated external defibrillator.
- Request advanced life support (ALS) (when available) to continue the chain of survival.
- Use a bag–valve–mask device with oxygen.
- Lift and move patients.
- Suction a patient's airway.
- Use airway adjuncts (oropharyngeal and nasopharyngeal airways).
- Interview bystanders and family members to obtain facts related to the arrest.

Remember that stress causes tunnel vision. This can be counteracted by simply looking left and right and taking time to see the entire scene. Good communication with team members also helps defeat this perceptual narrowing.

A Coordinated Resuscitation Team

High-performance resuscitation is the sum of excellent teamwork. As the chain of survival suggests, it requires multiple interventions to be coordinated into a single purpose and works best when teamwork is emphasized. Consider the need for additional resources early. High-quality CPR requires providers to switch roles as compressors to avoid fatigue. Take time immediately to be sure you have appropriate personnel on hand. High-performance resuscitation also integrates both BLS and ALS care. It may be appropriate to ensure that ALS resources are on the way.

As you begin the resuscitation, consider how best to facilitate the teamwork necessary to achieve high-performance results. Not every situation will have a well-practiced, highly coordinated response, but there are measures that can improve teamwork even in unpracticed situations.

If possible, a team leader should be assigned immediately. The job of the team leader is to control quality for the resuscitation team. Typically, a team leader assigns roles, provides timing (such as when to switch chest compressors), and offers performance feedback. Some systems utilize CPR checklists that the team leader can use to manage team performance better. (See Figure 21-9.)

If naming a team leader is not possible, coordinate the actions of the team using a preresuscitation huddle. Take just a moment to verbally express the desired outcome (uninterrupted compressions and early defibrillation, for example) and ensure that all those involved know what job they are doing. Consider the following example:

Madi and Shannon staff an EMT ambulance dispatched to a "man down" call. Dispatchers note that ALS and fire units have been dispatched and that pre-arrival CPR instructions are in progress. As they arrive on scene, a police unit joins them. Although Madi and Shannon have never trained with that officer, Shannon takes a moment before entering the house to confirm that Madi will attach the AED while Shannon and police officer handle compressions. Shannon states, "Let's make sure we keep hands on the chest as much as possible." Madi and the police officer verbally agree.

Coordination does not necessarily require extensive training or practice. In this example, a short pre-resuscitation huddle, closed-loop communication, and a quick confirmation of roles made sure resources were allocated to the appropriate purpose. Coordination may also keep team members from performing redundant or unnecessary actions.

If this situation were to proceed in an ideal fashion, when additional resources arrived, Shannon could step back into a team leadership role. Additional firefighters could be deployed to assist with compressions, and a provider could be assigned to manage the airway and provide ventilations. When paramedics arrived, they could step in to provide their

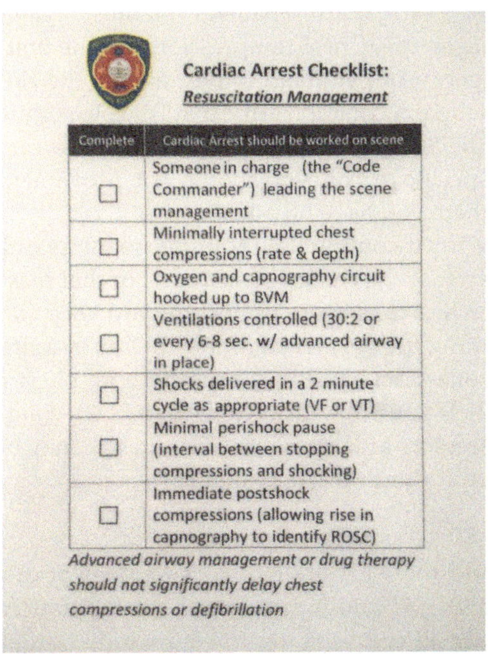
Cardiac Arrest Checklist:
Resuscitation Management

Complete	Cardiac Arrest should be worked on scene
☐	Someone in charge (the "Code Commander") leading the scene management
☐	Minimally interrupted chest compressions (rate & depth)
☐	Oxygen and capnography circuit hooked up to BVM
☐	Ventilations controlled (30:2 or every 6-8 sec. w/ advanced airway in place)
☐	Shocks delivered in a 2 minute cycle as appropriate (VF or VT)
☐	Minimal perishock pause (interval between stopping compressions and shocking)
☐	Immediate postshock compressions (allowing rise in capnography to identify ROSC)

Advanced airway management or drug therapy should not significantly delay chest compressions or defibrillation

FIGURE 21-9 CPR checklist.

advanced procedures and medications without interrupting the flow of the call. Of course, no situation is ever simple, but if coordination begins early, optimal care is possible.

The Steps of Resuscitation

High-performance resuscitation is a series of steps designed to ensure that the key elements of cardiac arrest care are provided. By thinking of the resuscitation scene in a step-by-step process, it is easy to coordinate efforts and add resources as they become available. In this section, we will describe the details of each step and discuss how to best integrate them within the larger resuscitation effort. Depending on resource availability, your sequencing may be slightly different, and steps may be combined. It is appropriate to tailor the steps of resuscitation to meet the individual needs of a situation as long as the key elements of cardiac arrest care (quality CPR and rapid defibrillation) are the end goals. Be wary of shifting focus to objectives outside of these key elements. Consider the previously discussed example:

Shannon and Madi find the cardiac arrest patient in a back bedroom at the end of a long hallway. They begin chest compressions and deploy the AED immediately.

Suggestion: "Let's move the patient to the living room so that access to the front door would be simpler."	**Resolution:** Shannon, the team leader, decides to stay in the bedroom because the move to the living room would lead to a pause in chest compressions.
Suggestion: "Stop compressions for a moment while I place the AED pads."	**Resolution:** Madi, who is doing compressions, replies, "Just work around my hands while compressions keep going."
Suggestion: "Should we move the patient to the ambulance before we defibrillate? It might be safer."	**Resolution:** In this case, there is no indication of a safety issue, so Shannon decides not to move the patient. Using an AED is a very safe procedure if completed correctly. If safety were a real issue, such as if an angry bystander or menacing dog were present, it might be reasonable to move the patient. The benefit of movement must outweigh the risk of the delay in defibrillation and the pause in compressions.
Suggestion: The paramedic tells Madi to pause compressions while he inserts an endotracheal tube.	**Resolution:** Advanced airways have little proven benefit in resuscitation success, so Madi respectfully reminds the paramedic that continuing compressions is more important.

Step 1: Identify Cardiac Arrest and Begin the Resuscitation

Once you have identified a cardiac arrest patient, you must organize the team, call for appropriate resources, and begin care. Chest compressions are the first treatment priority. Unless there is a specific danger or impediment to performing the skill, begin the resuscitation where the patient has fallen. A common error that leads to significant delays and pauses in chest compressions is the assumption that you must move a cardiac arrest patient. In fact, unless there is a very specific reason, you should not. Movement should be the exception, limited to situations where you have no other choice.

Chest compressions must continue without pause for as much of the resuscitation as possible. All pauses decrease the chance of success. For that reason, remember the concept of compression fraction and take every opportunity to keep compressions going.

If you are alone waiting for the arrival of an AED, as in a first-response situation, you may need to provide one-rescuer CPR, managing both chest compressions and rescue ventilations (Scan 21-2). If you are with a team (Scan 21-3), compressions should continue with a switch in compressors at least every 2 minutes. It may be appropriate to deploy a mechanical CPR device at this point, if available.

Step 2: Integrate the AED

Chest compressions and the AED are two cornerstones of cardiac arrest management. These interventions must go hand in hand in any resuscitation plan. Although we have described the initial step in resuscitation to be the initiation of chest compressions, the

SCAN 21-2 One-Person CPR

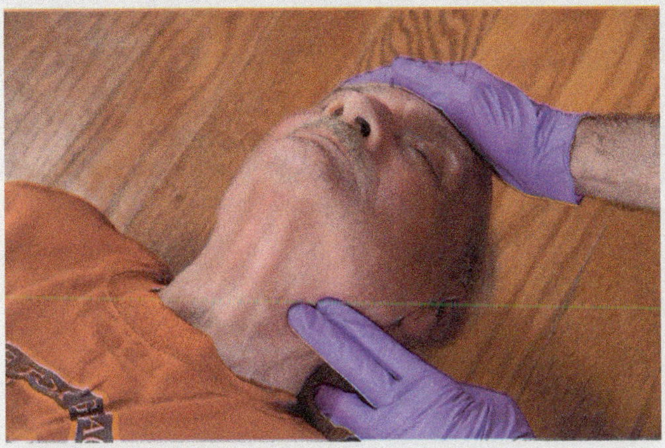

1. Verify cardiac arrest. (Assess responsiveness, check breathing, and check a pulse for no longer than 10 seconds.)

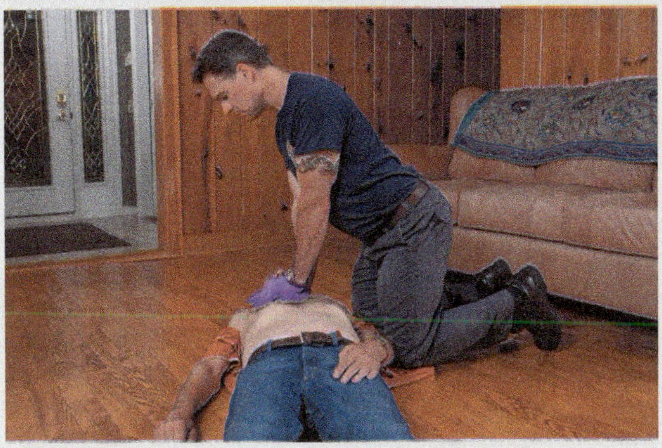

2. Begin chest compressions. (Place hands over lower third of the patient's sternum, lock elbows, pivot at the waist.)

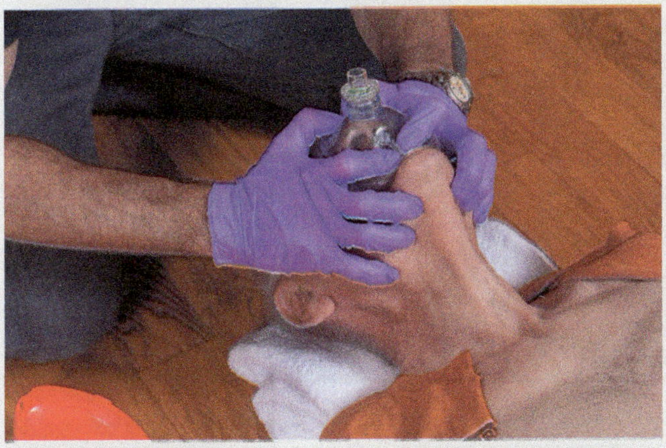

3. Deliver 30 compressions at an appropriate rate and depth; then deliver 2 rescue breaths.

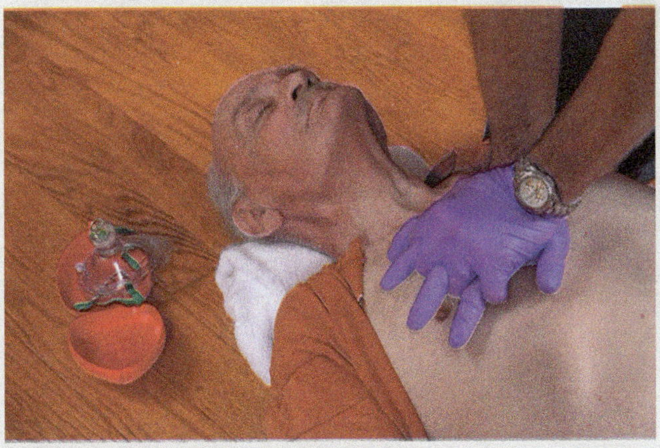

4. Continue chest compressions.

SCAN 21-3 High-Performance Team CPR

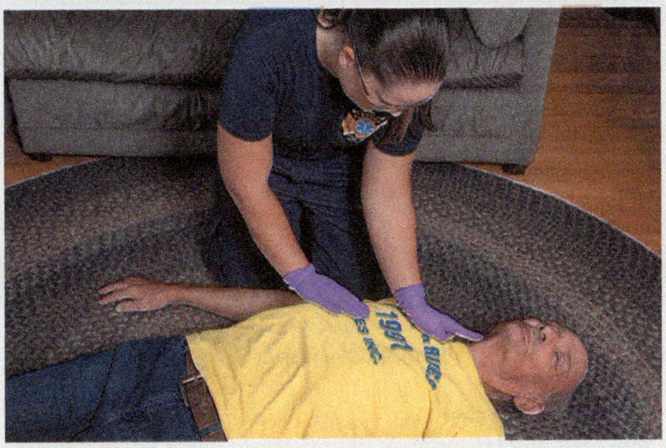

1. Verify cardiac arrest. (Assess responsiveness, check breathing, and check for a pulse for no longer than 10 seconds.)

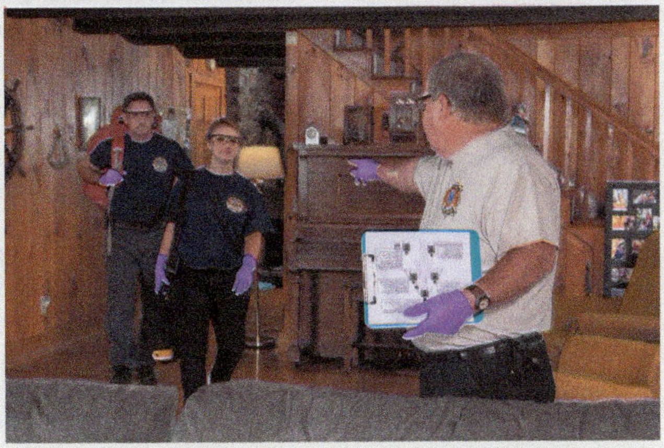

2. If not already planned, the team leader assigns the roles of the "triangle of life."

(continued)

SCAN 21-3 High-Performance Team CPR *(continued)*

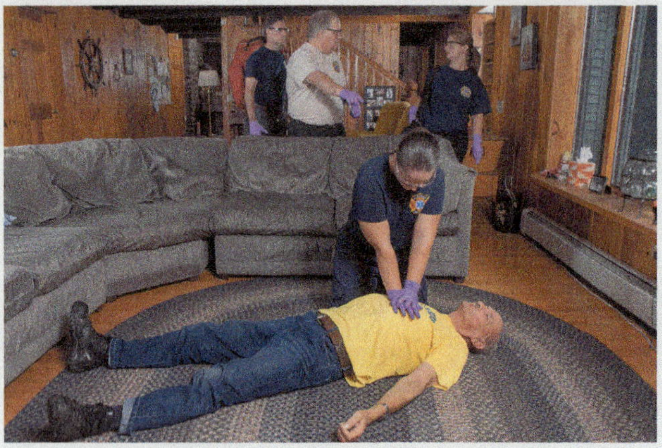

3. Provider 1 moves to the patient's side and begins quality chest compressions.

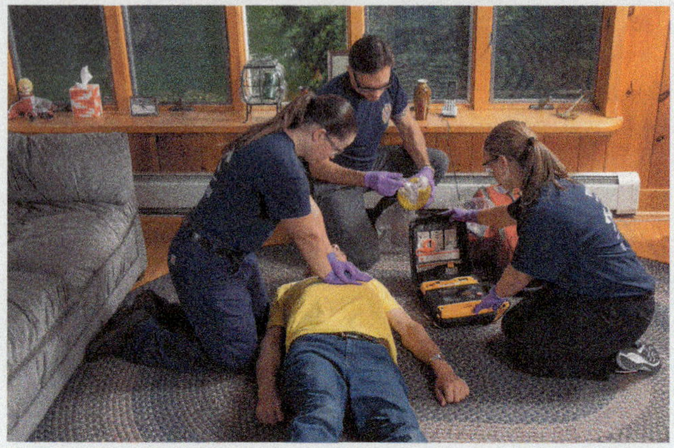

4. Provider 2 moves to the patient's head to manage the airway and provide rescue breathing.

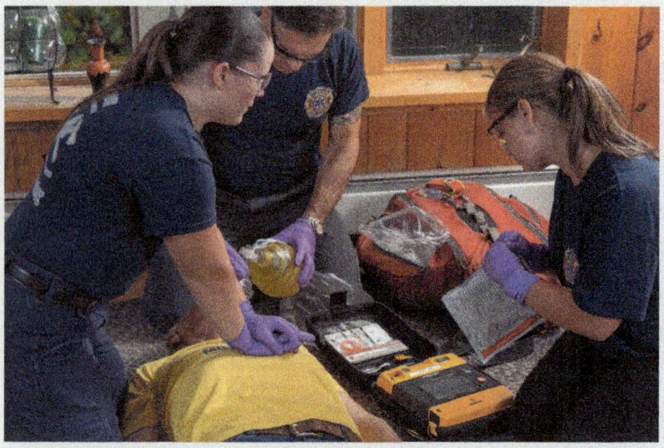

5. Provider 3 prepares the AED.

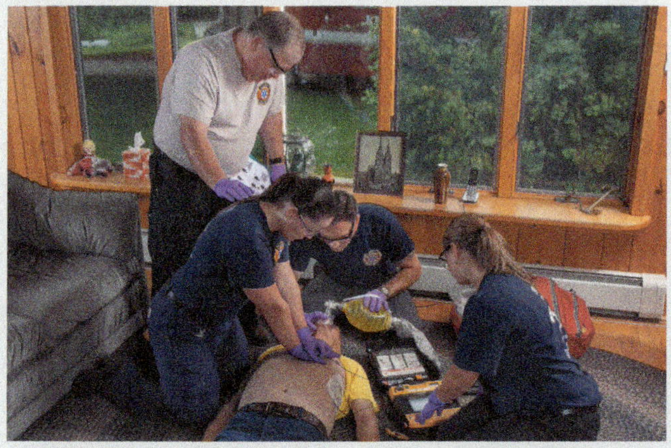

6. The team leader provides timing and ensures quality.

deployment of an AED will generally occur at the same time. In an optimal situation, one provider would start compressions while a second attached an AED. There are some systems that require chest compressions to be initiated and continued for a specified period of time prior to attaching the AED. However, recent research has demonstrated that there is no benefit in purposefully delaying the application of an AED even in patients with an unknown down time. Unless directed otherwise by local protocols, you should apply the AED to the patient as soon as it becomes available.

Responding Alone

When responding alone, as in a first-response situation, you may have to make a choice whether to place the AED immediately or begin CPR first. Although in most resuscitation situations, this is not a necessary decision, the first-response setting poses a unique challenge. Here the answer depends on the age of the patient.

ADULT PATIENT	CHILD OR INFANT PATIENT
In an adult patient, you should attach the AED first. Although chest compressions are important, the odds would suggest that a sudden dysrhythmia was the most likely cause of the arrest. Applying the AED first, when no other options are available, allows you to address the most likely pathology.	In a pediatric patient, you should begin CPR first. Although the AED is important, most pediatric arrests are asphyxial in nature. This means that the patient is likely to be profoundly hypoxic, so the importance of immediate chest compressions and ventilations may outweigh the benefit of defibrillation. In this situation, you would provide 2 minutes of CPR and then attach the AED.

When applying the AED, you should not interrupt chest compressions. The AED provider should, when possible, work around the hands of the compressor to place the pads. Chest compressions should continue until the AED is ready to analyze.

The integration of an AED into the resuscitation sequence is detailed in Figure 21-10 and Scan 21-4, but first consider the following key points:

- The AED should be turned on first. Modern AEDs utilize a voice prompt that directs the rescuer on the appropriate sequence of events. By turning the device on first, you have an immediate backup reminder if the situation is particularly stressful.
- The success of defibrillation depends on pad contact. AED electrode pads should be placed per manufacturer's recommendation against bare skin. Any clothing, jewelry, or medication patches that might interfere with pad contact should be removed prior to placement. Excessive hair should be quickly trimmed with a safety razor. Sweat or other liquids should be wiped away. If an indwelling device such as a pacemaker or internal defibrillator is visualized beneath the skin, placement of the AED pad should be offset to avoid the device.

FIGURE 21-10 AED cardiac arrest treatment sequence.

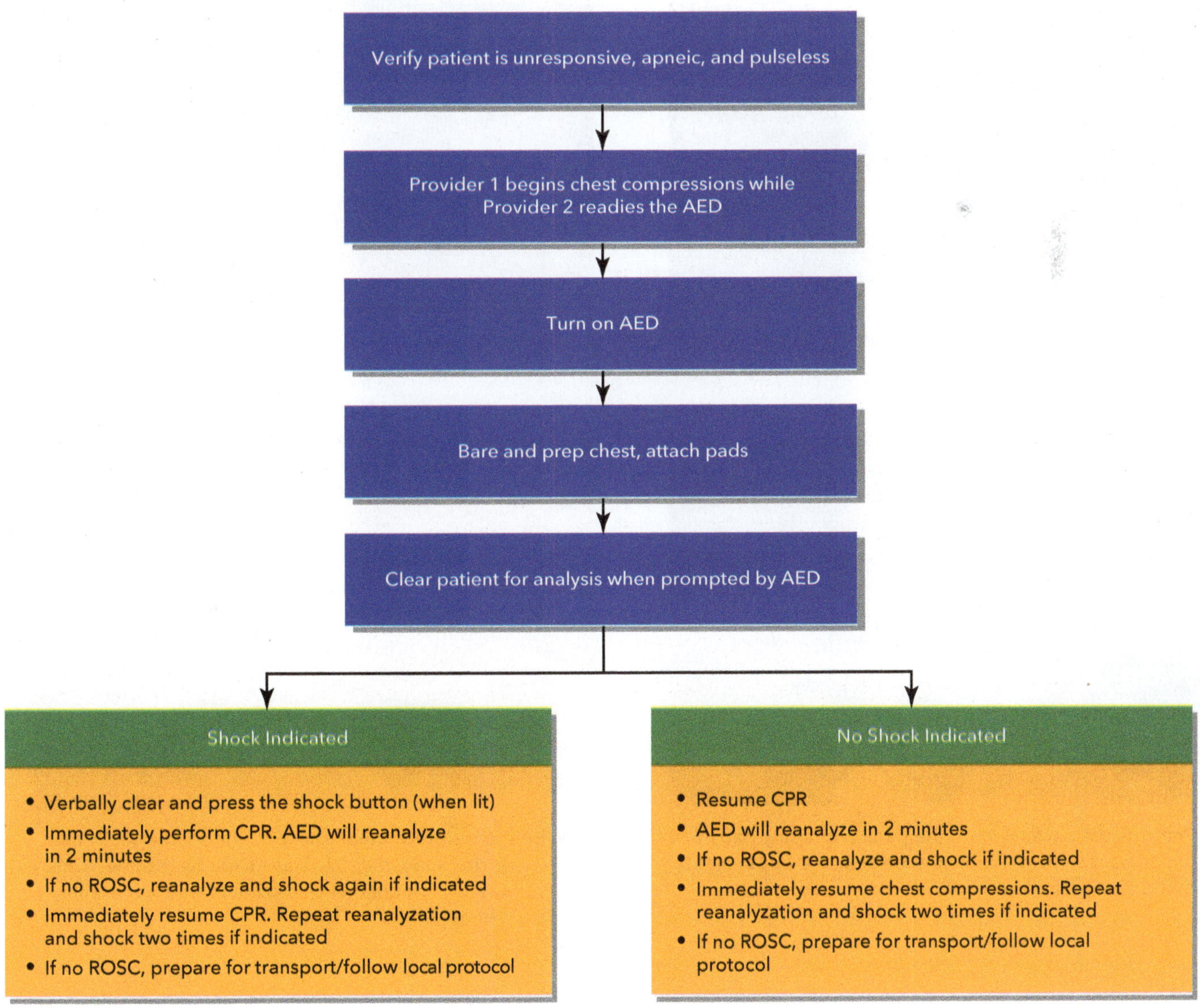

SCAN 21-4 Assessing and Managing a Cardiac Arrest Patient

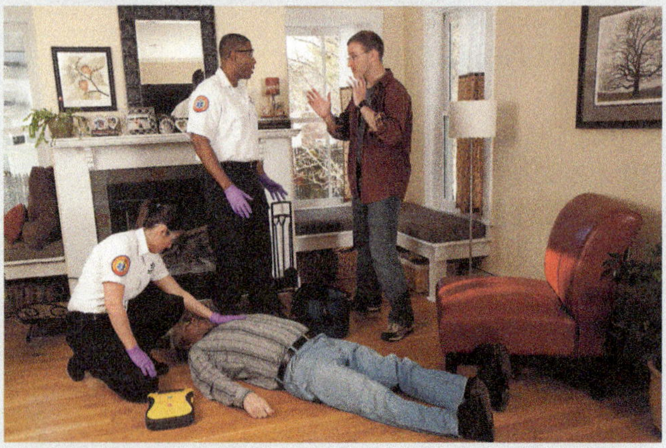

1. If the patient appears lifeless, do a quick scan for breathing. Obtain a quick history of events from family or bystanders.

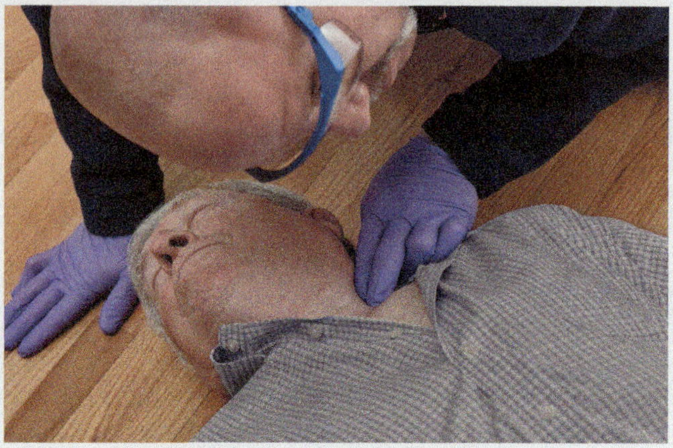

2. Verify the absence of a spontaneous pulse. Check for no longer than 10 seconds.

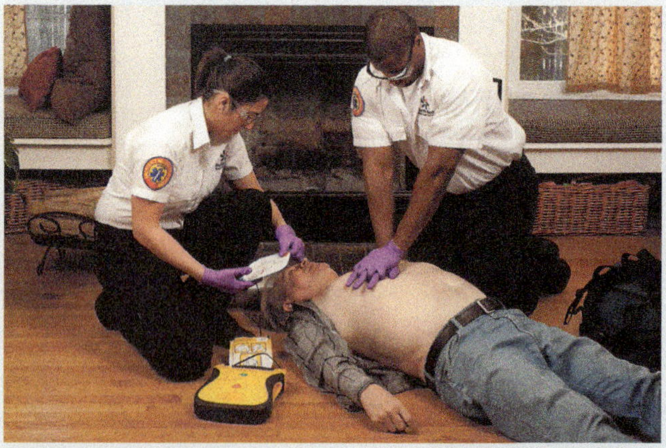

3. Begin chest compressions while another EMT sets up the AED.

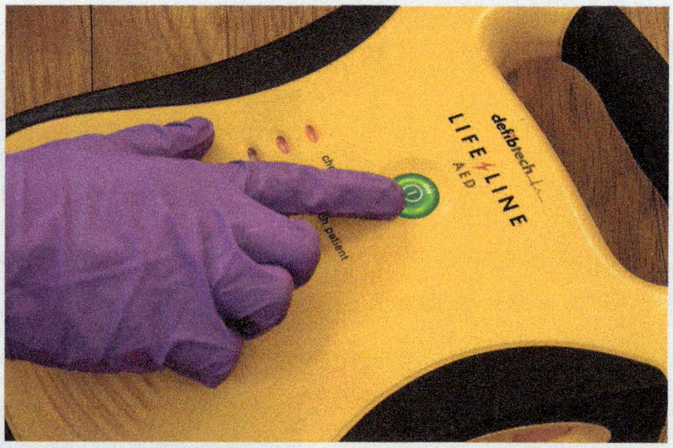

4. Turn on the AED.

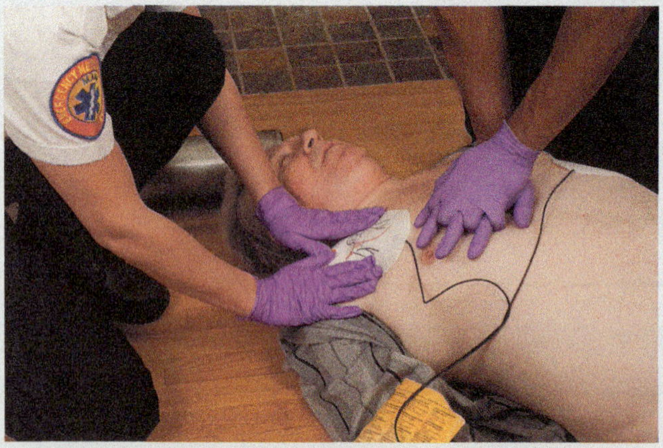

5. Remove the backing from the pads and apply pads to the patient's chest. Place one pad on the upper right chest, one on the lower left ribs.

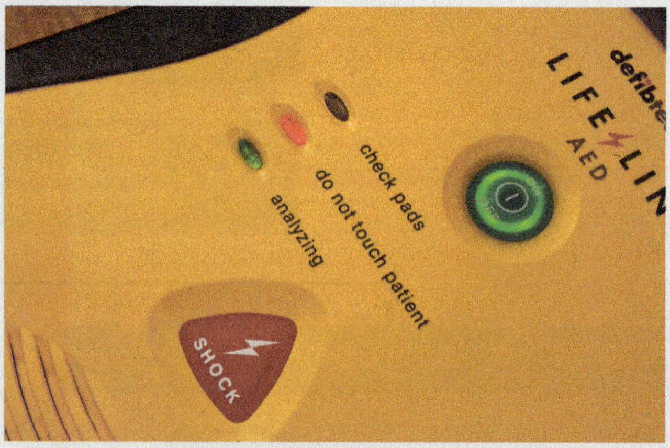

6. When prompted, clear the patient so the AED can analyze the heart rhythm. Stay ready to resume compressions, but ensure that all providers are clear in anticipation of defibrillation.

SCAN 21-4 Assessing and Managing a Cardiac Arrest Patient *(continued)*

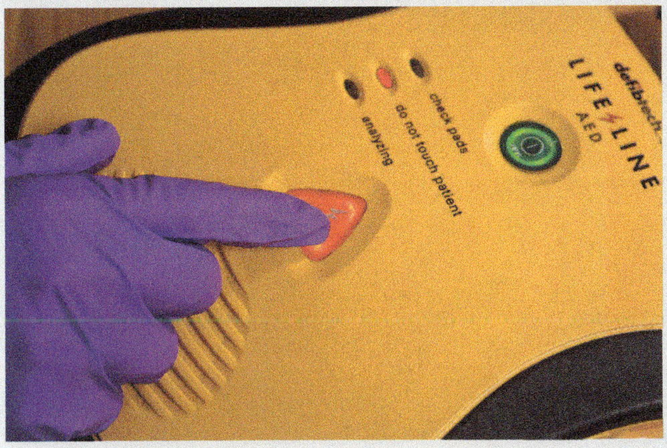

7. If advised by the AED, press the button to deliver a shock. Immediately resume CPR.

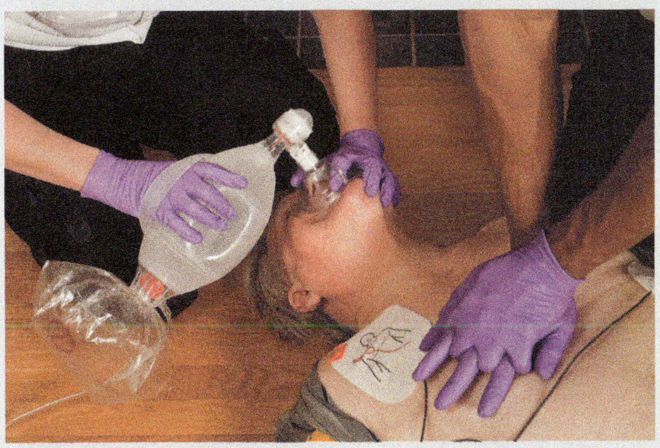

8. Perform CPR for 2 minutes (five cycles), unless the patient wakes up, moves, or begins to breathe. Follow AED prompts.

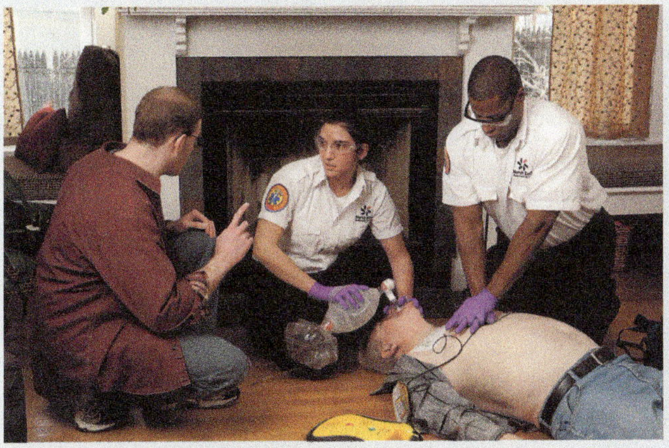

9. Gather additional information on the arrest events.

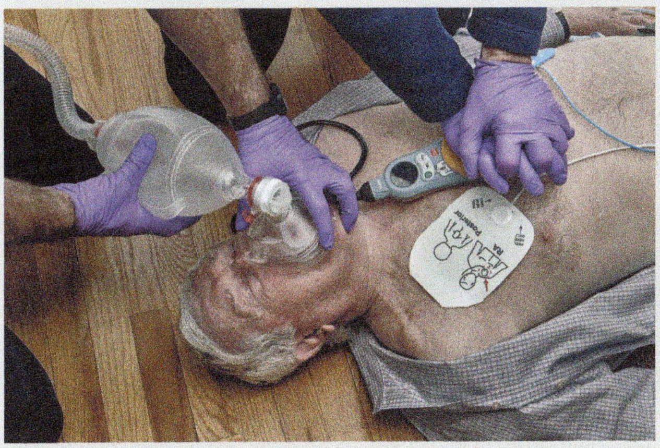

10. Check the patient's pulse during CPR to confirm the effectiveness of compressions.

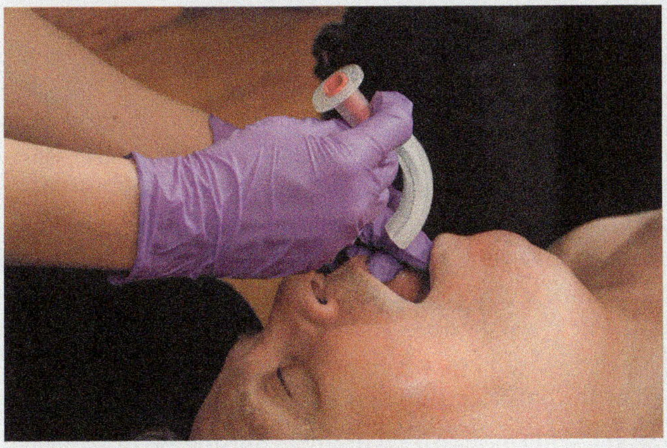

11. Direct insertion of the airway adjunct.

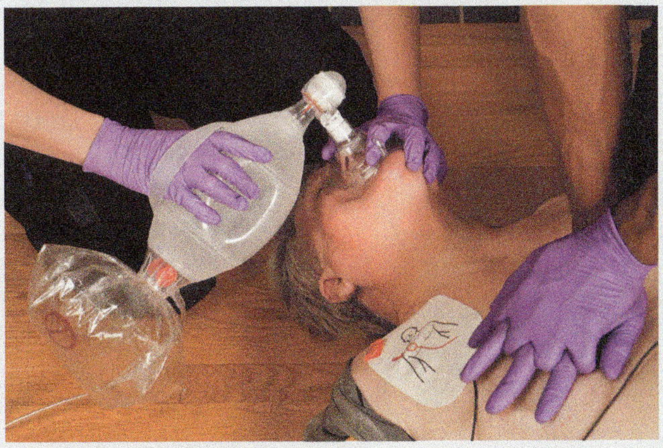

12. Direct ventilation of the patient with high-concentration oxygen.

(continued)

SCAN 21-4 Assessing and Managing a Cardiac Arrest Patient *(continued)*

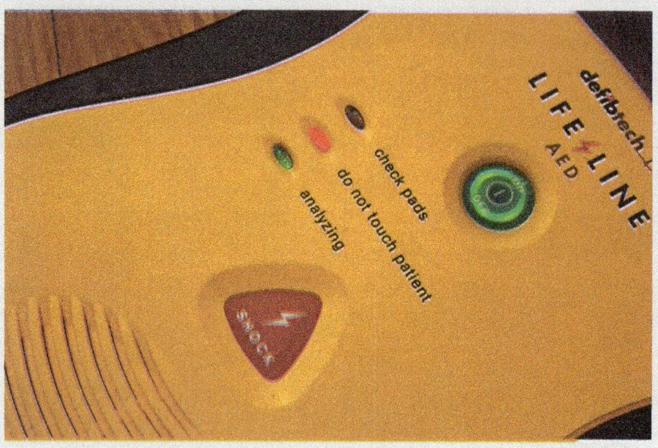

13. After 2 minutes of CPR, the AED will prompt to clear for the next analysis. Remain ready, but clear the patient.

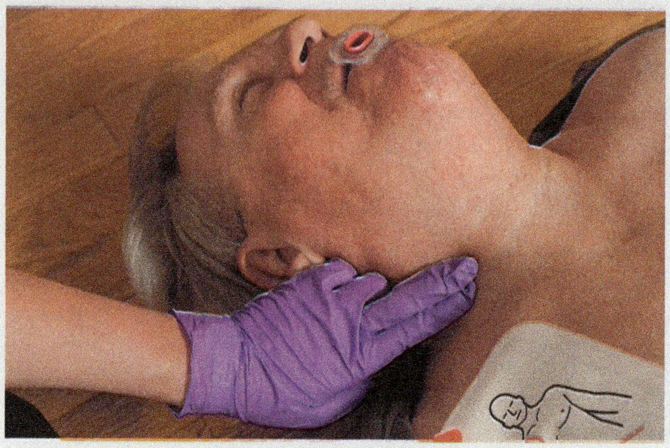

14. If prompted by the AED or if spontaneous respirations are present, check the patient's pulse.

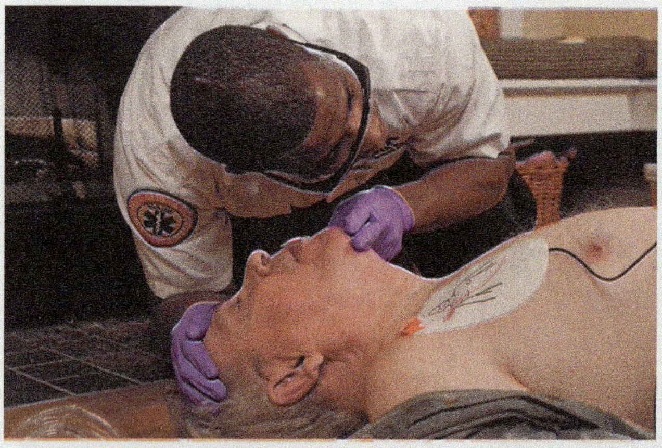

15. If there is a spontaneous pulse, check the patient's breathing and initiate postarrest care. Note that in many cases, even when a pulse has returned, the patient will require ventilatory assistance.

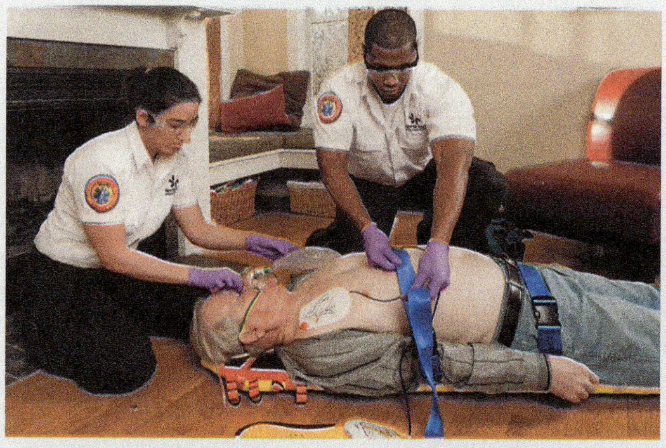

16. If breathing is adequate, provide high-concentration oxygen by nonrebreather mask. If breathing is inadequate, ventilate the patient with high-concentration oxygen. Transport without delay.

- Once pads are placed, the device will analyze the cardiac rhythm. Although there are monitors and AEDs that can analyze a rhythm while compressions are ongoing, most devices prompt rescuers to stop compressions for the 15–20 seconds necessary to analyze. Touching the patient while the AED is analyzing the rhythm can create interference from the electrical impulses of your heart and from movement of the patient's muscles. For this reason, no one should ventilate, do chest compressions, or touch the patient in any way when the rhythm is being analyzed or a shock is being delivered. However, the person in the role of chest compressor should maintain CPR position. Hands should hover 18–20 inches (45–50 cm) off the chest in a state of readiness to resume compressions as soon as the shock is delivered.
- During the analyzation phase, the AED looks for ventricular fibrillation or ventricular tachycardia. If either dysrhythmia is found, the AED will verbally announce "Shock advised" and a red or orange shock button will light up on the device. If ventricular fibrillation or ventricular tachycardia is not found, the prompt will be "No shock advised—resume CPR."
- While providers are prompted to stop compressions during analyzation, the AED provider should make sure all rescuers are clear of the patient so that a defibrillation can be

delivered without pause as soon as the AED is ready. Clearing the patient is typically accomplished with a verbal warning such as "Everyone off the patient—be sure you're clear," and then a visual inspection to confirm all providers are actually clear. A second verbal "Clear!" should be made prior to depressing the shock button.

- When possible, chest compressions should resume *as soon as the defibrillation has been delivered*. Do not wait for the AED's prompt. A defibrillation can be seen by witnessing the brief muscle spasm that accompanies the shock. Resume compressions immediately after this spasm.
- Once a "Shock" or "No shock advised" prompt has been given, the AED will count down a 2-minute cycle. At the end of this cycle, the AED will automatically prompt providers to clear the patient for the next analyzation phase. During the "clear" interval, compressors should switch, to prevent fatigue.

Decision Points

- Does my patient have signs of life?
- Do I have a defibrillator immediately available? How will I integrate defibrillation?

NOTE: *If the patient already has an AED attached when you arrive, your actions will be slightly different. You will need to evaluate the performance of the person operating the machine. If the person is operating it properly, allow the person to continue until the next reasonable time to switch operators. If the person's actions are improper or less than optimal, you must either offer suggestions to correct those actions or take over control of the device. Patient care is your highest priority, keeping in mind that roughly interrupting a smoothly functioning operation does not benefit the patient or the layperson trying to assist.*

Step 3: Continue the Resuscitation

Quality chest compressions and defibrillation offer the patient the best opportunity for successful resuscitation. Now that both elements are combined, you must focus on high-quality teamwork and integrate additional resources as they become available.

Pediatric Note

It is appropriate to deploy an AED on any presumed cardiac arrest patient, regardless of age. Although infants and children have fewer "shockable" rhythms in cardiac arrest, around 20 percent will present with ventricular fibrillation or ventricular tachycardia. Using an AED on a pediatric patient requires slight modification for size and age. If the child is less than 8 years old, the American Heart Association recommends using pediatric defibrillator pads. These pads are typically smaller and designed to deliver a slightly lower defibrillation dose than are adult pads. Most pediatric pads are placed in an "anterior-posterior" configuration (Figure 21-11), meaning that one pad is placed on the anterior chest of the infant or child while the second pad is placed in the center of the patient's back. If the child is large enough, it may be appropriate to place pads in a more traditional "apex-sternum" (top right and bottom left of the anterior chest) configuration. Some AEDs utilize a pediatric key or switch designed to change internal settings to a pediatric level. Always know the specific manufacturer's recommendations for your AED and its guidance for pediatric use.

If the AED has no pediatric capabilities, it is still appropriate to use it on a pediatric patient in cardiac arrest. If no pediatric-specific device is available, you should use an adult AED with the idea that it is better to administer too high a level of defibrillation than no defibrillation at all. If an adult AED is used, consider attaching the adult pads in an anterior-posterior configuration. Never overlap or cut AED pads. Use the AED in the manner and procedure detailed in this section.

FIGURE 21-11 Anterior-posterior positioning for AED pads on a pediatric patient.

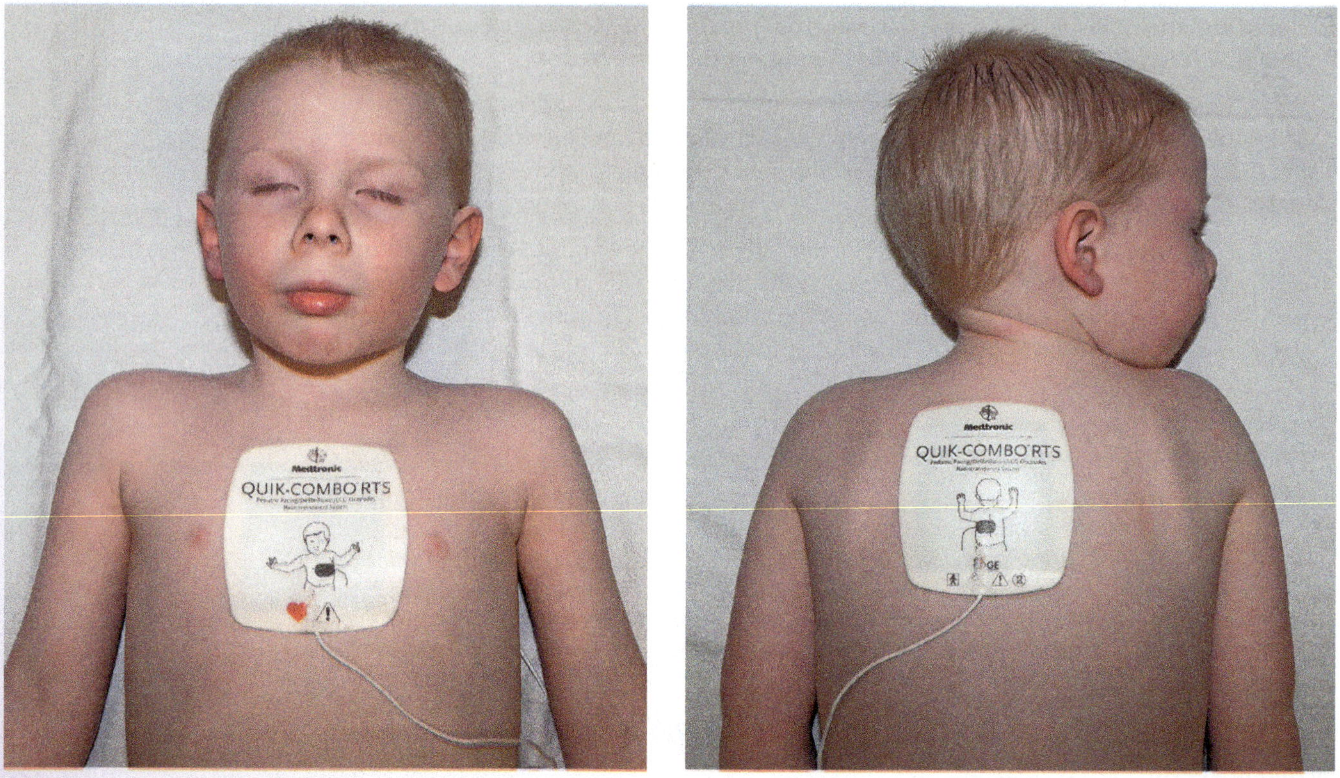

A B

The sequence of resuscitation is entirely predictable. Once the AED has analyzed for the first time and offered a "Shock" or "No shock advised" message, it will automatically reanalyze every 2 minutes. That means that for the 2 minutes between analyzations, your team will perform CPR, offer advanced life support interventions when appropriate, and prepare for the next opportunity to defibrillate. The team leader may track this time and offer prompts as the analyzation time approaches. This allows team members to position themselves properly, to prepare for a compressor switch (Figure 21-12), and to ready the next intervention. When the AED prompts to clear the patient for analyzation, the team should be ready and prepared to resume chest compressions as soon as the defibrillation is delivered.

FIGURE 21-12 Preparing for a switch of chest compressors in high efficiency CPR.

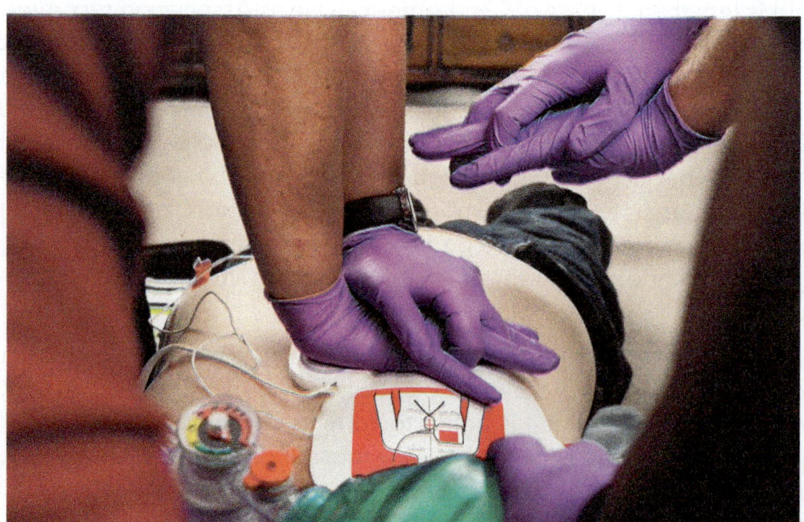

A return of spontaneous circulation might not come after the first shock. Many successful resuscitations occur after the second, third, or even fourth defibrillation. Remember that a "No shock advised" message in the first analyzation may become a "Shock advised" message in the next. Teams should be ready for these changes to occur.

If resources are available, a team member should be detailed to obtain patient information. Although the immediate priority is the resuscitation, there is valuable information to be obtained in the patient history and the history of the present illness. If time allows, consider the elements of the secondary assessment. Use SAMPLE and OPQRST to identify information about the events that led up to the cardiac arrest. In many cases, specific historical findings may help identify correctible causes of cardiac arrest, such as a tension pneumothorax or a pulmonary embolism. Interventions for these may not be in the EMT scope of practice, but your efforts to identify them can shorten the treatment gap. Remember also to review physical findings. Although there may not be time to perform a full head-to-toe examination, a brief review of any obvious physical findings as well as a quick overview of the patient's surroundings can provide valuable clues to the nature of the cardiac arrest. Even when extra team members are not available, you may be able to utilize the pauses during analyzation to ask questions of family members or to inspect the area. Keep in mind the priority of not interrupting compressions, however.

Consider also the extended trauma imposed upon family members witnessing the arrest. Although resources will dictate your actions here as well, it is entirely appropriate to detail a team member to look after the needs of the family.

Should the Family Watch the Resuscitation? The question of whether family members should be present during resuscitation is a complicated one. On the one hand, there may be a post-traumatic stress reduction value in being in the room when resuscitative efforts are ongoing. Allowing family members to be present may offer them a better understanding of the great efforts made to save their loved one or provide an important sense of closure if the efforts are unsuccessful. On the other hand, some family members are unprepared to witness such a difficult moment and can get in the way of the resuscitation effort. It is reasonable then, to offer the option of remaining in the room, but also be ready to relocate the family if necessary. In either case, remember that family members are patients in this situation as well. While the resuscitation effort itself should take precedence for resources, do not forget about their needs.

Step 4: Transitioning Resuscitation

As mentioned previously, the most likely indicator of successful resuscitation is the return of breathing. Other signs may include consciousness, purposeful movement, or a pulse. If these or any other signs of spontaneous circulation are present, your team goals must shift rapidly from resuscitation to postarrest care. Now, instead of focusing on CPR and defibrillation, you must focus on rapid, appropriate transport; airway management; and access to ALS. Remember also that cardiac arrest is a symptom of acute coronary syndrome.

A patient who has been resuscitated from cardiac arrest is at high risk of going back into arrest. This change may be difficult to detect, since most patients who have just been resuscitated are unconscious, and many of them will need assisted ventilation. Since you are breathing for the patient, you may not notice that the patient no longer has a pulse. This is why, on unconscious patients who have recovered a pulse, you should continue to check the pulse about every 30 seconds. The AED may alert you that the patient has a shockable rhythm. If you get such a prompt from the defibrillator, check for a pulse immediately. If you find that there is no pulse, follow these steps:

1. If you are en route, stop the vehicle.
2. Have someone else start CPR if the AED is not immediately ready.
3. Analyze the rhythm.
4. Deliver a shock, if indicated.
5. Continue with two shocks separated by 2 minutes (five cycles) of CPR or as your local protocol directs.

If resuscitation continues, it may be appropriate to consider the next steps beyond CPR and defibrillation. Some systems set time frames and initiate transport to the hospital if initial resuscitative efforts are unsuccessful. Other systems have developed protocols that allow EMTs (or EMTs and advanced life support providers) to terminate efforts after a predetermined period of CPR and defibrillation. It will be important to understand and follow local protocol in these situations.

Terminating Resuscitation

If you are in doubt as to when or whether to terminate resuscitation efforts, seek a physician's advice. Once you have started resuscitation, you must continue to provide resuscitation (CPR, defibrillation) until:

- Spontaneous circulation occurs. Then provide rescue breathing as needed.
- Spontaneous circulation and breathing occur.
- Another trained rescuer can take over for you.
- You turn care of the patient over to a person with a higher level of training.
- You are too exhausted to continue.
- You receive a "cease resuscitation" order from a physician or other authority per local protocols.

If you turn the patient over to another rescuer, this person must be trained to the same or a greater level of proficiency as you. If there are ALS providers on the scene, they may also receive a termination order from their medical direction if the patient has failed to respond to BLS and ALS interventions such as drug administration and advanced airway intervention.

Death Notification

More and more, EMTs are being tasked with managing family after termination of resuscitation. Although we typically take a clinical approach to patient care, the emotional care provided in these situations is also important. Although there is no universal approach for making a tragic situation better, there are strategies that can be used to offer the best care under the circumstances. Consider the following:

- If notifying the family of an unsuccessful resuscitation, be straightforward and use direct language. Do not attempt to soften the moment with vague terms. For example, "I'm very sorry, but your father has died" is much more appropriate than saying "I'm sorry, we've lost him."
- When possible, allow the family time with the deceased patient. Make sure to offer privacy and space.
- Take time and be patient. Remember that this moment may be the worst day that family member has ever had. Your desire to get back in service or to get back to the station for dinner is inconsequential by comparison. Provide assistance in contacting additional resources for the family and do what you can to help in the moment.
- Do not suggest that you "know how they feel." Grief is unique to every individual. Although empathy is very important in this situation, sometimes this statement can be taken the wrong way.
- Most importantly, be yourself. If you are sad, it is okay to be sad. Do not fake emotions. Your deception will be obvious.

Special Considerations in Resuscitation

Coordination with Others Who Defibrillate Before You Arrive

Emergency medical responders, police officers, security officers, and others may defibrillate the patient before you arrive. If this happens, you should let the operator of the AED complete the shock before you take over care of the patient. After the shock is delivered or a

"No shock advised" message is received, work with the operator to bring about an orderly transfer of care.

In some areas, you may need to take the first AED to the hospital with the patient so that data can be retrieved from the machine. Your protocols should address this. They also should tell you whether to switch from the first AED to your own.

Resuscitation in the Ambulance

In general, the initial steps of resuscitation in a moving vehicle should be avoided. Although the idea of reaching a hospital quickly is, in most cases, a good idea, the unstable work platform of an ambulance moving through traffic often hinders the key components of a successful resuscitation. Research has shown that a moving vehicle increases the likelihood of pauses and reduces the effectiveness of chest compressions. Inappropriate rate and depth and residual leaning on the chest during compressions have also been reported. In addition, some AEDs are unable to analyze a rhythm accurately in a moving emergency vehicle.

If your patient goes into cardiac arrest during transport, stop the vehicle to perform CPR and deploy the AED. Local guidelines may indicate that transport be resumed after a certain period of time or after a designated number of CPR cycles and/or AED shocks. Follow your local protocols.

Cardiac Arrest Care for Hypothermia and Submersion Injuries

Hypothermia (very low body temperature) and submersion (drowning) injuries present a unique challenge to cardiac arrest. Prolonged exposure to cold and the dropping body temperatures associated with submersion injuries change our approach to cardiac arrest care. Keep in mind that accurate measurement of hypothermia is difficult in the field. Although most priorities remain the same, consider the following necessary adaptations:

- Current recommendations are to attempt defibrillation once in a hypothermic cardiac arrest patient, then wait until the core temperature is at least 86°F (30°C) before attempting defibrillation again. Some systems recommend additional shocks in the event of cardiac arrest. If this does not work, the patient should be transported immediately.
- Hypothermia may change local guidelines associated with transport and termination of cardiac arrest. Because of low body temperatures, the period of survivability in a cardiac arrest associated with hypothermia may be much longer than that in a normal cardiac arrest. In general, hypothermic patients should be transported to a facility capable of rewarming while resuscitation is ongoing. Resuscitation of hypothermic patients *should not be terminated in the field*.

Except for hypothermia considerations, treating a submersion-injury patient in cardiac arrest is essentially the same as treating any other cardiac arrest patient. In addition to numerous scene safety issues, the water environment can create specific challenges. Keep in mind that most submersion-related cardiac arrest is caused by asphyxia. Unlike a typical acute coronary syndrome patient, these patients need oxygen and ventilations. While quality compressions and defibrillation are still the most important priorities, you should be aggressive with airway management and rescue breathing.

Defibrillation can be challenging in a water environment. When you defibrillate a patient, you are delivering electrical current through the patient's chest. Although it is unlikely, electrical current can theoretically be carried or conducted to you under certain conditions. Modern biphasic defibrillation technology is unlikely to cause you significant harm, but you should take precautions to make every defibrillation safe for you and your team. Water is a very good conductor of electricity. Do not defibrillate a soaking-wet patient. Dry the patient's chest or move the patient out of the wet environment (if it can be done quickly). See Figure 21-13.

If you see a medication patch on the patient's chest, remove it carefully before defibrillating. The plastic in the patch can burn and may impede conduction. Be absolutely sure that before every shock, you say "Clear!" and ensure that, from head to toe, no one is touching the patient or any conductive material that is touching the patient.

FIGURE 21-13 Be alert to safety hazards when using an AED. Do not defibrillate a patient who is soaking wet. Before defibrillation, remove all clothing, dry the chest, and remove any medication patches you find. Do not defibrillate until everyone is clear of the patient.

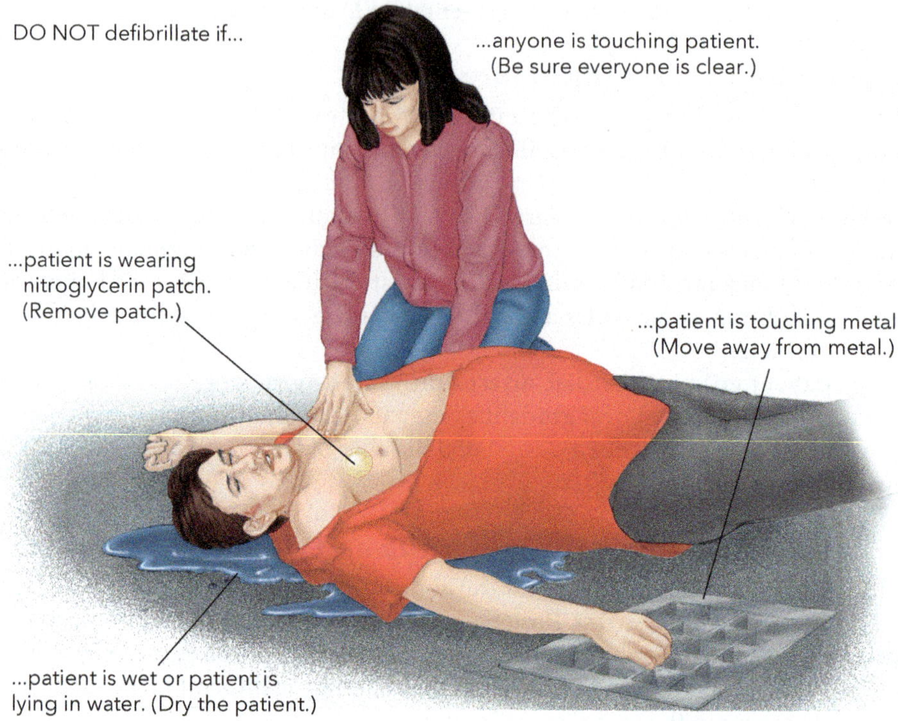

Implants and Surgeries

With the rapidly expanding medical technology available, the EMT may be presented with patients who have undergone surgeries or had special devices implanted in the body. The ABCs, including CPR and appropriate oxygen delivery, will not change because of prior surgery or conditions, with rare exceptions. Defibrillation can be performed on such a patient, although the positioning of defibrillation pads on the patient's chest may need to be adjusted to avoid contact with an implanted device.

Some of the devices and surgical implants you may observe in the field include the following:

- **Cardiac pacemaker.** (See Figure 21-14A.) When the heart's natural pacemaker does not function properly, an artificial pacemaker can be surgically implanted to perform the same function. This pacemaker helps the heart beat in a normal, coordinated fashion. It is often placed below one of the clavicles, is visible as a small lump, and can be palpated. If you notice a lump under a clavicle, do not put a defibrillation pad over it. Try to put the pad at least several inches away while staying in the general area where you want the pad.

  Occasionally, pacemakers malfunction. Although this situation is rare, it is life-threatening when it occurs. A malfunctioning pacemaker usually results in a slow or irregular pulse. The patient may have signs of shock due to the fact the heart is not beating properly. Remember that care for patients with implanted pacemakers and signs of a cardiac emergency is the same as for those without a pacemaker. You should arrange for an ALS intercept and transport the patient immediately.

- **Implanted defibrillator.** Cardiologists are sometimes able to identify patients who are at high risk of going into ventricular fibrillation. These patients sometimes receive a miniature defibrillator surgically implanted in the chest or abdomen. When the patient develops a lethal cardiac rhythm, the implanted defibrillator detects it and shocks the patient. Since the implanted defibrillator is directly attached to the heart, low energy

FIGURE 21-14 (A) An implanted pacemaker is visible in this patient's left chest. (B) A combination implanted cardioverter defibrillator/pacemaker is noticeable in this patient's left chest. *(Photos: © Edward T. Dickinson)*

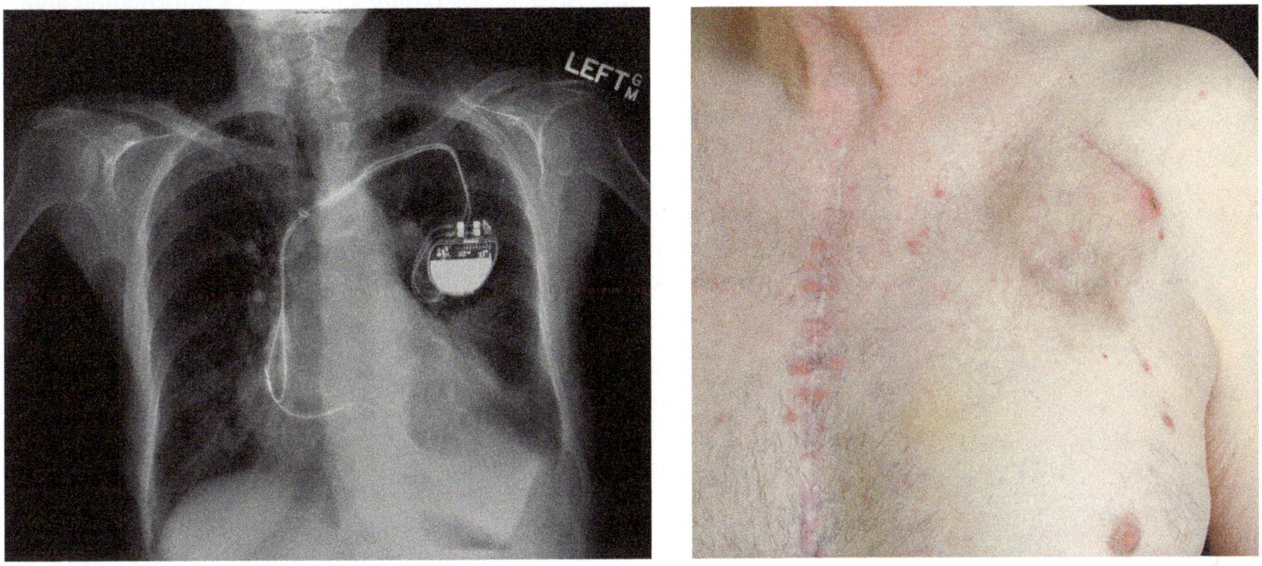

A   B

levels are needed for each shock. These are sometimes combined with a pacemaker. (See Figure 21-14B.) Patients can sometimes anticipate this situation, and the muscle contraction caused by the internal defibrillation is often visible. Often EMS is called to care for patients whose internal defibrillators have fired. Remember that this is a good thing and likely lifesaving, even though it may cause great discomfort to the patient. You should transport these patients immediately and call ALS for more advanced cardiac care. The presence of the implanted defibrillator should not pose a threat to the EMT.

A patient with an implanted defibrillator can still go into cardiac arrest. Occasionally, these devices fail, or the cardiac arrest could be caused by a nonshockable dysrhythmia. If this occurs, treat the patient like any other cardiac arrest patient. You should use your AED and just remember to offset your pads to avoid placing them over the implanted defibrillator.

- **Ventricular assist device.** When one or both ventricles of the heart are very weak, a patient may receive a ventricular assist device (VAD), a mechanical device that pumps blood for the heart. Typically, the device consists of a pump in the patient's chest connected to a battery power source outside the patient. Outside of the hospital, a left ventricular device (LVAD) is more common than a right VAD. The LVAD takes blood out of the left ventricle and pumps it to the aorta, providing blood to the systemic circulation. Instead of repeatedly pushing blood into the aorta the way the heart normally does, the pump often provides a continuous flow of blood.

  Since there is no variation in the pressure in the arteries, the patient will not have any palpable pulses or blood pressure. This can be confusing for the EMT or other health care provider who is trying to determine whether the patient is alive. In this situation, you will have to rely on the patient's level of consciousness and breathing.

  The decision to begin CPR on a VAD patient is not simple. If a VAD is running normally, as evidenced by the motor's humming and the device's not sounding an alarm, CPR may not be needed. However, if the patient is unconscious with signs of poor perfusion (cyanosis), it may be reasonable to assume that the device is not functioning properly and to begin chest compressions. The American College of Cardiology suggests that if you are in doubt, provide CPR. However, you should follow local protocols and procedures created for the specific needs of the patient. Transport the patient promptly.

A patient who has an LVAD typically has severe heart disease and either is waiting for a heart transplant or has a heart so weak that the patient would not be able to function without the device. The patient and family should have information about the device.

- **Cardiac bypass surgery.** The coronary artery bypass has become a relatively common procedure in cardiac surgery. A blood vessel from another part of the body is surgically implanted to bypass an occluded coronary artery. This helps restore blood flow to a section of the myocardium. Should a patient with a suspected myocardial infarction report a history of bypass surgery, or if you observe a midline surgical scar on the chest of an unconscious patient, provide the same emergency care, including CPR and defibrillation, as for any other patient.

Chapter Review

Key Facts and Concepts

- Cardiac arrest occurs when the pumping of the heart stops. This is commonly caused by lethal dysrhythmias including:
  - Ventricular fibrillation
  - Ventricular tachycardia
  - Asystole
  - Pulseless electrical activity
- Cardiac arrest causes an immediate drop in coronary and cerebral perfusion pressure. Without immediate care, the cells of the heart and brain will die.
- Most cardiac arrest is sudden in nature, most commonly caused by acute coronary syndrome. Some cardiac arrest is caused by asphyxial causes (especially in pediatric arrest).
- Cardiac arrest is recognized by unresponsiveness, apnea, and pulselessness.
- To provide excellent care and the maximum chance of survival for patients in cardiac arrest, EMS agencies must strengthen their performance of the five elements of the chain of survival:
  - Recognition and activation of the emergency response system
  - Immediate high-quality CPR
  - Rapid defibrillation
  - Basic and advanced emergency medical services
  - Advanced life support and postarrest care
- Successful resuscitation is a product of teamwork and quality management.

Key Decisions

- Is the patient in cardiac arrest?
- What kind of cardiac arrest is this—respiratory (making airway and breathing top priorities) or cardiac (making circulation and compressions top priorities)?
- Are we providing quality CPR (i.e., compressing fast and hard, changing compressors often, avoiding hyperventilation, and minimizing interruptions)?
- How can we improve our resuscitation capabilities?

Chapter Glossary

agonal breathing irregular, gasping breaths that precede apnea and death.

apnea (AP-ne-ah) no breathing.

asphyxial cardiac arrest (aus-fix-ial) a cardiac arrest caused by systemic hypoxia, typically due to a respiratory disorder.

asystole (ay-SIS-to-le) a condition in which the heart has ceased generating electrical impulses. Commonly called *flatline*.

cardiac arrest a state in which the heart is no longer pumping blood.

cardiopulmonary resuscitation (CPR) actions taken to revive a person by keeping the person's heart and lungs working.

chain of survival a metaphor that describes the key elements of cardiac arrest management. Each link in the chain describes a different but interconnected intervention; when combined, these interventions offer optimal care.

commotio cordis a cardiac arrest caused by acute blunt force trauma to the anterior chest.

compression fraction the amount of time chest compressions are being performed compared with the total time of patient contact.

defibrillation delivery of an electrical shock to stop the fibrillation of heart muscles and restore a normal heart rhythm.

dysrhythmia (dis-RITH-me-ah) a disturbance in heart rate and rhythm.

pulseless electrical activity (PEA) a condition in which the heart's electrical rhythm remains relatively normal, yet the mechanical pumping activity fails to follow the electrical activity, causing cardiac arrest.

return of spontaneous circulation (ROSC) the heart beating again after successful resuscitation

sudden cardiac arrest a cardiac arrest occurring due to the abrupt onset of a dysrhythmia.

ventricular fibrillation (VF) (ven-TRIK-u-ler fib-ri-LAY-shun) a condition in which the heart's electrical impulses are disorganized, preventing the heart muscle from contracting normally.

ventricular tachycardia (V-tach) (ven-TRIK-u-ler tak-i-KAR-de-uh) a condition in which the heartbeat is quite rapid; if rapid enough, ventricular tachycardia will not allow the heart's chambers to fill with enough blood between beats to produce blood flow sufficient to meet the body's needs.

Preparation for Your Examination and Practice

Short Answer

1. List the three indications of cardiac arrest.
2. Describe the appropriate depth of chest compression for adults, children, and infants.
3. List three safety measures to keep in mind when using an AED.
4. List the steps in the application of an AED.

Thinking and Linking

Think back to the chapter Cardiac Emergencies. *If acute coronary syndrome is the most common cause of cardiac arrest in adults, what symptoms might a patient complain of that might identify the potential for cardiac arrest?*

Think back to the chapter Medical, Legal, and Ethical Issues *and link information from that chapter with information from this chapter as you consider the following situation:*

- You are called to treat an unconscious person in a local park. He is unresponsive when you arrive. How would you obtain consent to treat this patient if no family member were available?

Critical Thinking Exercises

The chain of survival as defined by the American Heart Association has five factors: immediate recognition and activation, early CPR, rapid defibrillation, effective advanced life support, and integrated post-cardiac arrest care. The purpose of this exercise is to apply these factors to the system where you work or live.

1. Evaluate the system you work or live in with respect to the chain of survival. Which links are strong, and which need work?
2. How successful is your system in resuscitating patients from cardiac arrest?

Pathophysiology to Practice

The following questions are designed to assist you in gathering relevant clinical information and making accurate decisions in the field.

1. A 10-year-old male was struck in the chest by a lacrosse ball. The blunt trauma was transmitted through his heart and caused ventricular fibrillation. He collapsed immediately and remains unresponsive. How will the current condition affect the patient's heart and brain? What is the most important treatment priority to correct the current problem?
2. A 16-year-old male was pulled from the water after a submersion injury. On arrival, he is unresponsive and not breathing. His skin is cold to touch. How would this condition change your typical resuscitation management, and why?

Street Scenes

Kerry is an active 80-year-old who lives alone in an upstairs apartment. She hasn't been feeling well all day. She has noticed that she is more tired than normal and that she is much more out of breath while climbing the stairs than usual. Kerry doesn't care much for going to the doctor, but she called her son because she suddenly got "all sweaty."

Her son arrives and finds her looking very unwell. Although Kerry denies it, she appears out of breath and very gray. She says that she will be fine and just needs to rest. She asks for a cup of tea. The son is very concerned but knows how stubborn his mother can be.

He calls to Kerry from the kitchen to ask her where the sugar is. He gets no response. He calls again . . . nothing. He rushes into the small living room and finds his mother unresponsive. He calls 911.

An emergency medical dispatcher recognizes the potential cardiac arrest situation and guides the son through chest compressions. The second dispatcher alerts your BLS ambulance as well as the ALS engine company for support. Your initial dispatch notes that CPR is in progress.

You arrive at the same time as the fire engine. You've trained with this team in the past, but before rushing in, you stop briefly to make a coordinated plan. You will be the team leader. The engine company will handle CPR, and your partner will deploy the AED. You gather equipment and enter.

You find the son doing chest compressions. His mother is lying on the couch, unresponsive.

Street Scene Question

1 **Since you have already established incident command, what is the first priority you will direct your team to complete?**

The team moves the patient to the floor. The patient is not responsive, and she does not appear to be breathing. One of the team members reports that no pulse is palpable.

NOTE: *Some of the material in this chapter on defibrillation and the AED has been adapted from material written by Kenneth R. Stults, M.S., former Director of the University of Iowa Hospitals and Clinics, Emergency Medical Services Learning Resources Center.*

Street Scene Questions

2 **What are the two most important treatment priorities for this patient?**

3 **Describe how you will deploy your five-person team.**

Chest compressions are initiated and ventilations are being performed. Your partner is cutting away clothes to attach the AED pads when the patient gasps.

Street Scene Question

4 **What does this finding tell you? How should you respond?**

Once the defib pads have been placed, the AED prompts to clear the patient by stating "Analyzing." The team leader ensures that no team member is touching the patient, but the compressor stays in place, with hands hovering over the patient's chest. Your partner verbally and visually clears the patient while the device analyzes. The AED prompts "Shock advised." After quickly announcing "Clear!" your partner hits the Shock button. You witness the patient's muscles contract with defibrillation.

Street Scene Question

5 **Now that the patient has been defibrillated, what should the team do next?**

The paramedic starts an intravenous line and administers medication. The patient starts to breathe on her own. You prepare for transport, and 20 minutes later you arrive in the emergency department with a conscious patient. A few weeks later, you learn from your agency's quality improvement coordinator that Kerry has recovered fully and is expected to return to an active lifestyle.

Diabetic Emergencies and Altered Mental Status

22

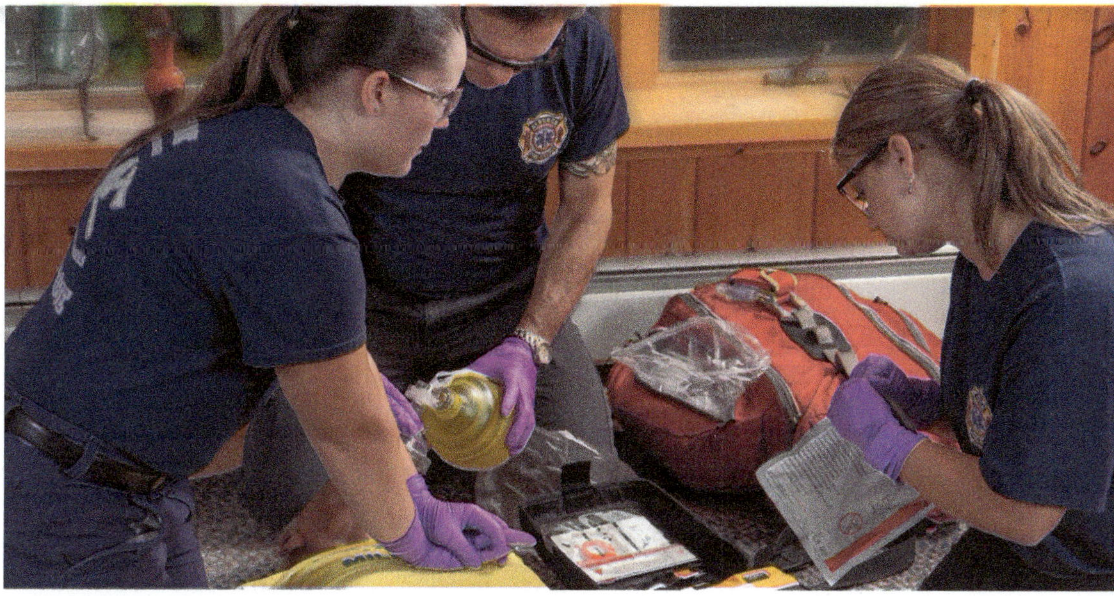

Related Chapters

The following chapters provide additional information related to topics discussed in this chapter:

- 4 Medical, Legal, and Ethical Issues
- 12 Primary Assessment
- 13 Vital Signs and Monitoring Devices
- 14 Principles of Assessment
- 15 Secondary Assessment
- 16 Reassessment
- 18 General Pharmacology
- 36 Obstetric and Gynecologic Emergencies

Standard

Medicine (Endocrine Disorders; Neurology)

Competency

Applies fundamental knowledge to provide basic emergency care and transportation based on assessment findings for an acutely ill patient.

Core Concepts

- General approaches to assessing the patient with an altered mental status
- Understanding the causes, assessment, and care of diabetes and various diabetic emergencies
- Understanding the causes, assessment, and care of seizure disorders

- Understanding the causes, assessment, and care of stroke
- Understanding the causes, assessment, and care of dizziness and syncope

Outcomes

After reading this chapter, you should be able to:

22.1 Explain the concepts of altered mental status (AMS). (pp. 622–624)

- Recall the role of the reticular activating system in level of responsiveness.
- List factors that can interfere with the function of the reticular activating system.
- Identify the range of changes that are considered alterations in mental status.
- Recognize the reason why a patient presenting with altered mental status is considered an emergency.
- Describe the emphasis on using the AVPU mnemonic in patients with AMS.
- Describe how the determination to use blood glucose monitoring is made in the assessment of a patient with AMS.
- Compare the assessment of the level of responsiveness in pediatric patients with limited verbal skills with that of adults.
- State the importance of interpreting trends in repeated assessments of the level of responsiveness.

22.2 Summarize the application of concepts of diabetes to patient care. (pp. 624–634)

- Describe the physiology of normal glucose breakdown and use by the body.
- Compare the pathophysiology of type 1 and type 2 diabetes.
- Describe causes of diabetic emergencies.
- Compare the effects of hypoglycemia on the body with those of hyperglycemia.
- Describe the pathophysiology of diabetic ketoacidosis.
- Differentiate through assessment findings between hypoglycemia and hyperglycemia.
- Describe the determination of blood glucose levels by glucometer.
- Interpret glucometer readings.
- Identify the indications and contraindications for administering oral glucose.
- Describe how to prioritize the administration of oral glucose with other interventions for a diabetic patient with AMS.
- Recall the key pharmacology of oral glucose.
- Describe the decision-making process in giving oral glucose to a diabetic patient in whom the EMT cannot distinguish between hypoglycemia and hyperglycemia.

22.3 Summarize the application of concepts of seizures to patient care. (pp. 634–638)

- Differentiate between partial and generalized seizures.
- Describe the phases of tonic-clonic generalized seizures.
- Identify common causes of seizures.
- Apply knowledge of causes of seizures to assessment findings to identify correctible causes of seizures.

- Explain why status epilepticus requires priority transport.
- Formulate questions to ask of witnesses about a patient who has had a seizure.
- Use the information attained in the clinical reasoning process to establish the patient's priority for transportation.
- Identify situations in which requesting advanced life support providers should be considered in the management of a patient having a seizure.
- Justify a treatment plan based on assessment findings.
- Compare the nature of pediatric seizures with that of seizures in adults.

22.4 Summarize the application of the concepts of stroke to patient care. (pp. 639-643)

- Compare the mechanisms of stroke caused by blood vessel obstruction and by hemorrhagic stroke.
- Describe how a stroke scale, such as the Cincinnati Prehospital Stroke Scale, is used to identify patients whose signs and symptoms may be caused by a stroke.
- Use clinical reasoning to determine whether your patient is likely to be having a stroke.
- Describe considerations in transporting a patient to a stroke center.

22.5 Summarize the application of concepts of dizziness and syncope to patient care. (pp. 643-647)

- Give examples of questions to ask a patient to clarify whether what was experienced was dizziness or syncope.
- Recognize potentially life-threatening causes of dizziness and syncope.
- Outline specific steps in the care of a patient with dizziness or syncope.

Key Terms

aura, *635*
diabetes mellitus, *624*
diabetic ketoacidosis (DKA), *626*
epilepsy, *636*
generalized seizure, *634*
glucose, *624*
hyperglycemia, *625*
hypoglycemia, *625*
insulin, *624*
partial seizure, *634*
postictal phase, *635*
reticular activating system (RAS), *622*
seizure, *634*
status epilepticus, *638*
stroke, *639*
syncope, *643*
tonic-clonic seizure, *634*

Altered mental status is a term used to describe a broad spectrum of abnormal responsiveness, clarity of thought, or mood that ranges from slight anxiety to unconsciousness. These changed mental states can result from structural damage to the brain, such as a traumatic brain injury; chemical changes to the brain, such as might be caused by exposure to a toxin; or metabolic changes to the brain caused, for example, by a lack of oxygen or glucose. Regardless of the cause, altered mental status represents a change in the way the brain is functioning that should always be considered a serious finding. A mental condition generally considered abnormal may be a normal state, or chronic condition, in a particular patient. However, altered mental status can often be the first and possibly only sign of a life-threatening condition.

A thorough assessment should be employed in all patients with altered mental status not only to differentiate acute changes from chronic conditions but also to identify the subtle indicators that point to life-threatening underlying problems. It may not always be possible to identify the cause of altered mental status, but recognizing its dangerous potential and treating any associated immediate life threats are key elements of a successful strategy of patient care.

Pathophysiology

reticular (ruh-TIK-yuh-ler) ***activating system (RAS)*** series of neurologic circuits in the brain that control the functions of staying awake, paying attention, and sleeping.

Normal consciousness is regulated by a series of neurologic circuits in the brain that comprise the ***reticular activating system (RAS)***. The RAS is essentially responsible for the functions of staying awake, paying attention, and sleeping.

The brain tissue of the RAS has simple requirements to function properly and thereby keep a person alert and oriented. Oxygen is needed to perfuse brain tissue, glucose is needed to nourish brain tissue, and water is needed to keep brain tissue hydrated. A lack of any of these can lead to rapid and serious alterations of function and result in altered mental status. In addition to deficiencies in any of these basic needs, other causes such as trauma, infection, and chemical toxins (as in overdoses and substance abuse) can also harm brain tissue.

Altered mental status can result from a primary brain problem, such as a stroke, but it may also be a symptom of a problem within another system, such as hypoxia due to an asthma attack. Often altered mental status is rapidly correctable by treating the underlying cause.

Assessing the Patient with Altered Mental Status

CORE CONCEPT
General approaches to assessing the patient with an altered mental status

Later in the chapter, we will discuss the assessment of specific disorders that may lead to altered mental status. However, there are some general approaches to assessing the patient with altered mental status that are important regardless of the cause.

Safety

A patient with altered mental status often can be dangerous to responders. Always consider the safety of yourself and your team prior to approaching a patient who is not acting appropriately. Use law enforcement when necessary.

"Altered mental status cases are the detective cases of EMS."

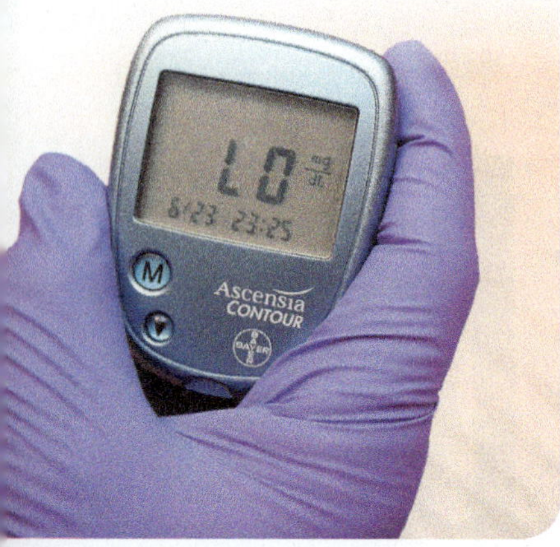

(© Daniel Limmer)

Primary Assessment

Among the most common causes of altered mental status are hypoxia and retention of carbon dioxide due to inadequate respiratory efforts. Even simple anxiety and combativeness may be the result of a failing respiratory system. Always consider the possibility of an airway and/or breathing problem in a patient with altered mental status. Although you should complete a thorough primary assessment on every patient, be especially attentive in the event of altered mental status.

Remember that the purpose of the primary assessment is to identify and treat life-threatening problems as found. As you assess the airway and breathing of a patient with altered mental status, you should carefully watch for any indication of inadequate breathing. Remember that as mental status decreases, so may the patient's ability to control and keep the airway open. Position may be very important to keeping an airway open in a semiconscious patient. Be alert to the possible need for suction, and use airway adjuncts if necessary.

When examining a patient who is breathing, look for the signs of respiratory failure and begin positive pressure ventilations as needed. Consider the administration of oxygen if you suspect hypoxia. Remember also that hypoperfusion associated with shock can cause mental status changes. Be alert for indicators such as rapid heart rate, absent radial pulses, pale skin, and delayed capillary refill time. Aggressively treat for shock if you identify its indicators.

During the primary assessment, you will determine a baseline mental status for your patient. This process does not need to be formal; it is typically accomplished simply by saying hello and assessing the patient's ability to respond. The acronym *AVPU* (as detailed in the *Primary Assessment* chapter) is a way to categorize the patient's initial response rapidly:

Alert: Patient responds with appropriate words when you introduce yourself.

Verbal: Patient responds by opening the eyes to the sound of your voice.

Painful: Patient opens the eyes only upon the application of an uncomfortable sensation such as a finger pinch.

Unresponsive: Patient does not respond at all.

AVPU is not a precise assessment of altered mental status, but it can be used as a quick reference point in the primary assessment. As the assessment progresses, the results of the quick AVPU check may be replaced by a more detailed Glasgow Coma score.

Secondary Assessment

Often altered mental status is a subtle sign. Although you may rule out immediate life threats, even a slightly altered mental status indicates serious underlying issues. Any patient exhibiting new, unusual behavior must be examined thoroughly. A body-systems exam and complete history may reveal important information about the suspected cause of the altered mental status. Based on this exam, you may find that field treatments are available, including administering glucose in the case of hypoglycemia, or prompt transport to an appropriate facility for stroke. Consider interviewing family members and bystanders, who may be able to tell you whether the patient's behavior and mental condition are normal and provide information the patient may not be able to provide. Review the patient's medicines to point to relevant medical history. Look for clues such as medic alert bracelets and other health-related items at the scene.

Consider also the need to document the patient's level of consciousness accurately over time. Although documentation should never stand in the way of urgent treatment needs, it is important to provide evidence of any changes in the level of consciousness as the call progresses. Consider using the Glasgow Coma Scale (which will be explored in further detail in the chapter *Trauma to the Head, Neck, and Spine*) to provide a precise measurement of the patient's responses. The Glasgow Coma Scale provides a numeric measure of various patient responses. This score can be compared with later measurements to help identify trends. It is particularly helpful because it uses a language that is common throughout the branches of health care; it is the same measuring tool that the emergency department, the operating room, and the critical care units will use. This standardization of terminology allows for a smooth transition as the patient progresses from one level of health care to another.

Pediatric Note

Young children may not be able to answer questions in the same manner as adults, and therefore their mental status is often difficult to establish. In these cases, use parents or caregivers to identify children's baseline level of consciousness by asking, "Are they acting differently than normal?" Most often, parents are the best judge of their child's current mental status.

CORE CONCEPT

Understanding the causes, assessment, and care of diabetes and various diabetic emergencies

Diabetes

Glucose and insulin are key elements in human physiology. The condition known as diabetes mellitus occurs as a result of the body's inability to maintain a balance between these substances or the interaction between them.

Glucose and the Digestive System

glucose (GLU-kos) a form of sugar, the body's basic source of energy.

Glucose, a form of sugar, is the body's basic source of energy. The cells of the body require glucose to remain alive and create energy. We take sugars into our body from the foods we eat, either sugar itself or other carbohydrates that the body's digestive system will convert to glucose. After the digestive system converts sugar and other carbohydrates into glucose, the glucose is absorbed into the bloodstream. The glucose molecule is large and will not pass into most of the cells without the assistance of insulin (described next). The pancreas secretes insulin when the blood glucose rises above about 90 mg/dL. Insulin binds to receptor sites on cells—especially those in the liver and muscles—and allows the large glucose molecule to pass into the cells. Normal glucose levels in the bloodstream are an essential part of maintaining normal mental status because glucose is essential for proper brain functioning.

Patients with diabetes (1) don't produce insulin, (2) don't produce enough insulin, and/or (3) have a body that has become resistant to the insulin that is produced. Medications taken by diabetics are designed to overcome these conditions.

Insulin and the Pancreas

insulin (IN-suh-lin) a hormone produced by the pancreas, or taken as a medication by many diabetics.

The pancreas is an organ found along the midline of the upper abdomen. The pancreas has a variety of functions, but one of its most important roles is the production of the hormone ***insulin***. Within the pancreas, specialized clusters of cells called the islets of Langerhans secrete insulin. Brain cells do not require insulin to move glucose from the bloodstream, but most other body cells use the insulin secreted by the pancreas to help transfer glucose from the blood across cell membranes into the cells. The insulin–glucose relationship has been described as a "lock and key" mechanism. Consider insulin the key. Without the insulin "key," glucose cannot enter the locked cells (Figure 22-1). When sugar intake and insulin production are balanced, the body can effectively use sugar as an energy source.

Diabetes Mellitus

diabetes mellitus (di-ah-BEE-tez MEL-i-tus) also called *sugar diabetes* or just *diabetes*, the condition brought about by decreased insulin production or the inability of the body cells to use insulin properly. The person with this condition is a diabetic.

About 30 million Americans, or roughly 1 in 11 people, have a condition called ***diabetes mellitus***. Generally speaking, this condition results either from an underproduction of insulin by the pancreas or from an inability of the body's cells to use insulin properly.

There are two primary types of diabetes, type 1 and type 2. *Type 1 diabetes* (formerly known as *juvenile* or *insulin-dependent* diabetes) occurs when pancreatic cells fail to function properly and insulin is not secreted normally. A person with type 1 diabetes simply does not produce enough, or in some cases any, insulin to transfer circulating glucose into

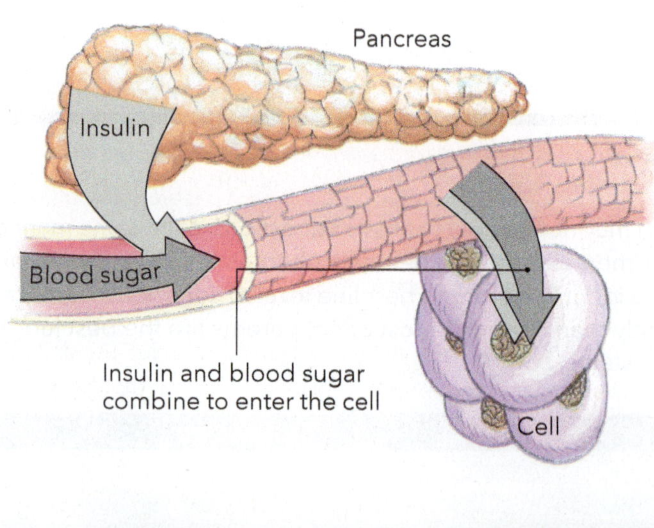

FIGURE 22-1 Insulin is needed to help the cells take in glucose.

the cells. If left untreated, glucose levels will build up in the blood while the cells of the body starve for sugar—too much glucose in the blood, not enough in the cells. A type 1 diabetic would be prescribed synthetic insulin to supplement inadequate naturally occurring insulin.

Type 2 diabetes (formerly known as non–insulin-dependent diabetes) occurs when the body's cells fail to use insulin properly. The pancreas may be secreting enough insulin, but the body is unable to use it to move glucose out of the blood and into the cells. Patients with type 2 diabetes can often control their condition with diet, oral antidiabetic medications, and sometimes insulin.

Diabetic Emergencies

Hypoglycemia

The most common medical emergency for the diabetic is ***hypoglycemia***, or low blood sugar. (*Hypo-* means "less than normal" or "deficient." *Glyc* means "sugar.") Hypoglycemia occurs when the person with diabetes does any one of the following:

hypoglycemia (HI-po-gli-SEE-me-ah) low blood sugar.

- Takes too much insulin (or, less commonly, takes too much of an oral medication used to treat diabetes), thereby transferring glucose into the cells too quickly and causing a rapid depletion of available sugar.
- Reduces sugar intake by not eating.
- Over-exercises or over-exerts, thus using sugars faster than normal.
- Vomits a meal, emptying the stomach of sugar as well as other food.
- Increases the metabolic rate in conditions such as fever or shivering.

When blood sugar is reduced, brain cells, as well as other cells of the body, starve. Even when the cause is too much insulin, the rapid uptake of sugar into the cells soon depletes the available supply in the bloodstream. Altered mental status, possible unconsciousness, and even permanent brain damage can occur quickly if the sugar is not replenished.

The brain and body do not tolerate low levels of sugar. Because of this fact, hypoglycemia typically has a very rapid onset. Abnormal behavior that often mimics a drunken stupor is very common. The body also responds to hypoglycemia with a fight-or-flight response. The sympathetic nervous system signals the liver to release glycogen (a form of stored sugar) in an attempt to raise blood glucose levels. Signs of this sympathetic discharge, which are very common, include pale, sweaty skin; tachycardia; and rapid breathing. Seizures can also occur as a result of altered brain function. Quick replenishment of blood sugar, often in the form of oral glucose, is critical to this patient's outcome. When it can be given without threatening the patient's airway, oral glucose should be administered promptly, before the patient becomes unconscious.

Inside the body of a hypoglycemic patient, the cells are starving for sugar. Brain cells, particularly the cells of the reticular activating system, are in need of glucose and, therefore, energy. As the body attempts to compensate, the fight-or-flight mechanism of the autonomic nervous system is engaged. Blood vessels constrict, the heart pumps faster and harder, and breathing accelerates.

Outside of the body, we see these changes in the form of signs and symptoms. Starving brain cells result in altered mental status. Confusion, stupor, unconsciousness, and seizures are common. Constricted blood vessels give the patient pale and sweaty skin. The fight-or-flight response increases the pulse rate and the respiratory rate.

Hyperglycemia

Hyperglycemia is high blood sugar. (*Hyper-* means "more than normal" or "excessive." *Glyc* means "sugar.") Hyperglycemia is usually caused by a lack of sufficient insulin, which leaves sugar in the bloodstream rather than helping it to enter the cells. The insulin deficiency may be due to the body's inability to produce insulin or may exist because insulin injections were forgotten or not given in sufficient quantity. Infection, stress, or increasing dietary intake can also be factors in hyperglycemia.

hyperglycemia (HI-per-gli-SEE-me-ah) high blood sugar.

Hyperglycemia typically develops over days and even weeks—in contrast to the typically rapid onset of hypoglycemia. Glucose levels in the blood creep up while the cells of the body begin to starve for sugar. As blood sugar levels increase, the patient may complain of chronic thirst and hunger. Some diabetics who are less attentive to managing their glucose can almost always be hyperglycemic, with glucose routinely running in the 200 -300 mg/dL range.

As blood sugar increases, water is pulled away from cells, causing systemic dehydration and potentially hypovolemic shock. Brain cells are damaged by dehydration, leading to a profound change in mental status. The overall dehydration results in the signs and symptoms of shock, including tachycardia, rapid respirations, and dropping blood pressure.

As a last resort, cells begin to break down fats and proteins, giving off ketones and other waste products. These waste products build up and combine with dehydration to cause a condition called ***diabetic ketoacidosis (DKA)***. The production of ketones can result in a fruity smell on the breath, similar to nail polish remover. A person with this complication will breathe rapidly as the body works to expel these by-products. If untreated, DKA can lead to death.

diabetic ketoacidosis (di-ah-BET-ic KEY-to-as-id-DO-sis) ***(DKA)*** a condition that occurs as the result of high blood sugar (hyperglycemia), characterized by dehydration, altered mental status, and shock.

In an attempt to rid the blood of excess sugar, the body will increase urination. Nausea is also a frequent complaint.

In some patients, on the other hand, production of ketones plays no role, or only a minor role, in the physiologic processes that are occurring. This condition is called *hyperglycemic hyperosmolar nonketotic syndrome.* (Some authorities don't include the word *nonketotic* in this name.) These patients typically have type 2 diabetes, but some have not yet been diagnosed and do not know they have diabetes. Patients who develop this condition tend to be older adults. Like patients with DKA, these patients look very sick. They are very dehydrated and have an altered mental status. The major difference in presentation is that with HHNS, there might be no unusual breath odor. Prehospital treatment is the same for both conditions.

Remember that it is not part of the scope of practice for an EMT to determine exactly which condition has caused a diabetic emergency. However, a later section of this chapter, Hypoglycemia and Hyperglycemia Compared, provides more information on these conditions.

Patient Assessment

Diabetic Emergencies

Prehospital diabetic treatment depends on rapid identification of the patient with an altered mental status and a history of diabetes. To assess the patient:

- Ensure a safe scene. People with diabetic emergencies can be agitated and sometimes violent. Always ensure the safety of yourself and your crew before approaching a patient with altered mental status.
- Perform a primary assessment. Identify altered mental status.
- Perform a secondary assessment. Gather the history from the patient or bystanders:
- Gather a history of the present episode. Ask about how the episode occurred, time of onset, duration, associated symptoms, any mechanism of injury or other evidence of trauma, and whether there have been any interruptions to the episode, seizures, or a fever.
    - During the SAMPLE history, ask the patient or bystanders if the patient has a history of diabetes. Look for a medical identification bracelet, wallet card, or other item suggesting a diabetic condition, such as a home-use blood glucose meter. Look in the refrigerator and elsewhere for medications such as insulin, a medication with a trade name for insulin (e.g., Humulin®), or an oral medication used to treat diabetes (such as metformin, Glucotrol®, Glucophage®, or Micronase®) (Figure 22-2). Cartridges containing an inhaled form of insulin do not need to be refrigerated if they are going to be used within a short time, so they may not be in a refrigerator. Some diabetic patients use an insulin pump. These small pumps are about the size of a deck of cards and are usually found worn on the belt. The pump will have a small catheter that enters into the abdomen or thigh (Figure 22-3). Also ask about the patient's last meal, last medication dose, and any related illnesses.

FIGURE 22-2 (A) Look for indications that the patient may have a history of diabetes, including medications in the refrigerator. (B) Victoza®, a daily noninsulin medication. (C) Trulicity® and Bydureon BCise®, weekly noninsulin medications.

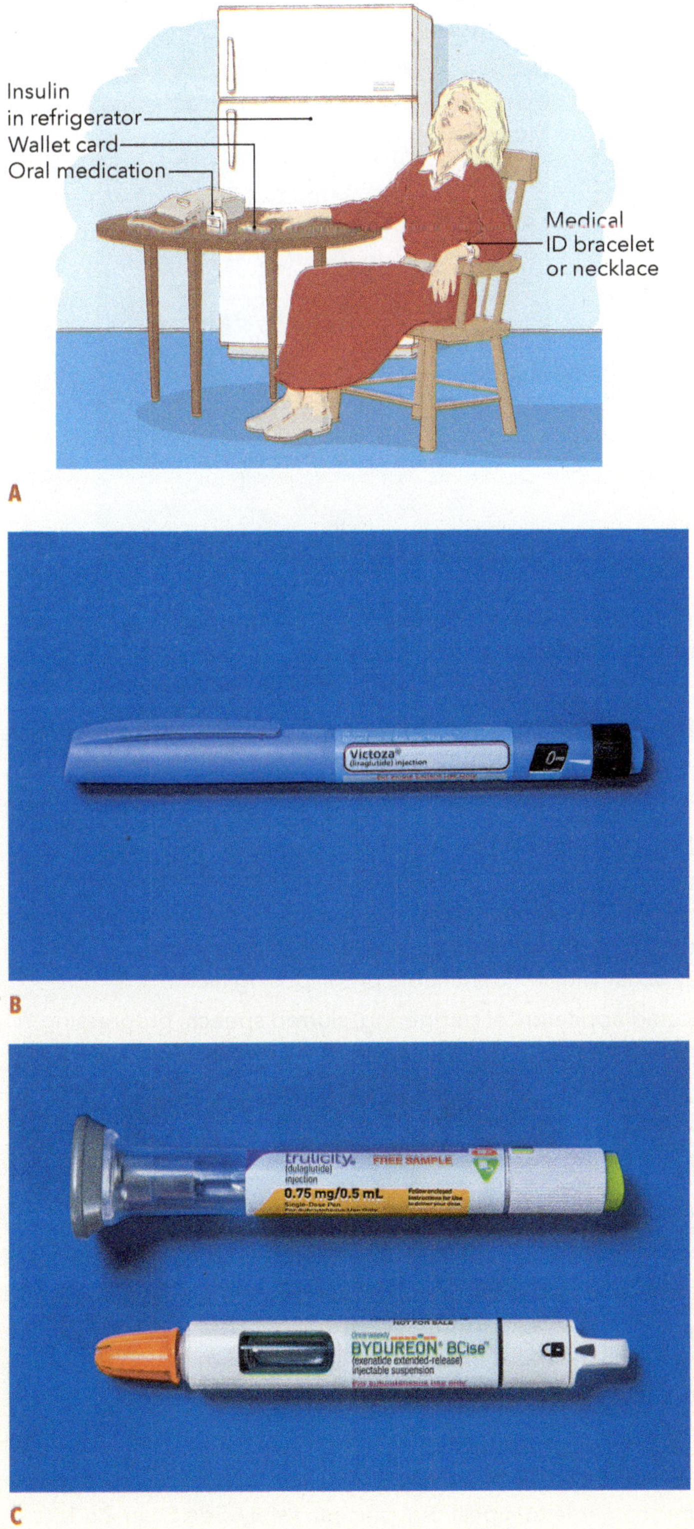

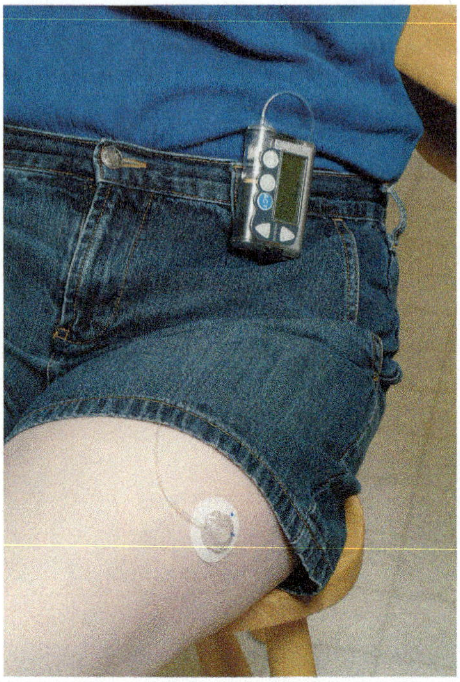

FIGURE 22-3 Some diabetics use an insulin pump.

  - Perform blood glucose monitoring if local protocols permit you to do so. (See the information in the next section.)
- Determine if the patient is alert enough to be able to swallow.
- Take baseline vital signs. (In some jurisdictions, oral glucose will be administered before the vital signs are taken.)

The following signs and symptoms are associated with a diabetic emergency:

- Rapid onset of altered mental status:
  - After missing a meal on a day the patient took prescribed insulin
  - After vomiting a meal on a day the patient took prescribed insulin
  - After an unusual amount of physical exercise or work
  - May occur with no identifiable predisposing factor
- Intoxicated appearance, staggering, slurred speech, progressing to unconsciousness
- Cold, clammy skin
- Elevated heart rate
- Hunger
- Uncharacteristic behavior
- Anxiety
- Combativeness
- Seizures

Decision Point

Is My Patient Hypoglycemic?

This is important because there is an effective field treatment for the patient who is hypoglycemic and able to ingest oral glucose safely. See Scan 22-1.

SCAN 22-1 Management of a Diabetic Emergency

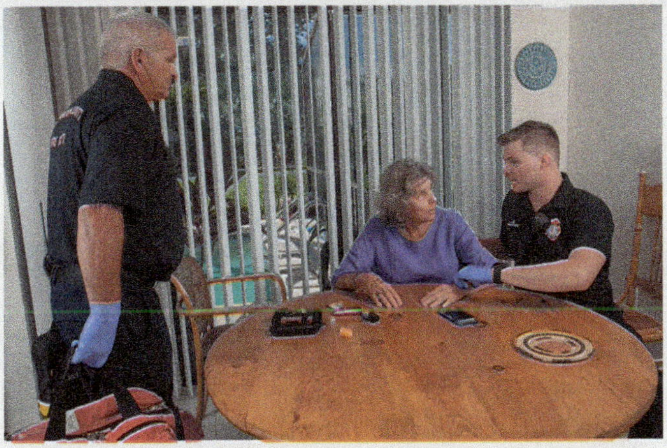

1. Perform a primary assessment. Determine if the patient's mental status is altered.

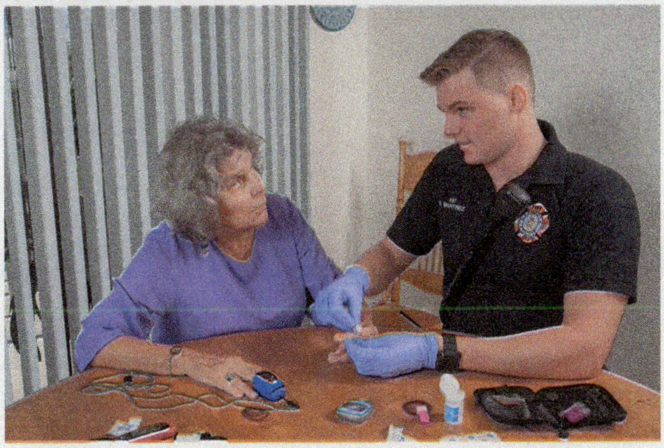

2. Perform a secondary assessment and take the patient's vital signs. Be sure to find out if the patient has a history of diabetes. Observe for a medical identification device.

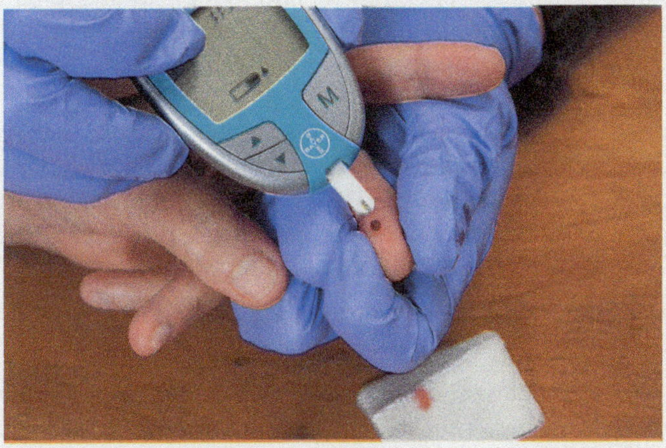

3. If your protocols allow, check the patient's blood glucose level. (See the *Vital Signs and Monitoring Devices* chapter.)

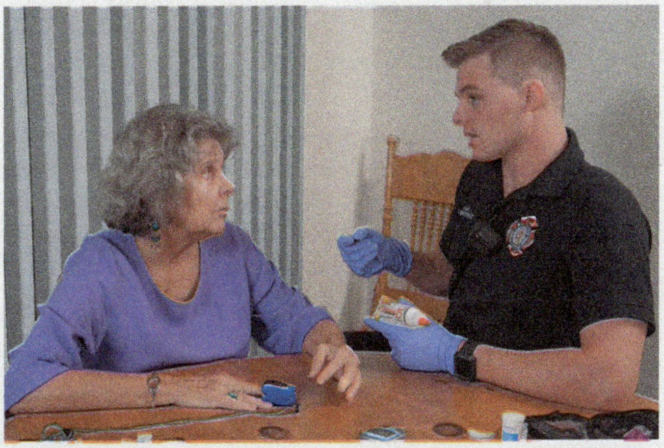

4. If the patient has a history of diabetes, has an altered mental status, and is alert enough to swallow, check the expiration date and prepare to administer oral glucose.

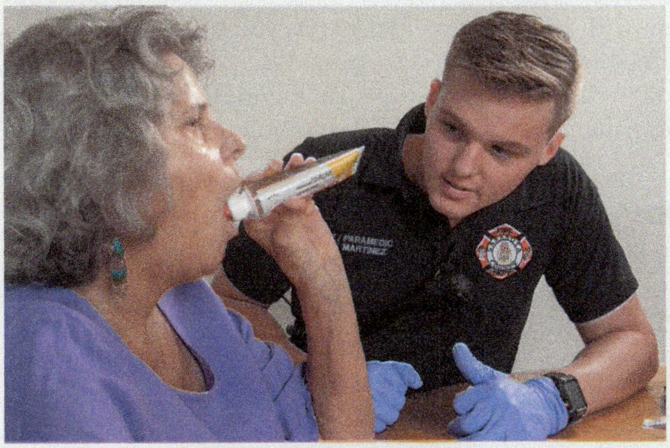

5. Assist the patient in accepting oral glucose.

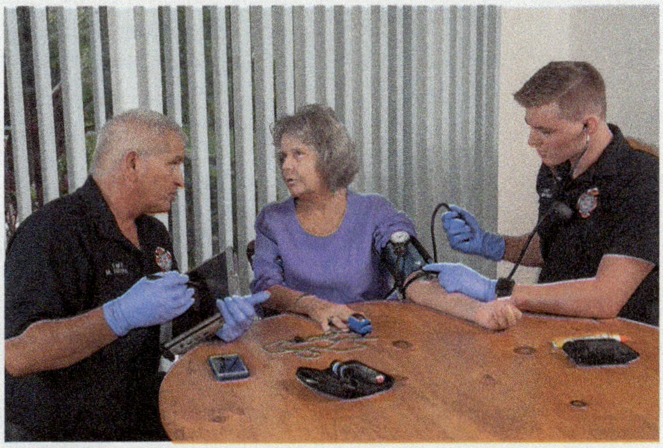

6. Reassess the patient. Document oral glucose administration.

Pediatric Note

Type 1 diabetes often presents for the first time during childhood. Children with diabetes are more at risk for medical emergencies than diabetic adults. Children are more active and may exhaust blood sugar levels by playing hard—especially if they have taken their prescribed insulin. Children are also less likely to be disciplined about eating correctly and on time. As a consequence, children are more at risk of hypoglycemia.

Blood Glucose Meters

One of the many advances in managing diabetes has been the development of portable, reliable blood glucose meters (Figure 22-4). People with diabetes now routinely test the level of glucose in their blood at least once a day and sometimes as often as five or six times a day. By measuring the amount of glucose in their blood, they can determine very precisely how much insulin they should take and how much and how often they should eat. Keeping blood glucose levels as close to normal as possible leads to significantly fewer diabetes-related complications (like heart disease, blindness, and kidney failure, to name a few), so people with diabetes have a strong motivation to keep their blood glucose level within the normal range. The chapter *Vital Signs and Monitoring Devices* discussed blood glucose meters and steps for their use.

Another advance in the management of diabetes is the continuous glucose monitor. This device includes several parts: a sensor that goes just under the skin, a transmitter that sends data from the sensor, and a receiving device, like a smart phone, that records and displays the data. This allows someone with diabetes to get glucose readings as often as every 5 minutes.

NOTE: *EMTs must have permission from medical direction or local protocol to perform blood glucose monitoring using a blood glucose meter.*

If the patient has a glucose meter, the patient or a family member can use it to determine the patient's blood glucose level. Generally, EMTs should not use a patient's glucose meter. There are many different types of these devices on the market, each with its own instructions for use that vary from device to device. In addition, there is no way for the EMT to know whether the test strips have been stored properly or when the device was last calibrated. These facts are very important if the reading is to be accurate. Similarly, if the patient has a continuous glucose monitor, you may be able to view the data, but if you encounter a diabetic patient with an altered mental status, you should use your own blood glucose meter to determine the patient's blood sugar.

A value lower than 60 mg/dL (milligrams per deciliter) in a symptomatic diabetic (i.e., a patient with a mild alteration in mental status or who is diaphoretic [sweaty]) is typical

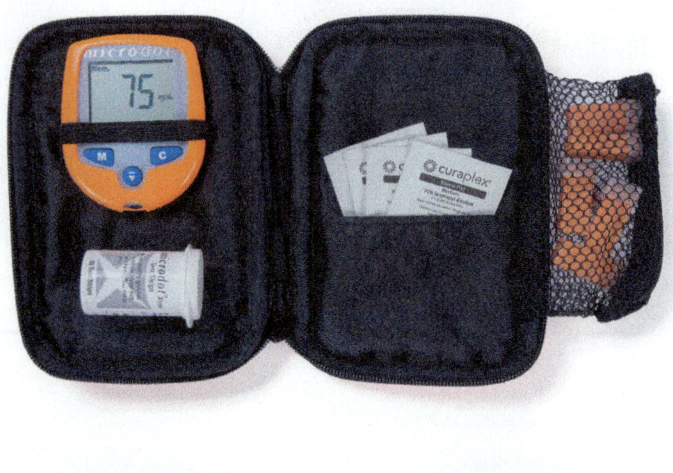

FIGURE 22-4 Most diabetics use home glucose meters to test their blood glucose levels.

of hypoglycemia and indicates the need for prompt administration of glucose. Some protocols use slightly different thresholds for the definition of hypoglycemia, so be sure to become familiar with your system's guidelines. Patients with values lower than 50 mg/dL will typically have significant alterations in mental status. They may be unable to focus or perform simple tasks. They may become completely unresponsive. Patients with a blood glucose level that is this low will often be unable to receive oral glucose safely.

Generally, a reading greater than 140 indicates hyperglycemia. Patients with glucose levels in the mid and high 100s often do not have acute symptoms. However, over time hyperglycemia can cause damage to various body organs. Patients with blood glucose levels greater than 300, especially for a prolonged time, may experience dehydration and other more serious symptoms, and they should receive medical care.

A reading inconsistent with the patient's symptoms (such as 25 mg/dL in a patient who is alert and oriented) should make the EMT question the result. There are many potential causes of inaccurate results, including insufficient blood on the test strip, a strip past its expiration date or not stored properly, or a meter that needs calibration. Although many people use blood glucose meters appropriately and accurately, it is quite common to get an inaccurate reading, especially when the device is not used properly. It is critical that any health care provider using a blood glucose meter to test a patient's blood have the proper training in use of the device and be thoroughly familiar with its care and maintenance. Calibration and testing on a regularly scheduled basis are essential if the device is to give accurate results.

On occasion, the glucometer will display the word *HIGH* rather than a number. Depending on the manufacturer, a "High" or "HI" reading indicates an extremely high glucose level, usually in excess of 500 mg/dL. The word *LOW* usually indicates blood glucose levels that are extremely low (often less than 15 mg/dL).

Remember that the blood glucose monitor is just one tool used in your assessment of a patient with an altered mental status. Blood glucose monitoring, and any other examination, should never be done before a thorough primary assessment has been performed. Some areas recommend that the blood glucose measurements be done while en route to the hospital.

Patient Care

Care of the Patient with a Diabetic Emergency

Fundamental Principles of Care

It is important to recall that excessively low blood glucose is a more life-threatening emergency than excessively high blood glucose. Administering glucose can help a hypoglycemic patient and will cause no long-term harm in a hyperglycemic patient being transported to a health care facility that will provide definitive diagnosis and treatment.

Emergency care of a patient with a diabetic emergency includes the following, generally in this order (see Scan 22-1 and Scan 22-2):

- Occasionally a person with only mild hypoglycemia and minor altered mental status can be treated simply by giving the patient something to eat. It may be more appropriate to ask a person who is only slightly confused to drink a glass of juice or eat a piece of toast than to ingest a tube of oral glucose. You must understand that food treatment will take longer to resolve the hypoglycemia than tube glucose and that food will raise glucose levels in a patient who has severe hyperglycemia. Always use good clinical judgment to determine whether your patient needs more aggressive care.
- Determine if all of the following criteria for administration of oral glucose are present: The patient has a history of diabetes, has an altered mental status, and is awake enough to swallow safely.
- If the patient meets the criteria for administration of oral glucose, let the patient squeeze the glucose from the tube directly into the mouth.
- Reassess the patient. If the patient's condition does not improve after administration of oral glucose, consult medical direction about whether to administer more. If at any time the patient loses consciousness, do not administer further oral glucose, and take steps to ensure an open airway.

If the patient is not awake enough to swallow, treat as you would any other patient with an altered mental status—that is, secure the airway, provide artificial ventilations if necessary, and be prepared to perform CPR if needed. Position the patient appropriately. If the patient does not need to be ventilated, place the patient in the recovery position (on one side) so there is less likelihood of choking on or aspirating fluids or vomitus into the lungs. Request an ALS intercept if available.

Decision Point

Should I Give Oral Glucose?

The most important decision point in choosing to give oral glucose is the patient's ability to swallow. Although a severely hypoglycemic patient may desperately need sugar, if the patient is unable to protect the airway, administration of oral gel may be the worst thing you can do. Only administer oral glucose to those patients who can swallow it and protect their airway from aspiration.

A few EMS systems allow administration of intranasal glucagon to patients who are unable to swallow oral glucose safely. Glucagon is a naturally occurring hormone that signals the liver to convert stored glycogen into glucose and release it into the bloodstream. This is the same compensatory action that occurs with the fight-or-flight nervous system response. To use an intranasal medication, the appropriate dose of glucagon is drawn into a syringe, which is then attached to an atomizer device. The atomizer is inserted into the patient's nostril, and the medication is administered rapidly. The mist that is ejected from the atomizer clings to the highly vascular mucous membrane of the nose, and the medication is absorbed into the bloodstream. Intranasal glucagon is not commercially available and has not been approved by the Food and Drug Administration, but some EMS systems may be administering it under a research protocol.

SCAN 22-2 Oral Glucose

MEDICATION NAME

Generic: Glucose, oral
Trade: Glutose®, Insta-glucose®

INDICATIONS

Patients with altered mental status and a known history of diabetes mellitus

CONTRAINDICATIONS

- Unconsciousness
- Known diabetic who has not taken insulin for days
- Unable to swallow

MEDICATION FORM

Gel, in toothpaste-type tubes

DOSAGE

One tube

ADMINISTRATION

1. Ensure signs and symptoms of altered mental status with a known history of diabetes.
2. Ensure patient is conscious.
3. Administer glucose by one of these two methods:
   a. Place on tongue depressor between cheek and gum.
   b. Have patient self-administer between cheek and gum.
4. Perform reassessment. Document administration.

ACTIONS

Increases blood sugar.

SIDE EFFECTS

None when given properly. May be aspirated by the patient without a gag reflex.

REASSESSMENT STRATEGIES

If patient loses consciousness or has a seizure, remove the tongue depressor from the mouth.

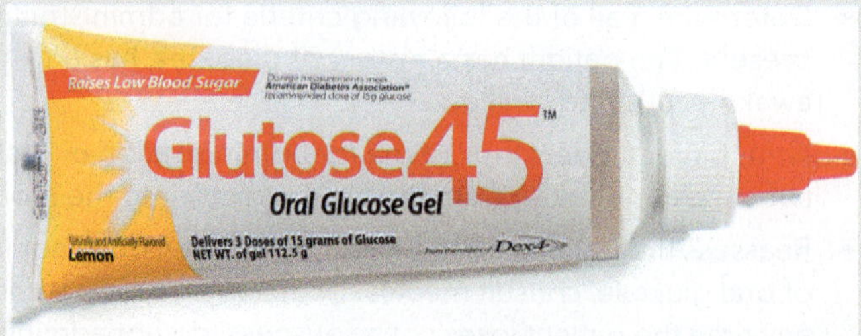

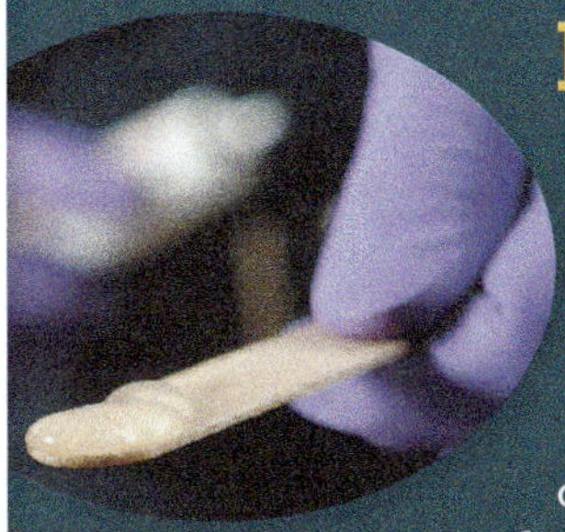

Point of View

"You'd think after you've been a diabetic most of your life that the meter needles wouldn't bother you. Actually, they've gotten better and need less blood.

"Despite how much I try to keep my blood sugar regulated, no matter how much I see my doctor, I end up needing an ambulance a couple of times a year. It is almost embarrassing. I see the same people time after time, and they are always so nice to me.

"I remember the days before we could check my blood sugar. I'd just have to get some sugar. If it wasn't low, it would take days to get me back regulated again after all that sugar. When the EMTs came today, they were right on the ball. They checked my sugar, and it was the lowest I have ever seen it. They put a blob of that goop on a tongue depressor and put it in my mouth, and I was better pretty quickly.

"But I still get sick of the needles sometimes."

Hypoglycemia and Hyperglycemia Compared

Many students find that they confuse hypoglycemia and hyperglycemia. Fortunately, the use of reliable blood glucose monitoring in the field has made this distinction much easier. It is also important to note that it is not necessary to distinguish between the two conditions to give emergency treatment. There are three typical differences between hypoglycemia and hyperglycemia:

1. **Onset.** Hyperglycemic emergencies usually have a slower onset, whereas hypoglycemia tends to come on suddenly. This is because sugar still reaches the brain in hyperglycemic (high–blood sugar) states. With hypoglycemia (low blood sugar), it is possible that no sugar is reaching the brain. Seizures may occur.

Think Like an EMT

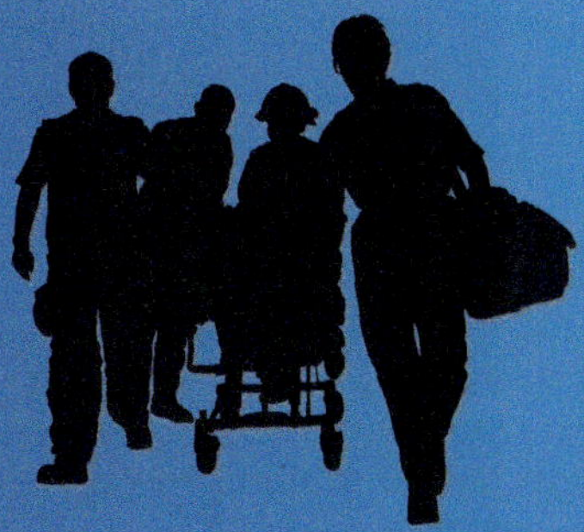

The Sweet Taste of Success

For each of the following patients, determine if the general criteria are met for you to administer glucose to the patient. Oral glucose is carried on your ambulance. For the purposes of this exercise, assume that your blood glucose monitor is not available. (It is sometimes important to make decisions independent of devices.)

1. Your patient is confused. She doesn't know what day it is and is talking but not making any sense. Her nurse's aide tells you the patient has diabetes and has been having trouble managing her blood sugar levels. She will occasionally take insulin but not eat, and vice versa.
2. At a facility for disabled youth, a 19-year-old man recovering from a head injury was seizing prior to your arrival, but the seizure has stopped. He responds to loud verbal stimulus. He has a history of diabetes.
3. You respond to a motor-vehicle collision and find a patient sitting behind the wheel of his car, rocking back and forth, muttering incoherently. The accident was low-speed, with a very minor impact. You observe a medical identification bracelet that indicates the patient has diabetes.

2. **Skin.** Hyperglycemic patients often have warm, red, dry skin. Hypoglycemic patients have cold, pale, moist, or "clammy" skin.
3. **Breath.** The hyperglycemic patient often has acetone breath (like nail polish remover), whereas the hypoglycemic patient does not. However, you should keep in mind that not all hyperglycemic patients will exhibit this sign.

Also, patients who are hyperglycemic frequently breathe very deeply and rapidly, as though they have just run a race. Dry mouth, intense thirst, abdominal pain, and vomiting are all common signs and symptoms of this condition. The proper treatment is given under close medical supervision in a hospital.

There appear to be clear-cut differences between the signs and symptoms of hyperglycemia and those of hypoglycemia, but distinguishing between them in the field can be difficult and is not necessary. If your system allows the use of blood glucose monitoring, that may provide the patient's actual blood glucose level. This can be used to identify someone with hypo- or hyperglycemia. Remember that this is just one tool in your assessment, which—when combined with the patient's history (e.g., food intake and medications taken) and your protocols—will aid in your decision-making process. Always consult medical direction if questions or concerns arise.

Giving glucose will help the hypoglycemic patient by getting needed sugar into the bloodstream and to the brain. Although the hyperglycemic patient already has too much sugar in the blood, the extra dose of glucose will not have time to cause damage in the short time before reaching the hospital, where the patient can receive a definitive diagnosis and treatment. This is why "sugar (glucose) for everyone" is the rule of thumb for diabetic emergencies, whether the patient is hypo- or hyperglycemic, and why you do not need to distinguish between the two conditions.

NOTE: *Some hyperglycemic and hypoglycemic patients will appear to be intoxicated. Always suspect a diabetic problem in cases that seem to involve no more than intoxication. Remember that the patient intoxicated on alcohol may also be a diabetic, with the alcohol breath covering the acetone odor of diabetic ketoacidosis. Alcoholic diabetics are good candidates for a diabetic emergency because they tend to neglect eating and taking insulin during prolonged drinking.*

Other Causes of Altered Mental Status

In addition to diabetic emergencies, there are many other causes of altered mental status. Examples include hypoxia; sepsis; drug and alcohol use; brain injuries, both traumatic and medical; metabolic abnormalities; brain tumors; and infectious diseases such as meningitis. In all cases, use a thorough primary assessment to identify immediate life threats. Gather a careful history; then calm the patient and transport to the hospital.

The following sections provide additional information on three causes of altered mental status: seizure disorders, stroke, and dizziness or syncope. Other chapters describe more fully other conditions that can cause or lead to altered mental status.

seizure (SEE-zher)
a sudden change in sensation, behavior, or movement. The most severe form of seizure produces violent muscle contractions called convulsions.

partial seizure
a seizure that affects only one part or one side of the brain.

generalized seizure
a seizure that affects both sides of the brain.

tonic-clonic (TON-ik-KLON-ik) ***seizure***
a generalized seizure in which the patient loses consciousness and has jerking movements of paired muscle groups.

Seizure Disorders

If the normal functions of the brain are upset by injury, infection, or disease, the brain's electrical activity can become irregular. This irregularity can bring about a sudden change in sensation, behavior, or movement, called a ***seizure*** (also called a *fit*, *spell*, or *attack* by nonmedical people). A seizure is not a disease in itself but rather a sign of some underlying defect, injury, or disease.

There are two types of seizures: partial and generalized. ***Partial seizures*** affect only one part or one side of the brain. Often these seizures affect only one area of the body, and the patient usually does not lose consciousness. ***Generalized seizures*** affect the entire brain, and as a result affect the consciousness of the patient. EMS is most likely to be called for a type of generalized seizure characterized by unconsciousness and major motor activity, called a ***tonic-clonic seizure***. A tonic–clonic seizure often comes without warning, although a person may cry out before it begins. The patient will thrash about wildly, and the entire body is involved. The convulsion usually lasts only a few minutes and has three distinct phases:

- **Tonic phase.** The body becomes rigid, stiffening for no more than 30 seconds. Breathing may stop, and the patient may bite the tongue (rare) and could lose bowel and bladder control.
- **Clonic phase.** The body jerks about violently, usually for no more than 1 or 2 minutes. (Some can last 5 minutes.) The patient may foam at the mouth and drool. The face and lips often become cyanotic.
- **Postictal phase.** The ***postictal phase*** begins when convulsions stop. The patient usually regains consciousness quickly and enters a state of drowsiness and confusion that gradually clears. Some postictal patients may remain unconscious for more prolonged periods. Headache is common. Some postictal patients may show temporary strokelike unilateral weakness.

postictal (post-IK-tul) ***phase***
the period of time immediately following a tonic-clonic seizure in which the patient goes from full loss of consciousness to full mental status.

The length of the postictal phase may vary greatly from patient to patient. A few patients come around immediately, but most take much longer. It is important to remember that some patients may become combative and even violent toward rescuers during this phase. Safety should always be a priority.

Some seizures are preceded by an aura. An ***aura*** is a sensation the patient has when a seizure is about to happen. Often the patient notes a smell, a sound, or even just a general feeling right before the seizure begins. It is important to document this finding when it exists.

aura
a sensation experienced by a seizure patient right before the seizure, which might be a smell, sound, or general feeling.

Not all seizures you will see are generalized tonic–clonic seizures. Although infrequent, partial seizures may require your assistance. In this type of seizure, you may see uncontrolled muscle spasm or convulsion in a patient with a fully alert mental status. You may also see a patient who has only a brief loss of consciousness, without muscle convulsions. These seizures may be very difficult to distinguish from other disorders. Always use a thorough patient assessment to guide your care.

Causes of Seizures

The most common cause of seizures in adults is failure to take prescribed antiseizure medications. The most common cause of seizures in infants and children 6 months to 3 years of age is high fever (febrile seizures). Other causes include:

- **Hypoxia.** A lack of oxygen frequently causes seizures. These seizures often immediately precede respiratory and/or cardiac arrest.
- **Stroke.** Clots and bleeding in the brain are frequent causes of seizure. We will discuss this topic in greater detail later in this chapter.
- **Traumatic brain injury.** Acute brain injuries can cause seizures. Some patients with a previous history of brain injury can develop chronic seizures disorders.
- **Toxins.** Drug or alcohol use, abuse, or withdrawal can cause seizures. Other poisons can also alter brain function to cause a seizure.
- **Hypoglycemia.** As we discussed earlier in this chapter, hypoglycemia (low blood sugar) is a frequent cause of seizures.
- **Brain tumor.** A brain tumor may occasionally cause seizures.
- **Congenital brain defects.** Seizures due to congenital defects of the brain (defects one is born with) are most often seen in infants and young children.
- **Infection.** Swelling or inflammation of the brain caused by an infection can cause seizures.
- **Metabolic.** Seizures can be caused by irregularities in the patient's body chemistry (metabolism).
- **Idiopathic.** This means occurring spontaneously with an unknown cause. This is often the case with seizures that start in childhood.

In addition, seizures may be seen with:

- Epilepsy
- Measles, mumps, and other childhood diseases
- Eclampsia (a severe complication of pregnancy)
- Heat stroke (resulting from exposure to high temperatures)
- Briefly, with the onset of syncope

epilepsy (EP-uh-lep-see) a medical condition that causes seizures.

Epilepsy is perhaps the best known of the conditions that result in seizures. Epilepsy is not a disease itself but rather an umbrella term used when a person has multiple seizures from an unknown cause. Some people are born with epilepsy, whereas others develop epilepsy after a head injury or surgery. Conscientious use of medications allows most epileptics to live normal lives without seizures of any type. However, it is common for epileptic patients to seize if they fail to take their medications properly or if an illness interferes with the normal medication routine. Remember that although a patient with seizures may be epileptic, epilepsy is only one condition that causes seizures.

Patient Assessment

Seizure Disorders

It is very important to be able to describe the seizure to emergency department personnel. If you have not observed the seizure (usually EMS is called after the seizure has taken place), always try to find out what it was like by asking the following questions of bystanders. Be sure to record and report your findings.

- What was the person doing before the seizure started? Was there an aura?
- Exactly what did the person do during the seizure–movement by movement–especially at the beginning? Was there loss of bladder and/or bowel control?
- How long did the seizure last?
- What did the person do after the seizure? Was the person asleep? For how long? Was the person awake? Was the person able to answer questions? (If you are present during the seizure, use the AVPU scale to assess mental status.)

NOTE: *Multiple patients seizing at the same time is a major scene safety red flag. If this occurs, consider the possibility of a chemical weapon or similar weapon of mass destruction or hazardous material exposure, and take appropriate precautions.*

Patient Care

Care of the Patient with a Seizure Disorder

Fundamental Principles of Care

Most seizures are brief, lasting no more than minutes, so a patient who is still seizing when you arrive is a priority transport. Establishing and maintaining a patent airway at the scene and en route to the hospital is essential.

Emergency care of a patient with a seizure disorder includes the following.

If You Are Present When a Convulsive Seizure Occurs:

- Place the patient on the floor or ground. If there is no possibility of spine injury, position the patient on the side, to allow drainage from the mouth.
- Loosen restrictive clothing.
- Remove objects that may harm the patient.
- Protect the patient from injury, but do not try to hold the patient still during convulsions (Figure 22-5).

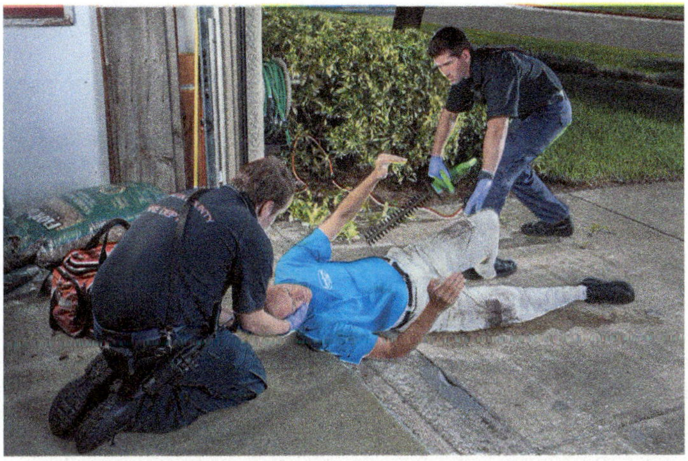

FIGURE 22-5 Protect the seizure patient from injury.

- If the patient has a vagus nerve stimulator (a watch-sized device implanted in the chest with a wire that can send electrical impulses to the left vagus nerve in the neck), allow family members familiar with the device to apply their magnet to the device (Figure 22-6). These impulses can reduce the frequency or intensity of seizures when medications are not able to control them fully.

After Convulsions Have Ended:

- Protect the airway. A patient who has just had a generalized seizure will sometimes drool and will usually be very drowsy for a little while, so you may need to suction the airway. If there is no possibility of spine injury, position the patient on one side, to allow drainage from the mouth.
- If the patient is cyanotic (blue), ensure an open airway and provide artificial ventilations with supplemental oxygen. Patients who are breathing adequately may be given oxygen by nasal cannula or nonrebreather based on pulse oximetry readings. Hypoxia is common after long periods of seizure activity.
- Treat any injuries the patient may have sustained during the convulsions, or rule out trauma. Head injury can cause seizures, or the patient may have sustained injuries from striking objects during the seizure. Immobilize the neck and spine if trauma is suspected.
- Transport to a medical facility, monitoring vital signs and respirations closely.

NOTE: *Never place anything in the mouth of a seizing patient. Objects can be broken and could obstruct the patient's airway.*

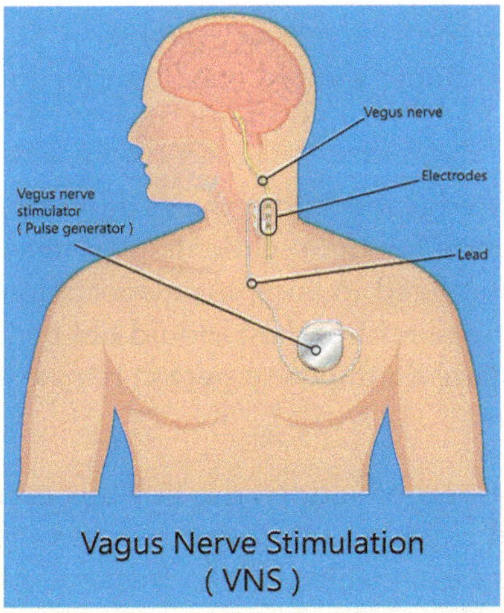

FIGURE 22-6 Illustration of the positioning of a vagal nerve stimulator. (rumruay/Shutterstock)

status epilepticus (STAY-tus or STAT-us ep-i-LEP-ti-kus) a prolonged seizure or situation when a person suffers two or more convulsive seizures without regaining full consciousness.

NOTE: *Seizures usually last no more than 2 or 3 minutes. When the patient has two or more convulsive seizures in a row without regaining full consciousness, or has a single seizure lasting more than 10 minutes, it is known as* ***status epilepticus****. Some systems consider all patients who are still seizing when EMS arrives on the scene to be in status epilepticus. This is a high-priority, life-threatening emergency requiring immediate transport to the hospital and possible ALS intercept (having an advanced life support team meet your ambulance en route). The paramedics must open and maintain the airway at the scene and while en route. In a person with status epilepticus, oxygen and other support for breathing; intravenous fluids; and emergency medications will be needed.*

Types of Seizures

It is beyond the EMT's scope of practice to identify the type of seizure the patient is having. The EMT's job is to treat immediate life threats, gather a history, and provide other normal assessment and care as previously described. However, some additional background information about types of seizures can provide perspective.

Partial Seizures. In a simple partial seizure (also called a *focal motor*, *focal sensory*, or *Jacksonian seizure*), there is tingling, stiffening, or jerking in just one part of the body. There may also be an aura, which is a sensation such as a smell, bright lights, a burst of colors, or a rising sensation in the stomach. There is no loss of consciousness. However, in some cases the jerking may spread and develop into a tonic–clonic seizure.

A complex partial seizure (also called *psychomotor* or *temporal lobe seizure*) is often preceded by an aura. This type of seizure is characterized by abnormal behavior that varies widely from person to person. It may involve confusion, a glassy stare, aimless moving about, lip smacking or chewing, or fidgeting with clothing. The person may appear to be drunk or on drugs. The patient is not violent but may struggle or fight if restrained. Very rarely, such extreme behavior as screaming, running, disrobing, or showing great fear may occur. There is no loss of consciousness, but there may be confusion and no memory of the episode afterward. In some cases, the seizure may develop into a tonic–clonic seizure. For a simple or complex partial seizure, do not restrain the person; simply remove nearby objects and gently guide the patient away from danger.

Generalized Seizures. When we think of generalized seizures, we think of the tonic–clonic seizure. However, there are other types of generalized seizures we should know about.

An absence seizure (also called a *petit mal seizure*) is brief, usually less than 10 seconds. There is no dramatic motor activity, and the person usually does not slump or fall. Instead, there is a temporary loss of concentration or awareness. An absence seizure may go unnoticed by everyone except the person and knowledgeable members of the person's family. A child may suffer several hundred absence seizures a day, severely interfering with the ability to pay attention and do well in school. Absence seizures often stop before adulthood but sometimes worsen and become tonic–clonic seizures.

Patient care for the generalized tonic–clonic seizure was described earlier. For an absence seizure, if you are aware that it has occurred, simply provide any information the patient may have missed.

Patients with epilepsy are often knowledgeable about their condition, medications, and history. Since seizures may be common for these patients, they may refuse transportation. These patients should be encouraged to accept transportation to a hospital for examination. Should patients continue to refuse, they should not be left alone after the seizure, and they must not drive. Be sure a competent person remains with patients in these cases.

Pediatric Patients with Seizures. High fevers or sudden rise in temperature is the most common cause of seizures in infants and children. Idiopathic seizures (with no known cause) are also common in children. Seizures in children who frequently have them are rarely life-threatening. However, as an EMT, you should treat any seizure in an infant or child as if it is life-threatening. Parents or caregivers of children with first-time seizures will often need emotional support by the EMT, as these events can be very frightening.

Stroke

One of the many causes of altered mental status may be a ***stroke***. Formerly called a *cerebral vascular accident (CVA)*, *stroke* refers to the death or injury of brain tissue that is deprived of oxygen. This can be caused by blockage of an artery that supplies blood to part of the brain, or by bleeding from a ruptured blood vessel in the brain. A stroke caused by a blockage, called an *ischemic stroke*, can occur when a clot or embolism occludes an artery. This mechanism is responsible for most strokes. A stroke caused by bleeding into the brain, called a *hemorrhagic stroke*, frequently is the result of long-standing high blood pressure (hypertension). It also can occur when a weak area of an artery (an aneurysm) bulges out and eventually ruptures, forcing the brain into a smaller-than-usual space within the skull.

stroke
a condition of altered function caused when an artery in the brain is blocked or ruptured, disrupting the supply of oxygenated blood or causing bleeding into the brain. Formerly called a *cerebrovascular accident (CVA)*.

CORE CONCEPT
Understanding the causes, assessment, and care of stroke

Different patients experiencing a stroke may have very different signs and symptoms, depending on the size and location of the arteries involved. One of the most common signs is one-sided weakness (hemiparesis). Stroke patients commonly note difficulty moving one side of their body or report changes in their ability to do common tasks such as hold a pen or walk normally. Because the left side of the brain controls movement on the right side of the body (and vice versa), someone with right-sided weakness from a stroke actually has a problem on the left side of the brain. However, the nerves that control the face muscles do not necessarily cross over in the same way, so sagging or drooping on one side of the face is not a reliable sign of injury to the opposite side. Difficulty speaking or a complete inability to speak is also a common finding in stroke patients. Your patient may be unable to form words, and might be speaking incomprehensibly. You might also find a patient forming words but using inappropriate phrasing or a jumbled pattern of speech.

A less common but very important sign of stroke is a headache caused by bleeding from a ruptured vessel. If you find in gathering a history that the patient cried out in pain, clutched the head, and collapsed, this is very important information to relay to the hospital staff. This patient may have had a particular kind of bleeding from an artery under the arachnoid layer of the meninges. (The meninges are several layers of tissue that surround the brain and spinal cord.) This is called a *subarachnoid hemorrhage*. Fortunately, most stroke patients are not hemorrhaging and do not experience headaches.

Other less common signs of stroke include deviation of the eyes and inability to recognize parts of the patient's own body. These signs are more often associated with strokes involving clots in the large arteries in the brain, a condition sometimes referred to as a *large vessel obstruction* (LVO). In a patient with eye deviation, the eyes are looking off to the side rather than directly in front. This can take two forms. The patient with a gaze preference can move the eyes when asked to do so, but the patient with forced deviation is unable to.

Some patients with an LVO may be completely unaware that they are unable to control part of their body. If you ask them "Are you weak anywhere?" they may respond "No," even though they are slumped over to one side. Similarly, if you touch their arm and ask "Whose arm is this?" they may say "I don't know." These findings suggest a severe stroke.

In many cases you will find it difficult to communicate with stroke patients. The damage to the brain sometimes causes a partial or complete loss of the ability to use words. Patients may be able to understand you but will not be able to talk, or will have great difficulty with speech. Sometimes patients will understand you and know what they want to say, but will say the wrong words. This difficulty in using words is known as *expressive aphasia*. *Aphasia* is a general term that refers to difficulty in communication. Another form of it is *receptive aphasia*. In this case, patients can speak clearly but cannot understand what you are saying, so they will clearly say things that do not make much sense or are inappropriate for the situation.

Transient Ischemic Attack

A common occurrence is for an EMT to respond to a patient described as being confused, weak on one side, and having difficulty speaking. The EMT arrives only to find an elderly patient who is alert, oriented, and perfectly normal, without any evident weakness or speech difficulties. This patient may have had a *transient ischemic attack* (TIA), sometimes called a "ministroke" by laypeople. When this condition occurs, a patient appears to be having a stroke because the typical signs and symptoms of the condition are present. However, unlike stroke, a patient with a TIA has complete resolution of these symptoms without treatment within 24 hours (usually much sooner).

With TIA, small clots may be temporarily blocking circulation to part of the brain. When the clots break up, the patient's symptoms resolve because the affected brain tissue had only a short period of hypoxia and did not sustain permanent damage. However, this patient is at significant risk of having a full-blown stroke. If the patient refuses transport, you have a responsibility to attempt to persuade the patient to be evaluated as soon as possible, so a subsequent stroke can be prevented. Contact medical control to see if they can persuade the patient to agree to transport.

Mental status may fluctuate, and signs and symptoms may come and go with stroke patients, too, so do not assume that a patient who seems to be getting better is having "just a TIA." Always remember that if symptoms are present, it is impossible to distinguish between a stroke and a TIA in the field. Always assume the worst and treat as if it were a stroke.

Patient Assessment

Stroke

A very good way to assess conscious patients for stroke is to evaluate three items that constitute the Cincinnati Prehospital Stroke Scale (Figure 22-7 and Scan 22-3):

- Ask the patient to grimace or smile. (Demonstrate what you want the patient to do, making sure that you show your teeth. This allows you to test control of the facial muscles.)

FIGURE 22-7 The Cincinnati Prehospital Stroke Scale.

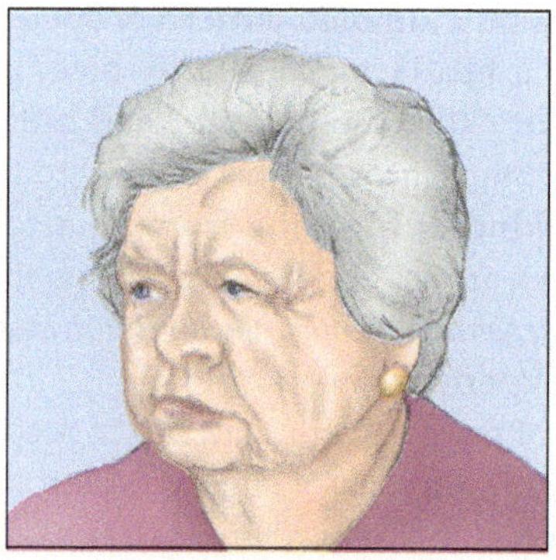

Facial Droop

Normal: Both sides of face move equally.

Abnormal: One side of face does not move at all.

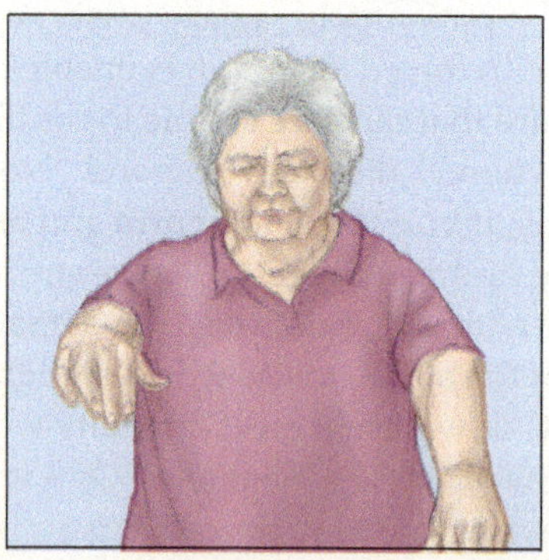

Arm Drift

Normal: Both arms move equally or not at all.

Abnormal: One arm drifts compared with the other.

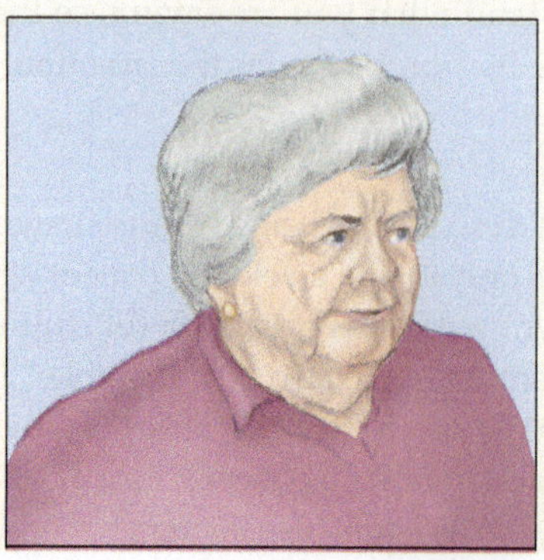

Speech

Normal: Patient uses correct words with no slurring.

Abnormal: Slurred or inappropriate words or mute.

A normal response is for patients to move both sides of their face equally and to show you their teeth. An abnormal response is unequal movement or no movement at all.

- Ask the patient to close the eyes and extend the arms straight forward with the palms facing upward. Have the patient hold this position for 10 seconds. A normal response is for the patient to move both arms at the same time. An abnormal response is for one arm to drift down or not move at all, or for the arms to turn downward so that the palms face the opposite direction.
- Ask the patient to say, "You can't teach an old dog new tricks." An uninjured person's speech is usually clear. A stroke patient is more likely to show an abnormal response to the test, such as slurred speech, the wrong words, or no speech at all.

Other signs and symptoms of stroke, which will often fluctuate in severity while you observe the patient, include:

- Confusion
- Dizziness
- Numbness, weakness, or paralysis (usually on one side of the body)
- Loss of bowel and/or bladder control
- Impaired vision
- High blood pressure
- Difficult respiration or snoring
- Nausea or vomiting
- Seizures
- Unequal pupils
- Headache
- Loss of vision in one eye
- Unconsciousness (uncommon).

Other conditions can mimic the signs of a stroke. Hypoglycemia is a notorious imitator. If your system allows, you should always assess the blood glucose level of a suspected stroke patient. This simple intervention quickly rules out an immediately treatable problem and can help decrease the time necessary to initiate later hospital therapies for treating stroke. Patients who are postictal after a generalized seizure may have transient one-sided weakness that mimics findings in a stroke. Infections and sepsis, especially in older

SCAN 22-3 Cincinnati Prehospital Stroke Scale

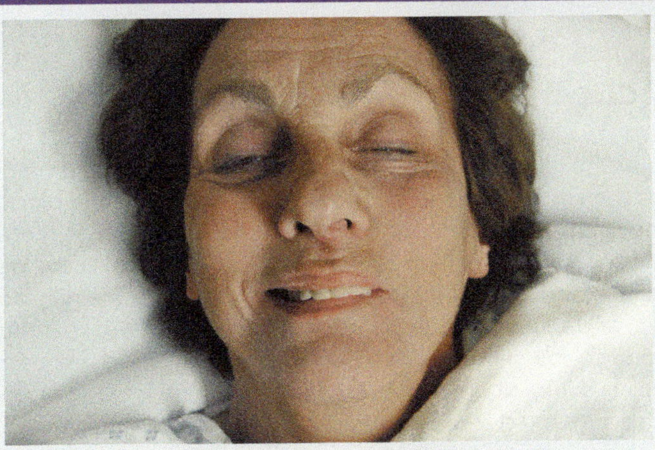

1. Assess for facial droop. The face of a stroke patient often has an abnormal drooped appearance on one side. *(© Edward T. Dickinson, MD)*

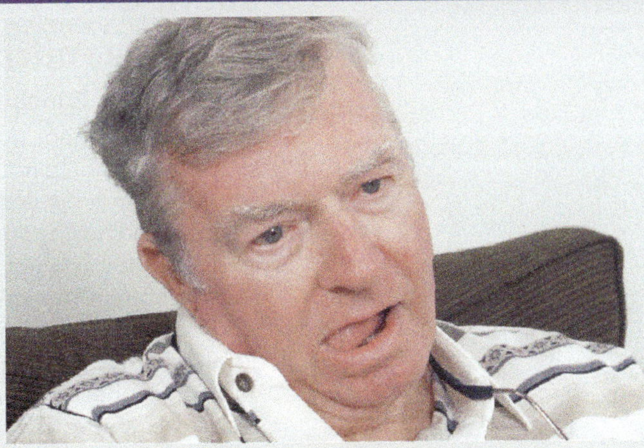

2. Assess for speech difficulties. A stroke patient will often have slurred speech, use the wrong words, or be unable to speak at all.

(continued)

SCAN 22-3 Cincinnati Prehospital Stroke Scale *(continued)*

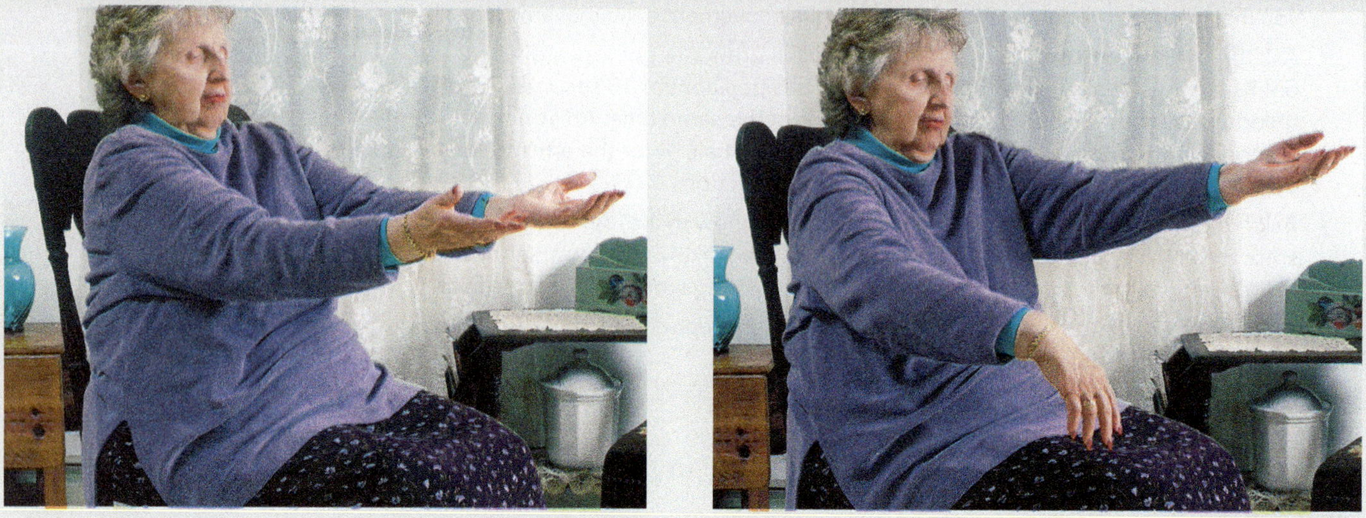

3. Assess for arm drift by asking the patient to close both eyes and extend the arms, palms up, for 10 seconds. (A) A patient who has not suffered a stroke can usually hold the arms in an extended position with eyes closed. (B) A stroke patient will often display arm drift or palm rotation–that is, one arm will remain extended, but the arm on the affected side will drift downward or turn over.

patients, can also cause signs and symptoms that resemble a stroke. Taking the patient's temperature can help you and the emergency department in determining the best care.

Decision Point

Is My Patient Having a Stroke?

Identify patients who appear to be having a stroke. These patients should be transported promptly to an appropriate facility.

NOTE: *A patient who demonstrates any one of the three findings of the Cincinnati Prehospital Stroke Scale has a 70 percent chance of having had an acute stroke.*

Patient Care

Care of the Patient with a Stroke

Fundamental Principles of Care

The most important treatment step in caring for a stroke patient is recognition of the stroke. EMTs should not underestimate their value in making this possible. Rapid communication of findings, and steps such as the Cincinnati Prehospital Stroke Scale and blood glucose readings, are truly important components of overall stroke care. As vital as these steps are, they may not be enough to determine that a stroke has taken place. There are many problems that can mimic strokes, including tumor or infection in the brain, head injury, seizures, hypoglycemia, and bacterial or viral infections that cause weakness or paralysis of facial nerves. Although you should conduct a thorough patient assessment and do your best to identify likely stroke situations, you should also not fear being incorrect. It is far better to overtreat a suspected stroke patient than to ignore an actual stroke.

Stroke is a time-sensitive disorder–that is, the longer a vessel is blocked, the more damage occurs. You should keep this in mind when thinking about your overall treatment plan. Although there may be life threats that need immediate attention, commonly the most important treatment priority will be rapid transport to an appropriate destination.

Take the following steps when caring for patients with potential stroke:

- For conscious patients who can maintain their airway, provide a calm and reassuring presence, monitor the airway, and administer oxygen if the oxygen saturation is below 94 percent or if signs of hypoxia or respiratory distress are present.
- For unconscious patients or patients who cannot maintain the airway, maintain an open airway, provide enough oxygen for adequate oxygen saturation, and transport.
- Transport to a hospital with the capability of managing a stroke patient (CT scan at a minimum). Your destination choice may be guided by a local stroke-care protocol, so follow local guidelines.
- Some EMS systems recommend keeping the acute stroke patient's head at 30 degrees or less on the stretcher during transport to assist with optimal blood flow to the brain. Follow local protocols.

Depending on the hospitals and resources nearby, you may have special protocols for management and transport of patients with signs and symptoms of stroke. Time is of the essence if any treatments is to be effective. There appears to be a narrow window within which assessment must be completed and treatment started.

The most widespread advance in stroke care is the use of clot-busting (thrombolytic) drugs in cases of ischemic stroke. This therapy can potentially reverse the symptoms of stroke, but patients must meet very specific criteria:

- Definite onset of stroke symptoms less than 3 hours (less than $4\frac{1}{2}$ hours in some systems) prior to the administration of the thrombolytic drug
- An emergency CT scan of the brain confirming that there is no evidence of a hemorrhagic stroke
- Blood pressure that is not excessively high at the time the drug is administered

One of the most important things the EMT can do to optimize the care of stroke patients who are potential candidates for thrombolytics is to determine and document the exact time of onset of symptoms. If that is not possible, determine the time the patient was last known to be well. If the person who provides you with this information is someone other than the patient, it is a good idea to document who that person is and how the person can be contacted (e.g., cell phone number) if the physician in the emergency department should have to verify any information. In cases where the exact time of onset is not known, the patient will not be able to receive thrombolytics. For example, the patient who awakens at 7 a.m. and is immediately noted by the family to have new stroke symptoms but who was last seen in a normal condition at 11:30 the night before cannot get thrombolytic therapy, because it is not known when during the night the stroke occurred.

Another more recent advance in the treatment of stroke is thrombectomy, the removal of a clot obstructing one of the large cerebral arteries. In this procedure, physicians thread a catheter into the obstructed artery and mechanically remove the clot, thereby reestablishing perfusion to that part of the brain. At the moment, it is only certain large arteries for which this procedure is safe and effective. Fortunately, the window of opportunity for this procedure seems to be larger—as much as 24 hours after onset of symptoms. Only a minority of ischemic stroke patients are eligible for this treatment, however, since most clots are not in the large arteries where a catheter can retrieve them. Although most emergency departments can administer thrombolytic therapy for acute strokes, thrombectomy is only available in specialized stroke centers. Know the specific resources available for stroke patients in your EMS system.

NOTE: *If you suspect the patient has had a stroke, it is important to transport promptly, and to notify the hospital of symptoms you see and the results of the Cincinnati Prehospital Stroke Scale. If you have a choice of hospitals, your protocols may direct you to a hospital capable of providing the most recent stroke treatments.*

Dizziness and Syncope

Dizziness and ***syncope*** (another term for fainting) are common reasons EMS is called. They can occur in patients of any age, but are more common among older adults. These complaints might seem to be harmless, but in fact they can be indicators of serious or even

syncope (SIN-ko-pee) fainting.

CORE CONCEPT

Understanding the causes, assessment, and care of dizziness and syncope

life-threatening problems. In many cases you will not be able to diagnose the true cause of the syncope. However, you should use your assessment to rapidly identify and treat life threats and to gather important information that will assist in the overall treatment of the patient.

Dizziness and syncope are separate problems that are sometimes related. It is not uncommon for someone to complain of dizziness before fainting. Because these two conditions are often caused by the same problems, we will consider them together in this chapter.

Dizziness is a common term that means different things to different people. It is important in your assessment to find out what the patient means by "dizziness." Does this mean weakness, as in a sensation of loss of strength? Does the patient feel vertigo? Vertigo is the sensation of your surroundings spinning around you. Is it light-headedness, the sensation that one is about to pass out (sometimes called *presyncope* or *near syncope*)? Is it something else?

Syncope is a brief loss of consciousness with spontaneous recovery. Typically, it is very short, from a few seconds to at most a few minutes. The patient usually regains consciousness very soon after being allowed to lie flat (Figure 22-8).

Patients will often have some warning that a syncopal episode or fainting spell is about to occur. This may include such symptoms as light-headedness, dizziness, nausea, weakness, vision changes, sudden pallor (loss of normal skin color), and sweating. Occasionally incontinence of bladder and/or bowel occurs as part of the episode, but this is more common with seizures.

Patients may be able to describe specific signs or symptoms that indicate certain causes of the episode are more likely than others. These may include fluttering in the chest (palpitations), a sensation of a racing heart (tachycardia), a slow heart rate (bradycardia), or headache.

Causes of Dizziness and Syncope

The factors that cause dizziness and syncope are generally related to the brain. Problems such as hypoxia, hypoglycemia, and hypovolemia all interfere with normal brain function. These events may happen rapidly, such as blood flow to the brain being reduced by a cardiac dysrhythmia; or they may happen slowly, such as slow gastrointestinal bleeding that finally reaches the point where the patient is unable to stand without losing consciousness.

There are many causes of dizziness and syncope. The more common ones can be grouped into four categories: cardiovascular, hypovolemic, structural/metabolic, and environmental/toxicologic. In general, syncope that occurs with no warning, syncope associated with a headache or another neurologic finding (altered mental status, focal weakness, etc.), and syncope in the older adult patient are all associated with the more serious causes of syncope. Similarly, vertigo and dizziness tend to be more serious in older patients.

Cardiovascular Causes. Cardiovascular causes of dizziness and syncope should be an immediate consideration. Frequently these symptoms are caused by electrical changes in

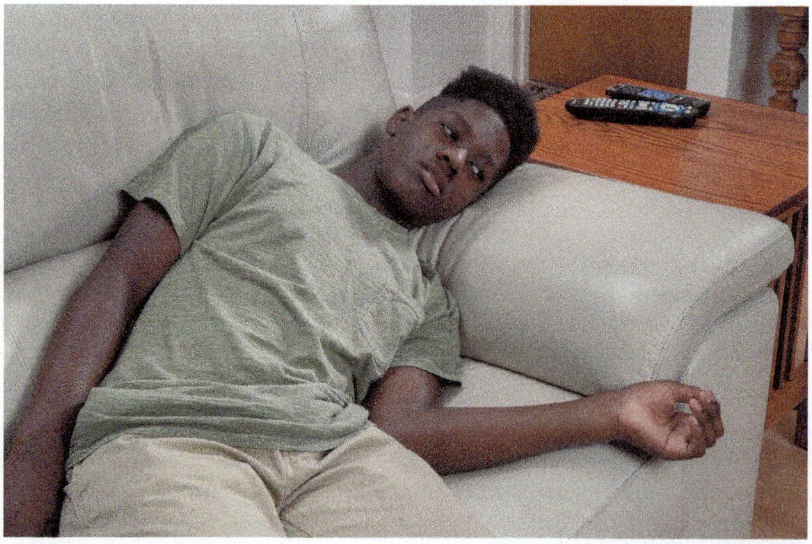

FIGURE 22-8 Loss of consciousness with syncope is usually brief. The patient usually regains consciousness very soon after being allowed to lie flat.

the heart that result in abnormal heart rates. A cardiac dysrhythmia in which the heart beats extremely fast (a tachycardia) can lead to either dizziness or syncope. You should remember that syncope can also be a sign of acute myocardial infarction and can be caused by an alteration in the heart's ability to pump. Ordinarily, increases in the heart rate result in more blood being pumped out of the heart (greater cardiac output). However, when the heart beats extremely rapidly, the ventricles do not have time to fill before they pump blood out again. So even though the heart is beating much more rapidly than normal, it is actually pumping out less blood than usual. A very slow heart rate (a bradycardia) may also lead to dizziness or syncope through reduced cardiac output, in this case because the heart is not beating rapidly enough to pump out sufficient blood. Certain structural heart problems may also cause syncope. Abnormal heart anatomy may result in obstruction of normal blood flow from the heart, resulting in syncope. This type of syncope often occurs during exertion.

Stimulation of the carotid sinus is a cardiovascular cause of syncope that is not a result of a problem with the heart's electrical system. This area is located in the carotid artery under the mandible. When stimulated, it sends signals to the heart to slow down. Some people have a very sensitive carotid sinus. All that may be needed to stimulate it in some sensitive individuals is turning the head while wearing a shirt with a tight collar.

One of the most common types of syncope is *vasovagal syncope*, or simple fainting. This is thought to be the result of stimulation of the vagus nerve, which in turn signals the heart to slow down. When someone is suddenly frightened or put under significant emotional stress, this nerve can be stimulated, leading to reduced cardiac output, which in the upright individual can quickly result in syncope. When the patient reaches a horizontal position, the brain regains perfusion and the patient regains consciousness.

Hypovolemic Causes. Hypovolemia, or low fluid/blood volume, can cause dizziness or syncope when the patient attempts to sit up or stand. In this case there is enough blood to perfuse the brain when the patient is lying down. However, when the patient tries to get up, the body is unable to quickly divert enough blood from the legs to the brain. There are several common causes of hypovolemia, including dehydration, internal bleeding, and trauma. The most serious cause of hypovolemia is bleeding.

In a patient with dizziness or syncope, the source of the bleeding may not be obvious. A woman of childbearing age can have a ruptured ectopic pregnancy that results in significant blood loss. (See the chapter *Obstetric and Gynecologic Emergencies* for more information about ectopic pregnancy.) This is usually accompanied by lower abdominal pain. A slowly bleeding ("leaking") abdominal aortic aneurysm can also lead to life-threatening blood loss. Such an aneurysm often causes the patient to experience abdominal pain radiating to the back. Gastrointestinal bleeding, with or without associated abdominal pain, is fairly common, especially among the older population.

There are other ways to become hypovolemic besides bleeding. Dehydration results from losing more fluid than the patient takes in. This is very common in hot weather, when the patient sweats a great deal but does not drink enough liquid to keep up with this fluid loss (heat exhaustion). It can also happen when someone becomes ill with diarrhea. Because eating or drinking anything is followed by a painful, watery bowel movement, the patient is reluctant to drink any fluids at all and becomes dehydrated. Sometimes, with severe diarrhea, this happens despite the patient's efforts to drink liquids.

Structural/Metabolic Causes. Because a properly functioning brain is necessary to maintain consciousness, alterations in the brain structure or chemistry can lead to a diminished level of consciousness, the sensation of dizziness, and even syncope. Similarly, because the inner and middle ears must be properly functioning for a person to maintain a sense of balance, a problem in this region can lead to dizziness and vertigo. Inflammation of this area is a very common cause of vertigo. A patient who has been diagnosed with such a problem may be taking a medication called meclizine. Occasionally a stroke will present with either dizziness or syncope. In this case, there may be other neurologic signs and symptoms present, such as one-sided weakness, drooping of one side of the face, or slurred speech. A seizure, too, can cause a temporary loss of consciousness. You learned about managing a patient having a seizure earlier in this chapter.

Hypoglycemia deprives the brain of glucose, which it needs all the time to function properly. An interruption in this supply can lead to both dizziness and syncope. If the patient remains unconscious more than a few minutes, however, it is not considered syncope, or fainting, but rather "unresponsiveness." There is likely to be a more serious cause of the episode.

Environmental/Toxicologic Causes. Environmental and toxicologic imbalances can lead to alterations in consciousness. Alcohol is the most commonly used drug, and when a patient drinks too much, it can lead to an altered level of consciousness. Many people who are intoxicated display a fluctuating level of consciousness that can appear to be syncope. Other drugs that are central nervous system depressants can cause similar effects. Syncope and near syncope also commonly occur with carbon monoxide poisoning.

Panic attacks and anxiety attacks can lead a patient to become so anxious that the patient hyperventilates by breathing faster and deeper. When a patient breathes this hard, it can change the blood chemistry in a way that constricts the blood vessels supplying the brain with oxygen. Fortunately, when the patient loses consciousness, the hyperventilation ceases and things return at least partly to normal.

Other Causes. The causes previously discussed are just a few of the origins of dizziness and syncope. There are many others. In some cases, you will gather information that suggests one of them is the culprit. In many cases you will not. Determining the cause can be extremely difficult. In half of the cases of dizziness or syncope, no cause is ever found, despite thorough evaluation by emergency physicians and other specialists.

Patient Assessment

Dizziness and Syncope

Syncope is usually easily recognized by the patient's complaint of a brief loss of consciousness. The secondary assessment for a patient with dizziness or syncope includes an appropriate history and vital signs. Questions to ask include:

- Describe what you mean by "dizziness." (Let patients use their own words.)
- Did you have any warning? If so, what was it like?
- When did it start?
- How long did it last?
- What position were you in when the episode occurred?
- Have you had any similar episodes in the past? If so, what cause was found?
- Are you on medication for this kind of problem?
- Did you have any other signs or symptoms? Nausea? Vomiting (is there blood or material resembling coffee grounds)? Black, tarry stools (digested blood)?
- Did you witness any unpleasant sight, or experience a strong emotion?
- Did you hurt yourself?
- Did anyone witness involuntary movements of the extremities (like seizures)?

Patient Care

Care of Patients with Dizziness and Syncope

Fundamental Principles of Care

The greatest danger for a client with syncope is from falls. Ensure that the environment will not cause harm to the patient. If possible, assist the patient to a safe, protected position on the floor or a bed with siderails.

When a patient has experienced dizziness or syncope, provide the following care after attending to any threats to life, generally in this order:

- Lay the patient flat.
- Loosen any tight clothing around the neck.
- Administer oxygen based on oxygen saturation levels (goal is 94 percent) and patient's level of distress. Some patients will not receive oxygen.
- Call for ALS if it is available in your area and the patient has signs of instability.
- Treat any associated injuries the patient may have incurred from the fall.

Decision Point

Is my patient stable? Is my patient likely to remain stable?

The urgency of your treatment and transport will depend on these decisions.

In most cases, syncope should be evaluated by advanced life support. Although many cases of syncope are benign, cardiac causes should always be considered. ALS has the ability to initiate cardiac monitoring and rule out certain dysrhythmias as a cause. Consider blood glucose monitoring (if your system allows) to rule out hypoglycemia as a cause. Finally, do not underestimate shock and sepsis as a potential underlying problem associated with these findings.

Chapter Review

Key Facts and Concepts

- Diabetic emergencies are usually caused by ineffective management of the patient's diabetes.
- Diabetic emergencies are often brought about by hypoglycemia, or low blood sugar.
- The chief sign of hypoglycemia is altered mental status.
- Whenever a patient has an altered mental status and a history of diabetes and is able to swallow, administer oral glucose.
- Seizures may have a number of causes. Assess and treat for possible spinal injury, protect the patient's airway, and provide oxygen as needed.
- You should gather information about the seizure to give to hospital personnel.
- A stroke is caused when an artery in the brain is blocked or ruptures.
- Signs and symptoms of a stroke commonly include an altered mental status, numbness or paralysis on one side, and difficulty with speech.
- For stroke patients, ensure an open airway and, if appropriate, provide supplemental oxygen. Determine the exact time of onset of symptoms and transport promptly.
- Dizziness and syncope (fainting) may have a variety of causes.
- In the case of syncope, loosen clothing around the neck, and place the patient flat with raised legs if there is no reason not to. Administer oxygen if appropriate. Treat any injuries and transport.
- In all patients with altered mental status, your decision to administer oxygen will be based on the pulse oximetry readings as well as the patient's level of respiratory distress and other signs of hypoxia.

Key Decisions

- Is this patient's altered mental status being caused by hypoxia?
- In a hypoglycemic emergency, does the patient have a mental status that would allow the administration of oral glucose?
- Does the seizure patient need artificial ventilation?
- When did the symptoms of the stroke begin?

Chapter Glossary

aura a sensation experienced by a seizure patient right before the seizure that might be a smell, sound, or general feeling.

diabetes mellitus (di-ah-BEE-tez MEL-i-tus) also called *sugar diabetes* or just *diabetes*, the condition brought about by decreased insulin production or the inability of the body cells to use insulin properly. The person with this condition is a diabetic.

diabetic ketoacidosis (di-ah-BET-ic KEY-to-as-id-DO-sis) ***(DKA)*** a condition that occurs as the result of high blood sugar (hyperglycemia), characterized by dehydration, altered mental status, and shock.

epilepsy (EP-uh-lep-see) a medical condition that causes seizures.

generalized seizure a seizure that affects both sides of the brain.

glucose (GLU-kos) a form of sugar, the body's basic source of energy.

hyperglycemia (HI-per-gli-SEE-me-ah) high blood sugar.

hypoglycemia (HI-po-gli-SEE-me-ah) low blood sugar.

insulin (IN-suh-lin) a hormone produced by the pancreas or taken as a medication by many diabetics.

partial seizure a seizure that affects only one part or one side of the brain.

postictal (post-IK-tul) ***phase*** the period of time immediately following a tonic-clonic seizure in which the patient goes from full loss of consciousness to full mental status.

reticular (ruh-TIK-yuh-ler) ***activating system (RAS)*** series of neurologic circuits in the brain that control the functions of staying awake, paying attention, and sleeping.

seizure (SEE-zher) a sudden change in sensation, behavior, or movement. The most severe form of seizure produces violent muscle contractions called convulsions.

sepsis a life-threatening condition resulting from an abnormal and counterproductive response to infection by the body that causes damage to tissues and organs.

status epilepticus (STAY-tus or STAT-us ep-i-LEP-ti-kus) a prolonged seizure or situation when a person suffers two or more convulsive seizures without regaining full consciousness.

stroke a condition of altered function caused when an artery in the brain is blocked or ruptured, disrupting the supply of oxygenated blood or causing bleeding into the brain. Formerly called a *cerebrovascular accident (CVA).*

syncope (SIN-ko-pee) fainting.

tonic-clonic (TON-ik-KLON-ik) ***seizure*** a generalized seizure in which the patient loses consciousness and has jerking movements of paired muscle groups.

Preparation for Your Examination and Practice

Short Answer

1. List the chief signs and symptoms of a diabetic emergency.
2. Explain how you can determine a medical history of diabetes.
3. Explain what treatment may be given by an EMT for a diabetic emergency and the criteria for giving it.
4. Tell whether treatment for a diabetic emergency should be given before or after baseline vital signs are taken. (Answer according to your local protocol.)
5. Explain the care that should be given to a patient who has had a seizure.
6. Explain the care that should be given to a conscious and to an unconscious patient with suspected stroke.
7. Explain the care that should be given to a patient who has experienced dizziness or syncope.

Thinking and Linking

Think back to the sections about medical patients in the chapter Secondary Assessment *and link information from that chapter with information from this chapter as you consider the following question:*

1. What parts of the patient's SAMPLE history will provide clues to the cause of the patient's altered mental status?

Think back to the chapters Medical, Legal, and Ethical Issues *and* Communication and Documentation *as you consider the following situation:*

2. You have given a diabetic patient glucose. The patient is now oriented and does not want to be transported to the hospital. After you have made diligent efforts to persuade the patient to go, the patient still refuses transportation. What do you tell the patient? What do you document in relation to the refusal and your interaction with the patient?

Critical Thinking Exercises

Patients suffering a diabetic emergency are sometimes thought to be drunk. The purpose of this exercise will be to consider how to treat such a patient.

- You are dispatched to a "man behaving oddly" at a train station. When you arrive, you find that the man is unconscious. "He's drunk," a bystander tells you. "He was staggering and slurring his words." As you assess the patient, you find a medical identification bracelet that tells you he is diabetic. Do you administer oral glucose? How do you proceed?

Pathophysiology to Practice

The following questions are designed to assist you in gathering relevant clinical information and making accurate decisions in the field.

1. How might you differentiate a patient who had a seizure associated with hypoxia from a patient who had a seizure associated with epilepsy?
2. What assessment elements would be important in making this decision?

Street Scenes

While on your day off, you receive a telephone call about working a shift at the county fair. It sounds like fun, so you agree. That Friday night, you and your partner are on stand-by with an ambulance at the first aid tent. It is 10 p.m., and the evening has been quiet. Just when you think that it will also remain uneventful, you receive a call on the radio that security has an intoxicated person they want you to examine on the midway. Upon arrival, you find a male patient in his twenties, sitting and talking with slurred speech to a deputy sheriff. A security guard tells you that the patient was wandering down the midway and talking incoherently. "I'm sure he's drunk," he tells you, "but the rules say you have to take a look before we transport to the security office."

Street Scene Questions

1. Does this patient need a thorough assessment?
2. What is the first concern when starting to assess this patient?
3. What types of underlying medical problems might make a patient appear to be drunk?

As your partner approaches the patient, he is met with what appears to be an angry man, who says, "That's all I need—another cop." The patient then pushes the deputy sheriff away, and he turns to you. "This guy is just another drunk," your partner says, "and we are out of here." You almost buy into your partner's hasty evaluation, but you notice a bracelet on the patient's wrist. You approach, introduce yourself, and ask the patient if you can check him out. He reluctantly agrees, and as you take a pulse, which is rapid, you see that his bracelet indicates he has diabetes.

Street Scene Questions

4. Does your assessment plan change at this point?
5. How will you get a SAMPLE history if the patient is alone?
6. What is the priority level of this patient? Is there a need to call for ALS assistance?

After primary and secondary assessments, you find the patient's airway is open with no mucus or other secretions noted, his breathing is at 24 breaths per minute, and his pulse rate is 110.

Just as you finish taking vital signs, a person approaches who says he is a friend of the patient. He confirms that your patient is diabetic and that he took his insulin before they left for the fair. "He expected to eat here," the friend tells you, "but he was trying to win at the midway games and must have forgotten." You and your partner agree that he could tolerate oral glucose. You explain to your patient what you are doing and apply some to the inside of his cheek. In a few minutes, he starts to become more alert, and soon he says he feels fine.

The ALS unit is now on the scene and has checked his sugar level. It is in a normal range. The patient does not want to be transported, and after you talk to medical direction, he is allowed to leave with his friend, who promises to take him directly to a diner for something starchy to eat.

You call back in service and, as you walk to the ambulance, you remind your partner that you can never assume anything. Every patient needs an assessment.

23 Allergic Reaction

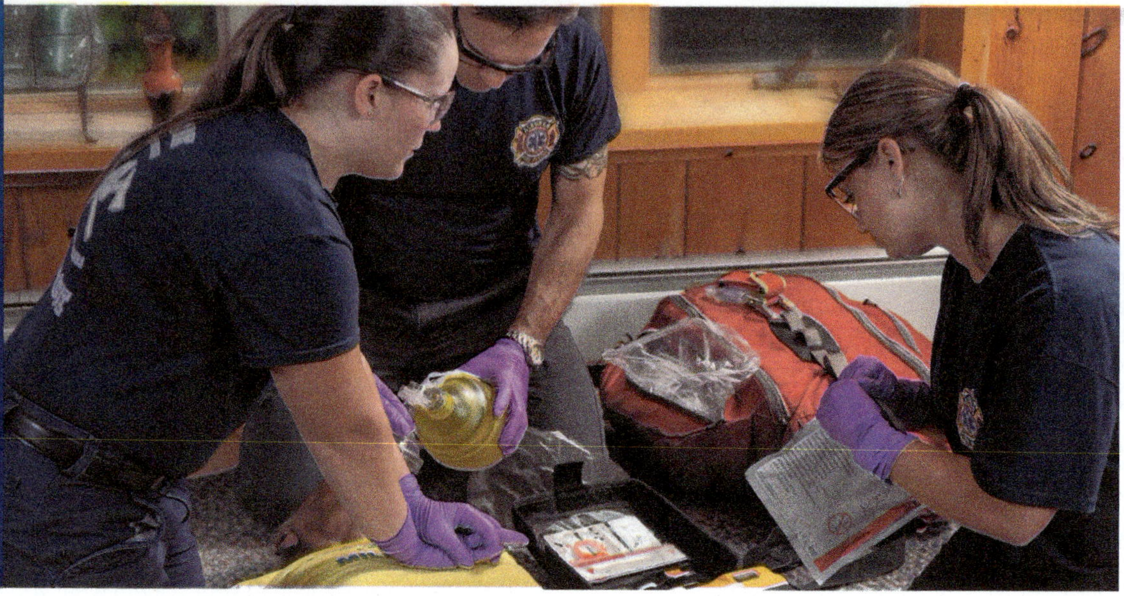

Related Chapters

The following chapters provide additional information related to topics discussed in this chapter:

Standard

Medicine (Immunology)

Competency

Applies fundamental knowledge to provide basic emergency care and transportation based on assessment findings for an acutely ill patient.

Core Concepts

- How to identify a patient experiencing an allergic reaction
- Differences between a mild allergic reaction and anaphylaxis
- How to treat a patient experiencing an allergic reaction
- Who should be assisted with an epinephrine auto-injector

Outcomes

After reading this chapter, you should be able to:

23.1 Summarize the concepts of the spectrum of mild allergic reactions to anaphylactic shock. (pp. 651-656)

- Describe how the interaction of the immune system with a substance leads to allergic reactions.
- List substances commonly implicated in allergic reactions.
- Describe the special considerations involved with latex allergies.
- Relate the signs and symptoms of allergic reactions to their underlying pathophysiologic processes.

23.2 Summarize the application of prehospital management for patients with allergic reactions. (pp. 656-666)

- Recognize assessment findings that point toward an allergic reaction.
- Distinguish the severity of patient allergic reactions.
- Explain the importance of communicating with medical direction based on the patient's history and current presentation.
- Describe decision making for assisting a patient with a prescribed epinephrine auto-injector.
- Describe decision making for administering epinephrine carried by the EMT.
- Outline the pharmacology of epinephrine.
- Compare the features of different kinds of epinephrine auto-injectors patients may have.
- List the priority of the administration of epinephrine with other patient interventions.
- Determine whether calling for paramedic assistance will benefit a patient.

Key Terms

allergen, *651*	anaphylaxis, *652*	epinephrine, *660*
allergic reaction, *651*	auto-injector, *656*	hives, *653*

Allergic reactions can be mild or extremely severe. A seemingly mild allergic reaction can rapidly develop into a severe reaction. A severe allergic reaction can quickly become life-threatening. For these reasons, prompt recognition and appropriate assessment and treatment of allergic reactions can be critical.

Allergic Reactions

A natural response of the human body's immune system is to react to any foreign substance—in other words, to defend the body by neutralizing or getting rid of the foreign material. Sometimes the immune response is exaggerated; this exaggerated reaction is called an ***allergic reaction***. Almost any of a wide variety of substances can be an ***allergen***, something that causes an allergic reaction. For example, cat dander can be an allergen. A person who is allergic to cat dander will itch and sneeze whenever a cat is nearby. The reaction is unpleasant but not dangerous.

allergic reaction
an exaggerated immune response.

allergen
something that causes an allergic reaction.

anaphylaxis (an-ah-fi-LAK-sis) a severe or life-threatening allergic reaction in which the blood vessels dilate, causing a drop in blood pressure, and the tissues lining the respiratory system swell, interfering with the airway. Also called *anaphylactic shock*.

"Anaphylaxis is a life-threatening condition that involves shock and/or respiratory compromise."

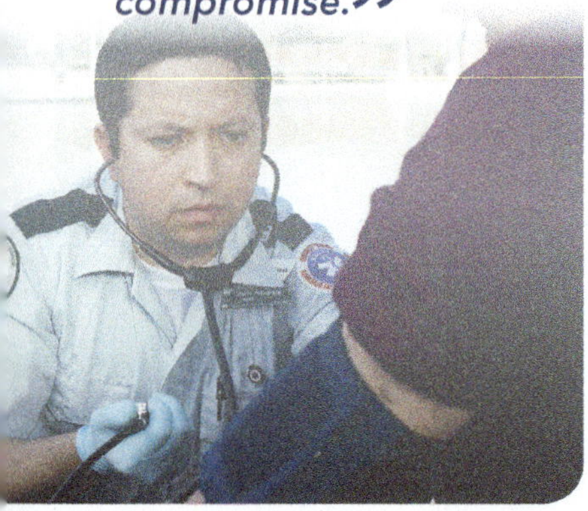

In some people, however, contact with certain foreign substances triggers an immune response that gets out of hand. Consider bee stings. Most people have no reaction to a bee sting other than pain and some swelling at the sting site. However, some people have very severe, life-threatening reactions to bee stings. This kind of severe allergic reaction is called ***anaphylaxis***, or *anaphylactic shock*. In anaphylaxis, exposure to the allergen triggers an overwhelming immune response that causes blood vessels to dilate rapidly and cells to leak fluid, which causes a drop in blood pressure (hypotension). Many tissues may swell, including those that line the respiratory system. This swelling can obstruct the airway, leading to respiratory failure.

There are many causes of allergic reactions (in some individuals), such as (Figure 23-1):

- **Insects.** The stings of bees, yellow jackets, wasps, and hornets can cause rapid and severe reactions.
- **Foods.** Foods such as nuts, eggs, milk, and shellfish can cause reactions. In most cases the effect is slower than that seen with insect stings. An exception is peanuts. Peanut allergies are frequently very severe and very rapid in onset. Many people with allergies to one food will have allergies to related foods (e.g., someone who is allergic to almonds is more likely to be allergic to walnuts). Again, peanuts are an exception. People who are allergic to peanuts do not necessarily have any other allergies, including to nuts (in part because peanuts are legumes, not nuts).
- **Plants.** Contact with certain plants such as poison oak, poison ivy, and poison sumac (Figure 23-2) can cause a rash that is sometimes severe. The rash associated with poison ivy is actually an allergic reaction. Approximately two-thirds of the population is allergic to the oil on poison ivy leaves. Plant pollen also causes allergic reactions in many people but rarely anaphylaxis.

FIGURE 23-1 Substances that may cause allergic reactions.

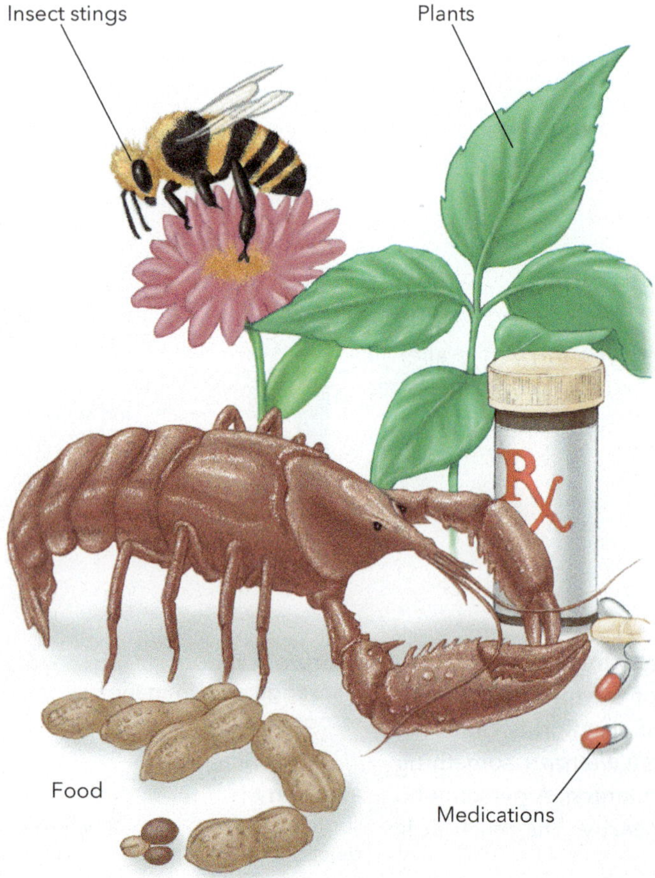

FIGURE 23-2 Contact with poison oak (shown here), poison ivy, or poison sumac can cause a rash that may be severe.

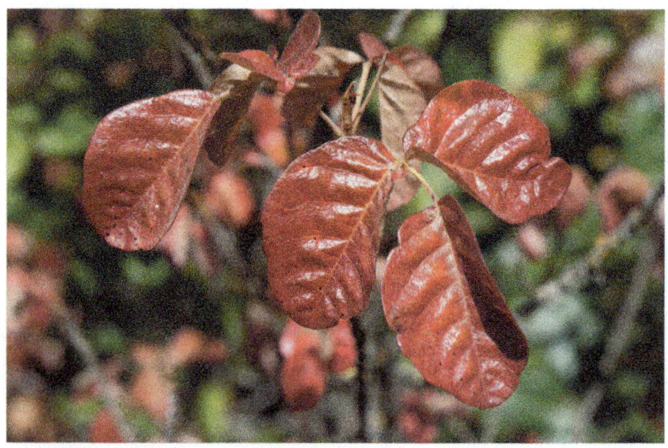

- **Medications.** Certain drugs, especially antibiotics such as penicillin, may cause severe reactions. Just as with foods, people who are allergic to one kind of antibiotic can be allergic to related antibiotics. In the course of evaluating patients, you will hear many of them say they are allergic to penicillin or other antibiotics. Many of them are wrong because they confuse side effects, such as nausea or diarrhea, with an allergic reaction.
- **Others.** Dust, chemicals, soaps, makeup, and a variety of other substances can cause allergic reactions, which are occasionally severe, in some people.

One particular product EMTs should be aware of as a possible allergen is latex. Two groups of people are especially likely to be allergic to latex. One is patients with conditions that require multiple surgeries. Even though most health care facilities have worked hard to reduce the amount of exposure patients have to latex, repeated exposure to the latex in gloves and other items is probably the reason many such patients develop a severe allergy to latex. This is very important to understand because if you wear latex gloves when treating a patient with a latex allergy, you may actually cause an allergic or anaphylactic reaction in the patient.

The other group that is becoming more sensitive to latex is health care professionals, including EMTs. Again, this increased sensitivity is probably because of more frequent exposure to latex as a result of practicing Standard Precautions. Fortunately, it is now possible to find virtually all medical equipment and supplies in forms that do not contain latex. Many hospitals and EMS agencies maintain latex-free environments to avoid causing reactions in latex-sensitive individuals.

Something that all allergic reactions share is that people do not have them the first time they are exposed to an allergen. This is because the body's immune system has not "learned" to recognize the allergen yet. The first time someone is exposed to an allergen, the immune system forms antibodies in response. These antibodies are the body's attempt to attack the foreign substances. A particular antibody will combine with only the allergen it was formed in response to (or with another allergen very similar to the original one).

The second time the person is exposed to the allergen, the antibodies already exist in the person's body. This time, the antibody combines with the allergen, leading to the release of histamine and other chemicals into the bloodstream. Together these substances have several effects that may lead to a spectrum of allergic reactions including, at times, the life-threatening condition known as *anaphylaxis*. They dilate blood vessels, decrease the ability of capillaries to contain fluid, cause bronchoconstriction, and promote the production of thick mucus in the lungs.

The dilation of blood vessels reduces the amount of blood returning to the heart, leading to decreased cardiac output and an increased risk of shock. Skin also becomes flushed, as blood vessels near the surface open up. When capillaries become leaky, fluid moves into the tissue and appears as swelling (angioedema), especially around the site of an injection (or sting) (Figure 23-3A) and the face (Figure 23-3B), including the eyes, lips, ears, tongue, and airway. If the area around the vocal cords becomes swollen, the patient may have a muffled voice or display stridor on inspiration. Urticaria, also called ***hives***—red, itchy, possibly raised blotches on the skin (Figure 23-3C)—is another result of the release of histamines and related substances in response to allergens. Bronchoconstriction causes decreased movement of air in the lungs, leading to wheezing and difficulty breathing. Thick mucus worsens this effect. Irritation of nerve endings results in itching.

hives
red, itchy, possibly raised blotches on the skin that often result from allergic reactions; also known as urticaria.

There is no way to predict the exact course of an allergic reaction. Severe reactions most often take place immediately, but they are occasionally delayed 30 minutes or more. A mild allergic reaction may turn into more serious anaphylactic shock in a matter of minutes. When a patient with an exposure to a known allergen is displaying only minor signs and symptoms, you must closely monitor the patient for signs of the condition's becoming more serious. This patient's airway may swell and close off in just a few minutes. Be prepared to manage the airway and to administer epinephrine if so advised by medical direction.

FIGURE 23-3 Signs of an allergic reaction may include (A) local angioedema, (B) facial swelling, and (C) hives.
(Photos A, B, and C: © Edward T. Dickinson, MD)

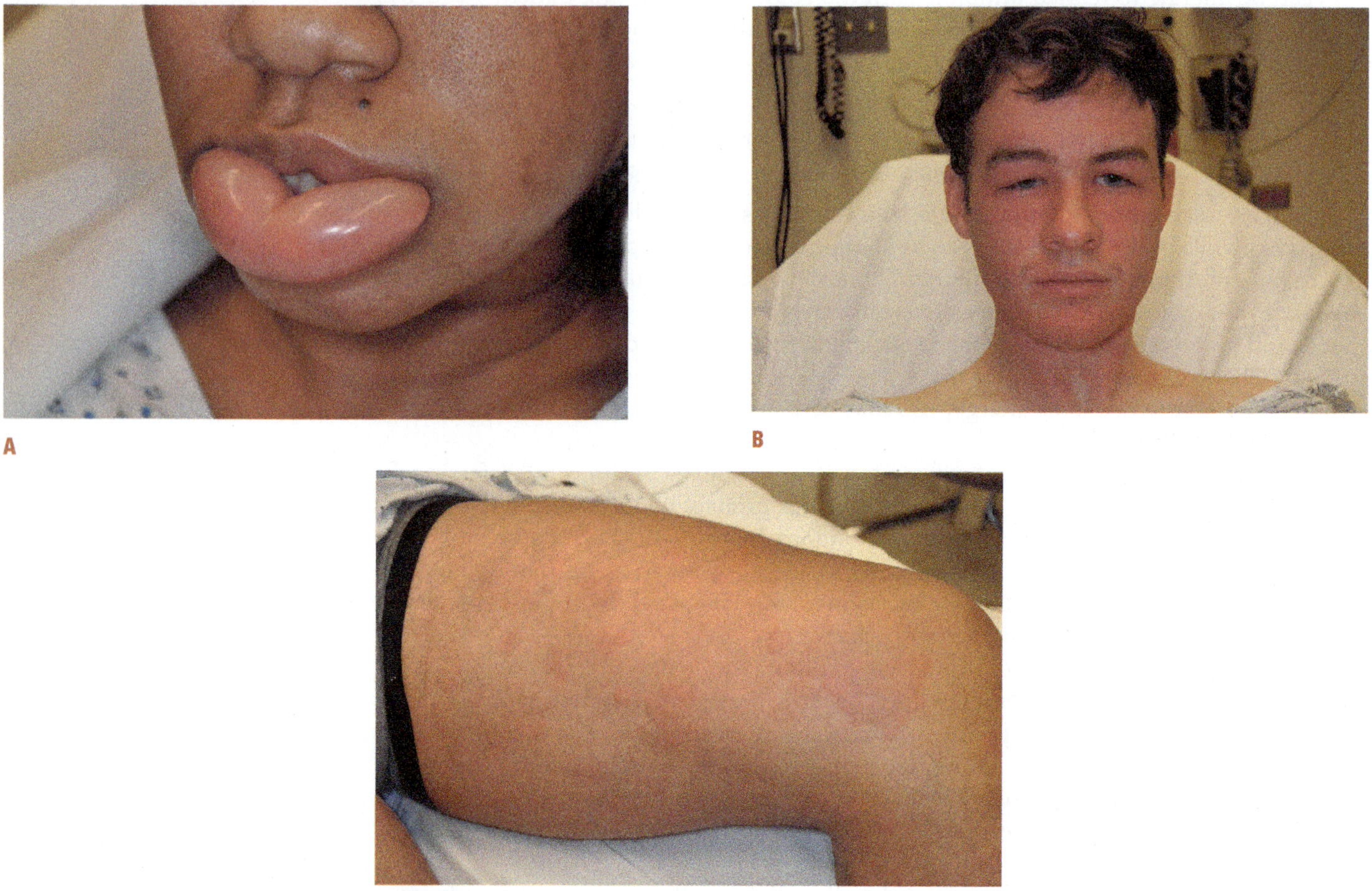

A

B

C

CORE CONCEPT
How to identify a patient experiencing an allergic reaction

The signs and symptoms of an allergic reaction or anaphylactic shock can include:

Skin:

- Itching
- Hives (may be localized—especially around an insect sting—or generalized over wide areas of the body)
- Flushing (red skin)
- Swelling of the face (especially the eyes and lips), neck, hands, feet, or tongue
- Warm, tingling feeling in the face, mouth, chest, feet, and hands

Respiratory:

- Patient report of a feeling of tightness in the throat or chest
- Cough
- Rapid breathing
- Labored, noisy breathing
- Hoarseness, muffled voice, or loss of voice entirely

- Stridor (harsh, high-pitched sound during inspiration)
- Wheezing (audible without a stethoscope)

Cardiac:

- Increased heart rate
- Decreased blood pressure

Generalized Findings:

- Itchy, watery eyes
- Headache
- Runny nose
- Patient-expressed sense of impending doom

Signs and Symptoms of Shock:

- Altered mental status
- Flushed, dry skin or pale, cool, clammy skin
- Nausea or vomiting
- Changes in vital signs: increased pulse, increased respirations, decreased blood pressure

CORE CONCEPT

Differences between a mild allergic reaction and anaphylaxis

Distinguishing Anaphylaxis from Mild Allergic Reaction

Any of the signs and symptoms discussed previously can be associated with an allergic reaction. *To be considered a severe allergic reaction, or anaphylaxis, the patient must have either respiratory distress or signs and symptoms of shock.*

Patient Assessment

Allergic Reaction or Anaphylaxis

Conduct the usual assessment sequence, as follows:

- Perform the primary assessment and care for any immediately life-threatening problems with the patient's airway, breathing, or circulation.
- Perform a secondary assessment. Inquire about:
  - History of allergies
  - What the patient was exposed to (what triggered the reaction)
  - How the patient was exposed (contact, ingestion, and so on)
  - What signs and symptoms the patient is having
  - Progression (What happened first? Next? How rapidly?)
  - Interventions (Has any care been provided? Has the patient taken any medication?)
- Assess baseline vital signs and get the remainder of the past medical history.

Suspect an allergic reaction whenever the patient has come in contact with a substance that has caused an allergic reaction in the past; whenever the patient complains of itching, hives, or difficulty breathing (respiratory distress); or when the patient shows signs or symptoms of shock (hypoperfusion).

Table 23-1 lists specific signs and symptoms and their likely association with either a non-life-threatening allergic reaction or a life-threatening anaphylactic reaction.

TABLE 23-1 Distinguishing Allergic from Anaphylactic Reactions

Signs and symptoms in the "Allergic" column are more likely to be associated with allergic reactions that are not life-threatening. Signs and symptoms in the "Anaphylactic" column are more likely to be associated with anaphylactic reactions that are life-threatening.

SYSTEM	ALLERGIC	ANAPHYLACTIC
Respiratory complaints	Sneezing, cough	Dyspnea, tightness in chest
Respiratory sounds	Normal	Wheezing, muffled voice, stridor
Skin findings	Local hives, local redness	Widespread hives, pallor, diffuse redness
Swelling	Local swelling	Swelling of face, lips, eyes, tongue, mouth, injection site
Vital signs	Normal or nearly normal vital signs	Tachycardia, hypotension, tachypnea, decreased oxygen saturation
Mental status	Normal, may be anxious	Syncope, altered mental status, feeling of impending doom

CORE CONCEPT

How to treat a patient experiencing an allergic reaction

Decision Points

- Is this an allergic reaction or anaphylaxis?
- Does it have the potential to become anaphylaxis?
- Do I need to administer epinephrine?

Patient Care

Patient with Allergic Reaction or Anaphylaxis

Fundamental Principles of Care

Manage the patient's airway and breathing. Apply high-concentration oxygen through a nonrebreather mask if the patient is in distress or in some other way appears to be having an anaphylactic reaction. Mild allergic reactions do not require oxygen. If you are not sure, apply oxygen and reassess the patient later to see if it is still necessary. If the patient has or develops an altered mental status, open and maintain the patient's airway. If the patient is not breathing adequately, provide artificial ventilations.

The management of the patient's A-B-Cs is essential care. However, in the setting of an anaphylactic reaction, it is the prompt administration of epinephrine that is the most important life-saving intervention.

auto-injector a syringe preloaded with medication that has a spring-loaded device that pushes the needle through the skin when the tip of the device is pressed firmly against the body.

You may be able to assist the patient in administering an epinephrine ***auto-injector***, or you may be allowed to carry epinephrine on your ambulance and administer it under local protocol. To find out if epinephrine is appropriate, consider each of the following:

- Contact medical direction if the patient has come in contact with a substance that caused an allergic reaction in the past, and the patient has signs or symptoms of respiratory distress, has tongue or lip swelling, or exhibits signs and symptoms of shock, and the patient has a prescribed epinephrine auto-injector (or if your protocols allow you to carry and give epinephrine). If ordered by medical direction, assist the patient with the prescribed auto-injector or administer epinephrine you carry on the ambulance Scan 23-1). Record the administration of the epinephrine. Transport. Reassess 2 minutes after epinephrine administration and record reassessment findings.

- If the patient has come in contact with a substance that caused an allergic reaction in the past, but the patient is not wheezing or showing signs of respiratory distress or shock (hypoperfusion), then continue with the assessment. Consult medical direction; if the patient has an epinephrine auto-injector (or if you carry and can administer epinephrine) and medical direction so orders, administer epinephrine. Some patients have histories of very rapid onset of severe symptoms, so the physician may wish you to give the medication even though the patient does not appear to need it.
- If the patient has come in contact with a substance that caused an allergic reaction in the past, and the patient complains of respiratory distress or exhibits signs and symptoms of shock, but the patient *does not* have a prescribed epinephrine auto-injector available or has never had one prescribed, and your protocols do not allow you to carry and use epinephrine auto-injectors, then perform care for shock and transport the patient immediately. If you carry and can administer epinephrine, give it in accordance with local protocol.

If the patient meets the criteria just listed but does not have an epinephrine auto-injector and your protocols do not allow you to carry and give epinephrine, consider requesting an ALS intercept. Paramedics and advanced EMTs carry and can administer epinephrine.

You probably will not see many patients with allergic reactions. However, most of those you do see will be able to give you a history of their allergies. Once in a while, you will see patients who have no history and are having their first allergic reaction. In these cases, the patients will not be carrying epinephrine auto-injectors, because their physicians have not prescribed them. Treat the patients for shock and transport immediately. Consider requesting ALS intercept.

Think Like an EMT

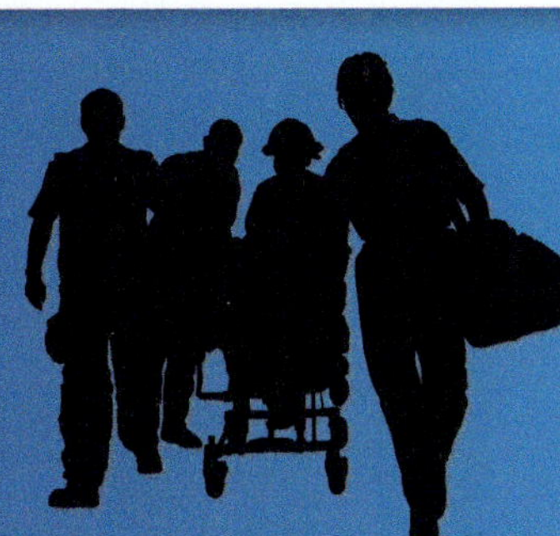

Allergic Reaction or Anaphylaxis?

For each of the following patients, decide whether the presentation is an allergic reaction or anaphylaxis:

1. A patient who has a history of allergy to bee stings and feels her throat "closing up" after a bee sting
2. A patient who suspects an allergic reaction and feels like his skin is "just itching all over"
3. A patient who has an "allergy" to dairy products and reports an upset stomach and diarrhea
4. A patient who is allergic to peanuts and has swelling of the face and neck, difficulty breathing, and a rapid pulse
5. A patient who is allergic to penicillin but accidentally took a medication containing penicillin; the patient is dizzy but has stable vital signs.

Review Scan 23-1 for a summary of assessment and care of patients with allergic or anaphylactic reactions.

SCAN 23-1 Assessing and Managing an Allergic Reaction

First Take Standard Precautions.

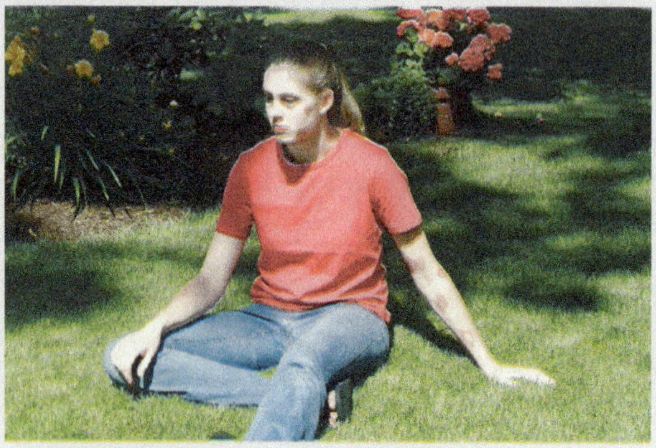

If a patient suffers a severe allergic reaction:

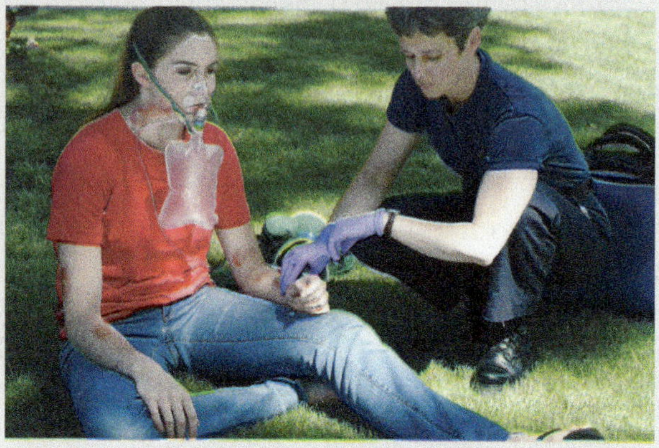

1. Perform a primary assessment. Provide high-concentration oxygen by nonrebreather mask if the patient appears to be having an anaphylactic reaction. For a mild allergic reaction, there is no need to give oxygen.

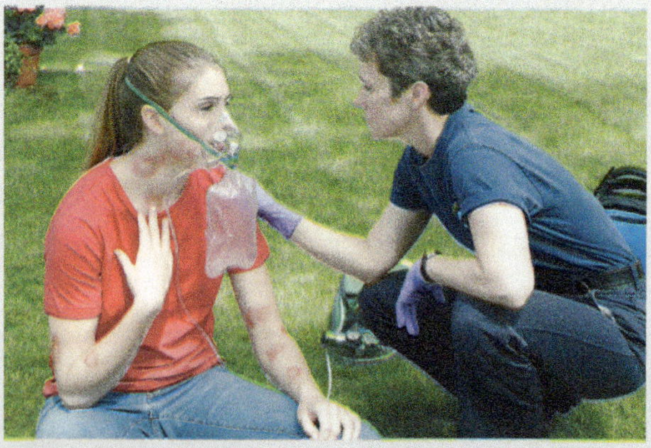

2. Perform a secondary assessment. Obtain a SAMPLE history (see this mnemonic in the chapter *Principles of Assessment*.

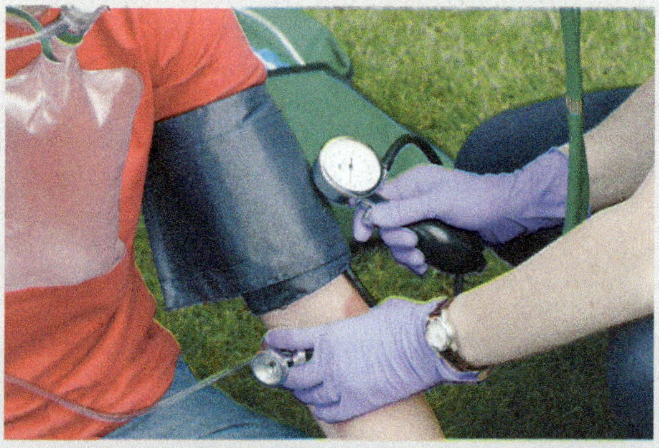

3. Take the patient's vital signs.

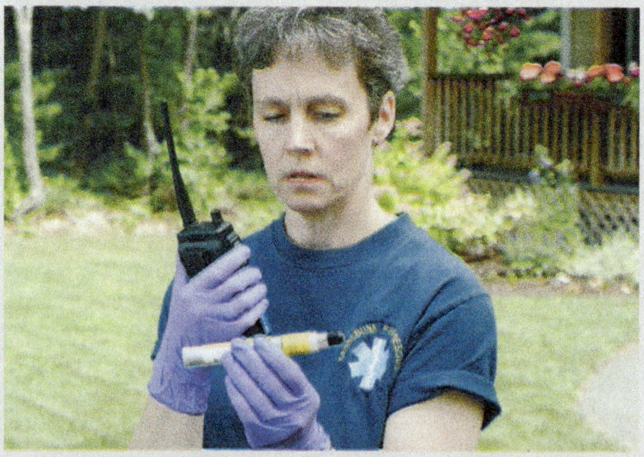

4. Find out if the patient has a prescribed epinephrine auto-injector and if it is prescribed for this patient, or ensure that your protocols allow administering an epinephrine auto-injector you carry on the ambulance. Then check the expiration date and check for cloudiness or discoloration, if liquid is visible. Contact medical direction if required to do so by local protocol.

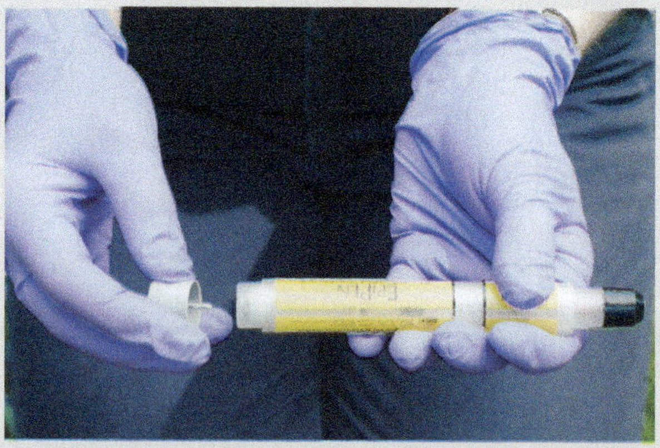

5. If medical direction orders use of the epinephrine auto-injector, prepare it for use by removing the safety cap. (Photo shows the EpiPen®.)

SCAN 23-1 Assessing and Managing an Allergic Reaction *(continued)*

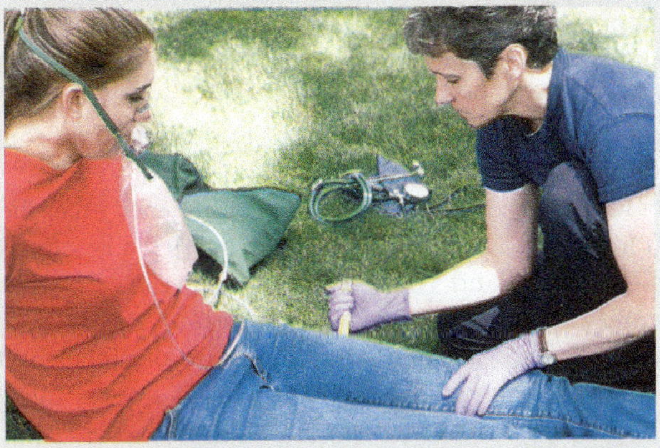

6. Press the injector against the patient's thigh to trigger release of the spring-loaded needle and inject the dose of epinephrine into the patient. Hold the device in place for 10 seconds. (*Note:* All epinephrine injectors will work through clothing.)

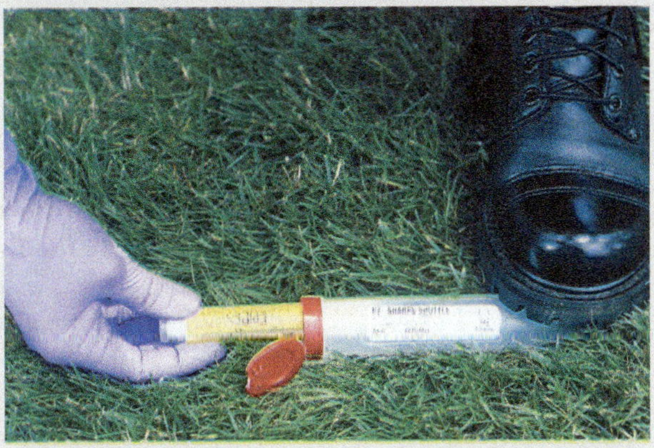

7. Dispose of the used single-dose injector in a portable biohazard container.

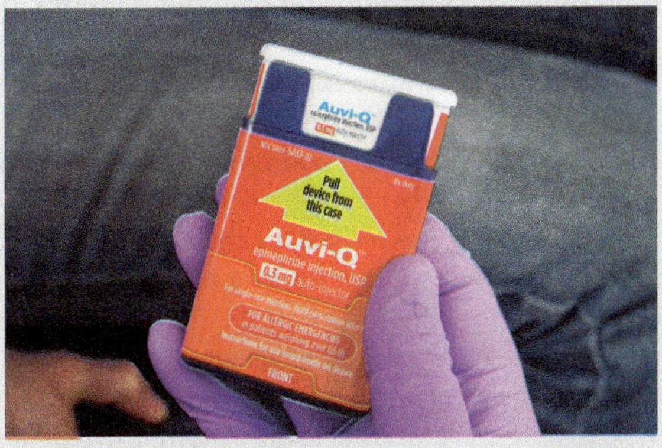

8. If using an Auvi-Q™ device, remove the outer case and follow the voice instructions: Pull off the red safety guard, place the black end against the outer thigh, press firmly, and hold in place for 10 seconds. Put the outer case back on before disposing of the device in a biohazard container.

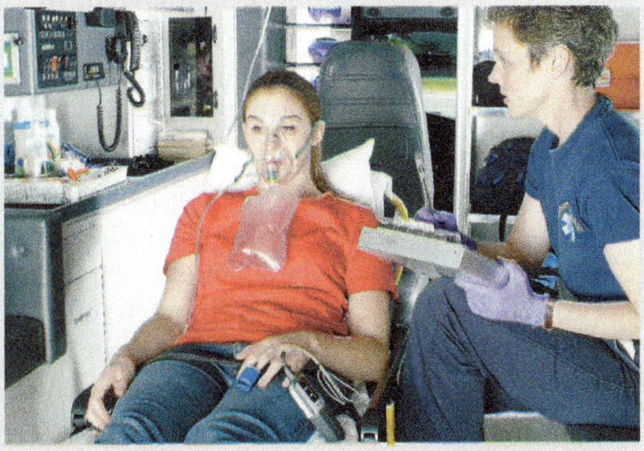

9. Document the patient's response to the medication.

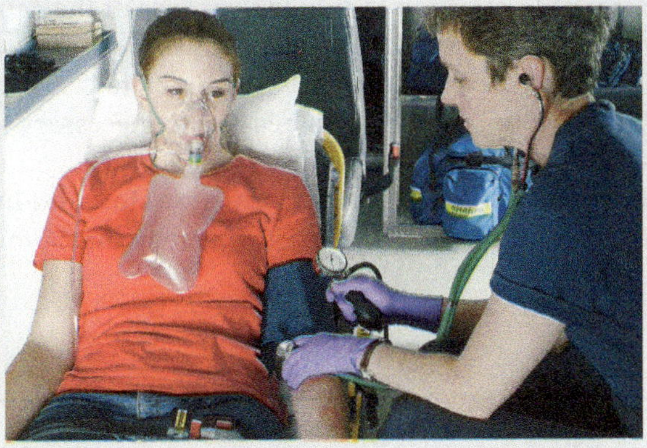

10. Perform a reassessment, paying special attention to the patient's ABCs and vital signs, en route to the hospital. Be prepared to administer a second dose of epinephrine if the patient's condition worsens.

Self-Administered Epinephrine

epinephrine (EP-uh-NEF-rin) a hormone produced by the body. As a medication, it constricts blood vessels and dilates respiratory passages, and is used to relieve severe allergic reactions.

Physicians have long prescribed ***epinephrine*** in bee sting kits, such as Ana-Kit® or EpiPen®, for patients who are susceptible to severe allergic reactions. Epinephrine is a hormone produced by the body. When administered as a medication, it will constrict blood vessels (helping to raise the blood pressure and improve perfusion) and dilate the bronchioles (helping to open the airway and improve breathing).

Many people who are subject to severe allergic reactions are prescribed an epinephrine auto-injector by their physician to carry with them and use when such a reaction occurs. An auto-injector is a spring-loaded needle and syringe with a single dose of epinephrine that will automatically release and inject the medication. The reason it is important for a patient with severe allergic reactions to carry an epinephrine auto-injector is that an allergic reaction can become life-threatening so quickly that there is not enough time to transport the patient to a hospital to receive the medication.

When authorized by medical direction, you may administer or help the patient administer a dose of epinephrine from an auto-injector that has been prescribed for the patient by a physician. Some states allow EMTs to carry epinephrine auto-injectors on the ambulance to administer with approval from medical direction. After you have checked the expiration date and made sure that the liquid is clear (if you can see it), remove the cap and press the injector firmly against the patient's thigh. (Injection on the outside of the thigh midway between the waist and knee is recommended.) Hold it there until the entire dose is injected. On reassessment 2 minutes after the epinephrine is administered, in addition to some relief of symptoms, expect the patient's pulse to have increased.

The procedure for administering an epinephrine auto-injector was shown in Scan 23-1. Information about epinephrine auto-injectors is summarized in Scan 23-2.

Epinephrine is a very powerful medication. One of the good things epinephrine does for patients is make the heart beat more strongly. This is beneficial when the patient is hypoperfusing (i.e., when the patient is in shock) because one reason for the hypoperfusion is that the patient's blood vessels are dilated and blood is not returning to the heart as quickly. Unfortunately, once you give a drug, you cannot take it back. If the dose of epinephrine in the auto-injector is more than the patient needs, the patient's heart will be working harder than it needs to. This can be potentially dangerous in a patient with a heart condition.

The power of epinephrine and its possible adverse effects are among the reasons EMTs have traditionally been taught to *give epinephrine only to patients who have been prescribed auto-injectors by their physicians*. These patients have been evaluated by physicians who have considered the patients' history and physical condition, were satisfied that the patients were good candidates for epinephrine, and wrote prescriptions. More recently, a number of high-profile cases where people died when epinephrine was not available have led to a reconsideration of this approach. Many EMS systems now allow EMTs to carry and administer epinephrine under certain conditions, which are described later in this chapter.

Although some patients receive instruction from their physicians in how to use the auto-injector, others will be uncomfortable or afraid to use one because of their unfamiliarity with the device and will prefer to have you help them with it. Ordinarily when a health care provider gives an injection, the clothing over the injection site is rolled up or down and the area is cleansed with an alcohol pad. These steps are not necessary with an epinephrine auto-injector. The risk of giving a patient an infection because you did not take those steps is so small, in fact, that the manufacturer's instructions for auto-injectors do not advise patients to take those steps. However, your protocols may direct you to act differently. Follow your local protocols.

SCAN 23-2 Epinephrine Auto-Injector

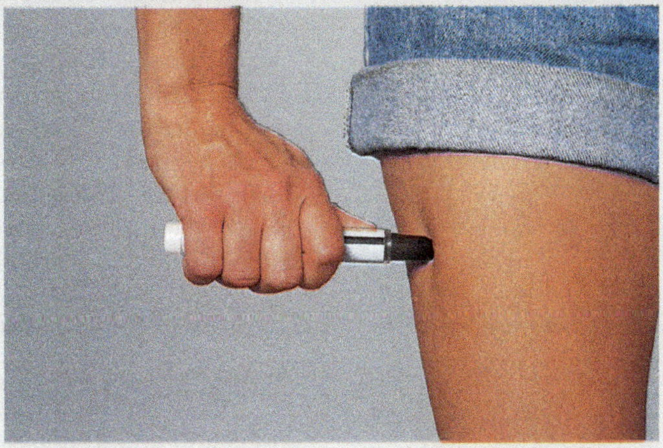

MEDICATION NAME

- Generic: epinephrine
- Trade: Adrenalin®
- Delivery system: EpiPen® or EpiPen Jr.®, or Auvi-Q™ (adult or child size)

INDICATIONS

Must meet the following three criteria:

1. Patient exhibits signs of a severe allergic reaction, including either respiratory distress or shock (hypoperfusion).
2. Medication is prescribed for this patient by a physician or is carried on the ambulance.
3. Medical direction authorizes use for this patient.

CONTRAINDICATIONS

No contraindications when used in a life-threatening situation

MEDICATION FORM

Liquid is administered by an auto-injector–an automatically injectable needle-and-syringe system.

DOSAGE

1. Adult: one adult auto-injector (0.3 mg)
2. Infant and child: one infant/child auto-injector (0.15 mg)

ADMINISTRATION

1. Obtain patient's prescribed auto-injector. Ensure:
   a. "Five rights" of medication administration
   b. Prescription is for the patient who is experiencing the severe allergic reaction, or your protocols permit carrying the auto-injector on the ambulance
   c. Medication is not discolored (if visible)
   d. Medication has not expired
2. Obtain an order from medical direction, either on-line or off-line.
3. Remove the safety cap(s) from the auto-injector.
4. Grasp the center of the auto-injector (to avoid accidentally injecting yourself).
5. Place the tip of the auto-injector against the patient's thigh.
   a. Lateral portion of the thigh
   b. Midway between waist and knee
6. Push the injector firmly against the thigh until the injector activates.
7. Hold the injector in place until the medication is injected (at least 10 seconds for the EpiPen® and at least 5 seconds for the Auvi-Q™).
8. Document medication administration and time.
9. Dispose of the injector in a biohazard container.

ACTIONS

1. Dilates the bronchioles.
2. Constricts blood vessels.
3. Makes the capillaries less permeable (leaky).

SIDE EFFECTS

1. Increased heart rate
2. Pallor
3. Dizziness
4. Chest pain
5. Headache
6. Nausea
7. Vomiting
8. Excitability, anxiety

REASSESSMENT STRATEGIES

1. Transport.
2. Continue secondary assessment of airway, breathing, and circulatory status.

If the patient's condition continues to worsen (decreasing mental status, increasing breathing difficulty, decreasing blood pressure):

a. Obtain medical direction for an additional dose of epinephrine.
b. Treat for shock (hypoperfusion).
c. Prepare to initiate basic life support procedures (CPR, AED).

If the patient's condition improves, provide supportive care:

a. Continue oxygen.
b. Treat for shock (hypoperfusion).

One of the most difficult things you may have to do is distinguish between the patient with an allergic (localized) reaction, who should not receive epinephrine, and the patient with an anaphylactic (generalized) reaction, who should be given epinephrine. Patients can and do present in many different ways. One patient in anaphylaxis may have severe difficulty breathing, with no hives or decreased blood pressure, whereas another patient may have a rapid heartbeat and decreased blood pressure, with no difficulty breathing. The important thing to recognize in any patient is the presence of *either signs or symptoms respiratory distress or signs and symptoms of shock (hypoperfusion)*. Very often, both of these—indications of respiratory distress and indications of shock—are present. However, only *one* of these needs to be present for the patient to be in anaphylaxis.

Pediatric Note

Signs and symptoms of anaphylaxis in children are not substantially different from those in adults. However, the treatment can differ because of the smaller size of these patients. Epinephrine auto-injectors come in two different sizes. The adult size contains an adult dose of 0.3 mg. The child size (for a child weighing less than 66 pounds [30 kg]) has 0.15 mg. Infants rarely experience anaphylactic reactions, because their immune systems have not matured enough to develop the kinds of antibodies that cause anaphylactic reactions. Allergic reactions are common in older children, though. Fortunately, many children "grow out of" their allergies as they mature. Parents frequently will have a great deal of useful information about the child's medical history.

FIGURE 23-4 Epinephrine auto-injectors: (A) EpiPen® and EpiPen Jr.®; (B) generic epinephrine auto-injector. (C) The Auvi-Q® provides voice instructions.

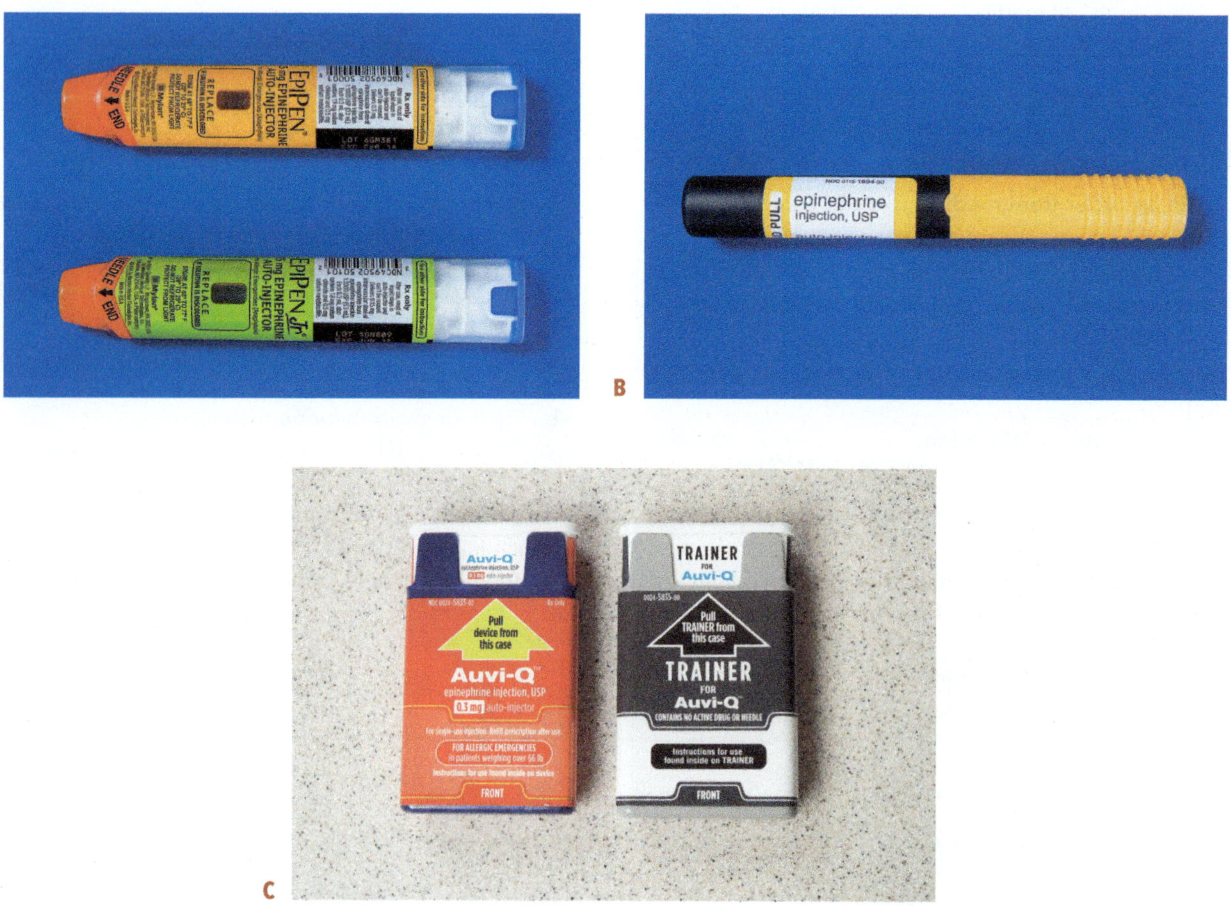

A

B

C

Additional Doses of Epinephrine

A patient with an allergic reaction may have a compromised airway or respiratory function, or these conditions may develop as the allergic reaction progresses. Carefully monitor the patient's airway and breathing throughout your care and transport.

In your reassessment, you will frequently find that the patient's condition improves, although sometimes it will deteriorate. You may need to give additional doses of epinephrine in these cases. You will be able to do this only if the patient has one or more extra auto-injectors and you have remembered to ask the patient to bring them in the ambulance, and you obtain permission for the second dose from medical direction (Figure 23-4). Don't forget: If a patient has an extra epinephrine auto-injector, bring it along.

CORE CONCEPT
Who should be assisted with an epinephrine auto-injector

EMT-Administered Epinephrine

For many years, EMTs have learned to assist patients in administering their own prescribed epinephrine. This approach has begun to change in recent years, particularly with the onset of extreme price increases in auto-injectors. Some ambulance services are simply no longer able to afford the cost of stocking all of their vehicles with epinephrine auto-injectors that typically expire before they are used. As a result, many EMS systems have moved to a system that trains EMTs to draw up and administer epinephrine with a hypodermic needle and syringe and allows them to carry epinephrine on the ambulance. This system is much less expensive (hundreds of dollars less per dose) and, when carried out under certain conditions, is safe and effective.

One of the commonly used systems for accomplishing this is called Ready-Check-Inject. It includes a number of safety measures:

- The only epinephrine allowed to be carried is 1 mL of the appropriate concentration (1:1,000, which has 1 mg epinephrine in 1 mL). A vial is preferred, but an ampule is acceptable in some systems. Containers with more than 1 mL are not allowed, preventing potentially harmful megadoses from being administered.
- A second provider must verify that the proper dose has been drawn up into the syringe (0.3 mL for adults and 0.15 mL for children less than 66 pounds [30 kg]). This decreases greatly the chance that a patient will get an improper dose.
- The syringe and needle are the proper size for intramuscular injection.
- All of the needed supplies are packaged in one container with a review card.
- EMTs are required to complete additional training on use of the kit, including determination of the proper dose and practice in drawing up the correct volume.
- EMTs are required to demonstrate competency in the technique of drawing up the proper volume and administering an IM injection.
- The agency maintains records of initial and review training.

If you work in a system where this approach is used (although it's possible it goes by a different name), you will need to complete the steps above in order to be authorized to administer epinephrine. You will also need to be sure you are completely familiar with your system's protocols, including whether you need to obtain on-line medical direction. Scan 23-3 demonstrates the steps involved in Ready-Check-Inject.

SCAN 23-3 Ready-Check-Inject

First, Take Standard Precautions.

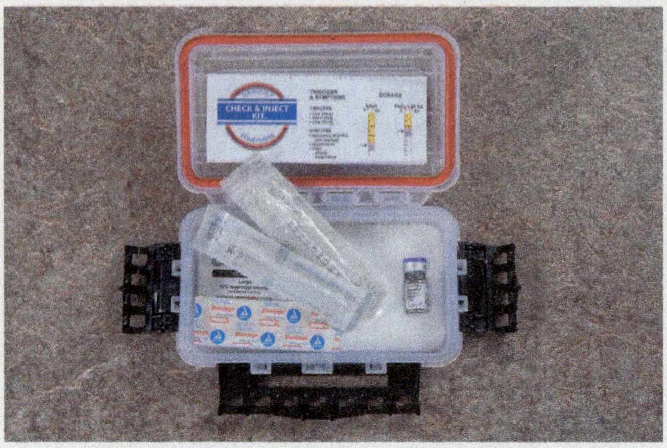

1. Open the kit, verify all components are present, and verify the expiration date of the epinephrine has not passed.

FOR EPINEPHRINE FROM VIAL:

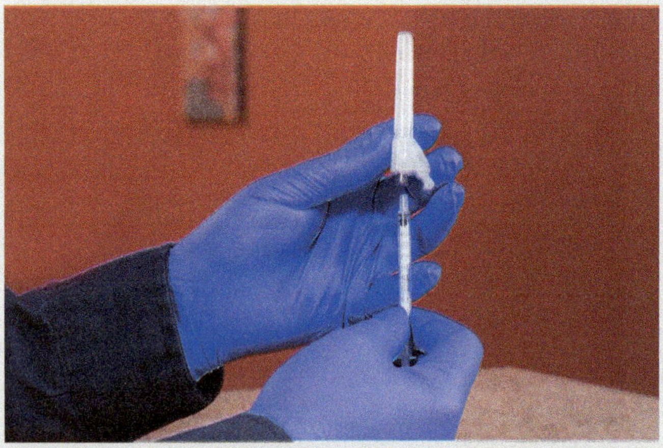

2A. Attach needle to syringe, maintaining aseptic technique.

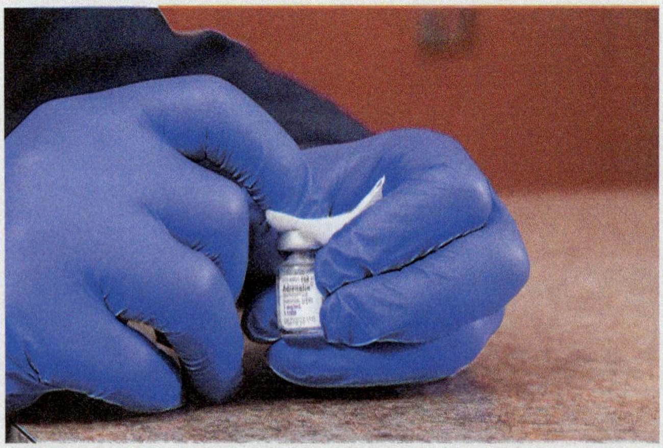

2B. Remove the cap from the medication vial and clean the top of the vial with an alcohol prep pad.

FOR EPINEPHRINE FROM AMPULE:

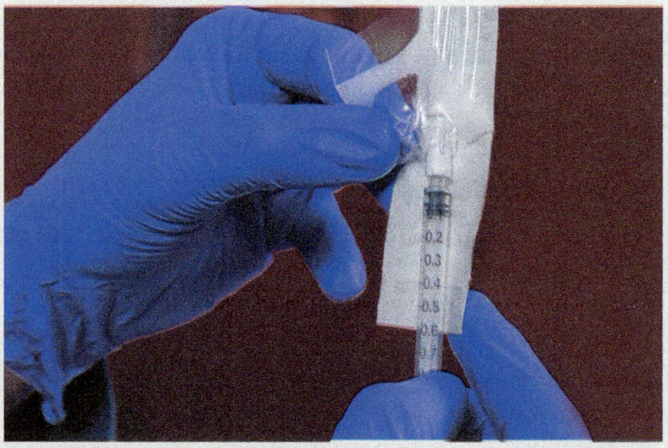

3A. Attach a filter straw to a syringe, maintaining aseptic technique.

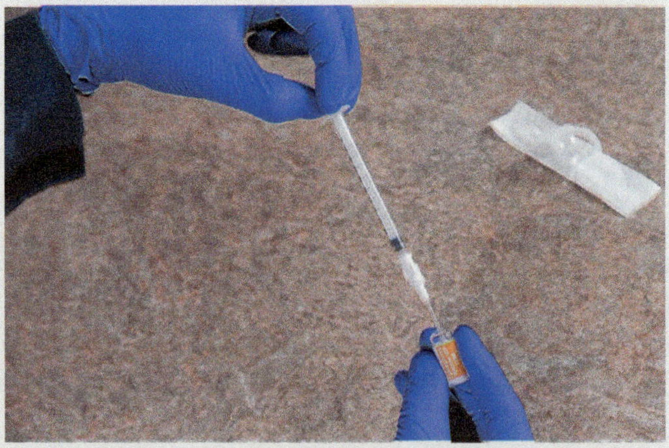

3B. Remove the top from the medication ampule, insert the filter straw into the epinephrine ampule, and withdraw the appropriate volume of medication.

SCAN 23-3 Ready-Check-Inject *(continued)*

FOR EPINEPHRINE FROM VIAL:

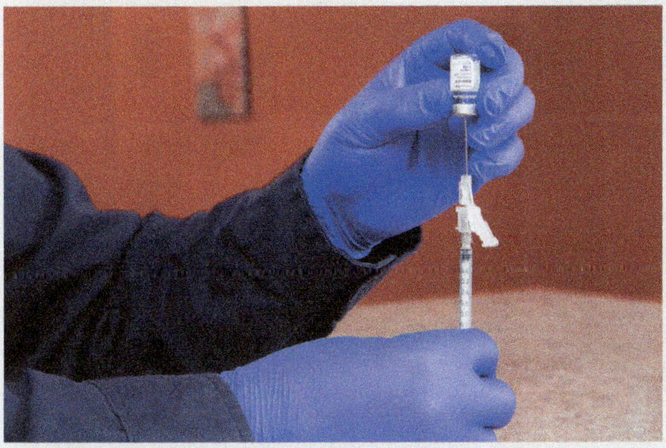

2C. Insert the needle into the epinephrine vial and withdraw the appropriate volume of medication.

FOR EPINEPHRINE FROM AMPULE:

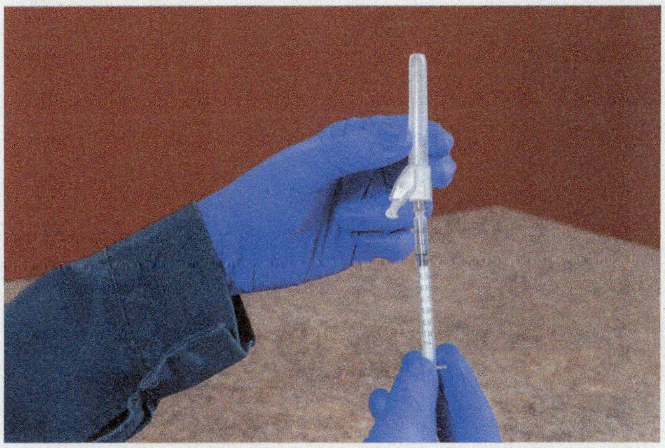

3C. Remove the filter straw and attach the needle.

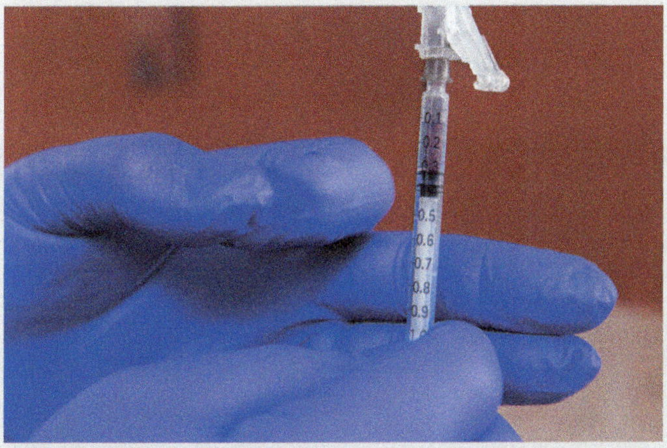

4. Remove air bubbles from the syringe and expel any additional air and fluid to reach the correct volume.

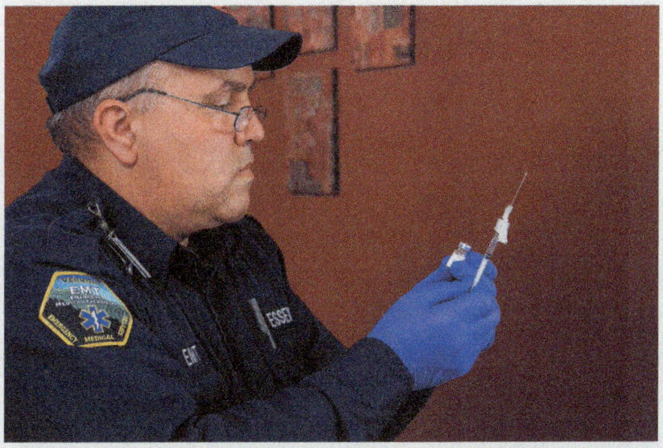

5. Confirm the five rights, including correct medication (epinephrine 1 mg/1 mL), correct dose and volume (0.3 mg [0.3 mL] for an adult or 0.15 mg [0.15 mL] for a child less than 66 pounds [30 kg]), and ensure no air bubbles are present.

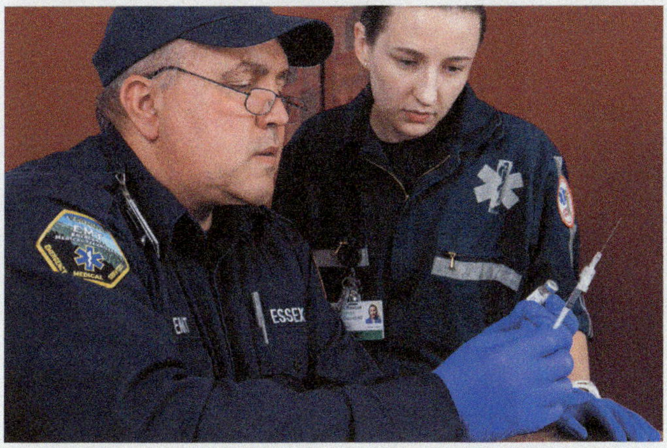

6. Have person 2 visually inspect and confirm: correct medication (epinephrine 1 mg/1 mL), correct dose and volume, and no air bubbles.

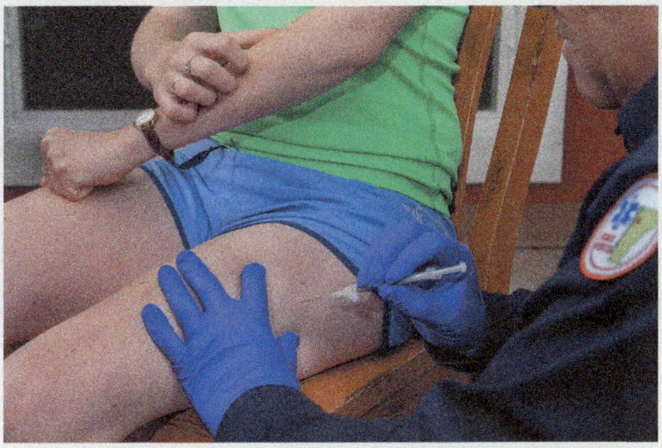

7. Identify the proper site for injection, flatten the skin with a thumb and forefinger, and insert the needle quickly at a 90-degree angle to the skin.

(continued)

SCAN 23-3 Ready-Check-Inject *(continued)*

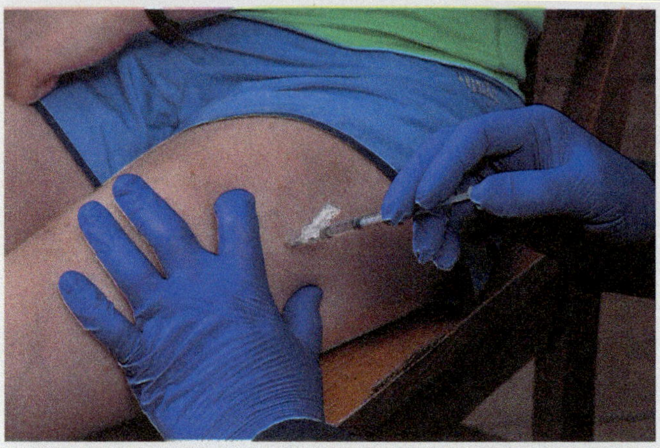

8. Draw back the plunger quickly to ensure you have not entered a blood vessel. Depress the plunger slowly to inject.

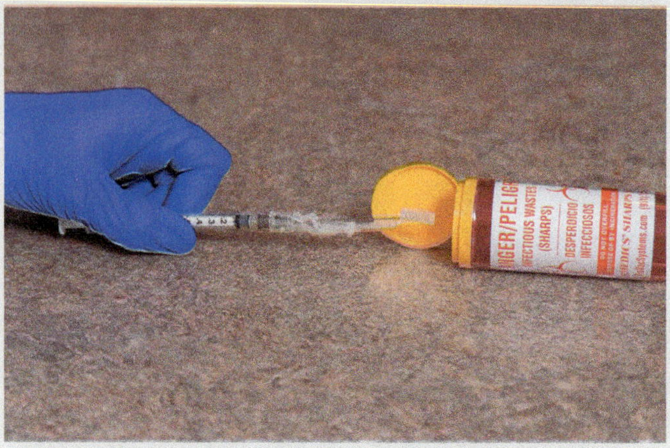

9. Remove the syringe and activate the needle safety mechanism. Dispose of the needle and syringe in a proper sharps container.

10. Document medication administration.

Point of View

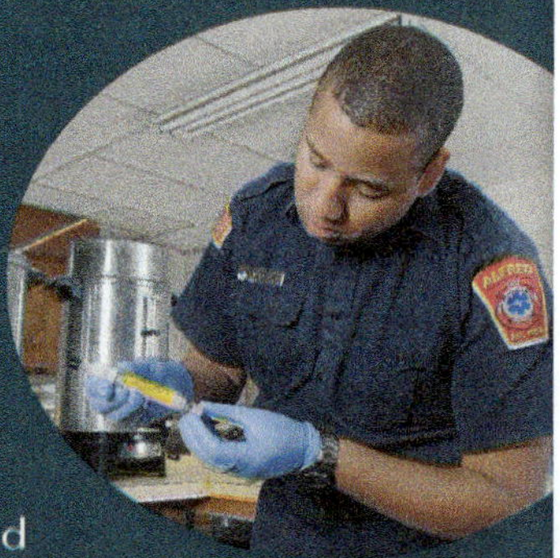

"I was at the lodge the other day. We were preparing for the holiday festival, our biggest fundraiser of the year. It is held during tourist season. We have a dinner and bake sale. I've worked it for the past twenty years, since I was a kid.

"Most people there know I have an allergy to nuts. It seems like all I have to do is look at them sometimes and I blow up and can't breathe. Someone brought some in, and the next thing I know, it started. It seemed like seconds, and I was wheezing and swelling up.

"My friends knew right away something was wrong. Mikey called 911 while Drew went out to my car to get my EpiPen®. The ambulance must have been right around the corner. They walked in with Drew. They took one look at me, and I could see the concern in their eyes. I've seen it before.

"Fortunately, they didn't waste time. They were putting me on oxygen and getting the stretcher while the EMT in charge got the EpiPen®. It saved my life before. It did again today. They actually had to use my second EpiPen® in the ambulance because it was such a bad reaction.

"The guys joked with me when I got out of the hospital. They were going to name the lodge after me if I died. They like to joke. But I'm not sure they know just how close it was."

Chapter Review

Key Facts and Concepts

- Allergic reactions are common. Anaphylaxis, a true life-threatening allergic reaction, is rare.
- The most common symptom in is itching. Patients with anaphylaxis, though, will also display life-threatening difficulty breathing and/or signs and symptoms of shock (hypoperfusion). These patients will also be extremely anxious. Their bodies are in trouble and are letting the patients know it.
- The signs and symptoms of anaphylaxis are a result of physiologic changes: vasodilation, bronchoconstriction, leaky capillaries, and thick mucus.
- By quickly recognizing the condition, consulting medical direction, and administering the appropriate treatment, you can literally make the difference between life and death for these patients.

Key Decisions

- Is the patient's breathing adequate, inadequate, or absent?
- Is the patient having an allergic reaction, or is the patient having a life-threatening anaphylactic reaction? Does the patient have respiratory difficulty or shock?
- Should I assist the patient with or administer epinephrine?

Chapter Glossary

allergen something that causes an allergic reaction.

allergic reaction an exaggerated immune response.

anaphylaxis (an-ah-fi-LAK-sis) a severe or life-threatening allergic reaction in which the blood vessels dilate, causing a drop in blood pressure, and the tissues lining the respiratory system swell, interfering with the airway. Also called *anaphylactic shock*.

auto-injector a syringe preloaded with medication that has a spring-loaded device that pushes the needle through the skin when the tip of the device is pressed firmly against the body.

epinephrine (EP-uh-NEF-rin) a hormone produced by the body. As a medication, it constricts blood vessels and dilates respiratory passages, and is used to relieve severe allergic reactions.

hives red, itchy, possibly raised blotches on the skin that often result from allergic reactions.

Preparation for Your Examination and Practice

Short Answer

1. What are the indications for administration of an epinephrine auto-injector?
2. List some of the more common causes of allergic reactions.
3. List signs or symptoms of an anaphylactic reaction associated with each of the following:
   - Skin
   - Respiratory system
   - Cardiovascular system

Thinking and Linking

Think back to the Cardiac Emergencies *chapter, and link information from that chapter with information from this chapter as you consider the following situation:*

- Your patient is a 60-year-old who used his friend's EpiPen® and is now complaining of chest pain. He thought he might have been stung and, although he wasn't sure, his friend had said, "Here, I can help you with that," handed him the EpiPen®, and helped him inject himself with epinephrine. You know that one action of epinephrine is making the heart beat more strongly. Could this be causing the patient's chest pain? How? And how should you proceed at this point to assess and care for this patient?

Critical Thinking Exercises

Anaphylactic reactions are truly life-threatening. Fortunately, many patients carry their own epinephrine auto-injectors. Many ambulances also carry epinephrine. Yet not all patients who have allergic reactions have anaphylaxis. The purpose of this exercise will be to determine the difference between an allergic reaction and anaphylaxis, and to determine whether epinephrine should be administered.

1. Your 24-year-old patient ate a meal that he believes contained shellfish. He is allergic to shrimp. While the kitchen staff rushes to determine if shrimp was used in or near the preparation of the patient's meal, you perform an examination. The patient is sweating and nervous. He appears to be breathing adequately. You do not note any wheezing or stridor. His face is slightly red. His pulse is 88, strong and regular; respirations 24; blood pressure 108/74; and skin warm and moist.
2. You are called to a 50-year-old woman who received a narcotic pain reliever after minor dental surgery. She believes she is allergic to some pain medication but can't remember which one. She has vomited twice. One time, she believes, she saw blood in her vomit. Her vital signs are pulse 92, strong and regular; respirations 22 and adequate, without wheezes or stridor; blood pressure 148/86; skin warm and dry; pupils equal and reactive to light.
3. Your patient is a parent who came into his daughter's kindergarten class as a helper. After eating a cookie, he developed a funny feeling in his tongue that progressed to swelling. He is anxious and sweaty when you see him. His pulse is 126 and regular, respirations 32 and slightly labored, blood pressure 96/58, skin cool and moist, pupils equal and reactive to light.

Pathophysiology to Practice

The following question is designed to assist you in gathering relevant clinical information and making accurate decisions in the field.

- Anxiety is a common symptom in anaphylactic reactions, but anxiety alone can produce symptoms that resemble an anaphylactic reaction. What would be the effect of epinephrine on a person who appeared to be having an anaphylactic reaction but was really having an anxiety attack with no anaphylaxis?

Street Scenes

As you respond to a remote neighborhood in your district for an unknown problem, your dispatcher gives you further information about the call. She states that an elderly male has been stung several times by hornets but has not developed difficulty breathing. The dispatcher also tells you there is an ALS unit responding from the other side of town.

As you arrive on scene, you see an older woman coming out to greet you. She appears upset as she tells you that her 68-year-old husband was doing some work in their storage shed. "I was working in the kitchen when I heard him yelling my name. As I ran outside, I could see him waving his arms around, trying to scare away the hornets."

You find Mr. Meeker sitting forward on a lawn chair at the rear of the house. You notice immediately he is using accessory muscles to breathe and that his face and neck appear flushed. He attempts to explain what has happened but is unable to speak in complete sentences.

Street Scene Questions

1. What is your impression of Mr. Meeker's condition?
2. What do you think might be happening to him?

As you apply a nonrebreather mask to the patient, Mrs. Meeker tells you that he has an allergy to hornet stings and that the last time he was stung was shortly after he returned from the war in southeast Asia in the 1970s. You ask, "Does your husband carry an EpiPen®?" She tells you no. He has no other allergies, takes an aspirin daily, and had a heart attack nine years ago.

You suspect the patient might be experiencing an allergic reaction to the insect stings and that this could be a life-threatening reaction.

As you place Mr. Meeker in the ambulance, your partner reassures the patient's wife and advises her to be careful as she follows the ambulance to the hospital. En route, you assess vital signs and find that the patient's pulse is 136 and thready, his respirations are 28 and shallow, oxygen saturation (SpO_2) is 93 percent on 15 liters per minute O_2, and he has a blood pressure of 92/60. You notice the patient's respiratory count is falling and that he has become extremely fatigued by breathing.

Street Scene Questions

3. What do you suspect is beginning to happen to your patient?
4. What further treatment should you render?

When you reassess the patient's breathing more closely, you notice his respiratory rate has dropped significantly, to about 12. Although that number is in the normal range for an adult, you realize that the depth of the patient's respirations is so shallow that he is not breathing adequately. You connect the bag-valve-mask (BVM) to the oxygen tank and ventilate Mr. Meeker about 12 times a minute, making sure you ventilate him deeply enough to make his chest rise. After a few breaths, you are able to match your ventilations to the patient's so he is not fighting against the BVM.

As it happens, the ALS intercept is delayed in a traffic snarl, and you reach the hospital before the intercept can happen. You advise the emergency department staff that you have a 68-year-old male who has been stung by several hornets and that you suspect a severe allergic reaction. The staff relieves you of patient care and thanks you for the report.

Infectious Diseases and Sepsis

24

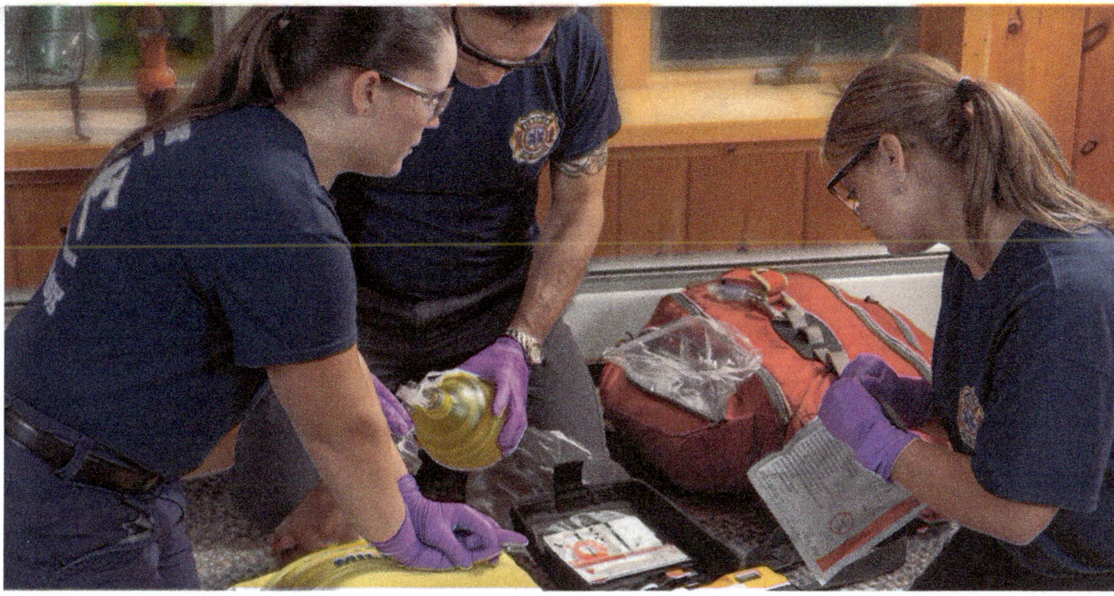

Related Chapters

Standard

Medicine (Infectious Disease)

Competency

Applies fundamental knowledge to provide basic emergency care and transportation based on assessment findings for an acutely ill patient.

Core Concepts

- Pathophysiology of infectious disease and sepsis
- How infectious diseases spread
- Recognition and management of patients with infectious diseases
- Recognition and management of the possibly septic patient

Outcomes

After reading this chapter, you should be able to:

24.1 Identify key factors involved in transmission of infectious diseases. (pp. 671–674)

- Describe the factors that determine whether exposure to a communicable disease results in infection.
- Define the terms incubation period, bacteria, viruses, sepsis, and septic shock.
- List the two most effective methods of preventing the spread of disease.

24.2 Explain the pathophysiology and progression of sepsis. (pp. 674–677)

- Describe how exposure to a disease can progress to septic shock.
- Identify common causes of sepsis.
- List criteria for recognizing sepsis using the systemic inflammatory response syndrome criteria.
- Given a patient description, determine whether you should notify the emergency department of a sepsis alert.

24.3 List the common patient presentation, treatment, standard precautions and postexposure actions for each of the following diseases: (pp. 677–691)

- Chickenpox
- Measles
- Mumps
- Hepatitis
- HIV/AIDS
- Influenza
- Croup
- Pertussis
- Pneumonia
- Tuberculosis
- Meningitis
- Sexually transmitted infections (STIs)
- Diseases carried by ticks

24.4 Discuss reactions among the public and health care providers when a potentially deadly infectious disease is discovered or rediscovered. (p. 691)

Key Terms

infectious diseases, *671*

communicable diseases, *671*

sepsis, *675*

Although infectious diseases have been recognized for thousands of years, it is only in modern times that we have come to understand them and have developed effective treatments against them. The discovery of germ theory and the development of antibiotics in the 20th century brought great advances in understanding, prevention, and treatment of infectious diseases, but new diseases are being discovered (or rediscovered) at an increasing rate. In many cases, the antibiotics that used to be effective against the most serious infectious diseases have become less effective, as bacteria have developed resistance to these antibiotics. Sepsis used to be considered an untreatable and, most often, fatal complication of an infectious disease when it led to septic shock. Over the last two decades, the early recognition and aggressive treatment of sepsis have changed that. In recent years, the mortality rate for sepsis has been cut in half thanks to these efforts, especially by physicians and health professionals who staff emergency departments. Even as we celebrate these advances, we have come to realize there is much more to be learned and more that can be done to improve patient outcomes. This chapter describes these topics and the steps EMTs can take to continue those efforts.

There is another dimension to infectious diseases that EMTs must consider—what risks (if any) do patients with infectious diseases pose to you personally as an EMT, and how do you reduce those risks? This chapter will also discuss exposure to infectious diseases and related issues (such as the importance of vaccination) to better prepare you as an emergency responder. EMTs should stay current on the types of infectious diseases that are prevalent at any given time (such as flu season). The Centers for Disease Control and Prevention (CDC) has excellent resources on infectious diseases that provide up-to-date information and are easily available at their website.

Infectious Diseases

Many of the conditions you encounter as an EMT occur because of poor life choices, like driving under the influence, or genetic tendencies, such as a familial tendency toward heart disease. In this chapter, we look at diseases that can be spread by bacteria, viruses, and other microbes, i.e., ***infectious diseases***. In particular, we focus on ***communicable diseases*** that can be passed from one individual to another, either through direct contact or contact with secretions from an infected person. These two terms sound similar, but they are very different. Lyme disease, for example, is infectious because a tick transmits it to a person by a bite, but it is not communicable, because one person cannot give it to another. See Table 24-1 for specific information about infectious and communicable diseases.

infectious diseases diseases that can be spread by bacteria, viruses, and other microbes.

communicable diseases diseases that can be passed from one individual to another, either through direct contact or contact with secretions from an infected person.

How Diseases Spread

There are many kinds of microbes that transmit disease. *Bacteria* are living organisms that consist of a single cell. They are found both inside and outside of the body and can reproduce in either environment. *Viruses*, on the other hand, are not cells, and have a protein coat or shell that encloses what they need to reproduce, either DNA or RNA. They need to be inside a host to reproduce. Bacteria are much larger than viruses and consist of both good and bad types. Although some bacteria cause infection that leads to illness, our bodies contain many good bacteria that are necessary for us to survive. Viruses, on the other hand, have few, if any, beneficial uses.

There are other types of microbes that can cause illness, like fungi that cause yeast infections, protozoa that can cause malaria, and parasites that live off the body without providing any benefit, like tapeworms. This chapter emphasizes common infections that EMTs need to be able to recognize, so it will focus on bacteria and viruses.

TABLE 24-1 Communicable Diseases

DISEASE	MODE OF TRANSMISSION	INCUBATION PERIOD	PERIOD OF COMMUNICABILITY	SIGNS AND SYMPTOMS
Chickenpox (varicella)	Airborne droplets. Can also be spread by contact with open sores.	10-21 days	1-2 days before rash until 5 days after	Fever and rash, especially on chest, abdomen, back, and proximal extremities
Measles	Airborne droplets and direct contact with nasal and throat secretions	3-7 days	4 days before rash to 4 days after	Fever, cough, eye irritation, rash
Mumps	Droplets of saliva or contact with objects contaminated by saliva	16-18 days	2 days before swelling to 5 days after	Muscle aches, loss of appetite, headache, painful swelling of parotid gland
Hepatitis A	Fecal-oral route	28-30 days	2 weeks after infection until 3 days after jaundice appears	Fever, nausea, loss of appetite, malaise, abdominal pain, jaundice
Hepatitis B	Blood, semen, CSF, amniotic fluid, vaginal secretions	60-90 days	As long as hepatitis B surface antigen test is positive	Nausea, loss of appetite, malaise, abdominal pain, jaundice
Hepatitis C	Blood, semen, CSF, amniotic fluid, vaginal secretions	6-9 weeks	From 1 week before symptoms appear; chronic carriers can transmit the virus forever.	Nausea, loss of appetite, malaise, abdominal pain, jaundice, but most patients don't show symptoms.
Human immunodeficiency virus (HIV)/Acquired immunodeficiency syndrome (AIDS)	Blood, semen, CSF, amniotic fluid, vaginal secretions, breast milk	Less than 1 year; might never progress to AIDS with proper treatment.	Most easily transmitted when viral load is high	Fever, sore throat, fatigue within a few weeks of being infected; opportunistic infections later
Influenza	Airborne droplets and direct contact	1-4 days	1 day before symptoms appear to 7 days after	Fever, nonproductive cough, severe muscle aches, sore throat, headache and severe weakness
Croup	Airborne droplets and direct contact	2-3 days	During incubation period to 10 days after symptoms start	Symptoms of upper respiratory infection, dyspnea, bark-like cough in children
Pertussis	Airborne droplets	9-10 days	Up to 3 weeks (5 days if on antibiotics)	Symptoms of upper respiratory infection, then severe uninterrupted coughing followed by a whooping sound on inspiration
Pneumococcal pneumonia	Droplets	1-3 days	Until 24 hours after antibiotics	Fever, chills, shortness of breath, tachypnea, pleuritic chest pain, productive cough
Tuberculosis	Airborne droplets	2-10 weeks	Until 2-4 weeks after antibiotics	Cough, fever, night sweats, weight loss
Meningococcal meningitis	Direct contact	3-4 days	3 days after infection to 24 hours after antibiotics	Abrupt onset of fever, nausea, vomiting, severe headache, nuchal rigidity, photophobia, petechiae

TREATMENT	PREVENTION	POSTEXPOSURE ACTIONS	SPECIAL CONSIDERATIONS
Isolation and anti-viral medication	Vaccine, Standard Precautions	If not immunized, receive vaccine.	The virus can reactivate in an adult who experiences severe pain along a dermatome (herpes zoster). A vaccine is available.
Isolation and supportive treatment	Vaccine, Standard Precautions	If not immunized, receive vaccine and possibly immune globulin.	Check to see if your health department requires you to report cases.
Isolation and supportive treatment	Vaccine, Standard Precautions	No specific actions	Adult males can develop orchitis (inflammation of testicles).
Supportive treatment	Vaccine, Standard Precautions	Vaccine, possible hepatitis A immune globulin	Hepatitis E is similar to hepatitis A, but is caused by a different virus.
Supportive treatment	Vaccine, Standard Precautions	Wash exposure site, get vaccinated if not immune, get evaluation for whether hepatitis B immune globulin is appropriate.	If you have hepatitis B, you can get infected with hepatitis D.
Several medication regimens are safe and effective.	Standard Precautions	No specific actions	Chronic untreated infection can lead to cirrhosis and liver cancer.
Anti-viral medications to suppress the virus	Standard Precautions	Wash exposure site, get evaluation for whether postexposure prophylaxis (anti-viral medication regimen) is appropriate.	HIV/AIDS is a chronic disease; patients can experience discrimination out of fear or ignorance.
Anti-viral medication, supportive treatment	Vaccine, Standard Precautions	Possibly anti-viral medication	Different strains of flu virus circulate each year, so EMTs should get vaccinated each year
Supportive treatment	Standard Precautions	No specific actions	ALS personnel may be able to administer medications to help the child.
Isolation antibiotics and supportive treatment	Vaccine, Standard Precautions	For pregnant women, possibly antibiotics; otherwise, no specific actions	Pertussis can be fatal to infants, so vaccination of adults is very important to prevent spread of infection.
Antibiotics, supportive treatment	Vaccine, Standard Precautions	No specific actions	Pneumonia is a common cause of sepsis in the young and the old.
Antibiotics, supportive treatment	Standard Precautions and airborne disease precautions	Report exposure to receiving hospital and get tested for TB. If positive, you will get antibiotics.	EMTs should wear N-95 respirators when treating a patient who may have TB.
Antibiotics, supportive treatment	Vaccine and Standard Precautions	No specific actions	Viral meningitis is less severe than the bacterial form.

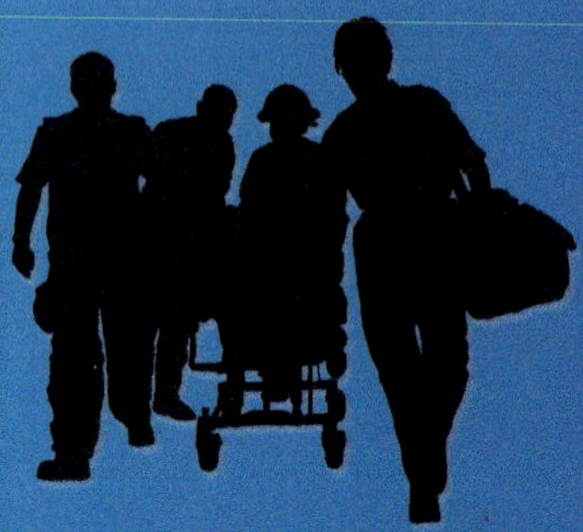

Think Like an EMT

What's Going On?

It may be difficult to recognize an infectious disease because you may never have seen it. In the developed world, most people have received immunizations, making some diseases that were common in the twentieth century uncommon or rare today.

A factor that makes recognition even harder is that different infectious conditions can look very similar. Consider the following situations, and determine what infectious diseases may be present, as well as conditions that may mimic them:

1. A 4-year-old boy broke out this morning in a rash that covers his body and is now scratching all over. He doesn't appear sick and has no fever.
2. A 36-year-old woman is complaining of the sudden onset of headache, nonproductive cough, muscle aches, and fever of 103° F.
3. A 65-year-old homeless man complains of a deep cough that produces a lot of mucus. He reports that the cough started "a month or two ago" and has gotten so bad that he's now having severe shortness of breath.

An important consideration to keep in mind when discussing infectious diseases is that infection may not always produce any outward signs of an illness. People who have an infection have a microbe inside their body, but they are not necessarily ill, although they may become ill with time. If the organism multiplies enough to be widespread or gets into certain tissues or organs, it may cause illness, but this often does not happen because of the body's natural defenses or for other reasons. When an infection does cause illness, the time from exposure to development of the first symptoms is called the *incubation period*. The interval when the patient is shedding or releasing infectious material is the *communicable period*, when the microbe can be potentially transmitted.

Whether a microbe causes infection and illness in a person after exposure depends on several factors. *Virulence* is the strength of the microbe in combating the body's defenses. Hepatitis B virus, for example, is very strong and can survive outside a human body for at least a week. The human immunodeficiency virus, HIV, though, is very weak and dies as soon as the fluid it is in begins to dry. The *dose* of the pathogen has a lot to do with whether infection occurs. The greater the number of microbes introduced, the more likely the patient will become ill. The *route* by which the pathogen enters the body is critical. Rabies virus infection, for example, is almost always fatal if the virus enters the body through the bloodstream, most often from the bite of an infected animal. However, swallowing the virus will not cause infection, because stomach acids and digestive juices will deactivate the virus before it can get into the bloodstream. The body's *resistance* plays an extremely important role in determining whether infection or illness occurs. A person with a functioning immune system can fight off many infections that patients with compromised immune systems, like chemotherapy patients, will not be able to fight off.

Sepsis

Infections are common events that we usually associate with a wound that got dirty and then started oozing pus. This is just one example in a broad range of ways in which an infection can occur. When an infection worsens, it can spread to the bloodstream or certain organ systems and cause life-threatening changes in the body. (See stages of sepsis in Figure 24-1.) Sepsis is what your grandparents may have referred to as "blood poisoning."

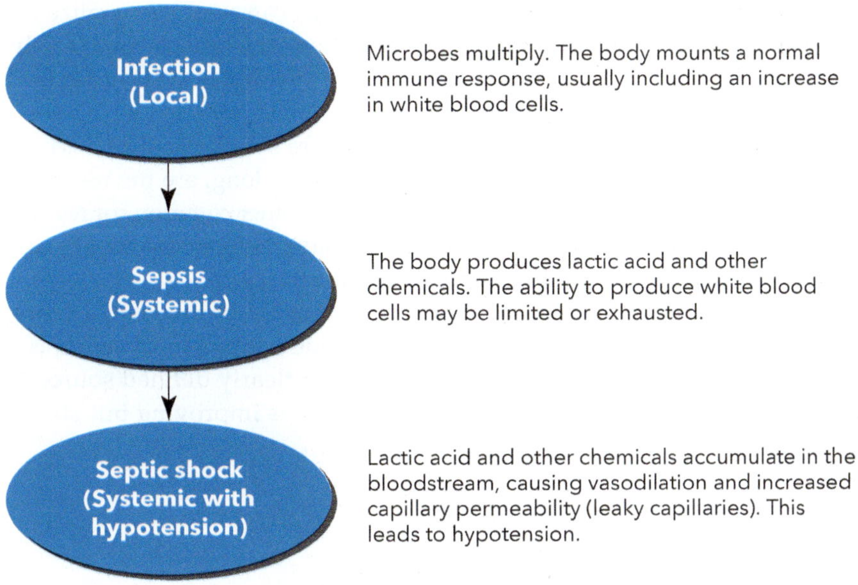

FIGURE 24-1 Stages of sepsis.

But it is not simply the presence of microbes such as bacteria in the bloodstream that can cause even more severe illness. The body's reaction to advanced infection can further worsen the illness. This is when sepsis can occur. The situation can deteriorate even further to a point where the patient goes into shock and becomes hypotensive. Septic shock is a common cause of death, but thanks to greater attention to sepsis detection and management, fewer patients are dying from it.

Pathophysiology

An infection occurs when bacteria, viruses, or parasites that are not usually present enter the body and multiply. Minor infections might not have any symptoms or might remain restricted to just one area. When those organisms spread, sepsis can develop. ***Sepsis*** is a life-threatening condition resulting from an abnormal and counterproductive response by the body that causes damage to tissues and organs. The body overreacts and secretes substances that, instead of helping, hurt cells, tissues, and organs. *Septic shock* occurs when these changes result in shock and hypotension that do not respond to intravenous fluids. Shock is often a result of both loss of fluid internally from increased capillary permeability ("leaky" blood vessels) and chemicals that cause vasodilation that prevents blood from returning to the heart. How much of a role each of these mechanisms plays depends in large part on the source, location, and type of infection.

sepsis
a life-threatening condition resulting from an abnormal and counterproductive response by the body that causes damage to tissues and organs. The body overreacts and secretes substances that, instead of helping, hurt cells, tissues, and organs.

The term "severe sepsis" was used until recently to indicate someone who had an infection and met certain criteria. This term is not used any longer because it does not help differentiate one patient from another in any useful way or predict who is at higher risk of death.

Common Causes

There are many locations in the body where infection can occur, but some are much more likely to be associated with sepsis. One of the most common you will see as an EMT is in the lungs, especially in cases of pneumonia. Very young and elderly patients are at high risk for pneumonia, as are those with compromised immune systems. Gastrointestinal infections are also a risk factor for development of sepsis. An infection can occur after abdominal surgery, or a patient can develop pancreatitis, an inflammation of the pancreas, with either leading to development of sepsis. A third area of origin for sepsis is the genitourinary tract. Infections of the kidney or prostate, for example, can easily generalize into sepsis. A urinary catheter allows microbes to enter the urinary tract much more easily and is a common source of sepsis. Additionally, any significant opening of the skin can lead to infection that generalizes. For example, a long-term intravenous catheter, a tracheostomy, or a gastrostomy tube can all lead to this condition. Pressure sores (also called *decubitus ulcers* or *bedsores*), which result from staying in one position too long, are the result of skin and tissue breaking down and can easily become infected. Another common source is the central nervous system, specifically the brain. Meningitis, inflammation of the tissues surrounding the brain and spinal cord, is a well-known cause of death.

Despite what we have learned about sepsis, especially in the last 20 years, there is much we still do not know. The exact pathway for development of sepsis is not clear. Many, perhaps even most, cases of sepsis do not have clearly defined sources. Even the definition of the condition is changing, and treatment is improving but still in need of improvement.

Patient Assessment

Many attempts have been made to find criteria that accurately separate patients with sepsis from those without sepsis. No one has been able to come up with such a list that is even close to perfect, even in the emergency department. One system relies on signs of *systemic inflammatory response syndrome (SIRS)*. In an adult with a documented or suspected infection, there is a higher risk of sepsis if the patient has two or more of the following:

- Temperature lower than 96.8° F (36° C) or higher than 101° F (38.3° C)
- Heart rate over 90
- Respiratory rate greater than 20
- Systolic blood pressure lower than 90 mmHg
- New-onset altered mental status or worsened mental status compared with normal

Although patients with serious infections usually have a fever, some patients with sepsis are actually slightly hypothermic, so do not ignore the possibility of sepsis in a patient with a lower-than-normal temperature.

Unfortunately, the SIRS criteria are fairly vague, and many patients without sepsis will have two or more abnormal findings, as in the case of trauma patients. Similarly, there are a number of patients with sepsis who will not have two or more abnormal findings.

Another system, the *qSOFA score*, has been proposed for this purpose. The acronym *qSOFA* stands for *quick sepsis-related organ failure assessment*. The qSOFA score is an abbreviated version of a score that was developed in the intensive care unit. When there are more abnormal findings, the score is higher. Such factors include the following:

- Altered mental status
- Respiratory rate greater than 22
- Systolic blood pressure lower than 100 mmHg

Obviously, this resembles the SIRS criteria. The qSOFA score, though, does not predict whether someone is septic. Instead, it predicts whether a septic patient will have a longer stay in the ICU or be more likely to die. Unfortunately, there is no way presently to identify in the field with 100 percent accuracy which patient has (or will develop) sepsis. Unless and until such a set of criteria is developed, you will need to follow your local protocols in combination with your clinical judgment.

Some EMS systems use capnography, the measurement of exhaled carbon dioxide, to help in the detection of sepsis. Because sepsis results in increased acid in the blood, and the body can excrete acid through exhalation, this is potentially a way to determine if the patient is at risk for sepsis. Other conditions can lead to abnormal end-tidal carbon dioxide ($ETCO_2$) levels, so if your agency uses capnography, follow your local protocols with regard to what threshold to use and how to interpret it.

Patient Care

Care of the Patient with Possible Sepsis

Fundamental Principles of Care

When you determine a patient may have an infection, you should look for signs of sepsis. Provide good supportive care, including administering oxygen to maintain a saturation of at least 94 percent, maintaining a normal body temperature, and calling for advanced life support as available and appropriate. Many EMS systems and hospitals have adopted either the SIRS criteria or something similar. If your patient meets those criteria, let the emergency department (ED) know. Many EDs call this a *"sepsis alert."* This will give the staff advance warning so that they can focus resources on this patient. One thing has become clear as we have learned more about sepsis: Earlier diagnosis leads to earlier treatment, which leads to higher survival rates. In the stable septic patient, probably the most important thing you can do is notify the ED.

Selected Common Communicable Diseases

You learned in the chapter on *Well-Being of the EMT* how to protect yourself and your patients from infectious diseases. We will summarize here the important things to remember about these steps.

- Get the appropriate vaccinations.
- Use Standard Precautions, including appropriate use of disposable gloves, eyewear, face protection, and respiratory protection.

Patient Assessment

Before the appearance of diseases like severe acute respiratory syndrome (SARS) and Ebola, the only health care providers who routinely asked patients about their travel history were infectious disease specialists. When you encounter patients with a fever, vague symptoms, or an ill-defined complaint, ask them where they have traveled in the previous several weeks. This may help the emergency department staff track down the cause of the patient's condition and can protect you from infection.

Another question that will sometimes be appropriate to ask is whether the patient has had the recommended vaccinations. Although people who have been vaccinated against a disease occasionally develop that disease, it is usually less severe than in an unvaccinated individual and complications are less common.

Patient Care

The descriptions of specific diseases in this chapter include any special treatment steps to keep in mind when you encounter a patient likely to have one of them.

An important part of patient care is understanding how the patient feels. This is particularly true in cases where some infectious diseases carry a stigma that can affect the patient's daily life. People have lost their jobs, housing, and even their families because they had a particular disease. You may be able to make a difference by letting the patient know of social workers in the hospital who can help.

It is very easy to feel frightened and anxious when you are treating a patient with an infectious disease, especially one you have never encountered. Keep in mind that you have all the tools you need to keep yourself safe in the form of personal protective equipment. The world's leading experts in infectious disease have made recommendations on how you can avoid becoming sick in these cases. Hospitals also have an obligation to notify EMS providers when their in-hospital evaluation has revealed that a patient has a communicable disease that requires an EMT, as a provider who came in contact with the patient, to have further testing, or to receive preventative prophylactic antibiotics.

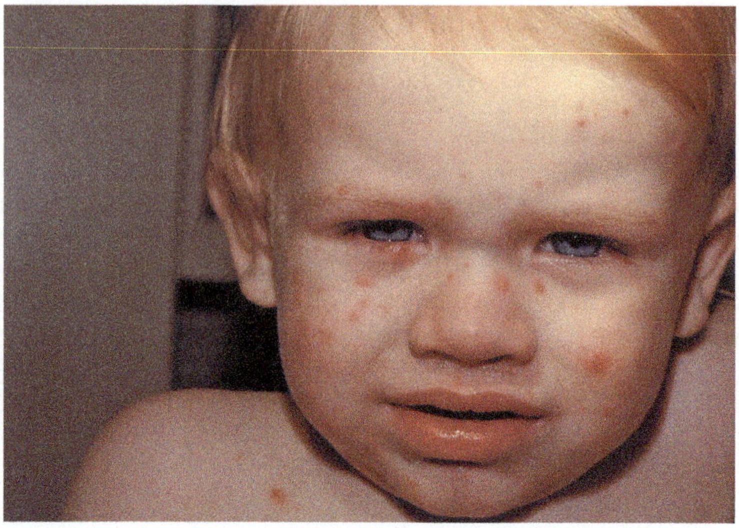

FIGURE 24-2 Child with chickenpox.
(© David Effron, MD)

Chickenpox

Chickenpox is caused by the varicella-zoster virus (VZV) and typically starts with vague symptoms resembling a cold, followed by fever and a rash that itches and looks like blisters (Figure 24-2). Symptoms start within 10–21 days of exposure, usually within 10–16 days. The rash tends to be more common on the chest, abdomen, back, and proximal extremities, although it can occur on the scalp, armpits, and mucous membranes of the mouth and throat. In the early 1990s. the chickenpox vaccine became a standard part of childhood immunizations in the United States. Other countries, such as Japan, had required the vaccine before that. Thanks to the childhood vaccine, the incidence of chickenpox has steadily declined over the past few decades.

Transmission, Incubation, and Communicability. Chickenpox is very contagious and easily spread by direct person-to-person contact, as well as airborne spread of the fluid from the rash on the skin or from the mucous membranes. Dried scabs do not spread the disease. A patient with varicella can spread it to other people from 1 to 2 days before the rash appears until all the lesions are dried and crusted, which usually take about 5 days after the rash starts.

Treatment and Prevention. Patients with chickenpox are isolated to prevent spread of the disease until all of the lesions have dried and have crusts on them. Antiviral medications may be given to shorten the course of the disease and prevent complications. A vaccine is available, and EMTs should take advantage of it if they have not had the disease or been previously immunized. EMTs should take opportunities to ask parents whether children have been vaccinated for infectious diseases and to encourage their parents to do so.

Postexposure Actions. If you are not immunized and you become exposed to a patient with varicella, you should receive the vaccine within 3 days of the exposure.

Special Considerations. Varicella is traditionally a childhood disease, but it can return in adults in a different form. Some people who had chickenpox as children experience herpes zoster, also known as shingles, when the virus reactivates years later. After the patient is ill with chickenpox, the virus becomes dormant in certain nerves and can be reactivated later in life, often in response to stress. It appears as a very painful rash on one side of the body along a dermatome, an area along the skin supplied by nerves from a spinal root, e.g., along a rib. (See Figure 24-3.) The rash most commonly appears along one of the thoracic or cervical dermatomes, although it can also affect the eye. The rash persists for 7–10 days and heals within a month.

FIGURE 24-3 (A) A shingles rash often appears as a narrow, beltlike band around the torso. (B) A shingles rash can appear anywhere on the body, including the face. *(Photos A and B: © Edward T. Dickinson, MD)*

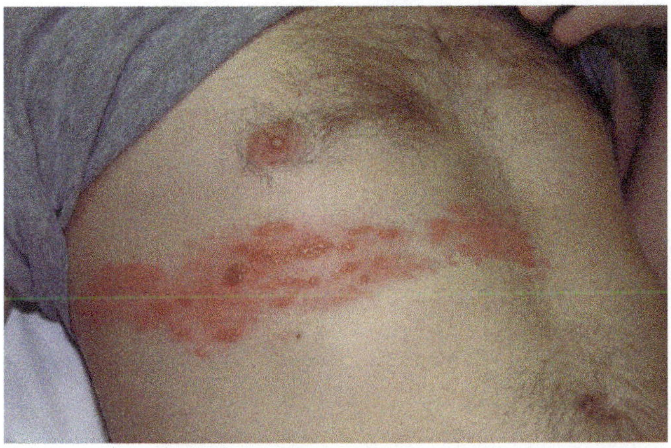

A

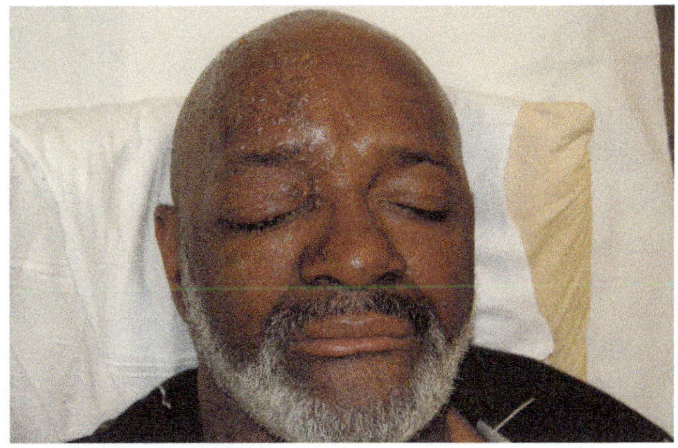

B

Point of View

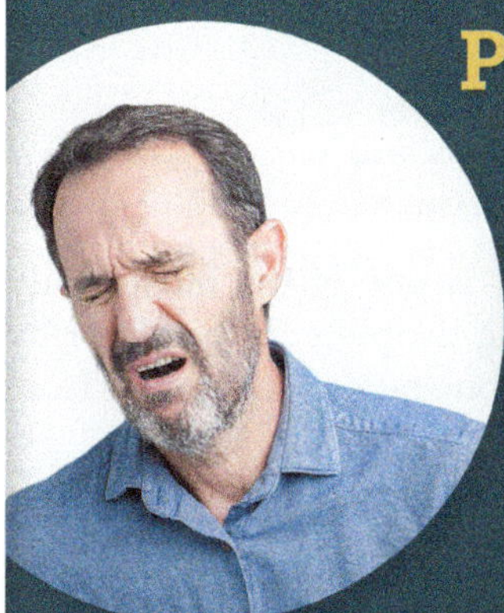

(Aaron Amat/Shutterstock)

"It was the worst pain I've ever had in my life. It felt like what I'd heard a kidney stone feels like—excruciating, burning pain on the left side of my back that came around to my side. I really didn't feel bad otherwise, but the pain was so overwhelming it was hard to think of anything else. Any contact with the area, even putting on a shirt, was agonizing.

"The provider who saw me said it was probably shingles. How could I have shingles? That's something old people get and I'm only 40. The PA explained that middle-aged people can get shingles, too, probably as a result of stress weakening the immune system. He also explained that in a day or two, if it was shingles, I'd get little painful bumps in that area. Sure enough, that's exactly what happened. It was another week before I began to feel normal again."

A small but significant number of people who get shingles experience postherpetic neuralgia, which is characterized by chronic pain long after the rash disappears. There is an adult vaccine for prevention of shingles, and antiviral medication may help to reduce the risk of postherpetic neuralgia.

Measles

Measles, or rubeola, is a highly infectious viral disease that starts with a fever, cough, and eye irritation. You may also see small white or bluish-white spots on the inside of the cheek, which are called *Koplik spots*. Within 3–7 days, a red, blotchy rash appears on the face and then spreads to the trunk and the rest of the body (Figure 24-4). The rash typically lasts 4–7 days. In areas of the world where the measles vaccine is not available or used, more than a hundred thousand children die of the disease each year.

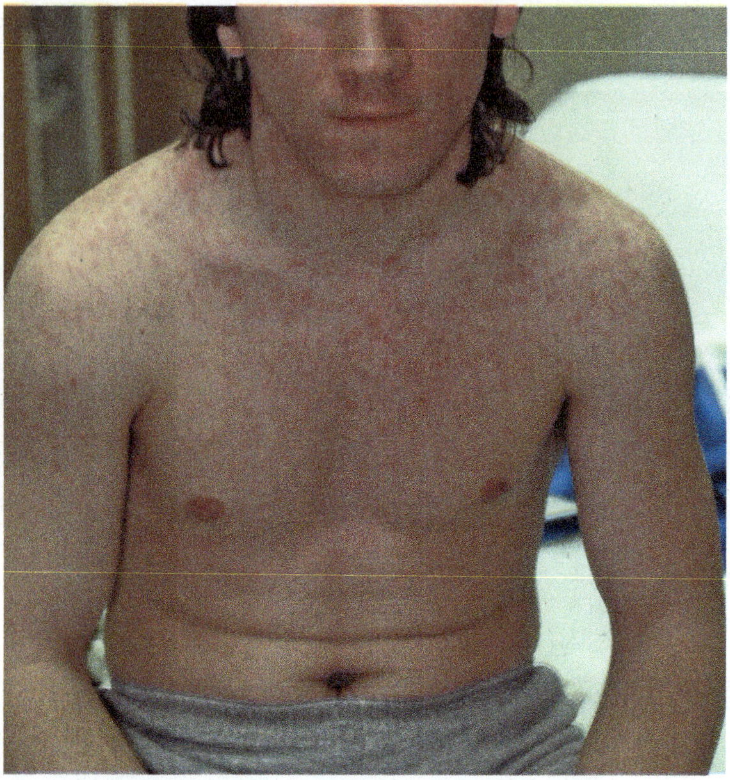

FIGURE 24-4 Measles rash.
(© David Effron, MD)

Transmission, Incubation, and Communicability. Measles is one of the most easily spread diseases known to humanity. It is spread by inhaling droplets in the air or by contact with nose and throat secretions. It can be spread from one person to another from 4 days before the rash starts until 4 days after.

Treatment and Prevention. There is no specific treatment for measles, so care is focused on the symptoms and preventing spread of the disease. This is accomplished primarily through vaccination and quarantining patients, as well as attention to hand hygiene.

Postexposure Actions. People who are at high risk of complications (e.g., infants less than 1 year old, pregnant women, and immunocompromised individuals) may be candidates for receiving immune globulin, which gives some protection from the disease. Those who are not vaccinated should receive the vaccine.

Special Considerations. There have been increasing numbers of measles outbreaks in recent years. Most of these cases are among patients who were not immunized against the disease by proper vaccination. Measles is a reportable disease—i.e., some health care providers are required to report cases to the local health department. This does not usually apply to EMS providers, but you should check state and local rules and regulations to be sure, especially if you encounter a patient with this disease but you do not transport the patient. On average, there are a few hundred cases of measles in the United States each year.

If you come across a patient you believe may have measles, you should determine which hospital the patient may go to and contact the facility before you transport to be sure the hospital will be able to handle the patient properly. Many patients in hospitals have compromised immune systems. Before you bring a patient with measles into such a facility, certain precautions are needed, like having a negative pressure room available that vents outside and minimizes the risk of spreading the disease.

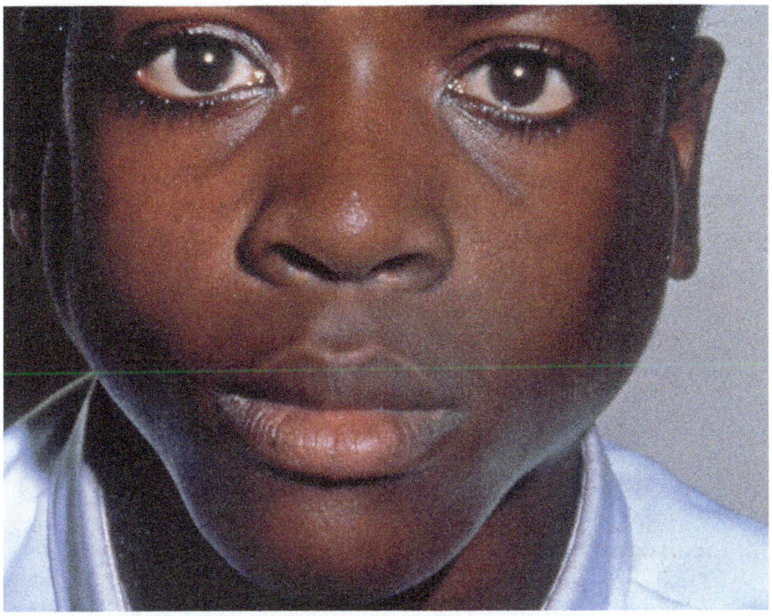

FIGURE 24-5 Mumps showing characteristic parotid gland swelling. *(© David Effron, MD)*

Mumps

Mumps is a disease caused by paramyxovirus that typically starts with vague symptoms like muscle aches, loss of appetite, and headache. This progresses to swelling and inflammation of the salivary glands, usually one or both parotids (the largest salivary glands) in front of the ear (Figure 24-5). This parotitis lasts 7–10 days.

Transmission, Incubation, and Communicability. Mumps is spread through droplets and direct contact with a patient's saliva. The incubation period is typically 16–18 days, though this can be extended a few days at either end of this period. The patient is most infectious from 2 days before the swelling appears until 5 days after.

Treatment and Prevention. There is no specific treatment for mumps, so treat the symptoms the patient is experiencing. Mumps can be prevented by vaccination. Sick patients should avoid contact with other people for 5 days after the swelling appears.

Postexposure Actions. There is no specific action to take if you are exposed.

Special Considerations. Approximately a quarter of adult males who get mumps will get orchitis, inflammation of a testicle. Sterility has resulted in a few cases, but this is extremely rare.

Hepatitis

Hepatitis is a general term that means inflammation of the liver. Many causes of hepatitis exist, including poisons, alcohol, and other drugs, but this section focuses on the most common forms of hepatitis transmitted by viruses. Five main types have been recognized, but more may be identified in the future.

Hepatitis A

Hepatitis A starts suddenly in adults with fever, nausea, loss of appetite, malaise, and abdominal pain. A few days later, jaundice (yellowish coloring of the skin and the white part of the eye) appears (Figure 24-6). Older patients generally have worse symptoms and may take some time to recover, but in general patients make a complete recovery.

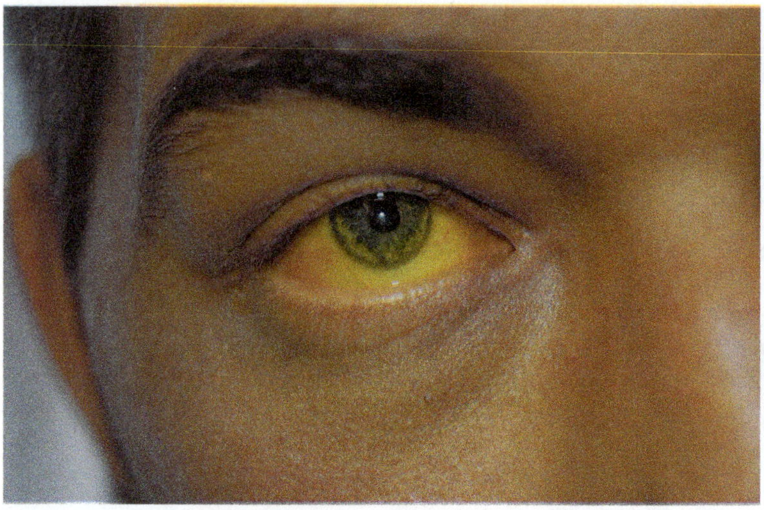

FIGURE 24-6 Jaundice from hepatitis A. *(© Edward T. Dickinson, MD)*

Transmission, Incubation, and Communicability. Hepatitis A is spread from person to person by the fecal–oral route; e.g., a person gets the disease by ingesting something touched by an infected patient who leaves the virus on food or food-serving utensils. This happens periodically in restaurants when food-preparation workers get the disease and fail to wash their hands. The incubation period of hepatitis A averages 28–30 days, although it can take 15–50 days in some cases. A hepatitis A patient is most likely to spread the disease to others approximately from two weeks after becoming infected until several days after jaundice appears. Children may be asymptomatic, so they can spread the disease easily and unknowingly.

Treatment and Prevention. There is no specific treatment for hepatitis A, so treatment is supportive and focuses on preventing the spread of the disease through attention to hand hygiene and proper food-preparation techniques. There is a vaccine, which EMS providers should receive if they have not already received it.

Postexposure Actions. If you are exposed to hepatitis A, you should receive the vaccine if you have no immunity to the disease through prior infection or vaccination. A health care provider may also decide, depending on the circumstances, to provide immune globulin, which provides passive immunity for a significant period.

Special Considerations. Like many infectious diseases, especially those transmitted through the fecal–oral route, hepatitis A may spread easily when people are crowded together, especially under unplanned circumstance, e.g., at an emergency shelter.

Hepatitis E

Hepatitis E is spread by the same route (fecal-oral) but by a different virus, which has characteristics very similar to those of hepatitis A. It is much more common outside of the United States and Europe and is often spread through contaminated drinking water. There is no approved vaccine, and immune globulin does not help.

Hepatitis B

Hepatitis B is very different from hepatitis A. It is a more serious disease with sometimes life-threatening consequences. Infection with the hepatitis B virus (HBV) is very common in many parts of the world. Before development of a vaccine and changes in injection practices, hundreds of health care workers (including EMS providers) died every year in the United States from occupationally acquired hepatitis B.

Patients usually present with nausea, vomiting, loss of appetite, and vague abdominal pain, which later progresses to jaundice. As with some other types of hepatitis, younger patients have fewer symptoms and may even have none, but they are much more likely to develop chronic infection. This carries a significant risk, because many of these patients will die young from cirrhosis or liver cancer. Approximately half of the world's cases of liver cancer are the result of HBV chronic infection.

Transmission, Incubation, and Communicability. HBV infection is spread through blood, semen, cerebrospinal fluid, amniotic fluid, vaginal secretions, any fluid that contains blood, and a few other fluids that EMS is not typically exposed to. For a person to become infected, the material must get into the body through percutaneous (injection through the skin) or mucous membrane exposure. The incubation period averages 60–90 days, but can be as short as 45 days or as long as 180 days. Individuals with hepatitis B can spread the disease as long as they are hepatitis B surface antigen (HBsAg)–positive (by blood test). Ways in which HBV has been transmitted include blood transfusion (before screening of donors and testing of blood were routine), sharing needles during injection of drugs, sexual intercourse, close household contacts, reuse of lancets for glucose testing in skilled nursing facilities, and childbirth (mother to neonate). Hepatitis B virus is very hardy and can survive for a week on surfaces outside the body, such as your trauma scissors or the bench seat of your ambulance. This fact highlights the importance of proper decontamination of your equipment and rig after each call.

Treatment and Prevention. There is no specific treatment for HBV infection, so treatment is supportive. In some countries, antiviral medications are administered to infected patients, but the safety and efficacy of this approach are not clear. Fortunately, there is a vaccine, which all EMS providers should receive if they have not already received it as part of their childhood vaccination series.

Postexposure Actions. If you sustain a significant exposure to blood or other body fluids ("significant" usually meaning via a direct injection of blood or a mucous membrane's being exposed to one of the fluids listed above), wash the site with soap and water (just water for an eye exposure) and see a health care provider right away. If you have not been immunized, the provider will arrange for vaccination and possibly an injection of hepatitis B immune globulin, which will give you some immunity until your body can develop its own from the vaccine. Intact skin is a very good barrier, so if you got some blood on unbroken skin and washed it off, or if there is other reason to believe the risk of infection is very low, the provider will probably not give you the immune globulin.

Special Considerations. Hepatitis D can occur only in patients who have HBV infection. Its signs and symptoms are very similar, but usually more sudden in onset, and the incubation period is shorter (2–8 weeks). There is no vaccine for hepatitis D, but if you are immunized against hepatitis B, you cannot be infected with hepatitis D. There is a treatment, but it is administered over the course of almost a year. About 5 percent of people with HBV have been infected with hepatitis D.

Hepatitis C

Hepatitis C is very similar to hepatitis B in many ways, but jaundice is less common, and more patients get infected without showing symptoms (approximately three-quarters). When symptoms do occur, nausea, vomiting, loss of appetite, and vague abdominal pain are most common.

Transmission, Incubation, and Communicability. Hepatitis C is transmitted through the same bloodborne mechanism as HBV, e.g., sharing needles, but is less commonly a result of sexual intercourse or childbirth. The incubation period is 6–9 weeks, with symptoms in some patients appearing as early as 2 weeks or as late as 6 months. An infected patient can spread the disease at least 1 week before symptoms appear, and hepatitis C may be communicable forever in those who have chronic infection.

Treatment and Prevention. There are several safe and effective medication regimens for eradicating the virus from a patient, but there is no vaccine. Prevention consists of taking Standard Precautions, including careful attention to proper use and disposal of sharps.

Postexposure Actions. If you are exposed to blood or other body fluids, take the same precautions that you would for any other exposure. There is no specific treatment to prevent or reduce the risk of developing the disease.

Special Considerations. Since hepatitis C can linger in the body for decades before it causes cirrhosis or liver cancer, development of safe and effective treatments has allayed the anxiety of many patients and prevented these conditions from occurring.

HIV/AIDS

Human immunodeficiency virus (HIV) has caused a great deal of fear among the lay public and the health care provider community since it was first discovered in the 1980s. Decades of experience with the disease has changed widespread panic to a low level of fear interrupted by occasional alarm. Some patients experience flu-like symptoms like fever, sore throat, and fatigue within a few weeks of being infected. Acquired immunodeficiency syndrome (AIDS), the end result for some patients with the virus, is characterized by infections that take advantage of the body's weakened immune system and may manifest as a particular form of pneumonia (*pneumocystis carinii*), a formerly rare form of skin cancer (Kaposi's sarcoma) (Figure 24-7), tuberculosis, or other opportunistic infections. AIDS is still one of the few diseases for which people experience discrimination, but treatments that have reduced the level of infectivity have made tremendous differences in the length and quality of life for these patients.

Transmission, Incubation, and Communicability. The most common routes of transmission in the developed world are sharing of needles and unprotected sex between men, though any penetrative activity involving blood or semen, including heterosexual sex, is also a route for spread of the virus. Mothers can also transmit the virus to their newborns during delivery or through breastfeeding. Less than a month after exposure, patients develop antibodies to the virus. Progression to AIDS can take less than a year or may never occur at all, thanks to treatment. Communicability depends primarily on how much the virus has multiplied in the blood (viral load), which usually rises early in the course of the disease and when the patient becomes ill with an opportunistic infection. Treatment has led to many patients having undetectable viral loads, making it virtually impossible for them to transmit the virus.

Treatment and Prevention. Antiviral medications are used to reduce and suppress a patient's viral load. Health care providers can avoid infection by using Standard Precautions. Effective measures for the public include use of condoms for penetrative sex and not sharing needles among intravenous drug users.

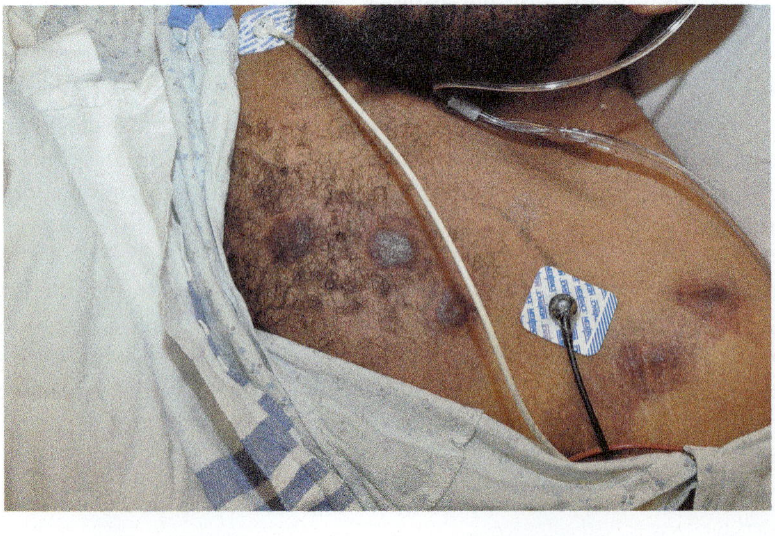

FIGURE 24-7 Kaposi's sarcoma. *(© Edward T. Dickinson, MD)*

Postexposure Actions. If you sustain a significant exposure to blood or other body fluids, wash the area as directed above, then consult a health care provider. Postexposure prophylaxis (PEP) in the form of certain antiviral medication can be prescribed for 28 days. This may reduce the risk of seroconverting (developing antibodies to the virus, a sign of infection).

Special Considerations. The panic that accompanied the discovery of HIV and AIDS has lessened significantly but persists in some areas and communities, even though HIV has become, for all practical purposes, a chronic disease that can be managed very well. You can help to reduce fear of HIV/AIDS even further by letting laypeople know that it is easy to avoid this disease with simple precautions, and all patients deserve respect and courtesy.

Influenza

Influenza, or flu, is a common viral illness that tends to occur at certain times of the year, but can occur at any time. More than two dozen viruses can cause influenza. Patients typically have fever, nonproductive cough, severe muscle aches, sore throat, headache, and severe weakness (Figure 24-8).

Transmission, Incubation, and Communicability. Influenza is spread by droplets and direct contact. The incubation period ranges from 1 to 4 days but is typically 2. Most symptoms resolve within 5–7 days, but the cough can persist for 2 or more weeks. An infected person can spread the disease from 1 day before symptoms appear to 7 days after.

Treatment and Prevention. Unlike with most viral illnesses, there are antiviral medications that patients can take to lessen the severity of influenza or shorten its duration (typically by about a day). These medications must be started within 48 hours of symptom onset. If they are started later, they have little or no effect. Since the disease is spread through droplets, attention to hand hygiene and using surgical masks limit spread of the disease.

Each year, an influenza vaccine is released which works against several of the viruses that scientists believe will be the most common that season. Some years their educated guesses are better than others, but there are very few serious adverse effects, and EMTs, like other health care providers, should get vaccinated to prevent spreading influenza to their patients.

Postexposure Actions. If you are exposed to someone with influenza, your health care provider may decide it is prudent for you to take an antiviral medication.

Special Considerations. When the CDC identifies a new strain of influenza, they recommend health care providers take respiratory precautions, including the use of N-95 respirators, until they can confirm that droplet precautions are sufficient to prevent

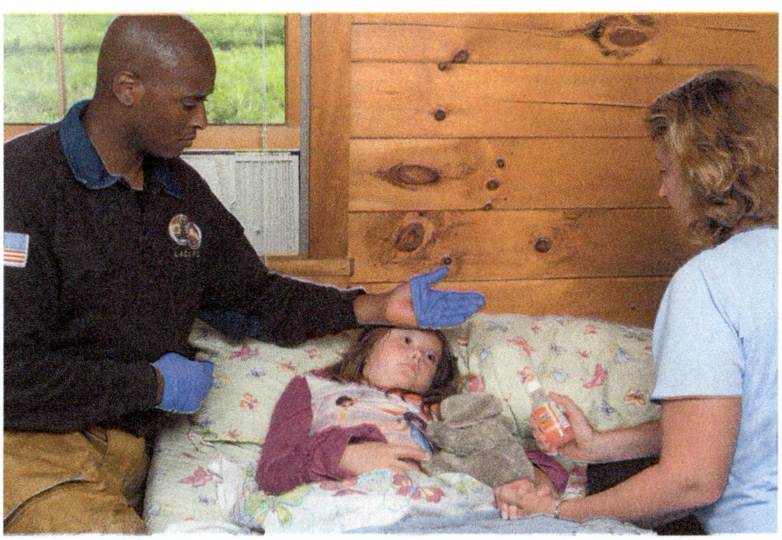

FIGURE 24-8 Child with influenza showing signs of a fever.

spread of the disease. To date, all forms of influenza have been spread by droplets, which can be handled with standard surgical masks. The very young, the elderly, and patients with chronic conditions are more prone to influenza and can die from it. EMS providers have a responsibility to prevent infecting them by being vaccinated and taking Standard Precautions.

Croup

Croup, also known as laryngotracheobronchitis, results from infection with a human parainfluenza virus (HPIV). Despite the resemblance of their names, parainfluenza and influenza are completely separate organisms and cause different signs and symptoms. A patient with croup gets inflammation and swelling of the larynx, trachea, and bronchi, which is uncomfortable and can make breathing difficult. Children between 6 months and 3 years are most susceptible to croup, and typically present with a history of an upper respiratory infection (a cold) that later produces a characteristic cough that sounds like a seal barking. Symptoms often get worse at night and may alarm parents who hear their child coughing loudly from another room.

Transmission, Incubation, and Communicability. The virus that produces croup is passed from one person to another in two ways. An infected patient who coughs or sneezes can infect others who inhale the infected air. Droplets can also survive on objects and be passed to another person who touches those objects and then touches the nose, eyes, or mouth. Symptoms typically appear 2–3 days after exposure. A patient can infect others during the incubation period and until 10 days after symptoms start.

Treatment and Prevention. Most cases of croup are more frightening than they are dangerous. Assess the child the same way you would for any patient with a chief complaint of shortness of breath. Treatment is symptomatic. There is no vaccine against the virus that causes croup, and it is possible to be reinfected. Because croup is caused by a virus, antibiotics do not help. Prevent passing the disease by washing your hands frequently and refraining from touching your nose, eyes, and mouth.

Postexposure Actions. There are no specific actions to take if you are exposed.

Special Considerations. ALS providers may be able to nebulize epinephrine, which may reduce swelling in the airway, and to administer a steroid, which will further reduce inflammation. A few patients with croup have enough inflammation and swelling of their airways to be admitted to a hospital, so look for signs of hypoxia.

Pertussis (Whooping Cough)

Whooping cough is a respiratory infection caused by *Bordetella pertussis* bacteria. It begins like a typical upper respiratory infection (a cold), but does not resolve within the usual 7–10 days, and proceeds to worsen into "fits" of uninterrupted coughing followed by a "whooping" sound on inspiration. Infants may not display this last sign, because their respiratory muscles are not that well developed. The disease gradually develops over 1–2 weeks and then resolves after 1–2 months. To be diagnosed with whooping cough, the patient must have a cough for at least 2 weeks with at least one of these: coughing paroxysms ("fits"), inspiratory whooping, or post-tussive vomiting (vomiting after coughing).

Transmission, Incubation, and Communicability. Pertussis is spread through large droplets in the air from infected patients. The incubation period is usually 9–10 days, although this may extend to several days on either side of these limits. The disease is very easily spread in the initial cold-like stage and for the first 2 weeks of the whooping stage. Within 3 weeks, the patient is no longer communicable. If patients are put on the appropriate antibiotics, they are no longer able to transmit the disease after 5 days.

Treatment and Prevention. Certain antibiotics can reduce the period of communicability, but they do not usually make the patient feel any better unless they are given early (before the coughing phase). Since patients at this stage believe they have just a cold, it is very unlikely they will receive antibiotics. The disease can be prevented through vaccination.

Additional booster doses of the pertussis vaccine are usually given at the same time as a tetanus booster. Patients who are ill are isolated to prevent spread of the disease to others.

Postexposure Actions. Antibiotics may be considered for women in the last 3 weeks of pregnancy and for infants younger than 1 year old. Getting the vaccine after you have been exposed does not seem to be an effective way to prevent becoming sick in the short term, although it will help in the long term.

Special Considerations. Whooping cough has had a big recurrence, perhaps because the immunization received in childhood seems to be less effective over time. This disease can be fatal to infants, who are too young to have completed their immunizations, so prevention in adults is the best way to avoid illness in the very young.

Pneumonia

Pneumonia is the result of infection by any one of a number of different microbes. This section focuses on pneumococcal pneumonia, one of the types an EMT is more likely to see, and which is caused by the bacterium *Streptococcus pneumoniae*. Signs and symptoms include fever, chills, shortness of breath, tachypnea, chest pain that worsens on inspiration (pleuritic pain), and a productive cough. A chest X-ray typically shows an area where inflammation has consolidated in part of the lung (Figure 24-9). In young children and infants, the fever may be high enough to cause febrile seizures. In the elderly, altered mental status is a common sign of pneumonia. Pneumococcal pneumonia is a frequent cause of sepsis.

Transmission, Incubation, and Communicability. Pneumococcal pneumonia is spread through droplets, but close contact for long periods is usually required for the infection to spread to a healthy person. The incubation period is not certain, but appears to be 1–3 days. A patient can spread the disease until 24 hours after appropriate antibiotics are begun.

Treatment and Prevention. Antibiotics are effective since pneumococcal pneumonia is the result of a bacterial infection. Prevention consists of vaccination, hand hygiene, and cough etiquette (when coughing or sneezing, turning away from others and using a disposable tissue or one's sleeve).

Postexposure Actions. There are no specific actions to take after exposure to a patient with pneumococcal pneumonia.

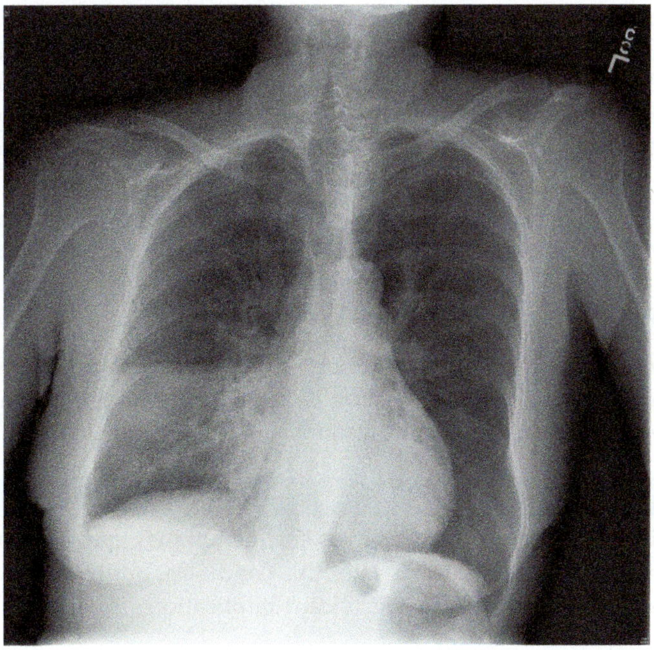

FIGURE 24-9 Chest X-ray showing inflammation in the lung. Note the area in the lower right lung that appears cloudy. This is where the pneumonia is located. *(© David Effron, MD).*

"If you encounter a patient who you suspect to have tuberculosis, it is important to protect yourself with an N-95 respirator or equivalent piece of PPE. A surgical mask is not enough in this case."

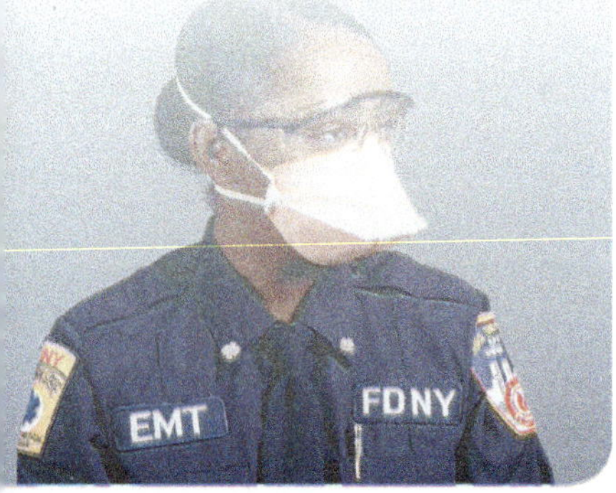

Special Considerations. There are many different causes of pneumonia, including viral infections, against which antibiotics are ineffective. Pneumonia is a common cause of sepsis in patients at the extremes of age or with compromised immune systems.

Tuberculosis

Tuberculosis (TB) is a bacterial illness caused by *Mycobacterium tuberculosis* that has been recognized for centuries; in the past, it was sometimes called "consumption" because of the way the disease seemed to consume patients as they lost weight and got progressively sicker. Latent TB is common in people who are exposed and means they have an infection but no symptoms. Patients with active TB typically have a cough, fever, night sweats, and weight loss. The cough is initially dry, but later produces purulent (pus-filled) sputum. This refers to pulmonary tuberculosis, although many other organs and tissues can be infected by the disease.

Transmission, Incubation, and Communicability. Patients with active pulmonary TB exhale the bacillus that causes tuberculosis when coughing, sneezing, and singing. Within 2–10 weeks of exposure, a person who develops latent TB will show evidence of the infection on laboratory testing. About 90 percent of people with latent TB will never develop active TB, but it is not possible to predict who will develop the active form of the disease. A patient with active TB who takes the appropriate antibiotics for 2–4 weeks is no longer able to spread the disease.

Treatment and Prevention. People with latent TB confirmed by skin or blood testing will be put on one or more antibiotics for 6–9 months. This prevents the disease from progressing to active TB in most people. Patients with active TB will receive several antibiotics for at least 6 months. If the patient is not likely to be compliant with treatment, public health officials may directly observe the patient taking the medication each day.

Prevention consists primarily of having a high index of suspicion in a patient with respiratory symptoms and taking airborne disease precautions, i.e., using an N-95 respirator. A surgical mask does not filter out the small particles that spread the disease.

Although there is a vaccine for TB (the BCG vaccine), it is not that effective, so its use is usually restricted to areas where TB is very common.

Postexposure Actions. If you are exposed to someone with active TB or believe you may have been exposed, report it to the hospital where you transported the patient. The hospital is required by federal law to notify the transporting ambulance service when it discovers that a patient transported by ambulance has an airborne communicable disease. This is true even if you do not notify the hospital, but it is prudent to notify them nonetheless.

If you have been exposed to TB, you should follow your agency's procedures for evaluation by a qualified health care provider. The provider will take a careful history, perform a physical exam, and obtain confirmation that the source patient actually has active TB. You will generally undergo skin testing to see if you have had been previously exposed to TB (baseline testing), and then receive a second skin test in several weeks to assess if you have become infected from the exposure. If you do develop a positive skin test, you will receive one or more prescriptions for antibiotics to prevent the infection from becoming active.

Depending on the prevalence of TB in the area where you provide EMS, you may need to undergo testing on an annual basis (higher-prevalence areas) or just when you may have been exposed (low-prevalence areas).

Special Considerations. TB is more common in settings where people with poor health are gathered together, e.g., nursing homes, jails, and homeless shelters. Patients with HIV, because of their compromised immune systems, are at higher risk for TB.

Meningitis

Meningitis is an inflammation of the meninges, the membranes that surround the brain and spinal cord. There are a number of causes of this condition, but this section will focus on meningococcal meningitis, which has significant implications for both patient and health care provider. Patients, especially at the extremes of age or with compromised immune systems, can sustain serious complications, including brain damage and even death.

Meningococcal meningitis is caused by the bacterium *Neisseria meningitidis* and typically starts with an abrupt onset of fever, nausea, vomiting, severe headache, nuchal rigidity (neck stiffness), and photophobia (sensitivity to light). The neck stiffness is an indication of inflammation of the meninges. Petechiae, pinpoint hemorrhages under the skin (Figure 24-10), may also be present. You can differentiate petechiae from other rashes by pressing on them. Petechiae will not blanch or turn white when pressed. Complications include shock, multiple-organ failure, and blood-clotting problems. Some patients suffer from brain damage, deafness, or loss of one or more limbs.

Transmission, Incubation, and Communicability. Meningococcal meningitis typically spreads through direct contact. The incubation period is usually 3–4 days, though it can be as short as 2 days or as long as 10. An infected patient can transmit the disease from 3 days after infection until 24 hours after appropriate antibiotics are started. Groups at the highest risk of becoming ill with meningitis include infants before they are vaccinated and young adults, when immunity begins to fade from their vaccinations. People with compromised immune systems are also at increased risk.

Treatment and Prevention. Prompt administration of antibiotics is the mainstay of treatment, so EMS treatment is supportive. There are also viral causes of meningitis. Some, such as herpes meningitis, are treated with antiviral medications. Other forms of viral meningitis have no specific treatment other than supportive care. Vaccines can prevent infection by several strains of the bacterium that causes the disease.

Postexposure Actions. If you are exposed to a patient with meningococcal meningitis, you are very unlikely to become sick unless you had very close contact with the patient, like performing mouth-to-mouth. Standard Precautions should protect you. Some more virulent and communicable bacterial forms of meningitis may require you to be placed on prophylactic antibiotics. In case of doubt about your risk, consult a health care provider.

Special Considerations. Test the patient for nuchal rigidity by asking the patient to bring the chin down to the chest. Inability or difficulty in doing so suggests irritation of the meninges.

Another form of meningitis is caused by viruses. It typically results in much less severe disease and complications.

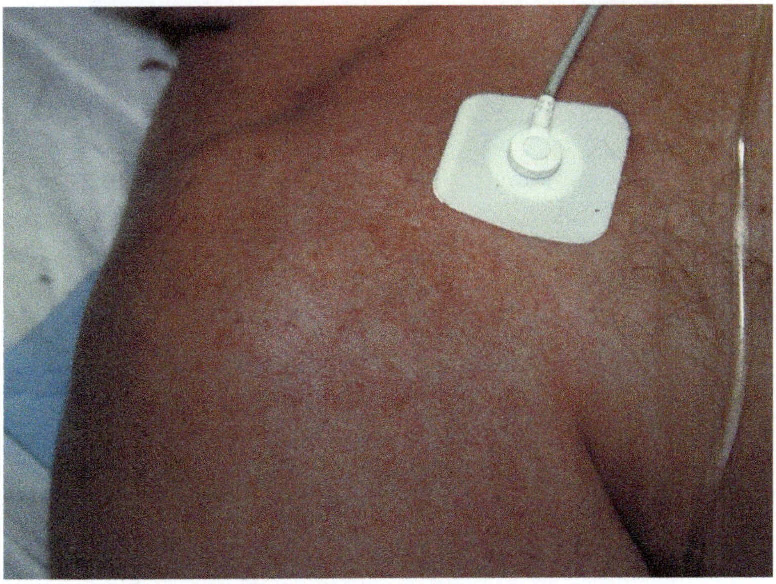

FIGURE 24-10 Petechial rash associated with meningitis. *(© Edward T. Dickinson, MD)*

Sexually Transmitted Infections (STIs)

Sexually transmitted infections are common in adolescents and adults. A wide variety of viral and bacterial diseases can be spread from one person to another as a result of vaginal, anal, or oral sex. Viral diseases include HIV; hepatitis A, B, and C; genital herpes; and human papilloma virus (HPV). HPV causes genital warts and is the causative agent of cervical cancer in women.

The most common sexually transmitted bacterial infections are chlamydia, gonorrhea, and syphilis. Many of these viral and bacterial diseases have long-term local (such as infertility) and even life-threatening systemic consequences if not treated. Bacterial infections are effectively treated with antibiotics. Viral STIs are generally more difficult to treat. For example, genital herpes and HIV are not presently "curable," but they can be treated with suppressive therapy medications to reduce the effects of the virus.

There are two primary ways to prevent the spread of STIs. First, and most importantly, is the use of a condom to prevent the passage of a pathogen from one person to another. Second, there are vaccinations available for several of the viral STIs, including HPV and hepatitis A and B.

In your role as an EMT, it will be unusual for you to encounter patients who access 911 emergency services for STIs. The exception are women who develop a widespread pelvic infection called pelvic inflammatory disease (PID). PID is most commonly caused by gonorrhea or chlamydia. Women with PID often develop severe lower abdominal pain that may or may not be associated with increased vaginal discharge.

Diseases Carried by Ticks

Lyme disease is transmitted through tick bites. Most, but not all, patients display a rash within a week that looks like a bull's-eye and is called *erythema migrans* (Figure 24-11). The rash fades, and months to years later, the patient can develop complications of the disease

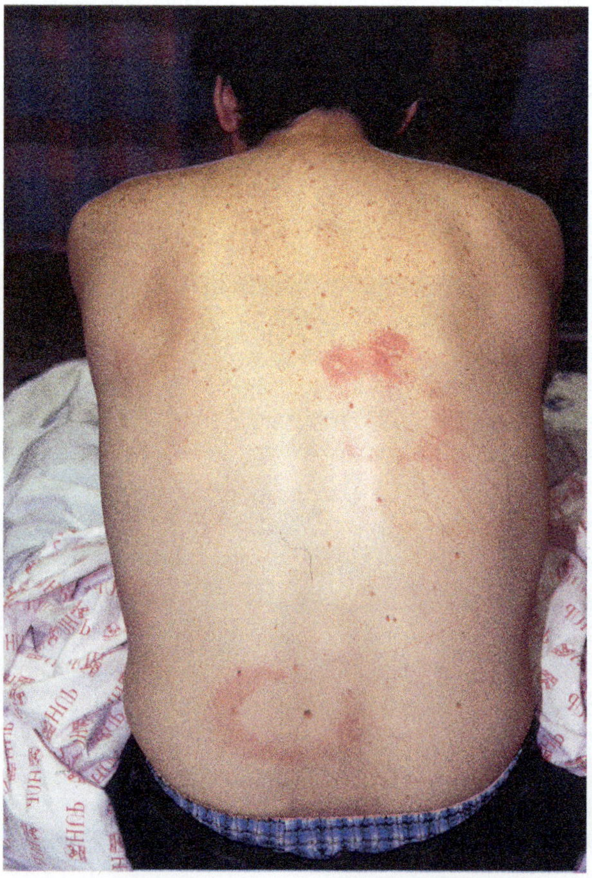

FIGURE 24-11 Several *erythema migrans* "bull's eye" skin lesions caused by Lyme disease. *(© Edward T. Dickinson, MD)*

including neurologic problems (especially Bells palsy), arthritis, or even electrical conduction problems in the heart. Fortunately, the disease can be treated with antibiotics, although they are most effective when administered early after exposure to the tick bite.

If you participate in a backcountry rescue team or are otherwise exposed to wooded areas where ticks are common, cover your arms and legs when in the area, check yourself frequently for ticks, and remove them with tweezers by pulling gently but steadily so that you don't leave the mouth parts of the tick in your skin. In the laboratory, it appears that ticks need at least 36 hours of feeding on a person to transmit Lyme, but consult a health care provider if you experience a tick bite.

Other diseases such as Rocky Mountain Spotted Fever are carried by ticks. If you live or work in an area with ticks, consider becoming familiar with which diseases are more common in your area.

Emerging and Newly Recognized Infectious Diseases

A problem in treating bacterial infections in the hospital is that in some cases, the antibiotics that used to be effective no longer work. This is a result of bacteria developing resistance. When an antibiotic is overused or used improperly, some bacteria can survive. Their offspring carry the ability to resist that antibiotic. As a result, a disease that once could be treated easily with a common antibiotic needs to be treated with a stronger antibiotic, which often has worse side effects than the original one. Additionally, as bacteria become immune to the new antibiotic, patients may get infections that are no longer treatable, and patients may die from diseases that were easily cured a few years ago.

This phenomenon has led to several conditions that EMTs deal with regularly, including methicillin-resistant *Staphylococcus aureus* (MRSA), vancomycin-resistant *Enterococcus* (VRE), and *Clostridium difficile* (C. diff). A less common but still important example is multidrug-resistant tuberculosis (MDR-TB). As bacteria evolve, this list will grow. You will not always know which patients have these conditions, so use Standard Precautions to protect yourself, your co-workers, and other patients.

Other diseases have emerged recently or been discovered after a period when they existed in just a corner of the world, like HIV/AIDS, which was only recognized toward the end of the twentieth century. In 2003, severe acute respiratory syndrome (SARS) caused panic when it seemed to explode around the globe. Outbreaks of Ebola virus disease (EVD) and Middle East respiratory syndrome (MERS-CoV) have led to similar reactions, as did the Zika virus.

Several common events occurred with all of these diseases. First, reports of outbreaks led to panic or near-panic states. Second, the CDC, the World Health Organization, and other national and international agencies worked diligently to discover the microbes that cause the diseases, effective treatment for them, and how to prevent their spread. Third, this information was disseminated to health care providers and institutions so that it could be implemented. Lastly, health care workers implemented appropriate steps and significantly reduced the number of people who became infected and ill.

When the next outbreak occurs, remain calm, understand that news reports may exaggerate the extent of the number of ill or the ease with which the disease is spread, and follow the recommendations of the CDC and your local health department. Because of the ease with which people can travel around the world, the only question about the next outbreak is not if, but when.

Chapter Review

Key Facts and Concepts

- Sepsis is a life-threatening condition resulting from an abnormal and counterproductive response by the body that causes damage to tissues and organs. Septic shock occurs when these changes result in shock and hypotension that does not respond to intravenous fluids.
- Common sources of infections that lead to sepsis include the pulmonary system, gastrointestinal system, genitourinary system, and central nervous system.
- The SIRS criteria are far from perfect, but may help in detecting sepsis. In a patient with an infection (either confirmed or suspected), look for:
  - Temperature lower than 96.8° F (36° C) or higher than 101° F (38.3° C)
  - Heart rate over 90
  - Respiratory rate greater than 20
  - Systolic blood pressure less than 90 mmHg
  - New-onset altered mental status or worsened mental status compared with normal
- In the septic patient who does not need resuscitation, the most important thing you can do is notify the receiving hospital of a sepsis alert.
- When evaluating a patient with a fever or other signs and symptoms suggestive of an infectious disease, ask the patient about recent travel.
- The most important and effective ways to avoid getting an infectious disease on an EMS call are to make sure you have the appropriate vaccinations and to use Standard Precautions.
- When new (or newly rediscovered) infectious disease outbreaks occur, follow the advice of the Centers for Disease Control and Prevention and your local health department.

Key Decisions

- Does this patient potentially have sepsis?
- What personal protective equipment do I need to wear to prevent infection?

Chapter Glossary

infectious diseases diseases that can be spread by bacteria, viruses, and other microbes.

communicable diseases diseases that can be passed from one individual to another, through either direct contact or contact with secretions from an infected person.

sepsis a life-threatening condition resulting from an abnormal and counterproductive response by the body that causes damage to tissues and organs. The body overreacts and secretes substances that, instead of helping, hurt cells, tissues, and organs.

Preparation for Your Examination and Practice

Short Answer

1. List the SIRS criteria.
2. What body systems are the most common sources of sepsis?
3. What is the difference between the incubation period and the period in which a disease is transmissible?
4. Have you had the vaccinations you need to take care of patients without getting sick yourself?
5. What are the differences in transmission routes, symptoms, severity of symptoms, prevention, and treatment among hepatitis A, B, and C?
6. What are the symptoms of meningococcal meningitis? What is unusual about the rash?

Thinking and Linking

Think back to the Well-Being of the EMT *chapter and link information from that chapter with information from this chapter as you consider the following situation:*

- A patient with abdominal pain tells you he is HIV-positive. He is not bleeding, but is nauseated and vomited twice before you arrived. Are there any special precautions you should take?

Critical Thinking Exercises

Children often become ill with communicable diseases since their immune systems have not yet fully developed. The purpose of this exercise will be to consider how such an illness affects the whole family.

- A 2-year-old girl wakes her parents one night with a very loud cough that sounds like a seal barking. They have never experienced anything like this before and are near panic. How should you deal with this situation?

Pathophysiology to Practice

The following questions are designed to assist you in gathering relevant clinical information and making accurate decisions in the field.

- The family of a 19-year-old college student calls EMS because their son suddenly became ill with fever, headache, nausea, and vomiting. What part of the physical exam that is rarely done might assist you in determining whether the patient's meninges are inflamed?

Street Scenes

Erwin McAuliffe is a 79-year-old retired engineer who has not been himself, according to his wife. Ordinarily "sharp as a tack," he now seems confused, she says. This started a day or two ago when he started asking for friends who died years ago. He denies chest discomfort, dyspnea, and abdominal pain, but has had some chills. His lung sounds are clear and equal, and you find he has a urinary catheter with a bag half full of normal-appearing urine. His vital signs are pulse 92, BP 108/70, respirations 22, oral temperature 100.4° F (38° C). He is oriented to person, but not to place or time.

Street Scene Questions

1. **What is the significance of the urinary catheter in the assessment of this patient?**
2. **How many SIRS criteria does this patient meet?**

Erwin doesn't object to going to the hospital by ambulance, so you move him into your vehicle and begin transport. Repeat vital signs are pulse 88, BP 100/78, respirations 18, oral temperature 100.4° F (38° C). His mental status remains unchanged.

Street Scene Questions

3. **How many SIRS criteria does this patient meet now?**
4. **Should you alert the hospital that this patient merits a sepsis alert?**

Just before you arrive at the ED, the patient's vital signs are pulse 108, BP 90/70, respirations 24. He is now very drowsy, although he does moan when you call his name loudly.

You discover later that the patient was diagnosed with septic shock from a urinary infection and was admitted to the ICU after intense treatment in the ED. The attending physician was grateful that you notified the hospital of a sepsis alert so that they could have extra personnel present. She can't be certain the patient will survive, but he has a better chance because of your actions.

25 Poisoning and Overdose Emergencies

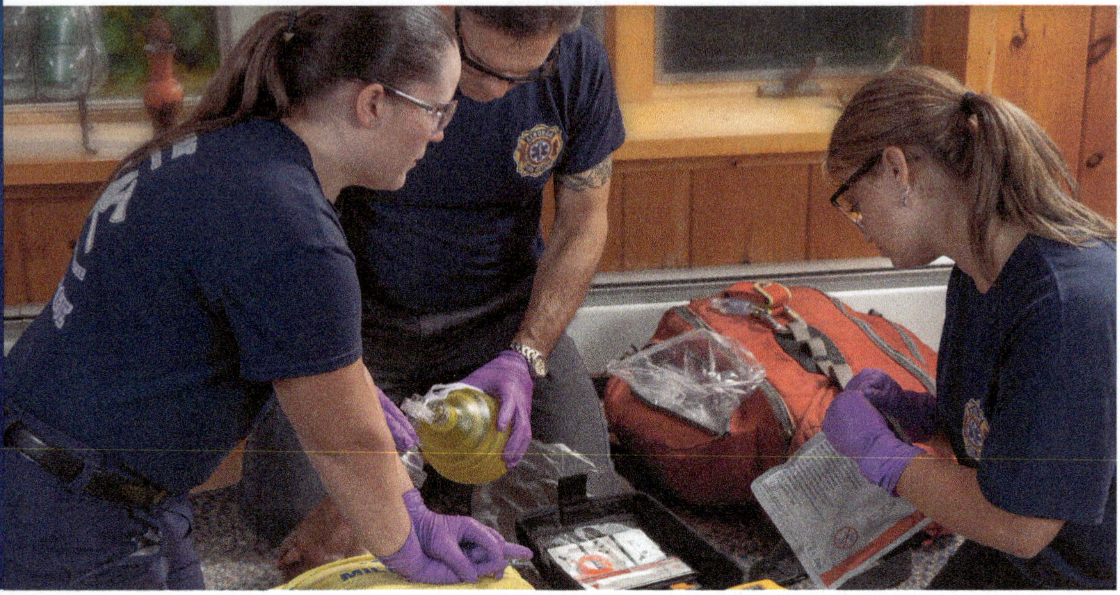

Related Chapters

The following chapters provide additional information related to topics discussed in this chapter:

- **11** Scene Size-Up
- **12** Primary Assessment
- **13** Vital Signs and Monitoring Devices
- **14** Principles of Assessment
- **15** Secondary Assessment
- **16** Reassessment
- **18** General Pharmacology
- **20** Cardiac Emergencies
- **29** Bleeding and Shock
- **33** Trauma to the Head, Neck, and Spine
- **35** Environmental Emergencies

Standard

Medicine (Toxicology)

Competency

Applies fundamental knowledge to provide basic emergency care and transportation based on assessment findings for an acutely ill patient.

Core Concepts

- How to know if a patient has been poisoned
- Assessment and care for ingested poisons
- Assessment and care for inhaled poisons
- Assessment and care for absorbed poisons
- Types of injected poisons
- Assessment and care for alcohol abuse
- Assessment and care for substance abuse

Outcomes

After reading this chapter, you should be able to:

25.1 Summarize concepts of poisoning. (pp. 697-699)

- Describe ways that poisons can damage the body.
- Describe the routes of exposure to poison.
- Explain the effects of commonly ingested poisons.
- Determine when a poisonous substance should be transported with the patient.
- Prioritize the specific steps in the care of patients with poisoning with other needed interventions.

25.2 Explain how to incorporate management relevant to ingested poisoning into the patient care process. (pp. 700-707)

- State the rationale for the specific questions that EMTs should ask of each type of poisoned patient.
- Identify the EMT's key decision points in the care of poisoned patients.
- Describe the steps that can minimize exposure to food poisoning.
- Outline the pharmacology of activated charcoal.
- Explain why syrup of ipecac is rarely used for ingested-poisoning emergencies.
- Explain the reason why many state legislatures have amended laws to allow laypeople to administer naloxone.
- Outline the process of using dilution as a treatment for ingested poisoning.
- Explain the extra consideration for avoiding direct mouth-to-mouth contact with a patient who has ingested poison and who requires positive pressure ventilation.
- State the reasons that the pediatric population is especially prone to ingested poisoning.
- Outline the pharmacology of naloxone.
- Paraphrase the concerns with acetaminophen overdose.

25.3 Explain how to incorporate management of inhaled poison into the patient care process. (pp. 708-712)

- Describe the observations that should make an EMT suspect carbon monoxide inhalation.
- Describe the special concerns associated with smoke inhalation.
- Recognize indications of hydrogen sulfide gas exposure.

25.4 Explain how to incorporate management of absorbed poison into the patient care process. (pp. 712–714)

- Describe the potential risks to EMTs of entering a scene involving absorbed poisons.
- Identify the additional resources that may be required at the scene before an EMT can provide treatment for a patient with absorbed poison.
- Describe the proper way of decontaminating patients of exposures to absorbed poisons.
- Describe special considerations in the scene size-up for poisoned patients.
- Recall sources of information about specific kinds of poisons.
- Identify situations in which additional resources are required for poisoning situations.

25.5 Summarize concepts of alcohol and substance abuse. (pp. 715–716)

- Describe the role of professionalism in increasing the substance abuse patient's cooperation with your interactions.
- Compare the acute and chronic effects of common substances of abuse.
- Explain the need for careful assessment of patients who are acutely intoxicated.
- Anticipate the potential for violence toward EMTs when caring for patients who have a substance abuse issue.
- Explain the considerations for restraining a substance abuse patient.

25.6 Apply knowledge of the effects of alcohol to the patient care process. (pp. 716–717)

- Explain clinical reasoning to identify problems that may be incorrectly attributed to alcohol intoxication.
- Recognize signs of alcohol intoxication.
- Recognize signs and symptoms of the spectrum of withdrawal from alcohol.
- Explain the reason why reassessment is especially important in the care of a patient with acute alcohol intoxication.
- Describe the risks of turning over an intoxicated patient without apparent injury or illness to law enforcement.
- Apply medical-legal and ethical principles to decision making regarding a patient's ability to consent under the influence of a substance.

25.7 Apply knowledge of the effects of a variety of substances of abuse to the patient care process. (pp. 717–722)

- Identify substance abuse as an illness.
- Outline the characteristics of the different categories of commonly abused substances.
- Relate a patient's presentation to the category of substance most likely to cause observed signs and symptoms.
- Recognize indications of substance withdrawal.
- Describe priorities in the care of patients with substance abuse.

Key Terms

absorbed poisons, *698*
activated charcoal, *702*
antidote, *704*
delirium tremens (DTs), *716*
dilution, *704*
downers, *719*
hallucinogens, *719*
ingested poisons, *698*
inhaled poisons, *698*
injected poisons, *699*
opioids, *718*
poison, *697*
toxin, *697*
uppers, *718*
volatile chemicals, *719*
withdrawal, *716*

The opioid epidemic has been in the forefront of the minds of EMTs, but this isn't the only type of substance than can cause an overdose or poisoning situation. As an EMT, how will you know that the patient you encounter at the scene of an emergency call has been poisoned? Family members or bystanders may report this fact when they call for help. There may be clues at the scene, such as empty pill bottles, syringes, or containers of toxic substances, and the patient's signs and symptoms may indicate poisoning or overdose. After you identify and treat immediately life-threatening problems, such as airway or breathing difficulties, you will turn your attention to the options you have to treat the patient's condition. Medical direction and the poison control center will help you in deciding what to do.

Poisoning

A ***poison*** is any substance that can harm the body, sometimes seriously enough to create a medical emergency—or cause death. In the United States, there are more than two million reported cases of poisoning annually. Although some of these result from murder or suicide attempts, most are accidental and involve young children. These incidents usually involve common substances such as medications, petroleum products, cosmetics, and pesticides. In fact, a surprisingly large percentage of chemicals in everyday use contain substances that are poisonous if misused.

poison
any substance that can harm the body by altering cell structure or functions.

CORE CONCEPT
How to know if a patient has been poisoned

We usually think of a poison as some kind of liquid or solid chemical that has been ingested by the poisoning victim. Although this is often the case, many living organisms are capable of producing a ***toxin***, a substance that is poisonous to humans. For example, some mushrooms and other common plants can be poisonous if eaten. These include some varieties of houseplants, including the rubber plant and certain parts of holiday plants, such as mistletoe and holly berries. In addition, bacterial contaminants in food may produce toxins, some of which can cause deadly diseases (such as botulism).

toxin
a poisonous substance secreted by bacteria, plants, or animals.

A great number of substances can be considered poisonous, with different people reacting differently to various poisons (Table 25-1). As odd as it may seem, what may be a dangerous poison for one person may have little effect on another. For most poisonous substances, the reaction is far more serious in the ill, the very young, and older adults.

Once on or in the body, poisons can do damage in a variety of ways. A poison may act as a corrosive or irritant, destroying skin and other body tissues. A poisonous gas can act as a suffocating agent, displacing oxygen in the air. Some poisons are systemic poisons, causing harm to the entire body or to an entire body system. These poisons can critically depress or overstimulate the central nervous system, cause vomiting and diarrhea, prevent red blood cells from carrying oxygen, or interfere with the normal biochemical processes in the body at the level of the cell. The actual effect and extent of damage are dependent on the nature of the poison, on its concentration, and sometimes on how it enters the body. These factors vary in importance depending on the patient's age, weight, and general health.

TABLE 25-1 Common Ingested Poisons

SUBSTANCE	SIGNS AND SYMPTOMS
Acetaminophen	No initial signs or symptoms. Nausea and vomiting. Jaundice is a delayed sign.
Acids and alkalis	Burns on or around the lips; burning in mouth, throat, and abdomen; vomiting
Antiarrhythmics (drugs to regulate electrical impulses and the speed of the heart)	Bradycardia, hypotension, syncope, decreased consciousness, respiratory depression
Antidepressants (selective serotonin reuptake inhibitors)	Tachycardia, hypertension, nausea, tremors
Antidiarrheals (medications to prevent diarrhea)	Used to get high when taken in significant quantity. Can cause an opioid-like high but have significant cardiac side effects and cause constipation.
Antihistamines and cough or cold preparations	Hyperactivity or drowsiness, rapid pulse, flushed skin, dilated pupils
Antipsychotics	Drowsiness, coma, tachycardia
Aspirin	Delayed signs and symptoms, including ringing in the ears, deep and rapid breathing, bruising
Food (contamination)	Different types of food poisoning have different signs and symptoms of varying onset. Most include abdominal pain, nausea, vomiting, and diarrhea, sometimes with fever.
Ibuprofen and other nonsteroidal anti-inflammatory drugs (NSAIDs)	Upset stomach, nausea, vomiting, drowsiness, abdominal pain, gastrointestinal bleeding
Insecticides	Slow pulse, excessive salivation and sweating, nausea, vomiting, diarrhea, difficulty breathing, constricted pupils
Petroleum products	Characteristic odor of breath, clothing, vomitus; if aspiration has occurred, coughing and difficulty breathing.
Plants	Wide range of signs and symptoms, ranging from none to nausea and vomiting to cardiac arrest

"Poisoning and overdose calls are like detective cases. Get a great history and examine the scene for clues."

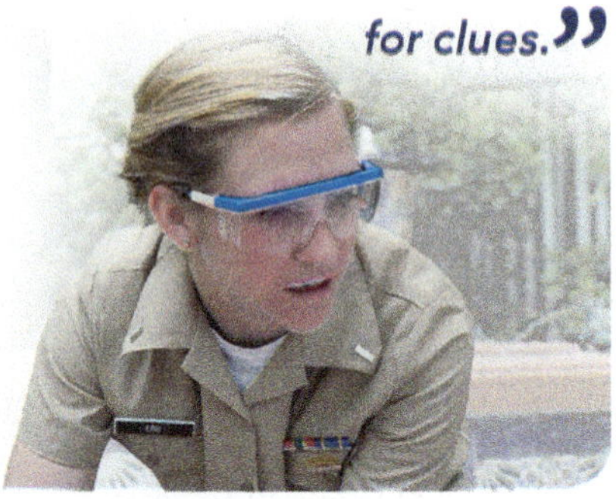

Poisons can be classified into four types, according to how they enter the body: ingested, inhaled, absorbed, and injected (Figure 25-1).

ingested poisons poisons that are swallowed.

inhaled poisons poisons that are breathed in.

absorbed poisons poisons that are taken into the body through unbroken skin.

- ***Ingested poisons*** (poisons that are swallowed) can include many common household and industrial chemicals, medications, improperly prepared or stored foods, cosmetic and personal care products, plant materials, petroleum products, and agricultural products made specifically to control rodents, weeds, insects, or crop diseases.
- ***Inhaled poisons*** (poisons that are breathed in) take the forms of gases, vapors, and sprays. Again, many of these substances are in common use in the home, industry, and agriculture. Such poisons include carbon monoxide (from car exhaust, wood-burning stoves, and furnaces), ammonia, chlorine, insect sprays, and the gases produced from volatile liquid chemicals. (*Volatile* means "able to change very easily from a liquid into a gas"; many industrial solvents are volatile.)
- ***Absorbed poisons*** (poisons taken into the body through unbroken skin) may or may not damage the skin. Many are corrosives or irritants that will injure the skin, then be slowly absorbed into body tissues and the bloodstream, possibly causing widespread

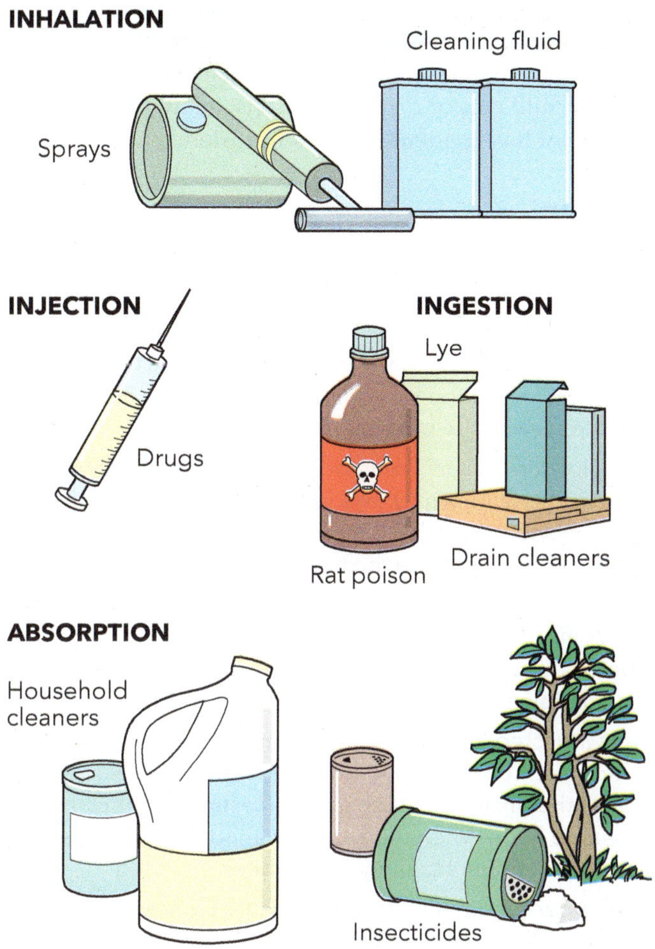

FIGURE 25-1 Poisons enter the body by way of ingestion, inhalation, absorption, and injection.

damage. Others are absorbed into the bloodstream without injuring the skin. Examples of these poisons include insecticides and agricultural chemicals. Contact with a variety of plant materials or certain forms of marine life can lead to skin damage and possible absorption into tissues under the skin.

- ***Injected poisons*** (poisons inserted through the skin) enter the body through a means that penetrates the skin. The most common injected poisons include illicit drugs injected with a needle and venoms injected by snake fangs or insect stingers. These will be discussed under Substance Abuse later in this chapter and in the *Environmental Emergencies* chapter.

injected poisons
poisons that are inserted through the skin—for example, by needle, snake fangs, or insect stinger.

NOTE: *If you suspect intentional poisoning or attempted suicide, approach the scene with caution and have police backup if indicated.*

Pediatric Note

Preventing poisoning is, of course, preferable to treating it. The EMT's own home and the squad building should be "childproofed" against poisoning by keeping medications and other dangerous substances out of children's reach. The EMT can also share poisoning-prevention information with members of the public during school visits and community outreach activities.

CORE CONCEPT
Assessment and care for ingested poisons

Ingested Poisons

Ingested poisons are poisons that have been swallowed. An ingested poison is often a toxic substance that a curious child eats or drinks. In adults, an ingested poison is often a medication on which the patient has accidentally or deliberately overdosed.

Patient Assessment

Ingested Poison

You must gather information quickly in cases of possible ingested poisoning. To determine if activated charcoal is appropriate, on-line medical direction will need certain information:

- What substance was involved? Many products have similar names. It is important to get the exact spelling of the substance. If it is possible and safe, bring the container to the hospital with the patient.
- When did the exposure occur? Some poisons act very quickly and will require immediate treatment. Others may take longer to affect the body, which may allow for other treatments to be used. It is important for emergency department personnel to know as closely as possible the time of ingestion, so that appropriate testing and treatment can be done.

  It is sometimes difficult to determine the time of the exposure from the reports of family members or witnesses. If you cannot get an exact time, determine the earliest and latest possible times of exposure.
- How much was ingested? This sometimes may be determined by simply counting the number of tablets left in a brand-new prescription. However, it can be difficult to determine in other instances, such as when estimating the amount of gasoline spilled on a garage floor. When the amount cannot be reliably estimated, determine the maximum amount that might have been ingested.
- Over how long a period did the ingestion occur? Someone who takes a certain medication chronically, then overdoses on it, may require very different hospital treatment from the patient who has the same overdose but has never taken that medication before.
- What interventions have the patient, family, or well-meaning bystanders taken? Many traditional home remedies for medical problems are harmful, particularly when someone has been exposed to too much of a substance. Product labels have been improved over the past few years, but some still contain inaccurate or even dangerous instructions for management of potentially toxic exposures.
- What is the patient's estimated weight? This estimate, in combination with the amount of substance ingested, may be critical in determining the appropriate treatment. Children experience greater effects of poison because of their lesser size.
- What effects is the patient experiencing from the ingestion? Nausea and vomiting are two of the most common results of poison ingestion, but you may also find altered mental status, abdominal pain, diarrhea, chemical burns around the mouth, and unusual breath odors.

Decision Points

- Is the scene safe from whatever poisoned my patient?
- Is my patient at risk for vomiting or other airway complications?
- Do I need to consult another source, such as poison control, medical direction, ALS, or the *DOT Emergency Response Guidebook*?

Food Poisoning

Another way someone can be poisoned is through food that becomes contaminated with bacteria or toxins because it has been improperly handled or cooked. Food poisoning can be caused by several different bacteria that grow when exposed to the right conditions. This frequently happens when raw meat, poultry, or fish is left at room temperature before being cooked, or the food does not reach a high enough temperature to kill the bacteria. Some food poisonings are the result of bacteria causing an infection in the patient (symptoms may occur a day or so after ingestion); other times, it may be the result of toxins formed by the bacteria that contaminate the food, and it is these toxins that result in symptoms (usually within hours of ingestion). Signs and symptoms vary somewhat, depending on the bacteria involved, but frequently include nausea, vomiting, abdominal cramps, diarrhea, and fever.

You can prevent food poisoning at home and at the station by washing your hands, utensils, cutting boards, and any surface the food touches before—and especially after—any contact with raw meat, fish, or poultry. (The bacteria can easily be spread to other foods from hands or surfaces.) You should also store and cook foods at appropriate temperatures and not leave raw or cooked foods at room temperature for long periods of time. To provide the proper emergency care for ingested poisons (Scan 25-1), follow the instructions given to you by medical direction or your regional poison control center.

SCAN 25-1 Ingested Poisons

First Take Standard Precautions.

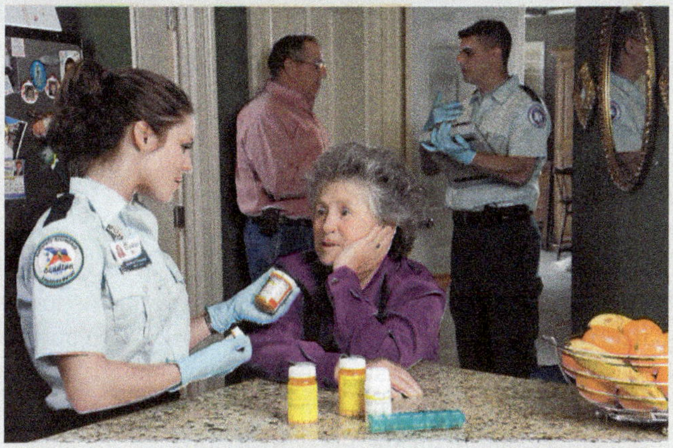

1. Quickly gather information.

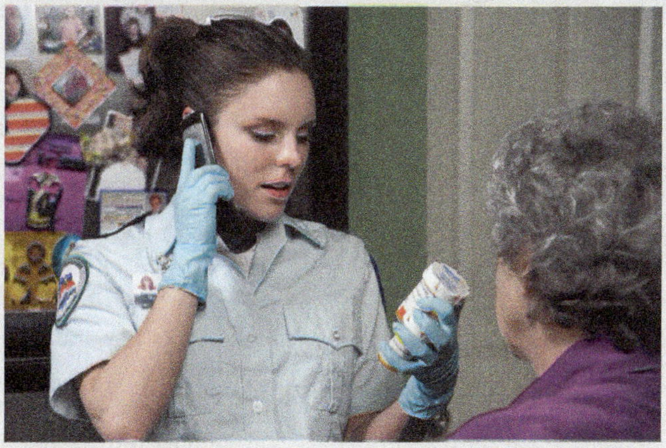

2. Call medical direction on the scene or en route to the hospital. Some protocols recommend contacting the poison control center instead of or in addition to medical direction.

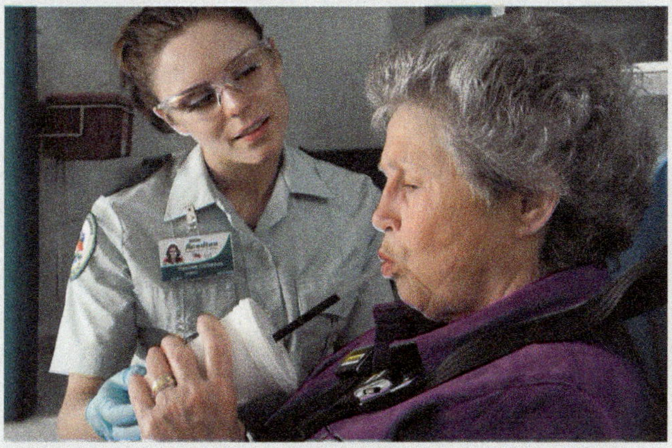

3. If directed, administer activated charcoal. You may wish to administer the medication in an opaque cup that has a lid with a hole for a straw.

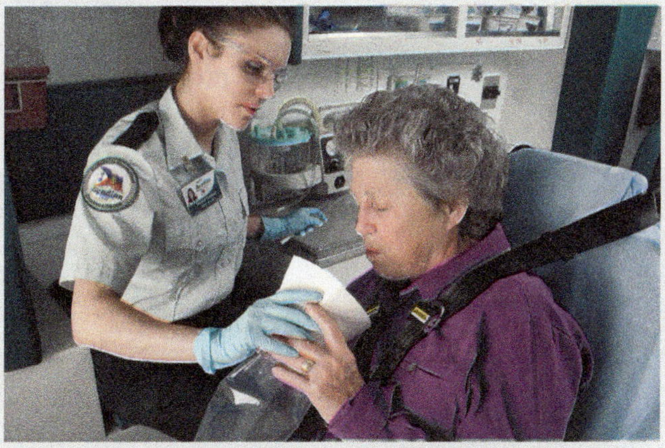

4. Position the patient for vomiting and save all vomitus. Have suction equipment ready.

NOTE: *When a patient has ingested a poison, it provides another reason to avoid mouth-to-mouth contact. Provide ventilations through a pocket face mask or other barrier device to prevent coming in contact with the poison.*

Point of View

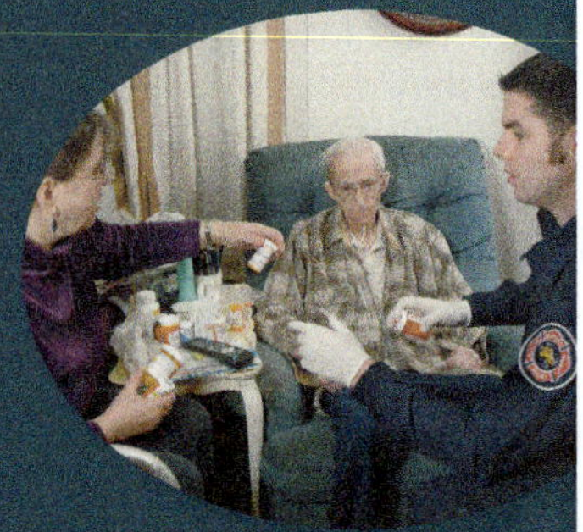

"We were sent to a call for an older patient with an altered mental status. We have a considerable older population in our community and a lot of assisted-living places.

"You read in the news that people are getting older and living longer. Medicine has helped people do this. I was on a call the other day. I looked at this nice older man. You wouldn't believe how many medications he had. It was crazy.

"I'm not saying he didn't need them. That's not my place. But with just a little confusion or disorganization, he could double up on powerful cardiac meds or change his blood sugar or blood pressure or thyroid levels. His daughter thought that is what happened.

"I guess, on the good side, the medications helped us figure out his medical history. We rarely get the full story from the patient and family.

"I know in this case it took five minutes just to get his history list of meds. It actually is an issue we see a lot."

Activated Charcoal

activated charcoal a substance that adsorbs many poisons and prevents them from being absorbed by the body.

In occasional cases of ingested poisoning, medical direction will order administration of ***activated charcoal*** (Scan 25-2).

Activated charcoal works through *adsorption*, the process of one substance's becoming attached to the surface of another. In contrast to ordinary charcoal, which adsorbs some substances, activated charcoal has been manufactured to have many cracks and crevices. As a result, activated charcoal has an increased surface area available for poisons to bind to (similar to corrugated cardboard, which, if you cut it open, has many more surfaces than you would expect by looking at the smooth outer surface). Activated charcoal is not an antidote; however, through the adsorption or binding process, in many cases it will prevent or reduce the amount of poison available for the body to absorb.

Some poisons are at least partially adsorbed by activated charcoal. Activated charcoal was once widely used to treat many ingestions. Now it is used only rarely for very specific overdoses and ingestions. The risk of activated charcoal use is largely that if the patient vomits (which is common) and then aspirates the charcoal, there can be devastating and even fatal consequences due to lung damage. Medical direction (often in consultation with a poison control center) will determine whether the use of activated charcoal is appropriate. Current medical practice balances the risks associated with activated charcoal with the potential benefit. While activated charcoal is carried on many ambulances and listed in protocols, the number of times it actually will be used is small.

SCAN 25-2 Activated Charcoal

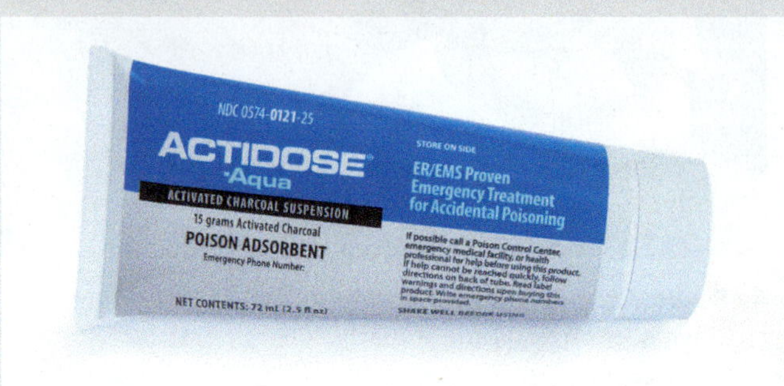

MEDICATION NAME

Generic: activated charcoal
Trade: SuperChar®, InstaChar®, Actidose®, Liqui-Char®, and others

INDICATIONS

Poisoning by mouth

CONTRAINDICATIONS

- Altered mental status
- Ingestion of acids, alkalis, or petroleum products
- Active vomiting
- Inability to swallow

SCAN 25-2 Activated Charcoal *(continued)*

MEDICATION FORM

- Premixed in water, frequently available in a plastic bottle containing 12.5 grams of activated charcoal
- Powder–should be avoided in the field

DOSAGE

- Adults and children: 1 g activated charcoal/kg of body weight
- Usual adult dose: 25-50 g
- Usual pediatric dose: 12.5-25 g

ADMINISTRATION

1. Consult medical direction.
2. Shake container thoroughly.
3. Since medication looks like mud, the patient may need to be persuaded to drink it. Providing a covered container and a straw will prevent the patient from seeing the medication and so may improve patient compliance.
4. If the patient does not drink the medication right away, the charcoal will settle. Shake or stir it again before administering.
5. Record the name, dose, route, and time of administration of the medication.

ACTIONS

- Activated charcoal adsorbs (binds) certain poisons and prevents them from being absorbed into the body.
- Not all brands of activated charcoal are the same. Some adsorb much more than others, so consult medical direction about the brand to use.

SIDE EFFECTS

- Some patients have black stools.
- Some patients may vomit, particularly those who have ingested poisons that cause nausea. If the patient vomits, and no contraindications have developed since the initial dose, repeat the activated charcoal dose once.

REASSESSMENT STRATEGIES

- Be prepared for the patient to vomit or for the patient's condition to deteriorate further.

You should know specific situations where the use of activated charcoal is contraindicated:

- Patients who cannot swallow obviously cannot swallow activated charcoal.
- Patients with altered mental status might choke on activated charcoal and aspirate it into the lungs.
- Patients who have ingested acids or alkalis should not take activated charcoal because the caustic material may have severely damaged the mouth, throat, and esophagus. Activated charcoal cannot help the damage that has already been done and swallowing it may cause further damage. Examples of such caustic substances are oven cleaners, drain cleaners, toilet bowl cleaners, and lye.
- Patients who have accidentally swallowed while siphoning gasoline should not be given activated charcoal. These patients will be coughing violently and possibly aspirating the gasoline. These patients will be unable to swallow activated charcoal.

In addition, activated charcoal is not indicated in cases of food poisoning.

Many brands of activated charcoal are on the market, but some have greater surface area than others. Medical direction can guide you in the selection of an appropriate brand.

Some patients, especially those who have taken an intentional overdose, may refuse to take activated charcoal. Never attempt to force a patient to swallow activated charcoal. If the patient refuses, notify medical direction and continue reassessment and care.

Activated Charcoal versus Syrup of Ipecac. A traditional treatment for poisoning used to be syrup of ipecac. This orally administered drug causes vomiting in most people with just one dose. When vomiting occurs, it results, on the average, in removal of less than one-third of the stomach contents. Because ipecac is slow, is relatively ineffective, and has the potential to make a patient aspirate vomitus, it is rarely used today (although occasionally you may encounter an actively vomiting patient who has taken or been given ipecac prior to your arrival).

Dilution

dilution (di-LU-shun) thinning down or weakening by mixing with something else. Ingested poisons are sometimes diluted by drinking water or milk.

Occasionally medical direction will give an order for ***dilution*** of a poisonous substance. This means an adult patient should drink one to two glasses of water or milk, whichever is ordered. A child should typically be given one-half to one full glass. Dilution with water may slow absorption slightly, whereas milk may soothe stomach upset. This treatment is frequently advised for patients who, as determined by medical direction or poison control, do not need transport to a hospital. Be alert for vomiting after providing water or milk for dilution.

Patient Care

Care of the Patient with Ingested Poison

Fundamental Principles of Care

There are a wide variety of substances that can be ingested. It is important to gather as much information as possible from the scene to assist in patient management at the hospital. Medical direction and poison control are the best resources. It is unreasonable for you to know what to do for every possible substance. Remember that airway control and reassessment are vital in the event the patient vomits or becomes unstable during your care.

Ensure an adequate airway and suction as needed. Poison control centers and/or medical direction will provide guidance based on the specific poison. Gather any specific information from the scene about the poison. Protect yourself from exposure to poisonous substances,

Emergency care of a patient who has ingested poison includes the following steps:

- Detect and treat immediately life-threatening problems in the primary assessment. Evaluate the need for prompt transport for critical patients.
- Perform a secondary assessment. Use gloved hands to carefully remove any pills, tablets, or fragments from the patient's mouth; package the material and transport it with the patient.
- Assess baseline vital signs.
- Consult medical direction or poison control. As directed, administer activated charcoal to adsorb the poison, or water or milk to dilute it. This can usually be done en route.
- Transport the patient with all containers, bottles, and labels from the substance if it is safe to do so.
- Perform reassessment en route.

NOTE: *Sometimes patients who have ingested poisons will require assisted ventilations. Direct mouth-to-mouth ventilation in such a case is dangerous, not only because of the danger of contracting an infectious disease, but also because of possible contact with poisonous substances remaining on the patient's lips, in the airway, or in vomitus. Use a pocket face mask with a one-way valve, a bag-valve-mask unit with supplemental oxygen, or positive pressure ventilation when providing ventilations to a patient who is suspected of ingesting a poison.*

Antidotes

antidote a substance that will neutralize the poison or its effects.

Many laypeople think that every poison has an ***antidote***, a substance that will neutralize the poison or its effects. This is not true. There are only a few genuine antidotes, and they can be used only with a very small number of poisons. Modern treatment of poisonings and overdoses consists primarily of prevention of absorption when possible (such as by administration of activated charcoal) and good supportive treatment (such as airway maintenance, administration of oxygen, and treatment for shock). In a small number of poisonings, advanced treatments are administered in a hospital (administration of antidotes and kidney dialysis).

Pediatric Note

It is the nature of infants and children to explore their world–and to get into and often taste whatever they find. Children will swallow substances adults cannot imagine swallowing, including horrible-tasting poisonous substances such as bleach or lye. The natural curiosity of children makes them the most frequent victims of accidental poisoning.

It is important to find out an infant or child's weight, which–in combination with the estimated amount of the poisonous substance that was ingested–will help medical direction determine appropriate treatment. Children's lesser weight increases the effect of any poison. As an EMT, always assume that the infant or child has ingested a lethal amount of the poison. Because it is usually extremely difficult or impossible to be sure exactly how much the child has taken in, always treat for the worst. Call medical direction, administer the recommended treatments, and transport the child to the hospital.

One antidote that has become increasingly important is naloxone (Scan 25-3). This is a medication that directly reverses narcotics' depressant effects on level of consciousness and respiratory drive. Because of an increase in the number of deaths from narcotic overdoses, a number of state legislatures have amended their laws to allow laypeople to administer naloxone to someone who may be in danger of dying from inadequate respirations from a narcotic overdose. Many EMTs are now permitted to administer this drug too. Naloxone has no effect if there is no narcotic in a patient's system. It can be administered through numerous routes. One route that requires no needle and is easy to use is intranasal, the spraying of a medication into the nasal passages. The rich blood supply in the capillaries of the nasal mucosa is able to absorb this medication, allowing it to be circulated to the rest of the body and reversing the effect of a narcotic (Scan 25-4).

Acetaminophen Poisoning

Acetaminophen overdose is a common cause of hospitalization of overdose patients. This is not surprising, given its effectiveness as an analgesic and its presence as an ingredient in many medications. It is relatively safe in recommended doses for healthy people who do not abuse alcohol or have liver problems, but acetaminophen is very dangerous in overdose. It is important to note that the toxic effects of acetaminophen do not appear right away. After someone takes too much of the drug, the liver becomes overwhelmed and unable to detoxify the substance. Over the next several hours, the liver sustains irreparable damage if nothing is done. If the antidote is given within the first 12 hours after an overdose, however, the patient should recover with a functioning liver.

Unfortunately, the signs and symptoms of acetaminophen overdose are delayed and not very specific. During the first 4–12 hours, the most the patient might experience are loss of appetite, nausea, and vomiting. It isn't until a day or two later, when it is too late for the antidote to work, that the patient typically experiences right upper quadrant pain and jaundice.

This points out the importance of several aspects of prehospital assessment and management:

- Suspect acetaminophen poisoning in conjunction with any other overdose.
- It may be appropriate to search medicine cabinets and garbage cans for empty pill bottles, depending on the circumstances.
- Deal with apparent threats to life first. Because the effects of acetaminophen poisoning are delayed, there is time to institute treatment in the hospital.

SCAN 25-3 Naloxone

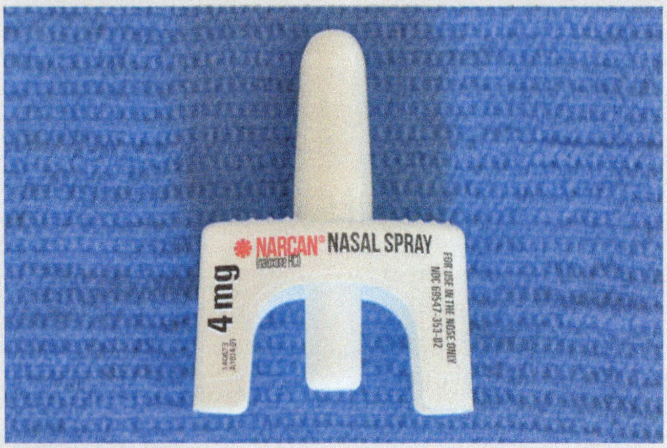

A A single dose nasal naloxone delivery device. *(© Edward T. Dickinson, MD)*

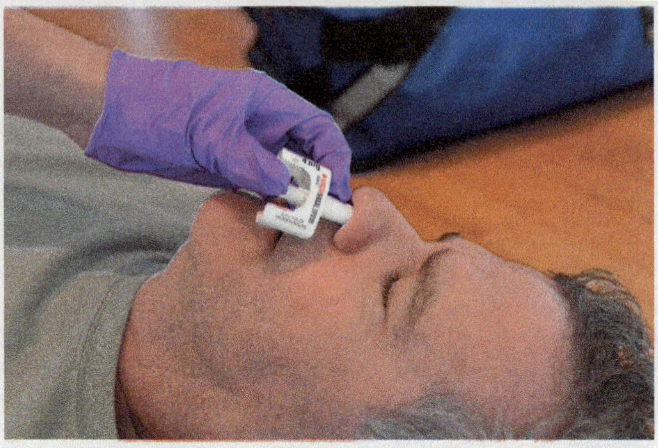

B Use of single dose nasal naloxone delivery device. *(© Edward T. Dickinson, MD)*

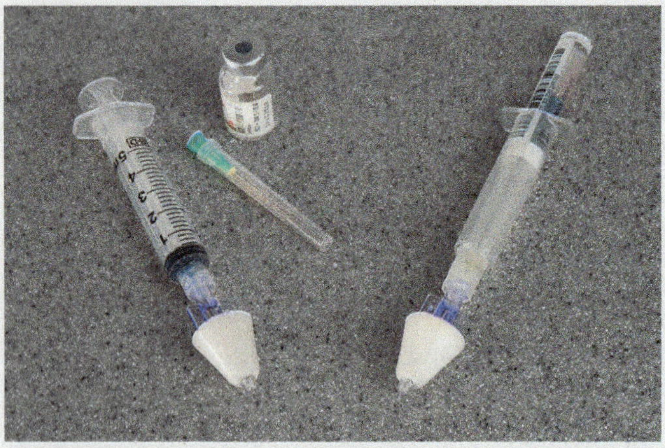

C Naloxone in prefilled syringe with a nasal atomizer tip (*right*), and naloxone drawn up from a vial with a needle into a syringe with a nasal atomizer tip (*left*).

MEDICATION NAME

Generic: naloxone
Trade: Narcan®

INDICATION

- Suspected opioid overdose

CONTRAINDICATION

- Patient breathing adequately and able to maintain own airway

MEDICATION FORM

- Liquid

DOSAGE

0.4–2.0 mg injection
2.0–4.0 mg preloaded atomizer

ADMINISTRATION

1. Ventilate the patient and suction as necessary.
2. Obtain medical direction, either on-line or off-line, as directed by your local protocols.
3. Inspect the patient's nostrils to be sure there are no obstructions to intranasal administration (excessive mucus, blood, etc.) or other reasons not to use this route (e.g., significant damage to or destruction of nasal membranes).
4. Attach the atomizer to the syringe containing the naloxone or remove the preloaded atomizer from the package.
5. Push the atomizer gently but firmly into the nostril opening.
6. Push the plunger of the syringe firmly but briefly until the desired amount of liquid has been expelled from the syringe. In preloaded naloxone devices (A & B above), you will administer the entire contents of the device. Limit the amount of fluid administered at one time to 0.5 mL per nostril. Follow local protocols.
7. Repeat as needed with the other nostril.
8. Record the name, dose, route, and time of administration of the medication.

ACTION

- Reverses the effects of narcotics, including depressed level of consciousness and respiratory depression.

SIDE EFFECT

- May precipitate withdrawal in patients dependent on narcotics. Symptoms of withdrawal include nausea, vomiting, abdominal pains, and agitation. Patients who have taken other medications (e.g., stimulants like methamphetamine or cocaine) with the opioids may become violent.

REASSESSMENT STRATEGY

- Evaluate level of consciousness and respiratory rate and depth frequently. The effects of naloxone do not last as long as those of some narcotics, so some patients may relapse into coma with respiratory depression.

SCAN 25-4 Naloxone Antidote for Narcotic Overdose

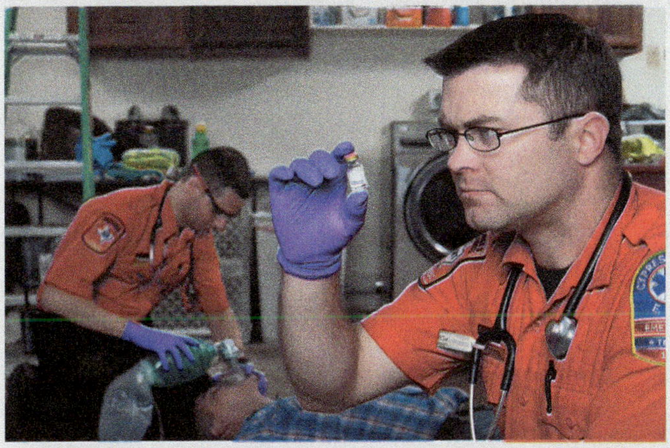

1. Confirm the indications for the medication and the "five rights." Provide ventilation while preparing the medication.

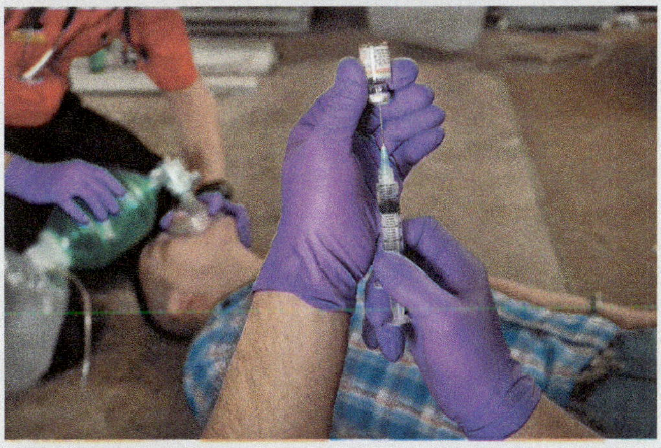

2. Prepare the naloxone. (Some packaging provides medication that is ready to use.)

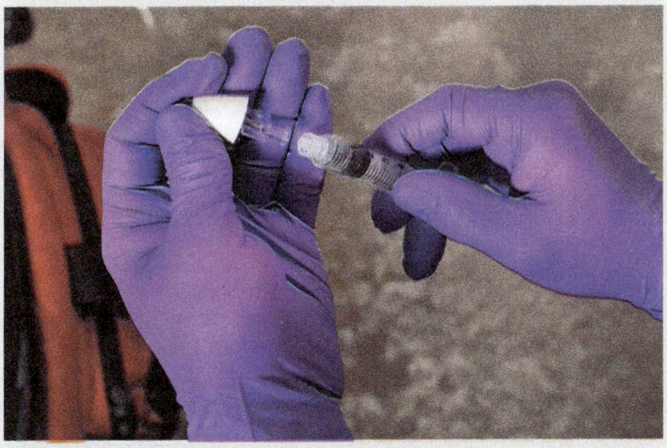

3. Attach the nasal atomization device.

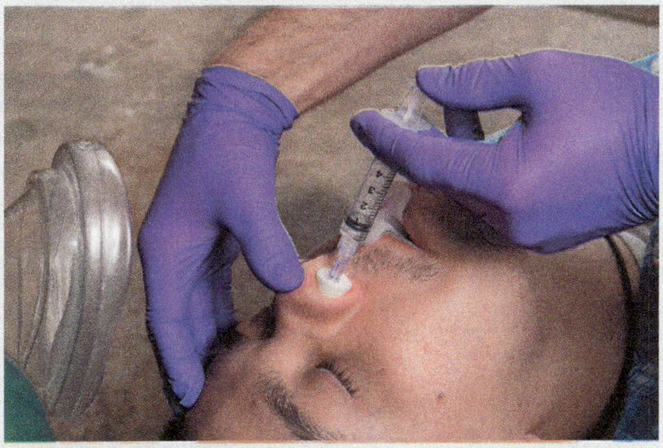

4. Administer naloxone into the nostril. Push firmly to ensure atomization of the medication.

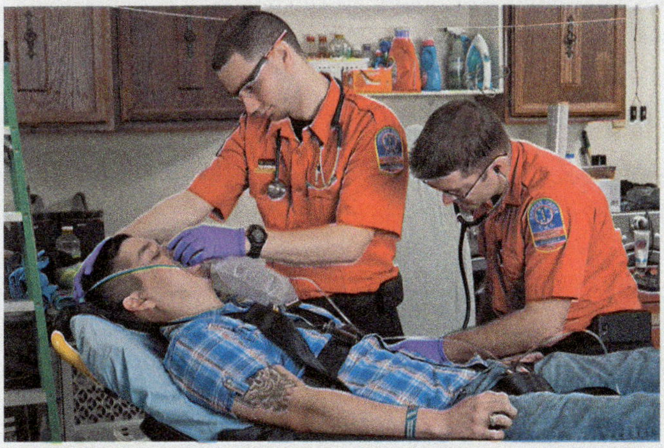

5. Reassess the patient and ensure adequate breathing. Readminister naloxone if respirations remain absent or inadequate and protocols allow.

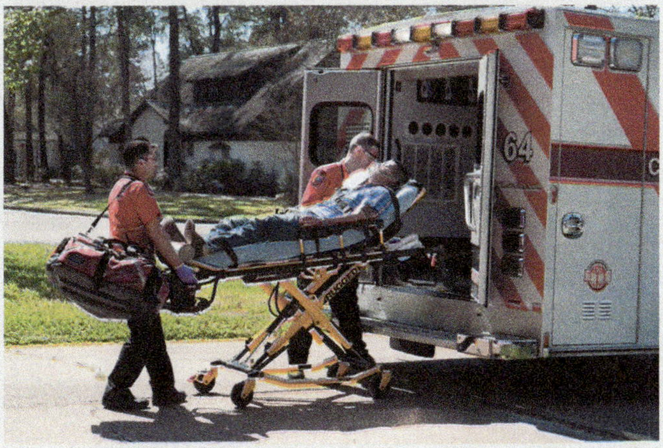

6. Transport the patient.

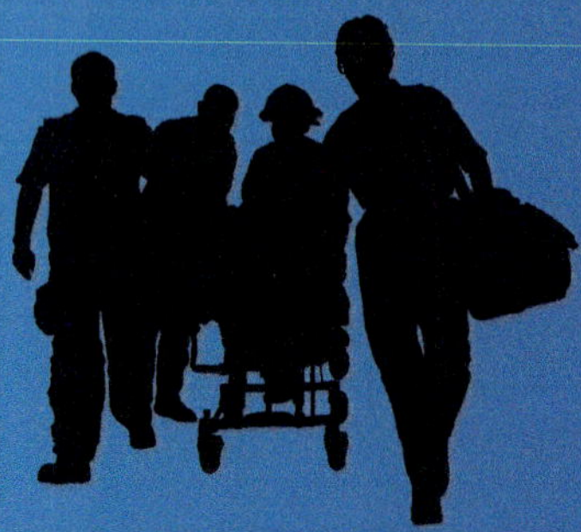

Think Like an EMT

Administer Naloxone?

For each of the following patients, decide whether you would administer naloxone. There is evidence of opioid use at each scene.

1. A 24-year-old male is found unresponsive with a pulse of 92 and regular and a respiratory rate of 16/minute.
2. A 56-year-old female is found unresponsive with a pulse of 128 and a respiratory rate of 6/minute.
3. A 44-year-old male is found without a pulse or respirations.
4. A 72-year-old female is cyanotic around her lips and moans to painful stimulus.
5. An 18-year-old male tells you he injected heroin 15 minutes ago and is concerned it contains fentanyl, like his friend's heroin did yesterday. His friend died.

Inhaled Poisons

CORE CONCEPT
Assessment and care for inhaled poisons

Inhaled poisons are those that are present in the atmosphere and that you, as well as the patient, are at risk of breathing. Carbon monoxide poisoning is a common problem. Other possible inhaled poisons include chlorine gas (often from swimming pool chemicals), ammonia (often released from household cleaners), sprayed agricultural chemicals and pesticides, and carbon dioxide (from industrial sources).

NOTE: *If you suspect that a patient has inhaled a poison, approach the scene with care. Some EMS systems provide training in the use of protective clothing and self-contained breathing apparatus (SCBA) to be used in a hostile environment (such as one containing chlorine gas, ammonia, or smoke). Remember that many inhaled poisons can also be absorbed through the skin. Go only where your protective equipment and clothing will allow you to go safely to perform your mission, and only after you have been trained in the use of this equipment. Do only what you have been trained to do, and go only where your protective equipment will allow you to go safely. If you do not have the necessary equipment or training, get someone there who is properly equipped and trained.*

Patient Assessment

Inhaled Poison

Gather the following information as quickly as possible:

- What substance was involved? Get its exact name if possible.
- When did the exposure occur? Estimate as well as you can when the patient was exposed to the poisonous gas by finding out the earliest and latest possible times of exposure.
- Over how long a period did the exposure occur? The longer someone is exposed to a poisonous gas, the more poison will probably be absorbed.
- What interventions has anyone taken? Did someone remove the patient or ventilate the area right away? When did this happen?
- What effects is the patient experiencing from the exposure? Nausea and vomiting are very common in poisoning of all types. With inhaled poisons, find out if the patient is having difficulty breathing, chest pain, coughing, hoarseness, dizziness, headache, confusion, seizures, or altered mental status.

Carbon Monoxide

Carbon monoxide (CO), one of the most commonly inhaled poisons, is usually associated with motor-vehicle exhaust and fire suppression. The number of carbon monoxide cases is a concern because of the carbon monoxide that can accumulate from the use of improperly vented wood-burning stoves and the use of charcoal for heating and indoor cooking in areas without adequate ventilation. Malfunctioning oil-, gas-, and coal-burning furnaces and stoves can also be sources of carbon monoxide. The indoor use of gasoline-powered small engines such as electrical generators or pumps is another common cause of CO poisoning. Situations such as this are often seen in natural disasters as people try to heat their home or generate electricity when the usual systems are down.

Since carbon monoxide is an odorless, colorless, and tasteless gas, you will not be able to directly detect its presence without special equipment (Figure 25-2). Look for indications of possible carbon monoxide poisoning such as wood-burning stoves, doors that lead to a garage, bedrooms above a garage where motor repair work is in progress, and evidence that suggests the patient has spent a long period of time sitting in an idling motor vehicle. When inhaled, carbon monoxide prevents the normal carrying of oxygen by the red blood cells. Long exposure, even to low levels of the gas, can cause dramatic effects. Death may occur as hypoxia becomes more severe.

The signs and symptoms of carbon monoxide poisoning are deceptive because they can resemble those of the flu. Specifically, you may see:

- Headache, especially "a band around the head"
- Dizziness
- Breathing difficulty
- Nausea
- Cyanosis
- Altered mental status; in severe cases, unconsciousness may result

Patient Care

Care of the Patient with Inhaled Poison

Fundamental Principles of Care

The principal prehospital treatment of inhaled poisoning consists of maintaining the airway and supporting respiration (Scan 25-5). In the case of inhaled poisoning, oxygen is a very important drug. Some inhaled poisons prevent the blood from transporting oxygen in the normal manner. Some prevent oxygen from getting into the bloodstream in the first place. In either case, your ability to keep the airway open, ventilate as needed, and give high-concentration oxygen may make the difference in the patient's survival and quality of life. Note that some inhaled poisons like carbon monoxide will provide falsely high pulse oximetry readings. In these cases, it may be prudent to administer oxygen even in the presence of adequate pulse oximetry readings.

Emergency care steps include the following:

- If the patient is in an unsafe environment, have trained rescuers remove the patient to a safe area. Detect and treat immediately life-threatening problems in the primary assessment. Evaluate the need to promptly transport critical patients.
- Perform a secondary assessment; obtain vital signs.
- Administer high-concentration oxygen. This is the single most important treatment for inhaled poisoning after the patient's airway is opened.
- Transport the patient with all containers, bottles, and labels from the substance.
- Perform reassessment en route.

SCAN 25-5 Inhaled Poisons

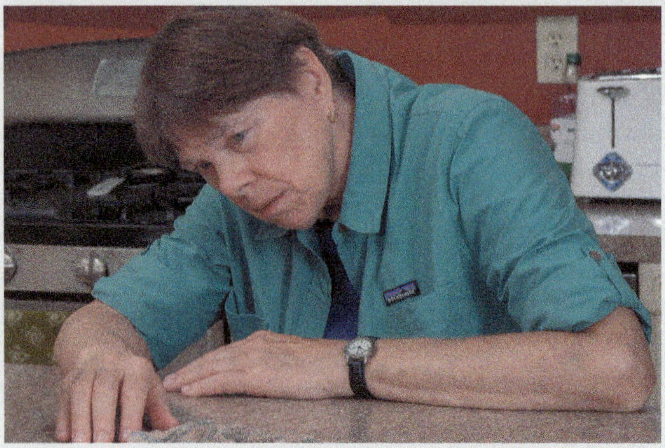

1. Remove the source of the poison.

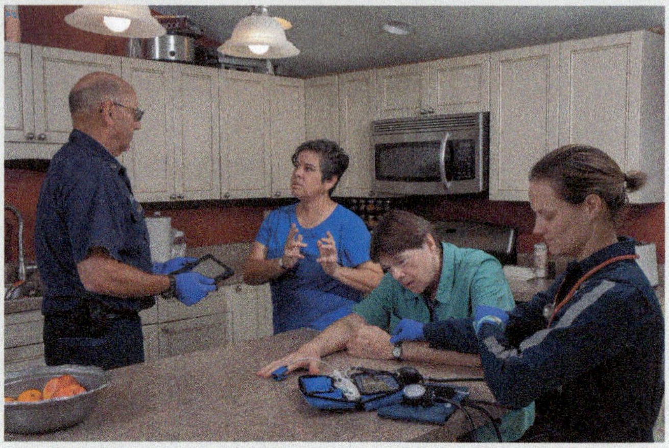

2. Perform a brief assessment and gather the patient's history.

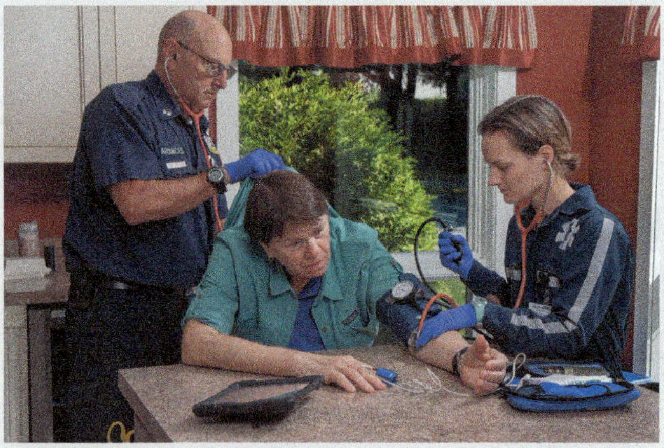

3. Take baseline vital signs and expose the thorax for auscultation.

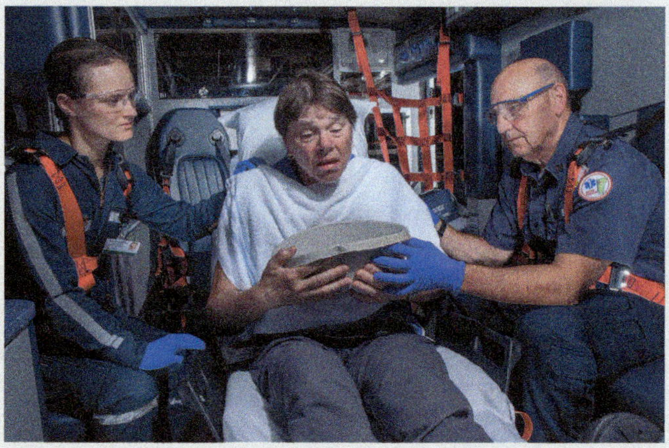

4. Position the patient upright, with a container to collect vomit.

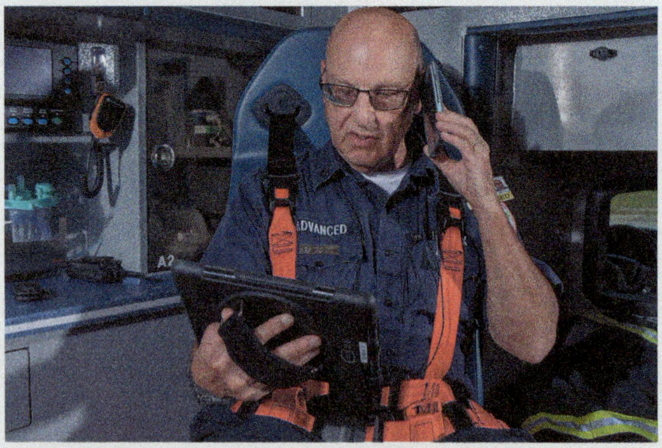

5. Contact medical direction and transport the patient.

NOTE: *In the presence of hazardous fumes or gases, wear protective clothing and self-contained breathing apparatus, or wait for those who are properly trained and equipped to enter the scene and bring the patient out.*

You should suspect carbon monoxide poisoning whenever you are treating a patient with vague, flulike symptoms who has been in an enclosed area. This is especially true when a group of people in the same area have similar symptoms. A patient with carbon monoxide poisoning may begin to feel better shortly after being removed from the

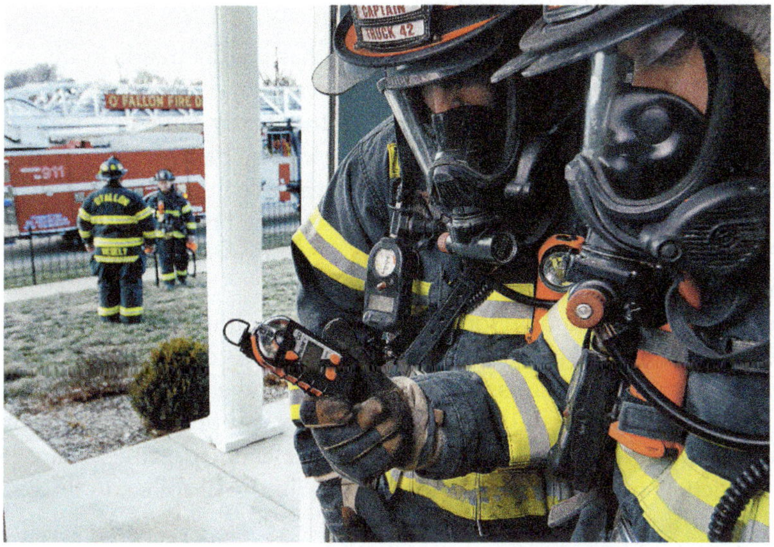

FIGURE 25-2 Special monitors are needed to detect the presence of carbon monoxide in the environment.

dangerous environment. However, it is still very important to continue to administer 100 percent oxygen and to transport these patients to a hospital. Oxygen is an antidote for carbon monoxide poisoning, but it takes time to "wash out" the carbon monoxide from the patient's bloodstream. These patients need medical evaluation because they can experience serious consequences, including neurologic deficits, from their exposure.

NOTE: *There is a commonly accepted idea that a patient exposed to carbon monoxide will have cherry-red lips. In fact, cherry-red skin is not typically seen in patients with carbon monoxide poisoning.*

Smoke Inhalation

Smoke inhalation is a serious problem associated with fire scenes. Smoke inhalation is often associated with thermal burns as well as with the effects of irritants and chemical poisons within the smoke. The smoke from any fire source contains many poisonous substances. Modern building materials and furnishings often contain plastics and other synthetics that release toxic fumes when they burn or are overheated. It is possible for the substances found in smoke to burn the skin, irritate the eyes, injure the airway, cause respiratory arrest, and in some cases cause cardiac arrest.

As an EMT, you will most likely find irritated (reddened, watering) eyes and, of far greater concern, injury to the airway associated with smoke.

The following signs indicate an airway injured by smoke inhalation:

- Difficulty breathing
- Coughing
- Breath that has a "smoky" smell or the odor of chemicals involved at the scene
- Black (carbon) residue in the patient's mouth and nose
- Black residue in any sputum coughed up by the patient
- Nose hairs singed from superheated air

Move the patient suffering from smoke inhalation to a safe area and provide the same care you would provide for any inhaled poison: Assess the patient, administer high-concentration oxygen, and transport. Someone with smoke inhalation is likely to have inhaled carbon monoxide, so administer high-concentration oxygen even if the pulse oximeter reading is 100 percent. Carboxyhemoglobin is red like oxyhemoglobin, and the two cannot be distinguished by pulse oximeters. Some EMS systems utilize co-oximeters that can identify elevated levels of carboxyhemoglobin.

NOTE: *The body's reaction to toxic gases and foreign matter in the airway can often be delayed. Convince all smoke-inhalation patients that they must be seen by a physician, even if they are not yet feeling serious effects.*

"Detergent Suicides"

A method of suicide that became popular in Japan has made inroads in the United States. By mixing two easily obtained chemicals, a person can cause the release of toxic hydrogen sulfide gas. In Japan, the chemicals involved are frequently toilet cleaner and bath salts, leading to the name "detergent suicide." The same kind of bath salts is not available in the United States, but using other chemicals that are available in the United States can lead to the same result. Typically, a source of acid, such as a strong household cleaner, and a source of sulfur, often a pesticide, will quickly release significant amounts of toxic hydrogen sulfide gas when mixed together.

Hydrogen sulfide is best known for its rotten egg odor, but less well known is that, even at moderate concentrations, it can be quite dangerous. Hydrogen sulfide not only takes the place of oxygen but also bonds with iron in cells, preventing oxygen from binding to those cells and getting to where it is needed. Mild exposure can result in coughing, eye irritation, and sore throat. More severe exposures can lead to dizziness, nausea, shortness of breath, headache, and vomiting. In severe cases, fluid will collect in the lungs (pulmonary edema), resulting in death.

The typical method of committing suicide in Japan with this toxic gas includes combining the chemicals in a small, enclosed space and posting warning signs advising people not to try to gain access to the subject but rather to call a hazardous materials team. Although this warning is common in Japan, it is not clear how often others attempting suicide in this manner will be so courteous toward rescuers.

Although this method of suicide has not yet become common in the United States, EMTs must be extremely careful when approaching a scene where a "detergent suicide" may have taken place. Warning signs to look for include a small, enclosed space, such as a car, with tape sealing the windows and doors. Any kind of sign or note warning people not to approach should be taken very seriously. Call the appropriate agency to open the space and remove the body. Do not become another casualty.

Absorbed Poisons

CORE CONCEPT
Assessment and care for absorbed poisons

Absorbed poisons frequently irritate or damage the skin. However, some poisons can be absorbed with little or no damage to the skin.

NOTE: *Just as poisonous substances can be absorbed by patients, they can also be absorbed by EMTs. It is critical that the EMT take protective measures to prevent exposure to these substances. Before touching an exposed patient, the EMT may need to wait for firefighters or HAZMAT team members to decontaminate the patient.*

Patient Assessment

Care of the Patient with Absorbed Poison

Fundamental Principles of Care

Poisons that are absorbed into a patient's body can also be absorbed into yours. Safety, always a primary concern, is very relevant here. Call any resources (e.g., HAZMAT teams, poison control, or medical direction) for help as needed. Follow the steps to remove the substance when it is safe to do so.

Do not allow contaminated patients into your ambulance, and do not transport contaminated patients to the hospital.

Emergency care of a patient with absorbed poisons includes the following steps:

- Detect and treat immediately life-threatening problems in the primary assessment. Evaluate the need for prompt transport of critical patients.
- Perform a secondary assessment; obtain vital signs. This includes removing contaminated clothing while protecting oneself from contamination.

- Remove the poison by doing one of the following:
  - Powders: Brush powder off the patient; then continue as for other absorbed poisons.
  - Liquids: Irrigate with clean water for at least 20 minutes and continue en route if possible.
  - Eyes: Irrigate with clean water for at least 20 minutes and continue en route if possible.
- Transport the patient with all containers, bottles, SDSs, and labels from the substance.
- Perform reassessment en route.

The most important part of the treatment of a patient with an absorbed poison is to get the poison off the skin or out of the eye (Scan 25-6). The best way to do this is by irrigating the skin or the eye with large amounts of clean water. A garden hose or fire hose can be used to irrigate the patient's skin, but care must be taken not to injure the skin further with high pressure.

SCAN 25-6 Absorbed Poisons–Hazmat–Illegal Meth Lab

First Take Standard Precautions.

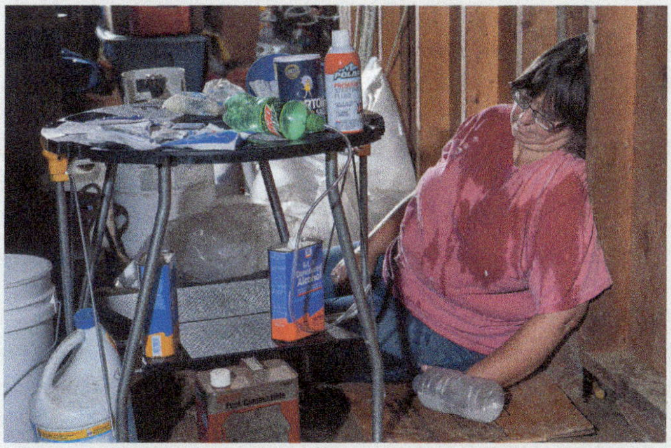

1. Scene size-up indicates poison (meth lab) and need for HAZMAT team.

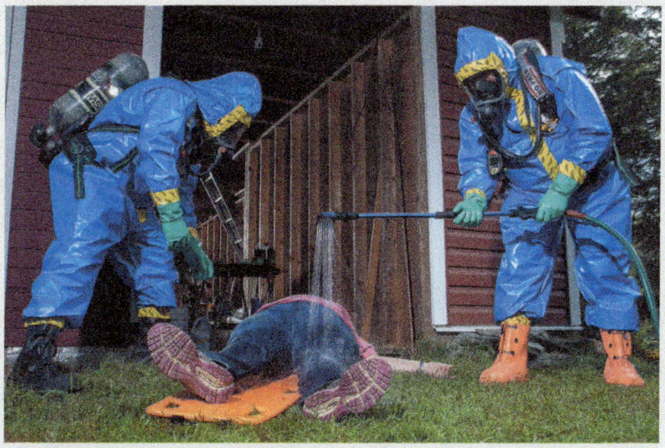

2. HAZMAT team performs the initial decontamination on the patient.

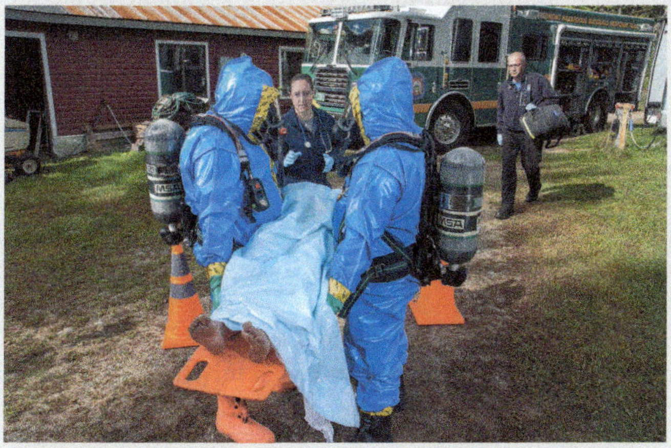

3. HAZMAT team takes the patient from the hot zone into the "warm zone." EMS takes over the decontaminated patient.

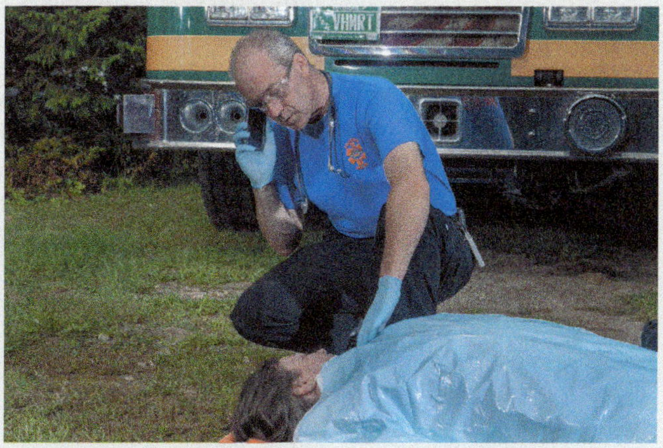

4. Contact medical direction and transport the patient.

NOTE: *Take care to protect your skin from contact with poisonous substances. Wear protective clothing. If necessary, have firefighters or others who are properly protected hose off the patient before you touch the patient.*

"Neutralizing" acids or alkalis with solutions such as dilute vinegar or baking soda in water should *not* be done. When poisoning incidents such as these occur, such substances are almost never readily available. Even if they were, they would not be appropriate. They have never been shown to help, and there is good reason to believe they would make matters worse. When an acid is mixed with an alkali, it is true that the two may be neutralized. It is also true, though, that this reaction produces heat. Skin that has been injured already by an acid or alkali may be further damaged by attempts to neutralize the chemical.

Injected Poisons

CORE CONCEPT
Types of injected poisons

The most common injected poisons are illicit drugs injected with a needle (which will be discussed later in this chapter) and the venom of snakes and insects (which will be covered in the *Environmental Emergencies* chapter).

Poison Control Centers

Emergency care in poisoning cases presents special problems for the EMT. Signs and symptoms can vary greatly. Some poisons produce a characteristic set of signs and symptoms very quickly, whereas others are subtle and slow to appear. Poisons that act almost immediately usually produce obvious signs, and the particular poison or its container is often still nearby. Slow-acting poisons can produce effects that mimic an infectious disease or some other medical emergency.

There will be times when you will not know the substance that caused the poisoning. In some of these cases, an expert may be able to tell, based on the combination of signs and symptoms. Even when you know the source of the poison, correct emergency care procedures may still be uncertain. Ideas about proper care keep changing as more research is done on poisoning. This constant change makes it impossible to print guides and charts for poison control and care that will be up-to-date when you use them. Although manufacturers have improved the instructions on many container labels, some still have inaccurate or even dangerous advice.

Fortunately, a network of poison control centers exists to provide information and advice to both laypeople and health care providers. Throughout the United States, it is possible to reach a poison control center 24 hours a day. Dialing 1-800-222-1222 connects you with the poison center covering the area the call is coming from. Your EMS agency may also have a local number for your regional poison center. Either number will work.

An EMT should consult a poison control center only when directed by local protocol. In most cases, EMTs get medical direction from physicians or nurses who are in hospital emergency departments. Unless special arrangements have been made, the poison control center staff do not have the authority to provide on-line medical direction. If the poison control center staff do have the authority to do so, they can tell you what should be done for most cases of poisoning.

If you are permitted to communicate directly with the poison control center in your area, do so by telephone. Even if you have radio contact with your local poison control center, the telephone is the preferred way to communicate. The staff member may need to talk to you for several minutes—far too long a period to monopolize the airwaves. The telephone will also allow you to maintain patient confidentiality. Make certain that you have memorized the number and/or that you carry the poison control center number with you into the residence—perhaps pasted inside your kit—so you do not have to return to the rig to get it.

To help the poison control center staff, gather all of the information you need before you call.

Many people have the impression that the poison control center should be called for only cases of ingested poisonings. However, the center's staff can provide valuable care information for all types of poisoning.

Your community may have special poisoning problems. For example, not every community is exposed to rattlesnakes, jellyfish, or powerful agricultural chemicals. Many EMS systems have compiled lists of poisoning problems specific for their areas. Check to see if this has been done for the area in which you will be an EMT.

Think Like an EMT

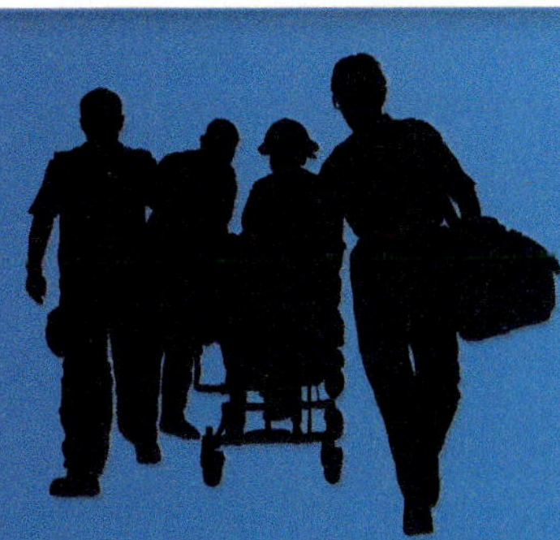

Find the Clues

Poisoning and overdose emergencies are challenging in that you will need to figure out what toxin caused the patient's current signs and symptoms. Your ability to examine the scene and report accurate findings to poison control is vital to the patient's well-being. In each of the following scenarios, decide what information you will need to gather and where to obtain it to ensure proper treatment for the patient.

1. Your patient states he has taken an overdose of prescription medications.
2. Your patient is found in a closed garage with the car running.
3. Your patient is found in the garden, confused and drooling.

Alcohol and Substance Abuse

Many patients' conditions are caused directly or indirectly by alcohol or drug abuse—problems that cross all geographic and economic boundaries.

Alcohol Abuse

CORE CONCEPT
Assessment and care for alcohol abuse

Many persons consume alcohol without having any problems. However, others occasionally or chronically abuse alcohol. Even though adults can legally drink alcohol, it is still a drug that can have a potent effect on a person's central nervous system. Emergencies arising from the use of alcohol may be due to the effect of alcohol that has just been consumed, or it may be the result of the cumulative effects of years of alcohol abuse.

EMTs often do not take alcohol-abuse patients seriously. This may be due to some such patients' belligerent or unusual behavior, frequent calls to EMS when intoxicated, or less-than-desirable hygiene. Nevertheless, you should provide care for the patient suffering from alcohol abuse the same as you would for any other patient. Patients who appear intoxicated must be treated with the same respect and dignity as those who are sober.

Above all, you must not neglect your duty to provide medical care. Not only do alcohol-abuse patients often have injuries from accidents and falls, but they are also candidates for many medical emergencies. Chronic drinkers (alcoholics) often have derangements in blood sugar levels, poor nutrition, the potential for considerable gastrointestinal bleeding, and other problems. A person can be both intoxicated and having a heart attack or hypoglycemia. If the patient has ingested alcohol and other drugs, this can produce a serious medical emergency. When alcohol is combined with other depressants such as antihistamines and tranquilizers, the effects of alcohol can be more pronounced and, in some cases, lethal.

Since EMT safety is a critical part of all calls, do not hesitate to ask for police assistance with any patient who appears intoxicated or irrational, or exhibits potentially dangerous behavior. The nature of intoxication is such that a passive person may suddenly become aggressive. Always be prepared for this event.

Patient Assessment

Alcohol Abuse

Keep in mind that although alcohol abuse may be the patient's apparent problem, another problem may be present. Conduct a complete assessment to identify any medical emergencies. Remember that diabetes, epilepsy, head injuries, high fevers, hypoxia, and other medical problems may make a patient appear to be intoxicated. Also, look for injuries. Do not allow the presence of alcohol or the signs and symptoms of alcohol abuse to override your suspicions of other medical problems or injuries.

Since a history from any patient who appears intoxicated will be difficult to get and perhaps unreliable, your powers of observation and resourcefulness will be tested. Family members and bystanders may provide important information.

The following list contains signs and symptoms of alcohol abuse:

- Odor of alcohol on the patient's breath or clothing. By itself, however, this is not enough to conclude alcohol abuse. Be certain that the odor is not "acetone breath," as with some diabetic emergencies.
- Swaying and unsteadiness of movement
- Slurred speech, rambling thought patterns, or incoherent words or phrases
- A flushed appearance to the face, often with the patient sweating and complaining of being warm
- Nausea or vomiting
- Poor coordination
- Slowed reaction time
- Blurred vision
- Confusion
- Hallucinations, visual or auditory ("seeing things" or "hearing things")
- Lack of memory (blackout)
- Altered mental status

withdrawal
referring to alcohol or drug withdrawal, in which the patient's body reacts severely when deprived of the abused substance.

delirium tremens (DTs) (duh-LEER-e-um TREM-uns)
a severe reaction that can be part of alcohol withdrawal, characterized by sweating, trembling, anxiety, and hallucinations. Severe alcohol withdrawal with the DTs can lead to death if untreated.

The patient who is an alcoholic might not be under the influence of alcohol but, instead, may be suffering from alcohol ***withdrawal***. This can be a severe condition occurring when the alcoholic patient cannot obtain alcohol, is too sick to drink alcohol, or has decided to quit drinking suddenly. The patient with alcohol-withdrawal may experience seizures, or ***delirium tremens (DTs)***, a condition characterized by sweating, trembling, anxiety, and hallucinations. In some cases, alcohol withdrawal can be fatal. Signs of alcohol withdrawal include:

- Confusion and restlessness
- Unusual behavior, to the point of demonstrating "insane" behavior
- Hallucinations
- Gross tremor (obvious shaking) of the hands
- Profuse sweating
- Seizures (common and often very serious)
- Hypertension
- Tachycardia

Be on the alert for signals—such as depressed vital signs—that the patient has mixed alcohol and drugs (prescribed, over-the-counter, or illegal). Also, when interviewing the intoxicated patient or the patient suffering from alcohol withdrawal, do not begin by asking if the patient is taking *drugs*. Your patient may react to this question as if you are gathering evidence of a crime. Ask if any medications have been taken while drinking. If necessary, when you are certain that the patient knows you are concerned about the patient's well-being, you can repeat the question using the word *drugs*.

NOTE: *All patients with seizures or DTs must be transported to a medical facility as soon as possible.*

Patient Care

Care of the Patient with Alcohol Abuse

Fundamental Principles of Care

Since alcohol-abuse patients often vomit, take Standard Precautions, including gloves, mask, and protective eyewear as necessary. Monitor the airway carefully. The behavior of an intoxicated person may be unpredictable. Take steps necessary to remain safe throughout the call. Intoxicated patients may have a variety of hidden medical and traumatic conditions. Never assume someone is simply/only intoxicated.

To provide basic care for the intoxicated patient or the patient suffering acute intoxication, follow these steps:

- Stay alert for airway and respiratory problems. Be prepared to perform airway maintenance, suctioning, and positioning of the patient should the patient lose consciousness, seize, or vomit. Help the patient so vomitus will not be aspirated. Have a rigid-tip suction device ready. Provide oxygen and assist respirations as needed.
- Assess for trauma the patient may be unaware of because of the patient's intoxication.
- Be alert for changes in mental status as alcohol is absorbed into the bloodstream. Continue to talk in an effort to keep the patient as alert as possible.
- Monitor vital signs.
- Treat for shock.
- Protect the patient from self-injury. Use restraint as authorized by your EMS system. Request assistance from law enforcement if needed. Protect yourself and your crew.
- Stay alert for seizures.
- Transport the patient to a medical facility.

Note that in some systems, patients under the influence of alcohol who are not suffering from any apparent medical emergency or injury are not transported. They are given over to the police. This may not be wise, since some patients having an alcohol-related emergency may die if they don't receive additional care. EMS personnel could potentially miss a medical problem or injury, or the patient's condition may worsen as the alcohol continues to be absorbed by the patient's system. Be especially careful of patients with even minor head injuries, since development of a subdural hematoma with minor or moderate head trauma (see the chapter *Trauma to the Head, Neck, and Spine*) is not uncommon in alcoholics.

NOTE: *A PATIENT UNDER THE INFLUENCE OF ALCOHOL CANNOT MAKE AN INFORMED REFUSAL OF TREATMENT OR TRANSPORT. However, if the patient refuses treatment or transport, you should contact medical direction and/or law enforcement personnel before transporting a patient against the patient's will. Document this in your prehospital care report.*

Substance Abuse

Substance abuse is a term that indicates a chemical substance is being taken for other-than-therapeutic (medical) reasons. Many substances have legitimate purposes when used properly. When these same substances are abused, however, the results can be devastating. Not only are substance-abuse patients at risk for dangerous effects of the substances they abuse, but they are also at increased risk of trauma as a result of their impaired judgment when under the influence and of the inherent risks of violence related to "drug deals."

Historically, marijuana was considered a drug of abuse. In the last decade many states have legalized "pot" and the active chemicals found in marijuana. One of the results of

CORE CONCEPT
Assessment and care for substance abuse

this increased availability has been an increase in the incidence of patients suffering from vomiting and abdominal pain syndromes associated with chronic marijuana use.

Individuals who abuse drugs and other chemical substances should be considered to have an illness. Therefore, they have the right to the same professional emergency care as any other patient.

The most common drugs and chemical substances that are abused and can lead to problems requiring an EMS response (Figure 25-3) can be classified as opioids, uppers, downers, hallucinogens, or volatile chemicals.

opioids
a class of drugs that affects the nervous system and changes many normal body activities. Their legal use is for the relief of pain. Illicit use is to produce an intense state of relaxation.

- ***Opioids*** are drugs that bind to opioid receptors in the body. Sometimes called *narcotics*, these drugs have a depressant effect on the body and cause an intense state of relaxation and a feeling of well-being. Opioids can be prescribed for pain (codeine, oxycontin, Percocet), but are also found as illegal drugs such as heroin. Many people who are addicted to heroin began using opioid medications for pain relief. This leads to addiction. Heroin is an illegal substance that can be injected or snorted. It is sometimes mixed with another substance called fentanyl which is more potent than heroin. This often results in a rapid and devastating overdose. Narcotic overdoses are generally characterized by three signs: coma (or depressed level of consciousness), pinpoint pupils, and respiratory depression (slow, shallow respirations). Together these are sometimes referred to as the "opioid triad."

uppers
stimulants such as cocaine and methamphetamine that affect the central nervous system and excite the user.

- ***Uppers*** are stimulants that affect the nervous system and excite the user. Many abusers use these drugs in an attempt to relieve fatigue or to create feelings of well-being. Examples are caffeine, methamphetamine, Ritalin, and cocaine. Cocaine may be "snorted," smoked, or injected. Other stimulants are frequently taken in pill form. Also included in this category are so-called "bath salts." These are synthetic drugs that have very potent stimulant effects and sometimes hallucinogenic effects as well.

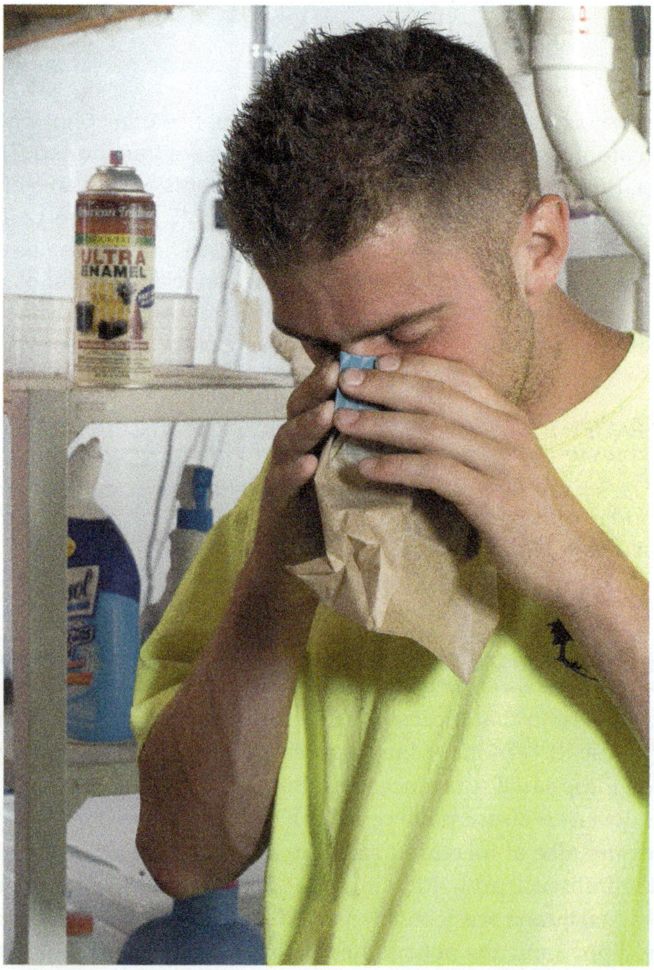

FIGURE 25-3 Volatile chemicals produce vapors that can be inhaled. Methods of inhaling substances include "huffing" (breathing fumes directly or from a substance-impregnated fabric) and "bagging" (breathing fumes from a substance sprayed into a bag).

- ***Downers*** have a depressant effect on the central nervous system. This type of drug may be used as a relaxing agent, sleeping pill, or tranquilizer. Benzodiazepines are an example. Valium (diazepam) and Xanax (alprazolam) are commonly abused medications. These are usually found in pill or capsule form. One example of a downer that you may encounter on an EMS call is Rohypnol (flunitrazepam), also known as "roofies." The effects of Rohypnol include sedation, confusion, and blackouts. Because it is colorless, odorless, and tasteless, it has been put into unsuspecting people's drinks and has become known as a "date rape" drug. Another downer you may see is GHB (gamma hydroxybutyrate), also known as Georgia Home Boy or goop. In addition to depressing the central nervous system, it produces a sense of euphoria and sometimes hallucinations. It has caused respiratory depression so severe that patients have required assisted ventilations even though some of them were still breathing.

downers
depressants, such as benzodiazepines, that depress the central nervous system, and which are often used to bring on a more relaxed state of mind.

- ***Hallucinogens*** such as LSD, PCP, and certain types of mushrooms are mind-affecting drugs that act on the nervous system to produce an intense state of excitement or a distortion of the user's perceptions. This class of drugs has few legal uses. They are often eaten or dissolved in the mouth and absorbed through the mucous membranes. Another hallucinogen is ecstasy, also known as XTC, X, or MDMA (because it is methylenedioxymethamphetamine). This hallucinogen also has the stimulant properties of uppers and is popular in the club scene.

hallucinogens
(huh-LOO-sin-uh-jens)
mind-affecting or mind-altering drugs that act on the central nervous system to produce excitement and distortion of perceptions.

- ***Volatile chemicals*** produce vapors that can be inhaled (see Figure 25-3). They can give an initial "rush" and then act as a depressant on the central nervous system. Cleaning fluid, glue, model cement, and correction fluids used to correct ink-based errors are commonly abused volatile chemicals.

volatile chemicals
vaporizing compounds, such as cleaning fluid, that are breathed in by the abuser to produce a "high."

Designer drugs are another type of commonly abused drug. There are substances that chemically resemble traditional drugs but have a slight difference in their molecular formula or composition. Designer drugs produce effects similar to (or greater than) the drugs they are based on but, because of their slight chemical differences, did not fall under the traditional legal definitions of prohibited drugs. Because of this, states have changed their laws to include these designer drugs.

Designer drugs are not actually one class of drugs, because they are based on drugs in all the categories discussed in this chapter. Their specific effects depend on many different factors, and new drugs are always being invented.

Patient Assessment

Substance Abuse

As an EMT, you will not need to know the names of the many abused drugs or patients' specific reactions to them. It is far more important for you to be able to detect possible drug abuse at the overdose level and to relate certain signs to certain types of drugs and to drug withdrawal. Table 25-2 provides some of the names of commonly abused drugs. Do not worry about memorizing this list. Read it through so you can place some of the more familiar drugs into categories in terms of drug type.

The signs and symptoms of substance abuse, dependency, and overdose can vary from patient to patient, even for the same drug or chemical. The problem is made more complex by the fact that many substance abusers take more than one drug or chemical at a time. Often you will have to carefully combine the information gained from the signs and symptoms, the scene, bystanders, and the patient to determine if you may be dealing with substance abuse. In many cases, you will not be able to identify the substance involved.

When questioning the patient and bystanders, you will get better results if you begin by asking if the patient has been taking any medications. Then, if necessary, ask if the patient has been taking drugs.

TABLE 25-2 Commonly Abused Drugs

UPPERS	DOWNERS	NARCOTICS	MIND-ALTERING DRUGS	VOLATILE CHEMICALS
AMPHETAMINE (Benzedrine®, bennies, pep pills, ups, uppers, cartwheels) BIPHETAMINE (bam) COCAINE (coke, snow, crack) DESOXYN (black beauties) DEXTROAMPHETAMINE (dexies, Dexedrine®) METHAMPHETAMINE (speed, crank, meth, crystal, diet pills, methedrine) METHYLPHENIDATE (Ritalin®) PRELUDIN®	BENZODIAZEPINES VALIUM® (diazepam), XANAX® (alprazolam), RESTORIL® (temazepam), KLONOPIN® (clonazepam) BARBITURATE AMOBARBITAL (blue devils, downers, barbs, Amytal®) PENTOBARBITAL (yellow jackets, barbs, Nembutal®) PHENOBARBITAL (goof-balls, phennies, barbs) SECOBARBITAL (red devils, barbs, Seconal®) ***Other downers***: CHLORAL HYDRATE (knockout drops, Noctec®) METHAQUALONE (Quaalude®, ludes, Sopor®, sopors) NONBARBITURATE SEDATIVES (various tranquilizers and sleeping pills: Miltown®, Equanil®, meprobamate, Thorazine®, Compazine®, Librium® or chlordiazepoxide, reserpine)	CODEINE (often in cough syrup) DEMEROL® (meperidine) DILAUDID®, FENTANYL (Sublimaze®) HEROIN (H, horse, junk, smack, stuff) METHADONE MORPHINE, OPIUM (op, poppy) PAREGORIC (contains opium) ACETOMINOPHEN WITH CODEINE (1, 2, 3, 4)	***Hallucinogenic***: DMT LSD (acid, sunshine) MESCALINE (peyote, mesc) MORNING GLORY SEEDS, PCP (angel dust, hog, peace pills) PSILOCYBIN (magic mushrooms) STP (serenity, tranquility, peace) ***Nonhallucinogenic***: HASH, MARIJUANA (grass, pot, tea, weed, dope) THC	AMYL NITRATE (snappers, poppers) BUTYL NITRATE (Locker Room, Rush) CLEANING FLUID (carbon tetrachloride) FURNITURE POLISH, GASOLINE, GLUE, HAIR SPRAY, NAIL POLISH REMOVER, PAINT THINNER, CORRECTION FLUIDS

Some significant signs and symptoms related to specific types of drugs include those listed in the following text. These are offered to help you recognize possible drug abuse in general. Your patient care may not change as a result of this knowledge, but information you can gather about what kind of drug the patient may have been taking will be useful to hospital personnel.

The following list features signs and symptoms of drug abuse for various types of drugs:

- Uppers: People who abuse these drugs display excitement, increased pulse and breathing rates, rapid speech, dry mouth, dilated pupils, sweating, and the complaint of having gone without sleep for long periods. Repeated high doses can produce a "speed run." The patient will be restless, hyperactive, and usually very apprehensive and uncooperative.
- Downers: People who abuse these drugs are sluggish, sleepy patients lacking typical coordination of body and speech. Pulse and breathing rates are low, often to the point of a true emergency.
- Opioids: People who abuse these drugs have a reduced rate of pulse and reduced rate and depth of breathing, which are often seen with a lowering of skin temperature. The pupils are constricted, often pinpoint in size. The muscles are relaxed, and sweating is profuse. The patient is very sleepy and does not wish to do anything. In overdoses, coma is common. Respiratory arrest or cardiac arrest may rapidly develop.
- Hallucinogens: People who abuse these drugs have a fast pulse rate, dilated pupils, and a flushed face. The patient often "sees" or "hears" things, has little concept of real time, and may not be aware of the true environment. Often what the

patient says makes no sense to the listener. The user may become aggressive or be very timid.

- Volatile chemicals: People who abuse these drugs appear dazed or show temporary loss of contact with reality. The patient may develop a coma. The linings of the nose and mouth may show swollen membranes. The patient may complain of a "funny numb feeling" or "tingling" inside the head. Changes in heart rhythm can occur. This can lead to death.

When reading the just-listed signs and symptoms of drug abuse, you will have noticed that many of the indications are similar to those for quite a few other medical emergencies. As an EMT, you must never assume drug abuse is occurring by itself. You must be on the alert for medical emergencies, injuries, and combinations of drug-abuse problems with other emergencies.

In addition to the effects of long-term drug use and overdose, you may encounter cases of severe drug withdrawal. Withdrawal occurs when the long-term user of certain drugs such as narcotics suddenly stops taking the drug. As in reactions to the use of various drugs, withdrawal varies from patient to patient and from drug to drug.

In cases of drug withdrawal, you may see:

- Shaking
- Anxiety
- Nausea
- Confusion and irritability
- Hallucinations, visual or auditory ("seeing things" or "hearing things")
- Profuse sweating
- Increased pulse and breathing rates.

Patient Care

Care of the Patient with Substance Abuse

Fundamental Principles of Care

Your care for the drug-abuse patient will be basically the same for all drugs and will not change unless you are so ordered by medical direction. When providing care for substance-abuse patients, make certain that you are safe, and identify yourself as an EMT to the patient and bystanders. Since these patients often vomit, take Standard Precautions, including gloves, mask, and protective eyewear as necessary. Be aware of loose hypodermic needles or weapons on the scene that can pose significant risks to you as an EMT.

Emergency care includes the following:

- Perform a primary assessment. Provide basic life support measures if required.
- Be alert for airway problems and inadequate respirations or respiratory arrest. Provide oxygen and assist ventilations if needed.
- If the patient's mental status is depressed enough to cause respiratory failure and your local protocols allow, administer naloxone intranasally.
- Treat for shock. (Treatment for shock will be discussed in the chapter titled *Bleeding and Shock*.)
- Use talking to gain the patient's confidence and to help maintain a level of responsiveness. Use the patient's name often, maintain eye contact, and speak directly to the patient.
- Perform a physical exam to assess for signs of injury to all parts of the body. Assess carefully for signs of head injury.

FIGURE 25-4 Needle tracks on a patient's arm indicate a history of injected drug use. *(© Edward T. Dickinson, MD)*

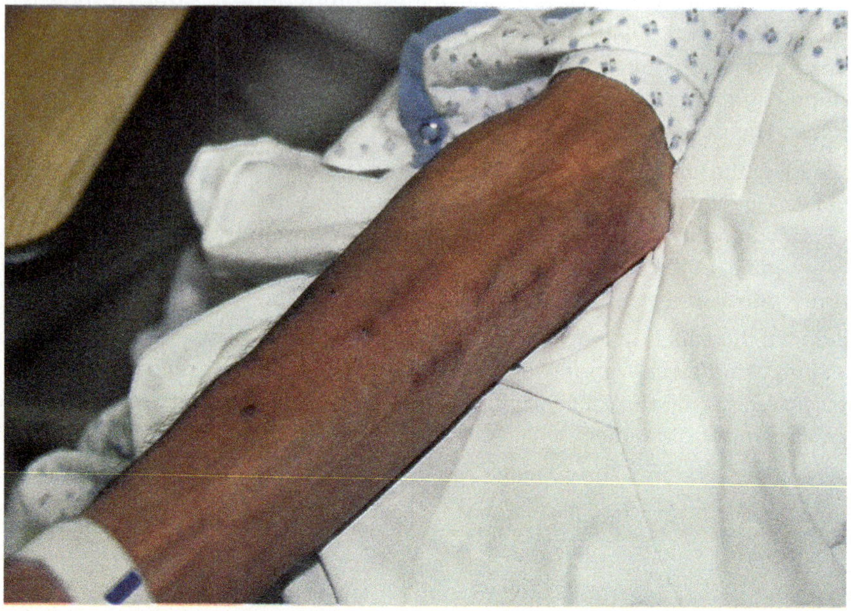

- Look for gross soft-tissue damage on the extremities resulting from the injection of drugs ("tracks"). Tracks usually appear as darkened or red areas of scar tissue or scabs over veins (Figure 25-4). Remember that drugs may be injected in places where track marks won't be visible (e.g., between the toes). Absence of track marks doesn't mean drugs haven't been injected.
- Protect the patient from self-injury and attempts to hurt others. Use restraint as authorized by your EMS system. Request assistance from law enforcement if needed.
- Transport the patient as soon as possible.
- Contact medical direction according to local protocols.
- Perform reassessment with monitoring of vital signs. Stay alert for seizures and be on guard for vomiting that could obstruct the airway.
- Continue to reassure the patient throughout all phases of care.

NOTE: *Many drug abusers may appear calm at first and become violent as time passes. Always be on the alert and ready to protect yourself. If the patient creates an unsafe scene and you are not a trained law enforcement officer, get out and find a safe place until the police arrive.*

When dealing with drug abuse, you must also protect yourself from the substance itself. Many hallucinogens can be absorbed through the skin and mucous membranes. Intravenous drug users may possess hypodermic syringes, which pose a hazard of infectious disease transmission through accidental punctures. Take Standard Precautions and follow all infection exposure-control procedures. Never touch or taste any suspected illicit substance.

Chapter Review

Key Facts and Concepts

- In a poisoned patient, perform a primary assessment and immediately treat life-threatening problems. Ensure an open airway. Administer high-concentration oxygen if the poison was inhaled or injected.
- Next perform a secondary assessment, including baseline vital signs. Find out if the poison was ingested, inhaled, absorbed, or injected; what substance was involved; how much poison was taken in; when and over how long a period exposure took place; what interventions others have already done; and what effects the patient experienced.
- Consult medical direction. As directed, administer activated charcoal or water or milk for ingested poisons.
- Remove the patient who has inhaled a poison from the environment and administer high-concentration oxygen. Remove poisons from the skin by brushing them off or diluting them.
- Transport the patient with all containers, bottles, and labels from the substance.
- Reassess the patient en route.
- Carefully document all information about the poisoning, interventions, and the patient's responses.

Key Decisions

- Is it safe for me to approach the scene and the patient?
- Is the patient breathing adequately?
- How much exposure did the patient have to the poison or drug?
- How is the patient reacting to the poison or drug?
- Are there any specific actions I need to take based on the identity of the poison or drug?

Chapter Glossary

absorbed poisons poisons that are taken into the body through unbroken skin.

activated charcoal a substance that adsorbs many poisons and prevents them from being absorbed by the body.

antidote a substance that will neutralize the poison or its effects.

delirium tremens (DTs) (duh-LEER-e-um TREM-uns) a severe reaction that can be part of alcohol withdrawal, characterized by sweating, trembling, anxiety, and hallucinations. Severe alcohol withdrawal with the DTs can lead to death if untreated.

dilution (di-LU-shun) thinning down or weakening by mixing with something else. Ingested poisons are sometimes diluted by drinking water or milk.

downers depressants, such as benzodiazepines, that depress the central nervous system, and which are often used to bring on a more relaxed state of mind.

hallucinogens (huh-LOO-sin-uh-jens) mind-affecting or mind-altering drugs that act on the central nervous system to produce excitement and distortion of perceptions.

ingested poisons poisons that are swallowed.

inhaled poisons poisons that are breathed in.

injected poisons poisons that are inserted through the skin–for example, by needle, snake fangs, or insect stinger.

opioids a class of drugs that affect the nervous system and change many normal body activities. Their legal use is for the relief of pain. Illicit use is to produce an intense state of relaxation.

poison any substance that can harm the body by altering cell structure or functions.

toxin a poisonous substance secreted by bacteria, plants, or animals.

uppers stimulants such as cocaine and methamphetamine that affect the central nervous system and excite the user.

volatile chemicals vaporizing compounds, such as cleaning fluid, that are breathed in by the abuser to produce a "high."

withdrawal referring to alcohol or drug withdrawal in which the patient's body reacts severely when deprived of the abused substance.

Preparation for Your Examination and Practice

Short Answer

1. Name four ways in which a poison can be taken into the body.
2. What is the sequence of assessment steps in cases of poisoning?
3. What information must you gather in a case of poisoning before contacting medical direction?
4. What are the emergency care steps for ingested poisoning?
5. What are the emergency care steps for inhaled poisoning? For absorbed poisoning?

Thinking and Linking

Patients who are exposed to poisons and drugs sometimes have preexisting medical problems. As you work on this exercise, combine what you have learned in this chapter with material from the assessment chapters and chapter titled Cardiac Emergencies.

1. A middle-aged woman who was in a house fire is out of the house and coughing quite a bit. She was exposed to smoke for up to 10 minutes because she was asleep when the fire started. How should you interpret her pulse oximeter reading? How should it affect your treatment?
2. A despondent older man took his recently deceased wife's medications. Medical direction advises you that one of the medications causes tachycardia. The patient has had a myocardial infarction and has congestive heart failure. He takes nitroglycerin as needed. What should you anticipate may happen to this patient? How should you manage it?

Critical Thinking Exercises

Many pesticides are highly toxic, yet many people who use them refuse to recognize the dangers. The purpose of this exercise will be to consider how you might manage a pesticide-poisoning patient who is in denial.

- A local farmer calls 911, concerned because one of his farmhands has tried to clean up some spilled pesticide powder with his hands. On arrival, you find that the patient insists he has brushed all the powder off, feels fine, and doesn't need to go to the hospital. As he talks, he continues to make brushing motions at his jeans, on which you can see the marks of a powdery residue. How do you manage the situation?

Pathophysiology to Practice

The following questions are designed to assist you in gathering relevant clinical information and making accurate decisions in the field.

1. A young man who kept a rattlesnake was handling it when it bit him on the hand. The area is swollen and discolored. When you call the poison center, the poison information specialist tells you that rattlesnake venom affects primarily the cardiovascular system. What signs and symptoms should you anticipate?
2. What if the snake were a coral snake, and the poison information specialist told you the venom affects primarily the nervous system? What signs and symptoms would you anticipate?

Street Scenes

You and your partner are assigned to the night shift when you are dispatched out for a "possible poisoning." You arrive on scene within 4 minutes to find a 20-year-old female sitting on the couch with a small child in her arms. The female, Anna Prince, states that she is the child's mother, and she believes the child has ingested some lamp oil. The child's name is Maria, and she is 8 months old. Anna states, "I was doing the dishes when I turned around and saw Maria with the oil candle in her hands. I don't know how much she drank or how much she spilled." Maria is crying and coughing excessively, but she is alert and responds to her mother. Her skin is warm, dry, and pink. You also notice that there is some lamp oil on the front of Maria's shirt.

Street Scene Questions

1. **What questions would you ask the patient's mother next?**
2. **What signs or symptoms should you inquire about?**

You continue to gather information about the situation and discover that the exposure occurred approximately 3–4 minutes before 911 was activated. Anna also reports that she neither has the original container that the lamp oil was purchased in nor remembers how much oil was left in the candle. You estimate the total container size to be 100 mL and determine that half of the oil is missing. Anna also reports that she gave Maria some water, but Maria vomited after drinking a small amount.

As you continue with your assessment, you find that Maria has a clear upper airway. Her mucous membranes are pink and moist, and her pupils are equal and reactive to light. Anna states that Maria has been sick lately and that she weighed 20 pounds (9 kg) at her last doctor's visit. Maria is currently taking Children's Tylenol® for fever reduction and has no known medical allergies. The only medical history that her mother reports is a recent fever and mild cough. Maria's current vital signs include a pulse of 140 that is strong and regular, respirations 36 with crying and coughing, and an oxygen saturation of 97 percent.

Street Scene Questions

3. **What treatments would you initiate?**
4. **Should you contact someone for advice? If yes, then whom?**

You provide the patient with blow-by oxygen, setting the flow rate at 10 liters per minute. You place the child in a car seat that is securely anchored to the ambulance stretcher for transport. The mother also is secured, in a seat inside the ambulance. You take the lamp oil candle with you.

You contact poison control, and they advise you that the main concern for Maria is related to aspiration of the oil into the lungs. They advise you that the oil may be a petroleum product with a hydrocarbon base, and that activated charcoal and syrup of ipecac are contraindicated. You also contact medical direction; they agree with the recommendations from poison control and order only supportive care.

During transport, you continually monitor your patient's airway and ventilatory status. When you repeat vital signs, respirations are 32 and slightly labored and pulse is 128, regular, and strong. As you arrive at the emergency department, Maria has stopped crying but continues to cough. No other changes occur during the transport.

Abdominal Emergencies

26

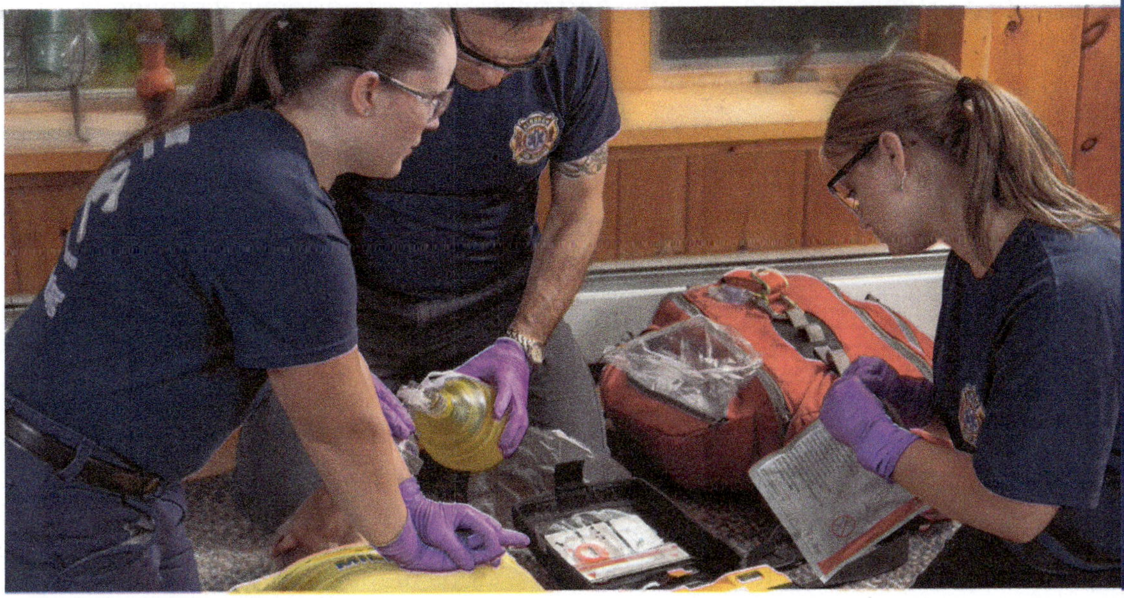

Related Chapters

The following chapters provide additional information related to topics discussed in this chapter:

12 Primary Assessment
15 Secondary Assessment
20 Cardiac Emergencies
29 Bleeding and Shock
30 Soft Tissue Trauma
36 Obstetric and Gynecologic Emergencies

Standard

Medicine

Competency

Applies fundamental knowledge to provide basic emergency care and transportation based on assessment findings for an acutely ill patient.

Core Concepts

- Understanding the nature of abdominal pain or discomfort
- Becoming familiar with abdominal conditions that may cause pain or discomfort
- How to assess and care for patients with abdominal pain or discomfort

Outcomes

After reading this chapter, you should be able to:

26.1 Summarize the anatomy and physiology of abdominal organs. (pp. 727–729)

- Describe the mechanism for visualizing abdominal quadrants.
- Describe the structure of the peritoneum.
- Match abdominal organs with their descriptions.
- Given a visual image, identify the abdominal organs.
- Differentiate between abdominal and retroperitoneal organs.
- List the internal female reproductive organs found in the pelvis.

26.2 Outline the pathophysiology of abdominal emergencies. (pp. 730–734)

- Compare the characteristics of different patterns of abdominal pain.
- Give examples of problems associated with describing abdominal pain.
- Describe characteristics of common causes of abdominal conditions.
- Identify nonabdominal causes of abdominal pain.

26.3 Explain how to prioritize specific steps of managing patients with abdominal pain. (pp. 734–742)

- Recognize elements of the scene size-up that can be clues to abdominal emergencies.
- Identify the significance of a patient's position in suspecting abdominal pain.
- Describe the reason why a thorough history and exam of the patient with abdominal pain are critical, despite limitations in identifying the exact problem.
- Anticipate complications of abdominal conditions that may change the sequence of an EMT's planned approach to care.
- Adapt the approach to history taking to account for a complaint of abdominal pain.
- Adapt the approach to history taking for abdominal complaints to a female patient.
- Recognize complicating factors when assessing geriatric patients with abdominal complaints.
- Outline the approach to physical examination of the abdomen.
- Describe the limitations of palpating for pulsating abdominal masses.
- Describe the approach to reassessment of the patient with abdominal complaints.
- Describe how to make a patient with abdominal pain as comfortable as possible.

Key Terms

parietal pain, *730*
peritoneum, *728*
referred pain, *730*
retroperitoneal space, *728*
tearing pain, *730*
visceral pain, *730*

Abdominal emergencies pose a particular challenge to EMTs. Not only are abdominal complaints somewhat commonplace, but they are occasionally life-threatening emergencies. The very real dilemma faced by today's prehospital professional is sorting out the merely uncomfortable problem from the deadly disorder. Abdominal emergencies can confound even the most sophisticated medical professionals. The sheer number of potential problems may seem overwhelming. Furthermore, unlike external injuries, problems within the abdomen are not visible, and in most cases, you will need to use patterns of symptoms to determine potential criticality and a likely problem.

Fortunately, these challenges can be overcome. The patient assessment process will help you identify those most emergent patients, and although pattern recognition will help you identify the most common abdominal disorders, reaching a diagnosis is often not a high priority. In most cases, the prehospital treatment for a wide range of abdominal conditions is relatively similar and does not require a specific diagnosis. Although you can and should attempt to identify the underlying problem, it is far more important to focus on more important lifesaving steps. This chapter will detail information about assessing and treating abdominal emergencies.

Abdominal Anatomy and Physiology

The abdomen—the area below the diaphragm and above the pelvis—contains a variety of organs that perform digestive, reproductive, endocrine, and regulatory functions. Although we may think the abdomen handles only the digestion of food, in reality, organs and structures within the abdomen do much more, including secreting insulin to regulate blood sugar (the islets of Langerhans of the pancreas), filtering blood and assisting with immune response (the spleen), and removing toxins from the body (the liver). Figure 26-1 shows the structures and organs of the abdomen. Table 26-1 lists the structures and organs of the abdomen with their functions.

The abdomen can be divided into quadrants. Imaginary lines drawn both vertically and horizontally through the umbilicus (the navel) create the four quadrants: right upper quadrant (RUQ), left upper quadrant (LUQ), right lower quadrant (RLQ), and left lower quadrant (LLQ). These quadrants are used to identify and describe areas of

FIGURE 26-1 The structures and organs of the abdomen.

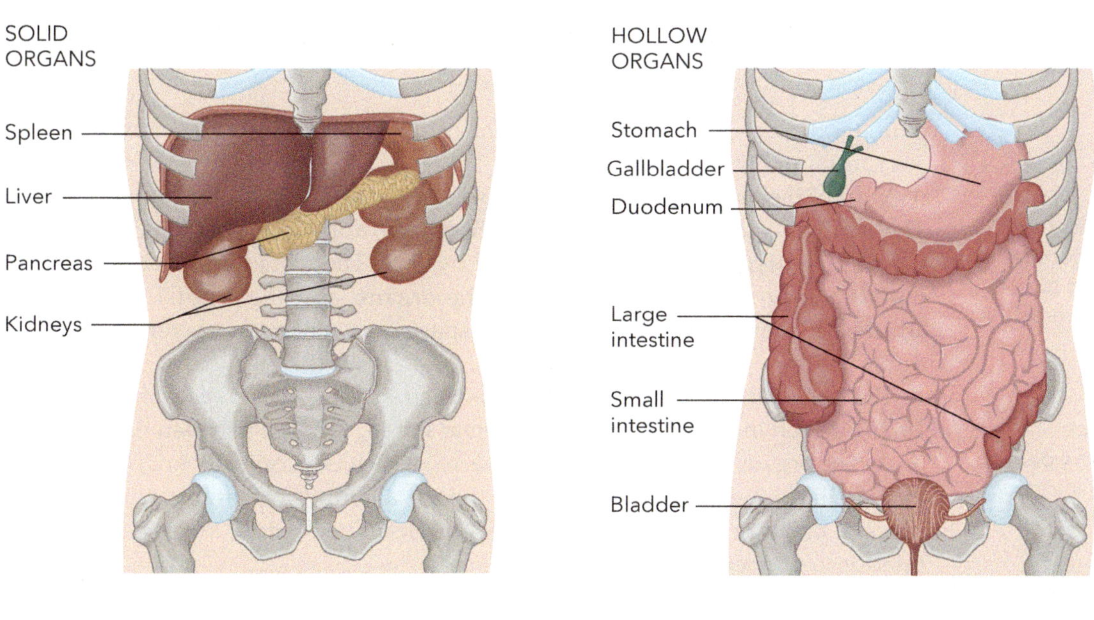

TABLE 26-1 Structures and Organs of the Abdomen

STRUCTURE OR ORGAN	TYPE OF STRUCTURE OR ORGAN	PURPOSE
Esophagus	Hollow digestive	This structure carries food from the mouth and pharynx to the stomach.
Stomach	Hollow digestive	This expandable organ, located below the diaphragm and connected to the esophagus and small intestine, begins the breakdown of foods.
Small intestine	Hollow digestive	The small intestine, consisting of the duodenum, jejunum, and ileum, takes stomach contents and removes nutrients as it passes its contents to the large intestine.
Large intestine (colon)	Hollow digestive	The large intestine absorbs fluid from its contents, creating fecal waste for excretion through the rectum and anus.
Appendix	Hollow lymphatic	This dead-ended sac of bowel rich in lymphatic tissue has no function in digestion. It may become infected (appendicitis), causing pain and requiring surgery.
Liver	Solid digestive; other functions with regulation of the blood and detoxification	This organ is involved in regulating levels of carbohydrate and other substances in the blood. It is involved in bile secretion for digestion of fats and has many other functions, including detoxification of the blood.
Gallbladder	Hollow digestive	This organ stores bile before its release into the small intestine.
Spleen	Solid lymphatic tissue	This organ removes abnormal blood cells and is involved in the immune response.
Pancreas	Solid digestive	This organ releases enzymes that assist in breaking down food in the small intestine into absorbable molecules. It also secretes the hormones insulin into the blood that regulate blood sugar levels.
Kidneys	Solid urinary	These organs filter and excrete waste. They also regulate water, blood, and electrolyte levels and assist the liver with detoxification.
Bladder	Hollow urinary	This organ collects urine from the kidneys prior to excretion (urination).

pain, tenderness, discomfort, injury, or other abnormalities. The abdominal quadrants are shown in Figure 26-2A.

peritoneum
the membrane that lines the abdominal cavity (the *parietal peritoneum*) and covers the organs within it (the *visceral peritoneum*).

retroperitoneal space
the area posterior to the peritoneum, between the peritoneum and the back.

Most of the organs of the abdomen are enclosed within the ***peritoneum*** (Figure 26-2B). These organs include the stomach, liver, spleen, appendix, small and large colon, and in women the uterus, fallopian tubes, and ovaries. There are two layers of the peritoneum: the *visceral peritoneum,* which covers the organs, and the *parietal peritoneum,* which is attached to the abdominal wall. A slight space between the two layers contains a lubricant fluid.

The area outside the peritoneum is called *extraperitoneal space* (refer again to Figure 26-2B), which includes the ***retroperitoneal space***, the area between the abdomen and the back. The organs in the retroperitoneal area, which is technically not part of the abdomen, include the kidneys, the pancreas, and the aorta. This information will be important when types of pain are discussed later in the chapter. The bladder and most of the rectum are inferior to the peritoneum.

FIGURE 26-2 (A) The abdominal quadrants. (B) The peritoneum and extraperitoneal (including retroperitoneal) space in a woman.

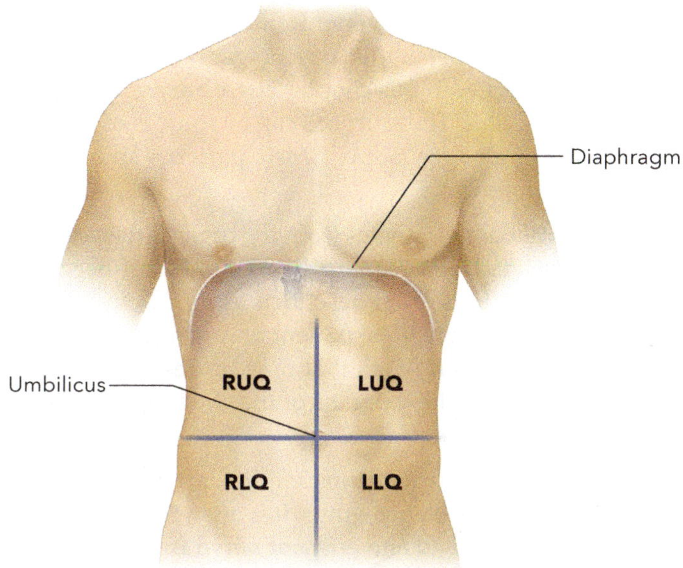

A

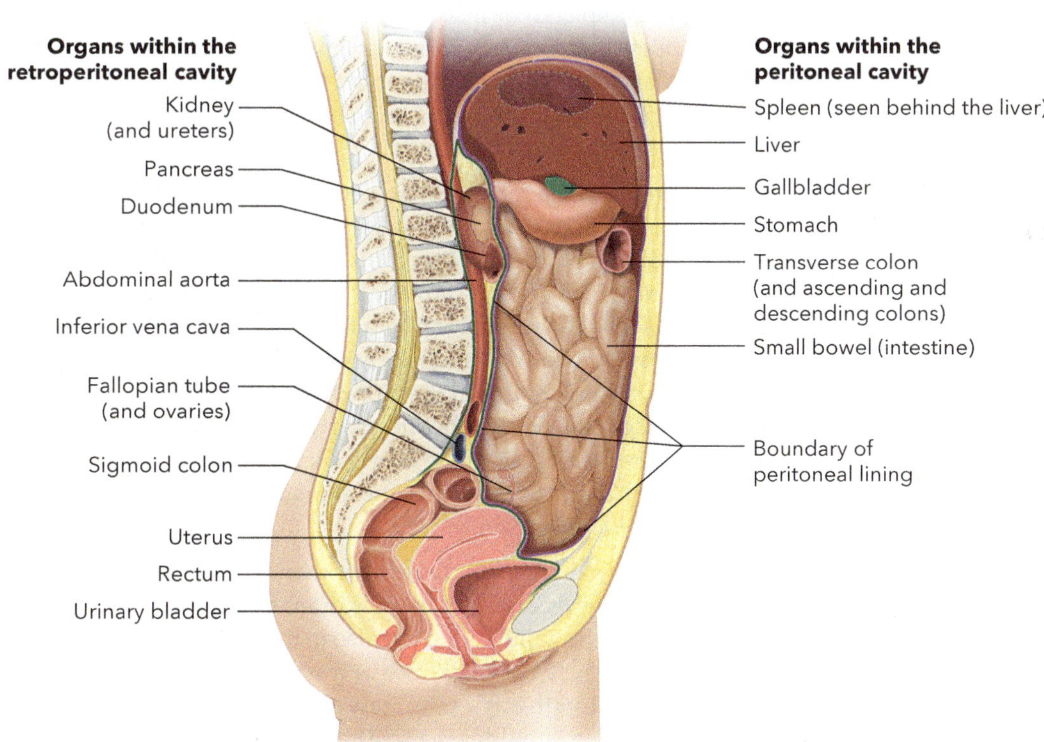

B

The female reproductive organs and structures also lie within the abdomen and pelvis. These include the ovaries, fallopian tubes, and uterus, which may be sources of abdominal pain. The anatomy of the female reproductive system and the assessment and care for related emergencies are discussed in detail in the chapter *Obstetric and Gynecologic Emergencies*.

It is important to remember also that some of the largest blood vessels in the body travel through the abdominal cavity. The aorta, the largest artery in the body, travels down through the diaphragm and traverses the retroperitoneal space. The inferior vena cava also can be found behind the peritoneum. These vessels branch further and form other large blood vessels such as the hepatic and splenic arteries, as well as the iliac artery and vein.

CORE CONCEPT

Understanding the nature of abdominal pain or discomfort

Abdominal Pain or Discomfort

The potential exists for both medical and traumatic emergencies to the abdomen. The traumatic emergencies are covered in the *Soft-Tissue Trauma* chapter. This chapter covers the most common acute (sudden or emergent) medical abdominal emergencies.

As noted earlier in this chapter, there are many organs within the peritoneal and retroperitoneal cavities. These organs can be sources of a wide range of problems or complaints in patients of all ages. Some classic patterns and types of pain involving the abdomen include the following:

visceral pain
a poorly localized, dull, or diffuse pain that arises from the abdominal organs, or viscera.

- ***Visceral pain*** originates from the organs (the *viscera*) within the abdomen. The organs themselves do not have a large number of nerve endings to detect pain. Therefore, visceral pain is often described as dull, achy, or intermittent, and may be diffuse or difficult to locate. (The patient may complain of abdominal pain but cannot point to a specific location.) Pain that may be described as *intermittent*, *crampy*, or *colicky* often comes from hollow organs of the abdomen. Pain that is *dull* and *persistent* often originates from solid organs.

parietal pain
a localized, intense pain that arises from the parietal peritoneum, the lining of the abdominal cavity.

- ***Parietal pain***, as the name implies, arises from the parietal peritoneum, the lining of the abdominal cavity—thus, it is often referred to as *peritoneal tenderness*. Because of its more widespread and efficient nerve endings, pain originating from the parietal peritoneum is easier to locate and describe than pain from the visceral organs.

  Parietal pain is the direct result of local irritation of the peritoneum. Such irritation may be caused by internal bleeding (as from blood leaking into the peritoneum from an injured spleen) or infection/inflammation (such as pain in the RLQ from an infected appendix). Parietal pain is often sharp and constant and is often localized to a particular area. When obtaining the history, you may find patients will describe this type of pain as worsening when they move and getting better when they remain still or lie with the knees drawn up.

tearing pain
sharp pain that feels as if body tissues are being torn apart.

- ***Tearing pain*** is not the most common type of abdominal pain. Most abdominal structures or organs do not have the ability to detect tearing sensations. The exceptions are the aorta and the stomach. In cases of an expanding abdominal aortic aneurysm (AAA), the inner layer of the aorta is damaged and blood leaks from the inner portions of the vessel to the outer layers. This causes a tearing of the vessel lining and pockets of blood resting in a weak area of the vessel. Much like a balloon, the area of collected blood creates an expanding pouch in the blood vessel wall. This is often described as a "tearing" pain in the back. (Remember that parts of the aorta are in the retroperitoneal space. This is why the pain is felt in the back.) Ulcers in the stomach can also cause pain like tearing as they erode or perforate the stomach wall. Patients with this problem also often report "burning" pain as well.

referred pain
pain that is felt in a location other than where the pain originates.

- ***Referred pain*** is pain felt in a place other than where the pain originates. For example, when a gallbladder is diseased, pain is often not just felt in the right upper quadrant (RUQ) area over the gallbladder, but also in the area of the right shoulder and shoulder blade. This is because nerve pathways from the gallbladder return to the spinal cord by way of shared pathways with nerves that sense pain in the shoulder area. Pain referred into the left shoulder is also a common complaint associated with an injury to the spleen.

Abdominal Conditions

Many types of abdominal problems lead to abdominal complaints. Remember that, as an EMT, it is far more important to provide proper assessment and management (including transport) than it is to try to diagnose specific conditions in the field. Although many conditions have "classic" signs and symptoms, there are many patients who do not display them. Some patients may be pain-free with a raging infection inside the abdomen, whereas others may be in agony from a minor irritant. That said, it is reasonable to recognize common features and assemble the pattern to help recognize common disorders. Although diagnosis may not be the most important element of care, often these disorders can be identified through common characteristics.

CORE CONCEPT

Becoming familiar with abdominal conditions that may cause pain or discomfort

Appendicitis

Appendicitis, an infection of the appendix, is the most common cause of a person's needing surgery. About 1 in 15 people will develop appendicitis at some time in their lives. Signs and symptoms include nausea and sometimes vomiting, pain in the area of the umbilicus (initially), followed by persistent pain in the right lower quadrant (RLQ). If the appendix ruptures, the patient will typically experience a sudden severe increase in pain. This is a result of the bowel contents' being let loose into the peritoneal cavity, leading to peritonitis.

Peritonitis

The peritoneum, the lining of the abdomen, is very sensitive to foreign substances. This is especially true with irritating substances such as gastric juices, bowel contents, and blood. The result of such an insult is peritonitis (an inflammation of the peritoneum). Peritonitis may be the result of a medical condition (such as the inflammation of a ruptured appendix) or the result of trauma (such as bleeding from a ruptured spleen). The abdomen typically becomes extremely painful and rigid. This rigidity is an involuntary response of the muscles over the peritoneum. Peritonitis can also be accompanied by fever and other signs of infection. Peritonitis represents a potentially life-threatening emergency. The patient needs prompt evaluation by a physician to determine the appropriate treatment, which is often surgery to control the source of the peritonitis.

Cholecystitis/Gallstones

Cholecystitis is an inflammation of the gallbladder, often caused by gallstones that block the normal flow of bile out of the gallbladder. The patient with this condition will experience severe and sometimes sudden right upper quadrant (RUQ) and/or epigastric (upper central abdomen just below the xiphoid process) pain, which may be referred to the right shoulder. Often this pain is confused with chest pain and may be difficult to distinguish from cardiac complaints. Cholecystitis pain may be caused or worsened by ingestion of foods high in fat and can sometimes end abruptly as a stone frees itself and is passed.

Pediatric Note

The pediatric patient poses a few challenges to abdominal complaints when compared with adults. The pediatric patient may not be able to relate an accurate history or description of the pain. Parents should be called to assist, although they may be upset because the child is sick.

Common conditions in the pediatric patient include gastroenteritis, constipation, urinary tract infection, and appendicitis. Some conditions may be age-dependent, as with young females who are past puberty but still considered children who may experience dysmenorrhea and pregnancy-related pain (e.g., ectopic pregnancy and pelvic inflammatory disease).

The EMT should look for bruising or other clues in the event a recent trauma is now causing pain. Active children may experience an injury but might not mention it to their parents until the pain becomes severe.

Pancreatitis

Pancreatitis, an inflammation of the pancreas, is common in patients with chronic alcohol problems. The pain from pancreatitis is found in the epigastric area. Because of the retroperitoneal location of the pancreas, behind the stomach, the pain may radiate to the back and/or shoulders. This is a serious condition, which in advanced cases can present with signs of shock.

Gastrointestinal (GI) Bleeding

Bleeding from within the GI system can occur anywhere from the esophagus to the rectum. Depending on the size of the source blood vessel, GI bleeding may be gradual or sudden and massive. Because this type of bleeding occurs inside the lumen of the esophagus, stomach, or intestines, blood eventually has to pass out through the rectum and/or through the mouth. Patients may report the passage of abnormal stools that are dark black or maroon in color and tarry in appearance, or they may simply pass frank blood without stool from the rectum. Patients who are bleeding from an upper GI source (the esophagus, stomach, or first portion of the small bowel) may also exhibit vomiting of frank blood or "coffee grounds" vomit. The coffee-grounds appearance is due to the partial breakdown of blood by digestive enzymes.

GI bleeding can be associated with pain but often occurs without pain. Painful GI bleeding most commonly occurs in patients with perforated ulcers in the stomach (gastric ulcers). These lesions are the result of acidic gastric juices wearing a hole in the upper gastrointestinal system. If the erosion eats into a blood vessel, GI bleeding will result. If the acid causes erosion all the way through the stomach or proximal small bowel wall, then this very acidic liquid leaks into the peritoneum, resulting in significant abdominal pain from chemical irritation and peritonitis.

Patients with GI bleeding may present in different ways. If the source vessel of the bleed is a small one, the patient may experience a slow loss of blood, referred to as chronic gastrointestinal hemorrhage. This results in the patient's becoming pale and weak over a period of days to weeks, unaware of the bleeding inside. The body can compensate for most of this blood loss over a period of time, but eventually the patient develops signs and symptoms of shock. If the source of bleeding is from a larger blood vessel, the patient may present with brisk bleeding from the rectum or vomiting of either bright red blood or material that resembles coffee grounds. This type of bleeding is associated with the sudden onset of signs and symptoms of hypoperfusion. The majority of patients with GI bleeding do not have associated abdominal pain.

Patients with esophageal bleeding (often from a condition called esophageal varices) present a particular challenge. The blood vessels of the esophagus can become vulnerable, often due to chronic alcohol ingestion or hypertension in the liver. If these blood vessels rupture, massive upper GI bleeding can occur. The blood from bleeding esophageal varices enters the stomach. The blood is an irritant to the stomach and causes vomiting of copious amounts of blood. This causes shock and can cause airway compromise.

Abdominal Aortic Aneurysm

An abdominal aortic aneurysm (AAA) is a ballooning or weakening in the wall of the aorta as it passes through the abdomen. When the aorta is weakened, it can rupture quite suddenly or leak relatively slowly. It can also dissect, which means that an inner layer of the aorta tears. The high pressures in the aorta spread apart the layers of the vessel, tearing the internal layer of the blood vessel and allowing blood to escape into the weaker, outer layers. As the pressure continues to exert force on the aorta, the area of dissection can spread. In some cases, the dissection spreads so far that it interferes with or even eliminates the blood flow to an artery that branches off the aorta. In this case, you may see decreased perfusion of an extremity with a decreased or absent pulse. Ruptured aneurysms are associated with an extremely high rate of death if they are discovered after they rupture.

You may encounter a patient who is aware of having an aneurysm. Fortunately, the incidence of ruptured AAAs has become less common in recent years with the advent of ultrasound aorta screening of high-risk patients (men over 50 years of age with a history of smoking). Not all are surgically repaired immediately, but they tend to enlarge over time. When patients tell you that they have an aneurysm and have abdominal pain, these are serious emergencies requiring prompt transportation to an appropriate hospital.

Patients with a slowly leaking AAA usually present with gradually developing abdominal pain, which can be described as sharp pain or tearing pain that may radiate to the back. The association of back pain with ruptured AAA is why back pain in older adults is considered a highest-priority dispatch in medical priority dispatch systems. A sudden rupture of the aorta typically causes rapid onset of excruciating abdominal and back pain. Signs of shock are usually present. Depending on the location of the AAA, there may be inequality between the femoral or pedal pulses.

Hernia

A hernia is a hole in the muscle layers of the abdominal wall, allowing tissue—usually intestine—to protrude up against the skin. This can be aggravated by heavy lifting or straining that causes the intestine to push through the weakened area in the abdominal wall. Such a hernia will cause a sudden onset of pain, usually after lifting. A hernia may be palpated as a mass or lump on the abdominal wall or in the creases of the groin (Figure 26-3). Although it may be very painful, it is a life-threatening condition only if the hernia causes an obstruction or twisting of the intestine.

Because pain at the site of a hernia may indicate obstruction or strangulation of the intestine, all patients with a painful hernia should be transported for further evaluation at the hospital.

Renal Colic

Under certain conditions the kidneys may form small, hard stones. If one of these stones begins to descend down the ureter on the way to the bladder, it can cause severe flank pain that often radiates anteriorly to the groin area. The visceral pain from such a "kidney stone" is often severe and may be associated with nausea and vomiting. Patients with this condition are typically described as "writhing" because they move around, trying unsuccessfully to find a position of comfort.

Cardiac Involvement

Pain from a heart attack (myocardial infarction) may be felt as abdominal discomfort. This pain, often described as indigestion or digestive discomfort, is commonly felt in the epigastric region (the area below the xiphoid, in the upper center of the abdomen). All epigastric abdominal pain should be considered cardiac in nature until proven otherwise. Care for this condition is described in the chapter *Cardiac Emergencies*.

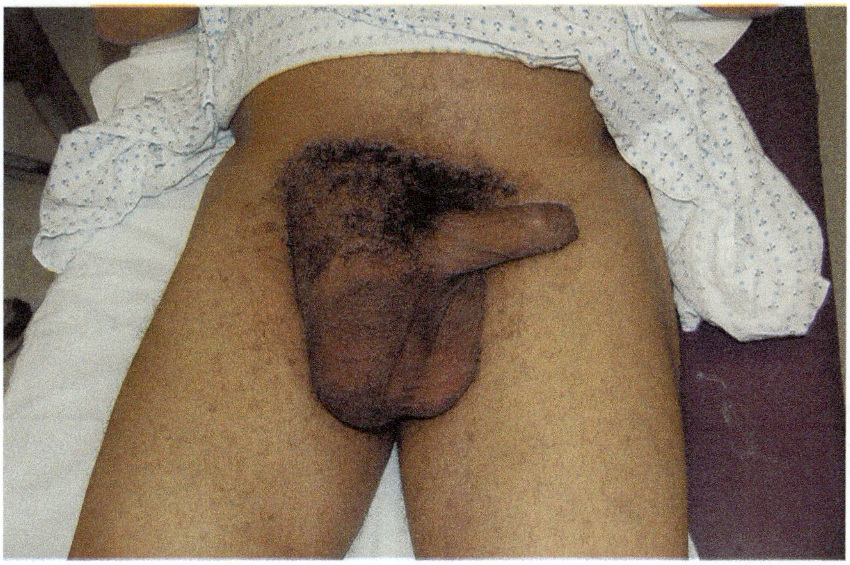

FIGURE 26-3 An inguinal hernia, a protrusion of abdominal-cavity contents through the inguinal canal into the lower right abdominal wall and scrotum. *(© Edward T. Dickinson, MD)*

Abdominal Pain Associated with the Female Reproductive System

Although abdominal pain associated with the female reproductive system will be discussed in the chapter *Obstetric and Gynecologic Emergencies*, it warrants mention here. The most serious cause of abdominal pain related to the female reproductive system is ectopic pregnancy. An ectopic pregnancy occurs when the fertilized embryo implants outside the uterus in the fallopian tube or abdominal cavity. As it grows, it eventually ruptures, frequently causing life-threatening internal bleeding. A rule of thumb is that "all women of childbearing age with lower abdominal pain have an ectopic pregnancy until proven otherwise" by testing at the hospital.

CORE CONCEPT
How to assess and care for patients with abdominal pain or discomfort

Assessment and Care of Abdominal Pain or Discomfort

There are so many potential causes of abdominal pain that the EMT should not be concerned with field-diagnosing a particular cause. Diagnosing can be difficult even in a hospital, where advanced diagnostic tests are available. The focus of your assessment process (Scan 26-1) will be to perform a secondary assessment to describe the condition accurately and identify potentially serious conditions such as shock.

For each of the steps in the assessment process, you may observe specific concerns and points of interest in the patient with abdominal pain.

SCAN 26-1 Assessment of the Patient with Abdominal Distress

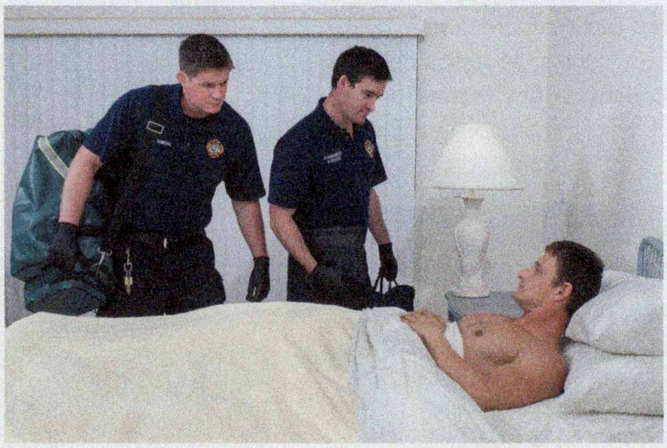

1. Perform a scene size-up.

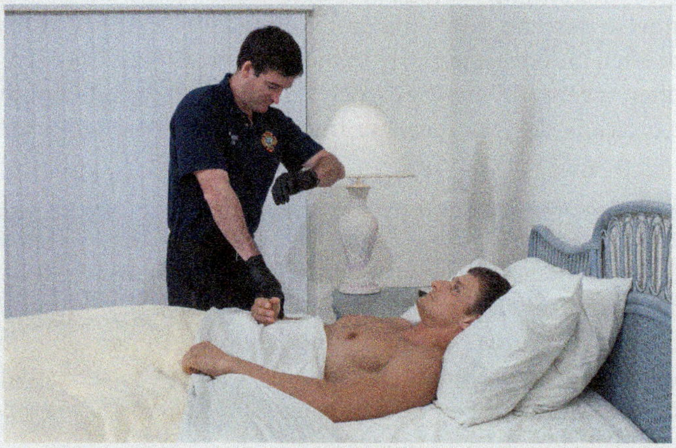

2. Perform a primary assessment and consider oxygen.

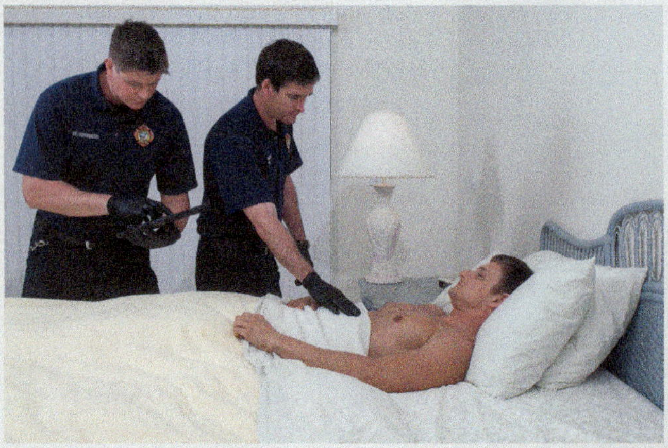

3. Take a patient history.

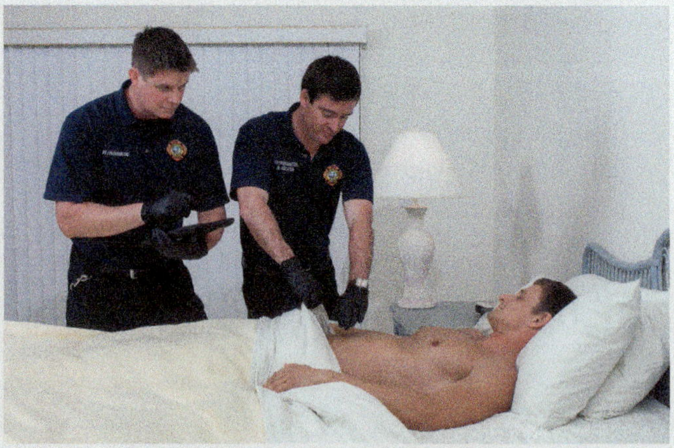

4. Expose the site.

SCAN 26-1 Assessment of the Patient with Abdominal Distress *(continued)*

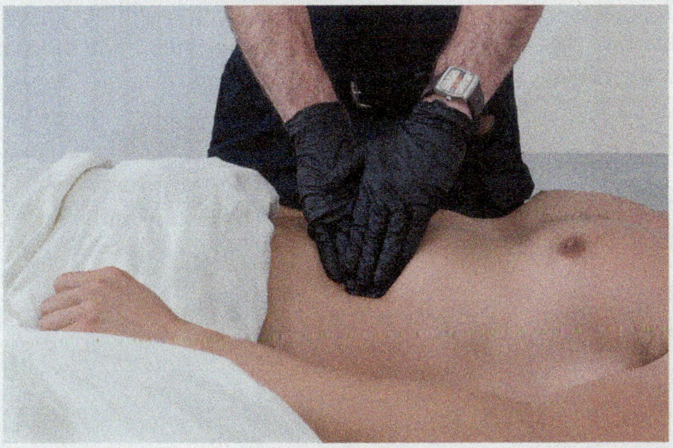

5. Palpate the abdominal quadrants and conduct other physical examinations as necessary.

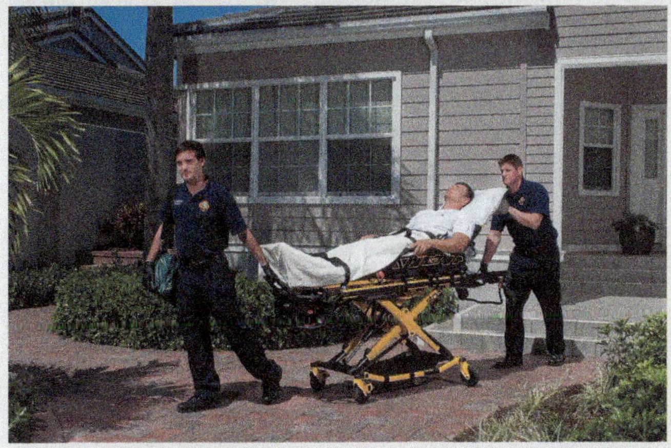

6. Transport the patient.

Scene Size-Up

As you approach and take the important scene size-up steps, be prepared to protect your face and clothes, in case vomiting occurs. Odors can be clinically important. For example, blood in vomit or feces creates a distinctly strong odor. Identifying this odor early will help you identify potential shock. Your search for a mechanism of injury may help you determine if this is a traumatic versus a medical condition.

"Don't forget the importance of the history in a patient with an abdominal complaint."

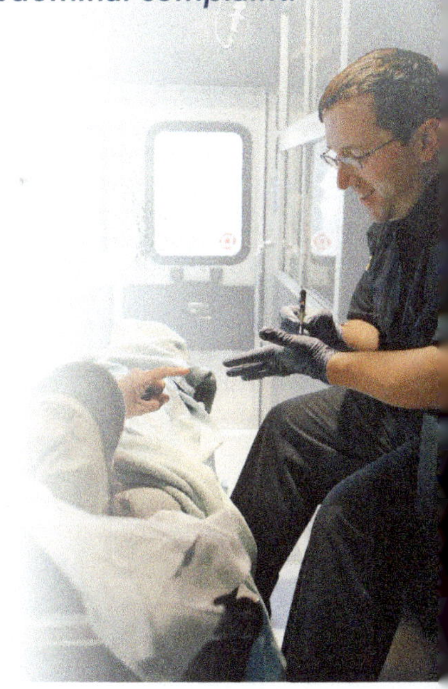

(© Daniel Limmer)

Primary Assessment

The general impression you obtain as you approach the patient will be valuable in determining the seriousness of the patient's condition and the urgency of your care. First, the patient's level of consciousness will help you determine the required airway care. If the patient is conscious, you will be able to begin talking to the patient to gain information. A patient who is talking has an open airway. Unconscious patients require airway care, and any history will be obtained from family or bystanders.

At this stage of assessment, you will be able to notice the early signs of shock. An altered mental status; anxiety; pale, cool, or moist skin; and rapid pulse and respirations will alert you to shock long before you would take a blood pressure or see trends in the blood pressure.

The position of the patient also provides important clues. Does the patient appear to be in pain? Is there guarding of the abdomen (Figure 26-4)? Is the patient in the fetal position?

Consider the application of supplemental oxygen to any hypoxic abdominal-pain patient (as evidenced by oxygen saturation less than 94 percent or signs of hypoxia) or in any situation where an oxygen saturation is deemed to be inaccurate. Maintain saturations of 94 percent using an appropriate oxygen-delivery device, such as a nasal cannula or a nonrebreather mask.

NOTE: *Abdominal pain or discomfort should always be considered an emergency—even if signs of shock are not present.*

History

The history is vital in the assessment of the patient with an abdominal emergency. Be systematic in your interviewing of the patient.

History of the Present Illness

Have the patient describe the pain in the patient's own words by answering your open-ended questions.

FIGURE 26-4 Patients with abdominal pain will often be found in a position of guarding (knees drawn up, arms across the abdomen). (A) Child with abdominal pain. (B) Man in guarding position.

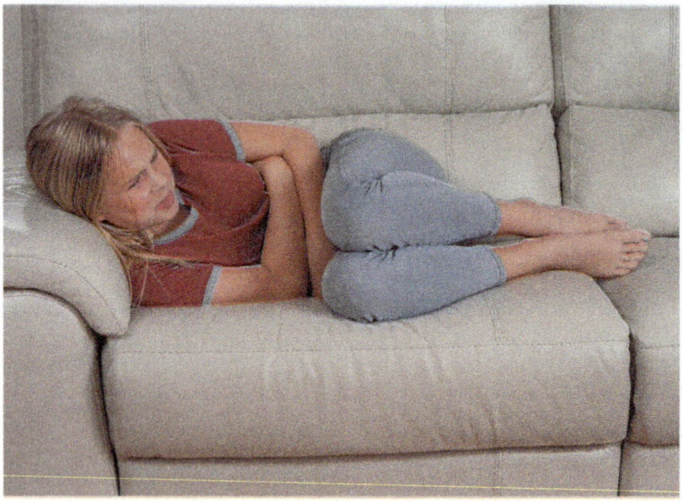

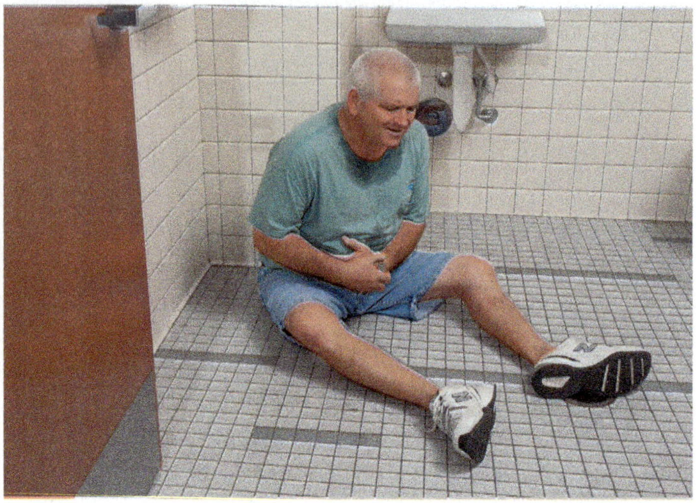

While gathering information about the patient's signs and symptoms, use the *OPQRST* mnemonic (onset, provocation/palliation, quality, region/radiation, severity, time) as a mental checklist to help you elicit information from the patient about the patient's pain or discomfort.

- **Onset.** *When did the pain or discomfort begin? Did it begin while at rest or during activity? How did the pain begin? Did it begin as steady and severe, or did it gradually build to this point?*
- **Provocation/palliation.** *What makes the pain better or worse? Does any position make the pain better or worse? Does movement affect the pain?*
- **Quality.** *Describe the sensation in your abdomen to me.*
- **Region/Radiation.** *Point to or show me where the pain or discomfort is.* (Remember that the patient's pain or discomfort may span more than one region or quadrant, or may be difficult for the patient to localize.) *Do you have pain anywhere else? Does the pain radiate or shoot to other parts of your abdomen, back, or body?*
- **Severity.** *How severe is the pain or discomfort?* Ask the patient to report the pain on a 0–10 scale, and be sure to give parameters, such as "ten being the worst pain you ever had and zero being no pain at all." In children, or in adults with verbal or cognitive deficits, consider the use of a visual pain scale that allows them to quantify pain without using complicated language (Figure 26-5).
- **Time.** *How long have you had the pain or discomfort? Has it changed over time? Is it better or worse?*

FIGURE 26-5 Sample visual pain rating scale. *(EgudinKa/Shutterstock)*

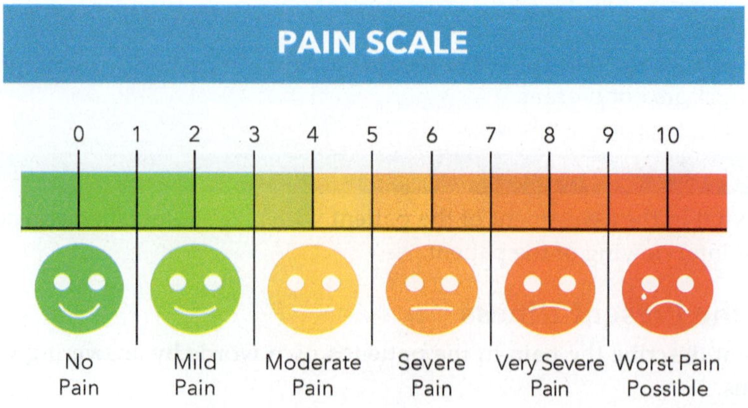

Keep in mind that using only the word *pain* in talking to the patient about the patient's symptoms may cause your history to be inaccurate. If you ask the patient if the patient has "pain" in the abdomen, the patient may reply, "No." The patient may have discomfort, pressure, bloating, cramping, or another sensation that the patient would not call "pain." This response will reduce the effectiveness of your exam, care for the patient, and subsequent reporting. The initial use of open-ended questions will help you to get accurate information in the patient's own words.

History Specific to Female Patients

When female patients, especially those within childbearing years, have abdominal pain, you must ask additional questions as part of the history.

As mentioned, ectopic pregnancy (a pregnancy developing outside of the uterus) can be life-threatening and must be considered in the history. Other conditions, such as ruptured ovarian cysts, pelvic inflammatory disease, and menstrual irregularities, can also cause significant pain.

The questions you will need to ask of a female patient in childbearing years who is suffering abdominal pain are highly personal but important to include in the history. Ask the questions directly, with the terminology taught in class. If the patient senses you are not at ease asking the questions, she will be uneasy answering them. Ensuring privacy for the patient while you ask these questions may help communication. Remember, this is important assessment information.

The following list includes important questions to ask when gathering a female patient's history:

Where are you in your menstrual cycle?

Is your period late?

Do you have bleeding from the vagina now that is not menstrual bleeding?

If you are menstruating, is the flow normal?

Have you had this pain before?

If so, when did it happen and what was it like?

If the patient is within childbearing years, ask if she believes she is pregnant or could be pregnant. If you ask questions such as "Is it possible you are pregnant?" or "Are you sexually active?" it leaves the answer to the patient's judgment.

Some patients may not be fully aware of how one becomes pregnant. Some may not realize that even if they have used birth control devices or techniques, they could be pregnant.

If the answer is "Yes" to any of these questions, suspect ectopic pregnancy. (Even if the answers are "No," pregnancy—with ectopic pregnancy being the potential cause of the patient's pain—is still a possibility.) An ectopic pregnancy is a serious emergency, requiring *immediate* transport to the hospital.

NOTE: *Ectopic pregnancy occurs at the beginning of pregnancy. A patient with an ectopic pregnancy will not "look pregnant"–that is, she will not have an abdomen that appears outwardly pregnant.*

Detailed information on emergencies related to the female reproductive system can be found in the chapter *Obstetric and Gynecologic Emergencies*.

Past Medical History

After you have elicited information about the patient's signs and symptoms (the OPQRST questions) already discussed under History of the Present Illness, continue with SAMPLE history questions pertaining to the patient's allergies, medications, pertinent past history, last oral intake, and events leading to the present emergency.

Allergies. Inquire if the patient has any allergies and, if so, what they are. Remember that the systemic inflammation associated with anaphylaxis can cause abdominal discomfort and diarrhea.

Medications. Ask if the patient takes any medications. This includes over-the-counter, herbal, and illegal medications or drugs. For example, aspirin used to prevent heart attack and stroke can cause bleeding in the stomach. Some illegal substances can cause abdominal distress in use and withdrawal. Diabetics can experience abdominal pain as a symptom of blood sugar abnormalities for which they may be taking prescribed medications.

Pertinent Past History. The patient's medical history may provide information about past problems that may be related to the current problem. If the patient has a history of abdominal problems, ask what these conditions are, whether the pain resembles past experiences with the condition, and what happened last time. (Was it serious? Was the patient in shock? Was surgery necessary?) Certain abdominal conditions that have been present in the past can present chronically. Kidney stones, cholecystitis, and hepatitis are conditions that will likely have a clear past history of similar complaints. A patient's cardiac history with epigastric discomfort may lead you to be concerned for heart attack.

Last Oral Intake. This is very important in patients with abdominal complaints. Determine the patient's last oral intake (liquids, meals, and snacks). In addition, determine if this intake and the intake over the past hours to days have been normal for this patient. Remember that intake of certain substances can be directly related to the current complaint. For example, cholecystitis is often aggravated by foods with high fat content. Chronic pancreatitis is often aggravated by the intake of alcohol.

Events Leading to the Emergency. The events leading up to the call for EMS (similar to the onset question in the OPQRST questions) can help you determine a timeline and progression of signs and symptoms. Ask again specifically about activity (even over the past few days) which seems related to the problem. Vomiting, nausea, diarrhea, and/or constipation are also important history items. Ask specifically if any dark red, bright red, or coffee-grounds–like substances were noted in the vomit or feces, indicating internal bleeding. You should inquire about recent bowel and urinary habits. Some conditions, such as kidney stones, cause painful or difficult urination. Abdominal pain can be caused by difficulty moving the bowels (constipation). Other conditions, such as bowel obstructions, make it impossible to move the bowels. Consider also the history of previous trauma that may have led to a delayed abdominal complaint.

Physical Examination of the Abdomen

Assessment of the abdomen involves two procedures for EMS personnel: inspection and palpation. You may see some health care providers in the hospital auscultating (listening to) bowel sounds. This can be a long process (listening 3 minutes per quadrant) that will not change prehospital care and is not recommended as part of prehospital assessment.

Geriatric Note

Geriatric patients may present some dilemmas when you are assessing abdominal pain. Older people may have a decreased ability to perceive pain. This, of course, makes obtaining a history and description of the pain or discomfort more difficult. It is also important to remember that older patients are likely to have a more serious cause of abdominal pain than younger patients typically have. Research has demonstrated that older adult patients with abdominal pain are up to nine times more likely to die than younger patients with the same cause of the abdominal pain.

Many geriatric patients also take medications (e.g., beta blockers such as atenolol or metoprolol) for high blood pressure or heart conditions, which will reduce the heart rate. These medications may prevent the patient's pulse from rising during shock. An EMT could find a pulse of 72 and think that shock is not present when in fact it is.

Before you physically assess the abdomen, you will have asked the patient where it hurts. The patient may have pointed to a spot or may have moved a hand around an area, indicating diffuse pain or discomfort. This will be important for your physical exam.

First, inspect the patient's abdomen. Look for distention, bloating, discoloration, abnormal protrusions, or other signs that appear abnormal or unusual. You may have to ask the patient or family members whether the current appearance of the abdomen is normal or changed, since body types and shapes vary widely.

Then palpate the abdominal quadrants. Always palpate the area that has pain or discomfort *last*. If this area is palpated first and causes additional pain, it will mask or alter the patient's response to palpation of the other quadrants.

To palpate the abdomen, use the fingertips of several fingers and gently press into the abdomen in each quadrant. While palpating, feel for rigidity or hardening, and ask or observe whether this causes pain for the patient. If the initial gentle palpation does not cause pain or discomfort, you may palpate a bit deeper. Once you have found pain, discomfort, or abnormality, there is no need to palpate further in that area.

You may observe that the patient is guarding the abdomen. The term *guarding* is used to describe two possible presentations: the patient's drawing arms down across the abdomen (review Figure 26-6) or the patient's tensing the muscles before you touch the abdomen. Guarding is a voluntary or involuntary attempt to protect the abdomen and prevent further pain.

In cases of abdominal aortic aneurysm, you may palpate a pulsating mass (abnormal bulge or lump). This mass may be found in conjunction with tearing or sharp pain in the back. This indicates an advanced aneurysm. If you gently palpate this mass, do not palpate it again. Instead, report this mass to the receiving hospital. Some patients may have knowledge of an aneurysm that, when first found, was not serious but has worsened, or was inoperable. This history is important.

Remember that the aorta normally creates a slight sensation of pulsing on deeper palpation of the abdomen, especially in very thin patients (Figure 26-7). The presence of the pulsating *mass* indicates an aneurysm. In larger patients, you will not be able to palpate a mass, even if an aneurysm is present. In this case, the patient's report of tearing pain may be the only indication of a possible aortic aneurysm.

NOTE: *A common assessment error is not assessing the lower quadrants properly. The lower quadrants extend from the umbilicus downward to the pelvis. In most people this extends well below the belt- or waistline and requires loosening of clothing to assess the lower quadrants.*

FIGURE 26-6 Guarding is a common response to abdominal pain.

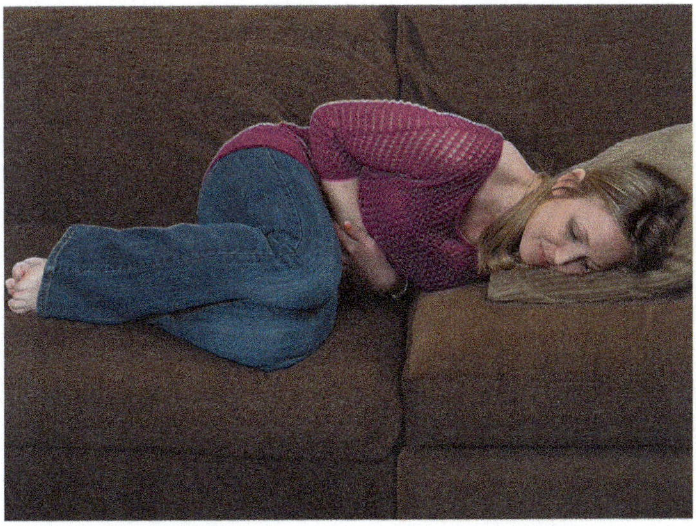

FIGURE 26-7 Palpating the upper quadrants. Adequate examination of the lower abdominal quadrants, well below the beltline or waistline, will require loosening of clothing.

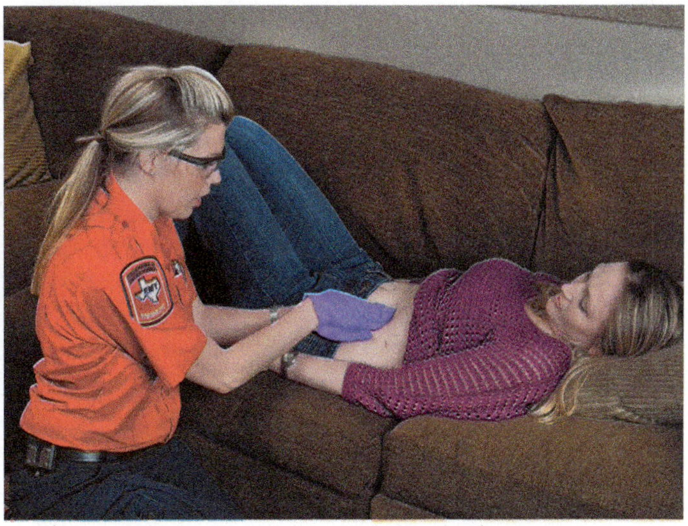

Vital Signs

Vital signs should be taken initially and every 5 minutes thereafter for a patient complaining of abdominal pain. These vital signs are pulse; respiration; blood pressure; skin color, temperature, and condition; and pulse oximetry. Mental status is also important to observe. Remember that shock will appear initially with increased pulse and respirations; pale, moist skin; and anxiety. Falling blood pressure will be a late sign. Shock will be discussed in detail in the chapter *Bleeding and Shock*.

Since patients with abdominal pain may have an increased pulse solely as a result of the pain, serial vitals taken over time will help identify potentially dangerous trends. Calming, placing the patient in a position of comfort, and administering oxygen may actually reduce the pulse, which is a good sign.

Respirations may also be affected by abdominal pain. If breathing worsens the abdominal pain, the patient may be breathing shallowly and sometimes more rapidly.

General Abdominal Distress

You may be called to evaluate patients who have complaints that appear nonspecific but involve the digestive system. Nausea, vomiting, and diarrhea are examples. Some of these complaints will result from digestive system disorders, whereas other causes could be cardiac issues, diabetic issues, food poisoning, or the flu.

Your assessment and care for these patients, like any others discussed in this chapter, will involve performing a proper scene size-up and primary assessment with appropriate airway care. Your history, physical exam, and vital signs assessments will be critical for determining the patient's priority and condition (stable versus unstable).

The assessment techniques discussed previously in the chapter will apply in the same manner to these patients. Determining if there is pain, tenderness, discomfort, or any associated complaints; asking about the time of onset (sudden versus over a period of time); asking about fever and malaise; and abdominal inspection and palpation are all appropriate.

Patient care will involve monitoring for airway problems if the patient is vomiting. Place the responsive patient in a position of comfort. Place the unresponsive patient or the patient who is having difficulty maintaining an airway in a left lateral recumbent position for drainage from the mouth.

You should always work to calm the patient and reduce anxiety. Patients who are in pain will require calming and reassurance.

Never give anything by mouth to a patient with a complaint of abdominal pain or discomfort.

NOTE: *This chapter has talked in great detail about assessment of the abdomen, searching for abnormal findings. Keep in mind, however, that the absence of abnormal findings does not mean the patient's condition is not serious. Patients with abdominal pain should always be considered at least potentially unstable and transported promptly.*

Point of View

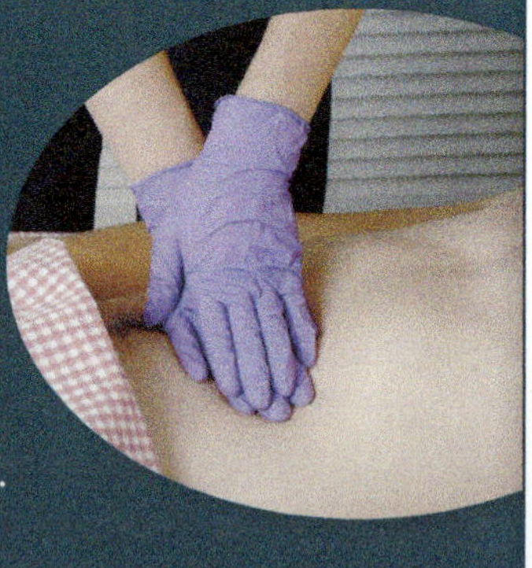

"I went to bed feeling like I had a stomachache. But I woke up with some really bad pain. It was so bad, I could barely roll over and call 911 for the ambulance.

"The EMTs came and started to take care of me. They asked me questions and took my blood pressure. Then they pressed on my belly. Whoa! Did that hurt like a . . . well, I won't use those words here. Trust me. It hurt a lot. I yelled and almost startled the EMT. I know he had to do it to check me out.

"I found out the reason I was in so much pain. It was my appendix. They said if I hadn't gotten to surgery when I did, it may have burst. I'm thankful for what the EMTs did–even if it did almost send me through the roof."

Patient Assessment

Abdominal Distress

To assess a patient suffering from abdominal pain or distress:

1. Perform a scene size-up, looking for clues to a possible mechanism of injury while taking Standard Precautions as well as safety precautions.
2. Perform a primary assessment including the general impression of the patient's level of distress, mental status, airway, breathing, and circulation. Consider oxygen. Make a transport/priority decision. Vomiting may cause airway compromise, so be prepared to suction.
3. Assist the patient to a position of comfort. Calm and reassure the patient. Relaxing the patient will help you complete your next assessment steps.
4. Perform a history, physical examination, and vital signs.
5. Perform a reassessment every 5 minutes en route.

NOTE: *Vomiting and diarrhea will require both strict attention to Standard Precautions during patient care and careful cleaning and disinfection of the equipment and ambulance after the call.*

Decision Point

- Is my patient in shock or developing shock?

Patient Care

Care of the Patient with Abdominal Distress

Fundamental Principles of Care

Although there are many types of abdominal emergencies, the care you will provide for all abdominal conditions is generally the same. You may find patients who appear unstable and obviously have a serious condition as well as others who are in pain yet appear stable. Look for signs of criticality, including pale skin, diaphoresis, and other signs of shock. Severe abdominal pain should also be considered serious until proven otherwise. Remember that abdominal pain may cause the pulse rate to rise.

Much of what we can do for the patient with abdominal pain is supportive care. In every case, despite the differences in patient presentation, you should follow these steps when treating a patient with an abdominal emergency:

- While performing the primary assessment, maintain the patient's airway. If the patient has an altered level of responsiveness, this will compromise the airway. Keep in mind that patients with abdominal emergencies may vomit. Suction whenever necessary.
- Consider the need for oxygen. Administer oxygen to any patient who is hypoxic (as evidenced by a saturation of less than 94 percent or signs of hypoxia). Consider oxygen for any complaint complicated by respiratory distress, or when pulse oximetry is unobtainable or unreliable (such as in shock conditions). Maintain oxygen saturations of 94 percent using an appropriate oxygen delivery device such as a nasal cannula.
- Place the patient in a position of comfort (Figure 26-8). However, if shock and/or airway problems are present, position the patient to treat these conditions. The left lateral recumbent position will help maintain the airway.
- Transport the patient promptly to an appropriate facility.

FIGURE 26-8 Place the responsive patient without airway problems or signs of shock in a position of comfort, and transport the patient to an appropriate facility.

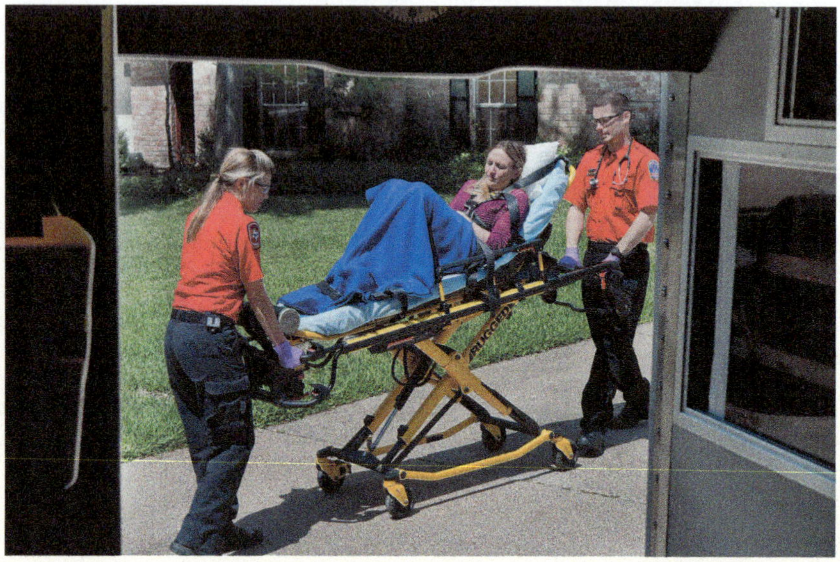

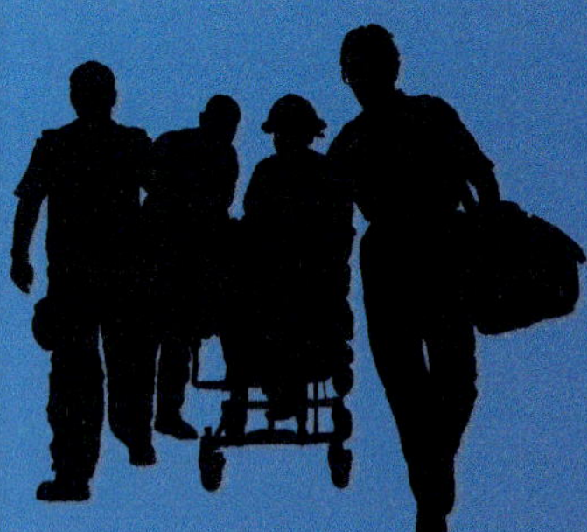

Think Like an EMT

Assessing a Patient with Abdominal Pain

Each patient with abdominal pain will receive a history and physical examination. In the following patient presentations, determine what part or parts of the history or physical examination are missing.

1. A 26-year-old female patient complains of pain in her left lower abdominal quadrant. The pain radiates from the left to the right lower quadrant. She denies allergies or medications. The pain came on while she was sitting at her desk earlier in the day. Her vital signs are pulse 104 and slightly irregular, respirations 22, blood pressure 128/90, skin warm and dry.
2. A 14-year-old boy complains of abdominal pain. It began slowly over a day or two and has gradually become more severe. His parents are present. The patient denies medical history, allergies, or meds. He hasn't eaten since yesterday because of the pain. His vital signs are pulse 96, strong and regular; respirations 20 and adequate; blood pressure 104/72; skin warm and dry.
3. A 56-year-old man complains of severe pain in both lower quadrants of his abdomen, which developed suddenly and without apparent provocation. The pain is intermittent and comes in waves. He has a history of high blood pressure and high cholesterol, and takes medications for both. His pulse is 88, strong and regular; respirations 18 and adequate; blood pressure 158/104; skin cool and moist.

Chapter Review

Key Facts and Concepts

- All patients with complaints of abdominal pain or distress should be transported to the hospital. These cases are difficult to diagnose without the testing resources that are available at the hospital.
- As an EMT, your responsibility is primarily to assess the patient and report your findings. Diagnosing the cause of an abdominal complaint in the field is often more difficult and time-consuming than diagnosing in the emergency department, where there are many more resources.
- Your assessment should include a thorough patient history, physical exam, and vital signs.
- Look for signs and symptoms that can signal serious trouble. These include the sudden onset of tearing pain radiating to the back; vomiting blood or coffee grounds-like material; the presence of black, tarry stools; and signs and symptoms of shock.
- Emergency care will consist of protecting the patient's airway; oxygen as needed; placing the responsive patient in a position of comfort, or placing the unresponsive patient or patient with difficulty maintaining an airway in the left lateral recumbent position; and transporting the patient to the hospital.
- Take all appropriate Standard Precautions and carefully clean and disinfect equipment and the ambulance, especially if the patient has vomited or had diarrhea.

Key Decisions

- Is the patient's airway at risk because of vomiting?
- Is supplemental oxygen necessary?
- Is the patient displaying signs and symptoms of shock?
- Does the patient's presentation suggest any critical problems (e.g., tearing abdominal pain radiating to the back)?
- Do I need to transport this patient immediately for definitive care in a hospital?

Chapter Glossary

parietal pain a localized, intense pain that arises from the parietal peritoneum, the lining of the abdominal cavity.

peritoneum the membrane that lines the abdominal cavity (the *parietal peritoneum*) and covers the organs within it (the *visceral peritoneum*).

referred pain pain that is felt in a location other than where the pain originates.

retroperitoneal space the area posterior to the peritoneum, between the peritoneum and the back.

tearing pain sharp pain that feels as if body tissues are being torn apart.

visceral pain a poorly localized, dull, or diffuse pain that arises from the abdominal organs, or viscera.

Preparation for Your Examination and Practice

Short Answer

1. List five signs and symptoms of abdominal distress.
2. Describe the difference between visceral and parietal pain and describe a condition that may be responsible for each.
3. Describe the emergency care for a patient experiencing abdominal pain or distress.
4. Name the four abdominal quadrants and explain how the quadrants are determined.

Thinking and Linking

Think back to the chapter Cardiac Emergencies, *and link information from that chapter with information from this chapter as you consider the following situation:*

- Your patient is an older adult male with a history of cardiac problems. He is complaining of central chest pressure without radiation. En route to the hospital, he says, "I'm going to be sick." He then vomits approximately a cup of material that looks like coffee grounds. How could the patient's bleeding be connected to his chest pain? What treatment available in an ambulance might help this patient?

Critical Thinking Exercises

Abdominal pain can have many causes and can vary significantly in severity. The purpose of this exercise will be to consider some elements of the history and management for such a patient.

- You are called to a patient with abdominal pain. You arrive to find him sitting on the couch, doubled over with pain. He describes the pain as severe and says it began as "on and off" over the past several days. It became severe within the last hour. What additional questions would you ask the patient? What position would he likely be most comfortable in?

Pathophysiology to Practice

The following question is designed to assist you in gathering relevant clinical information and making accurate decisions in the field.

- Although it is sometimes difficult to determine the cause of abdominal pain in young and middle-aged patients, it is even more difficult for older patients. They often have vague symptoms of abdominal problems rather than the traditional presentations of particular diseases. Describe two of the more likely causes for an elderly patient to have generalized abdominal pain with sustained life-threatening internal bleeding.

Street Scenes

You are dispatched to the Shop-Till-You-Drop supermarket for a "sick woman." You arrive at a scene that appears safe and observe store workers standing around an approximately 75-year-old woman who appears sweaty and somewhat pale. She is sitting in a chair that was brought over by a store employee. The employee tells you that the woman was standing in the checkout line and told the cashier that her stomach hurt and she felt ill. She vomited into the trash can the employee provided, then began to feel a bit weak and dizzy. She was placed in the chair to await EMS.

You introduce yourself and find the woman oriented but looking tired, breathing adequately but a bit rapidly, and having a slightly increased radial pulse. You ask the clerk to bring you the trash can the patient used to vomit. She thinks your request is kind of weird but she complies.

Street Scene Questions

1. What is your initial impression of this patient?
2. What is the significance of the patient's initial presentation?
3. Why would you want to see the trash can?

You ask your partner to administer oxygen and get a set of vitals while you get a history. The trash can contains a considerable amount of a reddish-brown substance you believe may be partially digested blood. You radio for advanced life support before you begin the history and realize the patient must be transported promptly.

Street Scene Questions

4. Why would you request advanced life support?
5. What findings convinced you to request advanced life support and make the patient's transport a high priority?

The patient reports diffuse pain across the upper abdominal quadrants that has been increasing slightly over the past few days. It is not worsened or made better by anything in particular and is slightly tender to palpation. No rigidity is noted. She has eaten and drunk normally over the past several days and has no history of abdominal problems. She had one "mini-stroke" a few months ago. She takes an unknown blood pressure medication and an aspirin a day to prevent further strokes. Her pulse is 104, respirations 26, blood pressure 102/68, skin pale and moist.

You promptly move the patient to the stretcher and into the ambulance. An ALS engine arrives and a paramedic arrives with her equipment. You explain that you are concerned about a potentially serious condition and shock. The paramedic agrees.

Street Scene Questions

6. Do you believe this patient is in shock? Explain your reasoning.
7. What effect might her history have on her current condition?
8. In what position should this patient be placed?

Because of the patient's apparent history of high blood pressure, you think that the blood pressure of 102/68, which would usually not be considered low, may actually indicate shock for this patient. The paramedic thinks that the aspirin taken for stroke prevention may have caused bleeding in the patient's stomach.

The paramedic begins advanced care, including an IV and electrocardiogram. As a precaution, she checks the patient's blood sugar level and finds it is within normal limits. The paramedic obtains a second set of vital signs: pulse 112, respirations 28, blood pressure 100/64, skin unchanged. The patient insists on sitting up because she feels she may vomit again.

You arrive at the hospital a short time later and make a report to the physician. The patient is, in fact, bleeding internally, and will be admitted for further care.

Behavioral and Psychiatric Emergencies and Suicide

27

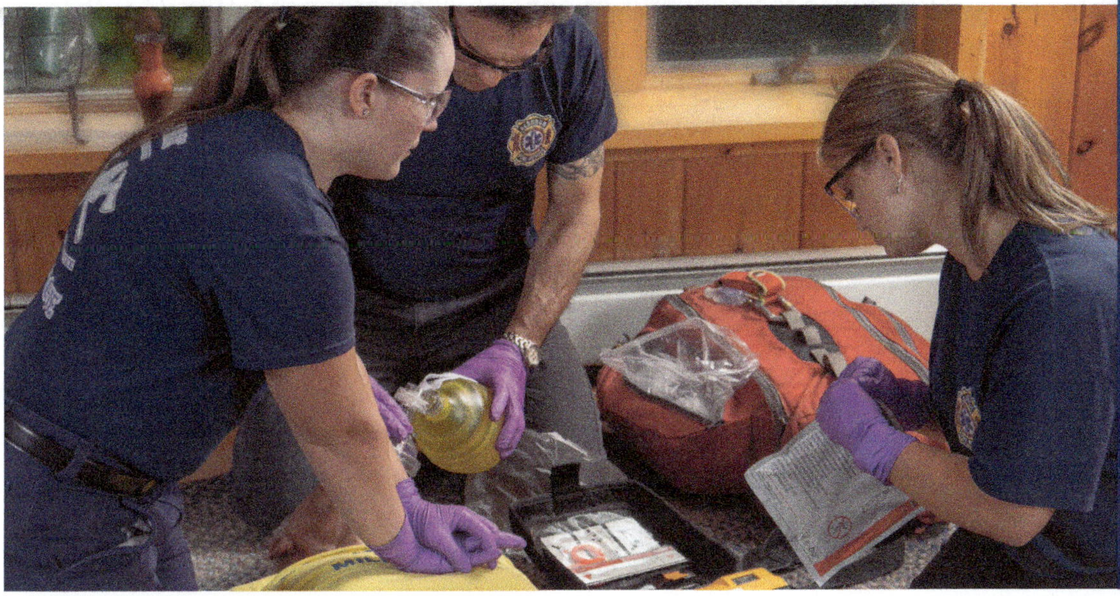

Related Chapters

The following chapters provide additional information related to topics discussed in this chapter:

Standard

Medicine (Psychiatric)

Competency

Applies fundamental knowledge to provide basic emergency care and transportation based on assessment findings for an acutely ill patient.

Core Concepts

- The nature and causes of behavioral and psychiatric emergencies
- Emergency care for behavioral and psychiatric emergencies
- Emergency care for potential or attempted suicide
- Emergency care for aggressive or hostile patients
- When and how to restrain a patient safely and effectively
- Medical/legal considerations in behavioral and psychiatric emergencies

Outcomes

After reading this chapter, you should be able to:

27.1 Summarize the concepts of behavioral emergencies. (pp. 747-751)

- Describe the factors that interact to determine if a patient's behavior constitutes an emergency.
- Identify the contribution of psychiatric conditions to the incidence of behavioral emergencies.
- Identify the rationale for prescribing drugs that affect neurotransmitters.
- Describe the pathophysiology by which physical conditions can result in altered behavior.
- Recognize signs of hostility and potential for violence against the patient's self or others.
- Describe approaches to preventing patients who are hostile or violent from harming themselves or others.
- Recognize common presentations that indicate psychiatric emergencies.

27.2 Integrate knowledge of behavioral emergencies into the overall care of specific patients. (pp. 751-755)

- Explain how to safely and compassionately treat a patient with behavioral emergencies.
- Give examples of how a thorough history can contribute to determining the underlying cause of a behavioral emergency.
- Recognize risk factors for suicide.
- Describe the priorities of care for patients who have attempted suicide.
- Explain the decision making related to care of a patient with a behavioral emergency.

27.3 Explain the decision-making process in the use of patient restraints. (pp. 755-760)

- Identify public safety personnel who may be required to assist with restraint procedures.
- Describe the concept of using reasonable force in restraint.
- Explain the phenomenon of excited delirium.
- Distinguish between safe and unsafe restraint procedures.
- Describe how restraint can lead to positional asphyxia.
- Describe the actions to be taken after a patient is restrained.
- Identify reasons the EMT should avoid being alone with patients with behavioral and psychiatric emergencies.

Key Terms

behavior, *747*
behavioral emergency, *747*
excited delirium, *757*
neurotransmitters, *748*
positional asphyxia, *757*
schizophrenia, *750*

How would you define normal behavior? For most of us, this is a very complicated question with no simple answer. Acting "normal" is quite dependent on the circumstances and setting that you are in. Although someone would not normally burst into tears while at the office, we might think this response was quite reasonable if that person had just received word that a close family member passed away. Similarly, your instructor might think it was quite abnormal for you to fall asleep halfway through class but would have an easier time understanding if you let him know you had been up all night caring for a sick child. The bottom line is that the way we act is heavily influenced by the challenges we face and our capability to respond to environmental stimuli or stress.

Occasionally, a person's ability to interact with the person's environment and to handle challenges is impaired. As you learned in previous chapters, this often results from illness or injury, or even substance abuse. However, there are times when a patient becomes impaired not because of a physical problem, but rather because that person's brain has lost its capacity to respond to the world around it in a manner we have come to expect. In these cases, responses may be inappropriate, unusual, and sometimes even dangerous to themselves or others.

These patients can be particularly challenging. They can be difficult to interact with and even pose a safety risk to the EMT. In addition, behavioral problems can sometimes be difficult to distinguish from the effects of other illnesses and injuries, and can often mask very real and very dangerous underlying medical conditions.

As an EMT, you are first and foremost an advocate for your patient, and it must be remembered that regardless of how challenging these situations can be, behavioral emergencies are *true emergencies* and represent very real crises for your patients. You must take steps to properly and carefully assess and treat both physical and emotional issues. It is the responsibility of all health care professionals to recognize the very real danger to the patient associated with psychiatric emergencies, and to understand that these issues are no less important or real than the more common medical complaints.

Behavioral and Psychiatric Emergencies

What Is a Behavioral Emergency?

We all exhibit behavior. ***Behavior*** is defined as the manner in which a person acts or performs. It involves any or all activities of a person, including physical and mental activity. Of course, behavior differs from person to person and from situation to situation. In fact, normal behavior is quite dependent on the circumstances a person faces. Everyone has good and bad days. We face tragedy and wonderful situations that require very different responses. We judge "normal" behavior based on the appropriateness of response in any given setting. Behavior is largely defined by those around us and based on the way we usually act. For example, grief would be an appropriate response to a tragedy but would be deemed abnormal when, after months or years, it continued to interfere with day-to-day activity and disrupted the patient's ability to interact with others.

behavior
the manner in which a person acts.

CORE CONCEPT
The nature and causes of behavioral and psychiatric emergencies

A ***behavioral emergency*** exists when a person exhibits abnormal behavior within a given situation that is unacceptable or intolerable to the patient, the family, or the community. Frequently, behavioral emergencies involve behavior that is potentially harmful to the patient or to the people that interact with the patient.

behavioral emergency
when a patient's behavior is not typical for the situation; when the patient's behavior is unacceptable or intolerable to the patient, the patient's family, or the community; or when a patient may harm self or others.

A key part of that definition is "within a given situation." You may have observed, in your own life or in those of friends or family, that behavior varies, depending on the situation at hand. For example, if a person is notified unexpectedly of the death of a loved one, common reactions might include screaming, crying, throwing things, or other emotional outbursts. In the context of the situation, this behavior would not be unusual. If the same behaviors were exhibited for no apparent reason in the middle of an ordinary shopping trip, they might indicate a behavioral emergency.

Remember that you will be exposed to persons from other cultures and people with different lifestyles. Some behaviors may seem unusual to you but might be quite normal to the person performing them. Behavioral conditions require full patient assessment, including primary and secondary assessments, just as with any other emergency. Remain objective. Do not judge patients hastily or solely on the way they look or act.

Behavior and Brain Chemistry

neurotransmitters chemicals within the body that transmit a message in the brain from the distal end of one neuron to the proximal end of the next neuron.

The behavior you see on the outside is largely controlled by ***neurotransmitters*** inside the body—specifically the brain. Medications that target these behavioral conditions help maintain proper levels and interactions of neurotransmitters.

The nervous system works through the use of neurotransmitters. Electrical impulses travel along neurons until they reach a synapse—a space between nerve cells. Neurotransmitters are chemicals within the body that transmit messages from the distal end of one neuron (the presynaptic neuron) to the proximal end of the next neuron (postsynaptic neuron). Although it sounds like a complicated process, it actually takes only milliseconds to occur.

Neurotransmitters are released from a neuron, then travel across the synapse to the next neuron. The receptors on the postsynaptic neuron receive the neurotransmitter. This is the mechanism by which the impulse is moved along the nervous system. After the impulse is transmitted, the neurotransmitter goes through a process called *reuptake,* in which the neurotransmitter is returned to the presynaptic neuron.

Neurotransmitters—or the lack of neurotransmitters—have been implicated in depression and other behavioral and psychiatric disorders. Medications prescribed for these conditions are designed to affect the relevant neurotransmitters. One commonly prescribed class of drugs is the *selective serotonin reuptake inhibitor (SSRI).* This medication is believed to elevate mood by preventing the reuptake of the neurotransmitter serotonin in the synapse. Prozac® (fluoxetine), Paxil® (paroxetine), Zoloft® (sertraline), Celexa® (citalopram), and Lexapro® (escitalopram) are trade and generic names, respectively, of commonly prescribed SSRI medications.

Newer medications offer reuptake inhibition of more than one neurotransmitter. In addition to serotonin, neurotransmitters include norepinephrine, epinephrine, and dopamine.

Psychiatric Conditions

Some, but not all, behavioral emergencies are caused by psychiatric conditions, which may also be called mental disorders.

According to the National Institute of Mental Health's 2016 statistics, 44.7 million adults suffer from a mental illness of some kind. That translates to approximately one in five adults in the United States About 9.2 million adults have concurrent mental health and addiction disorders. Based on these statistics, it is clear you will be called to deal with people experiencing psychiatric crises. Because of declining or overcrowded mental health services in some areas, more patients with mental illness are in the community with minimal treatment. This makes it more likely they will be seen as a patient by EMS systems.

This chapter will help you understand and care for this significant patient population.

Physical Causes of Altered Mental Status

It is helpful to consider patients who are exhibiting crises or unusual behaviors to be having an altered mental status from a *non*psychiatric cause until proven otherwise. Many medical and traumatic conditions are likely to alter a patient's behavior. These problems may include:

- Low blood sugar, which may be the cause of rapid onset of erratic or hostile behavior (similar to alcohol intoxication), dizziness and headache, fainting, seizures, sometimes coma, profuse perspiration, hunger, drooling, and rapid pulse but normal blood pressure (See the chapter *Diabetic Emergencies and Altered Mental Status.*)

- Lack of oxygen, which may cause restlessness and confusion, cyanosis (blue or gray skin), and altered mental status
- Stroke or inadequate blood to the brain, which may cause confusion or dizziness, impaired speech, headache, loss of function or paralysis of extremities on one side of the body, nausea and vomiting, and rapid full pulse
- Head trauma, which can cause personality changes ranging from irritability to irrational behavior, altered mental status, amnesia or confusion, irregular respirations, elevated blood pressure, and decreasing pulse (See the chapter *Trauma to the Head, Neck, and Spine.*)
- Seizures, which cause varied levels of abnormal movement from inattention to lip smacking to tonic–clonic motion. Postictal states may present as altered mental status.
- Mind-altering substances, which can cause highly variable signs and symptoms depending on the substance ingested (See the chapter *Poisoning and Overdose Emergencies.*)
- Environmental temperature extremes. Excessive cold may cause shivering, feelings of numbness, altered mental status, drowsiness, staggering walk, slow breathing, and slow pulse. Excessive heat may cause decreased or complete loss of consciousness. (See the chapter *Environmental Emergencies.*)

When dealing with someone who appears to be having a behavioral emergency, always consider the possibility that the patient's unusual behavior is caused by something other than a psychological problem (Figure 27-1). Use a thorough patient assessment to try to identify findings consistent with medical or traumatic causes before assuming a psychiatric condition exists. Remember also that medical conditions can coexist with

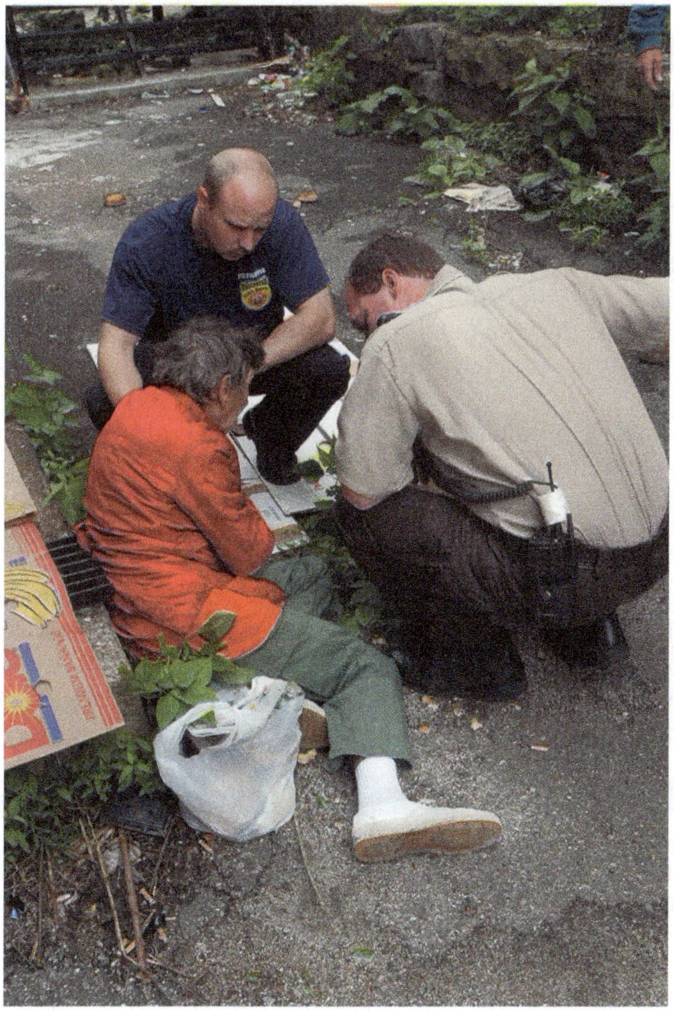

FIGURE 27-1 There are many reasons a patient may experience an altered mental status. *(Mark Ide/Science Source)*

underlying psychiatric or behavioral issues, sometimes making chronic behavioral symptoms worse. The *Diabetic Emergencies and Altered Mental Status* chapter discussed many of the common causes of altered mental status.

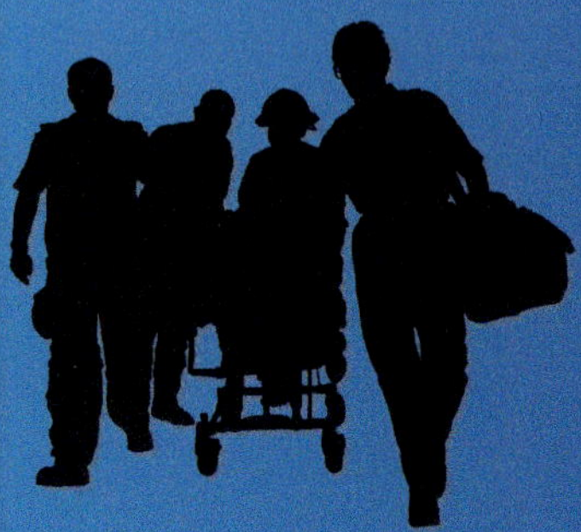

Think Like an EMT

Psych Condition or Hidden Medical Condition?

You will respond to many behavioral emergencies during your EMS experience. Sometimes patients with medical problems appear to be psychiatric patients, but they actually aren't. Other times patients with a psychiatric history have medical problems that aren't related to their psychiatric condition. For each of the following patients, describe how your assessment would determine whether the patient is suffering from a medical problem or a psychiatric problem.

1. Your patient is a 56-year-old man who was found to be "talking to God" and generally mumbling at the grocery store.
2. Your patient is a 21-year-old student who was found on the outskirts of his campus, acting strangely, with a slight smell of alcohol on his breath.
3. Your patient is an 84-year-old woman who is in a nursing home. She has a history of depression and cardiac problems. This morning she became agitated and angry with the staff.

Situational Stress Reactions

When faced with severe, unexpected stress, most patients will display emotions such as fear, grief, and anger. These are typical stress reactions at an accident scene and common reactions to serious illness and death. In the vast majority of cases, as you begin to take control of the situation and treat the patient as an individual, your personal interaction with the patient will inspire confidence in your ability to help. The patient will begin to calm down and may even feel able to cope with the emergency.

Be as unhurried as you can. If you rush your patient assessment and interview, patients may feel as if the situation is out of control. Patients also may believe that you are concerned about the problem but not about them. Let patients know that you are there to help.

Whenever you care for a patient who is displaying typical stress reactions, act in a calm manner, giving the patient time to regain emotional control. Quietly and carefully evaluate the situation, keeping your own emotions under control. Communicate that you are listening to what the patient is saying, and honestly explain things to the patient. Stay alert for sudden changes in behavior.

By acting in this manner, you are applying crisis management techniques to help the patient deal with stress. If the patient does not begin to calm down, and if there are no apparent medical causes for the behavior, you must assume that there is a problem of a more serious psychiatric nature. Proceed according to the recommendations in the following segments of this chapter.

schizophrenia
a chronic mental disorder that affects how a person thinks, feels, and behaves. People with severe or untreated schizophrenia may seem like they have lost touch with reality.

Acute Psychosis

Some emergencies are psychiatric rather than just behavioral, involving a severe break in patients' abilities to process information and interact with their environments. This kind of psychiatric emergency is often associated with a psychiatric disorder such as ***schizophrenia***. *Acute psychosis* occurs when the patient develops one or more of the following symptoms: hallucinations, delusions, catatonia, or a profound thought disorder. *Hallucinations* are inappropriate sensory observations such as visions or voices. Auditory hallucinations (hearing voices) are typical in acute psychosis from a psychiatric cause. Visual hallucinations can occur with acute psychosis, but they can also be associated with medical causes such as drug intoxication and alcohol withdrawal. *Delusions* are falsely held beliefs such as paranoia, the belief that one is being persecuted when that is not the case. *Catatonia* is characterized by either an almost complete noninteraction with the environment or wild and completely inappropriate movements and interactions. Finally, *thought disorders* impact a patient's ability to process information and to communicate, and can cause unusual speech patterns or strange writing.

Patients suffering acute psychosis can be particularly challenging, as they do not interact or respond as we would normally expect. Stimuli from hallucinations or delusions can cause severely erratic behavior. Great care should be taken not only to ensure the safety of the patient and responders but also to provide a sense of calm and gentle control to an otherwise out-of-control situation.

Emergency Care for Behavioral and Psychiatric Emergencies

Assessment and Care for Behavioral and Psychiatric Emergencies

CORE CONCEPT
Emergency care for behavioral and psychiatric emergencies

Behavioral and psychiatric problems have a wide variety of manifestations and presentations. One patient may be withdrawn and might not wish to communicate, whereas another may be agitated, talkative, or exhibiting bizarre or threatening behavior. Some patients may act as if they wish to harm themselves or others.

It is absolutely essential that you ensure scene safety before approaching a patient suffering from a behavioral emergency. Psychiatric and substance-abuse issues make predicting behavior extremely difficult, and sometimes unusual responses to the environment manifest as dangerous acts. Always take steps to protect yourself and your crew before interacting with any unusual behavioral situation. Enlist law enforcement if there is any question regarding safety.

Although every behavioral emergency is slightly different, it is generally important to provide a professional and calm atmosphere. In many cases your actions will serve to de-escalate an otherwise out-of-control situation. Providing a caring and compassionate setting while maintaining control is essential. Here are key techniques to consider:

- Identify yourself and your role.
- Speak slowly and clearly. Use a calm and reassuring tone.
- Make eye contact with the patient.
- Listen to the patient. You can show you are listening by repeating part of what the patient says back to the patient.
- Do not be judgmental. Show compassion, not pity.
- Use positive body language. Avoid crossing your arms or looking uninterested.
- Acknowledge the patient's feelings.
- Do not enter the patient's personal space. Stay at least 3 feet from the patient. Making the patient feel closed in can cause an emotional outburst.
- Be alert for changes in the patient's emotional status. Watch for increasingly aggressive behavior, and take appropriate safety precautions.
- Use restraint to prevent harm if necessary.

Patient Assessment

Behavioral or Psychiatric Emergency

To assess a patient who appears to be suffering a behavioral or psychiatric emergency:

- Perform a careful scene size-up. If there are indications at the time of dispatch that the call may involve a potentially violent or agitated patient, then police should be requested to respond to the scene, arriving ahead of EMS units to ensure the scene is safe ("secure") for EMS to enter (Figure 27-2).
- Identify yourself and your role. It may not be obvious to the patient who you are and what you intend to do.
- Complete a primary assessment, including assessment of the patient's mental status (level of responsiveness; orientation to person, place, and time). Remember that altered mental status can frequently be caused by hypoxia and shock.
- Perform as much of the detailed examination as possible. Be alert for medical and traumatic conditions that could be causing the patient's behavior.
- Gather a thorough patient history. This will alert you to past psychiatric problems, or psychiatric medications the patient may be taking (or not taking, causing the agitation). This may also alert you to conditions such as diabetes that can closely mimic a psychiatric condition. Consider the possibility of toxins or substance abuse.

The following are common presentations, or signs and symptoms, of patients experiencing psychiatric emergencies:

- Panic or anxiety
- Unusual appearance, disordered clothing, or poor hygiene
- Agitated or unusual activity, such as repetitive motions, threatening movements, or withdrawn stance
- Unusual speech patterns, such as too-rapid or pressured-sounding speech (as if being forced out), or an inability to carry on a coherent conversation
- Bizarre behavior or thought patterns
- Suicidal or self-destructive behavior
- Violent or aggressive behavior with threats or intent to harm others

Decision Points

- Is the scene safe?
- Is my patient having a behavioral/psychiatric crisis, or is this an altered mental status from a physical cause?

FIGURE 27-2 **Suicide scenes involving poisonous gas (carbon monoxide or other) can present dangers to emergency responders.**

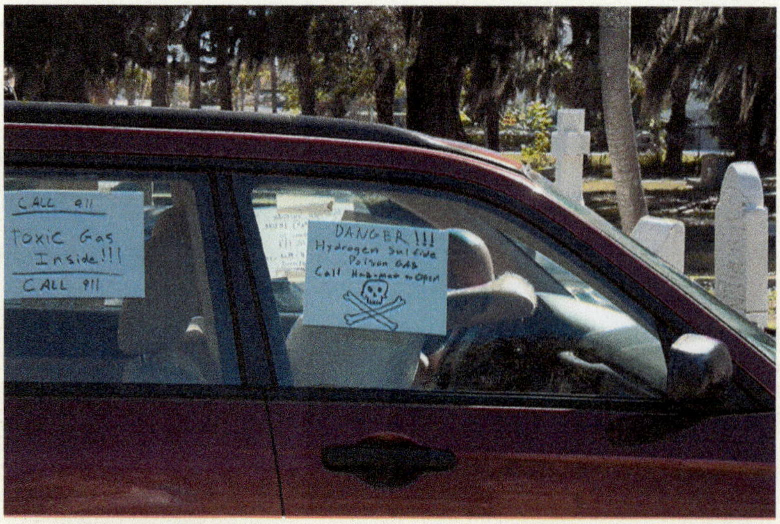
CALL 911
Toxic Gas
Inside!!!
CALL 911
DANGER!!!
Hydrogen Sulfide
Poison Gas

Patient Care

Care of the Patient with a Behavioral or Psychiatric Emergency

Fundamental Principles of Care

Be aware of the need for treatment of both medical and psychiatric conditions. Psychiatric conditions generally require time, compassion, and a steady approach to calm and reassure the patient for a safe and therapeutic transport.

Emergency care of a patient having a behavioral or psychiatric emergency involves these steps:

- Be alert for personal or scene-safety problems throughout the call.
- Treat any life-threatening problems during the primary assessment.
- Be alert for medical or traumatic conditions that could mimic a behavioral emergency. Treat conditions you identify (e.g., low blood sugar level, head injury).
- Be prepared to spend time talking to the patient. Use the skills listed in the Assessment and Care section when dealing with the patient. Remember to talk in a calm, reassuring voice. Use positive body language and good eye contact. Avoid unnecessary physical contact and quick movements.
- Encourage the patient to discuss what is troubling the patient, but do not dwell on stressors or situations that escalate the current behavior.
- Never play along with any visual or auditory hallucinations that a patient may be experiencing. Do not lie to the patient.
- If it appears it will help, involve family members or friends in the conversation. Evaluate the patient's response to the presence of others. If it agitates the patient, ask the others to leave.

Suicide

CORE CONCEPT
Emergency care for potential or attempted suicide

Each year in this country, tens of thousands of people commit suicide. Suicide is the tenth-leading cause of death in the United States, and the incidence of suicides continues to rise (Figure 27-3) Depression coupled with successful suicide has also reached alarming levels in combat veteran and senior citizen populations. Many more people suffer both physical and emotional injuries in unsuccessful suicide attempts. Anyone may become suicidal if emotional distress is severe, regardless of sex; age; or ethnic, social, or economic background.

People attempt suicide for many reasons, including depression caused by chemical imbalance, the death of a loved one, financial problems, the end to a love affair, poor health, loss of esteem, divorce, fear of failure, and alcohol and drug abuse. People attempt to end

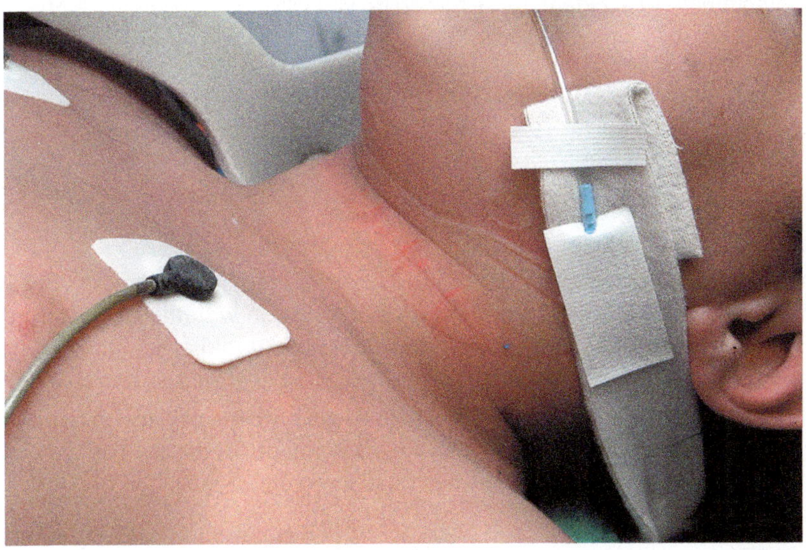

FIGURE 27-3 Child with ligature marks from a noose on the neck during an attempted suicide. *(© David Effron, MD)*

their lives by any one of a variety of methods. You may observe suicides or attempted suicides by drug overdose, hanging, jumping from high places, ingesting poisons, inhaling gas, wrist-cutting, self-mutilation, stabbing, or shooting.

Patient Assessment

Potential or Attempted Suicide

Factors often associated with a risk for suicide appear in the following list. Although some or even all of them may be present in a patient, it is not possible to use these characteristics to predict who will and who will not commit suicide:

- Depression: Take seriously a patient's feelings and expressions of despair or suicidal thoughts.
- High current or recent stress levels: If these are present, take the threat of suicide seriously.
- Recent emotional trauma: This could be job loss, loss of a significant relationship, serious illness, arrest, or imprisonment.
- Age: High suicide rates occur at ages 15–25 and over age 40. The elderly are a population in which suicide rates are increasing. This is often fueled by isolation and depression, death of one's spouse and friends, financial difficulties, and debilitating health problems.
- Alcohol and drug abuse.
- Threats of suicide: Patients may have told others that they were considering suicide. Take all threats of suicide seriously.
- Suicide plan: A patient who has a detailed suicide plan is more likely to commit suicide. Look for a plan that includes a method to carry out the suicide, notes, giving away personal possessions, or getting affairs in order.
- Previous attempts or suicide threats: These could include a history of self-destructive behavior. Often patients who have attempted suicide on a previous occasion are considered to be "looking for attention" and are not taken seriously on subsequent attempts. However, statistics reveal that a person who has attempted suicide in the past is more likely to commit suicide than one who has not.
- Sudden improvement from depression: A patient who has made the decision to commit suicide may actually appear to be coming out of a depression. The fact that the decision has been made and an end is in sight can cause this apparent "improvement." You may find family members and friends of suicidal patients who will report that the patient had seemed "better" in the past few days.

NOTE: *Whenever you are called to care for a patient who has attempted or may be about to attempt suicide, your first concern must be your own safety. Not all patients will wish to harm you, but the mechanism used to attempt suicide will be capable of causing death. It could intentionally or accidentally be turned on you.*

Patient Care

Care of the Patient with Potential or Attempted Suicide

Fundamental Principles of Care

Patients who are in an emotional, psychiatric, or attempted-suicide emergency are cared for in similar ways. In all cases, your personal interaction with the patient is key. Try to establish visual and verbal contact as soon as possible. Avoid arguing. Make no threats and show no indication of using force.

Remember that you are the first professional to begin both the physical and mental health care of the patient. The more reassurance you can provide for the patient, the easier it will be for the hospital emergency department staff to continue care.

Emergency care for patients who have a potential for or have attempted suicide includes the following components:

- Treatment must begin with scene size-up. Make sure it is safe to approach the patient. One-half of suicides in this country involve a firearm–these are high-risk scenes. If the scene is not safe, request assistance from the police, and wait until they have secured the scene. Do not leave the patient alone unless you are at risk of physical harm. Try to talk with the patient from a safe distance until the police arrive. Take Standard Precautions.
- When the scene is secure, look for and treat life-threatening problems to the extent that the patient will permit it. Seek police assistance in restraining the patient if necessary for care of life-threatening problems.
- Perform a secondary assessment and provide emergency care.
- Perform a detailed physical exam only if it is safe and you suspect the patient may have an injury.
- Perform a reassessment. Watch for sudden changes in the patient's behavior and physical condition.
- Contact the receiving hospital and report on the patient's current mental status and other essential information.

NOTE: *A physical exam may be difficult with the emotional or psychiatric patient. Be sure to balance the need for an exam to uncover important clinical conditions with the behavior problems the exam may cause.*

Throughout your interaction with the patient, speak slowly and patiently await answers to your questions. As you gain the patient's confidence, explain what questions must be answered and what must be done as part of the physical exam and taking vital signs. Let the patient know that you think it would be best if the patient goes to the hospital, and that you need cooperation and help. Back off if necessary. If the patient's fear or aggression increases, do not push the issues of the examination and transport. Instead, try to reestablish the conversation and give the patient more time before you again suggest that going to the hospital is a good idea.

CORE CONCEPT
Emergency care for aggressive or hostile patients

Transport all suicidal patients. Seek police assistance, if necessary. Report any attempted suicide or expression of suicidal thoughts to the medical facility, police, or government agency designated by your state law and local protocols.

Aggressive or Hostile Patients

Aggressive or disruptive behavior may be caused by trauma to the brain and nervous system, metabolic disorders, stress, alcohol, other drugs, or psychological disorders. Sometimes you will know that your patient is aggressive from the information you receive from dispatch. Other times, the scene may provide quick clues (such as drugs, yelling, unkempt conditions, or broken furniture). Neighbors, family members, or bystanders may tell you that the patient is dangerous or angry or has a history of aggression or combativeness. The patient's stance (tense muscles; fists clenched; or quick, irregular movements, for example) or the patient's position in the room may give you an early warning of possible violence. On rare occasions, you may start with an apparently calm patient who suddenly turns aggressive.

"Stay safe out there. Don't rush in if it may be dangerous. Your own safety is your first responsibility."

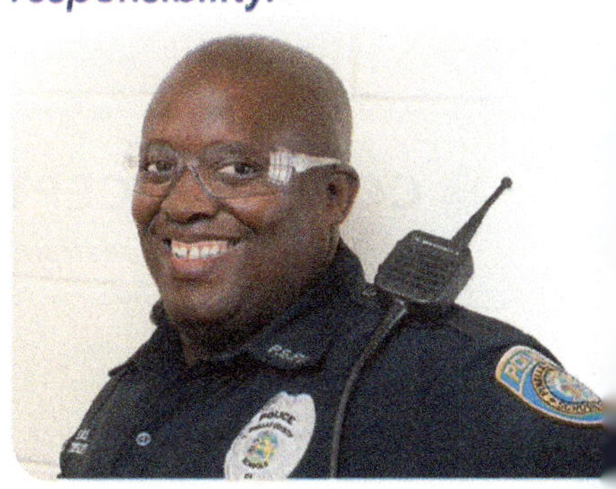

As already noted, when patients act as if they may hurt themselves or others, your first concern must be your own safety. Take the following precautions:

- Do not isolate yourself from your partner or other sources of help. Make certain that you have an escape route. Do not let patients come between you and the door. If a patient should become violent, retreat and wait for police assistance.

- Do not take any action that may be considered threatening by patients. To do so may bring about hostile behavior directed against you or others.
- Always be on the watch for weapons. Stay out of kitchens, as they are filled with dangerous weapons. Stay in a safe area until the police can control the scene.

Patient Assessment

Aggressive or Hostile Patient

Your assessment of the aggressive or hostile patient might not go beyond the primary assessment phase until the patient is appropriately calmed or restrained. Most of your time might need to be spent trying to calm the patient and ensuring everyone's safety. However, aggression or hostility in a patient should never be used as an excuse for not assessing the patient as thoroughly as possible. Aggressive or hostile patients:

- Respond to people inappropriately.
- Try to hurt themselves or others.
- May have a rapid pulse and breathing.
- Usually display rapid speech and rapid physical movements.
- May appear anxious, nervous, or "panicky".

Patient Care

Care for an Aggressive or Hostile Patient

Fundamental Principles of Care

Patients who may pose a danger to you are, in most cases, dealt with by the police. Restraint of the patient may be necessary. When dealing with the patient, be sure to remain calm and use a reassuring tone as a means of de-escalation while maintaining your personal safety.

Follow these guidelines for the emergency care of an aggressive or hostile patient:

- Treatment begins with scene size-up. Make sure it is safe to approach the patient. If needed, request assistance from law enforcement before approaching. Practice Standard Precautions.
- Seek advice from medical direction if the patient's behavior prevents normal assessment and care procedures.
- As part of reassessment, watch for sudden changes in the patient's behavior. An agitated patient who suddenly becomes silent may be experiencing a serious medical emergency. Complete reassessments involve rechecking the primary assessment frequently and on any change in mental status.
- Seek assistance from law enforcement, as well as from medical direction, if restraint seems necessary.

Reasonable Force and Restraint

CORE CONCEPT
When and how to restrain a patient safely and effectively

Reasonable force is the force necessary to keep patients from injuring themselves or others. Reasonableness is determined by looking at all circumstances involved, including the patient's strength and size, type of abnormal behavior, mental status, and available methods of restraint. Understand that you may protect yourself from attack, but otherwise you must avoid actions that can cause injury to the patient.

In addition, in most localities an EMT cannot legally restrain patients with a behavioral emergency, move such patients against their will, or force such patients to accept emergency care—even at the family's request. The restraint and forcible moving of patients is usually within the jurisdiction of law enforcement. The police (and, in some areas, a physician) can order you to restrain and transport a patient to the appropriate medical facility. However, the physician is not empowered to order you to take action that could place you in danger. If the police order restraint and transport for the patient, they must perform or assist with these procedures as necessary. Remember to follow local protocol.

At times, a patient with a medical or traumatic emergency may display violent behavior to the extent that restraint is necessary before receiving the medical treatment the patient needs. For example, a diabetic patient with hypoglycemia may be acting abnormally and even aggressively. If the patient's behavior interferes with or prevents treatment and the EMT can safely restrain the patient, the EMT should do so to initiate treatment. Similarly, a patient with a head injury may be hypoxic and acting abnormally. Again, if it can be done safely, the EMT should institute the needed treatment, which in this case includes restraint so the patient can be safely transported to a facility where the head injury can be treated.

Determining whether a particular patient has a medical or traumatic emergency that is causing the patient's abnormal behavior can be difficult. Consider whether the patient is capable of giving or refusing informed consent, consult medical direction, and administer the care that is in the patient's best interest without endangering yourself.

Never try to assist in restraining a patient unless there are sufficient personnel to do the job. You must be able to ensure your safety as well as the patient's safety. If you help the police or a physician to restrain a patient, make certain that the restraints are humane. For example, handcuffs and plastic "throwaway" criminal restraints should not be used, because of the soft-tissue damage they can inflict. Initially, the police may have to use such restraints. However, in some states they can be replaced with soft restraints such as leather cuffs and belts. If authorized in your state and by local protocol, an ambulance should carry leather cuffs, a waist-sized belt, and at least three short belts. Restraints for the wrists and ankles can be made from gauze roller bandages.

NOTE: *The medical literature refers to a condition called **excited delirium** (also called agitated delirium). In this situation, a patient begins to act extremely agitated or psychotic. The triggers for this condition can include uncontrolled psychiatric illness and/or drug intoxication. These patients frequently develop significant and even life-threatening cardiovascular and metabolic stress. Patients with excited delirium can suddenly cease struggling, and often within minutes the patient is found to have inadequate or absent respirations, and suddenly suffers cardiac arrest. It is important for the EMT to be alert for this sequence of events if patients exhibit this behavior and to monitor the patient constantly throughout the call.*

excited delirium bizarre and/or aggressive behavior, shouting, paranoia, panic, violence toward others, insensitivity to pain, unexpected physical strength, and hyperthermia, usually associated with cocaine or amphetamine use. Also called *agitated delirium*.

Do not remove police restraints until you and the police are certain that soft restraints will hold the patient. To ensure everyone's safety once they are on, do not remove soft restraints, even if the patient appears to be acting rationally.

Follow these guidelines when a patient must be restrained (Scan 27-1):

- Be sure to have adequate help.
- Plan your activities; have a well-delineated plan of action before initiating the restraint.
- Estimate the range of motion of the patient's arms and legs, and stay beyond that range until ready.
- Once the decision to restrain the patient has been reached, act quickly.
- Have one EMT talk to and reassure the patient throughout the restraining procedure.
- Approach with a minimum of four persons, one assigned to each limb, all to act at the same time. (Five rescuers would allow an extra person to control the head. However, the rescuer at the head should use caution to prevent being bitten.)
- Secure all four limbs with restraints approved by medical direction.
- Position the patient faceup. *Patients should never be restrained in a prone position or in any position that threatens movement of the chest wall.* Monitor the patient's airway. Never "hog-tie" the patient or restrain the patient in any manner that will impair breathing. Patients who have been improperly restrained have died as a result of a condition often referred to as ***positional asphyxia***. Carefully monitor all restrained patients.

positional asphyxia inadequate breathing or respiratory arrest caused by a body position that restricts breathing.

SCAN 27-1 Restraining a Patient

NOTE: *A fifth rescuer, if available, can control the patient's head—taking special care, however, not to be bitten.*

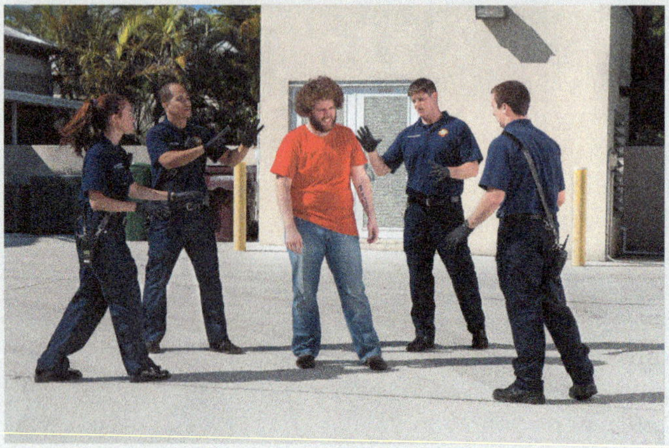

1. Plan your approach to the patient in advance and remain outside the range of the patient's arms and legs until you are ready to act.

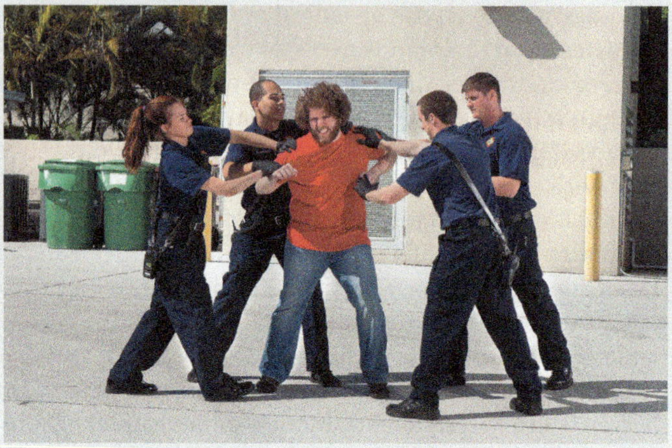

2. Have all the EMTs approach the patient at the same time.

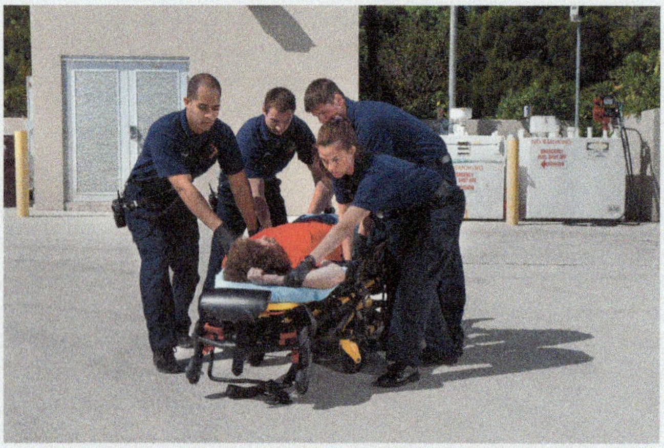

3. Place the patient on the stretcher as the patient's condition and local protocols indicate. Do not let go until the patient is properly secured.

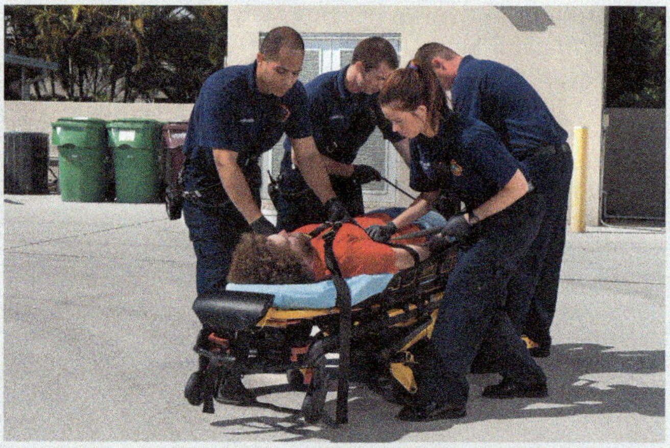

4. Use multiple straps or other soft restraints to secure the patient to the stretcher. When the patient is secure, assess distal circulation and continually monitor airway and breathing.

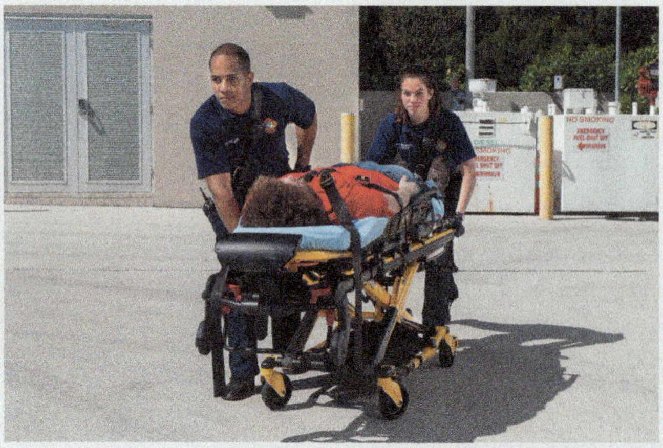

5. Transport. En route, frequently reassess distal circulation, airway, and breathing.

Remember that in some cases of substance abuse, such as with stimulants, the drugs will cause the body to continue to fight despite the fact that the extremities have been restrained. Although the arms and legs are being held in place, the muscles are still contracting. The heart and lungs work at their highest capacity. This can result in rapid decompensation as the ability to fight burns through energy stores. If a patient is being restrained in such a situation, you should contact ALS. Higher levels of care may be able to add chemical restraint by administering drugs that calm the patient to slow down the fighting response. Many times in an agitated restraint, a patient will become quiet and stop fighting, leading EMTs and police officers to relax because the patient appears to have calmed down. In some cases, the patient has stopped breathing and dies. It can't be repeated enough: *Monitor your restrained patient constantly throughout the call.*

- Use multiple straps or other restraints to ensure that the patient is adequately secured. Anticipate that the patient's behavior may turn more violent, and be sure that restraint is adequate for this possibility.
- If the patient is spitting on rescuers, place a surgical mask on the patient if the patient has no breathing difficulty or likelihood of vomiting and if local protocols permit, or have rescuers wear protective masks, eyewear, and clothing.
- Reassess the patient's distal circulation frequently, and adjust restraints as safe and necessary if distal circulation is diminished.
- Use sufficient force but avoid unnecessary force.
- Advanced life support providers may be able to administer medications to help sedate the highly agitated and restrained patient.
- Document the reasons the patient was restrained and the technique of restraint.

Transport to an Appropriate Facility

Your medical protocols or procedures should direct you to the most appropriate medical facility within your service area. Not all hospitals are prepared to treat behavioral emergencies.

Medical/Legal Considerations

CORE CONCEPT
Medical/legal considerations in behavioral and psychiatric emergencies

A patient who refuses emergency care or transport is a significant medical/legal risk for EMS agencies and EMTs. What should you do when a behavioral-emergency patient refuses or resists your efforts to provide care?

Most states have a provision in law that will allow patients to be transported against their will if they are a danger to themselves or others. This is an exception to the rule that patients must provide consent for their care and transportation. Know your state laws on treating patients without consent. Many states give this authority to law enforcement personnel. It will always be beneficial to have the police present if the patient must be restrained as a matter of safety.

You may also be required to contact medical direction about psychiatric patients who refuse care. Many communities have mental health teams that will respond to the scene to help with the care of patients with behavioral problems. This team will also help evaluate the need for transporting patients against their will.

Emotionally disturbed patients sometimes accuse EMS personnel of sexual misconduct. If possible, EMTs of the same sex as the patient should attend to the emergency care of disturbed patients. For the aggressive or violent patient, make sure law enforcement officers accompany you to the hospital to protect you and the patient. In the event of a legal problem, they can serve as third-party witnesses.

For more information on this topic, review the *Medical, Legal, and Ethical Issues* chapter.

Point of View

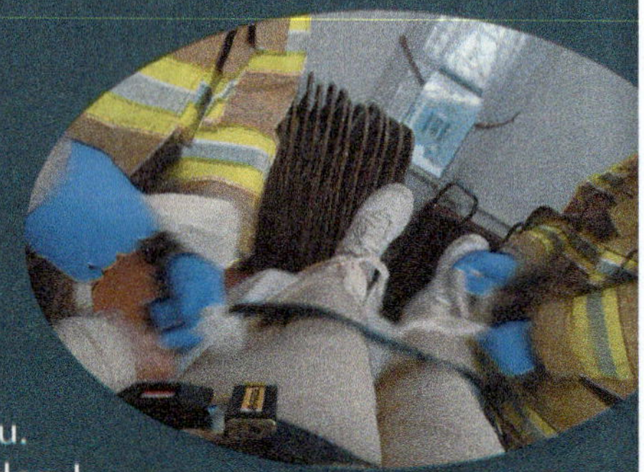

"I was at a group therapy session when I started noticing people were watching me. They did that for a while. When I would talk, they would whisper and giggle and point. I heard voices. They whispered too. I couldn't see the people, but I heard the voices very clearly. They were talking about me.

"I stood up and yelled, 'Don't say those things! Oh, yes, you. Stop it right now!' They kept going. The voices got louder. I started pushing people and throwing chairs. They had no right to do this to me. The voices just laughed. People pointed and whispered. I knew what they were thinking.

"The ambulance came. The police came. I got tied down and taken to the hospital.

"Some of what I tell you is based on what my counselor told me. I don't remember it all. You see, I am schizophrenic. I guess you could say reality isn't my strong point sometimes. I can joke about it now. What I experienced are called paranoid delusions. I get them a lot. I can usually control them. But sometimes when I can't afford my pills or I get fed up with the fact that I feel groggy all the time or when I can't have sex, I stop taking them.

"That's when I hear voices and get restrained and taken to the hospital. Man, there has got to be a better way."

Chapter Review

Key Facts and Concepts

- As an EMT, you will respond to many behavioral emergencies. Be sure to ensure your own safety before entering a scene or caring for a violent or potentially violent patient.
- A considerable portion of the population has a diagnosable psychiatric condition. However, not all patients are violent. It is important to remember that patients in crisis are patients—and people—who need your compassion as well as your care.
- Always consider patients acting in an unusual or bizarre fashion to be experiencing an altered mental status; this will help you to avoid overlooking a medical or traumatic cause for the patient's problem.
- Because the treatment for these patients usually requires long-term management, little medical intervention can be done in the acute psychiatric situation. However, the way you interact with the patient during the emergency and assess your patient throughout the call is crucial for the patient's continued well-being.

Key Decisions

- Is the patient a danger to me, my crew, or bystanders?
- Is the patient a threat to self?
- Is the patient experiencing a medical or traumatic condition (e.g., diabetic emergency, head injury) that may explain the patient's behavior?
- Does the patient require restraint?
- Have I assessed my patient thoroughly and frequently?
- Could my patient be experiencing a worsening of the patient's condition because of the restraints?

Chapter Glossary

behavior the manner in which a person acts.

behavioral emergency when a patient's behavior is not typical for the situation; when the patient's behavior is unacceptable or intolerable to the patient, the patient's family, or the community; or when the patient may harm self or others.

excited delirium bizarre and/or aggressive behavior, shouting, paranoia, panic, violence toward others, insensitivity to pain, unexpected physical strength, and hyperthermia, usually associated with cocaine or amphetamine use. Also called *agitated delirium*.

neurotransmitters chemicals within the body that transmit a message in the brain from the distal end of one neuron to the proximal end of the next neuron.

positional asphyxia inadequate breathing or respiratory arrest caused by a body position that restricts breathing.

schizophrenia a chronic mental disorder that affects how a person thinks, feels, and behaves. People with severe or untreated schizophrenia may seem like they have lost touch with reality.

Preparation for Your Examination and Practice

Short Answer

1. Name several conditions that can alter a person's mental status and behavior.
2. List several methods that can help calm the patient who is suffering a behavioral or psychiatric emergency.
3. Describe the signs and symptoms of a behavioral or psychiatric emergency.
4. Describe what you can do when scene size-up reveals that it is too dangerous to approach the patient.
5. List several factors that can help you assess the patient's risk for suicide.
6. Research your state law. Then describe the circumstances that must exist for you to treat and transport a behavioral-emergency patient without consent.

Thinking and Linking

Think back to the chapter Cardiac Emergencies *as well as the chapter* Allergic Reactions *and link information from those chapters with information from this chapter as you consider the following situation:*

- You are called to a patient who is acting bizarrely. List some indications (clues at the scene, signs and symptoms) that might indicate the abnormal behavior was actually due to a diabetic condition or overdose emergency.

Think back to the chapter Lifting and Moving Patients *and link information from that chapter with information from this chapter as you consider the following situation:*

- The police have subdued a violent psychiatric patient. They ask you to transport the patient to the hospital. What would you use to restrain the patient's extremities? What transport device would you use? How would you secure the patient's extremities to that device?

Critical Thinking Exercises

Behavioral and psychiatric emergencies come in a wide variety of presentations. The purpose of this exercise will be to consider an assessment issue, a management issue, and a transport issue associated with such behavioral and psychiatric patients.

1. You are transporting a psychiatric patient who was restrained by the police. The patient was highly agitated but now begins to act sleepy. Should you reassess the patient? If so, how?
2. You are called to respond to an intoxicated minor who is physically aggressive and who threatens suicide, and whose parents permit you to treat but not transport. How would you manage this patient?
3. You are treating a patient who has attempted suicide but appears stable. It is the patient's fourth attempt. Your partner says, "He's just looking for attention; we shouldn't even take him to the hospital." What do you think? What should you say to your partner?

Pathophysiology to Practice

The following questions are designed to assist you in gathering relevant clinical information and making accurate decisions in the field.

1. Why could a diabetic patient appear to be having a psychiatric emergency?
2. Why could a patient with a head injury appear to be having a psychiatric emergency?
3. Why does hypoxia cause unusual behavior?

Street Scenes

It's a sunny and relatively quiet summer afternoon when you are dispatched to a small manufacturing company for an individual "acting in a bizarre manner." The dispatcher is trying to get additional information, but it is difficult. Your response time is 5 minutes, and you are met outside by the manager. He tells you that about 15 minutes ago, a worker kicked a table and disrupted some of the equipment. When he was approached by coworkers, he said, "Stay away or I will hurt myself." The manager says the patient claims to have a knife, but no one has seen it.

Street Scene Questions

1. **What is your first and most important concern?**
2. **How should you handle the matter of scene safety?**
3. **When should you approach the patient?**

You contact the dispatcher, who informs you that two police officers are responding and should be on scene in 3 minutes. You make sure that your crew and bystanders are in a safe position, in case the patient exits the building. When the officers pull up, you tell them what you know. The police tell you to wait outside. They enter the building and find the patient still very agitated. While you wait outside, a coworker of the patient approaches and says that she might have some information that could help. Supposedly the patient is on antidepressant drugs and his wife recently left him. She believes that he could hurt himself, but she doubts he will hurt anyone else. At this point, one of the police officers tells you that the patient is calm and that they have frisked him.

Street Scene Questions

4. **How should the patient be approached?**
5. **What are the safety concerns when working with an agitated patient?**
6. **Does this patient need a medical assessment?**

You decide that only you should approach the patient, so as not to overwhelm him. There is already a police officer standing next to him. As you approach, you introduce yourself and tell the patient that you need to ask some questions and get some medical information. You listen to him and, during the medical history, ask if he has taken more medication than he should. He says that he took his morning dose, but that is all. You take a set of vital signs and continue to listen. After a few minutes, the patient agrees to go to the hospital with you.

You ask your partner to move the ambulance to a back door so the patient doesn't have to pass coworkers on the way out. You have discussed the situation with the police officers, and you feel confident that there is no longer a safety issue and that they won't be needed for the transport. The police searched the patient for weapons and found none. The patient is placed on the stretcher with all safety straps applied. You listen to the patient all the way to the hospital, being compassionate and acknowledging the patient's feelings as well as you can. Your partner calls the hospital on the radio and gives an ETA of 5 minutes.

Later, as you walk away from the patient in the emergency department, he smiles and thanks you for listening.

Hematologic and Renal Emergencies

28

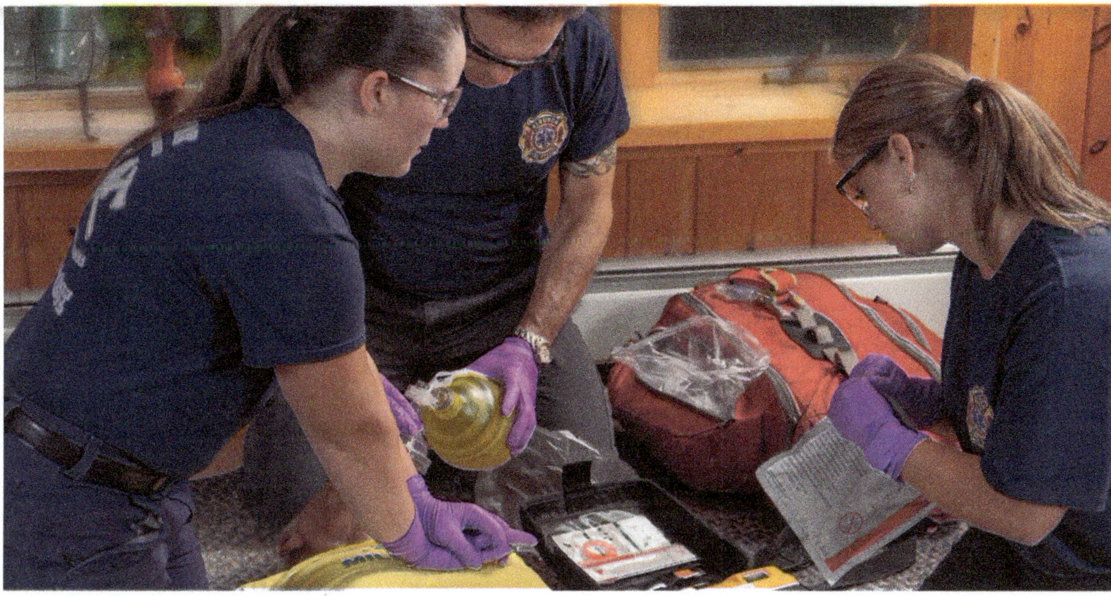

Related Chapters

The following chapters provide additional information related to topics discussed in this chapter:

Standard

Medicine (Content Area: Hematology)

Competency

Applies fundamental knowledge to provide basic emergency care and transportation based on assessment findings for an acutely ill patient.

Core Concepts

- Disorders of the hematologic system
- Disorders of the renal system

Outcomes

After reading this chapter, you should be able to:

28.1 Explain the anatomy and physiology of the blood as an organ. (pp. 765–766)

- Describe the overall functions of the blood.
- Identify the elements required for normal blood clotting.

28.2 Summarize the characteristics of disorders of the blood. (pp. 766–767)

- Describe the spectrum of coagulopathies.
- Recognize causes of coagulopathies.

28.3 Describe the EMT care approach to patients with coagulopathies. (pp. 767–770)

- Identify patients in whom coagulopathies may be a factor in their stability.
- Describe EMT decision making that provides coagulopathy patients with the best potential outcomes.
- Compare the characteristics of different types of anemia.
- Relate the pathophysiology of sickle cell anemia to presentations of the disease.

28.4 Describe the EMT care approach to patients with sickle cell anemia. (p. 770)

- State the importance of clarifying whether a patient has sickle cell anemia or sickle cell trait.
- Identify the signs and symptoms of sickle cell anemia emergencies.
- Identify the role of oxygen in treating sickle cell emergencies.
- Recognize factors that influence an EMT's decision to request ALS when caring for a patient with sickle cell anemia.

28.5 Summarize the anatomy and physiology of the kidneys. (pp. 771–772)

- Describe the function of each structure of the renal system.
- Describe the role of the kidneys in maintaining the proper balance of substances in the blood.
- Explain the kidneys' reactions to differences in hydration.

28.6 Summarize features of diseases of the renal system. (pp. 771–776)

- Identify the risk associated with inadequately treated urinary tract infections.
- Identify the circumstances when kidney stones become painful.
- Recognize reasons why patients may use urinary catheters.
- Describe the pathophysiology of renal failure.
- Recognize causes of acute renal failure.
- State causes of chronic renal failure.
- Compare the processes of hemodialysis and peritoneal dialysis in patients with renal failure.

28.7 Summarize the EMT care approach to patients with medical emergencies related to end-stage renal disease. (pp. 776–779)

- List complications of end-stage renal disease.
- Explain the consequences of missing dialysis appointments.

- Recognize complications of dialysis.
- Propose care plans for a variety of portrayals of dialysis complications.
- Describe the considerations in caring for a kidney transplant patient.

Key Terms

anemia, *768*

coagulopathy, *766*

continuous ambulatory peritoneal dialysis (CAPD), *776*

continuous cycler-assisted peritoneal dialysis (CCPD), *776*

dialysis, *773*

end-stage renal disease (ESRD), *773*

exchange, *775*

peritonitis, *777*

pyelonephritis, *771*

renal failure, *771*

sickle cell disease (SCD), *768*

sickle cell anemia (SCA), *769*

thrill, *775*

urinary catheter, *771*

Our good health depends on the human body's multiple organ systems working seamlessly together. As an EMT, you will focus much of your medical attention on acute emergencies that can be attributed to the cardiovascular and respiratory systems. In this chapter we will discuss patients who have diseases or problems with their *hematologic system* (pertaining to blood) or *renal system* (pertaining to the kidneys). (*Hematology* is the medical specialty concerned with blood disorders. *Nephrology* is the medical specialty concerned with renal/kidney diseases.) Dozens of medical conditions can arise from diseases involving these two body systems. However, certain patients with certain diseases in these groups are most likely to require EMS services as a result of their illnesses.

The Hematologic System

CORE CONCEPT
Disorders of the hematologic system

Our blood—although central to the function of our cardiovascular system—actually represents its own organ system. As you learned in the chapter *Anatomy and Physiology*, each component of the blood has specific functions that, when all are working properly, are critical to a patient's health and survival, such as:

- Control of bleeding by clotting
- Delivery of oxygen to the cells
- Removal of carbon dioxide from the cells
- Removal and delivery of other waste products to organs that provide filtration and removal, such as the kidneys and liver

Blood is made up of solid components (including red blood cells, white blood cells, and platelets) suspended in a liquid called *plasma*. The solid components of blood are created in the bone marrow that forms the specialized core of many of the body's bones. Red blood cells, white blood cells, and platelets survive in the circulation for only a finite period of time. Under normal circumstances, an RBC remains in the circulation for about four months, whereas platelets remain in the circulation for a little more than a week. There are several types of white blood cells and their life spans vary. The solid components of the blood are removed from the circulation by means such as filtration by the spleen or liver.

Each component of the blood has specialized functions:

- **Red blood cells (RBCs).** RBCs make up the majority of the cells in the circulation and give blood its characteristic red color. These cells contain specialized molecules called *hemoglobin* that bind to oxygen and are responsible for oxygen delivery to the cells. The amount of RBCs in a patient's circulation is measured by a blood test called a hemoglobin count.

- **White blood cells (WBCs).** WBCs are critical blood cells that respond to infection and are major mediators of the body's immune response. There are different types of white blood cells. For example, neutrophils are the major WBC type responsible for fighting bacterial infections, and eosinophils are associated with allergic conditions. (See the chapter titled *Allergic Reactions*.)
- **Platelets.** Platelets are actually fragments of larger cells, and are crucial to the formation of clots. Clumping (called *aggregation*) of platelets is the body's most rapid response to stop bleeding from an injured site. However, the clumping of platelets is not desirable in some situations, such as when plaque in a coronary artery ruptures. In this situation, the rapid clumping of platelets can cause a clot that then completely blocks the coronary artery and results in a heart attack (myocardial infarction). One of the most effective and widely available drugs to prevent the aggregation of platelets is aspirin. That is why patients who are having an acute heart attack or a potential heart attack are routinely given an aspirin.
- **Plasma.** Plasma is the liquid in which the blood cells and platelets are suspended. Plasma contains dissolved nutrients and also carries certain crucial proteins, such as the clotting factors.

Blood Clotting

When internal or external bleeding occurs as a result of a medical condition or injury, the body must mobilize its clotting system to control the bleeding, or the patient could bleed to death. There are two major components within the blood that are responsible for clotting: platelets and clotting factors. Clumping of platelets is the body's most rapid and initial response to stop bleeding.

Clotting factors are a group of proteins that are produced in the liver and released into the bloodstream. Clotting factors circulate in the bloodstream in inactive forms but are activated to initiate clotting when damage occurs to the lining of a damaged blood vessel. Once activated, clotting factors form clots though specific steps that are described as clotting cascades. These clotting factors form the most stable clots, replacing the initial efforts of the platelets to stop bleeding.

Coagulopathies

coagulopathy
loss of the normal ability to form a blood clot with internal or external bleeding.

The term ***coagulopathy*** is defined as abnormal clotting of blood. Coagulopathy can occur when the body forms clots too readily or (and most relevant to the EMT) when the patient clots too slowly, resulting in uncontrolled bleeding. Coagulopathies that result in abnormally slow clotting can occur due to problems with the clotting cascade, or as a result of too few platelets or platelets that are not functioning correctly. Some patients may even be coagulopathic for more than one of those reasons. By far, the most common reason for a coagulopathy encountered by the EMT is because the patient is on a prescribed medication designed to slow normal clotting in certain medical conditions.

Certain diseases make patients prone to poor clotting. Because clotting factors are manufactured in the liver, patients with advanced liver disease, such as cirrhosis, may not make adequate clotting factors to form stable clots. There are also certain inherited genetic disorders that result in coagulopathies. Hemophiliacs, for example, have inherited disorders that prevent them from producing certain clotting factors. Similarly, von Willebrand's disease is the most common inherited blood disorder, occurring in about one in a thousand persons. In this common disease, although the patient has a normal number of platelets circulating in the bloodstream, the patient's platelets are functionally defective, thus allowing for excessive bleeding when injury occurs.

FIGURE 28-1 (A) This patient on Plavix® was thought to have a minor head injury. However, the patient's CT scan (B) revealed significant intracranial bleeding. *(Photos A and B: © Edward T. Dickinson, MD)*

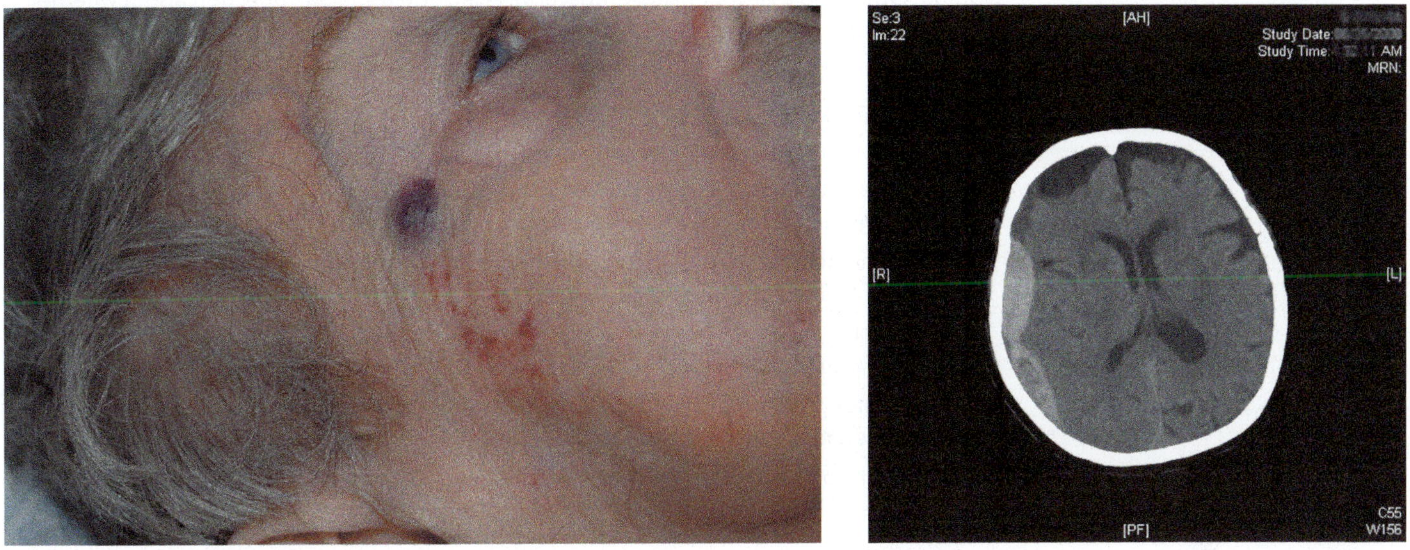

A

B

There are certain medical conditions in which the normal ability to form clots can worsen the patient's disease; for example, in those at risk for heart attacks or strokes, or those with abnormal cardiac rhythms such as atrial fibrillation. For this reason, millions of patients are on prescription drugs commonly referred to as "blood thinners." Drugs such as Coumadin® (warfarin), Pradaxa® (dabigatran), Eliquis® (apixaban), Xarelto® (rivaroxaban), and Lovenox® (enoxaparin) inhibit certain clotting factors. Other drugs, such as aspirin and Plavix® (clopidogrel), inhibit platelet aggregation. Patients on these medications are more prone to life-threatening bleeding when they are injured than patients who are not on these medications. In some EMS systems, injured patients taking these medications are frequently upgraded to trauma center transport, even with apparently minor injuries, because of their increased risk of uncontrolled bleeding. Follow your local protocols (Figure 28-1).

Identifying Patients with Coagulopathies

A thorough patient history becomes most important when assessing patients with suspected clotting disorders. A critical aspect of being able to manage patients with potential coagulopathies is identifying that the patient is in fact at risk for abnormal bleeding based on past medical history of the medications being taken. For example, patients with a history of the dysrhythmia called *atrial fibrillation* are commonly on blood thinners. Many EMTs have traditionally not made a priority of obtaining a *SAMPLE* history during the assessment of trauma patients. In fact, it is particularly important to ask all trauma patients you care for if they are on any blood thinner as part of your assessment.

Patient Care

Patient with Coagulopathy

Fundamental Principles of Care

Patients on prescription blood thinners have emerged as a vulnerable population prone to major complications in both trauma and certain medical emergencies, such as stroke and gastrointestinal bleeding. The first step in treating a patient with a medication-induced coagulopathy is confirming that the patient is actually on a medication that causes delayed clotting. Obtaining a proper history must always include a specific question about whether the patient takes any blood-thinning medication.

Emergency treatment of a patient with a potential coagulopathy includes the following:

- Take appropriate Standard Precautions.
- Perform a primary assessment and care for any immediate life threats.
- Obtain a history from the patient and identify which specific blood-thinning medication the patient is taking, or which bleeding disorder the patient suffers from.
- Notify the hospital as early as possible so they can prepare to manage the specific cause of the patient's bleeding disorder.
- Monitor the patient for the development of the signs and symptoms of shock or decreasing mental status.
- Administer supplemental oxygen if the patient appears to be in shock or has a decreased mental status.
- Transport to an appropriate receiving hospital. The patient may require large amounts of blood products not available in smaller hospitals. Follow local protocols.

Anemia

anemia deficiency in the normal number of red blood cells in the circulation.

Deficiency in the normal number of red blood cells (low hemoglobin count) in the circulation is called ***anemia***. There are many reasons a patient can become anemic. *Acute anemia* may be the result of trauma or of sudden massive bleeding from the gastrointestinal tract. These patients may rapidly exhibit signs and symptoms of shock (hypoperfusion), such as a rapid pulse rate; cool, clammy skin; and eventual hypotension. *Chronic anemia* occurs over time and can be caused by conditions such as recurrent heavy menstrual periods, slow gastrointestinal blood loss, or diseases that affect the bone marrow or the structure of the hemoglobin molecule itself. Patients with chronic anemia will often appear more pale than normal (from a lack of circulating red blood cells) and often complain of fatigue and shortness of breath with exertion (because of a lack of adequate oxygen being delivered to the body's cells). Only after a prolonged period of time will patients with chronic anemia exhibit signs and symptoms of shock. One of the best ways to assess for chronic anemia is to examine the color of the patient's conjunctiva on the lower eyelid. Anemic patients will have very pale conjunctiva, as opposed to the red/pink color seen in normal patients (Figure 28-2).

Sickle Cell Disease

sickle cell disease (SCD) an inherited disease in which patients have a genetic defect in their hemoglobin that results in an abnormal structure of the red blood cell.

Sickle cell disease (SCD) is an inherited disease in which patients have a genetic defect in their hemoglobin that results in an abnormal structure of the red blood cells. Sickle cell disease most

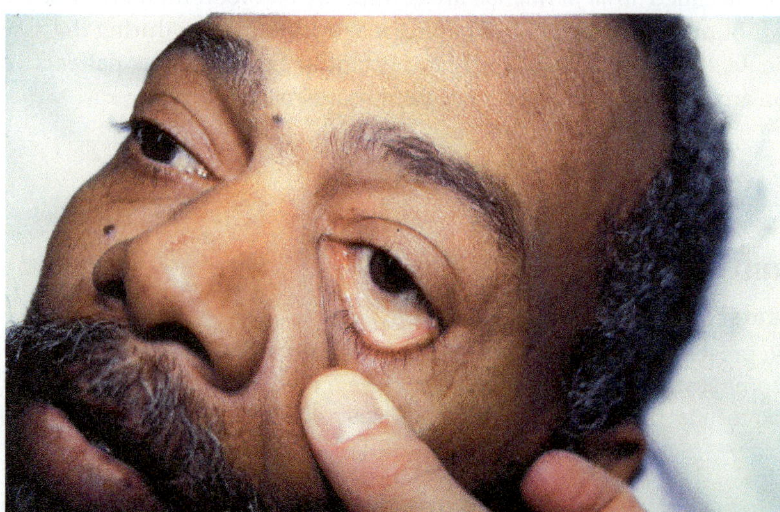

FIGURE 28-2 Pale conjunctiva in a patient with severe chronic anemia. *(© Edward T. Dickinson, MD)*

commonly occurs in patients of African descent, occurring in about 1 out of every 365 African American births. Sickle cell disease results in ***sickle cell anemia (SCA)***, because the abnormal structure of the RBCs results in their premature destruction in the circulation.

sickle cell anemia (SCA) an abnormally low number of RBCs in the circulation due to sickle cell disease.

A normal red blood cell is doughnut-shaped, with a depression rather than a hole in the center. Normal red blood cells are able to be compressed as they move and squeeze through small capillaries to deliver oxygen to the cells of the body's organs. Patients with sickle cell disease have red blood cells composed of defective hemoglobin that causes them to lose their ability to have a normal shape and compressibility. These abnormal RBCs resemble the shape of a sickle when observed under a microscope (Figure 28-3). Because of their abnormal shapes, these RBCs do not survive in the circulation as long as normal RBCs do. This results in chronic anemia.

The complications of SCA are generally attributed to the sludging of the abnormally shaped red blood cells, which causes blockages within the body's small blood vessels. The complications of sickle cell anemia include:

- **Destruction of the spleen.** The spleen, as it filters the blood, becomes blocked by the abnormal RBCs. Because the spleen is important in fighting infections, its loss places patients with SCA at higher risk for severe, life-threatening infections.
- **Sickle cell pain crisis.** Sickle cell crisis is caused by the sludging of sickled RBCs in capillaries, which results in severe pain in the arms, legs, chest, and/or abdomen.
- **Acute chest syndrome.** Acute chest syndrome is characterized by shortness of breath and chest pain associated with hypoxia (low oxygen saturation) when blood vessels in the lungs become blocked.
- **Priapism.** Painful prolonged erections in males occur because sludging RBCs prevent normal blood drainage from the erect penis.
- **Stroke.** Stroke can occur when sludging RBCs block blood vessels that supply the brain.
- **Jaundice.** The liver becomes overwhelmed by the breakdown in red blood cells, resulting in yellowish pigmentation of body tissues.

Despite advances in modern medical care, patients with SCA still have an abnormally short life span. In addition, some sickle cell patients suffer so persistently from painful vaso-occlusive crises that they may become dependent on narcotic pain medications.

NOTE: *Some patients may tell you that they have sickle cell trait as part of their past medical history. These patients carry the gene for sickle cell disease but do not have the disease. Therefore, these patients do not suffer the complications of sickle cell disease, and they have normal life spans. It is estimated that 1 in 13 African Americans have sickle cell trait.*

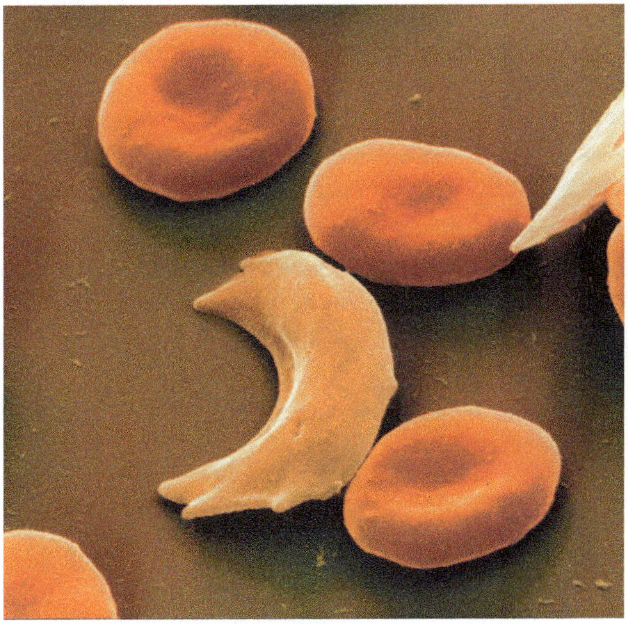

FIGURE 28-3 Scanning electron photomicrograph of normal red blood cells contrasted with a sickle cell. *(Eye of Science/ Science Source)*

TABLE 28-1 External Manifestations and Internal SCD Complications

OUTSIDE	INSIDE
Infections and fevers	The spleen may be so damaged from the sickled red blood cells that it no longer functions. This means that the spleen's normal role in immune function is lost, predisposing the sickle cell patient to more frequent and severe infections.
Pain in bones, joints, abdomen, soft tissues	A vaso-occlusive crisis is a condition in which sickled red blood cells block microcirculation. This causes hypoxia and severe pain in the affected organs. This often occurs in bones and joints but can also involve the abdomen and soft tissues.
Difficulty breathing, chest pain, cough, fever	When vaso-occlusive crisis occurs in the lungs, it can result in acute chest syndrome. Patients will complain of difficulty breathing (often severe), chest pain, cough, and sometimes fever.
Prolonged penile erection	Sickled red blood cells are believed to block blood that is trying to exit the corpus spongiosum (erectile tissue), causing the prolonged, painful erection of the penis, called priapism.
Stroke symptoms	Sickle cell patients (adults and children) are more likely to experience ischemic stroke. The exact mechanism for this isn't known. While sickled cells may affect the microcirculation of the brain and cause stroke, many strokes involve larger vessels in the arterial circulation.
Yellowed skin, yellowed eye whites	The liver is overwhelmed with the massive breakdown of red blood cells. This lack of normal liver function causes jaundice (a yellowish pigmentation of the skin, whites of the eyes, and other body tissues and fluids).

Manifestations and Pathophysiology

We have just listed some common complications of sickle cell anemia. As you assess your patient, what outside signs and symptoms are associated with which inside complications? Table 28-1 outlines the connections.

Patient Care

Patient with Sickle Cell Disease

Fundamental Principles of Care

Patients with SCD frequently interact with emergency medical services due to recurrent painful sickle cell crisis episodes. Never assume that the SCD patient is "just having another pain crisis." These patients are at high risk for developing life-threatening infections, strokes, and chest crises.

Emergency treatment of a patient with sickle cell anemia is as follows:

- Administer supplemental oxygen if the patient is short of breath, has chest pain, or has an oxygen saturation below 95 percent.
- Monitor patients with acute chest syndrome for signs of inadequate respiration, and provide bag-valve-mask ventilation as necessary.
- Monitor patients with high fever for signs of hypoperfusion, and treat for shock as necessary.
- Transport patients with acute stroke symptoms to a designated stroke center if available. Follow local protocols.

Decision Point

- Should I request ALS to provide pain control for my SCA patient?

The Renal System

The renal system is made up of two kidneys, two ureters (to carry urine from each kidney to the bladder), and a single urethra (to carry urine from the bladder to the outside of the body) (Figure 28-4).

CORE CONCEPT
Disorders of the renal system

As you learned in the chapter *Anatomy and Physiology*, the kidneys are responsible for the filtration of the blood and the removal of certain waste products, excessive salts, and excessive fluid from the body. In addition, in times of dehydration, the kidneys also help the body retain needed fluid. Because they perform these critical functions, the kidneys are essential to life.

Diseases of the Renal System

Many diseases involve the renal system. They affect different portions of the renal system and can range from minor, easily treated problems to life-threatening conditions.

Urinary Tract Infections

Urinary tract infections (UTIs) are perhaps the most common disease process that afflicts the renal and urinary system. UTIs are caused by bacteria, and most UTIs are limited to the bladder, causing symptoms of painful and frequent urination. If left untreated, an infection in the bladder can ascend up the ureter and into the kidney, a condition known as ***pyelonephritis***. Patients with pyelonephritis will often complain of unilateral flank pain in addition to normal UTI symptoms, and generally will appear more ill than those with uncomplicated bladder infections. A urinary tract infection can be a serious and life-threatening disease (especially in the elderly) if bacteria spread into the bloodstream.

pyelonephritis
an infection that begins in the urinary tract and ascends up the ureter into the kidney.

Kidney Stones

Kidney stones are a painful and common condition related to the renal system. Kidney stones are usually made of calcium and are formed within the kidney. If they remain in the kidney, they usually cause no symptoms. However, kidney stones can cause severe unilateral flank pain that radiates to the groin area when the stone descends from the kidney, becomes lodged in the ureter, and is unable to pass into the bladder (Figure 28-5). Patients with kidney stone pain often have associated nausea and vomiting.

Patients with Urinary Catheters

As an EMT, you will encounter certain patients who have lost the ability to urinate normally. This can be the result of obstruction of the outflow from the bladder (such as a tumor or enlarged prostate) or because of a neurologic disorder that has caused them to lose the ability to initiate normal urine flow. These patients commonly use a ***urinary catheter*** to drain their urine.

urinary catheter
a drainage tube placed into the urinary system to allow the flow of urine out of the body.

The most common placement for a urinary catheter is into the patient's urethra. Some catheters are in place for the long term, while other patients place a catheter into their own urethra each time they urinate (self-catheters). In certain cases, a urologist or surgeon may place a urinary catheter directly through the skin into the kidney or bladder to drain a patient's urine for either the short or long term.

Acute and chronic urinary tract infections and local trauma at the site of the catheter insertion are the most common complications encountered with urinary catheters.

Renal Failure

The most serious disease of the kidneys is ***renal failure***. Renal failure occurs when the kidneys lose their ability to adequately filter the blood and to remove toxins and excess fluid from the body.

renal failure
loss of the kidneys' ability to filter the blood and to remove toxins and excess fluid from the body.

There are many reasons patients develop renal failure. Some causes for renal failure are sudden (acute) and some develop gradually over time (chronic). *Acute renal failure* can occur as a result of shock, toxic ingestions, and other causes. Some patients who experience

FIGURE 28-4 The renal system.

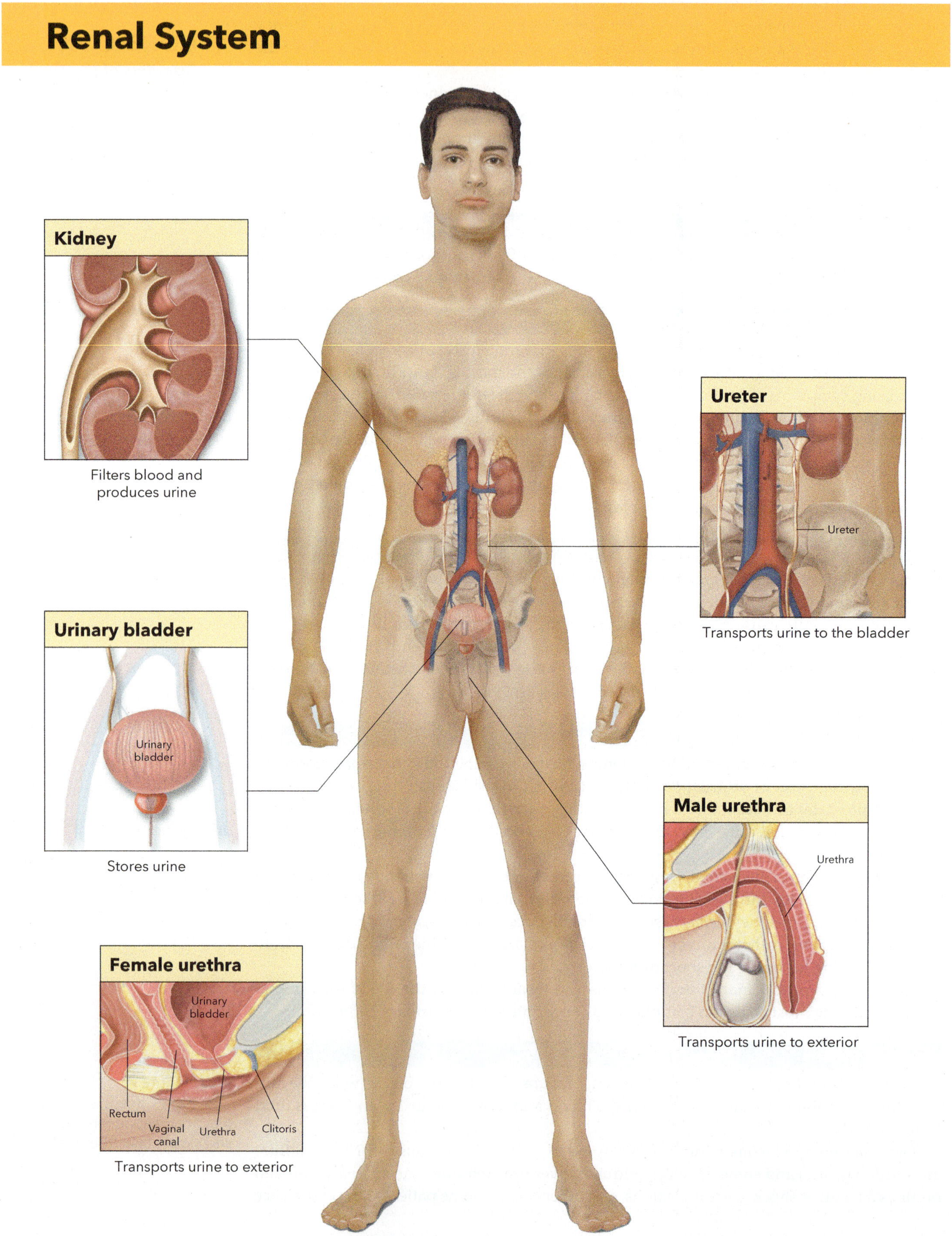

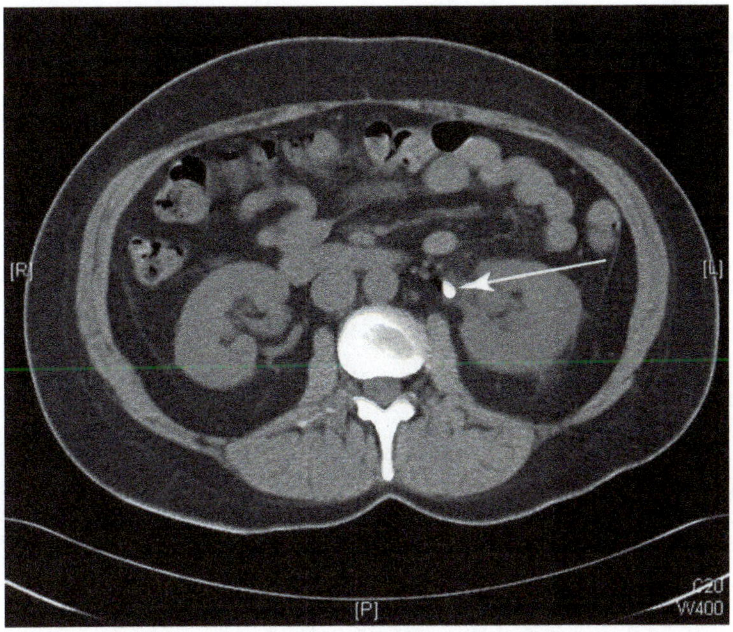

FIGURE 28-5 CT scan showing a kidney stone (see arrow) lodged in the proximal left ureter. *(© Edward T. Dickinson, MD)*

acute renal failure can recover normal kidney function if the underlying cause of the insult to the kidneys is rapidly identified and corrected. An example of this would be severe dehydration in a patient trapped in a building collapse for several days; with aggressive treatment with intravenous fluids, the patient can recover normal renal function over time. However, others who suffer acute renal failure never recover normal kidney function. Causes of *chronic renal failure* can include inherited diseases such as polycystic kidney disease. More commonly, however, long-term damage is caused by diabetes, or by high blood pressure that is not well controlled by diet and medication and that results in loss of normal renal function.

Patients who go on to develop irreversible renal failure—to the extent that their kidneys can no longer provide adequate filtration and fluid balance to sustain life—are defined as patients with ***end-stage renal disease (ESRD)***. Patients with ESRD usually require ***dialysis*** to survive. Approximately 900,000 Americans are being treated for ESRD, and more than 450,000 of these patients are on chronic dialysis.

end-stage renal disease (ESRD)
irreversible renal failure to the extent that the kidneys can no longer provide adequate filtration and fluid balance to sustain life; survival with ESRD usually requires dialysis.

dialysis
the process by which toxins and excess fluid are removed from the body by a medical system independent of the kidneys.

Dialysis is the process by which an external medical system independent of the kidneys is used to remove toxins and excess fluid from the body. There are two general types of dialysis: *hemodialysis* and *peritoneal dialysis*. More than 90 percent of ESRD patients who require dialysis get hemodialysis in specialized outpatient dialysis centers rather than peritoneal dialysis. Only 8 percent of U.S. dialysis patients treat themselves at home with hemodialysis or peritoneal dialysis. The vast majority of the more than 450,000 Americans on dialysis who are treated in dialysis centers undergo three treatments a week, each lasting 3 or 4 hours. Although some patients get to their dialysis appointments by their own means, many others use medical transport to get to and from dialysis. This need for medical transport has created a frequent interface between EMTs and patients with ESRD.

Hemodialysis

In hemodialysis (HD), the most common form of dialysis in the United States, a patient is connected to a dialysis machine that pumps the blood through specialized filters to remove toxins and excess fluid (Figure 28-6). A patient is connected to a dialysis machine by two large catheters. One catheter allows blood to flow out of the body into the dialysis machine, and the other catheter returns blood to the body after filtration. This creates a circuit by which the blood is removed from the body, filtered, and returned to the body continuously over several hours while the patient is connected to the machine.

Because HD requires a large blood flow from the body, ESRD patients on this type of chronic dialysis have specialized means of access to the body's blood circulation.

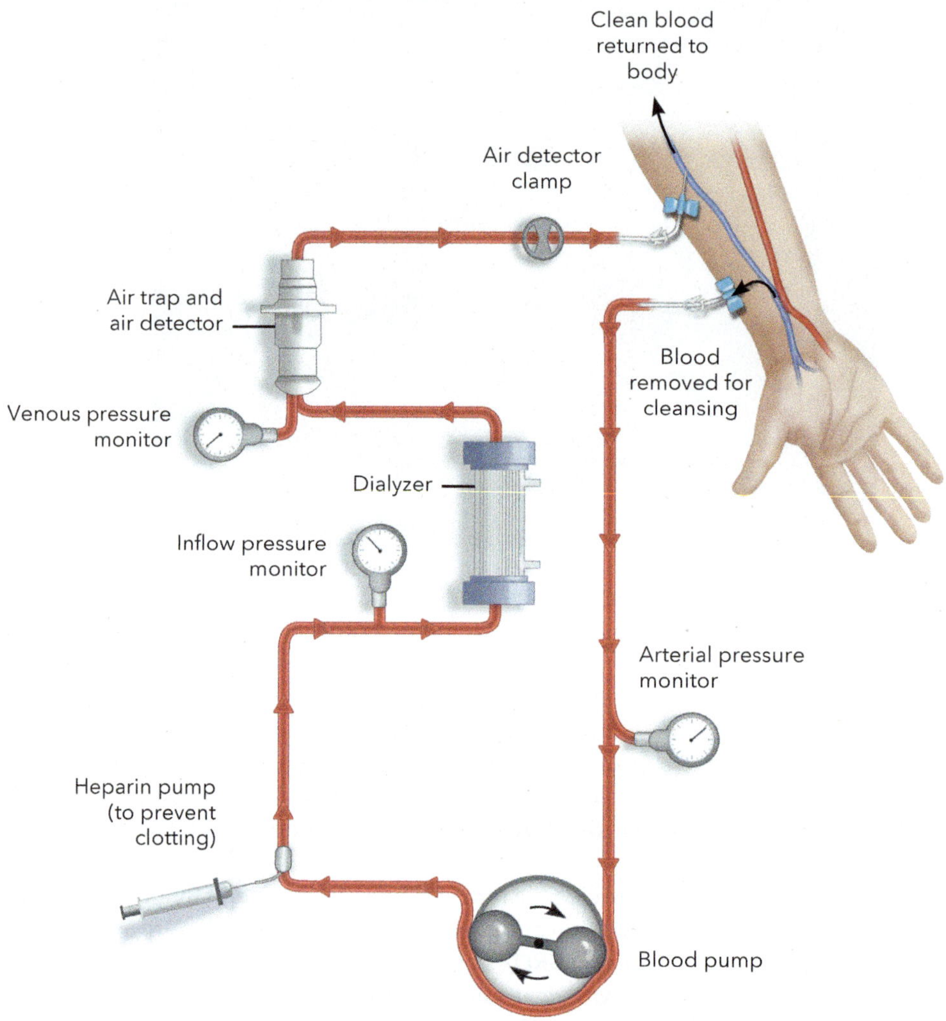

FIGURE 28-6 How hemodialysis works. *(Adapted from Treatment Methods for Kidney Failure, National Institute of Diabetes and Digestive and Kidney Diseases; U.S. Centers for Disease Control and Prevention.)*

Hemodialysis patients will have either a specialized two-port catheter that is inserted in one of the major veins of the torso (Figure 28-7) or a surgically created fistula in one of their extremities that connects arterial and venous blood flow (Figure 28-8). Because a fistula contains turbulent flow between a surgically connected artery and vein (A-V), a properly functioning A-V fistula will have a characteristic vibration,

Point of View

"I have a friend who is on dialysis. She is young—not someone you would think of as sick. Three times a week she goes for her treatments. Sometimes I go to keep her company—or I stop by when we are on a call at the hospital next door. It sure has made me more aware of dialysis and the people who get it. It seems like a miracle sometimes that dialysis is even possible. She has told me how it keeps her alive—and what happens when she misses her appointment."

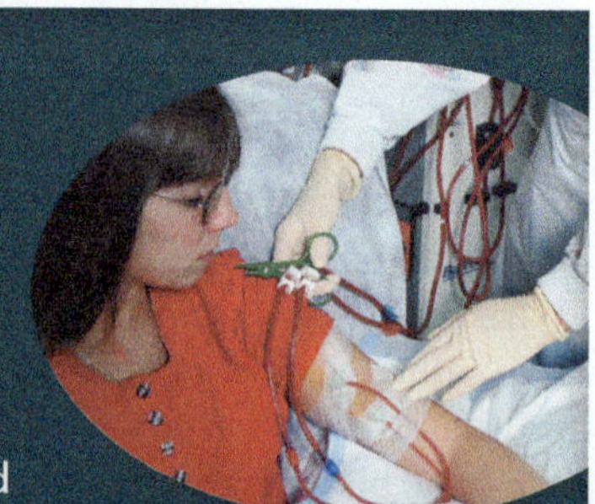

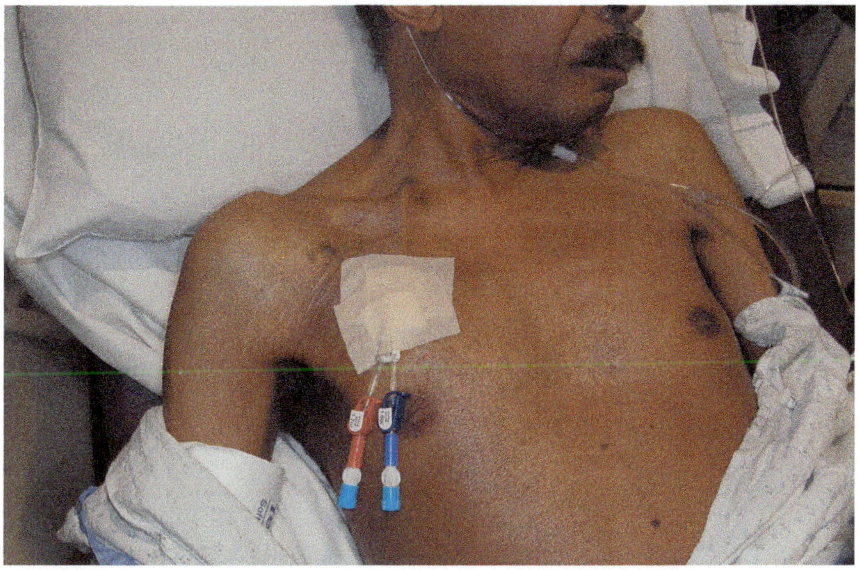

FIGURE 28-7 A two-port catheter for hemodialysis inserted into a major vein of the torso. *(© Edward T. Dickinson, MD)*

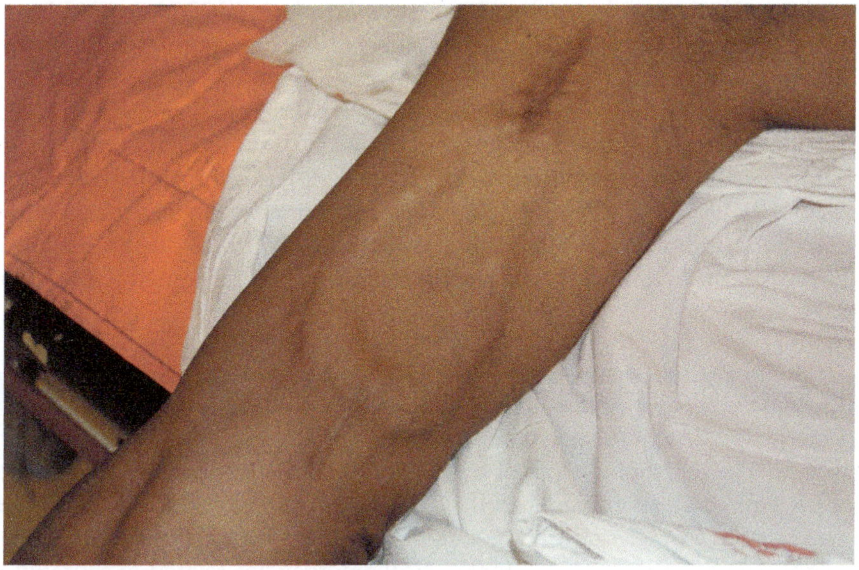

FIGURE 28-8 A fistula surgically connects an artery and a vein in an extremity. *(© Edward T. Dickinson, MD)*

called a ***thrill***, when gently palpated. ESRD patients are very protective of their fistulas, and will insist that you use another extremity to obtain a blood pressure. This is appropriate, given the importance and vulnerability of the fistula.

thrill
a vibration felt on gentle palpation, such as that which typically occurs within an arterial-venous fistula.

Peritoneal Dialysis

Patients who manage their ESRD with peritoneal dialysis (PD) usually do so in their own homes. PD is a slower process than HD, and requires multiple treatments every day for most patients. Despite requiring more frequent treatments, many patients prefer PD over HD because it allows them to be treated at home. Outside the United States and Canada, PD is the most common form of dialysis.

Peritoneal dialysis works by using the large surface area inside the peritoneal cavity that surrounds the abdominal organs as a means of removing toxins and excess fluid from the body. ESRD patients on PD have a permanent catheter that is implanted through their abdominal wall and into the peritoneal cavity (Figure 28-9). Several liters of a specially formulated dialysis solution are run into the abdominal cavity and left in place for several hours, where it absorbs waste material and excess fluid; then the fluid is drained back out into the bag and is discarded. The PD fluid setup looks much like a large IV bag and tubing. Each cycle of filling and draining the peritoneal cavity is called an ***exchange***.

exchange
one cycle of filling and draining the peritoneal cavity in peritoneal dialysis.

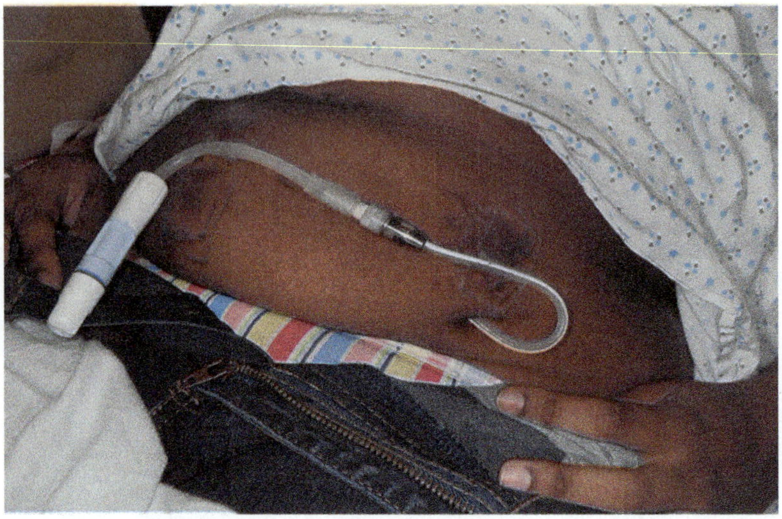

FIGURE 28-9 Peritoneal dialysis catheter. *(© Edward T. Dickinson, MD)*

continuous ambulatory peritoneal dialysis (CAPD) a gravity exchange process for peritoneal dialysis in which a bag of dialysis fluid is raised above the level of an abdominal catheter to fill the abdominal cavity and lowered below the level of the abdominal catheter to drain the fluid out.

continuous cycler-assisted peritoneal dialysis (CCPD) a mechanical process for peritoneal dialysis in which a machine fills and empties the abdominal cavity of dialysis solution.

There are two types of peritoneal dialysis: ***continuous ambulatory peritoneal dialysis (CAPD)*** and ***continuous cycler-assisted peritoneal dialysis (CCPD)***. In CAPD, the most common type of PD, the fluid is left in the peritoneal cavity by clamping the catheter for 4–6 hours. The patient then repeats the exchange several times a day. This is a simple gravity exchange process where the bag is elevated above the abdominal catheter to run dialysis fluid in, then lowered below the level of the abdomen to drain the fluid out.

Continuous cycler-assisted peritoneal dialysis (CCPD) uses the same type of peritoneal catheter as CAPD. However, rather than relying on gravity exchange, a machine is used to fill and empty the abdominal cavity with dialysis fluid 3–5 times during the night while the person sleeps. In the morning, the last fill remains in the abdomen with a dwell time that lasts the entire day.

Medical Emergencies with End-Stage Renal Disease

Medical emergencies encountered in patients with ESRD can be broadly divided into two groups: those that arise from the loss of normal kidney function and those that are complications of patients' dialysis treatments. In addition, never forget that the vast majority of dialysis patients have other underlying serious diseases such as diabetes and high blood pressure, so these patients are at risk for medical emergencies related to those diseases as well, independent of their renal failure.

Complications of ESRD

The most serious complications of ESRD seen by the EMT occur when patients fail to be dialyzed. Bad weather, illness, and poor compliance are all common reasons patients with ESRD miss their dialysis appointments.

Because they lack the ability to rid the body of excess fluid, patients who have missed dialysis will often present with signs and symptoms similar to those seen in congestive heart failure. (See the *Cardiac Emergencies* chapter.) These include shortness of breath because of fluid buildup in the lungs and the accumulation of fluids elsewhere, such as the ankles, hands, and face. In addition, because patients with ESRD can no longer balance and clear excess electrolytes as well as other toxins, patients who have missed dialysis may suffer from electrical disturbances of the heart (dysrhythmias). This is because the proper functioning of the heart's electrical system requires that the balance of electrolytes in the bloodstream be kept within a certain tight range. Elevated levels of the electrolyte potassium are particularly dangerous and can result in patient death from dysrhythmias.

Patient Care

ESRD Patient Who Has Missed Dialysis

Fundamental Principles of Care

Patients who have missed their normal dialysis sessions(s) may have done so because of an acute illness superimposed on their ESRD. Always be alert for illnesses such as stroke, sepsis, or cardiorespiratory emergencies, and be prepared to treat these conditions in addition to the complications of missed dialysis.

When encountering an ESRD patient who has missed dialysis and is experiencing problems, follow these steps:

- Assess the A-B-Cs.
- When you obtain vital signs, obtain a blood pressure on an arm that does not have a fistula.
- Place the patient in a position of comfort; this is usually sitting upright on the stretcher.
- Administer high-flow oxygen by nonrebreather mask for those in respiratory distress.
- Consider the use of noninvasive positive pressure ventilation (CPAP) in cases of severe respiratory distress. Follow local protocols.
- Monitor the patient's vital signs carefully and be prepared to attach and use the automatic external defibrillator (AED) if the patient becomes unresponsive and pulseless. Be aware that ESRD patients who suffer cardiac arrest might not respond to defibrillation. Paramedics carry certain drugs that can be administered in the field to help stabilize ESRD-induced dysrhythmias. Consider ALS backup, but do not delay transport to the hospital.
- Transport the patient to a hospital with renal dialysis capabilities.

Decision Point

- Should I request ALS for management of this patient's side effects of missed dialysis?

Complications of Dialysis

The major direct complications for patients on hemodialysis have to do with the fact that they must have large blood vessels accessed multiple times each week for their hemodialysis treatments. Other complications include:

- Bleeding from the site of the A-V fistula when the dialysis needles are removed while being disconnected from the machine
- Clotting and loss of function of the A-V fistula. This results in the fistula's feeling hard to the touch and in loss of the normal thrill felt on palpation.
- Bacterial infection of the blood due to contamination at the A-V fistula or dialysis catheter site during machine connection and disconnection

The most common serious complication of ESRD patients on peritoneal dialysis is acute ***peritonitis***, a bacterial infection within the peritoneal cavity. Patients on PD who develop peritonitis may develop abdominal pain, fever, and the telltale sign that their dialysis fluid appears cloudy when it is drained from the peritoneal cavity rather than displaying its normal clear appearance. Infected peritoneal dialysis fluid is much like chicken broth in color and turbidity.

peritonitis
bacterial infection within the peritoneal cavity.

Patient Care

ESRD Patient with Complications of Dialysis

Fundamental Principles of Care

Thousands of hemodialysis patients with ambulatory difficulty are transported to and from their appointments three times a week by EMTs. Always be alert for complications of dialysis even during these "routine" transports.

When encountering an ESRD patient who is experiencing complications of dialysis, follow these steps:

- Assess the A-B-Cs.
- Immediately control any serious bleeding from the site of the A-V fistula. Use direct pressure, elevation, and hemostatic dressings as needed. Generally, a tourniquet should be avoided in this situation, as it may damage the A-V fistula. But if life-threatening bleeding cannot be controlled by any other means, a tourniquet should be applied as proximally as possible on the limb and not directly over the fistula site.
- Administer supplemental high-flow oxygen by nonrebreather mask for dialysis patients in respiratory distress.
- Be aware that ESRD patients with peritonitis or a bacterial infection in their blood may present in shock with signs of hypoperfusion. Treat for shock by keeping the patient supine and warm.
- If peritonitis is suspected in a patient on peritoneal dialysis, transport the bag of exchanged dialysis fluid with the patient so it may be tested for bacteria at the hospital to confirm the diagnosis.

"When in doubt, you can call and talk to the doc. There is nothing wrong with that."

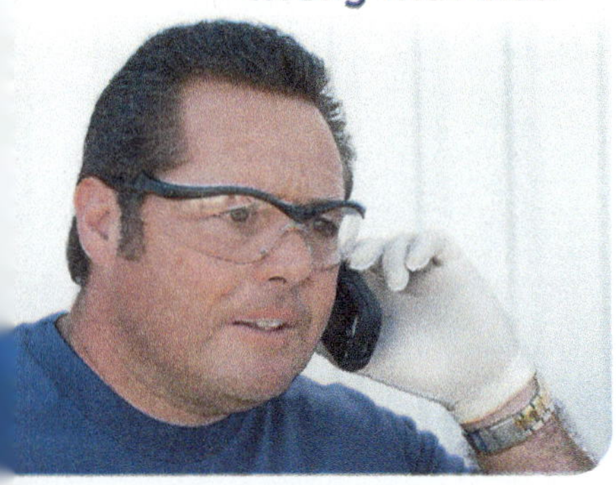

Finally, never forget that the vast majority of dialysis patients have other underlying diseases such as diabetes and high blood pressure, so they are at increased risk for medical emergencies related to those diseases as well, independent of their renal failure.

Kidney Transplant Patients

Kidneys are the most commonly transplanted organs. Patients with end-stage renal disease may be candidates for renal transplant, which, if successful, can provide the patient with a normally functioning kidney and end the need for dialysis.

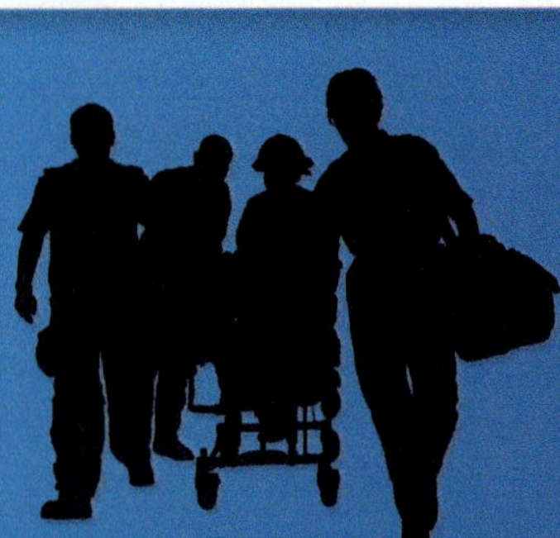

Think Like an EMT

Should You Request Advanced Life Support?

Determine if you would request advanced life support for the following patients and, if so, why.

1. A 29-year-old patient with sickle cell anemia who has severe pain in his arms and chest
2. A 42-year-old patient who recently completed his peritoneal dialysis and complains of severe abdominal pain that is worsened by movement
3. A 55-year-old female who refused to leave her house to go to her hemodialysis appointments and now complains of severe difficulty breathing, has a rapid pulse, and is anxious
4. A 37-year-old sickle cell anemia patient who complains of extreme fatigue

There are approximately twenty-one thousand kidney transplants performed by specialized surgeons in the United States each year. Thanks to the kindness of organ donors, a renal transplant places a single healthy kidney in the lower abdomen of the patient with ESRD. The surgeon then connects a blood supply and a ureter to the transplanted kidney, allowing the patient the opportunity to regain normal renal function.

Patients with kidney transplants spend the rest of their lives on a special class of drugs that prevent organ rejection by suppressing the body's immune system. However, these same drugs that help protect the transplanted kidney also make these patients more susceptible to serious infections, including sepsis. (See the chapter titled *Infectious Diseases and Sepsis.)*

Chapter Review

Key Facts and Concepts

- Blood delivers oxygen to the cells, removes carbon dioxide from the cells, and controls bleeding by clotting.
- Blood consists of red blood cells, white blood cells platelets, and plasma.
- Anemia is a deficiency of red blood cells in circulation.
- Sickle cell disease is an inherited disease in which a defect in the hemoglobin results in a sickle shape to red blood cells. This misshaping inhibits movement of the red blood cells through capillaries, causing "sludging" and blockages in smaller blood vessels, and causes chronic anemia.
- The renal system is composed of the kidneys, the ureters, the bladder, and the urethra.
- The kidneys perform a vital filtering of the blood to remove waste products. They also help maintain a water balance within the body.
- Problems with the renal system include infection, kidney stones, and renal failure.
- Renal failure is a condition in which the kidneys are unable to normally filter waste and to provide a balance of fluids and electrolytes in the body.
- Dialysis removes excess fluid and electrolytes from the body by filtration. Dialysis may be performed in either of two ways: hemodialysis or peritoneal dialysis. Hemodialysis at dialysis centers is generally performed three times per week. Peritoneal dialysis is done at home and is usually done several times daily.
- Major complications in patients with end-stage renal disease can occur after the patient has missed dialysis appointments, from infections, or as a result of bleeding from hemodialysis access sites.

Key Decisions

- Does my patient have a history of sickle cell disease or end-stage renal disease?
- Does my patient have an A-V fistula?
- Will I need to make an early request for advanced life support because of complications from a missed dialysis appointment?

Chapter Glossary

anemia deficiency in the number of red blood cells in the circulation.

coagulopathy loss of the normal ability to form a blood clot with internal or external bleeding.

continuous ambulatory peritoneal dialysis (CAPD) a gravity exchange process for peritoneal dialysis in which a bag of dialysis fluid is raised above the level of an abdominal catheter to fill the abdominal cavity and lowered below the level of the abdominal catheter to drain the fluid out.

continuous cycler-assisted peritoneal dialysis (CCPD) a mechanical process for peritoneal dialysis in which a machine fills and empties the abdominal cavity of dialysis solution.

dialysis the process by which toxins and excess fluid are removed from the body by a medical system independent of the kidneys.

end-stage renal disease (ESRD) irreversible renal failure to the extent that the kidneys can no longer provide adequate filtration and fluid balance to sustain life; survival with ESRD usually requires dialysis.

exchange one cycle of filling and draining the peritoneal cavity in peritoneal dialysis.

peritonitis bacterial infection within the peritoneal cavity.

pyelonephritis an infection that begins in the urinary tract and ascends up the ureter into the kidney.

renal failure loss of the kidneys' ability to filter the blood and remove toxins and excess fluid from the body.

sickle cell anemia (SCA) an inherited disease in which a genetic defect in the hemoglobin results in abnormal structure of the red blood cells.

sickle cell disease (SCD) an inherited disease in which patients have a genetic defect in their hemoglobin that results in an abnormal structure of the red blood cell.

thrill a vibration felt on gentle palpation, such as that which typically occurs within an arterial-venous fistula.

urinary catheter a drainage tube placed into the urinary system to allow the flow of urine out of the body.

Preparation for Your Examination and Practice

Short Answer

1. What is sickle cell anemia?
2. What is *sludging* in a patient with sickle cell anemia?
3. What is a *thrill*?
4. What is the difference between *hemodialysis* and *peritoneal dialysis*?
5. What are the complications that may be seen if a patient misses a dialysis appointment?

Thinking and Linking

Think back to the Cardiac Emergencies *chapter, and link information from that chapter with information from the section on end-stage renal disease in this chapter as you consider the following situations:*

1. You are treating a patient who has missed dialysis. Because of a fluid buildup, the patient has signs and symptoms similar to those of congestive heart failure. What are these signs and symptoms?
2. Your patient, who has missed several dialysis treatments, says he is having palpitations. Why?

Critical Thinking Exercises

Renal diseases and sickle cell anemia can result in life-threatening emergencies. The purpose of this exercise is to analyze the complaints of two such patients.

1. You have a patient who is transported routinely for dialysis three times per week. She was sick and cancelled the trip yesterday. Now she calls saying she can't breathe and feels like she is going to die. Is it possible that she has a legitimate complaint after missing dialysis by only one day?
2. You have a patient with a history of sickle cell crisis who is complaining of severe pain in his legs. The patient refuses to move because it hurts so much. Your partner thinks the patient is being overdramatic and falsely complaining of pain to get drugs from the hospital. Do you agree with your partner? Why or why not? What should you do for the patient?

Pathophysiology to Practice

The following questions are designed to assist you in gathering relevant clinical information and making accurate decisions in the field.

- You are treating a patient who is complaining of stroke symptoms. He has a history of sickle cell disease. Does sickle cell disease make the diagnosis of a stroke more likely or less likely in this patient? Why?
- A patient with sickle cell disease tells you of severe, recurring infections. Why would an SCA patient have this problem?

Street Scenes

You are sent to a "routine transfer" nonemergency call to transport a 64-year-old patient from a long-term care facility to a dialysis appointment. You arrive to find the patient with an altered mental status and "not feeling well."

You note the patient has poor color, which the staff tells you is normal for the patient. The patient is somewhat anxious, and her skin is warm to the touch.

Street Scene Questions

1. What are your initial steps in assessing this patient?
2. How does the dialysis history fit into the patient picture at this point?

You complete a primary assessment and find the patient is breathing somewhat rapidly but adequately at 28 per minute. The patient has peripheral pulses and no obvious external bleeding. Pulse oximetry reveals a saturation of 94 percent. The patient will respond to questions but is sleepy and a little confused. The staff says this is a new development in the patient, who is usually quite oriented.

Street Scene Questions

3. What assessments should you perform next?
4. Do you believe the patient's condition is related to her dialysis?

The patient's pulse and respirations are slightly elevated. Her blood pressure is 108/58, her skin is warm and dry, and her pupils are equal and reactive to light. The patient has a slight difficulty breathing, and some fluid is noticeable around her ankles. Her lungs show some mild crackles (also known as rales) in the bases. Blood glucose is 102. The patient cannot follow instructions for the stroke scale, but she does not have facial droop or slurred speech. The staff says she seemed fine when she went to bed last night.

Street Scene Question

5. **The staff asks you to take the patient to her dialysis appointment and says they think "she'll be fine by the time she gets back." Should you transport her to dialysis or to a hospital?**

5 SECTION

Trauma

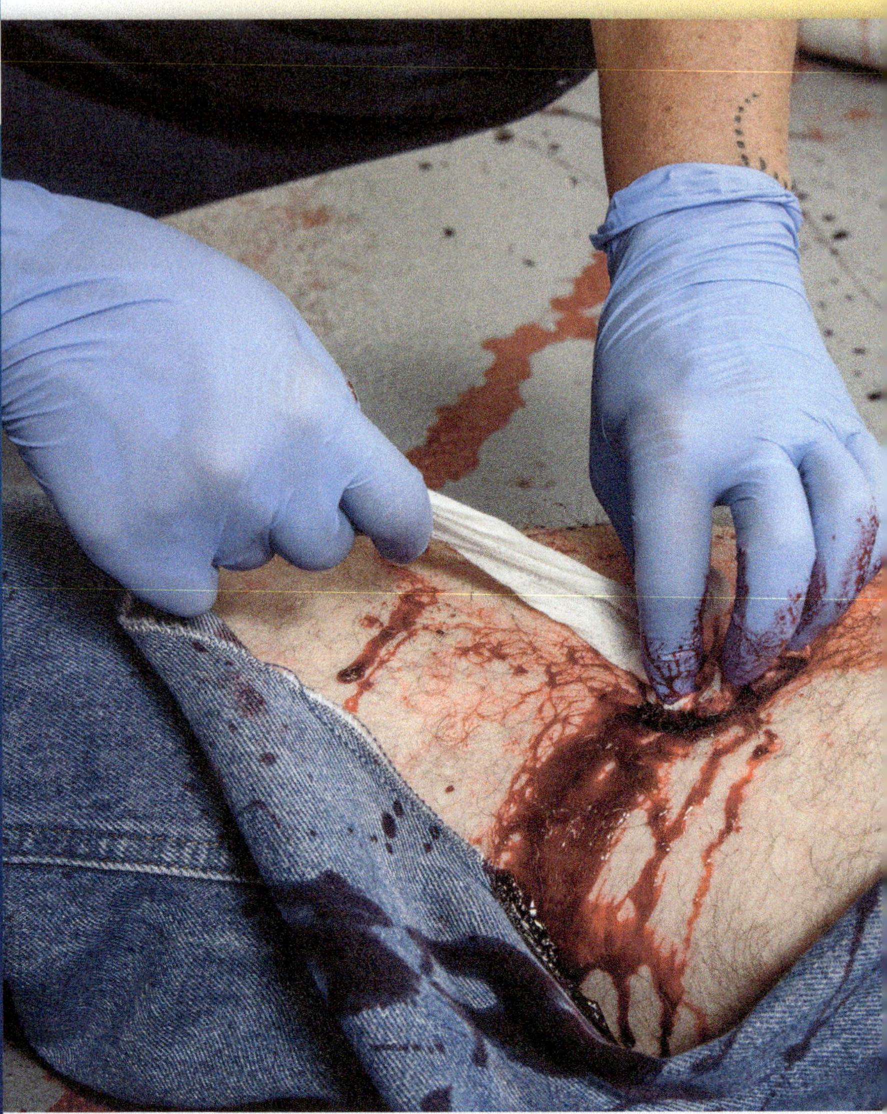

Trauma is another word for *injury*. Falls, vehicle collisions, and violence are just a few causes of trauma. The loss of blood during trauma, either externally or internally, can cause serious complications, the most critical of which is shock.

The first chapter in this section, *Bleeding and Shock*, covers these conditions as life-threatening emergencies. Other kinds of trauma are covered in *Soft Tissue Trauma*, *Chest and Abdominal Trauma*, *Musculoskeletal Trauma*, and *Trauma to the Head, Neck, and Spine*. The trauma section concludes with *Multisystem Trauma* and *Environmental Emergencies*.

Bleeding and Shock

29

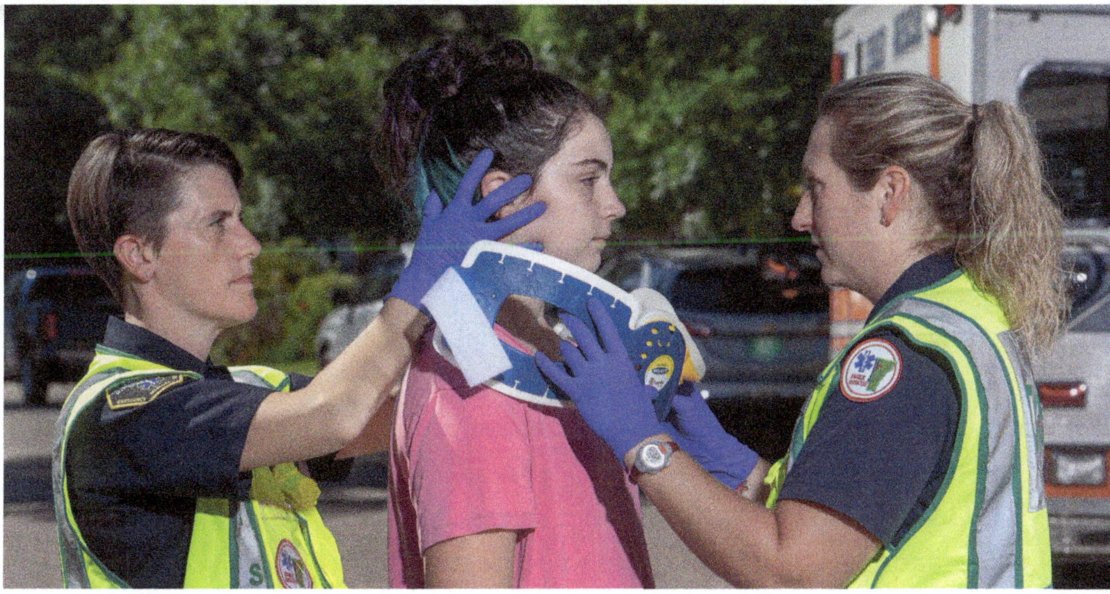

Related Chapters

The following chapters provide additional information related to topics discussed in this chapter:

6 Anatomy and Physiology
7 Principles of Pathophysiology
11 Scene Size-Up
12 Primary Assessment
13 Vital Signs and Monitoring Devices
14 Principles of Assessment
15 Secondary Assessment
16 Reassessment
19 Respiratory Emergencies
20 Cardiac Emergencies
22 Diabetic Emergencies and Altered Mental Status
23 Allergic Reactions
25 Poisoning and Overdose Emergencies
26 Abdominal Emergencies
27 Behavioral and Psychiatric Emergencies and Suicide
28 Hematologic and Renal Emergencies
32 Musculoskeletal Trauma

Standards

Shock and Resuscitation; Trauma (Bleeding)

Competency

Applies fundamental knowledge of the causes, pathophysiology, and management of shock, respiratory failure or arrest, cardiac failure or arrest, and post-resuscitation management.

Applies fundamental knowledge to provide basic emergency care and transportation based on assessment findings for an acutely injured patient.

Core Concepts

- Signs, symptoms, and care of a patient with shock
- Recognizing hemorrhage
- How to evaluate the severity of external bleeding
- How to control external bleeding
- Signs, symptoms, and care of a patient with internal bleeding

Outcomes

After reading this chapter, you should be able to:

29.1 Summarize the significance of bleeding in trauma. (pp. 786-788)

- Explain the impact on the body when a significant amount of blood escapes the vascular system due to injury.
- Explain the impact of modern battlefield injuries on the importance of immediate hemorrhage control in saving lives.
- Describe the interaction of the components of the circulatory system to maintain perfusion.

29.2 Summarize concepts of shock. (pp. 788-797)

- Describe how failure of any of the components of the cardiovascular system can lead to hypoperfusion.
- Describe the characteristics of the major classifications of shock.
- Compare compensated and decompensated shock.
- Compare the pediatric patient's presentation in shock with that of adults.
- Explain the role of time to definitive care in survival from hemorrhagic shock.
- Relate signs and symptoms of shock to the body's attempts to compensate for the amount of blood lost.

29.3 Summarize the EMT care approach to the patient in shock. (pp. 798-799)

- Prioritize the interventions for specific portrayals of patients in shock.
- Describe the decision-making process for transporting a patient in shock.

29.4 Summarize the EMT care approach to the patient with external bleeding. (pp. 799-818)

- Distinguish the characteristics of venous, arterial, and capillary bleeding.
- Identify assessment procedures required to ensure all external bleeding is found.
- Describe the team approach to caring for a patient with massive external bleeding.

- Explain the prioritization of external bleeding control in the overall context of the patient's presentation.
- Identify the rationale for selecting methods of controlling external hemorrhage.
- Outline the steps of the various approaches to external bleeding control.
- Describe the modified approaches to managing bleeding from head injuries and nose bleeds.

29.5 Summarize the EMT care approach to the patient with internal bleeding. (pp. 818–820)

- Recognize indications of internal bleeding.
- Outline the priorities of care for a patient with internal bleeding.

Key Terms

arterial bleeding, p. *800*
capillary bleeding, p. *801*
cardiogenic shock, p. *790*
compensated shock, p. *792*
decompensated shock, p. *793*
distributive shock, p. *790*
hemorrhage, p. *799*
hemorrhagic shock, p. *789*
hemostatic agents, p. *810*
hypoperfusion, p. *786*
hypovolemic shock, p. *789*
neurogenic shock, p. *790*
obstructive shock, p. *790*
perfusion, p. *786*
pressure dressing, p. *809*
shock, p. *786*
tourniquet, p. *811*
venous bleeding, p. *800*

In 2018 in the United States, more than three million people were injured by intentional or accidental trauma, and 150,000 of those patients died. Trauma deaths included more than 40,000 homicides and more than 43,000 fatal car crashes. In fact, trauma was the leading cause of death for persons between the ages of 1 and 45, and the fourth-leading cause of death overall. But the important fact that you should remember is that a great many of these deaths were preventable.

Although trauma may be a fact of life, EMS plays a vital role in the fight to lower its impact. Chief among these actions is prevention. We know that many trauma patients will die instantly because of their injuries. When a person sustains a lethal gunshot wound to the brain, for example, no amount or level of trauma care can change the outcome. Far too many of our trauma patients fall into this "nonsurvivable" category. To effect change, we must stop these injuries from happening, and the EMT's role in prevention is vitally important. From bicycle safety, to car seat installation, to "Stop the Bleed" campaigns, prevention strategies may offer the best avenue to lowering the toll of trauma deaths. With the emergence of mobile integrated health care and an increasing partnership between EMS and public health, prevention is not only an opportunity to save lives, but a growing responsibility of our profession. However, despite all the prevention strategies EMTs may put in place, patients will still need our immediate care.

If a trauma patient is not killed immediately, the numbers above suggest that they will survive. However, the impact of these injuries and the overall course of the patient's recovery depend greatly upon the care provided immediately after the initial trauma. In these situations, the immediate actions and competent care of EMS make a significant difference and can change that life-or-death equation.

Although all trauma care is important, very few interventions are more important than stopping hemorrhage and treating shock. As you know from the chapter *Principles of Pathophysiology*, the constant flow of oxygenated blood to body structures is essential to support life. In many trauma patients, this flow, or ***perfusion***, is interrupted. When blood escapes from the cardiovascular system or when it cannot be efficiently pumped to tissues, the cells become insufficiently oxygenated, a state known as ***hypoperfusion***, or ***shock***. Without sufficient oxygen and nutrients, the basic functions of cells cannot take place.

One of the core tenets of trauma care is to maintain or restore perfusion. There are many steps that need to be taken to make sure this happens. Your assessment skills must be up to date, and you must be ready to identify hypoperfusion quickly and move immediately to intervene.

The treatment steps you will take are actually very simple but nevertheless important. If the patient has life-threatening bleeding, you must stop it. If you cannot stop it, you must rapidly transport that patient to a setting with the capabilities to stop it. While doing this, you also must be mindful of the underlying hypoperfused state, known as shock. In shock, hypoperfused cells are not functioning normally. In a fight for life, these cells are producing energy inefficiently and creating more waste products than normal. Because metabolism has been affected, they are also not generating as much heat. By recognizing the warning signs of shock, you can intervene and take steps to assist the body's efforts to stay alive and prevent shock from worsening.

Most important, we know these steps work. As tragic as the battlefields of Iraq and Afghanistan have been, they have taught civilian medicine great lessons in trauma care. They have dispelled previously held myths and taught us new steps to fight against trauma death. Bleeding and shock have been particular focuses of attention, and we now know a great deal more about them than we did even 10 years ago. The simple steps used by the military to control hemorrhage and to treat shock have shown very real promise and have significantly advanced care in the civilian world. We will discuss those interventions in this chapter.

The Circulatory System

Main Components

The circulatory (or cardiovascular) system is responsible for the distribution of blood to all parts of the body. This system has three main components: the heart, blood vessels, and the blood that flows through them. All components must function properly for the system to remain intact (Figure 29-1). (You may wish to review the information about the heart and the circulatory system in the chapters titled *Anatomy and Physiology* and *Principles of Pathophysiology*.)

The heart is a muscular organ that lies within the chest, behind the sternum. Its job is to pump blood, which supplies oxygen and nutrients to the body's cells. To provide a sufficient supply of oxygen and nutrients to all parts of the body, the heart must pump at an adequate rate and rhythm.

The blood is circulated throughout the body through three major types of blood vessels (Figure 29-2):

1. **Arteries.** The arteries carry freshly oxygenated blood away from the heart. They are under a great deal of pressure during the heart's contractions. (Taking the patient's blood pressure is a means of measuring arterial pressure.) An artery has a thick, muscular wall that enables it to dilate or constrict, depending on the amount of oxygen and nutrients needed by the cells or organs it feeds.
2. **Capillaries.** Oxygen-rich blood is emptied from the arteries into microscopically small capillaries, which supply every cell of the body. In areas where capillaries and body cells are in contact, a vital exchange takes place. Oxygen and nutrients are given up

perfusion
the supply of oxygen to and removal of wastes from the body's cells and tissues as a result of the flow of blood through the capillaries.

hypoperfusion
(HI-po-per-FEW-zhun)
the body's inability to adequately circulate blood to the body's cells to supply them with oxygen and nutrients. *See also* shock.

shock
the body's inability to circulate blood adequately to the body's cells to supply them with oxygen and nutrients, which is a life-threatening condition. Also known as *hypoperfusion*.

FIGURE 29-1 The circulatory system.

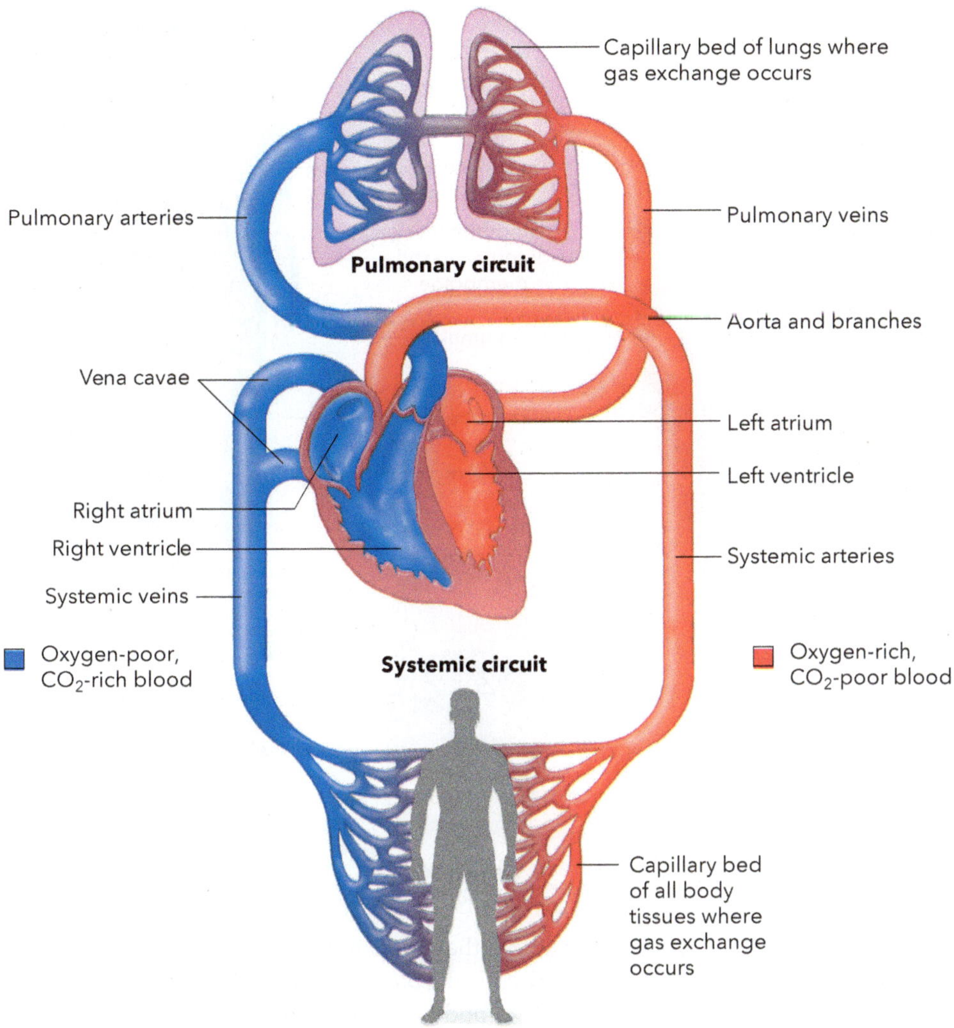

by the blood and pass through the extremely thin capillary walls into the cells. At the same time, carbon dioxide and other waste products given up by the cells pass through the capillary walls and are taken up by the blood.

3. **Veins.** Blood that has been depleted of oxygen and loaded with carbon dioxide and other wastes in the capillaries empties into veins that carry it back to the heart. Veins have one-way valves that prevent the blood from flowing in the wrong direction. Blood in a vein is under much less pressure than blood in an artery.

The blood has several functions:

- **Transportation of gases.** Oxygen is diffused into the blood at the alveoli in the lungs and is carried to the body's cells. In a similar fashion, carbon dioxide is diffused into the blood at the body's cells and is carried back to the alveoli, where it is offloaded and then exhaled.
- **Nutrition.** Blood circulates nutrients from the intestines or storage tissues (such as fatty tissue, the liver, and muscle cells) to the other body cells.
- **Excretion.** Blood carries waste products from the cells to organs, such as the kidneys, that excrete (eliminate) the waste products from the body.
- **Protection.** Blood carries antibodies and white blood cells, which help fight disease and infection. Blood also contains platelets and clotting factors that work to control bleeding from damaged blood vessels by forming blood clots.

FIGURE 29-2 Comparative structure of arteries, capillaries, and veins.

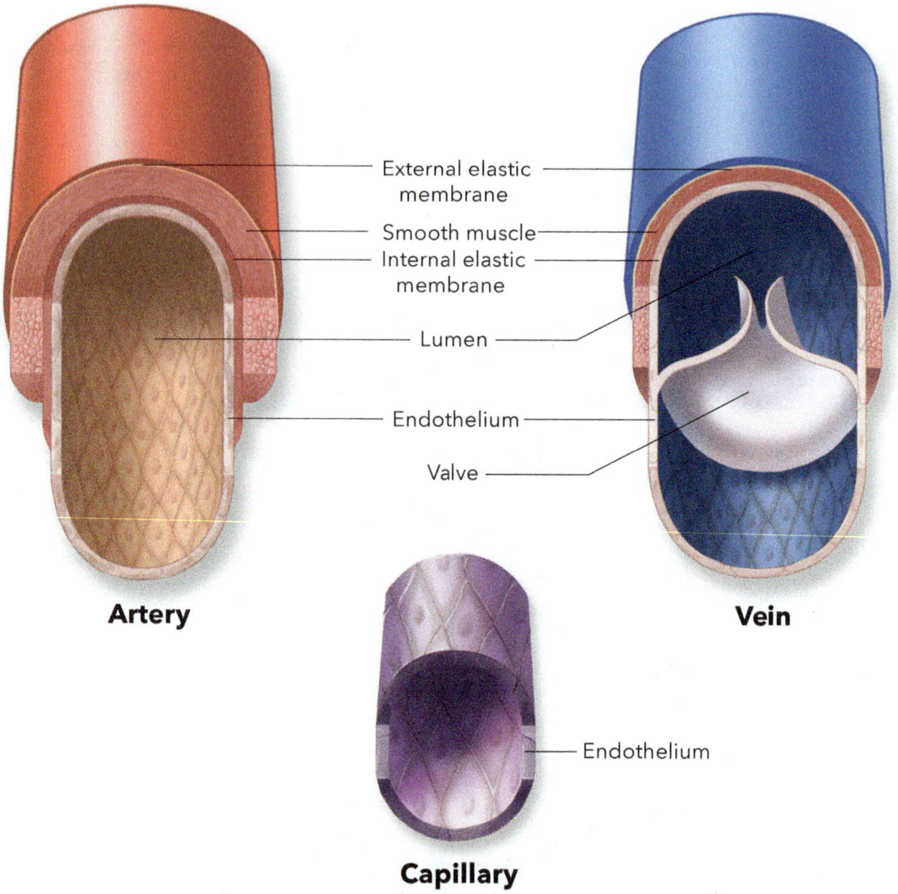

- **Regulation.** Blood carries substances that control the body's functions, such as hormones, water, salt, enzymes, and chemicals. Blood also plays an important role in regulating body temperature by carrying body heat to the lungs and skin surface, where it is dissipated. Dilation (expansion) of blood vessels increases blood flow to the skin, which increases heat loss from the skin surface. Conversely, constriction (narrowing) of blood vessels decreases blood flow to the skin, which decreases heat loss so core temperature can be preserved.

As mentioned earlier, the adequate circulation of blood throughout the body, which fills the capillaries and supplies the cells and tissues with oxygen and nutrients, is called perfusion. If, for some reason, blood is not adequately circulated, some of the body's cells and organs do not receive adequate supplies of oxygen, and dangerous waste products build up. Inadequate perfusion of the body's tissues and organs is called hypoperfusion. (*Hypo-* means "low," so *hypoperfusion* means "low perfusion.")

Recall that the heart, blood vessels, and blood are the three main components of the circulatory system. These components may be likened to a pump, pipes, and fluid in the pipes. For the circulatory system to function properly, all three components must function properly. If any component fails, or "leaks," the body will try in various ways to compensate and maintain adequate perfusion. However, if the problem is not corrected, adequate perfusion cannot be maintained, and shock (hypoperfusion) will result.

Shock

Shock is the inadequate perfusion of body cells, and it occurs when the circulatory system fails. Although we will describe several different classifications of shock, the overall condition is actually caused by only four potential problems: volume loss, pump failure, loss of blood vessel tone, and obstruction of blood flow. In each of these situations, blood is prevented from reaching the body's cells, and hypoperfusion occurs as the cells go without the oxygen and nutrients they desperately need. The further classifications of shock, which will be described later, address the individual and larger causes of the shock condition. For example, septic shock is a blood vessel tone problem, but that issue is caused by the larger problem of a systemic inflammatory response to infection. Although there are many classifications of shock, hypoperfusion in each case can be traced to one of the four root causes.

Hypoperfusion of the cells is a deadly problem. When cells fail to receive oxygen and glucose, they are unable to convert nutrients into energy, and cell function fails. If hypoperfusion persists, the cell itself will die. We know some cells can sustain a hypoperfused state longer than others. For example, skin and bone cells can stay alive even after hours of hypoperfusion. Conversely, the cells of the brain and the heart, which require a constant supply of oxygen, will die within minutes if that supply is fully interrupted (as in stroke or MI). Cells that make up larger organ systems like the kidneys and liver are more tolerant to hypoperfusion, but they often fall victim to prolonged hypoxia associated with shock states.

Consider the following example: A 6-year-old male is struck by a car while crossing the street. The initial trauma lacerates his liver, and he is losing blood rapidly into his abdomen. Blood leaving the circulatory system causes a volume problem, and hypovolemic shock occurs.

The young boy's body will fight to stay alive. His circulatory system will adjust to keep the remaining blood flowing to organs that need it the most. Blood vessels will constrict to restore pressure, and blood will be shunted away from the periphery and toward the brain, heart, and lungs. Although this compensation may keep the boy alive temporarily, other cells and organ systems will be affected. If the bleeding is not corrected and hypoperfusion persists, organs receiving decreased amounts of blood will begin to shut down and die. The longer shock continues, the more the damage will become irreversible.

The Pathophysiology of Shock

As mentioned, four specific pathophysiologies lead to the presentation of shock: volume problems, pump problems, blood vessel tone problems, and obstruction of blood flow. It is important to understand how these problems affect the body.

CORE CONCEPT

Signs, symptoms, and care of a patient with shock

Volume Problems

Volume problems, also known as hypovolemia, occur when blood is lost, or the liquid portion of the blood is removed from the circulatory system. In cases of *absolute hypovolemia,* like internal or external hemorrhage, blood physically leaves the circulatory system. When hemorrhage occurs, the circulatory system loses the hemoglobin, platelets, and nutrients that are normally transported by the blood. Cells must do without. Volume problems can also be caused by *relative hypovolemia.* In this instance, blood is not actually lost from the circulatory system, but conditions like dehydration or burns shift the liquid portion of blood, called plasma, out of the blood vessels and therefore out of the circulatory system. In these cases, even though blood is not lost, volume can be significantly depleted. When hypovolemia occurs (both absolute and relative), there is simply not enough volume within the blood vessels, so pressure within the circulatory system falls. This dropping pressure creates a circumstance in which the pumping of the heart is no longer capable of moving blood. Hypoperfusion results. Hypovolemic states also are worsened by the loss of blood products. When platelets are lost, clotting is affected. When hemoglobin is lost, the blood's oxygen-carrying capacity is reduced. Each of these issues contributes to the already serious problem of shock.

The categories of shock associated with volume problems include hypovolemic shock. ***Hypovolemic shock*** refers simply to an insufficient volume in the circulatory system, and applies to both relative and absolute hypovolemia. More specifically, ***hemorrhagic shock*** refers specifically to a loss of blood. In addition, both septic shock and anaphylactic shock also can cause fluid-shifting hypovolemic problems, but their underlying causes are more commonly associated with blood vessel tone issues.

hypovolemic (HI-po-vo-LE-mik) ***shock***
shock resulting from blood or fluid loss.

hemorrhagic (HEM-or-AJ-ik) ***shock***
shock resulting from blood loss.

Pump Problems

Shock can be caused by a failure of the heart to pump blood. Typically, a mechanical problem, like a rupture in a heart ventricle, or a failure of the papillary muscles that close a valve, causes the heart to pump inadequate amounts of blood. Like hypovolemia, the pump failure drops pressure within the circulatory system, and blood cannot be moved. Hypoperfusion of the cells follows. Pump problems are notoriously dangerous, as the heart is one of the key components of compensation in shock states. When it is the cause of shock, as with MI, the condition is frequently fatal. Pump problems are categorized as ***cardiogenic shock***, referring to the root cardiac cause of the hypoperfusion state.

cardiogenic shock
shock, or lack of perfusion, brought on not by blood loss but by the heart's inadequate pumping action. It is often the result of a heart attack (MI) or congestive heart failure.

Blood Vessel Tone Problems

Blood vessels play an important role in the development of shock (if they are *not* functioning properly) and in the body's ability to compensate for shock (if they are functioning properly). Blood vessels can change their diameter, either by dilating or constricting. These changes in size are governed by the need for blood in various areas of the body. In an area of the body that is doing more work, blood vessels dilate to allow more blood to flow to that area. At the same time, in another area of the body that is not working as hard, vessels will constrict. For example, if you are running, blood flow to the muscles in the legs increases through dilated arteries. At the same time, blood flow to the digestive system lessens because vessels supplying these organs have been constricted to compensate for the dilation of the arteries in the legs. Since the amount of blood in the body does not change, this balance between dilation of some vessels and constriction of others is necessary to keep the system full. The same amount of blood is in the body, but it is distributed differently. If all the blood vessels in the body dilated at one time, there would not be enough blood to fill the entire circulatory system. Circulation would fail, tissues would not be adequately perfused, and the patient would develop shock.

Hypoperfusion caused by failed blood vessel tone is broadly referred to as ***distributive shock***. Distributive shock describes numerous specific conditions caused by the massive *drop in pressure associated with systemic dilation. These include:*

distributive shock
hypoperfusion due to a lack of blood vessel tone. Blood vessel dilation leads to decreased pressure within the circulatory system.

Anaphylactic shock In anaphylaxis, a severe allergic reaction causes systemic vasodilation and massive drops in blood pressure. As noted earlier, increased capillary permeability is also a side effect of anaphylaxis and can cause volume-related issues as well. For more information on anaphylaxis, refer to the chapter titled *Allergic Reactions*.

Neurogenic shock ***Neurogenic shock*** occurs as a result of a spinal cord injury. When the cord is damaged, key messages to the sympathetic nervous system, the part of the nervous system that normally manages constriction of the blood vessels, get interrupted. Without these important messages, a systemic vasodilation dominates. Blood pressure can drop rapidly.

neurogenic shock
hypoperfusion caused by a spinal cord injury that results in systemic vasodilation

Septic shock Septic shock is a very dangerous form of distributive shock that also incorporates elements of hypovolemic and cardiogenic shock. In septic shock, a body infection causes a systemic inflammatory response to occur. This inflammatory response causes blood vessels to dilate and capillary membranes to become permeable. Dilation causes huge drops in blood pressure, and permeability robs the circulatory system of volume. In some infections, toxins are also released that affect the pumping ability of the heart. This combination of problems translates to a particularly deadly form of shock. For more information on septic shock, refer to the chapter titled *Infectious Diseases and Sepsis*.

Obstruction of Blood Flow

Some shock states are caused not by the circulatory system itself, but rather by problems that cause the flow of blood to be blocked (***obstructive shock***). Conditions like a pulmonary embolism, cardiac tamponade, and a tension pneumothorax obstruct the flow of blood in and out of the heart and lungs and cause hypoperfusion to the body cells. For example, in a pulmonary embolism, a clot blocks blood flow in a large blood vessel in the lungs. This clot stops blood from reaching the lung tissue and therefore reduces the ability

obstructive shock
a term commonly used to describe the different conditions that block the flow of blood and cause hypoperfusion.

of the lung to exchange oxygen and carbon dioxide. Although the circulatory system is not to blame, the net effect of hypoperfusion is the same.

Fight or Flight

When baroreceptors in the aorta and carotid artery sense decreased pressure, they stimulate release of epinephrine and norepinephrine into the bloodstream. This causes blood vessels to constrict, especially in skin, kidneys, and gastrointestinal tract. The skin becomes cool and pale. Sweat glands empty their contents, causing the sweaty skin so commonly seen in these situations. When blood vessels in the kidneys constrict, the kidneys produce less urine, thus preventing the loss of more fluid. Constriction of blood vessels in the GI tract causes the stomach to try to empty its contents, leading to nausea and vomiting. Finally, epinephrine triggers increased heart rate and contractility. These reactions are all part of the fight-or-flight response the body experiences when under extreme stress.

Compensation

The body is a remarkably resilient organism that can adapt to seemingly massive insults. When shock occurs, the body undertakes a series of predictable steps to make up for the underlying hypoperfusion. These steps are called *compensation*. Remember that shock occurs when the cells of the body cannot obtain an adequate supply of oxygen-rich and nutrient-rich blood. Compensation is aimed at restoring that blood flow, and its measures occur both locally and systemically.

The body has sensors strategically placed throughout the circulatory system to constantly measure the adequacy of perfusion. Baroreceptors, also known as "stretch receptors," sense pressure within the large vessels of the circulatory system and provide feedback to the brain. They sense both rising and falling pressure. When arterial pressure becomes too low, as in shock, the brain responds by initiating constriction in the blood vessels, essentially making the circulatory system smaller. In a similar way, the body also uses chemoreceptors. Chemoreceptors sense changes in oxygen, carbon dioxide, and body acid–base status (pH). When deficiencies are identified, urgent messages are transmitted via the nervous system, and similar responses are engaged.

The body compensates for shock in very predictable ways. These compensatory measures span the systems of the body. They include regulation of volume, vasoconstriction, and cardiopulmonary response (Table 29-1).

Regulation of Volume—In shock states, the body will take immediate steps to regulate volume within the circulatory system. The body signals the kidneys to retain fluid. Excretion is reduced to manage total body water and blood volume. In the hospital, shock patients are carefully monitored for urinary output as a measure for assessing volume. Sometimes this can be assessed in the field. For example, when assessing a dehydrated infant, it may be helpful to ask the caregiver about diaper routine. Has the caregiver had to change a normal number of diapers? Dehydration and associated hypovolemic shock would be associated with dry diapers and a diminished need to change them.

TABLE 29-1 The Signs and Symptoms of Shock

INSIDE	OUTSIDE
Hypoperfusion affecting sensitive body cells and disrupting function	Altered mental status: anxious, confused, or lethargic; changes in mentation
Regulation of volume, reduction of excretion	Decreased urinary output (not a common EMS assessment, but a key hospital finding)
Vasoconstriction	Pale skin, delayed capillary refill time, narrowing pulse pressure (as a trend in blood pressure measurements)
Cardiopulmonary response (increased heart rate and contractile force, increased respiratory rate)	Increasing pulse rate, increasing respiratory rate

Vasoconstriction—Probably the most effective immediate compensatory step is vasoconstriction, or the narrowing of blood vessel diameter. When baroreceptors sense a drop in pressure in the circulatory system, the brain signals the release of epinephrine and norepinephrine. These chemical mediators cause blood vessels throughout the body to constrict. Constriction moves blood away from small, peripheral blood vessels and into larger, more central blood vessels. This "shunt to the core" ensures that vital organs like the heart, lungs, and brain maintain blood flow while reducing blood flow to areas that can tolerate hypoperfusion longer. Vasoconstriction also reduces the overall size of the circulatory system and therefore increases pressure within the blood vessels. This pressure is essential to the ability to move blood with each pump of the heart. In shock patients, vasoconstriction is often seen in the form of pale skin and delayed capillary refill time, as both findings indicate shunting of blood. Remember that this compensatory effort is not always possible, especially in distributive shock. In those cases, a lack of constriction is actually causing the problem.

Cardiopulmonary Response—Epinephrine and norepinephrine, which are released in shock states, regulate the heart and lungs. When hypoperfusion is sensed, the brain signals the heart to beat faster and more forcefully. Faster heart rates and increased contractility (strength of contraction) typically improve cardiac output and maximize the remaining circulatory function. The brain also increases respiratory rates to optimize oxygen exchange. These changes are visible in shock patients in the form of increased pulses and increased respiratory rates.

The body buys time for itself during shock with compensation. Vasoconstriction and the cardiopulmonary responses can restore adequate pressure for prolonged, but limited, periods while the body attempts to heal. We refer to this collective set of compensatory actions as ***compensated shock***. The measures used to compensate cannot continue indefinitely. However, in the short run, compensation efforts such as vasoconstriction can effectively restore the arterial pressures necessary to maintain perfusion to vital organs. In some cases, compensation can be a very effective means of staying alive. As an EMT, it is very important to identify the signs and symptoms associated with compensation because they demonstrate an opportunity to intervene to prevent further progression of shock. Some shock states can be very difficult to detect, but compensatory changes like tachycardia and tachypnea are often excellent indicators that the fight is on.

compensated shock
period when the patient is developing shock but the body is still able to maintain perfusion.

Pediatric Note

Pediatric patients are excellent compensators. Children and infants often can compensate for massive insults and sustain this compensation for prolonged periods of time. Vasoconstriction is especially effective. Pediatric patients shunt blood to the core much more effectively than adults do. Small blood vessels narrow and maintain normal blood pressures, even as up to 40 percent to 50 percent of blood volume is lost. This is a key factor in the struggle for life, but it can also present a challenge to the recognition of shock. Although a drop in blood pressure is a sign of shock, you should never wait for low blood pressure to identify shock. This is especially true in pediatric patients.

Pediatric patients also rely much more on heart rate to compensate for shock. The ability of the heart to contract more forcefully in compensation is developed with age. Young hearts often have fewer contractile heart cells than do the hearts of adults. As a result, they rely more upon rate and less upon contractility. Fast heart rates during compensation in children are a key indicator of shock.

Decompensation

Compensation in shock is sustained by muscle use. Smooth muscle in the blood vessels constricts to cause vasoconstriction. Heart muscle strains to increase pumping rates and contractility. Muscles of the chest wall work harder to increase respiratory rate. Although each of these measures is an effective compensatory step, none can be sustained indefinitely.

When muscles work harder, they require more fuel. Oxygen and glucose are required to maintain the metabolism that drives muscle function. Remember that compensated shock is occurring because of a hypoperfusion issue. Underlying all these steps is a problem that likely arose because cells could not obtain the required amounts of oxygen and nutrients. Now, as muscle use increases, these demands increase.

If the underlying problem is not corrected and hypoperfusion persists, the muscles of compensation will simply run out of fuel. The timing of this decompensation varies greatly depending on the nature of the illness or injury and the severity of the problem, but in all cases, compensatory measures are temporary. In addition to running out of fuel, compensation has other ill effects. As blood is shunted to the vital organs, that blood is robbed from other systems that also need oxygenation and nutrients. If vasoconstriction is left uncorrected over time, those other systems can be damaged and die. The liver and kidneys are particularly vulnerable to this problem.

Other problems can also overwhelm the body's ability to compensate. For example, massive hemorrhage can be compensated for briefly, but as blood continues to be lost, there is a point of no return. The body can vasoconstrict and vasoconstrict, but if there is simply no blood in the system, that vasoconstriction will be ineffective. Similarly, in cardiogenic shock, the heart is the root cause of the hypoperfusion problem. It cannot participate in compensatory measures. Without the ability of the heart to increase cardiac output, this condition swiftly overcomes the body's ability to self-correct. When compensation fails, compensated shock becomes ***decompensated shock***.

decompensated shock period when the body can no longer compensate for low blood volume or lack of perfusion. Late signs such as decreasing blood pressure become evident.

Like compensatory shock, decompensated shock also has its indicators. A drop in blood pressure is frequently the hallmark. Remember that compensatory measures are used to maintain arterial pressure. As long as this pressure is maintained, blood pressure measurements remain normal. Falling blood pressure therefore indicates that compensatory measures are no longer adequate. Mental status is also a key finding. Compensation is designed to ensure blood flow to the brain. During decompensation, that blood flow drops. In this phase we typically see more severe mental status changes.

The heart and lungs can also be important indicators of decompensation. As muscles struggle in hypoperfused states, they eventually fail. Fast heart rates slow down and become bradycardic. Tachypnea changes over to irregular respiratory patterns and eventually slows as well. If the shock states are uncorrected, poorly perfused respiratory muscles will eventually stop.

Irreversible Shock and Death

If hypoperfusion states are left unchanged, cellular hypoxia will cause damage. Some body cells are more sensitive to hypoperfusion than others, but overall this damage is a predictable outcome. Prolonged vasoconstriction will lead to a progression of organ-system damage and death over time. As organ systems begin to fail, a condition called *irreversible shock* begins. It is called irreversible because at this point, even if the patient survives, the underlying problem of organ damage will likely be uncorrectable.

If hypoperfusion is sustained over a prolonged period, or if the underlying problem simply overwhelms the body's ability to compensate, the brain and heart will eventually be affected. Hypoperfusion of the heart frequently leads to life-threatening dysrhythmias. Apnea and cardiac arrest typically follow.

It is important to recognize the trends that indicate decompensation. In the chapter titled *Resuscitation*, you learned about signs that cardiac arrest is approaching (the peri-arrest state). The signs of decompensation, such as slowing heart rates, irregular respiratory rates, and falling blood pressures, suggest that the patient is very close to cardiac arrest. Remember that rarely is this peri-arrest condition observed as a single snapshot.

Rather, the trend is identified by comparing sets of assessment findings and vital signs. When a downward, decompensating trend is recognized, it is essential that you intervene to prevent the commonly associated cardiac arrest phase.

Experts often describe this progression of shock as a cycle or downward spiral. As an EMT, your most important role will be to interrupt this progression. Trauma systems are designed to intervene in shock patients before decompensation occurs and before the damage becomes irreversible. The role of EMS within this equation is to recognize the problem, support perfusion, and transport the patient rapidly to definitive care.

Patient Assessment

Assessing Client for Shock

The hypoperfusion that causes shock can be associated with a wide range of problems, and shock can occur in both medical and trauma patients. The most important assessment elements will be to identify the underlying problem that is causing shock (bleeding, anaphylaxis, an infection, etc.) and to recognize the signs and symptoms of compensation. A thorough patient assessment will incorporate both elements and is designed to gather the indicators of hypoperfusion rapidly.

The scene survey is an important part of shock recognition. In trauma patients, shock is often caused by internal bleeding. Considering the mechanism of injury will often help you predict the potential for this type of problem. A scene survey is also important in medical shock patients. Anaphylactic shock is caused by some form of environmental stimulus, so the scene survey can often help identify the trigger. Did the patient take a new medication or get stung by a bee? Although these considerations are not traditionally thought of as mechanisms of injury, they are certainly mechanisms of *illness*.

The primary assessment will offer the most critical information on shock patients, and will be used to differentiate compensated from decompensated shock. The primary assessment will start with a quick scan to identify massive hemorrhage. If this is found, you will correct this problem immediately. Although at that point you might not be thinking about the overall condition of shock, those initial corrective actions are key steps in preventing and treating it. An early assessment of mental status is also a key finding, as it will indicate how well (or how poorly) the brain is being perfused. As you then progress through airway, breathing, and circulation, you will review vital elements of compensation and identify immediate treatment needs. Each of these is especially relevant to the shock patient.

Airway

Although airway problems are not commonly a specific cause of shock, any deficit should be corrected immediately. Remember that shock is essentially an oxygenation problem, and any problem in bringing air into the body exacerbates its effects. Occasionally, anaphylactic shock can cause swelling in the upper airway and can be identified by voice changes (hoarse voice) and/or stridor associated with the reaction. Be aggressive in managing airway problems and be diligent in any effort to keep an airway open.

Breathing

EMTs must always be sensitive to the hypoxia traditionally associated with shock. No shock patient should ever be allowed to become or remain hypoxic. Low pulse oximetry and signs of hypoxia should be treated aggressively with supplemental oxygen. Remember that tachypnea is a key indicator of compensation. Any patient with an unexplained fast respiratory rate should be assumed to be in shock until proven otherwise (*particularly pediatric patients*). A breathing assessment can also indicate underlying shock conditions. Breathing issues, like wheezing, can sometimes indicate conditions like anaphylaxis. Also, consider tension pneumothorax as an underlying cause of obstructive shock. Absent lung sounds on one side (or sometimes both sides) of the chest are important indicators of this life-threatening condition.

Circulation

Shock is most readily identified in the circulation phase of the primary assessment. Here you will visualize skin color, check distal pulses and capillary refill time, and measure at least a brief snapshot of heart rate. These are all key findings associated with the onset and progression of shock. Although not all forms of shock cause pale skin (distributive shock frequently causes flushing, mottling, or a rash), this sign of vasoconstriction is quite important, especially if you have reason to suspect hypovolemia. Capillary refill time is also important. Typically, capillary refill is restored within 2 seconds after blanching the skin. Unfortunately, this finding is notoriously inaccurate in adults, but it is a much more reliable indicator in children. Fast heart rates should make you suspect shock. Changes in heart rate can reflect either compensation or decompensation. As patients compensate for shock, heart rates generally go up. As they decompensate, heart rates often fall (particularly in children, where very sudden decompensation may be encountered).

Any problem found in the primary assessment should be treated immediately. This is especially true in shock patients, particularly when it comes to external bleeding control and management of hypoxia. The assessment does not end there, though, and there are many other indicators of shock to be found as the assessment continues.

Shock is frequently identified by the trends in vital signs (called *trending*). As previously mentioned, sometimes a snapshot of heart rate, respiratory rate, or blood pressure can be telling; however, more often it is the trend that tells the tale. The progression of shock typically causes a predictable pattern of changing vital signs. As patients compensate, heart rates and respiratory rates rise. The more severe the problem, the faster these rates will be (to a point). As patients decompensate, these rates become irregular and slow. Blood pressure typically holds steady; it falls only once the patient begins to decompensate. However, a pattern of narrowing pulse can suggest systemic vasoconstriction. (A pulse pressure is the difference between the systolic and diastolic blood pressure. Since the diastolic pressure measures pressure in the circulatory system prior to the squeeze of the heart, an increasing value over time points to blood vessel constriction. Systolic pressure is frequently maintained by vasoconstriction but can slowly drop as the underlying problem—for example, bleeding—continues to have an effect. These combined effects cause pulse pressures to narrow as a trend. An example of narrowing pulse pressure would be this sequence of readings: 100/66, 100/74, 100/77, 100/84.) In any suspected shock patient, blood pressures should be repeated over time to help recognize a trend indicating compensation.

Physical examination will be used in trauma patients to identify bleeding and injuries that would likely be associated with shock. In medical patients, physical assessment will be used to identify specific patterns associated with shock-causing conditions. For example, a distributive shock condition caused by anaphylaxis would likely be associated with a skin rash, systemic swelling, and wheezing or stridor.

History taking in secondary assessment is equally important in identifying shock. Mechanism of injury and the history of the present illness help identify conditions frequently associated with hypoperfusion and shock states. The chief complaint and patterns of symptoms can also point to common shock types. For example, patients with anaphylactic shock frequently complain of GI distress including vomiting and diarrhea. Past medical history, allergies, and medications can all point to prior conditions that could be the root cause of shock today. Remember also that medications can change the way the body compensates. Blood thinners can make clotting much more difficult. Certain medications, like beta blockers, can also limit heart rate even when it is necessary for compensation.

The assessment of shock incorporates a wide range of potential underlying conditions, from anaphylaxis to sepsis, and from cardiogenic shock to bleeding. The recognition of shock largely will be tailored to identifying the specific patterns associated with the underlying conditions. However, if these underlying conditions are unclear, as they sometimes

"Don't wait for blood pressure to drop before you figure out your patient is developing shock."

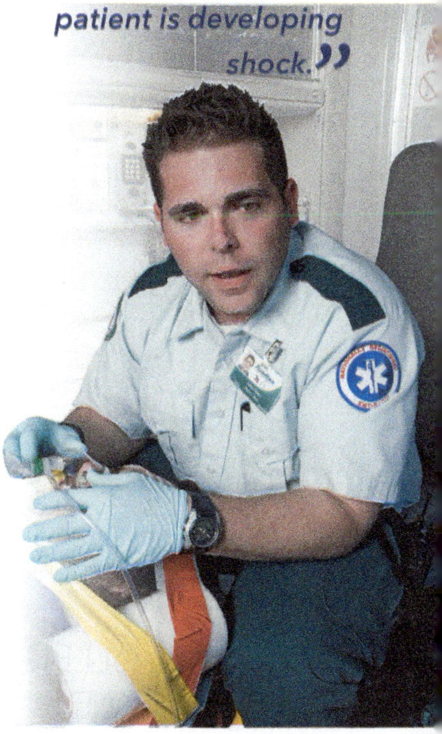

can be, you should focus on recognizing the signs of compensation and should assume shock is present. The signs and symptoms of shock are illustrated in Figure 29-3 and are described in Table 29-2.

When considering shock, it may also be helpful to keep in mind the very common causes. For example, hypovolemia is a very common cause of shock. If you are seeing an assessment pattern that suggests hypoperfusion, look first for situations that might cause hypovolemia. Is the patient bleeding (internally or externally)? Is the patient dehydrated? Dehydration is a common cause of hypovolemic shock, especially in children. Watch out for any child with reported vomiting or diarrhea, as these conditions rapidly deplete circulating volume.

In patients with allergies, consider anaphylaxis first. Is there any reason to believe they were exposed to an allergen? In patients with a history of infection, consider sepsis. This is especially true if they have an indwelling catheter or medication port, as these are common sources of dangerous infections. Patients who have undergone organ transplants are also at high risk for sepsis due to the medications they take, which suppress the normal immune system's response to infection.

FIGURE 29-3 Signs of shock will be detectable during the patient assessment.

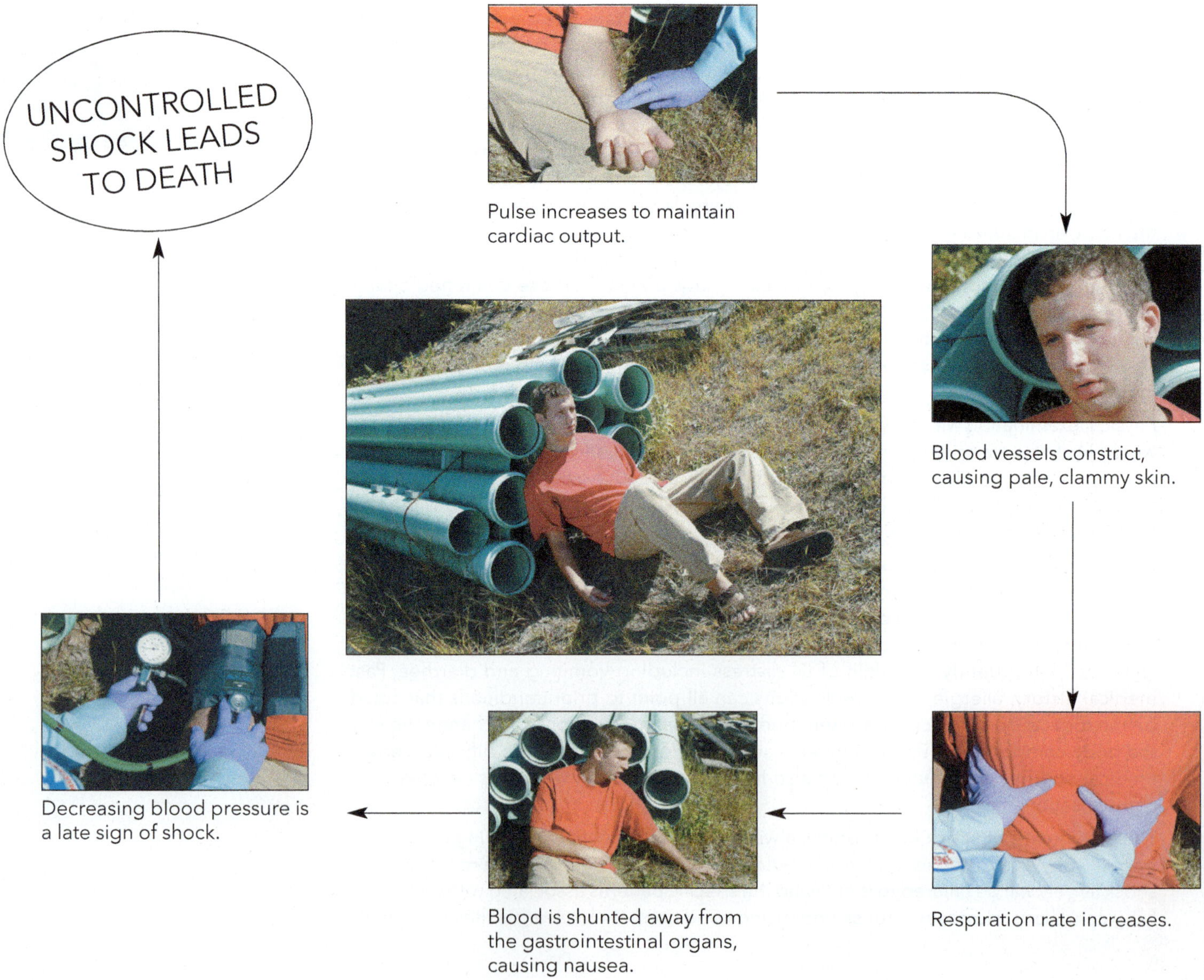

TABLE 29-2 Signs of Shock

SIGNS	DESCRIPTION
Altered mental status	Altered mental status occurs because the brain is not receiving enough oxygen. The brain is very sensitive to oxygen deficiencies. When it is deprived of oxygen, even slightly, behavioral changes may be noted. These changes may begin as anxiety and progress to restlessness and sometimes combativeness.
Pale, cool, and clammy skin	When the body senses low blood volume, natural mechanisms take over in an attempt to correct the problem. One of these mechanisms is to divert blood from nonvital areas to vital organs. Blood is quickly directed away from the skin to such organs as the brain and heart. This results in the loss of color and temperature in the skin. Infants and children may exhibit capillary refill times of more than 2 seconds. **NOTE:** *In anaphylactic and neurogenic shock (rare), the skin is typically warm, flushed, and dry because the circulatory system has lost the ability to constrict blood vessels in the skin.*
Nausea and vomiting	In the body's continuing effort to keep blood perfusing the vital organs, blood is diverted from the digestive system. This causes feelings of nausea and occasional vomiting.
Vital sign changes	The first vital signs to change are the pulse and respirations: • The pulse will increase in an attempt to pump more blood. As the pulse gradually increases, it becomes weak and thready. Most patients will become tachycardic with significant blood loss; however, a significant number will not, so you cannot rely solely on this sign. Remember also that as decompensation occurs, the heart rate can slow. • Respirations also increase, in an attempt to increase the amount of oxygen in the blood. The respirations will become shallower and labored as shock progresses. • Blood pressure is one of the last signs to change. When blood pressure drops, the patient is clearly in a state of serious, life-threatening shock. • A narrowing of the pulse pressure may also occur. This means that the difference between the systolic and diastolic pressures will progressively decrease.
Late signs	Late signs of shock that you may encounter include, in some cases, cyanosis around the lips and nail beds.

Think Like an EMT

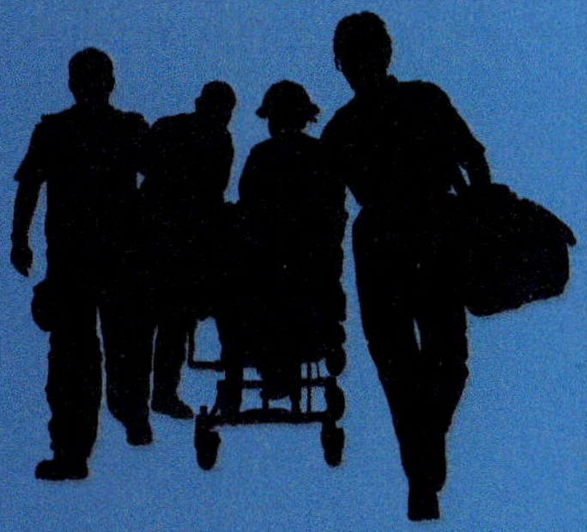

In Shock or Stable?

Falling blood pressure is a late sign of shock. In the following patients, use material you learned in this chapter to determine if your early decision making would lead you to expedite the call because you suspected shock or if, instead, you believe the patient will likely be stable. You will not be provided a blood pressure, but in each patient, you will find enough information to make a proper early decision without a blood pressure reading.

1. Your patient was working on scaffolding that collapsed, causing him to fall one story (about 10 feet [3 meters]). He is conscious, is alert but anxious, and complains of pain in the right side of his chest. His pulse is 102 and regular, respirations 26, skin cool and moist, and pupils equal and reactive to light.
2. Your patient is found sitting in a bathroom stall at an upscale restaurant. She is pale, sweaty, and leaning against the wall. She tells you she has recently had a problem with bleeding hemorrhoids. There is bright red blood in the toilet bowl. When you stand the patient up to move her to the stretcher, she says she thinks she is going to pass out.
3. You are called to an assault. A 25-year-old man was struck in the head by his girlfriend. She used a telephone to strike him once in the nose and again in the forehead. The police called you to evaluate his nosebleed. The patient's shirt has blood streaked down it. His nose is oozing blood now. He is alert and oriented. His pulse is 78, strong and regular; respirations 14; and skin warm and dry.

Treating Shock

The treatment of shock largely depends on the underlying cause. In most cases, the best way to resolve hypoperfusion is to stop whatever is causing it. That may mean surgery to stop internal bleeding; it may mean antibiotics to treat an infection; but it may also mean the patient needs immediate intervention. You should use your primary assessment to identify urgent interventions, and the larger patient assessment to identify the most appropriate treatment needs.

When considering shock treatment, it is reasonable to consider the "deadly triad of trauma." This name describes three conditions that significantly contribute to mortality in shock patients. The deadly triad consists of acidosis, hypothermia, and coagulopathy.

In shock, inadequate perfusion translates to inadequate removal of waste products. In addition, diminished oxygen delivery also causes the cells to shift to different forms of metabolism to maintain cell function. Both conditions lead to increased acid buildup and decreasing body pH. Acidosis (low pH) is particularly dangerous to hemorrhagic shock patients because it changes the body's ability to clot. As patients become more and more acidotic, this clotting deficiency, also known as *coagulopathy*, is increased.

Cellular metabolism is an important element of heat production for the body. When cells slow and stop metabolism due to hypoperfusion, they also lose this valuable source of heat. Even in hot outside environments, body temperature can plummet rapidly, and hypothermia can become a challenge. Hypothermia in this situation is significant because it also contributes to clotting problems. When patients are cold, they simply bleed more.

In severe trauma, clotting disorders can also occur naturally. Typically, the larger the insult, the more often coagulopathies become a problem. Considering that shock in many patients is caused by bleeding, conditions that lead to coagulopathy are dangerous, and they should be prevented as best we can with aggressive treatment. Although some shock care will be addressed by specific root cause, it is important to consider general treatment steps that address the deadly triad:

- *Initiate transport to an appropriate destination*—Although there are some shock interventions that are best completed prior to transport, in general, shock should be considered a time-sensitive disorder, and transport should be initiated as soon as possible. Particularly with shock caused by trauma, you should minimize scene times and always weigh the benefit of an intervention against the potentially greater good of getting the patient to more definitive care. Consider the destination as well. Is the destination hospital capable of managing the condition of the patient? For example, trauma patients are best managed at a dedicated trauma center. Weigh the value of lights and siren response carefully. Consider air transport when indicated.

- *Prevent hypoxia*—Managing the airway and preventing hypoxia reduces the effects of acidosis and its associated coagulopathies. We know that mortality rates increase when trauma patients become hypoxic. To best treat shock patients, be aggressive with airway management and treat any evidence of hypoxia with supplemental oxygen. The evidence remains unclear whether all shock patients should receive high-concentration oxygen. Follow local protocols. You should definitely apply supplemental oxygen to any patient with a low oxygen saturation and any patient with undifferentiated signs of potential hypoxia. Be aware that hypoperfused, vasoconstricted states often cause pulse oximetry to be inaccurate. When in doubt, it may be reasonable to err on the side of giving oxygen rather than withholding it.

- *Prevent heat loss*—Hypothermia is linked to coagulopathy. Temperature regulation should be considered in all shock patients, regardless of ambient environmental temperatures. Remove wet or bloody clothing. Insulate the patient with blankets and ensure that both the head and feet are covered. Consider external heat sources such as warmed blankets.

- *Consider shock positioning*—It is logical that blood is distributed throughout the body with less difficulty when a patient is in a supine position. Without the force of gravity, pumping blood to the superior aspects of the body may take less effort. Although the

TABLE 29-3 Categories of Shock and Key Interventions

SPECIFIC SHOCK STATE	KEY INTERVENTION
Hypovolemic shock	Bleeding control, rapid transport
Cardiogenic shock	Request ALS; certain medications and efforts to support blood pressure may be critical.
Distributive shock (anaphylaxis)	Administration of epinephrine
Distributive shock (sepsis)	Recognize and notify receiving hospital; rapid transport. Sepsis is a truly time-sensitive disorder. Early recognition reduces mortality.

evidence is not particularly strong, it may be reasonable to lay shock patients flat for transport. This is a longstanding practice in most areas. Laying the patient flat may not always be possible, however, especially in patients with breathing challenges. In those cases, you may have to use a more upright position. Always follow local protocol.

- *Consider advanced life support (ALS)*—In some cases, advanced life support will be very important in the treatment of the shock patient. In anaphylaxis, in sepsis, and with obstructive shock conditions like tension pneumothorax, ALS interventions can be lifesaving. Contact this resource early and consider intercept if waiting for their arrival will delay transport. Remember also that sometimes the closest advanced life support is the hospital.

For specific types of shock, more precise interventions may be necessary. For example, later in this chapter we will discuss bleeding control as a measure to prevent and treat shock. However, there are other specific interventions associated with different categories of shock. For more information, consult the specific chapters that discuss those conditions. For a general overview you may consider Table 29-3.

Patient Care

Care of the Patient with Shock

Fundamental Principles of Care

Patients with shock are priority transport and are in a life-threatening situation. Care is supportive.

In patients with signs and symptoms indicating shock:

- Initiate rapid transport to an appropriate destination.
- Manage specific underlying causes of shock. Consider the need for hemorrhage control in hypovolemia, epinephrine in anaphylaxis, and early recognition and transport for sepsis.
- Manage the airway and breathing to prevent hypoxia. Consider supplemental oxygen if the patient is hypoxic or demonstrating potential signs of hypoxia.
- Take steps to prevent heat loss. Remove wet clothing and insulate the patient.
- If possible, place the patient in a supine position.
- Request ALS.

Bleeding

Severe bleeding, or ***hemorrhage***, is the major cause of shock (hypoperfusion) in trauma. The body contains a certain amount of blood to circulate through the blood vessels. If enough blood volume is lost, perfusion will not occur in all cells. Inadequate perfusion of the body's cells will eventually lead to the death of tissues and organs. The cells and tissues of the brain, the heart, the spinal cord, and the kidneys are the most sensitive to inadequate perfusion.

hemorrhage (HEM-o-rej) bleeding, especially severe bleeding.

Bleeding, or hemorrhage, is classified as either external or internal, and can be either minor or severe, as explained in the next sections.

External Bleeding

CORE CONCEPT
Recognizing hemorrhage

External bleeding, or hemorrhage, is bleeding that occurs outside the body. It is typically visible on the surface of the skin. It occurs after force penetrates the skin and lacerates or destroys underlying blood vessels. Simple or minor bleeding is common, but occasionally bleeding can be so severe that it can very quickly threaten life.

How much a person bleeds is a function of several factors. The size and severity of a wound are major considerations. The amount of bleeding is also a function of the size and pressure of the blood vessel that has been ruptured (Figure 29-4) as well as of the person's ability to clot and stop the bleeding.

Massive Hemorrhage

Massive hemorrhage occurs when extensive wounds open up large blood vessels or many smaller blood vessels. ***Arterial bleeding*** can sometimes be recognized by its bright red color. (Blood coming from the heart is generally well oxygenated; the iron atoms in hemoglobin turn bright red when they bind with oxygen.) Often bleeding from an artery can be seen spurting with each beat of the heart. Keep in mind, however, that as pressure decreases in the cardiovascular system, spurting will decrease, and may not be noticeable.

arterial bleeding bleeding from an artery, which is characterized by bright red blood that is often spurting, profuse, and difficult to control.

Wounds to large veins, such as the jugular veins in the neck, can also cause massive bleeding. Although ***venous bleeding*** has less pressure behind it than arterial bleeding does, the sheer volume of blood carried by some veins is enough to create immediately life-threatening hemorrhage in some patients. Venous bleeding can sometimes be differentiated from arterial bleeding, as it tends to be darker in color and to flow steadily from a wound rather than spurt.

venous bleeding bleeding from a vein, which is characterized by dark red or maroon blood and a steady, easier-to-control flow.

Massive bleeding can occur in many places on the body, but some large blood vessels are particularly vulnerable to trauma. *Junctional hemorrhage* occurs where the appendages of the body connect to the trunk. In these locations, large arteries and veins tend to be less well protected and particularly vulnerable to traumatic forces. In the neck, the carotid arteries and the jugular veins are close to the surface of the skin. In the axillae, or armpits, the brachial arteries and veins are also superficial. In the groin, the very large femoral arteries and veins are relatively exposed and vulnerable. Each of these sites is a location where an injury is likely to cause massive bleeding.

Massive external bleeding is rare in civilian life, but when it occurs, you must treat it as soon as possible. Massive external bleeding is not subtle, so you will most often notice it when you form your general impression. If you encounter massive hemorrhage, there is no higher treatment priority than stopping the bleeding. Large arterial or venous bleeds can be life-threatening in a matter of minutes.

FIGURE 29-4 Three types of external bleeding.

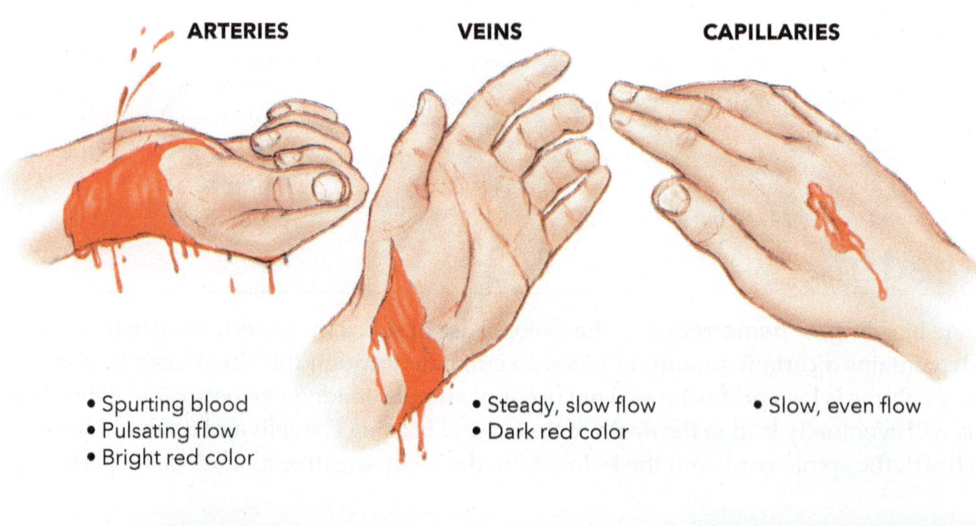

Other External Hemorrhage

The vast majority of external hemorrhage is not massive. Most penetrating injuries rupture smaller vessels that are under far less pressure and can be easily controlled. Superficial wounds to the surface of the skin often produce ***capillary bleeding***. This bleeding is under very low pressure and produces only a slow ooze from the wound. It typically ceases without any intervention at all. However, this type of bleeding sometimes occurs over large areas, so the risk of infection is high. Nonmassive bleeding can also come from veins and even small arteries.

capillary bleeding bleeding from capillaries, which is characterized by a slow, oozing flow of blood.

You will have to use clinical judgment to differentiate serious bleeding from massive bleeding, and you should consider two points. Keep in mind that all bleeding is bad for the patient and should be stopped, although when to do so will depend on what other threats to life a patient may have. Whether bleeding is high-pressure with blood escaping rapidly or low-pressure with blood escaping slowly, red blood cells on clothing or the ground cannot be used to perfuse cells. Another important point to keep in mind is that identifying the type of bleeding that is occurring is almost irrelevant and potentially time-consuming. Whether the bleeding is arterial, venous, or even capillary does not significantly change your treatment approach and should be a minor concern.

Bleeding can also be accelerated by underlying conditions. A growing number of patients are on prescription medications designed to limit the body's natural ability to form blood clots. Often referred to as blood thinners, these medications are commonly prescribed to patients with a history of stroke, irregular heartbeat (atrial fibrillation), heart attack, or artificial heart valves. These medications—which include aspirin, warfarin (Coumadin®), clopidogrel (Plavix®), dabigatran (Pradaxa®), apixaban (Eliquis®), and rivaroxaban (Xarelto®)—act to prevent strokes or heart attacks, but in the setting of external or internal bleeding can result in life-threatening bleeding from injuries that might have been relatively minor for a patient who was not on one of these medications. When treating patients with external or internal bleeding, it is important, if possible, to determine whether they are on blood thinners as part of the past medical history.

We know that hypothermia (reduced body temperature) also affects the body's ability to clot. The colder a patient gets, the more likely coagulopathy, or impaired ability to clot, will be a concern. Keep in mind that as patients become hypoperfused, their ability to generate heat through metabolism and their ability to conserve heat through blood flow can be affected. Hypothermia, therefore, must be an immediate and ongoing concern in any patient with bleeding.

For the most part, external hemorrhage is "compressible"; that is, it can be controlled by compressing the tissue around the wound or the vessel that is bleeding or both. If this intervention is performed in a timely fashion, bleeding generally can be controlled. Patients should never die from external bleeding. Unfortunately, many still do.

As an EMT, rapid identification of external bleeding and immediate bleeding control will likely be on your shoulders, and in many cases, your actions may decide the outcome for the bleeding patient.

Precautions with External Hemorrhage

Whenever bleeding is anticipated or discovered, you must use Standard Precautions to avoid exposure of your skin and mucous membranes. Blood and open wounds pose a risk of infection to the EMT. Therefore, you must wear protective gloves when caring for any bleeding patient. You should also wear a mask and protective eyewear if there is a chance of encountering splattered blood. In addition, you should wear a mask when assisting a patient suffering from profuse or spurting (arterial) bleeding, or one who is spitting or coughing up blood. Consider wearing a gown if clothing may become contaminated.

Although Standard Precautions decrease the possibility of exposure to blood and body fluids, you should nevertheless *always* wash your hands with soap and water immediately after each call. Gloves may develop tears or small holes without your knowledge. Always remove the gloves carefully, turning them inside out as you take them off. This reduces the possibility of blood or fluid on the gloves coming in contact with your hands.

CORE CONCEPT
How to evaluate the severity of external bleeding

Patient Assessment

Identifying Massive External Bleeding

Massive hemorrhage must be identified and controlled within the first seconds of the primary assessment. In most cases identification will be quite easy, because you will see the bleeding. Keep in mind the vulnerable junctional areas and look for any hemorrhage in those locations.

Not all bleeding may be obvious, though, and clothing can soak up a great deal of blood, particularly if the patient is wearing bulky clothing or many layers of clothing. The ground or carpeting beneath the patient can also soak up a lot of blood. In those cases, use a gloved hand to assess void spaces and detect bleeding. In low light, rapidly "feeling for the wet spots" with your gloved hands is an important assessment technique.

Immediate identification of massive bleeding is critical, and so is immediate treatment. If you recognize life-threatening hemorrhage, you must take immediate steps to correct it before you perform any other assessment or treatment. Continue the rest of the primary assessment only after you have controlled massive bleeding. If massive bleeding is difficult to control, you may find that you are unable to complete any other steps before transferring care to a higher level.

Assessing the Bleeding Patient

As mentioned, massive external bleeding in civilian life is rare. Most of the bleeding you will see in your career as an EMT will be nonmassive and far less imminently life-threatening. In this setting, proceed through the primary assessment as normal. *Airway* will be first and most important. Ensuring adequate *breathing* will be next. Finally, bleeding will be addressed in "C," the *circulation* phase, only after assessing and treating the prior elements. Remember always to seek out bleeding in clothing and surroundings, and use a gloved hand to detect blood in void spaces.

Sometimes external blood loss can be examined by looking at the amount of blood on the ground. This assessment technique is notoriously inaccurate, however, and usually useful only for differentiating "a lot" from "a little."

Estimating external blood loss is difficult, and it is equally important for you to watch for signs and symptoms of shock, which were listed in Table 29-2. Fortunately, the body responds to blood loss in a predictable fashion. The steps the body takes to stay alive are often visible from the outside. You can use these findings to judge the impact bleeding has had on the body and to recognize the warning signs of shock.

No matter how small blood loss appears to be, if the patient shows any signs or symptoms of shock, the bleeding must be considered serious. However, do not wait for signs and symptoms of shock to appear before you begin treatment. Any patient with significant blood loss should be treated to prevent the development of shock. Keep in mind that many of the signs and symptoms of shock appear late in the process. By the time they develop, it may be too late for the patient to recover.

Decision Points

- Does the patient have massive bleeding that must be controlled before I take any other assessment steps?
- Is the patient in shock or developing shock?

CORE CONCEPT
How to control external bleeding

Controlling External Bleeding

The control of external bleeding is one of the most important elements in the prevention and management of shock (hypoperfusion). If bleeding is not controlled, shock will continue to develop and worsen, leading to the patient's death.

Point of View

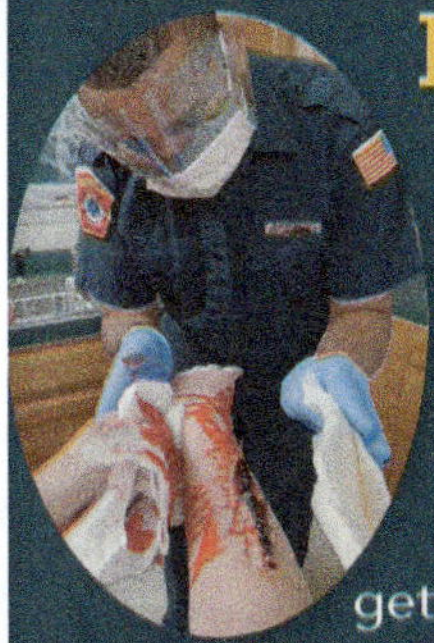

"I remember waiting to see if it would hurt.

"It wasn't the blood. That didn't bother me. I just sat there and waited for the pain. Things were in slow motion. The knife had gone into my forearm. Everyone stopped what they were doing and stared. I grabbed my arm and felt the warm blood drip down over my fingers. But it still didn't seem real.

"I heard someone scream. Someone else called 911. It took me a minute to get my head around what happened. It seemed like only a few seconds had gone by when the EMS people showed up. They put a bandage on my arm and made sure the bleeding had stopped.

"As I look back on it now, I am amazed at how detached I was from the whole thing. I guess some would call that shock.

"And for the record, once I got composed again, it hurt. Oh, yes, trust me. It hurt."

Patient Care

Care of the Patient with External Bleeding

Fundamental Principles of Care

Most external hemorrhage can be managed by direct pressure, and as an EMT, you will use compression techniques to control almost all of the bleeding you encounter. Controlling external bleeding can be thought of as a series of escalating steps designed to reduce blood flow through the ruptured vessel. These steps are typically sequential, but you should use the most appropriate technique for the situation at hand (Scan 29-1).

After ensuring that the scene is safe and donning appropriate personal protective equipment, determine how aggressive you need to be with bleeding control. If the bleeding is massive, you should make it your first priority. If not, continue through the airway and breathing steps, and correct those problems first. If the bleeding is massive, however, move immediately to the bleeding-control steps listed next.

The major methods of controlling massive external bleeding are:

- Direct pressure
- Hemostatic agents
- Wound packing
- Tourniquet use on extremities
- Specialized compression devices for junctional bleeding

Although control of major or massive bleeding is often accomplished by sequential interventions (direct pressure followed by wound packing with a hemostatic agent, etc.), there will be times when that progression is not in the patient's best interest. The best example of this situation is in the case of a proximal arm or leg amputation, where the most appropriate first intervention to control the massive bleeding is the immediate application of a tourniquet.

For any patient with significant bleeding or signs of shock, in addition to controlling external bleeding, consider the need to prevent hypoxia. Blood loss decreases perfusion. There are fewer red blood cells to carry oxygen because of blood loss, which means that less oxygen is delivered to the tissues. Any evidence of shock or hypoxia should be treated with supplemental oxygen immediately.

SCAN 29-1 Sequential Steps in The Control of External Bleeding

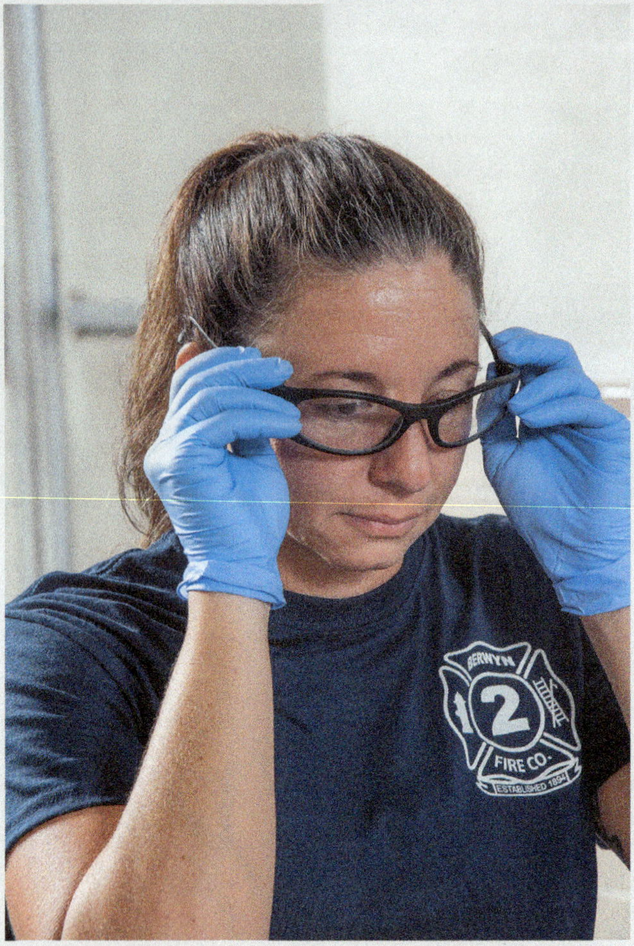

1. Take Standard Precautions.

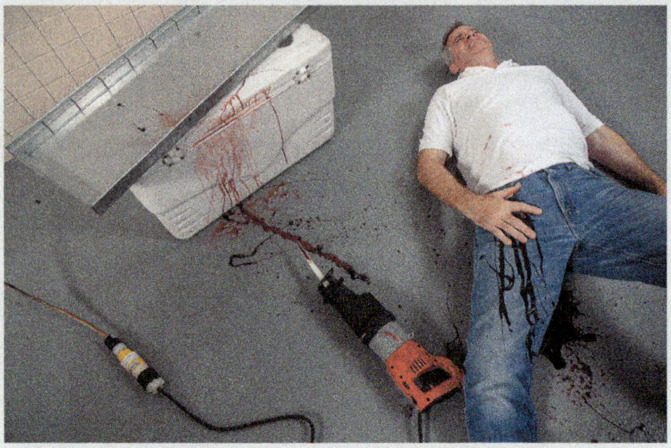

2. Assess the scene.

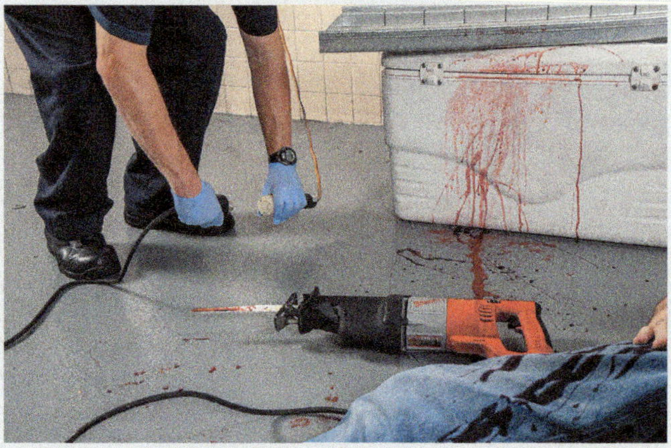

3. Assess scene safety.

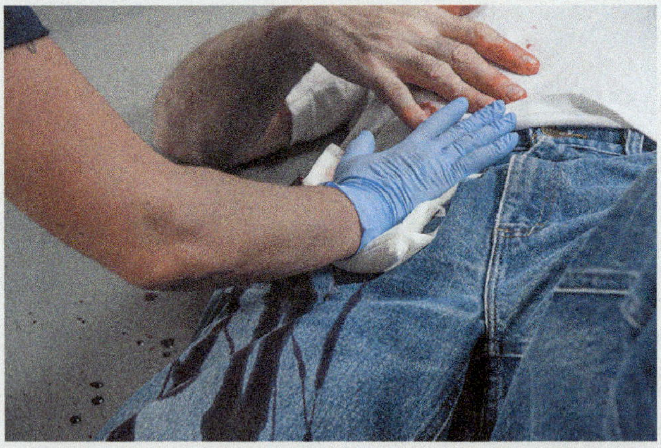

4. Apply firm direct pressure to the wound with a gloved hand.

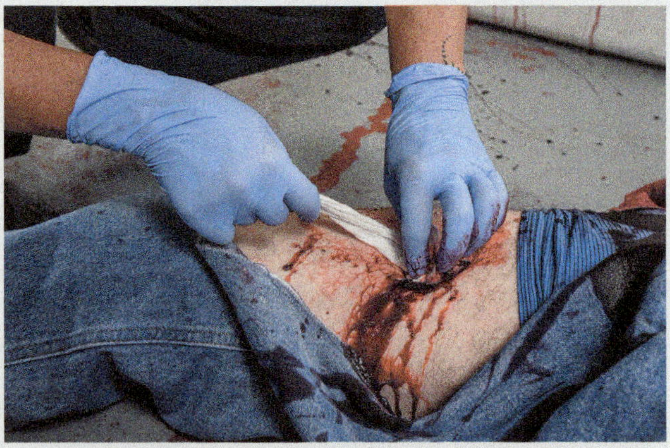

5. Pack the wound with hemostatic gauze if bleeding is not controlled by direct pressure.

SCAN 29-1 Sequential Steps in The Control of External Bleeding *(continued)*

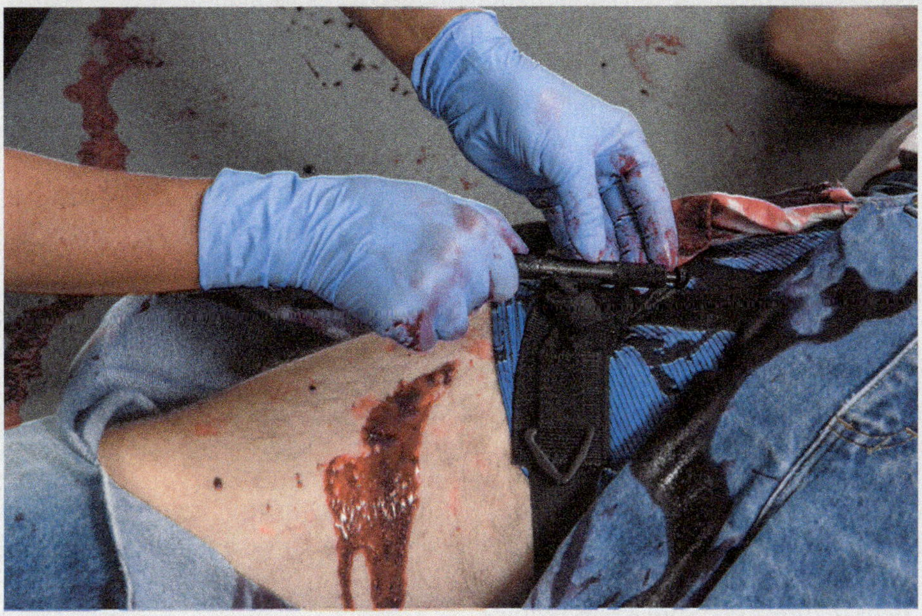

6. Apply a tourniquet proximal to the wound if bleeding remanis uncontrolled after wound packing, or if the wound is not controlled by direct pressure and the wound type cannot be packed effectively.

Standard Precautions are mandatory when attempting to control external bleeding. Always wear disposable gloves when caring for every patient with external bleeding. In cases of severe or massive external bleeding, eye protection (Scan 29-1 #1) and a disposable mask (Figure 29-5) should be used in addition to gloves.

Observing Standard Precautions and infection control practices is equally important when cleaning up after the call. Follow your local infection exposure control plan regarding the cleaning and disposal of contaminated bandages, sheets, and other materials and supplies.

FIGURE 29-5 Maintain safety by donning personal protective equipment before giving care to patients. EMT donning a disposable mask.

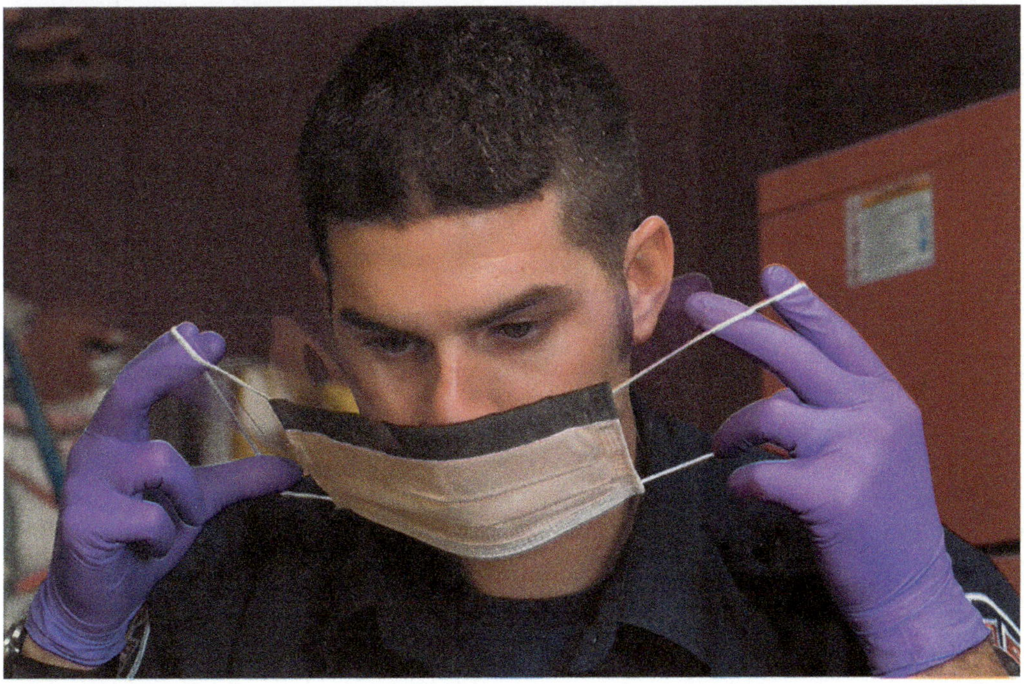

Strategies for External Bleeding Control

Control of external bleeding can be thought of as a series of escalating steps designed to reduce and stop blood flow through damaged blood vessels. In some cases, you will find wounds that have already formed a clot and stopped bleeding by themselves. In this case, simply applying gauze and securing it with a bandage will be your primary intervention, to prevent contamination of the wound. You will then observe the dressed wound for signs of bleed-through.

Many other wounds will exhibit active bleeding upon your assessment and will require your prompt intervention. You will utilize various strategies to control the bleeding.

Direct Pressure. In most cases, direct pressure is the first step in bleeding control. It works by compressing damaged blood vessels and stopping the flow of blood, which helps the body's own clotting mechanisms to start forming effective blood clots. In most cases, this will by itself control the external bleeding. This can be done with your gloved hand, a dressing and your gloved hand, or a pressure dressing and bandage. Direct pressure compresses the tissue around the wound and diverts blood flow from the affected blood vessels. It also compresses the local blood vessels and slows blood flow within their walls. This increase in pressure from outside reduces the force of bleeding and allows the blood to clot and plug the holes in damaged blood vessels within the wound.

The steps in direct pressure are as follows (Scan 29-2):

1. Apply firm pressure with the palm of your hand (or with your fingers, for a smaller wound). In the case of junctional hemorrhage, you may need to lean into the wound and apply body weight to enhance the pressure. See Figure 29-6A. The amount of pressure that should be used can be gauged by the severity of the wound. Minor bleeding can often be controlled with gentle pressure. If the bleeding is mild, use a sterile dressing between your gloved hand and the wound. If the bleeding is severe or spurting, immediately place your gloved hand directly on the wound. Do not waste time trying to find a dressing (Figure 29-6B and C). Consider aiming your direct pressure toward a bone. If the wound can be compressed between your hand and a bone, bleeding control will be more effective.
2. Hold the pressure firmly until the bleeding is controlled. Remember, your goal is limiting additional blood loss. If the bleeding is massive, direct pressure should be maintained until you arrive at the hospital. Every effort should be made to keep constant pressure on the wound. If the bleeding is not massive, it may be reasonable to check for bleeding after 5–10 minutes of pressure.
3. When applying direct pressure, resist the temptation to apply layers of "absorbent" dressings. Although absorption may be appropriate to prevent blood from spilling on clean surfaces, it does little to actually stop hemorrhage. In fact, layers of absorbent dressings can be counterproductive to direct pressure, as they can form a cushion between your hands and the wound. The exception to this rule would be wound packing, which will be discussed in the next section.
4. Once the bleeding has been controlled, bandage a dressing firmly in place to form a pressure dressing. (See the following explanation.)
5. Do not remove a dressing once it has been placed on the wound. Removal of a dressing may destroy clots or cause further injury to the site. If a dressing becomes soaked through with blood, it is a sign that what you are doing is ineffective. If the wound continues to bleed in this manner, you should move aggressively to other methods, such as wound packing with hemostatic agents or applying a tourniquet.

Wound Packing. Direct pressure is most effective in superficial wounds. However, in extremities and in junctional areas, a significant injury can result in the creation of a cavity and make direct pressure alone less effective. Certain areas of the body, such as

SCAN 29-2 Applying Direct Pressure

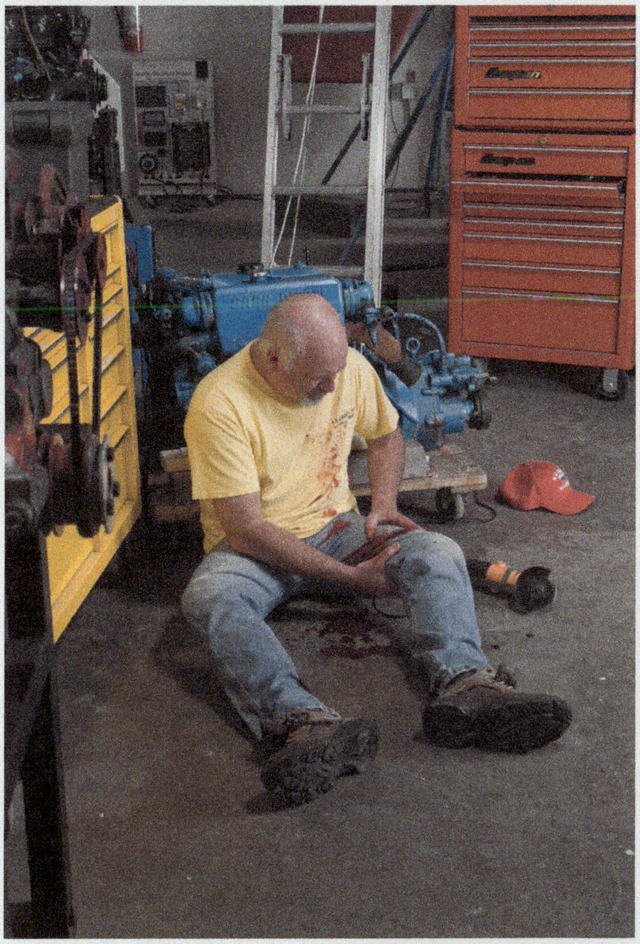

1. Perform a scene size-up and look for hazards.

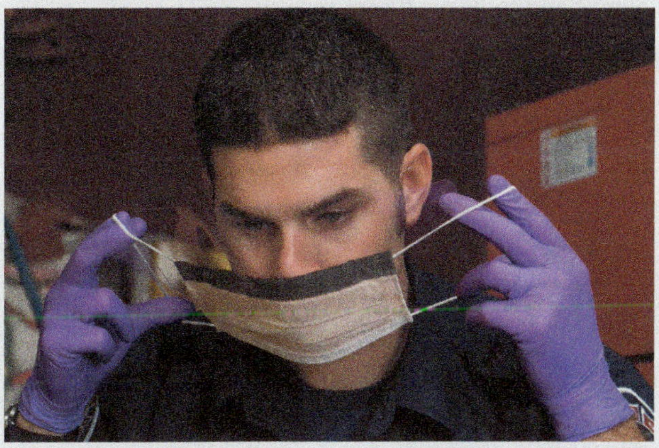

2. Take Standard Precautions.

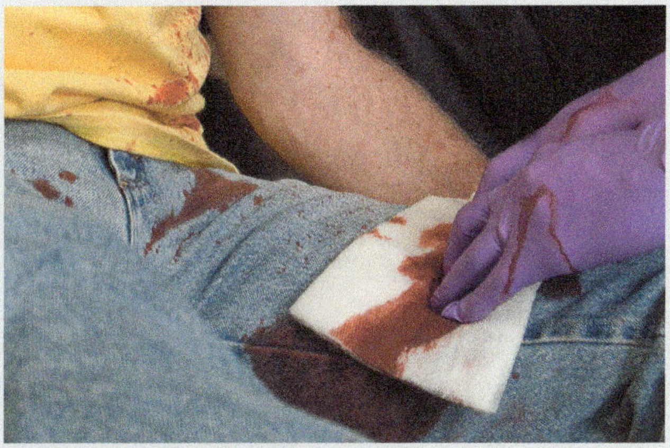

3. Begin with hand or palm pressure focused toward a bone. Remember that direct pressure is very effective in controlling bleeding and may be all you need.

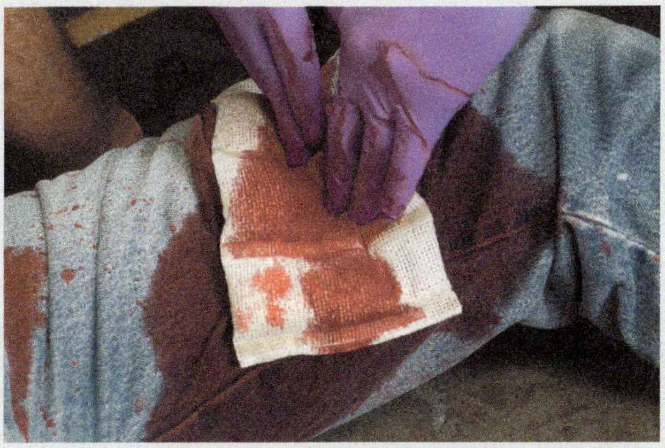

4. If another provider is available, and the patient continues to bleed, prepare additional hemorrhage-control materials. Once bleeding is controlled by direct pressure, secure the dressings with a bandage and monitor for any bleed-through. If bleeding is not controlled by direct pressure, move aggressively to other methods, such as wound packing with hemostatic agents or applying a tourniquet.

FIGURE 29-6 (A) In cases of junctional hemorrhage, you may need to lean into the wound and apply body weight to enhance wound pressure. (B and C) In cases of profuse bleeding, do not waste time finding a dressing. Instead, use your gloved hand to apply direct pressure.

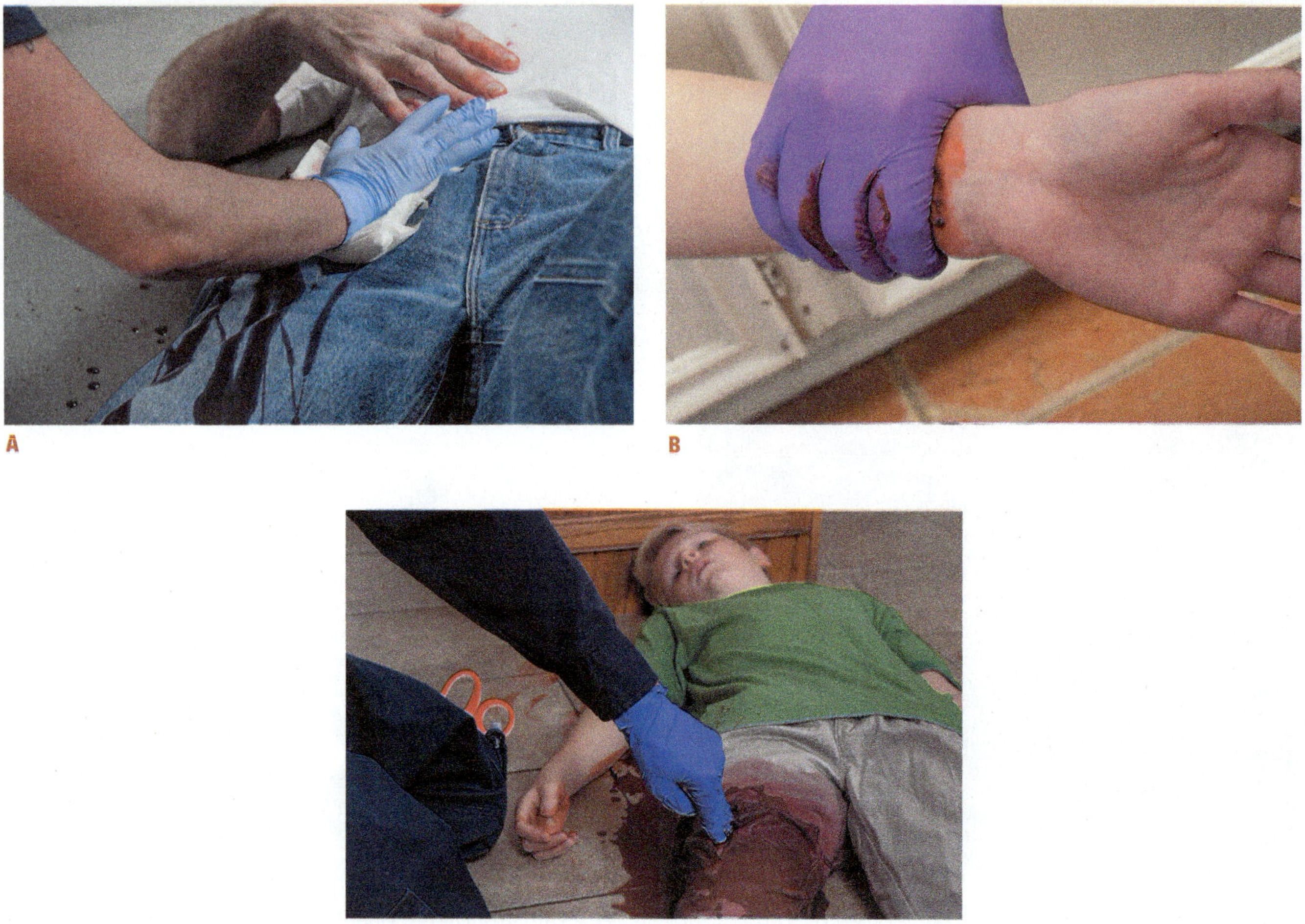

A B C

the armpit or the groin, also present natural cavities that promote profuse bleeding when massive hemorrhage occurs. In these situations, direct pressure should be augmented by wound packing.

Wound packing is accomplished by filling void spaces with gauze. It is most effective when hemostatic gauze is used, but it can still be effective using traditional gauze. Wound packing is used only in extremities and junctional areas and should *not* be utilized in chest or abdominal wounds. In optimal conditions, wound packing is an extension of the direct pressure sequence outlined above. In most cases, start with immediate palm pressure over the wound. If bleeding continues, have a partner prepare wound packing materials and expose the wound if necessary. Once the team and materials are ready, briefly visualize the wound. Here you are looking for the local source of the bleeding within the wound itself. Sometimes spurting or heavy flow can be seen. In some cases, however, neither might be apparent. Insert one end of a roll of gauze into the wound with the intent to place the gauze directly against the source of bleeding. If that site cannot be visualized, estimate as best you can. With one hand, keep the gauze firmly placed against the bleeding blood vessel. With the other hand, feed gauze into the cavity of the wound until that cavity is completely filled. Gauze should be fed in quickly, but in a controlled manner, to maintain the initial point of pressure. Once the cavity is filled, resume direct pressure on top of the wound and its packing.

FIGURE 29-7 Wound packing. (A) Feeding gauze into the wound. (B) Once the wound is packed, continue direct pressure and apply a bandage.

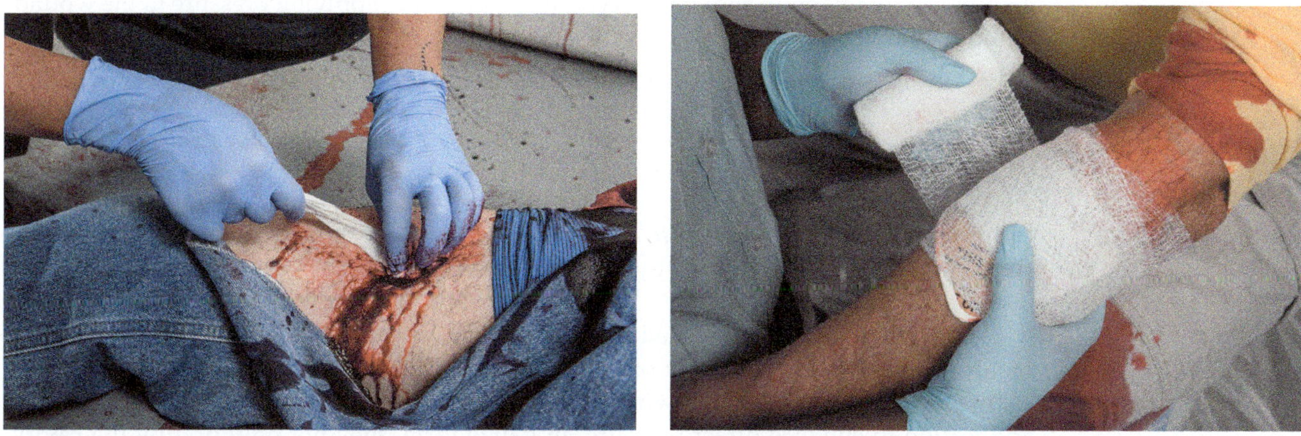

A B

Procedure for Wound Packing

1. Assess the scene and take Standard Precautions.
2. Begin with direct pressure.
3. If available, a second provider should remove clothing from the wound area and prepare packing materials (typically hemostatic gauze).
4. When ready, focus the team and expose the wound. Look for the specific site of bleeding.
5. Place the end of the gauze against the site of the bleeding. Begin feeding gauze into the wound cavity. Feed gauze into the cavity until the cavity is full (Figure 29-7A).
6. Once the cavity is full, resume direct pressure. Consider a pressure bandage (Figure 29-7B).

Several types of dressings may be used to control external bleeding (Figure 29-8). A ***pressure dressing*** will control most nonmassive external bleeding, and may be useful to maintain direct pressure once a wound has been packed. Be aware, however, that a pressure dressing should not take the place of direct pressure in serious hemorrhage situations. If bleeding is potentially life-threatening, use hand pressure first.

pressure dressing
a bulky dressing held in position with a tightly wrapped bandage, which applies pressure to help control bleeding.

Many commercial pressure dressings are available. To improvise a pressure dressing, place several gauze pads on the wound. Hold the dressings in place with a self-adhering roller bandage wrapped tightly over the dressings and above and below the wound site.

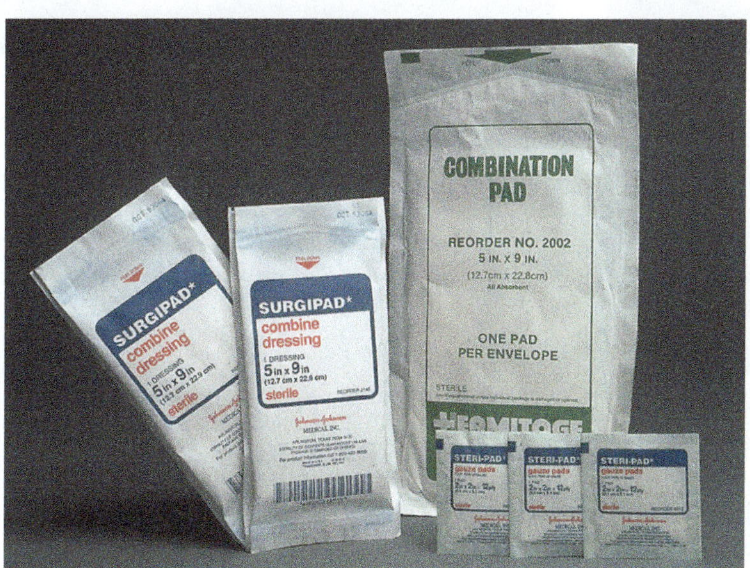

FIGURE 29-8 Various types of dressings.

You must create enough pressure to control the bleeding. Take care that the pressure dressing you are applying does not cut off blood flow and become a tourniquet. A pressure dressing should be snug enough to accomplish its goal of applying pressure to the wound without cutting off distal circulation. (See Figure 29-7B.)

> **NOTE:** *After controlling bleeding from an extremity using a pressure dressing, always check for a distal pulse to make sure that the dressing has not been applied too tightly. If you do not feel a pulse, adjust the pressure applied by the dressing to reestablish circulation. Check distal pulses frequently while the patient is in your care.*

hemostatic **(HEM-o-STAT-IK) *agents***
substances applied as powders, dressings, gauze, or bandages to open wounds to stop bleeding.

Hemostatic Agents. ***Hemostatic agents*** are products designed to enhance direct pressure's ability to control bleeding by way of various biochemical reactions when they come in contact with blood.

Hemostatic agents may be used in a variety of ways to control hemorrhage. Most commonly, agents come in the form of impregnated gauze or dressings. Ideally, hemostatic agents are best suited for the wound packing process described earlier or for topical application to enhance direct pressure. In gauze form, they not only occupy the cavity of the wound, but also apply hemostatic agent to the source of the bleeding. Although research is limited, there appears to be an advantage when these agents are used. Note that the U.S. military's Committee on Tactical Combat Casualty Care (CoTCCC) states that if hemostatic agents are used, they should be in combat gauze form (Figure 29-9).

Many myths persist regarding hemostatic agents, and we should take a moment to dispel some of them. While it is true that some original factor concentration agents did cause an exothermic (heat) reaction upon application and could cause burns, modern variants are prehydrated. Although they do get warm, they no longer reach dangerous

FIGURE 29-9 (A and B) Combat gauze. (C) "Tea bag"-type hemostatic agent. *(Photos A-C: © Edward T. Dickinson, MD)*

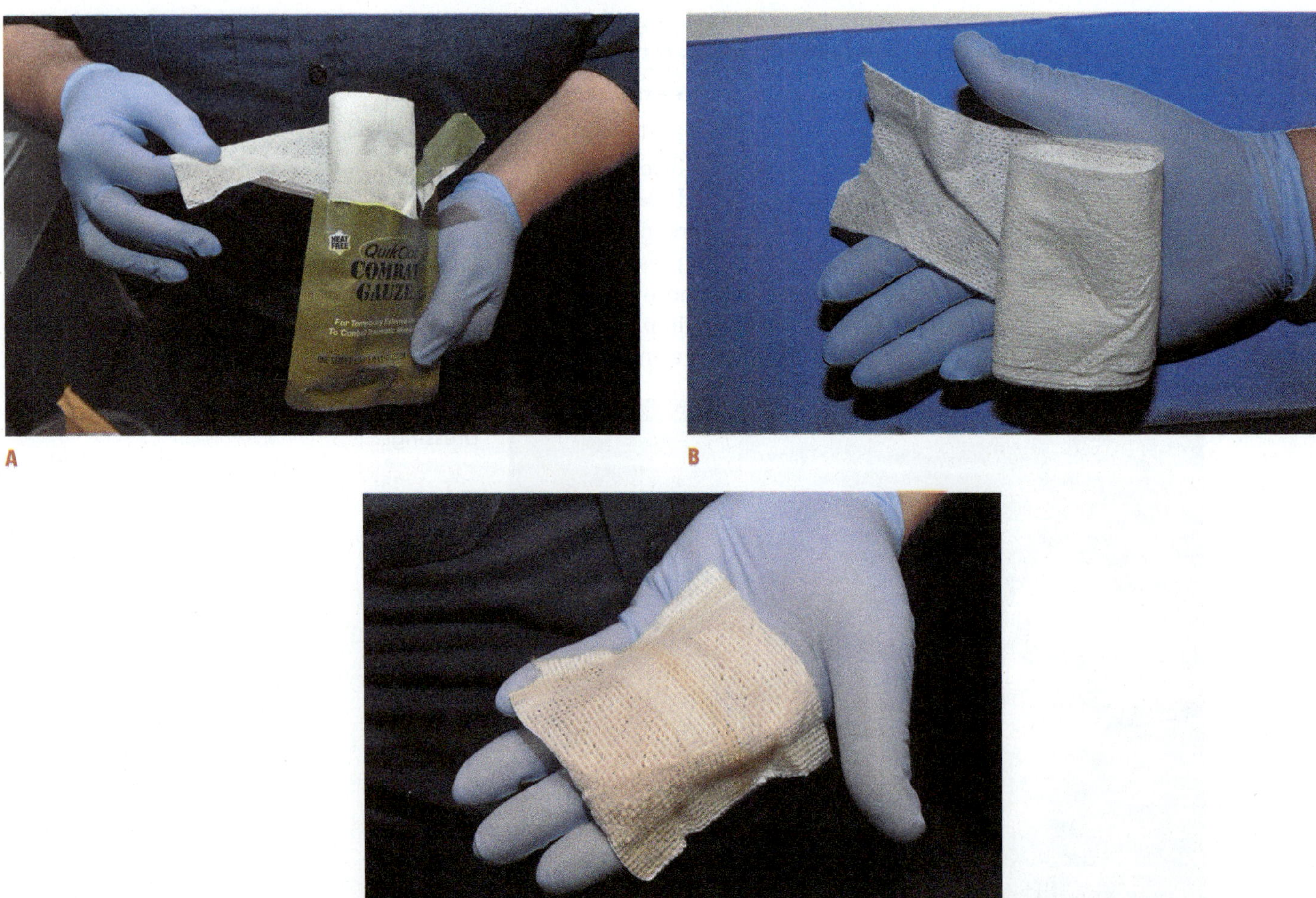

A B C

temperatures. It is also true that original agents were delivered in powder form and were theoretically able to cause an embolism. However, there is little evidence to suggest this complication actually occurred. Modern forms of hemostatic agents have small particles either impregnated in gauze (combat gauze form) or contained within a tea bag–type device. They can and should be applied directly into a wound without fear of causing embolism. These agents are also frequently augmented so that they appear on X-ray.

More recently available hemostatic agents include devices that insert multiple hemostatic tablets directly into deep extremity or junctional wounds (Figure 29-10). These products are designed to control bleeding not only using hemostatic agents but also by greatly expanding in size when they come in contact with blood (Figure 29-11). As always, follow local protocol.

It is important to remember that hemostatic agents aid direct pressure but do not replace it. Once the dressing or gauze is applied, you must apply direct pressure over the wound.

NOTE: *You should not push dressings or bandaging materials into a torso wound such as penetrating trauma to the abdomen or chest.*

Tourniquet. There are several situations in which direct pressure is not appropriate. Severe trauma to an extremity can cause multiple lacerations, penetrations, and anatomic destruction that may lead to bleeding in more than one area. Protruding broken bone ends and crush-type amputations can also prevent the ability to apply direct pressure. In these cases, it may be necessary to use a tourniquet as the initial means of bleeding control. In addition, sometimes direct pressure simply does not work. This will be evident when an extremity continues to bleed severely despite attempts at controlling the bleeding with direct pressure and hemostatic agents. Obvious bleeding and rapid soaking through of dressings are key indicators that your direct-pressure efforts have failed. In these cases, you must rapidly move to the next level of intervention, which is a tourniquet.

A ***tourniquet*** (Figure 29-12 and Scan 29-3) is a device that closes off all blood flow to and from an extremity. Previously believed to be an extreme last resort, tourniquets have moved into mainstream care for patients with severe bleeding that can't be controlled by direct pressure. At one point it was believed that the use of a tourniquet was a "life or limb" decision. It was felt that with blood flow cut off, the tissue of the limb would die and an amputation would be necessary. This is no longer assumed. In combat situations in Iraq and Afghanistan, many tourniquets have been placed with very few long-term injuries and, in fact, no tourniquet-related amputations.

tourniquet (TURN-i-ket) a device used for bleeding control that constricts all blood flow to and from an extremity.

Tourniquets are a rapid solution to massive bleeding in an extremity. Once they are applied, you can quickly move to address other pressing concerns such as airway and breathing issues. This is particularly helpful in an operational setting such as with tactical

FIGURE 29-10 X-Stat® device delivering hemostatic discs into the wound.

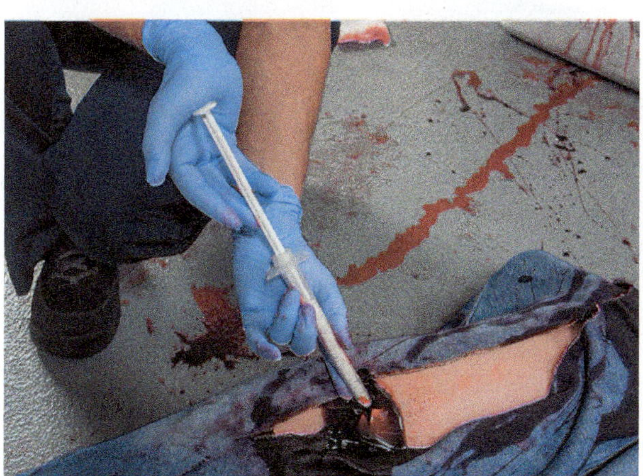

FIGURE 29-11 Dry hemostatic X-Stat® training disc (*left*); expanded wet hemostatic disc (*right*). *(© Edward T. Dickinson, MD)*

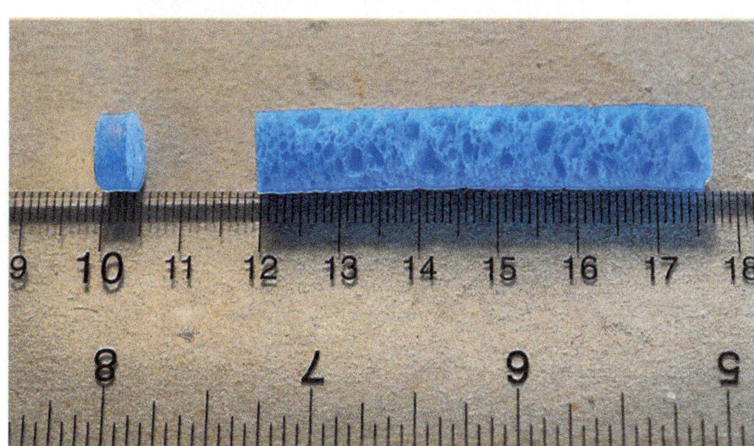

EMS or with military medics. However, its advantages are also useful in civilian trauma care (Figure 29-13).

The decision to use a tourniquet is an important one. You must recognize the situation as one in which direct pressure is inappropriate or one in which direct pressure efforts have failed. In these cases, you will apply, then tighten, a tourniquet.

FIGURE 29-12 (A) The mechanical advantage tourniquet (MAT®). (B) SOF-Tactical tourniquet® application and tightening.

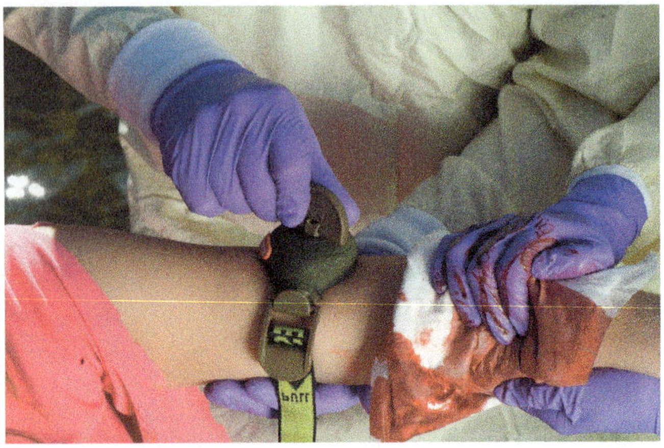

A

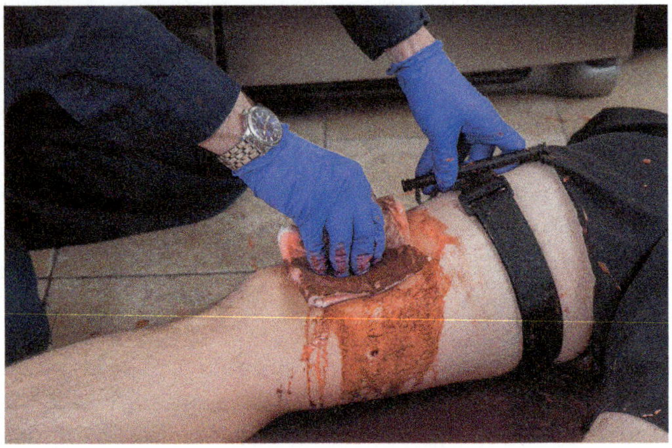

B

SCAN 29-3 Uncontrolled Extremity Bleeding that Requires Immediate Tourniquet Application

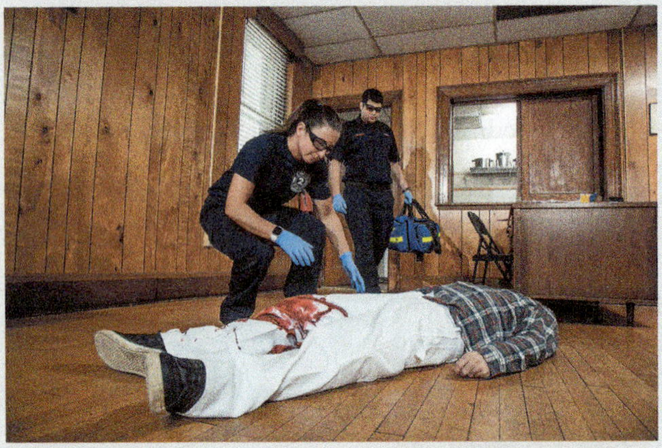

1. Take Standard Precautions and ensure scene safety. Assess the wound.

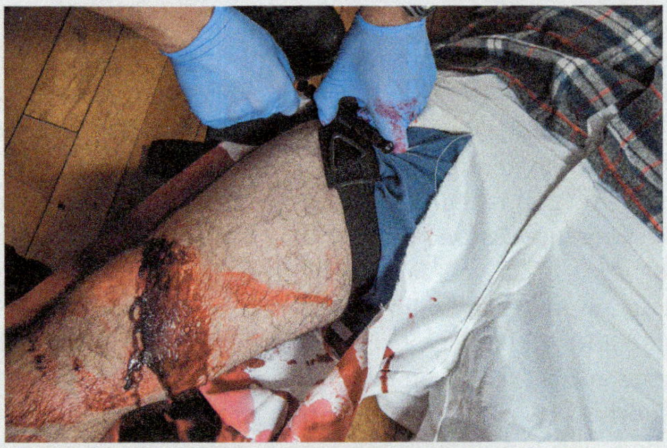

2. Apply the tourniquet proximal to the site(s) of bleeding and tighten until bleeding is controlled.

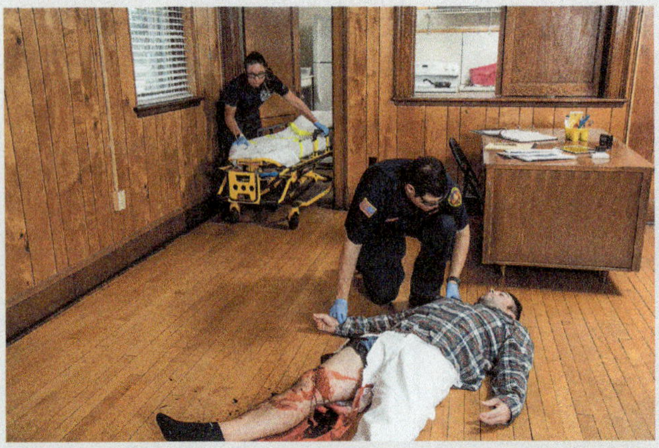

3. Assess and treat the patient for shock.

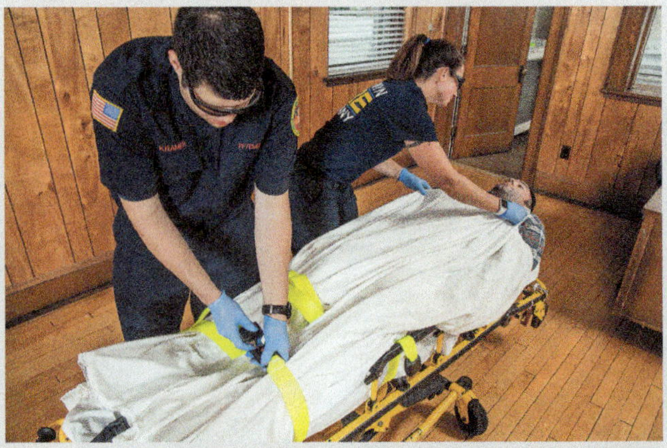

4. Initiate transport, minimizing excessive scene time.

SCAN 29-3 Uncontrolled Extremity Bleeding that Requires Immediate Tourniquet Application

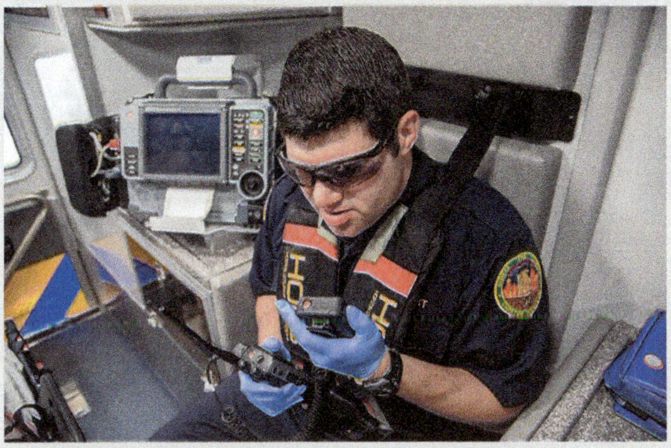

5. Notify the appropriate receiving facility (ideally a trauma center) including that a tourniquet has been used to control bleeding.

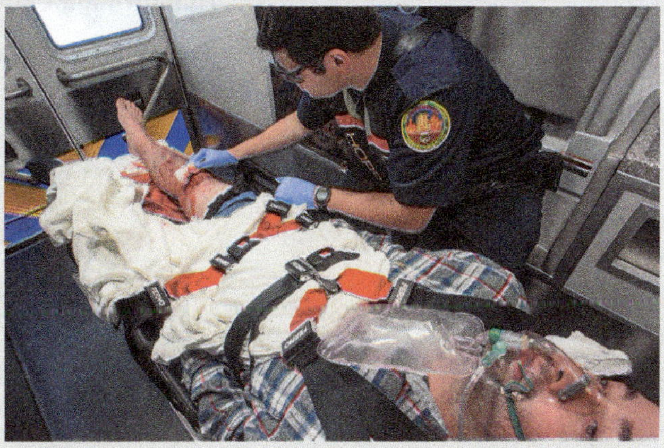

6. Reassess wound to ensure that bleeding remains controlled.

To determine when a tourniquet is appropriate, it may be reasonable to consider the American College of Surgeons Committee on Trauma's Evidence-Based Guideline for Prehospital Hemorrhage Control (Figure 29-14).

Tourniquets are used only on extremity injuries. A tourniquet must be placed between the heart and the wound to be effective. Experts disagree on where optimal placement of tourniquets should be. The National Association of State EMS Officials' National Model EMS Clinical Guidelines note that the tourniquet should be placed 2–3 inches (5–7.5 cm) proximal to the wound. The idea of this placement is to minimize potential damage associated with tourniquet use. Other experts will suggest that tourniquets should be placed as high as possible on the extremity, noting that in this location the arteries are most compressible, and that high placement makes the likelihood of missing a site of bleeding very low. Although more evidence is needed, it is likely that both answers have some logical basis. You should follow local protocol.

It is clear, however, that a tourniquet should not be applied directly over a joint (elbow or knee). There may also be evidence to suggest that a tourniquet is best placed proximal to the elbow or knee, as below these joints, the largest vessels travel between the two distal bones of the extremity.

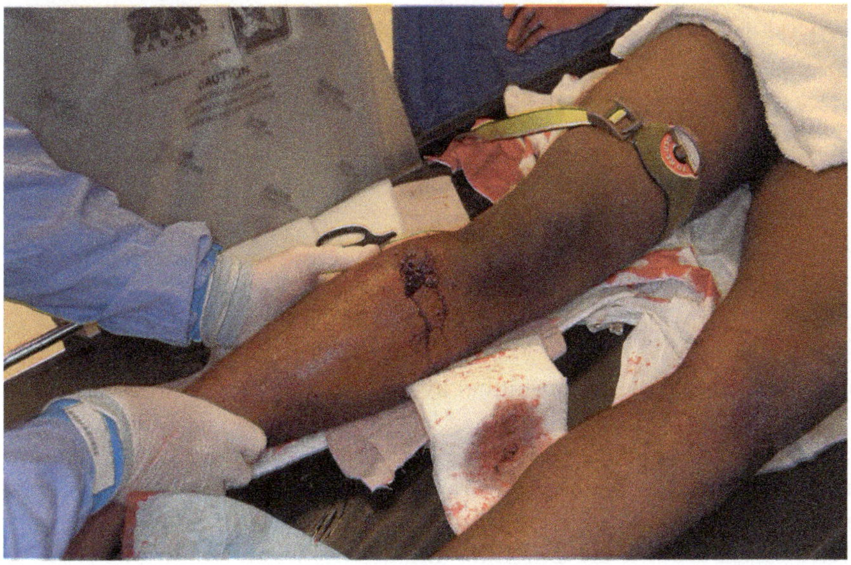

FIGURE 29-13 Commercial tourniquet in place to control bleeding from a gunshot wound. *(© Edward T. Dickinson, MD)*

FIGURE 29-14 Flow chart for bleeding control and tourniquet use.

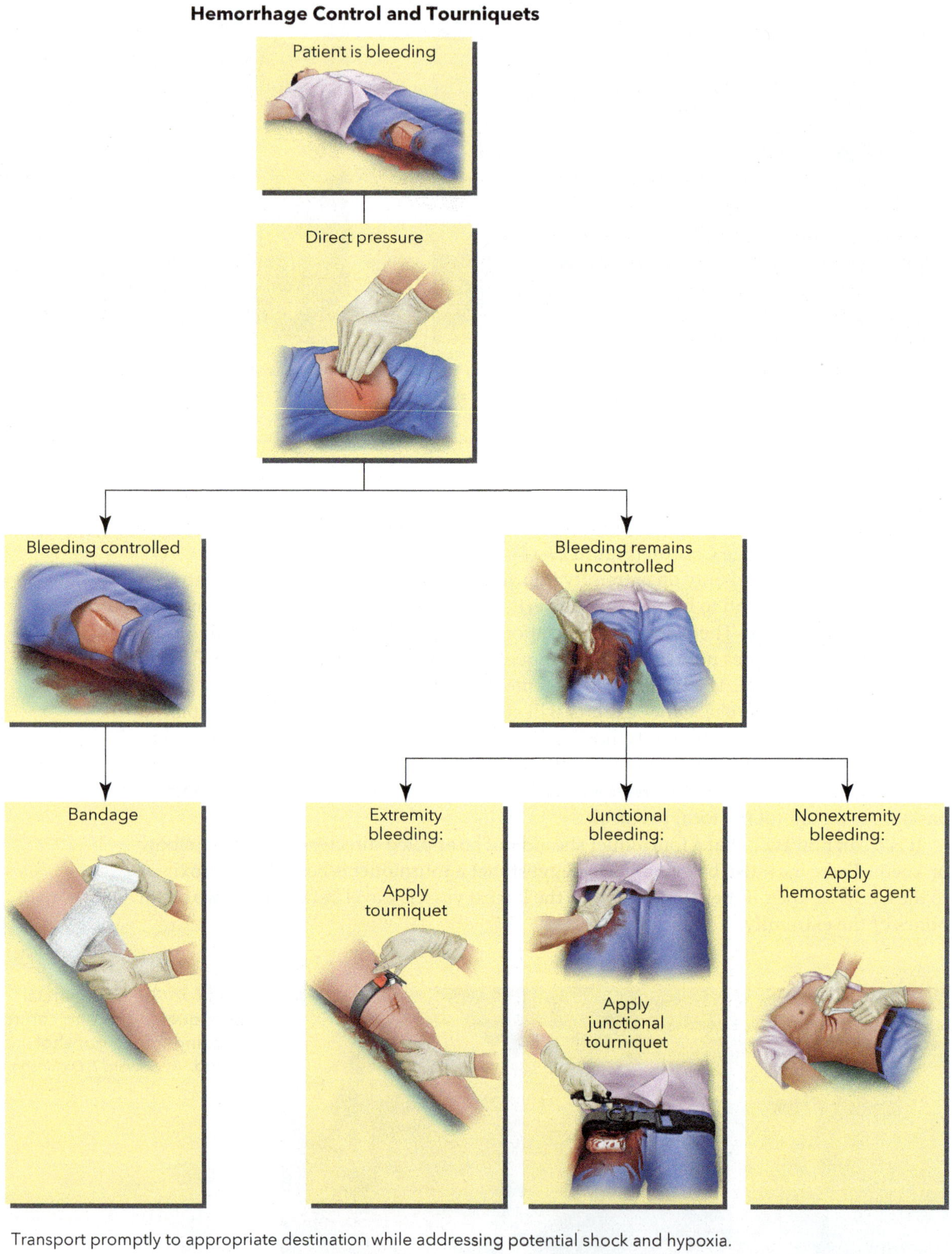

There are many different styles of tourniquet available. You should choose one that best suits your needs. The National Association of EMS Physicians, in its evidence-based guidelines, suggests that a commercially available tourniquet is preferred over an improvised tourniquet. Therefore, EMS should first use a tourniquet that is specifically designed for the purpose of being a tourniquet. Several brands of commercial tourniquets are available. These devices fasten around the extremity and are tightened by various types of turning, ratcheting, or twisting mechanisms. Although commercial tourniquets are superior, the reality of multi-casualty injury situations necessitates the need for EMTs to be proficient in improvising a tourniquet.

If a commercial tourniquet is not available, a tourniquet can be made from ambulance equipment or supplies such as a triangle bandage. Tourniquets improvised from materials such as this should be at least 2 inches (5 cm) wide and several layers thick. Never use narrow material such as a rope or wire that could cut into the skin.

Any tourniquet should be applied and tightened until the distal pulse has been lost in the affected extremity. Do not simply tighten a tourniquet until the bleeding stops, as this can create a situation where only venous blood flow is stopped. This means that arterial flow may be bringing blood into the extremity, but venous flow out has ceased. This condition can create high pressure in the vasculature extremity and is a key cause of long-term injury associated with tourniquet use. If a distal pulse is difficult to identify prior to tourniquet application, it may be reasonable simply to tighten the tourniquet until it cannot be tightened any more, with the idea that this technique is likely to result in arterial occlusion.

Once a tourniquet has been applied, do not remove or loosen it unless ordered by medical direction. Although evidence would suggest that it is reasonable to consider tourniquet removal after hours of application, for most EMS systems, this time frame is outside the range of patient contact. This could be a different consideration in remote care or prolonged extrication settings. If in doubt, contact medical control. While you are applying a tourniquet, have another rescuer apply direct pressure. This may slow the bleeding until the tourniquet is applied. To apply a tourniquet properly, follow these steps:

1. Select an appropriate site, following local protocols. The tourniquet should *always* be between the wound and the heart.

2. If using a commercial tourniquet, follow the manufacturer's instructions. In general, you should place the strap around the limb, pull the free end through the buckle or catch, and tighten this end over the pad. Ensuring that the original strap placement is tight before engaging the tightening mechanism is an important step in correct tourniquet placement. Prior to winding, you should make the band as tight as possible. Ideally, you should not be able to place a finger between the strap and the extremity prior to secondary tightening. Once you are sure the original band is tight, engage the mechanical tightening system (such as the windlass or ratcheting system). Tighten to arterial occlusion, as evidenced by loss of the distal pulse. Be aware that tightening a tourniquet causes great pain. You may need to prepare the patient for this and address the emotional aspects as the pain increases.

   If you are using an improvised tourniquet, wrap the tourniquet material around the injured limb tightly and tie a knot. It may be reasonable to insert a small dressing or pad beneath the area of the knot to minimize pinching of the skin. Do not delay tourniquet placement if padding materials are not immediately available. Slip a rigid device such as a pair of scissors, a large stick, or a metal tool into the knot and rotate to tighten the tourniquet. Resist the temptation to use a pencil, pen, or other fragile device, as these will frequently break when the tourniquet is tightened. Tighten to the point where a distal pulse can no longer be felt or until the tourniquet cannot be tightened any further. Secure the device in place with tape or by tying with the ends of the cravat.

3. Attach a notation to the patient to alert other rescuers and hospital staff that a tourniquet has been applied, and indicate the time of the application. Note this on your prehospital care report as well. Do not cover the extremity. You must visually monitor the wound site and the effectiveness of the tourniquet. Leave the tourniquet in open view. Advise hospital staff of the application of a tourniquet during your radio report and in person upon your arrival at the emergency department.

You may arrive at a scene to find that well-meaning bystanders have already applied a tourniquet to an injury, which may or may not have been necessary. If you or another EMT determines that the bleeding is not severe and other means would control it, medical direction may be contacted about removing the tourniquet. Always follow your local protocols for this situation. If you are directed to remove the tourniquet, have another rescuer

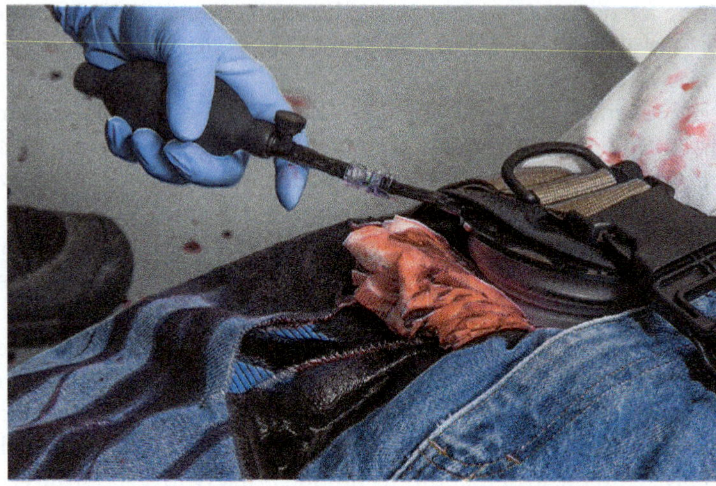

FIGURE 29-15 A junctional tourniquet. Because junctional tourniquets vary greatly in their application, you should follow the manufacturer's recommendations for use.

apply direct pressure to the wound while you release the tourniquet. If you find that the "tourniquet" applied by a layperson has not stopped the bleeding, immediately apply direct pressure and remove the tourniquet. Proceed to control the bleeding as you normally would.

In some cases, even the application of a tourniquet may not be enough to control bleeding. In these situations, consider applying a second tourniquet proximal to the first and/or using hemostatic agents and direct pressure as well as the tourniquet(s).

Junctional Tourniquets. We have previously discussed the idea that the areas where extremities join the torso are vulnerable to traumatic injury and are often the site of life-threatening hemorrhage. The groin area, in particular, houses the massive femoral artery and vein, and when injured can be a site of rapid exsanguination. These sites also pose notorious challenges to hemorrhage control. If the wound is close enough to the torso, it can be difficult to place a traditional tourniquet, leaving direct pressure as the only option to stop bleeding. A junctional tourniquet is a device designed specifically to control hemorrhage in these junctional areas. There are several different models available, but in general these devices are designed to place specific pressure on the axilla or groin regions. Most commonly a belt of band is used that places a semi-rigid or inflatable pad at the site of bleeding. (See Figure 29-15.) Various mechanical features, such as viselike screws or hand pumps, enable the user to adjust the pressure of these pads to control hemorrhage.

Although evidence is still lacking regarding their effectiveness, junctional tourniquets may be a viable tool to stop hemorrhage in areas where you have very few other options. As always, follow local protocols.

Other Methods of Bleeding Control

Although the methods of bleeding control listed previously in the chapter are the ones that most experts agree are the most effective, a variety of other techniques may have a benefit in limited or specific applications or may still be a part of the protocols in some areas. These methods include using elevation, splints, and cold applications.

Elevation. Elevation of an injured extremity to help control bleeding was for years taught as a key step in bleeding control. Recent research has proven that limb elevation is useful to decrease bleeding. Limb elevation can be done quickly and easily, so it makes sense to employ this method at the same time you apply direct pressure. When you elevate an injury above the level of the heart, gravity may help to reduce the blood pressure in the extremity, slowing bleeding. However, do not use this method if you suspect possible musculoskeletal injuries, impaled objects in the extremity, or spine injury. In such instances, the movement of broken bone ends or penetrating objects can further damage the tissues. To use elevation in controlling external bleeding, first apply direct pressure to the injury site; then elevate the injured extremity, keeping the injury site above the level of the heart.

Splinting. Bleeding associated with a musculoskeletal injury may be controlled by proper splinting of the injury. Since the sharp ends of broken bones may cause tissue and vessel injury, stabilizing them and preventing further movement of the bone ends prevents additional damage. There are several types of splints used for stabilizing injured extremities. (Splinting musculoskeletal injuries will be discussed in detail in the *Musculoskeletal Trauma* chapter.)

Inflatable splints, also called air splints, may be used to control internal and external bleeding from an extremity. This type of splint may be used to control bleeding even if there is no suspected bone injury. The splint produces a form of direct pressure. Air splints are useful if there are several wounds to the extremity or one that extends over the length of the extremity. Air splints are most effective for venous and capillary bleeding. However, they are not usually effective for the high-pressure bleeding caused by an injured artery—at least not until the arterial pressure has decreased below that of the splint. However, you may use an air splint to maintain pressure on a bleeding wound after other manual methods, such as a pressure dressing, have already controlled the bleeding.

Cold Application. A traditional method of controlling bleeding is the application of ice or a cold pack to the injury. The cold minimizes swelling and reduces the bleeding by constricting the blood vessels. Application of cold should not be used alone but rather in conjunction with other manual techniques. Application of cold will also reduce pain at the injury site.

NOTE: *Never apply ice or cold packs directly to the skin. This can cause frostbite and further damage to the tissue. Always wrap ice or a cold pack in a cloth or towel before applying it to the skin. Do not leave it in place for longer than 20 minutes at a time.*

Special Situations Involving Bleeding

Bleeding most often occurs from a wound caused by direct trauma (striking or being struck or cut by something, such as in a collision, a fall, a stabbing, or a shooting). However, you may also find external bleeding from other causes, such as bleeding from the ears caused indirectly by a head injury or a nosebleed caused by high blood pressure.

Head Injury. Traumatic injuries resulting in a fractured skull may cause bleeding or loss of cerebrospinal fluid (CSF) from the ears or nose. However, this fluid loss is not due to direct trauma to the ears or nose. Instead, the head injury results in increased pressure within the skull, which forces fluid out of the cranial cavity. You should not attempt to stop this bleeding or fluid loss, as doing so may increase the pressure in the skull. Do not apply pressure to the ears or nose. Allow the drainage to flow freely, using a gauze pad to collect it.

Nosebleed. Nosebleeds, also called *epistaxis*, may be caused by direct trauma to the nose. However, tiny capillaries in the nose may burst because of increased blood pressure (hypertension), sinus infection, or digital trauma (nose picking). Controlling bleeding from the nose is sometimes more difficult if the patient is taking certain medications, such as an anticoagulant like warfarin (Coumadin®). To stop a nosebleed, follow these steps:

1. Have the patient sit down and lean forward.
2. Apply or instruct the patient to apply direct pressure to the fleshy portion around the nostrils. Hold pressure for at least 5 minutes without checking to see if the bleeding has stopped.
3. Keep the patient calm and quiet and advise the patient not to snort or forcibly wipe the patient's nose once pressure is released. If residual blood drips from the nose, it is reasonable to dab with a tissue as long as the nose itself is not moved.
4. Do not let the patient lean back. This can allow blood to flow down the esophagus to the stomach as the patient swallows, resulting in nausea and vomiting.
5. If the patient becomes unconscious or is unable to control the patient's own airway, place the patient in the recovery position (on the patient's side), and be prepared to provide suction and aggressive airway management.

Patient Care

Care of the Patient with External Hemorrhage

Fundamental Principles of Care

Loss of blood can rapidly lead to death if not interrupted. The EMT must give prompt attention to stopping blood flow and must monitor for signs of shock.

In patients with external hemorrhage:

- If possible, begin hemorrhage control with direct pressure. If necessary, use body weight and angle pressure toward a bone. Maintain pressure for no less than 5 minutes or, in the case of massive hemorrhage, until you arrive at the hospital.
- Consider hemostatic agents to augment direct pressure.
- Consider the need for wound packing. If so, use hemostatic agents or regular gauze, if hemostatic agents are not available, and fill the wound cavity. Resume direct pressure once the cavity is filled.
- Consider the use of a junctional tourniquet to apply direct pressure to an injury in the groin or axilla.
- If direct pressure fails or is inappropriate, immediately apply a tourniquet.
- Initiate rapid transport.
- Consider the need for ALS.

Internal Bleeding

CORE CONCEPT
Signs, symptoms, and care of a patient with internal bleeding

Internal bleeding is bleeding that occurs inside the body. The bleeding itself is not visible, but many of the signs and symptoms are very apparent. There are several reasons internal bleeding can be very serious:

- Damage to the internal organs and large blood vessels can result in loss of a large quantity of blood in a short period of time.
- Blood loss cannot be seen. External bleeding is easy to identify, but internal bleeding is hidden. Patients may die of blood loss without exhibiting any external bleeding.
- Severe internal blood loss may even occur from injuries to the extremities. Sharp bone ends of a fractured femur can cause enough tissue and blood vessel damage to cause shock (hypoperfusion).

Patient Assessment

Internal Bleeding

Since internal bleeding is not visible and may not be obvious, you must identify patients who may have internal bleeding by performing a thorough history and physical exam. Suspicion of internal bleeding and estimates of its severity should be based on the mechanism of injury as well as clinical signs and symptoms. If a patient has a mechanism of injury that suggests the possibility of internal bleeding, treat as though the patient has internal bleeding.

Blunt trauma is the leading cause of internal injuries and bleeding. Mechanisms of blunt trauma that may cause internal bleeding are:

- Falls
- Motor-vehicle or motorcycle crashes
- Auto-pedestrian collisions
- Blast injuries

Penetrating trauma is also a common cause of internal injuries and bleeding. It is often difficult to judge the severity of the wound even when the size and length of the penetrating object are known. Always assess your patient for exit wounds. Mechanisms of penetrating trauma are:

- Gunshot wounds
- Stab wounds from a knife, ice pick, screwdriver, or similar object
- Impaled objects

Signs of Internal Bleeding

Many of the signs of internal bleeding that you will see are also signs of shock (hypoperfusion). These signs develop as a result of uncontrolled internal bleeding. They are late signs, indicating that a life-threatening condition has already developed. If you wait until signs of internal bleeding or shock are evident before beginning treatment, you have waited too long. Signs of internal bleeding are:

- Injuries to the surface of the body, which could indicate underlying injuries
- Bruising (Figure 29-16A), swelling, or tenderness over vital organs (especially in the chest and abdomen). Basic knowledge of anatomy is important for this reason.
- Painful, swollen, or deformed extremities
- Bleeding from the mouth, rectum, vagina, or other body orifice
- A tender, rigid, or distended abdomen
- Vomiting a coffee grounds–like substance or bright red vomitus, indicating the presence of blood. (Red blood is usually from an active, current, "new" bleeding. Dark blood is usually "old.")
- Dark, tarry stools or bright red blood in the stool. See Figure 29-16B.
- Signs and symptoms of shock. Remember that some of the signs listed in Table 29-2 are late signs. They will appear only after internal bleeding has already resulted in significant blood loss.

Remember, your best clue indicating the possibility of internal bleeding may be the presence of a mechanism of injury that could have caused internal bleeding.

FIGURE 29-16 Potential signs of internal bleeding. (A) Bruising. (B) Bright red blood and clots from the rectum due to gastrointestinal bleeding. *(Photo A: © Edward T. Dickinson, MD)*

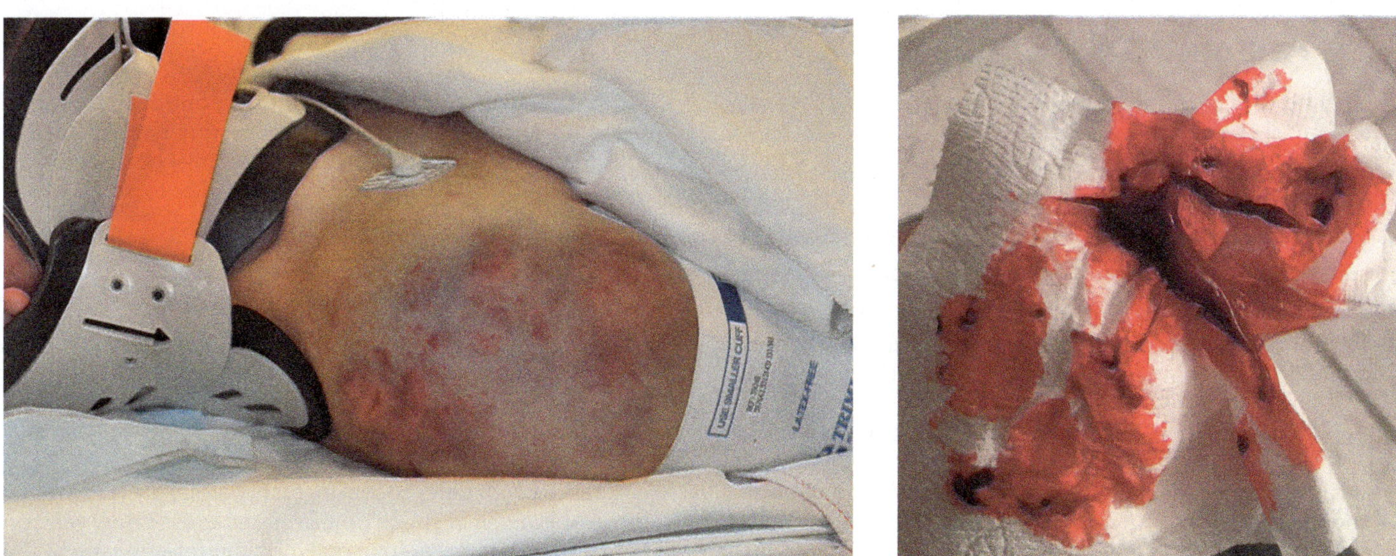

A B

Patient Care

Care of the Patient with Internal Bleeding

Fundamental Principles of Care

Care for the patient with internal bleeding centers on the prevention and treatment of shock (hypoperfusion). Definitive treatment for internal bleeding can only take place in the hospital. Patients with suspected internal bleeding must be considered serious, and warrant immediate transport to the hospital.

NOTE: *Unnecessary treatment for internal injuries will not harm the patient; however, death may result from not treating a patient who needs it.*

As with all patients, your first priority is the standard A-B-C; that is, ensure an open airway, adequate breathing, and circulation. Patients with internal bleeding may deteriorate quickly. Monitor the A-B-Cs and vital signs often. Be prepared to maintain the patient's airway, to provide or assist ventilations, or to administer CPR as needed.

- Maintain the A-B-Cs and provide support as needed.
- Consider the need for high-concentration oxygen. Treat low oxygen saturations or any potential indication of hypoxia.
- Control any external bleeding.
- If bleeding is significant, there are signs of hypoxia, or the patient's vital signs indicate or suggest the potential for shock, administer oxygen.
- If you suspect internal bleeding in an injured extremity, apply an appropriate splint.
- Take steps to preserve body temperature.
- Provide prompt transport to an appropriate medical facility. Internal bleeding must often be controlled in the operating room.

Chapter Review

Key Facts and Concepts

- Early signs of shock are often restlessness, anxiety, pale skin, and rapid pulse and respirations.
- If shock remains uncontrolled, the patient's blood pressure falls, a late sign of shock.
- Signs and symptoms of shock may not be evident early in the call, so treatment based on the mechanism of injury may be lifesaving.
- Treat shock by maintaining the airway, preventing hypoxia, controlling bleeding, and keeping the patient warm.
- Almost all external bleeding can be controlled by direct pressure and elevation. When these don't work, apply a tourniquet if the bleeding is on an extremity or a hemostatic dressing if the bleeding is from the head or torso.
- Emergency care for internal bleeding is based on the prevention and treatment of shock.
- One of the most important treatments is early recognition of shock and immediate transport to a hospital.

Key Decisions

- Has direct pressure controlled the patient's bleeding, or do I need to apply a tourniquet?
- What can I use for a tourniquet that will control bleeding but not damage tissue?
- Is a patient with pale, cool skin; tachycardia; and rapid, shallow respirations in shock or just under stress? How will continuing assessment help in making that determination?
- When treating a patient with shock, what should I do at the scene and what should I do en route to the hospital?

Chapter Glossary

arterial bleeding bleeding from an artery, which is characterized by bright red blood that is rapid, profuse, and difficult to control.

capillary bleeding bleeding from capillaries, which is characterized by a slow, oozing flow of blood.

cardiogenic shock shock, or lack of perfusion, brought on not by blood loss but by the heart's inadequate pumping action. It is often the result of a heart attack or congestive heart failure.

compensated shock when the patient is developing shock but the body is still able to maintain perfusion. *See also* shock.

decompensated shock when the body can no longer compensate for low blood volume or lack of perfusion. Late signs such as decreasing blood pressure become evident. *See also* shock.

distributive shock hypoperfusion due to a lack of blood vessel tone. Blood vessel dilation leads to decreased pressure within the circulatory system.

hemorrhage (HEM-o-rej) bleeding, especially severe bleeding.

hemorrhagic (HEM-or-AJ-ik) ***shock*** shock resulting from blood loss.

hemostatic (HEM-o-STAT-IK) ***agents*** substances applied as powders, dressings, gauze, or bandages to open wounds to stop bleeding.

hypoperfusion (HI-po-per-FEW-zhun) the body's inability to adequately circulate blood to the body's cells to supply them with oxygen and nutrients. *See also* shock.

hypovolemic (HI-po-vo-LE-mik) ***shock*** shock resulting from blood or fluid loss.

neurogenic shock hypoperfusion caused by a spinal cord injury that results in systemic vasodilation

obstructive shock a term commonly used to describe the different conditions that block the flow of blood and cause hypoperfusion.

perfusion the supply of oxygen to and removal of wastes from the body's cells and tissues as a result of the flow of blood through the capillaries.

pressure dressing a bulky dressing held in position with a tightly wrapped bandage, which applies pressure to help control bleeding.

shock the body's inability to adequately circulate blood to the body's cells to supply them with oxygen and nutrients, which is a life-threatening condition. Also known as *hypoperfusion*.

tourniquet (TURN-i-ket) a device used for bleeding control that constricts all blood flow to and from an extremity.

venous bleeding bleeding from a vein, which is characterized by dark red or maroon blood and steady, easier-to-control flow.

Preparation for Your Examination and Practice

Short Answer

1. Name the three main types of blood vessels, and describe the type of bleeding you would expect to see from each one.
2. List the patient care steps for external bleeding control.
3. Define *perfusion* and *hypoperfusion*.
4. List the signs and symptoms of shock. Which would you expect to see early? Which are late signs? Explain what causes each of them.
5. List the three major types of shock and what causes each one.
6. List the emergency care steps for treating a patient in shock.

Thinking and Linking

Think back to the chapters Scene Size-Up, Primary Assessment, Principles of Assessment, and Secondary Assessment, *as well as the chapters from the section* Medical Emergencies. *Link information from those chapters with information from this chapter as you consider the following questions:*

1. You respond to a shopping center parking lot for a motor-vehicle collision. You find an older male patient unresponsive in his vehicle. What facts could you gather at the scene that would help you determine whether the patient's unresponsiveness was caused by trauma and shock or by a medical condition?
2. What medical conditions can cause shock or present with signs and symptoms similar to shock?

Critical Thinking Exercises

Assessing and treating a patient at the scene of a collision is a challenge. The purpose of this exercise will be to consider assessment and care for such a patient.

- A patient has been involved in a motor-vehicle collision. There is considerable damage to his vehicle. The steering column and wheel are badly deformed. The patient complains of a "sore chest." You note no external bleeding. The patient's vital signs are pulse 116, respirations 20, blood pressure 106/70. How would you proceed to assess and care for this patient?

Pathophysiology to Practice

The following question is designed to assist you in gathering relevant clinical information and making accurate decisions in the field.

- A patient who was found unresponsive is in severe shock. She has no signs of trauma and has no medical history. How could an overdose of medication have caused her condition?

Street Scenes

Your ambulance is dispatched with an EMR unit from the fire department, Squad 31, to a 46-year-old male with injuries from a fall. Squad 31 is on scene first, gathering a history and taking a set of vital signs. You arrive about 3 minutes later. Arnold Johnson, your patient, is sitting in a chair and looking anxious.

Mr. Johnson likes to do odd jobs around the house. Today's project was to fix a loose shelf in the kitchen. He got out his ladder and tools and started to work. As he reached to hammer his first nail, he lost his footing and fell a few feet, hitting his left side on the corner of the kitchen table. It hurt, but he went back to finish the shelf. After a few minutes, he realized he was in considerable discomfort. As the pain increased and Arnold started to feel worse, he knew something was wrong, and called 911.

Street Scene Questions

1. **What is the priority for this patient? Does a primary assessment still need to be done?**
2. **What assessment information do you want to receive from Squad 31?**
3. **Is the mechanism of injury important information for this patient?**

You approach the patient as your partner gets the EMR information. You notice that Mr. Johnson is pale and seems to have an increased respiratory rate. Your partner gives you the patient history from Squad 31, including their impression that the patient may have broken some ribs. The EMR staff report the following vital signs: a thready pulse of 110, respiratory rate of 24 and labored, and a blood pressure of 130/85. As you move on to the secondary assessment, your partner prepares the stretcher. You are becoming more concerned. You ask Arnold's wife if this is his normal color, and she tells you he is very pale. At that point, the patient tells you he feels nauseated and thinks he might throw up.

Street Scene Questions

4. **What is the treatment priority for this patient?**
5. **How often should you get a new set of vital signs?**

You load the patient on the stretcher, ask him how he feels, and notice he is not as alert as when you arrived on the scene about 10 minutes ago. You administer oxygen by way of nonrebreather mask and move toward the ambulance, concerned that this patient may be bleeding internally. Once en route to the hospital, you get another set of vital signs and realize the pulse is weak and has increased by 10 beats per minute. The respiratory rate is now 28 and seems more labored. The blood pressure is 124/80. You do a detailed assessment of the abdomen, and the patient reacts with tenderness in the left upper quadrant. The closest hospital is a trauma center, and you tell your partner this is a high priority. You continue patient care with 15 liters per minute of oxygen by nonrebreather mask and keep the patient warm. You take another set of vital signs, followed by a radio report to the hospital. You end the transmission by advising ETA in 7 minutes.

A short time after you give your prehospital care report to ED personnel, you overhear a surgeon turn to a nurse and quietly say, "Get an operating room set up. This patient likely has a severe spleen injury."

Soft-Tissue Trauma

30

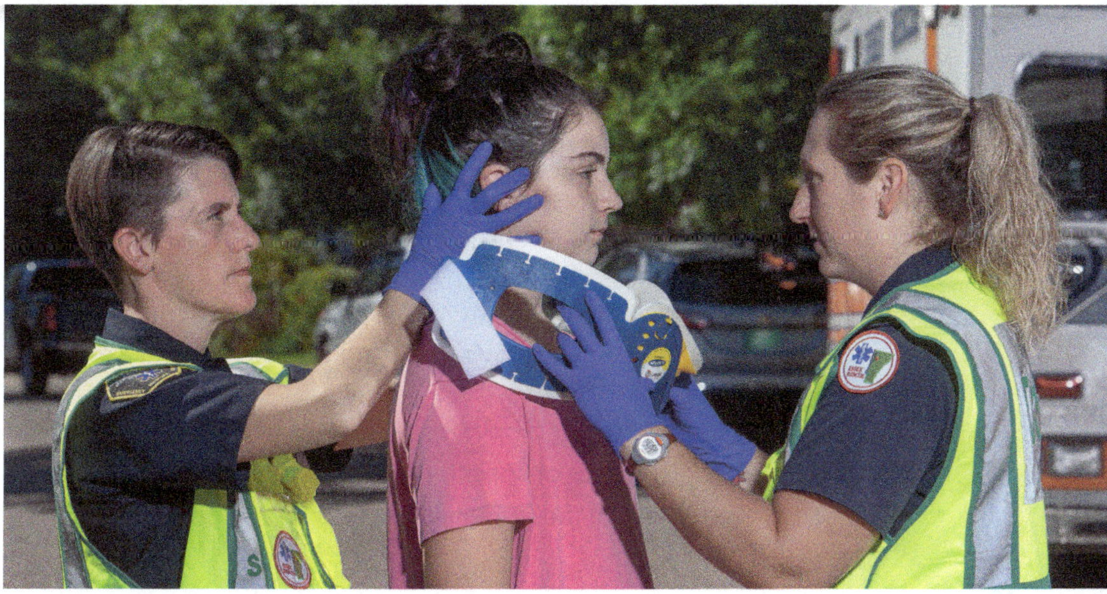

Related Chapters

The following chapters provide additional information related to topics discussed in this chapter:

1 Introduction to Emergency Medical Services
2 Well-Being of the EMT
11 Scene Size-Up
25 Poisoning and Overdose Emergencies
29 Bleeding and Shock
31 Chest and Abdominal Trauma
32 Musculoskeletal Trauma
33 Trauma to the Head, Neck, and Spine
40 Highway Safety and Vehicle Extrication

Standard

Trauma (Soft-Tissue Trauma)

Competency

Applies fundamental knowledge to provide basic emergency care and transportation based on assessment findings for an acutely injured patient.

Core Concepts

- Understanding closed wounds and emergency care for closed wounds
- Understanding open wounds and emergency care for open wounds

- Understanding burns and emergency care for burns
- Understanding electrical injuries and emergency care for electrical injuries
- How to dress and bandage wounds

Outcomes

After reading this chapter, you should be able to:

30.1 Summarize concepts of soft-tissue injuries. (pp. 825-835)

- List the soft tissues in the body.
- Describe the anatomy and physiology of the skin.
- Relate the potential for complications to the mechanisms that cause soft-tissue injuries.
- Distinguish between closed and open soft-tissue wounds.
- Recognize the characteristics of specific types of soft-tissue wounds.
- Relate soft-tissue injuries to the potential for trauma to underlying structures.

30.2 Integrate the steps of caring for soft-tissue injuries into the overall care of specific patients. (pp. 835-845)

- Relate the mechanism of injury to steps in caring for the patient.
- Compare the general approach to closed soft-tissue wounds with the approach to open soft-tissue wounds.
- Outline the specific considerations in managing a patient with penetrating trauma.
- Outline the specific considerations for treating an injury with an impaled object.
- Compare the approaches to managing partial and complete avulsions.
- Describe the care of amputations.
- Describe the approach to managing a patient with injuries to the genitalia.

30.3 Summarize the concepts of burn injuries. (pp. 845-863)

- Outline the prioritization for care for a variety of portrayals of burn patients.
- Identify the agents of burns.
- Identify the sources of burns.
- Classify portrayals of burn injuries by depth.
- Classify the severity of a variety of portrayals of burn injuries.
- Explain the classification of burn severity for patients of different age groups.
- Differentiate the steps in the approaches to treating specific types of burns.
- Explain complications commonly sustained with different types of burns.
- Match specific injury characteristics to the most appropriate dressing and bandaging techniques.

Key Terms

abrasion, *830*
amputation, *832*
avulsion, *832*
bandage, *858*
closed wound, *827*
contusion, *827*
crush injury, *829*
dermis, *827*
dressing, *858*
epidermis, *826*
full thickness burn, *847*
hematoma, *828*
laceration, *830*
occlusive dressing, *861*
open wound, *830*
partial thickness burn, *847*
pressure dressing, *861*
puncture wound, *831*
rule of nines, *848*
rule of palm, *849*
subcutaneous layers, *827*
superficial burn, *846*
universal dressing, *860*

EMTs are frequently called to deal with injuries to the soft tissues of the body. These injuries may range from minor scrapes and bruises to massive bleeding or amputations. Although most of these injuries are not life-threatening, your immediate care can make a significant difference in the outcome for the patient. Whether it be a lifesaving intervention, such as bleeding control, or simple emotional support in the setting of a disfiguring open wound, the immediate care provided for soft-tissue injuries does make a difference. This chapter will describe the various types of soft-tissue injury and discuss the range of treatment options to best handle these sometimes challenging injuries.

Soft Tissues

The soft tissues of the body include the skin, fatty tissues, muscles, blood vessels, connective tissues, membranes (tissues that line or cover organs), glands, and nerves (Figure 30-1). Teeth, bones, and cartilage are considered hard tissues.

The most obvious soft-tissue injuries involve the skin (Figure 30-2). Most people do not think of the skin as a body organ but in fact, it is the largest organ of the human body. The skin's total surface area is more than 20 square feet for an average adult. Its major functions are:

- **Protection.** The skin is a barrier that keeps out microorganisms (germs), debris, and unwanted chemicals. Underlying tissues and organs are protected from environmental contact. The surface of the skin also provides a home to millions of microorganisms designed to defend against unwanted germs. This population of helpful bacteria competes and balances against an overpopulation of harmful organisms.
- **Water balance.** The skin helps prevent water loss and stops environmental water from entering the body. This helps preserve the chemical balance of body fluids and tissues.
- **Temperature regulation.** Blood vessels in the skin can dilate (increase in diameter) to carry more blood to the skin, allowing heat to radiate away from the body. When the body needs to conserve heat, these vessels constrict (decrease in diameter) to prevent heat loss. The sweat glands found in the skin produce perspiration, which will evaporate and help cool the body. The fat that is part of the skin serves as a thermal insulator.
- **Excretion.** Salts and excess water can be released through the skin.
- **Shock (impact) absorption.** The skin and its layers of fat help protect the underlying organs from minor impacts and pressures.

In addition to these key functions, it is important to remember that the skin also plays a fundamental role in our interactions each day. Nerve endings provide us with sensory input in the form of tactile (touch) stimulation. We sense temperature and pleasurable

FIGURE 30-1 Soft tissues.

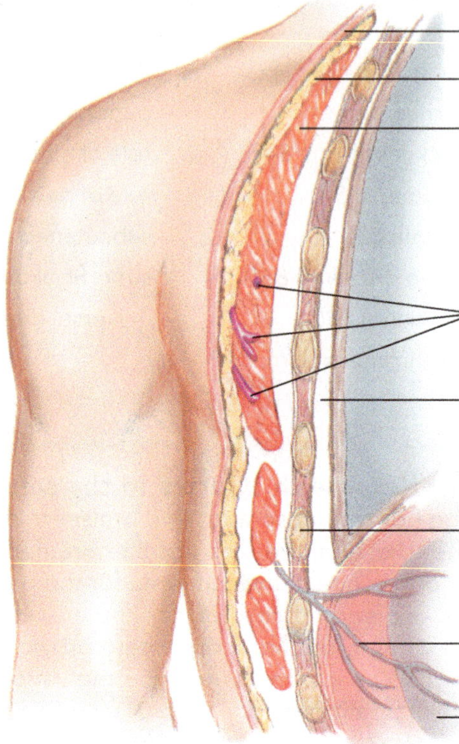

and painful stimuli. Most important, the skin defines who we are by creating many of our distinctive features and recognizable physical traits.

epidermis (ep-i-DER-mis) the outer layer of the skin.

The skin has three major layers: the epidermis, the dermis, and the subcutaneous layer. The outer layer of the skin is the ***epidermis***. The outermost epidermis is composed of dead cells, which are rubbed off or sloughed off and replaced. The pigment granules of the skin and living cells are found deeper in the epidermis. The cells of the innermost portion are actively dividing, replacing the dead cells of the outer layers. The epidermis contains no

FIGURE 30-2 The skin.

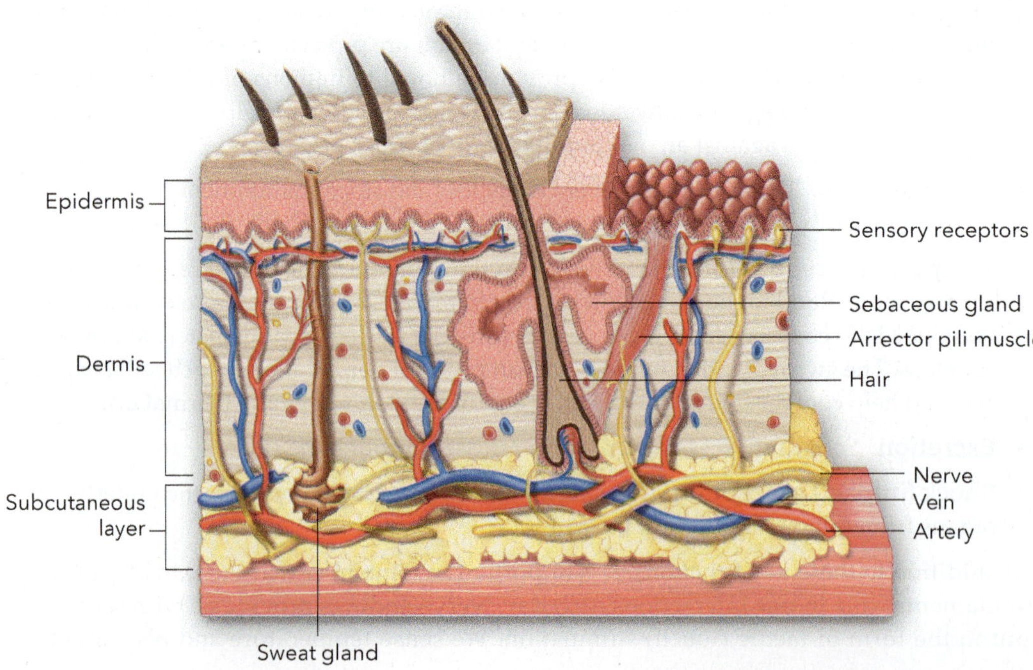

blood vessels or nerves. Except for certain types of burns and injuries due to cold, injuries of the epidermis present few problems in EMT-level care.

The layer of skin below the epidermis is the ***dermis***. This layer is rich with blood vessels, nerves, and specialized structures such as sweat glands, sebaceous (oil) glands, and hair follicles. Specialized nerve endings in the dermis are involved with the sense of touch that registers cold, heat, and pain. Once the dermis is opened to the outside world, contamination and infection become major problems. Such wounds can be serious, especially when accompanied by profuse bleeding and intense pain.

dermis (DER-mis)
the inner (second) layer of the skin found beneath the epidermis. It is rich in blood vessels and nerves.

The layers of fat and soft tissue below the dermis are called the ***subcutaneous layers***. Shock absorption and insulation are major functions of this layer. Again, when these layers are injured, there are problems of tissue and bloodstream contamination, bleeding, and pain.

subcutaneous (SUB-ku-TAY-ne-us) ***layers***
the layers of fat and soft tissues found below the dermis.

Soft-tissue injuries are generally classified as closed wounds or open wounds. The skin and its layers of soft tissue can be damaged in a variety of ways. Most commonly, mechanical force from trauma rips, crushes, stretches, and otherwise injures these relatively delicate cells. Soft tissue can also be injured chemically, thermally, and even electrically. In a broad sense, soft-tissue injuries can be categorized by type and by the cause of the injury.

Closed Wounds

A ***closed wound*** is an internal injury; that is, there is no open pathway from the outside to the injured site. In a closed wound, the skin can be damaged, but it remains intact. These wounds usually result from the impact of a blunt object. Although the skin itself may not be broken, there may be extensively crushed tissues beneath it. Closed wounds can be simple bruises, internal lacerations (cuts), or internal punctures caused by fractured bones, crushing forces, or the rupture (bursting open) of internal organs (Figure 30-3). Internal bleeding from a closed wound can range from minor to life-threatening.

closed wound
an internal injury with no open pathway from the outside.

CORE CONCEPT
Understanding closed wounds and emergency care for closed wounds

Types of Closed Wounds

The major types of closed wounds include contusions, hematomas, crush injuries, and primary blast injuries.

Contusions

A ***contusion*** is a bruise, the most frequently encountered type of closed wound (Figure 30-4). In a contusion, the epidermis remains intact, but cells and blood vessels in the dermis are damaged. A variable amount of internal bleeding occurs at the time of injury and may continue for a few hours. Pain, swelling, and discoloration occur at the wound site. Swelling and discoloration may occur immediately or may be delayed as much as 48 hours.

contusion (kun-TU-zhun)
a bruise.

Swelling is caused both by the collection of blood under the skin and by inflammation through fluid brought to the site of the injury by the immune system. Inflammation is helpful in that it cushions the injured area and helps dilute toxins, but it can also be

FIGURE 30-3 Examples of closed wounds.

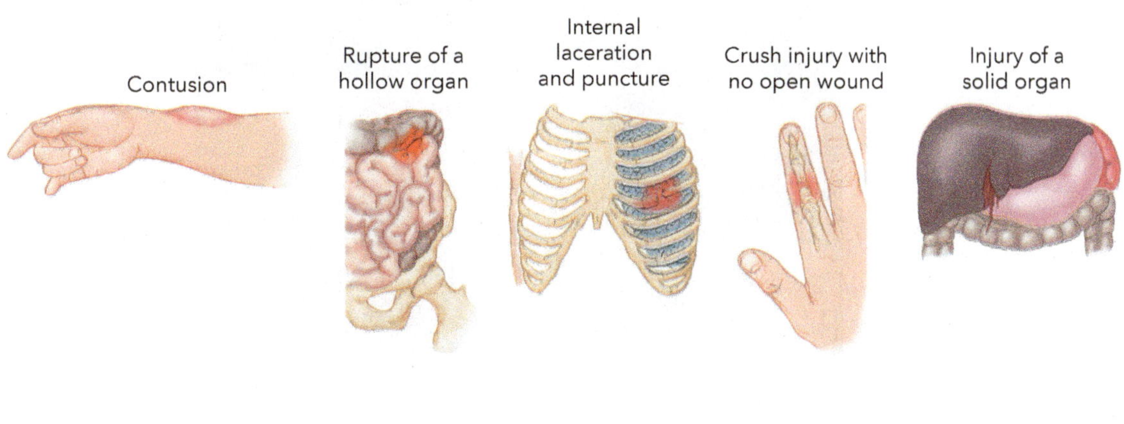

FIGURE 30-4 Contusions are the most common type of closed wound. (A) and (B) Injuries created by a seat belt. (C) Contusion from impact with airbag. *(Photos A and C: © Edward T. Dickinson, MD; photo B: © David Effron, MD)*

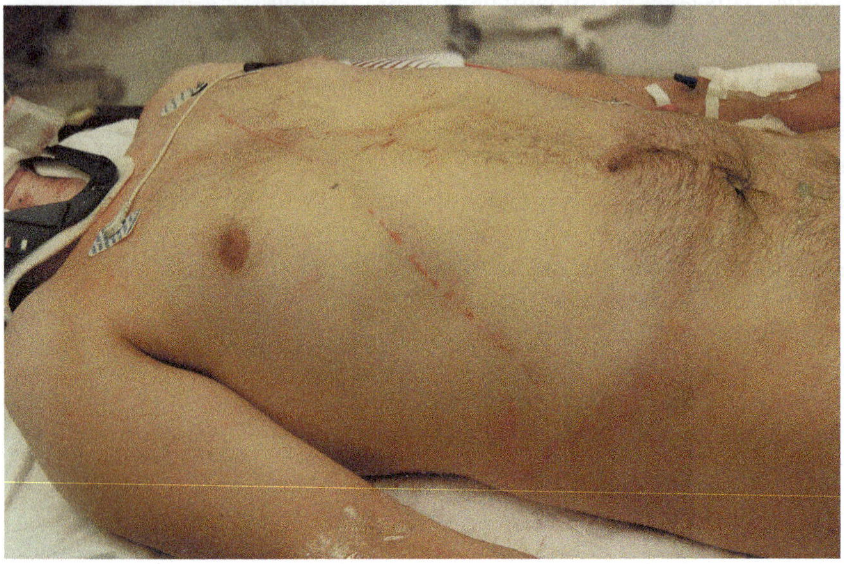

A

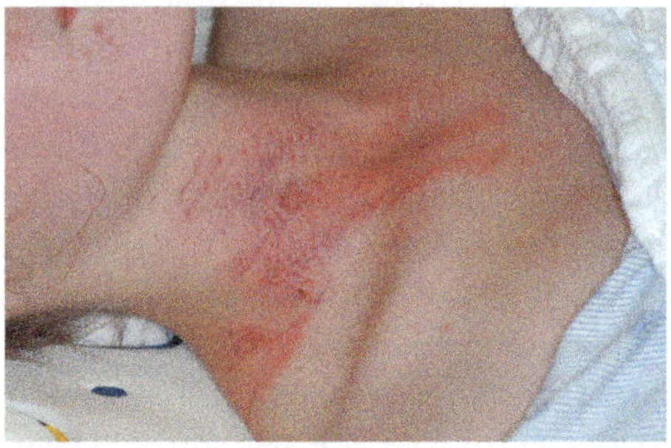

B

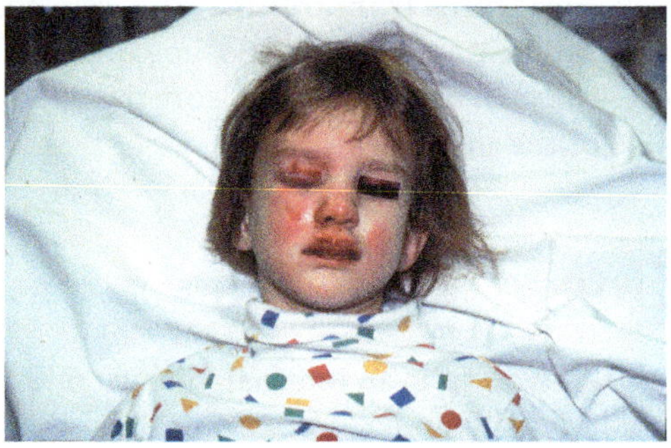

C

harmful, as it can cause tissues to occupy more space than usual. In closed containers such as to the skull, or in areas divided by non-stretching connective tissue, this increase in size can cause compression and even reduced blood flow. In addition to the skin, internal organs such as the brain, heart, lungs, and kidneys can also be contused and suffer similar injuries.

Hematomas

hematoma (hem-ah-TO-mah) a swelling caused by the collection of blood under the skin or in damaged tissues as a result of an injured or broken blood vessel.

A ***hematoma*** occurs when blood collects at the site of an injury (Figure 30-5). A hematoma differs from a contusion in that hematomas involve a larger amount of tissue damage, including damage to larger blood vessels, with greater internal blood loss. Where a contusion may cause some minor injury to small blood vessels, a hematoma is characterized by much more severe internal bleeding and the collection of a larger volume of blood beneath the skin. In fact, as much as a liter of blood may accumulate in a hematoma.

Closed Crush Injuries

Force can be transmitted from the body's exterior to its internal structures, even when the skin remains intact, and the only indication of injury is a simple bruise. This force can cause the internal organs to be crushed or ruptured, causing internal bleeding. This is called a

FIGURE 30-5 Abdominal wall hematoma from a dog bite. *(© Edward T. Dickinson, MD)*

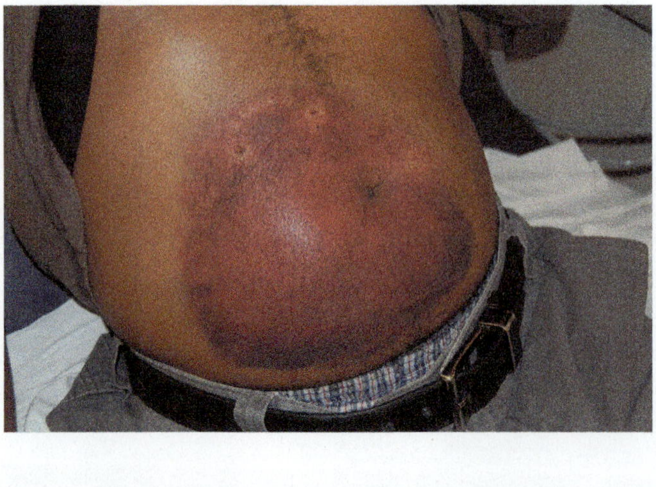

crush injury. Solid organs such as the liver and spleen normally contain considerable amounts of blood. When crushed, they bleed severely and cause shock. Contents of hollow organs, such as digested food or urine, can leak into the body cavities, causing severe inflammation and tissue damage.

crush injury
an injury caused when force is transmitted from the body's exterior to its internal structures. Bones can be broken; muscles, nerves, and tissues can be damaged, causing internal bleeding. In extreme cases where the torso is compressed, internal organs such as the stomach or urinary bladder can be ruptured, causing internal bleeding and allowing digested food or urine to spread into the abdominal cavities.

Emergency Care for Closed Wounds

Always take care to protect yourself when dealing with traumatic injuries. Be sure that what injured the patient cannot injure you. Many of the injuries discussed in this chapter result from violent trauma. Please be sure that the scene is secure before treatment begins. Use Standard Precautions, even though the patient's skin is not broken.

Patient Assessment

Closed Wounds

Bruising may be an indication of internal injuries and related internal bleeding (Table 30-1). In addition, consider the possibility of closed soft-tissue injuries whenever there is swelling, pain, or deformity, as well as a mechanism of blunt trauma. Internal head or brain trauma can present with bleeding from the ears and nose. Injuries to abdominal or pelvic organs can present as bleeding from the rectum or vagina. Similarly, coughing up blood in the setting of trauma indicates injury to the respiratory system. Always consider the mechanism of injury (MOI) when you examine a patient with a closed wound. Crush injuries may be difficult or impossible to identify during assessment, so you must rely on the MOI. Patients with a significant MOI should be considered to have internal injuries until they are ruled out in the emergency department.

TABLE 30-1 Contusions (Bruises) as Signs of Soft-Tissue Injury

SIGN	INDICATES
Swelling or deformity at the site of the bruise	Possible underlying fracture.
Bruise on the head or neck	Possible injury to the cervical spine or brain. Injury to major blood vessels in the neck. Search for blood in the mouth, nose, and ears.
Bruise on the trunk or signs of damage to the ribs or sternum	Possible chest injury. Determine if the patient is coughing up frothy red blood, which may indicate a punctured lung, and assess for difficulty breathing. Use your stethoscope to listen for equal air entry and any unusual breath sounds.
Bruise on the abdomen	Possible injury to underlying organs such as the spleen, liver, or kidneys.

Patient Care

Patient with Closed Wounds

Fundamental Principles of Care

Take the appropriate Standard Precautions and follow these steps for emergency care of a patient with closed wounds, generally in this order:

- Manage the patient's airway, breathing, and circulation. Consider the need for high-concentration oxygen by nonrebreather mask.
- *Manage as if there were internal bleeding* and *provide care for shock* if you believe that there is a reasonable possibility of internal injuries.
- Splint extremities that are painful, swollen, or deformed.

- Stay alert in case the patient vomits.
- Continue to monitor the patient for the development of shock and transport promptly.
- Apply cold packs to isolated injuries (avoid direct contact with skin) to manage pain and swelling.

NOTE: *Treatment for internal bleeding is discussed in the chapter* Bleeding and Shock; *treatment of chest and abdominal injuries is discussed in the chapter* Chest and Abdominal Trauma, *and head injury is discussed in the chapter* Trauma to the Head, Neck, and Spine.

Open Wounds

open wound an injury in which the skin is interrupted, exposing the tissue beneath.

An ***open wound*** is an injury in which the skin is interrupted, or broken, exposing the tissues underneath. The interruption can come from the outside, as with a laceration, or from the inside, as when a fractured bone end breaks the skin.

CORE CONCEPT
Understanding open wounds and emergency care for open wounds

Types of Open Wounds

There are numerous types of open wounds, including abrasions, lacerations, punctures, avulsions, amputations, crush injuries, blast injuries, and high-pressure-injection injuries.

Abrasions

abrasion (ab-RAY-zhun) a scratch or scrape.

The classification of ***abrasion*** includes simple scrapes and scratches in which the outer layer of the skin is damaged, but not all the layers are penetrated. Abrasions can range in severity (Figure 30-6). Skinned elbows and knees, road rash, mat burns, rug burns, and brush burns are examples of abrasions. With abrasions, there might be no detectable bleeding or only the minor ooze of blood from the capillary beds. The patient may be experiencing great pain, even if the injury is minor. Because of dirt or other substances ground into the skin, the opportunity for infection is great.

Lacerations

laceration (lass-er-AY-shun) a cut.

A ***laceration*** is a cut. It may be smooth or jagged (Figure 30-7). This type of wound is often caused by an object with a sharp edge, such as a razor blade, broken glass, a jagged piece of metal, or a chainsaw. However, a laceration can also result from a severe blow or impact with a blunt object. If the laceration has rough edges, it may tend to fall together and obstruct the view as you try to determine the wound depth. It is usually impossible to look at the

FIGURE 30-6 (A) Abrasions are usually the least serious type of open wound. (B) Some abrasions are more severe. *(Photos A and B: © Edward T. Dickinson, MD)*

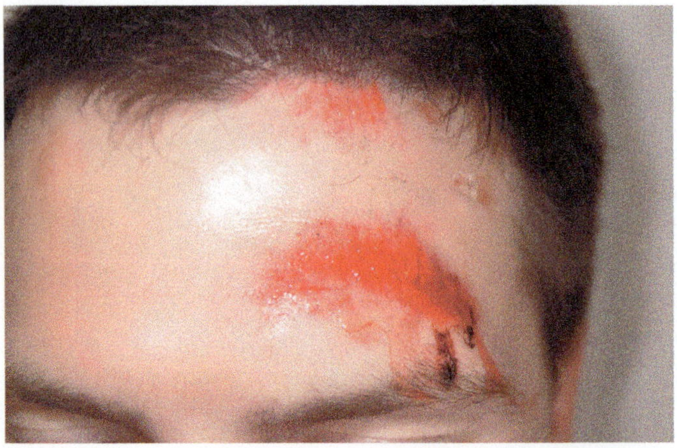

A

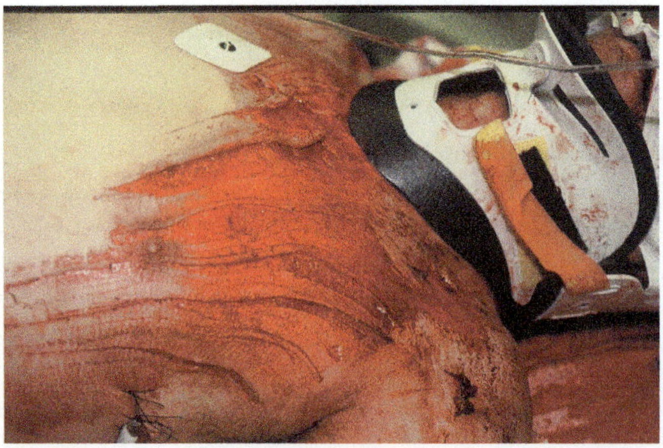

B

FIGURE 30-7 (A) Some lacerations have smooth edges, and (B) some have jagged edges. (C) Damage to tissue and tendon from a chainsaw injury. *(Photo A: © Edward T. Dickinson, MD; photos B and C: © David Effron, MD)*

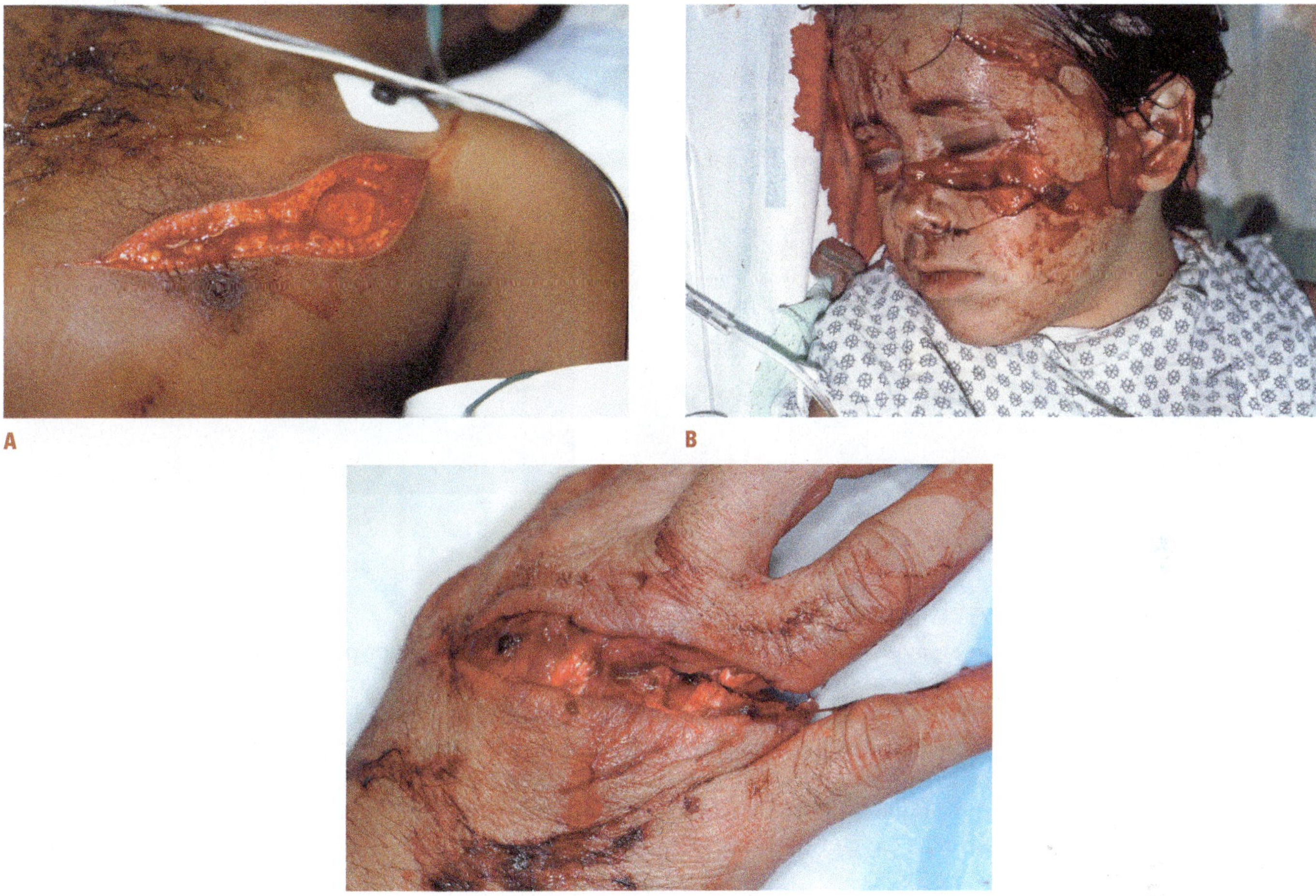

A B C

outside of a laceration and determine the extent of the damage to underlying tissues. If significant blood vessels have been torn, bleeding will be considerable. Sometimes the bleeding is partially controlled when blood vessels are stretched and torn. This is due to the natural retraction and constriction of the cut ends, which aid in rapid clot formation.

Penetrating Trauma and Punctures

When an object passes through the skin or other tissue, penetrating trauma occurs. A ***puncture wound*** results from the penetration of the skin. Typically, puncture wounds are caused by objects such as bullets, nails, ice picks, splinters, and knives (Figure 30-8). Blast injury can also cause penetrating trauma by launching high-velocity *shrapnel* (objects thrown by the blast, including bomb materials and debris), as discussed in more detail later. Penetrating trauma violates the skin and soft tissues by pushing objects through them. Often there is no severe external bleeding, although internal bleeding may be profuse. Common puncture wounds are relatively small and insignificant to look at but, depending on the depth of penetration, may cause devastating injuries. Your assessment may find only tiny external wounds on the surface of the skin, but the damage may prove to be deadly. Always consider a puncture wound a serious injury. The threat of contamination and subsequent infection is high.

puncture wound
an open wound that tears through the skin and destroys underlying tissues. A *penetrating puncture wound* can be shallow or deep. A *perforating puncture wound* has both an entrance and an exit wound.

A penetrating puncture wound can be shallow or deep. In either case, tissues and blood vessels are injured. If the object causing the injury passes through the body and out again, the exit wound may be more serious than the entrance wound, as in a gunshot wound.

In most cases the most significant damage from penetrating trauma will not be to the skin and external tissues. The most significant damage will occur in the structures beneath the skin. You should use your knowledge of anatomy and physiology to anticipate injuries to underlying organs and blood vessels and to treat accordingly.

FIGURE 30-8 (A) The knife penetrating this patient's back constitutes a serious puncture wound. (B) An X-ray of the same wound. *(Photos A and B: © Edward T. Dickinson, MD)*

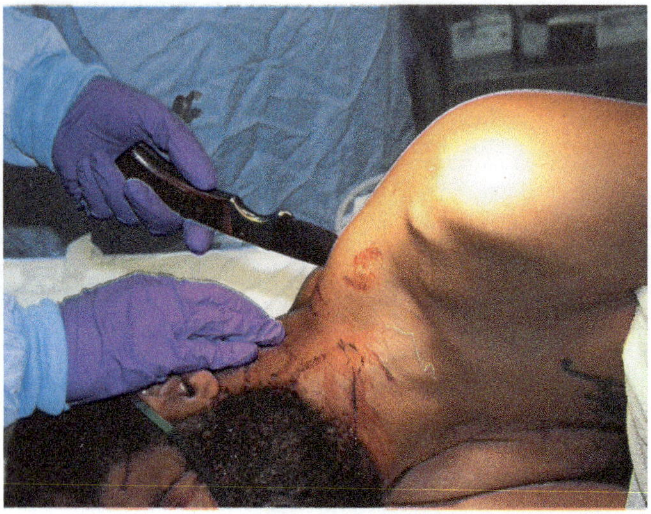

A

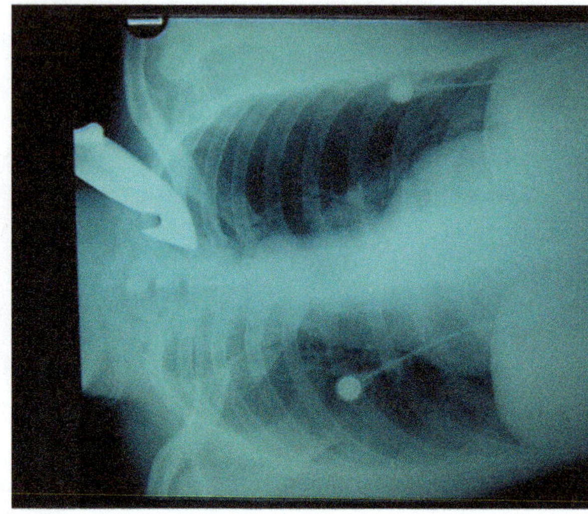

B

Avulsions

avulsion (ah-VUL-shun) the tearing away or tearing off of a piece or flap of skin or other soft tissue. This term also may be used for an eye pulled from its socket or a tooth dislodged from its socket.

In an ***avulsion***, flaps of skin and tissues are torn loose or pulled off completely. When the tip of the nose is cut or torn off, this is an example of an avulsion. The same applies to the external ear (Figure 30-9A). A degloving avulsion occurs when the hand is caught in a roller. In this type of incident, the skin is stripped off like a glove (Figure 30-9B). An eye pulled from its socket (extruded) is also a form of avulsion. The term *avulsed* is used in reporting the wound, as in "an avulsed eye" or "an avulsed ear." When tissue is avulsed, it is cut off from its oxygen supply and will soon die.

Amputations

amputation (am-pyu-TAY-shun) the surgical removal or traumatic severing of a body part, usually an extremity.

The extremities are sometimes subject to ***amputation***. Amputated fingers, toes, hands, feet, or limbs are completely cut through or torn off (Figure 30-10). Jagged skin and bone edges can sometimes be observed. There may be massive bleeding; or the force that amputates a limb may close off torn blood vessels, limiting the amount of bleeding. Often blood vessels collapse, or they retract and constrict, which limits bleeding from the wound site.

FIGURE 30-9 (A) An avulsion of the earlobe. (B) An avulsion injury that caused a degloving. *(Photos: © Edward T. Dickinson, MD)*

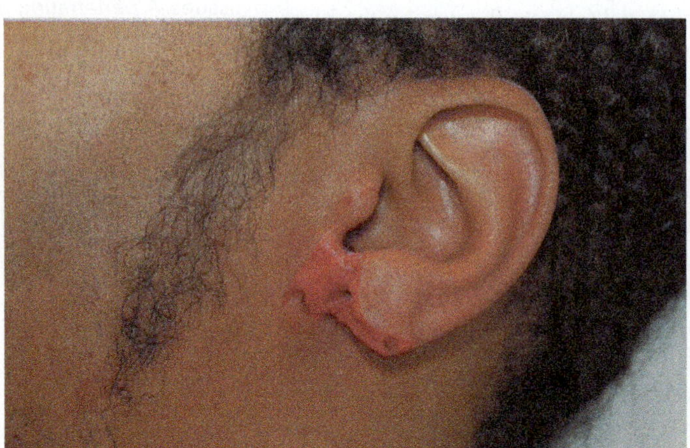

A

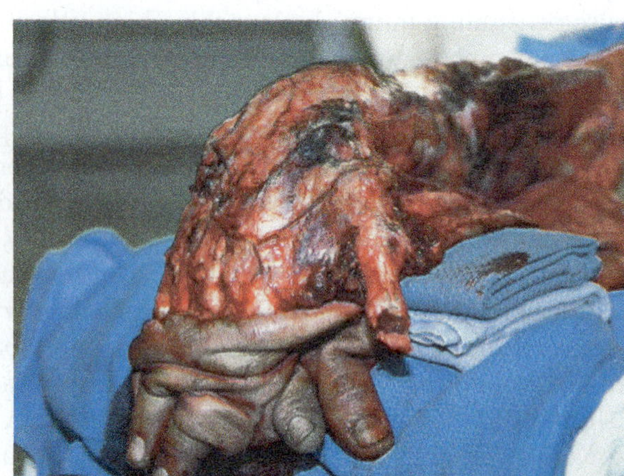

B

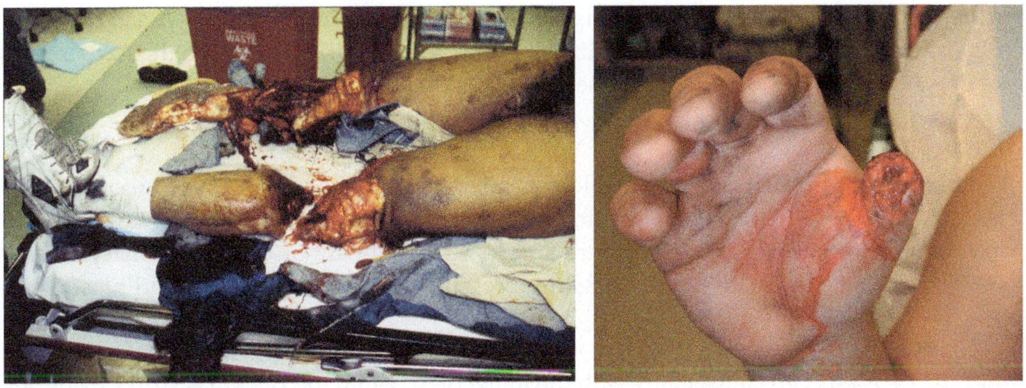

A B

FIGURE 30-10 (A) Amputated leg. (B) Hand with amputated thumb. *(Photos A and B: © Edward T. Dickinson, MD)*

Open Crush Injuries

Although crush injuries were discussed earlier in this chapter as closed wounds, crush injuries also can be open wounds. An open crush injury can result when an extremity is caught between heavy items, such as pieces of machinery. Blood vessels, nerves, and muscles are involved, and swelling may be a major problem, with resulting loss of blood supply distally. Bones are fractured and may protrude through the wound site. Soft tissues and internal organs can be crushed to produce profuse bleeding, both externally and internally (Figure 30-11).

Bite Wounds

Bite wounds (Figure 30-12) are also relatively common open soft-tissue injuries. Although for the most part they are assessed and treated like any other open wound, you should be

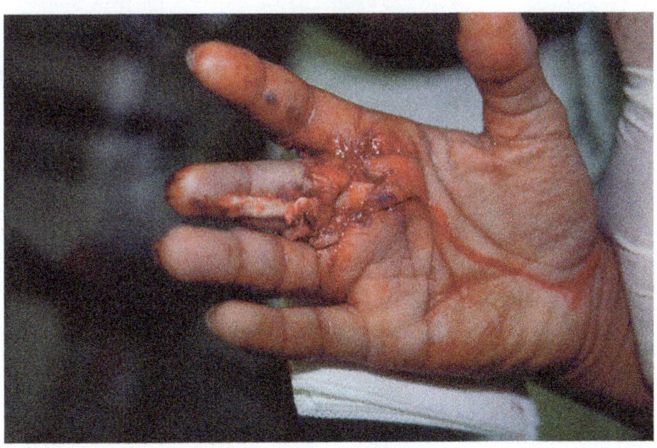

FIGURE 30-11 An open crush injury. *(© Edward T. Dickinson, MD)*

FIGURE 30-12 (A) Multiple bite wounds in young child. (B) Wound in cheek of adult from dog bite. *(Photo A: © David Effron, MD; Photo B: © Edward T. Dickinson, MD)*

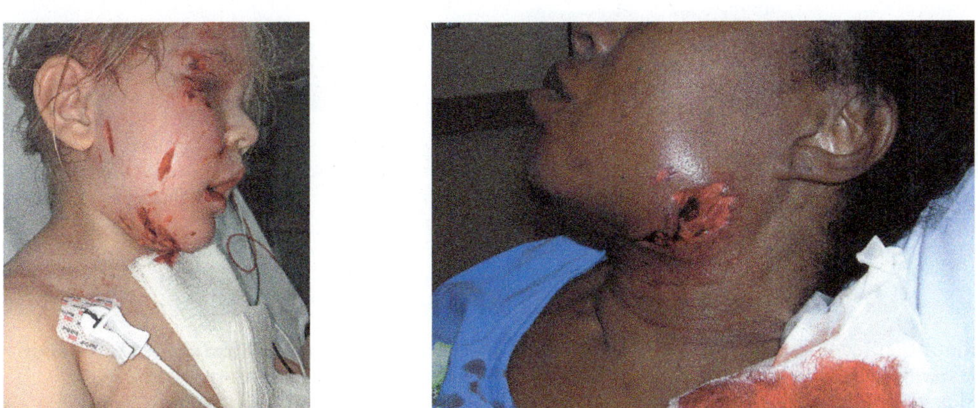

A B

aware that infection rates tend to be higher in these types of injuries, and human bites may be considered a sign of abuse or assault. In general, these injuries, although most commonly not life-threatening, should be taken seriously and evaluated by a physician.

Blast Injuries

A patient injured from a blast or explosion may sustain a combination of all of the injuries just described. The unusual characteristics of a blast mean that a mixture of open and closed injuries can be the result (Figure 30-13). As previously discussed, primary injuries occur because of the intense high pressure (pressure wave; overpressure) and blast winds

FIGURE 30-13 Blasts can cause injury with the initial blast, when the patient is struck by debris, or when the patient is thrown by the blast. In addition, the patient may sustain additional injuries, such as from exposure to chemicals or toxins or be injured by structural collapse.

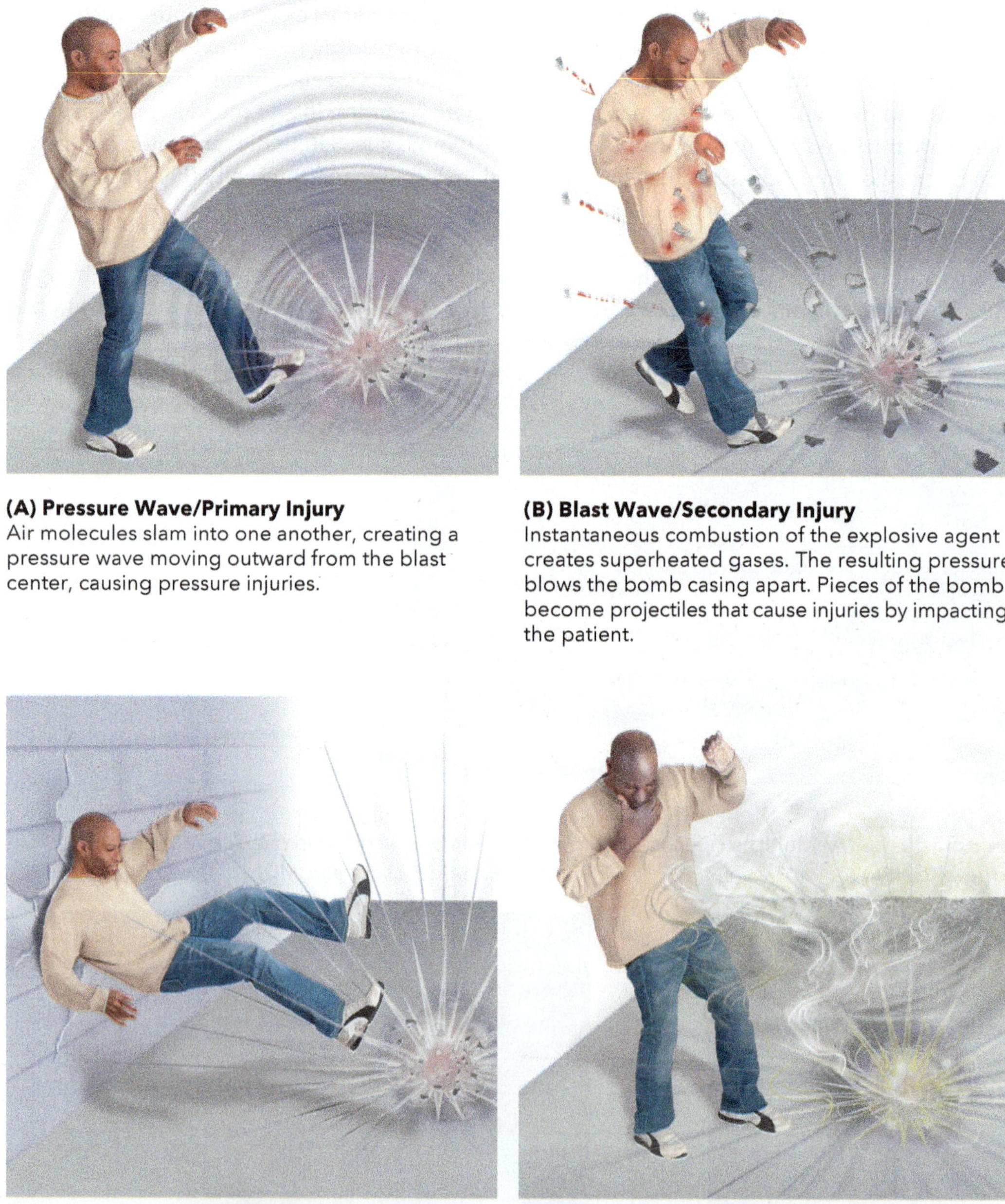

(A) Pressure Wave/Primary Injury
Air molecules slam into one another, creating a pressure wave moving outward from the blast center, causing pressure injuries.

(B) Blast Wave/Secondary Injury
Instantaneous combustion of the explosive agent creates superheated gases. The resulting pressure blows the bomb casing apart. Pieces of the bomb become projectiles that cause injuries by impacting the patient.

(C) Patient Displacement/Tertiary Injury
The blast wind may propel the patient to the ground or against objects, causing further injuries.

(D) Patient Exposed to Hazardous Material or Structural Collapse/Quaternary Injury
The patient may also be exposed to harmful chemicals or toxins or may be injured by structural collapse.

that hit the patient. Injuries can include damage to any air- or fluid-filled body organ or cavity, especially pressure injury to the lungs. Secondary injury is the result of projectiles (shrapnel) such as debris hitting the patient (blast wave), leading to open and penetrating wounds. Tertiary (third-level) injuries occur if the patient is thrown by the blast. Tertiary injuries occur both from the force of the blast and as a result of the violent landing after being thrown. These injuries can include not just soft-tissue injuries but also fractures, avulsions, and amputations. Finally, the patient may sustain additional injuries such as from exposure to chemicals or toxins, burns, and crush injuries. These are sometimes referred to as quaternary (fourth-level) injuries.

High-Pressure-Injection Injuries

An uncommon but important injury can occur when a patient is working with a machine that injects grease, paint, air, or some other substance under high pressure. If the nozzle injects the substance into the patient—typically into the finger—rather than the object it was intended for, this can lead to significant injury. These machines may use pressures of thousands of pounds per square inch, which results in a wound that is much worse than it looks. There is typically very little (or even no) injury apparent on inspection. The real damage is not visible, because it is under the skin. When the high-pressure device injects its solution, it can travel a significant distance; for example, it can move through most or all of a limb. The injected solution causes extensive tissue damage, both from the force of the pressure and from the toxic nature of some solutions. Over the course of the following few hours, tissue begins to die. If the patient does not get the appropriate treatment early enough, there is a high probability that at least part, and perhaps all, of the patient's limb will have to be amputated.

EMT treatment for high-pressure injection includes elevating and splinting the limb. Although the patient may complain of severe pain, do *not* apply cold. This causes vasoconstriction and can lead to further tissue damage and death from lack of perfusion. If the incident occurred just before your arrival, the patient might not have any pain and might not wish to go to an emergency department. It is, nonetheless, vital that you persuade the patient to be evaluated in an ED as soon as possible. If the patient delays treatment, the patient may end up losing a hand or forearm.

"Don't get distracted by wounds that are obvious and gross and miss the big things—the things (like airway or breathing problems or shock) that can kill your patient."

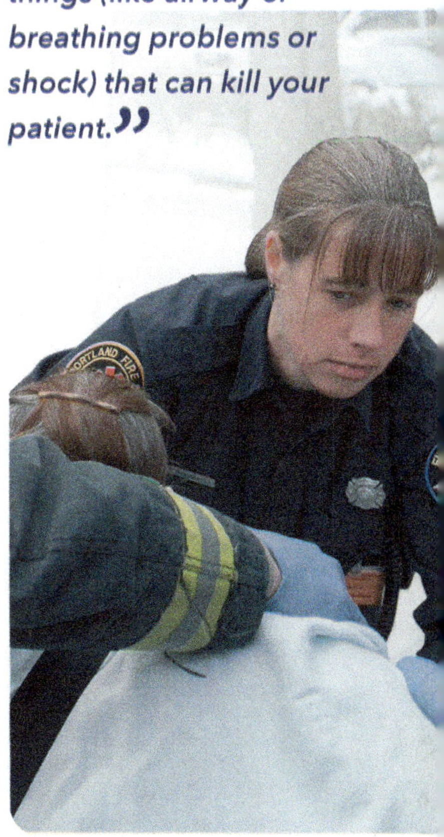

(© Daniel Limmer)

Emergency Care for Open Wounds

Open wounds require strict attention to Standard Precautions. In addition to wearing gloves, a gown and protective eyewear may also be required. Remember to properly dispose of all soiled materials and wash your hands after each call.

Patient Assessment

Open Wounds

Airway, breathing, circulation, and severe bleeding are identified and treated in the primary assessment. Once the primary assessment and the appropriate physical examination have been completed, care for the individual wounds begins.

Decision Point

- Does this injury affect my patient's airway, breathing, or circulation?

Patient Care

Patient with Open Wounds

Fundamental Principles of Care

When taking care of someone with open wounds, you need to protect yourself with Standard Precautions. Then stop the bleeding, expose the wound, consider the possibility of shock, prevent further contamination, and address the patient's fear and anxiety.

The following steps are general guidelines for emergency care of open wounds. Steps for specific kinds of open wounds appear on the following pages. Be sure to take appropriate Standard Precautions when performing these steps.

- Expose the wound. Clothing that covers a soft-tissue injury must be lifted, cut, or split away. (Avoid cutting through a hole left by a bullet or knife, cutting around it instead, to preserve evidence.) For some articles of clothing, this is best done with scissors or a seam cutter. Do not attempt to remove clothing in the usual manner, which can aggravate existing injuries and cause additional damage and pain. Take care in removing clothing if blood or debris has adhered it to the wound.
- Clean the wound surface. Do not try to pick embedded particles and debris from the wound. Simply remove large pieces of foreign matter from the surface. When possible, use a piece of sterile dressing to brush away large debris while protecting the wound from contact with your soiled gloves. Do not spend much time cleaning the wound. Control of bleeding is the priority.
- Control bleeding. Start with direct pressure or direct pressure and elevation. When necessary, apply a tourniquet. It may be important to remember that direct pressure may not be possible in certain crush-type injuries or amputations. Damage may be too widespread or bone ends may interfere with the ability to apply direct pressure. If direct pressure to an extremity is not appropriate or possible, move directly to the placement of a tourniquet. (See the chapter *Bleeding and Shock.*) Remember also that with penetrating trauma and puncture wounds, bleeding may be occurring internally without its being visible on the surface of the skin.
- For all serious wounds, provide care for shock, including administration of high-concentration oxygen. (See the chapter *Bleeding and Shock.*)
- Prevent further contamination. Use a sterile dressing to prevent infection later. When none is available, use the cleanest cloth material at the scene.
- Bandage the dressing in place after you have controlled the bleeding. If an extremity is involved, check for a distal pulse to make certain that circulation has not been interrupted by the application of a tight bandage. With the exception of a pressure dressing, bleeding must be controlled before bandaging is started. Periodically recheck the bandage to make certain that bleeding has not restarted.
- Keep the patient lying still. Any movement will increase circulation and could restart bleeding.
- Reassure the patient. This will help ease the patient's emotional response and perhaps lower the pulse rate and blood pressure. In some cases, this may help to reduce the bleeding rate. Also, a patient who feels reassured will usually be more willing to lie still, reducing the chances of restarting bleeding.

Treating Specific Types of Open Wounds

Treating Abrasions and Lacerations

In treating abrasions, take care to reduce wound contamination (Figure 30-14). Although bleeding from a long, deep laceration may be difficult to control, direct pressure over a dressing usually works well. Do not pull apart the edges of a laceration in an effort to see into the wound.

Most lacerations can be cared for by bandaging a dressing in place. Some EMS systems recommend using special wound-closure strips that are designed to bring the sides of a laceration together for minor lacerations. Place a gauze dressing and bandage over the laceration where wound-closure strips have been applied.

NOTE: *Do not underestimate the effects of a laceration. When evaluating a laceration, check the pulse as well as motor and sensory function distal to the injury. The patient may need stitches, plastic surgery, antibiotics, or a tetanus shot at the hospital, so do not put on bandages and leave the patient at the scene. Serious infection or scarring could result.*

FIGURE 30-14 (A) Lacerations in a child. (B) Deep laceration in a young child showing underlying tissue.
(Photos A and B: © David Effron, MD)

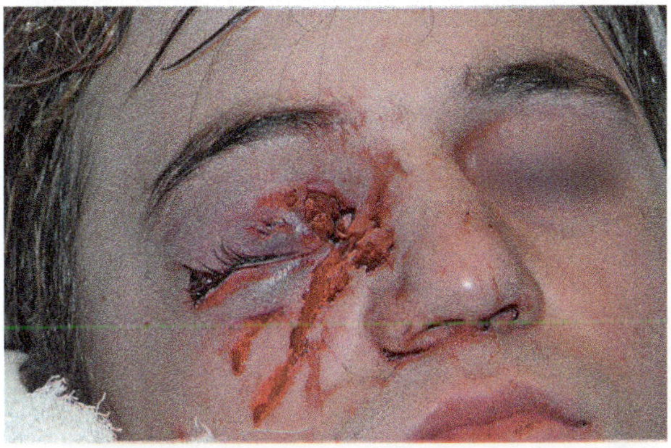

A

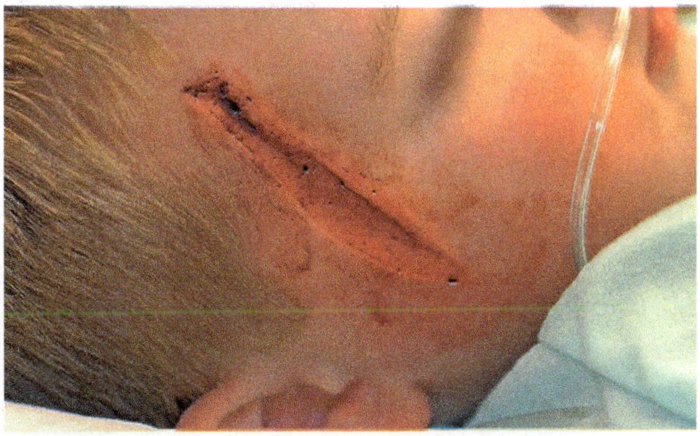

B

Treating Penetrating Trauma

Use caution when caring for puncture wounds. An object that appears to be embedded only in the skin may actually go all the way to the bone. In such cases, it is possible that the patient may not have any serious pain. Even an apparently moderate puncture wound may cause extensive internal injury with serious internal bleeding. What appears at first to be a simple, shallow puncture wound may be only part of the problem. There also could be a severe exit wound that requires immediate care, so be sure to search for one.

Gunshot wounds are puncture wounds that can fracture bones and cause extensive soft-tissue and organ injury. The seriousness of the wound cannot be determined by the caliber of the bullet or the point of entry and exit. The bullet may have tumbled through tissues, deflected off a bone, fragmented, or exploded inside the body (Figure 30-15A, Figure 30-15B, and Figure 30-15C). All bullet wounds are considered serious. If the bullet has penetrated the body, you must assume that there is considerable internal injury. Close-range shootings often have burns around the entry wound (Figure 30-15D). Remember that any gunshot wound to the face, no matter how minor, can create airway problems. Air guns fired at close range can cause serious damage by injecting air into the tissues.

All stab wounds should be considered serious, especially when they involve the head, neck, chest, abdomen, or groin, or are inflicted proximal to the knee or elbow.

Care for a patient with a moderate or serious puncture wound includes these steps. Assign a priority to each step that is appropriate to the severity of the injuries and to the environment.

- Reassure the alert patient. Such wounds can be frightening.
- Search for additional penetrations, including exit wounds, especially in the case of a gunshot wound. Control bleeding and provide adequate wound treatment to both the entry and exit wounds.
- Assess the need for basic life support whenever there is a gunshot wound. Look for and manage shock, administering high-concentration oxygen as appropriate.
- Follow your local protocols with regard to spinal motion restriction when the patient's head, neck, or torso is involved. (See the chapter *Trauma to the Head, Neck, and Spine.*) There is evidence to suggest that you should not immobilize a patient with penetrating trauma to the torso unless there is neurologic deficit. Doing so can harm the patient's ability to breathe and has proven to be of little value in the vast majority of cases. As always, follow your local protocols.
- Transport the patient. If the object that caused the puncture wound is available, and if the scene of the emergency is not a crime scene, take the object to the emergency department for examination as well.

FIGURE 30-15 (A) Bullets travel in an unpredictable path once they are inside the patient's body, and can therefore cause damage to multiple organs and bones. (B) A gunshot wound to the right flank. (C) X-ray of the same wound showing tumbling of the bullet within the body. (D) A close-range gunshot with burns around the entry wound. *(Photos B, C, and D: © Edward T. Dickinson, MD)*

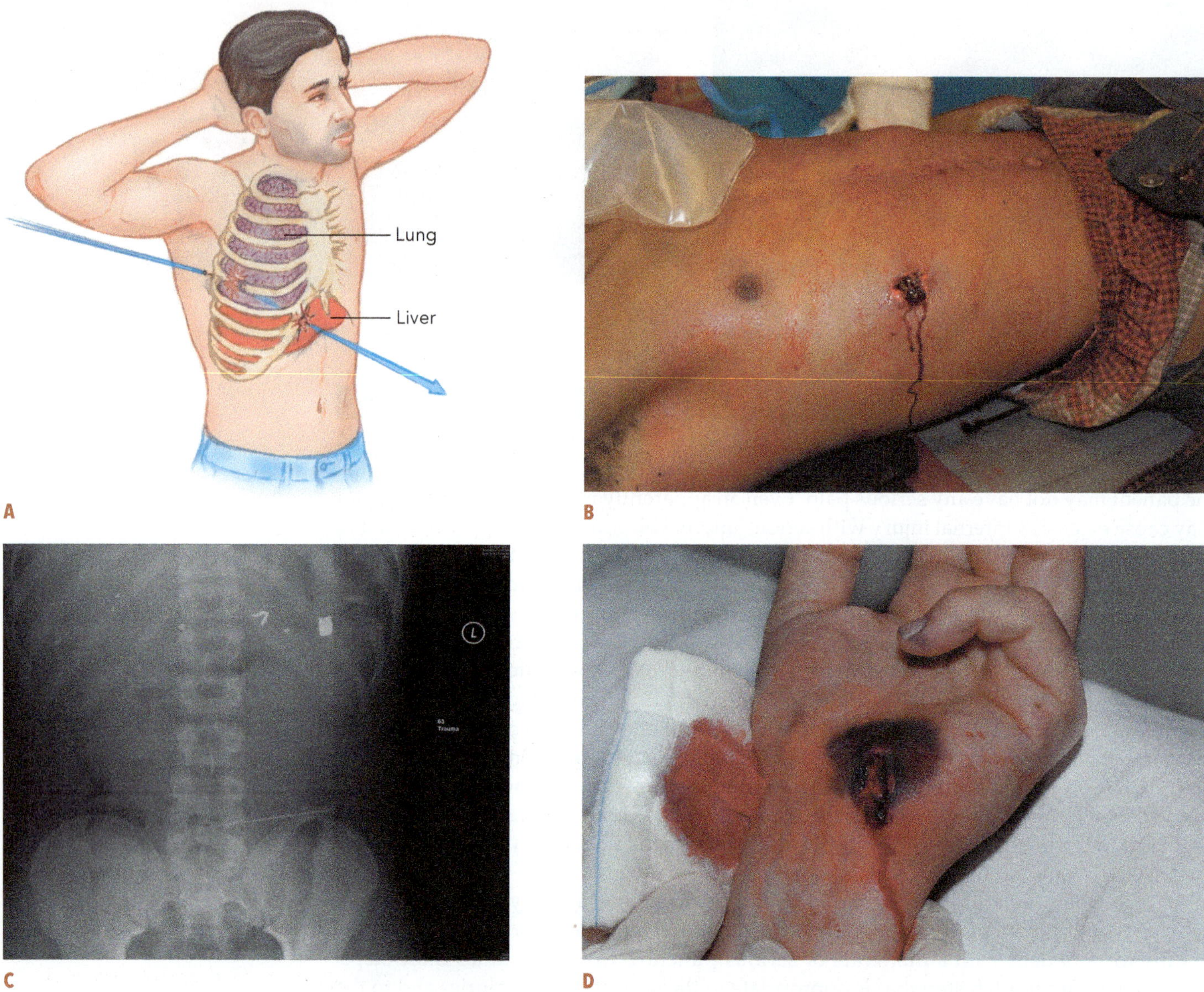

Treating Impaled Objects

A puncture wound may contain an impaled object. The object may be a knife, a fence post or guard rail, a shard of glass, or even a wooden stick—or part of any of these that has broken off in the wound (Figure 30-16), piercing any part of the body. Even though it is rare, you may be confronted with an impaled object that is long enough to make transport impossible unless the object is shortened. In such cases, contact the emergency department physician for specific directions. Usually someone must hold the object, keeping it very stable, while you gently cut through it at the desired length. A fine-toothed saw with rigid blade support (e.g., a hacksaw or reciprocating saw) should be used. In some cases, you may need to leave the object in place as found. The challenge in these cases is stabilization of the object.

In general, when caring for a patient with a puncture wound involving an impaled object, *do not remove the impaled object* (Figure 30-17). The object may be plugging bleeding from a major artery while it is in place. If you remove it, you may cause severe bleeding when the pressure is released. Removal of the object also may cause further injury to

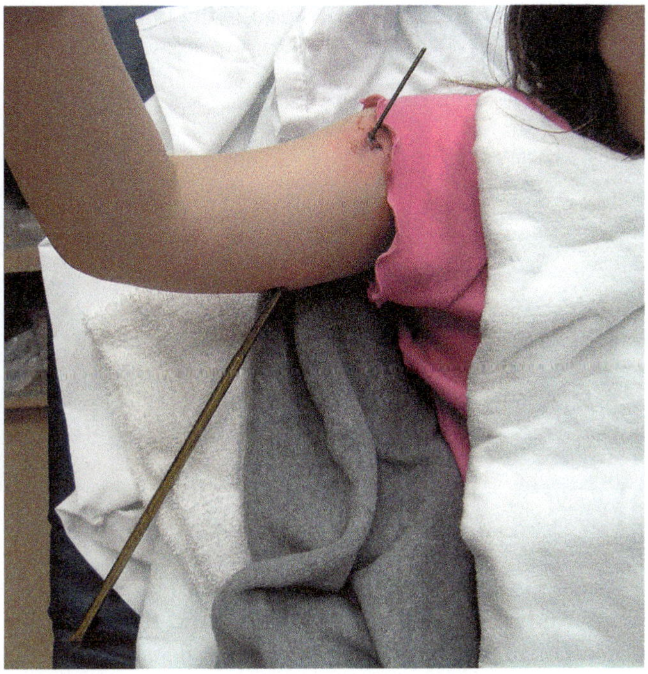

FIGURE 30-16 Child with object impaled through the soft tissue of the right arm. *(© David Effron, MD)*

nerves, muscles, and other soft tissues. Any movement of the impaled object at the skin's surface will be magnified several times in the inner tissues. Proceed as follows, generally in this order:

- Expose the wound area. Cut away clothing, taking great care not to disturb the object. Do not attempt to lift clothing over the object, as you may accidentally move it. Long impaled objects may have to be stabilized by hand during exposure, bleeding control, and dressing.
- Control bleeding by direct pressure, if possible. Be careful to position your gloved hands on either side of the object and exert pressure downward. *Do not put pressure on the object.* Apply pressure with great care if the object has a cutting edge, as with a knife or a shard of glass; otherwise, you may cause additional injury to the patient. Be careful not to injure your hands or damage your gloves.
- Get a description of the length and width of the object so that you can estimate how much of it may be inside the patient; you will relay this information later to the ED staff.

FIGURE 30-17 (A) Part of a knife impaled in a wound near the clavicle. (B) X-ray of the same impaled knife fragment. *(Photos A and B: © Edward T. Dickinson, MD)*

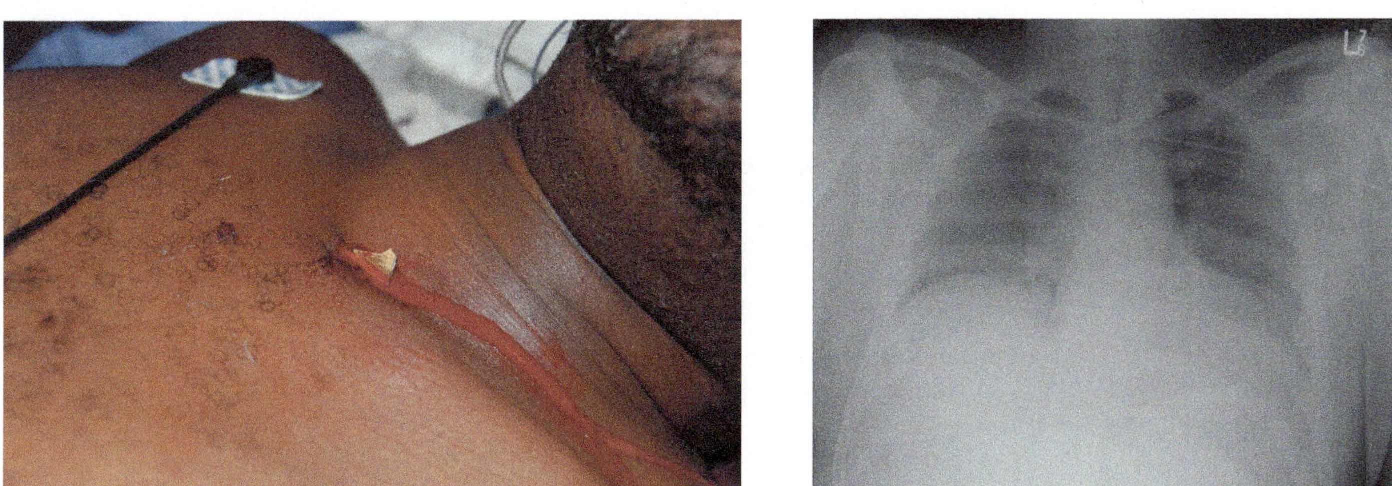

A

B

FIGURE 30-18 (A) Stabilize an impaled object with bulky dressings. (B) Bandage the impaled object and surrounding dressings in place.

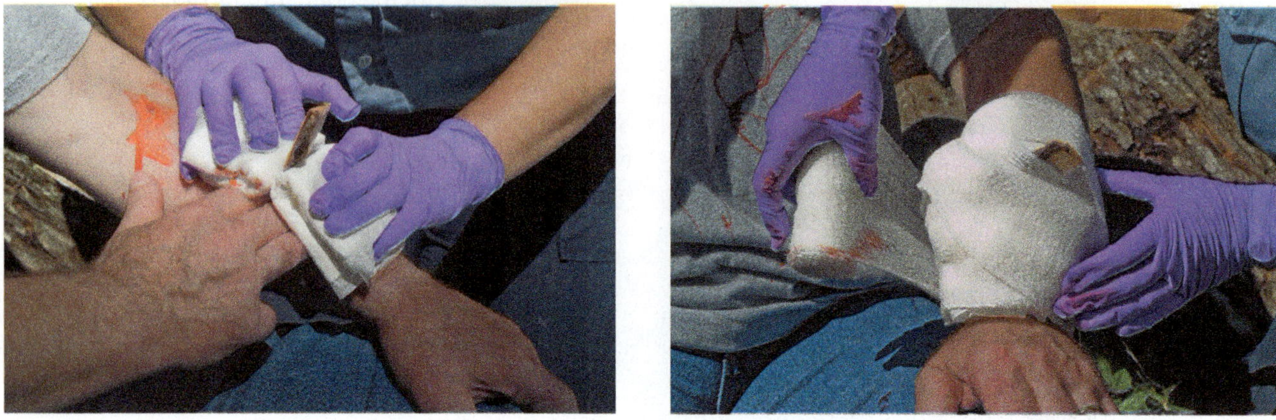

A B

- While you continue to stabilize the object and control bleeding, have another trained rescuer place several layers of bulky dressing around the injury site so the dressings surround the object on all sides (Figure 30-18). Manual stabilization must continue until the stabilizing dressings are secured in place.
- Have the other rescuer begin by placing folded universal pads or some other bulky dressing material on opposite sides of the object. For long or large objects, folded towels, blankets, or pillows may have to be used in place of dressing pads. Remove your hands from under the pads. Place them on top and apply pressure as each layer is placed in position. The next layer of pads should be placed on opposite sides of the object, perpendicular to the first layer. Continue this process until as much of the object as possible has been stabilized. Once bandaged in place, the dressings will stabilize the object and exert downward pressure on bleeding vessels. Keep in mind that there is a limited amount of time that can be given to stabilizing an impaled object. Stay in contact with the medical director for directions and recommendations.
- Secure the dressings in place. Although adhesive strips may hold the dressings in place, blood around the wound site, sweat, and body movements may not allow you to use tape. Triangular bandages folded into strips (cravats) can be applied by tying one above and one below the impaled object. The cravats should be wide (no less than 4 inches [10 centimeters] in width once folded). A thin, rigid splint can be used to push the cravats under the patient's back when they are needed to care for objects impaled in the trunk of the body.
- Care for shock. Provide oxygen as appropriate. When working by yourself, you may have to delay oxygen administration and heat conservation while you attempt to control bleeding.
- Keep the patient at rest. Position the patient for minimum stress. If possible, immobilize the affected area—for example, with a splint or a spine board. Provide emotional support.
- Transport the patient carefully and as soon as possible. Avoid any movement that may jar, loosen, or dislodge the object. If the object was removed by bystanders before you arrived, bring it to the hospital for examination.
- Reassure the patient throughout all aspects of care. An alert patient who is afflicted with an impaled object is usually very frightened.

Object Impaled in the Cheek

A dangerous situation exists when the cheek has been penetrated by a foreign object. First, the object may go into the oral cavity and create an airway obstruction, or it may stay

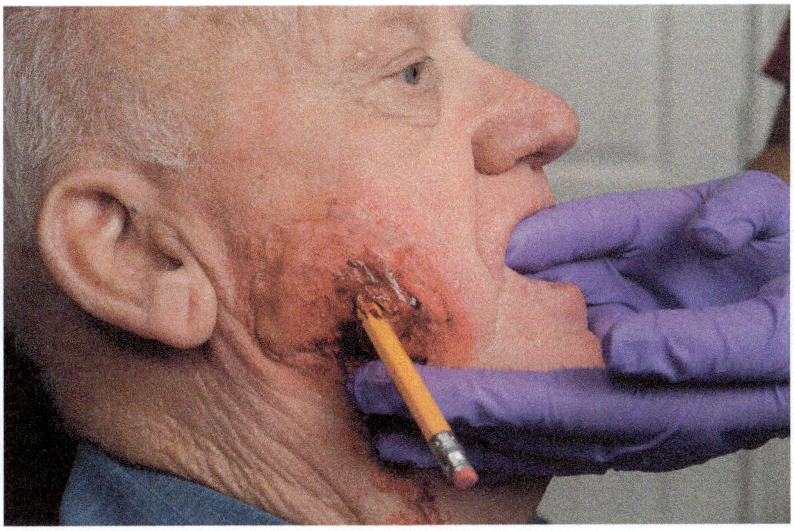

FIGURE 30-19 The process of removing an impaled object from the cheek.

impaled in the cheek wall but then work its way free and enter the oral cavity later. Second, when the cheek wall is perforated, bleeding into the mouth and throat can be profuse and interfere with breathing, or it may make the patient nauseated and induce vomiting. External wound care will not stop the flow of blood into the mouth.

If you find a patient with an object impaled in the cheek, you should follow these steps, generally in this order (Figure 30-19):

- Examine the wound site. Gently inspect both the external cheek and the inside of the mouth. Use your penlight and look into the patient's mouth. If need be, carefully use your gloved fingers to probe the inside cheek to determine if the object has passed through the cheek wall. This is best done with a dressing pad used to protect your fingers and any wound you touch.
- Remove the object *if* you find perforation and *you can see both ends* of the object. Pull it out in the direction that it entered the cheek. If this cannot be easily done, leave the object in place. Do not twist the object. *If* you find perforation but *the tip of the object is also impaled into a deeper structure* (e.g., the palate), *stabilize the object*. Do not try to remove it.
- Position the patient. Make certain that you allow for drainage. (The possibility of spine injuries may require you to immobilize the head, neck, and spine first, and to tilt the patient and the spine board as a unit if you use a spine board.)
- Monitor the patient's airway once the object is removed or stabilized. *Be prepared to suction as necessary*. Keep in mind that an object penetrating the cheek wall also may have caused teeth or dentures to break, creating potential airway obstruction. Pay close attention, especially if the patient is not alert. Blood in the patient's mouth can compromise the airway.
- Dress the outside of the wound using a pressure dressing and bandage, or apply a sterile dressing and use direct hand pressure to control the bleeding. You may be able to place gauze on the inside of the cheek to help control bleeding into the mouth, but only if the patient is alert and cooperative. Monitor the patient's mental status closely, and make sure the dressing does not work its way into the airway.
- Consider the need for oxygen and care for shock. You may have to use a nasal cannula if constant suctioning is required. If any dressing materials are placed in the patient's mouth, use of standard face masks can be dangerous unless you leave 3–4 inches (7.5–10 centimeters) of the dressing outside of the patient's mouth.

Puncture Wound or Object Impaled in the Eye

Use loose dressings for a puncture wound to the eye with no impaled object. If you find an object impaled in the eye, you should follow these steps, generally in the order described here (Figure 30-20).

FIGURE 30-20 Managing an object impaled in the eye. (*Right*) The object is contained and immobilized.

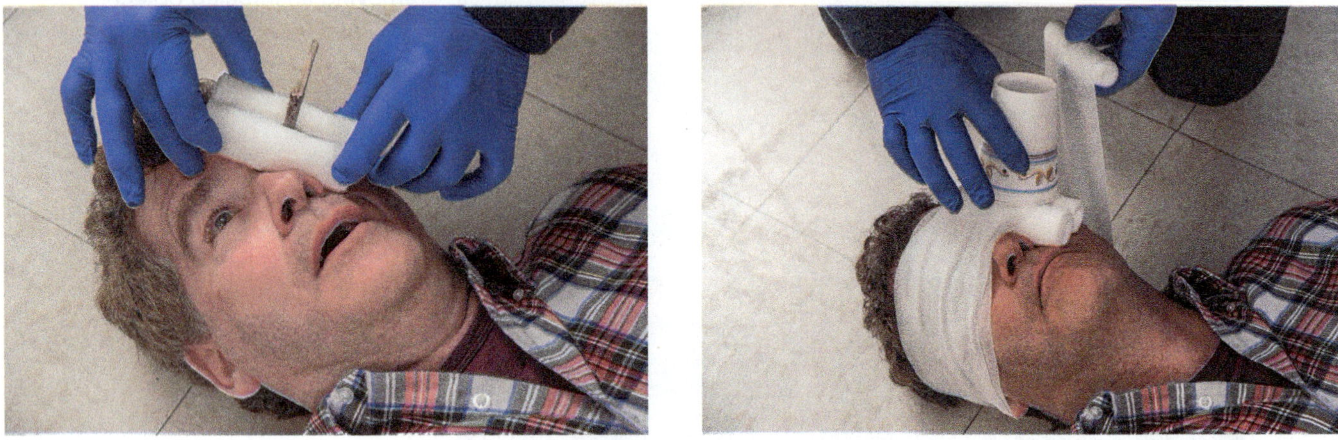

A B

- Stabilize the object. Place a roll of 3-inch (7.5-centimeter) gauze bandage or folded 4 × 4s on either side of the object, along the vertical axis of the head, in a manner that will stabilize the object.
- Apply rigid protection. Fit a disposable paper drinking cup or paper cone over the impaled object, and allow it to come to rest on the dressing rolls. Do not allow it to touch the object. Do not use a Styrofoam cup, which can flake.
- Whenever possible, have another rescuer stabilize the dressings and cup while you secure them in place with a self-adherent roller bandage or with a wrapping of gauze. Do not secure the bandage on top of the cup.
- Dress and bandage the uninjured eye. Because eyes move together, this will help to reduce eye movements in the injured eye.
- Consider the need for oxygen and care for shock.
- Reassure the patient and provide emotional support.

This method can also be used as a pressure dressing to control bleeding in the area of the eye.

NOTE: *In some EMS systems, dressing and bandaging the uninjured eye is not part of the recommended treatment when the other eye is injured. Covering both eyes often makes a patient anxious. Furthermore, covering the uninjured eye seems to make little, if any, difference in patient outcome. However, you should follow your local protocols.*

An alternative to the previous method calls for the rescuer to make a thick dressing with several layers of sterile gauze pads or universal dressings. A hole approximately the size of the impaled object is cut in the center of this pad. The rescuer then carefully passes this dressing over the impaled object and positions the pad so the impaled object is centered in the opening. The rest of the procedure remains the same as previously described. If your EMS system instructs you to use this technique, remember that you must take great care not to touch the object as the dressing is set in place.

Treating Avulsions

Emergency care for avulsions requires the application of large, bulky pressure dressings. In addition, you should make every effort to preserve any avulsed parts and transport them to the medical facility along with the patient. It may be possible to surgically restore the part or to use it for skin grafts.

In cases in which flaps of skin have been torn loose but not off, follow these steps:

- Clean the wound surface of gross contaminants (only).
- Fold the skin back to its normal position as gently as possible.
- Control bleeding and dress the wound using bulky pressure dressings.

If skin or another body part is torn from the body, control bleeding and dress the wound using a bulky pressure dressing. Save the avulsed part and wrap it in a sterile dressing kept moist with sterile saline. Make certain that you label the avulsed part with what it is, the patient's name, and the date and time the part was wrapped and bagged. Your records should show the approximate time of the avulsion. Be sure to keep the part as cool as possible, without freezing it, by placing it in a cooler or any other available container so it is on top of a cold pack or a *sealed* bag of ice. Do not use dry ice. Do not immerse the avulsed part in ice, cooled water, or saline. Label the container the same as the label used for the saved part.

NOTE: *The care of avulsed tissues is directed by local protocols, which are often written to coordinate with the reimplantation procedures of the hospitals in your EMS system. Some EMS systems prefer that the dressing used to wrap the avulsed part be moistened with sterile normal saline. (Sterile distilled water is not recommended.) This saline must be from a fresh, sterile source. Keep in mind that once a sterile source of saline has been opened, it is no longer considered sterile. Take great care if you use this method, since the saline may carry microorganisms from your gloved hand through the dressing to the avulsed part. During your care, remember that avulsions appear grotesque and will be frightening to your patient. Provide reassurance to your patient throughout the call.*

Treating Amputations

In many cases, the amputation may itself be less dangerous than the serious bleeding caused by the injury process. Always take steps to control hemorrhage immediately. Apply direct pressure first and use a tourniquet if direct pressure fails or if direct pressure is not possible. Consider the use of a pressure dressing over the site of the amputation.

Care for the amputated part (Figure 30-21). When possible, wrap it in a sterile dressing and secure the dressing with a self-adhesive gauze bandage. Wrap or bag the amputated part in a plastic bag, and keep it cool by cold packs. Do not immerse the amputated part directly in water or saline. In addition, do not let the part come in direct contact with ice, or it may freeze. Never complete an amputation.

NOTE: *This is the thumb that was amputated from the hand shown in Figure 30-10B.*

FIGURE 30-21 Care for an amputated part. The amputated digit sits on sterile gauze, awaiting re-implantation at the trauma center. *(© Edward T. Dickinson, MD)*

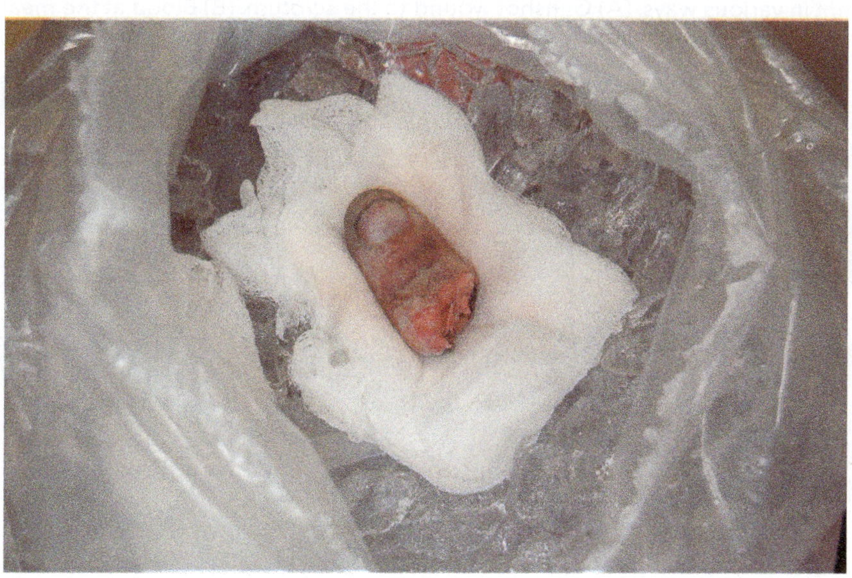

Treating Genital Injuries

Injuries to the genitals are not very common, but when they occur, they often bleed heavily and cause significant anxiety in patients. The genitals are very vascular (contain lots of blood vessels), so when they are injured, they bleed heavily. Because they are also part of the reproductive system, injuries in this area can affect a patient's ability to have children. Males tend to sustain trauma to the genitals more frequently than females because of the less-protected position of male genitalia, but anyone can sustain a genital injury.

Specific injuries that occur to the genitals are:

- Lacerations, contusions, and abrasions, which can result from either blunt or penetrating trauma (Figure 30-22A)
- Avulsions, including a degloving injury of the penis, in which the skin and tissue are pulled off and torn in the same way as in a degloving injury to the hand, as described earlier
- Blunt trauma, including straddle injuries in which the patient injures the perineum by landing heavily on a narrow structure
- Zipper injuries, which are especially common in uncircumcised boys. The foreskin may get caught in the zipper of the patient's pants.
- Foreign bodies and impaled objects in the vagina or penis
- Blood at the meatus (the external opening for urine flow) (Figure 30-22B), which is often an indication of a disruption of the urethra. In patients who have sustained blunt trauma, the cause of the urethral injury may be a fracture of the pelvis, which will be further discussed in the chapter *Musculoskeletal Trauma*.

Care for a patient with a genital injury includes these steps, generally in this order:

- Control bleeding as you would for other soft-tissue injuries.
- Preserve any avulsed parts as described in your local protocols.
- Consider whether the injury you see suggests another, possibly more serious, injury (e.g., blood at the meatus suggesting pelvic trauma).
- Display a calm, professional manner to maintain the patient's dignity. Although treatment is usually the same as for other soft-tissue injuries, the modest patient may need more reassurance.

FIGURE 30-22 Genital trauma can present in various ways. (A) Gunshot wound to the scrotum. (B) Blood at the meatus indicating disruption of the urethra, likely associated with significant pelvic trauma. *(Photos A and B: © Edward Dickinson, MD)*

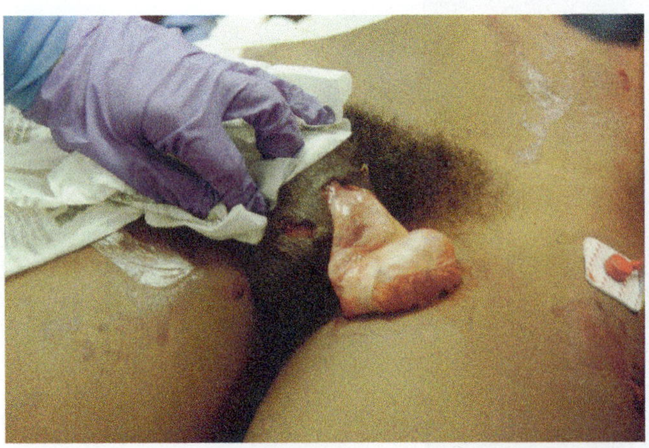

A

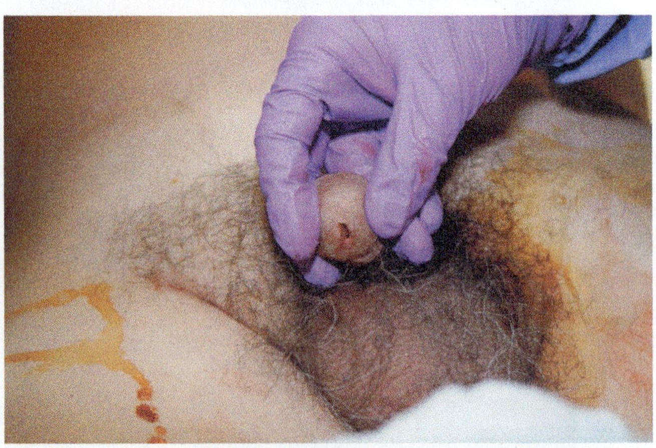

B

- If the patient is a child or another possibly vulnerable person, inquire in a nonthreatening way whether sexual abuse was involved.
- Dress and bandage the wound in accordance with the principles of bandaging (covered later in this chapter).
- Consider the possibility of sexual assault. Although not all genital injuries are caused by sexual assault, this mechanism of injury is a common cause. You should always consider this possibility and involve appropriate resources (law enforcement, sexual assault advocacy, etc.) in times of high suspicion.

Burns

CORE CONCEPT
Understanding burns and emergency care for burns

Most people think of burns as injuries to the skin, but burns can affect much more. Burn injuries often involve structures below the skin, including muscles, bones, nerves, and blood vessels. Burns can injure the eyes beyond repair. Respiratory system structures can be damaged, producing airway obstruction due to tissue swelling, and can even cause respiratory failure and respiratory arrest. In addition to the physical damage caused by burns, patients often suffer emotional and psychological problems that begin at the emergency scene and may last a lifetime.

When caring for a burn patient, always think beyond the burn. For example, a medical emergency or accident may have led to the burn. The patient may have had a heart attack while smoking a cigarette, and the unattended cigarette caused a fire. During the patient assessment, you should detect the heart problem even though the burn may be the most obvious injury. Conversely, a fire or burn may cause or aggravate another injury or medical condition. For example, someone trying to escape a fire may fall and suffer spinal damage and fractures. As an EMT, you should not only detect the burn but assess for spinal damage and fractures as well.

Patient Assessment

Burns

When your patient has been burned, patient assessment involves classifying, then evaluating, the burns. Burns can be classified and evaluated in three ways:

1. By agent and source
2. By depth
3. By severity

All three are important in deciding the urgency and the kind of emergency care the burn requires. These classifications are discussed in detail in the following text.

NOTE: Patient assessment should not be neglected to begin immediate burn care.

Classifying Burns by Agent and Source

Burns can be classified according to the agent causing the burn (e.g., chemicals or electricity). Noting the source of the burn (e.g., dry lime or alternating current) can make the classification more specific. You should report the agent and also, when practical, the source of the agent (Table 30-2). For example, a burn can be reported as "chemical burns from contact with dry lime."

Never assume the agent or source of the burn. What may appear to be a thermal burn could, in fact, be caused by radiation. You may find minor thermal burns on the patient's face and forget to consider light burns to the eyes. Always gather information from your observations of the scene, bystanders' reports, and the patient interview.

TABLE 30-2 Agents and Sources of Burns

AGENTS	SOURCES
Thermal	Flame; radiation; excessive heat from fire, steam, hot liquids, and hot objects
Chemicals	Various acids, bases, and caustics
Electricity	Alternating current, direct current, and lightning
Light (typically involving the eyes)	Intense light sources; ultraviolet light can also be considered a source of radiation burns
Radiological	Usually from nuclear sources; ultraviolet light can also be considered a source of radiation burns

Classifying Burns by Depth

superficial burn
a burn that involves only the epidermis, the outer layer of the skin. It is characterized by reddening of the skin and perhaps some swelling. A common example is a sunburn. Also called a *first-degree burn*.

Burns involving the skin are classified as superficial, partial thickness, or full thickness burns (Figure 30-23). These classifications are also sometimes called first-degree, second-degree, and third-degree burns, with first-degree burns corresponding to superficial burns and so on, as described next.

- A ***superficial burn*** (Figure 30-24) involves only the epidermis (the outer layer of the skin). It is characterized by reddening of the skin and perhaps some swelling. An example is a sunburn. The patient will usually complain about pain (sometimes severe) at the site. Typically, the burn will heal of its own accord, without scarring. Superficial burns are also called first-degree burns.

FIGURE 30-23 Burns are classified by depth.

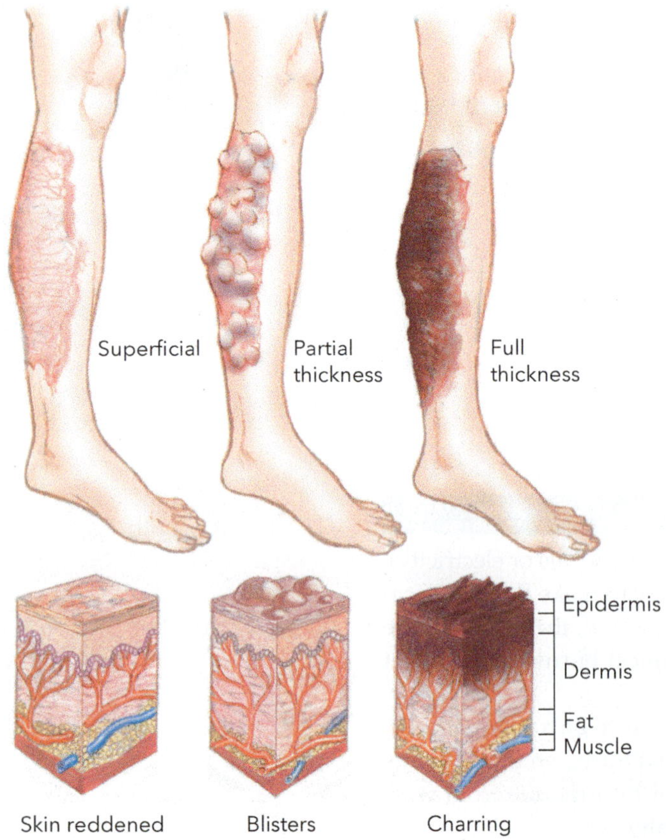

FIGURE 30-24 A superficial burn. *(© Edward T. Dickinson, MD)*

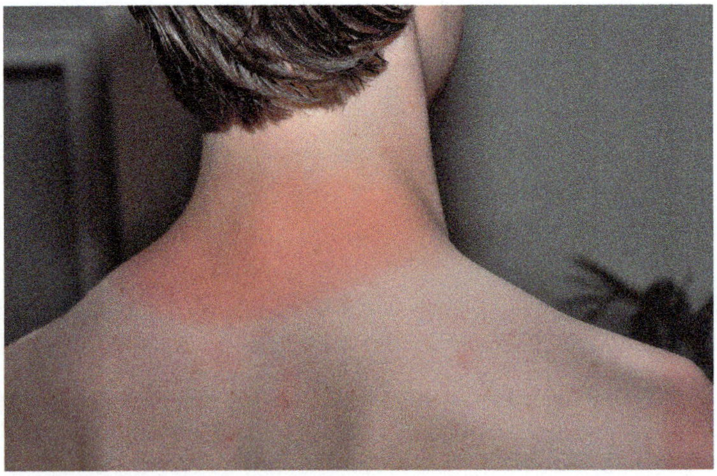

FIGURE 30-25 (A and B) Partial thickness burns. *(Photos A and B: © Edward T. Dickinson, MD)*

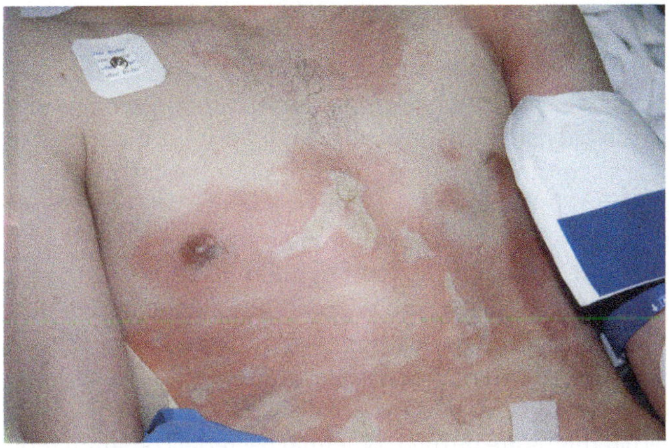

A

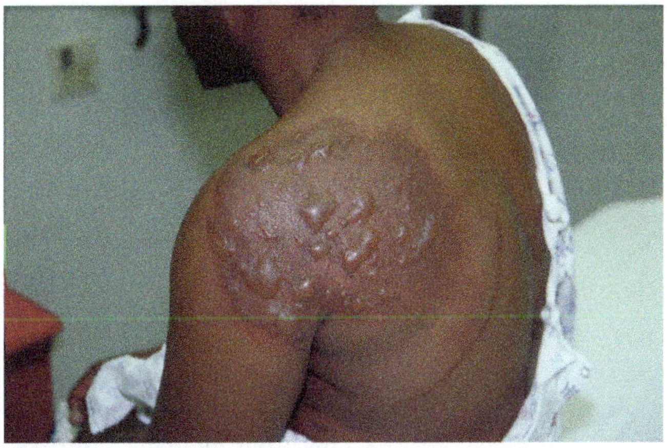

B

- In a ***partial thickness burn*** (Figure 30-25), the epidermis is burned through and the dermis (the second layer of the skin) is damaged, but the burn does not pass through to underlying tissues. There will be deep, intense pain; noticeable reddening; blisters; and a mottled (spotted) appearance to the skin. Burns of this type cause swelling and blistering for 48 hours after the injury, as plasma and tissue fluids are released and rise to the top layer of skin. When treated with reasonable care, partial thickness burns will heal themselves, producing very little or no scarring. Partial thickness burns are also called second-degree burns.
- In a ***full thickness burn*** (Figure 30-26), all the layers of the skin are damaged. Some full thickness burns are difficult to tell apart from partial thickness burns. There are usually areas that are charred black or brown, or areas that are dry and white. The patient may complain of severe pain or, if enough nerves have been damaged, may not feel any pain at all (except at the periphery of the burn, where adjoining partial thickness burns may be causing pain). This type of burn may require skin grafting. As these burns heal, dense scars form. Full thickness burns damage all layers of the skin and may damage subcutaneous tissue, muscle, bone, and underlying organs. These burns are sometimes called third-degree burns.

partial thickness burn
a burn in which the epidermis (first layer of skin) is burned through and the dermis (second layer) is damaged. Burns of this type cause reddening, blistering, and a mottled appearance. Also called a *second-degree burn*.

full thickness burn
a burn in which all the layers of the skin are damaged. There are usually areas that are charred black or areas that are dry and white. Also called a *third-degree burn*.

Determining the Severity of Burns

When determining the severity of a burn, consider the following factors:

- Agent or source of the burn
- Body regions burned
- Depth of the burn

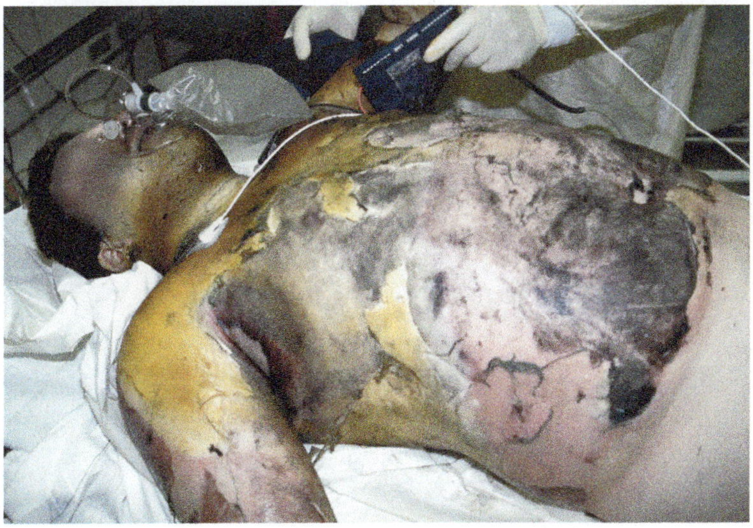

FIGURE 30-26 A full thickness burn. *(© Edward T. Dickinson, MD)*

- Extent of the burn
- Age of the patient
- Other illnesses and injuries

The agent or source of the burn can be significant in terms of patient assessment. A burn caused by electrical current may cause only small areas of skin injury but pose a great risk of severe internal injuries. Chemical burns are of special concern, since the chemical may remain on the skin and continue to burn for hours or even days, eventually entering the bloodstream. This is sometimes the case with certain alkaline chemicals.

When you are considering the body regions burned, keep in mind that any burn to the face is of special concern, since it may involve injury to the airway or the eyes (Figure 30-27). The hands and feet also are areas of concern, because scarring may cause loss of movement of fingers or toes. Special care is required to avoid aggravation to these injury sites when moving the patient and to prevent the damaged tissues from sticking to one another. When the groin, genitalia, buttocks, or medial thighs are burned, potential bacterial contamination can be far more serious than the initial damage to the tissues. Note that circumferential burns (burns that encircle the body or a body part) can be very serious because they constrict the skin. When they occur to an extremity, they can interrupt circulation to the distal tissues. When they occur around the chest, they can restrict breathing by limiting chest wall movement. In addition, the burn-healing process can be very complicated. This is particularly true when circumferential burns occur to joints, the chest, and the abdomen, where the encircling scarring tends to limit normal functions.

The depth of the burn is important to determine its severity. In partial thickness and full thickness burns, the outer layer of the skin is penetrated. This can lead to contamination of exposed tissues and the invasion of harmful chemicals and microorganisms into the circulatory system.

You also will need to roughly estimate the extent of the burn area. The amount of skin surface involved can be calculated quickly by using the ***rule of nines*** (Figure 30-28). For an adult, each of the following areas represents 9 percent of the body surface: head and neck, each upper extremity, chest, abdomen, upper back, lower back and buttocks, the front of each lower extremity, and the back of each lower extremity. These make up 99 percent of the body's surface. The remaining 1 percent is assigned to the genital region.

rule of nines
a method for estimating the extent of a burn. For an adult, each of the following areas represents 9 percent of the body surface: the head and neck, each upper extremity, the chest, the abdomen, the upper back, the lower back and buttocks, the front of each lower extremity, and the back of each lower extremity. The remaining 1 percent is assigned to the genital region.

In the rule of nines, the percentages are modified for infants and young children, whose heads are much larger in relationship to the rest of the body. An infant or young child's head and neck are counted as 18 percent; each upper extremity as 9 percent; chest and abdomen as

FIGURE 30-27 A singed face signals danger of airway burns or burns to the eyes. *(Left photo: © Edward T. Dickinson, MD; right photo: © David Effron, MD)*

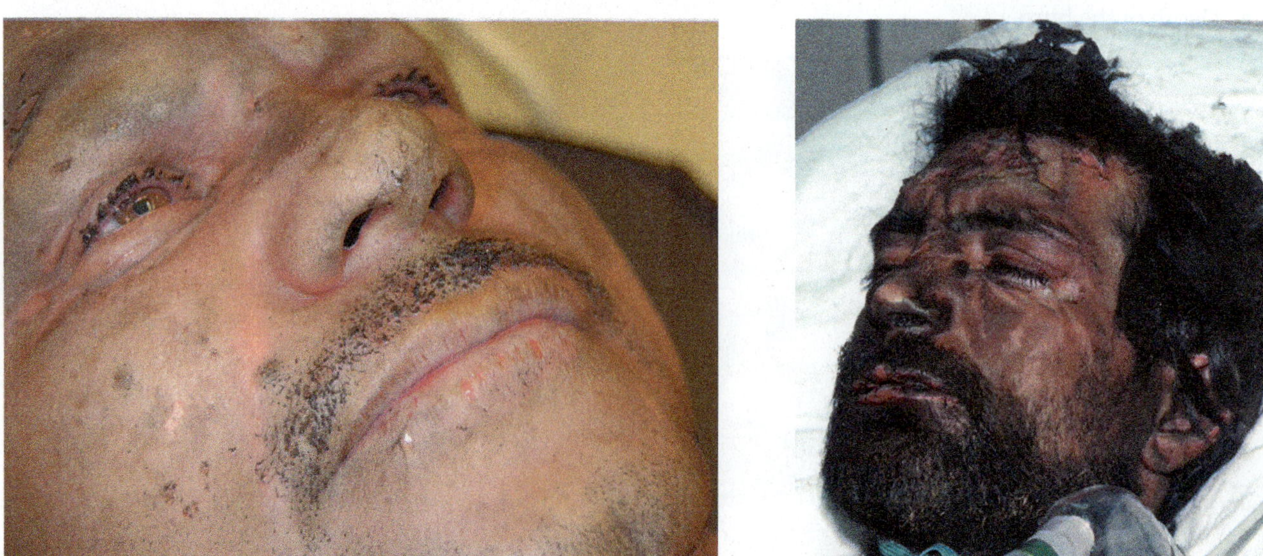

FIGURE 30-28 Rule of nines.

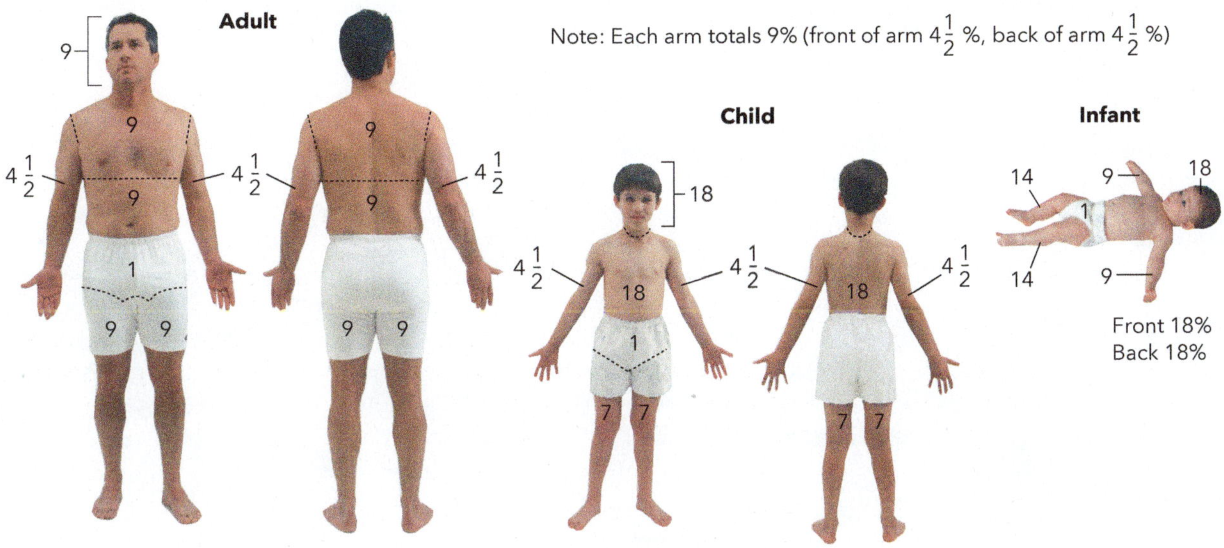

18 percent; the entire back as 18 percent; each lower extremity as 14 percent; and the genital region as 1 percent. (This adds up to 101 percent, but it is used to give only a rough determination. Some systems count each lower limb as 13.5 percent to achieve an even 100 percent.)

An alternative way to estimate the extent of a burn is the ***rule of palm***, also known as the *palmar method* or the *rule of ones*, which uses the patient's own hand to approximate the surface area. The rule of palm can be applied to any patient—infant, child, or adult. Since the palm and fingers of the hand equal about 1 percent of the body's surface area, mentally compare the patient's palm and fingers with the size of the burn to estimate its extent. (For example, a burn the size of five palms and fingers equals approximately 5 percent of the body.) The rule of palm may be easier to apply to smaller or localized burns, whereas the rule of nines may be easier for larger or more widespread burns. No matter which method you use to estimate the extent of a burn, keep in mind that it is only an estimate. It is very difficult to determine the exact area injured, and this may change over the first few days as the effects of exposure to heat make themselves more apparent.

rule of palm
a method for estimating the extent of a burn. The palm and fingers of the patient's own hand, which make up about 1 percent of the body's surface area, are compared with the patient's burn to estimate its size.

The patient's age is a major factor in considering the severity of burns. Infants, children under age 5, and adults over age 55, because of their anatomy and physiology, have the most severe responses to burns and the greatest risk of death. They also have different healing patterns than other age groups. Burns pose greater risks to infants and children than to adults. This is because their body surface area is greater in relation to their total body size. This results in greater fluid and heat loss than would occur in an adult patient. Infants have a higher risk of shock, airway problems, and hypothermia from burns. Burn intensity and body-area involvement that would be minor to moderate in a young adult could be fatal for an aged person. In late adulthood, the body's ability to cope with injury is reduced by aging tissues and failing body systems. The ability of tissues to heal from any injury is lessened, and the time of healing is increased.

When determining the severity of a burn, you also must consider the other illnesses and injuries a patient may have. Obviously, a patient with an existing respiratory illness will be especially vulnerable to exposure to heated air or chemical vapors. Likewise, the stress of a fire or other environmental emergency will be of particular concern for patients with heart disease. What may be a minor burn for a healthy adult could be of major significance to a patient with a preexisting medical condition. Patients with respiratory ailments, heart disease, or diabetes will react more severely to burn damage. Similarly, the stress of a burn added to other injuries sustained during the emergency may lead to shock or other life-threatening problems that would not have resulted from the nonburn injuries or the burn alone. Remember also that burns can sometimes mask more critical traumatic injuries, such as internal bleeding or internal organ damage. Complete a thorough patient assessment when possible.

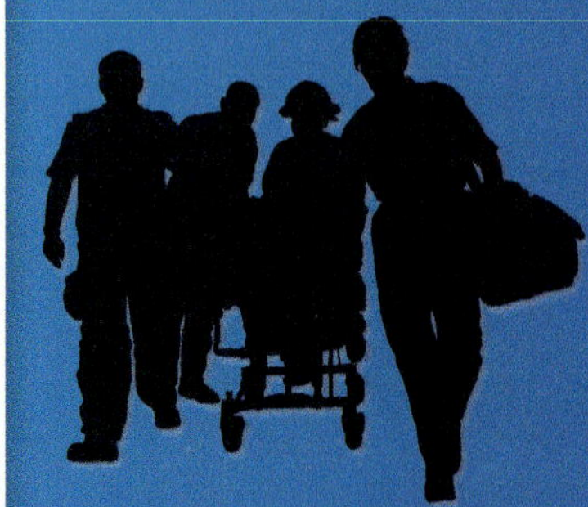

Think Like an EMT

Burns–By the Numbers

Burns are a type of soft-tissue injury. Decisions about burn care and transportation are often determined by an approximation of body surface area affected. For each of the following patients, determine the approximate body surface area burned and the degree of the burn.

1. Your patient fell asleep by the pool and was sunburned over the backs of both legs, his back, and the backs of both arms. The skin is bright red.
2. Your patient works at a fast food restaurant. She was by the fryer when someone threw in an ice cube as a joke to scare her. Hot grease splashed up and covered the anterior portion of her left forearm and her entire right hand. The skin is red and blistered.
3. Your patient fell asleep while smoking. He has circumferential burns on both legs and has burned the entire right arm. The legs are red and blistered. The patient's right arm is severely charred and peeling.

NOTE: *All burns are to be treated as more serious if accompanied by other injuries or medical problems. If you discover that the patient has a decreased blood pressure, always assume that the patient has other serious injuries. Attempt to determine the patient's problem through standard assessment techniques.*

Classifying Burns by Severity

The severity of burns must be classified to determine the order and type of care, to determine the priority for transport and the destination, and to provide maximum information to the emergency department. In some cases, the severity of the burn may determine if the patient is to be taken directly to a hospital with special burn-care facilities. In the past, the American Burn Association provided a list of conditions that determined whether a patient was classified as having a minor, moderate, or critical burn, but that was not very practical for EMS. They have now moved to a list of certain conditions that should be treated at a burn center. If you work in an area where a burn center is one of the transport choices available, you might transport some patients directly there. If there is no burn center near you, your protocols will assist you in determining the best destination for your patient. Box 30-1 lists the times when burn center treatment may help your patient.

BOX 30-1 Criteria for Burn Center Treatment

Some burn centers treat only adults, some treat only children, and some treat both. Local protocol will guide your decision making in determining whether to transport a patient directly to a burn center or to a closer hospital that will stabilize the patient and arrange for transfer.

Patients who should be treated at a burn center include those with:

- Second-degree (partial thickness) burns greater than 10 percent of total body surface area
- Burns involving the face (because of potential airway problems), genitalia or perineum, hands, feet, or major joints (because of the potential for infection and the importance of these areas in living a productive life)
- Third-degree (full thickness) burns
- Electrical burns (including those from lightning)
- Inhalation burns
- Other medical problems or trauma
- Other needs that a typical hospital will not be able to meet, e.g., rehabilitation

Additionally, children may need specialized equipment or personnel that some hospitals cannot provide, so protocols may direct you to particular hospitals that are able to provide these.

Treating Specific Types of Burns

First and foremost, take precautions to keep yourself safe. Burn injuries pose very significant scene-safety threats. What burned the patient could burn you! Be sure the burning process has stopped, and use specialized resources (fire and HAZMAT teams, and so on) if it has not. *Do not* approach a burn patient if there is a risk of electricity or a chemical/radiological threat.

Once the scene is safe, your immediate care will be especially important to the long-term outcome of the burn patient. There are special approaches to the care of thermal burns, general chemical burns, and chemical burns to the eyes (Figure 30-29).

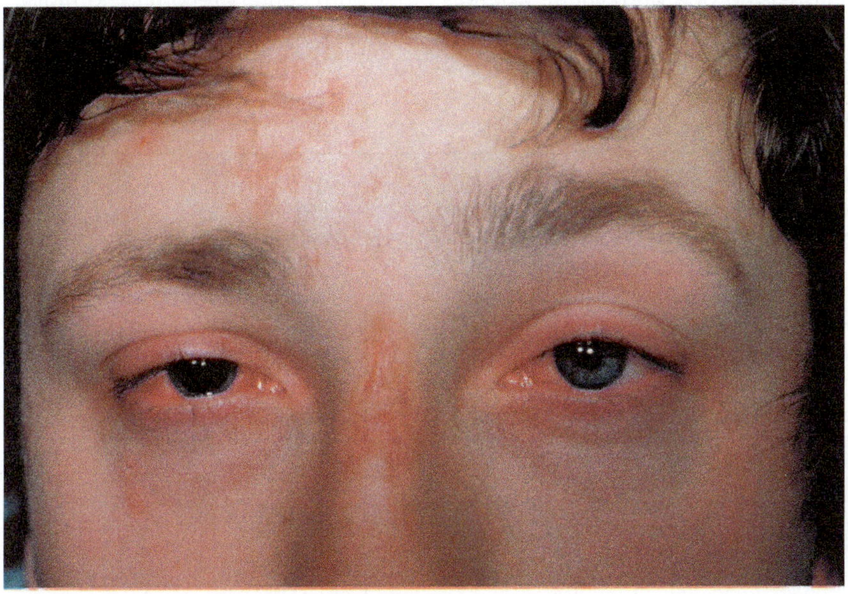

FIGURE 30-29 Chemical burns to the eyes. *(Western Ophthalmic Hospital/Science Source)*

Point of View

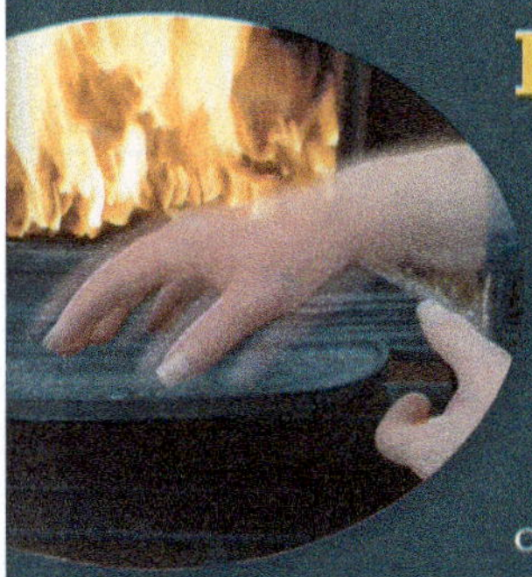

"I was tending the fire. I do it all the time. We were about to start a movie, so I may have gotten a bit greedy and wanted to load the fireplace up so it would burn long and hot.

"The wood was nice and dry, and a small fire had been going for a while. But like I said, I decided it would be a good idea to build up the fire, and I put too much wood in. The wood shifted. I moved to catch some of the pieces, and then I heard a whoosh. The shift must've created an airflow that fed the fire. Well, that fire certainly caught. And so did my hand.

"I didn't think my hand was in the fire for that long, but it must've been. I felt the heat first. I'm not sure why, but I noticed hairs burning on my wrist before I even noticed the pain . . . and redness . . . and blistering. It got most of my hand and up my wrist a little.

"The EMTs came and put a dressing on my hand. I knew it was bad by looking at it. They were even more concerned because they knew a burn to the hand can be really serious. They called the doctor on the radio, who said to go to a hospital different than my normal one. They took me to a hospital with a specialty in treating burns.

"I'll tell you this: I'll never try to overfeed a fire again. Burns hurt a lot–and for a long time."

Patient Care

Patient with Thermal Burns

Fundamental Principles of Care

As an EMT, you will have to care for thermal burns caused by scalding liquids, steam, contact with hot objects, flames, flaming liquids, and gases. Sunburn can also be severe in infants and young children, who may have other heat-related injuries.

The steps for basic care of thermal burns are given in Table 30-3. The standing orders for burn care are determined by your EMS medical director and the regional EMS system. Some EMS systems state that all partial thickness and full thickness burns are to be wrapped with dry sterile dressing or a burn sheet, whereas other burn centers recommend moist dressings for partial thickness burns to less than 10 percent of the body and dry dressings for more severe cases. The latter protocol is now being adopted by most EMS systems.

TABLE 30-3 Care for Thermal Burns

Stop the burning process!/Cool the burned area.

- Flame–Wet down, smother, then remove any affected clothing.
- Semi-solid (grease, tar, wax)–Cool with water. Do not remove the substance.
- Ensure an open airway. Assess breathing.
- Look for signs of airway injury: hoarse voice, stridor, soot deposits, burned nasal hair, or facial burns.
- Complete the primary assessment.
- Treat for shock. Provide high-concentration oxygen. Treat serious injuries.
- Evaluate burns by depth (see below), extent (rule of nines or rule of palm), and severity.

DEPTH OF BURN	OUTER SKIN LAYER IS BURNED	SECOND SKIN LAYER IS BURNED	TISSUE BELOW SKIN IS BURNED	COLOR CHANGES	PAIN	BLISTERS
Superficial	Yes	No	No	Red	Yes	No
Partial thickness	Yes	Yes	No	Deep red	Yes	Yes
Full thickness	Yes	Yes	Yes	Charred black or white	No	No

- *Do not* clear debris. Remove clothing and jewelry.
- Wrap with dry sterile dressing.
- Consider requesting ALS who can administer pain medications, especially in cases of partial thickness burns.
- *Burns to hands or feet*–Remove the patient's rings or jewelry that may constrict blood flow with swelling. Separate fingers or toes with sterile gauze pads.
- If allowed by local protocol, you may be able to reduce pain in a patient with a small burn by applying a cool, wet dressing to the area. This is ONLY for small, isolated burns. Cooling a burn that is large (greater than 10 percent body surface area) or in a patient who has other significant medical problems or trauma may make the patient hypothermic. The patient who is shivering is already too cold, and you should remove any wet clothing or dressings.
- *Burns to the eyes*–Do not open the patient's eyelids if burned. Be certain the burn is thermal, not chemical. Apply sterile gauze pads to *both* eyes to prevent sympathetic movement. (Some local protocols recommend covering only the injured eye. Follow your local protocols.) If the burn is chemical, flush the eyes for 20 minutes en route to the hospital.

FOLLOW LOCAL BURN CENTER PROTOCOLS AND TRANSPORT ALL BURN PATIENTS AS SOON AS POSSIBLE.

Remember also that some thermal burns, especially immersion burns and liquid scald burns, can be indicators of abuse. Always have a high index of suspicion when evaluating such burns, especially in children.

Note that EMTs must manage burns correctly until the patient can be transferred to the care of a medical facility's staff. Never apply ointments, sprays, or butter (which would trap the heat against the burn site and have to be scraped off by the hospital staff). Do not break blisters. Do not apply ice to any burn (as it can cause tissue damage). Keep the burn site clean to prevent infection. Keep the patient warm, as the temperature-regulation function of the skin may be affected by the burn.

A special consideration in thermal burns must be made for burns, or potential burns, to the airway. In addition to causing immediate damage to the mouth, trachea, and lungs, airway burns can be a very real long-term threat, as damaged tissues can swell and occlude the airway even hours later. Any evaluation of a burn patient should include special attention to the possibility of this type of injury. First consider the mechanism. Was the airway at risk? Steam and vapor injuries are considered high-probability mechanisms. Burns that occur in enclosed spaces also have a considerable likelihood to include the airway. Second, is there any evidence of airway involvement? Findings such as burns to the mouth and nose, soot in sputum or mucus, singed eyebrows or nose hairs, and difficulty speaking are all potentially dangerous. The development of a hoarse voice, particularly in a short-term setting, is especially ominous. If an airway burn is found, you should initiate rapid transport to an appropriate destination and consider an intercept with advanced life support to offer higher-level airway management techniques.

Airway-related burns can also expose patients to potentially harmful chemicals such as carbon monoxide and hydrogen cyanide. In general, any patient who has a potential airway burn or exposure to inhaled by-products of combustion should be monitored for the possibility of carbon monoxide and cyanide poisoning. At a minimum, these patients should be moved to fresh air and treated with high-concentration oxygen via nonrebreather mask. If your protocols allow, the application of humidified oxygen may slow down the swelling process. Safety of the rescuers on scene must always be a first priority when hazardous materials are expected.

NOTE: *Do not attempt to rescue persons trapped by fire unless you are trained to do so and have the equipment and personnel required. The simple act of opening a door might cost you your life. In some fires, opening a door or window may greatly intensify the fire or even cause an explosion.*

Patient Care

Patient with Chemical Burns

Fundamental Principles of Care

Chemical burns require immediate care, and in an ideal situation, people at the scene will begin this care before you arrive. At many industrial sites, workers and emergency medical responders are trained to provide initial care for incidents involving the chemicals in use at that facility. Most major industries have emergency deluge-type safety showers to wash dangerous chemicals from the body. However, this will not always be the case. Be prepared for situations in which nothing has been done and there is no running water near the scene. As always, take care to protect yourself from chemical injury. Use specialized response teams if the scene is not secure. Take care when coming into contact with contaminated clothing or with the patient if chemicals are still present.

Emergency care for a patient with chemical burns includes the following:

- The primary care procedure is to *wash* away the chemical with flowing water. If a dry chemical is involved, carefully remove any contaminated clothing, avoiding raising a cloud of the chemical agent. Simply wetting the burn site is not enough. Continuous flooding of the affected area is required, using a copious but gentle flow of water. Avoid hard sprays that may damage badly burned tissues. Continue to wash the area for at least 20 minutes, and continue the process en route to the hospital. Take steps as needed to avoid contaminating yourself with the chemical agent. Remove the patient's contaminated clothing, shoes, socks, and jewelry as you apply the wash. *Do not contaminate skin that has not been in contact with the chemical.*

- Apply a sterile dressing or burn sheet.
- Treat for shock.
- Transport.

Continue to be on the alert for delayed reactions that may cause renewed pain or interfere with the patient's ability to breathe. If the patient complains of increased burning or irritation, wash the burned areas again with flowing water for several minutes.

Treating Specific Chemical Burns

When possible, find out the exact chemical or mixture of chemicals that was involved in the incident. Most industrial sites will have a safety data sheet (SDS) that provides specific emergency information about the chemical agents being used. Although part of the treatment for both acid and alkali burns is irrigation, alkali burns should be irrigated longer because of the different ways in which these chemicals react with the human body.

When acids encounter tissue, they break down proteins. This results in coagulated tissue that limits further progression of the acid. There is a well-known exception to the principle of acids causing limited damage. Hydrofluoric acid not only causes burns like any other acid, but it also penetrates much more deeply. The fluoride released from the acid combines with calcium and magnesium in the tissue until the fluoride is used up. This typically results in significant tissue damage since there isn't that much calcium or magnesium outside of bone. Much of the damage is internal and not visible, especially with low concentrations. Higher concentrations will cause both internal damage and external damage. Hydrofluoric acid is used in industrial applications such as glass etching and electronics manufacturing, but it is also available in some rust removers intended for use around the home.

If you encounter a patient with a hydrofluoric acid exposure, you must irrigate copiously and for as long as you can or until medical direction tells you to stop. Hydrofluoric acid burns can cause great tissue damage with few external signs, so do your best to persuade a reluctant patient to go to the emergency department for further treatment.

Alkalis break down proteins too, but they also liquefy the damaged tissue. In fact, this process, called saponification, is how soap has been made for centuries. A strong alkali such as lye is mixed with fat or oil. The chemical reaction that occurs changes the two substances into soap. Because a strong alkali liquefies dead tissue, the alkali is able to eat into the tissue much farther than an acid can. Continued irrigation is the best method of diluting and removing the alkali and limiting the damage it causes.

Some special chemical burns require specific care procedures.

- **Mixed or strong acids or unidentified substances.** Many of the chemicals used in industrial processes are mixed acids, whose combined action can be immediate and severe. The pain produced from the initial chemical burn may mask any pain being caused by renewed burning due to small concentrations left on the skin.

  When the chemical is a strong acid (e.g., hydrochloric acid or sulfuric acid), a combination of acids, or an unknown, play it safe and continue washing even after the patient claims the patient is no longer experiencing pain.
- **Dry lime.** If dry lime is the burn agent, do not wash the burn site with water. To do so will create a corrosive liquid. Brush the dry lime from the patient's skin, hair, and clothing. Make certain that you do not contaminate the patient's eyes or airway.

  Use water only after the lime has been brushed from the body, contaminated clothing and jewelry have been removed, and the process of washing can be done quickly and continuously with running water.
- **Carbolic acid (phenol).** Carbolic acid does not mix with water. When available, use alcohol for the initial wash of unbroken skin, followed by a long steady wash with water. (Follow local protocols.)
- **Sulfuric acid.** Heat is produced when water is added to concentrated sulfuric acid, but it is still preferable to wash rather than leave the contaminant on the skin.

- **Hydrofluoric acid.** This acid is used for etching glass as well as many other manufacturing processes. Burns from it may be delayed, so treat all patients who may have come into contact with the chemical, even if burns are not in evidence. At high doses, hydrofluoric acid exposure can be fatal. Flood the affected area with water. Do not delay care or transport to find neutralizing agents. (Follow local protocols.)
- **Inhaled vapors.** Whenever a patient is exposed to a caustic chemical and may have inhaled the vapors, provide high-concentration oxygen (humidified, if available) and transport as soon as possible. This is very important when the chemical is an acid that is known to vaporize at standard environmental temperatures. (Examples include hydrochloric acid and sulfuric acid.)

Patient Care

Patient with Chemical Burns to the Eye(s)

Fundamental Principles of Care

A corrosive chemical can burn the globe of a person's eye before there is time to react and close the eyelid. Even with the lid shut, chemicals can seep through onto the globe.

To care for chemical burns to the eye, you should take the following steps:

- *Immediately* flood the eyes with water. Often the burn will involve areas of the face as well as the eye. When this is the case, flood the entire area. Avoid washing chemicals back into the eye or into an unaffected eye (Figure 30-30).
- Keep running water from a faucet, low-pressure hose, bucket, cup, bottle, rubber bulb syringe, IV setup, or other such source flowing into the burned eye. The flow should be from the medial (nasal) corner of the eye to the lateral corner. Since the patient's natural reaction will be to keep the eyes tightly shut, you may have to hold the eyelids open.
- If ALS is available, request them. Paramedics can often put anesthetic drops into the eyes that will make irrigation not only easier for the patient, but more effective.
- Start transport and continue washing the eye for at least 20 minutes or until the patient's arrival at the medical facility.
- After washing the eye, cover both eyes with moistened pads.
- Wash the patient's eyes for 5 more minutes if the patient begins to complain about renewed burning sensations or irritation.

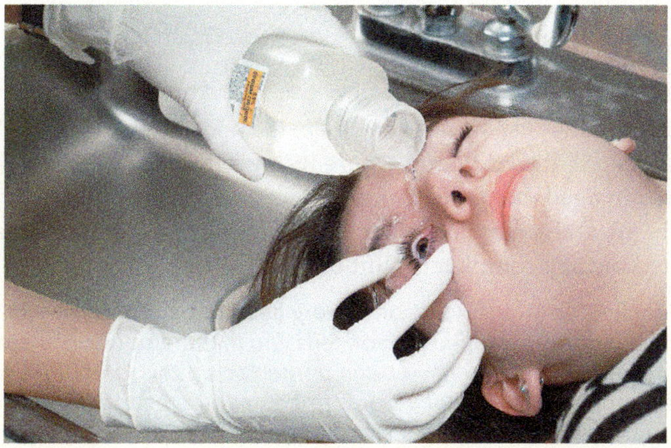

FIGURE 30-30 Emergency care of chemical burns to the eye.

NOTE: *Protect yourself during the washing process for a chemical burn. Wear protective gloves and eyewear and control the wash to avoid splashing.*

NOTE: *Do not use neutralizers such as vinegar or baking soda in a patient's eyes.*

NOTE: *Some scenes where chemical burns have taken place can be very hazardous. Always evaluate the scene. There may be large pools of dangerous chemicals around the patient. Acids could be spurting from containers. Toxic fumes may be present. If the scene will place you in danger, do not attempt a rescue unless you have been trained for such a situation and have the needed equipment and personnel at the scene.*

Radiation Burns

Radiation is a form of energy in which electromagnetic waves travel through space and through matter such as the human body. We are exposed to radiation every day from helpful sources such as sunlight. In fact, a sunburn is a specific type of relatively benign radiation burn. However, other types of radiation can be much more harmful. Processes, such as nuclear fission, and certain substances, known as radioactive materials, give off radiation in the form of radioactive waves and particles. These emissions can be harmful in many ways. Although a full explanation of how radiation affects the human body is beyond the scope of this chapter, you should know that exposures to high levels of radiation can harm the human body both immediately and in a delayed fashion. The immediate effects of high-dose radiation can be seen in the form of burns. The delayed effects develop in the form of radiation sickness and can cause a wide array of harmful side effects.

Radiation can be emitted from a great number of sources. Radioactive materials are used in medicine, in manufacturing, and in the production of electricity. In addition, radiation can be emitted from weapons of mass destruction such as nuclear weapons and so-called dirty bombs. Although nuclear weapons require high levels of technology to produce, low-technology dirty bombs could be a source of significantly harmful radiation as a result of a terrorist act.

Unfortunately, radiation is difficult to detect without specialized monitoring equipment. To identify injuries related to radiation, you would likely need either to have knowledge of the source or to be told by a specialized team, such as a hazardous materials team, that radiation was present.

Radiation can be extremely harmful, and contact with either the source of radiation or with a patient contaminated with radiological materials can pose a serious risk to your well-being. You should not approach a radiological injury without the proper protective equipment and specialized training. You may be called, however, to treat a patient with radiological injuries after that patient had been decontaminated. In the immediate setting, most radiological injuries will present like thermal injuries with damage to the various layers of the soft tissue. Care would be similar in these cases, and would consist of covering the burns and transporting to an appropriate facility. Know that radiation can also cause many other potentially harmful effects and that any patient with this type of injury should be carefully assessed and monitored for airway and breathing problems.

Electrical Injuries

CORE CONCEPT
Understanding electrical injuries and emergency care for electrical injuries

Electric current, including lightning, can cause severe damage to the body. In these cases, the skin is burned where the energy enters the body and where it flows into a ground. Along the path of this flow, tissues are damaged due to heat and to forceful contraction of muscle tissue. In addition, significant chemical changes take place in the nerves, heart, and muscles, and body processes are disrupted or may completely shut down.

NOTE: *The scenes of injuries due to electricity are often very hazardous. Assume that the source of electricity is still active unless a qualified person tells you that the power has been turned off. Do not attempt a rescue unless you have been trained to do this kind of rescue and have the necessary equipment and personnel. For information about electrical hazards at the scene of a vehicle collision, see the chapters* Scene Size-Up *and* Highway Safety and Vehicle Extrication.

Patient Assessment

Electrical Injuries

The victim of an electrical accident may have any or all of the following signs and symptoms (Figure 30-31):

- Burns where the energy entered and exited the body
- Disrupted nerve pathways displayed as paralysis
- Muscle tenderness, with or without muscular twitching
- Respiratory difficulties or respiratory arrest
- Irregular heartbeat or cardiac arrest
- Elevated blood pressure or low blood pressure with the signs and symptoms of shock
- Restlessness or irritability if conscious, or loss of consciousness
- Visual difficulties
- Fractured bones and dislocations from severe muscle contractions or from falling (can include the spinal column)
- Seizures (in severe cases)

FIGURE 30-31 (A) Injuries due to electrical shock; (B) entrance wound (right hand) and exit wound (left forearm) from an electrical shock; (C) electrical burn exit wound. *(Photos B and C: © Edward T. Dickinson, MD)*

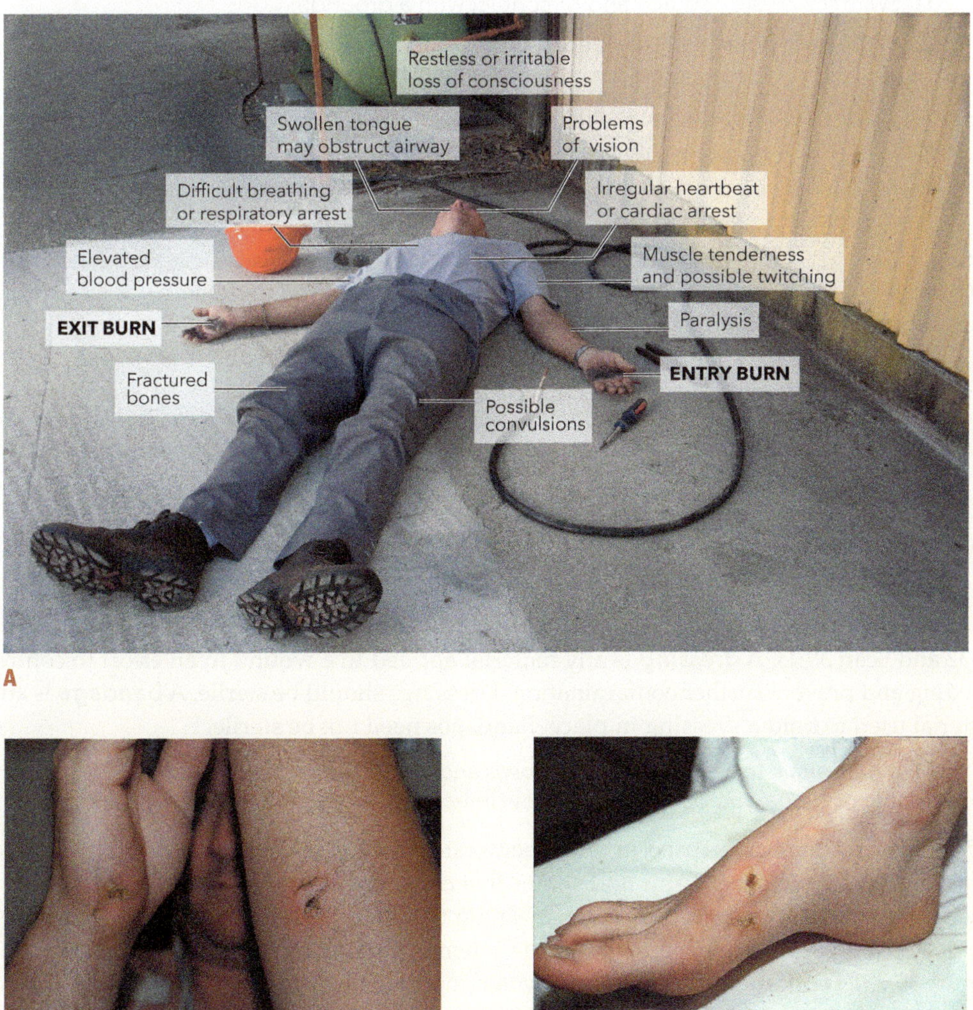

A

B

C

Patient Care

Patient with Electrical Injuries

Fundamental Principles of Care

When caring for electrical injuries, after you ensure airway, breathing, and circulation, be careful not to underestimate the severity of such a burn. You may see only a small wound or two, but the major damage is inside the body between those wounds.

Follow these steps to provide emergency care to a patient with electrical injuries, generally in this order:

- Provide airway and breathing care. Electrical shock may cause severe swelling along the airway and can cause respiratory failure. Be prepared to provide positive pressure ventilations.
- Provide basic cardiac life support as required. Since cardiac rhythm disturbances are common, be prepared to perform defibrillation if necessary.
- Care for shock and administer high-concentration oxygen as needed.
- Care for spine injuries, head injuries, and severe fractures. All serious electrical shock patients should be evaluated for spine injuries because electrical current can cause severe muscular contraction. Also, the patient may have been thrown by a high-voltage current. In either case there is the possibility of a spinal injury that requires spinal stabilization.
- Evaluate electrical burns, looking for at least two external burn sites: those of contact with the energy source and of contact with a ground.
- Cool the burn areas and smoldering clothing the same as you would for a flame burn.
- Apply dry sterile dressings to the burn sites.
- Transport as soon as possible. Some problems have a slow onset. If there are burns, there also may be more serious hidden problems. In any case of electrical shock, heart problems may develop.

Remember that the major problem caused by electrical shock is usually not the burn. Respiratory and cardiac arrest are real possibilities. Be prepared to provide basic cardiac life-support measures with automated defibrillation.

NOTE: *Make certain that you and the patient are in a safe zone (not in contact with any electrical source, and outside the area where downed or broken wires or other sources of electricity can reach you).*

Dressing and Bandaging

dressing
any material (preferably sterile) used to cover a wound that will help control bleeding and prevent additional contamination.

bandage
any material used to hold a dressing in place.

CORE CONCEPT
How to dress and bandage wounds

Most cases of open wound care require the application of a dressing and a bandage (Figure 30-32 and Scan 30-1). A ***dressing*** is any material applied to a wound in an effort to control bleeding and prevent further contamination. Dressings should be sterile. A ***bandage*** is any material used to hold a dressing in place. Bandages need not be sterile.

NOTE: *Be certain to wear disposable gloves and other barrier devices to avoid contact with the patient's blood and body fluids. Follow infection control procedures.*

Various dressings are carried in emergency care kits. These dressings should be sterile, meaning that all microorganisms and spores that can grow into active organisms have been killed. Dressings also should be aseptic, meaning that all dirt and foreign debris have been removed. Many EMS systems now also carry hemostatic dressings used to stop bleeding (Figure 30-33). Hemostatic dressings are covered more extensively in the chapter *Bleeding and Shock*. In emergency situations, when commercially prepared dressings are not available, clean cloth, towels, sheets, handkerchiefs, and other similar materials may be suitable alternatives.

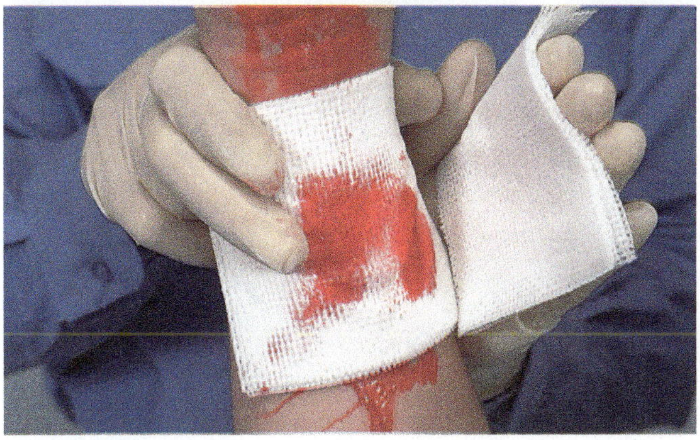

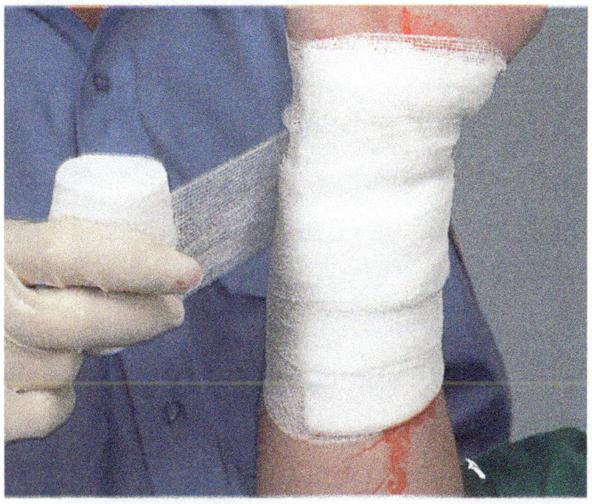

FIGURE 30-32 (A) Dressings cover wounds and (B) bandages hold dressings in place.

SCAN 30-1 Dressing and Bandaging

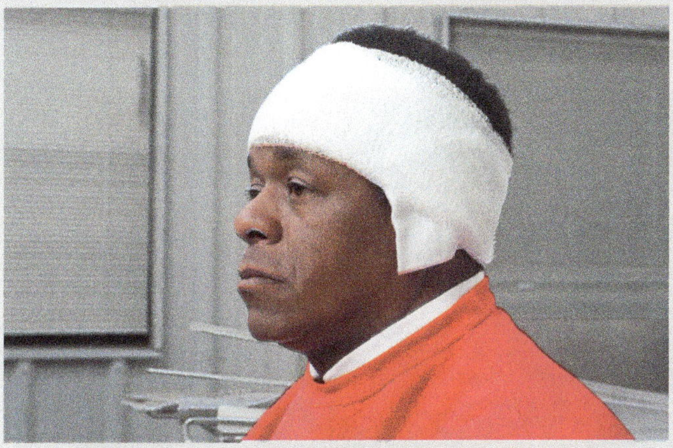

Forehead or Ear (No Skull Injury). Place the dressing and secure it with a self-adherent roller bandage.

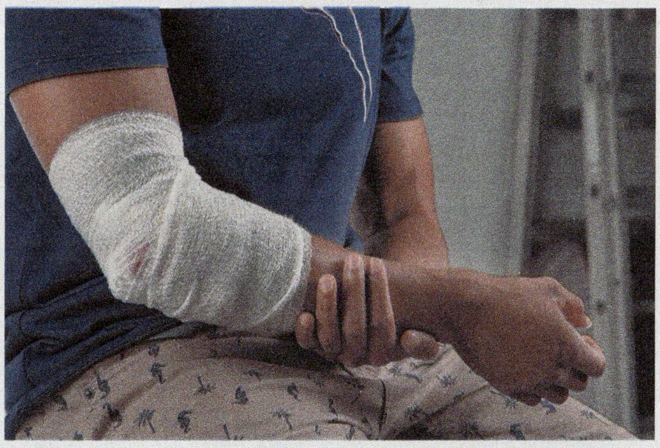

Elbow or Knee. Place the dressing and secure it with a cravat or roller bandage. Apply the roller bandage in a figure-eight pattern.

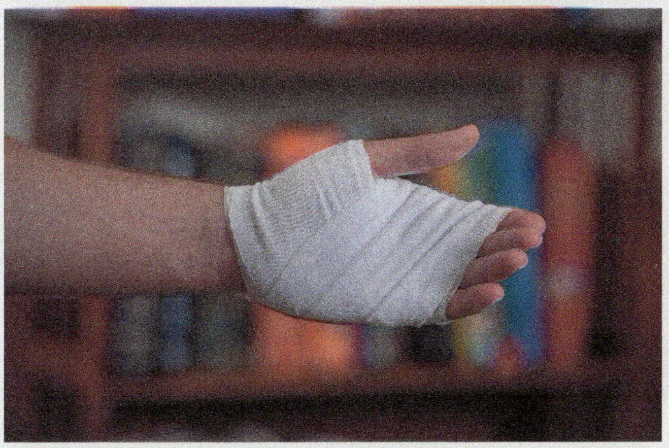

Hand. Place the dressing, wrap it with roller bandages, and secure it at the wrist. When possible, bandage it in the position of function.

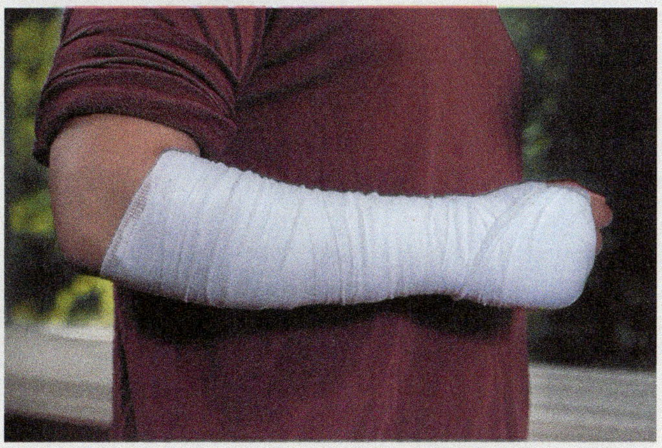

Forearm or Leg. Place the dressing and secure it with a roller bandage, distal to proximal. Better protection is offered if the palm or sole is wrapped.

(continued)

SCAN 30-1 Dressing and Bandaging *(continued)*

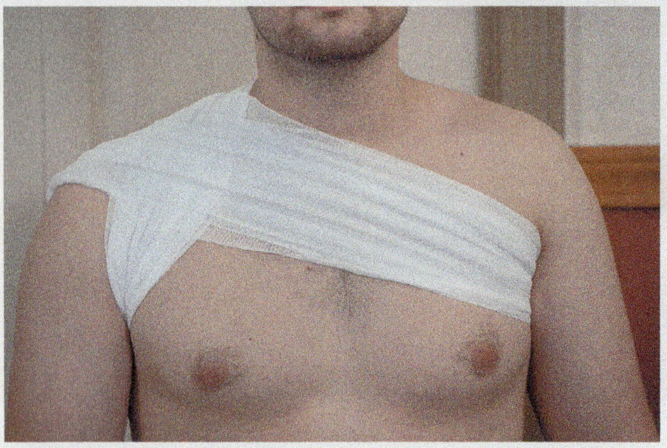

Shoulder. Place the dressing and secure it with a figure-eight of cravat or roller dressing. Pad under the knot if a cravat is used.

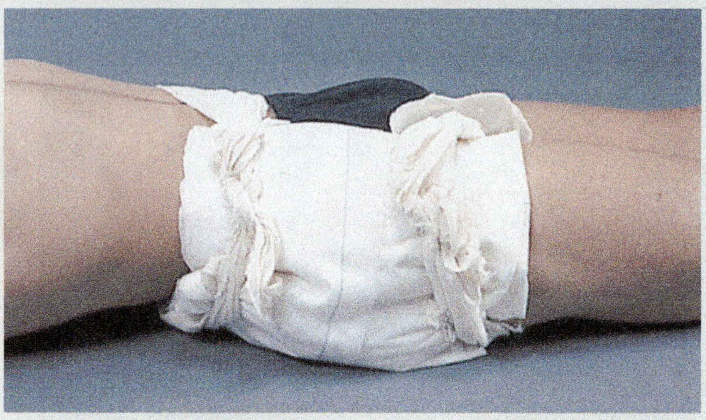

Hip. Place the bandage and use a large dressing to cover the hip. Secure it with the first cravat around the waist and second cravat around the thigh on the injured side.

FIGURE 30-33 (A and B) Application and bandaging of a hemostatic dressing. (C) Wound packing with hemostatic gauze on an extremity.

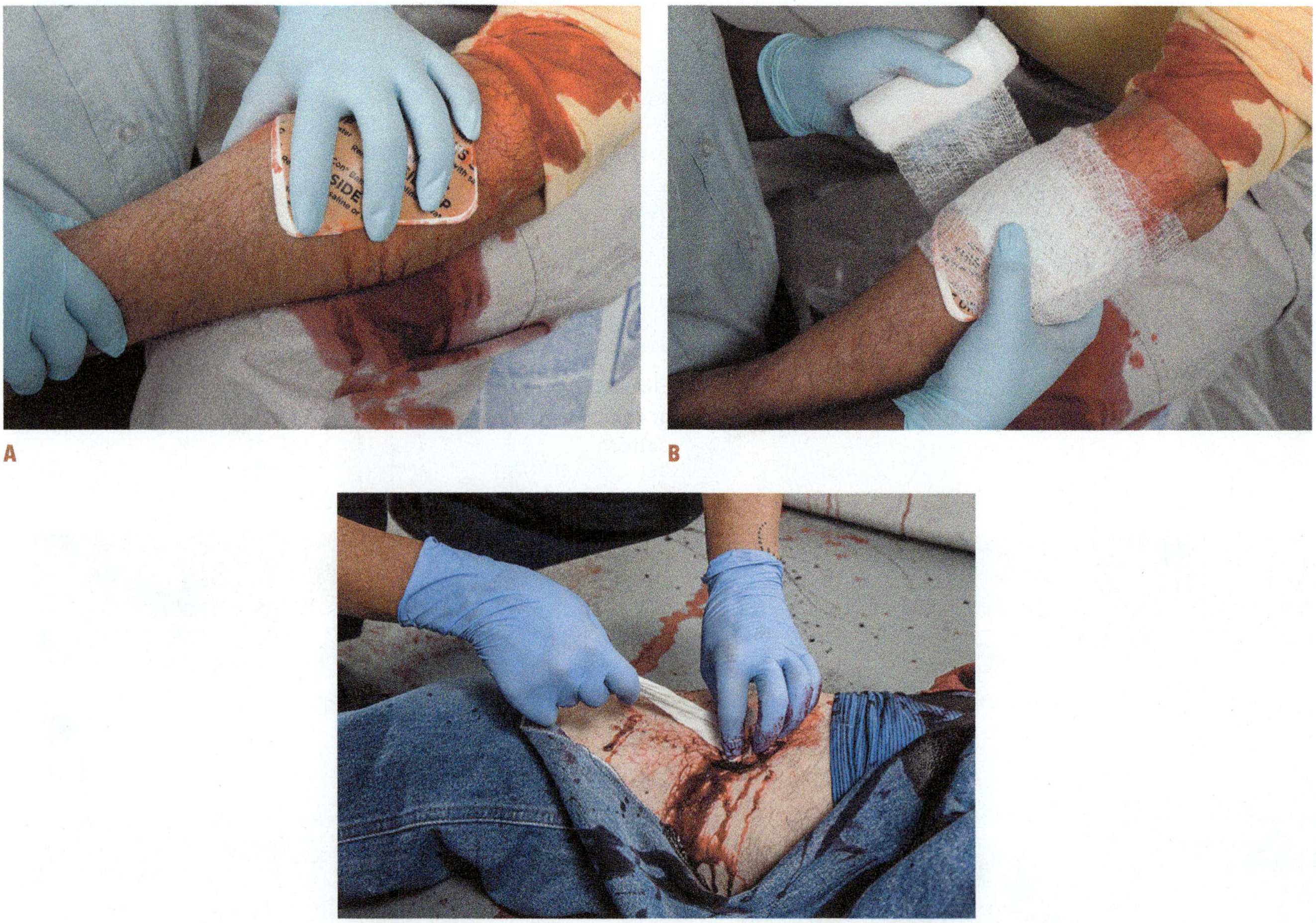

A

B

C

The most popular dressings are individually wrapped sterile gauze pads, typically 4 inches square. A variety of sizes are available, referred to according to size in inches, such as 2 × 2s, 4 × 4s, 5 × 9s, and 8 × 10s.

universal dressing a bulky dressing.

Large, bulky dressings, such as the multitrauma or ***universal dressing***, are available when bulk is required for profuse bleeding or when a large wound must be covered. These dressings are especially useful for stabilizing impaled objects. Sanitary napkins can sometimes be used in place of the standard bulky dressings. Although not sterile, they are separately wrapped and have very clean surfaces. (Do not apply any adhesive surface of the napkin directly to the wound.) Of course, bulky dressings can be made by building up layers of gauze pads.

A ***pressure dressing*** is used to control bleeding. Gauze pads are placed on the wound, and a bulky dressing is placed over the pads. A self-adherent roller bandage is then wrapped tightly over the dressing and above and below the wound. You must check and frequently recheck the distal pulse, and you may need to readjust the pressure to ensure distal circulation.

pressure dressing
a dressing applied tightly to control bleeding.

An ***occlusive dressing*** is used when it is necessary to form an airtight seal. This is done when caring for open wounds to the abdomen, for external bleeding from large neck veins, and for open wounds to the chest. Sterile, commercially prepared occlusive dressings are available in two different forms: plastic wrap and petroleum gel–impregnated gauze occlusive dressings. Local protocols vary as to which form to use. Nonsterile wrap also can be used in emergency situations. In emergencies, EMTs have been known to fashion occlusive dressings from plastic bags, sterile medical equipment wrappers, and defibrillator pads.

occlusive dressing
any dressing that forms an airtight seal.

Large dressings are sometimes needed in emergency care. Sterile, disposable burn sheets are commercially available. Bedsheets can also be sterilized and kept in plastic wrappers to be used later as dressings. These sheets can make effective burn dressings or may be used in some cases to cover exposed abdominal organs.

Bandages are provided in a wide variety of types. The preferred bandage is the self-adhering, form-fitting roller bandage (Figure 30-34). It eliminates the need to know many specialized bandaging techniques developed for use with ordinary gauze roller bandages.

FIGURE 30-34 To apply a self-adhering roller bandage, (A) secure it with several overlapping wraps, (B) keep it snug, and (C) cut and tape or tie it in place.

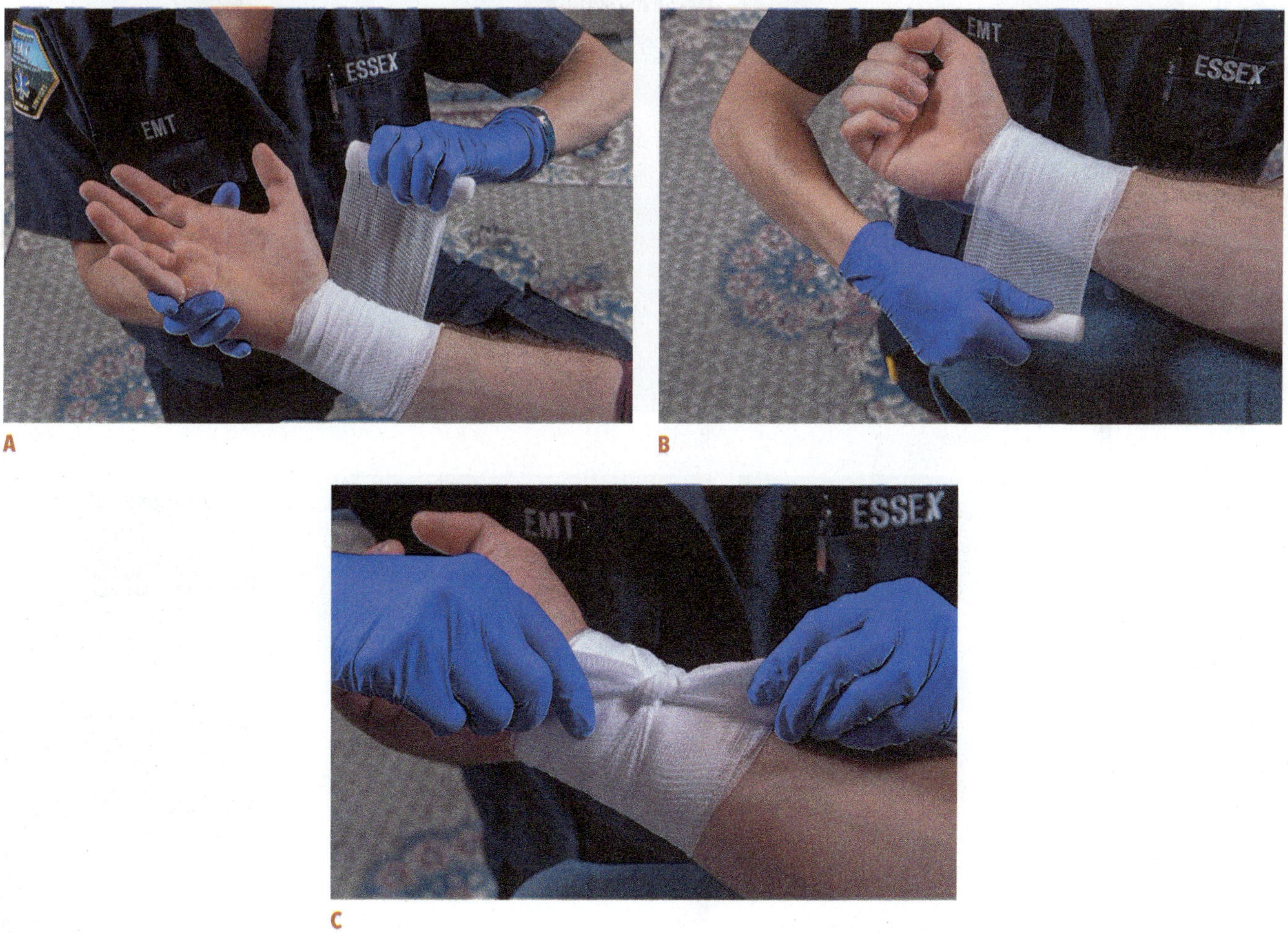

Dressings can be secured using adhering or non-adhering gauze roller bandages, triangular bandages, strips of adhesive tape, or an air splint. In a situation where none of these is available, you can use strips of cloth, handkerchiefs, or other such materials. Elastic bandages that are used in the general care of strains and sprains can be used to hold dressings in place, but care must be taken to prevent them from becoming constricting bands and interfering with circulation. Circulation deficits are especially likely to occur as the tissues around the wound site begin to swell after the bandage is in place. Always monitor distal pulses and circulation following bandaging.

Patient Care

Dressing Open Wounds

Fundamental Principles of Care

With open wounds, the primary concerns of the EMT are stopping bleeding and preventing infection.

The following principles apply to the general dressing of wounds (Figure 30-35):

- Take Standard Precautions.
- Expose the wound. Cut away any clothing necessary for the entire wound to be exposed.
- Use sterile or very clean materials. Avoid touching the dressing in the area that will come into contact with the wound. Grasp the dressing by the corner, taking it directly from its protective pack, and place it on the wound.

FIGURE 30-35 To dress an open wound, (A) expose the wound site, (B) control the bleeding, (C) dress and bandage the wound, and (D) keep the patient at rest and treat for shock if necessary.

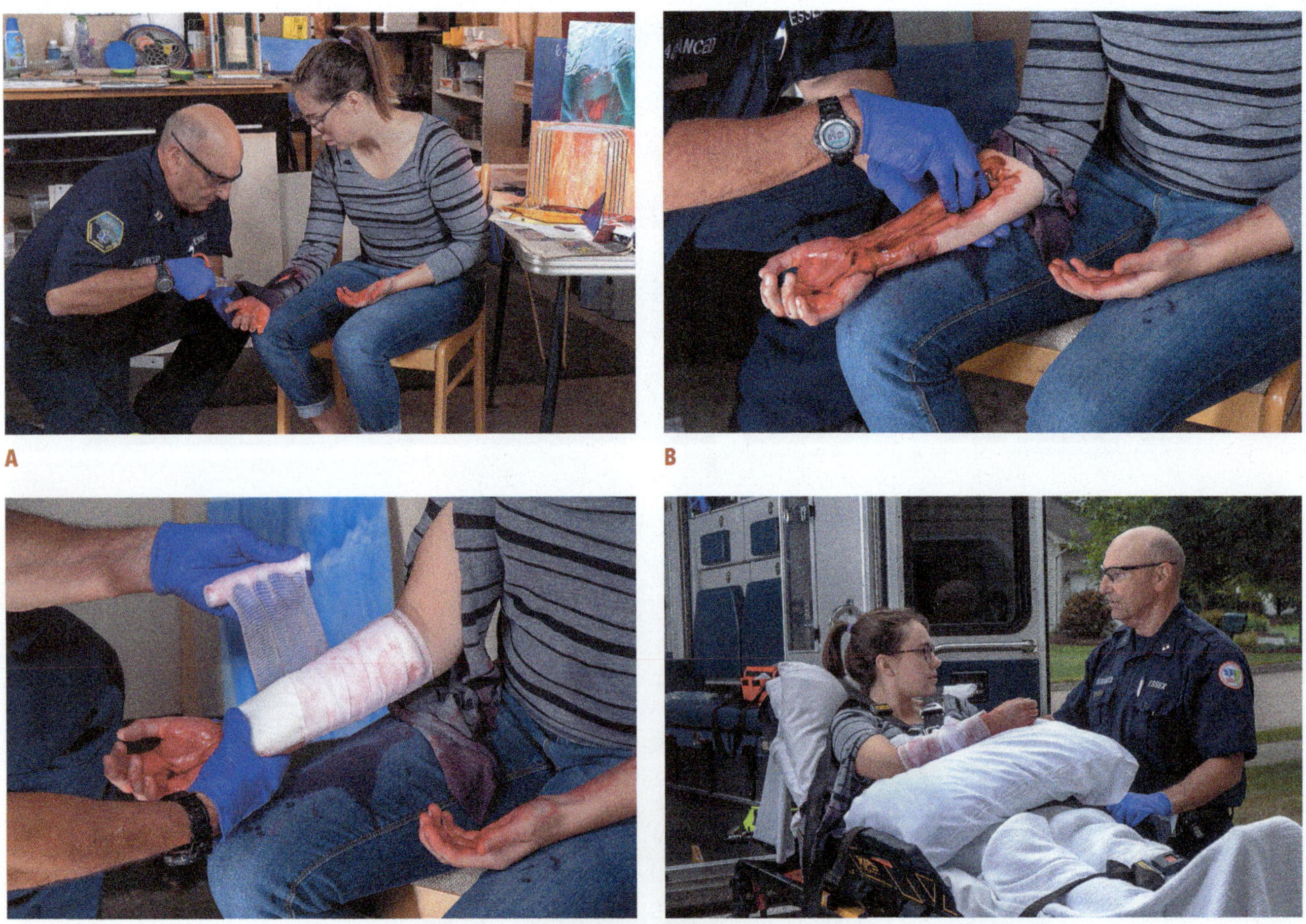

A B C D

- Cover the entire wound. The entire surface of the wound and the immediate surrounding areas should be covered.
- Control the bleeding. Use direct pressure and/or hemostatic agents or dressings to stop or slow the bleeding. With the exception of the pressure dressing, a dressing should not be bandaged in place if it has not controlled the bleeding. You should continue to apply dressings and pressure as needed for the proper control of bleeding.
- Do not remove dressings. Once a dressing has been applied to a wound, it must remain in place. Bleeding may restart and tissues at the wound site may be injured if the dressing is removed. If the bleeding continues, reapply pressure, apply additional hemostatic agent, and put new dressings over the blood-soaked ones.

There is an exception to the rule prohibiting the removal of dressings. If a bulky dressing has become soaked with blood, it may be necessary to remove the dressing so direct pressure can be reestablished or a new bulky dressing can be added and a pressure dressing created. Protection for the wound site is better maintained if one or more gauze pads are placed over the injured tissues before placing the bulky dressing. This will allow for the removal of a bulky dressing without disturbing the wound.

Patient Care

Bandaging Open Wounds

Fundamental Principles of Care

Most wounds are easy to bandage, but occasionally you may need to be a little creative with roller gauze or triangular bandages to keep dressings in place and maintain pressure on them.

The following principles apply to general bandaging:

- Do not bandage too tightly. All dressings should be held snugly in place, but they must not restrict the blood supply to the affected part.
- Do not bandage too loosely. Hold the dressing by bandaging snugly, so the dressing does not move around or slip from the wound. Loose bandaging is a common error in emergency care.
- Do not leave loose ends. Any loose ends of gauze, tape, or cloth may get caught on objects when the patient is moved.
- Do not cover the tips of fingers and toes. When bandaging the extremities, leave the fingers and toes exposed whenever possible to observe skin color changes that indicate a change in circulation and to allow for easier neurologic reassessment. Pain, pale or cyanotic skin, cold skin, numbness, and tingling are all indications that a bandage may be too tight. The exception is burned fingers or toes, which have to be covered.
- Cover all edges of the dressing. This will help to reduce additional contamination. The flutter-valve dressing for an open chest wound is an exception. (See the chapter *Chest and Abdominal Trauma.*)

Two special problems occur when bandaging an extremity. First, point pressure can occur if you bandage around a very small area. It is best to wrap a large area, ensuring a steady, uniform pressure. Apply the bandage from the smaller diameter of the limb to the larger diameter (distal to proximal) to help ensure proper pressure and contact. Second, the joints have to be considered. You can bandage across a joint, but do not bend the limb once the bandage is in place. Doing so may restrict circulation, loosen the dressing and bandage, or do both. In some cases, it may be necessary to apply an inflatable or rigid splint, or to use a sling and swathe to prevent the joint's movement.

Chapter Review

Key Facts and Concepts

- Soft-tissue injuries may be closed (internal, with no pathway to the outside) or open (an injury in which the skin is interrupted, exposing the tissues below).
- Closed injuries include contusions (bruises), hematomas, crush injuries, and blast injuries. Open wounds include abrasions, lacerations, punctures, avulsions, amputations, crush injuries, and blast injuries.
- For open wounds, expose the wound, control bleeding, and prevent further contamination.
- For both open and closed injuries, take appropriate Standard Precautions; note the mechanism of injury; protect the patient's airway and breathing; consider the need for oxygen by nonrebreather mask; treat for shock; and transport.
- Burn severity is determined by considering the source of the burn, body regions burned, depth of the burn (superficial, partial thickness, or full thickness), extent of the burn (by rule of nines or rule of palm), age of the patient (children under 5 and adults over 55 react most severely), and other patient illnesses or injuries.
- Care for burns includes stopping the burning process (using water for a thermal burn, or brushing away dry chemicals), covering a thermal burn with a dry sterile dressing, flushing a chemical burn with sterile water, protecting the airway, administering oxygen as appropriate, treating for shock, and transporting the patient to a medical facility.
- For treatment of electrical injuries, be sure that you and the patient are in a safe zone away from possible contact with electrical sources. Protect the airway, breathing, and circulation. Be prepared to care for respiratory or cardiac arrest. Treat for shock, care for burns, and transport the patient.

Key Decisions

- Does the patient have an adequate airway?
- Is the patient's breathing adequate, inadequate, or absent?
- If the wound is penetrating, are there additional penetrations, including exit wounds?
- What is the best way to immobilize an impaled object?
- Do I need to cool the burn area to stop the burning?
- Does the burn patient need to go to a special destination?
- Is there respiratory involvement with the burn?
- Have I sufficiently irrigated the chemical burn?
- Does the patient's electrical burn have an exit wound?
- Is the bandage on the patient's extremity snug enough without limiting circulation?

Chapter Glossary

abrasion (ab-RAY-zhun) a scratch or scrape.

amputation (am-pyu-TAY-shun) the surgical removal or traumatic severing of a body part, usually an extremity.

avulsion (ah-VUL-shun) the tearing away or tearing off of a piece or flap of skin or other soft tissue. This term also may be used for an eye pulled from its socket or a tooth dislodged from its socket.

bandage any material used to hold a dressing in place.

closed wound an internal injury with no open pathway from the outside.

contusion (kun-TU-zhun) a bruise.

crush injury an injury caused when force is transmitted from the body's exterior to its internal structures. Bones can be broken; muscles, nerves, and tissues damaged causing internal bleeding. In extreme cases where the torso is compressed, internal organs such as the stomach or urinary bladder can be ruptured, causing internal bleeding and allowing digested food or urine to spread into the abdominal cavities.

dermis (DER-mis) the inner (second) layer of the skin found beneath the epidermis. It is rich in blood vessels and nerves.

dressing any material (preferably sterile) used to cover a wound that will help control bleeding and prevent additional contamination.

epidermis (ep-i-DER-mis) the outer layer of the skin.

full thickness burn a burn in which all the layers of the skin are damaged. There are usually areas that are charred black or areas that are dry and white. Also called a *third-degree burn*.

hematoma (hem-ah-TO-mah) a swelling caused by the collection of blood under the skin or in damaged tissues as a result of an injured or broken blood vessel.

laceration (lass-er-AY-shun) a cut.

occlusive dressing any dressing that forms an airtight seal.

open wound an injury in which the skin is interrupted, exposing the tissue beneath.

partial thickness burn a burn in which the epidermis (first layer of skin) is burned through and the dermis (second layer) is damaged. Burns of this type cause reddening, blistering, and a mottled appearance. Also called a *second-degree burn*.

pressure dressing a dressing applied tightly to control bleeding.

puncture wound an open wound that tears through the skin and destroys underlying tissues. A *penetrating puncture wound* can be shallow or deep. A *perforating puncture wound* has both an entrance and an exit wound.

rule of nines a method for estimating the extent of a burn. For an adult, each of the following areas represents 9 percent of the body surface: the head and neck, each upper extremity, the chest, the abdomen, the upper back, the lower back and buttocks, the front of each lower extremity, and the back of each lower extremity. The remaining 1 percent is assigned to the genital region. For an infant or child, the percentages are modified so 18 percent is assigned to the head, 14 percent to each lower extremity.

rule of palm a method for estimating the extent of a burn. The palm and fingers of the patient's own hand, which equal about 1 percent of the body's surface area, are compared with the patient's burn to estimate its size.

subcutaneous (SUB-ku-TAY-ne-us) ***layers*** the layers of fat and soft tissues found below the dermis.

superficial burn a burn that involves only the epidermis, the outer layer of the skin. It is characterized by reddening of the skin and perhaps some swelling. A common example is a sunburn. Also called a *first-degree burn*.

universal dressing a bulky dressing.

Preparation for Your Examination and Practice

Short Answer

1. List three types of closed soft-tissue injuries.
2. List four types of open soft-tissue injuries.
3. Explain when you would remove an object impaled in the cheek and when you would, instead, stabilize an object impaled in the cheek.
4. Describe the three classifications (depths) of burns.
5. Differentiate between a dressing and a bandage.
6. List the qualities and purpose of an effective bandage. How can you tell if a bandage is improperly applied?

Thinking and Linking

Think back to the chapter Well-Being of the EMT *as you consider the following question:*

- What Standard Precautions are required for the following calls?
    a. An agitated person with a lip laceration and missing teeth
    b. A small cut to the left hand, which is oozing blood
    c. A laceration to the right forearm with bright red, spurting blood

Think back to the chapter Introduction to Emergency Medical Services *and the discussion of specialized trauma and other treatment centers in the* Components of the EMS System *section as you consider the following question:*

- Which specialty centers should the following patients be transported to (if the center is available in your region)?
    a. A patient with partial thickness burns on 35 percent of his body
    b. A patient with suspected internal bleeding and trauma
    c. A patient with an amputated hand

Critical Thinking Exercises

Assessing a wound that is covered can be tricky. The purpose of this exercise will be to consider one such situation.

- A 21-year-old male lacerated his anterior elbow when he fell through a window. There is a lot of blood around the patient. Bystanders have applied numerous towels and washcloths over the wound (at least 3 inches (7.5 centimeters) thick). There are so many dressings on the wound, in fact, that you can't tell if it is still bleeding. The patient is alert but pale and anxious. The radial pulse on his uninjured arm is weak and rapid. How much assessment of the wound should you do, and how do you do it without making things worse?

Pathophysiology to Practice

The following question is designed to assist you in gathering relevant clinical information and making accurate decisions in the field.

- Patients with extensive burns lose large amounts of fluid internally because of damage to vascular membranes. If you find a patient with a recent burn (less than 1 hour old) who is tachycardic, pale, and hypotensive, why should you look for a source of bleeding?

Street Scenes

Late Sunday evening, you respond to #4 Mountain View Apartments. You and your partner are met by the manager and a security guard, who lead you to Mary, a 42-year-old female sitting in a chair in the manager's office with a thick towel wrapped around her right forearm. Standard Precautions are in place. You greet the patient and identify yourself, then ask, "What happened?" You note the trail of blood spots on the floor leading to an outside door.

"I locked myself out of my apartment," she tells you, "so I wrapped my coat around my arm and broke the glass window above my kitchen sink. I thought the coat would protect me, but I was wrong."

Street Scene Questions

1. What is your general impression of this patient?
2. What priority would you assign to her?
3. What interventions are appropriate at this time?

Your general impression is of an alert female patient holding a blood-soaked towel to her right forearm. Primary assessment shows her airway open and clear, respirations normal, and a regular pulse in her right wrist. You assign her a low transport priority.

You ask Norma, your partner, to go to Mary's apartment accompanied by the security guard to see if she can learn anything more about the mechanism of injury. Meanwhile, you observe that the bleeding is being controlled, and you begin a secondary assessment. You gently remove the towel and note there is no active bleeding from a smooth and deep laceration with muscle and tendons visible. You dress and bandage the wound.

There are no other injuries or medical problems present. You do, however, detect an odor of alcohol on Mary's breath. "Have you had any alcohol today?" you ask.

"Yes, I drank two beers about three hours ago. That's all!" she exclaims. However, with the odor on her breath, you believe she must have had more than two beers. Focusing on her right arm, you find pulses still present in that extremity. Also, she is able to feel your finger touch her palm. However, when you ask her to wiggle her fingers, her ring and little fingers remain motionless. She also tells you it hurts to move her fingers. Norma returns and tells you there is a large pool of blood on Mary's patio.

Street Scene Questions

4. Would you change the priority of transport of this patient based on what you now know? Why or why not?
5. What interventions are appropriate for this patient?

While you continue with the patient history, Norma obtains baseline vital signs. You learn Mary is taking thyroid medication and a blood thinner for a medical condition. You ask when she received her last tetanus shot, and she tells you she cannot remember.

Norma informs you that Mary's pulse is equal in both extremities at a rate of 128 and regular; her blood pressure is 156/94; her respirations are 24 and unlabored; pupils are equal and reactive to light; and her skin is warm, dry, and a normal color.

You contact medical direction, concerned about the loss of movement in Mary's affected extremity. The doctor tells you that you should stabilize Mary's arm with a sling.

You apply a sling, reassess Mary's vitals, and find no significant changes. Reassessing her pulse, motor function, and sensation, you find Mary still unable to move her fourth and fifth digits on her right hand. You place her on your cot, load her into the ambulance, and transport her to the closest facility, monitoring her condition throughout the 15-minute ride. You find no other significant changes en route.

Chest and Abdominal Trauma

31

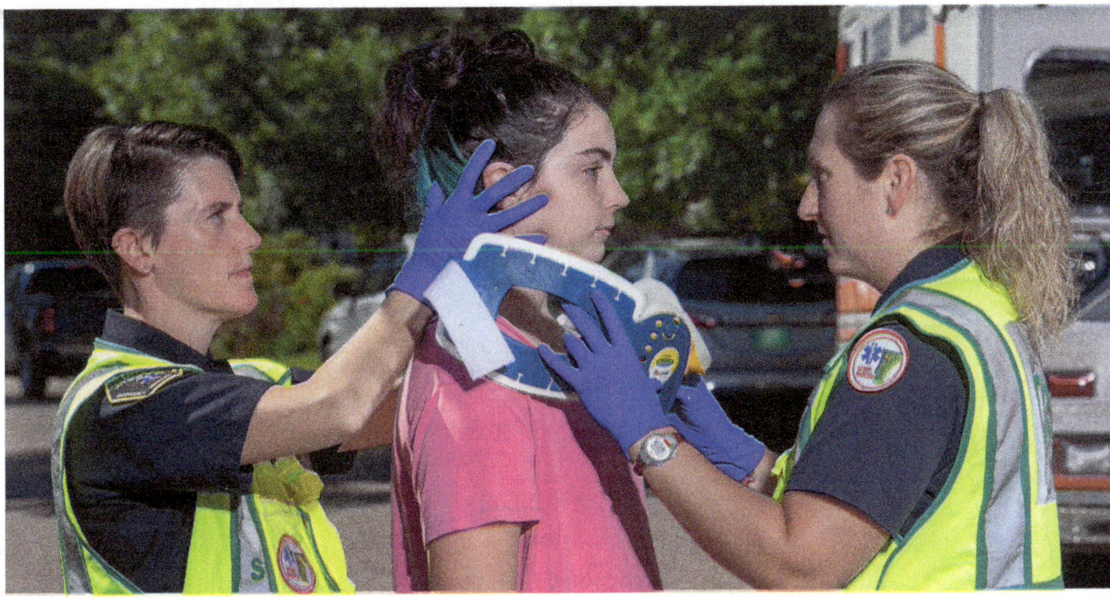

Related Chapters

The following chapters provide additional information related to topics discussed in this chapter:

2 Well-Being of the EMT
19 Respiratory Emergencies
20 Cardiac Emergencies
21 Resuscitation
26 Abdominal Emergencies
30 Soft-Tissue Trauma

Standard

Trauma (Chest Trauma; Abdominal and Genitourinary Trauma)

Competency

Applies fundamental knowledge to provide basic emergency care and transportation based on assessment findings for an acutely injured patient.

Core Concepts

- Understanding chest injuries and emergency care for chest injuries
- Understanding abdominal injuries and emergency care for abdominal injuries

Outcomes

After reading this chapter, you should be able to:

31.1 Summarize the concepts of chest injuries. (pp. 869–875)

- Review the anatomy and physiology of the chest.
- Review the anatomy and physiology of the abdomen.
- Relate mechanisms of injury to the potential for specific chest injuries.
- Compare the characteristics of closed (blunt) and open (penetrating) chest wounds.
- Relate the pathophysiology of specific types of chest injuries to patient assessment findings.

31.2 Summarize the management decisions required in the care of patients with chest injuries. (pp. 875–885)

- Select the approach to addressing gas exchange based on the adequacy of the patient's respiration.
- Describe how the treatment indicated for specific chest injuries helps mitigate the underlying problem.
- Outline the steps in designing the interventions for specific chest injuries.
- Explain how to prioritize management decisions for portrayals of a variety of patients with chest trauma.
- Compare the characteristics of pneumothorax, tension pneumothorax, hemothorax, and hemopneumothorax.
- Describe the processes by which specific types of chest injuries interfere with cardiopulmonary system function.

31.3 Summarize the concepts of abdominal injuries. (pp. 885–887)

- Relate mechanism of injury to the potential for closed or open abdominal injuries.
- Relate mechanism of injury to the potential for specific organ injury.
- Compare the characteristics of injury to solid abdominal organs with those of injury to hollow abdominal organs.

31.4 Summarize the management decisions required in the care of patients with abdominal injuries. (pp. 887–889)

- Prioritize the care of specific abdominal injuries among the other interventions for trauma patients.
- Use assessment findings to inform measures to minimize the pain of abdominal injuries.
- Describe how to address the concerns for vomiting by the patient with an abdominal injury.
- Describe the special bandaging techniques for specific open abdominal wounds.
- Apply assessment and EMS system characteristics to make decisions about patient transportation.

Key Terms

evisceration, *885*
flail chest, *874*
paradoxical motion, *875*
pneumothorax, *881*
sucking chest wound, *878*
tension pneumothorax, *881*

In 2018 in the United States, more than 150,000 people died from traumatic injury. Over 75 percent of those deaths were associated with chest and abdominal trauma. It is not difficult to understand why. The cavities of the chest and abdomen contain the body's most important and most vulnerable organs. From the heart and lungs to the liver, spleen, and kidneys, massive quantities of blood pass through these organs and sustain critical body functions. While abdominal and chest trauma accounts for a high percentage of trauma deaths, these types of injuries are also in many cases correctable. Conditions like tension pneumothorax are assuredly fatal if undiscovered, but very fixable if the patient can reach the right resources in a timely fashion. As an EMT, you will be the first point of contact and most often have the first opportunity to recognize, treat, and change the outcome of these chest and abdominal injured patients. Your assessment skills and immediate interventions will play a vital role in preventing death.

Anatomy and Physiology of the Chest and Abdomen

The most serious chest and abdominal injuries occur when internal organs are affected by trauma. That means, for a large portion of patients, all the actual damage will not be seen from the outside. Proper assessment will combine an examination of mechanism of injury, a physical examination, and an understanding of anatomy and physiology. Considering all three components will enable you to anticipate problems and to make the best and most accurate treatment decisions. This approach requires a basic understanding of the contents and the function of the organs contained within the cavities that make up the chest and abdomen.

Anatomy and Physiology of the Chest

The chest cavity extends from the collarbones to the dynamic lower border framed by the diaphragm. We use the term *dynamic* because depending upon the current stage of a patient's respiratory cycle, that lower border of the chest could be as high as the nipple line or as low as the umbilicus. When a person inhales, the diaphragm contracts and flattens. This process extends lung tissue inferiorly toward what we would consider the abdomen. Upon exhalation, the diaphragm relaxes and moves upward. This movement pushes lung tissue higher into the chest.

Although the chest cavity has some physiologic characteristics of a hollow cavity, it is fully packed with organs, major blood vessels, and lung tissue. In fact, there is little space for anything else in the chest. The heart and its great vessels, like the aorta and vena cava, occupy space along the midline, and lung tissue fills the remaining space. The great vessels extend outward and traverse the chest in multiple directions. The umbrella-shaped muscle called the *diaphragm* sits at the bottom of the lungs, in the inferior aspect of the chest, and separates chest contents from the abdominal cavity. See Figure 31-1.

The vital organs of the chest are well protected. Twelve sets of ribs, the anterior sternum, and the posterior thoracic spine vertebrae form the chest and guard vulnerable lung tissue from damage. Ten sets of ribs connect from the vertebrae to the sternum, while the last two sets connect only with the vertebrae and are often referred to as "free-floating."

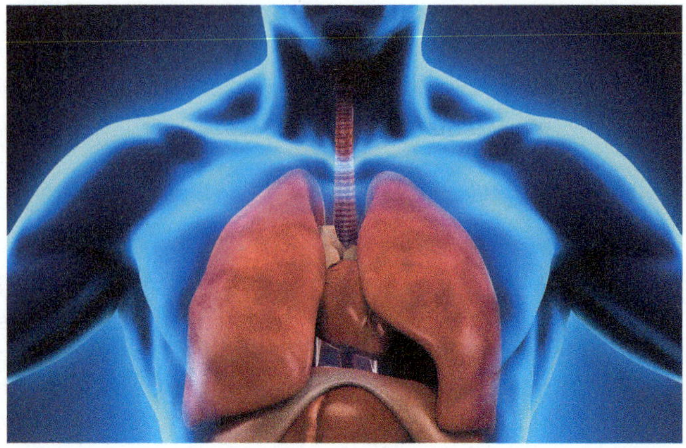

FIGURE 31-1 Anatomy of the chest. (Nerthuz/Shutterstock)

In addition to the ribs, the massive bones of the scapula offer the organs of the chest protection from the rear. Interlocking and overlapping muscles of the back and chest add an additional layer of protection.

Within the chest, several very important physiologic functions take place. In the center of the chest, the heart beats, providing a constant and vital blood flow to the rest of the body. Large blood vessels enter and exit the heart and traverse the chest in a variety of directions. A huge portion of the body's blood volume is contained within these vessels at any given moment, so trauma that violates these vessels can rapidly become fatal. In addition to cardiac circulation, the chest is also the home of respiratory function.

The Mechanism of Breathing

An essential physiologic activity that occurs in the chest is the mechanism of breathing. Here, the chest wall, diaphragm, and lungs work together to change pressure within the chest cavity and cause air to be moved in and out. Lung tissue that occupies space in the chest adheres to the chest wall due to small amounts of a clear, lubricating liquid, called *serous fluid,* and a constant, negative pressure. This adherence allows the lungs to expand and contract with movement of the chest wall and contraction of the diaphragm. Expansion and contraction of the lungs change pressure and lead to the movement of air. Consider the following sequence and review the chapter *Respiratory Emergencies,* especially Figure 19-1.

Inhalation—To inhale, the diaphragm contracts and flattens. At the same time, the muscles between the ribs, known as *intercostal muscles*, flex and expand the chest wall outward. These two actions together cause the chest cavity to increase in size. The lung tissue, which under normal circumstances adheres to the chest wall, expands as the chest grows larger. Expansion causes a negative pressure to be created within the lung spaces, and this negative pressure pulls air in through the trachea. Inhalation is generally referred to as an *active* process, as it requires muscle contraction and flattening of the diaphragm.

Exhalation—Exhalation generally reverses the movement of inhalation. It is most commonly thought of as a *passive* process, because it relies upon relaxation and the natural return of the chest to normal size. Exhalation starts when the diaphragm relaxes and curves upward. At the same time, the intercostal muscles also relax and allow the chest wall to contract and return to its normal position. As lung tissue is condensed, pressure inside the lung spaces is increased. Air is subsequently pushed out.

Understanding this physiology is important because many traumatic injuries can disrupt it.

Anatomy and Physiology of the Abdomen

The superior border of the abdomen is the diaphragm, and abdominal organs extend inferiorly to the lower regions of the pelvis. Many types of organs are housed within the abdominal cavity. The abdominal organs are often described in the context of their location relative

FIGURE 31-2 Anatomy of the abdomen.

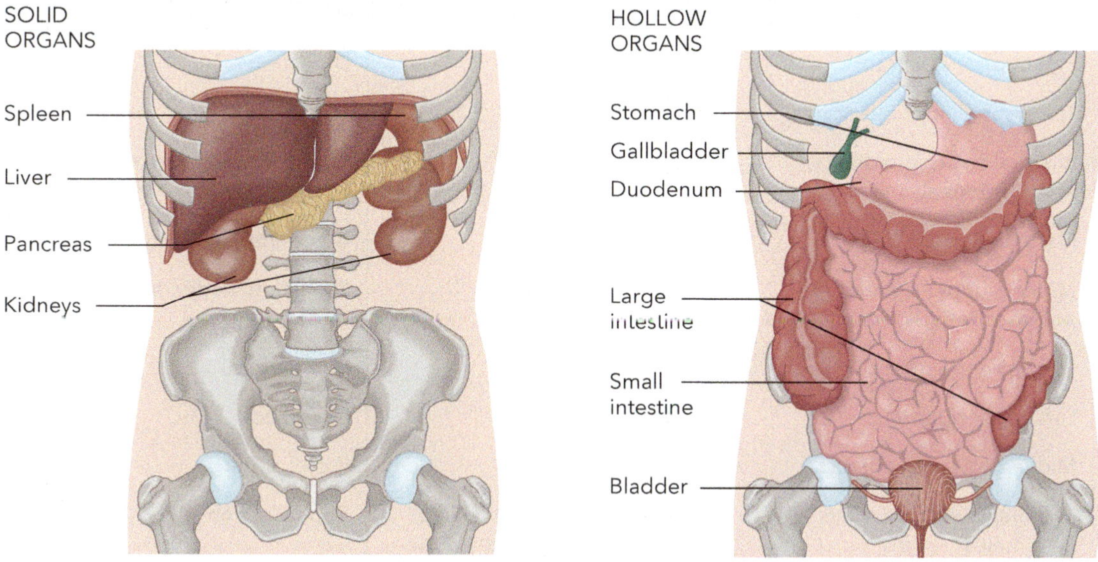

to the four abdominal quadrants. This anatomic distribution was described in detail in the chapter *Abdominal Emergencies*. It may be advisable to review that chapter before going any further. Figure 31-2 provides a general overview of abdominal anatomy.

Trauma assessment and care take into consideration both placement and function of abdominal organs. You will use mechanism of injury (MOI) to consider what, if any, abdominal organs could be injured, and will use physiology to better understand the impact of such an injury. For example, if a patient were shot in the right upper quadrant, you might immediately suspect an injury to the liver, gallbladder, or both. By remembering that the liver's principal responsibility is to filter blood, you would also understand that injury to that organ can lead to massive internal hemorrhage.

A simple consideration that can be helpful is to differentiate between hollow and solid organs. Hollow organs like the stomach, intestine, and urinary bladder usually tolerate trauma well. Although they certainly can be injured, they tend to compress and absorb trauma rather than be destroyed immediately. The danger of hollow-organ damage is that when hollow organs are violated, they often can spill their contents into the abdominal cavity and cause severe inflammation and infection later.

Solid organs, like the liver, spleen, and kidneys, do not tolerate trauma well at all. Relatively small traumatic forces can cause damage to these organs because they have little capacity to stretch or compress. Solid organs also tend to have large blood supplies. In particular, the liver and spleen pose a risk for life-threatening bleeding when injured.

Table 31-1 is a chart describing the location, type, and function of the most common abdominal organs.

The physiology of abdominal organs is dependent on individual function. Each organ contributes to body function in its own particular way. There are two important general considerations to keep in mind, however. First, the abdominal cavity is dynamic in nature, depending on the location of the diaphragm. Organs can shift locations depending on the cycle of breathing. These dynamic changes can also cause pressure within the abdominal cavity to change. High-pressure states, such as the pressure caused by rapid inhalation, can cause organs to be pushed outside the body if the abdominal wall is violated (Figure 31-3). Secondly, there is always a large volume of blood contained within the abdomen. Large blood vessels like the descending aorta, the inferior vena cava, and the iliac arteries—as well as veins of the pelvis—move large volumes of blood through the abdomen at any given moment. There is also a tremendous volume of blood contained within large solid organs like the liver and spleen. Between blood vessels and solid organs, a significant percentage of the body's blood volume can be found in the abdomen.

TABLE 31-1 Location, Type, and Function of the Abdominal Organs

ORGAN	LOCATION	TYPE	PRIMARY FUNCTION
Gallbladder	Right upper quadrant	Hollow	Digestion
Intestine (large and small)	Traverses all four quadrants	Hollow	Digestion
Kidneys	Bilateral upper quadrants, retroperitoneal	Solid	Blood filtration, excretion
Liver	Right upper quadrant	Solid	Blood filtration
Pancreas	Midline, upper quadrants, partial retroperitoneal	Solid	Digestion, endocrine functions
Spleen	Left upper quadrant	Solid	Blood filtration
Stomach	Left upper quadrant	Hollow	Digestion
Urinary bladder	Midline, lower quadrants	Hollow	Stores urine
Uterus and ovaries	Midline, lower quadrants (in females)	Solid in nonpregnant states, but can change greatly during pregnancy	Reproduction

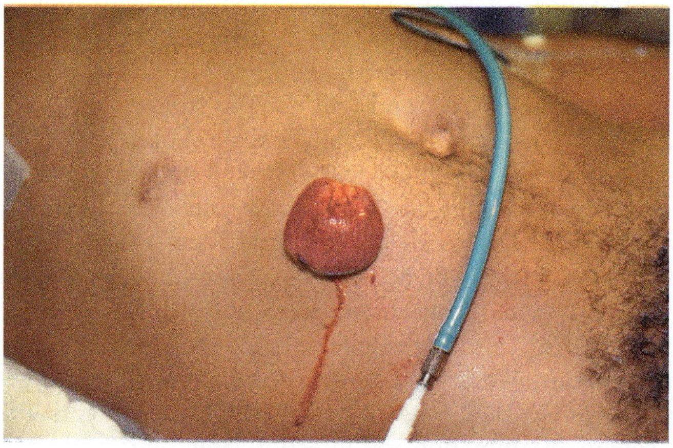

FIGURE 31-3 A section of small intestine forced out of the abdomen after a stab wound. *(© Edward T. Dickinson, MD)*

Pediatric Note

The anatomy and physiology of the chests and abdomens of pediatric patients is not significantly different than those of adults. However, there are subtle differences that should be considered. The chests of small children (typically those younger than 8 years old) are more pliable. The bones of their chests have less calcium compared with the more rigid calcified bones of adults, which means the protective capabilities of the ribs are not as developed as they are in adults. Ribs that would protect and typically break due to trauma in adults often remain intact but hide potentially devastating internal chest injuries in children. The abdominal organs in young children are also more exposed and vulnerable to injury. In adults, the lower ribs shield vital organs such as the liver and spleen, but in infants and small children, these organs are less well protected.

Pathophysiology of the Chest and Abdomen

The pathophysiology of the abdomen and chest in trauma can functionally be divided into three categories: disruption of breathing, hemorrhage and shock, and disruption of organ function. Infection is a factor that is integrally tied to traumatic injury.

Disruption of Breathing—When trauma occurs in the chest, often the immediate concern is breathing. Many forms of trauma can interfere with the physiology necessary to move air. If the chest wall is violated, such as in penetrating trauma, air and blood can occupy space and displace the lung tissue, causing it to collapse. Holes that allow air in through the chest wall or out through damaged lung tissue can also defeat the body's ability to create the negative and positive pressures that drive breathing. Injuries to the diaphragm can have a similar effect. Even seemingly minor injuries like rib fractures or blunt contusions can cause severe pain and inflammation in tissues, which can impair breathing.

Hemorrhage and Shock—Perhaps the largest threat in both chest and abdomen injuries is the risk of internal bleeding. Large vessels traverse the chest and abdomen and are vulnerable to trauma. Lacerating a vessel the size of the thoracic aorta in the chest or the iliac artery in the pelvis can be rapidly fatal. In addition, the solid organs and even some of the hollow organs discussed previously can have massive bleeding if damaged. Internal bleeding can quickly lead to shock. The difficulty of chest and abdominal bleeding is that both cavities can hold large volumes of blood without demonstrating external hemorrhage. Very often, shock states and internal hemorrhage have to be assumed based solely upon mechanism of injury and accompanying assessment findings.

Disruption of Organ Function—Trauma to specific thoracic and abdominal organs can cause problems related to those organs' functions. For example, trauma to the heart may result in bleeding, but it may also impair the specific pumping function. Bleeding within the pericardial sac and disruption of normal electrical conduction can cause disruption of the heart's ability to pump effectively in trauma.

Infection—Finally, infection is a delayed, but potentially large threat when chest and abdomen trauma occurs. Penetration of the walls of the chest and abdomen allows bacteria to enter. The rupture of hollow organs can spill unwanted contents into the thoracic and abdominal cavities, resulting in infection and related inflammation in those cavities. Although infection is rarely an immediate concern of EMS on a trauma scene, remember that often we are called to care for patients days after trauma has occurred. We may also manage the interfacility transport of patients in the postoperative phase following trauma.

Chest Injuries

CORE CONCEPT
Understanding chest injuries and emergency care for chest injuries

The chest can be injured in a number of ways:

- **Blunt trauma.** Defined as an injury that does not penetrate the chest wall, blunt mechanisms—including motor-vehicle crashes and falls—account for the majority of chest trauma incidents. A blow to the chest can fracture the ribs, the sternum, and the costal (rib) cartilages. Whole sections of the chest can collapse. With severe blunt trauma, the lungs, airway, great vessels (aorta and venae cavae), and the heart may be seriously injured. The effects of blunt trauma within the chest cavity can be difficult to detect. Chest wall bruising, signs of shock, and respiratory problems should raise concern about potentially serious unseen injuries deep in the chest.
- **Penetrating trauma.** Penetrating trauma is defined as a mechanism of injury that violates the integrity of the chest wall. The trauma physically penetrates. Although a much smaller proportion of chest trauma injuries are penetrating compared with blunt trauma, these injuries can easily be lethal. Bullets, knives, pieces of metal or glass, steel rods, pipes, and various other objects can penetrate the chest wall, damaging internal organs and impairing respiration.
- **Compression and shearing injuries.** Compression injuries develop from severe blunt trauma in which the chest is rapidly compressed, such as when a driver's chest

strikes the steering column or when a person is trapped in a trench-wall collapse. The sternum and ribs can be fractured due to the sudden compression, and breathing can be impaired by disruption of normal chest wall motion. Shearing injuries are seen due to sudden deceleration and seatbelt-related injuries. High-energy shearing injuries can damage the aorta and vena cava.

Chest injuries can also be classified as either *closed* or *open*. In a closed chest injury, the chest wall is not penetrated and trauma is usually caused by blunt mechanisms. Open chest injuries are associated with penetration of the chest wall and are typically caused by penetrating mechanisms.

"An injury that affects breathing could kill your patient. Never lose sight of that."

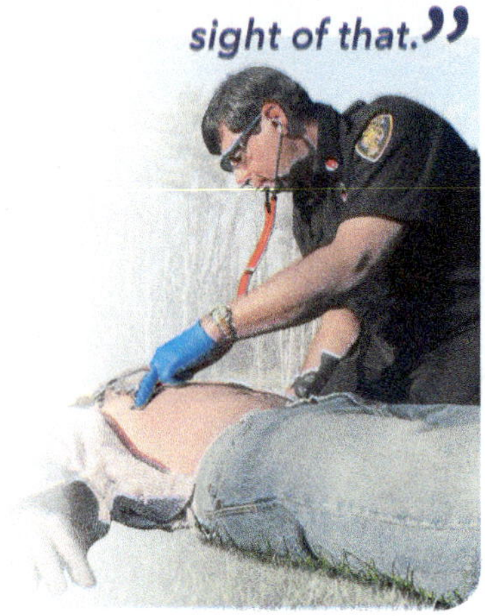

(© Daniel Limmer)

Blunt Chest Injuries

Blunt chest injuries are often considered less serious than penetrating injuries because they tend to be less visually dramatic. A bruise simply isn't as exciting as a bullet wound. However, certain patients with blunt trauma have higher mortality rates than patients with penetrating trauma. It is dangerous to make snap-assessment assumptions in patients with chest injuries.

In blunt trauma, minimal external evidence can distract from massive underlying problems. In many cases, especially in pediatrics, blunt force trauma can transmit energy through the intact chest wall and damage fragile underlying organs and tissues. Internal damage can be nearly impossible to estimate solely by looking at the chest. In these cases, injuries will be predicted by considering mechanism of injury and by performing a more comprehensive patient assessment.

The most common serious blunt chest trauma injuries are rib fractures. These injuries are particularly common in youth sports and geriatric patients. Although most are painful but not life-threatening, these injuries can have dangerous consequences (e.g., a punctured lung). Pain from rib fractures often makes breathing difficult. In more severe fractures, especially in ribs high in the chest, respiratory failure can occur. This happens when the pain of breathing overwhelms the need to move air. Because of that pain, patients simply do not breathe deeply enough. These injuries can require intervention with positive pressure ventilation. Rib fractures can also lacerate adjoining blood vessels and damage underlying lung tissue.

flail chest
fracture of two or more adjacent ribs in two or more places that allows for free movement of the fractured segment.

One type of severe rib fracture is a condition known as ***flail chest*** (Figure 31-4). This condition is defined as a fracture of two or more consecutive ribs in two or more places. (Some sources say three or more ribs in two or more places.) The most important factor to remember—even more than the number of broken ribs—is that flail chest leaves a portion

FIGURE 31-4 Flail chest occurs when blunt trauma creates a fracture of two or more adjacent ribs in two or more places.

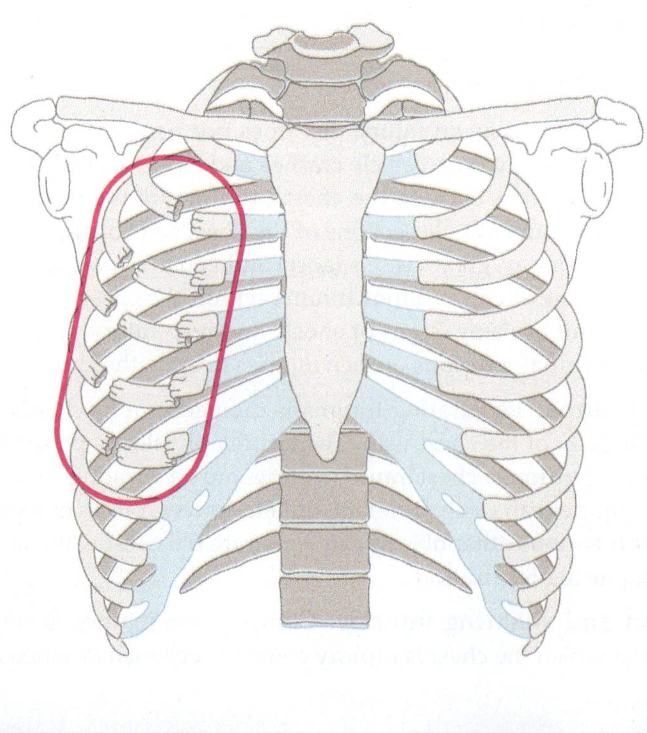

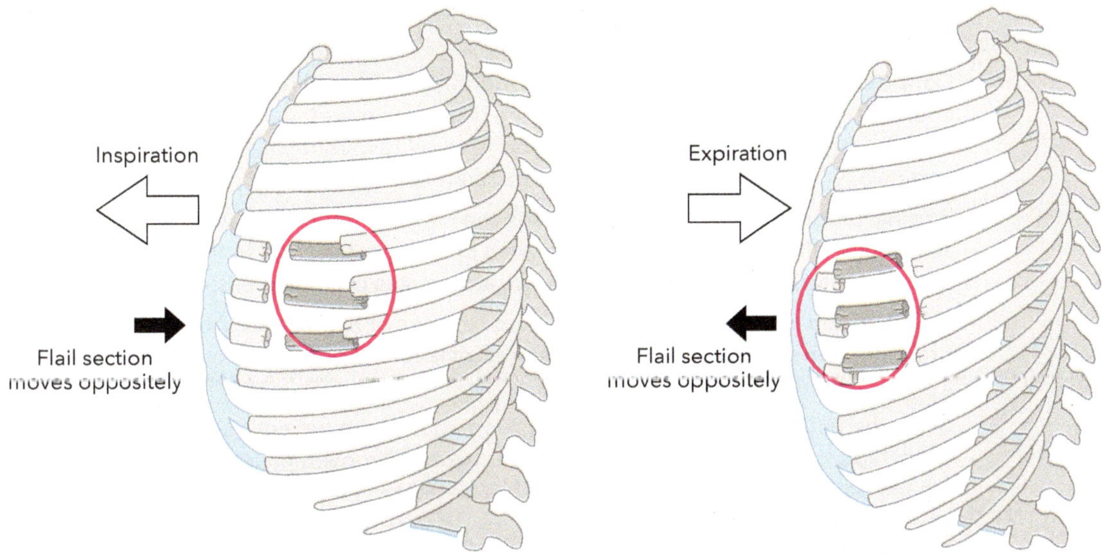

FIGURE 31-5 Paradoxical motion.

of the chest wall unstable, which impacts the mechanism of breathing and reduces lung expansion. This can lead to inadequate breathing and hypoventilation.

Because the flail segment is not attached, it is free to move independently. When the patient's chest expands to inhale, negative pressure draws air into the lungs. This negative pressure also draws the flail segment inward. When the patient's chest moves inward, positive pressure is created that pushes air out of the lungs, and this positive pressure also pushes the flail segment outward. Thus, the movement of the flail segment is opposite to the movement of the remainder of the chest cavity. This is called ***paradoxical motion*** (Figure 31-5).

paradoxical motion movement of ribs in a flail segment that is opposite to the direction of movement of the rest of the chest wall.

Patient Assessment

Rib Fracture

Rib fractures are most commonly identified by considering the mechanism of injury. Falls, sports injuries, and motor-vehicle crashes that cause blunt force trauma to the chest are likely culprits. The most common symptom of a rib fracture is pain at the site of injury. This pain will likely be increased with breathing. Patients with rib fractures may also complain of difficulty breathing. On examination, you will likely find tenderness in the injured area and you may observe redness, swelling, or bruising of the skin overlying the rib fracture. Respiratory distress, hypoxia, and even respiratory failure are fairly common. Patients with rib fractures will also frequently "self-splint," keeping an arm held tightly against their chest.

Flail Chest

The patient with flail chest will have a mechanism of injury capable of causing it, difficulty breathing, pain at the injury site, and likely signs of shock and hypoxia. Sometimes a flail chest will be obvious from the beginning, especially when a greater number of ribs are involved. At other times, the characteristic paradoxical motion may be difficult to observe in early stages, since the chest wall muscles will tighten and naturally splint the area. This muscle tightening, combined with efforts necessary to breathe, will eventually cause the patient to become fatigued. In turn, this can cause the flail segment to become more visible.

Patient Care

Care of the Patient with a Rib Fracture

Fundamental Principles of Care

Immediate care for chest injuries is aimed at maintaining the mechanism of breathing. A key element of all care will be to maintain oxygenation and ventilation.

Steps in caring for patients with rib fractures include the following:

- Consider the need for advanced life support (ALS). Often the most important intervention in a patient with a rib fracture is pain management. Taking away pain enables the patient to breathe easier and fend off respiratory failure. Call ALS early, particularly if there is any indication of respiratory impairment.
- If spinal precautions are not needed (see the chapter *Trauma to the Head, Neck, and Spine*), allow the patient to remain in a position of comfort. Most commonly, an upright seated position will be preferred, as it makes breathing easier.
- Treat hypoxia. If oxygen saturation is low or if signs of hypoxia are present, administer high-concentration oxygen. If respiratory failure is present, consider the need for positive pressure ventilation.
- Allow the patient to hold a pillow or cushion against the patient's chest. DO NOT strap, tape, or secure the pillow or restrict chest wall movement in any way. Allowing the patient to hold the pillow can make breathing more comfortable and aid as a basic pain management step.

Patient Care

Care of the Patient with a Flail Chest

Fundamental Principles of Care

The fundamental principles of treating a patient with a flail chest include maintaining oxygenation and ensuring ventilation. High-concentration oxygen should be administered to maintain an oxygen saturation of 95 percent. Do not restrict chest wall movement in any way. Consider ALS early for pain management. Transport immediately to an appropriate trauma destination. Steps to take in the care of a patient with flail chest follow:

- Perform a primary assessment. Flail segments should be identified as early in the assessment as possible, since they pose a threat to life.
- Administer high-concentration oxygen.
- If the patient is breathing inadequately, assist ventilations.
- Because maintaining positive thoracic pressure may reduce the degree of flail segment movement, some EMS systems allow the use of noninvasive positive pressure ventilation (NIPPV), such as CPAP, for patients with flail chest who have inadequate breathing. It is important to note that NIPPV can potentially worsen a collapsed lung (pneumothorax), which is often associated with a flail chest injury. If NIPPV is used in the trauma patient with a flail chest, careful monitoring for decompensation is mandatory. Follow your local protocols.
- Request ALS for pain management. (Remember that pain often reduces ventilation by causing the patient to limit chest wall movement.)
- Monitor the patient carefully.
- Watch the patient's respiratory rate and depth. If respirations become too shallow, assist ventilations with a bag-valve mask.
- Do not tape, pad, or in any way restrict chest wall movement, even if paradoxical movement is identified.

Penetrating Chest Injuries

Whenever the skin is broken, the patient has an open wound. However, the term *penetrating chest wound* implies that not only is the skin broken, but the chest wall is also penetrated, such as by a bullet or a knife blade (Figure 31-6).

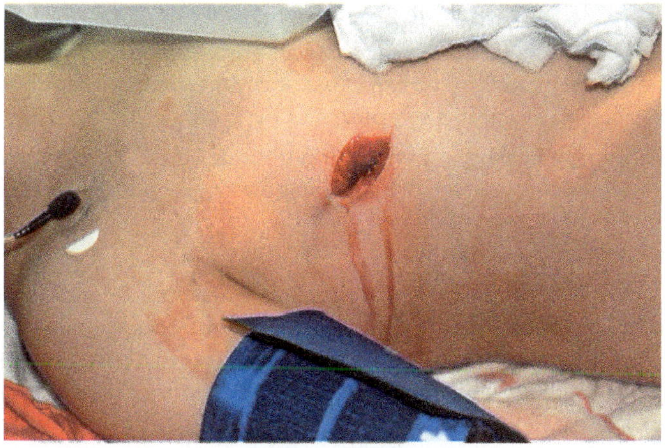

FIGURE 31-6 Child with knife wound in the chest. *(© David Effron, MD)*

An object can pass through the chest wall from the outside, or a fractured and displaced rib can penetrate the chest wall from within. The heart, lungs, and great vessels can be injured at the same time the chest wall is penetrated. Many penetrating injuries leave only small puncture wounds on the surface of the skin but can cause a lethal pathway of damage beneath the chest wall. In many cases, it can be difficult to tell if the chest cavity has been penetrated merely by looking at the wound.

You must consider all open wounds to the chest to be life-threatening wounds. Always presume any open wound on the chest wall penetrates into the chest cavity. Do not open the wound to determine its depth. An object producing such a wound may remain impaled in the chest, or the wound may be completely open.

When air enters the chest cavity through an open wound, the delicate pressure balance within the chest cavity is destroyed. This causes the lung on the injured side to collapse. (Injuries associated with air in the chest cavity are discussed in more detail in this chapter under the heading Injuries within the Chest Cavity.)

Patient Assessment

Penetrating Chest Trauma

Mechanism of injury will often point to penetrating chest trauma. The most frequent open chest wounds involve ballistic trauma such as knife and gunshot wounds. When assessing suspected penetrating chest trauma, it is helpful to consider the object that penetrated. For example, how big was the knife? What caliber was the bullet? How fast was the object traveling? You may not always be able to obtain this information, but when you can, these facts can help anticipate the pathway and severity of a penetrating wound.

Remember that penetrating wounds are not always visually dramatic. Consider the fact that a nine-millimeter bullet for the most part leaves only a nine-millimeter hole as it enters. Often you will need to look carefully for these injuries; if one is found, assume there are others. Although the concept of entry and exit wounds is frequently discussed in the context of gunshot wounds, there is little evidence to support the value of determining which hole is which. Rather, when two penetrating wounds are found, treat them simply as two penetrations of the chest. When mechanism of injury suggests penetrating trauma, be sure to visualize the entire chest (front, and sides) during your assessment. A quick scan to identify holes can be a life-saving step during the primary assessment, especially when life-threatening external hemorrhage is present. Consider also listening for the presence of lung sounds on both sides during the primary assessment in penetrating chest trauma. Although lung sounds are normally incorporated later in the physical exam, in penetrating trauma, a rapid evaluation of equality of lung sounds can help you immediately identify a potentially life-threatening pneumothorax or hemothorax, conditions that are best identified as early as possible to optimize patient survival.

Penetrating chest trauma is frequently accompanied by severe lung damage. This is frequently identified as difficulty breathing, absent or unequal lung sounds, coughing up blood (*hemoptysis*), and signs and symptoms of hypoxia.

Shock is also a common finding in penetrating trauma. Large thoracic blood vessels can be damaged, and the development of a tension pneumothorax can cause hypoperfusion. Beware tachycardia, tachypnea, pale skin, and low blood pressures, as they likely indicate serious injury within the chest cavity.

sucking chest wound a penetrating chest wound in which air is "sucked" into the chest cavity.

If a hole in the chest is large enough, the negative pressure of breathing can draw air in through the hole. This occasionally creates a dangerous condition known as a ***sucking chest wound***. The movement of air through a hole in the chest is a significant risk to the mechanism of breathing, and should be addressed immediately. The following signs indicate a sucking chest wound:

- The patient has a wound to the chest.
- There might or might not be the characteristic sucking sound associated with an open chest wound. There may simply be small air bubbles seen within the wound.
- The patient may be gasping for air.

Decision Points

- Does my patient have a chest injury that must be treated during the primary assessment?
- Does my patient have a penetrating chest injury that requires an occlusive dressing?
- Does my patient have an injury or injuries that require minimal scene time and prompt transport to a trauma center?

Patient Care

Care of the Patient with Penetrating Chest Trauma

Fundamental Principles of Care

The fundamental principles of care for a patient with penetrating chest trauma include maintaining oxygenation and ventilation. You should use the primary assessment to rapidly identify penetrating injuries. Any potentially open wound should be sealed immediately with an occlusive dressing. Administer high-concentration oxygen to maintain saturations between 94 and 95 percent. Request ALS early to address the potential for tension pneumothorax and rapidly transport to an appropriate trauma destination. Penetrating chest trauma is a *true emergency* that requires rapid initial care and immediate transport to an appropriate medical facility, ideally a trauma center.

For the patient with open chest trauma, follow these steps:

- Stay safe. Penetrating trauma is commonly caused by violence. Take care not to put yourself or your team in situations that make you vulnerable to similar trauma.
- Scenes involving penetrating trauma should be rendered safe and secure by law enforcement before EMS enters the scene.
- Consider the need for advanced life support. Penetrating trauma can cause a tension pneumothorax, a life-threatening condition that requires immediate intervention. ALS care can in some cases resolve this problem. Do not delay transport to wait for ALS. Consider intercept if ALS arrival is delayed. Remember also that in some cases, the hospital may be your nearest ALS.
- Maintain an open airway. Provide basic life support if necessary.
- Rapidly identify and seal any open chest wound as quickly as possible. If need be, use your gloved hand. Do not delay sealing the wound to find an occlusive dressing.
- Apply an occlusive dressing to seal any open chest wound. When possible, the dressing should be at least 2 inches (5 centimeters) wider than the wound. If there

are multiple penetrating wounds, apply occlusive dressings to them all. If commercial occlusive dressings are not available, or if you have more wounds than dressings, it may be reasonable to apply traditional gauze dressings in a best effort to cover and at least partially seal these wounds. Note that an occlusive dressing is preferred.

- If possible, allow the patient to remain in a position of comfort. Penetrating neck and chest trauma alone are not automatic indicators for spinal precautions. In many situations, laying a patient with penetrating chest trauma flat will significantly impair breathing and ultimately harm outcomes. There is no indication to perform spinal immobilization on a backboard in this situation unless the patient suffered blunt trauma as well (e.g., was shot, or fell off a roof and is now unconscious).
- Administer high-concentration oxygen.
- Treat for shock.
- Transport as soon as possible. Unless other injuries prevent you from doing so, keep the patient positioned on the injured side. This allows the uninjured lung to expand without restriction.

Occlusive and Flutter-Valve Dressings

The most important care for an open chest wound involves preventing air from entering the chest cavity. Most commonly, this involves sealing the wound with a dressing that stops any movement of air by creating a nonpermeable barrier. This type of dressing is called an occlusive dressing (Figure 31-7A). These dressings are commercially available and come in many forms. Some are simply airtight covers that physically block air movement, while others include a one-way valve to allow air to escape, but not to enter the wound. Occlusive dressings can also be improvised and can be created by using any airtight material. Most ambulances carry sterile disposable items that are wrapped in plastic. The inside surface of the plastic is sterile. If you do not have an occlusive dressing, use one of these wrappers or the wrapper from an IV bag. Keep in mind that household plastic wrap is generally not thick enough to make an effective occlusive dressing for a large open chest wound. If nothing else is available, plastic wrap can be folded several times to create the proper thickness. The military also has demonstrated that traditional bulky dressings, more commonly used for hemorrhage control, can be nearly as effective in preventing the movement of air. These should not take the place of specific occlusive dressings but may be used if better options are not available.

Some occlusive dressings have a one-way, or "flutter," valve designed to allow air to escape from the chest if pressure builds as a pneumothorax develops. In addition, some EMS systems suggest that if an occlusive dressing is improvised, it should be created by taping nonpermeable materials to the chest and leaving one side of the dressing untaped. It is suggested that this untaped side can mimic the effects of a flutter valve (Figure 31-7B). The importance of flutter (or exhalation) valves in occlusive dressings is debated among experts. While there is little evidence to demonstrate their effectiveness, the danger of a pneumothorax's developing into a tension pneumothorax (see the description of pneumothorax and tension pneumothorax under the heading Injuries within the Chest Cavity) is the reason medical authorities sometimes continue to recommend their use. Commercial devices, such as the Asherman Chest Seal™ (Figure 31-8), seal all the wound edges and have a valve that allows pressure relief.

You may have to maintain hand pressure over the occlusive dressing en route to the hospital. Also, the tape might not stick well to bloody skin or to skin that is sweaty from shock.

NOTE: *Once a chest wound is sealed, you must continue to monitor the patient and stay alert for complications. Even if you use a flutter valve or a commercial chest seal device, you still must monitor the patient for a buildup of pressure. Blood may accumulate under the dressing, or the dressing may be drawn into the wound, causing the valve to fail.*

FIGURE 31-7 (A) Occlusive dressing over a gunshot wound to the chest. (B) Creating a flutter valve to allow air to escape from the chest cavity.

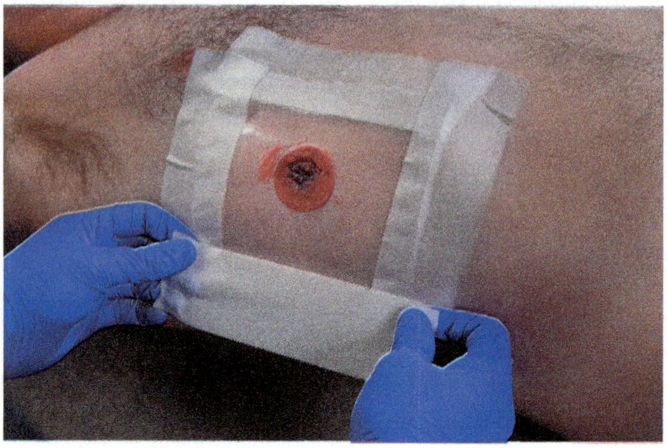

A

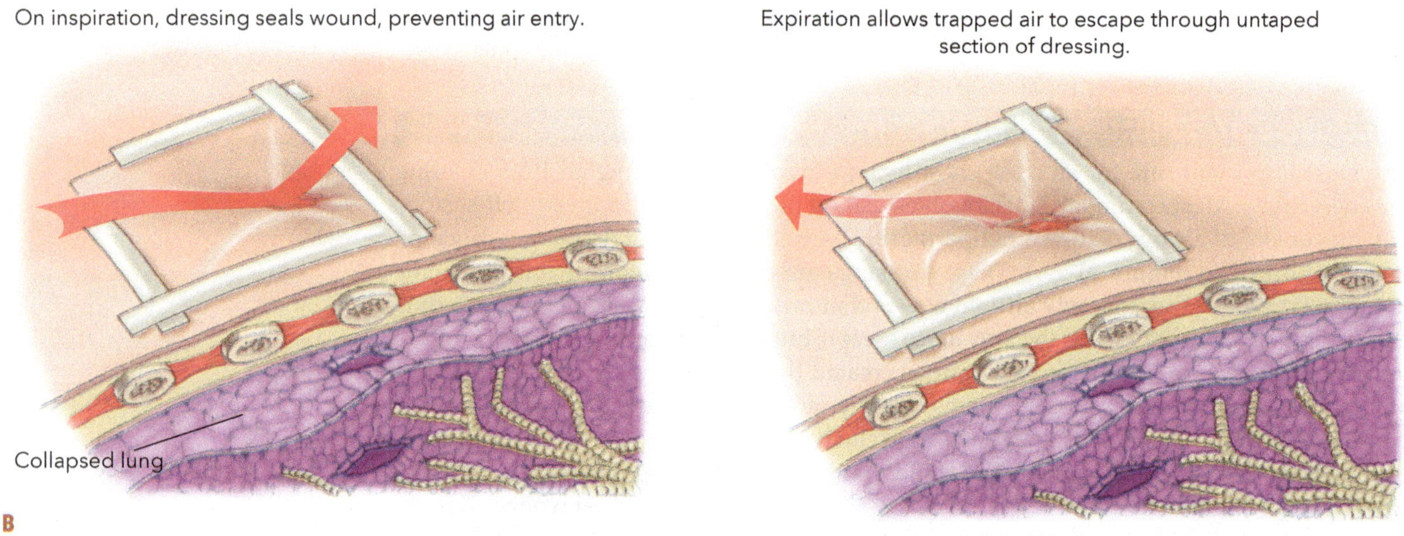

B

FIGURE 31-8 (A) An open chest wound from a gunshot. (B) An Asherman Chest Seal™ applied to the wound. *(Photos A and B: © Edward T. Dickinson, MD)*

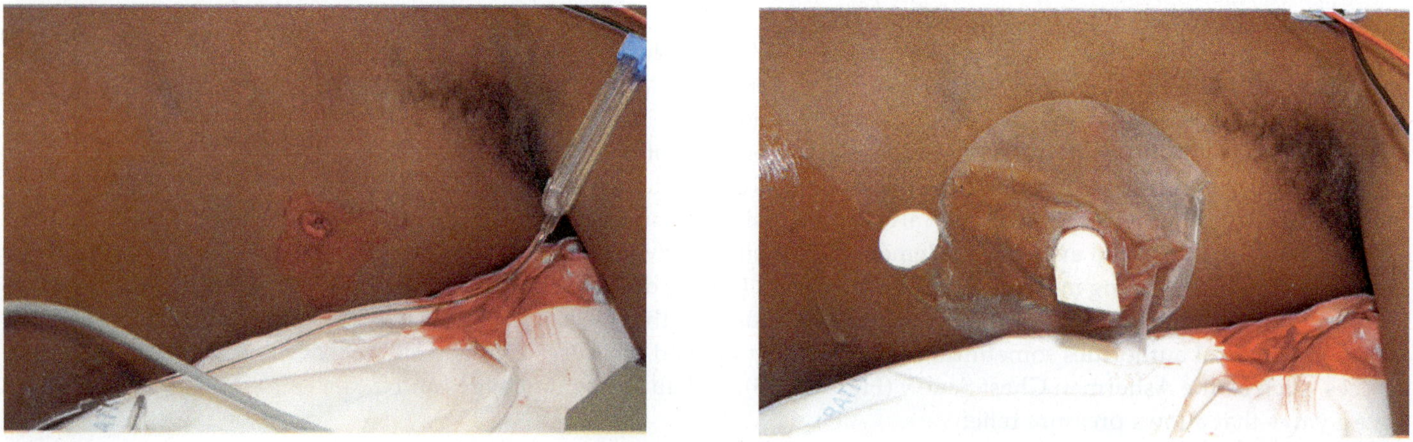

A B

Injuries within the Chest Cavity

Because each of the organs inside the chest cavity is vital to life, any chest injury has the potential to be serious. Since the blood vessels that run through the chest are the largest in the body, injury to these vessels is often fatal. In fact, the chest can hold more than 3 quarts

(3 liters) of blood. It is possible to bleed to death within the chest cavity and never spill a drop outside the body.

Since chest injuries have the potential to be serious—even fatal—it is important to describe some of the specific injuries that may occur within the chest cavity. The signs and symptoms of different chest injuries often overlap, so you may be able only to narrow the possibilities instead of determining the patient's exact problem. This is sufficient for you to assess and care for the patient effectively, as described at the end of this section.

- **Pneumothorax and tension pneumothorax.** ***Pneumothorax*** occurs when air accumulates in the potential space in the area where the lung tissue adheres to the chest wall. When air accumulates in this space, it pushes lung tissue away from the chest wall, causing collapse of the lung. Air can enter this space through an external wound (Figure 31-9) or through escape from a punctured lung. Occasionally both events may occur. ***Tension pneumothorax*** is especially critical. In this case, the buildup of air in the chest cavity becomes so severe that it puts pressure on the heart and vena cava. This pressure compresses the heart and prevents it from filling. It can also shift the position of the heart and blood vessels, causing a kinking effect of the vena cava. As a result, blood returning back to the heart can be significantly obstructed. These effects rapidly drop cardiac output and cause severe and abrupt shock.

  Patients with pneumothorax will typically have diminished or absent lung sounds on the affected side. As the pneumothorax progresses to a tension pneumothorax, the jugular veins in the neck may become distended (unless blood volume is low). Signs of shock will also be present. The trachea may shift to the opposite side, but this is a very late sign, and one which is difficult to detect.

pneumothorax
air in the chest cavity.

tension pneumothorax
a type of pneumothorax in which air accumulation puts pressure on the heart and vena cava and causes shock.

- **Hemothorax and hemopneumothorax.** *Hemothorax* is a condition in which the chest cavity fills with blood. With *hemopneumothorax*, the chest cavity fills with both blood and air. It is easy to distinguish between these two complications with pneumothorax if you remember that *pneumo* means "air" and *hemo* means "blood." In pneumothorax, there is a buildup of air in the thorax. In hemothorax and hemopneumothorax, blood creates or adds to the pressure (Figure 31-10).

  Hemothorax can be caused when lacerations within the chest cavity are produced by penetrating objects or fractured ribs. Blood will flow into the space around the lung, the lung may collapse, and the patient will experience a loss of blood, leading to shock. Hemopneumothorax involves a combination of blood and air that usually produces the same results: a collapsed lung and loss of blood, leading to shock. Patients with hemothorax will often present with signs of shock.

- **Traumatic asphyxia.** Traumatic asphyxia is associated with sudden compression of the chest. When this occurs, the sternum and the ribs exert severe pressure on the

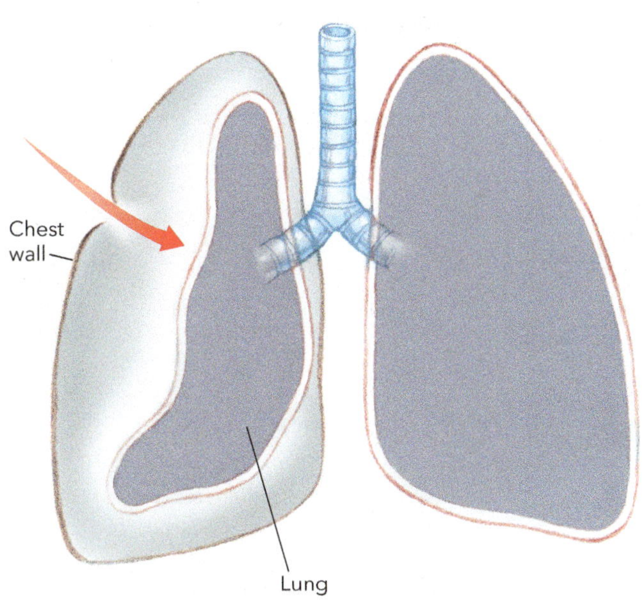

FIGURE 31-9 Air can enter the chest cavity through a puncture in the chest wall. This can cause the collapse of a lung and impaired breathing.

FIGURE 31-10 Pneumothorax, hemothorax, and hemopneumothorax.

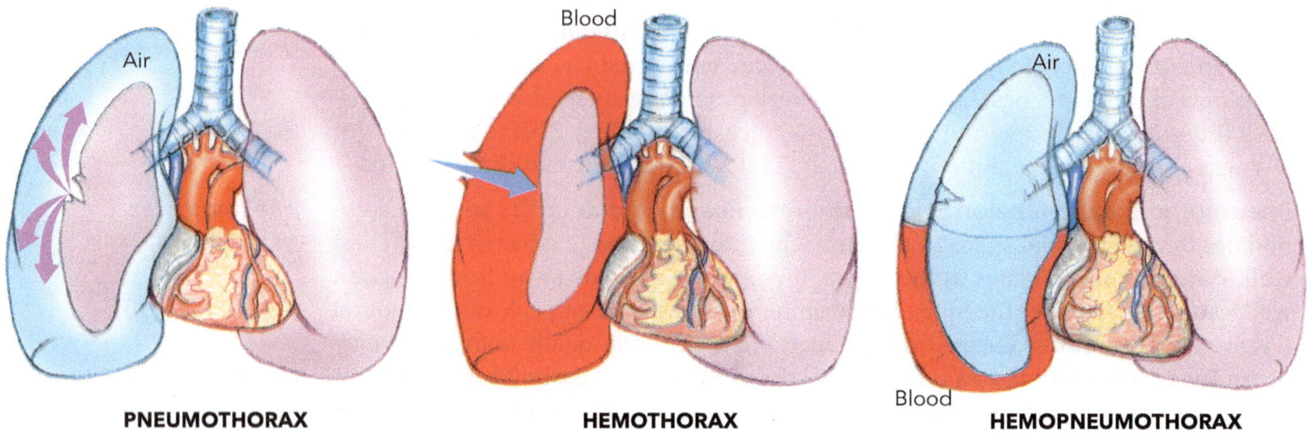

heart and lungs, forcing blood out of the right atrium and up into the jugular veins in the neck. The pressure of the blood being forced into the head and neck will usually result in blood vessels in and near the skin rupturing, causing extensive bruising of the face and neck (Figure 31-11).

Patients with traumatic asphyxia present with a mechanism of injury that can cause compression of the chest. The patient's neck and face will be a darker color (red, purple, or blue) than the rest of the body. Depending on the amount of pressure and how long the pressure was exerted on the torso, the patient may also have bulging eyes, distended neck veins, and broken blood vessels in the face.

- **Cardiac tamponade.** When an injury to the heart causes blood to flow into the surrounding pericardial sac and to compress the heart, the condition produced is cardiac tamponade. The heart's unyielding sac fills with blood and compresses the chambers of the heart to a point where they will no longer adequately fill, backing up blood into the veins. This is usually the result of penetrating trauma, such as a stab wound. The pericardium is very tough, with limited ability to quickly stretch.

  Patients who experience cardiac tamponade will usually have distended neck veins because blood cannot return to the right atrium as normal due to built-up pressure in the heart. The patient will also exhibit signs of shock. A finding commonly associated with tamponade is narrowed pulse pressure. Narrowed pulse pressure is a trend where the difference between the systolic blood pressure and the diastolic blood pressure becomes smaller over time. An additional finding that occasionally can be identified in the prehospital setting is muffled heart sounds. Although listening to heart sounds is beyond the scope of practice of EMTs, the fluid and pressure built up around the heart

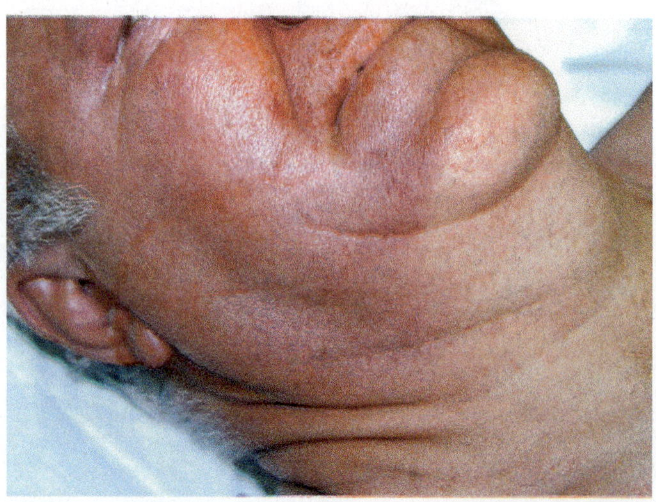

FIGURE 31-11 A patient suffering traumatic asphyxia. *(© Edward T. Dickinson, MD)*

can significantly change the normal sounds detectable by a stethoscope. In fact, the findings of distended neck veins, muffled heart sounds, and narrowing pulse pressure (sometimes listed as dropping blood pressure) are commonly known as *Beck's triad*, and are a well-known pattern frequently associated with tamponade.

- **Aortic injury.** Trauma can also cause injury to the aorta, the largest artery in the body. Damage to this large, high-pressure vessel causes massive bleeding that is often fatal. Penetrating trauma can cause direct damage to the aorta. Blunt trauma and shearing force, such as sudden deceleration from a severe motor-vehicle collision (e.g., head-on), can sever or tear the aorta.

The aorta can also be damaged without trauma in the medical patient. Degeneration of the aorta, often worsened by high blood pressure or other diseases, causes weakening of this large vessel. Aortic dissection is a condition where the inner layer of the wall of the aorta begins to tear. Aortic dissections most commonly occur in the chest. Blood from the interior of the vessel leaks into the outer layers, causing blood to flow between the layers of the aorta's wall, rather than down the lumen of the aorta. Aortic dissections, especially those involving the ascending aorta and the arch where major vessels branch off, are rapidly fatal without immediate treatment.

The wall of the aorta may also develop weakness that results in a balloon-like protrusion, called an *aneurysm*. This is most commonly seen in smokers and those with chronic high blood pressure. As pressure builds in the aneurysm, it expands in size and there is an increased risk of rupture, leading to the patient's death. The aorta runs from the left ventricle through the chest and abdomen, and aneurysms can occur anywhere along its path. In thin patients or those with a large aneurysm in the abdomen, the aneurysm may occasionally be palpated. Other than routine abdominal palpation, however, you should not probe the abdomen specifically for aneurysms, as it may cause injury to the patient, such as rupture of the aorta.

The patient with an aortic injury may complain of pain in the chest, abdomen, or back, depending on the injury's location. The patient will often exhibit signs of shock. The patient may have differences in pulse or blood pressure between the right and left arms (in proximal aortic injury) or differences in pulses between the arms and the legs, or between the legs themselves.

Commotio cordis is an uncommon condition that is easy to recognize and treat. When someone gets hit in the center of the chest, the result is usually a bruise or even perhaps a fracture. In *commotio cordis* (Latin for *commotion* or *disturbance of the heart*), however, the impact occurs just when the heart is electrically vulnerable. There are several hundredths of a second during each heartbeat when the heart, if sufficiently stimulated, will go into ventricular fibrillation (VF). A patient in *commotio cordis* experiences this condition. An example of this is the young athlete who tries to catch a baseball but misses. The ball strikes him in the center of the chest, and the patient can collapse in cardiac arrest.

If you obtain a history like this, treat the patient like any other patient in ventricular fibrillation. Do *not* treat the patient as a trauma patient, and do not delay defibrillation because of the concern about internal blood loss. If the patient receives defibrillation and CPR quickly enough, the patient has a very good chance of a full, neurologically intact survival and usually has a very healthy heart that will respond well to CPR and defibrillation.

Patient Assessment

Injuries within the Chest Cavity

The following are common signs of pneumothorax:

- Respiratory difficulty
- Uneven chest wall movement
- Reduction or absence of breath sounds on the affected side of the chest (Listen with a stethoscope.)

Signs of tension pneumothorax include those items discussed above and:

- Increasing respiratory difficulty and signs of hypoxia, including cyanosis
- Indications of developing shock, including rapid, weak pulse and low blood pressure due to decreased cardiac output
- Distended neck veins (unless the patient is hypovolemic)
- Tracheal deviation to the uninjured side (which is a late sign and difficult to observe)

The following sign may commonly indicate a hemothorax:

- Signs of pneumothorax plus coughed-up frothy red blood

The following are common potential signs of traumatic asphyxia:

- Distended neck veins
- Head, neck, and shoulders appearing dark blue or purple
- Bloodshot and bulging eyes
- Swollen and blue tongue and lips
- Chest deformity or tenderness

The following are common signs of cardiac tamponade:

- Distended neck veins
- Very weak pulse
- Low blood pressure
- Steadily decreasing pulse pressure (Pulse pressure is the difference between systolic and diastolic readings.)

The following are common signs of aortic injury or dissection:

- Tearing chest pain radiating to the back
- Differences in pulse or blood pressure between the right and left extremities or between the arms and legs
- A palpable pulsating mass (in the case of abdominal aortic aneurysm)
- Cardiac arrest

Patient Care

Care of the Patient with a Pneumothorax or Tension Pneumothorax

Fundamental Principles of Care

A tension pneumothorax is a life-threatening problem and must be dealt with immediately. Although the most important care may be to reach ALS or a hospital quickly, EMTs must rapidly identify the possibility of a tension pneumothorax and move quickly to enable definitive care.

Take the following steps when caring for a patient with a pneumothorax or tension pneumothorax:

- Contact advanced life support. If ALS will be delayed, consider intercepting them en route, and remember that occasionally the hospital is the closest ALS.
- Seal all open chest wounds with an occlusive dressing.
- If signs of a tension pneumothorax develop, consider opening the occlusive dressing to allow air to be expelled. If a flutter valve is present, check to be sure the valve is not clogged. (Note: Not all tension pneumothoraxes will be relieved by opening a dressing. In fact, most develop internally, regardless of the condition or placement of an occlusive dressing).
- Manage the patient's airway if necessary, and administer supplemental oxygen to treat hypoxia.
- If possible, allow the patient to remain in the position of comfort.

Care of the Patient with Other Injuries within the Chest Cavity

Fundamental Principles of Care

Treating chest injuries is about anticipating problems. Although a significant injury like a pneumothorax may not be present, you should still anticipate breathing problems and potential internal bleeding. In undifferentiated situations, care will focus on these areas.

The treatment is the same for all of the previously noted types of injuries within the chest cavity:

- Maintain an open airway. Be prepared to apply suction.
- Administer supplemental oxygen to treat hypoxia.
- Follow local protocols as to the preferred type of dressing for any open wound.
- Care for shock.
- Transport as soon as possible.
- Consider ALS intercept if it will not delay the patient's arrival at the hospital. ALS personnel can perform procedures such as chest decompression that can greatly benefit a patient suffering from certain chest injury complications.

Abdominal Injuries

CORE CONCEPT
Understanding abdominal injuries and emergency care for abdominal injuries

Like chest injuries, abdominal wounds can be either open or closed. In closed wounds, the abdominal wall is intact and unpenetrated. In an open abdominal wound, a penetration has occurred. Most closed abdominal wounds are caused by blunt trauma. Penetrating injuries typically result from ballistic trauma such as bullets and other high-energy penetrations, as well as from hand-driven or other low energy penetrations such as knives. The most serious concern with abdominal injuries is the potential for massive internal hemorrhage and shock. Solid organs like the liver, spleen, and kidneys each have a rich blood flow, and when damage occurs, the bleeding can be severe. Hollow organs in the abdomen pose a risk of rupture when trauma occurs. If these organs are damaged, their contents can be spilled into the abdominal cavity, creating a high risk for infection. Open wounds of the abdomen may be so large and deep that organs protrude through the wound opening. This is known as an ***evisceration*** (Figure 31-12).

evisceration (e-vis-er-AY-shun) an intestine or other internal organ protruding through a wound in the abdomen.

A more common condition than an evisceration is blunt trauma to one or more abdominal organs. The liver is the most commonly injured organ because of its relatively large size and its position in the right upper quadrant, under the lowermost ribs on the right side. The liver is very vascular; therefore, when it is injured, it can bleed profusely, often to the point of life-threatening blood loss. Another very vascular organ is the spleen, located in the left upper quadrant and under the lowermost ribs on the left. Like the liver, the spleen can produce life-threatening blood loss.

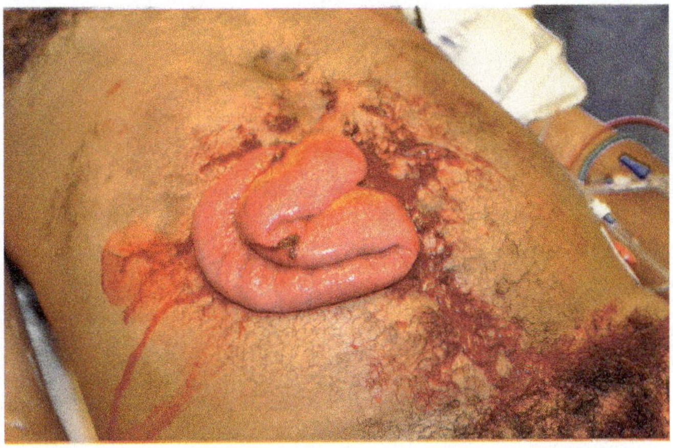

FIGURE 31-12 An abdominal evisceration from a stab wound. *(© Edward T. Dickinson, MD)*

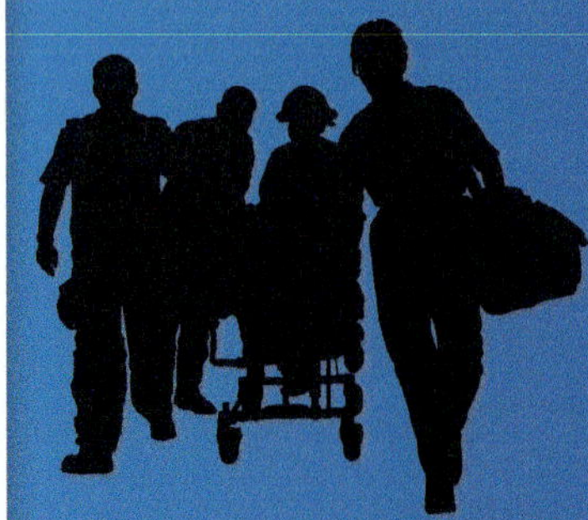

Think Like an EMT

What's the Likely Cause?

For each of the following patient presentations, determine what you believe is the likely cause:

1. You are called to a man who was jogging when he suddenly had a sharp pain in his right chest. He has difficulty breathing but is oriented, and he is in pain that changes when he breathes. He has diminished lung sounds in the upper right chest.
2. Your patient was stabbed in the right side of her chest. She is hypotensive, has distended neck veins, has no lung sounds on the right side of her chest, and has diminished sounds on the left side of her chest.
3. Your patient was shot in the chest near the fourth intercostal space on the left side. He has hypotension, distended neck veins, narrowing pulse pressure, and adequate lung sounds on both sides of the chest.

The diaphragm is occasionally injured, from either blunt trauma or penetrating trauma. If there is a sudden severe force applied to the abdomen, that pressure can be posteriorly and superiorly transmitted. This pressure can be so great that the diaphragm partially detaches, allowing abdominal contents to enter the thoracic cavity. A penetrating injury such as a stab wound can also injure the diaphragm. If the resulting wound is significant, abdominal contents can enter the thoracic cavity in this manner too.

Hollow organs in the abdomen include the stomach, small and large bowels, gallbladder, and urinary bladder. If these organs are injured, they often spill their contents into the abdominal cavity, leading to severe irritation and often peritonitis. This can cause the abdominal muscles to involuntarily contract, leading to rigidity of the abdominal wall.

Retroperitoneal organs, located in the posterior abdomen, are less commonly injured than are the organs inside the peritoneal cavity. The pancreas, for instance, lies across the spine. Unless a knife or bullet hits it or there is significant force to the center of the abdomen, this organ is rarely injured. The kidneys are also retroperitoneal, with protection from the muscles of the back and the lower ribs that cover their superior portion. If a kidney is injured, it is usually from a direct blow.

Information on abdominal emergencies from medical causes may be found in the chapter *Abdominal Emergencies*.

Point of View

"I was bringing in a patient with an altered mental status from a nursing home when our medical director called me over to one of the big trauma bays. She asked me if I had ever seen an evisceration. I said, 'You mean . . . ' and she smiled and motioned me inside. I am a pretty new EMT. I'm glad I saw it there at the hospital before I saw it on the street. It was like amazing and gross at the same time. She showed me how delicate the tissue is and why we handle the exposed organs gently. You certainly don't see that all the time."

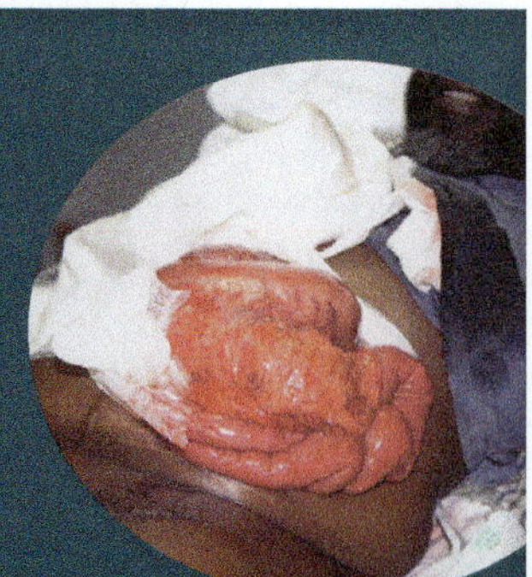

(© Edward T. Dickinson, MD)

Patient Assessment

Abdominal Injury

Gunshot wounds can cause serious abdominal damage. A misconception about bullet wounds is that internal damage can be easily assessed. On the contrary, any projectile entering the body can be deflected, or it can explode and send out pieces in many directions (Figure 31-13). Do not believe that only the structures directly under the entrance wound have been injured. Also, keep in mind that the bullet's pathway between the entrance wound and exit wound is seldom a straight line.

Further complicating the problem, penetrating abdominal wounds can be associated with wounds in adjacent areas of the body. For example, a bullet can enter the chest cavity, pierce the diaphragm, and cause widespread damage in the abdomen. A complete patient assessment is essential in determining the probable extent of injuries. Always assess for an exit wound.

The following are some common signs and symptoms of abdominal injury:

- Pain, often starting as mild pain and then rapidly becoming intolerable
- Cramps
- Nausea
- Weakness
- Thirst
- Obvious lacerations and puncture wounds to the abdomen
- Lacerations and puncture wounds to the pelvis and middle and lower back, or chest wounds near the diaphragm
- Indications of blunt trauma, such as a large bruised area or an intense bruise on the abdomen
- Indications of developing shock, including restlessness; pale, cool, and clammy skin; rapid, shallow breathing; a rapid pulse; and low blood pressure (Sometimes patients with abdominal injuries who are in extreme pain show an initial elevated blood pressure.)
- Coughing up or vomiting blood; the vomitus may contain a substance that looks like coffee grounds (partially digested blood)
- Rigid and/or tender abdomen, which the patient tries to protect (guarded abdomen)
- Distended abdomen
- A patient who tries to lie very still, with the legs drawn up, in an effort to reduce the tension on the abdominal muscles

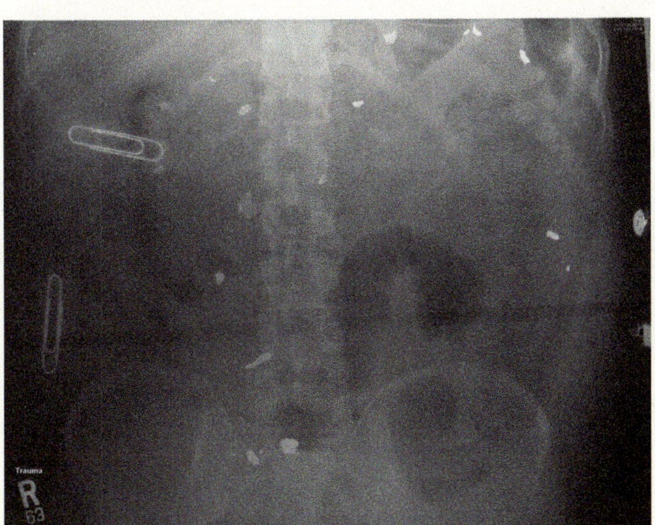

FIGURE 31-13 X-ray showing two bullets that entered the patient's abdomen on the right side (at the paper clips) and then fragmented throughout the abdomen. *(© Edward T. Dickinson, MD)*

Decision Points

- Does the patient have an abdominal injury that must be treated during the primary assessment?
- Does the patient have an open abdominal injury that requires an occlusive dressing?
- Does the patient have an injury or injuries that require minimal scene time and prompt transport to a trauma center?

The Path of the Bullet

A patient who has gunshot wounds in the lower ribs and at the same level in the back may appear to have a chest wound. In reality, you need to treat such patients for both a chest wound and an abdominal wound. It is obvious that the bullet may have penetrated the lung, but since the spleen and liver are posterior to the lowermost left and right ribs, you must assume they may have been injured at the same time. If a patient was inhaling deeply when shot (resulting in the abdominal organs' taking up less space in the chest), the spleen and liver might not have been in the direct path of the bullet. But bullets often take paths that are not straight. If the bullet tumbled or produced cavitation, the spleen or liver may very well have sustained serious injury. You will need to be alert to the possibility of both chest and abdominal injuries.

Patient Care

Care of the Patient with Abdominal Injury

Fundamental Principles of Care

Some emergency care steps apply to both closed and open abdominal injuries. However, other additional care steps are necessary for open abdominal injuries.

For both closed and open abdominal injuries:

- Stay alert for vomiting and keep the airway open.
- Place the patient on the back, legs flexed at the knees, to reduce pain by relaxing abdominal muscles.
- Administer supplemental oxygen to treat hypoxia.
- Treat for shock.
- Give nothing to the patient by mouth. This could induce vomiting or pass through open wounds in the esophagus, stomach, or intestine and enter the abdominal cavity.
- Constantly monitor vital signs.
- Transport as soon as possible.

Additional steps for open abdominal injuries:

- Control external bleeding and dress all open wounds.
- Do not touch or try to replace any eviscerated, or exposed, organs. Apply a sterile dressing moistened with sterile saline over the wound site. Some EMS systems may recommend that you apply an occlusive dressing as well. It may be necessary to remoisten the dressings with additional saline to ensure that the eviscerated organ or organs do not dry out. In cases of large eviscerations, maintain warmth by placing layers of bulky dressing over the moistened dressing (Scan 31-1).
- Do not remove any impaled objects. Stabilize impaled objects with bulky dressings that are bandaged in place (see the chapter *Soft-Tissue Trauma).* Leave the patient's legs in the position in which you found them, to avoid muscular movement that may move the impaled object.

NOTE: *Do not use aluminum foil as an occlusive dressing. Foil has been known to cut eviscerated organs.*

SCAN 31-1 Dressing an Open Abdominal Wound

First Take Standard Precautions.

Perform a scene size-up and use Standard Precautions.

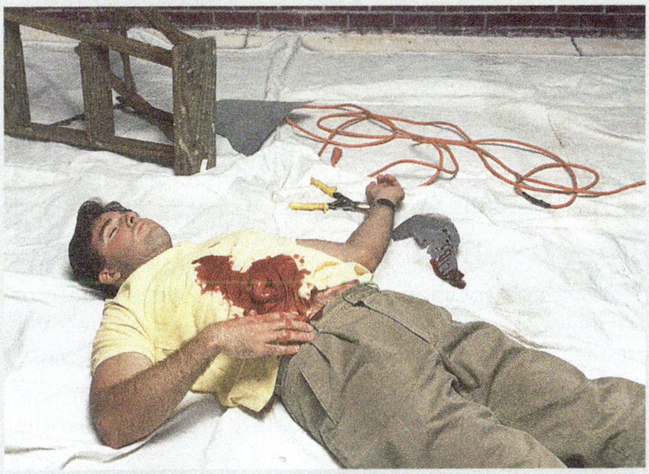

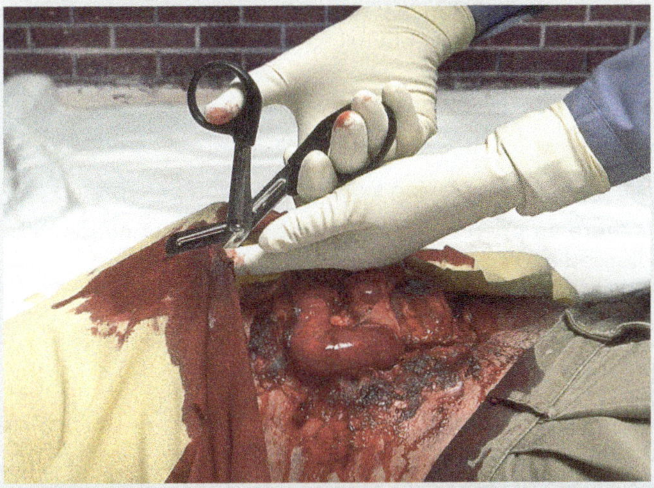

Open abdominal wound with evisceration.

1. Cut away clothing from the wound.

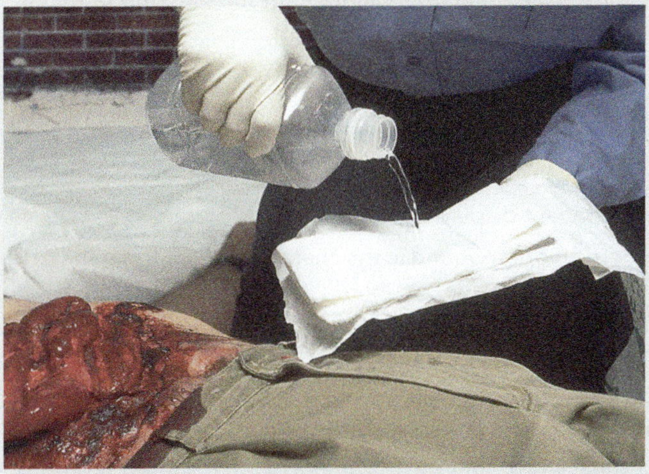

2. Soak a sterile dressing with sterile saline.

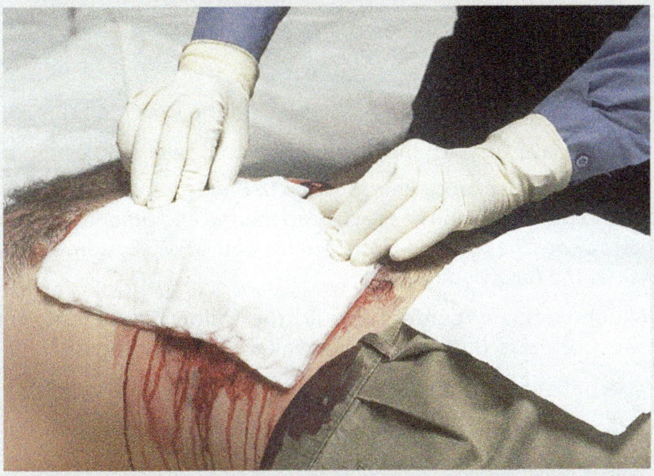

3. Place the moist dressing over the wound. It may be necessary to remoisten the dressing with additional sterile saline to keep the eviscerated organ or organs from drying out.

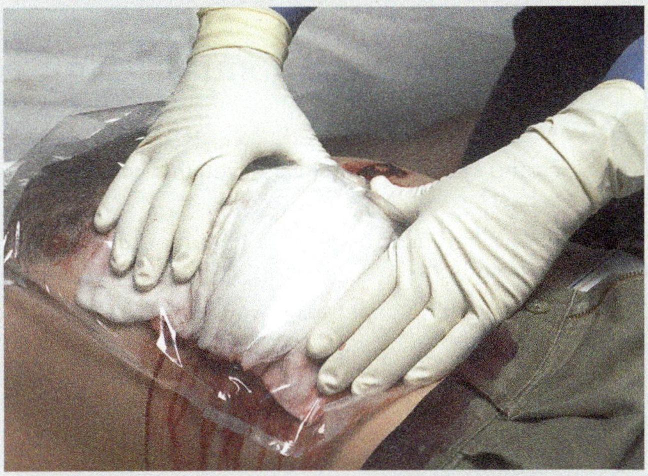

4. Apply an occlusive dressing over the moist dressing if your local protocols recommend taking this action Cover the dressed wound to maintain warmth. Secure the covering with tape or cravats tied above and below the position of the exposed organ.

Chapter Review

Key Facts and Concepts

- An open chest or abdominal wound is considered to be one that penetrates not only the skin but also the chest or abdominal wall to expose internal organs. Open chest and abdominal wounds are life-threatening. For both open and closed injuries, take appropriate Standard Precautions, note the mechanism of injury, protect the patient's airway and breathing, treat for shock, and transport. If there are signs of hypoxia, or the patient's vital signs indicate or suggest the potential for shock, administer oxygen.
- A flail chest can be characterized by paradoxical motion. If the patient is unable to adequately breathe, assist the patient's ventilations.
- Seal a penetrating chest wound with an occlusive dressing. Monitor the patient for changes, and be prepared to manually relieve any pressure in the chest.
- Closed chest wounds are sometimes difficult to distinguish or may occur together. Assess the patient, including breath sounds, and maintain ventilation, oxygenation, and perfusion.
- A patient who collapses in cardiac arrest after a force is applied to the center of the chest should receive CPR and defibrillation like any other patient in arrest from a cardiac cause.
- If a patient develops signs of a tension pneumothorax, arrange immediately for an ALS intercept or transport promptly to a facility that can treat this injury.
- When solid abdominal organs are injured, life-threatening amounts of blood loss can occur.
- When hollow abdominal organs are injured, their contents can spill into the abdominal cavity and cause irritation and peritonitis.

Key Decisions

- Is the patient's breathing adequate, inadequate, or absent?
- Is the patient displaying signs of shock?
- Is there an open wound in the chest that needs to be sealed?
- Is the patient displaying signs of a tension pneumothorax?
- Is there an open wound in the abdomen that needs to be dressed and covered?

Chapter Glossary

evisceration (e-vis-er-AY-shun) an intestine or other internal organ protruding through a wound in the abdomen.

flail chest fracture of two or more adjacent ribs in two or more places that allows for free movement of the fractured segment.

paradoxical motion movement of ribs in a flail segment that is opposite to the direction of movement of the rest of the chest cavity.

pneumothorax air in the chest cavity.

sucking chest wound an open chest wound in which air is "sucked" into the chest cavity.

tension pneumothorax a type of pneumothorax in which air that enters the chest cavity is prevented from escaping.

Preparation for Your Examination and Practice

Short Answer

1. What signs and symptoms would alert you that your patient has a flail chest?
2. What are the differences between a pneumothorax and a tension pneumothorax?
3. Describe the care for a penetrating wound to the chest.
4. Describe the care for an open abdominal wound.

Thinking and Linking

Think back to the chapter titled Well-Being of the EMT *as you consider the following question:*

- Which Standard Precautions are required for the following calls?
  a. An open wound in the chest that makes a sucking noise when the patient breathes
  b. A patient with paradoxical motion in the lower left ribs
  c. An evisceration of the abdomen with bowel visible

Think back to the chapter Introduction to Emergency Medical Services *and the discussion of specialized trauma and other treatment centers under the heading* Components of the EMS System *as you consider the following question:*

- Which specialty centers should the following patients be transported to (if the center is available in your region)?
  a. A patient with a collapsed lung
  b. A patient with suspected internal bleeding and trauma

Critical Thinking Exercises

Chest trauma can be difficult to assess and treat in the emergency setting. The purpose of this exercise will be to consider assessment and care for one severe chest injury.

- You have been caring for a patient who was shot in the chest with a nail gun, and you have applied an occlusive dressing around the wound. The patient is suddenly beginning to deteriorate. He is having extreme difficulty breathing, and his color has worsened. Breath sounds have become almost totally absent on the side with the impaled nail. What complication might you suspect is causing his worsening condition? How could this be corrected?

Pathophysiology to Practice

The following questions are designed to assist you in gathering relevant clinical information and making accurate decisions in the field.

1. Your patient, who sustained a blunt injury to the chest, is starting to have more difficulty breathing, and her respirations are not as deep as they were when you arrived. What factors should you consider in deciding whether to ventilate her? What condition might you cause if you ventilate her?
2. A 64-year-old male is tachycardic, pale, sweaty, and hypotensive. The only injury he has sustained was when he fell two days ago and struck his lower left ribs hard on some furniture. He hasn't been feeling well since then, and today he felt much worse. What injured organ is most likely the cause of his condition? Why did it take so long for the patient to develop shock?

Street Scenes

At the scene of a collision between two cars at an intersection, you find a 30-year-old male who was the driver of the car that was hit on the driver's door. He is able to tell you that his chest hurts "very bad" and that he has slight difficulty breathing. His skin is slightly pale and sweaty, he answers questions appropriately, and he is holding his arm across his lower chest.

Street Scene Questions

1. What is your general impression of this patient?
2. What priority would you assign to him?
3. What interventions are appropriate at this time?

Your general impression is of a 30-year-old male who appears to be injured. Your primary assessment reveals normal mental status, an open airway, slightly labored but adequate breathing, and a weak, rapid radial pulse, with no external bleeding visible. You assign him a high priority for now, with the understanding that you may change his priority later.

You apply a cervical collar and begin administering oxygen by nonrebreather mask. You also coordinate extrication activities with the fire department on the scene.

Assessment of the patient reveals significant tenderness over the middle ribs on the left side. Breath sounds are difficult to hear because of the noise of the extrication equipment. His upper abdomen on the left side is a little tender but not guarded or rigid.

Street Scene Questions

4. Would you change the priority of transport of this patient based on what you now know? Why or why not?
5. What interventions are appropriate for this patient?

You decide this patient is still a high priority because he is at high risk for internal bleeding in the chest, the abdomen, or both. You would like to get him out of the car as soon as possible because one of the most important interventions is prompt transport to a hospital capable of taking care of a serious trauma patient. If advanced life support is available, you will call for it. You continue administration of oxygen by nonrebreather mask and monitor the patient for signs of fatigue that might indicate a need for assisted ventilations.

Your partner obtains a pulse of 116, blood pressure 110/80, and respirations 22 and shallow. His oxygen saturation is 99 percent.

As soon as the patient is free from entanglement in the wreckage, you perform a rapid extrication and get him onto a backboard. En route to the hospital, you reevaluate the patient and find that although you have found no new injuries, his chest pain is getting worse and he is having more difficulty breathing. As you approach the hospital, you observe that his respirations are becoming shallower. They are still adequate by the time you arrive at the emergency department, but you can see a clear trend in the patient's condition that will require treatment soon.

You advise the trauma team of your observations as you give your report and turn over care of the patient.

32

Musculoskeletal Trauma

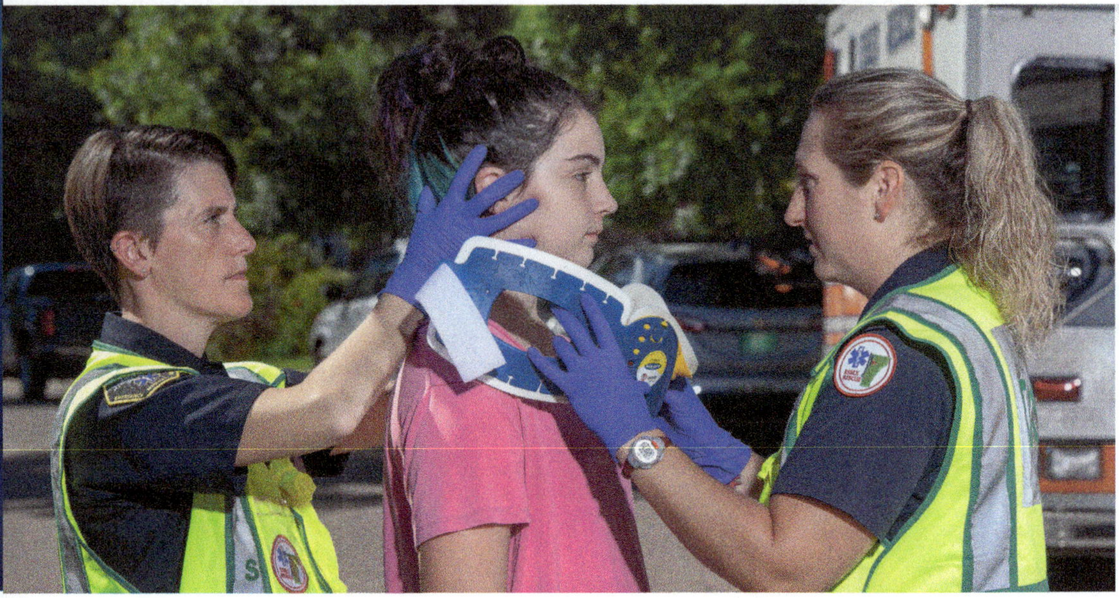

Related Chapters

The following chapters provide additional information related to topics discussed in this chapter:

15 Secondary Assessment

29 Bleeding and Shock

Standard

Trauma (Orthopedic Trauma)

Competency

Applies fundamental knowledge to provide basic emergency care and transportation based on assessment findings for an acutely injured patient.

Core Concepts

- Knowledge of bones, muscles, and other elements of the musculoskeletal system
- Knowledge of general guidelines for emergency care of musculoskeletal injuries
- Purposes and general procedures for splinting
- Assessment and care of specific injuries to the upper and lower extremities

Outcomes

After reading this chapter, you should be able to:

32.1 Summarize concepts of the musculoskeletal system. (pp. 894–904)

- Describe the functions of the musculoskeletal system.
- Identify the anatomy of bone.
- Relate the nature of bones as living tissue to the implications of skeletal injury.
- Describe the function of joints.
- Identify each of the bones of the skeletal system.
- Apply knowledge of the forces that produce musculoskeletal injuries to the anticipation of specific patterns of injury.
- Identify fractures with high potential for emergency complications.
- Distinguish the anatomy and physiology of muscles, cartilages, ligaments, and tendons.
- Relate the anatomy of musculoskeletal injuries to the potential for underlying organ injury.
- Match different types of musculoskeletal injuries to their descriptions.
- Relate the anatomy and physiology structures adjacent to bone to complications of musculoskeletal injury.

32.2 Summarize the management decisions required in the care of patients with musculoskeletal injuries. (pp. 904–943)

- Outline the general assessment findings associated with musculoskeletal injuries.
- Relate specific findings to the potential for specific types of musculoskeletal injuries.
- Explain the importance of serial checks of the distal circulation, sensation, and motor function (CSM) in the care of extremity injuries.
- Explain how to prioritize steps in caring for patients with musculoskeletal injuries.
- Explain how and when traction may be used in caring for patients with musculoskeletal injuries.
- Recognize the signs of compartment syndrome.
- Describe the role of splinting in managing musculoskeletal injuries.
- Identify the principles of splinting musculoskeletal injuries.
- Associate musculoskeletal injuries with the most appropriate type of splint.
- Explain how to make transport decisions by placing musculoskeletal injuries in the overall context of the patient's condition.

Key Terms

angulated fracture, *903*
bones, *894*
cartilage, *899*
closed extremity injury, *904*
comminuted fracture, *903*
compartment syndrome, *905*
crepitus, *906*
dislocation, *904*
extremities, *894*
fracture, *903*
greenstick fracture, *903*
joints, *894*
ligaments, *901*

manual traction, *909*	sprain, *904*	tendons, *901*
muscles, *899*	strain, *904*	traction splint, *903*
open extremity injury, *904*		

Musculoskeletal injuries are common. As an EMT, you will be called upon to treat injuries to muscles and bones which range from minor to life-threatening. Many musculoskeletal injuries can have a grotesque appearance. When called upon to fully evaluate the patient, do not be distracted from life-threatening conditions by a deformed limb.

Musculoskeletal System

CORE CONCEPT
Knowledge of bones, muscles, and other elements of the musculoskeletal system

The musculoskeletal system is composed of all the body's bones, joints, and muscles, as well as cartilage, tendons, and ligaments. As an EMT, you do not need to know every structure found in the body. However, you do need to remember how complex the structures are and what kinds of damage may be done in case of injury.

Review the skeleton (Figure 32-1) and its major divisions, the axial skeleton and the appendicular skeleton (Figure 32-2). The bones of the axial skeleton include the skull (including the cranium and face), the sternum, the ribs, and the spine, including the cervical, thoracic, and lumbar vertebrae; the sacrum; and the coccyx (Figure 32-3).

In this chapter, we will pay special attention to the appendicular skeleton, particularly the ***extremities***—the upper extremities (clavicles, scapulae, arms, wrists, and hands) and the lower extremities (pelvis, thighs, legs, ankles, and feet) (Figure 32-4).

extremities (ex-TREM-i-teez)
the portions of the skeleton that include the clavicles, scapulae, arms, wrists, and hands (upper extremities) and the pelvis, thighs, legs, ankles, and feet (lower extremities).

Anatomy of Bone

Bones are formed of dense connective tissue. As components of the skeleton, they provide the body's framework. They need to be strong to provide support and protection for the internal organs, but they also need to be somewhat flexible to withstand stress. The bones store salts and metabolic materials and provide a site for the production of red blood cells. Because of this, bones are very vascular—that is, they contain a rich supply of blood. It is important to know this because, simply stated, bones bleed. Although broken bone ends may cause damage to surrounding tissue and blood vessels, the bones themselves also bleed. This is why a patient with a fractured pelvis, hip, or femur—or multiple fractures—may actually develop shock from blood loss from the bone itself.

bones
hard but flexible living structures that provide support for the body and protection to vital organs.

Joints are the places where bones articulate, or meet, and are a critical element in the body's ability to move.

joints
places where bones articulate, or meet.

Generally, bones are classified according to their appearance—long, short, flat, or irregular (Figure 32-5). The bones found in the arm and thigh are examples of long bones. The major short bones of the body are in the hands and feet. The flat bones include the sternum, shoulder blades, and ribs. The vertebrae of the spinal column are examples of irregular bones.

The outward appearance of a typical long bone creates the impression that it is a simple, rigid structure made of the same material throughout. Actually, it is quite complex. Most people are aware that bone contains calcium, which helps to make it very hard. Bone also contains protein fibers that make it somewhat flexible. The strength of our bones is due to a combination of this hardness and flexibility. As we age, less protein is formed in the bones, and less calcium is stored. As a result, bones become brittle and break more easily.

Bones are covered by a strong, white, fibrous material called the *periosteum*. Blood vessels and nerves pass through this membrane as they enter and leave the bone. When bone is exposed as a result of injury, the periosteum becomes visible. Although you may

FIGURE 32-1 Human skeleton.

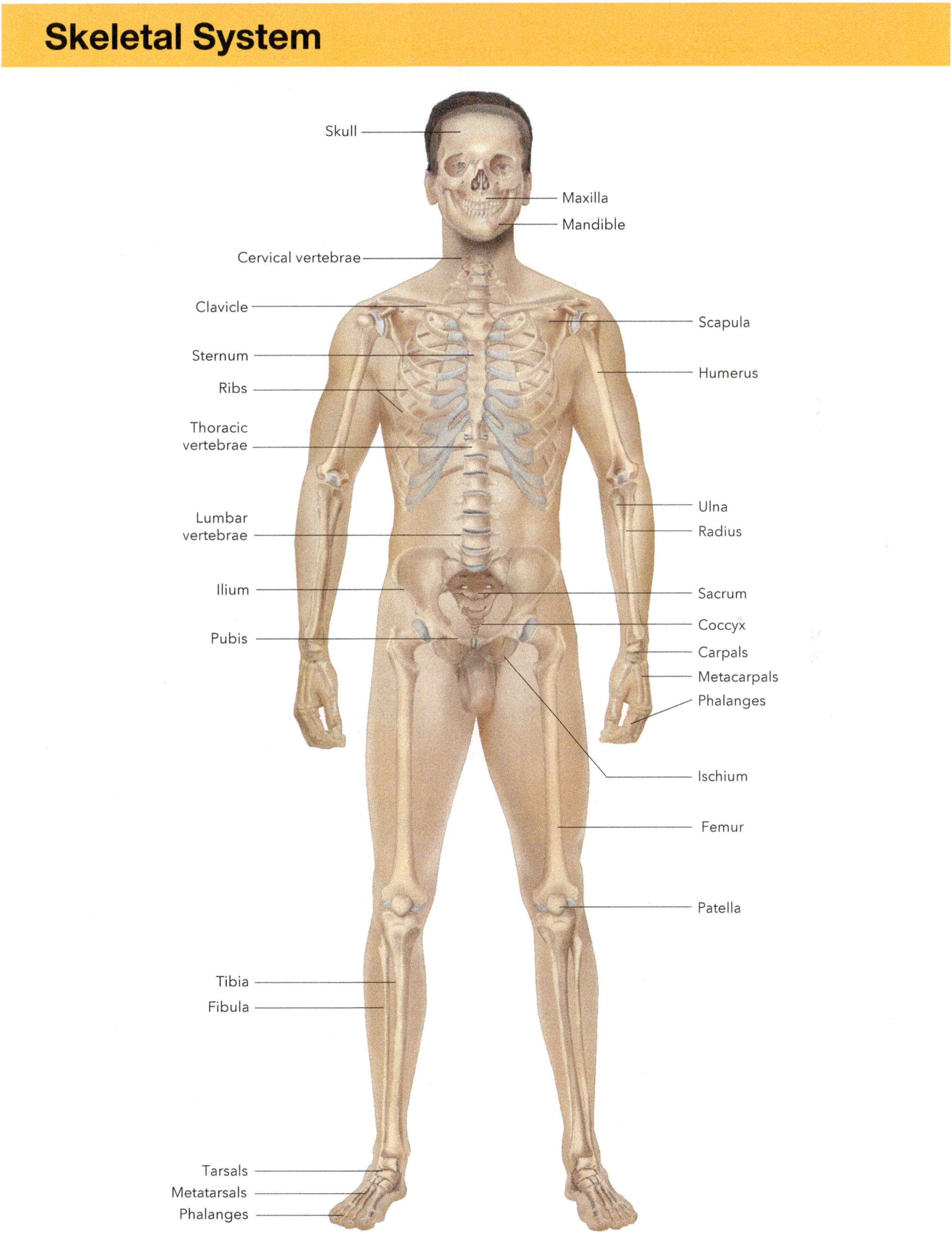

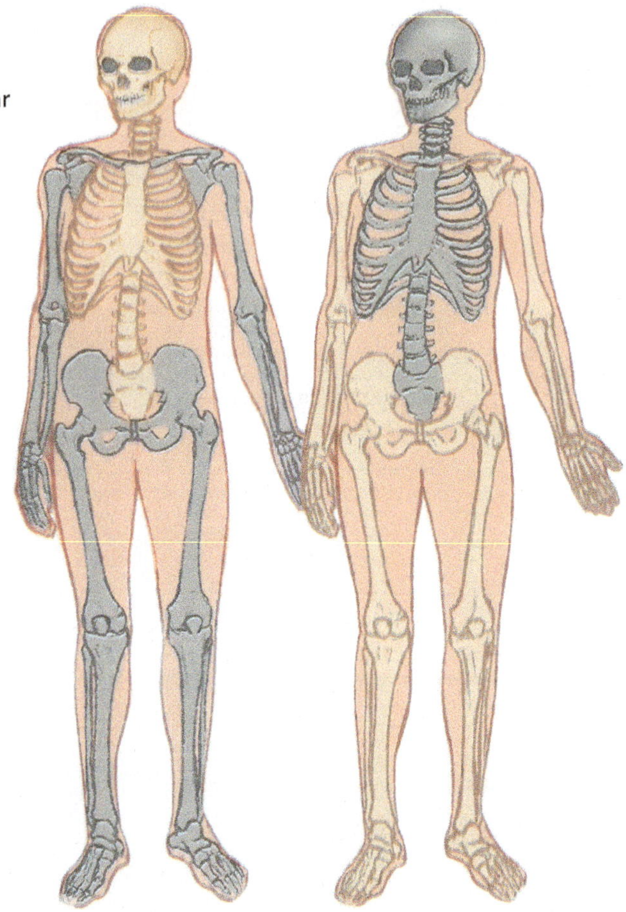

FIGURE 32-2 Highlighted in gray: The axial skeleton *(right)* comprises the skull, spine, ribs, and sternum. The extremities *(left)* comprise the appendicular skeleton.

see fragments of bones and foreign objects on this covering, do not remove them. If they have pierced the periosteum, the objects might be held firmly in place and might offer a great resistance to any pulling or sweeping efforts. In addition, you will not be able to tell if the object has entered the bone or is impaled in an underlying blood vessel or nerve.

Although the shafts of bones appear to be straight, each bone has its own unique curvature. When the end of a bone is involved in forming a ball-and-socket joint, it will be rounded to allow for rotational movement. This rounded end, called the head of the bone, is connected to the shaft by the neck of the bone. Bone marrow, which is contained in the center of bone, is the site of red blood cell production.

Self-Healing Nature of Bone

The most common bone injury is a break, or fracture (Figure 32-6). The first effects of a bone injury are swelling of soft tissue and the formation of a blood clot in the area of the fracture. Both the swelling and the clotting are due to the destruction of blood vessels in the periosteum and the bone as well as to loss of blood from adjacent damaged vessels.

Interruption of the blood supply causes death to the cells at the injury site. Cells a little farther from the fracture remain intact and, within a few hours, begin to more rapidly divide. They soon grow together to form a mass of tissue that completely surrounds the fracture site. New bone is generated from this mass to eventually heal the damaged bone. The whole process can take weeks or months, depending on the bone that has been fractured, the type of fracture, and the patient's health and age.

It is very important for a broken bone to be immobilized quickly and remain immobilized to properly heal. If the fractured bone is mishandled early in care, more soft tissue may be damaged, which would require a longer period for the formation of a tissue mass and replacement of bone. If the bone ends are disturbed during regeneration, proper

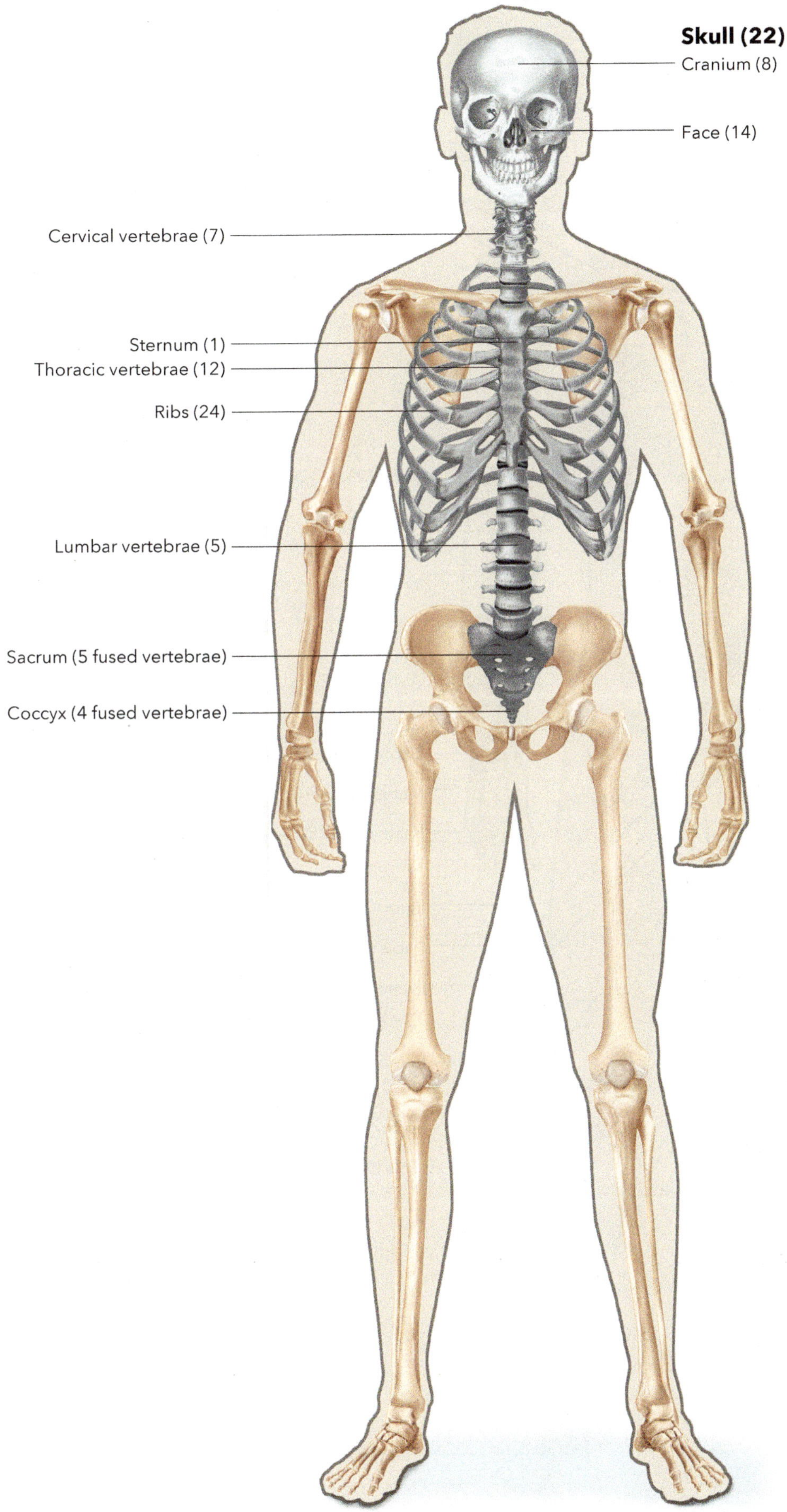

FIGURE 32-3 Bones of the axial skeleton (gray color).

FIGURE 32-4 Bones of the appendicular skeleton (light tan color).

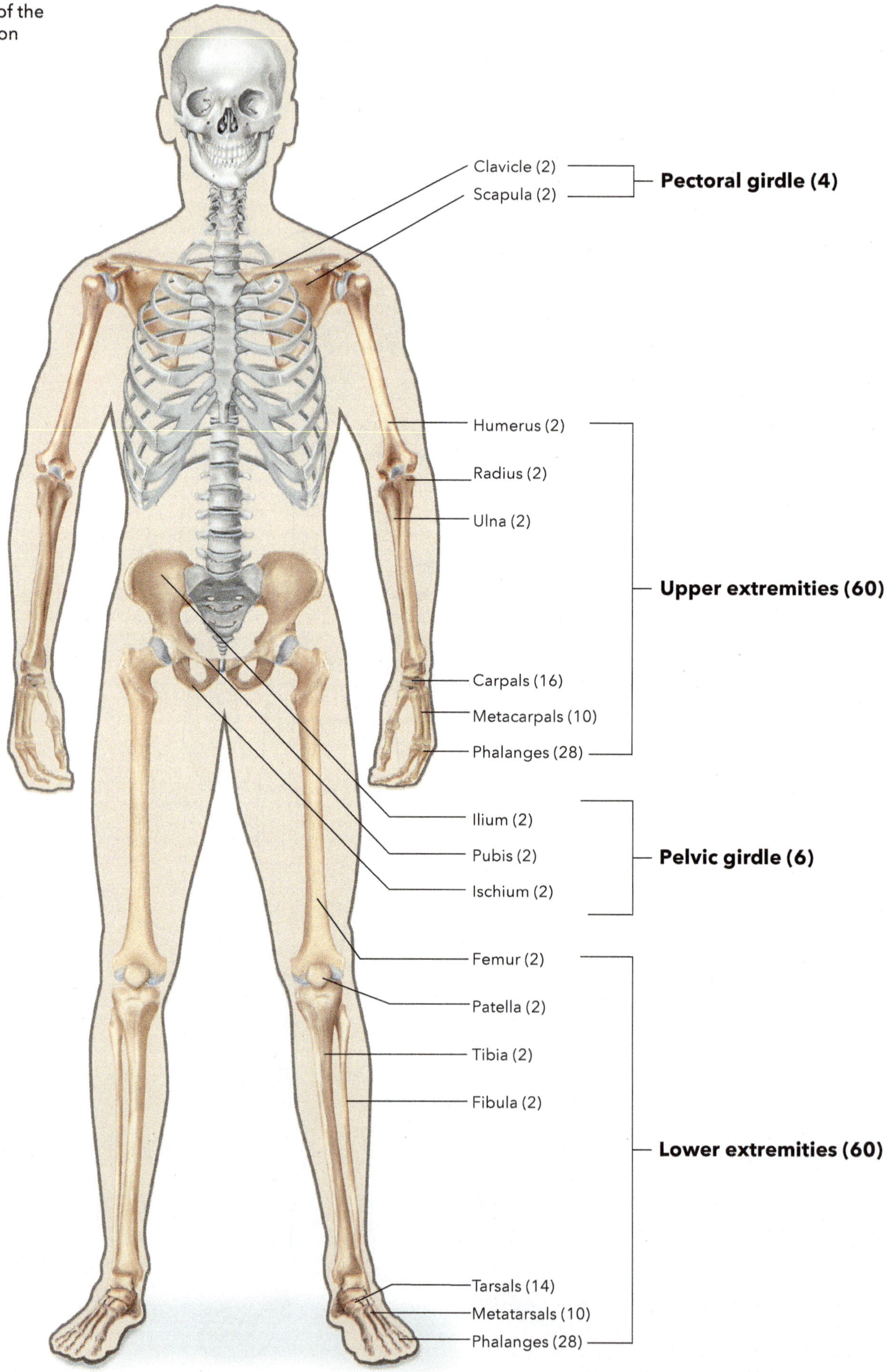

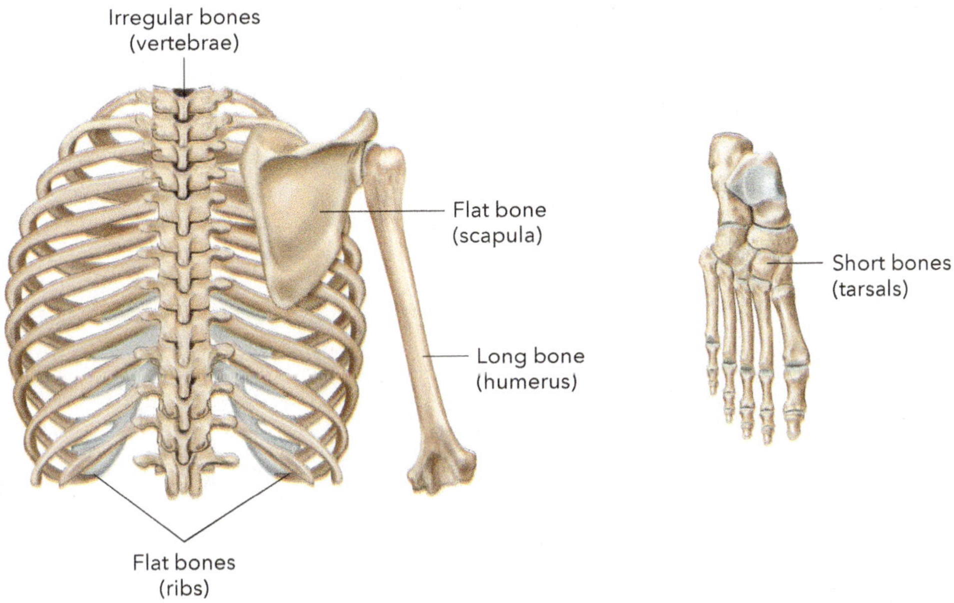

FIGURE 32-5 Bones are classified by shape.

FIGURE 32-6 (A) Open fracture and dislocation of the ankle. (B) X-ray of the same injury. *(Photos A and B: © Edward T. Dickinson, MD)*

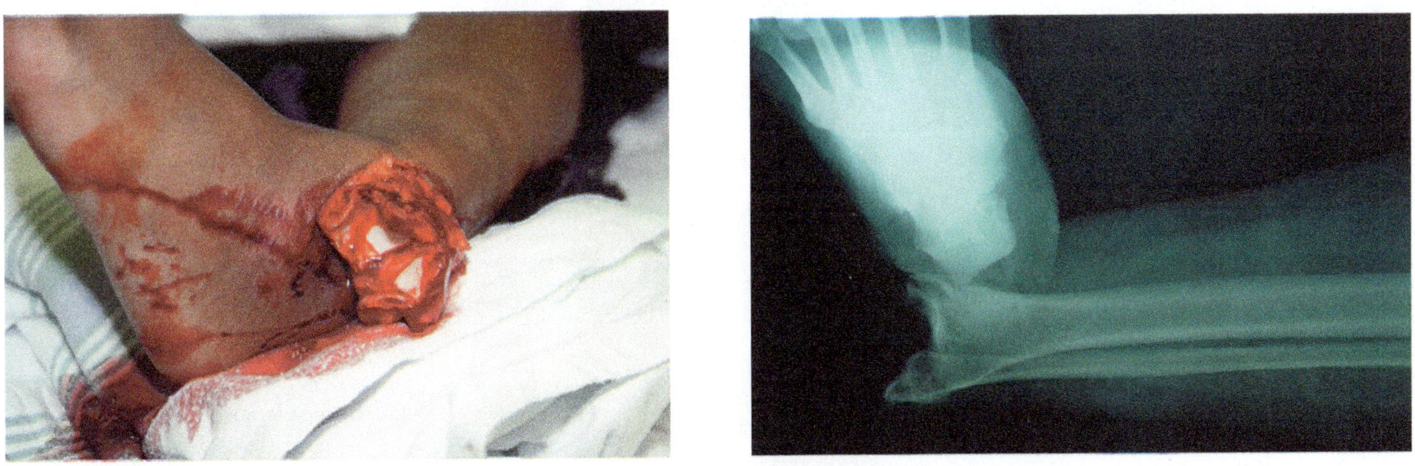

A B

healing will not take place and a permanent disability may result. In children, the majority of growth of a long bone occurs in the area known as the growth plate, which is near the end of the shaft. If a fracture in this area is not properly handled, the child may grow up with one limb shorter than the other.

Muscles, Cartilage, Ligaments, and Tendons

In addition to bones, the elements of the musculoskeletal system are the muscles, cartilage, ligaments, and tendons. ***Muscles*** (Figure 32-7A) are the tissues or fibers that cause movement of body parts or organs. There are three kinds of muscles: smooth (involuntary), cardiac (myocardial) and skeletal, (voluntary) (Figure 32-7B). Smooth muscles are found in the walls of organs and digestive structures. These muscles move food through the digestive system and perform other functions. Cardiac muscle is found in the walls of the heart. The muscles that are of chief concern in trauma and musculoskeletal injury are the skeletal, or voluntary, muscles. These muscles control all conscious or deliberate motions. The skeletal or voluntary muscles include all the muscles that are connected to bones as well as the muscles in the tongue, pharynx, and upper esophagus.

Cartilage is connective tissue that covers the outside of the bone end (epiphysis) and acts as a surface for articulation, allowing for smooth movement at joints. Cartilage, which

muscles
tissues or fibers that cause movement of body parts and organs.

cartilage
tough tissue that covers the joint ends of bones and helps to form certain body parts, such as the ear.

FIGURE 32-7 (A) The muscular system. (B) Three types of muscle.

Muscular System

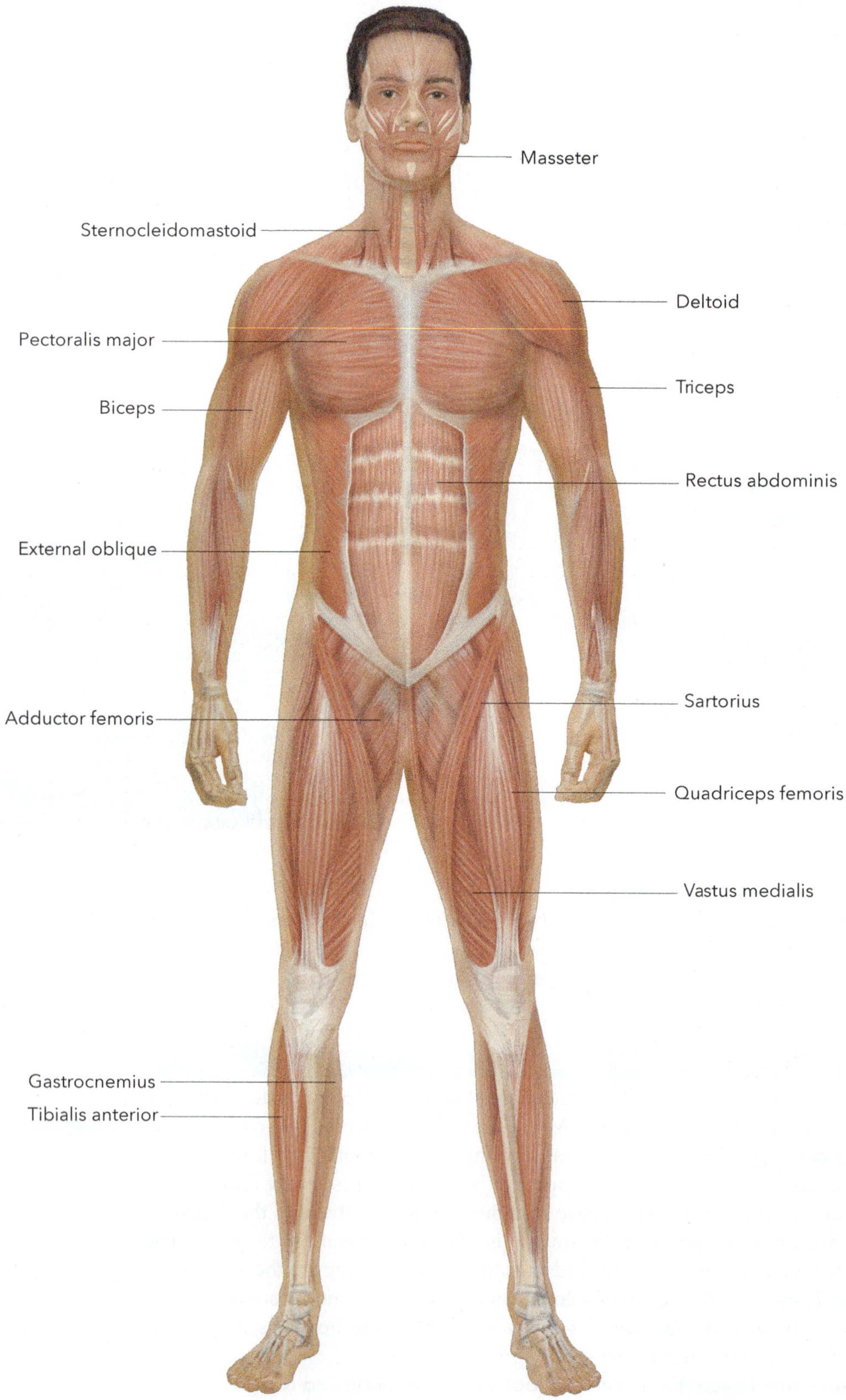

A

FIGURE 32-7 *(continued)*

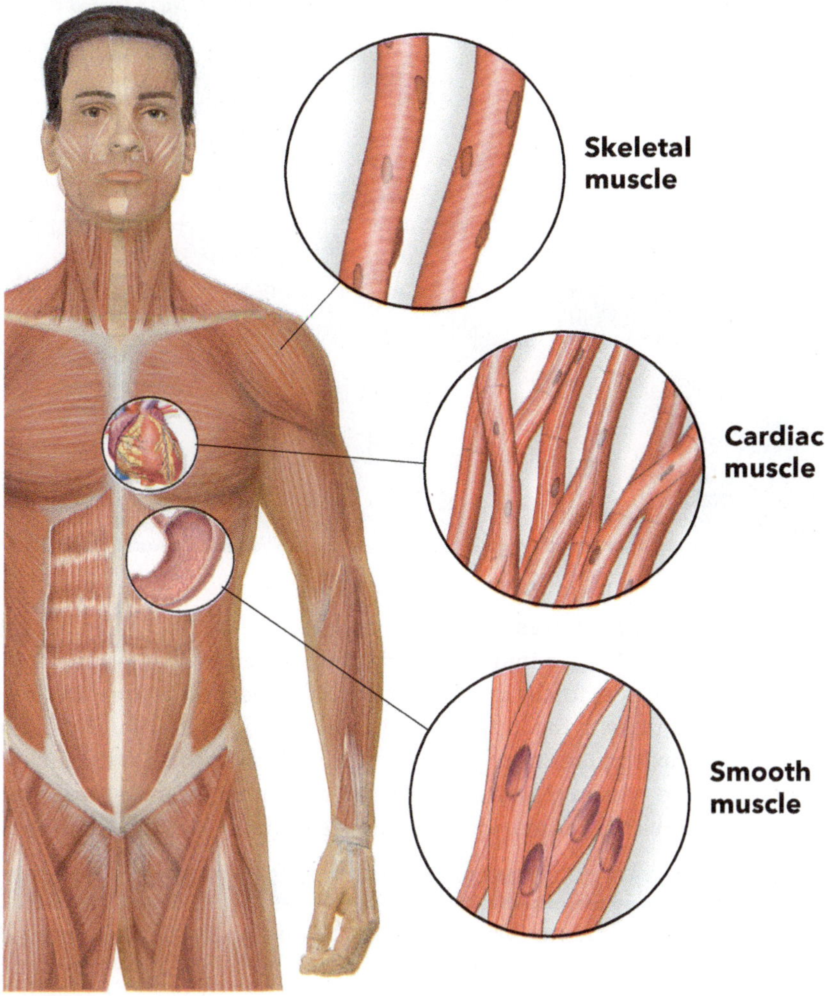

is less rigid than bone, forms or helps to form some of the more flexible structures of the body, such as the septum of the nose (the wall between the nostrils), the external ear, the trachea, and the connections between the ribs and sternum (breastbone).

Tendons are bands of connective tissue that bind muscles to bones. The tendons allow for the power of movement across the joints (Figure 32-8).

Ligaments are connective tissues that support joints by attaching the bone ends and allowing for a stable range of motion. Two mnemonics can help you distinguish between the connective functions of tendons and ligaments: MTB = muscle–tendon–bone; BLB = bone–ligament–bone (Figure 32-9).

tendons
tissues that connect muscle to bone.

ligaments
tissues that connect bone to bone.

General Guidelines for Emergency Care

Mechanisms of Musculoskeletal Injury

There are three types of mechanisms that cause musculoskeletal injuries: direct force, twisting force, and indirect force. An example of *direct force* is a person being struck by an automobile, causing crushed tissue and fractures. *Twisting* or *rotational forces* can cause stretching or tearing of muscles and ligaments, as well as broken bones, such as occur when a ski digs into the snow while the skier's body rotates. Sporting activities such as football, basketball, soccer, in-line skating, skiing, snowboarding, and wrestling—in addition to motor-vehicle collisions—account for many musculoskeletal injuries.

CORE CONCEPT
Knowledge of general guidelines for emergency care of musculoskeletal injuries

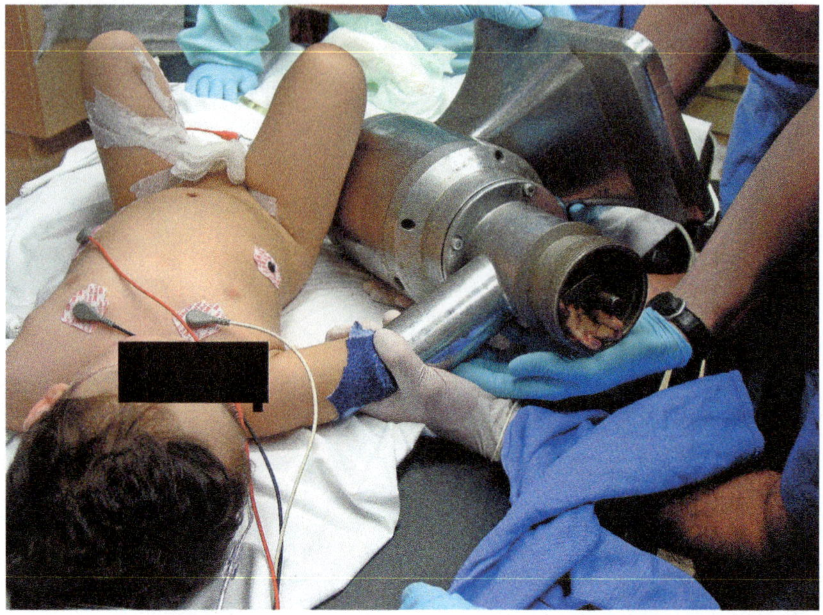

FIGURE 32-8 Meat grinder injury to soft tissue, tendons, ligaments, and bone in a child. *(© David Effron, MD).*

It is easy to see how direct forces cause injuries, but an *indirect force* can be just as powerful. For example, a well-known injury pattern occurs when people fall from heights and land on their feet. The direct forces cause injuries to the feet and ankles, whereas *indirect forces* usually cause injuries to the knees, femurs, pelvis, and spinal column. In fact, most injuries to the upper extremities are caused by forces applied to an outstretched arm. In the course of a fall, the person reaches out with an arm in an effort to break the fall and, in doing so, often breaks the radius, ulna, or clavicle or dislocates the shoulder.

Injury to Bones and Connective Tissue

A fracture is the breaking of a bone. Some fractures you may encounter are grossly deformed and painful. However, you may also encounter extremities that have minimal pain and deformity but are, in fact, fractured. Unless there is a very obvious deformity, it is not possible or even important for you to decide if a patient's injury is a fracture, a dislocation, a sprain, or a severe bruise. Most patients simply present with pain, swelling, and—sometimes—deformity. It will take an X-ray or other imaging process to precisely diagnose the injury. In the field, therefore, the worst must be assumed, and patients with signs and

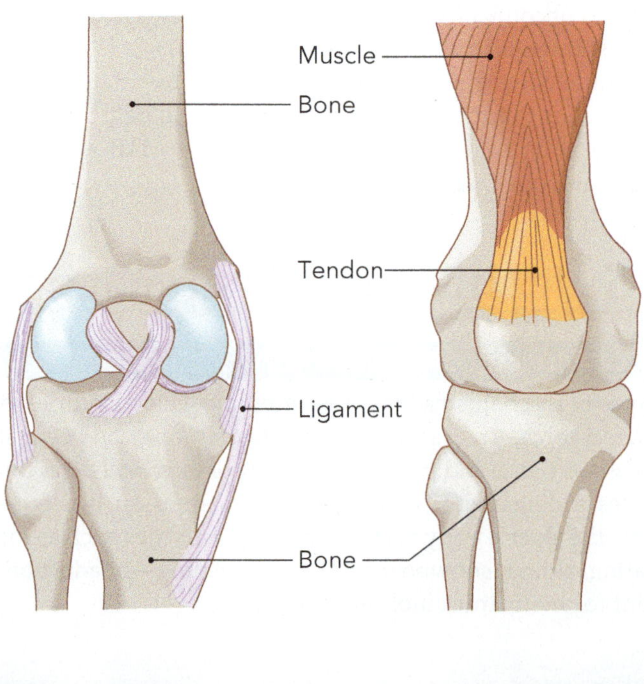

FIGURE 32-9 Ligaments tie bone to bone. Tendons tie muscle to bone.

symptoms of a fracture—a painful, swollen, or deformed extremity—should be treated as though they have a fracture. Although most fractures are not life-threatening, remember that bones are living tissue. Even in simple, uncomplicated fractures, bones bleed. For example, a simple closed tibia–fibula fracture typically causes a 1-pint (500-cc) blood loss. Fractures of the femur typically cause a 2-pint (1,000-cc) blood loss, and pelvic fractures cause a 3- to 4-pint (1,500- to 2,000-cc) blood loss (Figure 32-10).

In World War I, the battlefield death rate from closed fractures of the femur was about 80 percent, because of complications such as blood loss. Two surgeons noticed that large muscle groups in the thigh go into spasms (contract, or shrink), forcing the broken femoral ends to override each other, injuring the blood vessels. To correct the problem, they invented the ***traction splint***, a splint that applies constant pull along the length of the leg to help stabilize the fractured bone and reduce muscle spasms. With early application of a traction splint, the mortality rate from femur fractures dropped to less than 20 percent (and is much lower today).

Remember that splinting an extremity with a suspected fracture can prevent additional blood loss, pain, and complications from nerve and blood vessel injury. Therefore, treat for the worst (a fracture) and immobilize. Physicians in the hospital will diagnose the actual injury with an X-ray.

There are four types of musculoskeletal injury:

1. ***Fracture***. A fracture is any break in a bone. Fractures can be classified as open or closed (Figure 32-11) and are also classified by the way the bone is broken—a ***comminuted fracture*** if broken in several places (Figure 32-12A), a ***greenstick fracture*** if the break is incomplete (Figure 32-12B), or an ***angulated fracture*** if the broken bone is bent at an angle (Figure 32-13). Greenstick fractures are common in children, since their bones are more flexible than bones of adults. The name comes from what happens when you bend a green twig or branch. Instead of snapping in two the way a mature branch would, the twig bends and only part of it breaks.

traction splint
a splint that applies constant pull along the length of a lower extremity to help stabilize the fractured bone and to reduce muscle spasm in the limb. Traction splints are used primarily on femoral shaft fractures.

fracture (FRAK-cher)
any break in a bone.

comminuted fracture
a fracture in which the bone is broken in several places.

greenstick fracture
an incomplete fracture.

angulated fracture
a fracture in which the broken bone segments are at an angle to each other.

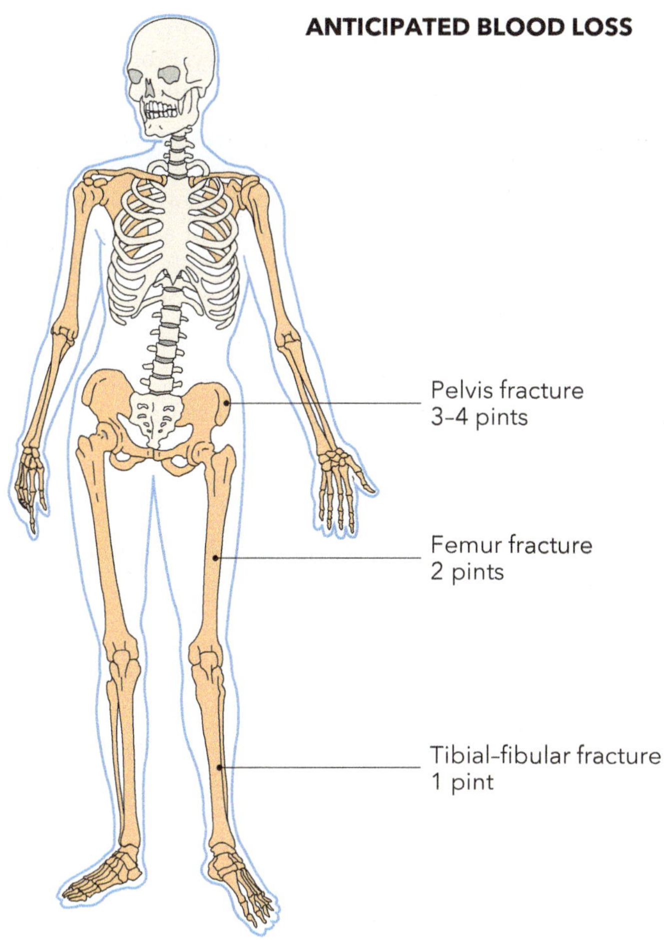

FIGURE 32-10 Bones bleed. In fact, there may be considerable blood loss, even from an uncomplicated closed fracture.

FIGURE 32-11 (A) Open fracture. (B) Closed fracture. *(Photos A and B: © Edward T. Dickinson, MD)*

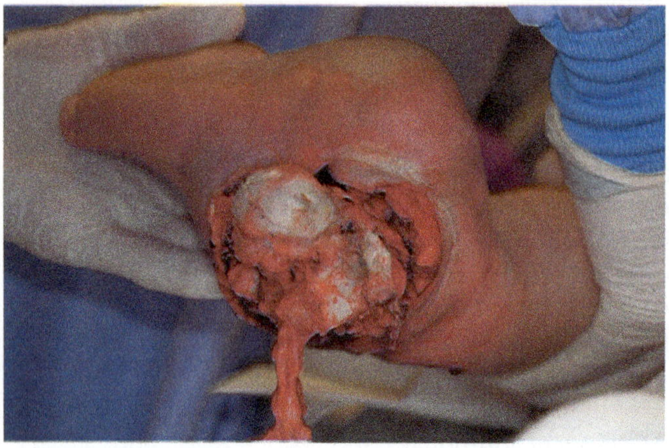

A

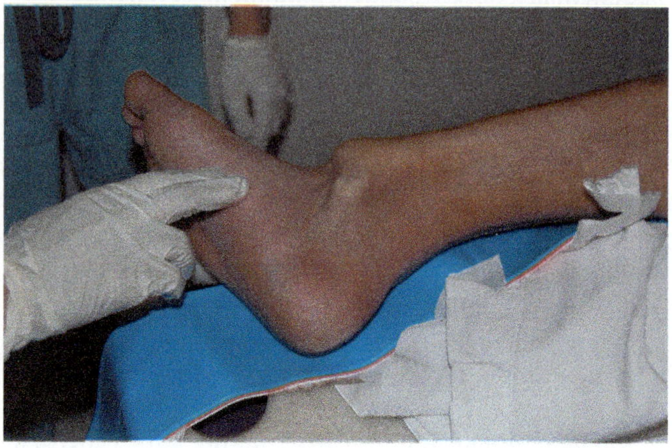

B

dislocation
the disruption or "coming apart" of a joint.

sprain
the stretching and tearing of ligaments.

strain
muscle injury resulting from overstretching or overexertion of the muscle.

closed extremity injury
an injury to an extremity with no associated opening in the skin.

open extremity injury
an extremity injury in which the skin has been broken or torn through from the inside by an injured bone, or from the outside by something that has caused a penetrating wound with associated injury to the bone.

2. ***Dislocation***. The disruption or "coming apart" of a joint is called a dislocation (Figure 32-14). For a joint to dislocate, the soft tissue of the joint capsule and ligaments must be stretched beyond the normal range of motion and torn.
3. ***Sprain***. A sprain is caused by the stretching and tearing of ligaments. It is most commonly associated with joint injuries.
4. ***Strain***. A strain is a muscle injury caused by overstretching or overexertion of the muscle.

A ***closed extremity injury*** is one in which the skin is not broken. An ***open extremity injury*** is one in which the skin has been broken or torn through from the inside by the injured bone or from the outside by something that has caused a penetrating wound with associated injury to the bone. An open injury is a serious situation because of the increased likelihood of contamination and subsequent infection.

Although many closed injuries can be handled simply in the hospital emergency department, patients with open fractures require surgery. Proper splinting and prehospital care of musculoskeletal injuries help prevent closed injuries from becoming open ones.

Assessment of Musculoskeletal Injuries

Examination involves your senses and the skills of inspection (looking), palpation (feeling), and auscultation (listening). One of the basic principles of assessment is that it is difficult to do a proper examination on patients when they are fully clothed. However, it often is difficult, impractical, or inadvisable to completely disrobe or cut away a patient's clothing

FIGURE 32-12 (A) Comminuted fracture. (B) Greenstick fracture.

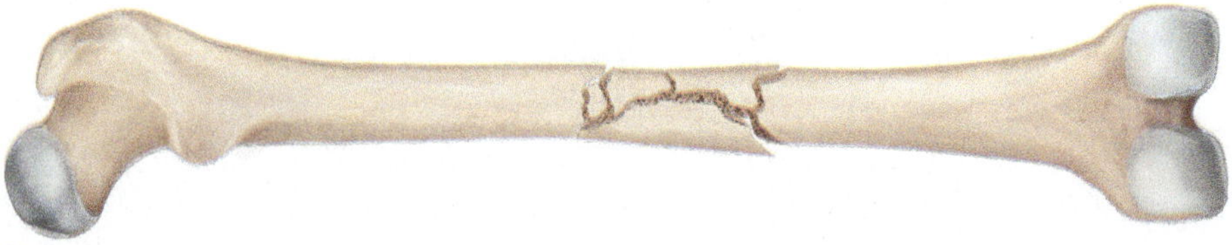

A

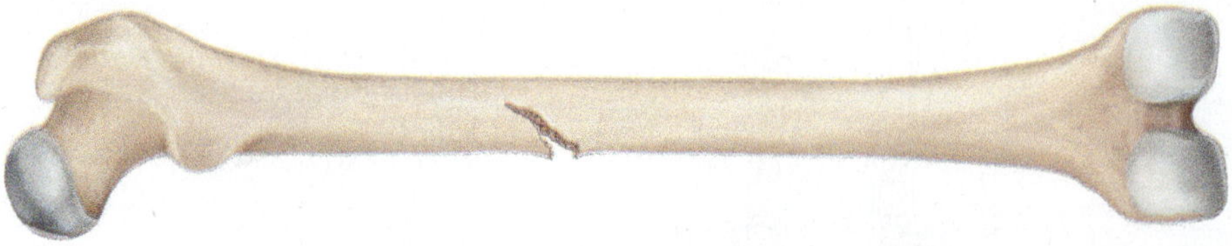

B

FIGURE 32-13 (A) A closed angulated fracture. (B) An X-ray of the same fracture. *(Photos A and B: © Edward T. Dickinson, MD)*

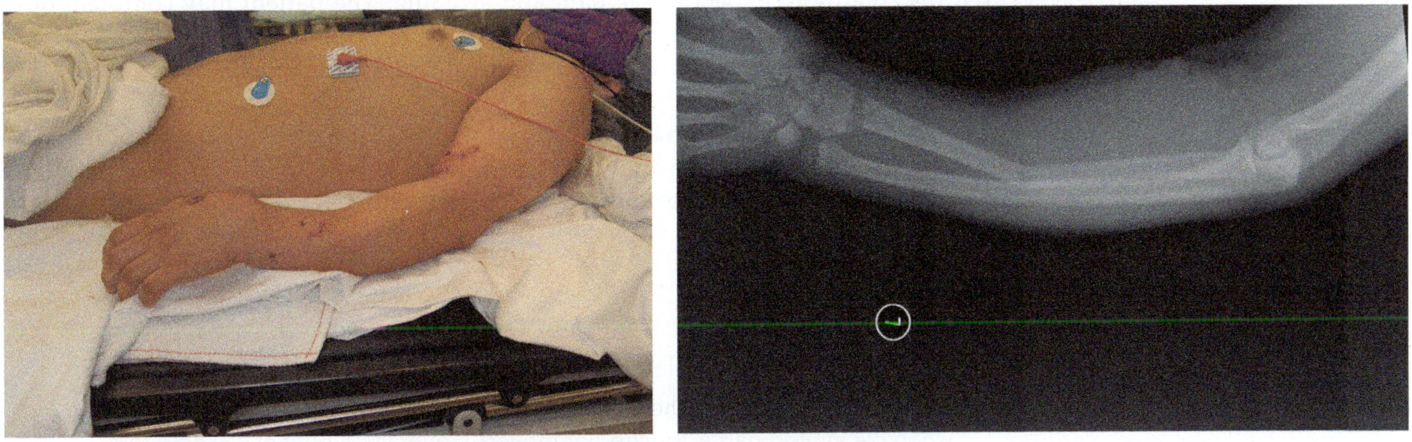

A

B

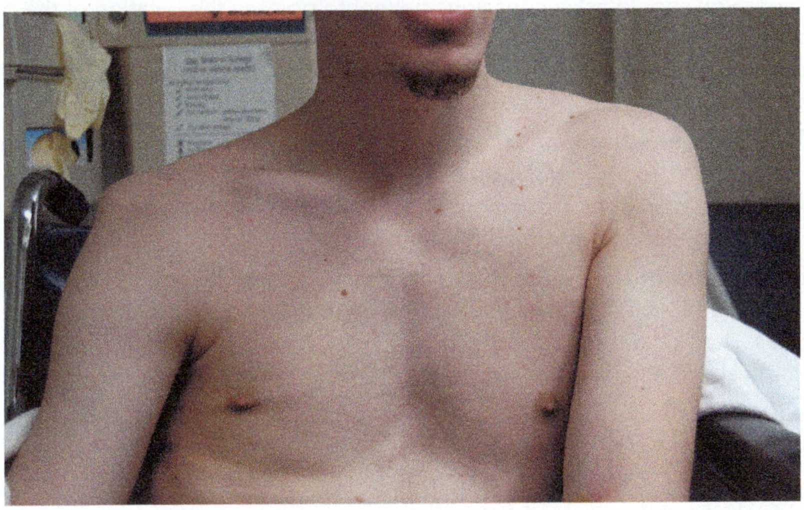

FIGURE 32-14 A right shoulder dislocation. *(© Edward T. Dickinson, MD)*

because of weather, the patient's modesty, or patient refusal. A good rule of thumb is to cut or remove clothing according to the environment and severity of the situation.

In cases of severe extremity trauma, injuries can be very obvious. However, when treating trauma patients, *your priority must be to rapidly identify and treat life-threatening conditions first*. Do not let a grotesque but relatively minor extremity injury sidetrack you—or the patient. The pain or terrible appearance of an extremity injury may distract the patient from awareness of other injuries or symptoms, such as abdominal pain from internal bleeding. Be sure to assess the patient fully and ask appropriate questions to avoid missing other injuries. Only after your primary assessment and rapid trauma assessment have ruled out obvious life-threatening airway, breathing, or circulation problems and injuries to the head, spine, chest, and abdomen should you focus your attention on musculoskeletal injuries to the extremities.

Compartment Syndrome

A critical complication of extremity fracture is ***compartment syndrome***. This is a serious condition caused by severe swelling in the extremity—in this case as the result of a fracture. Compartment syndrome progresses as follows:

1. A fracture or crush injury causes bleeding and swelling within the extremity.
2. Pressure and swelling caused by the bleeding within the muscle compartment become so great that the body can no longer perfuse the tissues against the pressure.
3. Cellular damage occurs and causes additional swelling.
4. Blood flow to the area is lost. The limb itself may be lost if the pressure is not relieved.

compartment syndrome injury caused when tissues such as blood vessels and nerves are constricted within a space, as from swelling or from a tight dressing or cast.

Signs and symptoms of compartment syndrome are similar to those of the injury that caused the condition. Expect to see pain and swelling. The patient may complain of a sensation of pressure. The extremity may feel hard on palpation when compared with the uninjured side, and distal circulation, sensation, and motor function (CSM) may be reduced or absent.

EMTs can best treat compartment syndrome by some of the same treatments as for fracture, including cold application and elevation of the extremity (if this can be done safely after splinting). Prompt transport to an appropriate facility is important.

Patient Assessment

Musculoskeletal Injuries

Signs and symptoms of musculoskeletal injuries in a patient include the following:

- **Pain and tenderness.** The patient with a fractured extremity experiences pain when the injured part is touched or moved. Generally, a patient will hold the injured part still, or guard it, in an effort to minimize pain. When examining such an injury, you should ask a conscious patient to point to the location of the pain, if possible. Then, initially avoiding that location, carefully examine the injured part to assess if there are any other painful or injured areas. With unresponsive patients, suspicion of injury must be based on other physical findings.
- **Deformity or angulation.** The force of trauma causes bones to fracture and become deformed, or angulated, out of the anatomic position. Note that when a patient has joint injuries, the deformity is sometimes subtle. When in doubt, look at the uninjured side and compare it with the injured one.
- **Grating,** or ***crepitus***. This is a sound or feeling caused by broken bone ends rubbing together. It can be painful for the patient, so never intentionally cause crepitus. The patient may report grating noises or sensations that occurred prior to your arrival and examination.
- **Swelling.** When bones break and soft tissue is torn, bleeding causes swelling that may increase the proportions of a deformity. Rings, watches, and other jewelry can easily constrict and injure underlying tissue. Therefore, slide or cut them off as soon as possible if swelling is likely to occur.
- **Bruising.** Ecchymosis, or large black-and-blue discoloration of the skin, indicates an underlying injury that may be hours or days old. Obvious bruises indicate the need for splinting.
- **Exposed bone ends.** Bone ends protruding through the skin indicate a fracture that requires splinting. Again, the more gruesome the appearance of the extremity, the greater the temptation is for you to treat that injury first. Remember that you should care for life-threatening injuries first. Extremity injuries rarely kill patients.
- **Joints locked into position.** When joints are dislocated, they may lock into normal or abnormal anatomic positions. Joint injuries usually need to be splinted as found.
- **Nerve and blood vessel compromise.** Examine for pulses, sensation, and movement distal to the injury site. This must be accomplished before and after splinting. Check for nerve injury by asking if the patient can sense your touch and can move all fingers or toes. Any problem of sensation or movement must be noted. Next feel for pulses in the wrist (radial), ankle (posterior tibial), or foot (dorsalis pedis). Obviously, to accurately examine for sensation, movement, and pulses, the patient's gloves and footwear must be removed.

crepitus (KREP-i-tus) a grating sensation or sound made when fractured bone ends rub together.

Another method of assessing compromise to an extremity when a musculoskeletal injury is suspected is to learn and follow the "six Ps":

Pain or tenderness

Pallor (pale skin or poor capillary refill)

Paresthesia, or the sensation of "pins and needles"
Pulses diminished or absent in the injured extremity
Paralysis, or the inability to move
Pressure

Decision Points

- Do the patient's musculoskeletal injuries add up to serious multiple trauma?
- Does the patient have circulation, sensation, and motor function (CSM) distal to the suspected fracture or dislocation?

Patient Care

Care for the Patient with Musculoskeletal Injuries

Fundamental Principles of Care

You will learn about management of specific injuries as you read this chapter. Emergency care of a patient with musculoskeletal injuries includes the following general principles:

- Take and maintain appropriate Standard Precautions.
- Perform the primary assessment. Remember, do not get distracted from your primary assessment and from determining patient priority by focusing on a dramatic-looking or painful extremity injury. Keep in mind, however, that multiple fractures, especially to the femurs, can cause life-threatening external or internal bleeding.
- During the secondary assessment, apply a cervical collar if you suspect a spine injury.
- After life-threatening conditions have been addressed, any suspected extremity fracture must be splinted. For a low-priority (stable) patient, splint individual injuries before transport. For a high-priority (unstable) patient, immobilize the whole body on a long spine board, then "load and go." If time and the patient's condition permit, you may be able to splint a specific injury en route.
- If appropriate, cover open wounds with sterile dressings, elevate the extremity, and apply a cold pack to the area to help reduce swelling.

NOTE: *If a primary assessment reveals that your patient is unstable, managing extremity injuries becomes a low priority. An unstable patient with "load and go" problems must have the A-B-Cs managed and the entire body splinted or immobilized on a long spine board. Do not take time to individually splint each injury. It is not in the patient's best interest for you to waste time treating minor injuries and delivering a perfectly packaged but unsavable patient to the hospital.*

Splinting

CORE CONCEPT
Purposes and general procedures for splinting

Emergency care for all suspected extremity fractures starts with splinting (Figure 32-15). *For any splint to be effective, it must immobilize adjacent joints and bone ends.* Effective splinting minimizes the movement of disrupted joints and broken bone ends, and it decreases the patient's pain. It helps prevent additional injury to soft tissues such as nerves, arteries, veins, and muscles. It can prevent a closed fracture from becoming an open fracture, a much more serious condition, and it can help to minimize blood loss. In the case of the spine, immobilization prevents injury to the spinal cord and helps to prevent permanent paralysis.

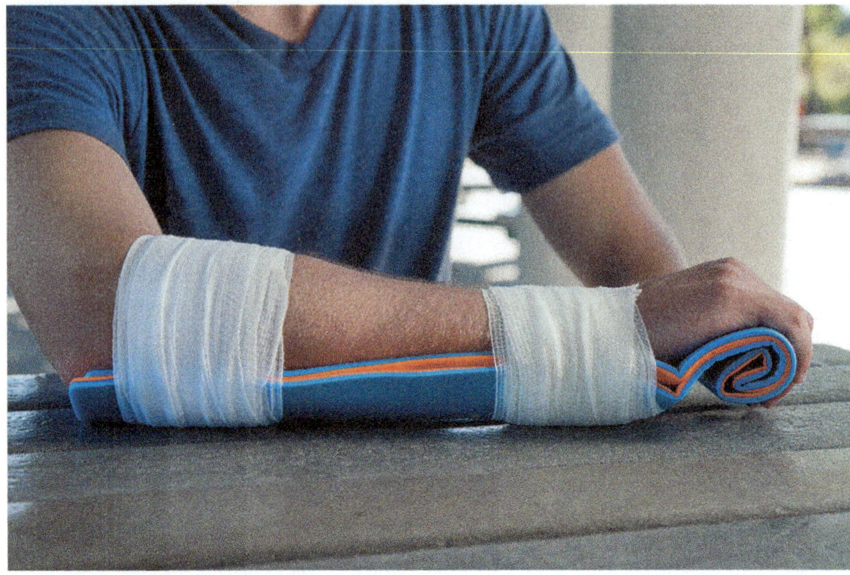

A

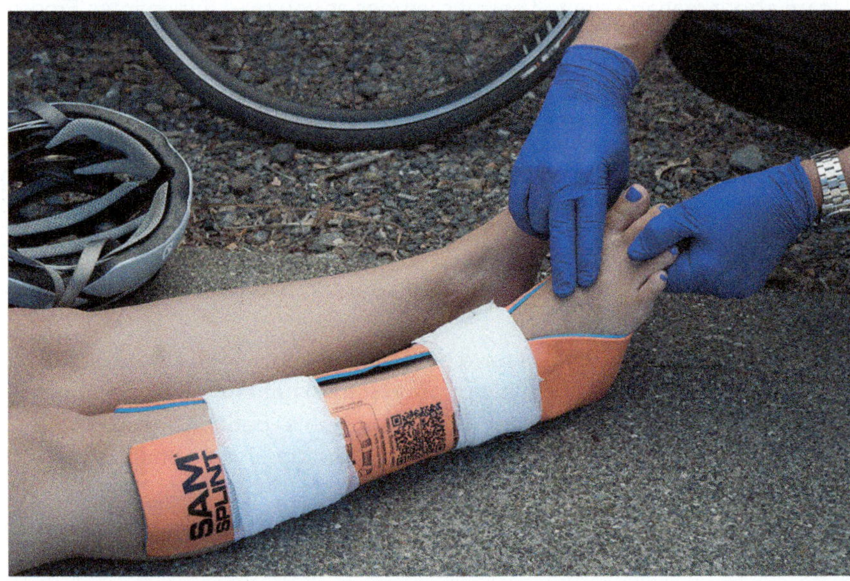

B

FIGURE 32-15 (A) SAM® splint on lower arm. (B) SAM® splint on lower leg.

"Take care when splinting. Have a good plan. Be gentle. Broken bones hurt."

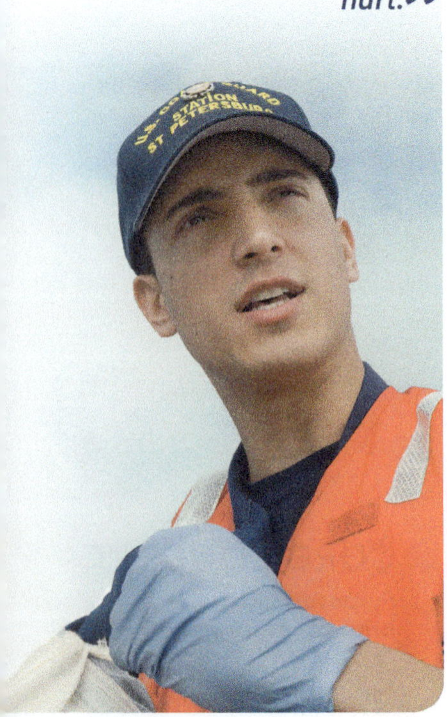

Realignment of the Deformed Extremity

The object of realignment (straightening) of a deformed extremity is to assist in restoring effective circulation to the extremity and to simplify splinting. For the EMT, realignment of a deformed extremity is generally limited to the angulated shafts of the long bones (the humerus, ulna, radius, femur, tibia, and the fibula).

The thought of realigning an angulated injury can be a frightening one. However, remember these points:

- If the extremity is not realigned, the splint may be ineffective, causing increased pain and possible further injury (including an open fracture) during transportation.
- If the extremity is not realigned, the chance of nerves, arteries, and veins being compromised increases. When distal circulation is compromised or shut down, tissues beyond the injury become starved for oxygen and die.
- Pain is increased for only a moment during realignment under traction. Pain is reduced by effective splinting.
- Generally, injured joints should be splinted in the position found unless the distal extremity is cyanotic or lacks pulses. If these conditions are present, try to align the joint to a neutral anatomic position using gentle traction, provided that no resistance is felt.

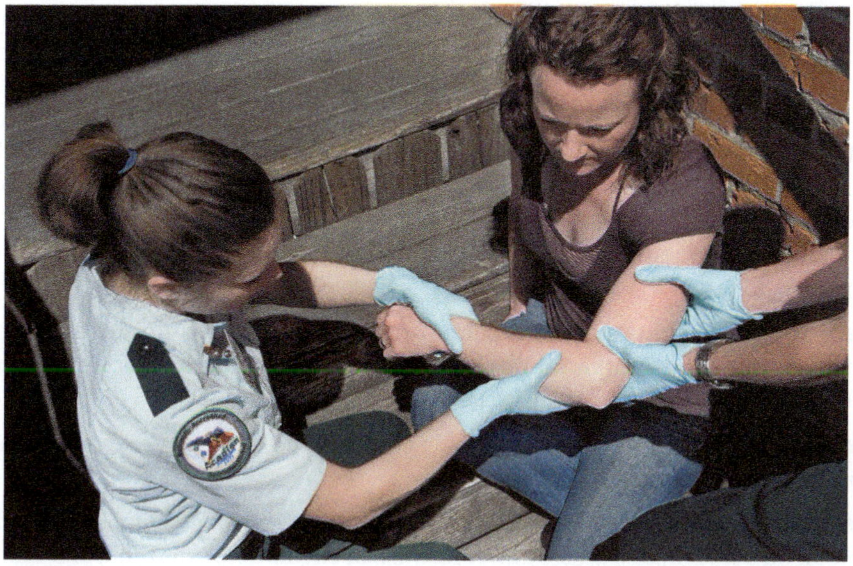

FIGURE 32-16 Realigning an extremity.

The general guidelines for realigning an extremity are as follows (Figure 32-16):

1. One EMT grasps the distal extremity while a partner places one hand above and one hand below the injury site.
2. The partner supports the site while the first EMT creates gentle ***manual traction*** in the direction of the long axis of the extremity. If you feel resistance or if it appears that bone ends will come through the skin, stop realignment and splint the extremity in the position found.
3. If no resistance is felt, maintain gentle traction until the extremity is properly aligned and splinted.

manual traction the process of applying tension to straighten and realign a fractured limb before splinting. Also called *tension*.

Strategies for Splinting

Effective splinting may require some ingenuity. Even though you carry different types of splinting devices, many situations will require you to improvise. In a pinch, you can use pillows or rolled blankets as soft splints. For rigid splints, you can use a piece of lumber, cardboard, a rolled newspaper, an umbrella, a cane, a broom handle, or a catcher's shin guard. For a finger, you can use a tongue depressor. A bystander can often rummage through the car trunk and find something suitable.

Splints carried on EMS units come in three basic types: rigid splints, formable splints, and traction splints (Figure 32-17). Rigid splints require the limb to be moved to the

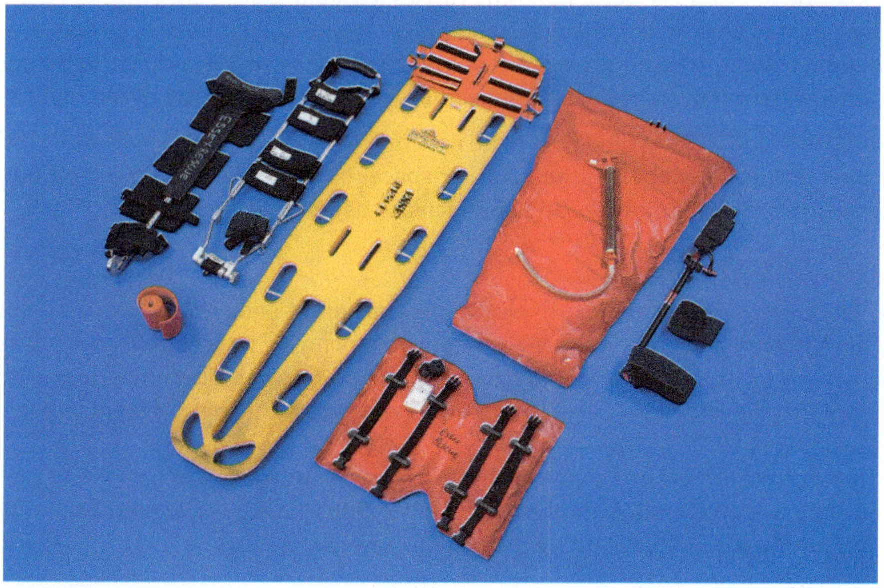

FIGURE 32-17 Splints and accessories for musculoskeletal injuries.

anatomic position. They tend to provide the greatest support and are ideally used to splint long-bone injuries. Examples are cardboard, wood, Velcro, pneumatic splints such as air splints and vacuum splints, and the pneumatic anti-shock garment. Formable splints are capable of being molded to different angles and generally allow for considerable movement. They are most commonly used to immobilize joint injuries in the position found. Examples are pillow and blanket splints. Traction splints are used specifically for femur fractures.

Regardless of the method of splinting, general rules that apply to all types of immobilization are as follows:

- **Care for life-threatening problems first.** If the patient is unstable, do not waste time with splinting. You can align the injuries in the anatomic position and immobilize the whole body to a long spine board.
- **Expose the injury site.** Before moving the injured extremity, expose the area and control any bleeding.
- **Assess distal CSM.** Because complications of musculoskeletal injury include nerve and blood vessel injury, assess and record distal circulation, sensation, and motor function (CSM) both before and after splinting. (Review the scan in the *Secondary Assessment* chapter that illustrates how to assess distal function.)
- **Align long-bone injuries to the anatomic position.** Do this under gentle traction if severe deformity exists or if distal circulation is compromised.
- **Do not push protruding bones back into place.** However, when you realign deformed open injuries, they may slip back into position under traction.
- **Immobilize both the injury site and adjacent joints.** For splints to be effective, they must keep the injury site and the joints above and below still. (If the joint is injured, splint to immobilize the joint and the adjacent bones.)
- **Choose a method of splinting.** This is always dictated by the severity of the patient's condition and the patient's priority level. If the patient is a high priority for "load and go" transport, choose a fast method of splinting. If the patient is a low priority for transport, choose a slower but better splinting method. The methods of splinting, from slowest to fastest, are:
  - Splint each site individually (slowest but best).
  - Secure the limb to the torso or an uninjured leg (a bit faster but second choice to individual splints).
  - Secure the entire body to a spine board (fastest but better only than no splint at all).
- **Splint before moving the patient to a stretcher or other location if possible.** A good rule of thumb is "least handling causes least damage." Sometimes patients must be extricated from where they are before ideal splinting techniques can occur. Attempt to immobilize the extremity as well as you can. (For example, prior to extrication, the injured extremity might be immobilized by securing it to the uninjured one.)
- **Pad the voids.** Many rigid splints do not conform to body curves and allow too much movement of the limb. Pad the voids, or spaces between the body part and the splint, to ensure proper immobilization and increase patient comfort.

Hazards of Splinting

By far, the most serious hazard of splinting is "splinting someone to death"—splinting before life-threatening conditions are addressed, or spending time splinting a high-priority patient instead of immediately getting the patient into the ambulance and to the hospital. Remember that deformed fractures look painful and grotesque. Do not let that distract you from your priorities.

Always ensure the patient's airway, breathing, and circulation before going on to care for other injuries. Remember, the method of splinting is always dictated by the severity of the patient's condition and by the priority for transportation.

Other hazards include improper or inadequate splinting. If a splint is applied too tightly, it can compress soft tissue and injure nerves, blood vessels, and muscles. If it is applied too loosely or inappropriately, it will allow so much movement that further soft-tissue injury or an open fracture may occur. In addition, because rescue workers may be insecure about realigning a deformed injury, they may attempt to splint it in a deformed position and actually do more harm than good. Remember, it can be very difficult to splint deformed long-bone injuries well enough to prevent excessive movement.

Splinting Long-Bone and Joint Injuries

Before you start the splinting process, select a splint appropriate to the severity of the patient's condition and method of transportation. Be sure to have cravats, padding, and roller bandages immediately at hand.

The splinting of joints usually requires considerable ingenuity. In most cases, formable splints are used to splint the joint in the position in which it is found. If the distal extremity is pulseless or cyanotic, try to align the joint to the anatomic position using gentle traction. As with long-bone splinting, get all of your equipment ready before starting the splinting process.

To splint long-bone or joint injuries, follow these guidelines (Scan 32-1 and Scan 32-2):

1. Take appropriate Standard Precautions, and if possible, expose the area to be splinted.
2. Manually stabilize the injury site. This can be done either by you or by a helper.
3. Assess circulation, sensation, and motor function (CSM). Check for pulses and see if the patient can feel your touch distal to the injury. Ask the patient to wiggle fingers or toes so you can assess movement. Do not ask the patient to grasp, press, or pull with an extremity you believe may be fractured. This will cause unnecessary pain and may aggravate the injury.
4. Realign the injury if deformed or if the distal extremity is cyanotic or pulseless. Be sure to attempt to realign an injured joint only if the distal extremity is pulseless or cyanotic.
5. Measure or adjust the splint and move it into position under or alongside the limb. Maintain manual stabilization or traction during positioning and until the splinting procedure is complete.
6. Apply and secure the splint to immobilize adjacent joints and the injury site.
7. Reassess CSM distal to the injury.

SCAN 32-1 Immobilizing a Long Bone

First Take Standard Precautions.

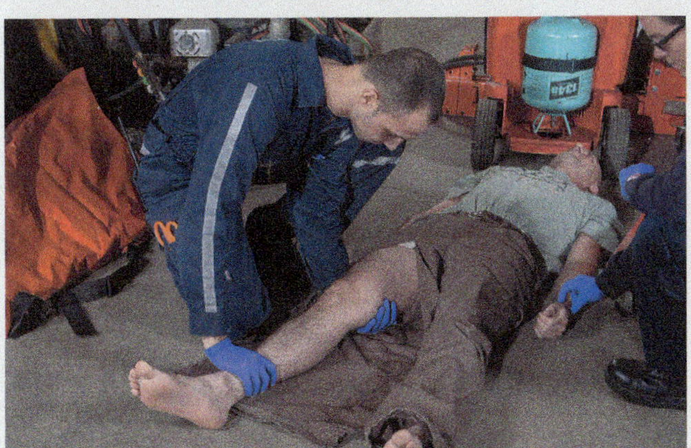

1. Manually stabilize the injured limb.

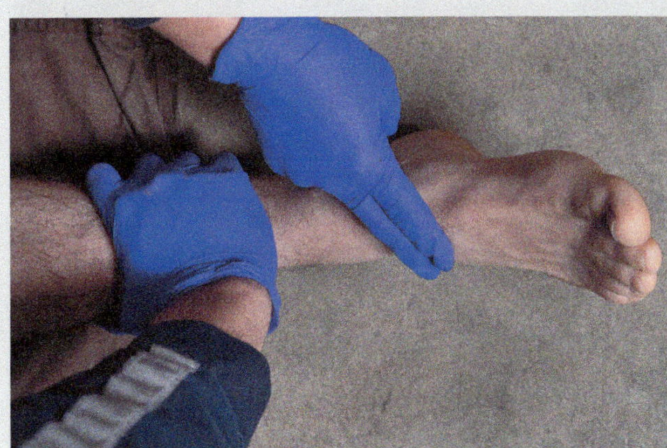

2. Assess distal circulation, sensation, and motor function (CSM).

(continued)

SCAN 32-1 Immobilizing a Long Bone *(continued)*

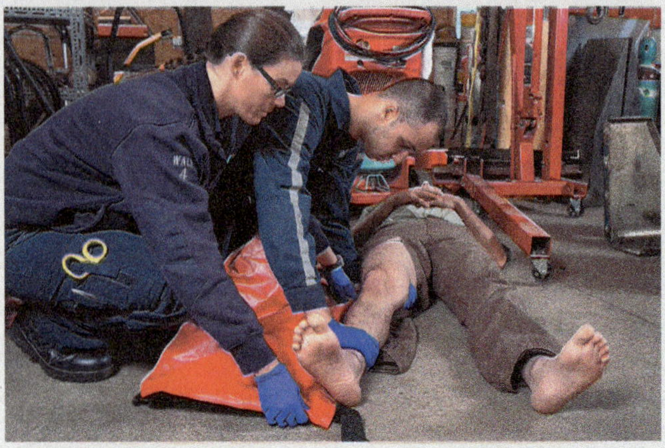

3. Measure the splint. It should extend several inches beyond the joints above and below the injury.

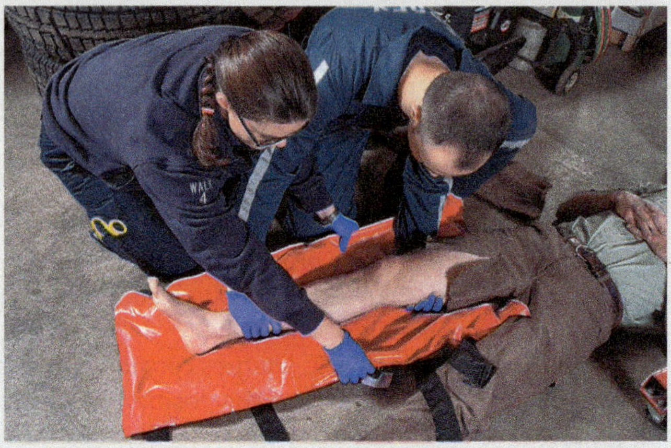

4. Apply the splint and immobilize the joints above and below the injury.

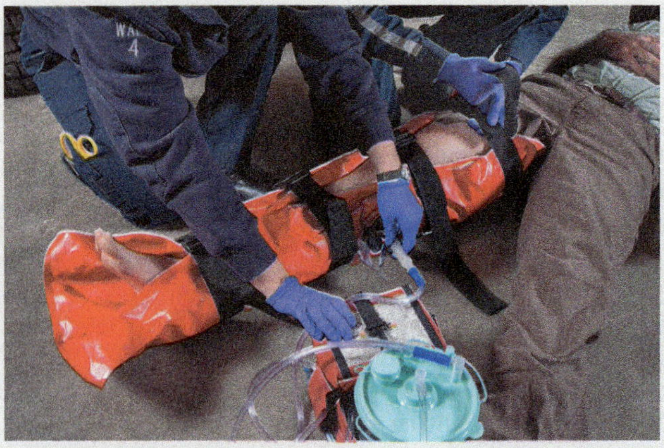

5. Secure the entire injured extremity.

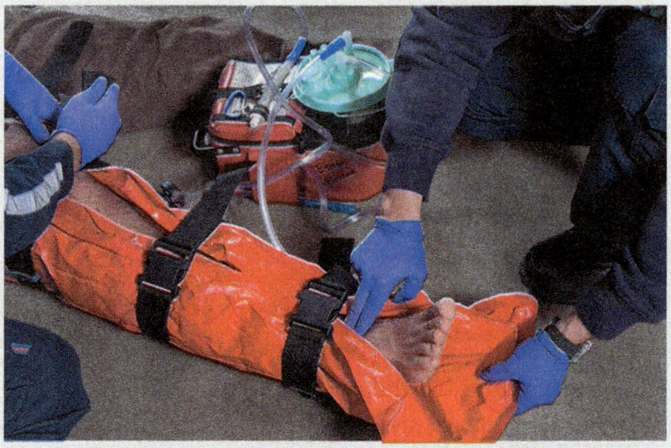

6. Secure the foot in the position of function.

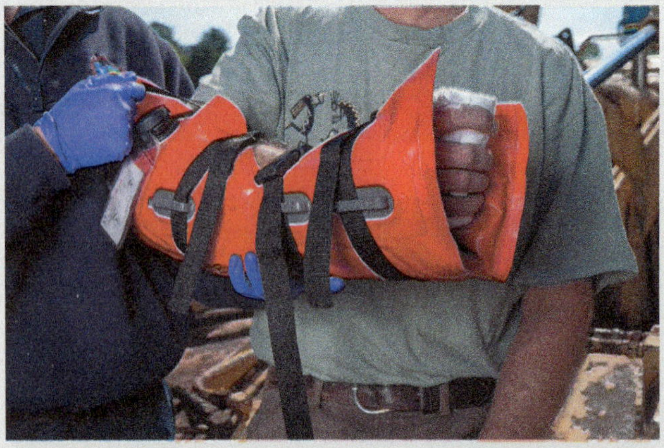

Or, if splinting an arm, secure the hand in the position of function. This is the position the hand would be in if the patient were holding a palm-sized ball. A roll of bandage can be placed in the patient's hand to help maintain the position of function.

7. Reassess distal CSM.

SCAN 32-2 Immobilizing a Joint

First take Standard Precautions.

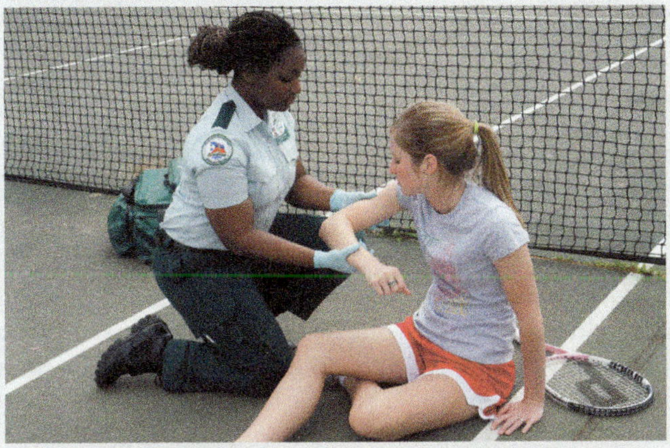

1. Manually stabilize the injured joint—in the case illustrated here, an injured elbow.

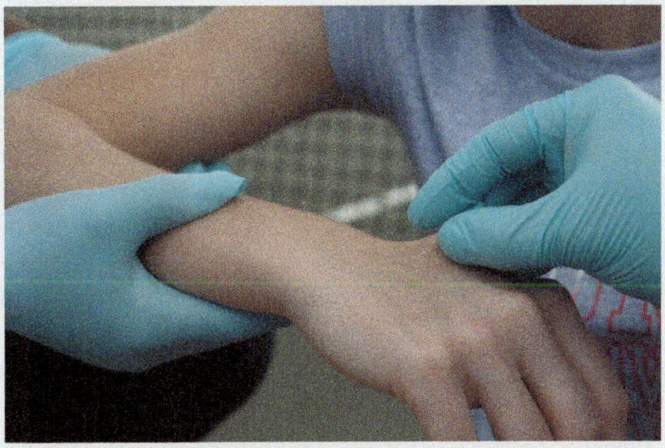

2. Assess distal pulse, sensation, and motor function (CSM).

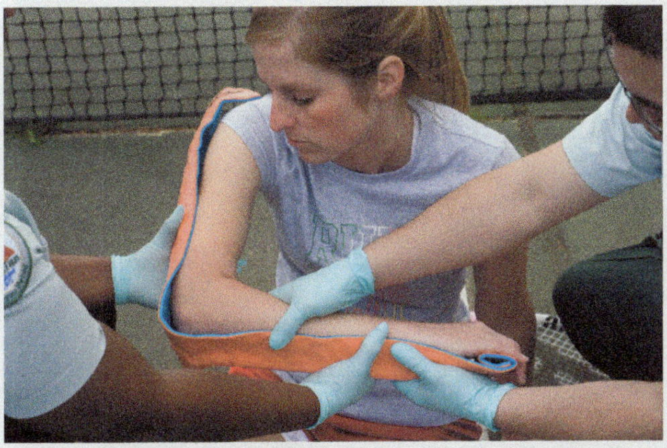

3. Select the proper splint material. Immobilize the site of injury and bones above and below.

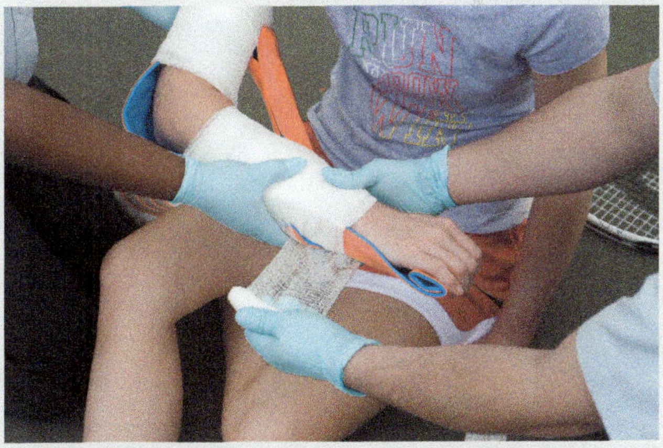

4. Secure the splint.

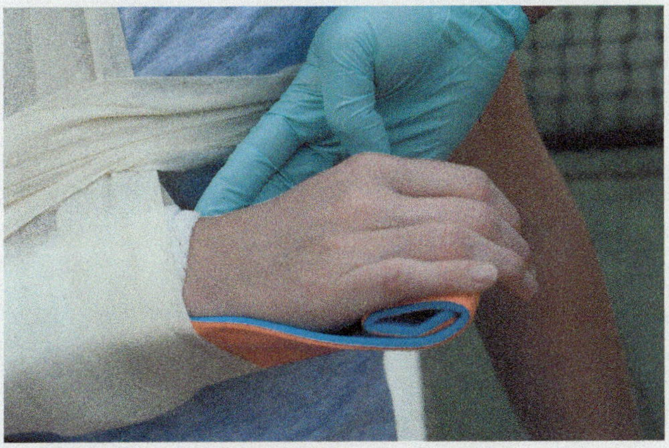

5. Reassess distal CSM.

If using a vacuum splint (Scan 32-3), use the previous steps to assess and prepare the extremity for splinting. Move the vacuum splint into position. Place the splint around the extremity, leaving the distal end (fingers or toes) exposed. Using the pump, withdraw the air from the splint until it is firm; then secure the Velcro straps. Monitor the patient.

Traction Splint

Splinting a femur injury is different from splinting other long-bone or joint injuries. The major problem with femur fractures is the tendency for the large muscle groups of the thigh (quadriceps and hamstrings) to go into spasm, forcing the bone ends to override each other, causing pain and further soft-tissue injury. A traction splint counteracts the muscle spasms and greatly reduces the pain.

Traction splints come in two basic varieties: bipolar and unipolar. A bipolar splint cradles the leg between two metal rods; a unipolar splint has a single metal rod that is placed alongside the leg. Examples of the bipolar splint are the half-ring splint, Hare, and Fernotrac. Examples of the unipolar splint are the Sager and the Kendrick traction devices.

SCAN 32-3 Applying a Vacuum Splint

First take Standard Precautions.

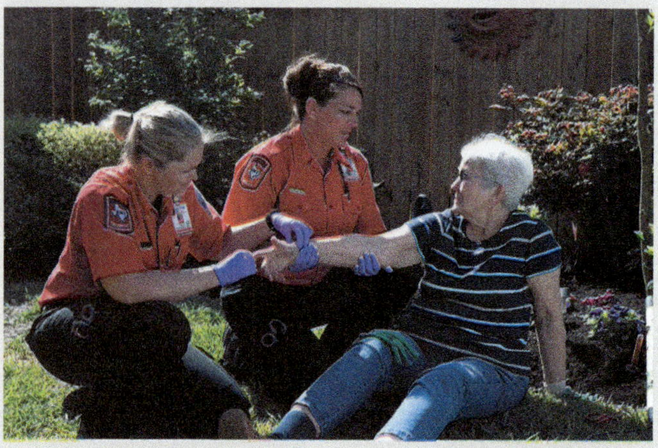

1. Stabilize the extremity and check distal circulation, sensation, and motor function (CSM).

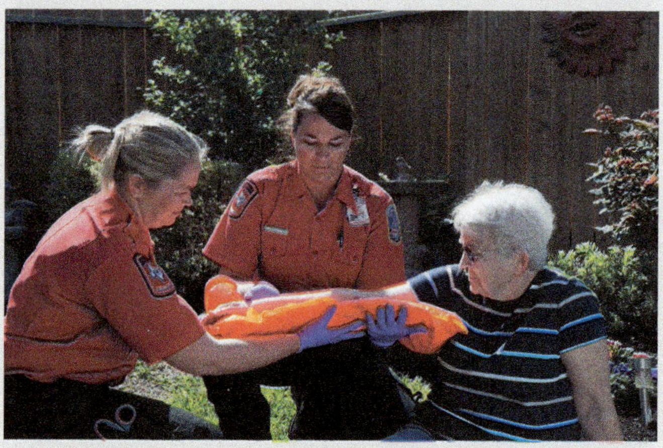

2. Apply the splint to the extremity and secure it with the straps.

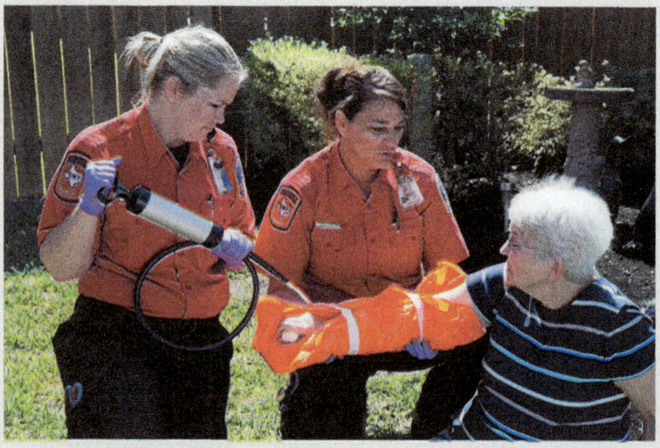

3. Remove the air from the splint with the pump provided by the manufacturer.

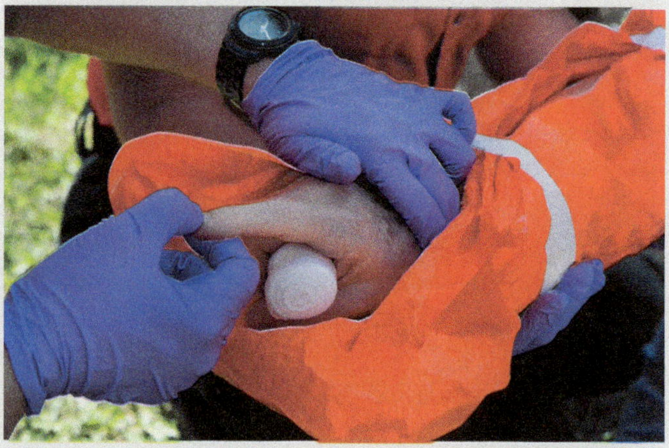

4. Reassess distal CSM.

Typically, traction splints increase the "length" of the patient only slightly. (Applying a bipolar traction splint will be shown later, in Scan 32-9. Applying a unipolar splint will be shown in Scan 32-10.)

One of the most common EMT questions is "How much traction should I pull?" An answer commonly given is "Pull enough traction to give the patient some relief from the pain." This answer can be misleading. When the thigh muscles begin to spasm and the bones begin to override, the patient is in real pain. When manual or mechanical traction is applied, you are pulling against a muscle spasm, and that hurts too. Most patients do not begin to feel relief with the traction splint until it has been applied for several minutes and the muscle spasms begin to subside. With the Sager unipolar splint, traction can be measured. The amount of traction applied should be roughly 10 percent of the patient's body weight and should not exceed 15 pounds (6.8 kg). With a bipolar splint, firm traction should be applied to align the limb. Exert and maintain a firm pull to prevent bones from continuing to override.

No traction splint applied in the field pulls true traction. Instead, all exert "counter-traction." The splint pulls on an ankle hitch and the splint frame is anchored against the pelvis. Once anchored, a pull is felt on the leg. With bipolar splints, any movement of the pelvis off the ground causes a shifting of the splint and loss of traction. Unipolar splints, such as the Sager, are anchored against the pubis between the legs and are less apt to shift and cause a loss of traction during patient movement.

The indications for a traction splint are a painful, swollen, deformed mid-thigh with no joint or lower leg injury. A traction splint is contraindicated if there is a pelvis, hip, or knee injury; if there is an avulsion or partial amputation where traction could separate the extremity; or if there is an injury to the lower third of the leg that would interfere with the ankle hitch.

When possible, use three rescuers to apply a traction splint. One can support the injury site when the limb is lifted to position the traction splint.

General guidelines for the application of a traction splint are as follows:

1. Take Standard Precautions and, if possible, expose the area to be splinted.
2. Manually stabilize the leg and apply manual traction.
3. Assess CSM distal to the injury.
4. Adjust the splint to the proper length and position it at or under the injured leg.
5. Apply the proximal securing device (ischial strap).
6. Apply the distal securing device (ankle hitch).
7. Apply mechanical traction.
8. Position and secure support straps.
9. Reevaluate the proximal and distal securing devices and reassess CSM distal to the injury.
10. Secure the patient's torso and the traction splint to a long spine board to immobilize the hip and to prevent movement of the splint.

Emergency Care of Specific Injuries

The specific injuries described in this section are usually identified as fractures or dislocations. Remember that you do not need to determine the exact nature of an extremity injury. You will simply immobilize any painful, swollen, or deformed extremity. Specific techniques are discussed on the following pages and illustrated later in Scans 32-4 through 32-15.

CORE CONCEPT

Assessment and care of specific injuries to the upper and lower extremities

Upper-Extremity Injuries

Patient Assessment

Shoulder Girdle Injuries

The following are common signs and symptoms of an injury to the shoulder girdle:

- Pain in the shoulder may indicate several types of injury. Look for specific signs.
- A dropped shoulder, with the patient holding the arm of the injured side against the chest, often indicates a fracture of the clavicle.
- A severe blow to the back over the scapula may cause a fracture of that bone. (All the bones of the shoulder girdle can be felt except the scapula. Only the superior ridge of the scapula, called its spine, can be easily palpated. Injury to the scapula is rare but must be considered if there are indications of a severe blow at the site of this bone.)

Check the entire shoulder girdle. Feel for deformity and tenderness where the clavicle joins the anterior scapula (the acromion). Feel and look along the entire clavicle for deformity from the sternum medially to the shoulder laterally. Note if the head of the humerus can be felt or moves in front of the shoulder. This is a sign of possible anterior dislocation or fracture.

Patient Care

Care for the Patient with Shoulder Girdle Injuries

Fundamental Principles of Care

Emergency care of a patient with a shoulder girdle injury includes the following steps:

- Assess distal CSM. If distal CSM is impaired, immobilize and transport as soon as possible, notifying the receiving facility.
- It is not practical to use a rigid splint for injuries to the clavicle, the scapula, or the head of the humerus. Use a sling and swathe (Scan 32-4). If there is a possible cervical-spine injury, do not tie a sling around the patient's neck.
- If there is evidence of a possible anterior dislocation of the head of the humerus (the bone head is pushed toward the front of the body), place a thin pillow between the patient's arm and chest before applying the sling and swathe.
- Do not attempt to straighten or reduce any dislocations.
- Reassess distal CSM.

NOTE: *Sometimes a dislocated shoulder will reduce itself (the displaced head of the humerus "pops" back into place). When this happens, check distal CSM. Apply a sling and swathe and transport the patient. Because the ligaments are weak or stretched, the joint is at high risk of dislocating again. The patient must be seen by a physician.*

Lower-Extremity Injuries

Patient Assessment

Pelvic Injuries

Fractures of the pelvis may occur with falls, in motor-vehicle collisions, or when a person is crushed between two objects. Pelvic fractures may be the result of direct or indirect force. The following are common signs and symptoms of a pelvic injury:

- Complaint of pain in the pelvis, hips, groin, or back. This may be the only indication, but it is significant if the mechanism of injury indicates possible fracture. Usually, obvious deformity is associated with the pain.
- Painful reaction when pressure is applied to the iliac crests (wings of the pelvis) or to the pubic bones.
- Complaint that the patient cannot lift the legs when lying supine. (Do not test for this, but do check for sensation.)
- Foot on the injured side may turn outward (lateral rotation). This also may indicate a hip fracture.
- Patient has an unexplained pressure on the urinary bladder and the feeling of having to empty the bladder.
- Bleeding from the urethra, rectum, or vaginal opening in the setting of a high-impact mechanism of injury. Blood at the meatus of the penis (opening of the urethra) is a finding unique to pelvic trauma/fracture (Figure 32-18).

FIGURE 32-18 (A) Blood at the meatus of the penis is a sign of a pelvic fracture. (B) A pelvic wrap can help to stabilize a fractured pelvis. Shown here is a commercial pelvic binding device placed on a severely injured patient with an open pelvic fracture. *(Photos A and B: © Edward T. Dickinson, MD)*

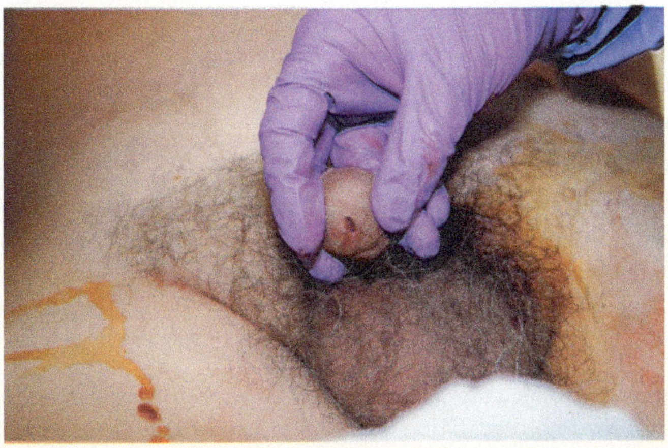

A

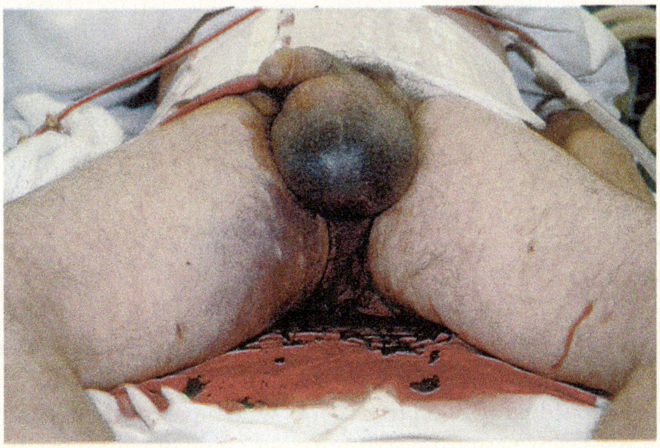

B

Patient Care

Care for the Patient with Pelvic Injuries

Fundamental Principles of Care

Emergency care for pelvic injuries includes the following steps:

- Move the patient as little as possible. If you must move the patient, move the body as a unit. Never lift the patient with the pelvis unsupported. Warning: Use caution when using a log roll to move a patient with a suspected pelvic fracture. Roll the patient gently to the uninjured side when possible.
- Determine CSM distal to the injury site.
- Straighten the patient's lower limbs into the anatomic position if there are no injuries to the hip joints or lower limbs, and if it can be done without meeting resistance or causing excessive pain.
- Prevent additional injury to the pelvis by stabilizing the lower limbs. Either apply a pelvic wrap or place a folded blanket between the patient's legs, from the groin to the feet, and bind them together with wide cravats. Thin, rigid splints can be used to push the cravats under the patient. The cravats can then be adjusted for proper placement at the upper thigh, above the knee, below the knee, and above the ankle.
- Assume that there are spinal injuries. Immobilize the patient appropriately. When securing the patient, avoid placing the straps or ties over the pelvic area.
- Reassess distal CSM.
- Care for shock, providing high-concentration oxygen as appropriate. Pelvic fractures are typically associated with significant internal blood loss.
- Transport the patient as soon as possible.
- Monitor vital signs.

Once the patient is in the ambulance, some EMTs are allowed to make adjustments to improve patient comfort and reduce muscle spasms of the abdomen and lower limb by gently flexing the legs and placing a pillow under the knees. If you are allowed to follow this protocol, be extremely careful not to move the spine since the patient may have associated spinal injuries.

NOTE: *It may be very difficult to tell a fractured pelvis from a fracture of the upper femur. When there is doubt, to protect blood vessels and nerves associated with the femur-pelvis (hip) joint, care for the patient as if there is a pelvic fracture. Remember, there may also be spinal injuries.*

Pelvic Wrap

One method of treating pelvic injuries is the pelvic wrap. Performed with commercially available devices or formed from a sheet (these steps are described in the following text), the wrap reduces internal bleeding and pain while providing stabilization to the pelvis. It may also prevent further injury. Since many systems no longer carry the pneumatic anti-shock garment (PASG), the pelvic wrap provides an alternative treatment for suspected pelvic fracture.

The pelvic wrap should be applied to patients who have pelvic deformity or instability (movement upon palpation) regardless of whether signs of shock are present. Some systems may also recommend use of the pelvic wrap with a mechanism of injury that would indicate pelvic injury (e.g., motorcycle crashes, auto–pedestrian collisions) even if obvious deformity is not present.

As already noted, you may carry a commercial pelvic splint (Figure 32-19A) on the ambulance for use with such injuries. If you do not have a commercial device available,

FIGURE 32-19 (A) A commercial pelvic splint. (B) To devise a pelvic wrap, lay a sheet, folded flat, approximately 10 inches (25 centimeters) wide onto the backboard. (C) Bring the sides of the sheet together. (D) Tie the sheet firmly without overcompression to complete the pelvic wrap.

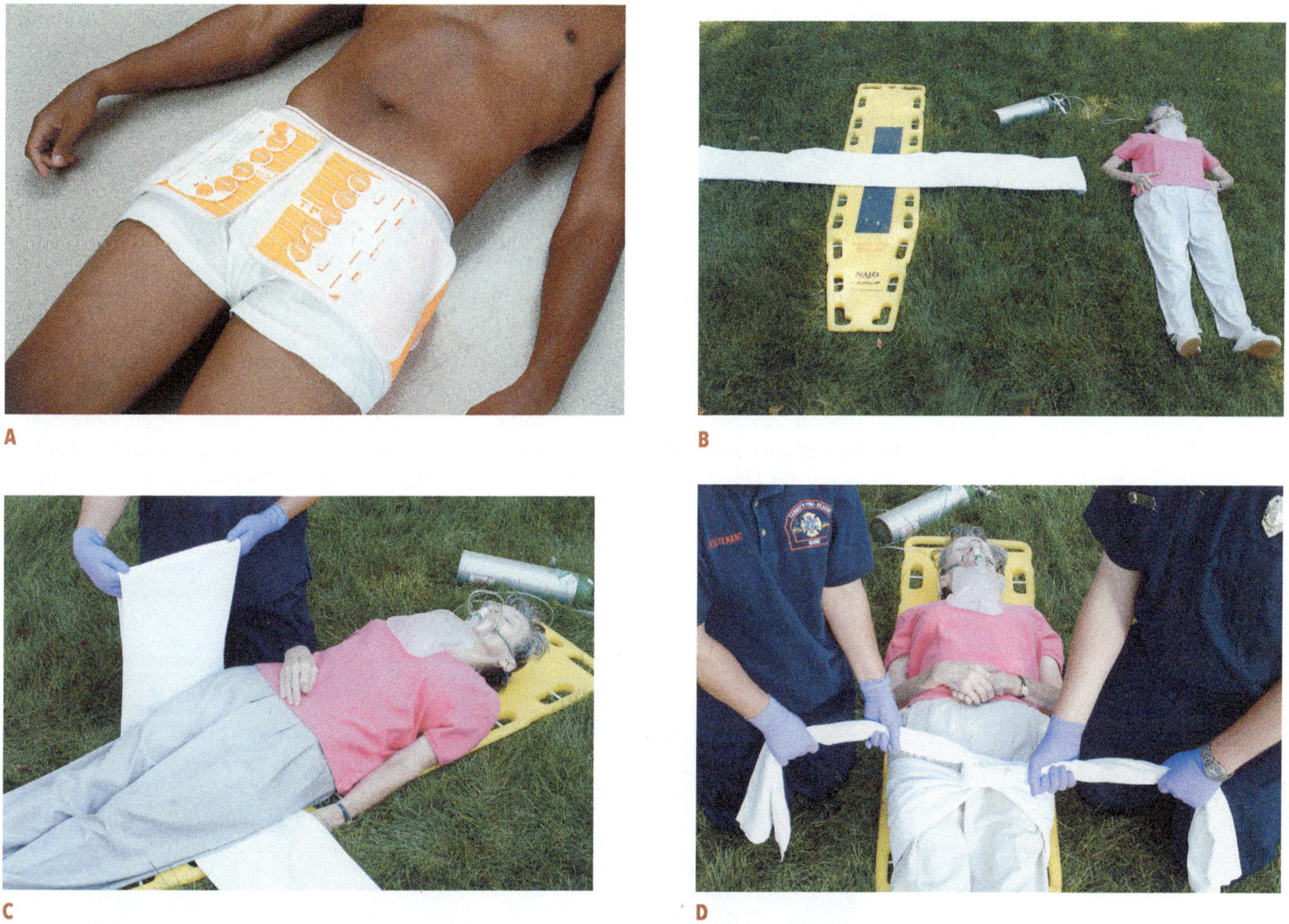

you can devise a pelvic wrap from a sheet (Figure 32-19B). You may place an open commercial pelvic splint or a sheet on the backboard before moving the patient to the backboard, even if you do not immediately secure it, in the event evidence of instability or shock develops. Always follow your local protocols.

To apply a sheet as a pelvic wrap:

1. Once you determine the patient is a candidate for pelvic stabilization (unstable pelvis with or without signs of shock or MOI), prepare a backboard with a sheet, folded flat, approximately 10 inches (25 centimeters) wide and lying across the backboard where the hips will be positioned.
2. Carefully roll the patient to the backboard. Center the sheet at the patient's greater trochanter (the bony prominence at the proximal end of the femur). This will position the sheet lower than the iliac "wings." This is the correct position.
3. Bring the sides of the sheet around to the front of the patient (Figure 32-19C). As you bring the sides of the sheet together and tie them, you will cause compression and stabilization of the pelvis. The sheet should feel firm enough on the pelvis to keep it in normal position without overcompression (Figure 32-19D).
4. Secure the sheet using ties or clamps so the compression is maintained.

NOTE: *Some EMS agencies prefer to apply the pelvic wrap to the patient before moving the patient to the backboard to reduce the pain of that move.*

Patient Assessment

Hip Dislocation

A hip dislocation occurs when the head of the femur is pulled or pushed from its pelvic socket. It can be difficult to tell a hip dislocation from a fracture of the proximal (uppermost portion of the) femur. Conscious patients will complain of intense pain with both types of injury. Patients who have had a surgical replacement of the hip joint are at increased risk of hip dislocation. Before hip replacements were common, this was a very uncommon injury that EMTs mainly saw in healthy young males who had sustained significant trauma. Now EMTs encounter hip dislocations regularly, particularly in middle-aged and older patients, because the hip prosthesis has malfunctioned and allowed the head of the femur to slip out of the socket in the pelvis. The hip can be either anteriorly or posteriorly dislocated.

The following are common signs and symptoms of a hip dislocation:

- **Anterior hip dislocation.** The patient's entire lower limb is rotated outward, and the hip is usually flexed.
- **Posterior hip dislocation (more common).** The patient's leg is rotated inward, the hip is flexed, and the knee is bent (Figure 32-20). The foot may hang loose (foot drop), and the patient is unable to flex the foot or lift the toes. Often there is a lack of sensation in the limb. These signs indicate possible damage, caused by the dislocated femoral head, to the sciatic nerve, the major nerve that extends from the lower spine to the posterior thigh. This injury often occurs when a person's knees strike the dashboard during a motor-vehicle collision.

FIGURE 32-20 A right posterior hip dislocation from dashboard impact.
(© Edward T. Dickinson, MD)

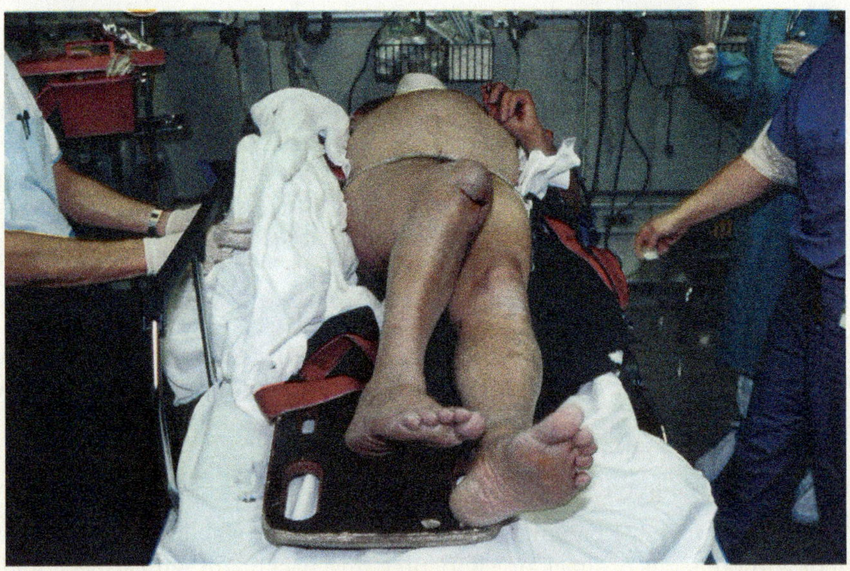

Patient Care

Care for the Patient with a Hip Dislocation

Fundamental Principles of Care

Emergency care of a patient with a hip dislocation includes the following steps:

- Assess distal CSM.
- Move the patient onto a long spine board. Some systems use a scoop-style stretcher. When this device is used, the limb should be immobilized.

- Immobilize the limb with pillows or rolled blankets.
- Secure the patient to the long spine board or scoop-style stretcher with straps or cravats.
- Reassess distal CSM. If there is a pulse, sensory, or motor problem, notify medical direction and immediately transport.
- Care for shock by providing high-concentration oxygen as appropriate.
- Transport carefully, monitor vital signs, and continue to check for nerve and circulation impairment.

NOTE: *If you find a painful, swollen, or deformed thigh, and the leg is flexed and will not straighten, the patient may also have a fractured femur.*

Patient Assessment

Hip Fracture

A hip fracture is a fracture of the proximal femur, not the pelvis. The fracture can occur to the femoral head, the femoral neck, or at the portion of the femur just below the neck of the bone. Sometimes the hip fractures after the patient—commonly an older female—falls on the floor and lands on the hip. Older adults are more susceptible to this type of injury because of brittle bones or bones weakened by disease. Some patients, though, sustain a fracture of a weak spot in the hip and then fall to the floor. Asking the patient about the sequence of events will often allow you to determine what happened and in what order.

The following are common signs and symptoms of a hip fracture:

- Pain is localized, although some patients also complain of pain in the knee.
- Sometimes the patient is sensitive to pressure exerted on the lateral prominence of the hip (greater trochanter).
- Surrounding tissues are discolored; however, discoloration may be delayed.
- Swelling may be evident.
- The patient is unable to move the limb while on his or her back.
- Patient complains about being unable to stand.
- Foot on injured side usually turns outward; however, it may rotate inward (rarely).
- Injured limb may appear shorter.

Patient Care

Care for the Patient with a Hip Fracture

Fundamental Principles of Care

Be certain to assess distal CSM before and after splinting and during transport. You should place the patient on a long spine board or orthopedic stretcher after splinting.

One of the following emergency care methods can be used to stabilize a hip fracture (Figure 32-21):

- **Bind the legs together.** Place a folded blanket between the patient's legs, and bind the legs together with wide straps, Velcro-equipped straps, or wide cravats. Carefully place the patient on a long spine board and use pillows to support the lower limbs. Secure the patient to the board. An orthopedic stretcher can be used in place of the long spine board.

- **Padded boards.** Use thin splints to push cravats or straps under the patient at the natural voids (such as the small of the back and backs of the knees) and readjust them so they will pass across the chest, the abdomen just below the belt, below the crotch, above and below the knee, and at the ankle. Splint with two long padded boards. Ideally, one should be long enough to extend from the patient's armpit to beyond the foot. The other should be long enough to extend from the crotch to beyond the foot. Cushion with padding in the armpit and crotch, and pad all voids created at the ankle and knee. Secure the boards with the cravats or straps.

FIGURE 32-21 Binding together the legs of a patient with a hip injury.

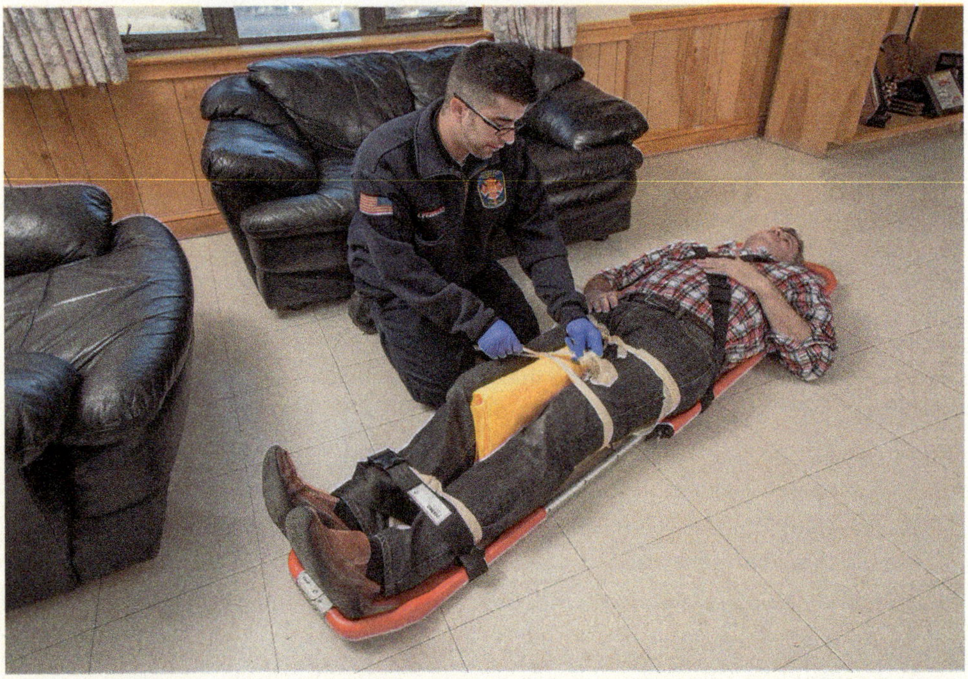

Patient Assessment

Femoral Shaft Fracture

Because the femur is a large, strong bone, considerable force is necessary to cause a fracture of the femoral shaft. Remember that muscle contractions can cause bone ends to ride over each other. The bone ends may or may not protrude from an open wound. Never assume that a wound on the thigh is superficial because you do not see bone ends. Always check for signs and symptoms that this wound may be an open fracture.

The following are common signs and symptoms of a femoral shaft fracture:

- The patient may complain of pain, which is often intense.
- Often there will be an open fracture with deformity, and sometimes with the end of the bone protruding through the wound. When the injury is a closed fracture, often there will be deformity with possible severe angulation.
- The injured limb may appear to be shortened because the contraction of the thigh muscles caused the bone ends to override each other.

Patient Care

Care for a Patient with a Femoral Shaft Fracture

Fundamental Principles of Care

Emergency care of a patient with a femoral shaft fracture includes the following steps:

- Control any bleeding by applying direct pressure (avoiding the possible fracture site) forcefully enough to overcome the barrier of muscle mass. If there is external bleeding that you cannot control with direct pressure, apply a tourniquet.
- If the patient is displaying signs of shock (hypoperfusion), treat for it, including providing high-concentration oxygen.
- Assess distal CSM.
- If the patient is stable, apply a traction splint. (See Scan 32-9 and Scan 32-10.) When pulling traction, do not try to make the legs the same length. Your goal is to overcome muscle spasm that makes the bone ends override. If a traction splint is not available, or the patient is not stable, bind the legs together after placing them in the anatomic position.
- When traction-splinting thigh injuries in children, be sure to use appropriate-sized splints.
- Reassess distal CSM.

NOTE: *The traction splint should not be applied if you suspect that there may be additional injuries or fractures to the area of the knee or to the tibia or fibula of the same limb.*

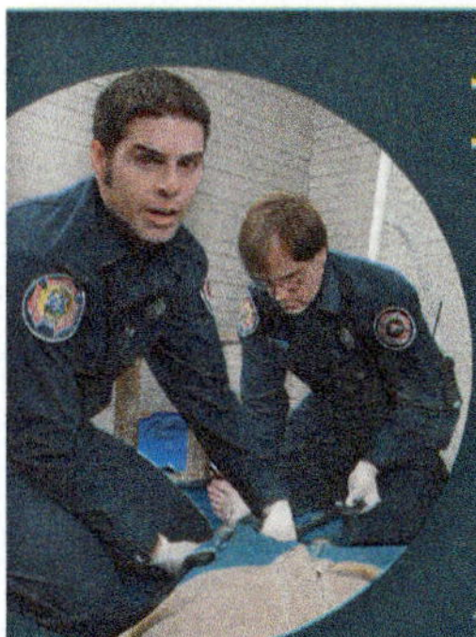

Point of View

"I was building this really cool indoor driving range in the loft over the barn. I put down green artificial turf. It was going to be great. I was hanging the net when the ladder gave way and I fell.

"It's funny but on the way down, I had time to get a sinking feeling: knowing it was going to hurt when I landed, hoping I didn't break anything, and thinking that probably no one would even hear me. I hit the floor and broke my leg. I knew because I heard–and felt–the twist, then the break.

"I yelled for about five minutes before a neighbor heard me. But then the EMTs came pretty quickly, and they were good guys. They didn't sugarcoat the situation. They said it might hurt when they put the splint on and when they carried me down the narrow barn stairs. I hadn't even thought of how they would get me downstairs. I'm not a small guy.

"But they did it. They did it well. They were right; it hurt some, but I appreciate them telling me the truth.

"I guess I've got about eight weeks before I get to take the first swing in my new driving range."

Patient Assessment

Knee Injury

The knee is a joint, and not a single bone. Fractures can occur to the distal femur, to the proximal tibia and fibula, and to the patella (kneecap). The following are common signs and symptoms of a knee injury:

- Pain and tenderness (Figure 32-22)
- Swelling
- Deformity with obvious swelling

FIGURE 32-22 EMT assessing knee injury in a child.

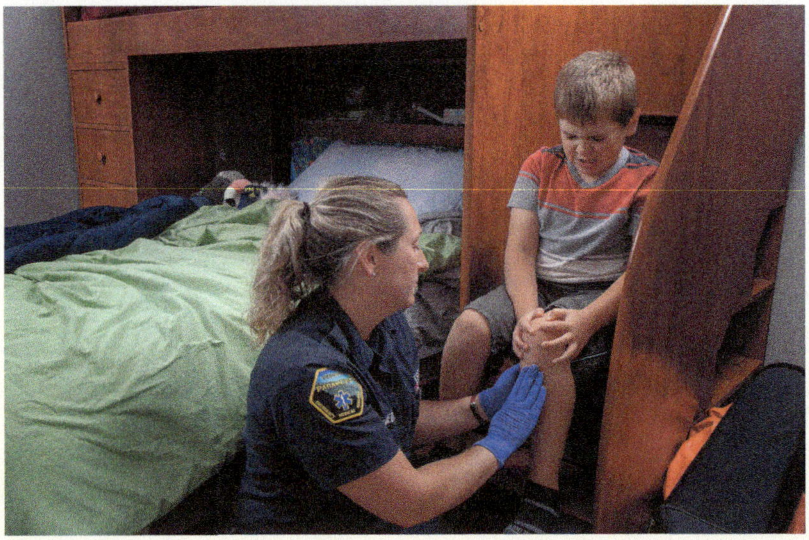

Patient Care

Patient with a Knee Injury

Fundamental Principles of Care

There are two general emergency care methods used for immobilizing the knee–one if the knee is bent, the other if it is straight:

- **Knee is bent.** Assess distal CSM. Immobilize the knee in the position in which the leg is found. Tie two padded board splints to the thigh and above the ankle so the knee is held in position. You can use a pillow to support the leg. Reassess distal CSM. (See Scan 32-11.)
- **Knee is straight or returned to the anatomic position.** Assess distal CSM. Immobilize the knee with two padded board splints or a single padded splint. When using two padded boards, placing one medially and one laterally offers the best support. Remember to pad the voids created at the knee and ankle. Reassess distal CSM. (See Scan 32-12 and Scan 32-13.)

Do not confuse a patella dislocation with a knee dislocation. The patella can become displaced when the lower leg and knee are twisted, as in a skiing or racquetball accident. In a patellar dislocation, the knee will be stuck in flexion and the kneecap will be displaced and laterally palpable. A knee dislocation occurs when the tibia itself is forced either anteriorly or posteriorly in relation to the distal femur. Always check for a distal pulse, since the dislocated knee joint can compress the popliteal artery and stop the major blood supply to the lower leg. If there is no pulse, this is a true emergency. Contact medical direction for permission to gently move the lower leg anteriorly to allow for a pulse, and immediately transport the patient.

What appears to be a dislocation may prove to be a fracture or a combined fracture and dislocation. Even if you believe that the patient has suffered a dislocated patella and the kneecap has repositioned itself, realize that other damage may be hidden. Whether you suspect a fracture, a dislocation, a sprain, or a strain, always splint the injury and transport the patient.

Once splinting is done, monitor the patient. If there is a loss of distal CSM, or if the foot becomes discolored (white, mottled, or blue) and turns cold, transport the patient without delay. Notify medical direction while en route.

Patient Assessment

Tibia or Fibula Injury

The following are common signs and symptoms of a tibia or fibula injury:

- Pain and tenderness
- Swelling
- Possible deformity (You might expect to see a deformity of the lower leg when the tibia or fibula is fractured. However, such deformity is often absent.)

Patient Care

Care of the Patient with a Tibia or Fibula Injury

Fundamental Principles of Care

Because immobilizing the leg can help to relieve pain and control bleeding, apply a splint using one of the following methods. Remember to assess distal CSM before and after application.

- **Vacuum splint.** Apply a vacuum splint. While maintaining manual traction, have your partner slide the splint under the injured limb. Your partner must make sure that the splint is relatively wrinkle-free and that it extends to adjacent joints (for a bone injury) or bones (for a joint injury). Continue to maintain traction while your partner deflates the splint. Test to see if the splint is firm and provides support. Remember to check periodically to see that the splint is still firm and doing its job.
- **Air-inflated splint.** Apply an air-inflated splint (Figure 32-23). Slide the uninflated splint over your hand and gather it in place until the lower edge clears your wrist. Using your free hand, grasp the patient's foot and leg just above the injury site. While maintaining manual traction, have your partner slide the splint over your hand and onto the injured leg. Your partner must make sure that the splint is relatively wrinkle-free and that it covers the injury site. Continue to maintain traction while your partner inflates the splint. Test to see if you can cause a slight dent in the plastic with fingertip pressure. Remember to check periodically to see that the pressure in the splint has remained adequate and has not decreased or increased.

- **Two-splint method.** You can immobilize the fracture using two rigid board splints (Scan 32-14).
- **Single splint.** A single splint with or without an ankle hitch can be applied (Scan 32-15).

FIGURE 32-23 An air splint may be used for a lower leg injury.

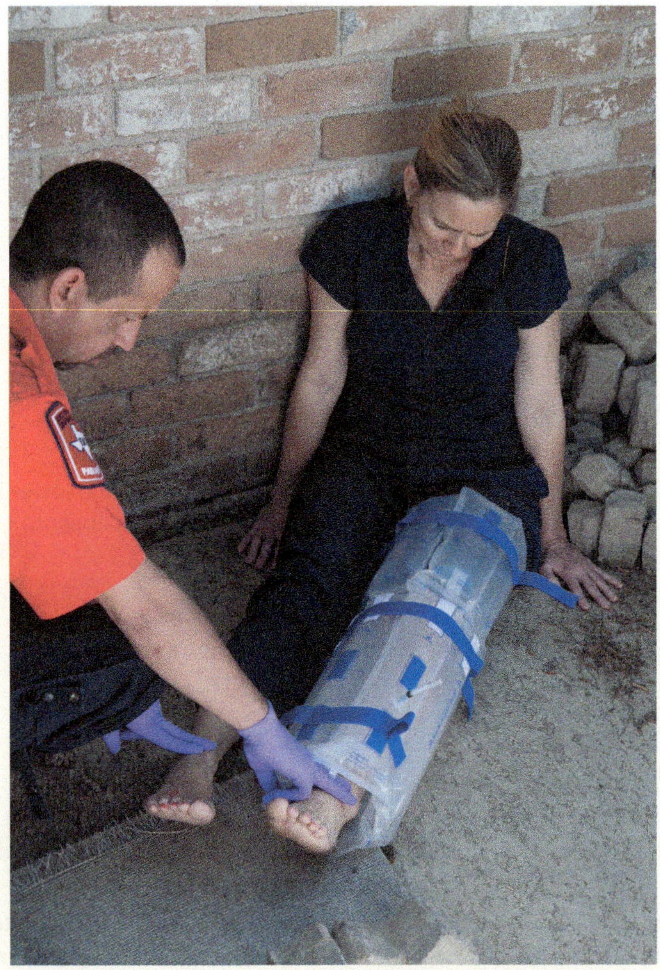

Patient Assessment

Ankle or Foot Injury

Sprains (torn ligaments) and fractures are the most common musculoskeletal injuries to the ankle and foot. It is often difficult to distinguish between them, so always treat for a fracture. The following are common signs and symptoms of an ankle or foot injury:

- Pain
- Swelling
- Possible deformity

Patient Care

Care of the Patient with an Ankle or Foot Injury

Fundamental Principles of Care

Long splints, extending from above the knee to beyond the foot, can be used. However, soft splinting is an effective, rapid method and is recommended for most patients (Figure 32-24).

FIGURE 32-24 A pillow splint may be used for an injured ankle.

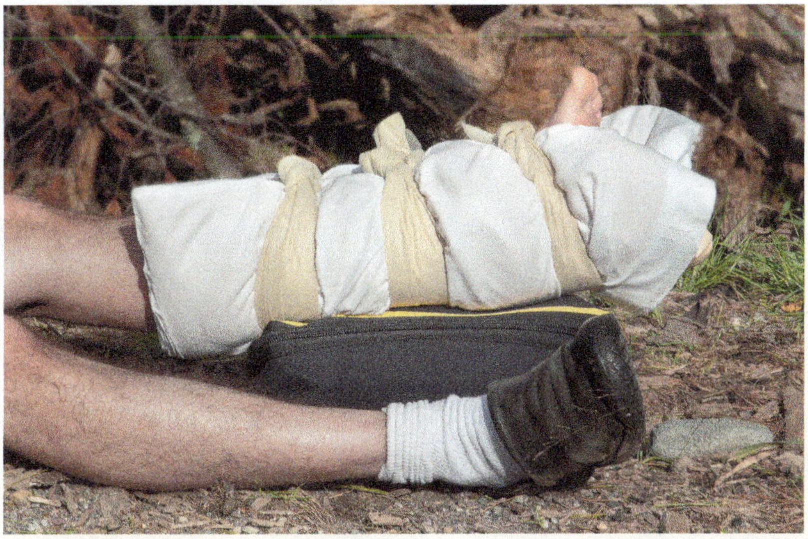

To soft splint, you should follow the emergency care steps described in the following list:

- Assess distal CSM.
- Stabilize the limb. Remove the patient's shoe if possible, but only if it removes easily and can be done with no movement to the ankle.
- Lift the limb but do not apply manual traction (tension).
- Place three cravats on the floor under the ankle. Then place a pillow lengthwise under the ankle on top of the cravats. The pillow should extend 6 inches (15 centimeters) beyond the foot.
- Gently lower the limb onto the pillow, taking care not to change the ankle's position. Stabilize by tying the cravats, and adjust them so they are at the top of the pillow, midway, and at the heel.
- Tie the pillow to the ankle and foot.
- Tie a fourth cravat loosely at the arch of the foot.
- Elevate with a second pillow or blanket. Reassess distal CSM.
- Care for shock (hypoperfusion) if needed. This is usually not necessary for an isolated injury.
- Apply a cold pack to the injury site to reduce bleeding and swelling if appropriate. Do not apply the pack directly to the skin.

Note that a commercial lower extremity splint that stabilizes the ankle and that extends above the knee may be better than a pillow since it will also immobilize the knee, the joint adjacent to the ankle.

SCAN 32-4 Applying a Sling and Swathe

A sling is a triangular bandage used to support the shoulder and arm. Once the patient's arm is placed in a sling, a swathe can be used to hold the arm against the side of the chest. Commercial slings are available. Velcro straps can be used to form a swathe. Use whatever materials you have on hand, provided they will not cut into the patient. Also, remember to assess distal circulation, sensation, and motor function (CSM) both before and after immobilizing or splinting an extremity.

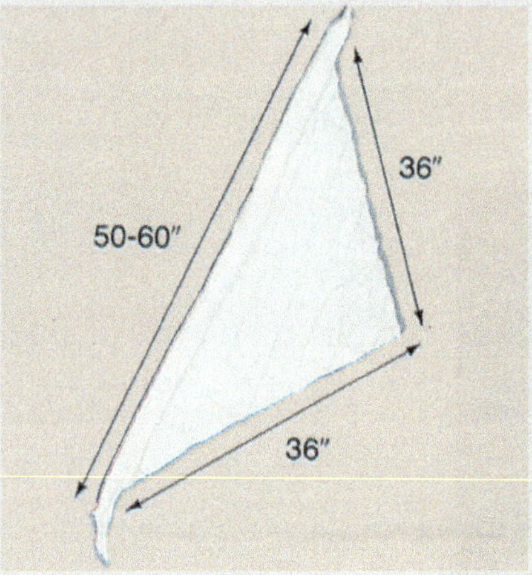

1. Prepare the sling by folding cloth into a triangle.

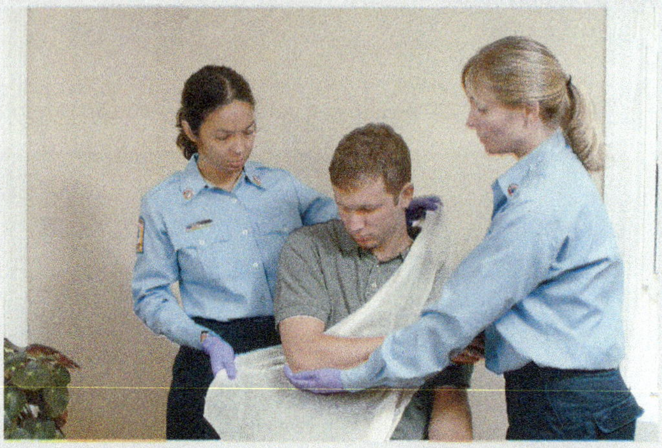

2. Position the sling over the top of the patient's chest as shown. Fold the injured arm across the patient's chest.

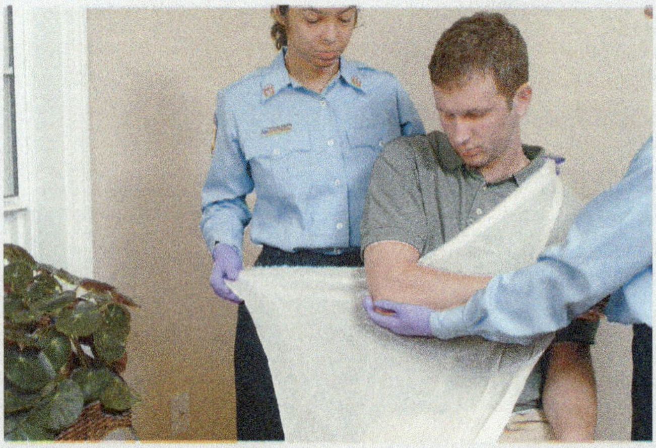

If the patient cannot hold the patient's arm, have someone assist until you tie the sling.

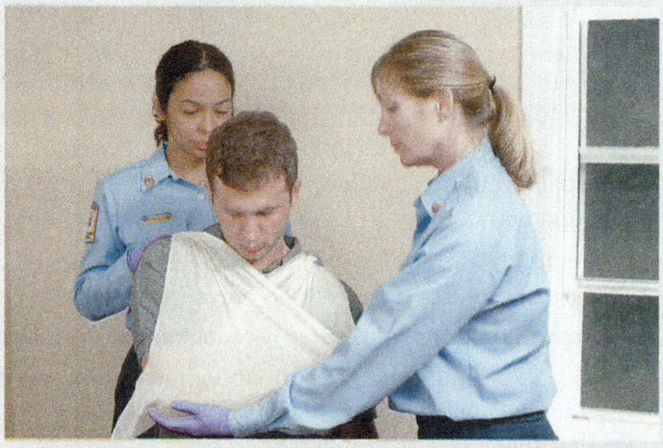

3. Extend one point of the triangle beyond the elbow on the injured side. Take the bottom point and bring it up over the patient's arm. Then take it over the top of the injured shoulder.

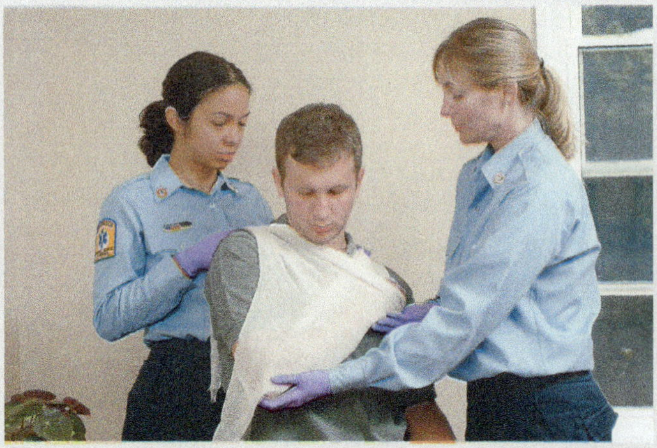

4. If appropriate, draw up the ends of the sling so the patient's hand is about 4 inches (10 centimeters) above the elbow.

SCAN 32-4 Applying a Sling and Swathe *(continued)*

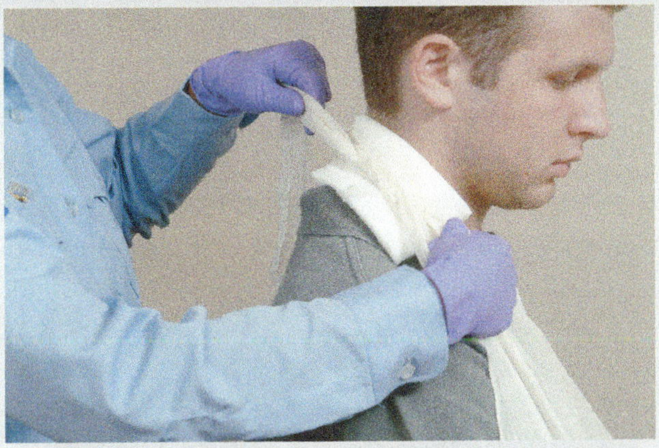

5. Tie the two ends of the sling together, making sure that the knot does not press against the back of the patient's neck. Pad with bulky dressings. (If spine injury is possible, pin the ends to the patient's clothing. Do not tie them around the neck.)

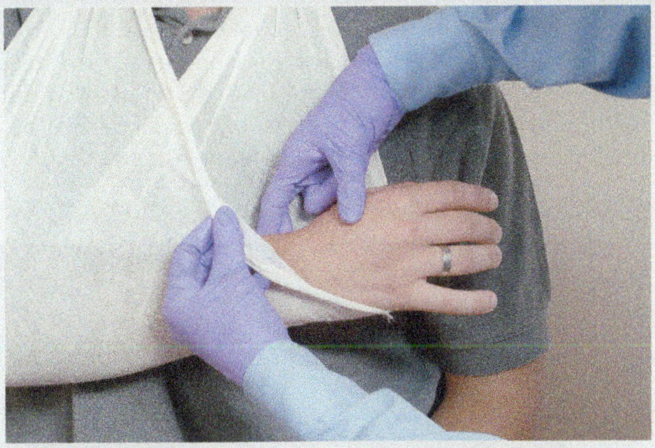

6. Check to be sure you have left the patient's fingertips exposed. Then assess distal circulation, sensation, and motor function (CSM). If the pulse has been lost, adjust or take off the sling and repeat the procedure. Then check again.

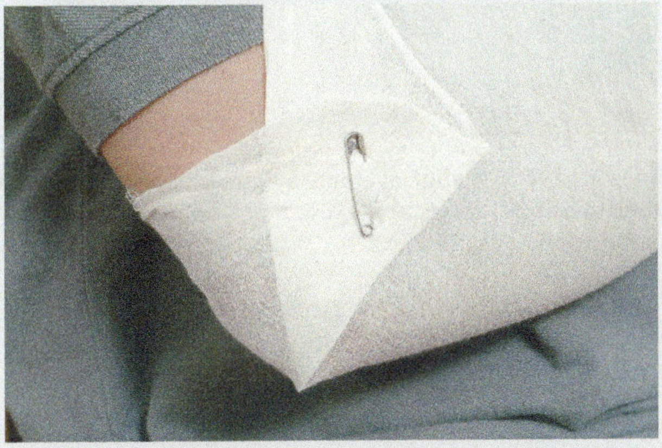

7. To form a pocket for the patient's elbow, take hold of the point of material at the elbow and fold it forward, pinning it to the front of the sling.

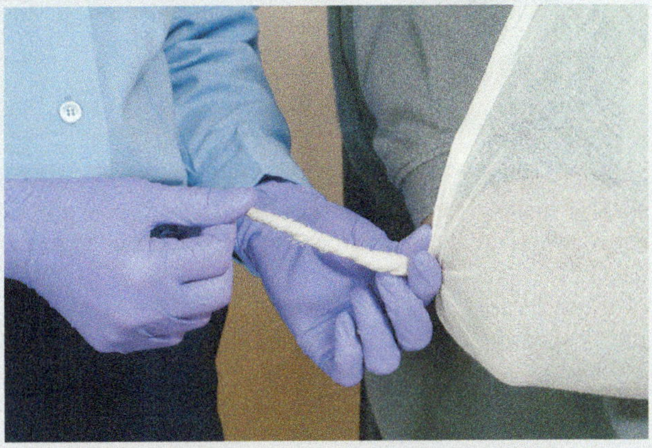

If you do not have a pin, twist the excess material and tie a knot in the point.

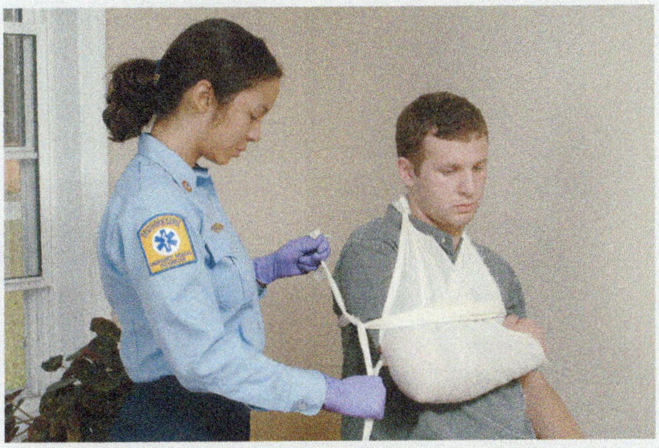

8. Form a swathe from a second piece of material. Tie it around the chest and the injured arm, over the sling. Do not place it over the patient's arm on the uninjured side.

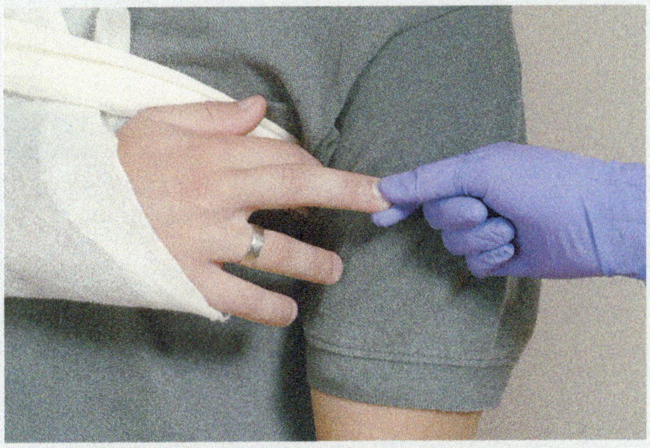

9. Reassess distal CSM. Take vital signs. Perform detailed assessments and reassessments as appropriate.

SCAN 32-5 Splinting an Injured Humerus

SIGNS: Injury to the humerus can take place at the proximal end (shoulder), along the shaft of the bone, or at the distal end (elbow). Deformity is the most obvious sign used to detect fractures to this bone in any of these locations; however, assess for all signs of skeletal injury, including pain or swelling. Follow the rules and procedures for care of an injured extremity.

NOTE: *Assess distal circulation, sensation, and motor function (CSM) both before and after immobilizing or splinting an extremity.*

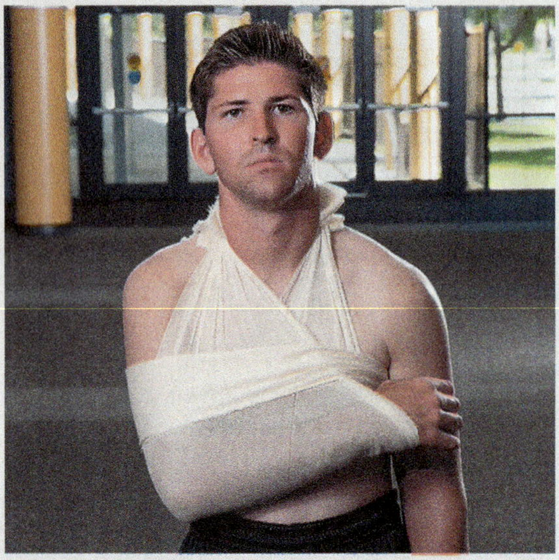

VARIATION ONE: Apply a sling and swathe. If you have only enough material for a swathe, bind the patient's upper arm to the body, taking great care not to cut off circulation to the forearm.

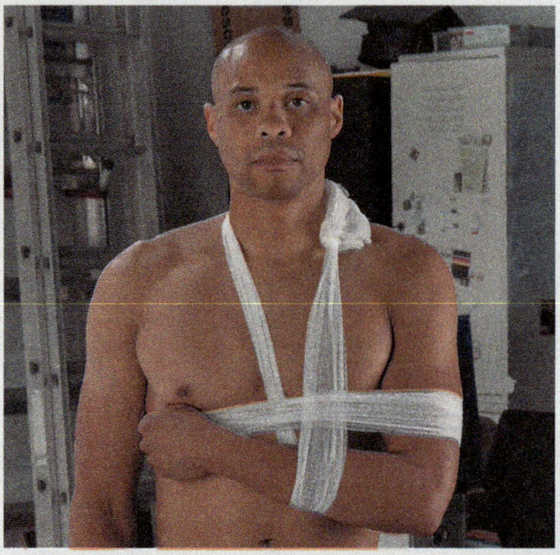

VARIATION TWO: If you have only a narrow or short length of material to use as a sling, apply it so that it supports the arm.

NOTE: *Before applying a sling and swathe to care for injuries to the humerus, check the patient's distal circulation, sensation, and motor function (CSM). If you do not feel a pulse, attempt to straighten angulation if the patient has a closed fracture. (Follow local protocol.) Otherwise, prepare for immediate immobilization and transport. If straightening of the angulation fails to restore the pulse or function, splint with a fixation splint, keeping the forearm extended. If there is no sign of circulation or of sensory or motor function, you will have to attempt a second splinting. If this fails to restore distal function, immediately transport the patient. Do not try to straighten angulation of the humerus if there are any signs of fracture or dislocation of the shoulder or elbow.*

SCAN 32-6 Splinting Arm and Elbow Injuries

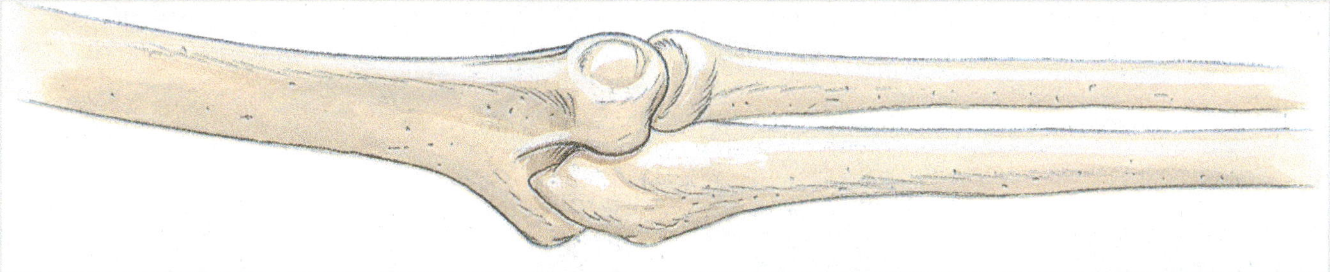

SIGNS: The elbow is a joint and not a bone. It is composed of the distal humerus and the proximal ulna and radius, which form a hinge joint. You will have to decide if the injury is truly to the elbow. The location of deformity and tenderness will direct you to the injury site.

CARE: If there is a distal pulse, the dislocated elbow should be immobilized in the position in which it is found. The joint has too many nerves and blood vessels to risk movement. When a distal pulse is absent, make one attempt to slightly reposition the limb after contacting medical direction. Do not force the limb into the anatomic position.

Elbow in STRAIGHT Position

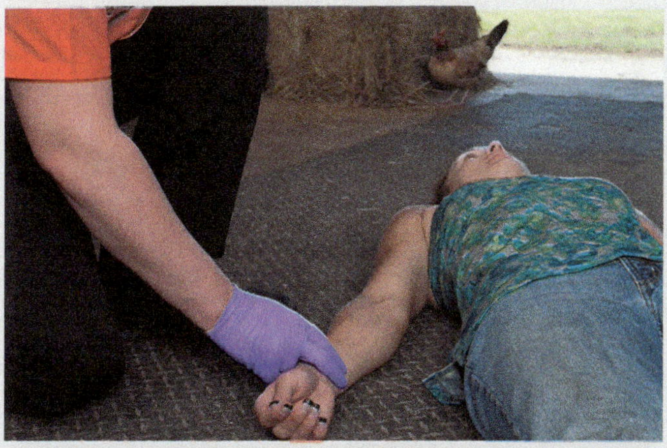

1. Assess the patient. Assess distal circulation, sensation, and motor function. Move the limb only if necessary for splinting or if the pulse is absent. *Stop* if you meet resistance or significantly increase the pain.

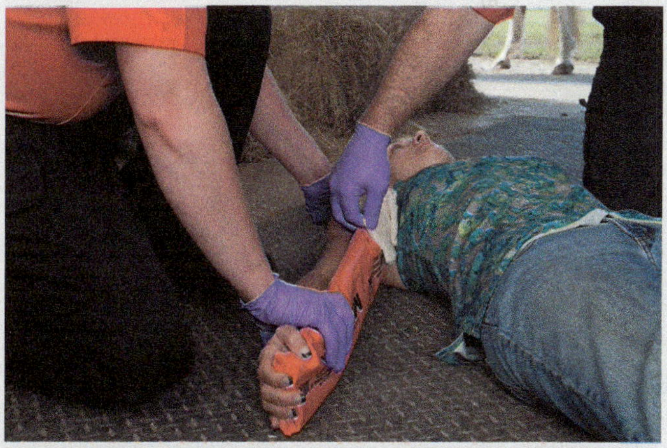

2. Use a padded board splint that will extend from the armpit to the fingers. Pad the armpit.

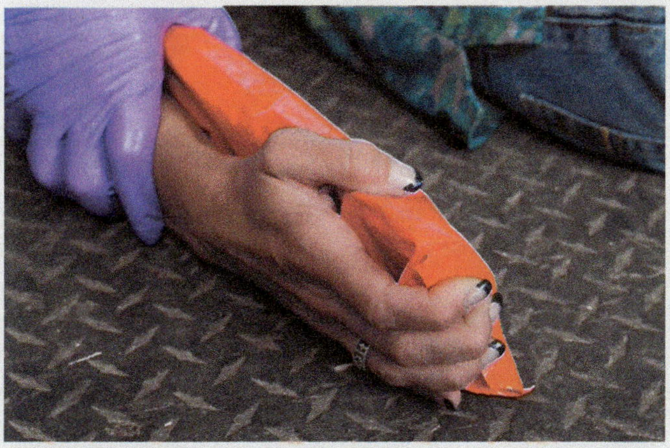

3. Make sure the distal end of the splint is placed so that the fingers curl around it in a natural way, approximating as nearly as possible the position of comfort.

NOTE: *Assess the distal CSM both before and after immobilizing or splinting an extremity.*

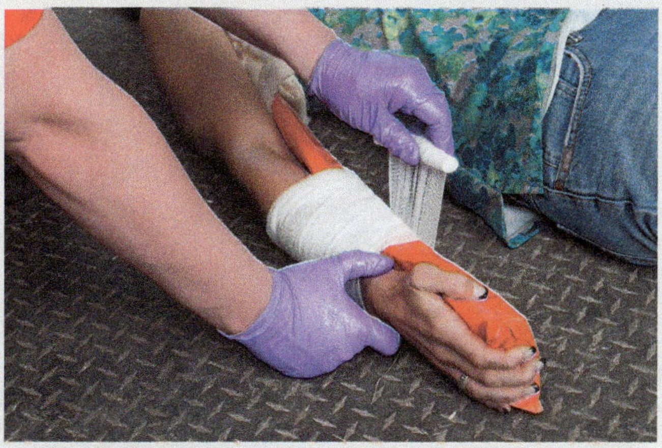

4. Secure the padded splint to the forearm with gauze bandaging.

(continued)

SCAN 32-6 Splinting Arm and Elbow Injuries (*continued*)

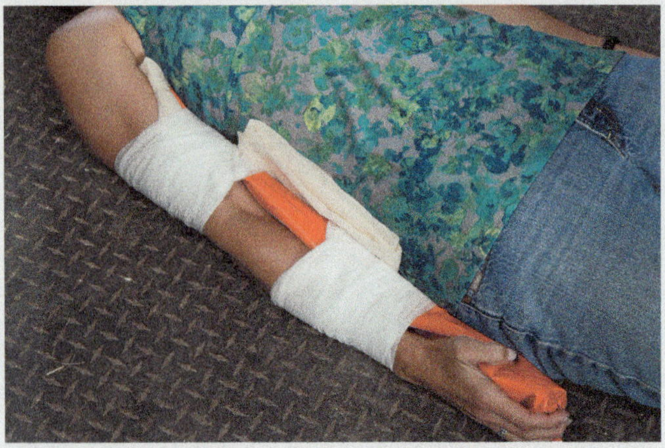

5. Secure the upper arm and place additional padding between the splint and the patient's body.

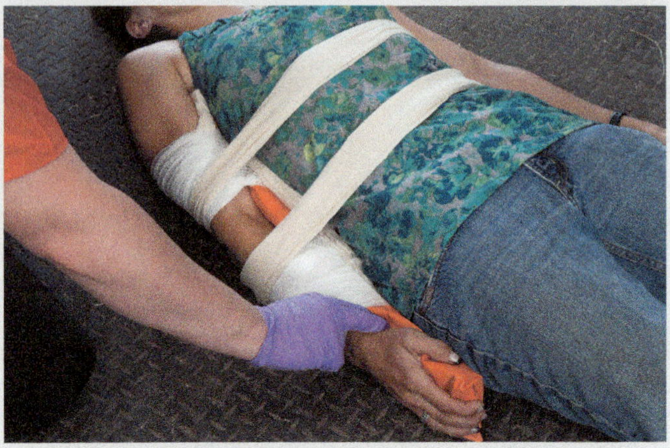

6. Secure the splinted limb to the body with two cravats. Avoid placing the cravats over the suspected injury site. Reassess the distal circulation, sensation, and motor function (CSM).

Elbow in BENT Position

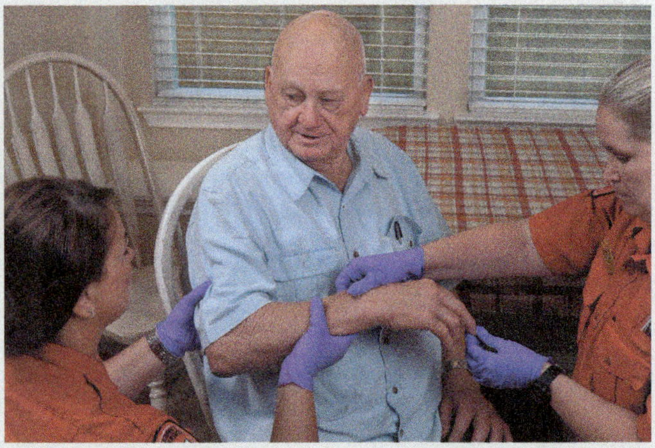

1. Assess the patient. Assess distal circulation, sensation, and motor function (CSM).

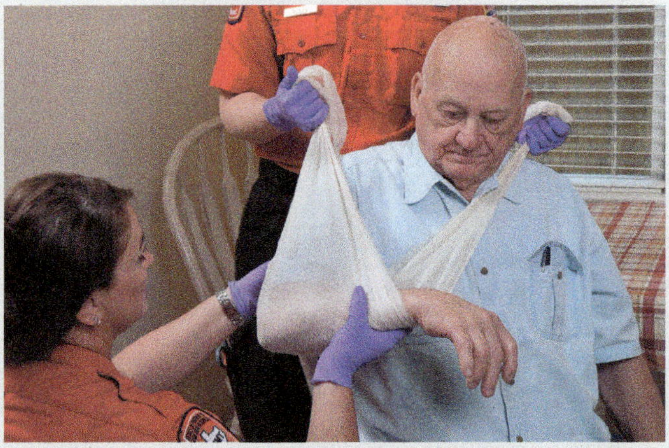

2. Support the injured arm with a sling, retaining the bent position of the elbow with as little movement as possible. Leave the fingertips exposed.

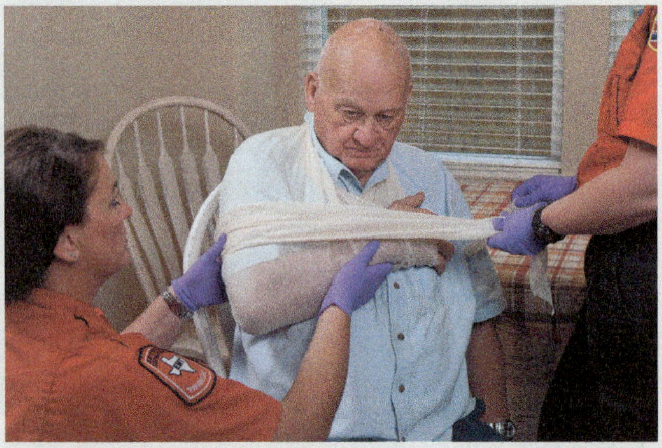

3. Secure the injured arm to the body with a swathe.

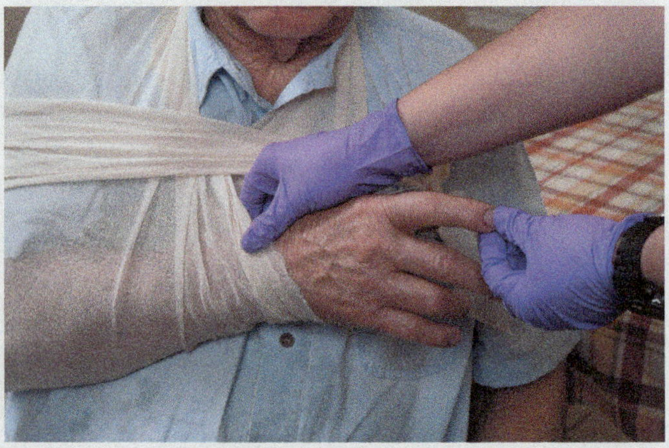

4. Reassess distal CSM.

SCAN 32-7 Splinting Forearm, Wrist, and Hand

SIGNS:

- ***Forearm.*** Deformity and tenderness. If only one bone is broken, deformity may be minor or absent.
- ***Wrist.*** Deformity and tenderness.
- ***Hand.*** Deformity and pain. Dislocated fingers are obvious.

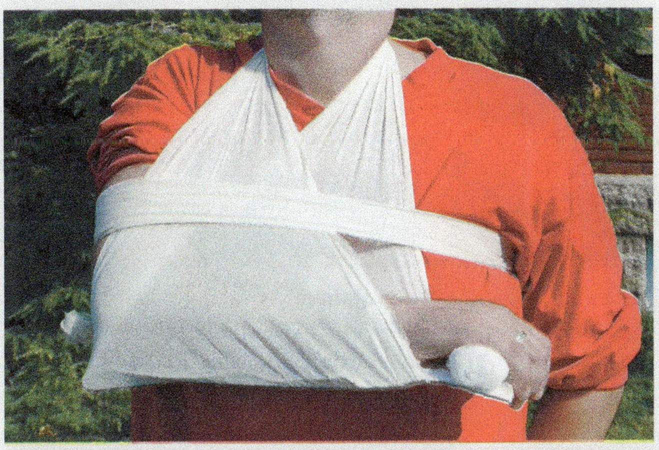

SPLINT, SLING, AND SWATHE: Injuries occurring to the forearm, wrist, or hand can be splinted using a padded rigid splint that gives support from elbow to hand. The patient's elbow, forearm, wrist, and hand all need the support of the splint. Tension must be provided throughout the splinting. A roll of bandages should be placed in the patient's hand to ensure the position of function. After rigid splinting, apply a sling and swathe.

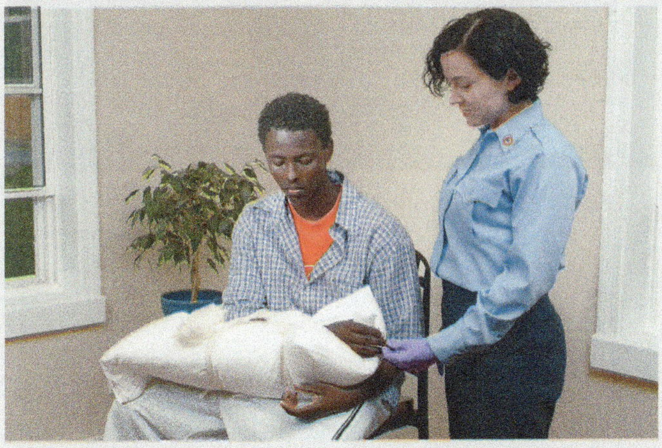

PILLOW SPLINT: Injuries to the hand and wrist can be cared for with soft splinting by placing a roll of bandages in the hand to maintain the position of function, then tying the forearm, wrist, and hand into the fold of one pillow or between two pillows.

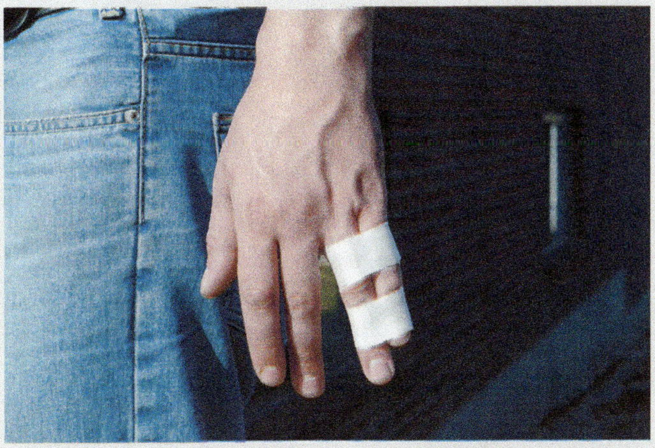

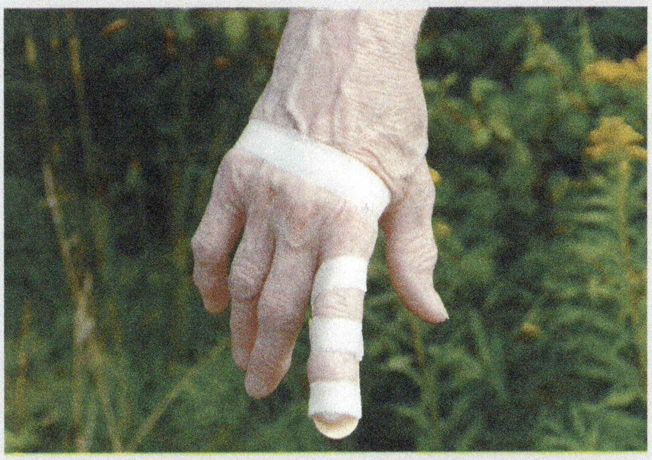

SPLINTING A FINGER An injured finger can be taped to an adjacent uninjured finger, which acts as a splint to the injured finger, or it can be splinted with a tongue depressor. Some emergency department physicians prefer that care to an injured finger be limited to a wrap of soft bandages. Do not try to "pop" dislocated fingers back into place.

NOTE: *Assess the distal circulation, sensation, and motor function both before and after immobilizing or splinting an extremity.*

SCAN 32-8 Applying an Air Splint

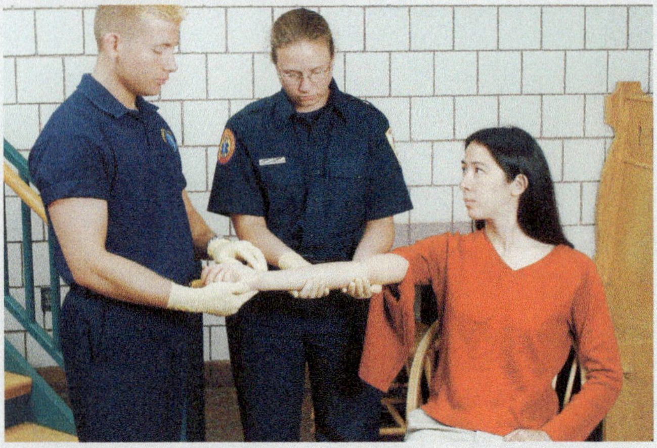

1. Check distal circulation, sensation, and motor function (CSM). Grasp the hand of the patient's injured limb as though you were going to shake hands and apply steady tension.

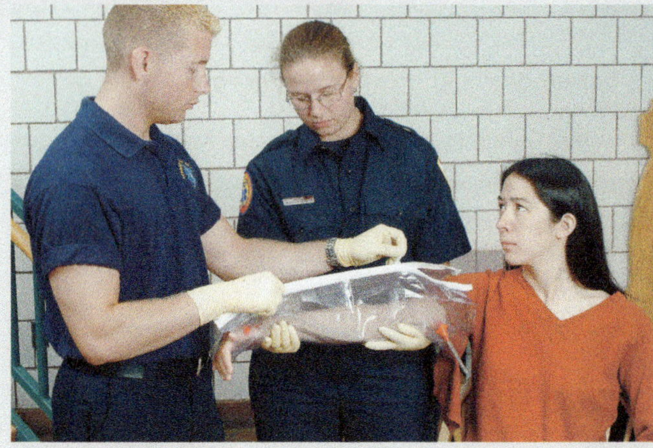

2. While you support the patient's arm, your partner gently slides the splint over your hand and onto the patient's injured limb. The lower edge of the splint should be just above the knuckles. Make sure the splint is free of wrinkles.

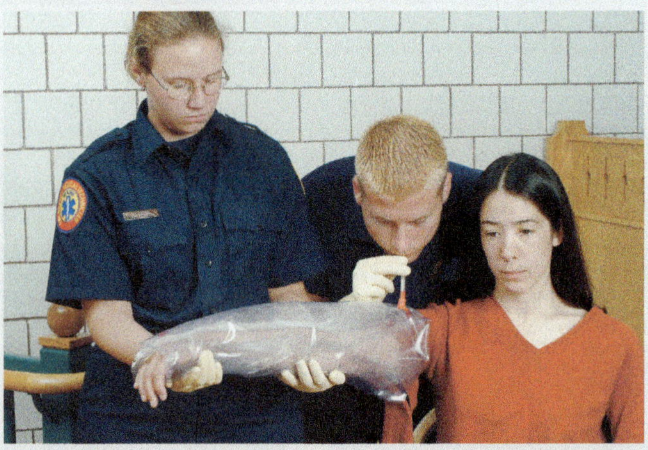

3. Continue to support the arm while your partner inflates the splint by mouth to a point where you can make a slight dent in the plastic when you press it with your thumb.

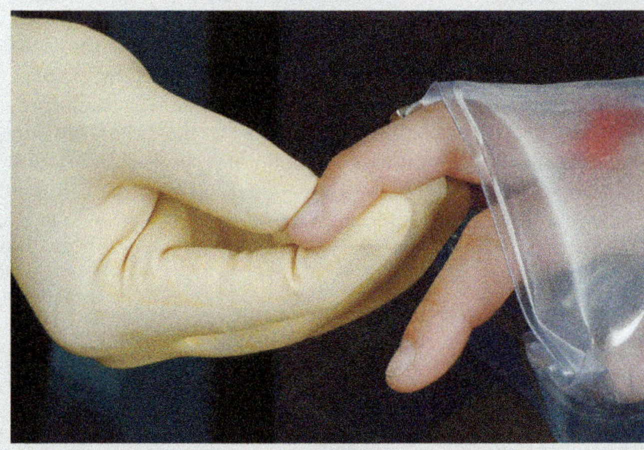

4. Continue to assess distal CSM.

NOTE: *Air-inflated splints may leak. When applied in cold weather, an inflatable splint will expand when the patient is moved to a warmer place. Variations in pressure also occur if the patient is moved to a different altitude. Frequently monitor the pressure in the splint with your fingertip. Air-inflated splints may stick to the patient's skin in hot weather.*

SCAN 32-9 Applying a Bipolar Traction Splint

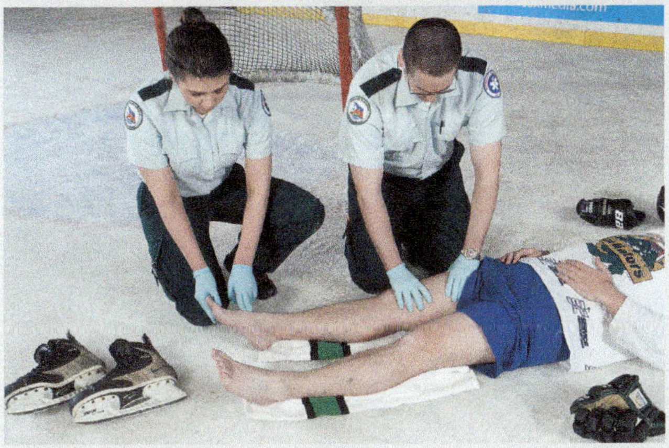

1. Take Standard Precautions. Begin by assessing the limb.

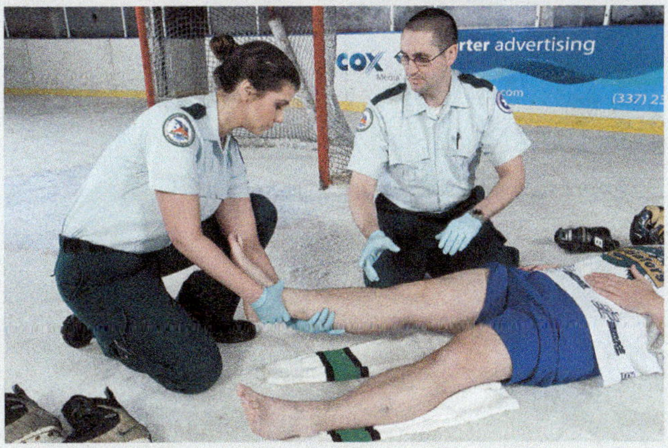

2. Manually stabilize the injured leg.

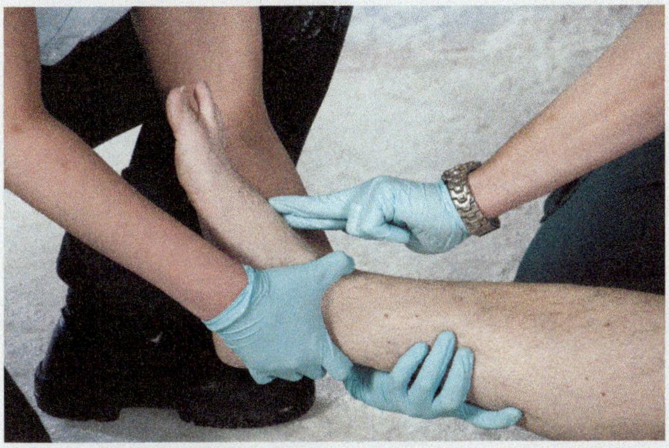

3. Assess circulation, sensation, and motor function (CSM).

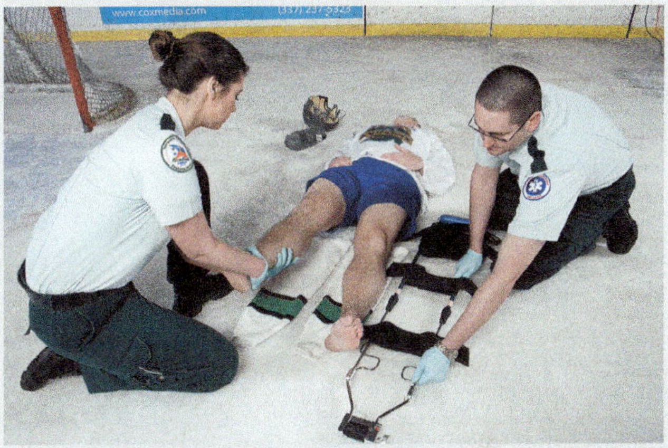

4. Adjust the splint to the proper length and position it next to the injured leg.

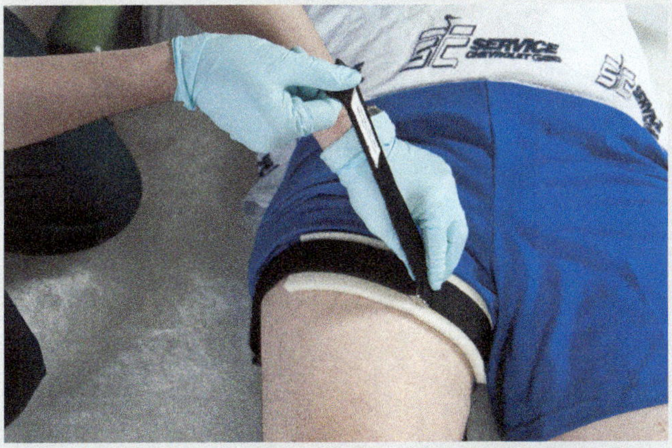

5. After lifting the extremity and positioning the splint under it, apply the ischial securing device.

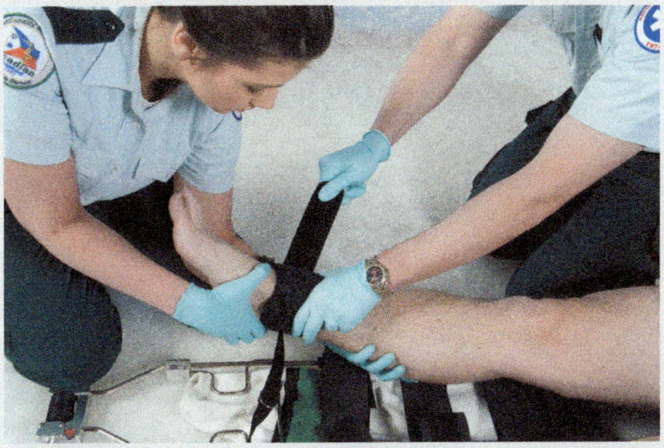

6. Apply an ankle hitch.

NOTE: *Assess the distal CSM both before and after immobilizing or splinting an extremity.*

(continued)

SCAN 32-9 Applying a Bipolar Traction Splint (*continued*)

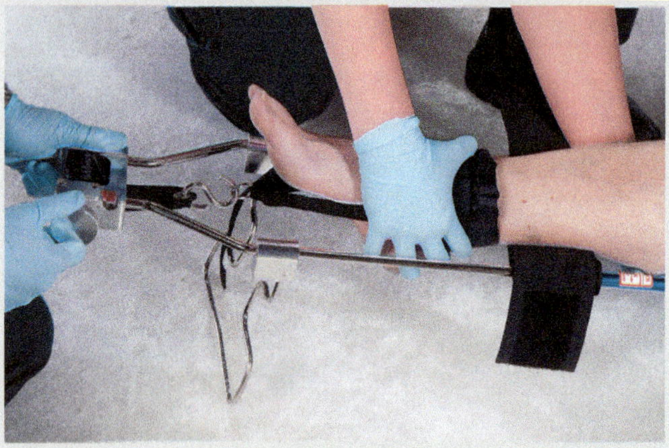

7. Apply manual traction, then mechanical traction.

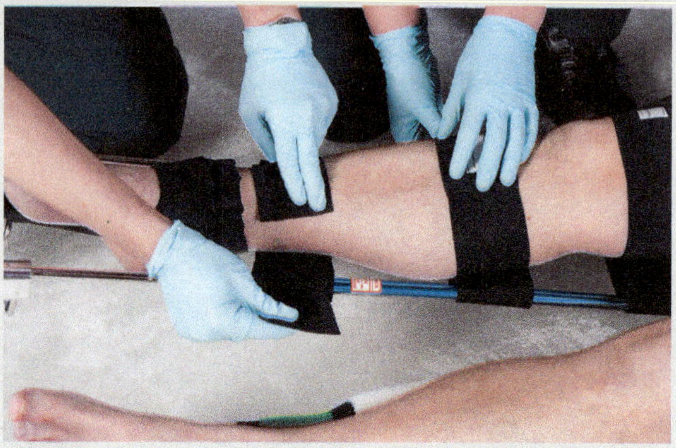

8. Secure support straps, as appropriate.

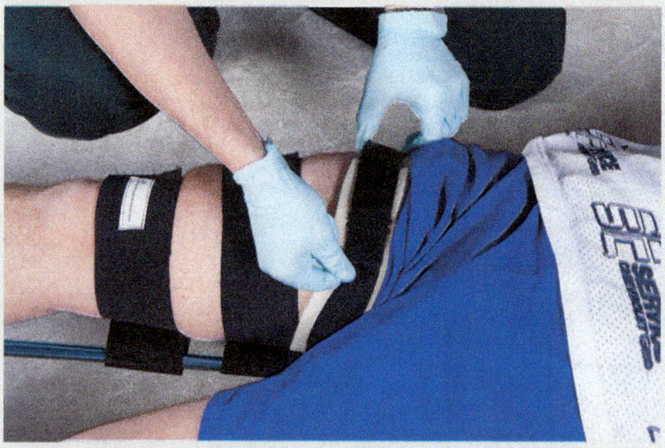

9. Reevaluate the ischial securing device.

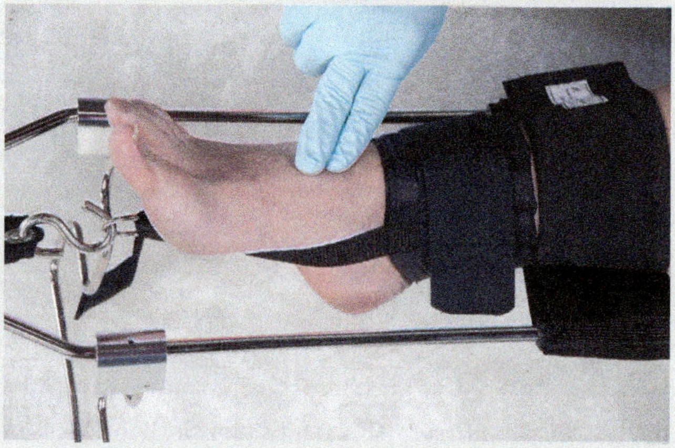

10. Reassess CSM function.

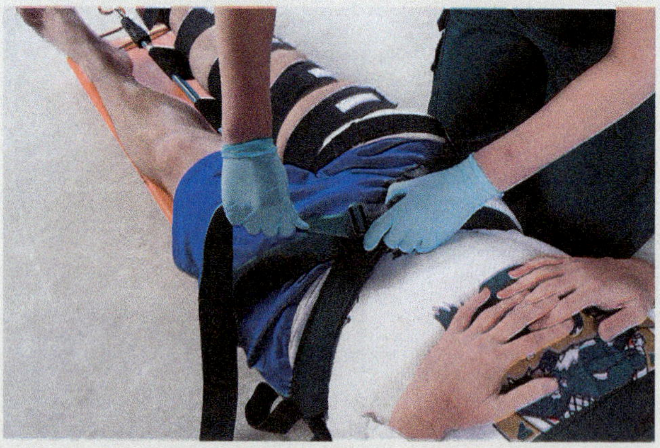

11. Secure the patient's torso to the long board to immobilize the hips.

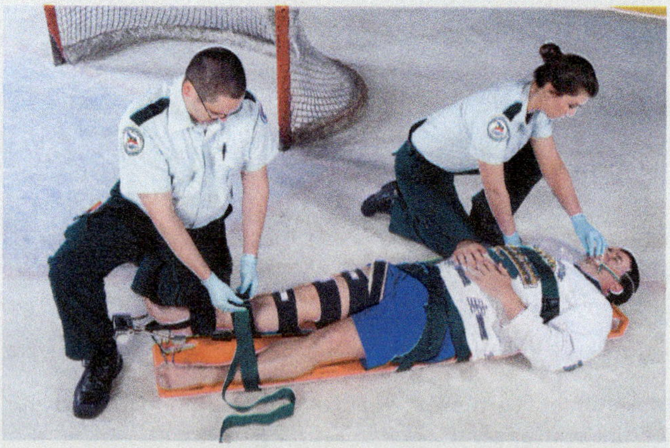

12. If the patient exhibits signs and symptoms of shock, administer oxygen. Secure the splint to the long board to prevent movement of the splint.

SCAN 32-10 Applying the Sager Traction Splint

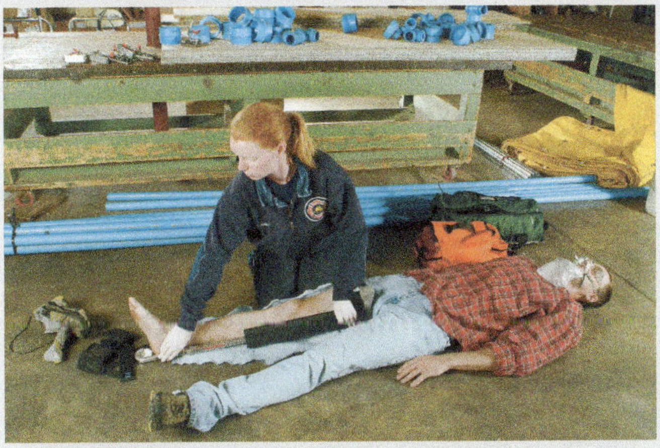

1. Place the splint medially.

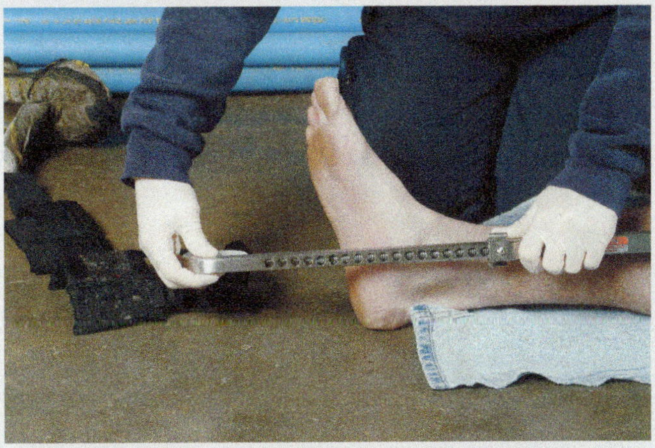

2. The length of the splint should be from groin to 4 inches (10 centimeters) below the heel. Unlock the clasp to extend the splint.

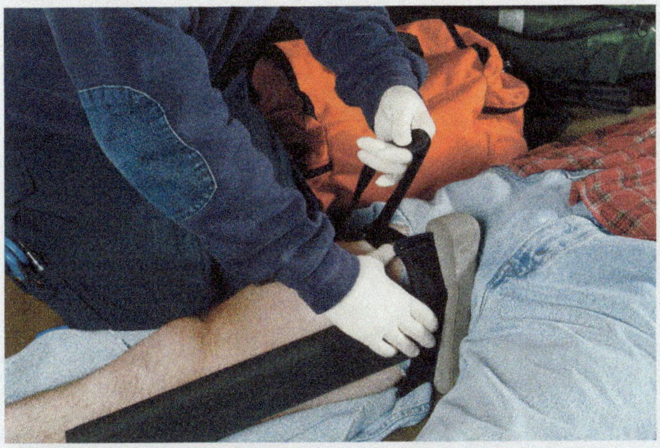

3. Secure the thigh strap.

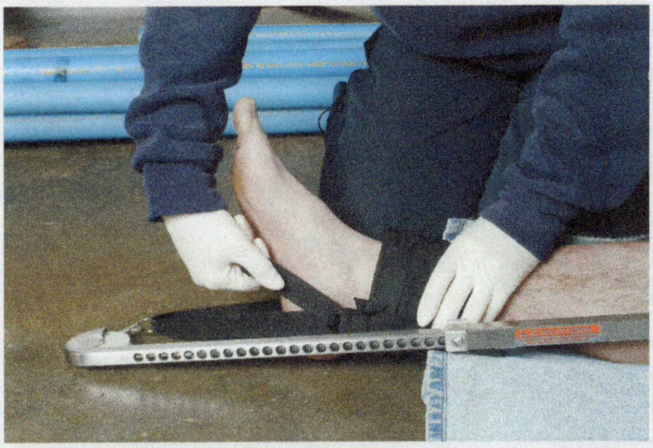

4. Wrap the ankle harness above the ankle (malleoli) and secure it under the heel.

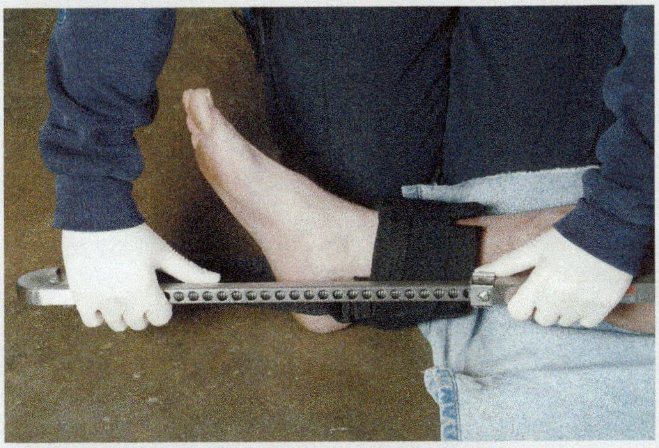

5. Release the lock and extend the splint to achieve the desired traction (in pounds on the pulley wheel).

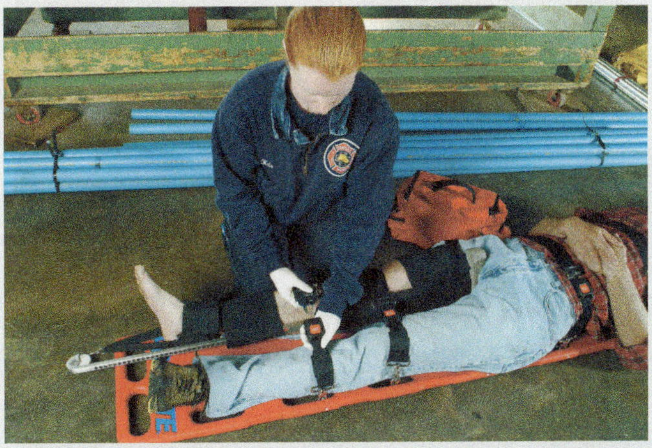

6. Secure the straps at the thigh, lower thigh and knee, and lower leg. Strap the ankles and feet together. Secure the patient to the spine board.

NOTE: *Assess distal CSM both before and after immobilizing or splinting an extremity.*

SCAN 32-11 Two-Splint Method–Bent Knee

If there is a distal pulse and nerve function, or the limb cannot be straightened without meeting resistance or causing severe pain, knee injuries should be splinted with the knee in the position in which it is found.

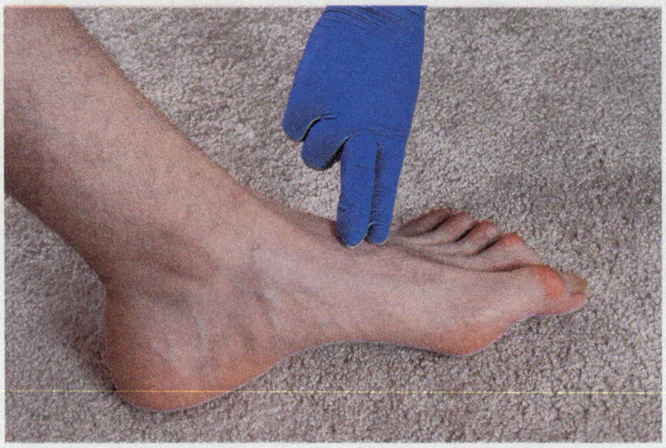

1. Assess distal CSM.

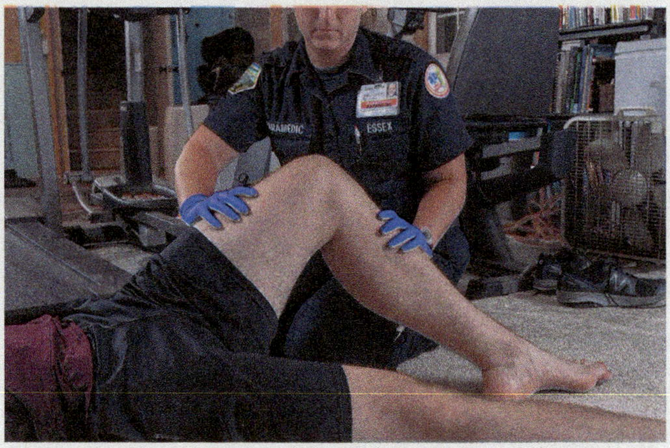

2. Stabilize the knee above and below the injury site.

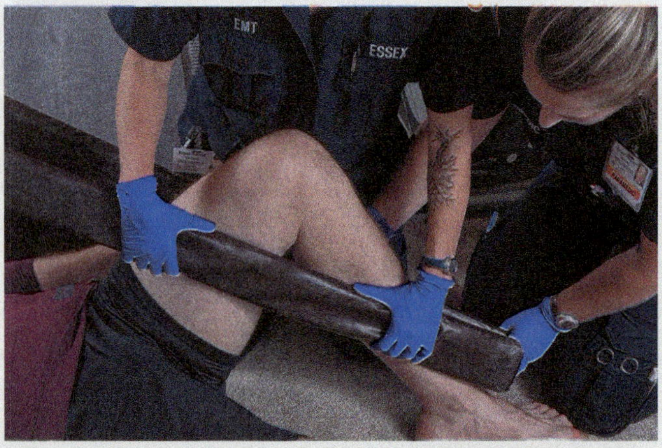

3. Place the padded side of the splints next to the injured extremity. Note that they should be equal in length and extend 6–12 inches (15–30 centimeters) beyond the mid-thigh and mid-calf.

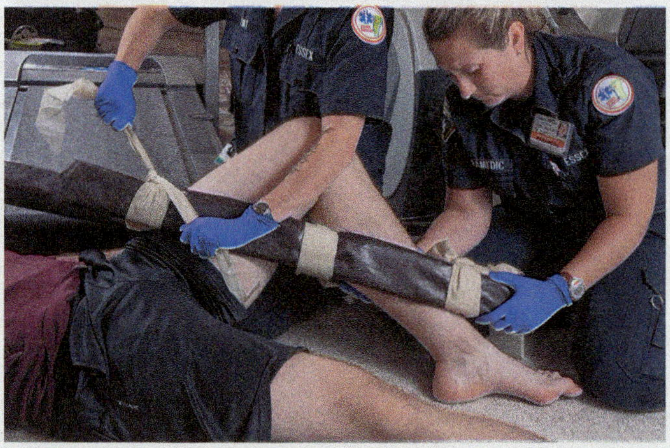

4. Place a cravat through the knee void and tie the boards together.

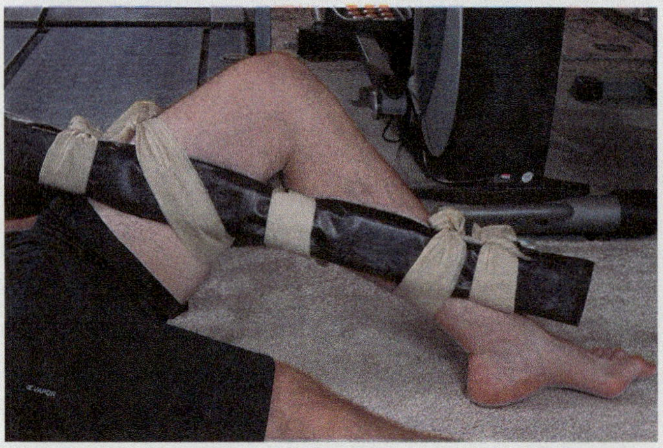

5. Using a figure-eight configuration, secure one cravat to the ankle and the boards and the second cravat to the thigh and the boards.

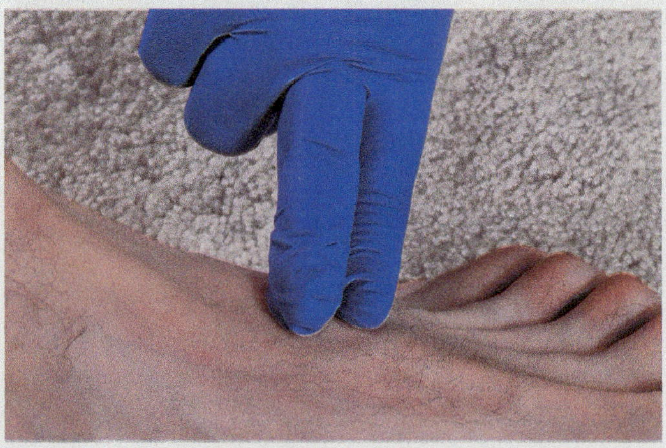

6. Reassess distal CSM.

SCAN 32-12 One-Splint Method–Straight Knee

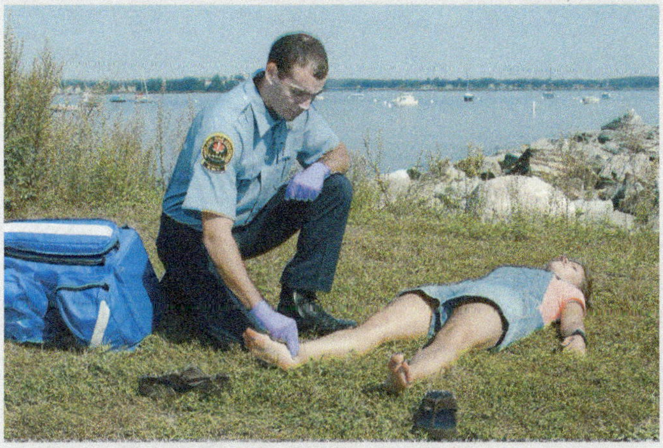

1. Assess distal CSM.

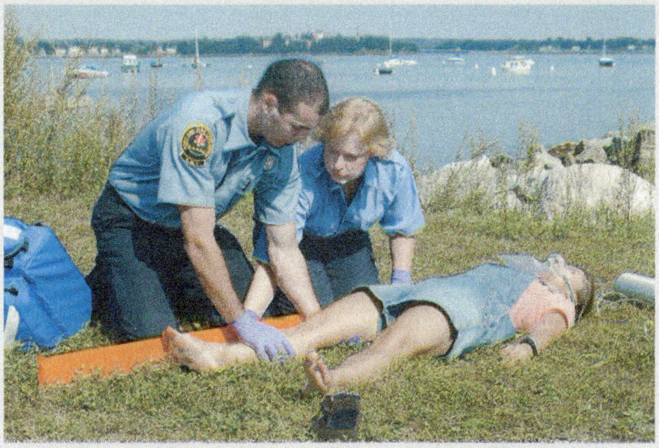

2. Stabilize. The padded board splint should extend from the buttocks to 4 inches (10 centimeters) beyond the heel.

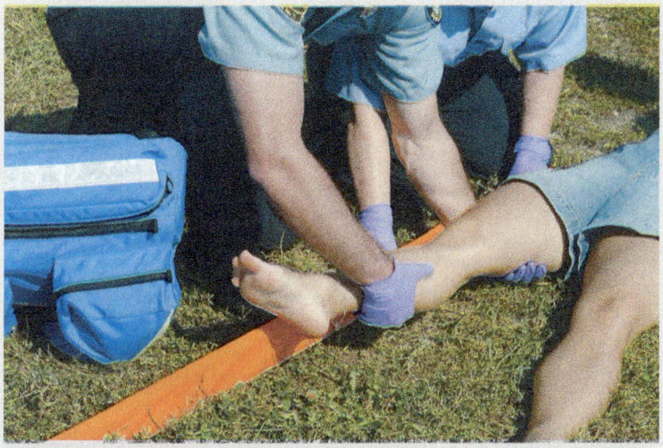

3. Maintain stabilization and lift the limb.

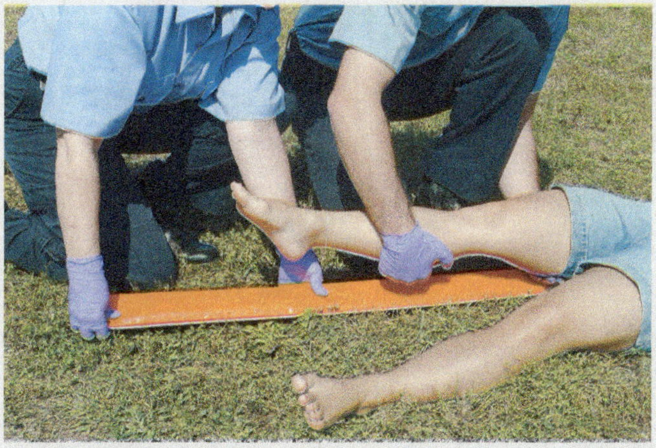

4. Place the splint along the posterior of the limb.

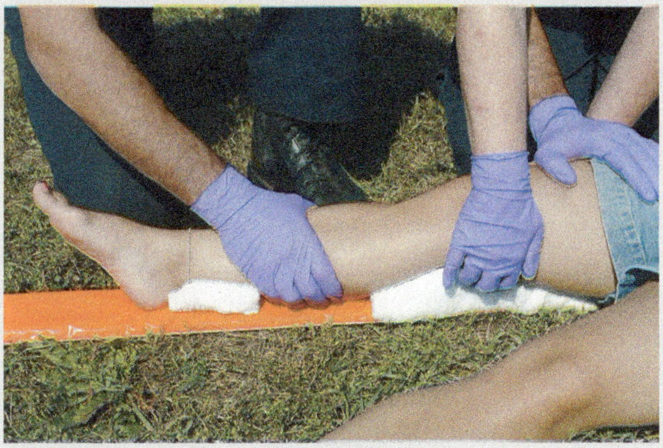

5. Pad the voids.

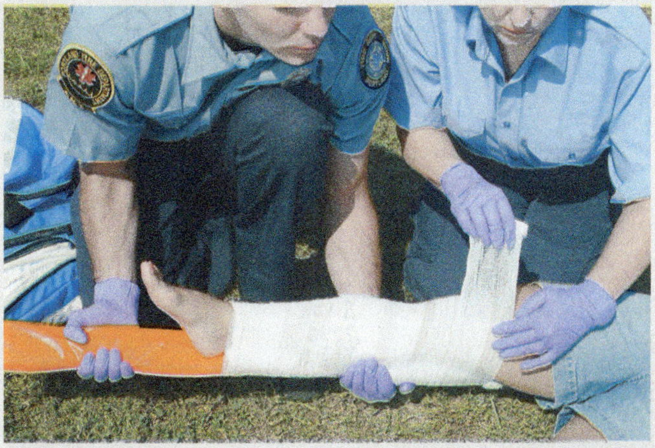

6. Use a 6-inch (15-centimeter) roller bandage or cravats to secure the injured leg to the splint.

(continued)

SCAN 32-12 One-Splint Method–Straight Knee *(continued)*

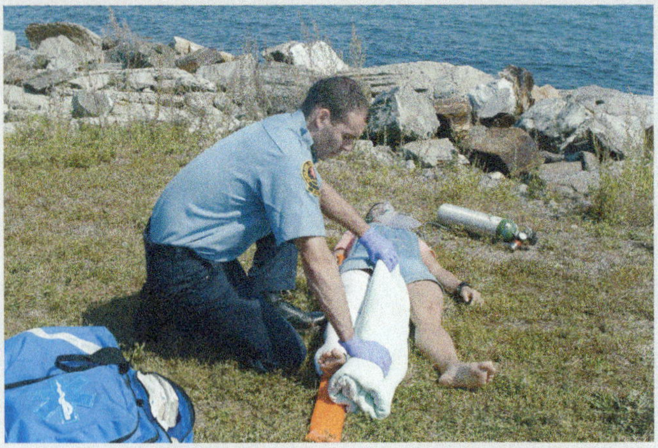

7. Place a folded blanket between the patient's legs, groin to feet.

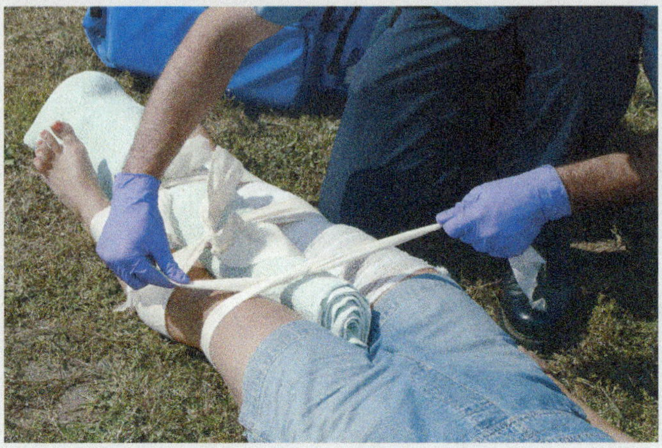

8. Tie the patient's thighs, calves, and ankles together. Do not tie a knot over the injured area.

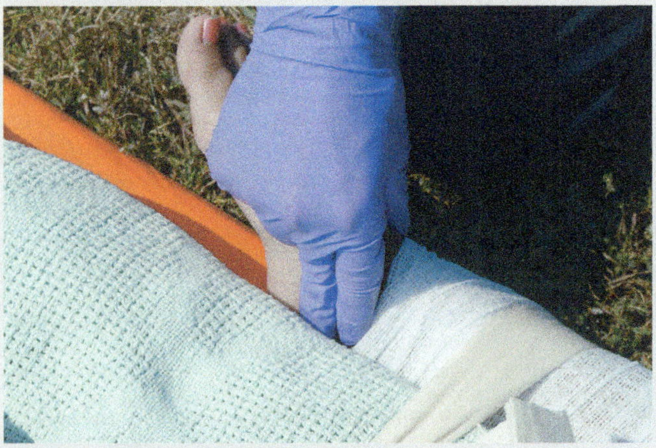

9. Reassess the distal CSM.

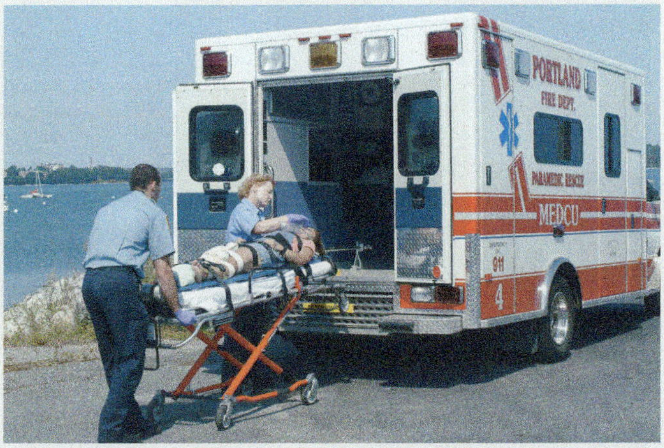

10. Provide emergency care for shock as needed.

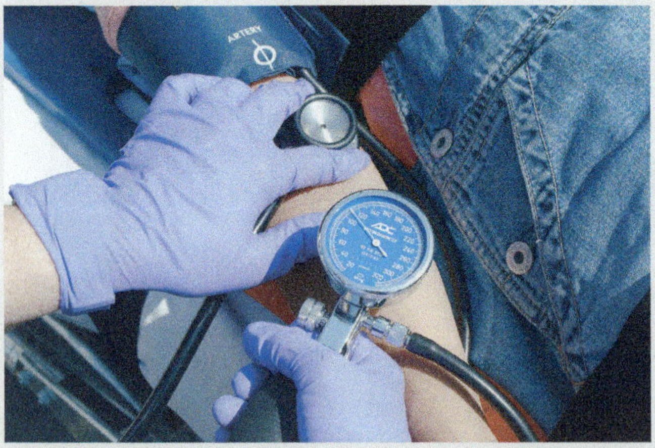

11. Monitor distal pulse and vital signs.

NOTE: *Assess distal CSM both before and after immobilizing or splinting an extremity.*

SCAN 32-13 Two-Splint Method–Straight Knee

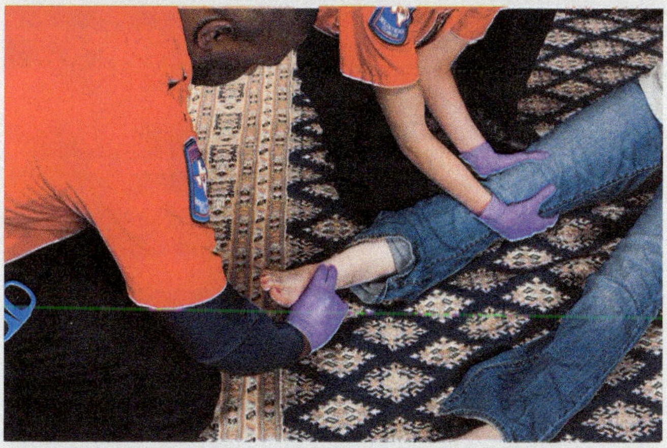

1. Stabilize the injured limb and assess distal CSM.

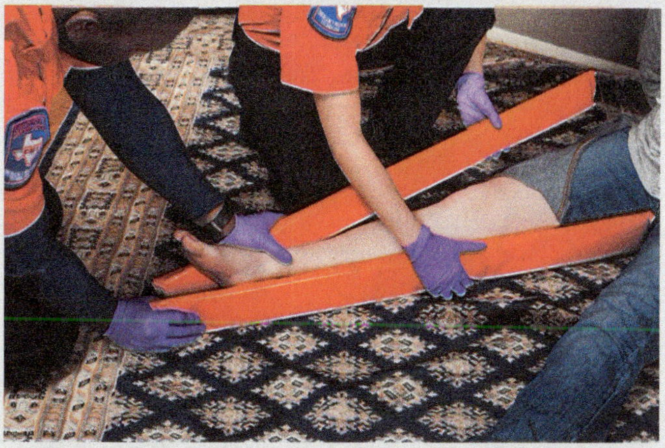

2. Measure the padded board splints, medial from the groin, lateral from the iliac crest, each to 4 inches (10 centimeters) beyond the foot.

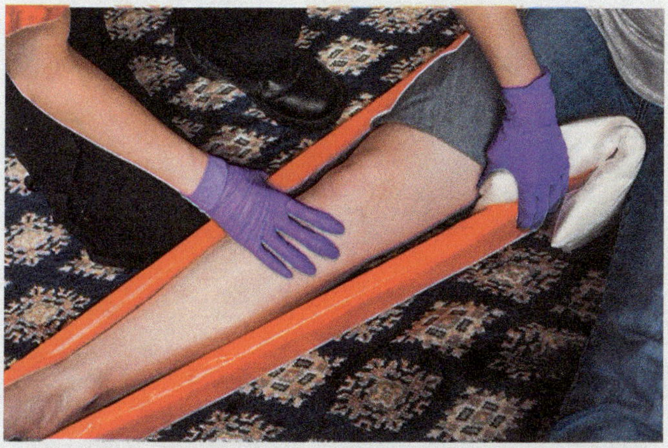

3. Position the splints.

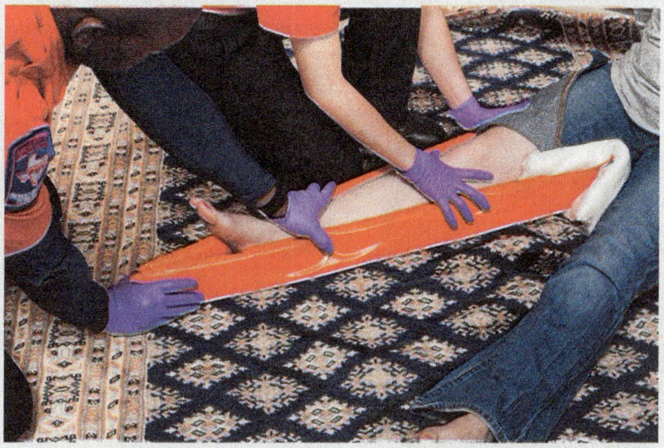

4. Pad the groin.

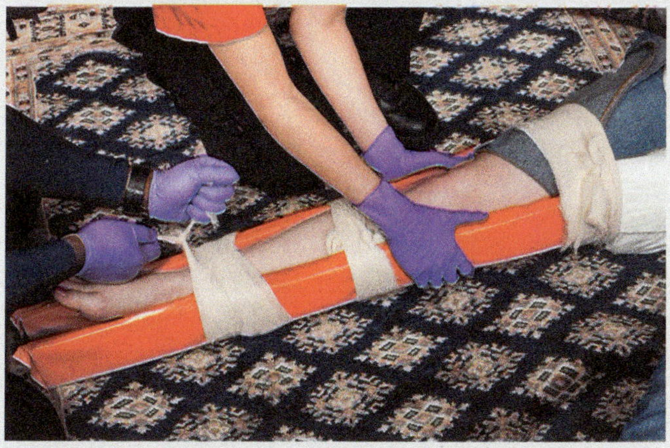

5. Secure the splints at the thigh, above and below the knee, and at mid-calf. Pad all voids.

NOTE: *Assess distal CSM both before and after immobilizing or splinting an extremity.*

SCAN 32-14 Two-Splint Method–Leg Injuries

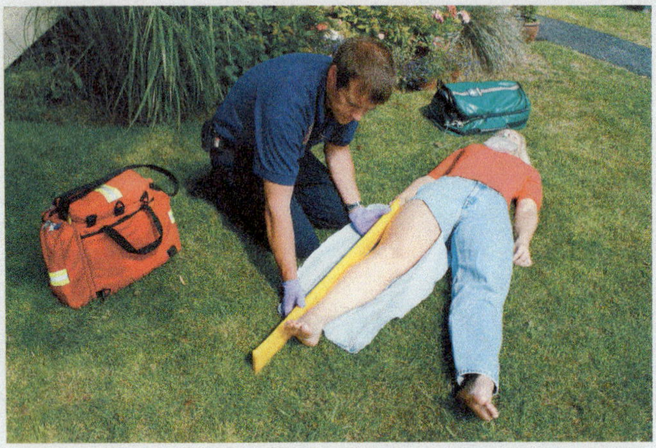

1. Assess the distal CSM. Measure the splints. They should extend above the knee and below the ankle.

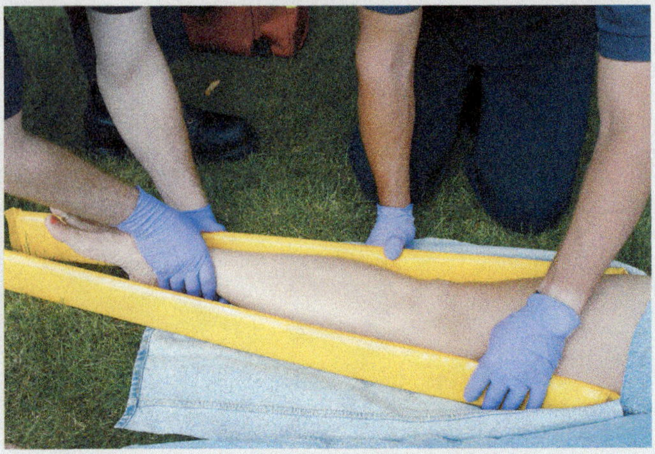

2. Apply manual traction (tension) on the leg; then place one splint medially and one laterally. Padding is toward the leg.

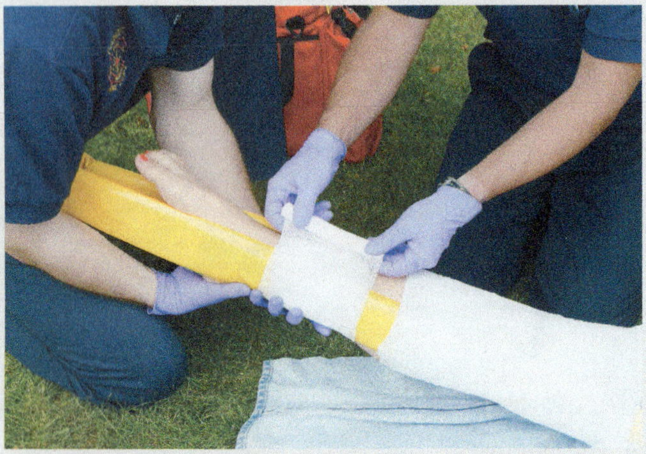

3. Secure the splints, padding the voids.

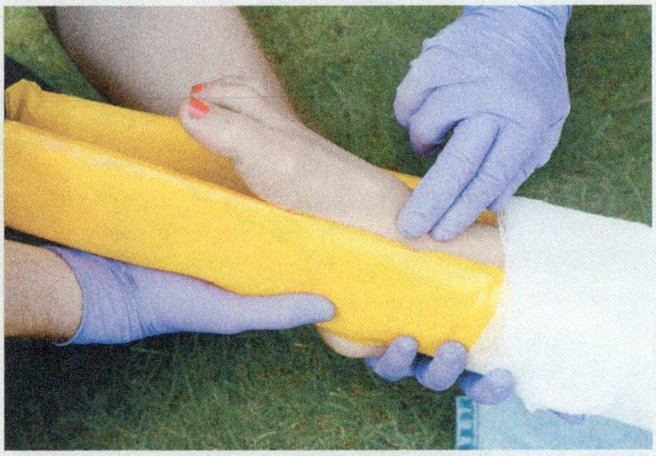

4. Reassess distal CSM.

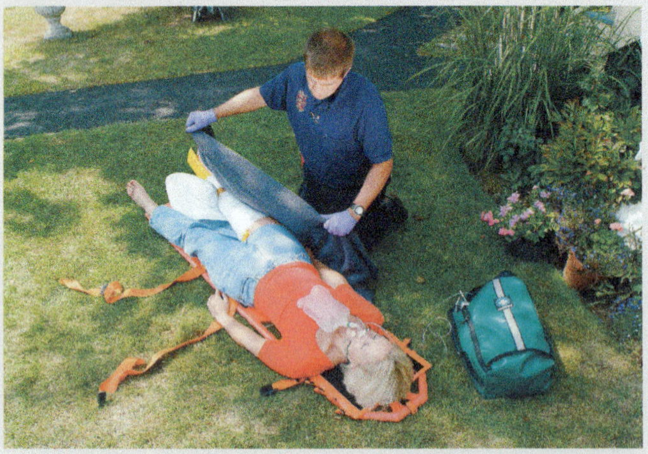

5. Reassess for shock and administer high-concentration oxygen as appropriate. Transport on a long spine board.

NOTE: *Assess distal CSM both before and after immobilizing or splinting an extremity.*

SCAN 32-15 One-Splint Method–Leg Injuries

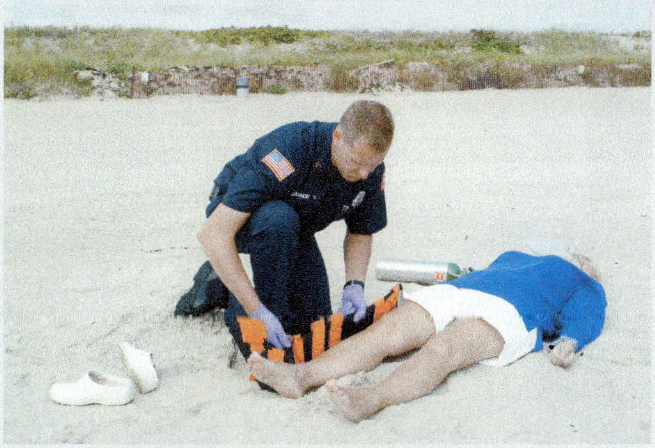

1. Assess distal CSM. Measure the splint.

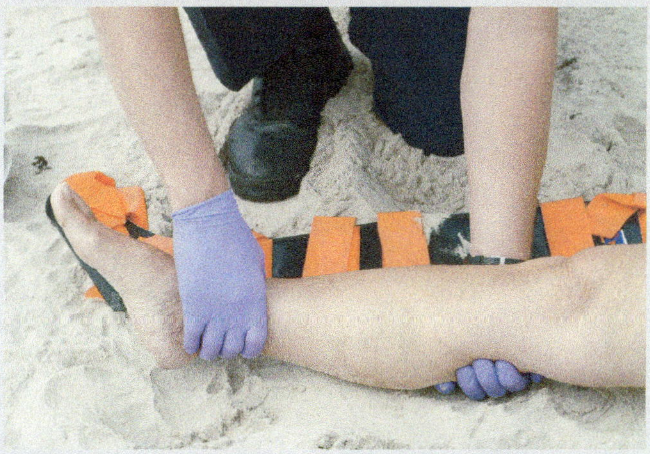

2. Apply manual traction (tension).

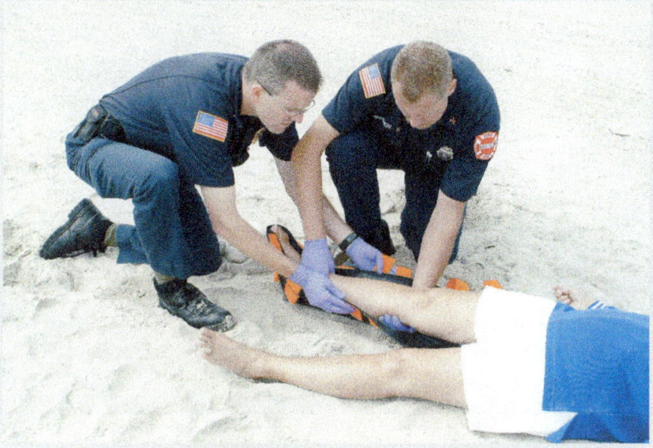

3. Lift the limb off the ground and place it in the splint.

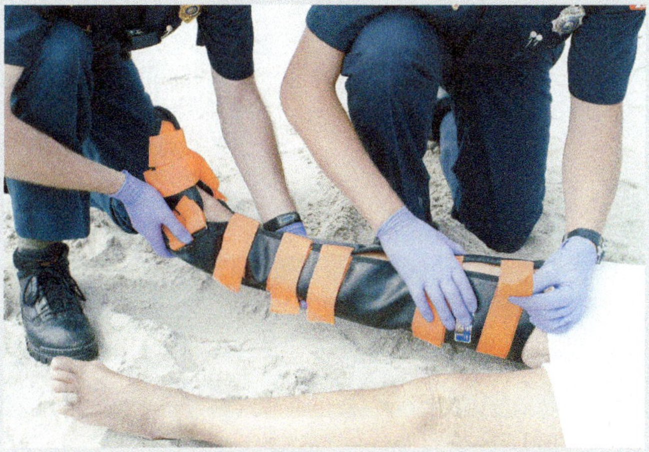

4. Secure the splint to the injured leg.

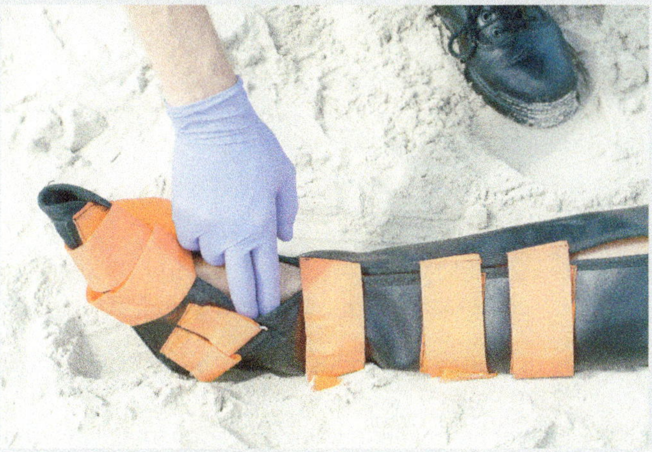

5. Reassess distal CSM.

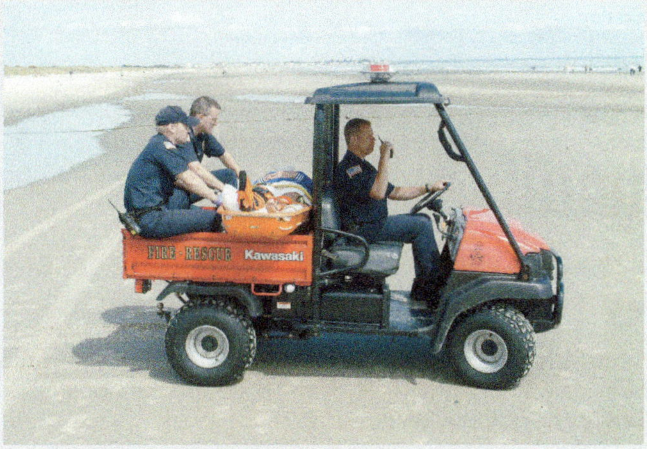

6. Reassess for shock. Package the patient and prepare to transport.

NOTE: *Assess distal CSM both before and after immobilizing or splinting an extremity.*

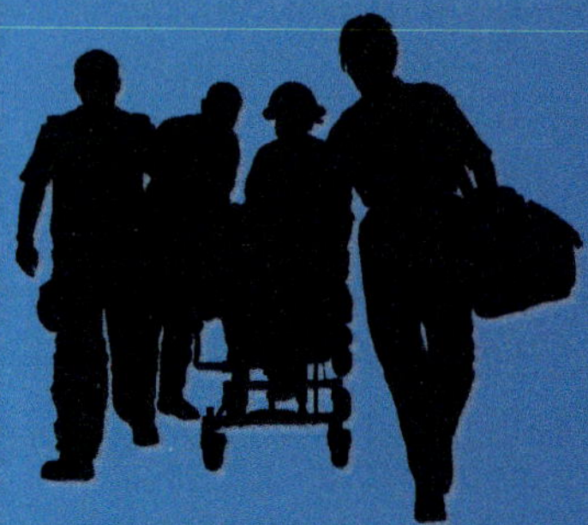

Think Like an EMT

Sticks and Stones May Break My Bones, but Trauma Centers Save Me

Care for patients with musculoskeletal injuries depends on each patient's overall condition. Patients with isolated fractures may routinely be splinted and transported, whereas those with multiple fractures are at an increased risk of shock and should be treated as multiple-trauma patients. For each of these patients, determine whether you would stay and splint or, as a higher priority, consider transport to a trauma center, using a backboard as the main splinting device.

1. You are called to a patient who tripped and tried to catch himself with an outstretched arm. He believes he broke his wrist and hit his head when he fell. He is alert and oriented. His vital signs are pulse 88, strong and regular; respirations 16; blood pressure 140/84; SpO_2 97%; skin warm and dry; and pupils equal and reactive to light.
2. You are called to an industrial complex where a large spool pinned a man by the legs. The workers are able to move the spool for you to safely access the patient. The patient is in extreme pain. Your physical examination reveals deformity in both thighs and in the patient's left lower leg. The patient is agitated. His pulse is 112 and regular, respirations 24 and adequate, blood pressure 108/64, SpO_2 97%, and pupils equal and reactive to light.
3. Your patient was ejected from a vehicle and found about twenty feet away. He complains only of a broken arm. Your physical assessment doesn't reveal any other injuries. The patient is alert and oriented. His pulse is 130 and weak, respirations 28 and adequate, blood pressure 88/56, SpO_2 97%, skin cool and moist, and pupils equal and reactive to light.

Chapter Review

Key Facts and Concepts

- Bones bleed. Fractures cause blood loss from within the bone as well as from tissue damage around the bone ends. Serious or multiple fractures can cause shock.
- Splinting of long-bone fractures involves immobilizing the bone ends as well as the adjacent joints.
- Splinting protects the patient from further injury, reduces pain, and helps control bleeding.
- You may need to be creative while splinting. There are many correct ways to splint the same extremity.
- Injuries to bones and joints should be splinted prior to moving the patient.
- If the patient has multiple trauma or appears to have shock (or a significant potential for shock), do not waste time splinting individual fractures. Place the patient on a long spine board and secure the limbs to the board. You can splint individual fractures en route if time and priorities allow.

Key Decisions

- Have I fully addressed life threats and maintained my priorities—even in the presence of a grossly deformed extremity?
- Does the patient have an injury that requires splinting?
- Does the patient have multiple fractures, multiple trauma, or shock?
- Does the patient have adequate CSM distal to the musculoskeletal injury?
- Should I align the angulated extremity fracture?

Chapter Glossary

angulated fracture fracture in which the broken bone segments are at an angle to each other.

bones hard but flexible living structures that provide support for the body and protection to vital organs.

cartilage tough tissue that covers the joint ends of bones and helps to form certain body parts, such as the ear.

closed extremity injury an injury to an extremity with no associated opening in the skin.

comminuted fracture a fracture in which the bone is broken in several places.

compartment syndrome injury caused when tissues such as blood vessels and nerves are constricted within a space, as from swelling or from a tight dressing or cast.

crepitus (KREP-i-tus) a grating sensation or sound made when fractured bone ends rub together.

dislocation the disruption or "coming apart" of a joint.

extremities (ex-TREM-i-teez) the portions of the skeleton that include the clavicles, scapulae, arms, wrists, and hands (upper extremities) and the pelvis, thighs, legs, ankles, and feet (lower extremities).

fracture (FRAK-cher) any break in a bone.

greenstick fracture an incomplete fracture.

joints places where bones articulate, or meet.

ligaments tissues that connect bone to bone.

manual traction the process of applying tension to straighten and realign a fractured limb before splinting. Also called *tension*.

muscles tissues or fibers that cause movement of body parts and organs.

open extremity injury an extremity injury in which the skin has been broken or torn through from the inside by an injured bone, or from the outside by something that has caused a penetrating wound with associated injury to the bone.

sprain the stretching and tearing of ligaments.

strain muscle injury resulting from overstretching or overexertion of the muscle.

tendons tissues that connect muscle to bone.

traction splint a splint that applies constant pull along the length of a lower extremity to help stabilize the fractured bone and to reduce muscle spasm in the limb. Traction splints are used primarily on femoral shaft fractures.

Preparation for Your Examination and Practice

Short Answer

1. Describe the basic anatomy of bone and its purposes.
2. Identify the signs and symptoms of musculoskeletal injury.
3. Describe basic emergency care for painful, swollen, or deformed extremities, including general guidelines for splinting long bones and joints.
4. Explain why angulated deformed injuries to the long bones should be realigned to the anatomic position.
5. List the basic principles of splinting.
6. Describe the hazards of splinting.
7. Describe the basic types of splints carried on ambulances.

Thinking and Linking

Think back to the chapter Bleeding and Shock, *and link information from that chapter with information from this chapter as you consider the following situations:*

Blood loss can be significant with a fracture—even with a closed fracture. For each of the following, describe the signs and symptoms of shock you might see and whether you would expect the patient to compensate or eventually decompensate for the blood loss:

a. Fractured tibia and fibula
b. Both tibias and fibulas fractured
c. Femur fracture
d. Pelvic fracture

Think back to the chapters Lifting and Moving Patients *and* Scene Size-Up, *and link information from those chapters with information from this chapter as you consider the following situation:*

- *You have a patient who was thrown from an ATV deep in the woods. He complains of pain in his thigh and hip. What treatment and transportation devices would you use? What assistance would you call for in the scene size-up?*

Critical Thinking Exercises

Shock and pain are often associated with musculoskeletal injuries. The purpose of this exercise will be to consider how you might deal with these factors when your patient has a musculoskeletal injury.

1. List three assessment findings that you would use to help determine if your musculoskeletal injury patient is in shock.
2. Patients who suffer fractures can be in extreme pain. Pain can cause anxiety and elevated pulse rates. How could you differentiate between a patient with a rapid pulse and anxiety from pain versus a patient with rapid pulse and anxiety from shock?

Pathophysiology to Practice

The following questions are designed to assist you in gathering relevant clinical information and making accurate decisions in the field.

1. Why do broken bones cause shock?
2. Why would you attempt to straighten an extremity that has no pulses distal to the extremity?
3. Can a patient have a fracture without obvious deformity? Explain your answer.

Street Scenes

You and your crew arrive for duty at the firehouse when you are called out for a "fall injury." A police unit is already on scene, and they inform you that it is safe. Exiting your engine and taking Standard Precautions, you observe a tall woman in her twenties in jogging clothes leaning on the front hood of a car. She is wincing. The police officer standing next to her approaches and introduces you to your patient. She says her name is Desta.

Your primary assessment reveals that Desta has a good airway and that she is breathing fine. "What happened, Desta, and why did you call EMS this morning?"

"I fell off that wall while trying to climb over it," she answers, simultaneously pointing to a 4-foot rock wall approximately 100 feet away. "When I landed, I heard something crack in my right leg. I hopped on one foot to this car and called for help." You quickly make a mental note that the surface she landed on is asphalt.

Street Scene Questions

1. **What priority would you assign to this patient? Why?**
2. **How would you continue your assessment?**

Desta's mental status seems normal. There are no signs of bleeding anywhere on her body. You assign a low priority to her and continue your assessment by performing a history and physical exam. Desta tells you that she is taking no medications. You ask if she has any allergies, and she smiles as she replies, "Rock walls, apparently." She laughs, then suddenly grimaces in pain as she unintentionally shifts her weight onto her right leg.

You obtain baseline vital signs and learn Desta's pulse is 88 and regular, respirations are 16 and unlabored, and blood pressure is 108/72. Her SpO_2 is 96%. Her pupils are equal and reactive. She states she has no pain anywhere but in her lower right leg.

Street Scene Questions

3. **What signs might you expect to find with a broken long bone?**
4. **What are your major concerns with possible broken bones in the extremities?**

You assist Desta from her standing position onto your cot, carefully supporting her right leg. Then you expose the extremity. About 2 inches (5 centimeters) above the ankle, you observe swelling and a noticeable, unnatural curve to her leg. The skin is not broken. You are concerned that she might have nerve and muscle damage below the injury, but she is able to move her toes and feel you touching her foot. You also detect a pulse below the injury site.

Street Scene Question

5. **What interventions are appropriate for this patient?**

A member of your crew brings a vacuum splint, which provides immobilization to the joint above and below the injury site. You maintain manual traction, being careful not to unnecessarily move the extremity, and apply the splint. After application, the patient states her leg feels more secure. You reassess her vitals as well as pulses, sensation, and motor function below the injury site. Everything appears to be normal. During transport, you continue to check distal pulses, sensation, and motor function on the affected extremity. Transport to the hospital is uneventful.

Trauma to the Head, Neck, and Spine

33

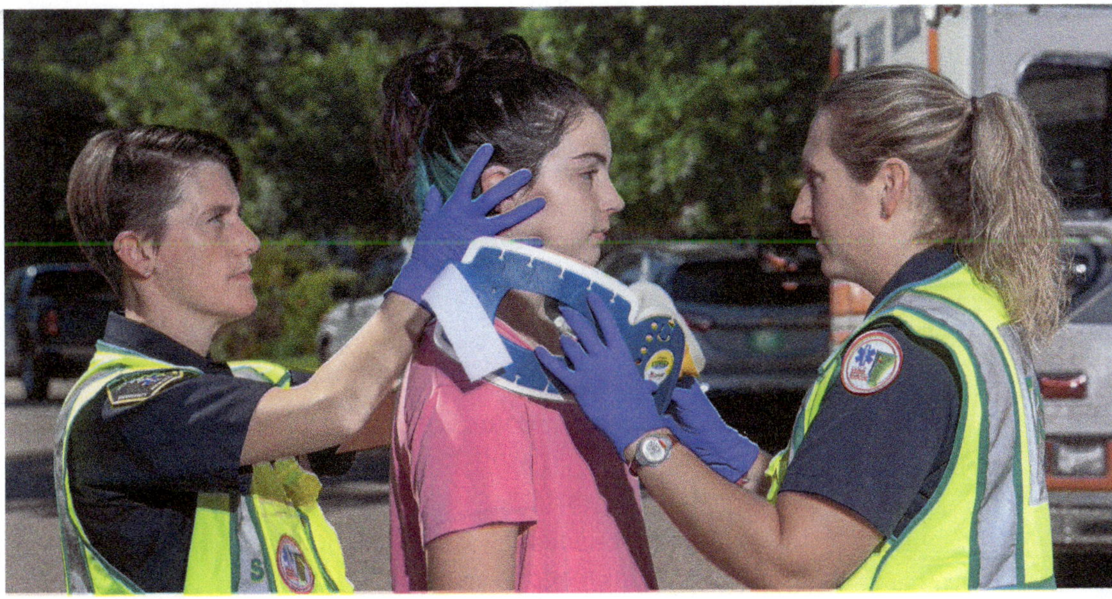

Related Chapters

The following chapters provide additional information related to topics discussed in this chapter:

- 3 Lifting and Moving Patients
- 6 Anatomy and Physiology
- 12 Primary Assessment
- 14 Principles of Assessment
- 15 Secondary Assessment
- 16 Reassessment
- 22 Diabetic Emergencies and Altered Mental Status
- 30 Soft-Tissue Trauma
- 31 Chest and Abdominal Trauma
- 32 Musculoskeletal Trauma

Standard

Trauma (Head, Facial, Neck, and Spine Trauma)

Competency

Applies fundamental knowledge to provide basic emergency care and transportation based on assessment findings for an acutely injured patient.

Core Concepts

- Understanding the anatomy of the nervous system, head, and spine
- Understanding skull and brain injuries and emergency care for skull and brain injuries

- Understanding wounds to the neck and emergency care for neck wounds
- Understanding spine injuries and assessment and emergency care for spine injuries
- Understanding spinal motion restriction issues and how to immobilize various types of patients with potential spine injury

Outcomes

After reading this chapter, you should be able to:

33.1 Summarize concepts of injuries to the head and spine. (pp. 950-958)

- State the consequences to society of brain and spine injuries.
- Explain the overall purposes served by the nervous system.
- Describe how the structures and functions of the central and peripheral divisions of the nervous system work together.
- Identify the anatomy of the skull.
- Explain the relationship between the components of the central nervous system and the structures that protect them.
- Describe the pathophysiologic consequences of injuries to the brain and spinal cord.
- Explain how the presence of injuries of the soft tissues, skull, and spinal column relates to injuries to the central nervous system.
- Relate mechanisms of injury to the potential for injuries to the head and spine.
- Categorize the features of different types of traumatic brain injuries.
- Describe the pathophysiology that increases intracranial pressure.

33.2 Summarize management considerations in the care of a patient with an injury to the head and spine. (pp. 958-963)

- Explain the attention required for the assessment of and intervention with a patient's airway and breathing.
- Relate abnormal assessment findings to the potential for central nervous system injury.
- Apply the Glasgow Coma Scale to the assessment of level of responsiveness.
- Explain how to prioritize the steps of management for patients who have sustained injuries to the head or spine.
- Justify transportation decision making with interpretation of the patient condition in the context of the EMS system.

33.3 Summarize concepts of injuries to the face, jaw, and soft tissues of the neck. (pp. 963-966)

- Recognize how injuries of facial and soft tissues of the neck are associated with potential brain and spinal cord injuries.
- Explain the relationship between injuries to the face, jaw, and soft tissues of the neck and life-threatening injuries of associated structures.
- Recommend a prioritized plan of treatment for patients with injuries to the face, jaw, and soft tissues of the neck.

33.4 Summarize concepts of spinal injuries. (pp. 966-993)

- Distinguish between spinal injury and spinal cord injury.
- Identify mechanisms of injury with potential for injury to the spine and spinal cord.
- Outline the steps for assessing for a suspected injury of the spine and spinal cord.
- Identify signs and symptoms of spine and spinal cord injuries.
- Describe the application of the NEXUS algorithm in assessing for spinal cord injury.
- Identify patients who are candidates for spinal motion restriction procedures.
- Prioritize spinal motion restriction among the patient's needs.
- Match various portrayals of patients with the devices most suited to achieve spinal motion restriction.
- Outline the steps of applying each type of spinal motion restriction device to a patient.
- Explain how to adapt steps of spinal motion restriction to special circumstances.

Key Terms

air embolism, *965*
ataxic respirations, *957*
autonomic nervous system, *950*
central nervous system, *950*
central neurogenic hyperventilation, *957*
cerebrospinal fluid (CSF), *951*
Cheyne-Stokes breathing, *957*
concussion, *954*
contusion, *955*
cranium, *950*
dermatome, *972*
foramen magnum, *951*
hematoma, *955*
herniation, *957*
intracranial pressure (ICP), *956*
laceration, *955*
malar, *951*
mandible, *950*
maxillae, *950*
nasal bones, *950*
nervous system, *950*
neurogenic shock, *974*
orbits, *951*
peripheral nervous system, *950*
pulmonary air embolism, *965*
spinal motion restriction, *977*
spinous process, *953*
temporal bones, *950*
temporomandibular joint, *950*
vertebrae, *951*

Brain and spinal injuries are among the most devastating injuries a patient can endure. Brain injuries alone account for more trauma-related death than any other traumatic injury. Survivors of these injuries also face severe and significant long-term and life-changing consequences. Brain-injured patients often see permanent changes to the basic functions that their brains perform. Spine-injured patients may face permanent paralysis. These injuries impact not only the patient but also society as a whole. The National Spinal Cord Injury Statistical Center estimates the cost of caring for a patient with complete quadriplegia is more than $120,000 per year.

The important fact to remember is that much of the devastation associated with these injuries is preventable. Not only can many of these injuries be prevented altogether with EMS-driven strategies, but more and more we are realizing that the care provided in the immediate postinjury setting is critical to interrupting the ongoing injury process and preventing initial problems from getting far worse.

Nervous and Skeletal Systems

The following segments briefly review the anatomy of the nervous system, head, and spine. For more information on these areas, review the chapter *Anatomy and Physiology*.

CORE CONCEPT
Understanding the anatomy of the nervous system, head, and spine

nervous system
provides overall control of thought, sensation, and the body's voluntary and involuntary motor functions. The components of the nervous system are the brain and the spinal cord as well as the nerves that enter and exit the brain and spinal cord and extend to the various parts of the body.

central nervous system
the brain and the spinal cord.

peripheral nervous system
the nerves that enter and exit the spinal cord between the vertebrae, the 12 pairs of cranial nerves that travel between the brain and organs without passing through the spinal cord, and all of the body's other motor and sensory nerves.

autonomic nervous system
controls involuntary functions.

cranium (KRAY-ne-um)
the bony structure making up the forehead, top, back, and upper sides of the skull.

temporal (TEM-po-ral) ***bones***
bones forming part of the sides of the skull and the floor of the cranial cavity.

mandible (MAN-di-bl)
the lower jawbone.

temporomandibular (TEM-po-ro-mand-DIB-yuh-lar) ***joint***
the movable joint between the mandible and the temporal bone, also called the TMJ.

maxillae (mak-SIL-e)
the two fused bones forming the upper jaw.

nasal (NAY-zul) ***bones***
the bones that form the upper third, or bridge, of the nose.

Nervous System

The components of the ***nervous system*** are the brain and the spinal cord as well as the nerves that enter and exit the brain and spinal cord and extend to the various parts of the body. The nervous system provides overall control of thought, sensations, and motor functions, whereas the skeletal system provides support and protection. The skull protects the brain, while the bones of the spine protect the spinal cord. Whenever the skull or the spine is injured, suspect possible nervous system damage as well.

The nervous system (Figure 33-1) is divided into two subsystems: the central nervous system and the peripheral nervous system. The ***central nervous system*** consists of the brain and the spinal cord. The ***peripheral nervous system*** includes the pairs of nerves that enter and exit the spinal cord between each pair of vertebrae, the 12 pairs of cranial nerves that travel from the brain without passing through the spinal cord, and all of the body's other motor and sensory nerves. *Neurons* are the specialized nerve cells that transmit nervous system impulses throughout the body.

Messages from the body to the brain are carried by sensory nerves. Messages from the brain to the muscles are carried by motor nerves. The motor nerves control voluntary movements, or those we consciously control, such as running or grasping. As the nerves exit the brain, prior to traveling down the spinal cord, they cross over to the opposite side of the body. This is why an injury to the left side of the brain may produce effects such as weakness or lack of sensation on the right side of the body.

Other nerves control involuntary functions—those we do not consciously control—including heartbeat, breathing, control of the diameter of the vessels, control of the round sphincter muscles enclosing the bladder and bowel, and digestion. These nerves are part of the ***autonomic nervous system***. (*Autonomic* means *automatic*.)

Anatomy of the Head

The skull is made up of the ***cranium*** and the facial bones (Figure 33-2). The cranium, the portion of the skull that encloses the brain, is formed by several distinct regions of bone. The frontal region forms the forehead. The parietal bones form the right and left superior skull. The ***temporal bones*** form the right and left inferior skull, and the occipital bone forms the posterior of the skull. The cranial floor is the inferior wall of the brain case, the bony floor beneath the brain. The cranial bones are fused together to form immovable joints, called *sutures*.

There are 14 irregularly shaped bones forming the face. The facial bones are fused into immovable joints, except for the ***mandible***, which joins on each side of the cranium at the temporal bones to form the ***temporomandibular joint***, sometimes referred to as the TM joint or TMJ.

The upper jaw is made up of two fused bones called the ***maxillae***. Each is known as a *maxilla*. The upper third, or bridge, of the nose contains two ***nasal bones***. There is a cheekbone on each side of the skull, which can be called the ***malar*** or *zygomatic bone*. The maxillae and the malars form a portion of the ***orbits*** (sockets) of the eyes.

The brain is held within the skull. The spinal cord exits the base of the brain and leaves the skull through a large hole called the ***foramen magnum*** (Figure 33-3). The brain is bathed in a fluid called ***cerebrospinal fluid (CSF)***, which also circulates down the spine around the spinal cord.

Anatomy of the Spine

The spine consists of the spinal cord and the spinal column. The spinal cord is a bundle of nervous tissue about the width of a thumb that extends about 18 inches from the brainstem down to the small of the back. It is the central pathway for messages to and from the brain, and all along its anatomy, spinal nerves branch out to the various regions of the body. At the lower end of the spinal cord, a fan of nerves that resembles a horse's tail, called the

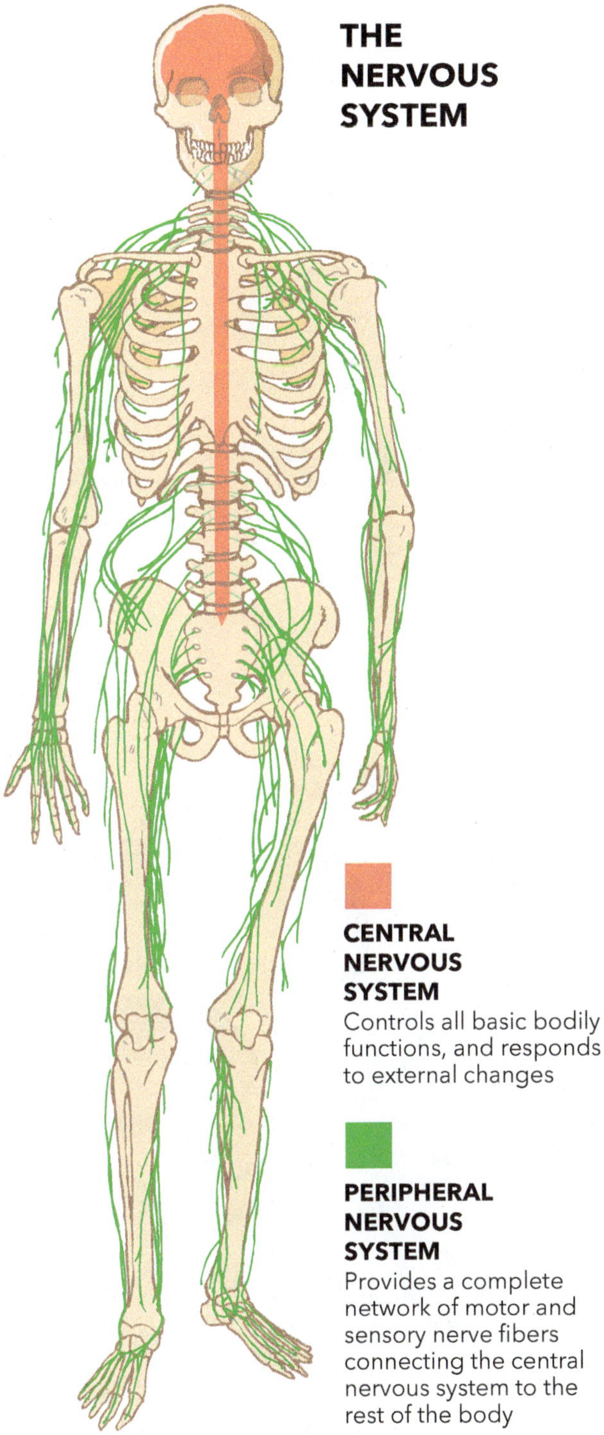

FIGURE 33-1 Nervous system.

cauda equina, emerges from the cord. The tissue of the spinal cord is like any other tissue in the body in that it requires oxygen and glucose to survive. It has a relatively soft consistency, making it vulnerable to injury, but it is *very* well protected by the bony spinal column.

The first layer of protection for the spinal cord consists of tough, fibrous membranes called *meninges*. These are the same layers that protect the brain inside the skull. In addition, 33 irregularly shaped bones, called ***vertebrae*** (singular *vertebra*), surround the cord and provide it with bony protection. The vertebrae are stacked one on top of another and interlock to form the spinal column. They are linked together with ligaments and are further supported and protected by several muscle groups in the back. A hollow space inside each bone, similar to a doughnut hole, allows the spinal cord to run through a channel down the center of the spinal column. Inside the channel, the cord is surrounded and

malar (MAY-lar)
the cheekbone. Also called the *zygomatic bone*.

orbits
the bony structures around the eyes; the eye sockets.

foramen magnum (FOR-uh-men MAG-num)
the opening at the base of the skull through which the spinal cord passes from the brain.

cerebrospinal (suh-RE-bro-SPI-nal) ***fluid (CSF)***
the fluid that surrounds the brain and spinal cord.

vertebrae (VERT-uh-bray)
the bones of the spinal column (singular *vertebra*).

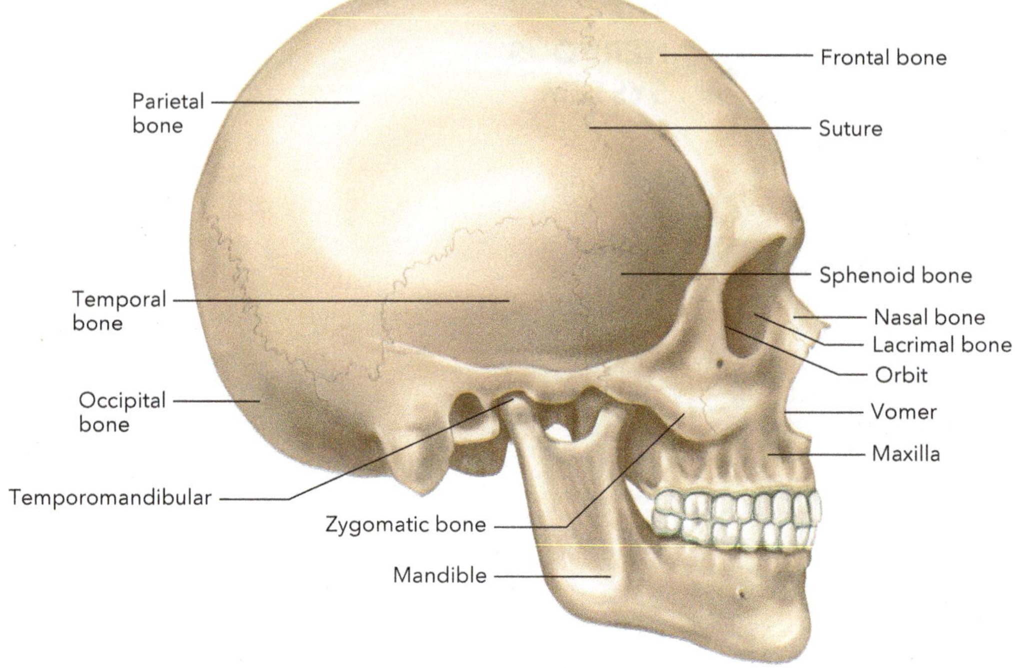

FIGURE 33-2 Bones of the cranium and face. *(Source: FREMGEN, BONNIE F.; FRUCHT, SUZANNE S., MEDICAL TERMINOLOGY: A LIVING LANGUAGE, 5th Ed., © 2013. Reprinted and Electronically reproduced by permission of Pearson Education, Inc., New York.)*

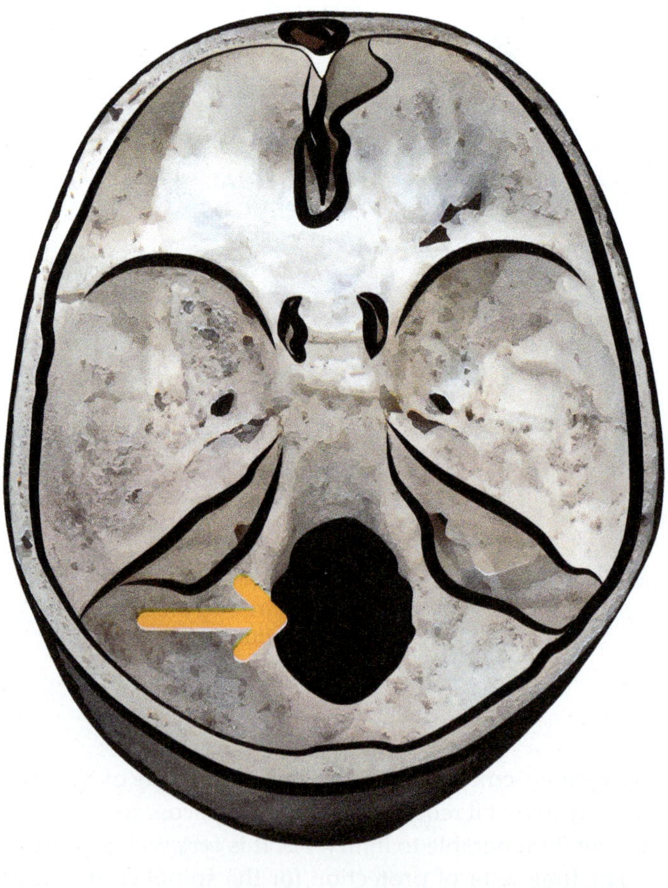

FIGURE 33-3 Foramen magnum at the base of the skull.

cushioned by cerebral spinal fluid. Vertebrae fit together like puzzle pieces, using their shape to allow specific movements and rotation of the column but also protecting against movements that would threaten the integrity of the channel. Small projections from the vertebrae allow ligaments to be connected to one another.

The vertebrae are divided into five areas (as shown in Figure 33-4A). From top to bottom, they are: 7 cervical (in the neck), 12 thoracic (to which the ribs attach), 5 lumbar (mid-back),

FIGURE 33-4 (A) Divisions of the spinal column. (B) A cervical vertebra.

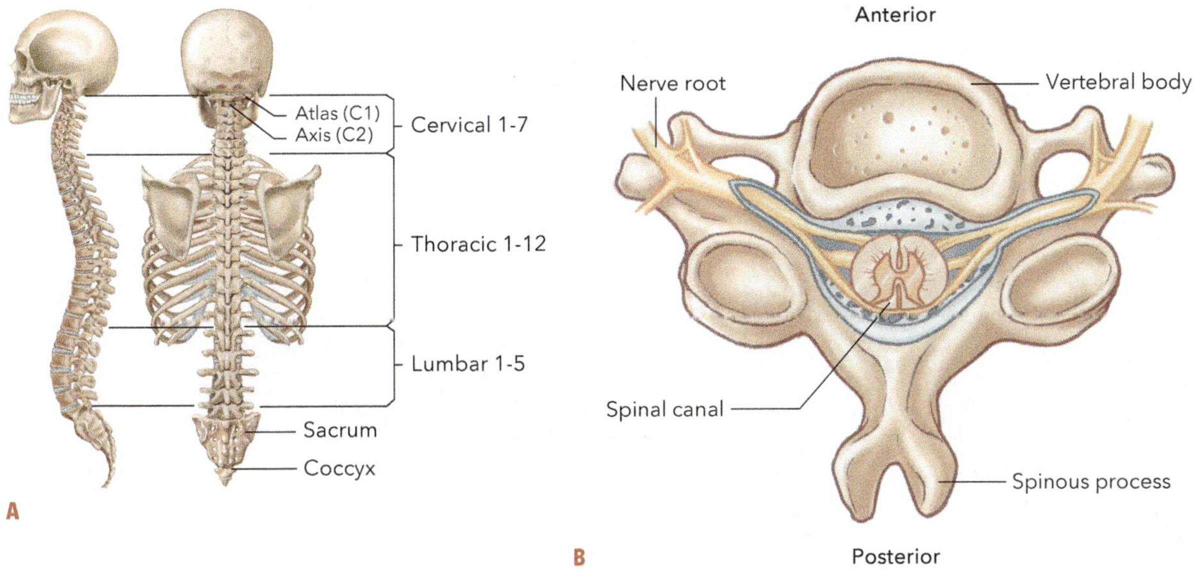

5 sacral (lower back), and 4 coccygeal (in the coccyx, or tailbone). Both the sacral and coccygeal vertebrae are fused together, forming the posterior portion of the pelvis. Each vertebra has a ***spinous process***, a bony bump you can feel along the center of a person's back (Figure 33-4B).

spinous (SPI-nus) ***process*** the bony bump on a vertebra.

Injuries to the Skull and Brain

Scalp Injuries

The scalp has many blood vessels, so any scalp injury may cause profuse bleeding. Control scalp bleeding by applying direct pressure. Dress and bandage scalp bleeding as you would other soft tissue injuries. However, be careful about applying direct pressure when there is a possible skull injury. Do not apply pressure if the injury site shows bone fragments or depression of the bone or if the brain is exposed. Instead, use a loose gauze dressing.

CORE CONCEPT
Understanding skull and brain injuries and emergency care for skull and brain injuries

Skull Injuries

Skull injuries include fractures to the cranium and the face. If severe enough, there can also be injuries to the brain.

Skull injuries can be either open or closed. With most injuries, the words *open* and *closed* refer to whether the skin and its underlying tissues have been broken. With head injuries, however, the words *open* and *closed* refer to the cranial bones. When the bones of the cranium are fractured, the patient has an *open head injury* (Figure 33-5). If the scalp is lacerated but the cranium is intact, it is considered to be a *closed head injury*. In practice, you may not be able to determine if a head injury is open or closed. It is safest to assume that there may be an open head injury beneath any contusion or laceration of the scalp. You should also be aware that a brain injury may be present with *no* external injury.

NOTE: *Whenever you suspect a skull or brain injury, also suspect spine injury.*

Brain Injuries

Brain injuries can be classified as direct or indirect. *Direct injuries* to the brain can occur in open head injuries, with the brain being lacerated, punctured, or bruised by the broken bones or by a foreign object such as a bullet. *Indirect injuries* to the brain may occur with either closed or open head injuries. In an indirect injury, the shock of impact on the skull is transferred to the brain. Indirect injuries to the brain include concussions and contusions.

FIGURE 33-5 (A) An open skull fracture. (B) Skull injury in a child. *(Photo A: © Edward T. Dickinson, MD. Photo B: © David Effron, MD)*

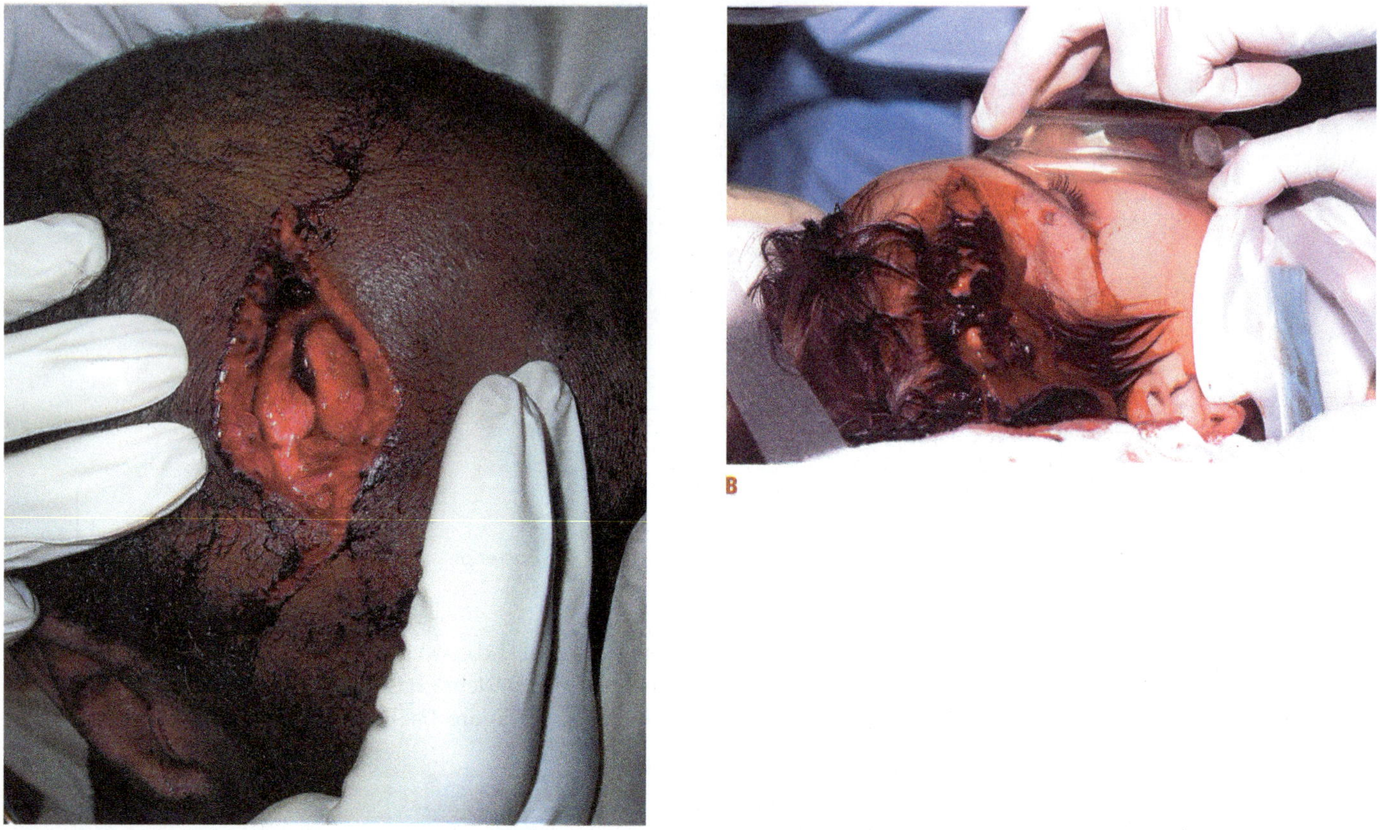

B

A

NOTE: *One of the first and most significant signs of head injury is altered mental status. In some patients, it would be easy to assume the patient was intoxicated or on drugs when the true underlying problem was a head injury. Never assume a patient with an altered mental status is simply intoxicated or on drugs. Always complete a thorough patient assessment.*

Traumatic Brain Injuries

A traumatic brain injury (TBI) is an injury that disrupts the normal functioning of the brain. It may be a brief (e.g., concussion) or long-term condition with permanent damage to the brain. The Centers for Disease Control and Prevention (CDC) estimates 1.7 million people sustain a traumatic brain injury each year in the United States, and traumatic brain injury accounts for slightly more than a third of all injury-related deaths.

The following sections describe types of traumatic brain injury. It is not necessary for you as an EMT to diagnose these specific conditions (this is done in the hospital), but knowing the types of brain injuries and how they may present will help you understand these conditions, identify critical patients, and make appropriate transport decisions.

concussion
mild closed head injury without detectable damage to the brain. Complete recovery is usually expected, but effects may linger for weeks, months, or even years.

Concussion. A ***concussion*** (Figure 33-6) may be so mild that the patient is unaware of the injury. When a person strikes the head in a fall or is struck by a blunt object, a certain amount of the force is transferred through the skull to the brain. Usually there is no detectable damage to the brain, and the patient might or might not become unconscious. Most patients with a concussion will feel a little "groggy" after receiving a blow to the head, and a headache is also common. If there is a loss of consciousness, it usually lasts only a short time and does not tend to recur. Sometimes, after a head blow, bystanders will say the patient "just sat there staring off into space for a few minutes." Some loss of memory (amnesia) of the events surrounding the incident is fairly common. A common saying is that a fighter did not see the punch that did him in. Actually, he probably did see the punch but then forgot it because of the concussion.

Despite their frequently short-term symptoms, concussions are true brain injuries and should be taken seriously. In many cases, very mild initial symptoms turn into far more significant problems hours later. Occasionally, EMTs are put into the difficult situation of evaluating patients with suspected concussions, and frequently, as in the case of athletes, there is pressure to make quick decisions following this evaluation. The CDC suggests that the following signs and symptoms indicate the presence of concussion: loss of consciousness (no matter how brief); amnesia and repetitive questioning; altered level of consciousness, including feeling sluggish and difficulty concentrating or "feeling off" or "not right"; slurred speech; headache; nausea; blurred or disrupted vision; and sensitivity to light or loud noises. It is also important to remember that a lack of a loss of consciousness does not rule out a concussion. The identification of any of these findings, whether paired with loss of consciousness or not, suggests the presence of a concussion and warrants further evaluation of the patient.

Contusion. A bruised brain, or brain ***contusion*** (see Figure 33-6), can occur with closed head injuries when the force of the blow is great enough to rupture blood vessels on or within the brain. A contusion is often caused by a collision or blow that causes the brain to hit the inside of the skull, bounce off the opposite side, then rebound to strike the first side of the skull again. When the bruising of the brain occurs on the side of the blow, it is called a coup injury; when it occurs on the side opposite the blow, it is called a *contrecoup injury*.

contusion
in brain injuries, a bruised brain caused when the force of a blow to the head is great enough to rupture blood vessels.

Laceration. A ***laceration***, or cut, to the brain can occur from the same forces that might cause a contusion. The inner skull has many sharp, bony ridges that can lacerate a moving brain. A laceration or a puncture wound can also be caused by an object penetrating the cranium.

laceration (las-uh-RAY-shun)
in brain injuries, a cut to the brain.

Hematoma. A ***hematoma*** is a collection of blood within tissue. A hematoma inside the cranium is named according to its location, which may be inside or outside the dura, the brain's protective outer covering (Figure 33-7), or within the brain itself. A *subdural hematoma* is a collection of blood between the brain and the dura. An *epidural hematoma* is blood between the dura and the skull. An *intracerebral hematoma* occurs when blood pools within the brain (Figure 33-8).

hematoma (HE-mah-TO-mah)
in a head injury, a collection of blood within the skull or brain.

FIGURE 33-6 Closed head injuries: concussion and contusion.

CONCUSSION
- Mild injury, usually with no detectable brain damage
- May have brief loss of consciousness
- Headache, grogginess, and short-term memory loss common

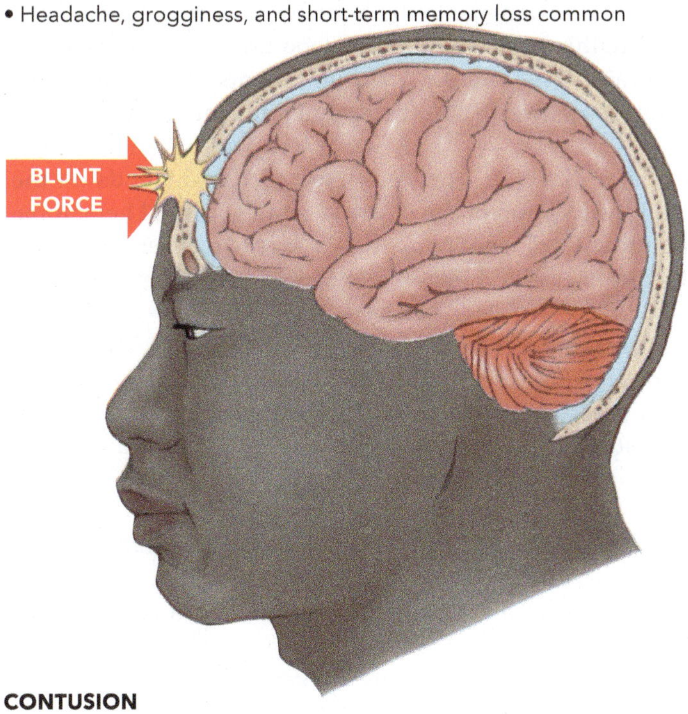

CONTUSION
- Unconsciousness or decreased level of responsiveness
- Bruising of brain tissue

FIGURE 33-7 Meninges (covering layers) of the brain.

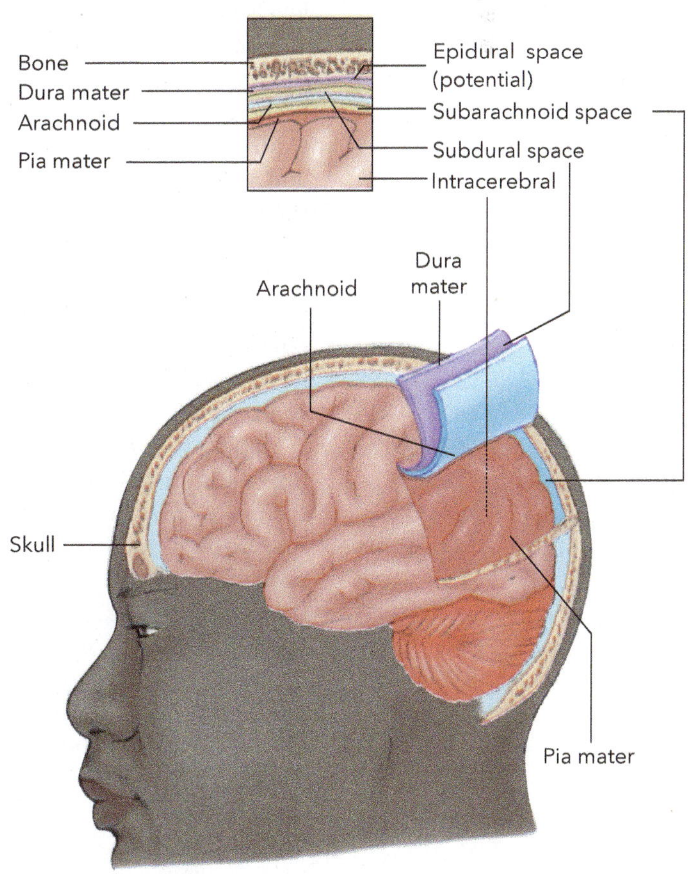

FIGURE 33-8 Hematomas within the cranium.

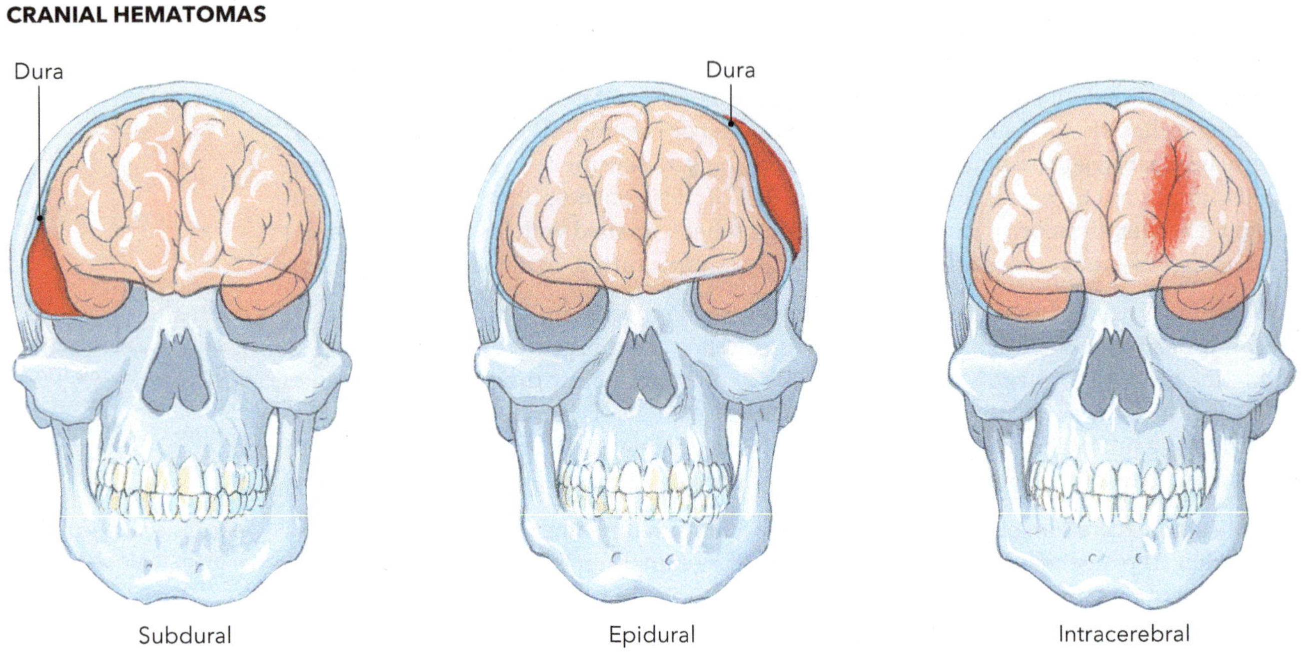

Intracranial Pressure

intracranial (IN-truh-KRAY-ne-ul) ***pressure (ICP)*** pressure inside the skull.

There is limited room for expansion inside the patient's hard skull. When a hematoma develops, pressure increases inside the skull. This is referred to as increasing ***intracranial pressure (ICP)***. There is a typical progression that is seen with this condition. As ICP builds and compresses the brain tissues, progressive neurologic abnormalities—such as decreasing levels of consciousness and one-sided (unilateral) weakness—develop.

The hematoma expands and places pressure on the brain, pushing and compressing the brain tissue. Since the cranium is a rigid container, pressure within this space begins to increase. This pressure can cause direct damage to the brain by compressing it against skull structures, but more important, this pressure reduces blood flow through the brain and can limit vital perfusion of brain tissue. As the pressure mounts, the brain can be forced downward toward the only space available—the foramen magnum, the opening at the base of the skull.

The time it takes for symptoms to develop from an increased ICP depends on the rate of bleeding into the skull and the location of the bleed. A small subdural hematoma obtained in an assault or a fall could take from hours up to two days before serious symptoms develop, whereas a brisk epidural bleed may almost instantly develop and show symptoms.

The body responds to rising intracranial pressure in a predictable manner. The body's highest priority is to perfuse the brain with oxygen. When intracranial pressure increases, the body must increase the blood pressure to overcome the resistance to blood flow in the cranium. Increased blood pressure is necessary to pump blood into the brain and to perfuse brain tissue. This is why you will see increasing blood pressure in patients with increased intracranial pressure.

The remainder of the body does not need this increase in blood pressure and responds to the hypertension by slowing the heart rate. As a result, you will frequently see a slowing heart rate paired with rising blood pressure in response to rising intracranial pressure. Heart rate can also be slowed in this case by compression of the vagus nerve as the brain swells. Increased blood pressure and decreased heart rate are key findings that indicate rising intracranial pressure, and together are known as *Cushing reflex*.

As ICP increases and cerebral perfusion decreases, carbon dioxide levels in the brain increase. This causes brain tissue to swell. The swelling worsens intracranial pressure and creates a vicious cycle in which the body increases blood pressure in an attempt to perfuse the brain while carbon dioxide builds and increases swelling.

As the hematoma continues to grow, swelling worsens, and the brain is pushed downward toward the foramen magnum, compressing the brainstem. The brainstem regulates our most vital functions, including breathing, heartbeat, and blood pressure. As this area is compressed, in addition to an altered mental status, you may see dilated pupils or sluggish pupil reaction, increased systolic blood pressure, and a decreased pulse rate. Brainstem compression also commonly results in abnormal respiration patterns. Patients may display tachypnea or more distinct patterns such as the quickening and deepening pattern followed by a period of apnea called ***Cheyne-Stokes breathing***. Other distinct patterns include ***central neurogenic hyperventilation***, which is a pattern of very rapid breathing associated with progressive damage to the brainstem. ***Ataxic respirations*** are a pattern characterized by irregular and unpredictable breathing. Any of these patterns of abnormal breathing can result from rising intracranial pressure and herniation, and should be assumed to be a sign of this type of injury.

As the brain and brainstem become severely compressed and pushed downward (***herniation***), the patient may exhibit decorticate or decerebrate posturing. There may be neurologic posturing, such as flexing the arms and wrists and extending the legs and feet (decorticate posture) (Figure 33-9A) or extension of the arms with the shoulders rotated inward and wrists flexed and the legs extended (decerebrate posture) (Figure 33-9B). These postures may be assumed spontaneously or in response to a painful stimulus.

Signs and symptoms of rising intracranial pressure may be immediate, but they may also present with a delayed onset. A patient who has a significant epidural or subdural hematoma (remember that there are variables such as the size and location of the bleed, as well as concurrent injuries) may present in the following sequence:

1. A woman falls and strikes her head. She appears all right at first or may have a brief loss of consciousness.
2. After about 10 minutes, she develops a slightly altered mental status. This is because the hematoma is beginning to place pressure on one or both cerebral hemispheres.
3. The altered mental status worsens. Soon the patient responds to loud verbal stimulus only by moaning. Her blood pressure begins to increase.
4. She has a generalized seizure. A seizure may occur at any time in the setting of significant brain injury or increasing intracranial pressure.
5. The patient is now totally unresponsive to any stimuli. Her blood pressure is 220/106. You notice her pulse beginning to drop. It had been 88 and now it is 54. Her pupils have become unequal or nonreactive.
6. Respirations become slightly irregular. Blood pressure continues to increase. The pulse now drops to 48 beats per minute.
7. The patient may begin to develop decorticate posturing, followed by decerebrate posturing. Death follows if the condition is uncorrected by intervention at a trauma center.

FIGURE 33-9 (A) Decorticate posturing. (B) Decerebrate posturing.

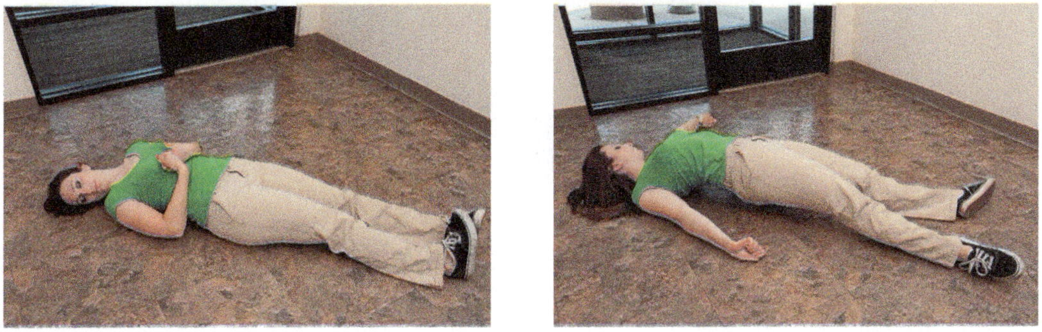

A B

Cheyne (CHAY-ne) ***-Stokes breathing***
a distinct pattern of breathing characterized by quickening and deepening respirations followed by a period of apnea.

central neurogenic hyperventilation
a pattern of rapid and deep breathing caused by injury to the brain.

ataxic (AY-taks-ic) ***respirations***
a pattern of irregular and unpredictable breathing commonly caused by brain injury.

herniation (her-ne-AY-shun)
pushing of a portion of the brain downward toward the foramen magnum as a result of increased intracranial pressure.

Subdural hematomas can present with delayed symptoms even 12–24 hours later. Remember that the mechanism of injury (MOI) for these patients may not be apparent. You will need to recognize the pattern of symptoms associated with rising intracranial pressure and use your patient assessment to identify an injury that occurred hours ago. Suspect traumatic injury in any patient with altered mental status, and be sure to ask questions about previous trauma.

Patient Assessment

Skull Fractures and Brain Injuries

The signs of skull fracture and of brain injury are very similar, as noted in the following list (see Figure 33-10):

- Although visible bone fragments and perhaps bits of brain tissue are the most obvious signs of skull fracture, most skull fractures do not produce these signs.
- The patient may have an altered mental status. Check mental status by using the AVPU scale (alert, verbal stimulus, painful stimulus, unresponsive). If the patient is alert, check for orientation to person, place, and time. Some EMS agencies also use the Glasgow Coma Scale (described later in this chapter).
- There may be a deep laceration or severe bruise or hematoma to the scalp or forehead. Do not probe or separate the wound opening to determine wound depth.
- Depressions or deformity of the skull, large swellings ("goose eggs"), or anything unusual about the shape of the cranium may be visible.
- Severe pain may exist at the site of a head injury. Pain may range from a headache to severe discomfort. Do not palpate the injury site with your fingertips, as you may push bone fragments into the injury.
- "Battle sign," a bruise behind the ear (late sign), may be present (Figure 33-11).
- Pupils are unequal or nonreactive to light (Figure 33-12).
- "Raccoon eyes," black eyes, or discoloration of the soft tissues (Figure 33-13) is present under both eyes (late sign).

FIGURE 33-10 Signs of cranial fracture or brain injury.

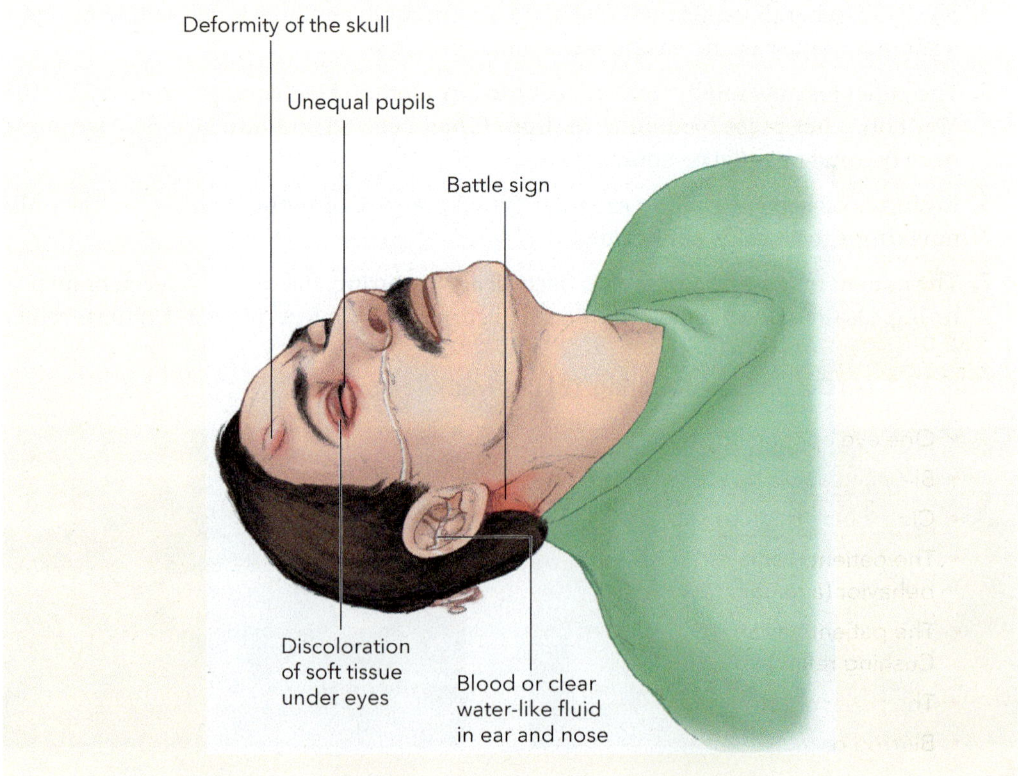

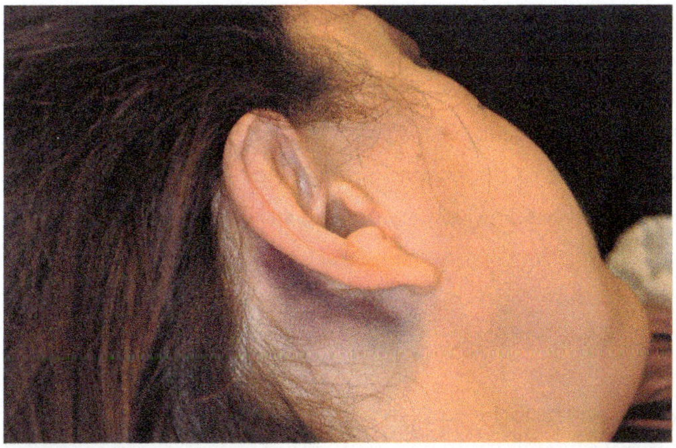

FIGURE 33-11 Battle sign. *(© Edward T. Dickinson, MD)*

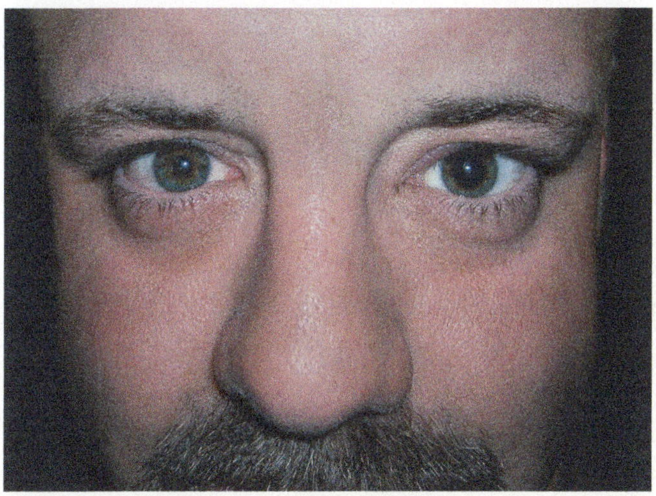

FIGURE 33-12 Unequal pupils. *(© Edward T. Dickinson, MD)*

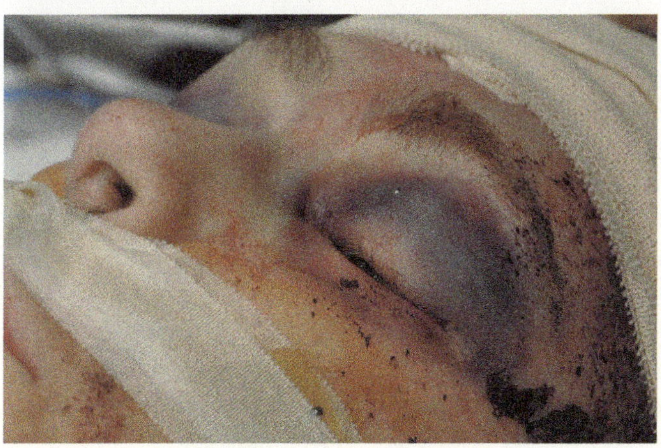

FIGURE 33-13 Raccoon eyes. *(© Edward T. Dickinson, MD)*

- One eye appears to be sunken.
- Bleeding exists from the ears and/or nose.
- Clear fluid flows from the ears and/or nose.
- The patient displays a personality change, ranging from irritable to irrational behavior (a major sign).
- The patient has an increased blood pressure and decreased pulse rate (also called Cushing reflex).
- The patient has irregular breathing patterns.
- Blurred or multiple-image vision is present in one or both eyes.

- Impaired hearing or ringing occurs in the patient's ears.
- Equilibrium problems exist. The patient may be unable to stand still with eyes closed or may stumble when attempting to walk. (Do not test for this.)
- Forceful or projectile vomiting may occur.
- The patient may exhibit decorticate or decerebrate posturing.
- The patient may experience paralysis or disability on one side of the body.
- Seizures may be present.
- There is a temperature increase (late sign due to inflammation, infection, or damage to temperature-regulating centers).
- The patient has deteriorating vital signs.

Note that shock (hypoperfusion) from blood loss is generally not a sign of head injury, except in infants. There simply is not enough room within the adult skull to permit enough bleeding to cause shock. If there is head injury with shock, look for indications of blood loss somewhere else on the body.

With so many factors to consider, possible skull or brain injury can be very difficult to determine definitively. So you must assume the patient has a skull or brain injury when the MOI and the location of the injury indicate a head injury.

Decision Points

- Does the patient have a serious or potentially serious head injury? Should the patient be transported to a trauma center?
- Do the patient's complaint and MOI indicate that spinal motion restriction is warranted?

Patient Care

Care of the Patient with a Skull Fracture or Brain Injury

Fundamental Principles of Care

It is important to recognize that a serious brain injury may be present. EMT care is based on prevention of hypoxia and inappropriate carbon dioxide levels from contributing to secondary injuries. By placing a high priority on airway and breathing management and on rapid transport, you can affect the outcome of even a significant brain injury.

Key elements of care include:

- Take appropriate Standard Precautions.
- Consider the possibility of a spine injury. If indicated, provide manual stabilization of the head on first patient contact, and use the jaw-thrust maneuver to open the airway.
- Open and maintain the airway. For the unconscious patient, insert an oropharyngeal airway. Have suctioning equipment ready since these patients are prone to vomiting. Remember that as mental status changes, so may the patient's ability to maintain an airway. Be vigilant and consider airway management to be an ongoing need.
- Monitor the unconscious patient for changes in breathing. Provide artificial ventilations if breathing is inadequate and take care to avoid hyperventilation. Maintain a ventilation rate of 10–12 breaths per minute. Administer high-concentration oxygen via a nonrebreather mask if the patient is breathing adequately. (Note that some advanced providers may use targeted hyperventilation to maintain a specific end-tidal CO_2 ($ETCO_2$) in a patient with brain injury. Uncontrolled or excessive hyperventilation can reduce perfusion to the brain and be harmful.)
- If indicated, apply a rigid cervical collar and initiate spinal motion restriction. If appropriate, determine the method of extrication, either normal or rapid (discussed later in this chapter).

- Control bleeding. Do not apply direct pressure if the injury site shows bone fragments or depression of the bone or if the brain is exposed. Do not attempt to stop the flow of blood or cerebrospinal fluid from the ears or the nose; if the skull is fractured, you might increase intracranial pressure and the risk of infection. Instead, use a loose gauze dressing.
- Keep the patient at rest. This can be a critical step.
- Talk to the conscious patient and provide emotional support. Ask the patient questions which require concentration to help you to detect changes in the patient's mental status.
- Dress and bandage open wounds. Stabilize any penetrating objects. (Do not remove any objects or fragments of bone.)
- Manage the patient for shock, even if signs of shock are not yet present.
- Be prepared for vomiting. Have a suction unit ready for use.
- Transport the patient promptly. When possible, transport to a trauma center or other facility capable of handling head trauma.
- Monitor vital signs every 5 minutes en route to the hospital.

Remember, it is not necessary for you to try to determine the exact type of brain injury that has occurred (such as epidural or subdural bleeding). What is crucial is that you recognize the signs and symptoms of a traumatic brain injury and treat them accordingly to prevent secondary brain injury.

Decision Point

- Does the patient have increasing intracranial pressure?

If there is evidence of spine injury or if the patient with a head injury is unconscious, then consider spinal motion restriction according to local protocols. Some patients with head injuries will vomit without warning. Many vomit without first experiencing nausea. The vomiting is likely to be projectile vomiting (forceful, explosive vomiting). Constant monitoring and frequent suctioning are required.

Glasgow Coma Scale

All head-injury patients must be constantly monitored during transport. Be prepared in case the patient vomits or has a seizure. What you observe and report can have a great bearing on the ED staff's initial actions on your arrival. The early signs of deterioration are subtle changes in mental status that may be overlooked if you are not watching for them.

Some EMS agencies use the Glasgow Coma Scale (GCS) (Figure 33-14), in addition to AVPU, for ongoing neurologic assessment. Some systems would immediately transport a patient with a GCS score of less than 14 directly to the trauma center if they were within 30 minutes' transport time. When using this score, keep the following considerations in mind:

NOTE: *Do not spend extra time at the scene calculating a GCS score. Calculate the score en route to the hospital to avoid prolonged scene times.*

- **Eye opening.** Spontaneous eye opening means that the patient opens the eyes without your having to do anything. If the patient's eyes are closed, say "Open your eyes" in a normal level of voice. If this fails, shout the command. Should the patient's eyes remain closed, apply an accepted painful stimulus (such as pinching a toe, scratching the palm or sole, or rubbing the sternum). Note any eye injuries or injuries to the face that prevent the patient from opening the eyes. If the injuries are more than minor ones, do not ask the patient to open the eyes.

FIGURE 33-14 Glasgow Coma Scale.

GLASGOW COMA SCALE

Eye Opening	Spontaneous	4	
	To Voice	3	
	To Pain	2	
	None	1	
Verbal Response	Oriented	5	
	Confused	4	
	Inappropriate Words	3	
	Incomprehensible Sounds	2	
	None	1	
Motor Response	Obeys Command	6	
	Localizes Pain	5	
	Withdraws (pain)	4	
	Flexion (pain)	3	
	Extension (pain)	2	
	None	1	
Glasgow Coma Score Total			

- **Verbal response.** When evaluating the patient's verbal responses, use the following criteria:
  - **Oriented.** Once aroused, a person who can answer all three of these questions appropriately is said to be alert on the AVPU scale: What is your name? Where are you (location)? and What day of the week is this?
  - **Confused.** The patient cannot answer the previous questions, but can speak in phrases and sentences.
  - **Inappropriate words.** The patient says or shouts a word or several words at a time. Usually this requires physical stimulation. The words do not fit the situation or a particular question. Often the patient curses.
  - **Incomprehensible sounds.** The patient responds with mumbling, moans, or groans.
  - **No verbal response.** Repeated stimulation, both verbal and physical, does not cause the patient to speak or make any sounds.
- **Motor response.** The following criteria are used to evaluate motor response:
  - **Obeys command.** The patient must be able to understand your instruction and carry out the request. For example, you may ask the patient (when appropriate) to hold up two fingers.
  - **Localizes pain.** If the patient fails to respond to your commands, apply pressure to one of the nail beds for 5 seconds or apply firm pressure to the sternum. Note if the patient attempts to remove your hand. Do not apply pressure over an injury site. Do not apply pressure to the sternum if the patient is experiencing difficulty breathing.
  - **Withdraws after painful stimulation.** Note if the elbow flexes, if the patient moves slowly, if there is the appearance of stiffness, if the patient holds a forearm and hand against the body, or if the limbs on one side of the body appear to be paralyzed (hemiplegic position).
  - **Posturing after painful stimulation.** Note if the legs and arms extend, if there is apparent stiffness with these moves, and if there is an internal rotation of the shoulder and forearm.
  - **No motor response to pain.** Repeated painful stimulation does not cause the patient to grimace or make any motions.

Cranial Injuries with Impaled Objects

If there is an object impaled in the cranium, do not remove it. Instead, stabilize the object in place with bulky dressings. (See information on stabilizing impaled objects in the chapter *Soft-Tissue Trauma*.) This, with care in handling, will minimize accidental movement of the object.

A lengthy impaled object can make transporting the patient impossible until the object is cut or shortened. Pad around the object with bulky dressings, then carefully (and rigidly) stabilize the object on both sides of where the cut will be made. Cutting should be done with a tool that will not cause the object to move or vibrate when it is finally severed. A hand hacksaw with a fine-tooth blade can be carefully controlled and produces only a small amount of heat. In any case in which you may have to cut an impaled object, seek advice from medical direction or the emergency department physician.

Injuries to the Face and Jaw

Facial fractures are usually caused by an impact, as when a child is struck in the face by a baseball bat or when someone is thrown against a windshield. Bone fragments may lodge in the back of the pharynx and cause airway obstruction. Blood, blood clots, dislodged teeth, or a separated palate may also block the airway. Figure 33-15 shows (A) a facial laceration and (B) signs of a facial fracture.

NOTE: *The face is part of the skull. Therefore, brain injury may accompany a blow of sufficient force to the face. Treat this patient as you would any patient with a suspected skull or brain injury.*

The mandible is subject to dislocation as well as to fracture. As with any facial injury, there may be pain, discoloration, swelling, and facial distortion. In addition, when the mandible is injured or dislocated, the patient may be unable to move the lower jaw or may have difficulty speaking. There may be an improper alignment of the upper and lower teeth, and bleeding around the teeth (Figure 33-16).

The primary concern with facial fractures is the patient's airway (Figure 33-17). Be prepared to suction to remove debris, including loose teeth and blood, from the airway. If a spinal injury is suspected, use the jaw-thrust maneuver to open the airway. Control profuse bleeding. (See the *Soft-Tissue Trauma* chapter for care of an object impaled in the cheek.) Consider the need for spinal motion restriction. If possible, position the patient to allow drainage from the mouth. Treat for shock.

FIGURE 33-15 Facial injuries: (A) a complex intraoral-facial laceration; (B) signs of facial fracture. *(Photo A: © Edward T. Dickinson, MD)*

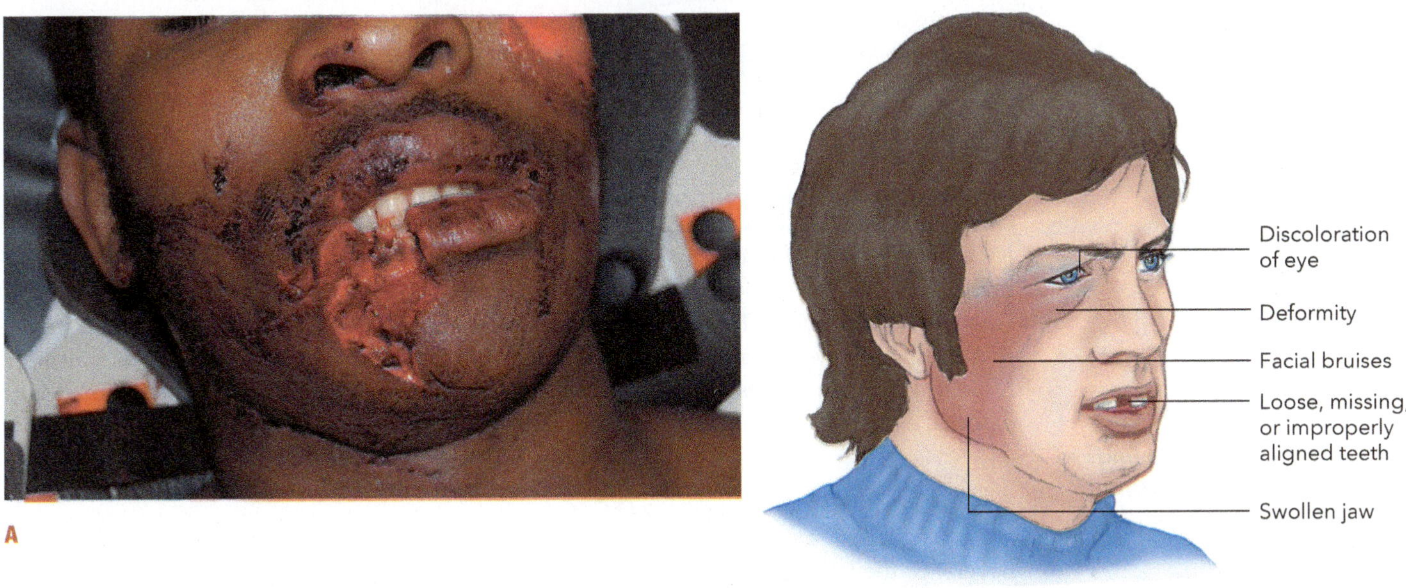

FIGURE 33-16 Facial injuries: (A) an open displaced mandible (jaw) fracture; (B) a CT scan of the injury shown in (A). *(Photos A and B: © Edward T. Dickinson, MD)*

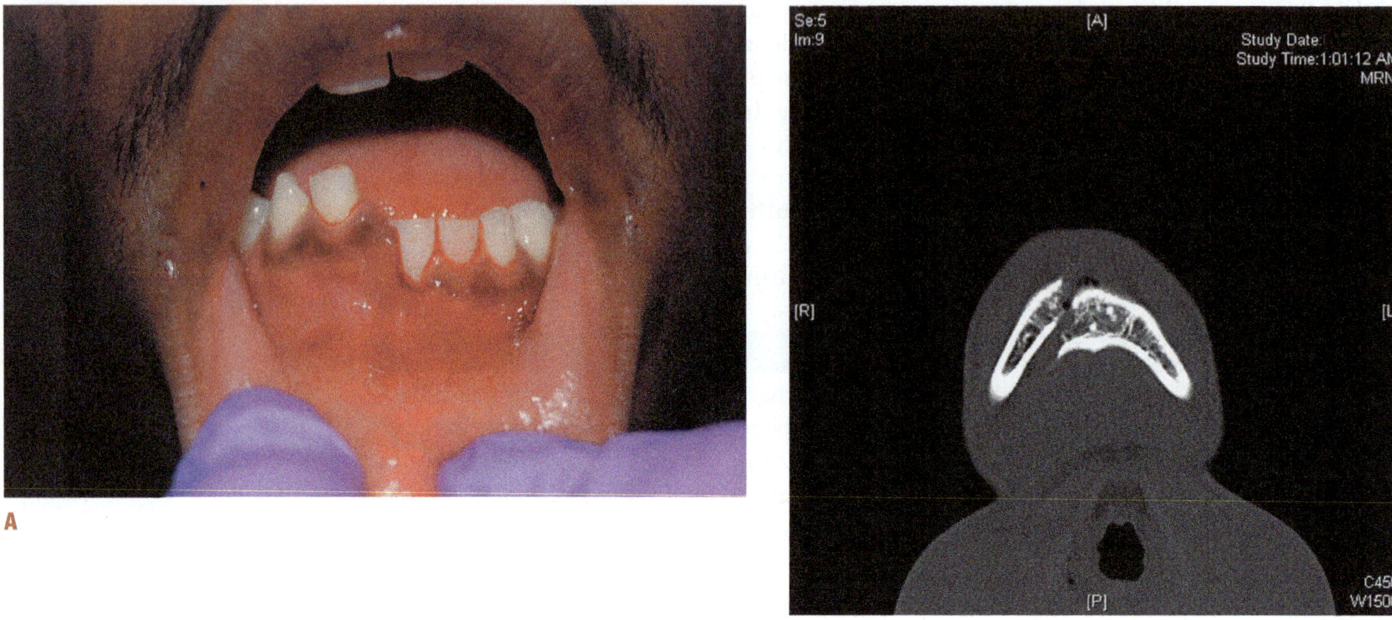

A

B

FIGURE 33-17 Complications of facial fracture.

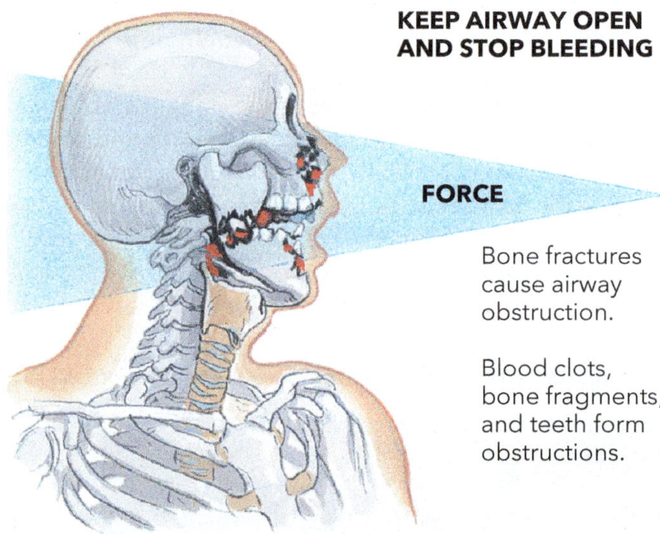

Nontraumatic Brain Injuries

Many of the signs of brain injury may be caused by an internal brain event such as a hemorrhage or blood clot. (See the information on stroke in the chapter *Diabetic Emergencies and Altered Mental Status*.) The signs of nontraumatic stroke will often differ from those of traumatic brain injury. Stroke is more apt to affect only one side of the body, whereas traumatic brain injury often causes a more generalized picture of altered mental status coupled with external signs of trauma.

CORE CONCEPT
Understanding wounds to the neck and emergency care for neck wounds

Wounds to the Neck

Several of the largest arteries and veins in the body lie close to the surface of the neck. As a result, bleeding from the neck can rapidly be life-threatening. Massive hemorrhage from a neck wound must be treated with the highest priority. In addition, the pressure in a large vein is likely to be lower than atmospheric pressure. Therefore, it is possible for air to be sucked into the vessel and cause an ***air embolism*** (air bubble). An air embolus can be carried to the lungs and interfere with the pulmonary circulation and with the body's ability to exchange oxygen and carbon dioxide. This condition, called a ***pulmonary air embolism***, can cause cardiac arrest.

Battlefield medicine has developed a reluctance to apply direct pressure to neck wounds. This error must be avoided. Although care should be taken not to interfere with breathing, direct pressure is a lifesaving step in treating hemorrhage from neck wounds. In the case of severe bleeding, care is centered on stopping the hemorrhage immediately, and secondarily on preventing the introduction of air into the large blood vessels.

air embolism (EM-boh-lizm) a bubble of air in the bloodstream.

pulmonary air embolism a blockage in the blood circulation of the lung caused by a blood clot or air bubble.

Patient Care

Care of the Patient with an Open Neck Wound

Fundamental Principles of Care

An injury that has severed a major artery or vein of the neck will produce severe and often life-threatening bleeding. There are three critical elements to consider when caring for a neck wound. These are bleeding control, managing the patient's airway, and preventing air from entering the vessels of the neck. (Scan 33-1).

Steps to take when caring for a patient with an open neck wound include the following:

- Ensure an open airway.
- Place your gloved hand over the wound.
- Apply an occlusive dressing to the wound. The dressing should be a thick material that will not be sucked into the wound, and must extend 2 inches (5 cm) past the sides of the wound. Seal the dressing on all four sides.
- If time allows, place a dressing over the occlusive dressing.
- Apply pressure as needed to stop the bleeding. Consider using hemostatic agents to aid in hemorrhage control. Be careful not to compress both carotid arteries at once.
- Once bleeding has stopped, bandage the dressing in place. Take care not to restrict the airway or the arteries and veins of the neck.
- If the MOI could have caused cervical injury, immobilize the spine.

SCAN 33-1 Dressing an Open Neck Wound

First Take Standard Precautions.

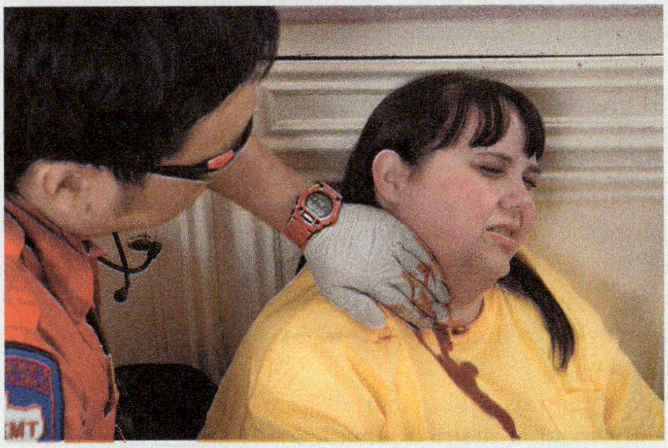

1. Do not delay! Place your gloved palm over the wound.

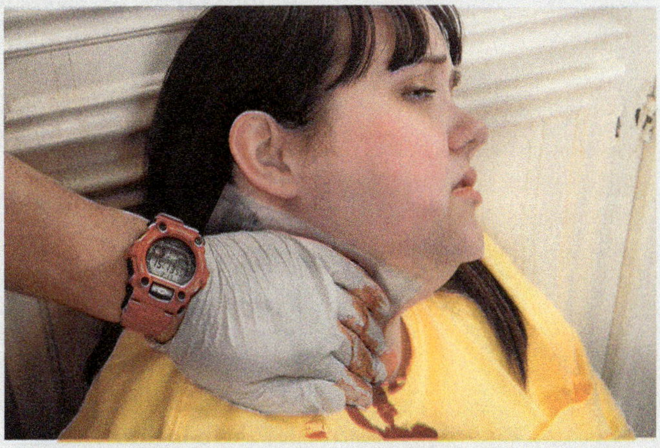

2. Place an occlusive dressing over the wound. It must be heavy plastic and sized to be 2 inches (5 cm) larger in diameter than the wound site. Continue to apply direct pressure to control the bleeding.

(continued)

SCAN 33-1 Dressing an Open Neck Wound *(continued)*

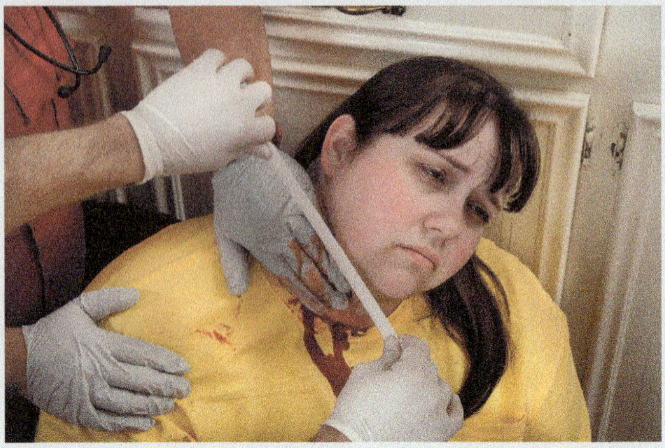

3. Seal the dressing with tape on all four sides.

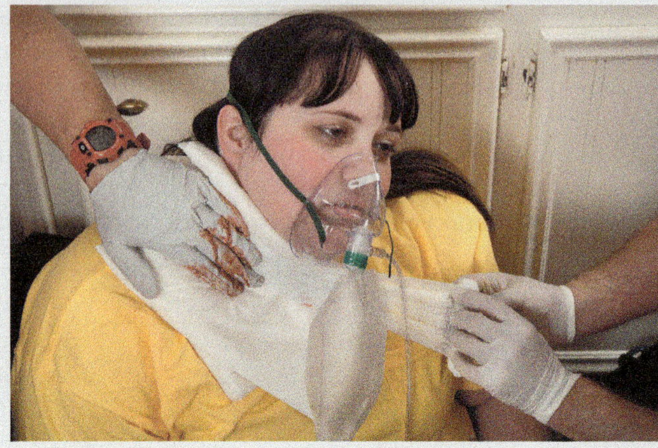

4. Cover the occlusive dressing with a large gauze dressing. Bring a bandage over the dressing, and wrap it in a figure-eight configuration, winding the bandage under the arm opposite the wound. Never wind the bandage around the patient's neck.

NOTE: *For demonstration purposes, the patient is upright. The patient would normally be in a supine position.*

Injuries to the Spine

CORE CONCEPT

Understanding spine injuries and assessment and emergency care for spine injuries

Injuries to the spinal column pose a unique challenge in terms of assessment and treatment. Although in many ways they are similar to any other musculoskeletal problem, the presence of the spinal cord running through the channel in the spinal column creates a special risk. When the bones, ligaments, and cartilage of the column are damaged, the spinal cord can be damaged as well. Although there are many examples of damage to vertebrae not resulting in injury to the spinal cord, this risk needs to be taken into consideration.

Specific injuries to the spinal column include fractures with and without bone displacement, dislocations, muscular strains, and disk injury, including compression. These injuries can occur without injury to the spinal cord, but when displaced fractures or dislocations occur, the cord, disk, and spinal nerves can be severely injured.

The spinal cord itself can be damaged in the same way that other tissue is damaged. It can be lacerated, contused, or impinged on. Injuries that occur immediately and as a result of direct force are called *primary injuries*. Unfortunately, primary injuries often lead to the irreversible outcomes we think of when we imagine spinal cord injuries. The nervous tissue of the spinal cord does not heal well, and when it is injured, interruption in nervous transmission tends to be permanent. Harm to the spinal cord can lead to ongoing loss of neurologic function, including paralysis. These potentially devastating consequences mean that injuries to the spine must be assessed and treated with specific care.

Secondary injuries to the spinal cord can be equally dangerous. These injuries occur after the initial insult but can cause the same or even more harm. It was once thought that secondary injuries were mostly the result of moving damaged bone ends into the spinal cord. In fact, there is very little evidence of this type of secondary problem. However, we know absolutely that hypoxia, shock, swelling of the cord, and even hypoglycemia can lead to devastating spinal cord damage.

Because of the risk of both primary and secondary injuries, your assessment must account for the possibility of spinal involvement in many traumatic injuries. This does not mean that every trauma patient has a spinal injury; in fact, there are relatively few. It does mean, however, that your assessment should evaluate specific physical findings in each patient to make appropriate decisions regarding the risk of potential spinal damage.

Injuries to the spine must be considered whenever there is serious trauma to any part of the body. Spine injury can be associated with head, neck, and back injuries—and with chest, abdominal, and pelvic injuries. Even injuries to the upper and lower extremities can be caused by forces intense enough to produce spine injury.

As an EMT, you will carefully evaluate the findings of your assessment and determine the relative need for spinal motion restriction. Unfortunately, there are no shortcuts, and good decisions are based on quality assessment.

Identifying Potential Spine and Spinal Cord Injuries

Spinal cord injuries have devastating consequences, and you should be vigilant for these types of injuries anytime you are assessing a trauma patient (Figure 33-18). Keep in mind, however, that there are roughly 6.2 million injuries to the head, neck, and back reported each year, but there are only about 12,000 new spinal cord injuries in that same time period. This means that many people injure the area around their spinal column without damaging their spinal cord. As an EMT, you must use patient assessment to identify high-risk patients and to make appropriate treatment decisions.

Identifying a potential spinal injury results from an assessment of the patient. This will be discussed later in the chapter. Mechanism is considered to identify the energy and forces that went into the injury—but in itself, it does not offer enough information to determine the presence of spinal injury. Reviewing these forces can help us identify scenarios where spinal injury may be *likely*. Mechanism of injury must be paired, however, with physical assessment. The mechanism alone is never enough to definitively identify an injury. You will use the mechanism to build suspicion, then confirm that suspicion through your physical assessment. (See Scan 33-2, Spinal Trauma Gallery.)

FIGURE 33-18 (A) Child with a facial injury in a cervical collar. (B) Child with facial abrasions and lacerations. *(Photo A: © David Effron, MD)*

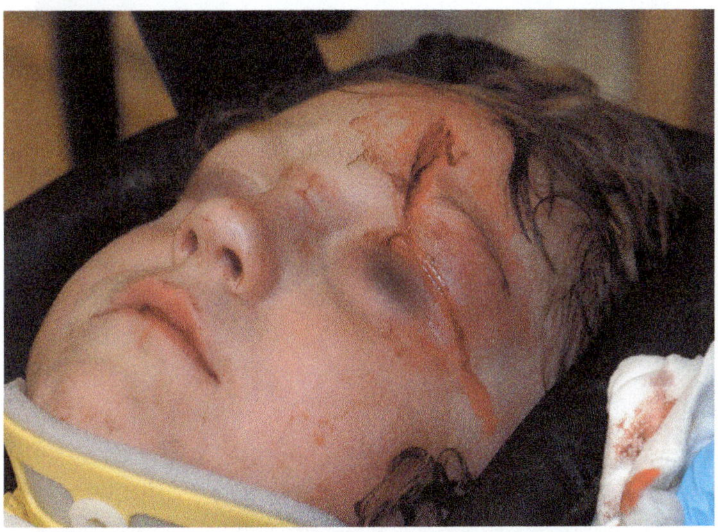

A

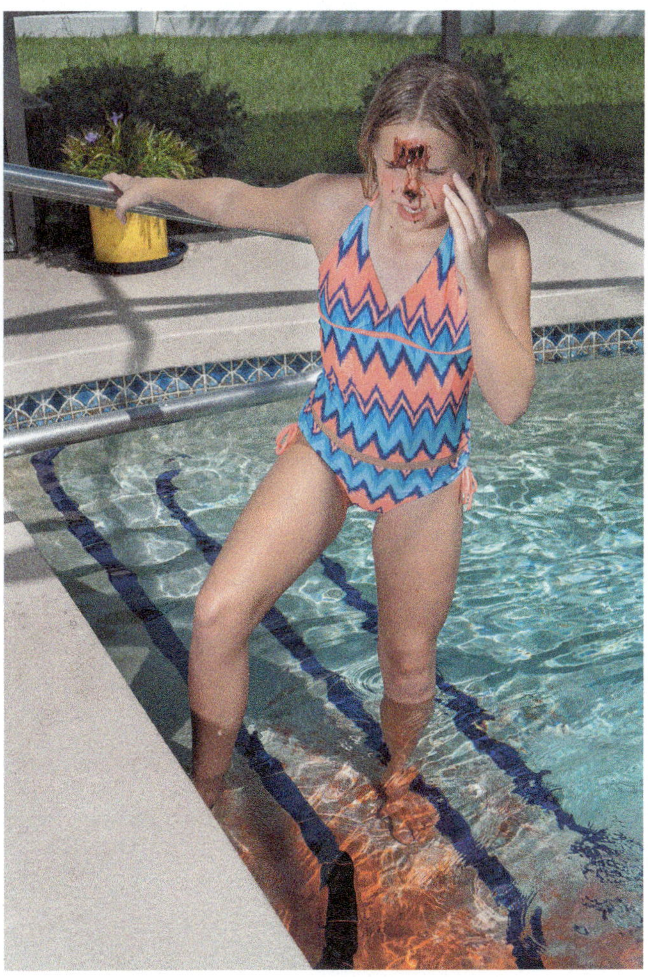

B

SCAN 33-2 Spinal Trauma Gallery

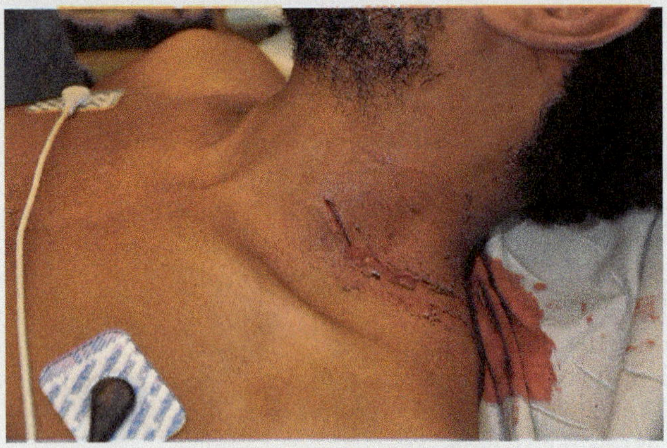

1. Penetrating trauma to the head or neck does not require spinal restriction unless neurologic signs or symptoms are present. Follow your local protocols. *(© Edward T. Dickinson, MD)*

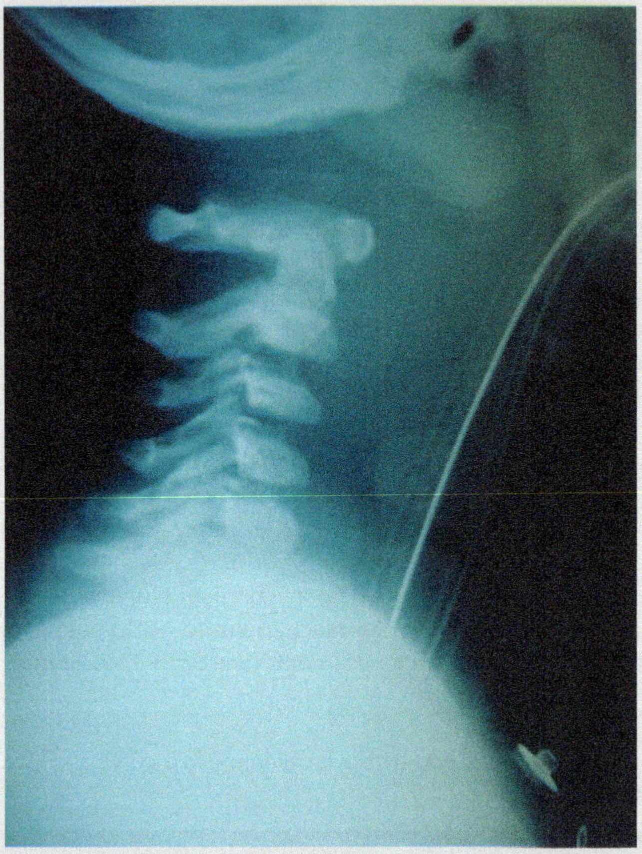

2. X-ray showing separation of the cervical spine from the skull of a child struck by the bumper of a car. *(© Edward T. Dickinson, MD).*

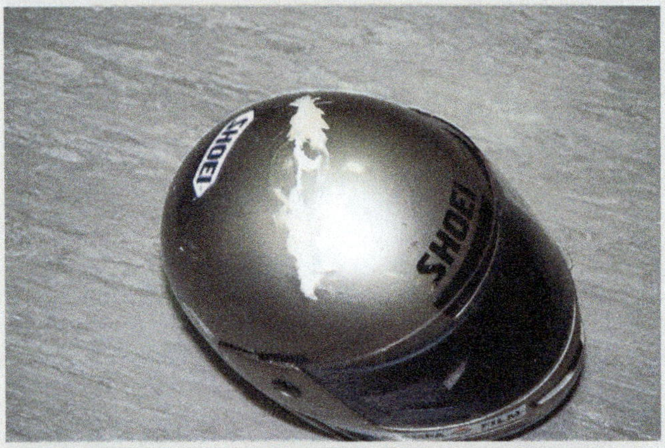

A

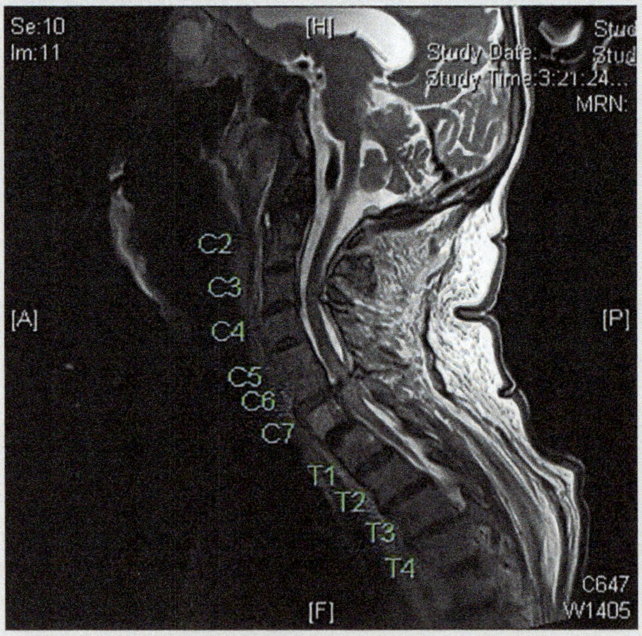

B

3. (A) Helmet from a motorcycle collision that caused cervical spine trauma. at the C6-C7 level. (B) MRI image showing cervical spine fracture and spinal cord damage at the C6-C7 level. *(Photo: © Edward T. Dickinson, MD)*

SCAN 33-2 Spinal Trauma Gallery *(continued)*

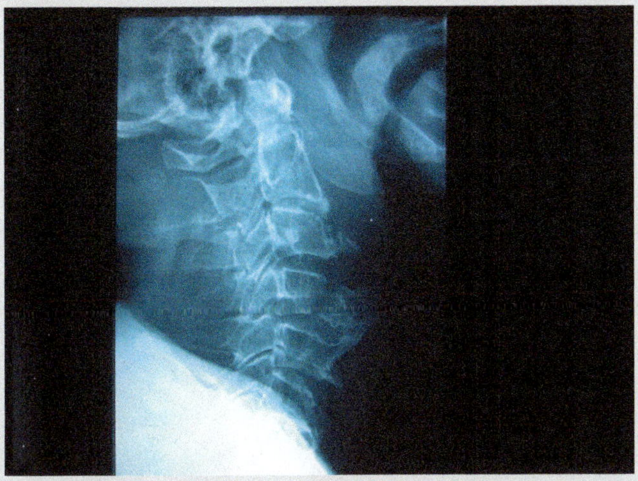

4. Cervical spine fractures in a geriatric patient. *(© Edward T. Dickinson, MD)*

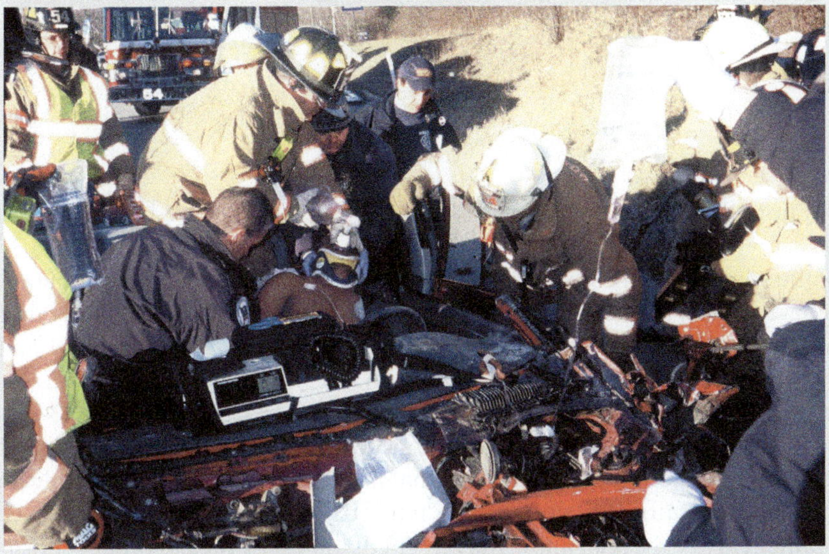

5. Critical patient with c-spine precautions in place during extrication from a high-energy motor-vehicle collision. *(© Edward T. Dickinson, MD)*

Mechanisms of Spine Injury

The spine is well protected, but the forces of trauma can sometimes overcome the defense mechanisms (Figure 33-19). In preparing to assess the likelihood of spinal cord injuries, it is helpful to think about the mechanisms by which the spinal column is injured.

The spine is most often injured by energy that forces movement of the spine beyond its normal range of motion. These movements can cause fracture and dislocation of the vertebrae or cause a disruption of the spinal canal by moving bone or bone fragments into the area where the spinal cord otherwise would be. Flexion and extension injuries are common. In these cases, the neck is either extended or flexed beyond its normal range of motion. This type of injury is very common in the cervical spine, as the heavy head exerts force on the relatively less protected neck. Whiplash injury is a common example of such a flexion and/or extension injury, and it occurs commonly in rear-end collisions that cause the head to accelerate/decelerate independently from the seatbelt-secured torso. The head is "whipped" forward or backward, causing abnormal motion in the neck (Figure 33-20). Sometimes the spine is over-rotated, as in a twisting sports injury, or excessively compressed (this is commonly referred to as *axial loading*), as in a shallow-water diving injury. When the spine is excessively pulled, it can cause a "distraction" injury. This mechanism of spine injury occurs in a hanging. Penetrating trauma can also cause destruction of vertebrae and damage to the spinal cord. Spinal injuries in EMS workers

FIGURE 33-19 Mechanisms that may cause spine injury.

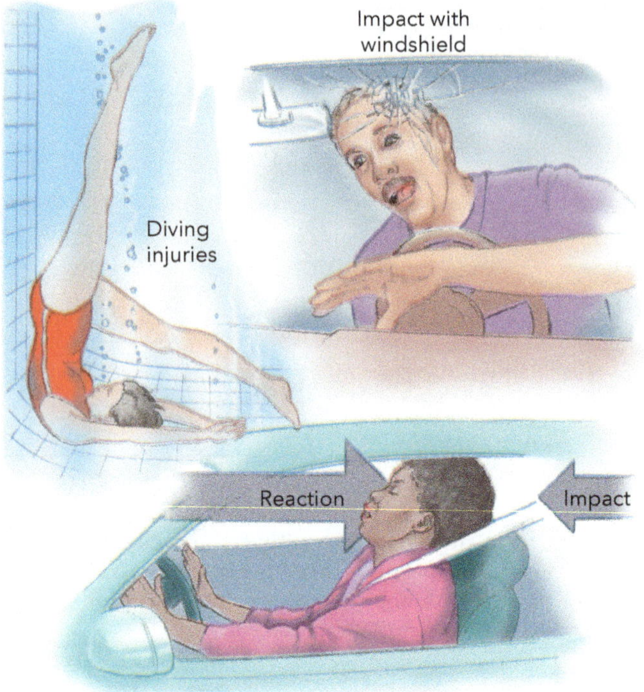

FIGURE 33-20 Usually whiplash is caused by a poorly adjusted or absent headrest during a rear-end collision.

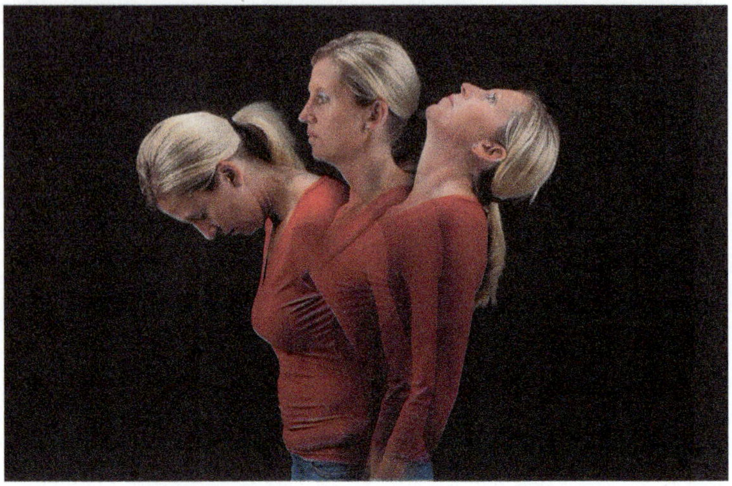

often result from not adhering to the proper lifting techniques, causing lateral bending or disk injuries.

Some parts of the spine are more susceptible to injury than others. Because it is somewhat splinted by the attached ribs, the thoracic spine is typically well protected against all but the most violent collisions and penetrating trauma. The pelvic–sacral spine attachment helps to protect the sacrum in the same way. However, the cervical and lumbar vertebrae are susceptible to injury because they are not supported by other bony structures (Figure 33-21).

Certain medical conditions also make the spine more vulnerable to injury. Many geriatric patients suffer from osteoporosis, a disease that causes bones to become brittle and weak. This condition can cause the spine to be injured with much less force. Certain patients have ligament laxity that can allow movement of the vertebrae beyond the normal range. This is common in pregnant women and in patients with Down syndrome. Other patients have conditions where the spine cannot move the way it normally would. Patients with fused vertebrae or fixed flexion deformities are at higher risk of injury. A condition called *ankylosing spondylitis* causes the vertebrae of the spine to essentially fuse together, creating great vulnerability of the spine to injury.

FIGURE 33-21 Various parts of the spine are vulnerable to injury. Running with the bulls may be one of the less common ways of injuring your spine. *(Kevin Link/Science Source)*

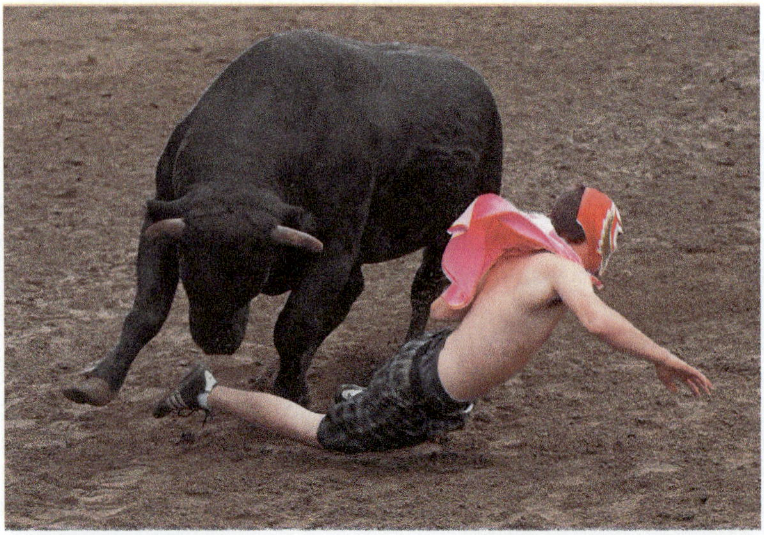

Certain mechanisms of injury (MOI) are associated with a high risk for spinal injury. These mechanisms of injury result in a higher proportion of spinal injuries than do others. Although they do not definitively predict injury, it is useful to have an even higher index of suspicion when they are present. These high-risk mechanisms include:

- Falls from higher than 3 feet (1 meter) or down more than five stairs
- Axial loading (compression) injuries, such as those that occur in diving injuries
- High-speed motor-vehicle crashes, especially with rollover or ejection of the patient
- Motorized recreational vehicle (ATV) crashes
- Bicycle collisions

Maintain a high degree of suspicion for a potential spine injury when your patient is a victim of a motor-vehicle or motorcycle collision, was struck by a vehicle, received blunt injury to the spine or above the clavicles, was involved in a diving incident, was found hanging by the neck, or was found unconscious from trauma. Geriatric patients may experience more severe injuries than would a younger patient with the same MOI.

As previously noted, diving incidents often produce injury to the cervical spine. When the diver strikes the diving board, the side or bottom of the pool, or an underwater object, the head can be severely forced beyond its normal limits of motion (flexion or extension), or be compressed. Cervical vertebrae may be fractured or dislocated, ligaments may be severely sprained, and the spinal cord may be damaged.

Just as there are high-risk mechanisms of injury, there are also low-risk mechanisms of injury. These are assessed using common sense. Generally speaking, low-energy mechanisms pose low threats of spinal injury. There are also, however, high-energy mechanisms that pose a low threat for spinal injury. Penetrating trauma, for example, was once thought to be a high-risk mechanism. However, research has proven this not to be the case. Today we can say that unless the penetrating trauma was to the spine itself, and unless it caused an immediate neurologic deficit, there is little risk in terms of spinal injury.

It is important to remember that many other mechanisms of injury, some obvious and some subtle, can cause spinal injuries. You should always use clinical judgment and evaluate the scene for clues that such injuries may have occurred. Consider also how underlying factors such as preexisting conditions could make otherwise minor mechanisms into very real threats. For example, a fall from a standing position is not a very significant MOI when considering a healthy adult, but it could be far more meaningful in a geriatric patient with a history of osteoporosis.

Physical Assessment for Spine and Spinal Cord Injuries

Mechanism alone does not identify injury. Although your scene assessment can help provide reasonable suspicion, spinal injuries are identified by physical examination. Your assessment, especially in times of high-risk MOI, should specifically look for the physical indicators of spinal injury. You may believe that you will always identify spinal injury from significant signs like paralysis. This is actually relatively rare. Sometimes the findings can be subtle or delayed and require a detailed physical examination to find. It helps to remember that most orthopedic injuries cause pain and tenderness in the area that has been injured. Therefore, pain and tenderness, particularly in the area of the spine, will be important findings.

Spinal assessment has been discussed in the chapter *Secondary Assessment*, and the components will be reviewed here. The flow chart (Figure 33-22) details the components of the spinal assessment. It is important to make assessments of each of the areas as well as assessments required by local protocols to make your decision on spinal motion restriction.

Relating Spinal Function to Injury

While a specific spinal assessment has been outlined, it is also helpful to relate the function of the spinal cord to what may be seen in specific injuries.

The spinal cord is a relay between most of the body and the brain. A large number of the messages to and from the brain are sent through the spinal cord. Therefore, damage

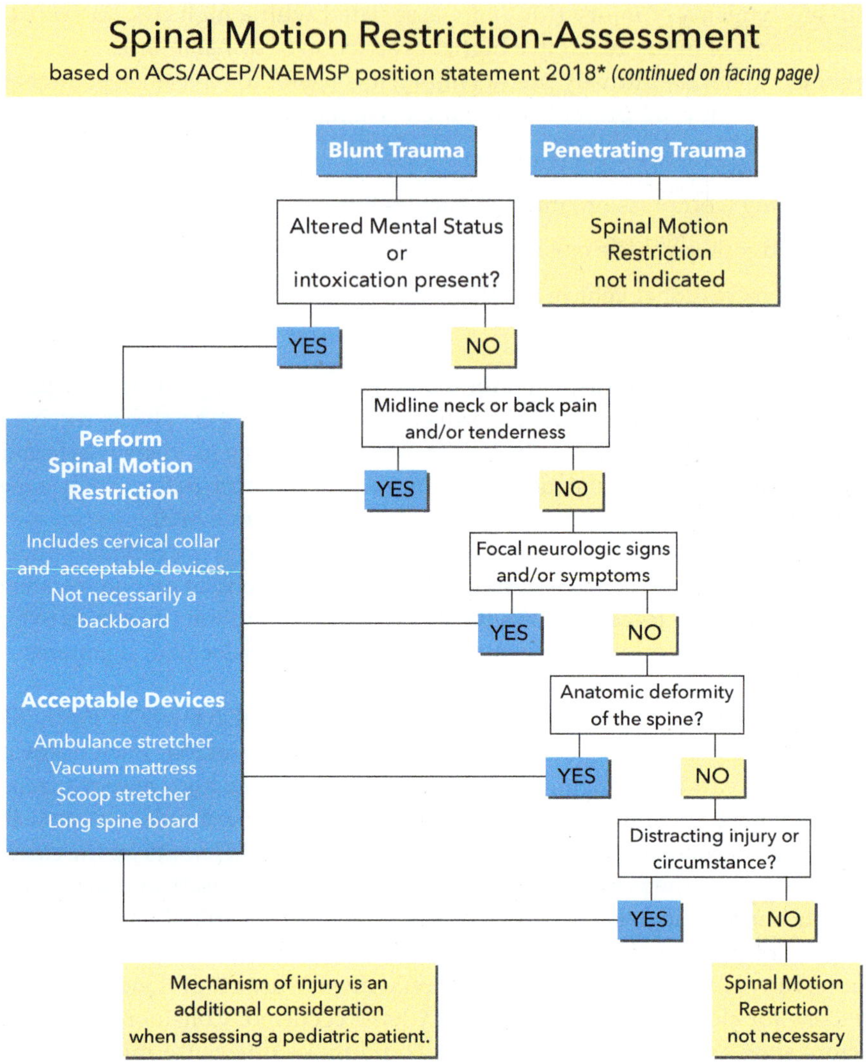

FIGURE 33-22 Flow chart for assessment for spinal restriction.

to the cord can isolate a part of the body from the brain, resulting in loss of function of this region—possibly forever.

dermatome (DERM-uh-tohm) an area of the skin that is innervated by a single spinal nerve.

A ***dermatome*** is an area of the body surface that is innervated by a single spinal nerve. Dermatomes can be used to identify loss of function that is associated with a particular area of the spinal cord. Sensation at the nipple level is considered to align with T4, while sensation at the umbilicus is T10. (Figure 33-23 provides an idea of how nerves that originate from the spine innervate specific parts of the body.)

The following are additional key indicators of spinal injury:

- **Paralysis of the extremities.** Paralysis of the extremities may occur. *Paralysis of the extremities is probably the most reliable sign of spinal cord injury in conscious patients.*
- **Changes in neurologic function.** These changes can include loss of sensation (as in paralysis) or loss of motor function. They might also include unusual sensations such as paresthesia, or "pins and needles." Remember that these findings might be different in upper versus lower extremities.
- **Pain with movement.** The patient normally tries to lie perfectly still to prevent pain. However, do not ask the patient to move just to determine if it will cause pain. If the patient experiences pain in the neck or back with voluntary movements, including spinal pain with movement in apparently uninjured shoulders and legs, this is a good indicator of possible spinal injury.

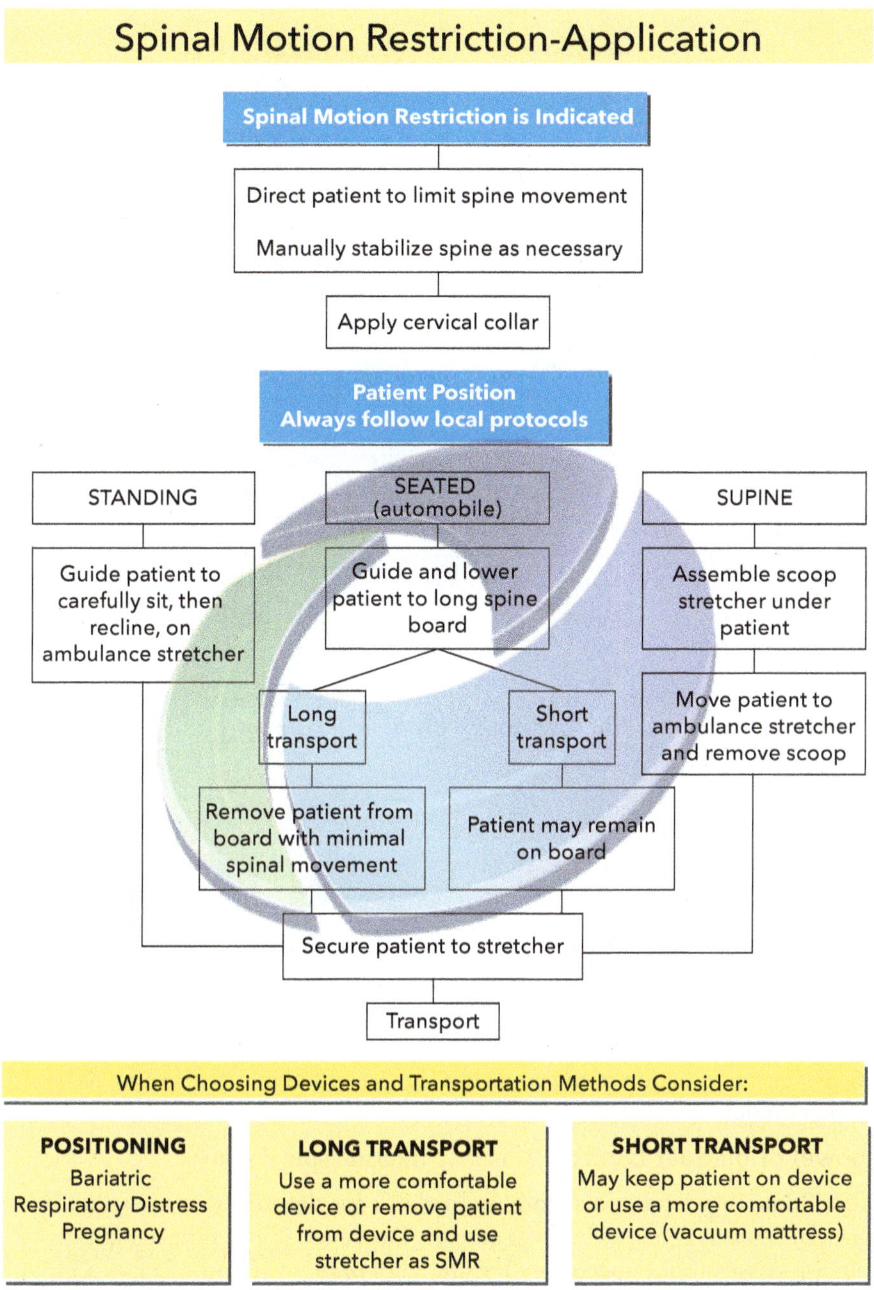

FIGURE 33-22 *(continued)*

- **Tenderness anywhere along the midline spine.** Gentle palpation of the injury site, when accessible, may reveal point tenderness.
- **Impaired breathing.** Watch the patient breathe. If there is only a slight movement of the abdomen, with little or no movement of the chest, it is safe to assume that the patient is breathing with the diaphragm alone (diaphragmatic breathing). This is also true if there is a reversal of normal breathing patterns, with the rib cage collapsing on inspiration and rising on expiration. Damage to the nerves that control the movement of the rib cage can cause this breathing pattern. The nerves that control the diaphragm are located high in the cervical area (the third, fourth, and fifth cervical nerves) and are often unharmed, but the intercostal (between the ribs) nerves that control the chest muscles are often damaged in cervical and thoracic injuries. As a result, when the diaphragm moves downward to pull in air, the ribs, instead of expanding, collapse. When the diaphragm relaxes and air is expelled, the rib cage rises—which is the opposite of the normal pattern. Impaired breathing is characteristic of spinal cord injury. Check abdominal movement from the side by placing your hand on the patient's abdomen and looking for reversed movements during respiration. Panting due to respiratory insufficiency may develop.

FIGURE 33-23 Dermatomes are areas of the skin that are innervated by various segments of the spinal cord. Those labeled "C" are innervated by levels of the cervical spine; "T," the thoracic spine; "L," the lumbar spine; and "S," the sacral spine.

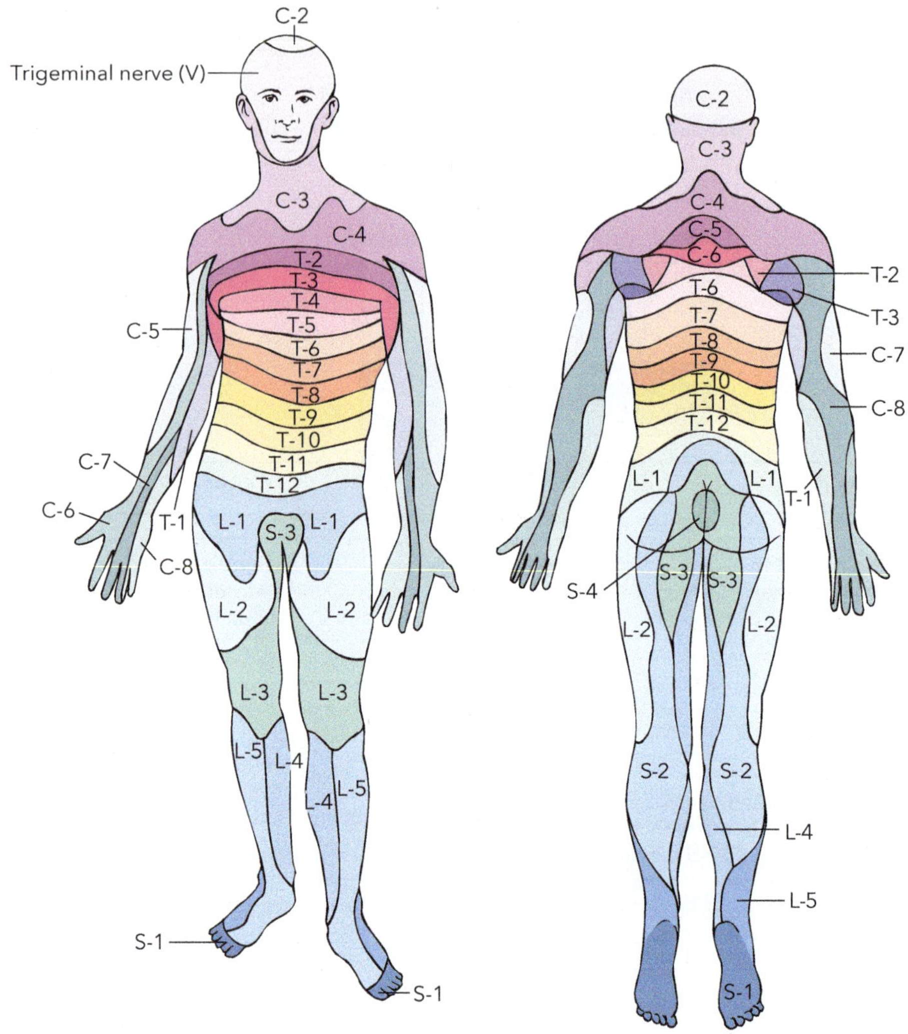

- **Priapism.** Persistent erection of the penis is a sign of spinal injury affecting nerves to the external genitalia.
- **Loss of bowel or bladder control.** This may indicate spinal injury.
- **Deformity.** Removing a patient's clothing to check for deformity of the spine is not recommended. *Obvious spinal deformities are rare.* However, if you note a gap between the spinous processes (bony extensions) of the vertebrae, or if you can feel a broken spinous process, you must consider the patient to have serious spinal injuries. It is also possible to feel tight muscles in spasm.
- **Neurogenic shock.** ***Neurogenic shock*** can be caused by the failure of the nervous system to control the diameter of blood vessels. The pulse rate may be normal—or even slow in the setting of a low or falling blood pressure—because a message to "speed up" the heart may be prevented from getting to the heart due to the cord injury. The patient's skin in neurogenic shock may be flushed and warm because of dilation of the blood vessels. (Other types of shock usually involve constriction of the blood vessels with resulting pale, cool, and clammy skin.)

neurogenic shock
a state of shock (hypoperfusion) caused by nerve paralysis that sometimes develops from spinal cord injuries.

These signs and symptoms are reliable indicators of possible spinal injury in the conscious patient. If any one of them is present, you have sufficient reason to suspect spinal injury.

Patient Assessment

Assessment of the Spine

Physician groups such as the American College of Surgeons, the American College of Emergency Physicians, and National Association of EMS Physicians have issued several position papers about spinal assessment–and how that spinal assessment is related to a need to restrict motion of the spine. Many of these position papers have their roots in the National Emergency X-Radiography Utilization Study (NEXUS). This study was published in 1998 and was designed to provide a validated assessment tool for physicians to use to make decisions about the need for spinal X-rays in the emergency department. What it also did, as a secondary benefit, was provide an evidence-based framework for assigning risk of spinal injury.

This spinal assessment method has been rolled out to the field with the following components:

- Is the patient reliable? Can the patient be depended upon to relay to you accurate information about personal injuries? The two most common reasons a patient may be unreliable are acute changes in mental status and intoxication with alcohol or drugs.
- Does the patient have any pain or tenderness anywhere along the spine? You must palpate the entire length of the spine for this pain or tenderness.
- Does the patient have any focal neurologic signs or symptoms? Does the patient have equal grip strength? Does the patient have any paralysis, numbness, or other signs of spinal injury as noted earlier in the chapter?
- Does the patient have a distracting injury or circumstance? Distracting injuries are painful or grotesque injuries that could distract the patient from recognizing spinal pain or tenderness. The most common of these are painful musculoskeletal injuries. Circumstances that may distract patients include fear or panic, as in situations in which a spouse or child is also injured, causing the patient to focus more on the other person's care.
- In pediatric patients, closer attention is paid to the MOI because younger children may not be able to reliably relate or describe feelings of pain on other portions of the examination. Thus, the MOI must play a greater part in decision making for spinal motion restriction in children. In addition, because the relatively soft vertebrae in the pediatric neck are less prone to fracture than are adults', children can suffer significant spinal cord injuries without the expected external findings of tenderness or deformity.

The NEXUS study reviewed more than 34,000 patients and showed that when the protocol was used appropriately, it had a 99.6 percent sensitivity to finding serious spinal injury. These results have been further reinforced by subsequent studies, such as the Canadian Cervical Spine Rule–which used similar criteria–and have been successfully deployed in a number of EMS systems without incident. It is reasonable, then, to use these best practices to formalize spinal assessment. See Scan 33-3 regarding spinal assessment.

SCAN 33-3 Selective Spinal Immobilization Assessment

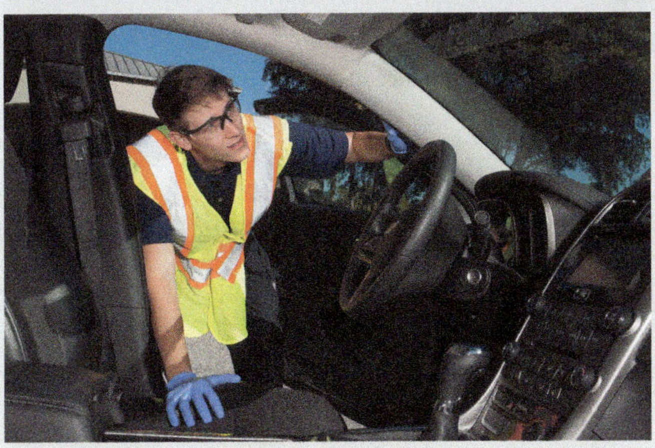

1. First take Standard Precautions. Assess the mechanisms of injury.

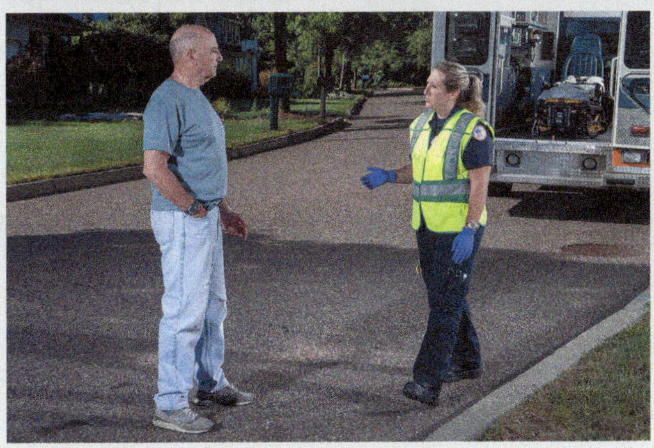

2. Assess mental status. Take cervical spine precautions if spinal injury is likely.

(continued)

SCAN 33-3 Selective Spinal Immobilization Assessment *(continued)*

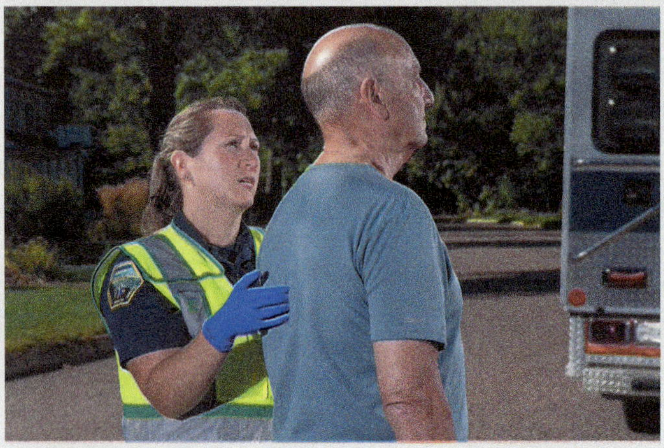

3. Assess midline spinal tenderness.

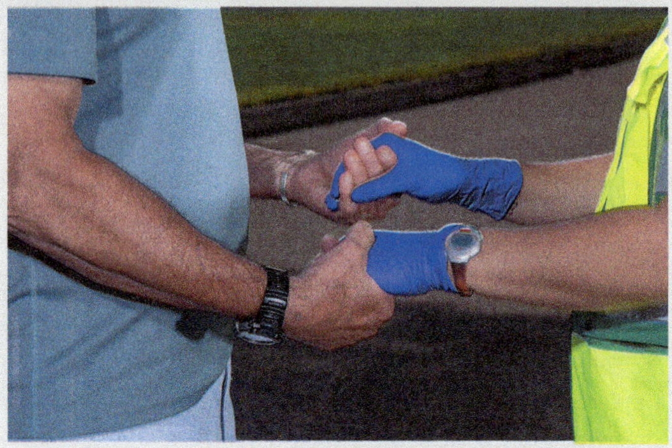

4. Assess for neurologic deficits—for example, by testing grip strength.

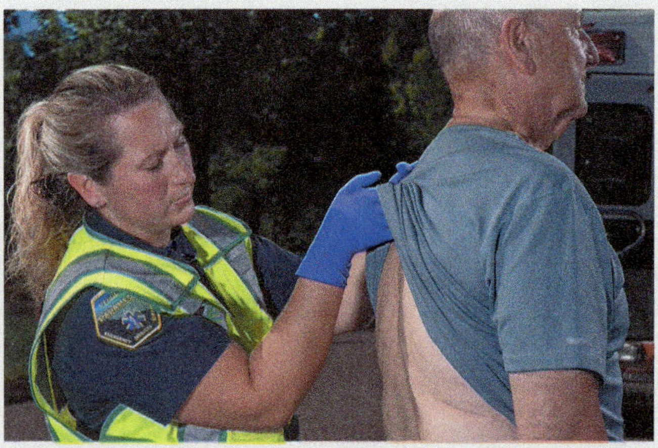

5. Inspection of the back for deformity, swelling, bruising or wounds.

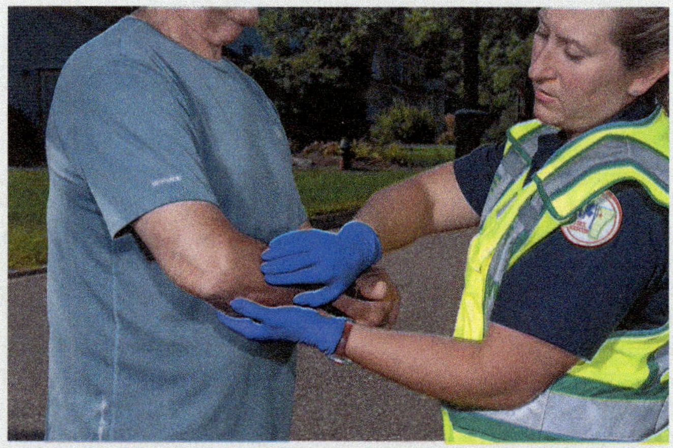

6. Assess distracting injuries, such as arm or rib cage injuries.

Geriatric Note

Keep in mind that fractured spines in the elderly are often caused by falls or by spontaneous fractures of brittle bones that, in turn, cause falls.

Decision Point

Has a spine injury affected the efficiency or function of the respiratory system or circulatory system? How can I support these vital functions?

Your spinal assessment has determined that your patient is a candidate for spinal motion restriction. The following section highlights various options for preventing movement of the spine.

The Evolution of Spinal Care

The origins of spinal care are rooted in a concept called *spinal immobilization*. Practically all trauma patients were assumed to have spinal injuries and were cared for based on MOI alone. Even low-risk patients were affixed to rigid spine boards and transported in very uncomfortable circumstances. Modern spinal care has adapted to place faith in the EMT's assessment. Patients are selected for spinal care through thoughtful assessment and good clinical decision making. We now realize that there can be harmful side effects of rigid spinal immobilization. For example, making patients with lung injuries lie flat creates a situation that is not only uncomfortable but also potentially deadly. Furthermore, we now recognize that even routine immobilization has consequences that must be addressed. Even a short time spent on rigid spine boards can cause hypothermia and pressure sores to soft tissue. What has evolved is a deliberate thought process that must weigh the value of spinal motion restriction against the potential risk.

It was once thought that the most important care for a patient with a spinal injury was to restrict movement and prevent broken bone ends from doing further damage to vulnerable spinal cord tissue. Although this is still theoretically true, we now know there are equally important treatment goals. Although broken bone ends need to be accounted for, we know that far more often, secondary injury is caused not by jagged bone but by hypoxia, shock, or hypoglycemia.

In this section, you will learn the details of spinal motion restriction, but you should consider airway, breathing, and hemorrhage control as important as any of the other steps that will be discussed. For any patient with a spinal injury, you must aggressively ensure oxygenation and normal ventilation. You should actively treat severe bleeding, and you should, if you have the capability, pay attention to blood glucose levels. Your primary assessment is intended not only to identify the potential for spinal injury but also to identify immediate interventions in the interest of preventing hypoxia and treating shock. Treating these concerns should be considered the same priority as spinal motion restriction.

In addition to preventing secondary injuries by managing the A-B-Cs, you should also consider the possibility of those broken bone ends. Although it is unclear how much of a risk is posed, a lack of evidence means that we should err on the side of caution and protect against such injuries until better research tells us otherwise. Because the spine is made up of 33 interconnected bones, the best way to prevent movement of an unstable vertebra is to limit movement of the entire spine. This concept is called ***spinal motion restriction*** and is the basic principle of prehospital spinal injury care.

spinal (SPI-nal) ***motion restriction***
limiting the movement of the spine to prevent additional injury.

It is now understood that there are different ways to restrict movement of the spine properly. In this section, we will review a variety of choices. However, these choices all have similar characteristics that you should keep in mind regardless of the method you choose.

Spinal motion restriction is designed to limit the movement of individual vertebrae to prevent their movement from causing secondary damage to the spinal cord. Because all of the vertebrae are interconnected, you should stabilize not just one section of the spine but rather all sections together.

Movement of the spine generally follows the largest areas of mass in the body—that is, when heavy things move, the spine moves with them. The three centers of mass in the body are the head, the shoulder girdle, and the pelvis. When these areas are prevented from moving, the spine generally remains stable.

Remember also that the spine is not aligned along a straight line. Rather, its natural anatomic position is an S-shaped curve. Spinal motion restriction uses the idea of *inline, neutral position*, which means that the vertebrae are kept in a position of function that best represents their natural anatomic position. Natural curvature should be taken into account.

Finally, there is no way to prevent absolutely any movement of the spine. In most cases, the patient will be limiting movement because it hurts to move. In the best-case situations, your efforts will reinforce the protective steps the patient is already taking.

For patients you have determined are at risk for spinal injury, and for all trauma victims when there is the possibility of spinal injury, spinal motion restriction is used to prevent further injury.

Spinal Motion Restriction—The Cervical Spine

The average head weighs 17 pounds (approximately 8 kg), and the neck is relatively poorly supported by muscles and other anatomy. As a result, the head and neck tend to move independently from the rest of the body. In spinal motion restriction, the objective is to keep the spine immobilized in an inline, neutral position. To achieve this, the head and neck must be managed by stabilization at the outset of patient care.

Manual stabilization of the head is one of the first steps of spinal motion restriction. You can begin by instructing the patient to focus on a point and use that focus to help limit head movement. You should physically restrict head movement by placing your hands on either side of the patient's head. Gentle guidance should be used to stop movement and to keep the cervical spine in an inline neutral position. If the cervical spine is found to be out of natural anatomic position (such as in a flexed position), you can attempt to return it to a neutral position unless the patient complains of pain or the head is not easily moved into that position. If that is the case, steady the head in the position in which it was found. Maintain manual stabilization until the assessment is complete or until further spinal precautions are taken.

Rigid cervical collars, or extrication collars, are frequently used to aid in the spinal motion restriction of the cervical spine. A collar is a device that wraps around the neck and provides rigid form to help prevent movement. Collars must be properly sized. A wrong-sized collar may do more harm than good by hyperextending the neck if it is too large or allowing flexion if it is too small. Also, the collar must not be applied in a way that will obstruct the airway. Maintain manual stabilization even after the collar is in place until the patient is secured to a backboard.

Once cervical spinal movement is restricted, it is important to establish a baseline for sensory, motor, and circulatory function in four extremities. This quick assessment allows you to identify existing deficits and to compare those findings after further steps in spinal motion restriction are achieved.

Spinal Motion Restriction Devices

Once the cervical spine has been immobilized, the remainder of the spinal column's motion needs to be restricted. As noted, rigid, long spine boards were commonly used to accomplish this goal; however, we are now realizing that there are many additional ways to accomplish similar spinal motion restriction. More modern methods are being adopted as evidence is examined. In their 2013 position paper and subsequent papers on EMS spinal precautions and use of the long backboard, the National Association of EMS Physicians and the American College of Surgeons stated that although backboards remain useful for extrication and for movement of patients, the ambulance stretcher is, in effect, a padded backboard and, in combination with a cervical collar and straps to secure the patient in a supine position, provides appropriate spinal protection for patients with spinal injury. Perhaps the key concept to understand is that there are many methods that can accomplish the goal of spinal motion restriction.

The orthopedic stretcher and vacuum mattresses are also devices that are acceptable to use for restricting spinal motion and patient movement.

Rigid Spine Board. The rigid spine board, a mainstay of spinal care for generations of EMS providers, has been significantly limited today because the spine board can cause significant pain and discomfort, pressure sores, and respiratory compromise. After a long transport to the hospital, it is sometimes difficult to assess what pain has been caused by the backboard and what pain has been caused by the injury itself.

However, there are still uses for the long spine board. In many cases, it is used to transport the patient from a scene or vehicle to the ambulance stretcher. The patient is then removed from the spine board, and the stretcher itself is used for spinal motion restriction, Consider the following when deciding on use of the long spine board:

- How long is the transport time to the hospital? If the time is short, you might decide to keep the patient on the spine board. Longer trips will cause pain and discomfort, and the spine board will generally not be used.
- Is the board necessary as a "big splint" because of multiple traumatic injuries that the spine board would support?
- Is the patient likely to require resuscitation, making the board necessary for effective CPR compressions?
- Are there clinical needs of the patient that would be affected by the board? This may be true of a patient who is in respiratory distress or a bariatric patient who will have difficulty breathing when lying flat. In these cases, a spine board would not be used.
- Would removing the patient from the spine board cause excessive movement? In this case, the patient may remain on the spine board for transport.

"It's great we don't use backboards as much as we used to. But now the spinal assessment and the decisions we make are really, really important."

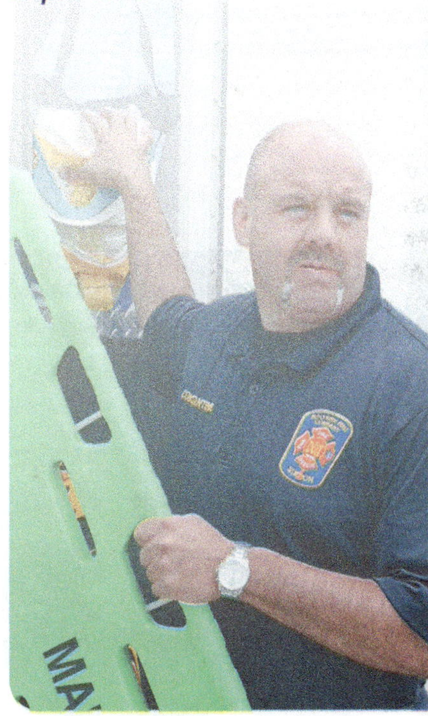

Scoop Stretcher. The scoop, or orthopedic, stretcher has a role in care of the patient with suspected spinal injuries. Since this device may be split and inserted under the patient with minimal movement, it is helpful when patients with potential spine injuries must be lifted from the floor to a stretcher. The scoop is easily removed once the patient has been placed on the ambulance stretcher.

Vacuum Mattresses. Vacuum mattresses also have a role in spinal motion restriction. These devices are essentially hollow bags that allow the air to be pumped out of them to create a rigid form. The benefit of these devices is that they can accomplish many of the objectives of a rigid spine board while conforming better to the patient's natural anatomic position. As a result, they tend to be more comfortable than rigid spine boards. Vacuum mattresses also have some disadvantages. They can leak, and thus they can lose their rigidity over time. Although they tend to be warmer than hard plastic spine boards, they also rob heat from the patient.

Scans 33-4 through 33-9 demonstrate the proper procedures to use based on the condition and position in which a patient is found.

Following the application of any spinal motion restriction device, you should reassess sensory and motor function in all four extremities if the patient is responsive. This assessment allows you to identify changes in neurologic function and compare function with the baseline assessment that was conducted before applying the device.

NOTE: *Do not spend much time trying to rule out spinal injury in an unresponsive patient. If there is a MOI associated with spinal injury, initiate spinal motion restriction immediately and treat as if there is a spinal injury.*

Spinal Motion Restriction Decision Making

CORE CONCEPT
Understanding spinal motion restriction issues and how to immobilize various types of patients with potential spine injury

Patients who may have been subject to spinal injury are, of course, found in different positions. Some are seated inside a crashed vehicle. Some are lying on the ground. Some are standing or walking around. In some instances, the patient may be found wearing a helmet that may or may not need to be removed. Before reading the following sections that deal with these specific situations, review the information on manual stabilization in the *Primary Assessment* chapter and on cervical-collar sizing and application in the *Secondary Assessment* chapter.

While the concept of spinal motion restriction has been around for some time, you will still notice some contradictions. For example, at the time of publication of this text, the National Registry of EMTs still tests certain spinal skills that are not often used in practice. Seated spinal immobilization using a vest-type extrication device is no longer recommended in the field. However, because it is still tested as a skill on the exam, it is included in this text.

Pediatric Note

For an infant or child, be sure to use a pediatric-sized collar. If you do not have the right pediatric size, use a rolled towel, maintaining manual support of the infant's or child's head.

Spinal Motion Restriction in a Seated Patient

When a patient is found in a sitting position, there are two basic options for maintaining spinal motion restriction. One is to place a long spine board under the patient's buttocks and then carefully lower the patient to the board in a supine position. The spine board is then used to transport the patient to the stretcher (where the spine board is often removed). The other possibility used in some systems is to have the patient self-extricate by standing and then sitting on the ambulance stretcher. Some believe that this is acceptable if the patient has been ambulatory after the injury and prior to your arrival. It may cause less stress on the spine than manipulating the patient to the spine board, from which the patient will have to be removed anyway. This technique would not be used if the patient complained of pain

SCAN 33-4 Applying a Vest-Type Extrication Device

First Take Standard Precautions.

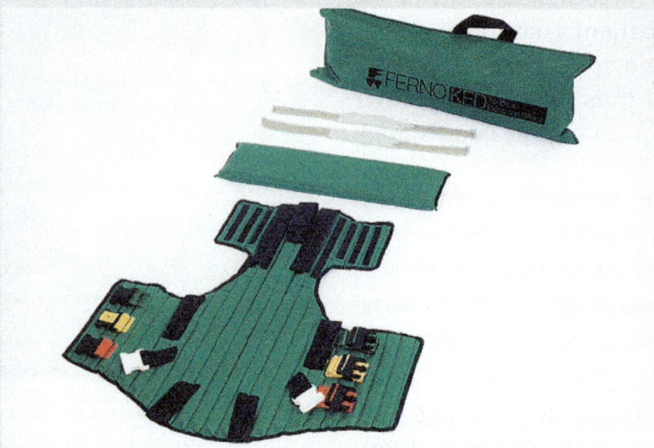

1. Select an appropriate spinal motion restriction device.

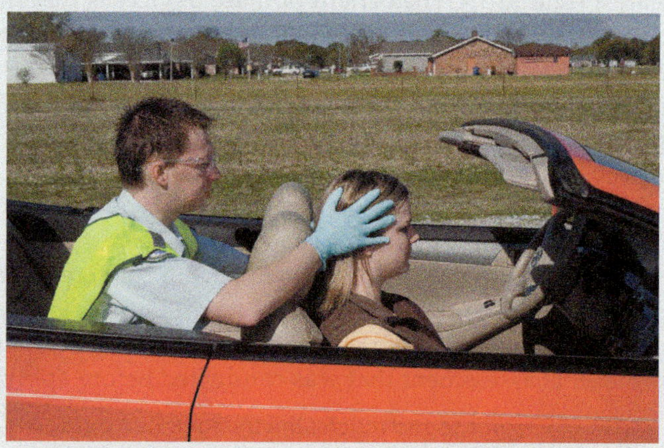

2. Manually stabilize the patient's head in a neutral, inline position.

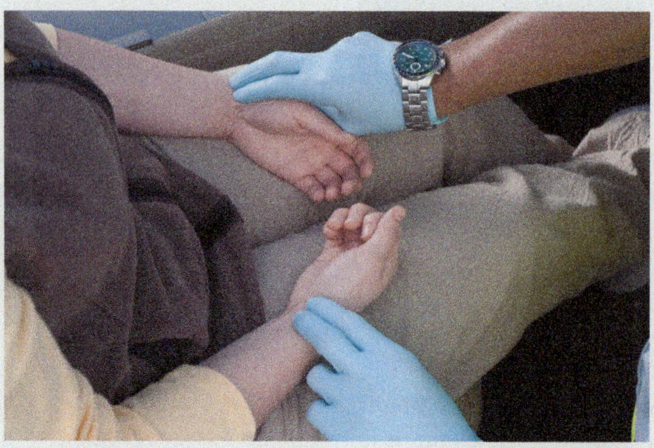

3. Assess distal circulation, sensation, and motor function (CSM).

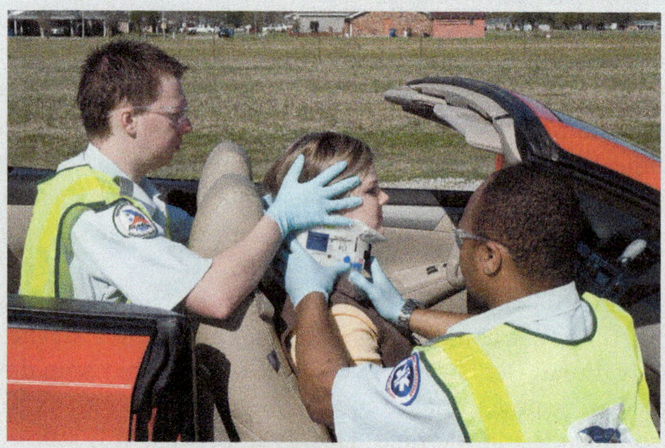

4. Apply the appropriately sized extrication collar.

SCAN 33-4 Applying a Vest-Type Extrication Device *(continued)*

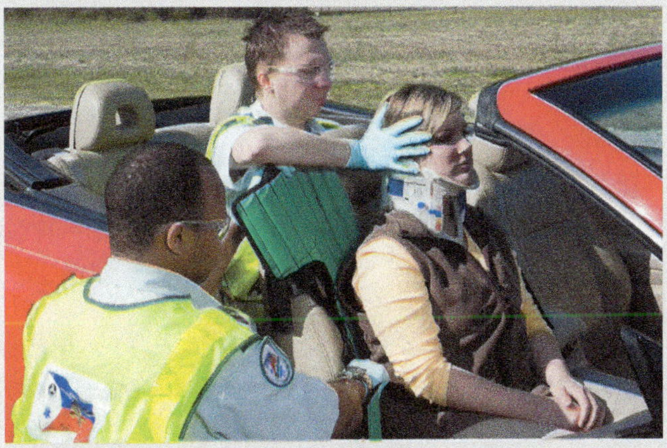

5. Position the immobilization device behind the patient.

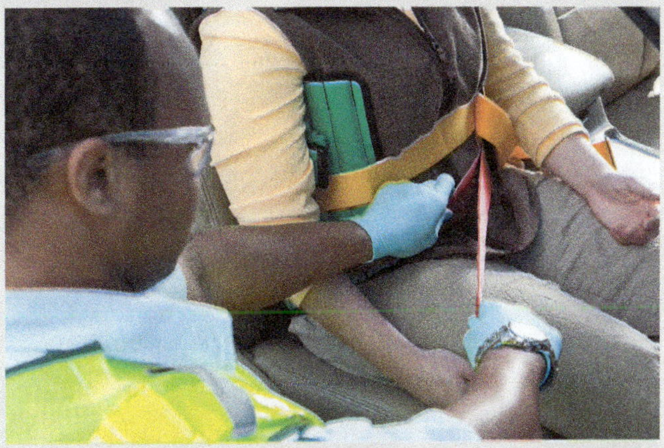

6. Secure the device to the patient's torso.

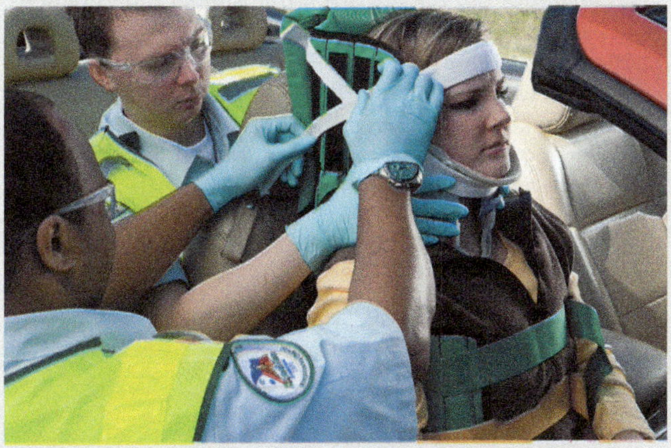

7. Evaluate and pad behind the patient's head as necessary. Secure the patient's head to the device.

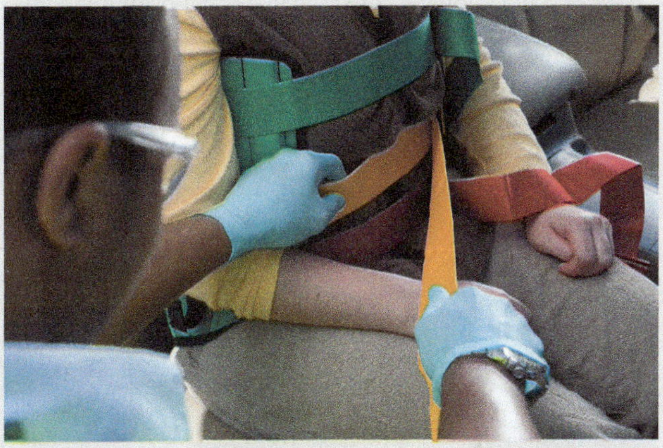

8. Evaluate and adjust the straps to be tight enough so the device does not move up, down, left, or right excessively, but not so tight as to restrict the patient's breathing.

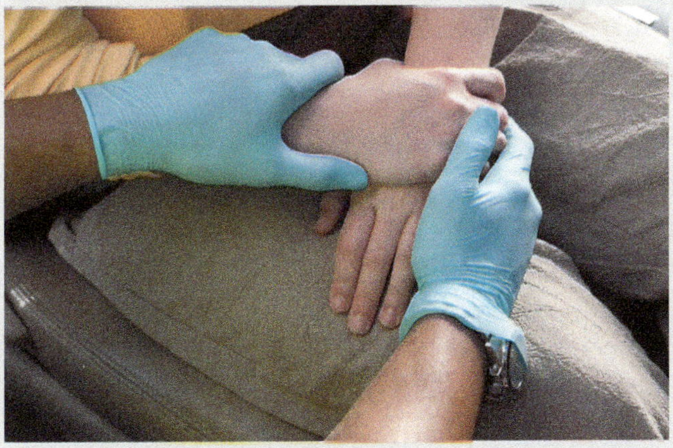

9. As needed, position or secure the patient's wrists and legs.

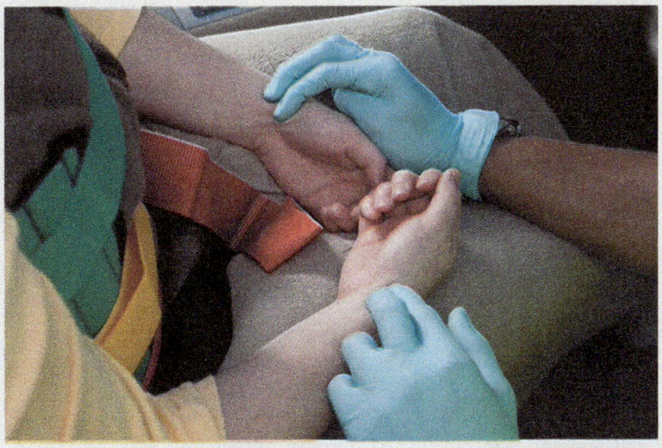

10. Reassess distal CSM, and transfer the patient to the long board.

NOTE: *Most EMS systems no longer use vest-type extrication devices, but it may be on your skills exam, so it is shown in the text. Follow your local protocols. In the photos, the roof of the vehicle has been removed to allow for easier illustration of the positions of the EMTs.*

SCAN 33-5 Extrication Procedures

Sitting Patient Extrication

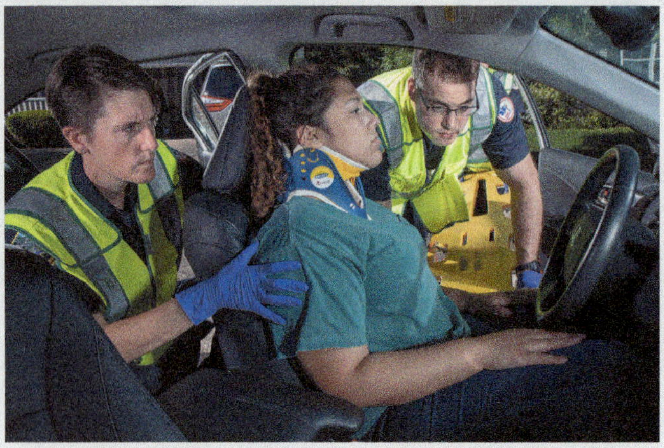

1. Manually stabilize the patient's head and neck. Have a second EMT apply a cervical collar and position the long board.

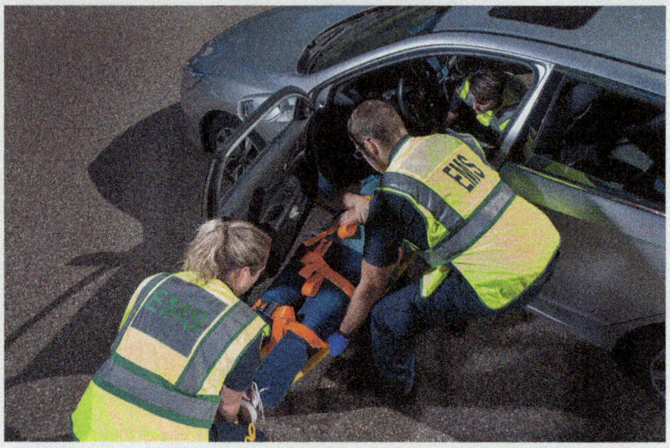

2. At the direction of the EMT holding the head and neck, carefully turn the patient a quarter turn so the patient's back is toward the door of the vehicle. As you move the patient from a sitting to a supine position, the spine must not bend, twist, or get jolted. Handle the patent very gently, and make sure you have enough assistance to perform the move correctly. Secure the patient to the long board and remove the patient from the vehicle.

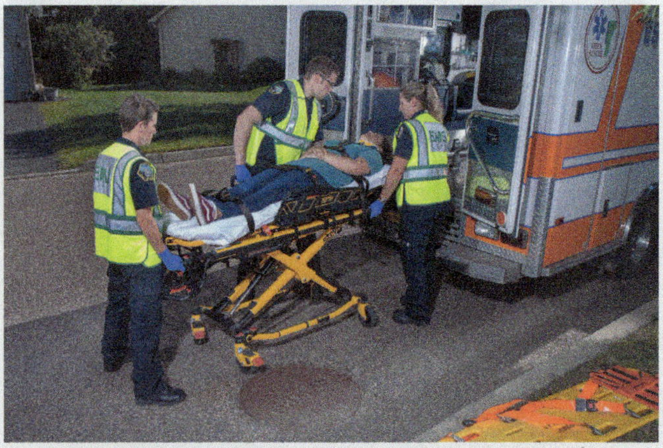

3. Move the patient from the spine board onto the stretcher, secure the patient, and place the stretcher in the ambulance.

Self-Extrication

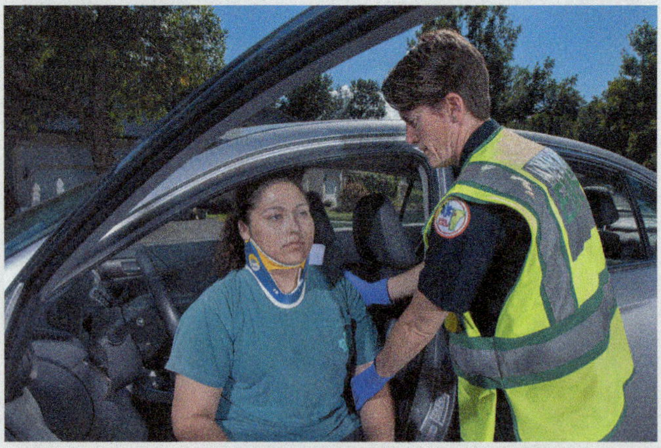

1. As guided by your assessment, the patient may be assisted in self-extrication from the vehicle.

on movement or had musculoskeletal injuries that would be worsened by movement, or if the spinal assessment showed deformity or focal differences.

A particular sequence must be followed in all applications, whether of a flexible extrication device or a short spine board. That sequence is: Secure the torso first and the head last. This ensures greater stability during the strapping process and may help prevent compression of the cervical spine. If the patient has suffered abdominal injuries or displays diaphragmatic breathing that prevents adequate securing of the torso, the torso straps will still be needed, but care must be taken so as not to interfere with breathing.

There are a number of special considerations when applying a short board to a patient:

- Assessment of the back, shoulder blades, arms, and collarbones must be done before the device is placed against the patient.
- The EMT applying the board must angle the short board behind the patient, without striking or jarring the patient or the arms of the rescuer who is stabilizing the head from behind the patient.
- To provide full cervical support, the uppermost holes must be level with the patient's shoulders. The base of the board should not extend past the coccyx.
- Never use a chin cup or chin strap, as it can prevent the patient from opening the mouth to vomit.
- Avoid applying the first torso strap too tightly. This could aggravate an abdominal injury or limit respirations for the diaphragmatic breathing patient.
- Some buckles have quick-release mechanisms. Be careful not to accidentally loosen these buckles when moving the patient.
- Do not pad between the collar and the board. This will create a pivot point that may cause the cervical spine to hyperextend when the head is secured. Instead, pad the occipital region, but only enough to fill any void. This will help keep the head in a neutral position. Sometimes when the shoulders are rolled back to the board, the head will come back to the board far enough that padding is not needed. Never use excessive padding behind the head, because when the patient is placed in a supine position, the shoulders will fall back but the head will not be able to. This will place the patient in an undesirable position of flexion.
- Follow the instructions provided by the manufacturer of the device you are using.
- After applying the short spine board, the packaging of the patient will be completed as shown in Figure 33-24.

Point of View

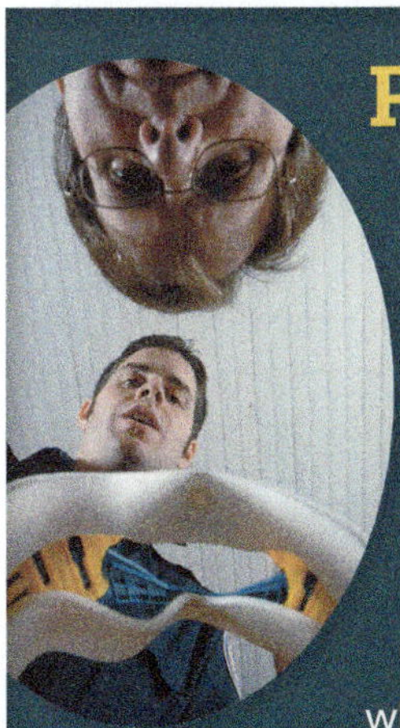

(© Edward T. Dickinson, MD)

"I was sitting on the sofa at my daughter's house, and when I got up to change the TV, I got dizzy and passed out–passed out good! When I woke up, there were these two cute young guys directly over me. Everything around them was white. I was confused. For a minute I thought I was in heaven.

"Then I felt my head. It hurt. I was trying to figure out what was going on. Nothing made sense. The EMTs were so kind. They stopped what they were doing and explained what had happened. They had to explain a couple of times. All I remember was my head hurting and being confused.

"My doctor had just changed my blood pressure medication, and I guess that's why I felt faint when I stood up fast. My daughter said that when I fell, I hit my head on the coffee table. Because of that, the EMTs put a collar around my neck and put me on the most uncomfortable board. They said it was necessary, and I believed them. But after the ride to the hospital on that board, my back hurt worse than my head.

"At 75 and with blood pressure problems, I have to learn to take my time. Now I get up slowly. I don't want to have that happen again!"

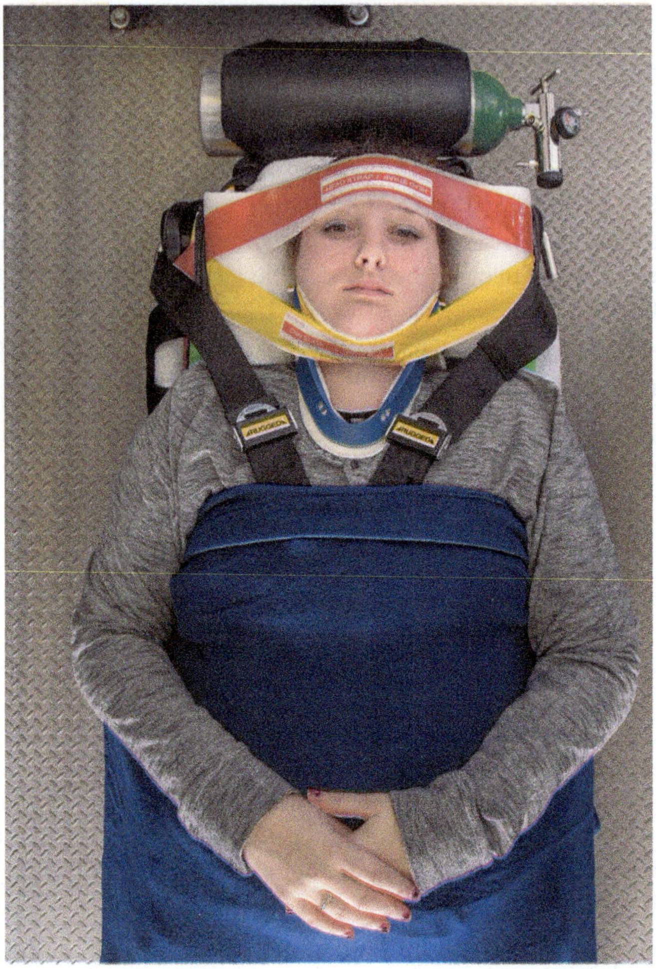

FIGURE 33-24 Spine-injured patient, "packaged."

It should be noted that the use of extrication vests and short spine boards is no longer recommended by national physician groups. In a very limited study, it was found that more movement of the spine was caused by applying a vest-type device than by simply having the patient self-extricate from the vehicle and lie down on the backboard. You should follow local protocols.

Tips for Applying a Long Backboard

The following tips relate to immobilization of the supine patient:

- You will need to log-roll the patient to apply the long backboard (Scan 33-6 and Scan 33-7). This procedure must be done carefully, keeping the patient's spine in alignment. Quickly assess the posterior body before rolling the patient back onto the board. Whenever a move is done involving neck stabilization, the EMT holding the head calls for the move. ("We will turn on three: One . . . two . . . three.")
- Pad voids between the patient's head and torso and the board. Be careful not to cause extra movement or to move the patient's spine out of alignment. The shoulder and pelvis are better at maintaining spinal alignment than movable parts like the upper arm.
- When a patient is secured to a long spine board (Figure 33-25), the head is secured last. Strapping is easier with Velcro or speed-clip straps.
- Additional immobilization for the head and neck can be provided with light foam-filled cushions, a commercial head-immobilization device (Figure 33-26) (such as the Ferno Washington head immobilizer, Bashaw CID, or the Laerdal Head Bed), or a blanket roll. If used, these are applied after securing the patient's body to the long backboard. Secure the head with 3-inch hypoallergenic adhesive tape. The tape offers support, especially if the patient and board are to be tilted to allow for drainage.

SCAN 33-6 Four-Rescuer Log Roll

First Take Standard Precautions.

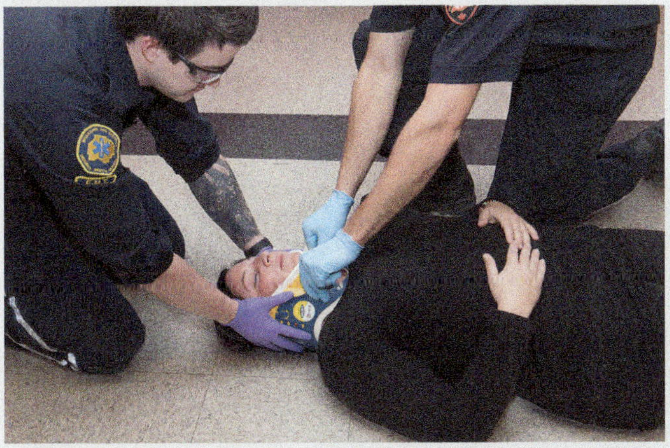

1. Stabilize the head and neck. Apply a rigid cervical collar.

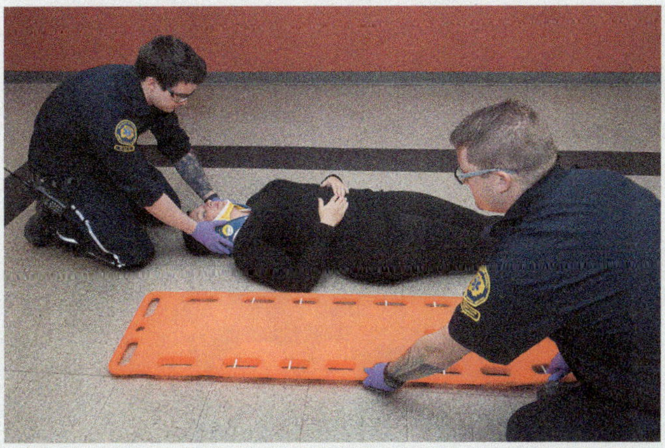

2. Place the board parallel to the patient.

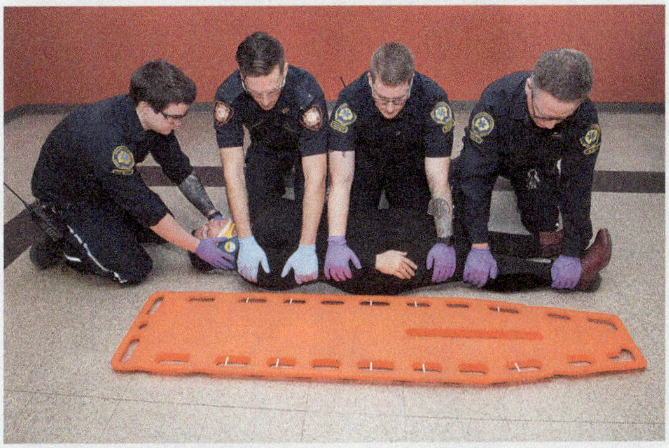

3. Have three rescuers kneel at the patient's side opposite the board, leaving room to roll the patient toward them. Place these rescuers at the shoulder, waist, and knee. The fourth EMT will continue to stabilize the head while the others reach across the patient to position their hands properly.

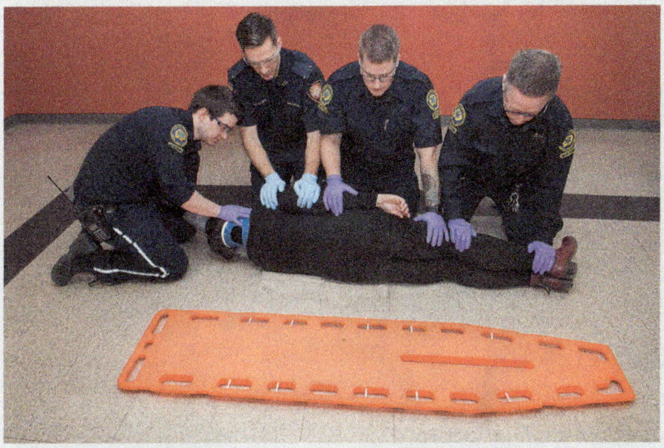

4. The EMT at the head and neck directs the others to roll the patient as a unit.

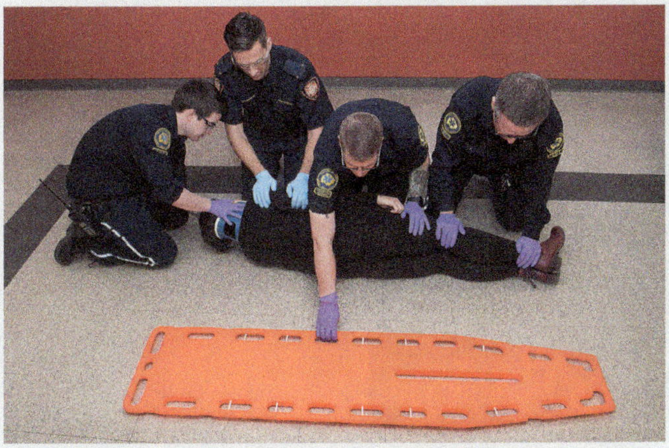

5. The EMT at the patient's waist grips the spine board and pulls it into position against the patient. (This can be done by a fifth rescuer.)

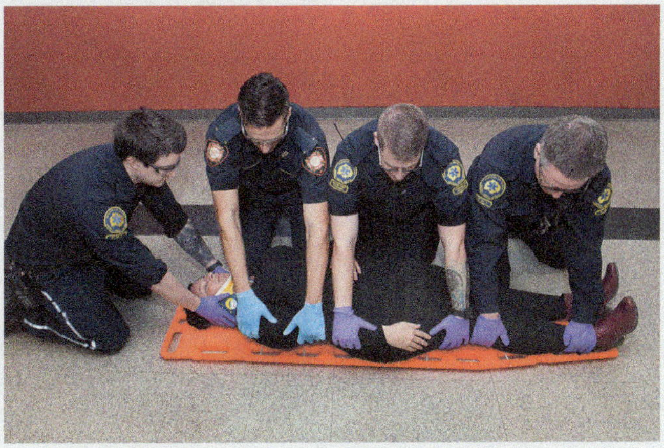

6. Roll the patient as a unit onto the board.

SCAN 33-7 Spinal Precautions for a Supine Patient Utilizing a Scoop Stretcher

First Take Standard Precautions.

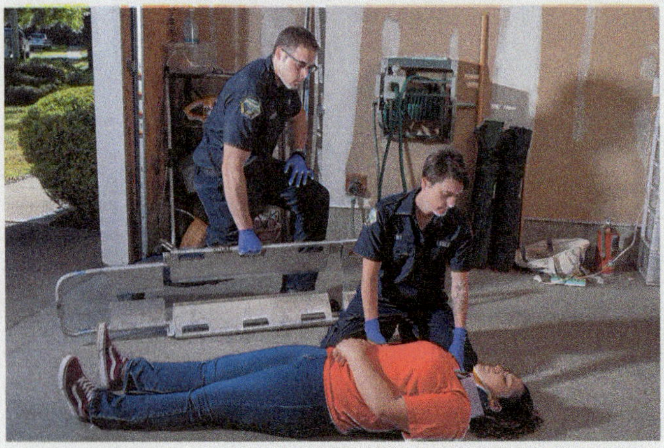

1. Place the patient's head in a neutral, inline position and maintain manual stabilization of the head and neck. Assess distal CSM. Apply an appropriate-sized cervical collar.

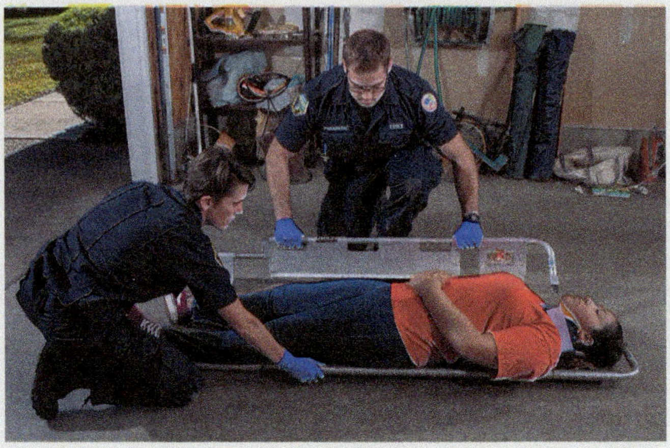

2. Position the scoop under the patient.

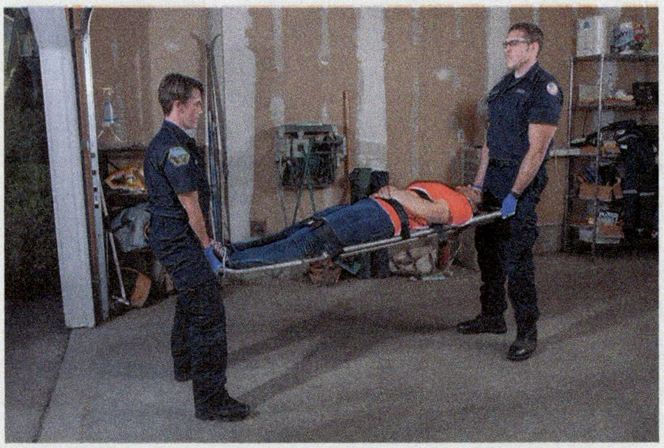

3. Keeping the back straight and using the muscles of the legs, lift the patient and carry the patient to the stretcher.

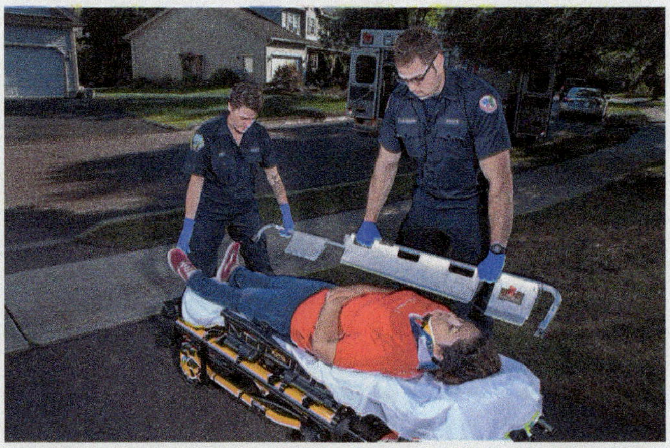

4. After placing the patient on the stretcher, remove the scoop.

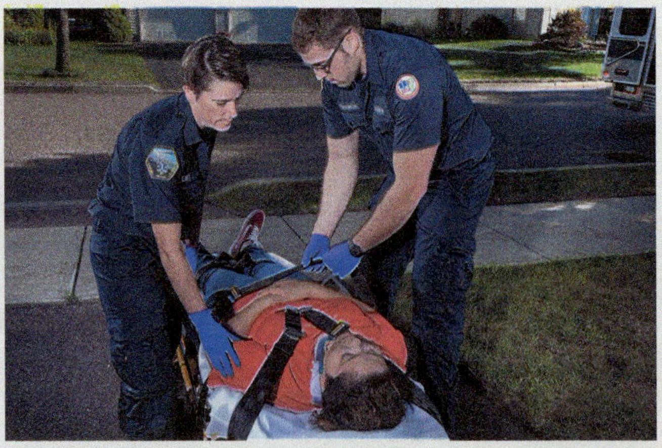

5. Secure the patient to the stretcher.

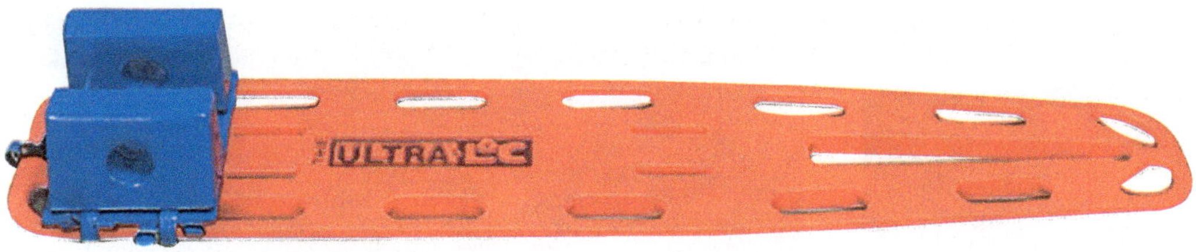

FIGURE 33-25 Long spine board with head immobilizer.

FIGURE 33-26 Disposable head immobilizer. *(Photos A and B: © Ferno-Washington, Inc)*

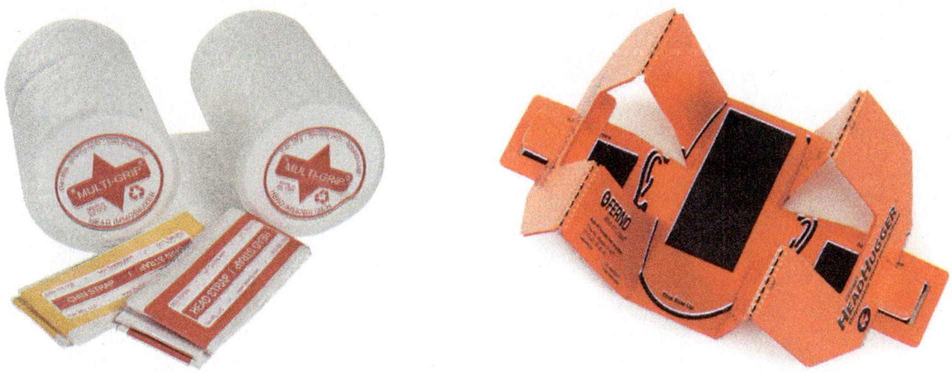

A

B

However, blood on the patient's skin and hair may make using tape impractical. You should learn to use cravats or self-adhering roller bandages as a backup method. Do not tape or tie the cravats across the patient's eyes.

- If the patient is a full-term pregnant woman, immobilize her on the backboard. Then tilt the board to the left by propping up the right side, to minimize the effect of the uterus's compressing the vena cava and causing hypotension and dizziness.
- Unless the spine board has straps specifically intended to crisscross the shoulders and chest, it is best to strap across the upper chest, the pelvis, and the thighs. If you will need to stand the patient up to carry the patient out of a tight building, up a basement stairwell, or into a small elevator, make sure the straps are secure under the patient's armpits and tight on the thighs.

Pediatric Note

When immobilizing a 6-year-old or younger child, provide padding beneath the shoulder blades to compensate for the child's proportionally larger head. Pad from the shoulders to toes as needed to establish a neutral position.

If you do not carry a pediatric long spine immobilization device, then practice immobilizing children using adult equipment and lots of towels or blankets to pad around the child. EMTs are usually very good at improvising. In this case, however, the first time you improvise should be in the classroom so that you will work quickly in the field! Occasionally EMTs are confronted at a motor-vehicle collision with an infant or young child who was riding in a child safety seat. At one time, it was recommended that if the child did not need immediate resuscitation or need to be placed supine for any reason, the child could be immobilized in the child safety seat. *Immobilizing a child in a child safety seat is no longer recommended because the integrity of a safety seat may have been compromised in the collision.*

The procedure for rapid extrication from the child safety seat is shown in Scan 33-8.

SCAN 33-8 Rapid Extrication from a Child Safety Seat

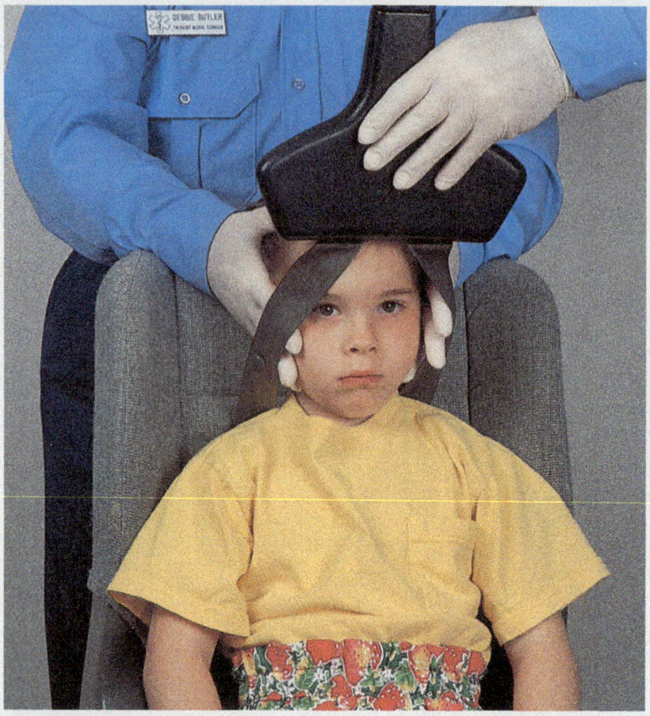

1. EMT 1 stabilizes the car seat in the upright position and applies manual stabilization of the patient's head and neck. EMT 2 prepares equipment, then loosens or cuts the seat straps and raises the front guard.

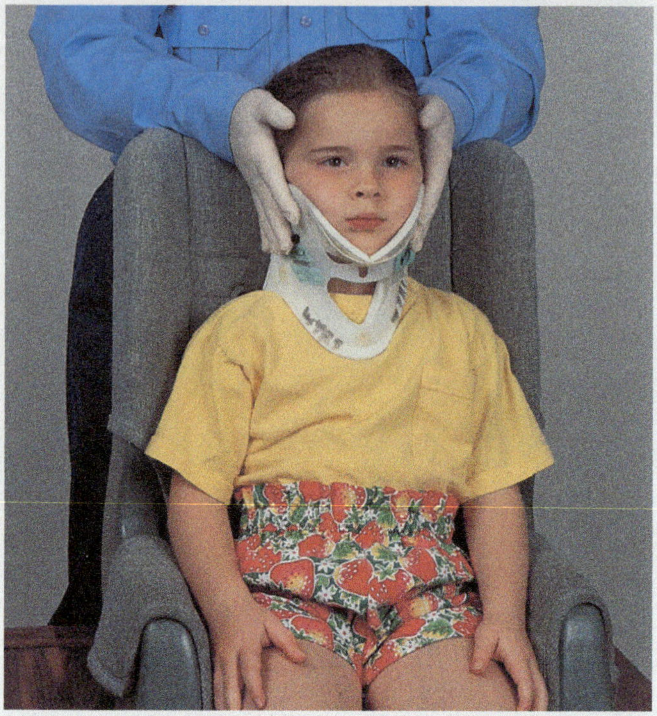

2. The cervical collar is applied to the patient as EMT 1 maintains manual stabilization of the head and neck.

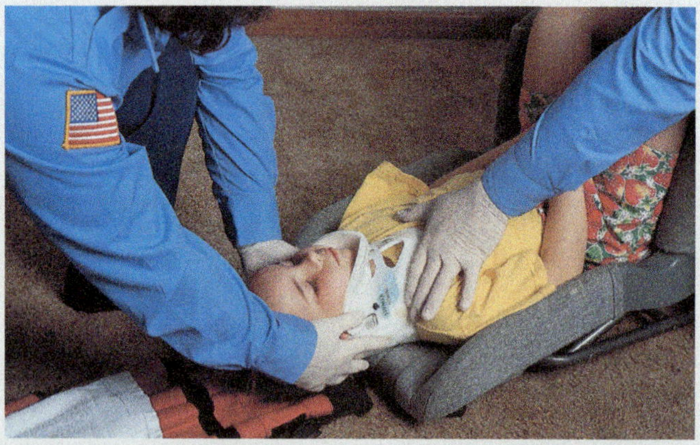

3. As EMT 1 maintains manual stabilization, EMT 2 places the child safety seat on the center of the backboard and slowly tilts it into the supine position. The EMTs are careful not to let the child slide out of the chair. For the child with a large head, place a towel under the area where the shoulders will eventually be placed on the board, to prevent the head from tilting forward.

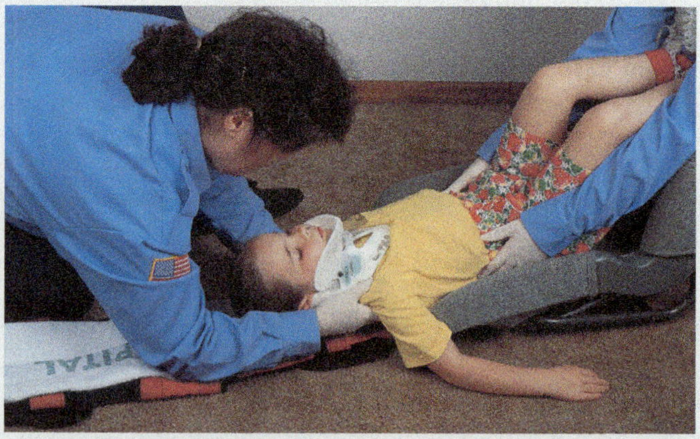

4. EMT 1 maintains manual stabilization and calls for a coordinated long axis move onto the backboard.

SCAN 33-8 Rapid Extrication from a Child Safety Seat *(continued)*

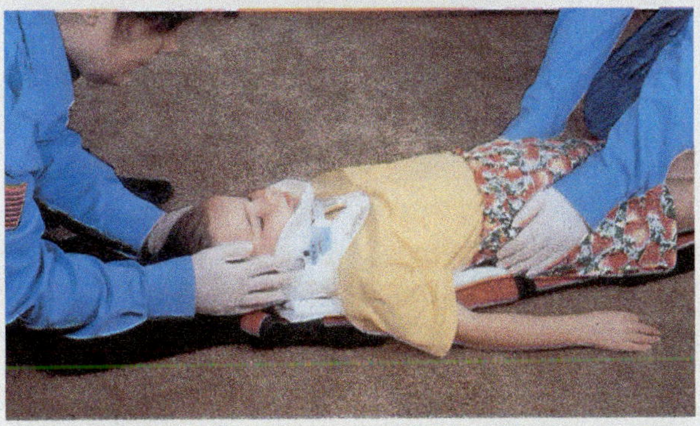

5. EMT 1 maintains manual stabilization as the move onto the board is completed, with the child's shoulders over the folded towel.

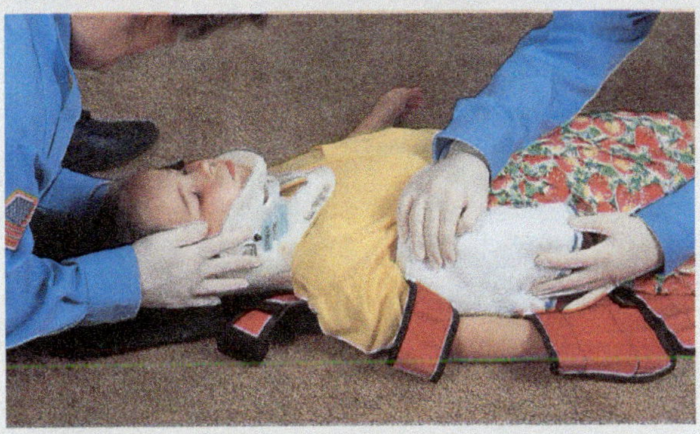

6. EMT 1 maintains manual stabilization as EMT 2 places rolled towels or blankets on both sides of the patient.

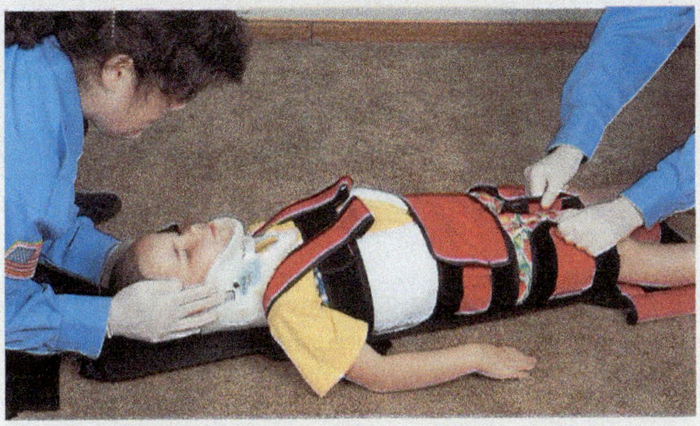

7. EMT 1 maintains manual stabilization as EMT 2 straps or tapes the patient to the board at the level of the upper chest, pelvis, and lower legs. *Do not strap across the abdomen.*

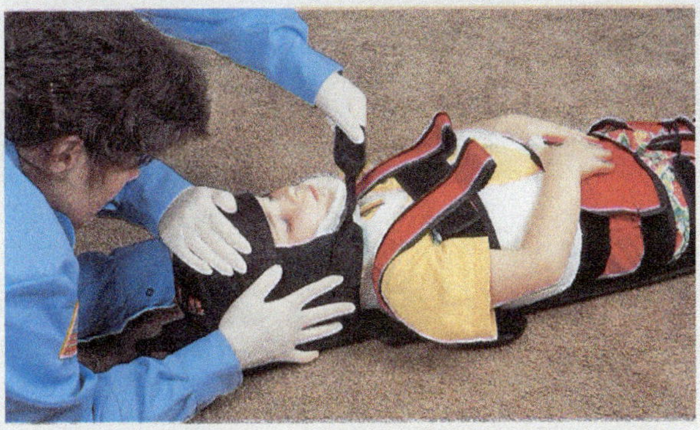

8. EMT 1 maintains manual stabilization, as EMT 2 places rolled towels on both sides of the head then tapes the head securely in place across the forehead and cervical collar. *Do not tape across the chin in order to avoid pressure on the neck.*

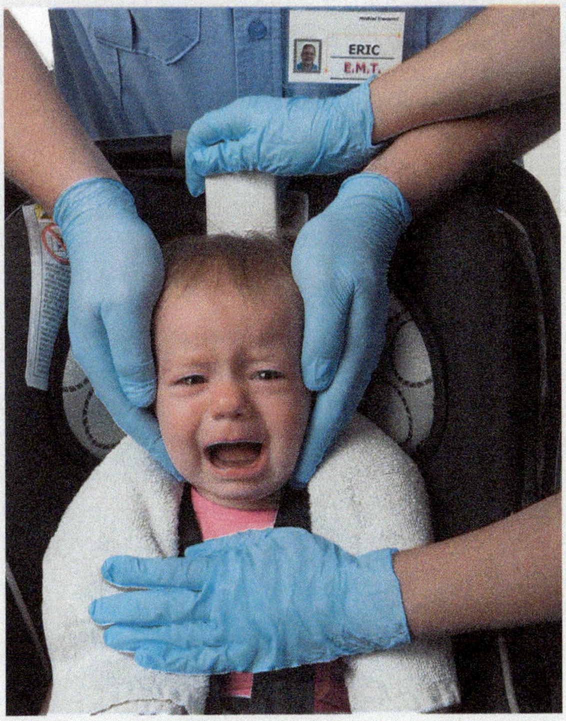

9. The newborn and infant procedure is exactly the same as for a child, except that an armboard is inserted behind the child in step 2. If the infant is very small, the armboard may actually be used as the spine board.

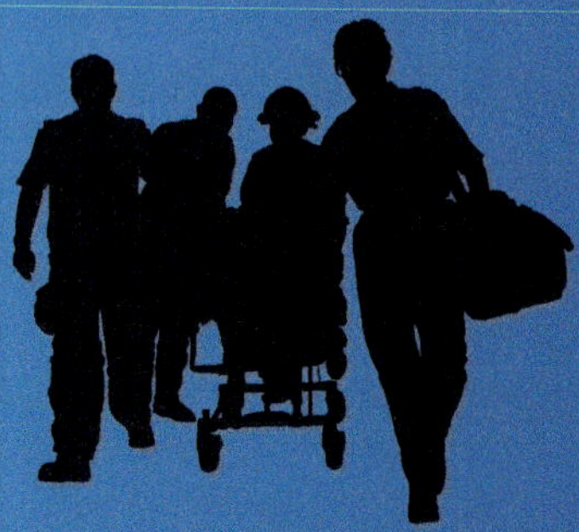

Think Like an EMT

More than a Pain in the Neck

You have learned the procedure for spinal precautions. However, the decision-making process that leads up to these precautions is equally important. Which patients require spinal motion restriction and which do not?

NOTE: *Use the general concepts from this chapter to make your determination. Your protocols in the field may vary.*

1. Your patient was the driver of a vehicle that was struck from behind while stopped at a light. The patient denies pain, but you observe her rubbing her neck and looking as if she may have some pain.
2. Your patient was in the backseat of a car that was hit broadside (T-bone). He doesn't complain of neck pain, but his head was knocked into the side of the car during the collision. He has a large hematoma on the right side of his head from the impact.
3. Your patient was a passenger in a car that was struck on the driver's side in a minor collision. She denies all injury and isn't sure she wants to go to the hospital.

- If your service transports to a helicopter, make sure that your backboard fits. There are some restrictions on the size or taper of the long backboard, depending on the helicopter's loading configuration, so find this out ahead of time.
- For a water rescue or diving injury, there are various specialty backboards, such as the Miller board, that are designed to float up beneath the patient and that use Velcro closures for ease of application.

Spinal Motion Restriction—Standing Patient

If a patient who requires spinal motion restriction is found standing, you will apply a cervical collar and have the patient carefully sit down on the stretcher. You will then guide the patient into a supine or semi-sitting position of comfort on the stretcher. The straps of the stretcher will secure the patient and help to limit movement. (See Scan 33-9.)

Patient Found Wearing a Helmet

Helmets are worn in many sporting events and by many motorcycle riders. Even ski resorts are advocating the use of helmets. Sporting helmets are typically open in the front, making it easier to access the patient's airway than when a patient is wearing a motorcycle helmet, which has a shield and often a full-face section that is not removable.

Face, neck, and spine care and airway management or resuscitation may call for the removal of the helmet, especially if the helmet will prevent you from reaching the patient's mouth or nose. If the helmet is left on, shields can be lifted and face guards removed. One EMT must manually steady the patient's head and neck while the other cuts, snaps off, or unscrews the guard. Do not attempt to remove a helmet if doing so causes increased pain or if the helmet proves difficult to remove, unless there is a possible airway obstruction or ventilatory assistance must be provided. Indications for leaving the helmet in place or for removing the helmet are summarized in the following text.

Indications for leaving the helmet in place:

- Helmet fits snugly, allowing little or no movement of the patient's head within the helmet.
- There are absolutely no impending airway or breathing problems or any reason to resuscitate or ventilate the patient.

SCAN 33-9 Patient in Standing Position with Possible Spine Injury

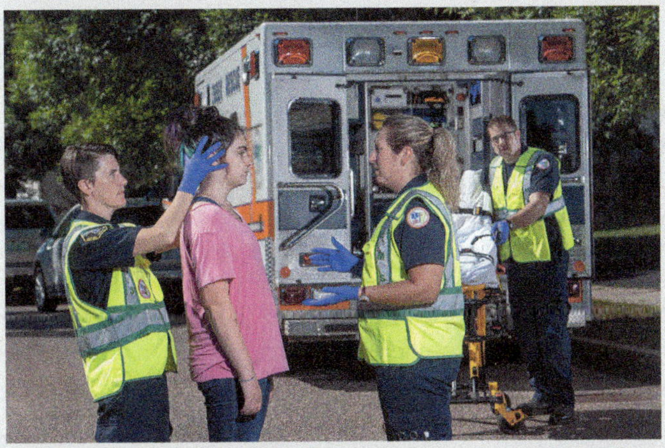

1. Stabilize the cervical spine.

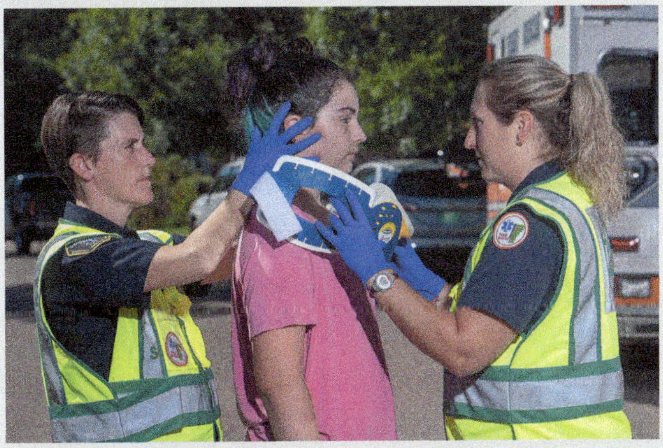

2. Apply a cervical collar.

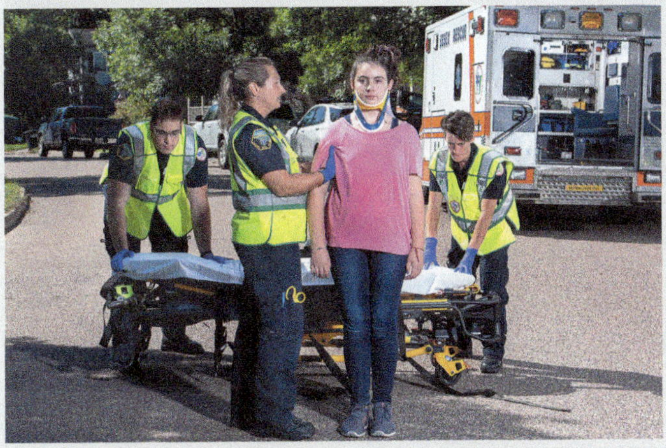

3. Position the stretcher.

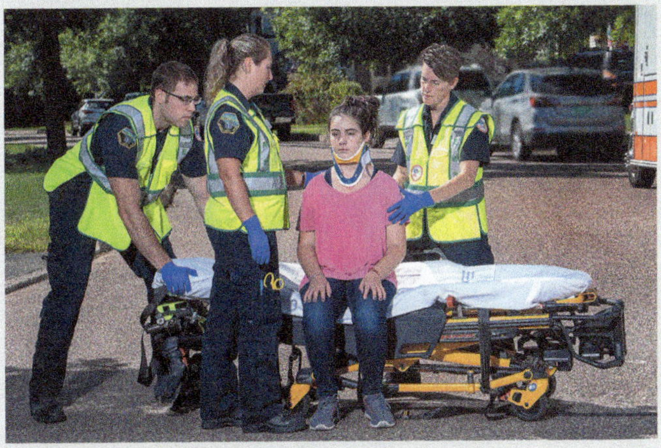

4. Assist the patient to sit on the stretcher.

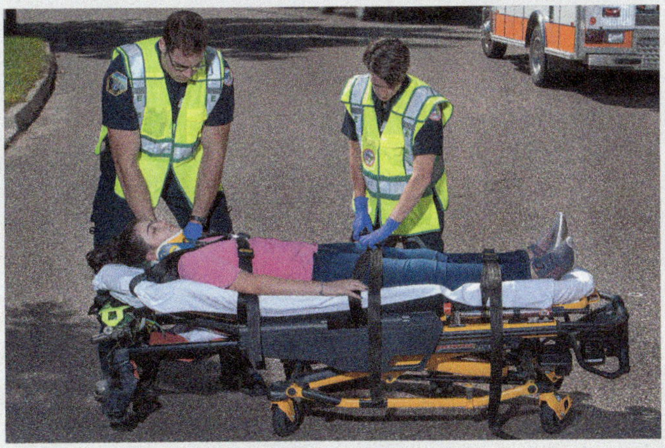

5. Secure the patient on the stretcher.

- Removal would cause further injury.
- Proper spinal immobilization can be done with the helmet in place.
- There is no interference with the EMT's ability to assess the airway or breathing.

Indications for removing the helmet:

- The helmet interferes with the EMT's ability to assess and manage airway and breathing.
- The helmet is improperly fitted, allowing excessive head movement.

- The helmet interferes with immobilization.
- Cardiac arrest is present.

Many experienced EMS providers put the controversy of removal versus nonremoval into the following perspective: If your son injured his neck playing football, would you want the trainer and the EMT to work together carefully to remove the helmet at the scene, or would you prefer this to be left to emergency department personnel, who probably will not have the help of the trainer or the benefit of lots of practice in the helmet-removal technique?

Note that if an athlete is wearing a helmet and structured shoulder pads, such as in football, hockey, or lacrosse, you should either remove the pads and the helmet or you should leave them both on. Taking off one but not the other will result in hyperflexion or hyperextension because of the space the pads occupy behind the patient's shoulders.

When a helmet must be removed, it is a two-rescuer procedure, as shown in Scan 33-10.

SCAN 33-10 Removing a Helmet from an Injured Patient

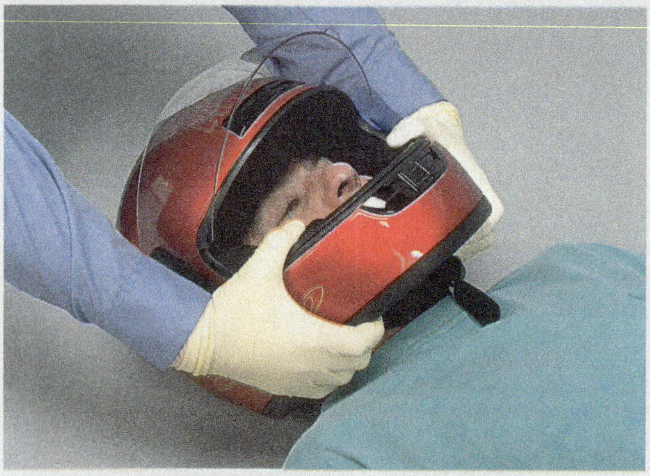

1. EMT 1 is positioned at the top of the patient's head and maintains manual stabilization. Two hands hold the helmet stable while the fingertips hold the lower jaw.

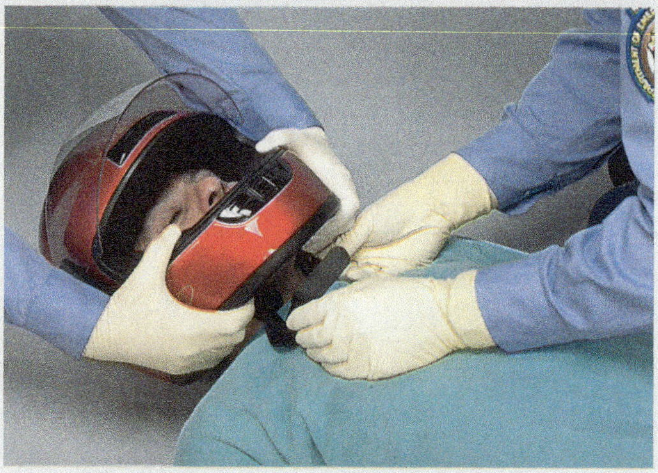

2. EMT 2 opens, cuts, or removes the chin strap.

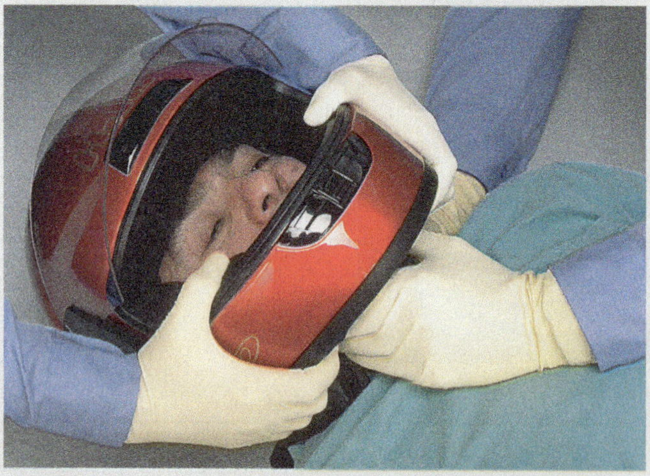

3. EMT 2 then places one hand on the patient's mandible and, using the other hand, reaches in behind the neck and stabilizes the occipital region. Using the combination of the hand in front of the chin and the hand behind the neck, EMT 2 should be able to securely hold the patient's head. If the patient is wearing glasses, these should be removed now, prior to removal of the helmet.

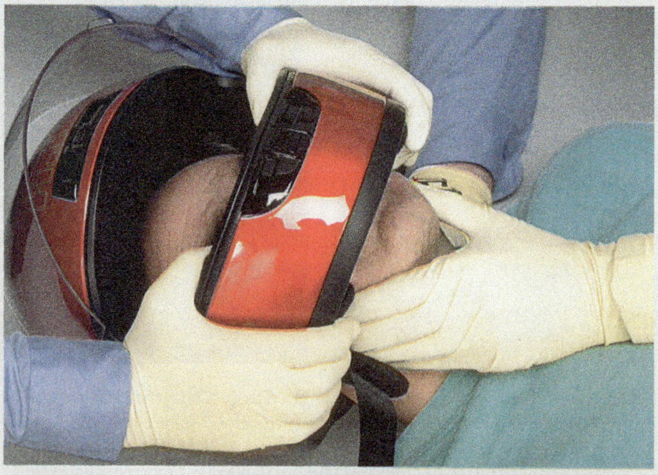

4. EMT 1 can now release manual stabilization and slowly remove the helmet. The lower sides, or ear cups, of the helmet will have to be gently pulled out in order for the helmet to clear the ears.

SCAN 33-10 Removing a Helmet from an Injured Patient *(continued)*

NOTE: *If the patient has shoulder pads and you are removing a football helmet, remember to remove the shoulder pads or pad behind the head first to keep it aligned. With either helmet-removal method, manual stabilization must be maintained until the patient is secured to a long spine board with full immobilization of the head.*

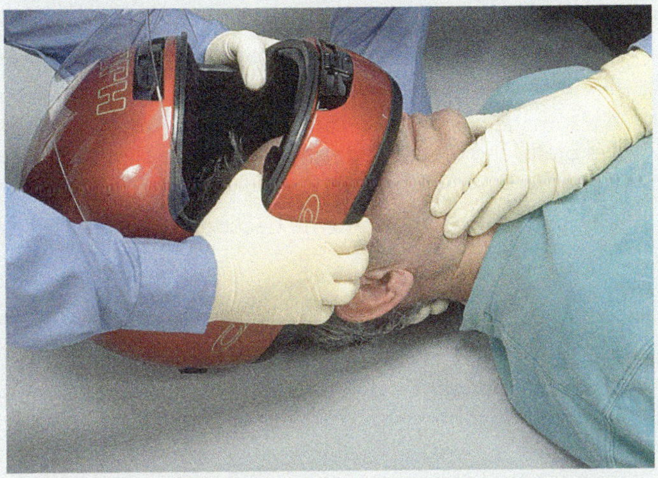

5. The helmet should come off straight, with no backward tilting. A full-face helmet may need to be tilted just enough for the chin guard to clear the nose. EMT 2 must support and prevent the head from moving as the helmet is removed.

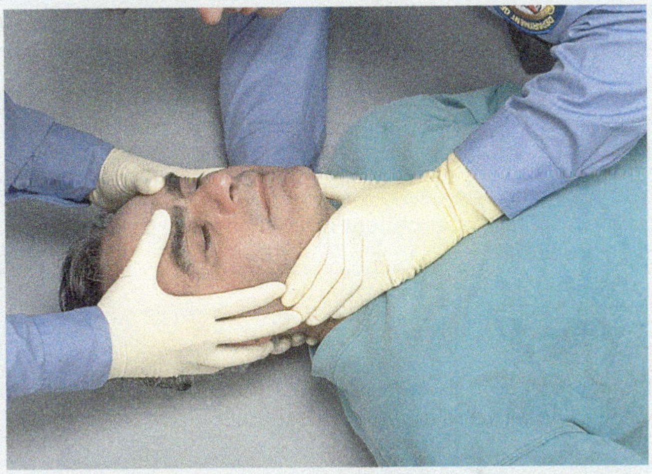

6. EMT 1, after removing the helmet, reestablishes manual stabilization and maintains an open airway by using the jaw-thrust maneuver.

Helmet Removal–Alternative Method

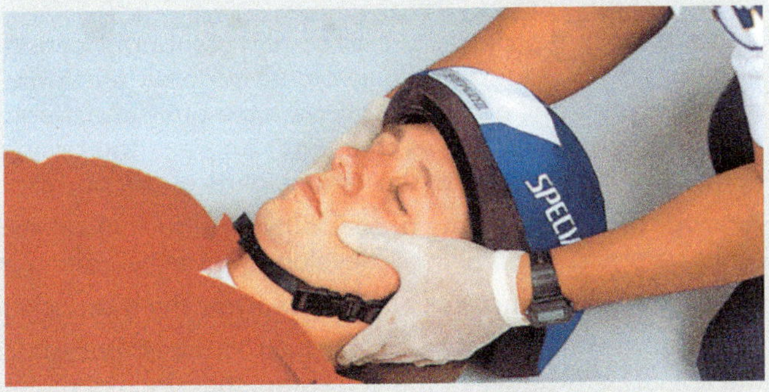

1. EMT 1 applies manual stabilization with the patient's neck in a neutral position.

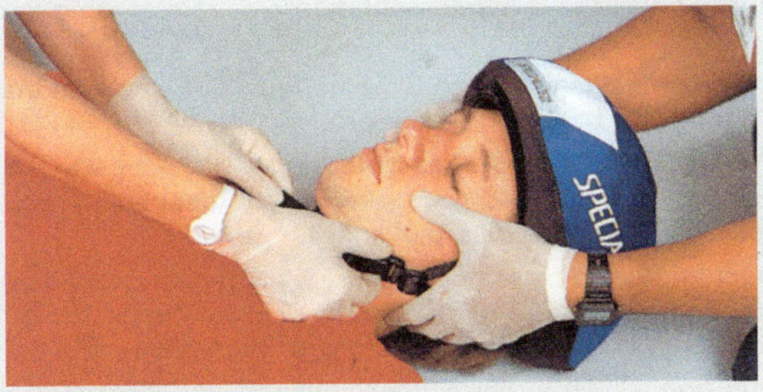

2. EMT 2 removes the chin strap.

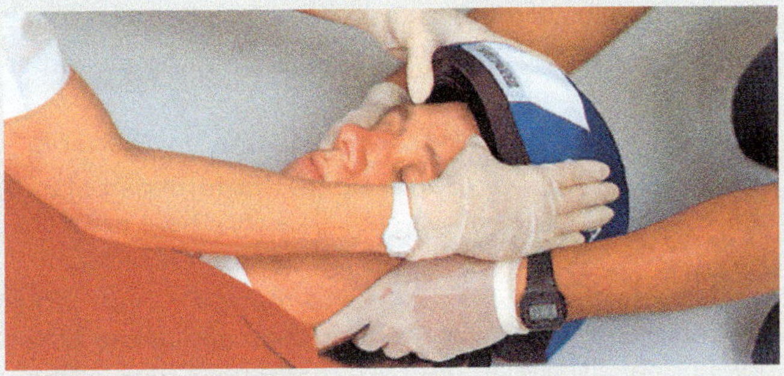

3. EMT 2 removes the helmet, pulling out on each side in order for the helmet to clear the ears.

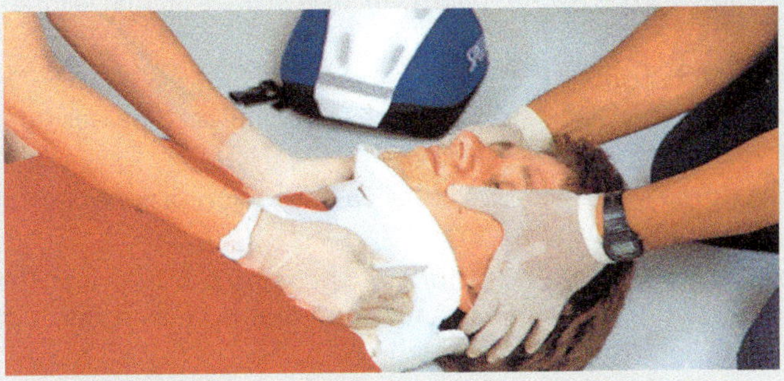

4. EMT 1 maintains manual stabilization as EMT 2 applies a cervical collar.

Chapter Review

Key Facts and Concepts

- The two main divisions of the nervous system are the central nervous system and the peripheral nervous system.
- You should maintain a high index of suspicion for head or spine injury whenever there is a relevant mechanism of injury (MOI).
- You must provide cervical spinal motion restriction before beginning any other patient care when head or spine injury is suspected.
- Altered mental status is an early and important indicator of head injury. Monitor and document your patient's mental status throughout the call.
- A traumatic brain injury is any injury that disrupts function of the brain, and may include anything from a slight concussion to a severe hematoma.
- Always secure the torso to the backboard before the head.

Key Decisions

- Does the patient have mechanism and assessment findings that would indicate the need for spinal motion restriction?
- Does the patient's potential head or spine injury require prompt transport to a trauma center?

Chapter Glossary

air embolism (EM-boh-lizm) a bubble of air in the bloodstream.

ataxic (AY-taks-ic) ***respirations*** a pattern of irregular and unpredictable breathing commonly caused by brain injury.

autonomic nervous system controls involuntary functions.

central nervous system the brain and the spinal cord.

central neurogenic hyperventilation a pattern of rapid and deep breathing caused by injury to the brain.

cerebrospinal (suh-RE-bro-SPI-nal) ***fluid (CSF)*** the fluid that surrounds the brain and spinal cord.

Cheyne (CHAY-ne) ***-Stokes breathing*** a distinct pattern of breathing characterized by quickening and deepening respirations followed by a period of apnea.

concussion mild closed head injury without detectable damage to the brain. Complete recovery is usually expected but effects may linger for weeks, months, or even years.

contusion in brain injuries, a bruised brain caused when the force of a blow to the head is great enough to rupture blood vessels.

cranium (KRAY-ne-um) the bony structure making up the forehead, top, back, and upper sides of the skull.

dermatome (DERM-uh-tohm) an area of the skin that is innervated by a single spinal nerve.

foramen magnum (FOR-uh-men MAG-num) the opening at the base of the skull through which the spinal cord passes from the brain.

hematoma (HE-mah-TO-mah) in a head injury, a collection of blood within the skull or brain.

herniation (her-ne-AY-shun) pushing of a portion of the brain downward toward the foramen magnum as a result of increased intracranial pressure.

intracranial (IN-truh-KRAY-ne-ul) ***pressure (ICP)*** pressure inside the skull.

laceration (las-uh-RAY-shun) in brain injuries, a cut to the brain.

malar (MAY-lar) the cheekbone. Also called the *zygomatic bone*.

mandible (MAN-di-bl) the lower jawbone.

maxillae (mak-SIL-e) the two fused bones forming the upper jaw.

nasal (NAY-zul) ***bones*** the bones that form the upper third, or bridge, of the nose.

nervous system provides overall control of thought, sensation, and the body's voluntary and involuntary motor functions. The components of the nervous system are the brain and the spinal cord, as well as the nerves that enter and exit the brain and spinal cord and extend to the various parts of the body.

neurogenic shock a state of shock (hypoperfusion) caused by nerve paralysis that sometimes develops from spinal cord injuries.

orbits the bony structures around the eyes; the eye sockets.

peripheral nervous system the nerves that enter and exit the spinal cord between the vertebrae, the 12 pairs of cranial nerves that travel between the brain and organs without passing through the spinal cord, and all of the body's other motor and sensory nerves.

pulmonary air embolism (EM-boh-lizm) a blockage in the blood circulation of the lung caused by a blood clot or air bubble.

spinal (SPI-nal) ***motion restriction*** limiting the movement of the spine to prevent additional injury.

spinous (SPI-nus) ***process*** the bony bump on a vertebra.

temporal (TEM-po-ral) ***bones*** bones that form part of the side of the skull and floor of the cranial cavity. There are right and left temporal bones.

temporomandibular (TEM-po-ro-mand-DIB-yuh-lar) ***joint*** the movable joint formed between the mandible and the temporal bone; also called the *TMJ*.

vertebrae (VERT-uh-bray) the bones of the spinal column (singular vertebra).

Preparation for Your Examination and Practice

Short Answer

1. Name the two components of the central nervous system, and discuss their functions.
2. List five signs of a brain injury, and explain why MOI is important in determining possible brain injury.
3. Describe the appropriate emergency treatment of a patient with a possible head or brain injury.
4. List five high-risk mechanisms of injury associated with high rates of spine injury.
5. Describe the appropriate emergency care for a patient with a possible spine injury.

Thinking and Linking

Think back to the Lifting and Moving Patients *chapter, and link information from that chapter with information from this chapter as you explain how you would provide spinal motion restriction and transport for the following patients found at the scene of an automobile collision.*

1. A patient seated on the driver's side of a car that was in a collision, complaining of neck pain
2. A patient who was thrown from one of the cars in the collision and is lying on his side in a ditch
3. A patient from one of the cars in the collision who is found on his feet and is wandering around the scene

Critical Thinking Exercises

Head and spine injuries are among the most dangerous issues to the patient and the most challenging to the EMT. The purpose of this exercise will be to consider how you might manage such patients.

1. Your 24-year-old patient has been involved in a serious motor-vehicle collision. He complains of back pain and presents with significant hypotension, but his pulse is normal and his skin is pink, warm, and dry. What condition involving the spine could account for this?
2. You are treating a patient with a brain injury. He has a decreased mental status, inadequate breathing, and a significant MOI to the head. During treatment, you identify your partner ventilating the patient too fast. What should you instruct your partner to do, and why?
3. You are called to the scene of a motor-vehicle collision. After ensuring scene safety and taking Standard Precautions, you approach the car, which has struck a bridge abutment, and note a deformed steering wheel. The driver's-side door is open and, out on the middle of the bridge, you see a person you presume to be the driver wandering erratically toward the opposite side of the bridge. How should you proceed?

Pathophysiology to Practice

The following question is designed to assist you in gathering relevant clinical information and making accurate decisions in the field.

- You encounter patients who experience pain in the areas listed below. From the three choices given for each, choose the dermatome associated with it.

  Nipple level (C4, T4, or L2)

  Navel (T10, L1, or S3)

  Little finger (C5, C8, or C2)

  Big toe (S1, L4, or T12)

Street Scenes

You and your partner are dispatched to the city park for a patient with a head injury. Arriving on scene, you determine the scene is safe and observe a group of teenage boys huddled around a person who is lying on the ground. Taking Standard Precautions, you grab your equipment and approach the patient. Your partner asks, "What happened?"

"We were jumping ramps on our bicycles when Lee tried to do a flip," states one of the boys. "He hit the ground headfirst. I told that fool he should be wearing a helmet!" You observe a young male lying supine on the asphalt parking lot, eyes closed, with blood oozing from the top of his head from what appears to be an abrasion.

One of the boys identifies himself as Lee's brother and tells you that Lee is 13 years old. He states he lives just around the corner. You ask if his mother is home, and he says she is. You ask him to go tell his mother what happened and to immediately come to the park.

Street Scene Questions

1. **What is your general impression of this patient?**
2. **What immediate treatment should be provided?**

Your general impression is of an unconscious male with head and possible spine injuries, so your partner provides manual stabilization of the head and neck. Lee's airway is patent, and he is breathing normally. You observe no other bleeding than from the laceration on the top of his head. You decide this is a high-priority trauma patient.

"Lee," you call out. "Lee, can you hear me?"

Lee opens his eyes and asks, "What happened?" Though the patient responds to verbal stimuli, it is apparent that he does not know what happened. He is able to tell you what day it is (Saturday), but not the date.

"Lee, I am going to give you a number to remember. It's number fifty-one. Can you say that?" you ask.

He replies, "Fifty-one." About this time, Lee's mother arrives. You briefly recount what you know. She seems concerned but not overly upset. You apply a rigid collar to further restrict the motion of the patient's neck. You learn that Lee is on no medications, has no allergies, and has no medical history. He ate lunch two hours ago. You obtain baseline vitals and find his pulse is 80 and normal; respirations are 24 and unlabored; blood pressure is 108/74; skin is pink, warm, and dry; and pupils are equal and reactive to light.

Street Scene Question

3. How should you monitor changing levels of responsiveness in a patient with a head injury?

"Lee, tell me what day it is today. Then tell me that number I asked you to keep in mind," you say.

"Saturday. But what number?" he responds.

You apply a loose dressing to the abrasion on his forehead. There is no other sign of injury on his body. Lee denies any neck pain and has good pulses, motor function, and sensation in all extremities.

The fire department rescue squad is now on scene, and they help you restrict motion of the patient's neck. This is done because Lee has an altered mental status and is "unreliable" in providing details. Lee is picked up from the ground and moved to the stretcher. The scoop is removed. Lee continues to have good pulses, motor function, and sensation in all extremities. When asked to recall the number again, he states, "I think it was thirty-seven." You tell him, "It was fifty-one," and ask him to repeat it. "Fifty-one," he says.

On-line medical direction has no other orders for you but tells you to keep an eye on his airway and mental status. You allow his mother to ride in the ambulance with you. You assess vitals once more en route, noting no significant changes. You once again ask Lee what day and what number, and this time he looks at you and says, "Saturday, and I think it's fifty-one." You tell him he's correct. He groans and states he has a headache. The rest of the transport is uneventful.

Multisystem Trauma

34

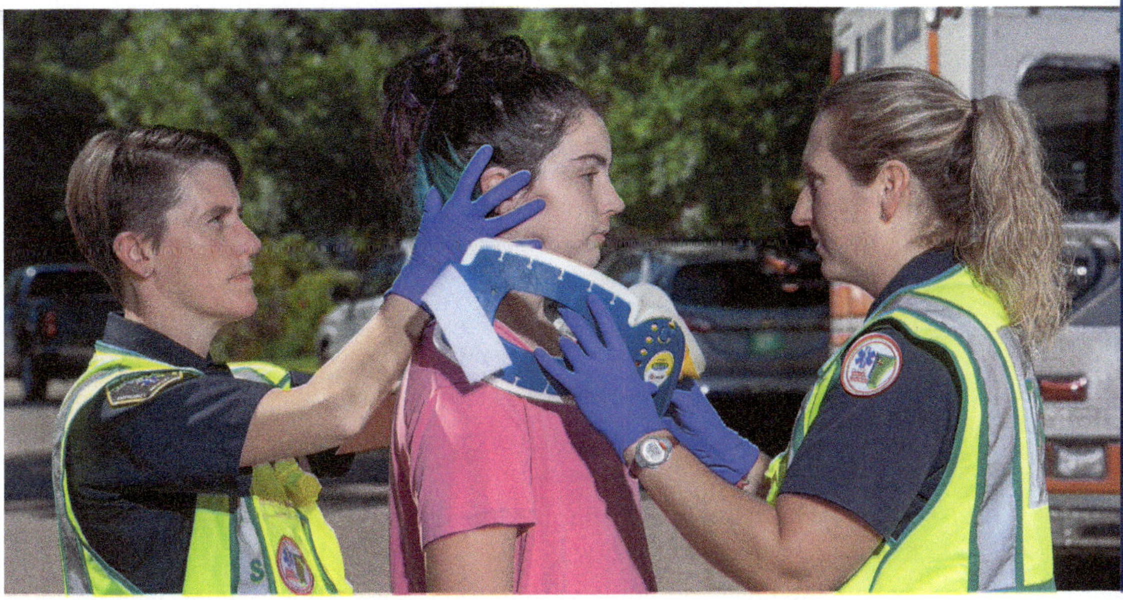

Related Chapters

The following chapters provide additional information related to topics discussed in this chapter:

Standard

Trauma (Multisystem Trauma)

Competency

Applies fundamental knowledge to provide basic emergency care and transportation based on assessment findings for an acutely injured patient.

Core Concepts

- How to balance the critical trauma patient's need for prompt transport against the time needed to treat all of the patient's injuries at the scene
- How to determine the severity of the trauma patient's condition, priority for transport, and appropriate transport destination

- How to select the critical interventions to implement at the scene for a multiple-trauma patient
- How to calculate a trauma score

Outcomes

After reading this chapter, you should be able to:

34.1 Summarize the approach to patients with multisystem trauma. (pp. 998–1009)

- Outline the key decisions that must be made with regard to treatment and transport priorities of patients with multisystem trauma.
- Analyze the combination of physiologic, anatomic, mechanism-of-injury, patient, and situational factors to estimate the patient's severity of injury.
- Relate specific assessment findings to a potential for critical internal injuries.
- Describe the emphasis on teamwork required for successful management of multisystem trauma patients.
- Apply the principles of managing multisystem trauma to descriptions of multisystem trauma situations.
- Explain the utility of trauma scoring tools in assessing trauma patients.

Key Terms

multiple trauma, *998* multisystem trauma, *998* trauma score, *1008*

There are many differences between trauma patients and medical patients. Medical patients generally call for a single complaint. In contrast, trauma patients often have more than one problem—a head injury and a broken leg, for example. When an emergency causes damage to more than one area of the body, this is referred to as *multisystem trauma* and is a serious condition.

Multisystem Trauma

CORE CONCEPT
How to balance the critical trauma patient's need for prompt transport against the time needed to treat all of the patient's injuries at the scene

multiple trauma more than one serious injury.

multisystem trauma one or more injuries that affect more than one body system.

The ***multiple-trauma*** patient has more than one serious injury. The ***multisystem-trauma*** patient has one or more injuries serious enough to affect more than one body system. For example, a patient with a gunshot wound to the chest and a fractured upper extremity is a multiple-trauma patient, having more than one serious injury. This patient is also likely to be a *multisystem*-trauma patient. The gunshot wound to the chest affects some or all of the heart and great blood vessels (cardiovascular system) and the lungs (respiratory system). If the bullet or its energy cross the diaphragm, nearby organs such as the spleen (immune system), pancreas (digestive and endocrine systems), and the stomach, liver, and intestines (digestive system) may be affected. Finally, the arm fracture will obviously affect the musculoskeletal system.

When the mechanism of injury (MOI) suggests that your patient has more than one serious injury or has an injury or injuries that are likely to affect more than one body system, decisions beyond what are called for on more typical EMS runs become necessary.

For example, consider the patient who has fallen 30 feet (9 meters) from some scaffolding and has an angulated forearm injury. Your primary assessment reveals the patient to be unresponsive, with the airway partially occluded by the tongue. Do you spend time applying a rigid splint to this patient's arm? The answer in this case is no.

This patient has life-threatening injuries, affecting at least the respiratory system, that can be treated only in a hospital emergency department or operating room. Spending additional time at the scene to treat an injury that is not life-threatening may reduce the patient's chances of survival.

Now consider an alert patient with no signs or symptoms of shock who has pain and tenderness in the middle of the thigh as well as an angulated forearm. In this case, the patient is stable enough to allow you a few minutes to apply a splint and prevent further injury. In each of these two examples, your actions as an EMT should provide the most benefit to the patient, while at the same time reducing risk as much as possible.

These decisions are made easier when your crew works well together and each member knows what to expect from one another. This is called *teamwork*. Crew members also must be aware of the importance of moving a multisystem-trauma patient to definitive care as soon as possible since it is rarely possible for EMS providers (even paramedics) to truly stabilize a trauma patient in the field. This is called *timing*. Finally, the appropriate destination must be chosen for the patient. This is a *transport* decision. In areas where some hospitals are designated trauma centers, it is important that protocols specify which patients need to be taken there and when it is (and is not) appropriate for EMS to bypass another hospital.

Determining Patient Severity

CORE CONCEPT

How to determine the severity of the trauma patient's condition, priority for transport, and appropriate transport destination

When you first approach a trauma scene, you will need to take in as much information as possible to make the best decisions. There will be times when you will come upon a horrific crash and see a patient standing there, seemingly uninjured, whereas after a similar crash on a different day, you will find a critically injured patient.

Although you have heard much about critical decision making, perhaps the most critical decisions you will make for any trauma patient are determining (1) patient priority/severity, (2) whether to limit scene time or not, and (3) which hospital and/or transport method is best for your patient.

These decisions are a foundation for the entire call. A wrong decision about patient severity or transport—especially one that delays transport of a patient who needs it—can result in a delay of necessary surgical care at the hospital and create a disorganized, chaotic scene while you try to play catch-up with a crashing patient.

It is also worthwhile to note that there are so many variables at trauma scenes that it is impossible to provide exact guidelines for each situation. The decisions you make will be based on several things, including your patient's condition, the proximity of hospitals, options available for transport (e.g., air medical evacuation), your protocols, and the advice of medical direction. Remember also that many EMTs partner with a paramedic on the ambulance.

Consider the following situations. The nature of the area where you provide care may fit one of these situations or be somewhere in between.

- The incident site is a suburban location with a 5-minute transport to a trauma center, so the EMT keeps scene time short and transports the patient expeditiously to the trauma center.
- Another EMT is 30 minutes from the trauma center and has a patient who is bleeding into the airway. The EMT is having trouble controlling the bleeding. In this case, getting ALS assistance en route or diverting the patient to a closer community hospital is necessary because it is unlikely the patient will survive the trip to the trauma center without someone's securing the airway.
- A third EMT works in a very rural community. It is 45 minutes to a community hospital and more than 2 hours to a trauma center. In this case, a helicopter is summoned to transport this EMT's patient to the trauma center.

You will need to consider many factors when making determinations about patient severity, priority, and transport destination. The next section will cover some of these issues.

TABLE 34-1 CDC Trauma Triage Guidelines: Physiologic Criteria

Glasgow Coma Scale	Below 14
Systolic blood pressure	Below 90
Respiratory rate	Below 10 or over 29 (< 20 in infants less than 1 year)

The Centers for Disease Control and Prevention (CDC) has released guidelines for trauma triage and transport to trauma centers. These take three main factors into consideration: physiologic determinants, anatomic criteria, and MOI.

You will encounter various determinants at different times in the call. You will notice the MOI as you size up the scene, observe specific injury patterns as you approach, and notice the patient's mental status and vital signs as you begin to assess the patient. Each of these factors will play into your transport decisions.

Finally, each of the categories of criteria discussed next—physiologic criteria, anatomic criteria, and MOI—should be considered separately and in sequence, addressing the first of these sets of criteria before the second and addressing the second before the third. For example, if you encountered a patient who was physiologically unstable, you would transport the patient to a trauma center. However, if your patient were physiologically stable, you would move on to consider the anatomic criteria, and so on.

Determining Severity: Physiologic Criteria

It is believed that the most valuable findings during an assessment are the patient's physiologic conditions (Table 34-1). Any time you have a patient with an altered mental status, hypotension, or an abnormally slow or rapid respiratory rate, you should place this patient at a high priority and initiate prompt transport to a trauma center when available and following your local protocols.

- Altered mental status (GCS below 14) is a significant indicator of head injury (which may present with unresponsiveness, confusion, or otherwise altered mental status) and hypoxia (which may present with anxiety and/or restlessness).
- Hypotension (systolic blood pressure less than 90 mmHg) is a definitive sign for shock and indicates some sort of internal bleeding or other circulatory disturbance.
- Abnormal respiratory rates are also indicative of serious injury. Rapid respiratory rates (above 29) usually indicate shock. Abnormally slow rates (below 10), in contrast, may indicate head injury or later stages of shock. In infants, respiratory rates below 20 are an extremely grave sign.

Determining Severity: Anatomic Criteria

Injuries of certain types or to specific areas of the body require care that is usually available in a trauma center only. For example, it makes sense that injuries to the head and chest could be serious. Other specific injuries require prompt surgical intervention for the patient to recover to the fullest extent possible. This list includes multiple musculoskeletal injuries (more than two long-bone fractures means multiple trauma), amputations, and severely mangled extremities. Pelvic injuries are associated with significant internal bleeding.

These specific anatomic criteria are listed in Box 34-1.

Determining Severity: Mechanism of Injury (MOI)

A significant mechanism of injury does not guarantee the patient has a serious injury. In the absence of physiologic or anatomic criteria, however, the fact that significant forces have acted on the body causes us, as EMTs, to act in a more cautious manner.

BOX 34-1 CDC Trauma Triage Guidelines: Anatomic Criteria

- All penetrating injuries to head, neck, torso, and extremities proximal to elbow and knee
- Chest wall instability or deformity (e.g., flail chest)
- Two or more proximal long-bone fractures
- Crushed, degloved, mangled, or pulseless extremity
- Amputation proximal to wrist or ankle
- Pelvic fractures
- Open or depressed skull fracture
- Paralysis

Some newer vehicles have the ability to transmit data after a crash (telemetry). In addition to notifying police and rescue personnel, the on-board computer in the vehicle may also transmit data such as vehicle speed at the time of the crash, whether the vehicle rolled over or had multiple impacts, which part of the vehicle was struck (e.g., front end), and whether or not the air bag was deployed.

Box 34-2 lists mechanism-of-injury criteria that may cause you to choose transport to a trauma center over transporting to other facilities.

Determining Severity: Special Patients and Considerations

You will read in subsequent chapters that not everyone responds to illness and injury the same way. For example, older adult patients do not compensate for shock efficiently. Children also respond differently, and may benefit from transport to a pediatric specialty facility. Protocols often consider MOI when evaluating the need for spinal motion restriction in children.

Patients with certain conditions, such as patients on anticoagulants (blood thinners) or those who are pregnant, may also require transport to a trauma center, but these decisions are generally made on a case-by-case basis.

One example of a patient who will likely require triage to a higher level of care is an older adult patient who has had a fall, is on anticoagulant medications, and has a head injury. Even if the patient appears fine after the fall, the risk of intracranial bleeding is high for this patient.

Box 34-3 lists trauma triage guidelines for special patient or system considerations.

Pathology of Internal Injuries

Multisystem trauma is serious and often involves internal organs. Understanding the pathophysiology of certain conditions helps you identify criticality when signs or symptoms appear.

BOX 34-2 CDC Trauma Triage Guidelines: Mechanism-of-Injury Criteria

Falls

- Adults: > 20 feet (6 meters) (One story is equal to 10 feet [3 meters].)
- Children: > 10 feet (3 meters) or 2–3 times the height of the child

High-Risk Auto Crash

- Intrusion (including roof) > 12 in. (30 cm) occupant site; > 18 in. (45 cm) any site
- Ejection (partial or complete) from automobile
- Death in same passenger compartment
- Vehicle telemetry data consistent with high risk of injury

AUTO VERSUS PEDESTRIAN/BICYCLIST THROWN, RUN OVER, OR WITH SIGNIFICANT (> 20 MPH [32 KPH]) IMPACT

MOTORCYCLE CRASH > 20 MPH (32 KPH)

INJURY	SIGNS AND SYMPTOMS
Pneumothorax–air enters the pleural space and collapses a lung or part of a lung.	• Diminished or absent lung sounds on one side • Respiratory distress • Elevated pulse • Possible injury on that side of the chest
Tension pneumothorax–a pneumothorax worsens; pressure in the pleural space collapses the vena cava, severely reducing blood flow to the heart.	• Very labored breathing • Absent lung sounds on one side • Distended neck veins • Altered mental status • Low blood pressure • Narrowing pulse pressure • Increased pulse and respirations • Possible injury (penetrating) to the chest • Tracheal deviation (very late sign)
Cardiac tamponade–blood collects in the pericardial sac around the heart. This creates pressure, which prevents adequate filling of the chambers, reducing cardiac output.	• Distended neck veins • Low blood pressure • Narrowing pulse pressure • Increased pulse and respirations • Penetrating injury to the chest
Solid organ damage occurs.	• Solid organs are vascular and can bleed profusely, causing shock. • A capsule around solid organs such as the liver can mask bleeding and pain, delaying diagnosis. • Injury to these vascular organs is often (although not always) sharp and in predictable patterns/locations (e.g., referred to shoulder).
Hollow organ damage occurs.	• Hollow organ damage (e.g., to the small intestine) may cause a spilling of contents into the surrounding abdominal tissue. This frequently causes severe and diffuse pain because of widespread irritation to surrounding structures.

BOX 34-3 CDC Trauma Triage Guidelines: Special Patient or System Considerations

AGE

- Older adults: Risk of injury or death increases after age 55.
- Older adults: Systolic blood pressure below 110 may represent shock after age 65.
- Older adults: Low-impact injuries (e.g., ground-level fall) may result in severe injury.
- Children: Should be triaged preferentially to pediatric-capable trauma centers.

ANTICOAGULANTS AND BLEEDING DISORDERS

BURNS

- Without other trauma mechanism: Triage to burn facility.
- With trauma mechanism: Triage to trauma center.

PREGNANCY > 20 WEEKS

EMS PROVIDER JUDGMENT

Managing the Multisystem-Trauma Patient

The following scenario describes a typical multiple-trauma call. As you read, ask yourself these questions: When does the EMT recognize that the patient has multiple injuries? What body systems would the EMT suspect have been affected by this patient's injuries? What is the EMT's first decision about managing those injuries, and why would you make it? What actions would you take to support the affected body systems? What priorities would you set for this patient?

CORE CONCEPT

How to select the critical interventions to implement at the scene for a multiple-trauma patient

A Typical Call

You receive a call for a motorcyclist who was hit by a car. The scene is safe, so you approach the patient, an adult male you estimate to be about 25 years old. He appears unresponsive in a pool of blood on the road, and is not wearing a helmet (Figure 34-1). Police point to the motorcycle he was riding about 20 feet (6 meters) away.

You and your partner recognize two concurrent serious problems: unresponsiveness with gurgling respirations and apparently severe bleeding from his thigh. After calling for an engine company for assistance, you each decide to address one of these fatal problems.

You quickly expose the leg and see blood flowing briskly from the wound. You recognize that while it is not "spurting," you must apply a tourniquet for two reasons. First, the blood loss is significant—especially when it may be combined with blood loss from internal injuries. His skin is pale and sweaty, so you already suspect shock. Secondly, you have much to do at this scene, and if you are tied up with prolonged direct pressure and bandaging, no one will be available to prepare this patient for transport.

The patient is making gurgling sounds with each breath, so your partner suctions blood out of the airway. He also is making snoring sounds, so your partner inserts an oropharyngeal airway, which the patient tolerates and which eliminates the snoring sounds. Breathing is shallow and labored at a rate of about 30, so your partner stabilizes the patient's head with her knees and ventilates the patient 12 times a minute with a bag–valve mask and high-concentration oxygen.

You assign this patient a high priority for rapid treatment and transport based on altered mental status, presence of shock, and the MOI. You request ALS intercept en route if it is available and will not delay transport.

You perform a trauma assessment. At the same time, a firefighter gets a long backboard for moving the patient from the scene. By the time the firefighter returns, you have finished the rapid trauma assessment and gained the following information: A hematoma (lump) is present on the right side of the patient's head; neck veins are flat; there is no deformity of the cervical spine; breath sounds are decreased on the right side of the chest; the abdomen

"Multisystem trauma will test you. If you want to do well with a severely injured patient, remember three vital factors: A . . . B . . . C."

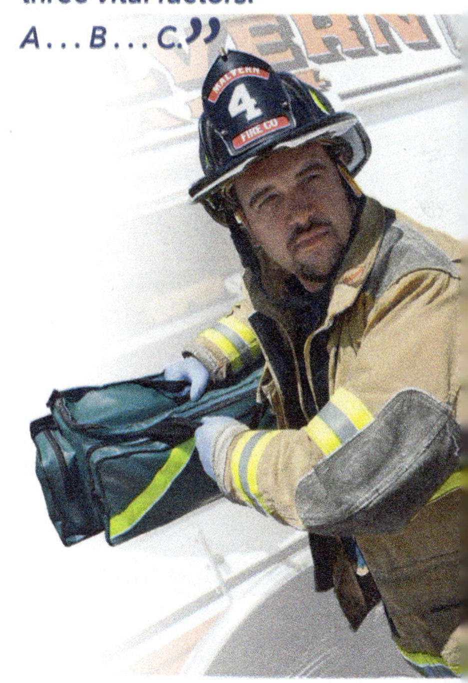

(© Edward T. Dickinson, MD)

FIGURE 34-1 Unresponsive adult male patient, victim of a motorcycle-passenger vehicle collision.

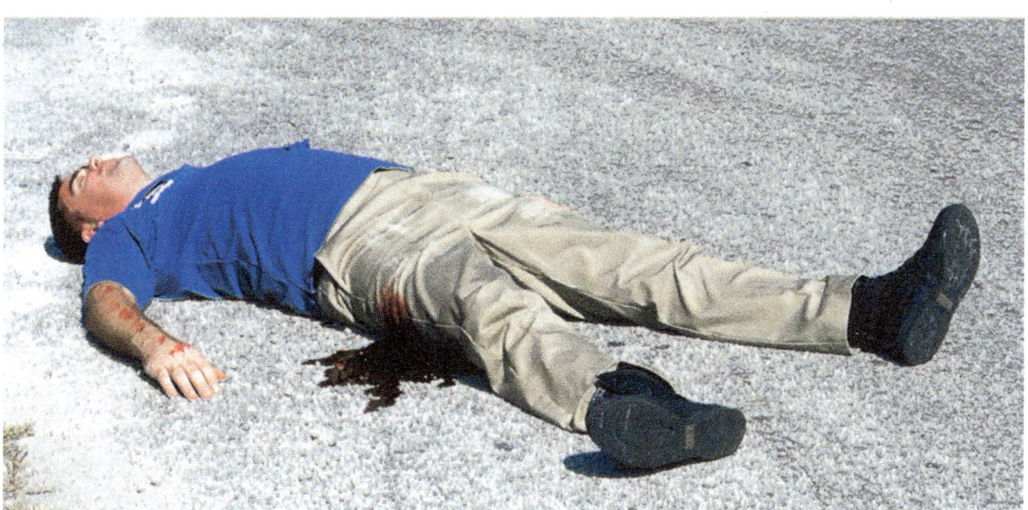

is soft; the pelvis seems stable; there is an obvious compound angulated midshaft femur fracture on the right side, from which the bleeding has been controlled with direct pressure; there are some nonbleeding lacerations on the right forearm and lower leg; and pulses are weak but palpable in all extremities except the leg with the tourniquet.

With a cervical collar in place on the patient, you quickly examine the spine and posterior trunk. You find no further injuries.

As you move the backboard to the stretcher, you make sure the firefighter is available to drive the ambulance, so that you and your partner can tend to the patient in back. You confirm that the firefighter knows you are to go to the trauma center, not to the community hospital that is 5 minutes closer. Your protocols specify that you are to go directly to the trauma center under conditions such as these because of the comprehensive care available there.

You move the patient and board onto the stretcher and into the ambulance, making sure your partner is able to continue ventilating him during the move. The board will stay in place as a splint for the femur and as a secure surface in the event CPR is necessary. Once inside the patient compartment, you repeat the primary assessment. Your general impression is of a young adult male with multiple injuries. His mental status remains unchanged: He tries to brush your hand away when you apply a painful stimulus. His tongue is prevented from obstructing his breathing by the oropharyngeal airway. There is a little bit of gurgling as you listen, so you suction some more blood out of his mouth. There are now no abnormal sounds as your partner ventilates him. Oxygen is flowing, and you see the patient's chest rise with each breath. The bleeding from the thigh remains controlled, and you see no other bleeding wounds. His radial pulse is rapid and weak. The patient is still a high priority.

With a second primary assessment completed, you call the trauma center and notify them of the patient's condition and your estimated time of arrival (10 minutes). You tell them you will give them vital signs as soon as you get them. With the hospital preparing for the patient's arrival, you turn to obtaining vital signs. The patient's pulse is 108, weak, and regular; blood pressure 92/56; respirations assisted at 12 per minute; and skin pale and sweaty. You relay this information to the trauma center.

You have a few minutes before you arrive, so you check that your partner is still able to ventilate the patient well before you perform a detailed head-to-toe physical exam. You find the patient has equal pupils that are slow to react, a hematoma (lump) on the right side of his head, nothing unusual in or behind the ears, deformity on both sides of the mandible (you conclude this is what is causing the bleeding into his airway), and flat neck veins. (You are unable to palpate the cervical spine because the cervical collar is in place.) His breath sounds are still decreased on the right side of his chest; his abdomen seems to be firmer than it was before; his pelvis seems stable; there is an obvious compound midshaft femur fracture on the right side (it is no longer angulated, because you straightened it when you put the patient on the board); and there are some nonbleeding lacerations on the right forearm and lower leg. It is more difficult now to palpate peripheral pulses.

You would like to apply a traction splint but realize you do not have enough time or personnel. With just a few minutes before you arrive at the trauma center, you repeat the primary assessment one more time. The patient responds purposefully to painful stimuli, but now he also opens his eyes briefly when you pinch him. You find no other changes. You get another set of vital signs: pulse 120, blood pressure 90 by palpation, respirations assisted at 12 per minute, and skin pale and sweaty.

You arrive at the emergency department and give a report to the trauma team as you transfer your patient to the bed. The patient becomes a bit more responsive in the emergency department, but is agitated. The staff stabilize his vital signs for the moment. The emergency department staff ask you and your partner to help apply a traction splint to the patient's fractured femur. You are able to quickly and efficiently do so. The patient is taken away for further tests and surgery.

Later you learn that the patient had a cerebral contusion (bruise of the brain), bilateral fracture of the mandible, right hemothorax (blood in the right side of the chest cavity), and a fractured femur.

After a lengthy stay, the patient is able to walk out of the hospital with some temporary assistance from a pair of crutches.

Analysis of the Call

The previous scenario about the injured motorcycle rider shows an example of a patient who has critical injuries. Immediate threats to life included significant external bleeding, shock, and bleeding into an airway that was partially obstructed by the tongue. Other serious injuries included an apparent head injury, inadequate ventilation, a presumed chest injury, a mandible injury, a compound angulated femur fracture, and a possible spine injury (based on the MOI). The EMT in the scenario gave the patient the best possible chance of survival by following the priorities determined by the assessments.

The primary assessment revealed several immediate life threats that the EMT could affect:

- Bleeding from the leg was quickly stopped.
- The airway was partially obstructed by blood, which was suctioned.
- The patient's tongue was partially blocking the airway, causing snoring sounds with breathing, for which an artificial airway was inserted.
- The patient's breathing was shallow and labored at a rate of about 30, for which the EMT's partner instituted assisted ventilations at a rate of 12 per minute with high-concentration oxygen.

The EMT realized the seriousness of the patient's condition and made the decision not to treat some injuries in the ordinary way. Instead of applying a traction splint, and dressing and bandaging the limb lacerations, the EMT realized that it would be a mistake to delay transport. A patient who has bleeding into the airway does not have any time to spare. Accordingly, the EMT used a backboard as a universal splint for the femur and did not bandage the lacerations, because they were not bleeding.

Some might say the EMT in the scenario was wrong and should have applied the traction splint in the field. After all, the emergency department staff later asked the EMT to do it,

Think Like an EMT

Determining Criticality

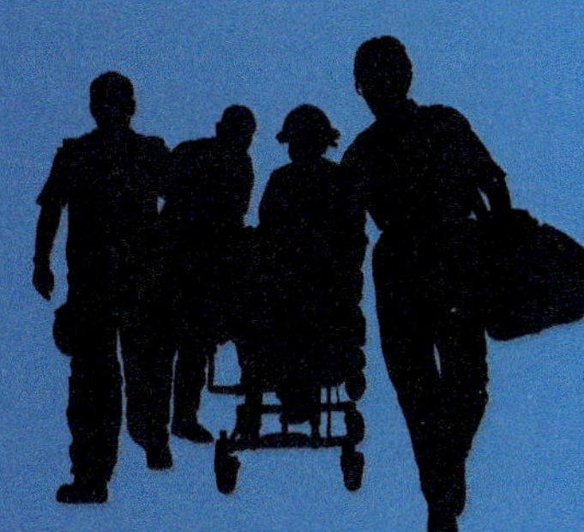

A determination of criticality (whether the patient has a serious condition or not) is one of the most important decisions you can make for the trauma patient. Just identifying when the *potential* for serious injury exists is vital. Your patient priority and transport decisions are based on these determinations. Assume you have a local hospital 15 minutes away and a trauma center 25 minutes away. Determine which of the following patients should be transported to the trauma center and which could be transported to the local hospital—and explain why.

1. Your 30-year-old patient fell 4 feet (1.2 meters) from a ladder and got his lower leg caught in a rung. He believes he broke his lower left leg. His pulse is 96, strong and regular; respirations 18 and adequate; blood pressure 126/86; pupils equal and reactive to light; and skin warm and dry. He is alert. There are distal pulses in the extremity.
2. Your patient is an 8-year-old male who fell 8–10 feet (2.4–3 meters) from a tree to the ground. He is holding his right wrist and says it hurts. As you talk with him and his parents, you note that he appears confused. As you move him to the ambulance, you believe his mental status is decreasing. His vitals are pulse 82, strong and regular; respirations 24; blood pressure 122/86; pupils equal and sluggishly reactive to light; and mental status as previously noted.
3. Your patient is a 32-year-old female who is 30 weeks pregnant and who fell down a flight of stairs. She struck her head and has pain in her left shoulder. Her main concern is the brisk vaginal bleeding that began after the fall.

right? In fact, the EMT showed good judgment. The appropriate place to apply a traction splint to this patient was in the emergency department, not in the field. When the emergency department staff asked the EMT to help apply the splint, it was because the patient was stable enough (and because the EMT was more familiar with the device than they were). If the patient's condition had not improved, they would not have asked the EMT to put the splint on. Instead, the patient would have been whisked away for surgery or further tests.

There were two additional ways in which the EMT showed good judgment: by postponing taking vital signs, and by giving the hospital staff time to prepare. The patient was ready to be put in the ambulance before the EMT was able to get vital signs, so the EMT appropriately postponed taking them until they were en route. As tempting as it might be to complete an assessment all at once, the EMT realized that vital signs were not going to change what could be done and that taking them would delay transport. The EMT also called the hospital and gave them an admittedly incomplete report so they could begin preparations, then gave them the patient's vital signs as soon as possible. This gave the hospital some additional time to notify the trauma team.

General Principles of Multisystem-Trauma Management

Prepare for a call to a multisystem-trauma patient by practicing for it. If you have a regular partner or crew, determine your individual roles beforehand. For example, someone should be designated to manually immobilize the patient's head and, if necessary, ventilate with a bag–valve mask. Depending on the number of people available, you may need to have each person handle several roles. En route to the call, if you have reason to believe you might care for a multisystem-trauma patient, review the roles each person will fill.

At the scene, follow the assessment steps as you learned them in your EMT course. Follow the priorities you discover in your primary assessment (airway, breathing, and circulation). Then balance the need for scene interventions with the time needed to perform them. As you may recall, the concept of the *golden hour* refers to the need for critical trauma patients to get to surgery within 1 hour of injury (not 1 hour from when you get to the patient). Although the time by which the patient has to get to surgery has not been scientifically proven to be within an hour, clearly some patients need surgical intervention earlier than others. Unfortunately, there is no reliable way to tell which patients need urgent transport. The concept of the golden hour is still a useful one in avoiding delays at the scene.

For most critical patients, limit scene treatment to:

- Stabilizing the cervical spine during all interventions
- Suctioning the airway
- Inserting an oral or nasal airway
- Restoring a patent airway by sealing a sucking chest wound
- Ventilating with a bag–valve mask
- Administering high-concentration oxygen
- Controlling bleeding
- Restricting spinal motion—especially when doing so won't significantly delay transport. A cervical collar is frequently used, and a backboard may be used in situations where spinal injury is detected or strongly suspected, or when the board serves other purposes—e.g., as a device for CPR or to immobilize the entire body.

Principles of multisystem-trauma management also include the following:

- **Scene safety is paramount.** Different kinds of trauma tend to pose different kinds of dangers. Blunt trauma, which is more common in rural and suburban areas, can be associated with such dangers as bent power poles, leaking fuel, sharp glass and metal edges, and passing traffic. Penetrating trauma, such as stab wounds and gunshot wounds, tend to occur more commonly in urban areas. Risks you will need to consider include the presence of the assailant (especially one who is upset because you are trying to save a person the assailant tried to kill), presence of multiple weapons (on the victim, assailant, and bystanders), absent or delayed police response, and angry crowds.

- **Ensure an open airway.** If you are unable to ventilate your patient without assistance, try other approaches until you find one that works. You might get another person to assist you en route, or you might have to switch places with your partner. Other alternatives include using a different device to ventilate, such as a pocket mask with supplemental oxygen, or you and your partner may have to work together to ventilate the patient.
- **Perform urgent or emergency moves as necessary.** For example, if a critical patient is sitting in a vehicle, you will need to perform a rapid extrication.
- **Adapt to the situation.** When a patient is trapped, for example, and part of the patient's body is not accessible, assess as much as you can. Keep in mind that when the patient is extricated, you will need to perform a complete examination.

For a multisystem-trauma patient, your overall goal is to treat immediate threats to life, which you can treat with prompt transportation to a facility that will provide definitive care (or as close to it as is available). Guard against the temptation in these cases to spend time at the scene treating all of the patient's injuries and immobilizing the patient perfectly. It is not good patient care to arrive at the hospital with the world's best-packaged corpse.

Multiple Trauma in the Pediatric Patient

All of the material you have learned about trauma applies to the pediatric patient. There are a few differences in assessment and care that are important to note in the context of multiple trauma.

Pediatric patients will need additional emotional support since younger patients may not understand what is occurring to them and around them. In situations where other family members are injured, the EMT must consider family dynamics such as separating parent and child, and parents who deny injury—even when seriously injured—so their children receive care first. When possible, transport family members together. If it isn't possible to transport them together, transporting them to the same facility when possible helps keep the family together in a time of crisis.

When deciding whether spinal motion restriction is necessary (Figure 34-2), many protocols add consideration of MOI. This is because children may not be able to fully or accurately describe pain or injury like an adult.

The chapters *Principles of Pathophysiology* and *Bleeding and Shock* discussed how pediatric patients may compensate more effectively, resulting in a sudden appearance of decompensated shock. Be alert for this in the pediatric population.

Remember that you may feel more emotion or urgency when treating a pediatric patient in a multiple-trauma situation. Be sure to focus and use the knowledge and skills you have learned for the best care of the pediatric patient.

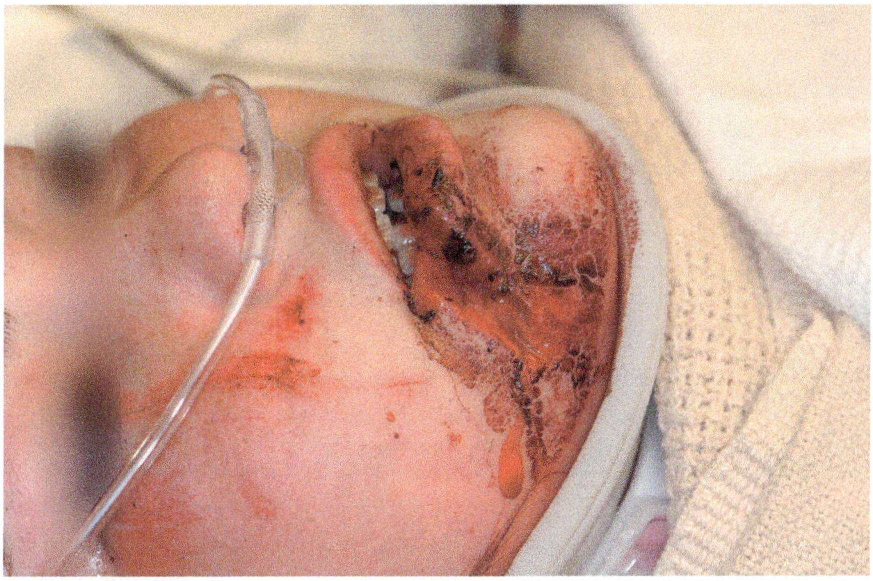

FIGURE 34-2 Child with jaw injury and potential spine injury. (*© David Effron, MD*)

CORE CONCEPT
How to calculate a trauma score

trauma score
a system of evaluating trauma patients according to a numerical rating system to determine the severity of the patient's trauma.

Trauma Scoring

In some EMS systems, hospitals ask EMTs and other providers not only to perform the usual assessment of trauma patients but also to evaluate trauma patients according to a numerical rating system. By evaluating certain patient characteristics and assigning a number to each of them, the provider can determine a ***trauma score*** that may do two things.

First, calculating the trauma score may help to determine whether a patient should go to a trauma center. A patient who needs the resources that a trauma center can provide (such as constant availability of trauma surgeons and nurses, operating rooms, and special intensive care beds) should be transported there as expeditiously as possible. In rural areas, this typically means EMS transports to the local hospital, where enough care can be provided to quickly stabilize the patient's condition before the patient is transferred to a distant trauma center. In more densely populated areas where some local hospitals are trauma centers and some are not, there will be local protocols describing when EMS should transport a patient directly to a trauma center, even if it is necessary to go past a hospital that is not a trauma center. This is where a trauma scoring system can help. By objectively describing the severity of a patient's condition, the score can direct more severely injured patients directly to trauma centers and allow less seriously injured patients to go to local hospitals.

The second major function of a trauma scoring system is to allow trauma centers to evaluate themselves in comparing the outcomes of trauma patients who have similar severity of injuries. In this way they can improve the quality of care their trauma patients receive and conduct research on trauma care.

Several systems are in use to achieve these purposes. One of the most useful and widely used is the Revised Trauma Score (RTS). The RTS evaluates three characteristics of the patient's condition: the Glasgow Coma Scale (GCS), which you learned about in the chapter on *Trauma to the Head, Neck, and Spine*, Figure 33-14; systolic blood pressure; and respiratory rate. The original trauma score included other characteristics that were difficult to evaluate consistently under field conditions and turned out to be unnecessary.

Point of View

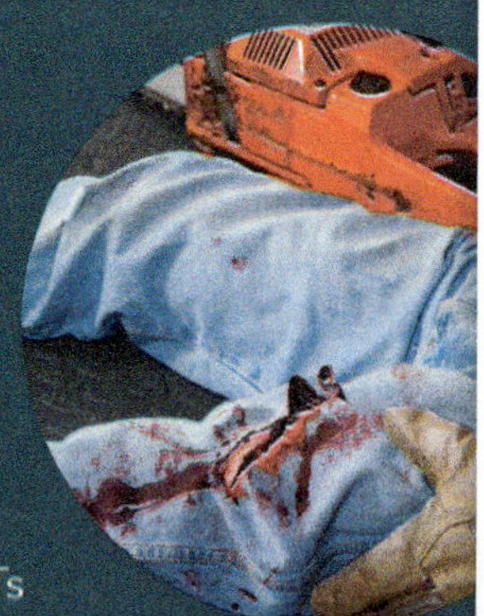

"I pulled the cord on my chainsaw. I really didn't think it would start. It had been in the garage for two or three years. Imagine my surprise when it fired up—which was nothing compared to my surprise when the saw slipped and cut into my leg.

"I don't remember much else, not even how I got to the ground. I do remember seeing blood and the room getting darker. Then I saw my wife . . . then the EMTs.

"As I came around, I figured it was just a bad cut on my leg. But the EMTs seemed pretty concerned. They were moving quickly. My wife looked worried. I heard the EMTs talking about my vital signs, and then they were moving me to the ambulance.

"On the way, I was a little more coherent. The EMTs told me that they were taking precautions because my pulse was a little high. The leg wound was pretty deep. They took me to a larger hospital close to the city—not my usual hospital. Turns out it was a good thing. I had a lot of muscle and nerve damage, and the hospital where they took me had the staff and equipment to deal with it.

"It was a tough day. My surgeon said the EMTs did a good job by realizing that my leg—and me—were in bad shape and deciding to take me to a hospital that could handle special surgery. They made a good decision—one I am very grateful for."

REVISED TRAUMA SCORE

Characteristic	Criterion	RTS Points	
Glasgow Coma Scale	13-15	4	
	9-12	3	
	6-8	2	
	4-5	1	
	3	0	
Systolic Blood Pressure	>89 mmHg	4	
	76-89 mmHg	3	
	50-75 mmHg	2	
	1-49 mmHg	1	
	0	0	
Respiratory Rate	10-29/min	4	
	>29/min	3	
	6-9/min	2	
	1-5/min	1	
	0	0	
Revised Trauma Score (Total)			

FIGURE 34-3 Revised Trauma Score. *(Data from Champion, H. R., Sacco, W. J., Copes, W.S., et al. "A Revision of the Trauma Score," The Journal Of Trauma 29(5): 623-9, 1989. Published by The Williams & Wilkins Co.)*

Figure 34-3 shows the values assigned to the EMT's assessment findings in the Revised Trauma Score. Between zero and four points are assigned for each of the elements of the RTS. The lower the score, the more serious are the injuries, and the less likely the patient is to survive, even with excellent care.

Follow your local protocols for use of a trauma scoring system, but do not let it interfere with patient care. Manage airway problems and control other immediate threats to life before trying to use a score. In some systems, EMTs are asked to determine the score en route. In others, they may be asked simply to gather all the elements used to calculate the score but not to assign numerical values. When you report this information, a physician or nurse at an emergency department can calculate the score and advise you on the appropriate destination for your patient. Follow your local protocols.

Chapter Review

Key Facts and Concepts

- Multisystem trauma is a serious condition in which two or more major body systems are injured or affected.
- Recognizing multisystem trauma, triaging properly, transporting promptly, and choosing the correct destination are vital for the survival of your patient.
- The CDC has issued guidelines for trauma triage and transport. These are a guide and should be used in conjunction with your protocols.
- The Revised Trauma Score (RTS) is one method of classifying trauma patients by severity, and includes the Glasgow Coma Scale (GCS), systolic blood pressure, and respiratory rate.

Key Decisions

- Is the patient seriously injured or potentially seriously injured?
- Should I expedite my scene time?
- Should I transport to a trauma center or ensure the patient can be transported to the trauma center (e.g., by contacting air medical evacuation services)?

Chapter Glossary

multiple trauma more than one serious injury.

multisystem trauma one or more injuries that affect more than one body system.

trauma score a system of evaluating trauma patients according to a numerical rating system to determine the severity of the patients' trauma.

Preparation for Your Examination and Practice

Short Answer

1. What considerations must the EMT weigh when considering whether to perform an intervention at the scene?
2. What are the interventions that should generally be performed for a critical trauma patient at the scene?
3. When might it be appropriate for EMTs to bypass a closer hospital for a trauma center?
4. When might it be appropriate not to apply a traction splint in the field to an obviously fractured femur?

Thinking and Linking

Think back to the chapter titled Cardiac Emergencies, *and link information from that chapter with information from this chapter as you consider the following situation:*

- Your patient is a 50-year-old male who has been electrocuted and knocked forcefully to the ground. He's an electrician who thought the power was off when it wasn't. You are taking his vital signs, which seem to be normal, when suddenly he goes into cardiac arrest. Should you use the AED and treat it as a medical arrest, or should you transport him immediately without using the AED, as for a trauma arrest? Why?

Critical Thinking Exercises

In a patient who has sustained significant trauma, making the correct transport decision is key. The purpose of this exercise will be to determine and explain the best transport decision for such a patient.

- You are called to a patient who has been involved in a crash in which the vehicle sustained significant intrusion into the area where the patient was sitting. The patient is alert and complains of pain in his ribs. His vital signs are pulse 96 and regular, respirations 30 and adequate, blood pressure 100/62, pupils equal and reactive, and skin cool and dry. Your partner says the patient is stable and could be easily transported to the community hospital nearby. You think the patient should be transported to the trauma center. How would you justify your decision to your partner?

Pathophysiology to Practice

For each of the following patients, explain why trauma triage guidelines place them at a higher priority:

1. Geriatric patients
2. Penetrating abdominal trauma patients
3. Patients who are on anticoagulants
4. Patients who have an amputated hand

Street Scenes

At 9:15 a.m. your BLS ambulance is dispatched to a busy intersection for a motor-vehicle collision. While responding, you are advised by dispatch that she has had several 911 calls regarding this collision and that there are two vehicles involved. As you arrive on scene, you observe that a full-size pickup truck apparently struck a smaller compact vehicle head-on. Your partner strategically places the ambulance to protect the scene. You notice two occupants slumped over inside the small vehicle, which has fluid draining from under the engine.

Street Scene Questions

1. What is your initial impression of the collision?
2. What additional resources will be necessary on scene?

The driver of the pickup truck walks over to you and says that he bumped his head but he feels okay. Since he can walk and talk, you move toward the smaller car. As you approach, you note that both air bags have deployed and that the leaking fluid appears to be antifreeze, which does not pose a danger. You call for additional ambulances and make sure the police are en route. The male driver is wearing a full shoulder-and-lap restraint and appears conscious but dazed. You notice his unrestrained passenger lying motionless on her left side across the console. Your primary assessment of the passenger reveals an approximately 25-year-old female responding to verbal stimuli who is verbally abusive and unaware of her surroundings. She is crying and complaining of pain to her right arm. Her airway appears clear, and you notice she has sustained severe facial trauma. Her respirations appear slightly labored and shallow. You note a strong and rapid radial pulse and warm and dry skin.

Street Scene Questions

3. **Which patient should be transported first?**
4. **What is your critical decision regarding the female patient?**
5. **What critical interventions should you perform on scene?**

You realize that the woman is the priority, because of her altered mental status and labored respirations. She has a large laceration, which extends from her upper lip up through her hairline, and you observe angulation to her right humerus. Because of the MOI and the patient's current status, you decide to perform a rapid extrication. You place a cervical collar on her and spin her onto a board. When she yells, "My baby! Don't hurt my baby!" you note her large abdomen, which is consistent with pregnancy. You place padding under the right side of the backboard, which moves the patient onto her left side. This prevents the baby from compressing the vena cava, which could lower the woman's blood pressure. You move the woman to the ambulance with 15 liters of oxygen by nonrebreather mask in place.

Once in the ambulance, you suction blood that has begun to drain into her mouth from the facial laceration. Her initial vital signs show a pulse rate of 122, slightly labored respirations at a rate of 28, and a blood pressure of 142/94. Her pupils appear equal and reactive, and you notice no fluid exiting the ears. Her neck veins are flat, and her trachea appears midline. You expose the patient, auscultate lung sounds, and find the right side sounds diminished, coinciding with tenderness to the right side of her chest. As you assess her abdomen, she winces and again yells about her baby. You recheck her arm and notice angulation and crepitus. You align it and secure her arm alongside her torso, which acts as a splint. Her remaining extremities appear unremarkable. Your patient's level of responsiveness is not reliable enough for a medical history, but you notice she is wearing a medical identification tag, which states she is allergic to sulfa medication.

Street Scene Questions

6. **What further information would you like to obtain about the female patient?**
7. **To what type of receiving facility should your patient be transported?**

While en route to the hospital, you notice the patient's heart rate has increased to 128, her blood pressure has fallen to 122/86, and she is now guarding her abdomen with her left arm. You have contacted medical direction and have been advised to transport the patient to the nearest trauma center. Upon arrival at the trauma center, you update the staff and transfer the patient to their care.

35

Environmental Emergencies

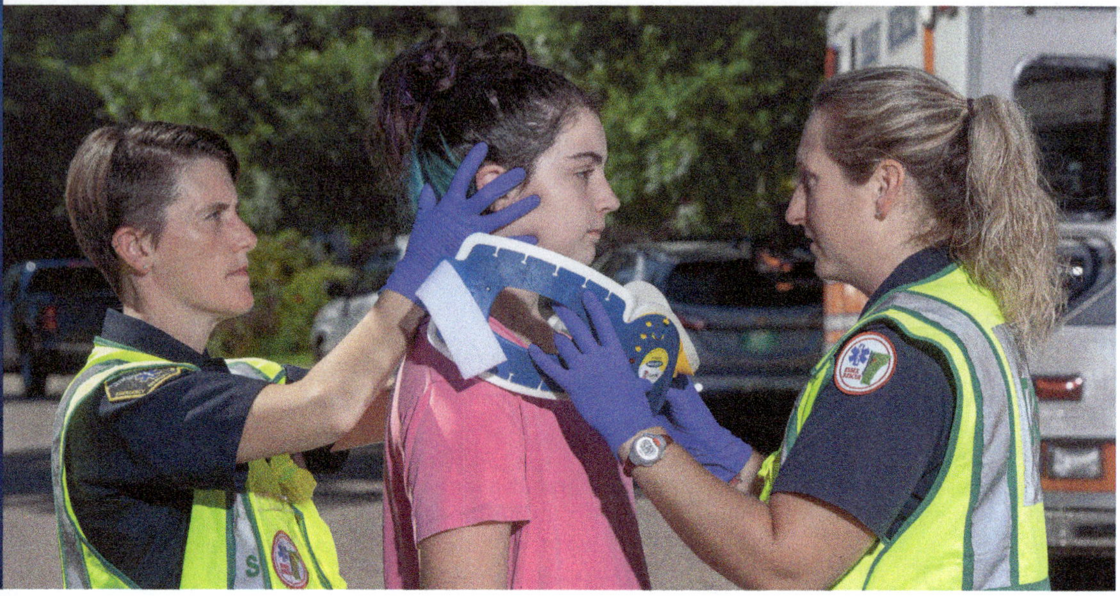

Related Chapters

The following chapters provide additional information related to topics discussed in this chapter:

1 Introduction to Emergency Medical Services
2 Well-Being of the EMT
17 Communication and Documentation
23 Allergic Reactions
25 Poisoning and Overdose Emergencies
29 Bleeding and Shock
36 Obstetric and Gynecologic Emergencies

Standard

Trauma (Environmental Emergencies)

Competency

Applies fundamental knowledge to provide basic emergency care and transportation based on assessment findings for an acutely injured patient.

Core Concepts

- Effects on the body of generalized hypothermia; assessment and care for hypothermia
- Effects on the body of local cold injuries; assessment and care for local cold injuries

- Effects on the body of exposure to heat; assessment and care for patients suffering from heat exposure
- Signs, symptoms, and treatment for drowning and other water-related injuries
- Signs, symptoms, and treatment for bites and stings
- Signs, symptoms, and treatment for high-altitude illness

Outcomes

After reading this chapter, you should be able to:

35.1 Summarize the scope of environmental emergencies. (p. 1015)

- Identify situations in which environmental emergencies may occur.
- List the general types of environmental emergencies.

35.2 Summarize the physiology and limitations of body temperature regulation. (pp. 1015–1016)

- Describe the mechanisms by which the body produces and conserves heat.
- Describe the mechanisms by which the body loses heat.
- Compare the mechanism of local cold injuries with that of generalized hypothermia.
- Describe the mechanisms underlying heat emergencies.

35.3 Recognize the presence of cold-related environmental emergencies. (pp. 1016–1018)

- Analyze environment, patient predisposing factors, and signs and symptoms to establish a suspicion for cold-related emergencies.
- Explain how age influences the suspicion for hypothermia.
- Recognize the potential for patients' becoming hypothermic as a result of another emergency or circumstance.
- Differentiate the characteristics of early and late localized cold injuries.

35.4 Summarize the approach to managing patients with cold emergencies. (pp. 1019–1025)

- Explain the significance in decision making of the finding of altered mental status in a patient with hypothermia.
- Explain how to prioritize rewarming procedures with other priorities for treatment as they are impacted by the presence of hypothermia.
- Compare the characteristics of active and passive rewarming techniques.
- Explain precautions in managing a hypothermic patient in proposed treatment plans.
- Explain the adaptation of resuscitative techniques to the severely hypothermic patient.
- Outline the management of localized cold injuries.

35.5 Recognize the presence of heat-related environmental emergencies. (pp. 1025–1026)

- Analyze environment, patient predisposing factors, and signs and symptoms to establish a suspicion for heat-related emergencies.

- Compare the heat-related emergencies most likely in patients who have moist, pale, and normal or cool skin; and those in patients who have hot, either dry or moist skin.

35.6 Summarize the approach to managing patients with heat-related environmental emergencies. (pp. 1027–1029)

- Recognize the importance of skin color and condition in the decision-making process for treating patients with suspected heat-related environmental emergencies.
- Compare the cooling techniques used for patients with cool, pale, moist, or normal skin with those used for patients with hot skin, whether dry or moist.

35.7 Explain the role of EMTs in the rescue of patients in water accidents. (pp. 1029–1031)

- List the conditions under which an EMT might reasonably consider making a water rescue.
- Describe the sequence of rescue attempts for reaching a patient in the water.
- Describe how EMTs may safely reach a patient requiring ice rescue.
- Describe considerations for starting rescue breathing with the patient still in the water.
- Describe the approach for caring for possible spinal injuries in the water.
- Anticipate injuries related to open-water diving emergencies.

35.8 Summarize the pathophysiology of a patient in a water accident. (pp. 1031–1039)

- Anticipate the types of problems that can accompany water-related accidents.
- Explain the mechanism by which drowning occurs.
- Compare the pathophysiology of air embolism and decompression sickness in scuba diving accidents.
- Compare the signs and symptoms of air embolism and decompression sickness in scuba diving accidents.

35.9 Summarize the pathophysiology of altitude illness. (pp. 1039–1041)

- Explain physiologic adaptations to high altitude.
- Describe the signs and symptoms of high-altitude illness.
- Discuss procedures to care for patients with high-altitude illness.

35.10 Differentiate the concepts of bites leading to anaphylaxis and those leading to venomous injection with localized or systemic reactions. (pp. 1041–1047)

- List information that should be gathered at the scene to determine the source of a bite.
- Recognize the assessment findings associated with dry and envenomated bites.
- Describe specific steps that are taken to manage the absorption of venom into the tissues and circulation.

Key Terms

active rewarming, *1019*
air embolism, *1035*
central rewarming, *1020*
conduction, *1015*
convection, *1015*
decompression sickness, *1035*
drowning, *1030*
evaporation, *1016*
hyperthermia, *1025*
hypothermia, *1016*
local cooling, *1022*
passive rewarming, *1019*
radiation, *1015*
respiration, *1016*
toxins, *1041*
venom, *1041*
water chill, *1015*
wind chill, *1015*

Environmental emergencies can occur in any setting—wilderness, rural, suburban, and urban areas. They include exposure to both heat and cold; drownings and other water-related injuries; high altitudes; and bites and stings from insects, spiders, snakes, and marine life. The keys to effective management are recognizing the patient's signs and symptoms and providing prompt and proper emergency care. However, as an EMT, you also must recognize that exposure may not be the only danger to the patient. Environmental emergencies can involve preexisting–or cause additional–medical problems and injuries.

Exposure to Cold

How the Body Loses Heat

If the environment is too cold, body heat can be lost faster than it can be generated. The body attempts to adjust to these temperature differences by reducing perspiration and circulation to the skin—shutting down avenues by which the body usually gets rid of excess heat. Muscular activity in the form of shivering and the rate at which fuel (food) is burned within the body both increase to produce more heat. At a certain point, however, not enough heat is generated to be available to all parts of the body. This may result in damage to exposed tissues and a general reduction or cessation of body functions.

To be able to prevent or compensate for heat loss, the EMT must be aware of the ways in which a body loses heat (Figure 35-1):

- **Conduction.** The transfer of heat from one material to another through direct contact is called ***conduction***. Heat will flow from a warmer material to a cooler one. Although body heat transferred directly into cool air is a problem, ***water chill*** is an even greater problem because water conducts heat away from the body 25 times faster than does still air. Patients with wet bodies or clothing are especially susceptible to water chill in cold environments. Heat loss through conduction can be a major problem when a person is lying on a cold floor or another cold surface. A person who is standing or walking around in cold weather will lose less heat than a person who is lying on the cold ground.
- **Convection.** When currents of air or water pass over the body, carrying away heat, ***convection*** occurs. The effects of a cold environment are worsened when moving water or air surrounds the body. ***Wind chill*** is a frequent problem. The faster the wind speed, the greater the heat loss. For example, if it is 10°F (-12.2°C) with no wind, the body will lose heat, but if there is a 20-mph (32-kph) wind, the amount of heat lost by the body is much greater.
- **Radiation.** In conduction and convection, heat is "picked up" by the surrounding (still or moving) air or water. In ***radiation***, the body's atoms and molecules send out rays of heat as they move and change. If you were in the vacuum of outer space with no air or

conduction
the transfer of heat from one material to another through direct contact.

water chill
chilling caused by conduction of heat from the body when the body or clothing is wet.

convection
carrying away of heat by currents of air, water, or other gases or liquids.

wind chill
chilling caused by convection of heat from the body in the presence of air currents.

radiation
sending out energy, such as heat, in waves into space.

FIGURE 35-1 Mechanisms of heat loss.

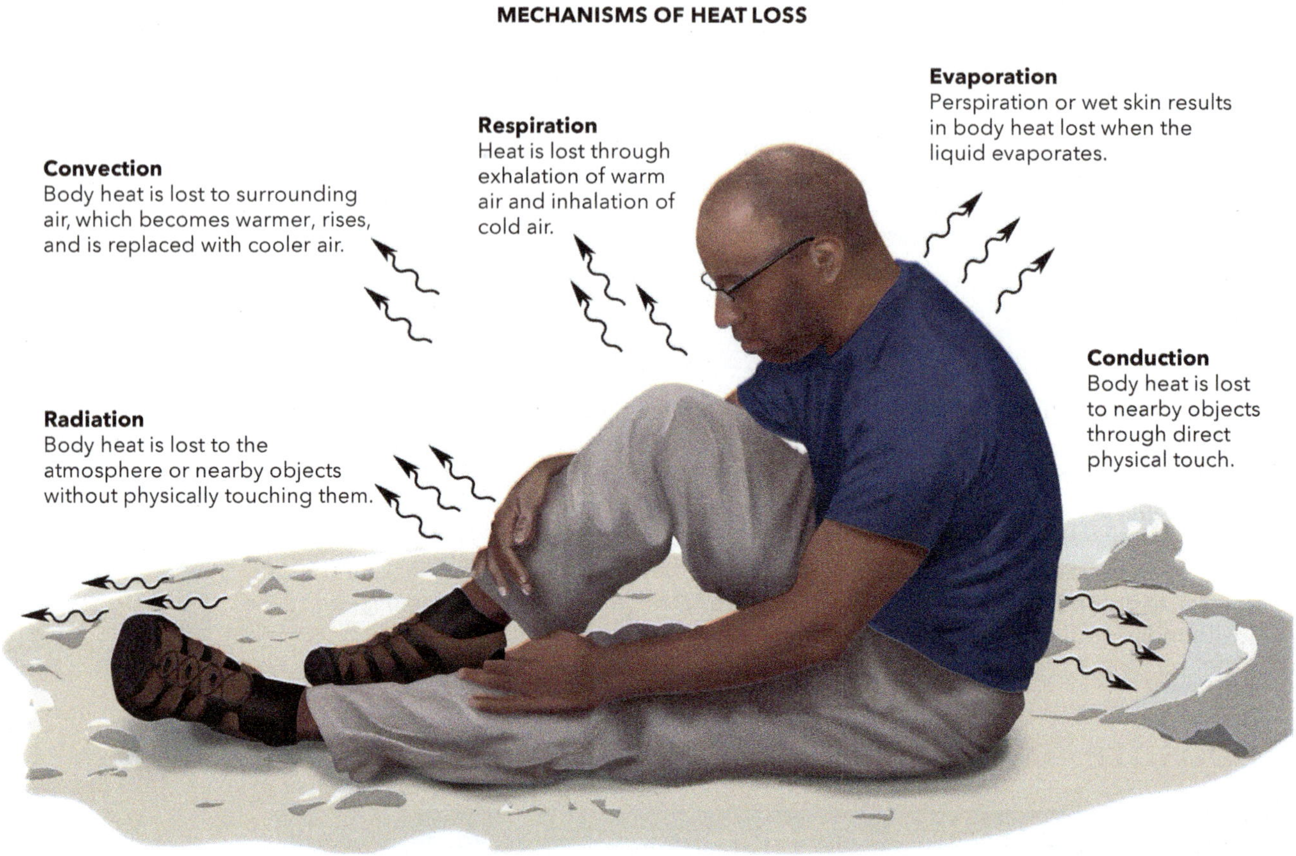

evaporation
the change from liquid to gas. When the body perspires or gets wet, evaporation of the perspiration or other liquid into the air has a cooling effect on the body.

respiration
breathing. During respiration, body heat is lost as warm air is exhaled from the body.

hypothermia
(HI-po-THURM-e-ah) generalized cooling that reduces body temperature below normal, which is a life-threatening condition in its extreme.

CORE CONCEPT

Effects on the body of generalized hypothermia; assessment and care for hypothermia

water around to pick up heat, you would still lose heat by radiating it out into space. Most radiant heat loss occurs from a person's head and neck, because other parts of the body are usually covered.

- **Evaporation.** ***Evaporation*** occurs when the body perspires or gets wet. As perspiration or water on the skin or clothing vaporizes, the body experiences a generalized cooling effect.
- **Respiration.** ***Respiration*** causes loss of body heat as a result of exhaled warm air. The amount of heat loss depends on the outside air temperature as well as the rate and depth of respirations.

Generalized Hypothermia

When cooling affects the entire body, a problem known as ***hypothermia***, or generalized cooling, develops. Exposure to cold reduces body heat. With time, the body is unable to maintain its proper core (internal) temperature. If this cooling is allowed to continue, hypothermia leads to death. The stages of hypothermia are described in Table 35-1. Although specific temperatures are listed for particular signs and symptoms, there is some variation in the temperatures at which these events occur. The sequence of signs and symptoms generally follows the signs and symptoms listed in the table.

Predisposing Factors

Patients with injuries, chronic illness, or certain other conditions will show the effects of cold much sooner than healthy persons. These conditions include shock (hypoperfusion), burns, head and spinal-cord injuries, sepsis, and diabetes with hypoglycemia. Those under the influence of alcohol or other drugs also tend to be affected more rapidly and more severely than others. The unconscious patient lying on the cold ground or another cold surface

TABLE 35-1 Stages of Hypothermia

CORE BODY TEMPERATURE		
FAHRENHEIT	**CELSIUS**	**SYMPTOMS**
99°F to 96°F	37.0°C to 35.5°C	Shivering
95°F to 91°F	35.5°C to 32.7°C	Intense shivering, difficulty speaking
90°F to 86°F	32.0°C to 30.0°C	Shivering decreases and is replaced by strong muscular rigidity. Muscle coordination is affected, and erratic or jerky movements are produced. Thinking is less clear, general comprehension is dulled, and total amnesia is possible. Patient generally is able to maintain the appearance of psychological contact with surroundings.
85°F to 81°F	29.4°C to 27.2°C	Patient becomes irrational, loses contact with the environment, and drifts into a stuporous state. Muscular rigidity continues. Pulse and respirations are slow, and cardiac dysrhythmias may develop.
80°F to 78°F	26.6°C to 20.5°C	Patient loses consciousness and does not respond to spoken words. Most reflexes cease to function. Heartbeat slows further before cardiac arrest occurs.

"Heat and cold can affect you too. Dress appropriately and plan for the weather you'll encounter out there."

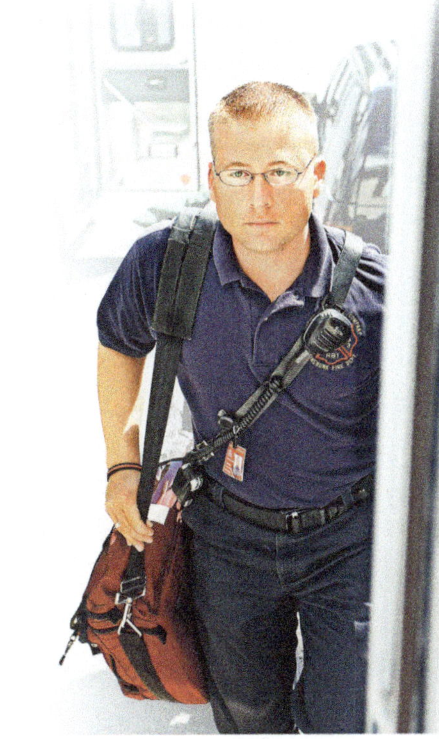

(© Daniel Limmer)

is especially prone to rapid heat loss through conduction and will tend to have greater cold-related problems than one who is conscious and able to walk around.

NOTE: *Be aware that hypothermia can develop in temperatures well above freezing.*

Obvious and Subtle Exposure

At times it is obvious that a patient has been exposed to cold and is probably suffering from hypothermia. With other patients, however, exposure is subtle—and not the first thing you might think about. The patient trapped in a wrecked auto is probably suffering a variety of injuries, but if the weather is cool and extrication from the vehicle takes a while, the patient can easily develop hypothermia as well. Consider, also, the older adult patient who has fallen during the night and is not discovered until morning. A broken hip or other injuries may claim your attention, but after being on the cold floor all night, the patient is probably also suffering from hypothermia.

Hypothermia is often an especially serious problem for older adults. The effects of cold temperatures on older people are immediate. During the winter months, older citizens on small, fixed incomes may live in unheated rooms or rooms that are kept too cool. Failing body systems, chronic illnesses, poor diets, certain medications, and lack of exercise may combine with the cold environment to bring about hypothermia.

At the other end of the spectrum of age, infants and young children have a great deal of skin surface area in relation to their total body mass and have little body fat, making them especially prone to hypothermia. Because of their small muscle mass, infants and children do not shiver very much or at all—another reason the very young are susceptible to the cold. You will learn in the chapter *Obstetric and Gynecologic Emergencies* that a crucial part of the care for newborn infants is to dry them (to prevent heat loss from evaporation) and cover their heads (to prevent heat loss by radiation and convection).

Consider the possibility of hypothermia in the following situations when another condition or injury may be more obvious:

- **Ethanol (alcohol) ingestion.** Has the intoxicated patient passed out on a cold floor or been wandering around outdoors in cool or cold weather?
- **Underlying illness.** Does the patient have a circulatory disorder or other condition that increases the patient's susceptibility to cold?

- **Overdose or poisoning.** Has the patient been lying in a cold garage or on a cold floor? Is the patient sweating heavily in a cool environment, with evaporation causing excessive heat loss?
- **Major trauma.** Has the patient been lying on the ground or trapped in wreckage during cold weather? Is shock (hypoperfusion, or inadequate circulation of the blood) preventing circulating blood from warming some parts of the body?
- **Outdoor resuscitation.** Is your patient getting too cold? If your patient is a drowning patient who has been in the water, has exposure to cool water caused hypothermia?
- **Decreased ambient temperature (for example, room temperature).** Is your patient living in a home or apartment that is too cold?

Remember that the injured patient is more susceptible to the effects of cold than would be a healthy individual. Protect the patient who is entrapped or who for any other reason must remain in a cool or cold environment for a period of time. The major course of action is to prevent additional body heat loss. It may be impractical or impossible to replace wet clothing, but you can at least create a barrier to the cold with blankets, a salvage cover, an aluminized blanket, a survival blanket, or even articles of clothing. A plastic trash bag can serve as protection from wind and water. Keep in mind that the greatest area of heat loss may be the head, so provide some sort of head covering for the patient.

When the patient's injuries allow, place a blanket between the patient and the cold ground, or between the patient's body and the wreckage. Rotate warm blankets from the heated ambulance to the patient. If the patient will remain trapped for a period of time, plug holes in the wreckage with blankets.

One way to understand the effect of wind on temperature is to look at the National Oceanic and Atmospheric Administration's National Weather Service wind chill chart (Figure 35-2). This demonstrates how even modest breezes not only have a significant impact on how temperature is perceived, but also remove heat from the body through convection. The chart has some limitations, so don't take it too literally, but look at it as a general guide to the effect of wind.

FIGURE 35-2 Wind chill chart from National Oceanic and Atmospheric Administration (NOAA's National Weather Service). With a wind speed of 5 mph, a temperature of 40°F feels like 36°F, but a temperature of 0°F feels like -11°F. Color bands indicate length of time before frostbite occurs at the different temperatures. *(National Oceanic and Atmospheric Administration)*

Wind Chill Chart

Wind (mph)	Temperature (°F)																	
Calm	40	35	30	25	20	15	10	5	0	-5	-10	-15	-20	-25	-30	-35	-40	-45
5	36	31	25	19	13	7	1	-5	-11	-16	-22	-28	-34	-40	-46	-52	-57	-63
10	34	27	21	15	9	3	-4	-10	-16	-22	-28	-35	-41	-47	-53	-59	-66	-72
15	32	25	19	13	6	0	-7	-13	-19	-26	-32	-39	-45	-51	-58	-64	-71	-77
20	30	24	17	11	4	-2	-9	-15	-22	-29	-35	-42	-48	-55	-61	-68	-74	-81
25	29	23	16	9	3	-4	-11	-17	-24	-31	-37	-44	-51	-58	-64	-71	-78	-84
30	28	22	15	8	1	-5	-12	-19	-26	-33	-39	-46	-53	-60	-67	-73	-80	-87
35	28	21	14	7	0	-7	-14	-21	-27	-34	-41	-48	-55	-62	-69	-76	-82	-89
40	27	20	13	6	-1	-8	-15	-22	-29	-36	-43	-50	-57	-64	-71	-78	-84	-91
45	26	19	12	5	-2	-9	-16	-23	-30	-37	-44	-51	-58	-65	-72	-79	-86	-93
50	26	19	12	4	-3	-10	-17	-24	-31	-38	-45	-52	-60	-67	-74	-81	-88	-95
55	25	18	11	4	-3	-11	-18	-25	-32	-39	-46	-54	-61	-68	-75	-82	-89	-97
60	25	17	10	3	-4	-11	-19	-26	-33	-40	-48	-55	-62	-69	-76	-84	-91	-98

Frostbite Times: 30 minutes; 10 minutes; 5 minutes

$$\text{Wind Chill } (^{\circ}F) = 35.74 + 0.6215T - 35.75(V^{0.16}) + 0.4275T(V^{0.16})$$

Where, T= Air Temperature (°F) V= Wind Speed (mph)

Effective 11/01/01

Patient Assessment

Hypothermia

Consider the impact of the following factors when assessing a patient: air temperature; wind chill and/or water chill; the patient's age; the patient's clothing; the patient's health, including underlying illness and existing injuries; how active the patient was during exposure; and possible alcohol or drug use.

The following list contains common signs and symptoms of hypothermia. Note that decreasing mental status and decreasing motor function both correlate with the degree of hypothermia:

- Shivering in early stages when the core body temperature is above 90°F (32°C). In severe cases, shivering decreases or is absent.
- Numbness, or reduced or lost sense of touch
- Stiff or rigid posture in prolonged cases
- Drowsiness and/or unwillingness or inability to do even the simplest activities. In prolonged exposures, the patient may become irrational, drift into a stuporous state, or actually remove clothing.
- Rapid breathing and rapid pulse in early stages, and slow or absent breathing and pulse in prolonged cases. (The patient's slow pulse and respirations require that you spend at least 60 seconds performing a check for a pulse and respirations.) Blood pressure may be low or undetectable.
- Loss of motor coordination, such as poor balance, staggering, or inability to hold things
- Joint/muscle stiffness, or muscular rigidity
- Decreased level of consciousness or unconsciousness. In extreme cases, the patient has a "glassy stare."
- Cool abdominal skin temperature (Place your hand inside the clothing, with the back of your hand against the patient's abdomen.)
- Skin may appear red in early stages. In prolonged cases, skin is pale or cyanotic. In most extreme cases, some body parts are stiff and hard (frozen).

During primary assessment, be sure to check awake patients' orientation to person, place, and time. (Can they tell you their name? Where they are? What day it is?) Perform a secondary assessment to help you estimate the extent of hypothermia. Assume severe hypothermia if shivering is absent.

Decision Point

- Does the patient have an altered mental status?

Passive and Active Rewarming

Passive rewarming allows the body to rewarm itself. It involves simply covering the patient and taking other steps, including removal of wet clothing, to prevent further heat loss. These actions allow the body to naturally regain its warmth. ***Active rewarming*** includes application of an external heat source to the body. All EMS systems permit passive rewarming. Although some allow the active rewarming of a hypothermic patient who is alert and responding appropriately, many do not. Follow your local protocols.

Active external rewarming is more complicated than simple passive rewarming. If you are allowed to rewarm a patient with hypothermia who is alert and responding

passive rewarming covering a hypothermic patient and taking other steps to prevent further heat loss and help the body rewarm itself.

active rewarming application of an external heat source to rewarm the body of a hypothermic patient.

appropriately, do not delay transport. Rewarm the patient while en route. The emergency care steps that follow assume a protocol that permits active rewarming of a patient who is alert and responding appropriately to your intervention. Follow your local protocols.

Patient Care

Care of the Hypothermic Patient Who is Alert and Responding Appropriately

Fundamental Principles of Care

All patients with hypothermia should have their wet clothes removed. When the patient is alert, hypothermia is mild, and it is safe to warm the patient actively.

For the hypothermic patient who is alert and responding appropriately, proceed with active rewarming, generally in the following order:

- Remove all of the patient's wet clothing. Keep the patient dry and dress the patient in dry clothing or wrap in dry, warm blankets. Keep the patient still and handle very gently. Do not allow the patient to walk or otherwise engage in physical activity. Do not massage the patient's extremities.
- During transport, actively rewarm the patient. Gently apply heat to the patient's body in the form of heat packs, hot water bottles, electric heating pads, warm air, radiated heat, and even your own body heat. Do not warm the patient too quickly. Rapid warming will circulate peripherally stagnated cold blood and rapidly cool the vital central areas of the body, possibly causing cardiac arrest. If transport is delayed, move the patient to a warm environment if at all possible.
- Give the alert patient warm liquids at a slow rate. When warm fluids are given too quickly, the patient's circulation patterns change. Blood is sent away from the core and instead routed to the skin and extremities. Do not allow the patient to eat or drink stimulants.
- Except in the mildest of cases (shivering), transport the patient. Continue to monitor vital signs. Never allow a patient to remain in or return to a cold environment.

Take the following precautions when actively rewarming a patient:

- Rewarm the patient slowly. Handle the patient with great care. Avoid rough handling such as a sudden stretcher drop or rough transfer to the emergency department stretcher.
- Use ***central rewarming***. Heat should be applied to the lateral chest, neck, armpits, and groin first. You must avoid rewarming the limbs. If they are warmed first, blood will collect in the extremities due to vasodilation (dilation of blood vessels), possibly causing shock. (See the chapter titled *Bleeding and Shock*).
- Keep the patient at rest. Do not allow the patient to walk. Since the blood is coldest in the extremities, exercise or unnecessary movement could quickly circulate the cold blood and lower the core body temperature.
- Avoid any rough handling of all hypothermic patients. Such activity may set off fatal dysrhythmias, especially ventricular fibrillation.

central rewarming
application of heat to the lateral chest, neck, armpits, and groin of a hypothermic patient.

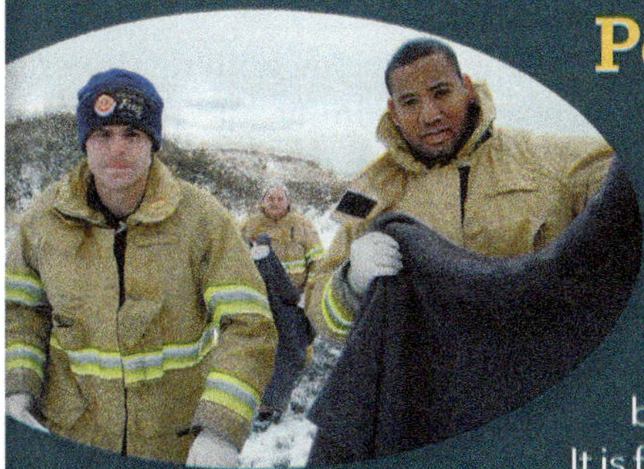

Point of View

"I was riding my horse on the beach. It is a wonderful feeling. Well, it was until I got thrown. Now, I've been thrown before, and you get back up. This time I broke bones.

"To make it worse, it was winter. No one was around.

"I shivered for a while. I yelled and yelled. I tried to move but no luck. Then I stopped shivering and started to get tired. It is funny looking back on that day. I kind of relaxed there at the end. Now I know that means I was on the final glide path. I was heading out.

"Someone finally saw the horse just standing there and came over to figure out why. By that time, I was like an ice cube.

"I remember the EMTs coming along and warming me up. Blanket after blanket and the heat in the ambulance was blasting. Those guys must've been boiling. I'm very thankful for them—and for the person that finally called for help. Without them, I wouldn't be telling this story."

Patient Care

Care of the Hypothermic Patient Who is Unresponsive or not Responding Appropriately

Fundamental Principles of Care

A patient who is unresponsive or not responding appropriately has severe hypothermia. For this patient, provide passive rewarming. Do not try to actively rewarm the patient with severe hypothermia. Remove the patient from the environment and protect from further heat loss. Active rewarming may cause the patient to develop ventricular fibrillation and other complications. Active rewarming can be initiated after arrival at the emergency department in a more monitored setting.

For the patient with severe hypothermia, you should take the following steps:

- Ensure an open airway.
- Provide high-concentration oxygen that has been passed through a warm-water humidifier. This promotes internal rewarming in addition to increasing the patient's blood oxygen level. If warmed oxygen is not available, follow your local protocols. Consulting medical direction may be helpful in determining whether to give regular oxygen (which can run the risk of cooling the patient further) or to allow the patient to breathe ambient air. Oxygen demands are considerably lower in a severely hypothermic patient, so ambient air may be the best treatment. Management of severe hypothermia is an area of continuing research, and local protocols vary.
- Wrap the patient in blankets. If available, use insulating blankets. Handle the patient as gently as possible, as rough handling may cause ventricular fibrillation. Do not allow the patient with altered mental status or unresponsive hypothermia to eat or drink. Do not massage the patient's extremities.
- Transport the patient immediately.

Extreme Hypothermia

In cases of extreme hypothermia, you will find the patient unconscious with no discernible vital signs. The heart rate can slow to fewer than 10 beats per minute, and the patient will feel very cold to your touch. (Core body temperature may be below 80°F [26.7°C].) Even so, it is possible that a patient in this condition is still alive! Provide emergency care as follows:

- Assess the carotid pulse for at least 60 seconds. If there is no pulse, start CPR immediately and prepare to apply the AED.
- If there is a pulse, follow the care steps for a patient who is unresponsive or not responding appropriately as previously listed.

When to start chest compressions in the extremely hypothermic patient remains controversial. Follow your local protocols and contact on-line medical direction for advice and other orders.

Because the hypothermic patient might not reach biological death for more than 30 minutes, the hospital staff will not pronounce a patient dead until after they have rewarmed the patient and applied resuscitative measures. This means you cannot assume that a severe hypothermia patient is dead on the basis of body temperature and lack of vital signs. As medical personnel point out, "You're not dead until you're warm and dead!"

Local Cold Injuries and Frostbite

local cooling
cooling or freezing of particular (local) parts of the body.

CORE CONCEPT
Effects on the body of local cold injuries; assessment and care for local cold injuries

Cold-related emergencies also can result from ***local cooling***. Local cooling injuries—those affecting particular (local) parts of the body—are classified as (1) early or superficial and (2) late or deep.

Local cooling most commonly affects the ears, nose, face, hands and fingers, and feet and toes. When a part of the body is exposed to intense cold, blood flow to that part is limited by the constriction of blood vessels. When this happens, tissues freeze. Ice crystals can form in the skin, and in the most severe cases, gangrene (localized tissue death) can set in, which may ultimately lead to the loss of the body part.

As you read the following pages, notice how the signs and symptoms of early or superficial cold injuries are progressive. First, the exposed skin reddens in light-skinned individuals. In dark-skinned individuals, the skin color lightens and approaches a blanched (reduced-color or whitened) condition. Regardless of skin color, as exposure continues, the skin takes on a gray or white blotchy appearance. Exposed skin becomes numb because of reduced circulation. If the freezing process continues, all sensation is lost and the skin becomes dead white.

Patient Assessment

Early or Superficial Local Cold Injury

Early or superficial local cold injuries (sometimes called frostnip) are brought about by direct contact with a cold object or exposure to cold air. Wind chill and water chill also can be major factors. In this condition, tissue damage is minor, and response to care is good. The tip of the nose, tips of the ears, upper cheeks, and fingers (all areas that are usually exposed) are most susceptible to early or superficial local cold injuries. The injury, as its name suggests, is localized, with clear demarcation of its limits. Patients are often unaware of the onset of an early local cold injury until someone indicates that there is something unusual about the person's skin color. The following list contains common signs and symptoms:

- The affected area in patients with light skin reddens; in patients with dark skin, it lightens. Both then blanch (whiten). Once blanching begins, the color change can take place very quickly.
- The affected area feels numb to the patient.

Patient Care

Care of the Patient with an Early or Superficial Local Cold Injury

Fundamental Principles of Care

Treating frostnip involves preventing further injury and rewarming the affected area.

Emergency care for early local cold injury is as follows:

- Get the patient out of the cold environment.
- Warm the affected area.
- If the injury is to an extremity, splint and cover it. Do not rub or massage the area, and do not re-expose it to the cold.
- Patients can often help warm affected areas of local cold injury. They can cup their warm hands over their ears, or if fingers are involved, they can blow warm air on the site or place them in their armpits for warmth. During recovery from an early local cold injury, the patient may complain about tingling or burning sensations, which is normal. If the condition does not respond to this simple care, begin to treat for a late or deep local cold injury.

Patient Assessment

Late or Deep Local Cold Injury (Frostbite)

Late or deep local cold injury (also known as frostbite) develops if an early or superficial local cold injury goes untreated. In late or deep local cold injury, the skin and subcutaneous layers of the body part are affected. Muscles, bones, deep blood vessels, and organ membranes can become frozen. The following list contains common signs and symptoms of this condition:

- Affected skin appears white and waxy. When the condition progresses to actual freezing, the skin turns mottled or blotchy, and the color turns from white to grayish yellow and finally to grayish blue (Figure 35-3A). Swelling and blistering may also occur.
- In deep cold injury, some soft-tissue death will occur. Several days after the injury, viable tissue will become evident as compared with the dark black (dead) necrotic tissue (Figure 35-3B). This condition will require surgery.

NOTE: *Do not squeeze or poke the tissue. The condition of the deeper tissues can be determined by gently feeling the area. Do the assessment as if the affected area had a fractured bone.*

FIGURE 35-3 (A) Foot showing tissue damage from acute frostbite. (B) Delayed tissue loss from frostbite four days after local cold injury *(Both photos: © Edward T. Dickinson, MD)*

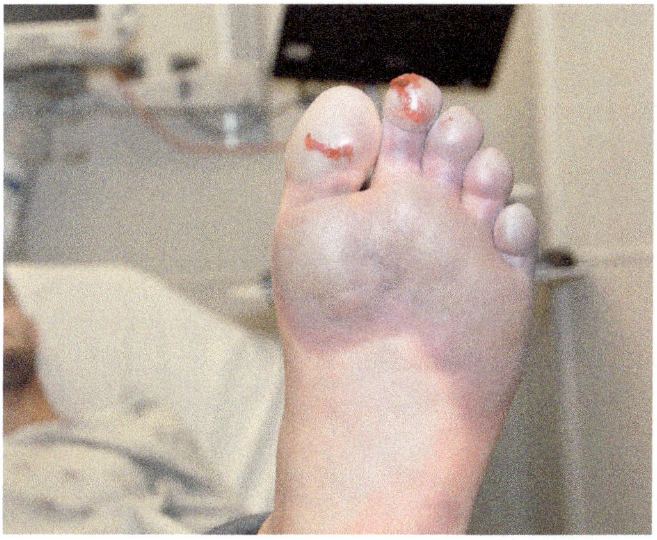

A

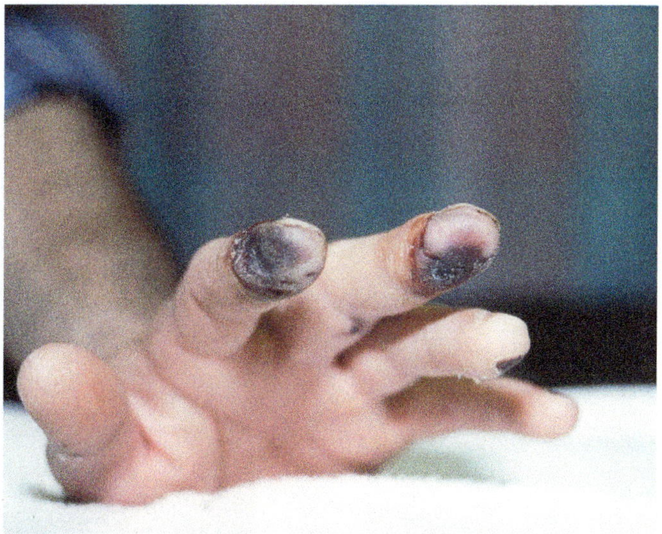

B

Patient Care

Care of the Patient with a Late or Deep Local Cold Injury

Fundamental Principles of Care

Treatment of frostbite focuses on prevention of further injury and transport to definitive care.

Initial emergency care for late or deep local cold injury–frostbite and freezing–is as follows:

- Oxygen. If there are signs of hypoxia, or the patient's vital signs indicate or suggest the potential for shock, administer oxygen.
- Transport to a medical facility without delay, protecting the frostbitten or frozen area by covering it and handling it as gently as possible.
- If transport must be delayed, get the patient indoors and maintain warmth. Do not allow the patient to drink alcohol or smoke, because constriction of blood vessels and decreased circulation to the injured tissues may result. Rewarm the frozen part as per local protocol, or request instructions from medical direction.

NOTE: *Never listen to myths and folktales about the care of frostbite. Never rub a frostbitten or frozen area. Never rub snow on a frostbitten or frozen area. There are ice crystals at the capillary level; rubbing the injury site may cause serious damage to the already-injured tissues. Do not break blisters or massage the injured area. Do not allow the patient to walk on an affected extremity. Do not thaw a frozen limb if there is any chance it will be refrozen.*

Active Rapid Rewarming of Frozen Parts

Active rewarming of frozen parts is seldom recommended. The chance of permanently injuring frozen tissues with active rewarming is too great. Consider it only if local protocols recommend it, if you are instructed to do so by medical direction, or if transport will be severely delayed and you cannot reach medical direction for instructions. If you are in a situation where you must attempt rapid rewarming without instructions from a physician, follow the procedure described here.

You will need warm water and a container in which you can immerse the entire site of injury without the limb touching the sides or bottom of the container. If you cannot find a suitable container, fashion one from a plastic bag supported by a cardboard box or wooden crate (Figure 35-4). Proceed as follows:

- Heat water to between 100°F and 105°F (37.8°C and 40.6°C). You should be able to put your finger into the water without experiencing discomfort. As you warm the water, request advanced life support. Rewarming a frostbitten extremity is extremely painful for the patient, and pain management is an important part of the treatment.

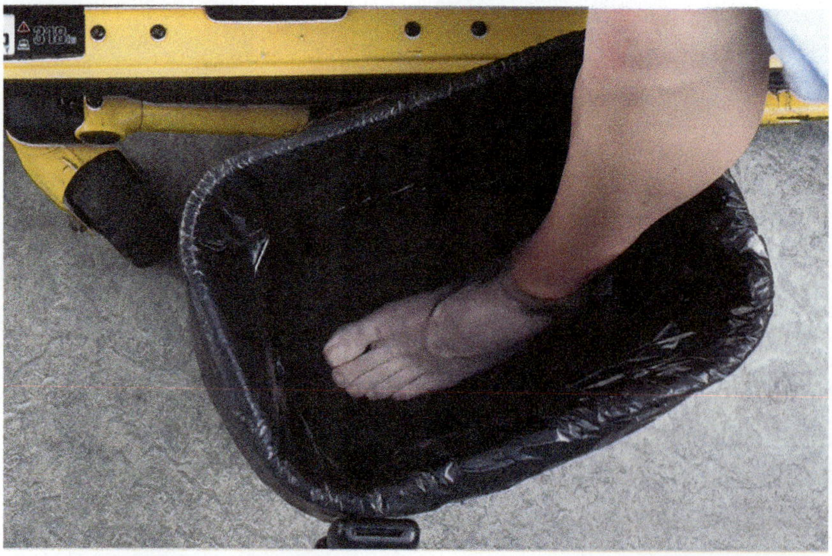

FIGURE 35-4 Rewarming the frozen part.

- Fill the container with the heated water, and prepare the injured part by removing clothing, jewelry, bands, or straps. Thawed areas often swell, so you need to remove potentially constricting items beforehand.
- Fully immerse the injured part. Avoid allowing the injured area to touch the sides or bottom of the container as much as possible. Do not place any pressure on the affected part. Continuously stir the water. When the water cools below 100°F (37.8°C), remove the affected part and add more warm water. The patient may complain of moderate or even intense pain as the affected area rewarms. Pain is usually a good indicator of successful rewarming.
- If you complete rewarming of the part (it no longer feels frozen and is turning red or blue), gently dry the affected area, and apply a dry sterile dressing. Place dry sterile dressings between the patient's fingers and toes before dressing the patient's hands and feet. Next, cover the site with blankets or whatever is available to keep the area warm. Do not allow these coverings to come in direct contact with the injured area or to put pressure on the site. First try to build some sort of framework on which the coverings can be placed.
- Keep the patient at rest. Do not allow the patient to walk if a frostbitten or frozen lower extremity has been rewarmed.
- Make certain that you keep the entire patient as warm as possible without overheating. Cover the patient's head with a towel or small blanket to reduce heat loss. Leave the patient's face exposed.
- Continue to monitor the patient.
- Do not allow the limb to refreeze.
- Transport as soon as possible with the affected limb slightly elevated.

Exposure to Heat

Effects of Heat on the Body

The body generates heat as a result of its constant internal chemical processes. A certain amount of this heat is required to maintain normal body temperature. Any heat that is not needed for temperature maintenance must be lost from the body. If it is not, the result is ***hyperthermia***, an abnormally high body temperature. If left unchecked, it will lead to death. Heat and humidity are often associated with hyperthermia.

As you learned earlier, heat is lost through the lungs or the skin. Mechanisms of heat loss include conduction, convection, radiation, evaporation, and respiration. Consider what can happen to the body in a hot environment. Air being inhaled is warm, possibly warmer than the air being exhaled. The skin may absorb more heat than it loses. When high humidity is added, the evaporation of perspiration slows. To make things even more difficult, all this can happen in an environment that lacks circulating air or a breeze which would increase convective and evaporative heat loss.

Since evaporative heat loss is reduced in a humid environment, moist heat can produce dramatic body changes in a short time. Moist heat usually tires people quickly and frequently stops them from harming themselves through overexertion. Dry heat, in contrast, often deceives people. They continue to work or remain exposed to excess heat far beyond what their bodies can tolerate.

A way to understand the impact of humidity on heat perception is to look at the NOAA's National Weather Service heat index chart (Figure 35-5). It shows how, especially at high temperatures, even a modest amount of humidity can make it significantly more difficult to get rid of excess heat. Like the wind chill chart, it has limitations, so don't take it too literally. Instead, view it as a way to understand some of the body's limitations in managing exposure to heat.

The same rules of care apply to heat emergencies as to any other emergency. You will need to perform the appropriate steps of assessment, remaining alert for problems other than those related to heat. Collapse due to heat exhaustion, for example, may result in a

CORE CONCEPT

Effects on the body of exposure to heat; assessment and care for patients suffering from heat exposure

hyperthermia
(HI-per-THURM-e-ah)
an increase in body temperature above normal, which is a life-threatening condition in its extreme.

FIGURE 35-5 Heat index chart from the NOAA's National Weather Service. Both relative humidity and temperature affect heat sensation. With a relative humidity of 40 percent, a temperature of 80°F feels like 80°F, but a relative humidity of 95 percent makes that same 80°F feel like 86°F. At relative humidity of 40, a temperature of 80°F feels like 80°F, but a temperature of 104°F feels like 119°F. *(National Oceanic and Atmospheric Administration)*

NWS Heat Index — Temperature (°F)

Relative Humidity (%)	80	82	84	86	88	90	92	94	96	98	100	102	104	106	108	110
40	80	81	83	85	88	91	94	97	101	105	109	114	119	124	130	136
45	80	82	84	87	89	93	96	100	104	109	114	119	124	130	137	
50	81	83	85	88	91	95	99	103	108	113	118	124	131	137		
55	81	84	86	89	93	97	101	106	112	117	124	130	137			
60	82	84	88	91	95	100	105	110	116	123	129	137				
65	82	85	89	93	98	103	108	114	121	128	136					
70	83	86	90	95	100	105	112	119	126	134						
75	84	88	92	97	103	109	116	124	132							
80	84	89	94	100	106	113	121	129								
85	85	90	96	102	110	117	126	135								
90	86	91	98	105	113	122	131									
95	86	93	100	108	117	127										
100	87	95	103	112	121	132										

Likelihood of Heat Disorders with Prolonged Exposure or Strenuous Activity

Caution | Extreme Caution | Danger | Extreme Danger

fall that can fracture bones. Preexisting conditions such as dehydration, diabetes, fever, fatigue, high blood pressure, heart disease, lung problems, and obesity may hasten or intensify the effects of heat exposure, as will ingestion of alcohol or other drugs.

Age, diseases, and existing injuries all must be considered. The elderly may be affected by poor thermoregulation, prescription medications, and lack of mobility. Newborns and infants also may have poor thermoregulation. Always consider the problem to be greater if the patient is a child or elderly person who is injured or living with a chronic disease.

Patient with Moist, Pale, and Normal or Cool Skin (Heat Exhaustion)

Prolonged exposure to excessive heat can create an emergency in which the patient presents with moist, pale skin that may feel normal or cool to the touch, a condition generally known as *heat exhaustion*. The individual perspires heavily, often drinking large quantities of water. As sweating continues, the body loses salts, bringing on painful muscle cramps (sometimes called *heat cramps*). A person who is strenuously exercising can lose more than a liter of fluid through perspiration per hour.

Healthy individuals who have been exposed to excessive heat while working or exercising may experience a form of shock brought about by fluid and salt loss. This condition is often seen among firefighters, construction workers, dockworkers, and those employed in poorly ventilated warehouses. It is a particular problem during prolonged heat waves early in the summer, before people have become acclimatized to summer heat.

Patient Assessment

Heat Emergency Patient with Moist, Pale, and Normal or Cool Skin

The following are common signs and symptoms of a heat emergency patient with moist, pale, and normal or cool skin:

- Muscle cramps, usually in the legs and abdomen
- Weakness or exhaustion, and sometimes dizziness or periods of faintness
- Rapid, shallow breathing
- Weak pulse
- Heavy perspiration
- Loss of consciousness is possible but is usually brief if it occurs.

Decision Point

- What is the color and condition of the patient's skin?

Patient Care

Care of the Heat Emergency Patient with Moist, Pale, and Normal or Cool Skin

Fundamental Principles of Care

Care of the patient with heat exhaustion centers on preventing further exposure to heat and on transport to definitive care. In very mild cases, if no nausea or vomiting is present, EMTs can start the rehydration process.

Emergency care of a heat emergency patient with moist, pale, and normal or cool skin includes the following steps, generally in this order:

- Remove the patient from the hot environment and place in a cool environment (such as in shade or an air-conditioned ambulance).
- If there are signs of hypoxia, or the patient's vital signs indicate or suggest the potential for shock, administer oxygen.
- Loosen or remove clothing and cool the patient by fanning without chilling the patient. Watch for shivering.
- Put the patient in a supine position. Keep the patient at rest.
- If the patient is responsive and not nauseated, and you will not transport, give the patient small sips of water to drink. If this causes nausea or vomiting, do not give any more water. Be alert for vomiting and airway problems. If the patient is unresponsive or vomiting, do not give water. Transport to the hospital with patient lying on the left side.
- If the patient experiences muscle cramps, apply moist towels over cramped muscles.
- Transport the patient.

Decision Point

- What is the color and condition of the patient's skin?

Patient with Hot Skin, Whether Dry or Moist (Heat Stroke)

When a person's temperature-regulating mechanisms fail and the body cannot rid itself of excessive heat, you will see a patient with hot skin that is either dry or moist. When the skin is hot—whether dry or moist—this condition, generally known as *heat stroke,* is a true emergency. The problem is compounded when, in response to loss of fluid and salt, the patient stops sweating, which prevents heat loss through evaporation. Athletes, laborers, and others who exercise or work in hot environments are especially at risk for this condition, as are elderly persons who live in poorly ventilated apartments without air conditioning, and children left in cars with the windows rolled up.

Patient Assessment

Heat Emergency Patient with Hot Skin, Whether Dry or Moist

The following are common signs and symptoms of a heat emergency patient with hot and dry or hot and moist skin:

- Loss of consciousness or altered mental status (Altered mental status must be present for a determination of heat stroke.)
- Rapid, shallow breathing
- Full and rapid pulse
- Generalized weakness

- Little or no perspiration
- Dilated pupils
- Potential seizures; no muscle cramps

Decision Point

- What is the color and condition of the patient's skin?

Patient Care

Care of the Heat Emergency Patient with Hot Skin, Whether Dry or Moist

Fundamental Principles of Care

Caring for a patient in heat stroke includes preventing further exposure to heat and providing immediate, aggressive cooling to prevent brain damage and other life-threatening consequences of this condition.

Emergency care of a heat emergency patient with hot and dry or hot and moist skin includes the following (Figure 35-6):

- Remove the patient from the hot environment, and place in a cool environment (in the ambulance with the air conditioner running on high).
- Remove the patient's clothing. Apply cool packs to the neck, groin, and armpits. Keep the skin wet by applying water by sponge or wet towels. Aggressively fan the patient. For infants or young children, start cooling with tepid (lukewarm) water. This water can then be replaced with cooler water at the recommendation of medical direction.
- Administer high-concentration oxygen.
- Transport immediately. If transport is delayed, continue to attempt to cool the patient with ice packs. In addition, you can cover the patient with a sheet, wet it, and fan the patient to enhance heat loss by evaporation.

FIGURE 35-6 Aggressively cool in a heat emergency where the patient's skin is hot and either dry or moist.

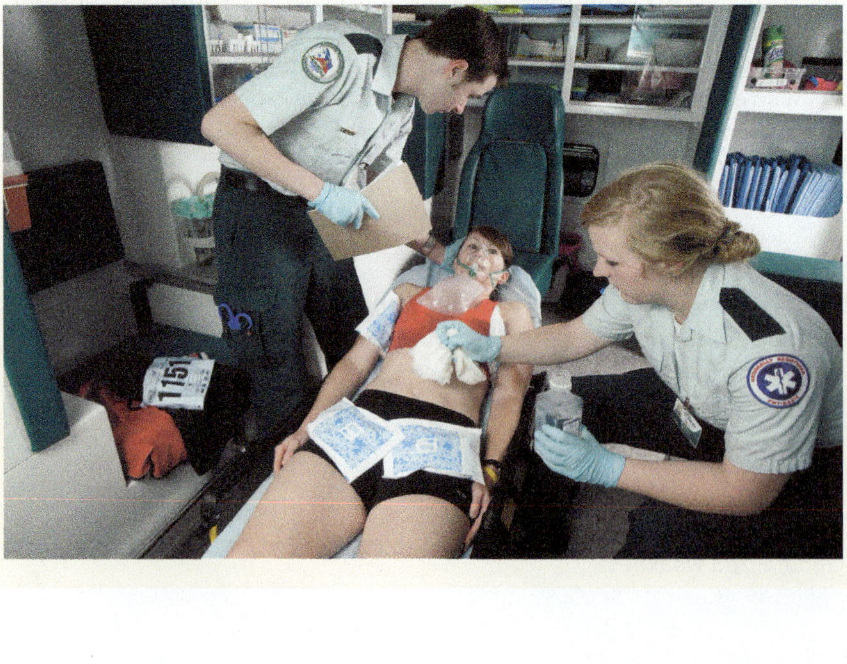

Beware of what you are told by some patients. They may not believe heat emergencies are serious. Many simply want to return to work once they are awake and feeling better. Nevertheless, conduct a thorough primary assessment plus a secondary assessment. If you have any doubts about the patient's condition, explain why transport to a hospital is important and seek permission to do so. You may have to spend a little time with some patients to gain their confidence.

The Dangers of Extreme Body Temperatures

Hypothermia and hyperthermia are serious conditions that, when not treated, can lead to death.

As a person's body temperature decreases, the body undergoes many changes. The cardiovascular and central nervous systems are perhaps the most affected by hypothermia, but the body attempts to prevent them from being affected. At first, the muscles shiver in order to increase heat production. Core temperature is generally preserved, with at most a drop of just a few degrees. This is reflected in hypothermia with normal mental status.

As heat continues to be lost, the heart becomes more irritable and prone to dysrhythmias. The central nervous system becomes more sluggish and less responsive. At about 91.5°F (33°C), electrical activity in the brain becomes abnormal. This is reflected in hypothermia with altered mental status.

When the problem is excess heat, on the other hand, the body at first prevents hyperthermia with sweating that leads to evaporation and then cool skin. Body temperature is balanced between inside and outside temperatures, and normal core temperature is preserved. This is reflected in cool skin.

At some point, if excess heat continues to build up, the body is no longer able to rid itself of that heat. Since the skin is the major cooling mechanism of the body, when it is hot, it indicates that this system is no longer able to dissipate enough heat to maintain a normal body temperature, and rapid cooling is necessary. A core temperature that has reached about 105.8°F (41°C) is at the critical point, though significant damage can occur before then. This is reflected in hyperthermia with hot skin.

Water-Related Emergencies

Water-Related Accidents

Drowning is the first thing people think of in connection with water-related accidents. However, there are many types of injuries resulting from many types of accidents that can occur on or in the water. Boating, water-skiing, wind-surfing, jet-skiing, diving, and scuba-diving accidents can produce fractured bones, bleeding, soft-tissue injuries, and airway obstructions. Even auto collisions can send vehicles or passengers into the water, resulting in any of the injuries usually associated with motor-vehicle collisions as well as the complications caused by the presence of water.

Medical problems such as heart attacks can also cause, or be caused by, water accidents, or can simply take place in, on, or near the water. Remember, too, that some water accidents happen far away from pools, lakes, or beaches. For example, bathtub drownings do occur. Adults as well as children can drown in only a few inches of water.

CORE CONCEPT
Signs, symptoms, and treatment for drowning and other water-related injuries

NOTE: *Do not attempt a rescue in which you must enter deep water or swim unless you have been trained to do so and are a very good swimmer. Except for shallow pools and open shallow waters with uniform bottoms, the problems faced in water rescue are too great and too dangerous for the poor swimmer or untrained person. If this bothers you—having to stand by, not being able to help—then take a course in water safety and rescue. (Both the American Red Cross and the YMCA offer water safety and rescue courses.) Otherwise, if you attempt a deep-water or swimming rescue, you will probably become a patient yourself.*

Patient Assessment

Water-Related Accidents

Learn to look for the following problems in water-related-incident patients:

- **Airway obstruction.** This may be from water in the lungs, foreign matter in the airway, or swollen airway tissues (which are common if the neck is injured in a dive). Spasms of the vocal cords may be present in some cases of drowning.
- **Cardiac arrest.** This often is related to respiratory arrest or occurs before drowning.
- **Signs of heart attack.** Some untrained rescuers too quickly conclude that chest pains are due to muscle cramps as a result of swimming.
- **Injuries to the head and neck.** These are expected to be found in boating, water-skiing, and diving accidents.
- **Internal injuries.** While doing the physical exam, stay on the alert for musculoskeletal injuries, soft-tissue injuries, and internal bleeding.
- **Generalized cooling, or hypothermia.** The water does not have to be very cold and the length of stay in the water does not have to be very long for hypothermia to occur.
- **Substance abuse.** Alcohol and drug use are closely associated with adolescent and adult drownings. Elevated blood alcohol levels have been found in more than 30 percent of drowning patients. The screening for drug use has not been as extensive as that done for alcohol, but research indicates that other drugs are a contributory factor in many water-related accidents.
- **Drowning.** Patients may be discovered under or facedown in the water. They may be unconscious and without discernible vital signs, or they may be conscious, breathing, and coughing up water.

Provide assessment and care for any of the previously noted problems as you have learned in other chapters of this text. Drowning is discussed in detail next.

Drowning

drowning
the process of experiencing respiratory impairment from submersion/immersion in liquid, which may result in death, morbidity (illness or other adverse effects), or no morbidity.

In 2002, the World Health Organization (WHO) adopted a definition of ***drowning*** that is different from the traditional one. According to the WHO, "Drowning is the process of experiencing respiratory impairment from submersion/immersion in liquid. Drowning outcomes are classified as death, morbidity, and no morbidity." *Morbidity* means the patient experiences illness or other adverse effects, such as unconsciousness or pneumonia. The American Heart Association has also adopted this definition of drowning. The WHO definition does not describe near drowning. Hence, the term *near drowning* is no longer used.

The process of drowning often begins as a person struggles to keep afloat in the water. The person gulps in large breaths of air while thrashing about. When individuals can no longer keep afloat and start to submerge, they try to take and hold one more deep breath. As they do, water may enter the airway. There is a series of coughing and swallowing actions, and the patient involuntarily inhales and swallows more water. As water flows past the epiglottis, it triggers a reflex spasm of the larynx. This spasm seals the airway so effectively that no more than a small amount of water reaches the lungs. Unconsciousness soon results from hypoxia (oxygen starvation).

About 10 percent of the people who die from drowning die just from the lack of air. In the remaining patients, the person typically attempts a final respiratory effort and draws water into the lungs, or the spasms subside with the onset of unconsciousness and water freely enters the lungs.

Some patients who drown in cold water can be resuscitated after 30 minutes or more in cardiac arrest. If the water temperature falls below 70°F (21.1°C), biological death may be delayed. The colder the water, the better the patient's chances for survival, unless generalized hypothermia produces lethal complications.

Rescue Breathing in or out of the Water

Transport for the drowning patient should not be delayed. You may initiate care when the patient is out of the water. At other times, you may need to initiate care while the patient is still in the water—especially rescue breathing and immobilization for possible spine injuries. Chest compressions will be effective only after the patient is out of the water.

If needed, rescue breathing should begin without delay. If you can reach the non-breathing patient in the water, provide ventilations as you support the patient in a semi-supine position. Continue providing ventilations while the patient is being removed from the water. If there are no signs of trauma, and there is no mechanism of injury (such as reported diving) to suggest a spinal injury, then avoid attempts at immobilization, as it may interfere with effective rescue breathing. If the patient is already out of the water, begin rescue breathing or CPR on the land.

You may encounter airway resistance as you ventilate the drowning patient. In this case, you will probably have to ventilate more forcefully than you would other patients. Remember, you must provide air to the patient's lungs as soon as possible.

A patient with water in the lungs usually has water in the stomach, which will add resistance to your efforts to provide rescue breathing or CPR ventilations. Since the patient may have spasm of the larynx or swollen tissues in the larynx or trachea, you may find that some of the air you provide will go into the patient's stomach. Remember, the same problem will occur if you do not properly open the airway or if your ventilations are too forceful.

If gastric distention interferes with artificial ventilation, place the patient on the left side. With suction immediately available, the EMT should apply firm pressure using a hand over the epigastric area of the abdomen to relieve the distention. This procedure should be done only if the gastric distention interferes with the EMT's efforts to artificially ventilate the patient in an effective manner.

Care for Possible Spinal Injuries in the Water

Injuries to the cervical spine can be encountered in water-related accidents. Most often, these injuries are received during a dive or when the patient is struck by a boat, skier, ski, surfer, or surfboard. Even though cervical-spine injuries are the most common of the spine injuries seen in water-related accidents, there can be injury anywhere along the spine. This is in contrast to simple immersion drownings without trauma involved, in which spinal injuries are very rare. Spinal motion restriction in simple immersion drownings may in fact do harm by delaying and impeding patient ventilation and other crucial interventions.

In water-related accidents, assume that the unconscious patient has neck and spinal injuries. If the patient has head injuries, also assume that there are neck and spinal injuries. Keep in mind that a patient found in respiratory or cardiac arrest will need resuscitation started before you can immobilize the neck and spine. Also, realize that you may not be able to carry out a complete assessment for spinal injuries while the patient is in the water. Take care to avoid aggravating spinal injuries, but do not delay basic life support. Do not delay removing the patient from the water if the scene presents an immediate danger. When possible, keep the patient's neck supported and in a straight line with the body's midline (Scan 35-1). Use the jaw-thrust maneuver to open the airway.

If the patient with possible spinal injuries is still in the water, you are a good swimmer with proper training, and you are able to aid in the rescue, secure the patient to a long spine board before removal from the water. This may help prevent permanent neurologic damage or paralysis. This type of rescue requires special training in the use of the spine board while in the water. This rigid device can "pop up" very easily from below the water surface. Make certain that you know how to control the board and how to work in the water.

SCAN 35-1 Water Rescue with Possible Spinal Injury

HEAD-CHIN SUPPORT

TWO RESCUERS IN SHALLOW WATER

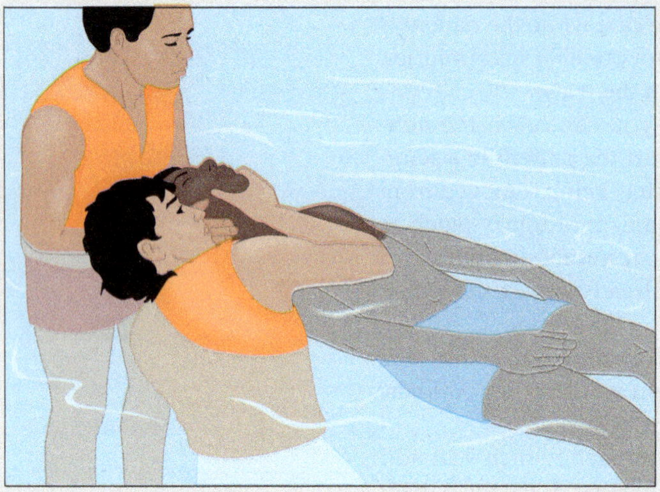

When there are two rescuers present, perform the head-chin support technique to provide in-line stabilization of a patient in shallow water.

HEAD-SPLINT SUPPORT

ONE RESCUER IN SHALLOW WATER

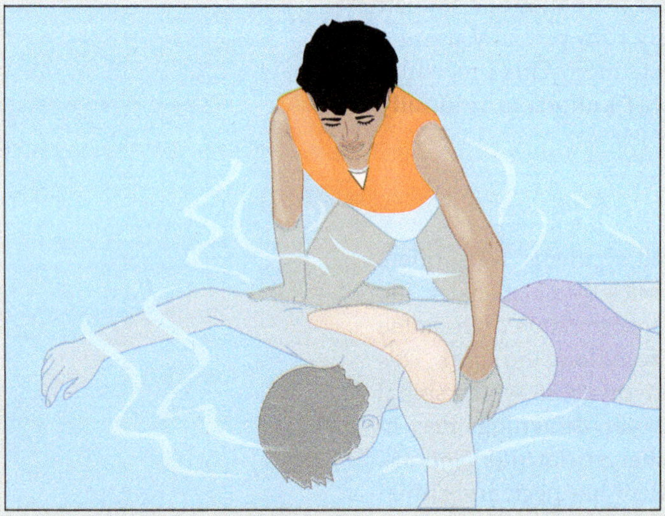

1. When you find a patient facedown in deep water, position yourself beside the patient. Support the patient's head with one hand and the mandible with the other.

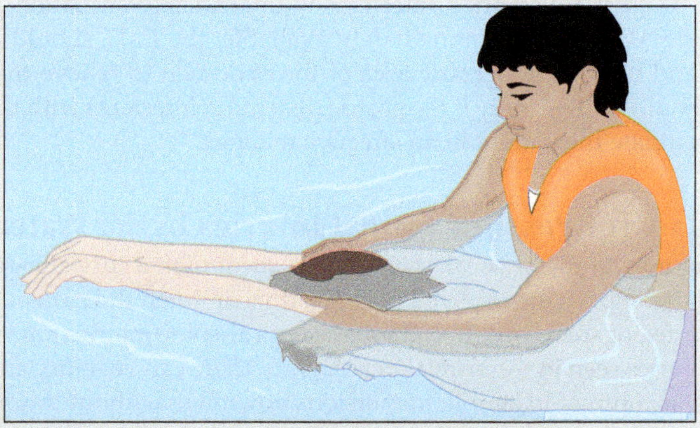

2. Extend the patient's arms straight up alongside the head to create a splint.

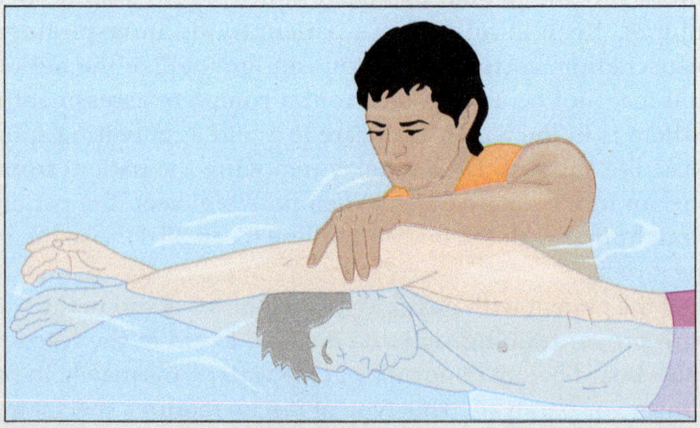

3. Begin to rotate the torso toward you.

NOTE: *Unless you are a very good swimmer and trained in water rescue, do not go into the water to save someone.*

SCAN 35-1 Water Rescue with Possible Spinal Injury *(continued)*

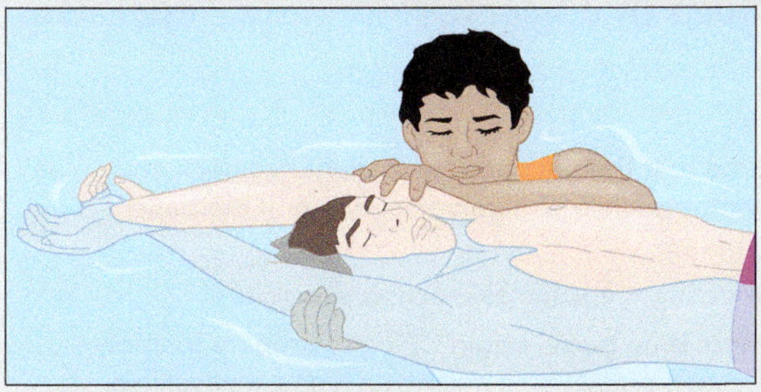

4. As you rotate the patient, lower yourself into the water.

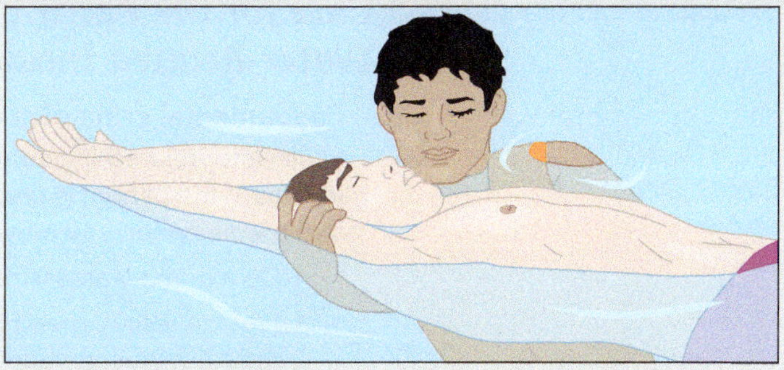

5. Maintain manual stabilization by holding the patient's head between the patient's arms.

HEAD-CHIN SUPPORT

ONE RESCUER IN DEEP WATER

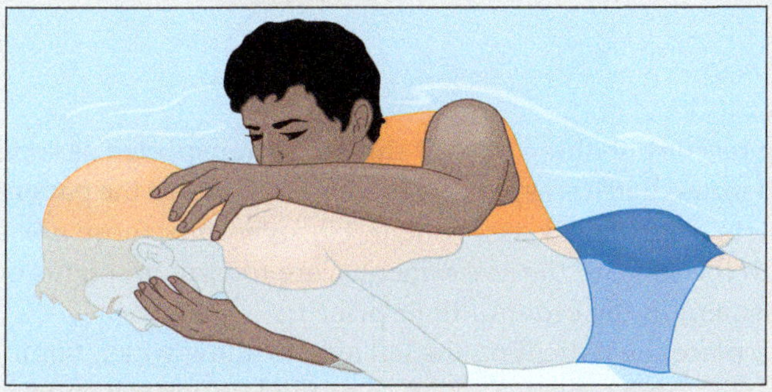

1. When you find a patient facedown in shallow water, position yourself alongside the patient.

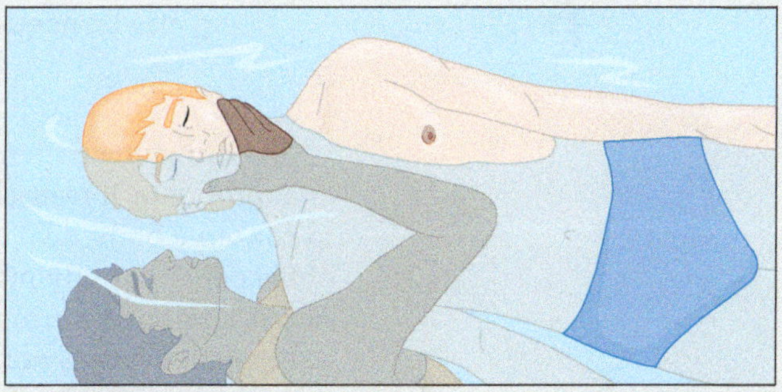

2. Rotate the patient by ducking underneath the patient's torso.

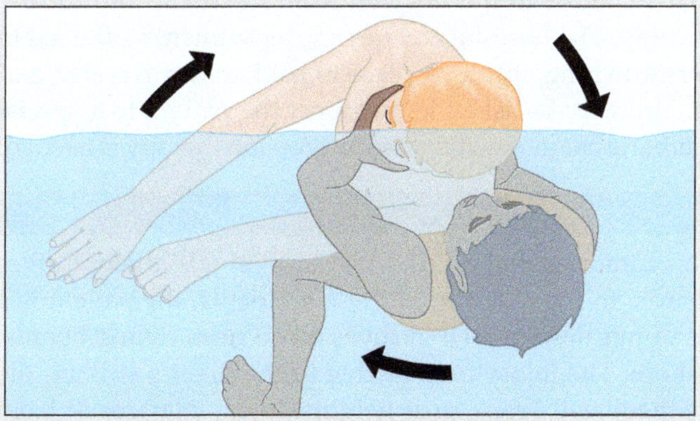

3. Continue to rotate until the patient is faceup.

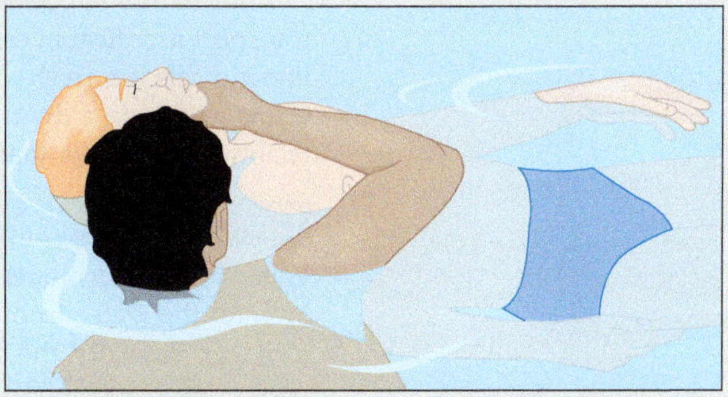

4. Maintain in-line stabilization until a backboard is used for spinal motion restriction.

Patient Care

Care for the Patient Involved in a Water-Related Incident

Fundamental Principles of Care

In all water-related incidents, assume that the unconscious patient has neck and spinal injuries. If the patient is rescued by others while you wait on shore, or if the patient is out of the water when you arrive, you should:

- Do a primary assessment, protecting the spine as much as possible.
- Provide rescue breathing. If there is no pulse, begin CPR and prepare to apply the AED. Protect yourself by using a pocket face mask with a one-way valve or bag-valve-mask unit.
- Look for and control profuse bleeding. Since the patient's heart rate may have slowed down, take a pulse for 60 seconds in all cold-water rescue situations before concluding that the patient is in cardiac arrest.
- Conserve heat, and if there are signs of hypoxia, or if the patient's vital signs indicate or suggest the potential for shock, administer oxygen.
- Continue resuscitative measures throughout transport. Initial and periodic suctioning may be needed.

The drowning patient receiving rescue breathing or CPR should be transported as soon as appropriate. If resuscitation and immediate transport are not required, cover the patient to conserve body heat and complete a secondary assessment. Uncover only those areas of the patient's body involved with the stage of the assessment. Care for any problems or injuries detected during the assessment in the order of their priority.

If spinal injury is not suspected, place the patient on the left side to allow water, vomit, and other secretions to drain from the upper airway. Suction as needed. When transport is delayed and you believe that the patient can be moved to a warmer place, do so without aggravating any existing injuries. Do not allow the drowning patient to walk. Transport the patient. A significant number of patients who appear normal after a drowning episode experience delayed effects, so persuade the patient to accept transport to a hospital.

Information supplied to the dispatcher or to the hospital from the scene and during transport is critical in cases of drowning. The hospital emergency department staff need to know if this is a fresh- or saltwater drowning, if it took place in cold or warm water, and if it is related to a diving accident. You may be asked to transport the patient to a special facility or to a center that has a hyperbaric chamber when decompression therapy is needed.

Diving Accidents

Water-related accidents often involve injuries that occur when individuals attempt dives or enter the water from diving boards. In the majority of these accidents, the patient is a teenager. Basically, the same types of injuries are seen in dives taken from diving boards, pool sides, docks, boats, and the shore. The injury may be due to the diver's striking the board or some object on or under the water. From great heights, injury may result from impact with the water.

Most diving accidents involve the head and neck, but you will also find injuries to the spine, hands, feet, and ribs in many cases. Any part of the body can be injured, depending on the position that the diver is in when striking the water or an object. This means that you must perform a primary assessment. You must also perform a secondary assessment on all diving-accident patients. Do not overlook the fact that a medical emergency may have led to the diving accident.

Emergency care for diving-accident patients is the same as for all accident patients if they are out of the water. Care provided in the water and during removal from the water is the same as for any patient who may have neck and spine injuries. Remember, you should assume that any unconscious or unresponsive patient has neck and spinal injuries.

Scuba-Diving Accidents

Diving accidents involving scuba (self-contained underwater breathing apparatus) gear have increased with the popularity of the sport, especially since many untrained and inexperienced persons are attempting dives. Today more than 2 million people scuba dive for sport or as part of their industrial or military jobs. Added to this are a large number who decide to "try it one time," without the benefits of lessons or supervision. Well-trained divers seldom have problems. However, those with inadequate training place themselves at great risk.

Scuba-diving accidents can involve any type of injury, as well as drowning. In many cases, scuba-diving accidents are brought about by medical problems that exist prior to the dive. There are two special problems seen in scuba-diving accidents: air emboli in the diver's blood and decompression sickness.

An ***air embolism***—more accurately called an *arterial gas embolism (AGE)*—is the result of gases leaving a damaged lung and entering the bloodstream. When you increase the pressure on a gas, its volume decreases, and when you decrease the pressure on a gas, its volume increases (Boyle's Law). You see this when you open a can of soda. The airtight, pressurized container holds the gas bubbles dissolved in the liquid, but when you open the can and decrease the pressure, the bubbles expand and come to the surface. If you scuba dive and descend to just 33 feet (10 meters), the pressure on your body doubles to 2 atmospheres. This pressure is transmitted to the gases in your body. A diver who comes up from this depth without exhaling has air in the lungs that wants to double in volume. This can cause rupture of the lung, which can then allow air to escape and lead to pneumothorax, pneumomediastinum (air in the area between the lungs, where the heart, trachea, esophagus, and great vessels are located), or arterial gas embolism (gas bubbles in the blood). These are most often associated with divers who hold their breath because of inadequate training, equipment failure, underwater emergency, or attempts to conserve air during a dive. However, a diver may develop an air embolism in very shallow water (as shallow as 4 feet (about 1.2 meters) deep). An automobile-collision patient who gulps air from air pockets while in a submerged vehicle also may suffer an air embolism. When freed, the patient may develop air emboli in the same way as a scuba diver.

air embolism
gas bubble in the bloodstream. The plural is *air emboli*. The more accurate term is *arterial gas embolism (AGE)*.

Decompression sickness occurs when a diver comes up too quickly from a deep, prolonged dive. The quick ascent causes nitrogen gas that was absorbed in body tissues during the dive to come out of solution rapidly and form gas bubbles in the bloodstream. Decompression sickness in scuba divers takes from 1 to 48 hours to appear, with about 90 percent of cases occurring within 3 hours of the dive. Scuba divers typically breathe compressed air that has approximately 21 percent oxygen and 79 percent nitrogen. As they go deeper and the pressure increases, these gases get pushed into the tissues. If they ascend slowly, the gases have time to go back into the bloodstream and get exhaled. This is the basis for dive computers that tell ascending divers how long to spend at a specific depth before going up any farther. (Written tables were used in the past before computers became small, efficient, and inexpensive.) When a diver comes up too quickly, the bubbles expand in the joints, skin (especially around the head and neck), lungs, brain, and spinal cord. Symptoms of decompression sickness, unlike arterial gas embolism, take at least an hour but rarely more than 12 hours to appear.

decompression sickness
a condition resulting from nitrogen trapped in the body's tissues, caused by coming up too quickly from a deep, prolonged dive. A symptom of decompression sickness is "the bends," or deep pain in the muscles and joints.

Divers increase the risk of decompression sickness if they fly within 18 hours of diving. Because of this, carefully consider all information gathered from the patient interview and reports from the patient's family and friends. This information may provide the only clues relating the patient's problems to a scuba dive.

The following are common signs and symptoms of scuba-diving problems:

Air Embolism (Rapid Onset–typically in less than 15 minutes–of Signs and Symptoms)

- Altered mental status
- Rapid loss of consciousness
- Blurred vision
- Seizures
- Paralysis or paresthesias in the extremities

- Stroke
- Frothy blood in the mouth or nose
- Incontinence
- Chest pain
- Stroke-like symptoms
- Myocardial infarction
- Respiratory arrest and cardiac arrest

Decompression Sickness (1- to 12-Hour Onset of Symptoms)

- Confusion, altered mental status, headache, visual disturbances, vertigo, nausea/vomiting, staggering gait
- Fatigue (may be extreme.)
- Pain in the muscles and joints (the "bends")
- Itchy blotches or mottling of the skin
- Numbness or paralysis
- Choking, coughing, dyspnea, substernal pleuritic chest pain
- Peripheral edema and swelling (usually in one region)
- Mottled/marbled skin; itching

For a patient with signs and symptoms of either air embolism or decompression sickness, follow the same emergency care steps:

- Maintain an open airway.
- Administer the highest possible concentration of oxygen by nonrebreather mask.
- Keep the patient warm.
- Position the patient either supine or on either side (Figure 35-7). Continue to monitor the patient. You may have to reposition the patient to ensure an open airway. Contact medical direction for specific instructions concerning where to take the patient. You may be sent directly to a hyperbaric trauma care center.
- Promptly transport all patients with possible air emboli or decompression sickness. If you are in an area with a hyperbaric facility, medical direction may tell you to transport the patient there directly.

The Diver Alert Network (DAN) was formed to assist rescuers with the care of underwater diving-accident patients. The staff, who are available on a 24-hour basis, can be reached by phoning the emergency contact number 1-919-684-9111. DAN can give you

FIGURE 35-7 Proper positioning of a scuba-diving accident patient. This patient is on her side because she is not awake enough to protect her airway.

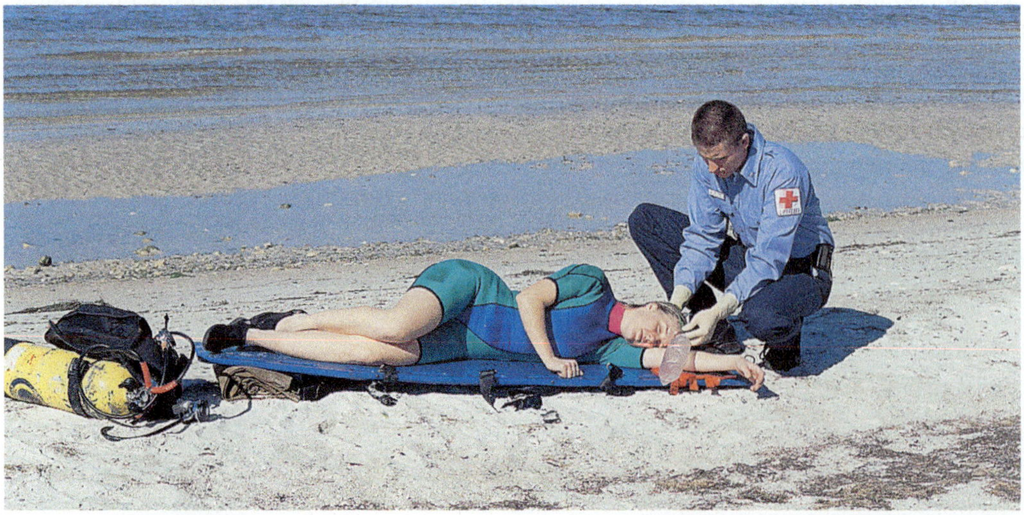

or your dispatcher information on assessment and care, and on whether and how to transfer the patient to a hyperbaric facility. For nonemergency medical information, call 1-919-684-2948.

NOTE: *The well-trained scuba diver makes use of a dive computer or chart. If it is available, it may provide you with useful information concerning the nature and duration of the dive. Transport the computer or chart with the patient.*

Water Rescues

The following is the order of procedures for a water rescue (Figure 35-8), most of which can be performed short of going into the water: Reach, throw and tow, row, and go.

- **Reach.** When the patient is responsive and close to shore or poolside, try to reach the patient by holding out an object for the patient to grab. Then pull the patient from the water. Make sure your position is secure. Line (rope) is considered the best choice. If no line is available, use a branch, fishing rod, oar, stick, or other such object—even a towel, blanket, or article of clothing. If no object is available, or you have only one opportunity to grab the person (e.g., in strong currents), position yourself flat on your abdomen and extend your hand or leg to the patient. (This is not recommended if you are a nonswimmer.) Again, make certain that you are working from a secure position.
- **Throw and tow.** If the person is conscious but too far away for you to reach and pull from the water, throw an object that will float (Figure 35-9). A personal flotation device (PFD or lifejacket) or ring buoy (life preserver) works best. Other buoyant objects include foam cushions, logs, plastic picnic containers, surfboards, flatboards, large beach

FIGURE 35-8 First try to reach and pull the patient from the water. (Note that the rescuer is low over the water and is kneeling, rather than squatting, so the base of support is broader and more secure.) If that fails, throw anything that will float to use as a way to tow the person from the water. If that fails, row to the patient.

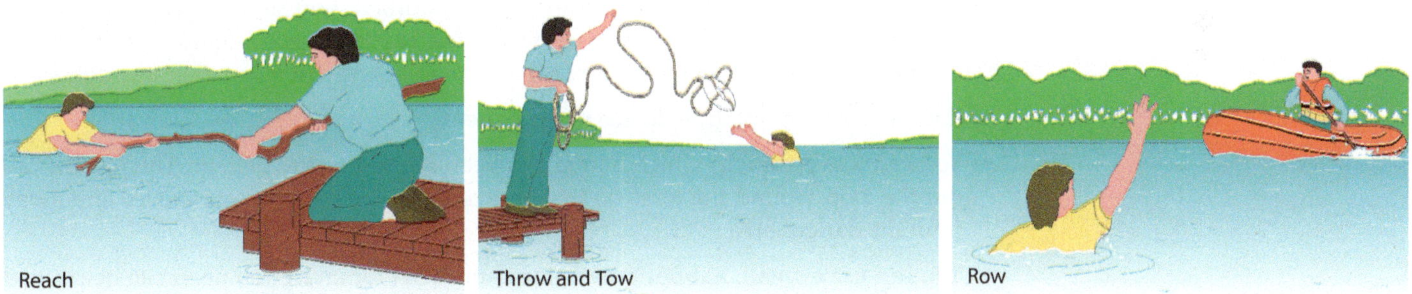

FIGURE 35-9 Throw the patient any object that will float.

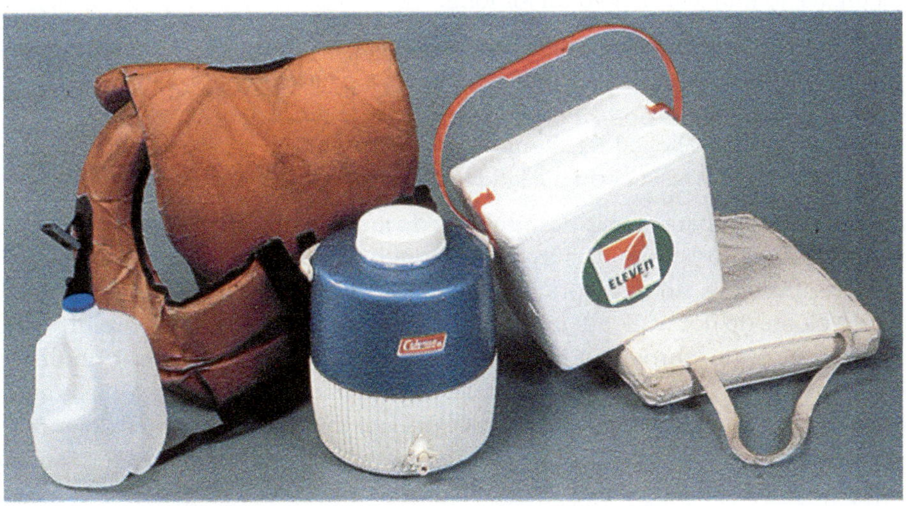

balls, and plastic toys. Two empty, capped plastic milk jugs can keep an adult afloat for hours. Inflatable splints can be used if there is nothing at the scene that will float.

Once the conscious patient has a flotation device, try to find a way to tow the person to shore. From a safe position, throw the patient a line or another flotation device attached to a line. If you are a good swimmer and you know how to judge the water, wade out no deeper than waist-high, wear a personal flotation device, and have a safety line that is secured on shore.

- **Row.** When the patient is too far from shore to allow for throwing and towing, or is unresponsive, you may be able to row a boat to the patient. However, do not attempt to row to the patient if you cannot swim. Even if you are a good swimmer, wearing a personal flotation device is required while you are in the boat.

  Tell a conscious patient in the water to grab an oar or the stern (rear end) of the boat. You must exercise great care when helping the patient into the boat. This is even trickier when you are in a canoe. If the canoe tips over, stay with it and hold on to its bottom and side. Most canoes will stay afloat.

- **Go.** As a last resort, when all other means have failed, you can go into the water and swim to the patient. However, you must be a good swimmer, trained in water rescue and lifesaving. Untrained rescuers can become patients themselves.

Decision Point

- What is the safest way to rescue the patient—considering safety for both the EMT and the patient?

Ice Rescues

Every winter, people fall through ice while skating or attempting to cross an ice-covered body of water. Often the scene becomes a multiple-rescue problem as other individuals fall through the ice while trying to reach the patient. The number-one rule in ice rescue is to protect yourself. Formal ice rescue training is available. In addition, you should wear a cold-water submersion suit and personal flotation device during any ice rescue attempt (Figure 35-10).

There are several ways in which you can reach a patient who has fallen through ice:

- You can throw a flotation device to the patient.
- You can toss a rope in which a loop has been formed to the patient. The patient can put the loop around the torso so that you can pull the patient onto the ice and away from the danger area.
- You can use a small, flat-bottomed aluminum boat for an ice rescue. It can be pushed stern (rear end) first by other rescuers and pulled to safety by a rope secured to the bow (front end). The primary rescuer will remain dry and safe if the ice breaks. The patient can be pulled from the water or allowed to grasp the side of the boat but may be unable to grasp or to hold on for long.
- A ladder is an effective tool often used in ice rescue. It can be laid flat and pushed to the patient, then pulled back by an attached rope. The ladder also can serve as a surface on which a rescuer can spread out body weight if it is necessary to go onto the ice to reach the patient. The ladder should have a line that can be secured by a rescuer in a safe position. Any rescuer on the ladder should have a safety line.

Remember that the patient may not be able to do much to help in the rescue process. In just a matter of minutes, hypothermia may interfere with both mental and physical capabilities.

Whenever possible, do not work alone when trying to perform an ice rescue. If you must work alone, do not walk out onto the ice. Never go onto ice that is rapidly breaking. Never enter the water through a hole in the ice to find the patient. Your best course of action will be to work with others from a safe ice surface or the shore. When there is no other choice, you and your fellow rescuers can elect to form a human chain to reach the patient. However, this is not the safest method to employ, even when all the rescuers are wearing personal flotation devices and using safety lines.

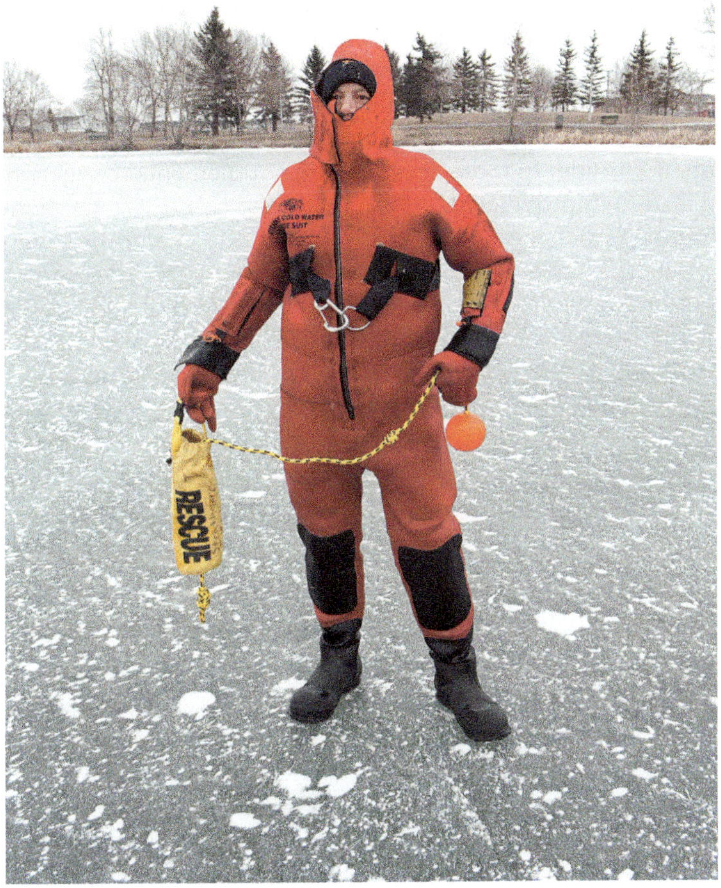

FIGURE 35-10 Safe ice rescues require proper equipment.

Expect to find injuries to most patients who have fallen through the ice. Treat for hypothermia according to local protocols, and treat for any injuries. Transport all patients who have fallen through ice.

High-Altitude Emergencies

High-Altitude Illness

Another kind of environmental emergency can occur when people go to high altitudes. Most of what we know about physiology we have learned from people who live at or near sea level. At higher altitudes, some of what we know has to be adjusted. The biggest difference in this environment is in the amount of oxygen available. Although the proportion of oxygen at high altitudes is the same as at sea level (21 percent), there is less air to breathe, because atmospheric pressure decreases as elevation increases (as the air becomes thinner). To compensate in the short term, a person breathes more rapidly and deeply. Over days to weeks at high altitude, the body increases its ability to use the limited oxygen in the atmosphere by increasing the number of red blood cells and therefore hemoglobin. The body also becomes accustomed to having less oxygen available. Normal, healthy people who have adjusted to high altitudes have a lower oxygen saturation than do those at sea level because there is less oxygen to breathe.

When the body is unable to adjust to the thinner air, a person can experience problems. The least serious of these is acute mountain sickness. Although this condition is more common above 8,000 feet (about 2400 meters), it can start at just 5,000 feet (about 1500 meters). Within 6 to 12 hours of arrival at a high altitude, the patient with acute mountain sickness experiences a diffuse headache and other symptoms that feel like a hangover. These symptoms can be accounted for by fatigue and dehydration, so it is not considered true acute mountain sickness unless at least two of the following signs or symptoms are present: nausea, vomiting, loss of appetite, lightheadedness, insomnia, paresthesia (prickling sensation, usually in the extremities), nosebleed, peripheral edema, shortness of breath, and tachycardia. If a person does not develop symptoms after 3 days at the same altitude, that person is not at risk of developing the condition, as the body has acclimated to the altitude.

In mild cases, all that may be needed to overcome acute mountain sickness is rest and rehydration at altitude. In more severe cases, supplemental oxygen and immediate descent should lead to improvement.

Two developments that may occur are high-altitude cerebral edema (HACE) and high-altitude pulmonary edema (HAPE). HACE is the worse form of acute mountain sickness, and produces symptoms related to swelling of the brain, including severe headache, altered mental status, and seizures.

CORE CONCEPT

Signs, symptoms, and treatment for high altitude illness

Patient Assessment

High-Altitude Cerebral Edema

The following are common signs and symptoms of high-altitude cerebral edema:

- Headache that worsens over time
- Loss of balance and coordination
- Severe fatigue
- Seizure
- Altered mental status
- Loss of consciousness

Decision Points

- Does the patient exhibit altered mental status, loss of balance, or loss of consciousness?
- Are the patient's signs and symptoms worsening over time?

Patient Care

Care of the Patient with High-Altitude Cerebral Edema

Fundamental Principles of Care

Caring for a patient with high-altitude cerebral edema includes preventing further exposure to high altitude and providing supportive treatment.

Emergency care of a patient with high-altitude cerebral edema includes the following:

- Arrange for immediate descent. All other treatments are secondary to this.
- Administer high-concentration oxygen.
- Provide supportive treatment.

An even more serious condition than high-altitude cerebral edema is high-altitude pulmonary edema (HAPE). This condition takes longer to develop, usually 2–3 days, probably because of the time it takes for fluids to accumulate in the lungs. Like all of the altitude illnesses, HAPE can be subtle at the start, but it is the most life-threatening of these conditions.

Patient Assessment

High-Altitude Pulmonary Edema

The following are common signs and symptoms of high-altitude pulmonary edema:

- Shortness of breath, initially just on exertion but later also at rest
- Dry cough that progresses to coughing up blood (hemoptysis)
- Tachypnea
- Tachycardia
- Mild fever up to 100.4°F (38.0°C)
- Oxygen saturation lower than other asymptomatic people in the same environment
- Respiratory failure and arrest

Patient Care

Care of the Patient with High-Altitude Pulmonary Edema

Fundamental Principles of Care

Caring for a patient with high-altitude pulmonary edema includes preventing further exposure to high altitude and providing supportive treatment.

Emergency care of a patient with high-altitude cerebral edema is as follows:

- Arrange for immediate descent. All other treatments are secondary to this.
- Administer high-concentration oxygen.
- Minimize physical activity, which uses oxygen needed for other organs.
- Provide supportive treatment.

Bites and Stings

Insect Bites and Stings

Insect stings, spider bites, and scorpion stings are typical sources of injected poisons, or **toxins**—substances produced by animals or plants that are poisonous to humans. (**Venom** is a term for a toxin produced by some animals, such as snakes, spiders, and certain marine life forms.) Commonly seen insect stings are those of wasps, hornets, bees, and ants. Insect stings and bites are rarely dangerous. However, 5 percent of the U.S. population will have an allergic reaction to them, which may result in shock. Those who are hypersensitive develop severe anaphylactic shock that is quickly life-threatening. (See the chapter *Allergic Reactions*).

toxins
substances produced by animals or plants that are poisonous to humans.

venom
a toxin (poison) produced by certain animals, such as snakes, spiders, and some marine life forms.

CORE CONCEPT
Signs, symptoms, and treatment for bites and stings

Although all spiders are venomous, most species cannot get their fangs through human skin. The black widow spider and the brown recluse, or fiddleback, spider (Figure 35-11) are two that can, and their bites can produce medical emergencies. Almost all brown recluse spider bites are painless, and patients seldom recall being bitten. The characteristic lesion appears in only 10 percent of cases and only after up to 12 hours (Figure 35-12). EMTs are seldom called to respond to a brown recluse bite. However, black widow bites cause a more immediate reaction.

Scorpion stings are common in the southwest United States. They do not ordinarily cause deaths, but one rare species (*Centruroides exilcauda*) is dangerous to humans and can cause serious medical problems in children, including respiratory failure.

Bites and stings belong in the class of injected poisons discussed in the chapter *Poisoning and Overdose Emergencies.*

FIGURE 35-11 (A) Black widow spider. (B) Brown recluse spider. *(Both photos: Centers for Disease Control and Prevention/Paula Smith)*

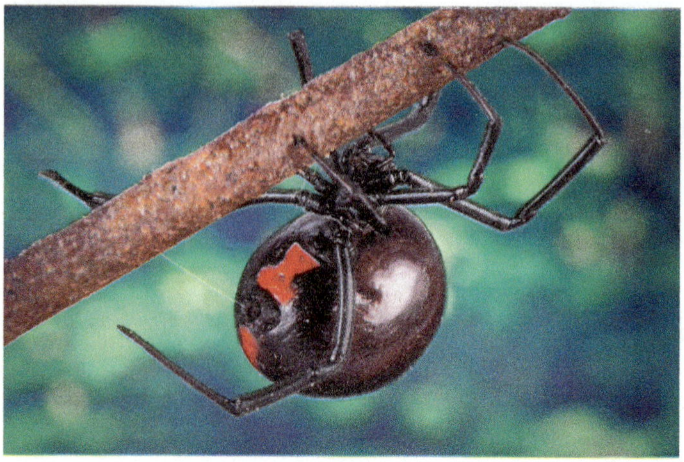

A

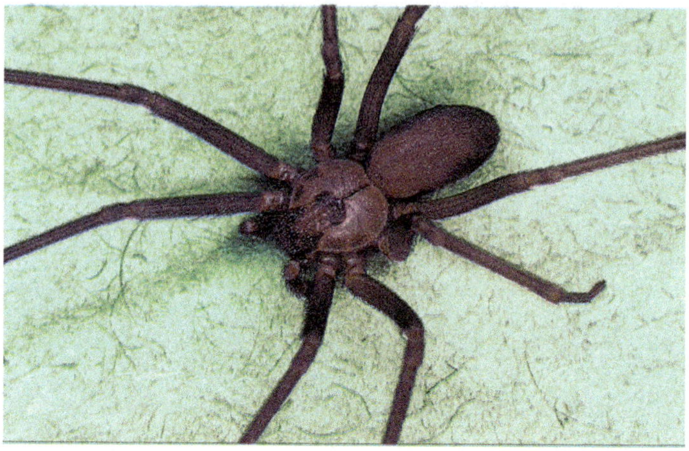

B

FIGURE 35-12 Brown recluse spider bite. *(Centers for Disease Control and Prevention)*

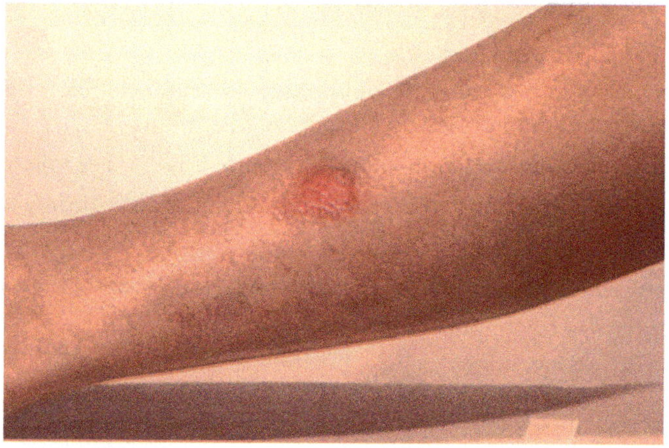

Patient Assessment

Insect Bites and Stings

Gather information from the patient, bystanders, and the scene. Find out whatever you can about the insect or other possible source of the envenomation (poisoning). The following are common signs and symptoms of injected envenomation:

- Altered mental status
- Noticeable stings or bites on the skin
- Puncture marks (especially note the fingers, forearms, toes, and legs)
- Blotchy (mottled) skin
- Localized pain or itching
- Numbness in a limb or body part
- Burning sensations at the site followed by pain spreading throughout the limb
- Redness
- Swelling or blistering at the site
- Weakness or collapse
- Difficult breathing and abnormal pulse rate
- Headache and dizziness
- Chills

- Fever
- Nausea and vomiting
- Muscle cramps, chest tightness, joint pain
- Excessive saliva formation, profuse sweating
- Anaphylaxis

NOTE: *Look for medical identification devices that identify persons sensitive to certain stings or bites. Some patients sensitive to stings or bites carry medication to help prevent anaphylactic shock. This situation is described in the* Allergic Reaction *chapter.*

Patient Care

Care of the Patient with Insect Bites or Stings

Fundamental Principles of Care

As an EMT, you are not expected to be able to identify insects and spiders. Proper identification of these organisms is best left to experts. If the patient's problem was caused by a creature that is known locally and is not normally dangerous (such as a bee, wasp, or puss caterpillar), your major concern regarding the patient will be anaphylactic shock. If anaphylactic shock does not develop, care is usually simple.

If the cause of the bite or sting is unknown or the organism is unknown, a physician should see the patient. Call medical direction or take the patient to a medical facility, and let experts decide on the proper treatment for the patient. If possible, transport the stinging object or organism in a sealed container, taking care not to handle it without proper protection, even if it is dead. If you can accomplish this safely, you may save precious minutes needed to identify the toxin.

Emergency care for injected toxins includes the following:

- Treat for shock, even if the patient does not present any of the signs of shock.
- Call medical direction. Skip this only if the organism is known and your EMS system has a specific protocol for care.
- Remove the stinger or venom sac. The traditional advice was to scrape the site with a blade or a card and to avoid pulling with tweezers. (It was thought using tweezers might squeeze more venom into the wound.) However, research indicates that how you remove the stinger or venom sac is far less important than doing so quickly. The venom sac is actually hard, not floppy, so the risk of squeezing venom into the wound is low.
- Remove jewelry from the patient's affected limb in case the limb swells, which would make removal more difficult later.
- If local protocols permit, and if the wound is on an extremity (not a joint), place constricting bands above and below the sting or bite site. This is done to slow the spread of venom in the lymphatic vessels and superficial veins. The bands should be made of $^3/_4$-inch to $1^1/_2$-inch-wide (about 2-cm to 4-cm-wide) soft rubber or another wide soft material. They should be placed about 2 inches (5 cm) from the wound. The bands must be loose enough to slide a finger under. They should not cut off circulation. Use of constricting bands is only necessary in the case of high-risk bites or stings, such as from a scorpion or black widow spider.
- Keep the limb immobilized and the patient still to prevent distribution of the venom to other parts of the body.

NOTE: *Some EMS systems recommend placing a cold compress on the wound. However, most EMS systems do not use cold for any injected toxin. Follow your local protocols.*

Snakebites

Snakebites require special care but are usually not life-threatening. Nearly fifty thousand people in the United States are bitten by snakes each year. Although more than eight thousand of these cases involve venomous snakes, on average, fewer than ten deaths each year are reported from snakebites. (In the United States, more people die each year from bee and wasp stings than from snakebites.) The signs and symptoms of snakebite envenomation may take several hours to appear. If death does result, it is usually not a rapidly occurring event unless anaphylactic shock develops. Most patients who die survive at least two days.

In the United States, there are two types of native venomous snakes—pit vipers (including rattlesnakes, copperheads, and water moccasins) and coral snakes (Figure 35-13). Up to 25 percent of pit viper bites and 50 percent of coral bites are "dry bites" without venom injection. However, the venomous bite from a diamondback rattler or coral snake is considered very serious. Since each person reacts differently to a snakebite, you should consider the bite from any known venomous snake or any unidentified snake to be a serious emergency. Staying calm and keeping the patient calm and at rest are critical.

NOTE: *Native snakes are not the only kind of venomous animals you may encounter. A number of people have decided to keep venomous reptiles, even though it is illegal to do so in most areas. So even if you live in an area where there are no native venomous snakes, you may encounter a patient who has sustained a bite from one.*

Patient Assessment

Snakebite

Unless you are dealing with a known species of snake that is not considered venomous, consider all snakebites to be from venomous snakes. The patient or bystanders may say the snake was not venomous, but they could be mistaken. The signs and symptoms of snakebite may include the following:

- Noticeable bite on the skin, which may appear as nothing more than a discoloration
- Pain and swelling in the area of the bite, which may be slow to develop, taking from 30 minutes to several hours
- Rapid pulse and labored breathing
- Progressive general weakness
- Vision problems (dim or blurred)
- Nausea and vomiting
- Seizures
- Drowsiness or unconsciousness

If the dead or captured snake is at the scene, your role as an EMT is not to identify the snake but to have a qualified person place it in a sealed container and transport it along with the patient. Arrange for separate transport of a live specimen. Do not transport a live snake in the ambulance.

If you see a live, uncaptured snake, take great care, or you may be its next victim. When possible, note its size and coloration. Getting close enough to look for details of the eyes or for a pit between the eye and mouth is foolish. The way you classify a snake, whether it is dead or alive, will probably have little to do with your subsequent care of the patient. The medical facility staff will arrange to have an expert classify a captured or dead specimen, and they have protocols to determine patient care if the snake has not been captured. Unless you are an expert in capturing snakes, do not try to catch the snake. *Never delay care and transport to capture the snake.*

FIGURE 35-13 The pit vipers include the (A) cottonmouth, (B) rattlesnake, and (C) copperhead. The coral snake (D) is also venomous. *(Photos A and B: Centers for Disease Control and Prevention/Edward J. Wozniak, DVM, PhD; Photo C: Centers for Disease Control and Prevention/James Gathany; Photo D: U.S. Fish and Wildlife Service/Luther C. Goldman)*

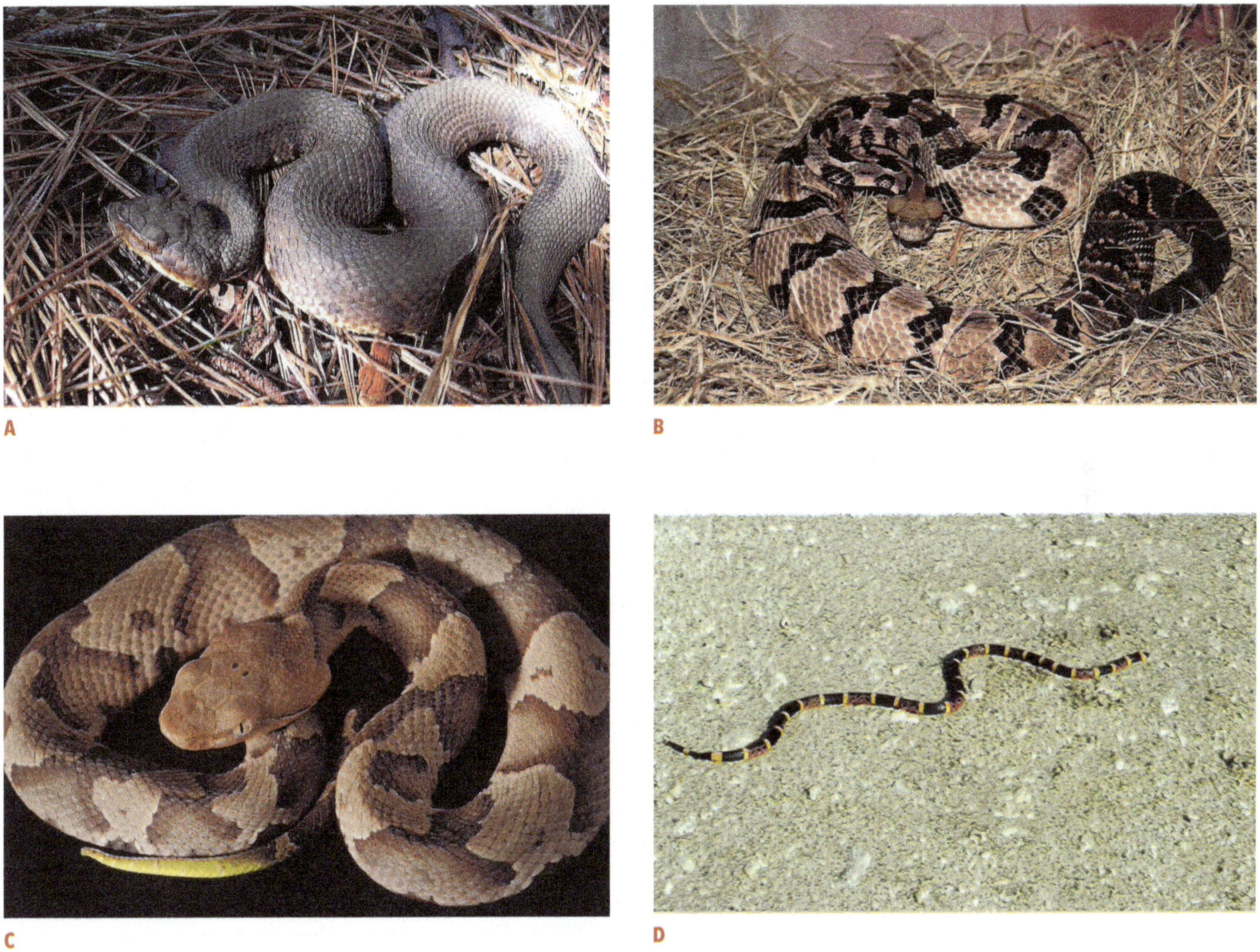

Patient Care

Care of the Patient with a Snakebite

Fundamental Principles of Care

Treatment of a patient with a snakebite is generally supportive and may include splinting to prevent or slow down absorption of venom.

Emergency care of a patient with snakebite includes the following:

- Call medical direction to determine the best receiving facility where antivenom will be most readily available to treat the patient. Rapid transport and the administration of antivenom are the most effective interventions for the treatment of life-threatening snakebite injuries.
- Treat for shock and conserve body heat. Keep the patient calm.
- Locate the fang marks. There may be only one fang mark.
- Remove any rings, bracelets, or other constricting items on the bitten extremity.
- Keep any bitten extremities immobilized—the application of a splint will help. Do not elevate the limb above the level of the heart.
- Transport the patient, carefully monitoring vital signs.

NOTE: *Do not place an ice bag or cold pack on the bite unless you are directed to do so by a physician or local protocols. Do not cut into the bite and suction or squeeze the bite site. Never suck the venom from the wound using your mouth. Instead, use a suction cup. However, suctioning is seldom done.*

Use of a *pressure immobilization bandage* may be the most effective technique to slow the spread of venom after a snakebite. This technique involves immediately wrapping the bitten extremity with an elastic (ACE-type) bandage and immobilizing the wrapped extremity with a rigid splint or a sling on the upper extremity. The wrap should be only as snug as if you were wrapping a sprained ankle. The purpose of the pressure immobilization bandage is to restrict the flow of lymph, not of blood. The wrap should be snug but not tight enough to cut off circulation. Monitor for a pulse at the wrist or ankle. Check to be certain that tissue swelling does not cause the constricting bands to become too tight.

Poisoning from Marine Life

Poisoning from marine life forms can occur in a variety of ways—from eating improperly prepared seafood or poisonous organisms to receiving stings and punctures from aquatic life forms. Patients who have ingested spoiled, contaminated, or infested seafood may develop a condition that resembles anaphylactic shock. Therefore, they should receive the same care as any patient in anaphylactic shock. During care, you must be prepared in case the patient vomits. Most patients will show the signs of food poisoning. The care for seafood poisoning is the same as for all other food poisonings.

It is extremely rare for someone in the United States to eat a poisonous variety of marine life, since creatures such as puffer fish and paralytic shellfish are not readily available. For all cases of suspected poisoning due to ingestion, call your on-line medical direction or the poison control center as local protocols direct you. Be prepared for the patient to display vomiting, convulsions, and respiratory arrest.

Venomous marine life forms producing sting injuries include the jellyfish, the sea nettle, the Portuguese man-of-war, coral, the sea anemone, and the hydra. For most victims, the sting produces pain with few complications. Some patients may show allergic reactions and possibly develop anaphylactic shock. These cases require the same care as rendered for any case of anaphylactic shock. Stings to the face, especially those near or on the lip or eye, require a physician's attention. Rinsing the affected area with vinegar will reduce the pain of the sting. However, be careful not to let vinegar get into the patient's mouth or eyes. Once the site has been rinsed with vinegar to inactivate the venom, immersion of the site in hot-but-nonscalding water (maximum temperature 113°F [45°C]) may further reduce the pain.

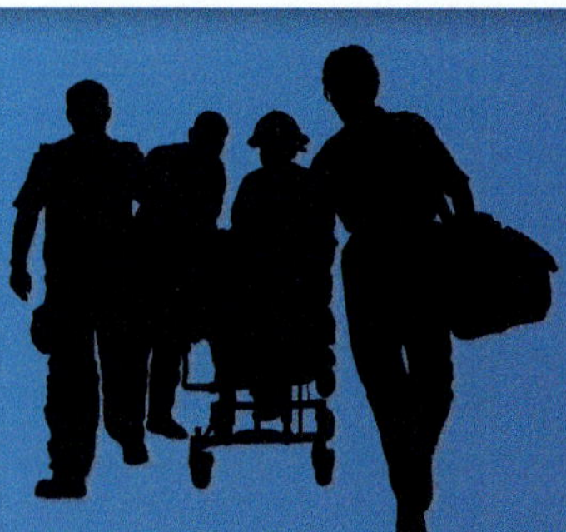

Think Like an EMT

Safety First

Environmental emergencies provide a variety of situations in which an EMT must act. Some patients need to be cooled, others warmed. However, before you even get to treat the patient, you must make some safety decisions. Consider the following situations, and identify the safety hazards:

1. You are taking a walk while on vacation. You hear a sound from the water and see that several hundred feet out in the water, a person is struggling to stay afloat.
2. You are ice skating with the family and hear screaming. Someone has fallen through the ice. A group of people have gathered around the hole, peering downward.
3. You are on a hiking path and hear screaming. A hiker has been bitten by a snake. He is in pain and holding his leg. He is sitting by an outcropping of rocks.

Puncture wounds can occur when someone steps on or grabs a stingray, sea urchin, spiny catfish, or other form of spiny marine animal. Although it is true that soaking the wound in nonscalding hot water for 30–90 minutes will break down the venom, you should not delay transport. Puncture wounds must be treated by a physician, and the patient may need a tetanus inoculation. Remember, the patient could react to the venom by developing anaphylactic shock.

Chapter Review

Key Facts and Concepts

- Patients suffering from exposure to heat or cold must be removed from the harmful environment as quickly and as safely as possible.
- Generalized cold injuries involve cooling of the entire body, also referred to as hypothermia. Treatment decisions are based on whether that patient has a normal or altered mental status.
- Patients who have hypothermia with an altered mental status are considered to have severe hypothermia; this indicates a life-threatening emergency.
- Local cold injury involves an isolated part or parts of the body. Early local injury sites may be rewarmed gently. Late local cold injury involves freezing of tissue (frostbite).
- Hyperthermia is a heat emergency. Its severity is determined by skin temperature. Skin that is normal to cool (heat exhaustion) is considered less severe than skin that is hot to the touch (heat stroke). All heat-emergency patients should be removed from the heat and cooled. Altered mental status in the setting of hyperthermia indicates a life-threatening emergency.
- Follow local protocols in reference to rewarming or cooling procedures.
- Immediate resuscitation of the water-related emergency patient may require quick and persistent intervention. Always ensure your own safety before attempting any sort of rescue.
- For injection or ingestion of the venoms of insects, spiders, snakes, and marine life, call medical direction and follow your local protocols.

Key Decisions

- Is the scene safe from heat, cold, and venomous creatures?
- How can I safely get the patient from the water?
- Hypothermia: Does the patient have an altered mental status?
- Hyperthermia: Is the patient's skin temperature cool to normal, or hot?

Chapter Glossary

active rewarming application of an external heat source to rewarm the body of a hypothermic patient.

air embolism gas bubble in the bloodstream. The more accurate term is *arterial gas embolism (AGE)*.

central rewarming application of heat to the lateral chest, neck, armpits, and groin of a hypothermic patient.

conduction the transfer of heat from one material to another through direct contact.

convection carrying away of heat by currents of air, water, or other gases or liquids.

decompression sickness a condition resulting from nitrogen trapped in the body's tissues, caused by coming up too quickly from a deep, prolonged dive. A symptom of decompression sickness is "the bends," or deep pain in the muscles and joints.

drowning the process of experiencing respiratory impairment from submersion/immersion in liquid, which may result in death, morbidity (illness or other adverse effects), or no morbidity.

evaporation the change from liquid to gas. When the body perspires or gets wet, evaporation of the perspiration or other liquid into the air has a cooling effect on the body.

hyperthermia (HI-per-THURM-e-ah) an increase in body temperature above normal, which is a life-threatening condition in its extreme.

hypothermia (HI-po-THURM-e-ah) generalized cooling that reduces body temperature below normal, which is a life-threatening condition in its extreme.

local cooling cooling or freezing of particular (local) parts of the body.

passive rewarming covering a hypothermic patient and taking other steps to prevent further heat loss and help the body rewarm itself.

radiation sending out energy, such as heat, in waves into space.

respiration breathing. During respiration, body heat is lost as warm air is exhaled from the body.

toxins substances produced by animals or plants that are poisonous to humans.

venom a toxin (poison) produced by certain animals, such as snakes, spiders, and some marine life forms.

water chill chilling caused by conduction of heat from the body when the body or clothing is wet.

wind chill chilling caused by convection of heat from the body in the presence of air currents.

Preparation for Your Examination and Practice

Short Answer

1. When is it appropriate to treat a cold emergency with active rewarming, and when should you perform passive rewarming?
2. List five situations in which a patient may be suffering from hypothermia along with another, more obvious medical condition or injury.
3. Name the signs and symptoms of a late or deep localized cold injury.
4. Describe the management of a patient suffering from heat emergency who has moist, pale, and cool skin.
5. Describe the management of a patient suffering from a heat emergency who has hot, dry skin.
6. Describe the proper care for a patient suffering from snakebite.

Thinking and Linking

Think back to the chapters titled Introduction to Emergency Medical Services, Well-Being of the EMT, *and* Communication and Documentation. *Link information from those chapters to information from this chapter as you consider the following situation:*

- You respond to a snakebite. At the scene, you find a patient and witnesses who describe a snake to you in great detail. Where would you find information on what type of snake this was, whether it was venomous, and how to treat the patient? What would you do if the snake were still present?

Think back to the chapters Introduction to Emergency Medical Services, Well-Being of the EMT, *and* Lifting and Moving Patients. *Link information from those chapters to information from this chapter as you consider the following situation:*

- You have a patient who is experiencing hypothermia, is half a mile into the woods, and is not accessible by ambulance. Do you have clothing available that would protect you and your crew/team from hypothermia during the trip in and out? If you will be an EMT in a warm climate, change the situation. It is hot and humid. A hiker has experienced a heat emergency. Can you and your crew/team get the patient out without experiencing a heat emergency yourselves? In either case, what transport device(s) and resources would you use to remove the patient from the woods?

Critical Thinking Exercises

Some environmental emergencies are dangerous for both the patient and the EMT. The purpose of this exercise will be to consider options for patient care in several such circumstances.

1. Your hypothermia patient has an altered mental status. How does this affect your care for the patient? What if you were several hours by snowmobile from the nearest road?
2. What is the underlying pathophysiology that makes hot skin more serious than having cool skin in a heat emergency? What are the implications of hot skin for the care you provide?
3. You are with your family at a local lake. You observe a boat capsize near the middle of the lake and can hear screams from the scene. You are a marginal swimmer. Several civilians begin swimming out to the site. Apply the concepts learned in the *Scene Size-Up* chapter to this scene.

Pathophysiology to Practice

The following questions are designed to assist you in gathering relevant clinical information and making accurate decisions in the field.

1. Why is an altered mental status a major factor in determining whether to actively or passively rewarm a hypothermia patient?
2. Explain why skin temperature (cool or warm versus hot) is a major factor in determining whether to aggressively cool a patient.

Street Scenes

It is very cold out, and it has been snowing for hours. Shortly after sundown, you get dispatched for an "unknown man down" call in a downtown area where homeless people often sleep outdoors. As you pull up to the scene, you are met by a police officer who tells you that the man sitting by the heater grate in the sidewalk was going to be taken to the shelter "but something didn't seem right." You get the first-in bag and approach the patient. You ask his name, and he says, "Frank." You ask for a last name, but he doesn't respond.

"Well, Frank, what's going on?" He just stares. "Do you have any pain?" Again, no response. He just sits with his arms folded over his chest and appears to be shivering. "Frank, we think you need to go to the hospital to get checked out."

"What?" he whispers. You ask the patient if he can stand up, but his response is unintelligible. You get the cot and load for transport. Your partner asks you what's wrong, and you tell him that you think the patient might be hypothermic.

Street Scene Questions

1. **What concerns might you have for this patient?**
2. **What assessment needs to be performed?**
3. **Should you rewarm this patient? If so, when should you start?**

When you get into the ambulance, you repeat your primary assessment, checking the patient's breathing closely and looking for any external bleeding. Again, you ask the patient if he knows where he is, but he responds with only groans. You notice that his clothing is wet, so you turn up the heat in the patient compartment, take off his wet jacket and shirt, and wrap him in more blankets. He is still shivering. You take a set of vital signs and determine his blood pressure is 90/60, pulse is 120, respiration rate is 28 and shallow, and skin is flushed. The pulse oximeter is unable to give you a reading. You are unable to get enough blood to determine his blood glucose level. When you feel the abdomen with the back of your hand, it feels cool. You do not smell any alcohol on the patient, and when you check distal pulses, motor function, and sensation, you find that he can move all extremities but it is difficult and seems painful. His pupils respond to light but appear sluggish. You decide to administer oxygen by nonrebreather mask. You also decide not to actively rewarm the patient but instead to keep him wrapped in blankets, covering his head and keeping the heater turned up.

Street Scene Questions

4. **How often should you take vital signs?**
5. **When moving the patient out of the ambulance and onto the hospital stretcher, what precautions should you take?**

You decide to take another set of vital signs after 5 minutes, because you think that this patient could be at risk for respiratory arrest or sudden cardiac death. You make sure the AED and the respiratory equipment are close at hand. His vital signs are about the same. You call the hospital, give your report, and advise an ETA of 5 minutes.

When you get there, you remind your partner that this patient needs to be handled gently. You get another blanket from the emergency department before you make the move. The patient seems to be warming up, and you don't want to put him at any additional risk. When you get into the emergency department, you smoothly move the patient to the stretcher and give the prehospital care report. As you are leaving, Frank looks at you and says, "Thanks. You're nice."

6 SECTION

Special Populations

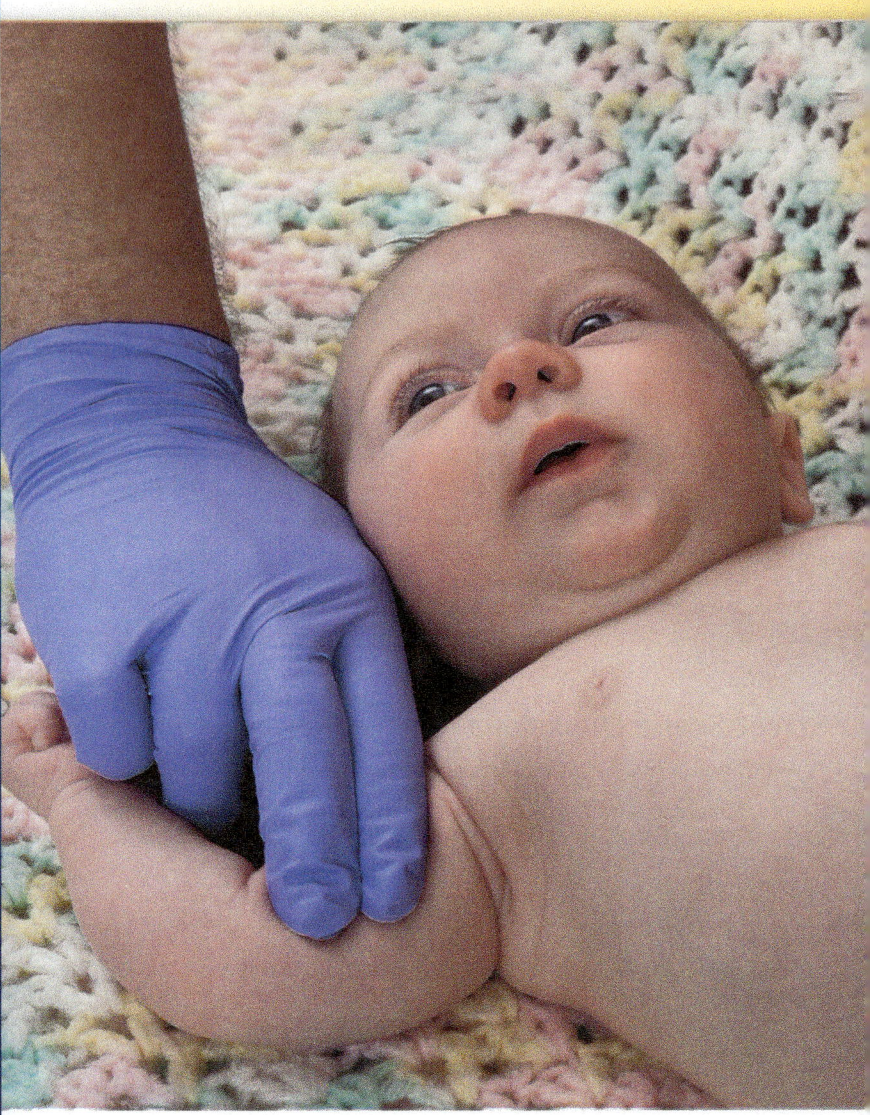

Special populations require special considerations. However, when assisting these patients, you will generally be able to adapt the basics of patient assessment and care that you have already learned.

Childbirth and emergencies associated with the female reproductive system are covered in Chapter 36, *Obstetric and Gynecologic Emergencies*. Chapter 37, *Emergencies for Patients with Special Challenges*, addresses the growing number of patients with advanced medical devices in their homes that enable them to live and function outside a hospital setting.

These patients require specialized considerations: understanding special aspects of their anatomy and physiology, ways that their signs and symptoms may differ from those of the general population, special communication challenges, and the need to treat these patients with respect and special concern for their emotional as well as physical needs.

Obstetric and Gynecologic Emergencies

36

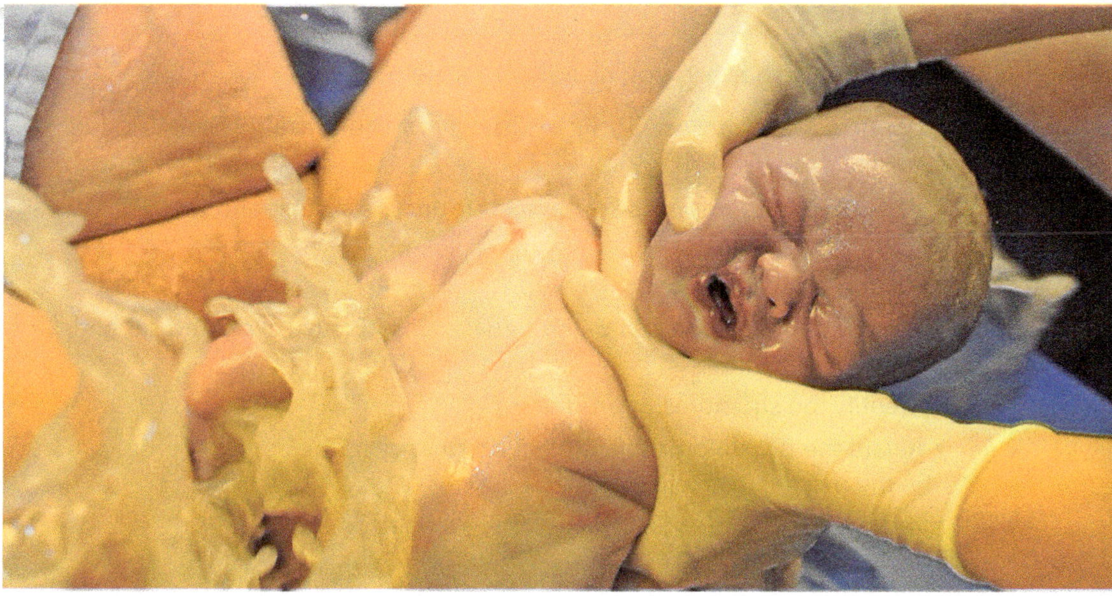

Related Chapters

The following chapters provide additional information related to topics discussed in this chapter:

2 Well-Being of the EMT
8 Life Span Development
21 Resuscitation

Standard

Medicine; Special Patient Populations (Gynecology; Obstetrics)

Competency

Applies fundamental knowledge to provide basic emergency care and transportation based on assessment findings for an acutely ill patient.

Applies a fundamental knowledge of growth, development, and aging, along with assessment findings, to provide basic emergency care and transportation for a patient with special needs.

Core Concepts

- Anatomy and physiology of the female reproductive system
- Physiologic changes in pregnancy
- Care of the mother and baby during labor and delivery
- Care of the neonate
- Postdelivery care of the mother
- Complications of labor and delivery

- Emergencies in pregnancy
- Gynecologic emergencies

Outcomes

After reading this chapter, you should be able to:

36.1 Describe the anatomy and physiology of the female reproductive system. (pp. 1054–1059)

- Describe structures of the female reproductive system and their functions.
- Identify female reproductive organs in diagrams.
- Describe the relationship of the female reproductive cycle and potential for pregnancy.
- Identify the structures of pregnancy.
- Relate the physiologic changes of pregnancy to the risks for complications in the mother and fetus.
- Explain the characteristics of the three stages of labor.
- Recognize indications of imminent delivery of the fetus.

36.2 Summarize the management of childbirth and immediate neonatal care. (pp. 1059–1078)

- Describe the evaluation of the pregnant patient in labor.
- Describe considerations to weigh in deciding whether to transport the patient or prepare for scene-delivery.
- State the steps in preparing for delivery at the scene.
- Describe the intended use of the items in an obstetric kit.
- Describe the importance of reassuring the mother.
- Outline the steps of assisting with a delivery.
- Explain findings that may indicate the need for neonatal resuscitation.
- Outline the steps of assessing a neonate.
- Outline the steps of caring for the neonate.
- Describe the procedure for clamping and cutting the umbilical cord.
- Describe the APGAR scale and Pediatric Resuscitation Triangle as they relate to decision making in the care of the neonate.
- Relate assessment findings to the specific interventions required for neonatal resuscitation.

36.3 Summarize the postdelivery care of the mother. (pp. 1078–1080)

- Describe decisions related to delivery of the placenta.
- Explain the risks of vaginal bleeding.
- Outline the steps of caring for vaginal bleeding.
- List comfort measures you can provide to the mother.
- Describe the reassessment of the mother during transport.

36.4 Summarize the approach to managing childbirth complications. (pp. 1080–1087)

- Name specific types of childbirth complications and their presentations.
- Outline the special care required for each type of childbirth complication.

36.5 Summarize the approach to managing pregnancy-related emergencies. (pp. 1087–1095)

- List specific types of pregnancy-related emergencies and their presentations.
- Outline the specific care required for each type of pregnancy-related emergency.

36.6 Summarize the approach to gynecologic emergencies. (pp. 1095–1097)

- Compare the steps in the approaches to nontraumatic vaginal bleeding and traumatic vaginal injury.
- Describe the special considerations required in the management of a situation in which a patient has been sexually assaulted.

Key Terms

abortion, *1091*
abruptio placentae, *1088*
afterbirth, *1059*
amniotic sac, *1057*
Braxton-Hicks contractions, *1060*
breech presentation, *1080*
cephalic presentation, *1063*
cervix, *1055*
crowning, *1063*
eclampsia, *1090*
ectopic pregnancy, *1089*
embryo, *1056*
fallopian tube, *1055*
fetus, *1056*
induced abortion, *1091*
labia, *1054*
labor, *1059*
lightening, *1060*
limb presentation, *1081*
meconium staining, *1061*
miscarriage, *1091*
mons pubis, *1054*
multiple birth, *1084*
neonate, *1071*
ovary, *1055*
ovulation, *1056*
perineum, *1054*
placenta, *1057*
placenta previa, *1088*
preeclampsia, *1090*
premature infant, *1085*
prolapsed umbilical cord, *1082*
spontaneous abortion, *1091*
stillborn, *1093*
supine hypotensive syndrome, *1059*
umbilical cord, *1057*
uterus, *1055*
vagina, *1055*

Understanding of the female reproductive system is an important element of your assessment and treatment of any female patient. As an EMT, you should know that the anatomy and physiology of this system can be vastly different from patient to patient. In a nonpregnant woman, the organs of reproduction are small and well protected, whereas in a pregnant woman these same organs are enlarged and therefore more vulnerable to injury. During pregnancy, a woman's reproductive system will undergo tremendous changes, leading up to the birth of a child.

Childbirth is a natural process that existed long before there were EMTs, and the vast majority of births are uncomplicated. However, you should always remember that if EMS has been called, something unexpected has occurred, and the likelihood of a problem has increased. With the potential for complications, the best place to deliver a baby is a hospital. Much of your assessment of the woman in labor will be geared toward making a decision about whether to transport the pregnant woman or prepare for an immediate delivery.

If an out-of-hospital delivery does become necessary, you should be prepared for many events to occur in rapid sequence. Delivery, neonatal resuscitation, and care of the mother often happen almost simultaneously, and in these often-unpracticed moments, preparation is key. This chapter is designed to help you better understand the sequence, necessary interventions, and potential complications involved in childbirth and neonate resuscitation. Although none of the concepts or actions described here is particularly complex, the stress of the moment is often the biggest challenge to optimal care. Remember that one of your main responsibilities will be to help calm the patient and family members through your unruffled, professional manner. Staying calm will also improve your ability to maintain situational awareness, prioritize, and approach neonatal emergencies with the organized and structured management plan so vital to positive outcomes.

Anatomy and Physiology

CORE CONCEPT

Anatomy and physiology of the female reproductive system

External Genitalia

A woman's external genitalia consist of three major structures: the labia, the perineum, and the mons pubis (Figure 36-1).

The ***labia*** consist of soft tissues that protect the entrance to the birth canal. The urethral opening and the nerve-rich center of sexual stimulation, called the clitoris, can be found in the anterior aspects of the labia. These tissues are highly vascular and prone to significant bleeding with trauma.

The ***perineum*** is the soft tissue and muscle found between the vaginal opening and the anus. This tissue is prone to tearing during childbirth. The ***mons pubis*** is a layer of soft tissue that covers and protects the pubic symphysis. It is the area where hair grows when a woman reaches puberty.

labia (LAY-be-uh)
soft tissues that protect the entrance to the vagina.

perineum (per-i-NE-um)
the surface area between the vagina and anus.

mons pubis
soft tissue that covers the pubic symphysis; area where hair grows when a woman reaches puberty.

"It may seem like an emergency to you, but childbirth is natural. It's happened long before EMTs were around!"

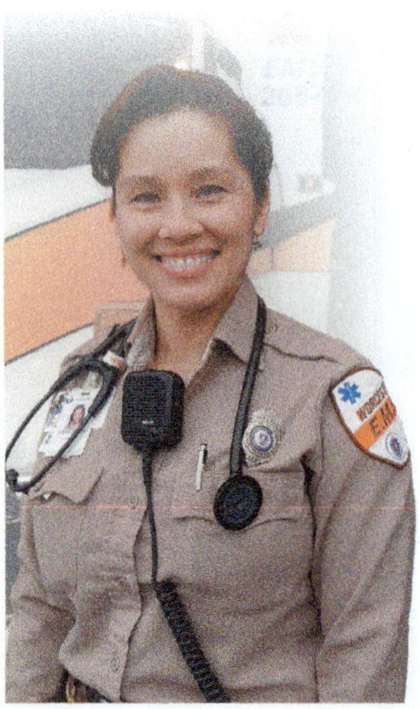

FIGURE 36-1 External female genitalia.

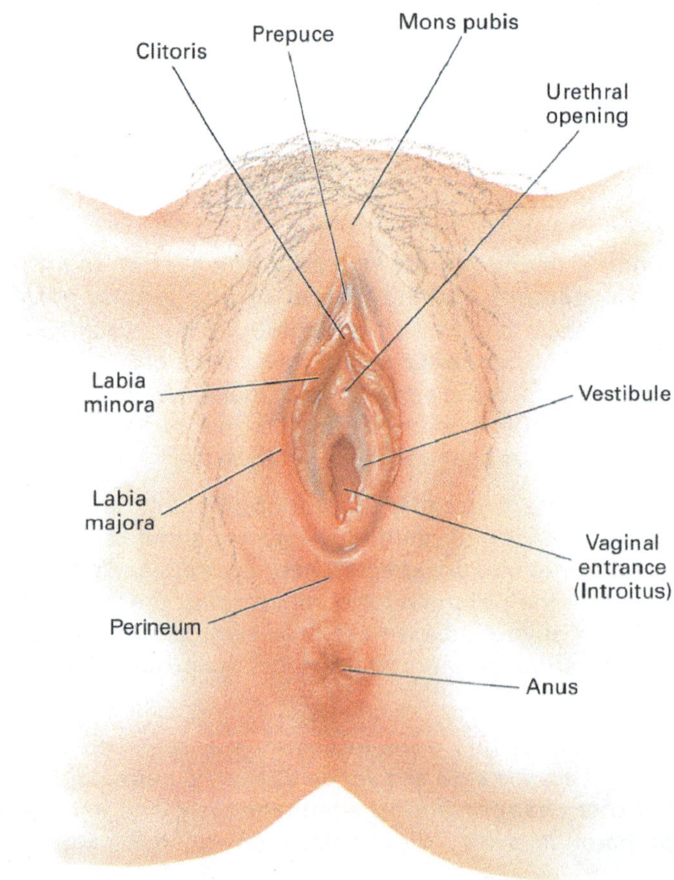

Internal Genitalia

A woman's internal genitalia consists of the vagina, the ovaries, the fallopian tubes, and the uterus (Figure 36-2).

The Vagina

The ***vagina*** is the birth canal. Made up of smooth muscle, it connects the uterus to the outside world and will stretch to accommodate passage of the fetus during delivery. It is also the passageway for menstrual waste products leaving the uterus at the conclusion of the menstrual cycle.

vagina (vah-JI-nah)
the birth canal.

The Ovaries and Fallopian Tubes

The ovaries are small, round organs that are located on either side of most women's lower abdominal quadrants. These organs are responsible for producing ova (eggs) for conception. They also produce many of the hormones necessary for the process of reproduction. An ovum that matures in the ovaries is transported through the fallopian tubes, or *oviducts*, to the uterus (the place where it may implant and develop if fertilized). Each ***ovary*** is connected to the uterus by a ***fallopian tube***. If fertilization occurs, it will most likely happen in these tubes. A dangerous condition called *ectopic pregnancy* can occur if the fertilized ovum implants in the fallopian tubes. Unlike the uterus, these tubes cannot expand as the fetus develops and are vulnerable to rupture and severe bleeding. (We will discuss ectopic pregnancy in greater detail later in this chapter.)

ovary (o-vu-RE)
the female reproductive organ that produces ova.

fallopian (fu-LO-pe-an) ***tube***
the narrow tube that connects the ovary to the uterus. Also called the *oviduct*.

The Uterus

The ***uterus*** (or womb) is a muscular, hollow organ located along the midline in most women's lower abdominal quadrants. This organ is the intended site for the fertilized ovum to implant and develop into a fetus. To accommodate that purpose, the uterus is able to stretch and grow as the fetus gets larger. The top, or fundus, of the uterus can be found as high as the xiphoid process (the lower anterior junction of the rib cage) in a late-term pregnant woman. The lower aspect of the uterus is connected to the vagina. A muscular ring called the ***cervix*** separates these two organs. In a nonpregnant female, the cervix is constricted

uterus (U-ter-us)
the muscular abdominal organ where the fetus develops; the womb.

cervix (SUR-viks)
the lower neck of the uterus at the entrance to the birth canal.

FIGURE 36-2 Internal female genitalia.

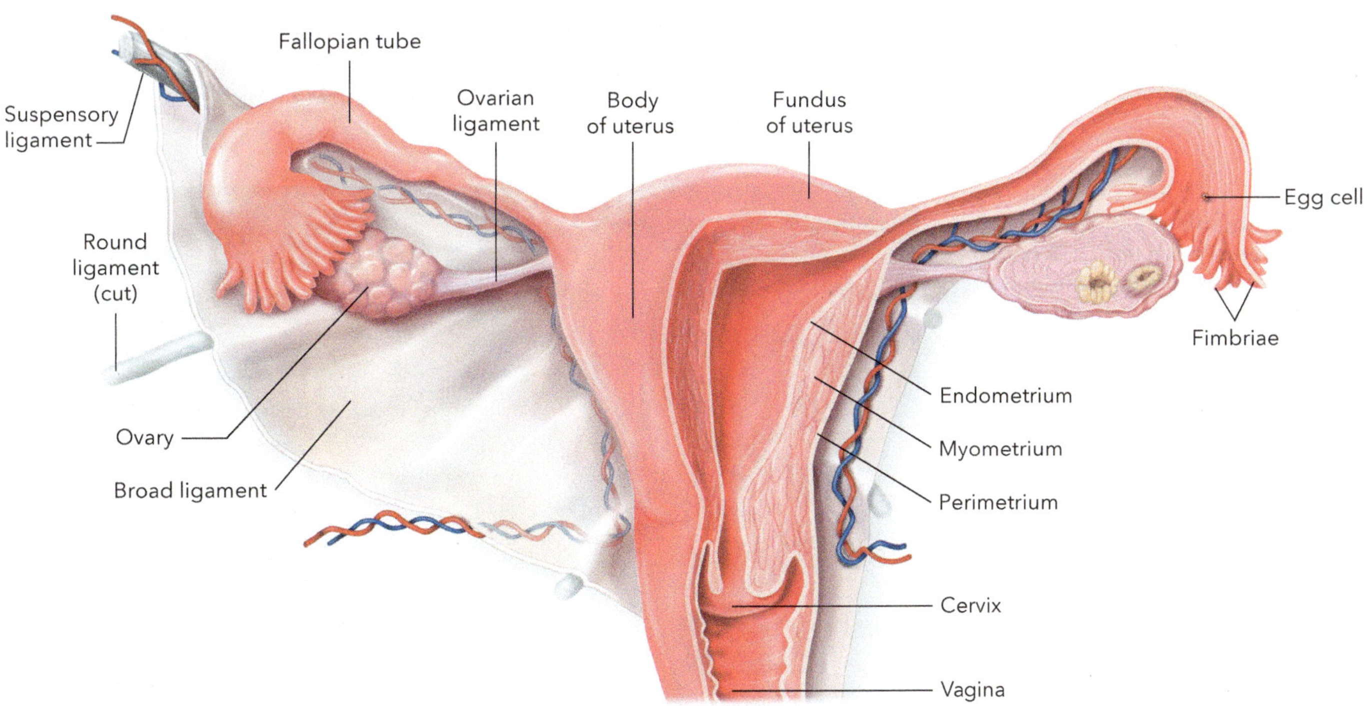

to close off the uterus. With labor, the cervix dilates and thins to allow the muscular walls of the uterus to contract and push the fetus out through the vagina and into the outside world. Cervical dilation is assessed in the hospital to predict the timing of delivery. (Note: This assessment is *not* conducted in the field by EMTs.) A patient will be described in terms of how many centimeters her cervix has opened. For example, a patient might be described as being 4 cm dilated. This means that her cervix has opened approximately 4 cm. As the cervix opens, it also begins to thin out. This thinning of the cervix is termed *effacement*. Cervical dilation and effacement are key factors in the progression of labor and delivery, and typically the timing of delivery correlates to the widening of the cervix and the degree of effacement.

The Female Reproductive Cycle

ovulation (ov-U-LA-shun) the phase of the female reproductive cycle in which an ovum is released from the ovary.

After a woman reaches the age of puberty, approximately every twenty-eight days, her uterus goes through a series of changes to prepare for the potential implantation of a fertilized egg. Hormones such as estrogen and progesterone stimulate these events. In the early phases, the ovaries are stimulated to release an ovum (egg) in a process called **ovulation**. At the same time, the walls of the uterus thicken in preparation for implantation of the egg if fertilization occurs.

The fallopian tubes now move the egg by peristalsis (waves of muscular contraction) toward the uterus. Fertilization typically occurs in the fallopian tubes. If fertilization does not occur, hormone levels once again change, and the uterus begins to change as well. Without fertilization, the thickened inner walls of the uterus begin to slough off and are expelled through the vagina. This process is called *menstruation* and is usually characterized by vaginal bleeding, typically totaling around 1.75 ounces (50 mL), for roughly three to five days. If the egg is fertilized and successfully implants, hormones induce other changes that occur with pregnancy.

Fertilization

embryo (EM-bree-o) the baby from fertilization to eight weeks of development.

fetus (FE-tus) the baby from eight weeks of development to birth.

If a woman has sexual intercourse that results in the release of sperm into the vagina in the period immediately following ovulation and sperm reaches the ovum, fertilization may occur. By combining with the sperm, an ovum becomes an **embryo** and the embryonic stage of pregnancy begins. The embryonic stage begins roughly from the point of fertilization and lasts eight weeks. During this stage, the embryo may implant in the lining of the uterus and develop basic connections between itself and the mother.

At eight weeks of development, the fetal stage begins. From this point until delivery, the developing baby is referred to as a **fetus** (Figure 36-3). The fetus will develop over the next 32 weeks (a typical pregnancy lasts about 40 weeks), during which time the woman's body will undergo significant changes.

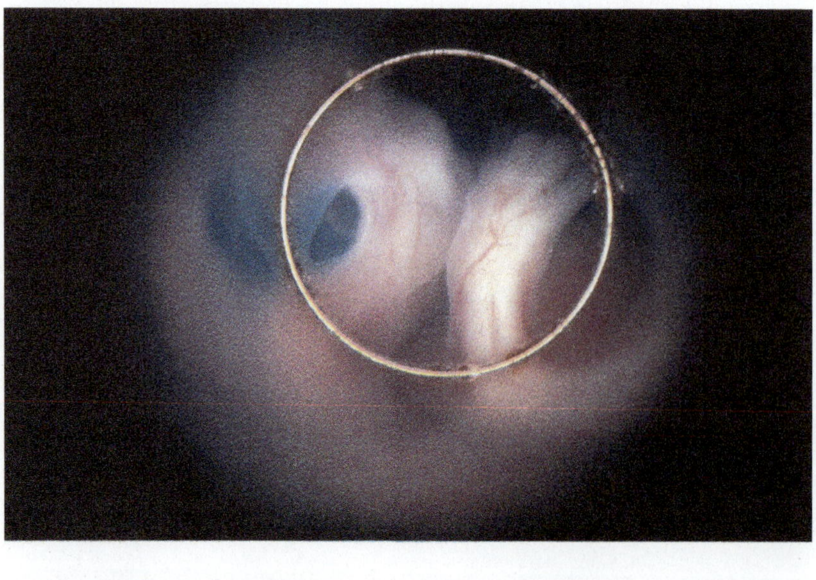

FIGURE 36-3 Endoscopic photograph of a 9-week-old live fetus in the uterus. A hand and eye are clearly visible. *(Petit Format/Science Source)*

Physiologic Changes in Pregnancy

Changes in the Reproductive System

CORE CONCEPT
Physiologic changes in pregnancy

Size is the most significant change that pregnancy brings to the reproductive system. As the fetus grows and develops, the uterus simply gets larger. It becomes thinner-walled and less protected by the abdominal cavity. Therefore, it becomes more vulnerable to injury.

The nine months of pregnancy are divided into three trimesters, or 3-month periods. During the first trimester, the fetus is being formed. Since the fetus remains quite small, there is little uterine growth during this period. After the third month, the uterus grows rapidly, reaching the umbilicus (navel) by the fifth month and the epigastrium (upper abdomen) by the seventh month.

As the fetus develops, other major changes occur in the reproductive system (Figure 36-4). In addition to the fetus, an organ called the ***placenta*** develops in the uterus. Composed of both maternal and fetal tissues, the placenta is attached to the wall of the uterus and serves as an exchange area between maternal and fetal blood. The mother's blood does not flow directly through the fetus's body. Instead, the fetus has its own circulatory system. Blood from the fetus is sent through blood vessels in the ***umbilical cord*** to the placenta, where, through diffusion, the blood picks up nourishment from the mother and offloads waste products, then returns through the umbilical cord to the fetus's body. The umbilical cord is approximately 1 inch (2.5 cm) wide and 22 inches (56 cm) long at birth, and has one vein (the umbilical vein) and two arteries (the umbilical arteries). Both the placenta and umbilical cord are expelled after the birth of the baby.

placenta (plah-SEN-tah) the organ of pregnancy where exchange of oxygen, nutrients, and wastes occurs between a mother and fetus.

umbilical (um-BIL-i-kal) ***cord*** the fetal structure containing the blood vessels that carry blood to and from the placenta.

The process of exchange between maternal and fetal blood is similar to the diffusion between the alveoli and pulmonary capillaries you read about in Chapter 10, *Respiration and Artificial Ventilation*. In the placenta, blood vessels from the mother come in close proximity to blood vessels from the fetus. Although blood does not mix, the proximity allows diffusion to transfer oxygen, nutrients, and waste products between the mother and fetus. Diffusion can also transfer unwanted substances such as opioids, nicotine, and alcohol. This process of diffusion allows the fetus to be oxygenated without breathing outside air.

While developing in the uterus, the fetus is enclosed and protected within a thin, membranous "bag of waters" known as the ***amniotic sac***. This sac contains almost 1 quart (just under 1 L) of liquid, called amniotic fluid. It allows the fetus to float during development,

amniotic (am-ne-OT-ik) ***sac*** the "bag of waters" that surrounds the developing fetus.

FIGURE 36-4 Structures of pregnancy.

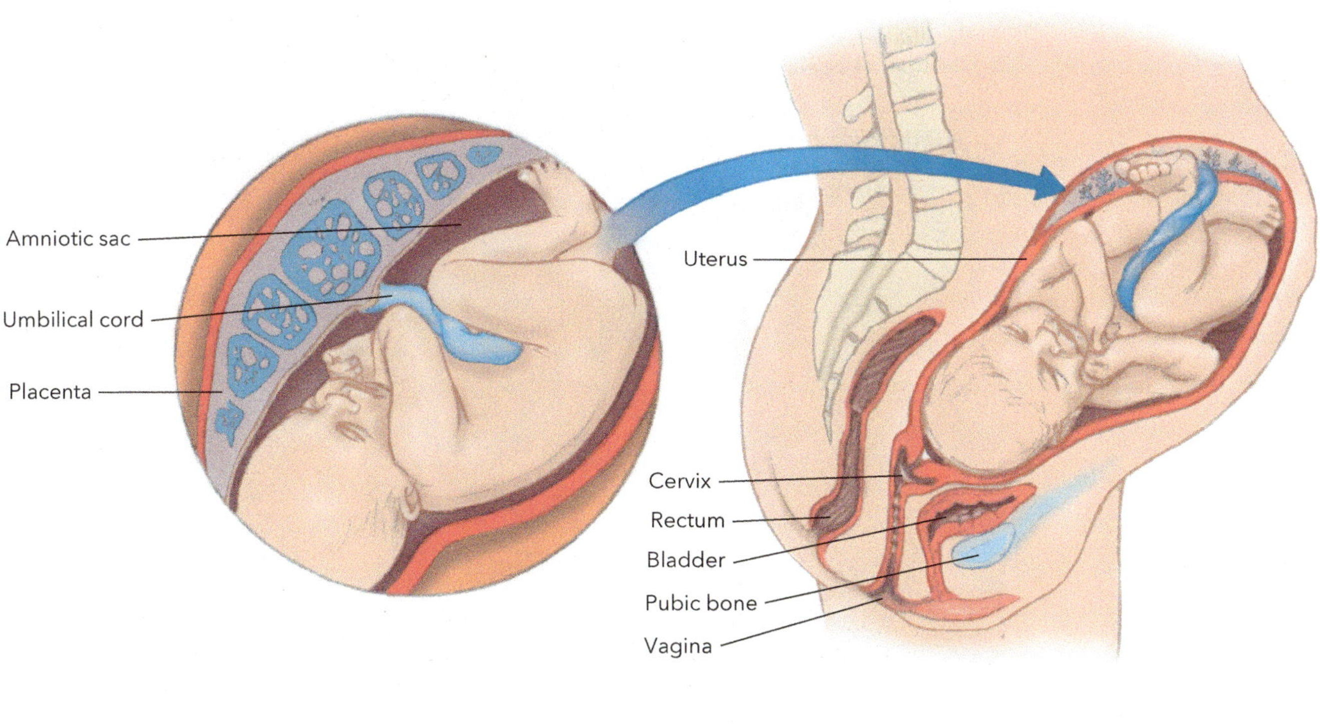

acts as a cushion between the fetus and minor injury, and helps maintain a constant fetal body temperature. In the vast majority of cases, the amniotic sac breaks during labor and the fluid gushes from the birth canal. This is a normal condition of childbirth that also provides a natural lubrication to ease the infant's progress through the birth canal.

Other Physiologic Changes in Pregnancy

In addition to reproductive system changes, other systems are also impacted by the developing fetus. The cardiovascular system responds to pregnancy by increasing blood volume, increasing cardiac output, and increasing heart rate. Although blood volume increases, the number of red blood cells remains the same. This causes a dilution of the blood, referred to as *anemia*, and it should be remembered that although there is more blood, its oxygen-carrying capacity is actually decreased. The blood pressure of a pregnant female is usually slightly decreased, but high blood pressure can occur as well. There is also a massive increase in vascularity (presence of blood and blood vessels) in the uterus and related structures.

Physiologic Changes of Pregnancy

Pregnancy causes numerous physiologic changes (Figure 36-5).

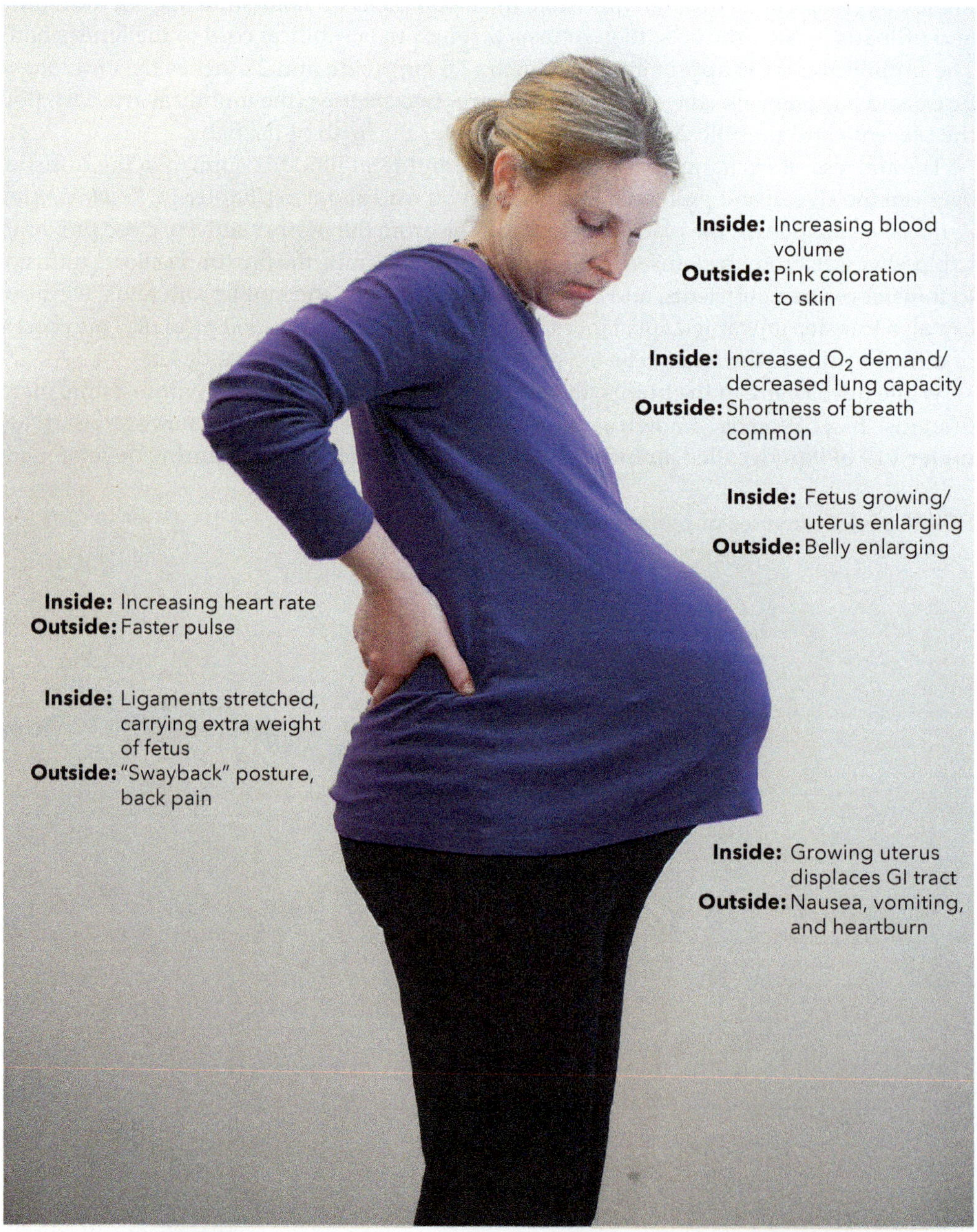

FIGURE 36-5 Physiologic changes in pregnancy.

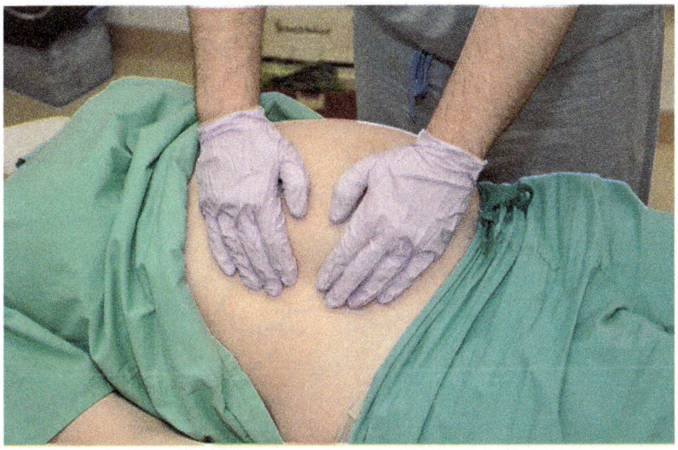

FIGURE 36-6 Gently displacing the pregnant patient's uterus toward her left side. *(© Edward T. Dickinson, MD)*

Pregnancy affects the respiratory system by increasing oxygen demand and consumption. In the later stages of pregnancy, the fetus can also put pressure on the woman's diaphragm and decrease the volume of air in her lungs.

In the gastrointestinal system, a growing fetus puts pressure on the stomach and intestines, which can slow digestion. Nausea and vomiting are also very common in pregnancy. Occasionally this nausea and vomiting can be severe and lead to dehydration and even hypovolemia.

Hormones released with pregnancy make the ligaments of a pregnant woman's musculoskeletal system more elastic and, therefore, more vulnerable to injury. The additional weight can also affect posture and lead to back pain as well as affect balance.

Pregnancy may also impact preexisting medical conditions in the mother. Asthma and diabetes both can be made worse with pregnancy.

Supine Hypotensive Syndrome

In the third trimester, near the time of birth, the weight of the uterus—combined with the weight of the infant, placenta, and amniotic fluid—totals approximately 20–24 pounds (9–11 kg). When the mother is in a supine position, this heavy mass will tend to compress the inferior vena cava, a major blood vessel, reducing return of blood to the heart, thereby reducing cardiac output. The resulting dizziness and drop in blood pressure constitute a set of signs and symptoms known as ***supine hypotensive syndrome***. This syndrome is also referred to as *vena cava compression syndrome*. When the body senses the drop in blood pressure, it compensates by contracting the uterine arteries and redirecting blood to the major organs of the mother. This can severely affect the fetus.

Although the drop in blood pressure signals shock, traditional methods of treating shock will not be effective in this instance. To take the weight off the vena cava and counteract or avoid the possible drop in blood pressure, *all third-trimester patients should be transported on their left sides*. A pillow or rolled blanket should be placed behind the back to maintain proper positioning. If the patient is not able to be moved to a lateral position, such as in cardiac arrest states, the uterus can also manually be displaced by gently pulling it toward the patient's left side (Figure 36-6).

supine hypotensive syndrome
dizziness and a drop in blood pressure caused when the mother is in a supine position and the weight of the uterus, infant, placenta, and amniotic fluid compress the inferior vena cava, reducing return of blood to the heart and cardiac output.

labor
the three stages of the delivery of a baby that begin with the contractions of the uterus and end with the expulsion of the placenta.

Labor and Delivery

The Stages of Labor

Labor is the entire process of delivery. There are three stages of labor (Figure 36-7):

- **First stage.** This stage starts with regular contractions and the thinning and gradual dilation of the cervix and ends when the cervix is fully dilated.
- **Second stage.** This stage begins when the baby enters the birth canal and lasts until the baby is born.
- **Third stage.** This stage begins after the baby is born and lasts until the ***afterbirth*** (placenta, umbilical cord, and some tissues from the amniotic sac and the lining of the uterus) is delivered.

CORE CONCEPT
Care of the mother and baby during labor and childbirth

afterbirth
the placenta, membranes of the amniotic sac, part of the umbilical cord, and some tissues from the lining of the uterus that are delivered after the birth of the baby.

FIGURE 36-7 Three stages of labor.

First stage:
beginning of contractions to full cervical dilation

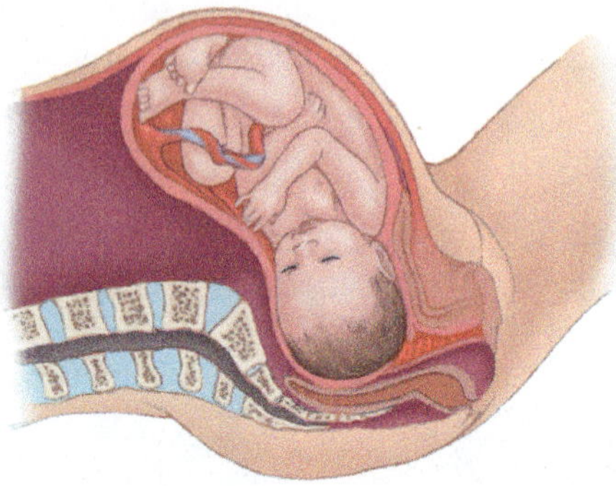

Second stage:
baby enters birth canal and is born

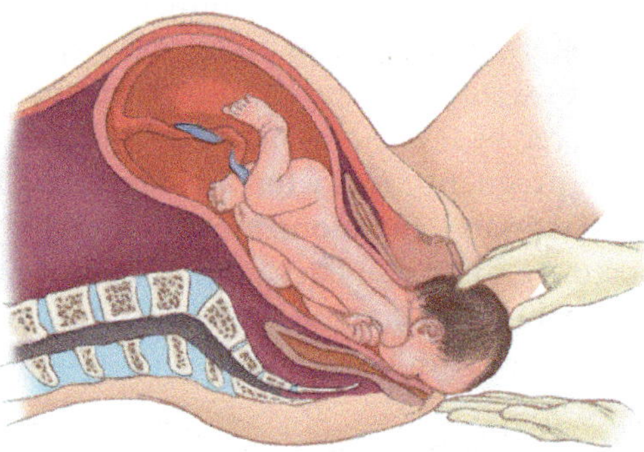

Third stage:
delivery of the placenta

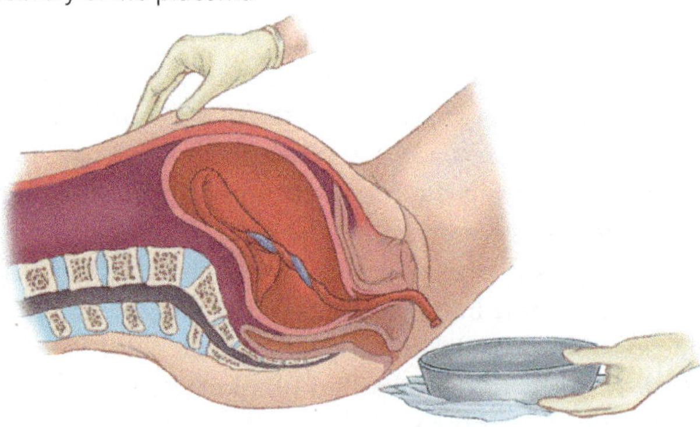

First Stage

The first stage of labor is also called the dilation period. Picture the uterus as a long-neck bottle. To expel the contents, the neck of the bottle must be stretched to the size of a wide-mouth jar. Before the cervix can fully dilate, the long neck of the cervix must be shortened and thinned (this process is called *effacement*) to the wide-mouth-jar shape.

Sometimes, several days or even weeks before the onset of actual labor, the uterine muscles begin mild contractions. These ***Braxton-Hicks contractions*** are usually irregular and not sustained, and they typically do not indicate impending delivery. In contrast, when actual labor begins, the uterus will begin to contract regularly, and the cervix will begin to dilate. As this happens, the fetus's head typically moves downward.

Lightening is a term used to describe the fetus's movement from high in the abdomen down toward the birth canal. Some women will experience this sensation. At times, this occurs well before the start of labor, but it can also be an indicator of the beginning of the labor process.

Braxton-Hicks (braks-tun-hiks) ***contractions***
irregular prelabor contractions of the uterus.

lightening
the sensation of the fetus moving from high in the abdomen to low in the birth canal.

When contractions begin, they may be up to 30 minutes apart. They progress to be 3 minutes or less apart near delivery.

The contractions of the uterus produce normal labor pains. Most women report the start of labor pains as an ache in the lower back. As labor progresses, the pain becomes most noticeable in the lower abdomen, with the intensity of pain increasing. The pains come at regular intervals, lasting from 30 seconds to 1 minute, and occur at 2- to 3-minute intervals. When the uterus starts to contract, the pain begins. As the muscles relax, there is relief from the pain. Labor pains may start, stop for a while, then start up again.

As an EMT, you should time the following characteristics of labor pains:

- **Contraction time, or duration.** This is the time from the beginning of a contraction to when the uterus relaxes (from start to end).
- **Contraction interval, or frequency.** This is the time from the start of one contraction to the start of the next.

Contractions that last between 30 seconds and 1 minute and those that are 2–3 minutes apart demonstrate that labor has progressed, and often indicate that delivery is imminent. However, contraction timing is not always an accurate indicator of the timing of delivery. Although contractions should be considered in decision making, more accurate indications will be discussed later.

As contractions continue, the cervix gradually shortens and thins enough (reaching wide-mouth-jar shape) to become flush with the vagina (fully open to the birth canal). The full dilation of the cervix signals the end of the first stage of labor. Women giving birth for the first time will remain in this first stage of labor for an average of sixteen hours. However, some women may remain in this stage as little as four hours, especially if this is not their first child.

NOTE: *There is no way to assess the dilation of the cervix externally. As an EMT, you will assess the progression of labor using other findings. EMTs do not do internal cervical examinations.*

As the fetus moves downward, and the cervix dilates, the amniotic sac usually breaks. This is commonly referred to as the "water breaking" or the "rupture of membranes." It is often felt by the woman as a gush or trickle of fluid exiting the vagina. Most commonly, it immediately precedes labor. However, it can also happen well before the onset of labor. This is called premature rupture of membranes; it can be a serious problem for the fetus.

Normally the amniotic fluid is clear. Fluid that is greenish- or brownish-yellow in color is due to fetal defecation and may be an indication of maternal or fetal distress, and is called ***meconium staining***.

meconium staining
amniotic fluid that is greenish- or brownish-yellow rather than clear, as a result of fetal defecation; an indication of possible maternal or fetal distress during labor.

There may also be a watery, bloody discharge of mucus (not bleeding) associated with the first stage of labor. Part of this initial discharge will be from a mucous plug that helped to keep the cervix closed during pregnancy. This is usually mixed with blood and is called the *bloody show*. Watery, bloody fluids discharging from the vagina are typical for all three stages of labor.

Second Stage

The second stage of labor begins after the full dilation of the cervix. During this time, contractions become increasingly frequent, and labor pains become more severe. In the second stage of labor, the cramping and abdominal pains associated with the first stage of labor are typically still present. As delivery approaches, most women will feel an urge to push or move their bowels. This occurs as the baby's body moves and places pressure on the rectum. The urge to push is a sign that birth is near, and the EMT will have to decide whether to transport the pregnant patient or keep the mother where she is and prepare to assist with delivery.

Third Stage

The third stage of labor begins immediately after the baby is born. In this stage, the placenta detaches itself from the wall of the uterus and is expelled. Contractions will resume and continue until the placenta is delivered. The contractions and labor pains may be as painful and severe during this stage as they were in the second stage. The third stage usually lasts 10–20 minutes and ends as the placenta is delivered.

Patient Assessment

Woman in Labor

Assessment of a woman in labor includes all the elements of a traditional patient assessment. Both the primary and secondary assessments are important. Remember that both the "airway, breathing, and circulation" issues of the primary assessment and the past medical history of the secondary assessment can have a major impact on the events of the moment. Begin by assessing the pregnant woman the same way you would any other patient. Ensure proper oxygenation, ventilation, and perfusion. Consider the chief complaint (especially if it is something other than the onset of labor). Consider medications and her past medical history. There are also a few assessment elements that are specific to pregnancy and to the onset of labor.

- **Ask what her expected due date is.** Due date is estimated by adding 40 weeks (the average time of development of a fetus) to the start date of the patient's last menstrual period. Identifying that last known menstrual period helps identify how far along her pregnancy is, but it can be inaccurate. Often a woman will have had an ultrasound during her pregnancy, which provides a more accurate determination of the pregnant woman's due date. A normal pregnancy lasts 40 weeks. But with intensive neonatal care in the hospital, a fetus can survive outside of the mother after 22–24 weeks' gestation.
- **Ask if this is her first pregnancy.** Learning about other pregnancies and deliveries can provide information relevant to the moment at hand. Has she previously had pregnancy-related problems? Were her previous deliveries rapid? Were they vaginal or by cesarean section? The number of prior deliveries can also help predict the timing of the one occurring now. The average time of labor for a woman having her first baby is about sixteen to seventeen hours. The time in labor is typically shorter for subsequent births.
- **Ask her if she has seen a doctor regarding her pregnancy.** This is called *prenatal care*, and is important in identifying such things as multiple gestations (twins, triplets, and so on), known complications or problems with the pregnancy, and possible medical issues with the mother. You should also ask specifically if she has had any issues with the current pregnancy or with her health during the pregnancy. This is a good opportunity to inquire respectfully if she has used any drugs such as stimulants or opioids, as both can affect the health of the fetus.

When an unexpected period of labor is occurring, you will use your assessment to determine if it is possible to reach the hospital before the birth occurs or if it would be better to stay in place and prepare for delivery on scene. This can be an exceptionally difficult decision. The best place for the mother to deliver the baby is in the hospital. There, the delivery can be controlled better and far more resources can be allocated to the safety of both mother and baby. However, precipitous deliveries, long transport distances, and even foul weather can often make reaching a hospital prior to delivery impossible. While it is preferable to transport immediately, delivering a baby in the back of the ambulance is the worst-case scenario. In that enclosed space, there is limited room to work, limited means to transport more than one patient, and a significant challenge to maintaining temperature. If a birth appears imminent, it may be more reasonable simply to stay in the patient's home and request additional resources. While there is no way to predict the exact timing of a baby's arrival, your assessment can provide valuable clues that delivery is about to occur.

A simple series of questions, an examination for crowning, and a determination of vital signs will help you to make the decision about whether to initiate transport or to prepare to deliver the baby where you are. Remember that this decision must also consider distance from the hospital, safety of the home-delivery situation, and available resources. It is also a best practice to consult medical control when making this decision. Although this can be a challenging situation, do not let the urgency of this decision upset the mother. Your patient needs emotional support at this time. Your calm, professional actions will help her feel more at ease and reassure her that you will provide the required care for both her and the unborn child.

In addition to the patient assessment discussed above, the following elements should be considered when making a transport decision:

- **Ask her when the labor pains started.** As discussed previously, the timing of contractions can indicate the progression of labor. As contractions become more frequent, typically the labor progresses. Contractions can be palpated as well. To do so, tell the patient what you are going to do, then place the palm of your gloved hand on her abdomen, above the navel. This can be done over the top of the patient's clothing. You should be able to feel her uterus contract. The uterus and the tissues between this organ and the skin will feel more rigid as the delivery of the baby nears. However, as mentioned, contraction timing can vary widely from delivery to delivery.
- **Ask her if her "water" has broken and if she has had any bleeding or bloody show.** The rupture of membranes (ROM), or release of the amniotic fluid, is usually a precursor to delivery. Like contractions, though, it is not always a reliable predictor of imminent delivery. Some women's water can break up to 24 hours prior to delivery.
- **Ask her if she feels the urge to push or if she feels as though she needs to move her bowels.** The urge to push is generally an accurate indicator of imminent birth and should be a serious finding when making a transport decision. As delivery begins, women will often note an urgency to push and sometimes describe a sensation that the baby has moved down. These sensations most commonly indicate that the baby has moved into the birth canal and is preparing its exit. The movement into the birth canal can also press the baby against the rectum, causing the mother to feel the urge to defecate. Do not allow the mother to go to the bathroom, as she may deliver the infant into the toilet.
- **Examine the mother for crowning (Figure 36-8).** This is a visual inspection to see if there is bulging at the vaginal opening or if the presenting part of the baby is visible. Such an examination requires clear and professional communication and careful explanation to the mother who is in labor. ***Crowning*** occurs when the *presenting part* of the baby first bulges from the vaginal opening, and is typically best seen during a contraction. The presenting part is defined as the part of the infant that is first to appear at the vaginal opening during labor. Usually the presenting part of the baby is the head. The normal headfirst birth is called a ***cephalic presentation***. If the buttocks or both feet of the baby deliver first, the birth is called a *breech presentation* or *breech birth*. If part of the baby's head or presenting part is visible with each contraction, then birth is imminent.
- **Take vital signs.** If you do not have a partner to do it, this is the point to check the patient's vitals.

NOTE: *Do not allow the mother to hold her legs together or use any other method to attempt to delay the delivery.*

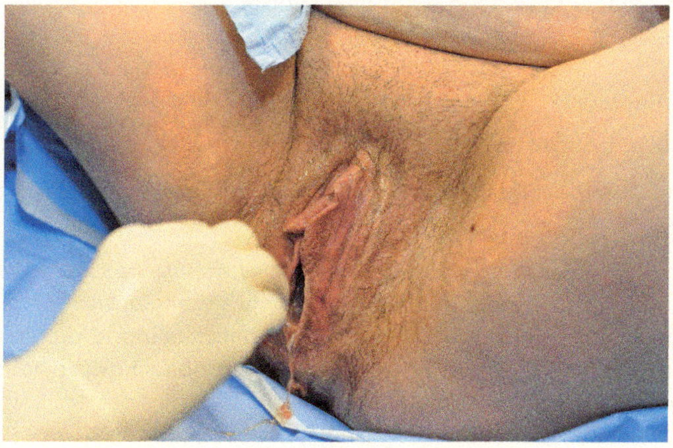

FIGURE 36-8 Crowning of the infant's head.

crowning
the point during childbirth when part of the baby is visible through the vaginal opening.

cephalic (se-FAL-ik) ***presentation***
normal birth presentation, where the baby's head appears first.

Point of View

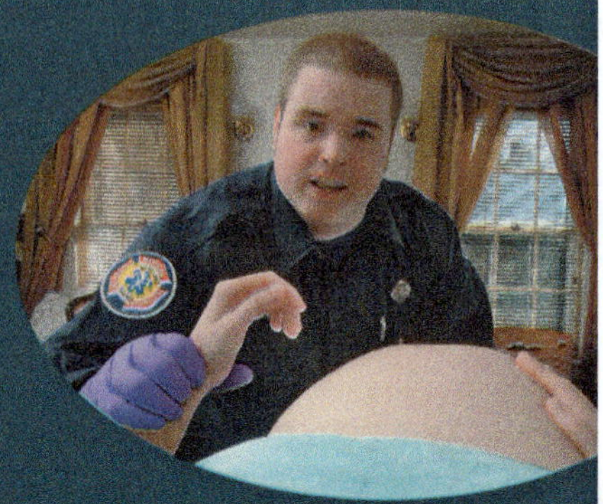

"I had planned to have a very controlled delivery. It was my first baby. And yes, maybe I was trying to micromanage a natural process . . . when all my plans went to hell. My contractions started, my water broke, and I felt like I was going to have the baby right there.

"My husband and I freaked. All the plans to call people and have a meaningful time together before the hospital went out the window. The only call we made was to 911.

"The EMTs arrived and were great. They calmed us down. Lord knows we needed that. After they asked a few questions and timed the contractions, they thought there would be time to get to the hospital before the baby was born.

"They were right. We did have time. About eight hours. Did I mention that we totally freaked out? If we ever do this again, it will be different. Honest!"

Examining for crowning may be embarrassing to the mother, the father, and any required bystanders. For this reason, it is important that you give full explanations of what you are doing and why. Be certain that you protect the mother from the stares of bystanders. In a polite but firm manner, ask everyone who does not belong at the scene to leave. Carefully help the patient remove enough clothing to allow you an unobstructed view of the vaginal opening.

If this is the woman's first delivery, she is not pushing, and there is no crowning, there is little reason she cannot be transported to a medical facility for delivery. (A first delivery typically takes longer than do subsequent ones.) However, if this is not her first delivery, and she is pushing, crying out, and complaining about having to go to the bathroom, birth will probably occur too soon for transport. If the mother is having labor pains from contractions that are about 2 minutes apart, birth may be very near. If you determine that delivery is imminent based on the presence of crowning or other signs, local protocol may require you to contact medical direction for the decision whether to commit to delivery on the site. If delivery does not occur within 10 minutes, contact medical direction again and request permission to initiate transport of the mother.

You may find a patient who is afraid of transport because she believes that her baby's birth will occur along the way. Assure her that you believe there is enough time to get to the hospital before delivery. Let her know that you are trained to assist with the delivery and that the ambulance is well equipped to handle her needs and care for the newborn in case she delivers en route. If crowning occurs during transport, stop the ambulance and prepare for delivery.

If your evaluation of the patient leads you to believe that birth is too near at hand for transport, you and your partner should prepare to assist the mother with delivery. Remember: As part of the preparation, the patient will need emotional support.

Decision Points

- Is delivery of the baby imminent?
- Should I prepare to deliver on scene or move to the ambulance?

NOTE: *It is best to transport an expecting mother unless, based on your evaluation, you expect delivery within a few minutes.*

Another important assessment goal is predicting the need for neonatal resuscitation. As you will learn in subsequent sections, neonatal resuscitation is a time-sensitive, rapid sequence of events that requires additional resources. Predicting its likelihood provides an advantage to be better prepared and to have the appropriate additional help on hand. Although the need for resuscitation can never be absolutely predicted, there are some assessment findings that indicate a higher probability of that need.

Findings That Might Indicate the Need for Neonatal Resuscitation

- No prior prenatal care. The patient has not seen an obstetrician and, therefore, has no idea regarding her health or the health of her unborn baby.
- Premature delivery. The earlier the labor, the higher the likelihood of resuscitation.
- Labor induced by trauma or medical conditions affecting the mother.
- Multiple births. Twins, triplets, or more babies significantly increase the likelihood of resuscitation.
- History of problems with the pregnancy, especially placenta previa and breech presentations. (We will discuss both these issues later in the chapter.)
- Labor induced by drug use, especially narcotics or stimulants.
- Meconium staining with the rupture of membranes (water breaking).

The most important outcome of anticipating a neonatal resuscitation is getting help. As you will read later in this chapter, a resuscitation requires a rapid series of actions, with full attention focused on the new baby. If resuscitation is necessary, you will need more help and probably ALS support if available. Good assessment will enable you to begin mobilizing these resources prior to delivering the baby.

Decision Point

- Do I need to prepare for neonatal resuscitation?

Normal Childbirth

Role of the EMT

Your primary role in a childbirth will be to determine whether the delivery will occur on scene and, if so, to assist the mother as she delivers her child.

NOTE: *EMTs do not deliver babies; mothers do!*

Think Like an EMT

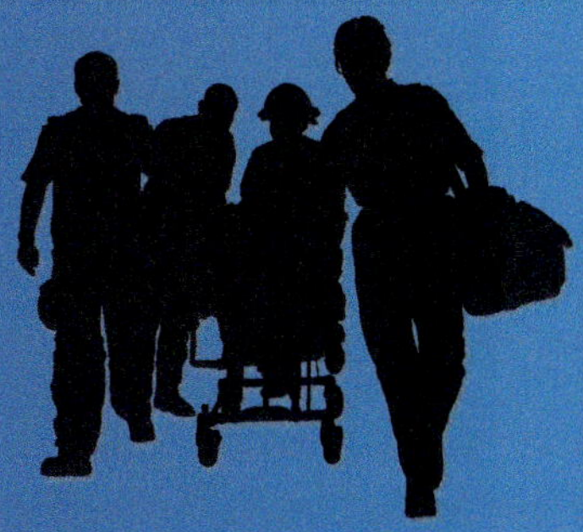

My Baby Won't Wait!

Childbirth in the field is a rare but very exciting call. For every baby you deliver, you may have dozens of maternity calls in which the mother is transported to the hospital before the baby is delivered. Being able to determine whether the birth is imminent is an important skill for an EMT. For each of the scenarios presented, determine whether you should stay and prepare for delivery or transport the patient to the hospital.

1. Your patient states her contractions are severe and about 30 seconds apart. She feels the need to push and suspects she has accidentally moved her bowels. There is significant bulging, and you can see the baby's head crowning. This is her fourth child.
2. Your patient reports that contractions are about 5–10 minutes apart but feel strong. This is her first child. You do not observe any crowning or bulging. She is not sure if her water has broken.
3. Your patient reports contractions that are about 2 minutes apart. They have been this way for about 8 hours. Her water broke when the contractions started. She doesn't feel she is progressing through labor and is concerned for her baby.

Preparing the Mother for Delivery

When your evaluation leads you to believe birth is imminent, you must immediately prepare the mother for delivery. To do so, you should:

1. Control the scene so the mother will have privacy. (Her birthing coach may remain.) If you are not in a private room and transfer to the ambulance is not practical (e.g., crowning is present), ask bystanders to leave.
2. In addition to surgical gloves, you and your partner should put on gowns, caps, face masks, and eye protection, since there is a high probability of splashing blood and other body fluids during delivery.
3. Place the mother on a bed, the floor, or the ambulance stretcher. Elevate her buttocks with blankets or a pillow. Have the mother lie with knees drawn up and spread apart. You will need about 2 feet (0.6 meters) of workspace below the woman's buttocks to place and initially care for the newborn. Having the patient positioned on the stretcher may speed transport if complications arise.
4. Remove any of the patient's clothing or underclothing that obstructs your view of the vaginal opening. Use sterile sheets or sterile towels to cover the mother, as shown in Figure 36-9. Clean sheets, clean cloths, towels, or materials such as tablecloths can be used if you do not have an obstetrics kit.
5. Position your assistant—your partner, the father, or someone the mother agrees to have assist you—at the mother's head. This person should stay alert to help turn the mother's head in case she vomits. In addition, this person should provide emotional support to the mother, soothing and encouraging her.
6. Position the obstetrics kit near the patient. All items must be within easy reach.
7. If possible, make the environment as warm as possible. If in the ambulance, turn the heat up to its highest setting. Cold is the most imminent danger for a newborn.

NOTE: *If delivery is to take place in an automobile, position the mother flat on the seat. Arrange her legs so she has one foot resting on the seat and the other foot resting on the floor.*

FIGURE 36-9 Preparing the mother for delivery. Numbers signify the order for placing linens and draping the mother.

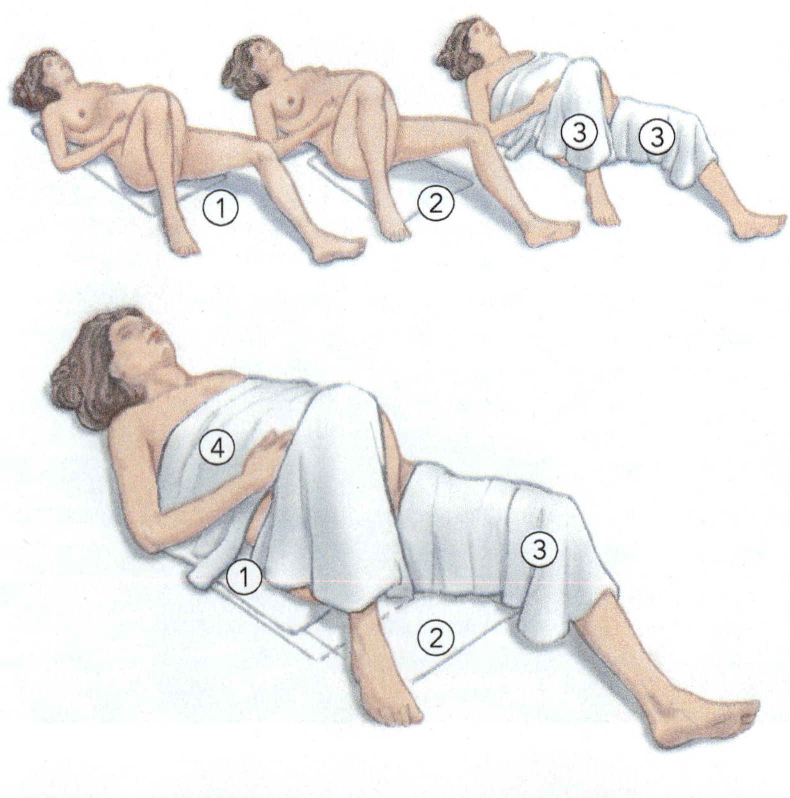

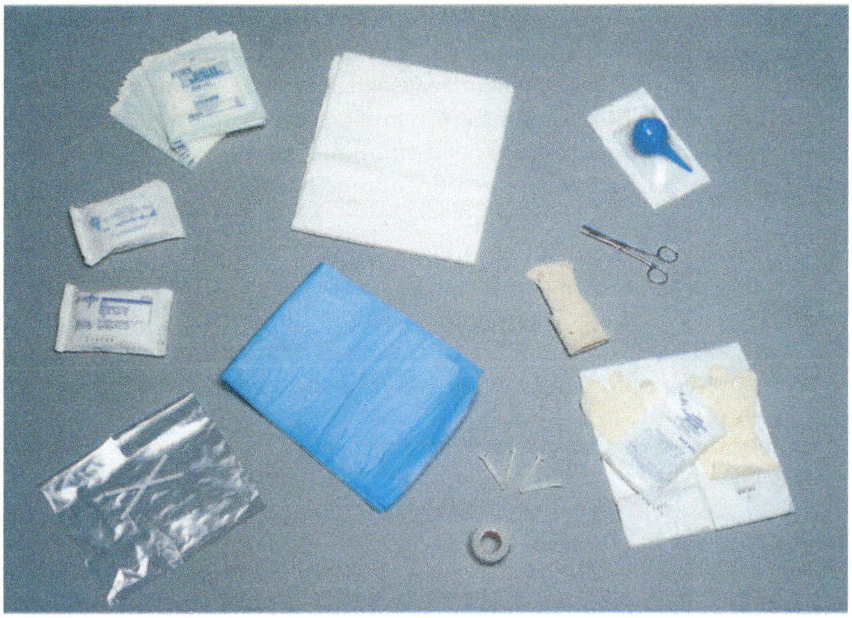

FIGURE 36-10 Contents of an OB (obstetrics) kit.

Preparing the Obstetrics (OB) Kit

A normal delivery requires some basic equipment that is typically kept in what is called an obstetrics (OB) kit (Figure 36-10). Although supplies will vary, this kit should include:

- Several pairs of sterile surgical gloves to protect you from infection
- Towels or sheets for draping the mother
- 1 dozen 2 × 2 (or 4 × 4) gauze pads (sponges) for wiping and drying the baby
- 1 small rubber bulb syringe (3 oz.) to suction the baby's mouth and nostrils if needed
- Cord clamps or hemostats to clamp the umbilical cord (plus extra clamps in case of a multiple birth)
- Umbilical cord tape to tie the cord
- One pair of surgical scissors to cut the cord
- Baby blankets and cap to dry and then wrap the baby (You should dry the baby with one set and wrap with a clean, dry set.)
- Several individually wrapped sanitary napkins to absorb blood and other fluids
- Plastic bag to wrap the placenta after it is expelled

Occasionally, in an off-duty situation, you may need to assist in the delivery of a baby without using a sterile delivery pack. In these cases, a few simple supplies can be used to assist the mother:

- Clean sheets and towels to drape around the mother and wrap the newborn
- Heavy flat twine or new shoelaces to tie the cord (Do not use thread, wire, or light string, since these may cut through the cord.)
- A towel or plastic bag to wrap the placenta after its delivery
- Clean, unused rubber gloves and eyewear to prevent exposure to infectious diseases
- A head covering for the baby may also be helpful, as it dramatically reduces heat loss.
- A neonatal-sized bag–valve mask (BVM) should also be prepared prior to the delivery.

Assisting the Delivery

Position yourself in such a way that you have a constant view of the vaginal opening. Be prepared for the baby to come at any moment.

In addition, be prepared for the patient to experience discomfort. Delivering a child is a natural process, but it is accompanied by pain. Your patient may also have intense feelings of nausea. If this is her first child, she may be very frightened. All these factors may cause your patient to be uncooperative at times. You must remember that the patient is in pain, and she may feel ill. Therefore, she will need emotional support.

Talk to the mother during the delivery. Encourage her to relax between contractions. Continue to time her contractions from the beginning of one contraction to the beginning of the next. Encourage her not to strain unless she feels she must. Remind her that her feeling of a pending bowel movement is usually just pressure caused by the baby moving into her birth canal. Encourage her to breathe deeply through her mouth. She may feel better if she pants, although she should be discouraged from breathing rapidly and deeply enough to bring on hyperventilation. If her water breaks, remind her that this is normal.

NOTE: *Unless there are signs of complications, consider the delivery to be normal if there is a cephalic presentation. Observe any unusual color in the amniotic fluid.*

NOTE: *Some deliveries are explosive. In these cases, do not squeeze the baby, but do provide adequate support. You can prevent an explosive delivery by using one hand to maintain slight pressure on the baby's head, thereby avoiding direct pressure to the infant's soft spots on the skull.*

To assist the mother with a normal delivery (Figure 36-11 and Scan 36-1):

1. Continue to keep someone at the mother's head to provide support, monitor vital signs, and be alert for vomiting. If no one is on hand to help, be alert for vomiting and check vital signs between contractions.
2. Position your gloved hands at the mother's vaginal opening when the baby's head starts to appear. Place your hand gently on the baby's head as it bulges out of the vagina, to prevent a sudden, uncontrolled expulsion of the newborn. Do not touch the area around the vagina except to assist with the delivery. For legal reasons, it is always preferable for both your protection and the patient's to have your partner present at all times when you are touching a woman's vaginal area.
3. Place one hand below the baby's head as it delivers. Spread your fingers evenly, remembering that the baby's skull contains "soft spots," or fontanelles. Support the baby's head, but avoid pressure to these soft areas at the top and sides of the skull. A slight, well-distributed pressure may help prevent an explosive delivery. Keeping one

FIGURE 36-11 (A) Delivering the infant's head. (B) Delivering the infant's shoulders.

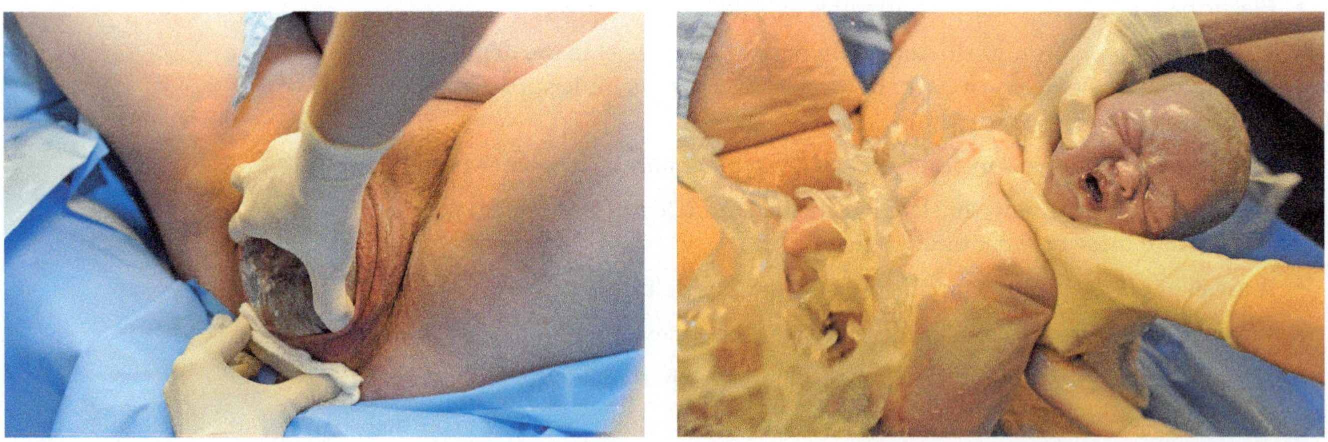

A B

SCAN 36-1 Assisting in a Normal Delivery

First Take Standard Precautions.

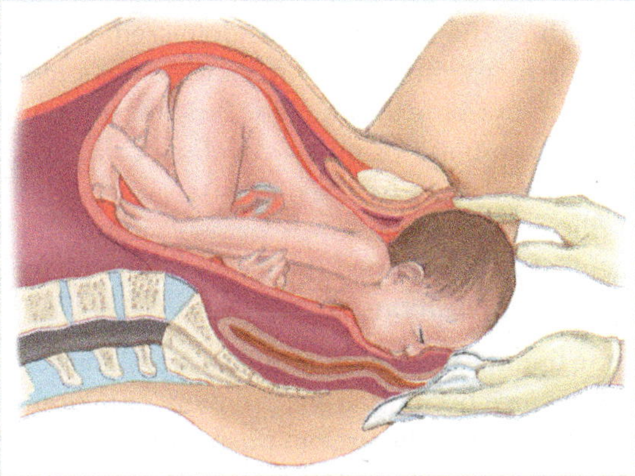

1. Support the infant's head. (Assist the mother by supporting the baby throughout the birth process.)

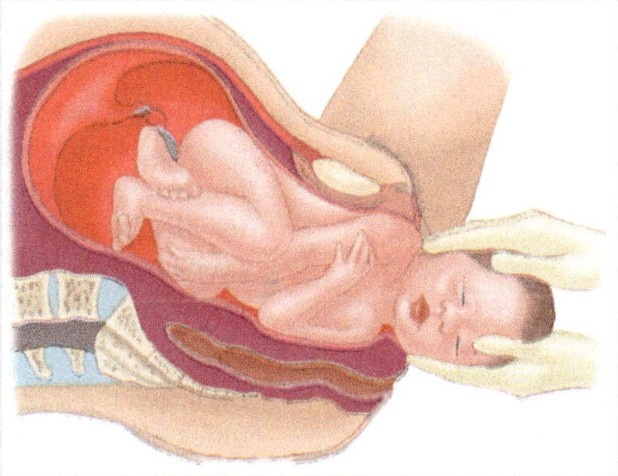

2. Aid in the birth of the upper shoulder.

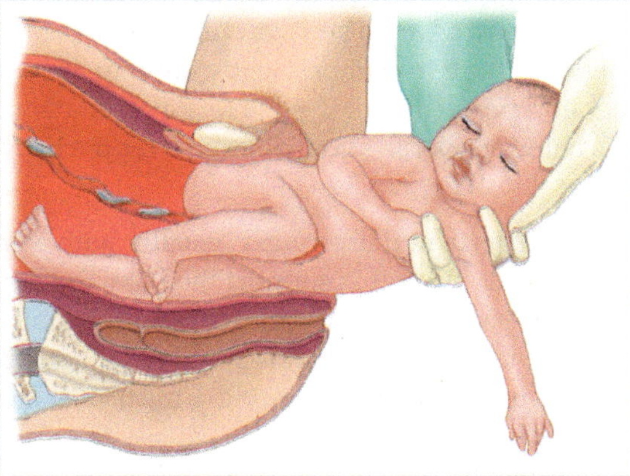

3. Support the trunk.

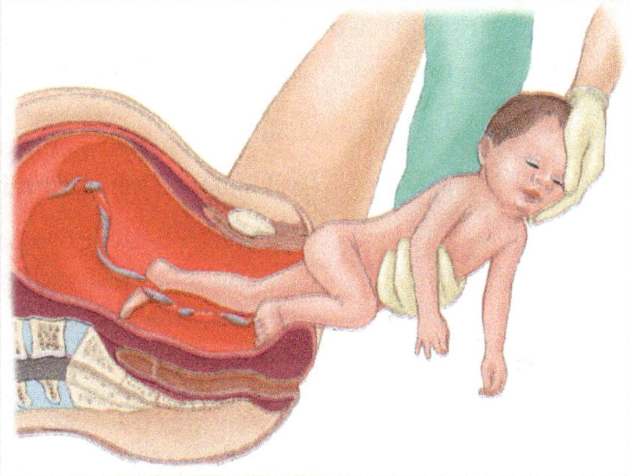

4. Support the pelvis and lower extremities.

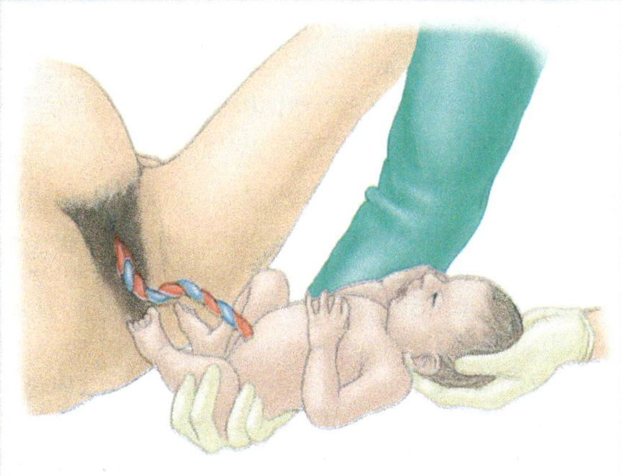

5. Keep the infant level with the vagina until the umbilical cord stops pulsating.

hand on the baby's head and using the other hand to hold a sterile towel to support the tissue between the mother's vagina and anus can help prevent tearing of this tissue during delivery of the head. *Do not pull on the baby!*

4. If the amniotic sac has not broken by the time the baby's head is delivered, use your finger to puncture the membrane. Pull the membranes away from the baby's mouth and nose. The amniotic fluid should be clear. Examine the amniotic fluid for meconium staining, which will appear to be a dark green-black or mustard yellow color. Meconium-stained amniotic fluid is caused by fetal feces (wastes) released during labor, usually because of maternal or fetal distress. If meconium is present, immediately prepare to suction the infant. If the meconium is aspirated (breathed in) by the fetus, the baby can develop pneumonia or other complications.

5. Once the head delivers, check to see if the umbilical cord is wrapped around the baby's neck. Tell the mother not to push while you are checking. If she can pant, or take short, quick breaths for just a moment, it may help relieve the urge to push while you check. Then gently loosen the cord, if necessary. Even though the umbilical cord is very tough, rough handling may cause it to tear. If the cord is wrapped around the baby's neck, try to place two fingers under the cord at the back of the baby's neck. Bring the cord forward, over the baby's upper shoulder and head.

   If you cannot loosen or slip the cord over the baby's head, or otherwise remove the cord, the baby cannot be delivered. Therefore, immediately clamp the cord in two places using the clamps provided in the obstetrics kit. Be very careful not to injure the baby. With extreme care, cut the cord between the two clamps. Gently unwrap the ends of the cord from around the baby's neck and proceed with the delivery. Fortunately, in most cases, a cord wrapped around the baby's neck can simply be slid over the baby's head. This option is always preferred.

6. Help deliver the shoulders. The upper shoulder will deliver next (usually with some delay), followed quickly by the lower shoulder. You must support the baby throughout this entire process. Gently guide the baby's head downward to assist the mother in delivering the baby's upper shoulder. If the lower shoulder is slow to deliver after the upper shoulder has delivered, assist the mother by gently guiding the baby's head upward.

7. Support the baby throughout the entire birth process. Remember that newborns are very slippery. As the lower extremities are born, grasp them to ensure a good hold on the baby. Never pick up babies by the feet, as they are very slippery, and you could drop the child. Once the feet are delivered, lay the baby on the side with the head slightly lower than the body. This is done to allow blood, fluids, and mucus to drain from the mouth and nose. Keep the baby at the same level as the mother's vagina until the umbilical cord stops pulsating. (Cutting the cord will be discussed later.) Dry the infant and then wrap the infant in a warm, dry blanket.

8. Assess the airway. Although most active babies will not require suctioning, for some it will be necessary. Suctioning will be important if positive pressure ventilations are necessary, or if secretions threaten the airway or obstruct normal breathing. If the baby is not moving or is not breathing, or if the airway is obstructed, use the rubber bulb syringe to suction the baby's mouth, and then the nose. Compress the syringe *before* placing it in the baby's mouth. Suction the mouth first, then the nostrils. Carefully insert the tip of the syringe about 1–1½ inches (2.5–3.75 cm) into the baby's mouth and release the bulb to allow fluids to be drawn into the syringe. Control the release with your fingers. Withdraw the tip and discharge the syringe's contents onto a towel. The tip of the syringe should not be inserted more than ½ inch (1.25 cm) into the baby's nostril.

9. Note the exact time of birth. Write the mother's last name and time of delivery on a piece of tape. Fold it so the adhesive does not touch the baby's skin, and place it around the baby's wrist.

Ongoing Assessment and Care of the Mother

Although care of the neonate following birth is extremely important and will be discussed in the section The Neonate, we cannot forget to continue to assess and care for the mother following birth. According to the Association of Women's Health, more than 100,000 women die during childbirth each year in the United States. It is estimated that more than 50 percent of these deaths are preventable.

Once the baby is delivered, be sure to reassess the mother. Like with any patient, use the primary assessment to rapidly identify life threats. Consider airway, breathing, and circulation issues of the highest priority. Remember that the delivery of the baby is not the end of labor for the mother. Contractions and pain will continue until the placenta is delivered, most commonly minutes later.

The most frequent risk for the mother in the immediate postpartum time frame (the time immediately following delivery) is bleeding. Vaginal bleeding can be severe, particularly if the placenta does not separate from the uterus fully as it is expelled. Postpartum hemorrhage is a true life threat and may need immediate intervention. Uterine massage will be discussed in an upcoming section, but be aware that this will be the time to initiate it. Other dangerous conditions such as seizures, pulmonary emboli, and clotting disorders are rare but possible.

Emotional care is also important. Be respectful of the mother's dignity and do your best to recognize the importance of the birth moment by allowing the mother to hold the infant and begin breastfeeding. Of course, medical issues will take priority, but often compromise is possible. More on maternal care is covered in the section of this chapter entitled Care after Delivery.

The Neonate

The term ***neonate*** is used for a newly born baby and infants less than 1 month old. A neonate is very different from other infants and must be treated accordingly.

neonate (NEE-oh-nate) a newly born infant or an infant less than 1 month old.

NOTE: *A number of terms are often used interchangeably. For clarity and uniformity, it is appropriate to use the following definitions: fetus–a baby as it develops in the womb; neonate–the baby at the time of birth to 1 month of age; infant–a baby in its first year of life.*

CORE CONCEPT

Care of the neonate

Assessing the Neonate

The neonate should be assessed immediately at birth. If you arrive on scene after the birth, it is still your responsibility to make the assessments based on your first observations. Remember, however, that care for the infant and the mother should not be delayed. The assessment is meant to take place while these other activities are being performed.

Your EMS system may call for a general or a specific evaluation protocol. A general evaluation usually calls for noting the neonate's ease of breathing, heart rate, crying, movement, and skin color. A normal neonate should have a pulse greater than 100 bpm, be breathing easily, be crying (vigorous crying is a good sign), be moving the extremities (the more active, the better), and show blue coloration at the hands and feet only (if at all). Five minutes later, these signs should still be apparent, with breathing becoming more relaxed. The blue coloration may or may not disappear, but it should not spread to other parts of the body.

A specific evaluation protocol that some EMS systems call for is an APGAR score. APGAR scores assign a number value to the neonate's assessment findings. Always remember that the APGAR score does not guide resuscitation efforts, and efforts to determine the APGAR score must never interfere with resuscitation efforts. Table 36-1 shows how an EMT assigns values to different aspects of a neonate's condition. The APGAR score is the total of the five values, and ranges from 0 to 10. It is traditionally determined 1 minute after birth and again 5 minutes after birth. APGAR first reviews **a**ppearance. Here skin color is assessed. Extensive cyanosis would be scored a "0." Cyanosis only in the extremities would be scored a "1" and pink skin all over would be scored a "2." Next the **p**ulse rate is assessed. Lack of pulse would be scored a "0." A rate less than 100 would be scored a "1" and a rate greater than 100 would be scored a "2." Next **g**rimace is assessed by flicking the

TABLE 36-1 The APGAR Score

APGAR SCORE			
	0	1	2
Appearance	Blue (or pale) all over	Extremities blue, trunk pink	Pink all over
Pulse	0	Less than 100	Greater than 100
Grimace (reaction to flicking of the feet or suctioning)	No reaction	Facial grimace	Sneeze, cough, or cry
Activity	No movement	Only slight activity (flexing extremities)	Moving around normally
Respiratory effort	None	Slow or irregular breathing, weak cry	Good breathing, strong cry

neonate's foot or, if necessary, suctioning. The grimace is the manner in which the neonate responds to this stimulus. Lack of reaction to the stimulus would be scored a "0." Facial changes (such as a grimace) in response to the stimulus would be scored a "1." If the neonate responds to the stimulus with a sneeze, cough, or cry, you would assign a "2." **Activity** is scored next. Here you will assess movement. Lack of movement would be scored a "0." Slight movement, such as flexion or extension of the extremities, would be scored a "1." If the patient moves normally, you would award a "2." Finally, you would assess **respiratory effort**. Lack of breathing would be scored a "0." Slow or irregular breathing, or a weak cry, would be assigned a "1." Good breathing and/or a strong cry would be awarded a "2." You should always follow the assessment protocol appropriate to your system.

Caring for the Neonate

Even with a normal delivery, each step in the care of the baby is essential for the baby's survival.

Keeping the Baby Warm

The most important aspect of caring for a neonate is keeping the baby warm. Newly born babies rapidly lose heat. This heat loss not only impacts their comfort but also can drop their glucose levels and even impact their ability to carry oxygen in their blood. For these reasons, you must consider heat retention a high priority. Dry the baby (Figure 36-12), discard any wet blankets, and wrap the baby in dry ones. Cover the baby's head. Commercially available infant swaddlers, known as "space blankets," are specially designed to retain warmth. Some systems utilize zip-type plastic bags to cover the blanket-wrapped neonate's body while leaving the covered head exposed. As soon as possible, move the baby to the mother's chest and encourage breastfeeding. In addition to making the mother happy, the close contact with the neonate helps prevent heat loss.

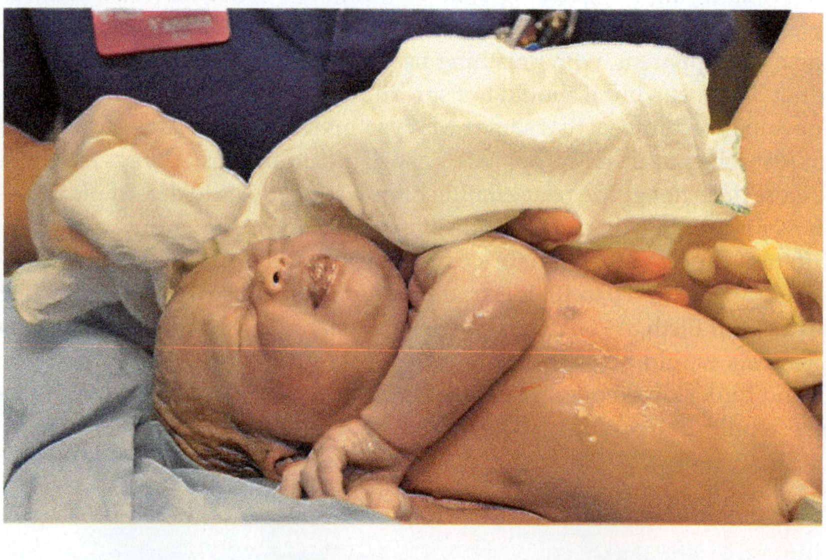

FIGURE 36-12 Dry and wrap the baby in a warm blanket or swaddler.

Cutting the Umbilical Cord

The timing of clamping and cutting the umbilical cord has historically been a heavily debated topic. You should always follow your local protocols. The current expert consensus, however, is that in uncomplicated childbirth the cord should not be cut any sooner than 30 to 60 seconds after birth. Do not cut a cord that is still pulsating.

In the world of EMS, the following circumstances would clearly necessitate prompt clamping and cutting of the cord:

- The cord is wrapped around the baby's neck and cannot be slipped over the head, the delivery is impeded, or the cord tightens around the neck, this is a critical situation that requires immediate clamping and cutting of the cord (discussed earlier).
- Attachment to the cord impedes a resuscitation effort.
- Attachment interferes with the urgent need for transport of the mother and/or the baby.
- Protocols require that the cord be cut.

In most cases, cutting the cord should be a relatively low priority, and there is no rush to complete this task. Before clamping and cutting the cord, palpate the cord with your fingers to make sure it is no longer pulsating. Pulsation typically stops shortly after delivery.

NOTE: *If the baby is not breathing without assistance, do not tie, clamp, or cut the cord of the baby unless you have to do so. Situations that would necessitate cutting a cord include removing the cord from around the baby's neck during birth and the immediate need for neonate resuscitation. Do not cut or clamp a cord that is still pulsating.*

The general procedure for umbilical cord care is as follows:

1. As already noted, keep the infant warm. Turn the heat up in the ambulance or the room. Dry off and then wrap the baby in a blanket or infant swaddler, clean towel, or sheet prior to clamping the cord. Do not wash the infant. Sometimes the mother may request you do so, but it is best to leave the protective coating (called the *vernix*) on the infant until you reach the medical facility with the baby.
2. Use the sterile clamps found in the obstetrics kit when cutting the cord.
3. Apply one tie or clamp to the cord about 10 inches (25 cm) from the baby. This leaves enough cord for intravenous lines to be used by paramedics or the staff at the hospital if they are needed.
4. Place a second clamp or tie about 7 inches (18 cm) from the baby. The proximal clamp should be about the width of four fingers from the distal clamp.
5. Cut the cord between the clamps using sterile surgical scissors (Figure 36-13). Use caution and protect your eyes when cutting the cord, as a spurt of blood is very common. Never unclamp a cord once it is cut. The placental end of the cord should be placed on the drape over the mother's legs to avoid contact with expelled blood, feces, and fluids. Examine the fetal end of the cord for bleeding. Do not attempt to adjust the clamp. If bleeding continues, apply another clamp as close to the original as possible.
6. Be careful when moving the baby so that no trauma is brought to the clamped cord. If the cord does not remain closed off completely, the baby may bleed to death from seemingly little blood loss. In most cases, the cord vessels will collapse and seal themselves.

If you are assisting at a birth when off duty, remember that there is no absolute need to cut the umbilical cord. If you do not have the proper equipment, unless there is an emergency, it would be reasonable for you to leave the cord intact and await better resources. That said, if there is an urgency, you will probably be able to find all the items you need to clamp and cut the cord. If no clamps are on hand, use clean shoelaces or similar soft, clean ties. If you tie the cord, believe it will be some time before you are able to transport and transfer the neonate, and do not have sterile scissors, soak scissors in alcohol for several minutes and use them to cut the cord. If the baby is still attached to the placenta when the organ is delivered, wrap the placenta in a towel and transport the infant and placenta as a unit. The placenta should be placed at the same level as the baby or slightly higher. Maintain careful monitoring of the baby.

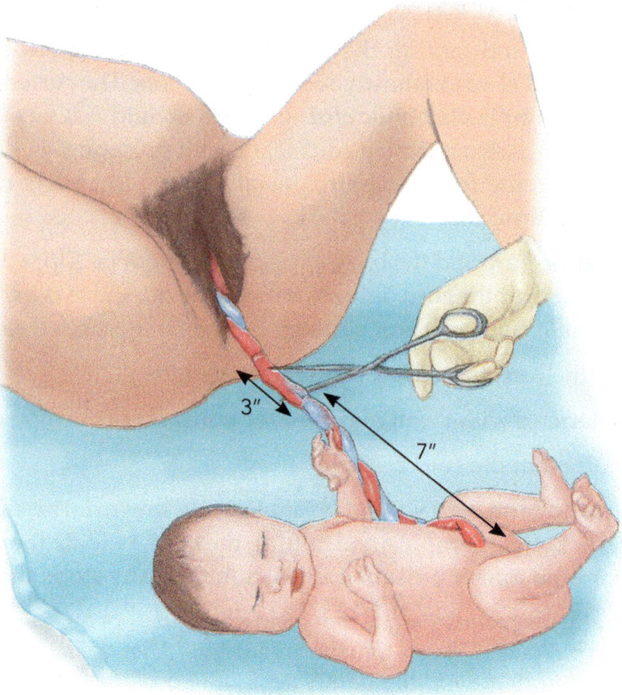

FIGURE 36-13 Cutting the umbilical cord.

Place the baby on the mother's abdomen (Figure 36-14), and allow the mother to begin breastfeeding (if your local protocols allow).

During the birth process, the fetus is passive. However, once born, the baby very quickly becomes active. Exposure to the air is usually enough to stimulate the infant to breathe. As you dry and warm the baby, the baby is stimulated even more. If the baby is breathing adequately and has a heart rate greater than 100 beats per minute but has central cyanosis (blue coloration of the torso), administer blow-by oxygen (Figure 36-15). If the neonate does not begin to breathe spontaneously after drying and warming for 30 seconds, begin neonate resuscitation.

Neonatal Resuscitation

Neonatal resuscitation follows an inverted pyramid (Figure 36-16). Most neonates with abnormal assessment findings respond to relatively simple maneuvers. Few require CPR or advanced life support measures.

FIGURE 36-14 Place the baby on the mother's abdomen.

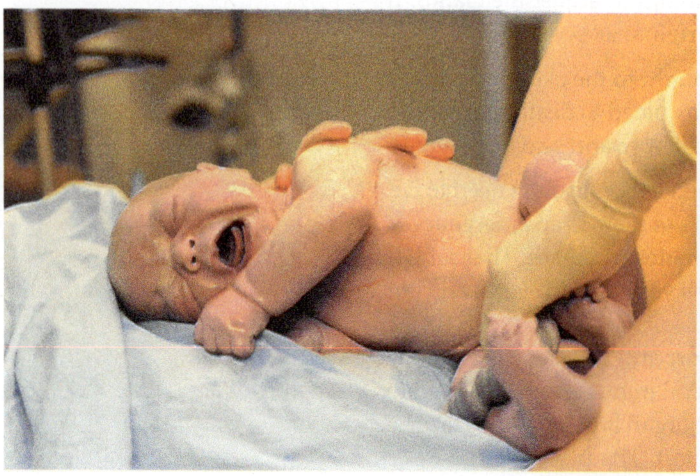

FIGURE 36-15 If the baby is breathing adequately and has a heart rate greater than 100 per minute but has a blue coloration to the torso, administer blow-by oxygen.

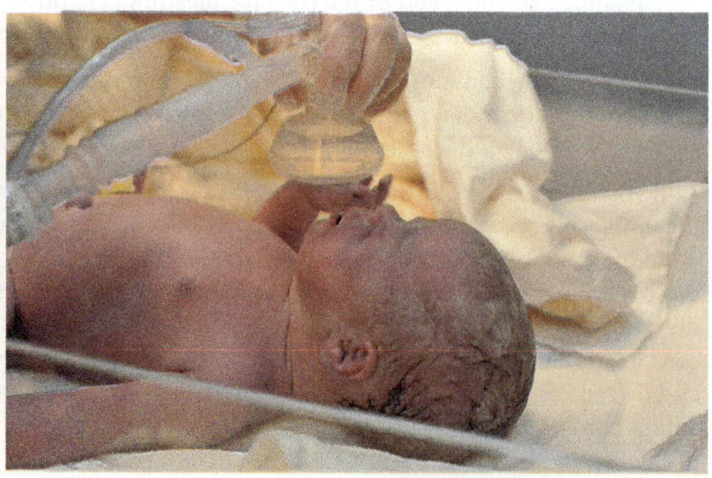

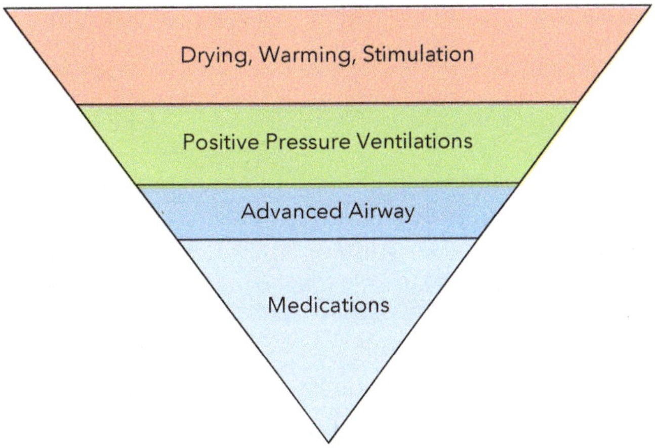

FIGURE 36-16 Inverted pyramid of neonatal resuscitation.

Neonate resuscitation consists of a series of assessments followed by interventions. Assessment identifies a need for an intervention, and each intervention is performed for 30 seconds. Once the intervention is complete, another assessment follows.

A normal neonate will be active, moving, and breathing on its own once born. Most commonly, the neonate will begin crying immediately. If the baby is breathing and active, the EMT dries and warms the neonate and provides routine care. On rare occasions, secretions and the byproducts of birth can obstruct normal breathing in an otherwise active neonate. If this occurs, clear the airway with suction immediately. If the baby is not active and breathing, the resuscitation must begin immediately and without hesitation.

The assessments and interventions involved in neonatal resuscitation are not complicated, but they do occur in a specific sequence and are initiated at a rapid pace. Neonatal resuscitation is also not a skill that is performed frequently. As such, it will be important to review and practice these steps often, and it is a best practice to utilize a checklist during an actual resuscitation. See Box 36-1 Putting it All Together: Neonatal Resuscitation Checklist, found at the end of this section.

Neonatal resuscitation combines assessment with intervention, as indicated in the following steps:

Step 1

ASSESSMENT		INTERVENTION
Is the neonate breathing? Is the neonate active? *If the answer is no, intervene.*	**Yes** →	**Dry, warm, and stimulate the neonate.**

Perform this intervention for 30 seconds and then reassess.

If the neonate is not active or not breathing, dry, warm, and stimulate the neonate for 30 seconds. (See Figure 36-17.) Physically dry the neonate with a soft towel. Remember that premature infants have very thin and fragile skin that can be damaged by aggressive friction. Use linens designed for neonates if possible. Rub the back. If the neonate does not respond, gently flick the sole of the foot. Perform this intervention for 30 seconds; then reassess.

Step 2

ASSESSMENT		INTERVENTION
Is breathing absent, or is the neonate gasping? **Is the heart rate less than 100?** *If apnea or gasping is present and/or if the heart rate is less than 100, intervene.*	**Yes** →	**Begin positive pressure ventilations.**

Perform this intervention for 30 seconds and then reassess.

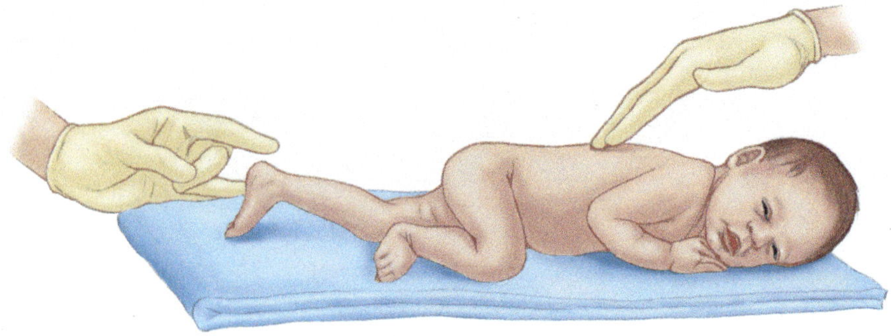

FIGURE 36-17 It may be necessary to stimulate the newborn to breathe.

After 30 seconds of drying, warming, and stimulating, reassess the neonate. Here you are looking to ensure that breathing has begun. Look for predictable rise and fall of the chest to indicate normal breathing. Beware of gasping, as this is likely to be a form of agonal breathing and is not likely to support life. You also should now assess heart rate. The most effective way to assess a pulse in a neonate is to place a stethoscope on the chest and listen. A pulse can also be found at the brachial artery and by palpating the base of the umbilical cord. At this time, the pulse should be greater than 100 beats per minute. If the infant is not breathing, is gasping, or has a pulse less than 100, you must begin positive pressure ventilations immediately with a bag–valve–mask device appropriately sized for the neonate.

To administer positive pressure ventilations, use a neonate-sized bag–valve–mask device. Open the neonate's airway and seal a properly fitting mask. Ventilate using just enough gentle pressure and volume to obtain chest rise. Neonates require 40–60 breaths per minute; this rate can be measured by saying out loud (or to yourself) *"breathe-two-three-breathe-two-three"* and repeating the sequence. It is not necessary to attach supplemental oxygen to the bag–valve–mask device during the initial stages of neonatal resuscitation. Use room air to deliver the ventilations, and consider supplemental oxygen only if oxygen saturation remains low following the resuscitation. This intervention should be performed for 30 seconds. You should then reassess.

Step 3

ASSESSMENT		INTERVENTION
Reassess heart rate. *If the heart rate is less than 100*	Yes	**Continue positive pressure ventilations. Ensure good chest rise.**
If the heart rate is less than 60		**Begin chest compressions.**
Perform this intervention for 30 seconds and then reassess.		

You will reassess after performing the initial 30 seconds of positive pressure ventilations. Now you will check the heart rate again. If the heart rate is less than 100, you should be concerned. Double-check to be sure that the airway is open and clear, and to make sure that your ventilations are achieving chest rise. Continue ventilations until the neonate begins breathing independently. If the heart rate is less than 60, you must begin chest compressions.

Chest compressions in the neonate are performed using the "two thumbs encircling" technique. (See Figure 36-18.) Your thumbs should be placed over the lower third of the patient's sternum and your fingers should encircle the chest to provide support from the back. Compress to a depth of one-third the anterior–posterior depth of the chest. Compressions should be delivered at a rate of 90 compressions per minute, working at a 3:1 ratio of compressions to breaths. The EMT should be delivering 120 "events" per minute (i.e., 90 compressions and 30 ventilations). It may be helpful to say out loud or to yourself "one-and-two-and-three-and-breathe" and to repeat the sequence. Take care to allow full recoil of the chest following each compression.

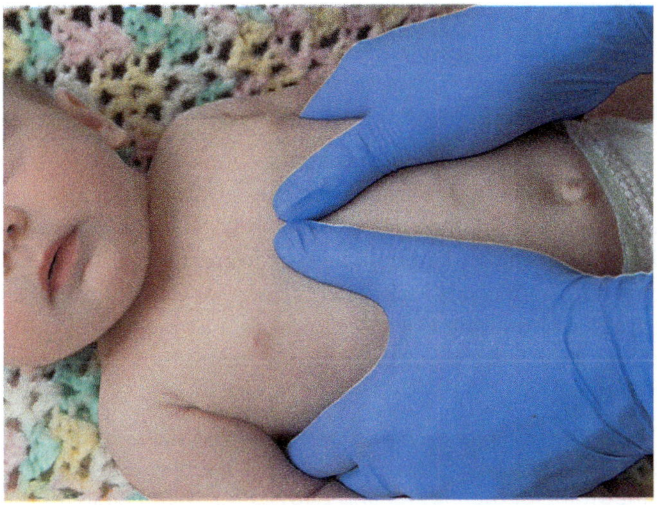

FIGURE 36-18 Deliver chest compressions mid-sternum with two thumbs, at a depth of one-third to one-half the depth of the chest. For a very small infant, the thumbs may be overlapped.

If CPR is initiated, initiate transport immediately and intercept with advanced life support if possible.

If at any point in the resuscitation the patient begins to breathe normally and the heart rate remains greater than 100, move to routine care. Keep the infant warm, transport, and reassess.

NOTE: *Consider heat loss when resuscitating a neonate. When lying the infant down, be sure to place dry blankets or towels under the infant to prevent heat loss through a cold surface.*

BOX 36-1 Putting It All Together: Neonatal Resuscitation Checklist

NEONATAL RESUSCITATION

- ☐ **Identify any need for resuscitation.**
  - ☐ Term gestation
  - ☐ Good tone? (If no, resuscitate.)
  - ☐ Crying? (If no, resuscitate.)
- ☐ **Call for ALS.**
- ☐ **Dry and warm neonate; clear secretions, position airway if needed. (30 seconds)**
- ☐ **Reassess breathing and heart rate.** (If apnea, gasping, or HR less than 100, continue resuscitation.)
- ☐ **Provide positive pressure ventilations.** (30 seconds)
  - ☐ *"Breathe-two-three-breathe-two-three"* (40-60 breaths per minute)
  - ☐ Ensure chest rise with each ventilation. *(Take ventilation corrective steps if necessary.)*
- ☐ **Reassess heart rate.**
  - ☐ If less than 100, double-check quality of ventilations and continue ventilations. (30 seconds)
- ☐ **If heart rate less than 60, begin CPR.**
  - ☐ Two-thumbs-encircling technique
  - ☐ Depth of compressions one-third anterior-posterior depth of chest
  - ☐ *"One-and-two-and-three-and-breathe"* at 30 breaths and 90 compressions (120 events) per minute
- ☐ **If resuscitation is successful, move to routine care.**
  - ☐ Warm, dry, and take steps to maintain neonate's temperature. (Wrap in dry towels and cover head).
  - ☐ Clear secretions if needed, and position airway.
  - ☐ Reassess frequently; record APGAR.

Care after Delivery

CORE CONCEPT
Postdelivery care of the mother

Caring for the Mother

Remember that you have two patients to care for following delivery: the infant and the mother. Although it is easy to make the baby your primary focus, remember that childbirth presents many risks for the mother. A woman who has just delivered a baby is at risk for serious bleeding, infection, and emboli. Be sure to treat her with the same attention you give the child. Care for the mother includes helping her deliver the placenta, controlling her vaginal bleeding, and making her as comfortable as possible. Note that in some circumstances, such as when performing neonatal resuscitation, you may need additional help to accomplish this goal.

NOTE: *Some EMS systems recommend transport without waiting for delivery of the placenta. There may be a condition in which the placenta does not separate from the uterine wall, and it is important for the mother and baby to get to the hospital. You can always stop the ambulance to deliver the placenta if it crowns en route.*

Delivering the Placenta

The third stage of labor is the delivery of the placenta with its umbilical cord section, membranes of the amniotic sac, and some of the tissues lining the uterus (Figure 36-19). (All of these together are known as the afterbirth.) Placental delivery begins with a brief return of the labor pains that stopped when the baby was born. You will notice a lengthening of the cord, which indicates the placenta has separated from the uterus. In most cases, the placenta will be expelled within a few minutes after the baby is born.

Although the process may take 30 minutes or longer, avoid the urge to put pressure on the abdomen over the uterus to hasten delivery of the placenta. If mother and baby are doing well and there are no respiratory problems or significant uncontrolled bleeding, transportation to the hospital can be delayed up to 20 minutes while awaiting delivery of the placenta.

Save all afterbirth tissues. The attending physician will want to examine the placenta and other tissues for completeness, since any afterbirth tissues remaining in the uterus pose a serious threat of infection and prolonged bleeding to the mother. Try to catch the afterbirth in a container. Place the container in a plastic bag, or wrap it in a towel, paper, or plastic. If no container is available, catch the afterbirth in a towel, paper, or a plastic bag. Label this material "placenta," and include the name of the mother and the time the tissues were expelled.

NOTE: *If the placenta does not deliver within 20 minutes of the baby's birth, transport the mother and baby to a medical facility without delay.*

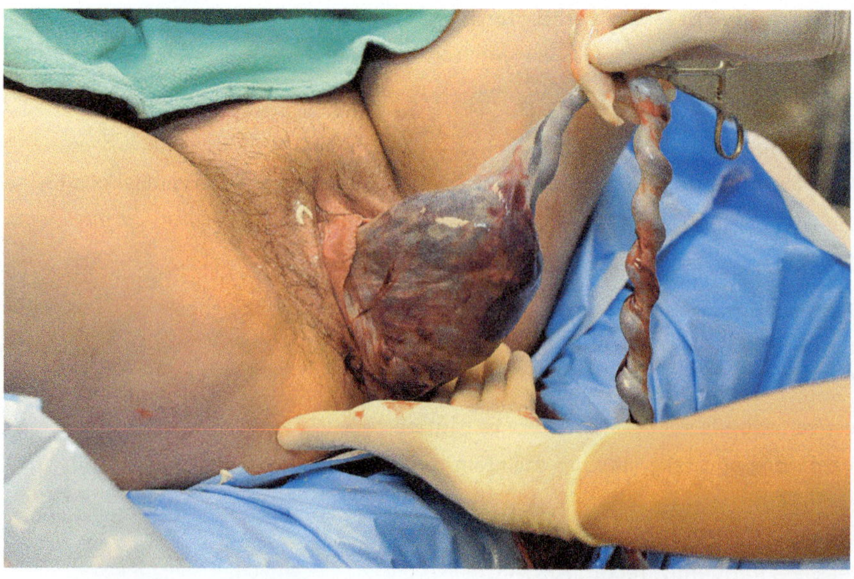

FIGURE 36-19 Guide the placenta out as it begins to appear at the vaginal opening.

Controlling Vaginal Bleeding after Birth

Delivery of the baby and placenta is *always* accompanied by some bleeding from the vagina. Although the blood loss is usually no more than 2 cups (500 cc), it may be profuse, which can lead to shock. Your reassessment of the mother must include evaluation of her bleeding and consideration of shock. To control vaginal bleeding after delivery of the baby and placenta, you should:

1. Place a sanitary napkin over the mother's vaginal opening. Do not place anything in the vagina.
2. Have the mother lower her legs and keep them together. Tell her that she does not have to squeeze her legs together.
3. Massaging the uterus will help it contract (Figure 36-20). This will help control the bleeding. To perform uterine massage, feel the mother's abdomen until you note a grapefruit-sized object. This is her uterus. Cup one hand on the inferior aspect, typically just above the pubic bone. Place the other hand at the superior aspect of the uterus, or fundus, to position the entire uterus between your hands. While supporting the uterus with the lower hand, gently massage the fundus in a circular fashion. In most cases, massage will lead the muscle of the uterus to contract. Contraction is the goal, as the tightening of this muscle diminishes bleeding. This action will be very painful for the mother, so you must explain that this procedure is necessary to stop serious bleeding.
4. Encourage the mother to begin nursing the baby. Nursing will stimulate the uterus to contract and may help decrease bleeding.

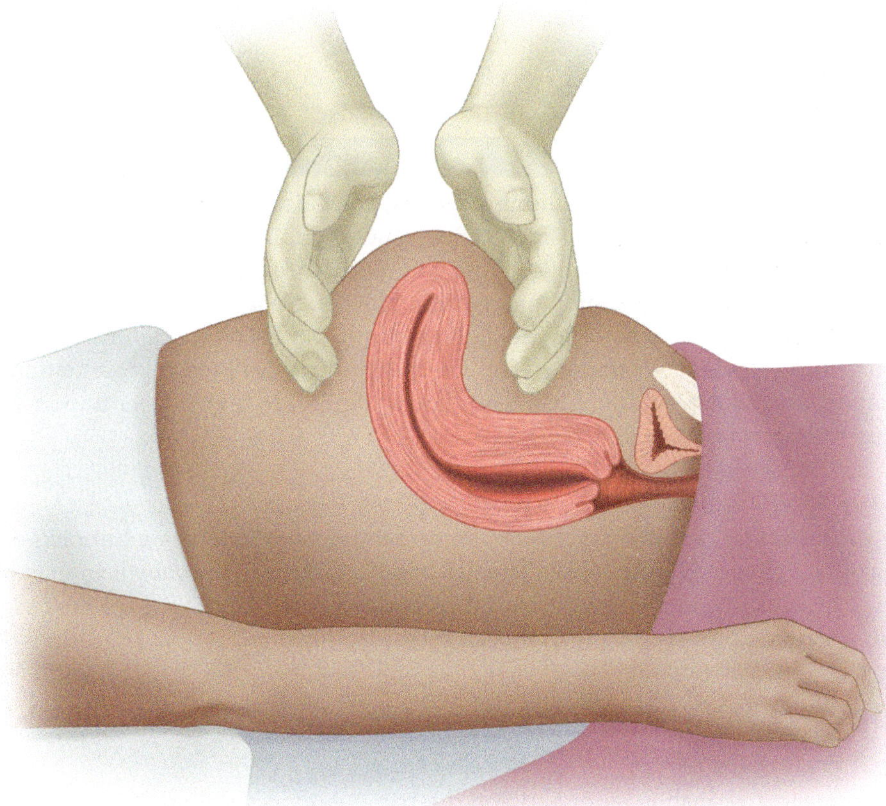

FIGURE 36-20 After delivery of the placenta, massage the uterus to help control vaginal bleeding.

A tearing of tissue can occur in the perineum at the vaginal opening during the birth process. The mother may feel the discomfort from this torn tissue. Let her know that this is normal and that the problem will be quickly cared for at the medical facility. Treat the torn perineum as a wound. Dress by applying a sanitary napkin and applying some pressure.

Providing Comfort to the Mother

Keep in contact with the mother throughout the entire birth process as well as after she has delivered. Your care for the mother does not end when you have completed your duties with the placenta and vaginal bleeding. Frequently take her vital signs. Be aware that she has just undergone a tremendous emotional experience and that small acts of kindness will be appreciated and remembered. Childbirth is a rigorous task, and a woman is physically exhausted at the conclusion of delivery. Wiping her face and hands with a damp washcloth and drying them with a towel will do wonders to refresh her and prepare her for the trip to the hospital. Replace blood-soaked sheets and blankets. Make sure that both she and the baby are warm.

When delivery occurs at home, ask a member of the family or a trusted neighbor to help you clean up. You should clean up whatever disorder EMS care has caused in the house; however, you should not delay transport to complete these activities. In some areas, local protocol may have you return to the house after transport to complete the cleanup process. If you do, you will have to be accompanied by a member of the family. Be sure to properly dispose of items that have been in contact with blood and other body fluids in a biohazard container.

NOTE: *Keep in mind that birth is an exciting and joyous event. Talking to the mother and paying attention to her new baby are part of total patient care. A good rule to follow is to treat your patient as you would wish a member of your family to be treated.*

Childbirth Complications

Complications of Delivery

CORE CONCEPT
Complications of delivery

Although most babies are born without difficulty, complications may occur during and after delivery. We have already considered three such complications: the cord around the neck, an unbroken amniotic sac, and infants who need encouragement to breathe. These problems can be handled by simple procedures. However, there are other complications that can threaten the lives of both mother and newborn and for which definitive treatment is beyond the EMT's level of training. For emergencies such as breech presentation, limb presentation, and prolapsed umbilical cord, you will provide high-concentration oxygen and rapid transport to the hospital.

Breech Presentation

breech presentation when the baby's buttocks or both legs appear first during birth.

Breech presentation, the most common abnormal delivery, involves a buttocks-first or both-legs-first delivery (Figure 36-21). The risk of birth trauma to the baby is high in breech deliveries. In addition, there is an increased risk of prolapsed cord. (See the next section.) Meconium staining often occurs with breech presentations.

Patient Assessment

Breech Presentation

If you evaluate a woman in labor and find the baby's buttocks or both legs presenting, rather than the head, this is a breech presentation. Breech presentations can spontaneously deliver successfully, but the complication rate is high.

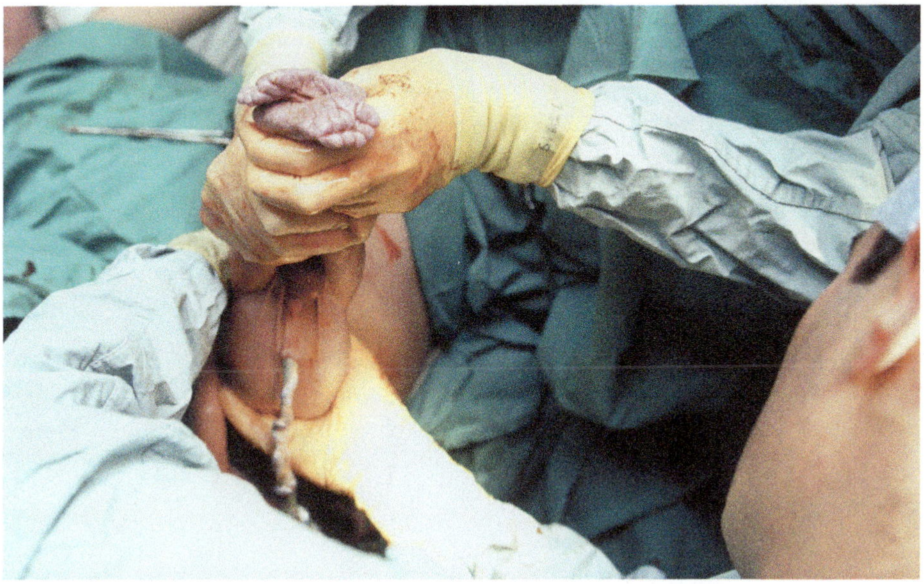

FIGURE 36-21 Breech delivery.
(Eddie Lawrence/Science Source)

Patient Care

Care of the Patient with a Breech Presentation

Fundamental Principles of Care

A breech birth can represent a true emergency. Although many babies are delivered normally despite a breech presentation, complication rates grow exponentially in this situation. If a breech presentation is suspected, every effort should be made to reach the hospital before the delivery occurs. If delivery is imminent, stay calm and hope the delivery proceeds normally. Be prepared, however, for complications. Start transport and get help.

Emergency care of a patient with a breech presentation includes the following steps:

- Initiate rapid transport upon recognition of a breech presentation.
- Never attempt to deliver the baby by pulling on the legs.
- Provide high-concentration oxygen to the mother.
- Place the mother in a head-down position with the pelvis elevated.
- If the body delivers, support it and prevent an explosive delivery of the head. If delivery is slow or delayed, keep the body aligned with the position of the head to prevent injury to the neck. Insert your gloved index and middle fingers into the vagina to form a *V* on either side of the baby's nose to lift it away from the vaginal wall in case the baby begins to breathe spontaneously.
- Care for the baby, cord, mother, and placenta as in after a cephalic delivery.

Limb Presentation

A ***limb presentation*** occurs when a limb of an infant protrudes from the vagina (Figure 36-22). The presenting limb is commonly a foot when the baby is in the breech position. Limb presentations cannot be delivered in the prehospital setting. In this case, rapid transport is essential to the baby's survival.

limb presentation
when an infant's limb protrudes from the vagina before the appearance of any other body part.

Patient Assessment

Limb Presentation

When checking for crowning, you may see an arm, a single leg, an arm and a leg together, or a shoulder and an arm. If one or more limbs present, there is often a prolapsed umbilical cord as well.

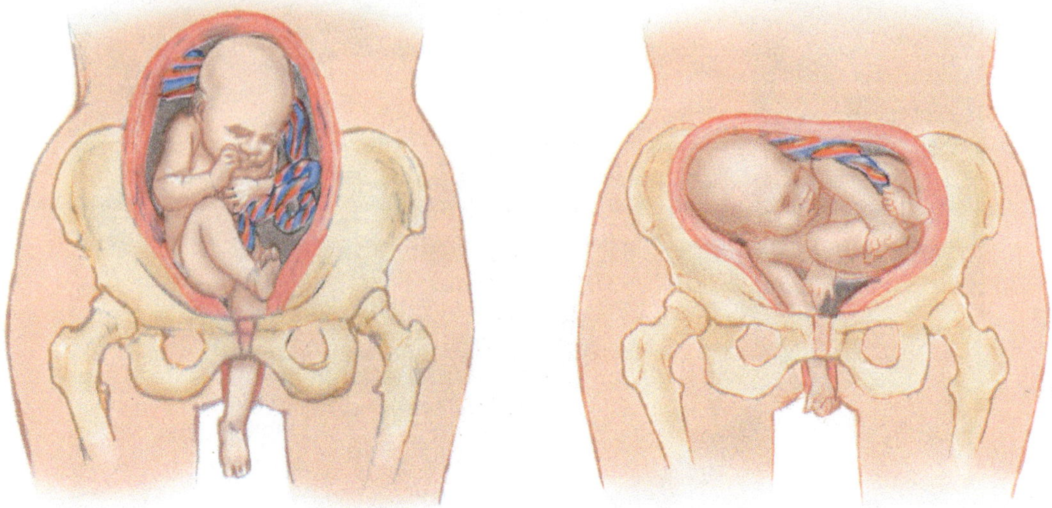

FIGURE 36-22 Limb presentation.

Patient Care

Care of the Patient with a Limb Presentation

Fundamental Principles of Care

Like breech deliveries, many limb presentations are delivered without complication. However, you should be prepared for this unusual presentation to delay or prevent normal delivery. As in a breech situation, do your best to get to the hospital before delivery. If delivery proceeds, stay calm, get help, and initiate transport as soon as it is safe to do so.

When you discover a limb presentation, take these emergency care steps:

- Transport the mother immediately to a medical facility.
- Place the mother in a head-down position with the pelvis elevated.
- Do not try to pull on the limb or replace the limb into the vagina.
- Do not place your gloved hand into the vagina unless there is a prolapsed cord.
- Administer high-concentration oxygen to the mother.
- Notify the receiving facility of the limb presentation so they can prepare the necessary obstetrical and neonatal resources.

Prolapsed Umbilical Cord

Sometimes during delivery, the umbilical cord presents first (this is most common in breech births) and the cord is squeezed between the vaginal wall and the baby's head. This occurrence is known as a ***prolapsed umbilical cord***. When this happens, the cord is pinched, and oxygen supply to the baby may be totally interrupted. This is a life-threatening condition to the neonate.

prolapsed umbilical cord when the umbilical cord presents first and is squeezed between the vaginal wall and the baby's head.

Patient Assessment

Prolapsed Umbilical Cord

If, upon viewing the vaginal area, you see the umbilical cord presenting, the cord is prolapsed.

Patient Care

Care of the Patient with a Prolapsed Umbilical Cord

Fundamental Principles of Care

A prolapsed cord is a dire emergency and an immediate life threat to the fetus. You must take immediate and aggressive action to maintain blood flow through the umbilical cord. Keep in mind that as the baby's head compresses the cord in the birth canal, oxygenated blood that is normally delivered via the umbilical cord is blocked. Fetal hypoxia and death are very real possibilities unless intervention occurs immediately.

Follow these steps when the umbilical cord is prolapsed (Figure 36-23):

- Position the mother with her head down and pelvis raised with a blanket or pillow, using gravity to lessen pressure on the birth canal.
- Provide the mother with high-concentration oxygen by way of a nonrebreather mask to increase the concentration carried over to the infant.
- Check the cord for pulses, and wrap the exposed cord, using a sterile towel from the obstetrics kit. The cord must be kept warm.
- Insert several fingers of your gloved hand into the mother's vagina so you can gently push up on the baby's head or buttocks to keep pressure off the cord. You will be pushing up through the cervix. This may be the only chance that the baby has for survival, so continue to push up on the baby until a physician relieves you. You may feel the cord pulsating when pressure is released.
- Keeping mother, child, and EMT as a unit, transport immediately to a medical facility. Be prepared to stay in this position until you reach the hospital.
- All patients with prolapsed cords require rapid transport. Have your partner obtain vital signs while en route to the hospital if possible.
- Notify the receiving facility of the limb presentation so they can prepare the necessary obstetrical and neonatal resources.

FIGURE 36-23 Prolapsed umbilical cord.

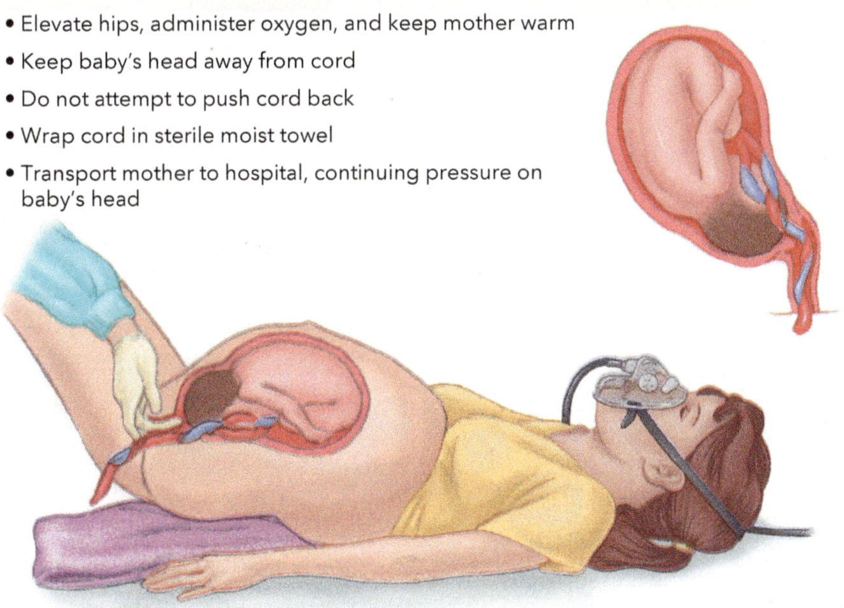

multiple birth
when more than one baby is born during a single delivery.

Multiple Birth

When more than one baby is born during a single delivery, it is called a ***multiple birth***. A multiple birth, usually twins, is not considered a complication, provided that the deliveries are normal. However, prematurity and other complications are common with multiple births. Twins are generally delivered in the same manner as a single delivery, with one birth following the other. However, if a multiple birth is encountered, you should have enough personnel and equipment available for multiple resuscitations. Call for assistance immediately.

When delivering twins, identify the infants as to order of birth (one and two, or A and B).

Patient Assessment

Multiple Birth

If the mother is under a physician's care, she will probably be aware that she is carrying more than one fetus. Without this information, you should consider a multiple birth to be a possibility if the mother's abdomen appears unusually large before delivery or it remains very large after delivery of one baby. If the birth is multiple, labor contractions will continue and the second baby will be delivered shortly after the first. The second baby may present in a breech position, usually within minutes of the first birth. The placenta(s) are delivered normally (Figure 36-24).

FIGURE 36-24 Multiple births.

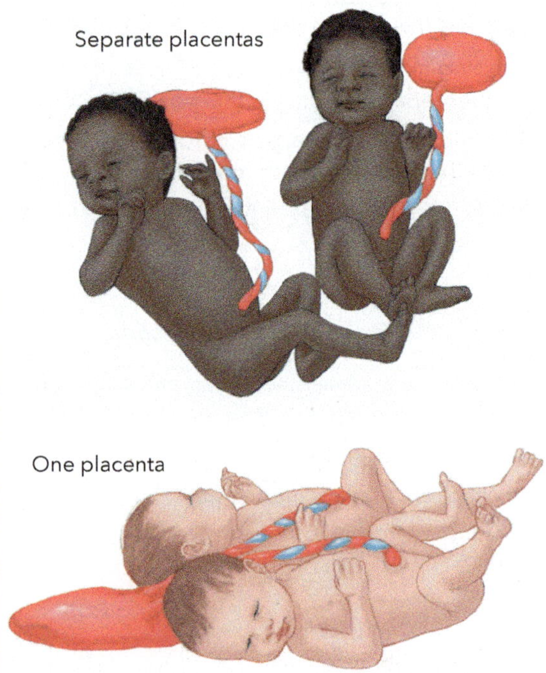

Patient Care

Care of the Patient with a Multiple Birth

Fundamental Principles of Care

Multiple births do not necessarily cause difficulty with the delivery. However, the probability of the need for neonatal resuscitation is much higher in this group than with single deliveries. The biggest need here is help. You should make every attempt to reach the hospital before delivery. If a multiple-birth delivery must take place outside the hospital, be sure to request additional resources early and be prepared to resuscitate more than one neonate at a time. Remember also that multiple-birth situations tend to be associated with earlier gestation (premature delivery) and smaller babies, which have their own unique risks.

When assisting in a multiple-birth delivery, follow these steps:

- Anticipate the need for neonatal resuscitation. Request additional assistance and ALS.
- Ensure you have appropriate resources on scene. Assume you will need to conduct multiple neonatal resuscitations simultaneously while still treating the mother.
- Clamp or tie the cord of the first baby before the second baby is born.
- The second baby may be born either before or after the placenta is delivered. Assist the mother with the delivery of the second baby.
- Provide care for the babies, umbilical cords, placenta(s), and the mother as you would in a single-baby delivery.
- The babies will probably be smaller than in a single birth, so take special care to keep them warm during transport.

Premature Birth

By definition, a ***premature infant*** is one who weighs less than 5½ pounds (2½ kg) at birth or one who is born before the thirty-seventh week of pregnancy.

premature infant any newborn weighing less than 5½ pounds (2½ kg) at birth or born before the thirty-seventh week of pregnancy.

Patient Assessment

Premature Birth

Since you probably will not be able to weigh the baby, make a determination as to whether the baby is full-term or premature based on the mother's expected due date and the baby's appearance. If the mother is unsure of her due date, you can make a rough estimate by asking her when she had her last menstrual period and adding 40 weeks. Assessment of the baby itself might indicate prematurity. By comparison with a normal full-term baby, the head of a premature infant is much larger in proportion to the small, thin, red body (Figure 36-25).

FIGURE 36-25 (A) Full-term newborn and (B) a premature newborn.

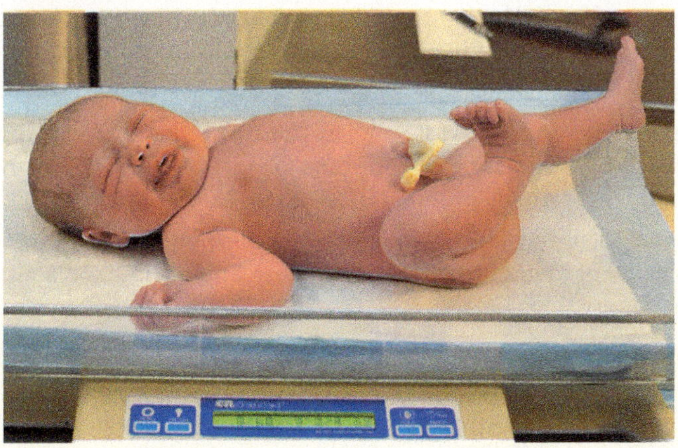

A

FIGURE 36-25 *(continued)*

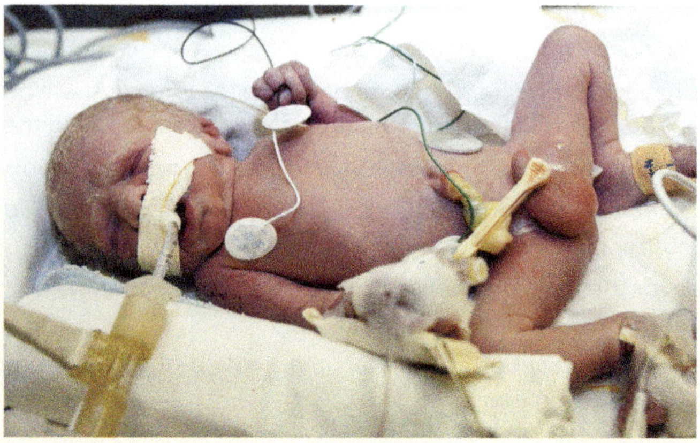

B

Patient Care

Care of the Patient with a Premature Birth

Fundamental Principles of Care

Premature babies need special care from the moment of birth. The smaller the baby, the more important is the initial care.

You should take the following steps when providing care for the premature infant:

- Anticipate the need for neonatal resuscitation. Request assistance and call for ALS.
- Keep the baby warm. Premature infants are at great risk of developing hypothermia. Once breathing, the baby should be dried with one blanket and wrapped snugly in another warm blanket. Additional protection can be provided by an outer wrap of plastic bubble wrap (keep this away from the infant's face) or a small reflective blanket. Premature babies lack fat deposits that would normally help keep them warm. Some EMS systems in cold regions use plastic, bubble wrap, or a bag for the infant, covered by a blanket. This helps maintain warmth and allows for easier visual inspection of the clamped cord to check for bleeding. A stockinette cap should be placed on the baby's head to help reduce heat loss.
- Keep the airway clear. Suction if necessary.
- Provide ventilations and/or chest compressions, as outlined earlier, based on the baby's pulse and respiratory effort. In some cases, resuscitation may not be possible if the baby is extremely premature.
- Watch the umbilical cord for bleeding. Carefully examine the cut end of the cord. If there is any sign of bleeding, even the slightest, apply another clamp or tie closer to the baby's body.
- Avoid contamination. The premature infant is susceptible to infection. Keep the infant away from other people. Do not breathe on the infant's face.
- Transport the infant in a warm ambulance. The desired ambient air temperature is between 90°F and 100°F (32°C and 38°C). Use the ambulance heater to warm the patient compartment prior to transport. In the summer months, the air conditioning should be turned off and all compartment windows should be closed or adjusted to keep the ambulance at the desired temperature.
- Call ahead to the emergency department, and consider transporting to a facility capable of caring for a premature infant.

Meconium

As noted earlier, meconium is a result of the fetus defecating (putting out wastes). It is a sign of fetal distress.

Patient Assessment

Meconium

Meconium is fetal stool that stains amniotic fluid greenish- or brownish-yellow in color. Infants born with meconium are at increased risk for respiratory problems, especially if aspiration of the meconium occurs at birth.

Patient Care

Care of the Patient with Meconium

Fundamental Principles of Care

The presence of meconium should be considered a concerning sign. Because a fetus in distress will often evacuate the bowels, meconium should be considered a flag that indicates something could be wrong with the baby. You should consider the presence of meconium—especially if it is evident when the woman's membranes rupture—a signal to prepare for a neonate resuscitation. Get help and make sure your equipment is ready. However, meconium's presence alone does not necessarily require any immediate treatment. If the baby is delivered normally and is responding as expected, you will simply clean and dry the neonate to remove the meconium. It is important that unnecessary suctioning of the nasopharynx be avoided as this may slow the neonate's heart rate due to vagal stimulation. In rare occasions, meconium can obstruct breathing. In these cases, you will act immediately to suction and clear the airway

If the baby requires resuscitation after birth and you see meconium staining in the amniotic fluid or on the baby itself, follow these steps:

- If meconium is present during the rupture of membranes (when the water breaks), anticipate the need for neonatal resuscitation. Request assistance and call for ALS.
- Warm the neonate and maintain normal temperature.
- Position the airway and check for obstruction.
- If suction is necessary to clear an airway obstruction caused by meconium, do not stimulate the neonate prior to suctioning in order to reduce the risk of aspiration.
- Maintain the open airway.
- Provide artificial ventilations and/or chest compression as indicated by the infant's effort of breathing and heart rate.
- Transport as soon as possible.
- Advise the receiving facility staff that meconium was identified at the scene.

Emergencies in Pregnancy

A number of predelivery emergencies can arise in the pregnant patient prior to labor or childbirth. When assessing a pregnant woman, consider the changes that have occurred to her body along with the pregnancy. Remember that you are really assessing two people, both the mother and fetus. Always complete a thorough assessment as you would for any other patient. You may also consider asking the woman about bleeding or other vaginal discharge as well as syncope, as these can indicate serious problems. Ask about the baby's movement.

CORE CONCEPT
Emergencies in pregnancy

Typically, after around twenty weeks, a mother will begin to feel movement of the fetus. Although this is not exact, movement or a lack thereof can be a helpful assessment finding.

When treating a pregnant woman (or a potentially pregnant woman), respect her modesty and privacy. Remember that she may be reluctant to share the information for which you are asking her.

Excessive Prebirth Bleeding

A number of conditions can cause excessive prebirth bleeding late in pregnancy. You should consider any bleeding in late pregnancy a serious emergency. Whether the vaginal bleeding is associated with abdominal pain or not, the risk to both the mother and the unborn child is great.

A pregnant woman does not have to be in labor to have excessive bleeding from the vagina. For example, bleeding in early pregnancy may be due to a miscarriage. If the bleeding occurs late in pregnancy, it may be due to problems involving the placenta.

placenta previa (plah-SEN-tah PRE-vi-ah)
a condition in which the placenta is formed in an abnormal location (low in the uterus and close to or over the cervical opening) that will not allow for a normal delivery of the fetus; a cause of excessive prebirth bleeding.

In one such condition, ***placenta previa***, the placenta is formed in an abnormal location, and this becomes concerning if it is implanted in an area of the uterus where it blocks the birth canal. If the placenta blocks or occupies space over the cervical opening, it can be damaged or torn as the fetus enters the birth canal. The placenta is a very vascular organ, and this damage can lead to severe bleeding. Placenta previa is most commonly diagnosed through the course of the pregnancy by ultrasound examination and will frequently be a known concern. Remember that not all women will have prenatal care, however, so this complication may not always be identified prior to delivery. Placenta previa occurs in the third trimester of pregnancy and usually presents with heavy vaginal bleeding often without associated abdominal pain.

abruptio placentae (ab-RUPT-si-o plah-SENT-ta)
a condition in which the placenta separates from the uterine wall; a cause of prebirth bleeding.

Another condition that causes prenatal bleeding is ***abruptio placentae***. In abruptio placentae, the placenta prematurely separates from the uterine wall. The most common cause of abruptio placentae is trauma, most often caused by falls and motor-vehicle crashes. Other causes include maternal hypertension and drug use, particularly of cocaine. Risk factors can be identified in patient history, and they include prior abruptions, history of trauma, smoking, drug use, and hypertension. An abruption can be partial or complete. A complete abruption separates the placenta fully from the uterine wall. This causes massive hemorrhage and is almost always fatal for the fetus. Partial abruptions separate a portion of the placenta from the uterine wall. They can also lead to severe bleeding. The most common assessment findings associated with abruption include abdominal or back pain and heavy vaginal bleeding. These findings become much more significant when paired with a history of trauma or other associated risk factors. Physical findings include vaginal bleeding, signs of shock, and uterine contractions. Like placenta previa, abruptio placentae occurs only in the third trimester of pregnancy.

Patient Assessment

Excessive Prebirth Bleeding

The following are considerations when assessing a pregnant woman who is having excessive prebirth bleeding:

- The main sign is usually profuse bleeding from the vagina.
- Consider mechanism of injury (MOI) if the bleeding follows any sort of trauma.
- The mother may or may not experience associated abdominal pain.
- During your primary assessment, you should look for signs of shock.
- Obtain baseline vital signs. A rapid heartbeat may indicate significant blood loss.

Patient Care

Care of the Patient with Excessive Prebirth Bleeding

Fundamental Principles of Care

Although prebirth bleeding can indicate any of a number of different pregnancy-related complications, your immediate concern will be the rapid identification and treatment of shock in the mother. Treating the mother aggressively is always the best way to keep the fetus alive. Consider how far along the pregnancy is because the length of gestation can help identify the cause. Consider underlying risk factors as well. Recognize that bleeding signifies risk for both the mother and fetus, so transport should be initiated immediately.

If there is excessive prebirth bleeding, take the following steps:

- If signs of shock exist, initiate rapid transport. Keep the patient warm. Administer high-concentration oxygen to prevent hypoxia.
- Place a sanitary napkin over the vaginal opening. Note the time of napkin placement. *Do not place anything in the vagina*. Replace pads as they become soaked, but save all pads for use in evaluating blood loss.
- Save all tissue that is passed.
- Rapidly transport to an appropriate medical facility. Notify the facility prior to arrival so then can mobilize the necessary obstetrical and neonatal resources to care for the mother and fetus.

Ectopic Pregnancy

In a normal pregnancy, the fertilized egg will begin to divide in the fallopian tube and eventually implant in the wall of the uterus. In an ***ectopic pregnancy***, the egg may implant outside the uterus—for example, in the fallopian tube, in the cervix, or in another area of the pelvic cavity. Ectopic pregnancies usually occur in the highly vascular fallopian tube, which will rupture as the fetus grows. This results in severe internal bleeding.

ectopic (ek-TOP-ik) ***pregnancy*** when implantation of the fertilized egg is not in the body of the uterus, occurring instead in the fallopian tube (oviduct), cervix, or abdominopelvic cavity.

Patient Assessment

Ectopic Pregnancy

The problems related to this condition are seen early in pregnancy. Indeed, some women with an ectopic pregnancy may be unaware that they are even pregnant when the signs and symptoms begin. Women may have a variety of signs and symptoms, including those indicating shock due to internal bleeding. This condition can be life-threatening. You should consider any woman of childbearing age with abdominal pain (and certainly any women of childbearing age with both abdominal pain and vaginal bleeding) to have an ectopic pregnancy until proven otherwise.

Be alert to recognize the following signs and symptoms as they develop:

- Acute abdominal pain, often beginning on only one side.
- Vaginal bleeding (often accompanies pain)
- Rapid and weak pulse (a later sign)
- Low blood pressure (a very late sign)
- Absent menstrual period, suggesting a possible pregnancy

Patient Care

Care of the Patient with an Ectopic Pregnancy

Fundamental Principles of Care

Ruptured ectopic pregnancy is a life-threatening condition that will rapidly lead to shock and death if untreated. If a woman of childbearing years complains of abdominal pain, this complication should come to mind first. Immediately treat shock if found. Remember that an ectopic pregnancy requires surgical intervention and should be considered a time-sensitive emergency. Initiate transport to an appropriate facility as soon as possible.

Emergency care includes the following steps:

- Initiate immediate transport.
- Administer oxygen if signs of hypoxia or shock are present.
- Do not give the patient anything by mouth.

eclampsia (e-KLAMP-se-ah) a severe complication of pregnancy that produces seizures and is very dangerous to the infant and mother.

preeclampsia (pre-e-KLAMP-se-ah) a complication of pregnancy in which the woman retains large amounts of fluid and has hypertension, and which may progress to eclampsia.

Seizures in Pregnancy

Seizures in pregnancy, sometimes caused by a condition called ***eclampsia***, tend to occur late in pregnancy. The seizures are typically a result of a condition called ***preeclampsia*** that has progressed to eclampsia. This condition is often related to pregnancy-induced hypertension, and may be well known to the patient. Preeclampsia can be recognized by altered mental status; swollen hands, feet, and/or face; and high blood pressure. Seizures in pregnancy pose a serious threat to both the mother and unborn baby.

Patient Assessment

Seizures in Pregnancy

A seizure may be associated with any of the following:

- Existing preeclampsia or pregnancy-induced hypertension
- Elevated blood pressure, which increases the risk of abruptio placentae
- Excessive weight gain
- Extreme swelling of the face, hands, ankles, and feet
- Altered mental status, headache, or other unusual neurologic findings

Patient Care

Care of the Patient with Seizures in Pregnancy

Fundamental Principles of Care

Seizures in pregnancy represent a risk to both mother and fetus and can be a devastating complication associated with labor and delivery. You should always be prepared for this possibility. Use your assessment to identify risk factors, and if warning signs are present, request ALS as soon as possible and initiate transport quickly. If a seizure occurs, stay calm. Most seizures stop in just a few minutes. Focus on maintaining oxygenation and ventilation, and care for the mother appropriately.

Emergency care of a pregnant patient with seizures includes the following steps:

- Ensure and maintain an open airway.
- Administer oxygen based on patient presentation. High-concentration oxygen may be appropriate because of the potential for hypoxia to the fetus.
- Transport the patient positioned on her left side.
- Keep the patient warm, but do not overheat.

- Have suction ready.
- Have an OB kit ready.
- Contact ALS for immediate assistance.
- Notify staff at the receiving facility so that they can mobilize appropriate resources.

Miscarriage and Abortion

For a number of reasons, the fetus and placenta may deliver before the twentieth week of pregnancy—generally before the baby can survive. This occurrence is referred to as an ***abortion***. When it happens on its own, it is called a ***spontaneous abortion***, more commonly known as a ***miscarriage***. An ***induced abortion*** is an abortion that results from deliberate actions taken to stop the pregnancy.

abortion
spontaneous (miscarriage) or induced termination of pregnancy.

spontaneous abortion
when the fetus and placenta deliver before the 20th week of pregnancy; commonly called a *miscarriage*.

miscarriage
see spontaneous abortion.

induced abortion
expulsion of a fetus as a result of deliberate actions taken to terminate the pregnancy.

Patient Assessment

Miscarriage and Abortion

Women having miscarriages that require them to seek emergency care generally have the following signs and symptoms:

- Cramping abdominal pains not unlike those associated with the first stage of labor
- Bleeding ranging from moderate to severe
- A noticeable discharge of tissue and blood from the vagina

Ask the patient about the starting date of her last menstrual period. If it has been more than 24 weeks, be prepared with an obstetrics kit. Premature infants may survive if they receive rapid neonatal intensive care.

Patient Care

Care of the Patient with a Miscarriage, or Spontaneous Abortion

Fundamental Principles of Care

Miscarriage represents both a physical and an emotional risk. Optimal care addresses both areas. First ensure that medical conditions such as bleeding and shock are addressed. If shock signs are present, initiate transport immediately. In addition to medical care, remember that a miscarriage is a devastating emotional moment. Be compassionate, be caring, and do your best to advocate for the patient's psychological needs.

For the patient with a miscarriage or an abortion, take the following steps:

- Obtain baseline vital signs.
- If signs of shock are present, keep the patient warm and prevent hypoxia. Treatment should be based on signs and symptoms.
- Help absorb vaginal bleeding by placing a sanitary napkin over the vaginal opening. Do not pack the vagina.
- Transport as soon as possible.
- Replace and save all blood-soaked pads.
- Save all tissues that are expelled. Do not attempt to replace or pull out any tissues that are being expelled through the vagina.
- Provide emotional support to the mother. Emotional support is very important. When speaking to the patient or her family, or in an area where bystanders may hear you, *always* use the term *miscarriage* instead of *spontaneous abortion*. Most people associate the word *abortion* with an induced abortion, not a miscarriage, and this is a taboo subject. It is essential to talk with the patient to gain her confidence and to allow you to provide emotional support.

Trauma in Pregnancy

Obviously, the pregnant patient, like any other patient, can sustain injury. However, especially during the last two trimesters, the uterus and fetus are also subject to injuries when the mother is injured. Injuries to the uterus may be blunt or penetrating. In either case, the greatest danger to the mother and baby is hemorrhage (bleeding) and shock.

The most common cause of blunt trauma is automobile collisions, although falls and assaults also account for many injuries. The uterus is well designed to protect the baby. The fetus is inside a muscular chamber filled with fluid. In this way, the uterus acts as an efficient shock absorber. Thus, most minor trauma to the abdomen, such as a blow or impact from a fall, typically does not harm the fetus.

Automobile collisions pose a high risk of injury, as the magnitude of forces in a collision is great. Because of its size and location, the uterus is frequently injured in these collisions. Sudden blunt trauma to the abdomen during the later months of pregnancy may cause uterine rupture or premature separation of the placenta (abruptio placentae). Other blunt-trauma injuries, such as a ruptured spleen or liver, may also occur. Rupture of the diaphragm may occur with blunt trauma during later pregnancy. Multisystem trauma with fractures of the pelvis can cause laceration or tearing of the vessels in the pelvis, leading to massive hemorrhage. The common problem with most blunt injuries to the pregnant woman's abdomen or pelvis is massive bleeding and shock.

Unfortunately, intimate partner violence also increases in frequency during pregnancy. Be mindful of any unexplained injury or evidence of past injury. If violence is suspected, contact law enforcement and be prepared to advocate for the patient. Remember that intimate partner violence is not limited to pregnancy. Any sign of genital trauma in a patient should raise a high index of suspicion.

If a pregnant woman is injured in an incident such as a motor-vehicle collision, intimate partner violence, or a fall, perform a patient assessment and treat her injuries as you would those of any other trauma patient. The best way to keep the fetus alive is to appropriately treat the mother.

Patient Assessment

Trauma in Pregnancy

During a trauma in pregnancy, follow these patient assessment steps:

- During primary assessment and assessment of vital signs, remember the following about the physiology of pregnant women:
    - The pregnant patient has a pulse that is 10–15 beats per minute faster than the nonpregnant female. Therefore, vital signs may be interpreted as being suggestive of shock when they are actually normal for the pregnant female.
    - A woman in later pregnancy may have a blood volume that is up to 48 percent higher than her nonpregnant state. With hemorrhage, 30 percent to 35 percent blood loss may occur before otherwise healthy pregnant females exhibit signs or symptoms.
    - Although shock is more difficult to assess in the pregnant patient, it is the most likely cause of prehospital fetal death from injury to the uterus.
- Question the conscious patient to determine if she has received any blows to the abdomen, pelvis, or back.
- Ask the patient if she has had bleeding or rupture of the bag of waters. When in doubt, examine the vaginal area for bleeding, being certain to provide privacy.
- Examine the unconscious patient for abdominal injuries, remembering to consider the MOI and being certain to provide privacy.

Patient Care

Care of the Patient with Trauma in Pregnancy

Fundamental Principles of Care

Remember that maintaining adequate breathing and ensuring adequate circulation are vital not only to the mother but also to the fetus. A developing fetus is critically dependent on the uninterrupted oxygenated blood supply that enters the placenta. What is good for the mother is good for the baby. The mother-to-be who has experienced trauma may have undetected internal bleeding, or the fetus may be injured.

Provide the following care to the injured mother:

- Provide resuscitation if necessary.
- Monitor saturation and aggressively treat any signs of hypoxia with high-concentration oxygen.
- Because of slowed digestion and delayed gastric emptying, there is a greater risk the patient will vomit and aspirate. Be ready with suction.
- Control external hemorrhage.
- Transport as soon as possible. Pregnant women in the late second or third trimester should be transported in the left lateral recumbent position, supported with pillows or blankets, unless a spinal injury is suspected. If so, first secure the mother to a spine board, then tip the board and patient as a unit to the left, relieving pressure on the abdominal organs and vena cava. Be sure to monitor and record the patient's vital signs.
- Provide emotional support. A pregnant woman who is a trauma victim will naturally worry about her unborn child. Reassure her that the developing baby is well protected in the uterus. Let her know that she is being transported to a medical facility that can take care of her needs and the needs of the unborn child.

Stillbirths

Some babies die in the uterus several hours, days, or even weeks before birth. Such a baby is called ***stillborn***.

stillborn born dead.

It is a tragic time for the parents and other family members when a baby is born dead or dies shortly after birth. Your thoughtfulness may provide the distraught parents with comfort. Never lie to the parents. Many death-and-dying experts believe that parents should be allowed to view the baby if they wish to.

Keep accurate records of the time of stillbirth and the care rendered, for completion of the fetal death certificate.

Patient Assessment

Stillbirth

When a baby has died some time before birth, death is obvious by the presence of blisters, foul odor, skin or tissue deterioration and discoloration, and a softened head. At other times, a baby may be born in pulmonary or cardiac arrest but in otherwise good condition. These babies have the possibility of being resuscitated.

Patient Care

Care of the Patient with a Stillbirth

Fundamental Principles of Care

Like miscarriage, a stillbirth represents both a physical and an emotional threat. First address any medical issues. Treat for shock if bleeding is present, and transport appropriately. A stillbirth can also pose an ethical dilemma for providers in that you must determine whether resuscitation is possible. Here consider gestational age, size, and physical findings. Consult medical control for assistance. Consider also the emotional needs of the patient.

Emergency care for a stillborn baby is as follows:

- Withhold resuscitative efforts from stillborn babies who have obviously been dead for some time before birth.
- Provide full resuscitation measures for any babies who are born in pulmonary or cardiac arrest.
- Prepare to provide life support when the baby is alive but respiratory or cardiac arrest appears to be imminent.

Cardiac Arrest in the Pregnant Patient

Cardiac arrest in a pregnant patient is a worst-case scenario. Here, not one but two patients face a potentially tragic outcome. Like in all cardiac arrests, survival rates are not good; however, you will proceed with resuscitation in the hope that quality CPR and early defibrillation could be the keys to spontaneous return of circulation. The unborn fetus is certainly a concern, but resuscitation efforts must focus on the mother if there is to be any hope of keeping the baby alive.

Cardiopulmonary resuscitation will proceed for the most part as described in the *Cardiac Emergencies* chapter. However, the changes that have occurred to the woman's body during pregnancy should be considered during the resuscitation effort. If the woman is estimated to be more than 20 weeks pregnant, the American Heart Association recommends that the uterus be displaced manually during CPR. This can be done by placing two hands on the side of the pregnant abdomen and pulling it toward the patient's left side. (See Figure 36-6.) Just as we transport pregnant women in the left lateral recumbent position to prevent supine hypotensive syndrome, this manual displacement prevents the pregnant uterus from compressing the large blood vessels of the abdomen and decreasing cardiac output. If resources or personnel are not available to manually displace the uterus, then it is reasonable to tilt the patient on a backboard to a left lateral angle of 27 degrees to 30 degrees. The evidence to support these maneuvers is acknowledged to be sparse, and you will have to use clinical judgment to assess the impact of the tilted position on the ability to perform quality compressions.

When performing chest compressions, you should reposition your hands 1–2 inches (2.5–5 cm) higher on the sternum to adjust for shifting of the heart by the large uterus. Because of the large uterus, there is higher risk for aspiration. Use good bag–valve–mask technique to deliver ventilations, and be aware that ventilation may require lower volumes because of the displaced diaphragm. Always be ready to suction the airway if needed. You should attach an AED, and pregnant patients can and should be defibrillated as needed.

Although in most cases you will not be immediately transporting a patient in cardiac arrest, pregnancy would be a special exception. Particularly if the arrest is witnessed or has happened less than 5 minutes prior to the arrival of EMS, there is at least a consideration that an emergency cesarean section could save the baby. Although data are scarce and outcomes are poor even in reported cases, it may be reasonable for you to consider early transport in the event that a caesarean section could be initiated. If transport is initiated, continue CPR on the mother until you are relieved in the emergency department. As always, follow local protocols and consult medical direction as necessary.

Gynecologic Emergencies

Not every emergency associated with the female reproductive system will be associated with pregnancy. Vaginal bleeding, trauma to the external genitalia, and sexual assault are all commonly encountered problems found in women of all ages. Although our focus thus far has been on pregnancy, it is important not to overlook specific reproductive complication in any woman you are assessing.

Vaginal Bleeding

CORE CONCEPT
Gynecologic emergencies

In the previous section, we discussed pregnancy-related vaginal bleeding, but it is important to remember that there are many other problems that can result in vaginal bleeding. Vaginal bleeding occurs normally due to the regular menstrual period, but excessive bleeding or unexpected bleeding can be a sign of a serious problem. Common nonpregnancy-related vaginal bleeding causes include trauma, sexually transmitted diseases, gynecologic cancers, and ovarian issues such as cysts and torsions. As we have discussed previously, you should also consider the possibility of pregnancy-related causes, especially ectopic pregnancy, in any woman of childbearing age with vaginal bleeding. Use a thorough assessment to identify the possibility of shock. Consider also the last menstrual period and the frequency and regularity of the woman's menstrual cycle to differentiate from normal menstrual bleeding. Treat any shock findings aggressively and initiate transport to an appropriate facility.

Patient Assessment

Vaginal Bleeding

Since it will be difficult for the EMT to determine a specific cause of the bleeding, it is important that all women who have vaginal bleeding be treated as though they have a potentially life-threatening condition. This is especially true if the bleeding is associated with abdominal pain. The most serious complication of vaginal bleeding is hypovolemic shock due to blood loss. If a woman has been using pads to absorb bleeding, consider asking her how many pads she has used. This count may be helpful in assessing blood loss.

Patient Care

Care of the Patient with Vaginal Bleeding

Fundamental Principles of Care

In any woman with vaginal bleeding, first consider pregnancy-related causes, especially ectopic pregnancy. If these causes are unlikely, consider nonpregnancy-related causes. Have a high suspicion for trauma. Aggressively assess for shock. If shock signs are present, take immediate action and initiate transport immediately.

For the patient with vaginal bleeding, take the following steps:

- Use Standard Precautions. Wear gloves, gown, protective eyewear, and mask as indicated.
- Ensure an adequate airway.
- Assess for signs of shock.
- Administer high-concentration oxygen if signs of shock are present or if shock is suspected.
- Transport.

Trauma to the External Genitalia

External genitalia have a high concentration of nerve endings and have a robust supply of blood. As a result, trauma to the genitalia causes severe pain and often significant bleeding. In addition, genital injuries require the exposure and examination of intimate areas, and often modesty is a major concern. As with any other traumatic injury, soft-tissue damage and bleeding should be your first concern. You should use basic hemorrhage-control and bandaging principles to manage external injuries, and you should be mindful of shock. External genital trauma should always be a warning sign for sexual assault. Although not every genital injury results from assault, statistically, it is a common cause. Although medical issues will take the first priority, remember that advocacy and emotional care will be necessary if sexual assault is the cause. Always be respectful and do your best to preserve patient dignity throughout the assessment and treatment phases.

Patient Assessment

Trauma to the External Genitalia

Injuries in this area tend to bleed profusely because of the rich blood supply provided to the area. Injuries to the female external genitalia are frequently the result of straddle-type injuries.

- Respect modesty and preserve patient dignity. Make every attempt to assess and treat with due regard to privacy.
- In sizing up the scene, observe for MOIs.
- During primary assessment, look for signs of severe blood loss and shock.
- Consider the potential for internal injuries.
- Consider the possibility of sexual assault.

Patient Care

Care of the Patient with Trauma to the External Genitalia

Fundamental Principles of Care

Injuries to the external genitalia are rarely life-threatening, but they certainly can be life-altering. These injuries carry with them a significant emotional weight, and assessment and treatment can quickly rob a patient of her dignity. Although you should always first consider life threats such as bleeding and shock, care here should most often focus on patient privacy, emotional needs, and the preservation of dignity. Always consider the possibility of sexual assault.

For the patient with trauma to the external genitalia, perform the following steps:

- Maintain a professional attitude.
- Control bleeding as you would any other external hemorrhage, with direct pressure over a bulky dressing or sanitary pad. (If the patient is alert, she will probably prefer to do this herself.) Do not remove the patient's undergarments unless necessary. Do not pack the vagina.
- If signs of shock are present, keep the patient warm and prevent hypoxia.
- Respect the patient's privacy. Remove unneeded bystanders and expose the patient's body only to the extent necessary to provide appropriate care.
- Consider the possibility of assault. Contact law enforcement and consider providing social service referrals if appropriate.

Sexual Assault

Situations in which a sexual assault has occurred are always a challenge to the EMT. Care of the patient must include both medical and psychological considerations. In addition, law enforcement agencies are also frequently involved.

There is no question that the sexual-assault patient is under tremendous stress. Because of this, you must be prepared to deal with a wide range of emotions that the patient may exhibit. The best approach is to be nonjudgmental and to maintain a professional but compassionate attitude. Unless it delays care, it is generally preferable for an EMT of the same sex as the patient to establish rapport and to be the primary provider of emergency care.

Patient Assessment

Sexual Assault

- Since you may be entering a potential crime scene, ensure that the scene is safe prior to entering. It may be necessary to "stage" your unit near the scene until it is rendered safe by police.
- Be professional and compassionate. Be nonjudgmental in your questioning, and do not make promises you cannot keep. For example, avoid saying things such as "It will be OK," or "He'll definitely go to jail."
- Be conscious of personal space. Explain your examinations and treatments beforehand. Be sensitive to the patient's fears and embarrassment.
- During assessment, identify and treat both the medical and the psychological needs of the patient.

Patient Care

Care of the Patient Who has Undergone Sexual Assault

Fundamental Principles of Care

In situations of sexual assault, remember that medical priorities always come first. Treat injuries, stop hemorrhage, and be mindful of shock. At the same time, consider that a sexual-assault situation requires consideration of other significant priorities, including emotional care, evidence preservation, and victim advocacy.

For the patient who has suffered sexual assault, take the following steps:

- Treat immediate life threats. Manage injuries, control hemorrhage, and treat for shock if necessary.
- Be careful not to disturb potential criminal evidence unless it is absolutely necessary for patient care.
- Examine the genitals only if severe bleeding is present.
- Consider crime scene preservation. If possible, avoid cutting the victim's clothes. Do not move items on scene, and limit the number of providers who access the scene.
- Discourage the patient from bathing, voiding, or cleansing any wounds, as this may result in loss of important evidence.
- Document the situation objectively and fulfill any reporting requirements that are locally mandated.
- Learn what social service resources are available in your area. Consider providing referrals.

Chapter Review

Key Facts and Concepts

- Although birth is a natural process that usually takes place without complications, the involvement of EMS usually indicates something unusual has happened.
- The EMT's role at a birth is generally to provide reassurance and to assist the mother in the delivery of her baby.
- During the normal delivery, the EMT will evaluate the mother to determine if there should be immediate transport to a medical facility or if birth is imminent and will take place at the scene.
- If birth is to take place at the scene, the EMT must prepare for the worst. Have equipment ready and appropriate resources on hand. Always be prepared for neonatal resuscitation.
- Complications of delivery represent a true emergency. An EMT must be prepared to initiate rapid transport in the case of breech presentation, prolapsed umbilical cord, limb presentation, premature birth, or meconium staining of the amniotic fluid.
- There may also be predelivery emergencies or emergencies associated with pregnancy (such as excessive bleeding, ectopic pregnancy, seizures, abortion, or trauma to the pregnant mother) that the EMT must be prepared to treat.
- Stillbirth, death of the mother, and sexual assault are difficult emergencies the EMT is occasionally called upon to manage. Emotional care for these issues may be as important as medical care.

Key Decisions

- Is there time to transport this woman in labor to the hospital, or should I prepare for delivery on scene?
- Should I anticipate a neonatal resuscitation after delivery? Do I have the necessary resources on scene?
- During neonatal assessment, are there necessary interventions I must perform?
- In a gynecologic emergency involving vaginal bleeding, how serious is the vaginal bleeding?

Chapter Glossary

abortion spontaneous (miscarriage) or induced termination of pregnancy.

abruptio placentae (ab-RUPT-si-o plah-SENT-ta) a condition in which the placenta separates from the uterine wall; a cause of prebirth bleeding.

afterbirth the placenta, membranes of the amniotic sac, part of the umbilical cord, and some tissues from the lining of the uterus that are delivered after the birth of the baby.

amniotic (am-ne-OT-ik) ***sac*** the "bag of waters" that surrounds the developing fetus.

Braxton-Hicks (braks-tun-hiks) ***contractions*** irregular prelabor contractions of the uterus.

breech presentation when the baby's buttocks or both legs appear first during birth.

cephalic (se-FAL-ik) ***presentation*** normal birth presentation, where the baby's head appears first.

cervix (SUR-viks) the lower neck of the uterus at the entrance to the birth canal.

crowning the point during childbirth when part of the baby is visible through the vaginal opening.

eclampsia (e-KLAMP-se-ah) a severe complication of pregnancy that produces seizures and which is very dangerous to the infant and mother.

ectopic (ek-TOP-ik) ***pregnancy*** when implantation of the fertilized egg is not in the body of the uterus, occurring instead in the fallopian tube (oviduct), cervix, or abdominopelvic cavity.

embryo (EM-bree-o) the baby from fertilization to 8 weeks of development.

fallopian (fu-LO-pe-an) ***tube*** the narrow tube that connects the ovary to the uterus. Also called the *oviduct*.

fetus (FE-tus) the baby from 8 weeks of development to birth.

induced abortion expulsion of a fetus as a result of deliberate actions taken to terminate the pregnancy.

labia (LAY-be-uh) soft tissues that protect the entrance to the vagina.

labor the three stages of the delivery of a baby that begin with the contractions of the uterus and end with the expulsion of the placenta.

lightening the sensation of the fetus's moving from high in the abdomen to low in the birth canal.

limb presentation when an infant's limb protrudes from the vagina before the appearance of any other body part.

meconium staining amniotic fluid that is greenish- or brownish-yellow rather than clear, as a result of fetal defecation; an indication of possible maternal or fetal distress during labor.

miscarriage *see* spontaneous abortion.

mons pubis soft tissue that covers the pubic symphysis; area where hair grows when a woman reaches puberty.

multiple birth when more than one baby is born during a single delivery.

neonate (NEE-oh-nate) a newly born infant or an infant less than 1 month old.

ovary (o-vu-RE) the female reproductive organ that produces ova.

ovulation (ov-U-LA-shun) the phase of the female reproductive cycle in which an ovum is released from the ovary.

perineum (per-i-NE-um) the surface area between the vagina and anus.

placenta (plah-SEN-tah) the organ of pregnancy where exchange of oxygen, nutrients, and wastes occurs between a mother and fetus.

placenta previa (plah-SEN-tah PRE-vi-ah) a condition in which the placenta is formed in an abnormal location (low in the uterus and close to or over the cervical opening) that will not allow for a normal delivery of the fetus; a cause of excessive prebirth bleeding.

preeclampsia (pre-e-KLAMP-se-ah) a complication of pregnancy in which the woman retains large amounts of fluid and has hypertension, and which may progress to eclampsia

premature infant any newborn weighing less than 5½ pounds or born before the thirty-seventh week of pregnancy.

prolapsed umbilical cord when the umbilical cord presents first and is squeezed between the vaginal wall and the baby's head.

spontaneous abortion when the fetus and placenta deliver before the twentieth week of pregnancy; commonly called a *miscarriage*.

stillborn born dead.

supine hypotensive syndrome dizziness and a drop in blood pressure caused when the mother is in a supine position and the weight of the uterus, infant, placenta, and amniotic fluid compress the inferior vena cava, reducing return of blood to the heart and cardiac output.

umbilical (um-BIL-i-kal) ***cord*** the fetal structure containing the blood vessels that carry blood to and from the placenta.

uterus (U-ter-us) the muscular abdominal organ where the fetus develops; the womb.

vagina (vah-JI-nah) the birth canal.

Preparation for Your Examination and Practice

Short Answer

1. Name and describe the anatomical structures of a woman's body that are associated with pregnancy.
2. Describe the three stages of labor.
3. Explain how to evaluate and to prepare the mother for delivery.
4. Name, in the order of the inverted pyramid, the steps that may be taken to resuscitate a newly born infant.
5. Name and describe several possible complications of delivery.
6. Name and describe several possible predelivery emergencies.

Thinking and Linking

Think back to the chapter Well-Being of the EMT, *and link information from that chapter with information from this chapter as you consider the following situation:*

- While assisting with an emergency out-of-hospital childbirth, you are sprayed with amniotic fluid. Afterward, you find out that the mother is HIV-positive. To whom should you go with this information? What should you do?

Critical Thinking Exercises

Your calm, professional demeanor is very important when you are called to care for a woman in labor. The purpose of this exercise will be to make a key decision for a particular patient: to prepare for delivery at the scene or to transport.

- You are called to respond to a woman who is in labor. During your evaluation, you find that this is the woman's first pregnancy, the baby's head is not yet crowning, and contractions are 10 minutes apart. You ask the mother if she feels like she needs to move her bowels, and she says she does not. Do you prepare for delivery at the scene, or do you transport the mother to the hospital? Explain your reasoning.

Pathophysiology to Practice

The following questions are designed to assist you in gathering relevant clinical information and making accurate decisions in the field.

1. How would you expect the vital signs to change in a late-term pregnant female as a result of the pregnancy?
2. How would the changes in pregnancy alter your ability to recognize shock?
3. How should you assess the severity of a vaginal bleed? Why should you assume the worst?
4. What are your priorities in assessing and treating a neonate?

Street Scenes

Your sleep is interrupted by the tones of the radio and the dispatcher saying, "Bravo 3, stand by for a call." You swing your feet onto the floor and grab the radio. "Go ahead, dispatch," you reply.

"Bravo 3, respond to 77 Maple Tree Lane for a pregnant patient in labor. The other dispatcher is still on the phone with the husband. Additional information to follow."

You and your partner head to the ambulance and start toward the scene. About 3 minutes from the patient's house, the dispatcher tells you that the baby appears to be crowning and the husband is still on the phone getting instructions. You and your partner decide you need a plan. You agree that both the adult and pediatric equipment need to be brought in, as well as the OB kit. You also agree that you will focus on the baby after delivery, and your partner will provide care to the mother.

Street Scene Questions

1. What should be the first priority when entering the scene?
2. Should ALS assistance be requested?
3. What questions should you ask the mother or the father?

As you move toward the house, you ask the dispatcher if ALS have responded. You are told they are already en route. When you walk into the room, you see the patient on the bed and the husband with the telephone cradled on his shoulder as he talks to the dispatcher. The husband immediately stands aside, and you and your partner see crowning and realize that the delivery will take place any minute. You put on gloves and set up the OB kit while getting assessment information from the mother. It is her second delivery, but it is two weeks early. Labor started about an hour ago, and the pains have been more frequent lately and very intense. The water broke just before they called 911. While your partner is obtaining a set of vital signs, the baby starts to deliver. The head comes out, and you notice that the umbilical cord is around the baby's neck. You are able to slip it over the baby's head, and the baby continues to deliver. The shoulders and the rest of the baby's body quickly follow.

Street Scene Questions

4. What immediate care should be provided to the newborn?
5. What care should your partner be giving to the mother?

You immediately start down the inverted pyramid for neonate resuscitation. You suction the mouth, then the nose. The baby immediately starts to cry. You dry the baby off and wrap the swaddling blanket around her, making sure that the top of the baby's head is covered. The baby is pink and actively moving. You check the pulse, and it is at least 150 beats per minute. Your partner clamps the cord and makes the cut. (In a routine, uncomplicated birth, some systems allow the father or patient's partner to cut the cord.) You call the dispatcher to log in the time of the delivery and announce that it is a girl. At that time, dispatch reports that ALS has been diverted to a cardiac arrest. After 20 minutes, the placenta still has not delivered, and you transport the patient to the hospital without any further delay.

When you arrive back at the station, there is still time to get a couple of hours sleep. However, since you are too excited, you turn on the television instead.

Emergencies for Patients with Special Challenges

37

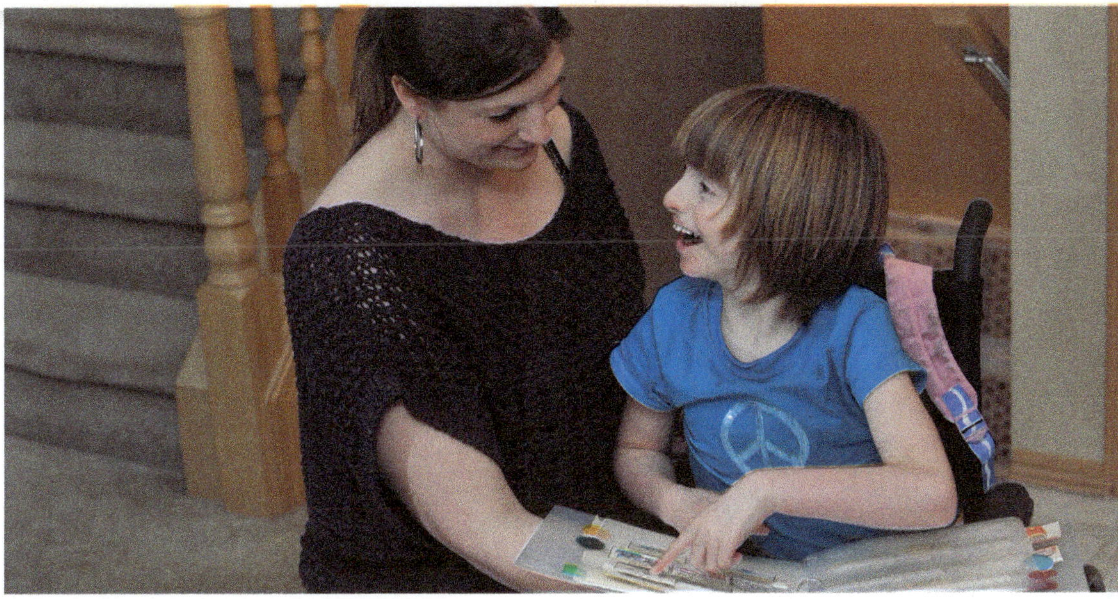

Related Chapters

The following chapters provide additional information related to topics discussed in this chapter:

- **2** Well-Being of the EMT
- **3** Lifting and Moving Patients
- **4** Medical, Legal, and Ethical Issues
- **10** Respiration and Artificial Ventilation
- **19** Respiratory Emergencies
- **28** Hematologic and Renal Emergencies

Standard

Special Patient Populations (Patients with Special Challenges)

Competency

Applies fundamental knowledge of growth, development, and aging and assessment findings to provide basic emergency care and transportation for a patient with special needs.

Core Concepts

- The variety of challenges that may be faced by patients with special needs
- Types of disabilities and challenges patients may have
- Special aspects of prehospital care for a patient with special challenges
- Congenital and acquired diseases and conditions

- Types of advanced medical devices patients may rely on
- How to recognize and deal with cases of abuse and neglect

Outcomes

After reading this chapter, you should be able to:

37.1 Summarize concepts related to patients who have special challenges. (pp. 1103–1107)

- Compare the characteristics of a disability and of a developmental disability.
- Outline the features of selected conditions associated with special challenges.
- Analyze terminal illness, obesity, homelessness, and poverty as special challenges.

37.2 Recommend approaches of care for patients with special needs. (pp. 1108–1111)

- State the key actions the EMT can use to improve interaction with patients who have autism.
- Recognize how to obtain information to troubleshoot unfamiliar medical devices in a patient's home.
- Match specific types of medical devices with the purposes for which patients have them.

37.3 Describe general considerations in responding to patients with special challenges. (pp. 1111–1116)

- Defend the rationale for a complete history and physical in the management of a patient who has special challenges.

37.4 Recognize physical impairments and common medical devices used in the home care of patients with special challenges, including respiratory devices, cardiac devices, gastrourinary devices, and central IV catheters, and discuss EMT assessment and transport considerations for each. (pp. 1116–1128)

- Explain how to improve interaction with patients who have hearing and vision impairments that interfere with their activities of daily living.

37.5 Explain why patients with special challenges are often especially vulnerable to abuse and neglect, and what the EMT's obligations are in such situations. (pp. 1128–1136)

- Identify the risk of abuse and neglect of patients with special challenges.

Key Terms

autism spectrum disorders (ASD), *1108*
automatic implanted cardiac defibrillator (AICD), *1120*
bariatrics, *1106*
central IV catheter, *1126*
continuous positive airway pressure (CPAP), *1116*
dialysis, *1125*
disability, *1103*
feeding tube, *1123*
obesity, *1106*
ostomy bag, *1125*
pacemaker, *1120*
stoma, *1117*
tracheostomy, *1117*
urinary catheter, *1124*
ventilator, *1119*
ventricular assist device, *1121*
wearable cardioverter defibrillator (WCD), *1121*

The principles of emergency medical care you have learned so far apply to a wide variety of patients. For some patients with special challenges, you will need to adapt these principles to meet their particular health care needs. Patients with special challenges include patients with sensory impairments, patients with developmental disorders, the terminally ill, patients who are very obese, those who are homeless or living in poverty, and patients who are dependent on advanced medical devices. The health problems associated with these special challenges increase the likelihood that these persons will need EMS at one time or another. In addition, like other vulnerable people, such as the elderly and children, some patients with special needs are at higher risk for abuse and neglect. This chapter focuses on meeting the unique emergency care needs of patients with special challenges.

Patients with Special Challenges

CORE CONCEPT
The variety of challenges that may be faced by patients with special needs

CORE CONCEPT
Types of disabilities and challenges patients may have

When we speak of patients with special challenges, sometimes referred to as special needs patients or patients with special needs, we are really referring to patients with many different types of challenges that require special considerations. As health care professionals, one of the few generalizations we can make about caring for such a diverse group is that empathy and respect for the patient, the patient's dignity, and the patient's rights are key factors in treatment.

Disability

Unfortunately, many special needs groups are discriminated against or viewed negatively by others. Because of the stigma that may be associated with certain conditions, and because we are often unsure about what descriptive terms are acceptable, we often feel uncomfortable with these patients or struggle to find the correct terminology to refer to their situations without causing offense.

The term ***disability*** is used to refer to a condition that interferes significantly with a person's ability to engage in activities of daily living, such as working and caring for oneself. Disabilities include vision impairment and loss (Figure 37-1), hearing impairment

disability
a physical, emotional, behavioral, or cognitive condition that interferes with a person's ability to carry out everyday tasks, such as working or caring for oneself.

FIGURE 37-1 (A) A blind patient may wish to touch the EMT's face. (B) If the blind patient has a guide dog, the EMT must never get between the dog and the patient. *(Photos A and B: © Michal Heron)*

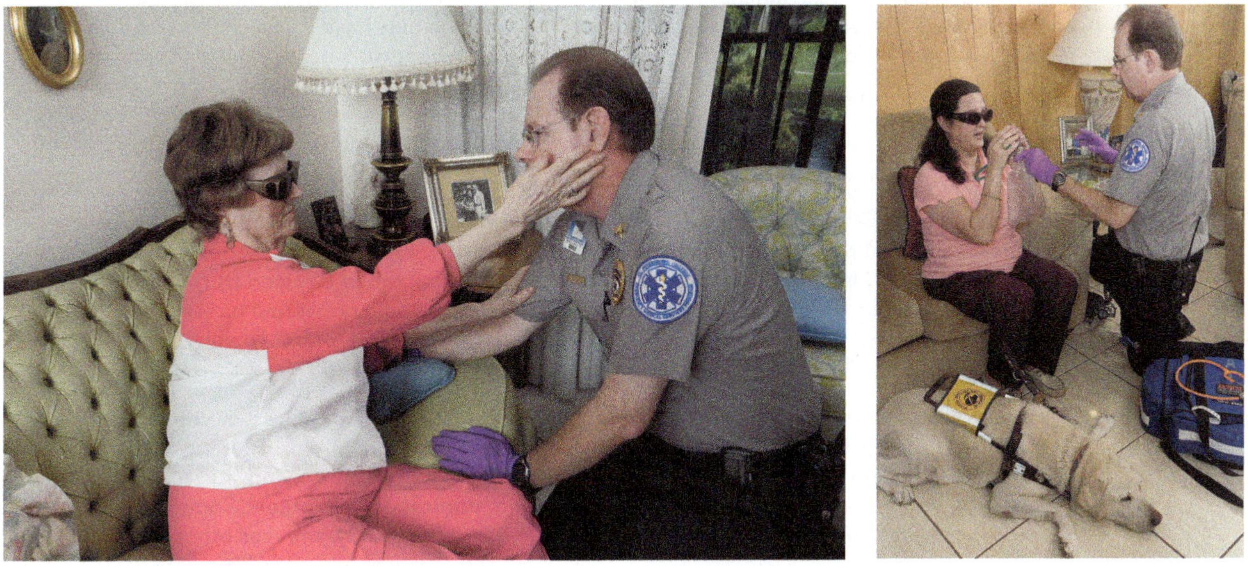

A B

and loss, loss of mobility, and emotional and cognitive impairments. It is preferable to speak of a person's having a disability, rather than using the term *handicapped*.

The Centers for Disease Control and Prevention (CDC) use the term *developmental disability* to mean a chronic (persistent or lasting) mental and/or physical impairment that begins at any age up until 22 years and causes significant impairment in the person's major life activities. Developmental disabilities include cerebral palsy and Down syndrome (Figure 37-2), among others. Other disabilities are not developmental in nature and may occur from traumatic injury or medical conditions. Multiple sclerosis, Parkinson's disease, stroke, traumatic brain injury, spinal cord injury, and other conditions can result in cognitive, emotional, and/or physical disability. Table 37-1 describes some impairments associated with particular conditions.

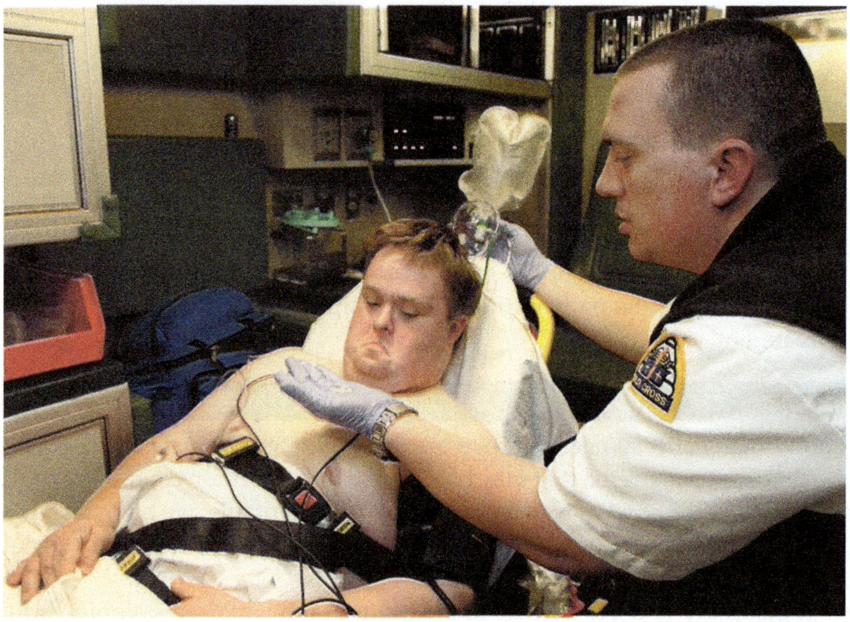

FIGURE 37-2 You may be called to care for a patient with a developmental disability, such as Down syndrome. *(© Daniel Limmer)*

TABLE 37-1 Selected Conditions for Patients with Special Challenges

CONDITION	DESCRIPTION	IMPLICATIONS
Autism	A developmental disorder in which the patient has impaired social functioning and communication. The patient may have repetitive or restricted behaviors.	There is a wide spectrum of autism disorders. Patients with what was called Asperger's syndrome may have social challenges and unusual behaviors but normal language and intellect. Patients with classic autism usually have language delays and communication problems, and often have intellectual disability.
Cerebral palsy	A permanent impairment in motor control, present at birth or within the first year of life. Cerebral palsy is not progressive. Movements are characterized by lack of coordination, exaggerated reflexes, and tightness of muscles.	Although some patients with cerebral palsy may also have cognitive impairment, do not assume this is the case. You should communicate with the patient as directed by the family or caregiver. Some nonverbal patients with CP can communicate with their eyes or assistive computers.
Cognitive disabilities	These may result from abnormalities of the brain due to a variety of genetic and congenital problems (e.g., Down syndrome, fetal alcohol syndrome). They may also result from stroke, dementia, or past traumatic brain injury.	Patients have varying levels of impairment in intellectual functioning, including learning, judgment, problem solving, social skills, and communication with others. Some patients may live independently, whereas others have only limited ability to interact with others.

TABLE 37-1 Selected Conditions for Patients with Special Challenges (*continued*)

CONDITION	DESCRIPTION	IMPLICATIONS
Hearing impairment	This condition may be congenital, due to trauma, or due to age. Hearing loss may be partial or complete.	Patients may have hearing aids, use TTY devices, or use sign language. Some patients can lip-read, so it is important to face the patient and talk to the patient directly, even if the patient has complete hearing loss.
Kidney (renal) failure	This condition may result from chronic illness such as diabetes, high blood pressure, or other medical problems, and can also be caused by traumatic injury. Patients can have varying levels of kidney function, and receive dialysis at different frequencies. (See the chapter *Hematologic and Renal Emergencies*.)	Patients are prone to a number of metabolic disturbances, especially if a dialysis appointment is missed. Dialysis access devices (shunts or fistulas) can malfunction and bleed. Do not take a blood pressure in an extremity with dialysis access. Patients with peritoneal dialysis will usually know the best way to manage their device.
Neuromuscular disorders	Examples include muscular dystrophy, multiple sclerosis, and Lou Gehrig's disease (amyotrophic lateral sclerosis or ALS).	Patients have varying levels of muscular weakness, which can be intermittent or progressive, resulting in paralysis. Complications can include bouts of severe pain, communication difficulties, urinary tract infections from associated catheters, and respiratory paralysis, in which the patient depends on a ventilator.
Stroke	Levels of disability vary from mild to incapacitating. Specific problems relate to the area of the brain affected and may involve emotional, behavioral, communication, intellectual, or physical limitations.	Don't make assumptions about a patient's ability to hear and understand, even though communication skills may be impaired.
Spinal cord injury	With complete spinal cord injury, patients experience lack of sensation and function below the level of injury.	Patients with high spinal cord injuries may be ventilator-dependent. This, combined with an inability to cough, increases the chances of pneumonia. Patients with urinary catheters are also prone to infection. Immobility may result in ischemia of compressed tissues, leading to breakdown of the skin and tissue beneath it (in the form of decubitus ulcer, pressure sore, or bedsore). Spinal cord-injured patients can also have difficulty regulating blood vessel tone. Changes in position (supine to seated) can drop blood pressure temporarily.
Vision impairment	This condition may be congenital or acquired, and may be either complete or partial.	Often, visually impaired patients cope well and are able to find their way through familiar surroundings. Ask the patient about the best way to help in navigating. Always explain what you are going to do before you do it. If the patient uses a cane or service animal, be sure to transport the cane or animal with the patient.

Many patients with disabilities live independently, often with some type of assistive equipment or accommodations. For example, wheelchair ramps, lowered countertops, handrails, and modified bathrooms can allow someone who relies on a wheelchair to live alone. Service animals can also be of great assistance to people with many different disabilities, increasing their independence. Some patients with more severe disabilities live at home but require special assistance, such as ventilators, feeding tubes, and home health care services. These patients may be independent, but often rely significantly on family and caregivers to support their special health care challenges. You may also encounter patients with special challenges in a variety of group home and institutional settings.

Terminal Illness

Terminally ill patients, such as patients with end-stage cancer, COPD, heart failure, or kidney failure, or those with progressive fatal diseases such as Huntington's disease or Lou Gehrig's disease, may prefer to stay at home under the care of family, possibly with assistance from hospice or home health care providers. Alternatively, they may spend the final weeks or days of their lives in a specially designated hospice facility. Terminally ill patients may be depending on technology to sustain life or relieve pain. Often, terminally ill patients have advance directives that specify what type of emergency care (if any) they are willing to accept. (See the chapter *Medical, Legal, and Ethical Issues*.)

Terminally ill patients and their families also have special emotional needs. (See Understanding Reactions to Death and Dying in the chapter *Well-Being of the EMT*.) Unfortunately, the cost of end-of-life care can also create financial problems, compounding the patient and family's concerns.

Obesity

bariatrics
the branch of medicine that deals with the causes of obesity as well as its prevention and treatment.

obesity
a condition of having too much body fat, defined as a body mass index of 30 or greater.

Bariatrics is the branch of medicine that deals with the causes, prevention, and treatment of obesity. ***Obesity*** is defined as a body mass index (BMI) of 30 or more. Body mass index is calculated by dividing your weight in pounds by the square of your height in inches, and multiplying by 703. For example, for a woman who weighs 135 pounds and is 5 feet, 5 inches tall (65 inches):

$$\text{BMI} = 135/(65 \times 65) \times 703 = 22.46$$

A BMI of up to 24.9 is considered healthy for people older than 20 years of age. A person with a BMI of 25–29 is considered overweight, while a person with a BMI of 30 or greater is considered obese. Keep in mind that BMI does not measure body fat directly and that an extremely muscular person could end up with a BMI of 30 or more without being obese. For most people, though, BMI is a good indicator of healthy weight range.

Obesity is a significant and growing health concern in the United States for both adults and children. Obesity increases the risk of some cancers, type 2 diabetes, hypertension, heart attack, stroke, liver and gallbladder disease, arthritis, sleep apnea, and respiratory problems. Because of the prevalence of obesity and because of the serious health issues related to obesity, you will frequently encounter obese patients.

As an EMT, you will need to take special measures to care for the obese patient. Very obese patients may have difficulty breathing when they are supine because of the extra weight that must be moved by the diaphragm during inspiration. If possible, allow the patient to assume a comfortable position for breathing. Monitor the patient's oxygen saturation, and provide oxygen and ventilatory assistance as needed. Bariatric patients are also associated with challenges to opening the airway during face mask ventilation, due to excessive body mass. The "ramp" technique detailed in the chapter *Respiration and Artificial Ventilation* is often the best approach to maintaining an open airway. Obese patients also have a lower threshold to allow air to enter their esophagus during positive pressure ventilation. This can lead to increased gastric insufflation when using a bag–mask device. Take care to use gentle pressure when ventilating and ventilate only with enough volume to achieve chest rise.

You will also need to take special care in lifting the obese patient to avoid injury to yourself, your coworkers, and the patient. Make sure you have enough assistance when lifting and moving obese patients, and use special equipment if the patient's weight exceeds the maximum load capacity of your stretcher. (See the chapter *Lifting and Moving Patients*.)

There has also been an increase in the rate of bariatric-related surgeries in the United States. These operations are specifically designed to promote weight loss in morbidly obese patients. There are different types of bariatric surgical procedures, including stomach stapling, the placement of a gastric sleeve over the stomach, and direct bypass of parts of the stomach and small bowel. These procedures can be effective in reducing weight but can also lead to complications that are encountered by EMS. Common postoperative complications include infection, leakage of digestive contents at surgical sites, bleeding (which may be internal or present as vomiting blood), nausea and vomiting, acid reflux, and obstruction. Bariatric surgery patients can also have issues with acute hypoglycemia as their systems adjust to the new process of digestion.

Homelessness and Poverty

Homelessness is a state of not having a regular place to live, often because of an inability to afford or otherwise maintain regular, safe, and adequate housing (Figure 37-3). The homeless may live in vehicles, in parks, on the street, in makeshift dwellings, or in abandoned buildings. In many communities, homeless shelters are available but may not have the capacity to provide for the number of homeless seeking shelter. In addition, many homeless individuals choose not to use shelters even when space is available. The homeless include men, women, children, and families. Disproportionate numbers of veterans and minorities make up the homeless population.

Several serious health problems are related to homelessness: mental health problems, malnutrition, substance abuse problems, HIV/AIDS, tuberculosis, bronchitis and pneumonia, environmental emergencies, wounds, and skin infections. The lack of access to health care means that conditions that begin as minor problems can go untreated until they become emergencies. Underlying chronic health problems and malnutrition can impair the body's ability to respond to injuries and acute illnesses, making these issues of more serious concern than they might be otherwise. Homeless women may be victims of domestic or sexual abuse. A large number of the estimated 1.4 million homeless children suffer from emotional problems.

Poverty, which may be a cause of homelessness, means that a person or family's income is not adequate to allow them a standard of living considered acceptable in society. For 2017 the U.S. Department of Health and Human Services determined the poverty guideline for a single person as an income of $12,060 or less, and $24,600 for a family of four. However, there are also large numbers of individuals and families whose incomes are above this yet are not enough to provide all their necessities, including health care, health insurance, prescription medications, and adequate nutrition. Therefore, the poor are prone to many of the same health issues as the homeless.

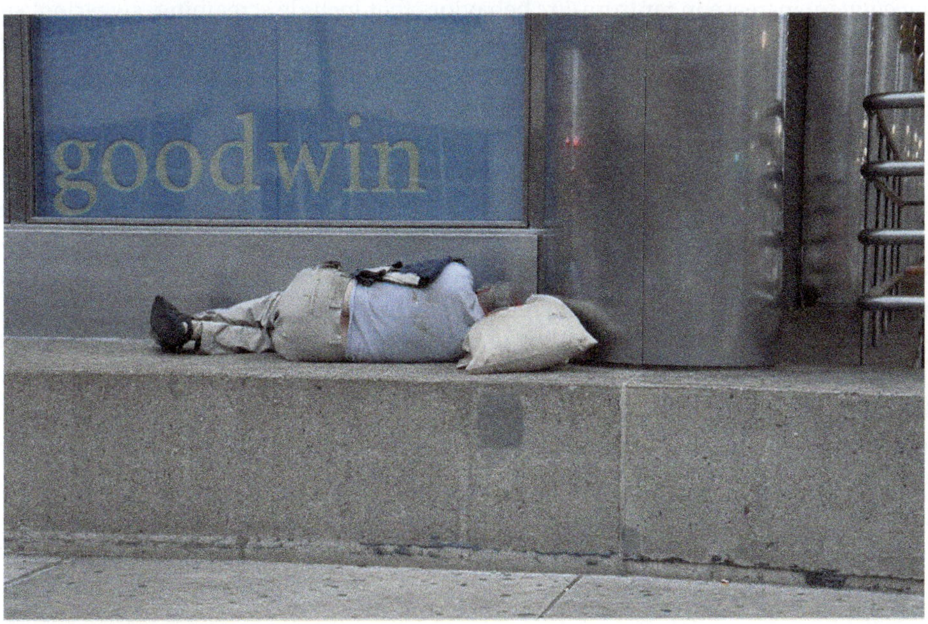

FIGURE 37-3 Homeless people often have complex medical and emotional issues.
(© Edward T. Dickinson, MD)

Approaches to Care of Patients with Special Needs

Autism

autism spectrum disorders (ASD)
Developmental disorders that affect, among other things, the ability to communicate, report medical conditions, self-regulate behaviors, and interact with others.

Autism spectrum disorders (ASD) are developmental disorders that affect, among other things, the ability to communicate, report medical conditions, self-regulate behaviors, and interact with others to get needs met. This can create serious problems for emergency responders. Traditional assessment techniques and treatment protocols may need to be modified for the ASD patient. With autism spectrum disorders affecting approximately 1 in 59 children, and 1.5 million Americans, you are likely to encounter a patient with an ASD. As recently as the year 2000, the autism spectrum prevalence was only 1 in 150 children.

A mnemonic to use when dealing with patients who have autism is *ABCS*: awareness, basic, calm, and safety.

Awareness

It is very important for EMTs to understand that people with an ASD will not behave or react in the same manner as most patients. Since these patients may not be able to adapt to the situation, EMTs will need to change their approach and strategies to meet the needs of the person with autism.

Persons with autism are susceptible to the same medical emergencies as the general population; often have coexisting medical conditions, such as seizure disorders; and are prone to sustaining certain types of injuries, all of which increase the likelihood of an EMS response. However, persons with autism also have rigid routines and a strong preference for things to be predictable and as expected. Disruption is not well tolerated.

Communication with the patient with an ASD can be challenging. Persons with autism often have literal perception and difficulty distinguishing patterns of speech—such as humor, slang, sarcasm, or idioms—from unambiguous statements. Body language, such as gesturing or facial expression, also might not be recognized. Approximately 25 percent to 30 percent of persons with ASD will stop speaking, usually between 15 and 24 months of age. About a quarter of those will remain nonverbal at age 9. In a stressful situation, even those with good verbal ability may be unable to speak. Consider using a picture card system, which can help patients express their needs and may assist you in explaining procedures and interventions to patients.

Escalation and meltdown, which can occur in a person with an ASD, can be described as an *involuntary* increase in tantrum-*like* behaviors that include screaming, swearing, stomping, throwing objects, hitting and/or kicking (people or objects), pushing, and biting. There are several causes of this behavior, with the most common involving sensory, emotional, or cognitive overstimulation; social skills deficits; excessive demands being placed on the individual; interruption of established routines; and being put in a situation that was unexpected or is unpredictable. If a person with an ASD is behaving aggressively or is escalated, it is rarely from what most of us would refer to as malicious or defiant behavior. It is much more likely that the individual is reacting to extreme stress and is out of control. These persons often know that they are out of control but do not have the ability to regain control effectively and may need your help to return to a calm sense of being. Simply put, they want circumstances to change, but do not know how to implement that change.

Basic

One of the most important aspects of interacting with persons with autism is to keep things basic. There are a few ways that this concept applies:

- **Keep your instructions basic.** Simple, clear, precise directions are easiest to follow for persons with autism. For example, say "Sit down here" (pointing at a chair), *not* "Why don't you have a seat?" Don't be sarcastic, use figures of speech, or tell jokes.

- **Ask basic questions.** Many people with autism will do better answering short, closed-ended questions than open-ended questions. Allow extra time to answer even simple questions. If the person still does not answer, the person may be nonverbal, may not understand the question, or may not know the answer. People who have an ASD have difficulty asking for clarification when they do not understand questions or instructions.
- **Basic means less "stuff"!** Our radios, pagers, cell phones, and even things such as flashlights and stethoscope covers may overstimulate the senses of a person with autism. They frequently have hyperacute responses to stimulations of one or more of the five senses that a majority of people tolerate well or don't even notice. For example, they may be able to see strobelike flickering in fluorescent lights when others don't. A gentle touch on the shoulder, intended to be reassuring, may feel like a powerful blow. They may also have difficulty separating loud foreground noise from faint background noise. Your radio, even if turned way down, may be perceived as being as loud as your speech. Sensory stimulus overload can easily be an antecedent to escalation and meltdown. Therefore, it is important to keep as much "stuff" as possible turned off and out of sight. If you are aware that your potential patient is autistic, it also is advisable to discontinue use of lights and siren as you approach the scene.
- **Keep your treatment basic.** Since persons with autism do not adapt well to sudden changes, it is best to minimize as many unplanned experiences as possible. In an emergency, the routines of these patients are interrupted, they are being bombarded with questions, things are being demanded of them from every direction, and an injury or illness may be causing significant pain or discomfort. Their already-heightened levels of anxiety, stress, and frustration are being pushed to the limit. The last thing they need is to be "attacked" by EMTs wanting to poke them here and put stickers there.

  Although you should not withhold absolutely necessary treatment, it is usually best to defer certain treatment interventions, such as obtaining a repeat set of vital signs in a very stable patient. Repeat vital signs are done routinely as precautions, but they may heighten the stress of the call for the patient. In other words, ask yourself "*Must this be done to get the patient to the hospital safely?*" before initiating specific treatments.

  It is critically important to remember, however, that the patient with autism may not offer typical complaints, may have very high pain thresholds (thereby tolerating injuries that most patients would describe as excruciating), and may choose to engage in a pleasurable activity (such as playing with a toy or listening to music) over dealing with an obvious injury or medical condition, despite the amount of discomfort it may be causing. In some cases, these traits may cause serious conditions to be missed. Therefore, careful assessment is always needed, and you should never withhold treatment the patient needs.

Calm

When dealing with a person with autism, particularly if the patient is escalating or having a meltdown, it is imperative that you remain calm. Posturing aggressively, commanding loudly, becoming aggravated—even telling the patient to "calm down"—will be either ineffective or counterproductive. Just because the individual has temporarily lost control of his or her behavior is no reason for you to do so. Remember: Calm creates calm.

Although a "show of force" may be an effective deterrent against aggressive behavior for many people, this strategy will likely be lost on the patient with autism. If anything, extra people add to confusion, increase frustration, and heighten anxiety, causing negative behaviors to escalate. A better approach is to allow one person to make direct contact with the patient with autism, preferably accompanied by a parent, family member, or caregiver. Keep your tone of voice clear and controlled. Offer empathy and compassion, and reassure the patient that you are there to help. Allow the patient to express concerns and frustrations.

Being calm means taking extra time—sometimes a lot of extra time. Don't force your agenda. Unless the patient has an immediately life- or limb-threatening condition, it's the patient's emergency and the patient's timeline. Forcing the patient to move on before the patient is ready likely will result in escalation and meltdown. If already escalated, it may increase the intensity and duration of the event and may break all trust that has already been established. Escalation could exacerbate medical emergencies such as asthma or heart problems. Since physical activity accompanies escalation, the patient's injuries could easily be aggravated.

Safety

Having a sense of safety and security is important to patients with autism. Often the environment where you find the patient offers a feeling of familiarity and security, even if it does not seem apparent to you. On the other hand, your ambulance is a strange and unfamiliar place, representing unpredictability to the patient with autism. Therefore, it is usually best to begin patient interaction where the patient is found. Remove things from the person's environment that may be aggravating (for example, turn off fluorescent lights), and disperse unnecessary personnel and bystanders.

Consider doing the physical exam in toe-to-head instead of head-to-toe order. Move slowly and do one thing at a time, such as assessing a leg or taking a blood pressure. Tell the patient *what* you are going to assess next and *how* you will assess it. Allow time for the patient to ask questions (e.g., some patients might want to know *why*), and make sure the patient is ready for you to do the next part of the assessment before you do it. If the patient begins to show signs of agitation or discomfort, and if this condition permits, consider taking a break before continuing the assessment. You may need to "segment" your exam and pause several times before completing it.

The concept of preparing the patient at each step along the way is essential to establish a sense of safety. The patient needs to know what to expect next. *What* can the patient expect to see? *When* will it occur? *How long* will it last? Use solid, descriptive terms to explain how an intervention will feel, as persons with autism often perceive pain quite differently than other people do. For example, when describing how it feels to have a blood pressure taken, don't say "It won't hurt." Instead, say "This cuff is going to squeeze your arm tight."

Allowing the patient to tell you when the patient is ready for you to perform procedures or treatments provides a much-needed sense of control. Let the patient tell you when he or she is ready to move to the ambulance. The patient may want to look around the ambulance, look in cabinets and drawers, and even handle equipment before settling down. The patient may want to sit in a specific seat, such as the captain's chair, or sit in various seats before deciding where to sit. Involving the patient in care and accommodating these needs, when possible, will likely build trust and increase compliance and cooperation.

Even if the person with autism is escalated or having a meltdown, restraining the individual is frightening and terrifying for the individual. It should be avoided, used only as a last resort, and performed only when the person is in imminent danger of causing harm to self or others.

Infants and Children with Medical Challenges

Over the years, medical expertise has improved significantly, allowing many children who formerly would have died to live. The following are some common groups of children with special challenges:

- Premature infants with lung disease
- Infants and children with heart disease
- Infants and children with neurologic disease
- Children with chronic disease or altered function from birth

Often these children are able to live at home with their parents. This means that you may receive calls to care for children who have complicated medical problems and are dependent on various technologies (Figure 37-4). Although pediatric emergency calls are relatively few, children with special challenges living at home constitute a significant percentage of those calls.

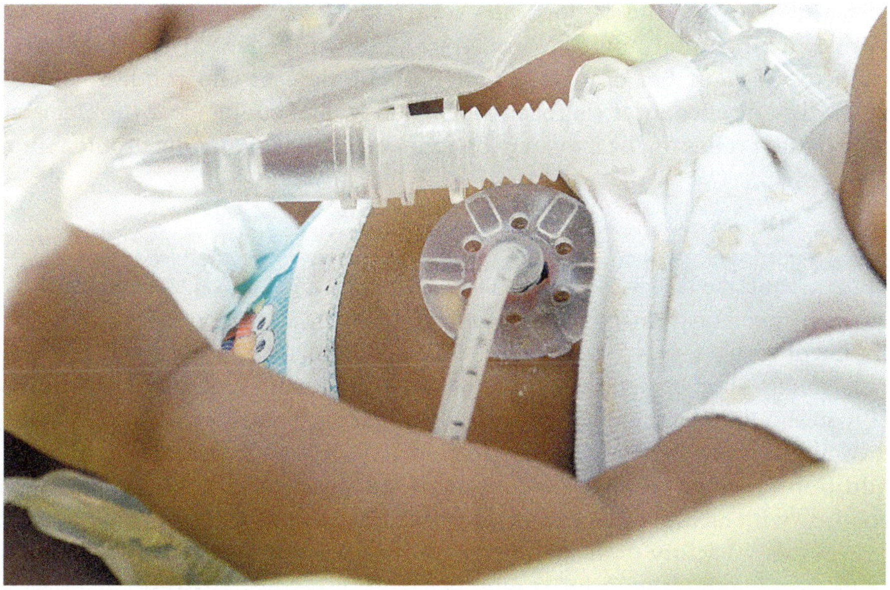

FIGURE 37-4 Children who have complicated medical problems are often dependent on various technologies, such as the gastric feeding tube implanted in this baby's stomach.

The children's parents will be familiar with the various devices used and can serve as a valuable resource. Common devices include tracheostomy tubes, home artificial ventilators, central intravenous lines, gastrostomy tubes and gastric feeding tubes, and shunts.

Emergency care of children with special challenges has often been complicated by the lack of information that EMTs and emergency department staff are able to quickly obtain about the children's medication, condition, history, precautions needed, and special management plans.

CORE CONCEPT
Special aspects of prehospital care for a patient with special challenges

NOTE: *In 1999, the American College of Emergency Physicians (ACEP) and the American Academy of Pediatrics (AAP) developed the* Emergency Information Form for Children with Special Needs, *which should be kept up to date and on hand by the patient's caregivers. If a copy of this form is available at the patient's home, it should be brought along if the child is transported to the hospital.*

"There will be times when you have no clue about some of the medical devices you will see. Ask the caregivers. It is amazing what they know—and how they can help."

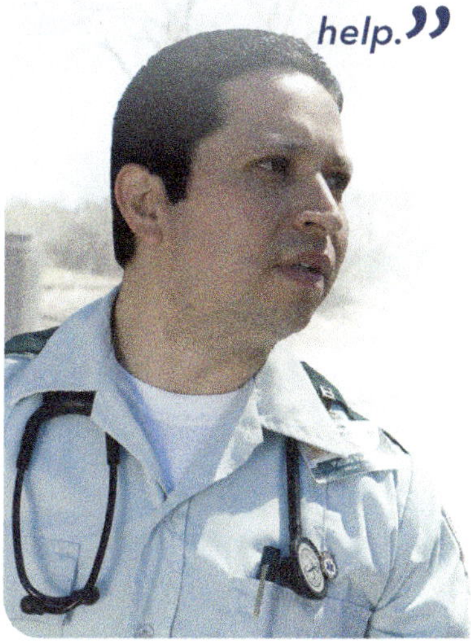

General Considerations in Responding to Patients with Special Challenges

In many respects, responding to and caring for a person with special challenges is like any other call for service, in that it may be for an emergency such as a fall, general illness, chest pain, seizures, or shortness of breath. What is different for you, the EMT, is that the patient's preexisting condition can complicate and quickly overwhelm your ability to assess and treat the patient. To ensure proper care for such a patient, you must be able to recognize, understand, and evaluate the patient's specific special health care needs in addition to the presenting problem or chief complaint that led to the 911 call. In addition to increasing your knowledge about patients with special challenges in general, you can take steps to be prepared for specific patients or types of patients in your response area.

Advanced Medical Devices in the Home

In recent years, medical advances and insurance-coverage changes have allowed more and more people to have medical devices and care at home that were formerly seen only in the hospital. Patients who previously may have been unable to survive at home are now afforded the opportunity and relative comfort of living and working in a normal, nonhospital environment. As a result, prehospital providers are faced with an increasing number of calls to patients with devices and conditions that EMTs previously did not encounter (Figure 37-5). These calls may be for a problem with the device the patient relies on, or they may be for a medical or traumatic problem unrelated to the device.

Variety of Health Care Settings

Patients with special care needs can be encountered in a variety of locations. With the proliferation of varied levels of health care settings, an EMT may respond to calls at private residences, nursing homes, specialty rehabilitation centers, and specialized care facilities. As an EMT, you should take the time to become familiar with any special health care settings in your community so you can be better prepared for calls of this nature.

In addition to identifying the locations of such facilities, EMTs should meet and develop plans with facility representatives to minimize confusion that could occur during an emergency call. Facility representatives may be able to arrange for you to see various medical devices in operation prior to any problems or medical distress.

Some communities have programs in place through their dispatch system to help identify people who may require additional help with medical devices in case of a disaster or evacuation from a building.

Families that care for patients with special health care challenges frequently have discussed a preplan with their primary care providers. Often EMS is involved in those preplans. Several health care organizations maintain standardized forms for use in preplanning special health care emergencies.

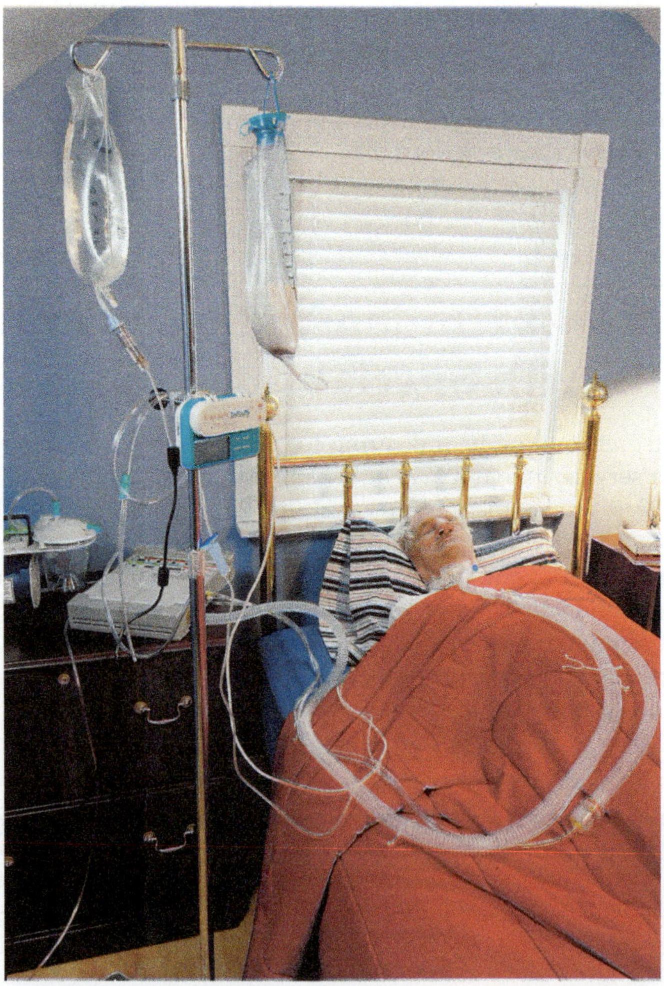

FIGURE 37-5 EMTs are increasingly called to assist patients who rely on advanced medical devices at home. This patient has a feeding line and a home ventilator connected to a tracheostomy.

These forms are often completed and kept on file in the patient's home. EMS agencies also use such materials when meeting with special health care patients living in their communities and create collaborative response plans that ensure optimal care.

Knowledgeable Caregivers

One of the advantages EMTs have when encountering patients with special challenges is that these patients will often have on site, or will be accompanied by, a person who has been trained in the use of the patient's devices and in the patient's conditions. This person may be medically trained, such as a registered nurse, a certified nursing assistant, or a home health aide; however, more often it will be a family member or friend.

Although family members may not have had formal medical training or certification, they are generally very familiar and comfortable with using the devices the patient relies on. Many learned about the equipment and techniques for using it from medical professionals before their family member (the patient) was discharged from a hospital. In most cases, emergency procedures have been explained and rehearsed. Because they have a vested interest in being competent with the devices, family members are very thorough and deliberate with their understanding and application of the devices and their features. Therefore, it is advisable to seek their input on any problem that may be occurring with devices the patient has and to ask if they have been in a similar situation before. Some general questions include:

Has this problem ever occurred before? If so, what fixed it?

Have you (or other family members/caregivers) been taught how to fix this problem?

Have you tried to fix the problem? If so, what happened?

In addition, asking questions such as "How do you normally move him?" or "Has she ever been transported by ambulance? What worked well for the transfer?" will allow family members to be part of the solution. Family members do not necessarily expect the arriving members of EMS to know or be familiar with the patient's medical device, and they can help guide the EMTs in the device's use and function. It is a good idea to assign a member of the EMS team to work with the family member regarding the medical device while others on the team concentrate on assessment, treatment, and moving the patient to the ambulance.

Although the family may have prior training, sometimes their capabilities fail when faced with an emergency involving a loved one. Often EMS has been called because the family is unable to manage the challenge at hand. Remember that family members may still be an important resource, and small amounts of coaching and prompting may be enough for them to overcome their initial stress response. Your calm and stable demeanor, combined with the family's particular expertise, is an important collaboration necessary to achieve a positive outcome. These difficult challenges may also be an opportunity to begin a discussion on future preplanning activities.

A Knowledgeable Patient

The patient may also be a great help to the EMT regarding the patient's condition, the patient's need for the device, the functioning of the device, and how the device operates. The patient has likely been using and/or watching the use of this device for some time and has most likely been trained by medical providers to correctly use the device. Ask about the device and any problems the patient may be having with it (Figure 37-6).

This approach will depend greatly on the patient's mental status and baseline level of functioning. If the patient has an altered mental status or if medical conditions dictate otherwise, the family will be the primary source of knowledge. Regardless of the patient's mental status or condition, always explain what you are doing. One of the last senses a patient might lose is hearing, so talking and explaining your actions to the patient may help alleviate any stress the patient may be feeling yet unable to show.

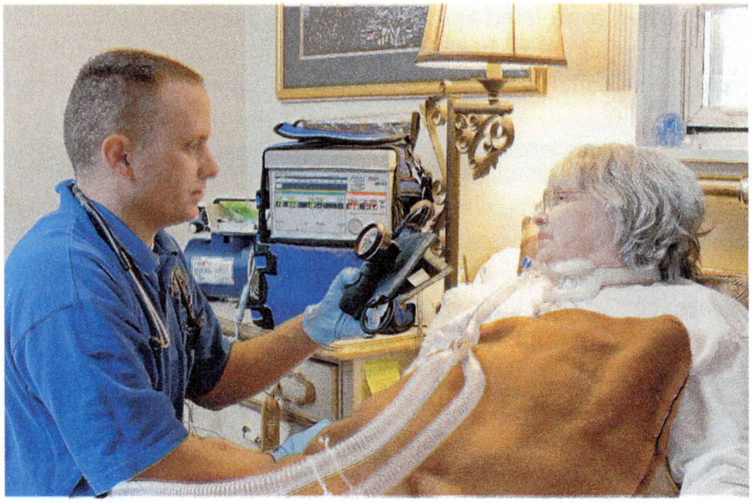

FIGURE 37-6 The patient is often an expert on the device or devices the patient depends on. Enlist the patient's advice as you discuss the condition, special devices, and the assessments and care you plan to perform.

Following Protocols

One note of caution is that as an EMT, your actions fall under specific regional and state scopes of practice. Thus, you should confer with medical direction if the treatment or skill required is not something you are trained in or allowed to do under these protocols. Specific considerations should be given, such as:

Is the problem with the device life-threatening?

Do I have the knowledge to fix this problem?

Do I have the supplies needed to fix this problem?

Is this within my protocols, or within medical control authorization?

Establishing the Baseline

There are thousands of diseases, conditions, and disabilities that could accompany a patient with special health care needs, and it would be impossible to discuss them all in a single text. This means that in many cases, you will encounter a situation or condition that you are unfamiliar with. That's okay. As an EMT, you don't have to know everything. It is important, however, to recognize that something is wrong with the patient, and the very fact that EMS has been called indicates that an unusual or untoward problem is at hand. It is now your job to assist the patient and caregivers to offer the best care possible.

One very important element of best-practice care is to establish the patient's baseline. Very often, traditional norms are not normal for a patient with special health care needs. For example, in a patient with cyanotic congenital heart disease, it is not reasonable to expect to see pink skin. On a good day, you may see only slight cyanosis around the eyes and fingernails. Cyanosis would not necessarily indicate a significant shift from the normal expectations of health in this patient. Patients with communication difficulties or cognition impairment might not be able to answer assessment questions in the same manner other patients would. Although you have been taught that cyanosis or an inability to answer questions properly is a serious deviation from the norm, in patients with special health care needs, you will need to adjust those expectations. It is your job, in these unusual situations, to determine exactly what normal expectations are for this patient and what, if anything, has changed to a point where EMS became necessary.

Patients are often the best source of baseline information, as they are typically well versed in their condition or disability. Simply asking what is different today or (respectfully) why they felt the ambulance was needed can provide volumes of information toward a care plan. A common answer might include something like "I'm usually able to get up and move with my walker, but today I just don't seem to have the energy." Remember that even patients who have baseline cognition problems or dementia can have acute changes. For example, a patient with Alzheimer's disease may have difficulty recalling facts and dates but may very well know what time of day it is, or when dinner is typically served. An acute alteration of mental status in a patient like this might be identified by a change in the normally expected routine (e.g., not coming to dinner on time).

Family and caregivers can also be very helpful in filling in assessment details. They often are very aware of what normal expectations are, and commonly are the ones who made the decision to call EMS. They are frequently well educated regarding the patient's special challenges and can be a great resource in determining the best care. In addition to aiding in your assessment, caregivers often are thoroughly educated in emergency procedures and may be able to offer actions that are outside of your scope of practice (like replacing a tracheotomy tube). The best care comes from engaging all of these resources.

Finally, consider any additional resources you may have access to. It is not unreasonable to take a moment and search for information on a specific disease or condition on your smart phone or computer. This isn't a sign of weakness, but rather a commitment to excellent patient care. Research should not replace more emergent actions such as airway management or ventilatory support, but for a stable patient, research can be part of an important commitment to doing your best. Remember also that medical control can be consulted for additional information and to help develop an appropriate treatment plan.

Don't Forget the Routine Care

Patients with special health care needs also have routine medical problems. Kids with chronic seizure disorders get influenza. People with renal failure fall and break their hip. Patients with Alzheimer's disease also may have diabetes and become hypoglycemic. It is very easy to become distracted by more complex or unusual disorders and lose sight of the fact that the same problems that harm everyday patients also harm patients with special health care needs.

The balance in assessing and managing a patient with special health care needs is to differentiate challenges associated with their unique, ongoing condition from routine problems associated with everyday life. Keep in mind that in many of these patients, routine issues exacerbate chronic conditions as well. The key is not to focus so much on the chronic condition that a simpler or expected problem is missed.

Although in many ways this is a complex dilemma, it can be simplified by starting with a standard patient assessment. Primary assessment problems that are life-threatening in everyday patients are life-threatening in patients with special health care needs. Massive hemorrhage is deadly regardless of whether it is coming from a simple laceration or a ruptured hemodialysis fistula. The treatment priorities are the same. Primary assessment issues, like airway obstruction and respiratory failure, are addressed first.

The secondary assessment will help better define the nature of today's problem. As previously discussed, it will be important to establish a baseline and better understand the expectations of the particular chronic health care challenge, but you must also pay attention to the routine patterns and suspicions that might offer an alternate diagnosis. For example, an Alzheimer's patient might have chronic dementia, but today might demonstrate an abrupt change in mental status. The change could be related to the Alzheimer's, but you should also inquire about the history of the present illness and past medical history conditions, like diabetes, that are commonly associated with altered mental status. Your physical exam should also include a blood glucose check.

Overall, you must keep a wide viewpoint in managing patients with special health care needs. Care needs to address specific challenges, but also incorporate day-to-day problems that you are already familiar with. Use as many resources as you can, and collaborate with caregivers as often as possible.

CORE CONCEPT

Congenital and acquired diseases and conditions

Diseases and Conditions

A disease or condition may be congenital or acquired. A *congenital disease* or condition is one that is present at birth. Some congenital diseases may be genetic; others might not. One example of a congenital disease is congenital heart disease (the most common birth defect), where the heart or large blood vessels of the heart are malformed. Other examples include cleft palates and congenital deafness.

An *acquired disease* or condition is one that occurs after birth and may be the result of exposure to a virus or bacterium, or the result of another medical condition or trauma. Examples of acquired diseases include COPD, AIDS, and traumatic spinal cord injury.

Some diseases or conditions may be either congenital or acquired. An example of this would be deafness. A patient may be congenitally deaf from a birth defect or may become deaf from a disease or from trauma (e.g., a loud explosion).

It is important to understand that a patient with a chronic disease, whether it is congenital or acquired, may develop a sudden, acute worsening of the disease that prompts a call to 911. In addition, the patient with a chronic disease may develop an acute illness, and this acute illness may be potentially more devastating than the same disease would be for a patient who did not have a coexisting chronic disease.

CORE CONCEPT

Types of advanced medical devices patients may rely on

Advanced Medical Devices

As an EMT, you may encounter patients of any age or physical condition who have advanced medical devices. Take into consideration what the device is doing for the patient and how important the device is to the patient's survival. Some devices are intended to allow the patient to improve quality of life or to have the fullest life possible, whereas others actually sustain life. Many patients who rely on such devices for life support have limited life expectancies. Even with proper use of the devices, their diseases or conditions may be terminal.

As already noted, you should include family caregivers, as appropriate, in care decisions and patient transportation.

Respiratory Devices

Noninvasive Positive Pressure Ventilation Devices (NIPPV)

continuous positive airway pressure (CPAP) a device worn by a patient that blows oxygen or air under constant low pressure through a tube and mask to keep airway passages from collapsing at the end of a breath.

We have discussed the use of CPAP in previous chapters. In addition to its emergent applications, you may find ***continuous positive airway pressure (CPAP)*** used to treat a variety of chronic medical conditions. CPAP is often prescribed to patients who suffer sleep apnea (periods when breathing stops during sleep) to help keep airway passages open (Figure 37-7). CPAP can help such patients prevent exacerbation of other medical conditions and conquer the chronic fatigue and irritability that are likely to result from interrupted sleep caused by the apneic periods, and may be especially helpful in moderating behavioral problems that can occur in children with sleep apnea. A related device is the biphasic continuous positive airway pressure (BiPAP) device, which provides assistance with both inhalation and exhalation. Collectively, CPAP and BiPAP fall under the generic term *noninvasive positive pressure ventilation (NIPPV)*.

Review the chapters *Respiration and Artificial Ventilation* and *Respiratory Emergencies* for a more complete discussion of CPAP and BiPAP.

EMT Assessment and Transport. A patient who uses a CPAP device at night is unlikely to have a medical emergency directly related to the device and will not need the device during transport. However, the patient may wish to bring the device along to the hospital. Hospital personnel should also be alerted that the patient uses a CPAP device during sleep.

FIGURE 37-7 A continuous positive airway pressure (CPAP) device provides constant pressure to keep airway passages open. It may be prescribed to (A) adults or (B) children.

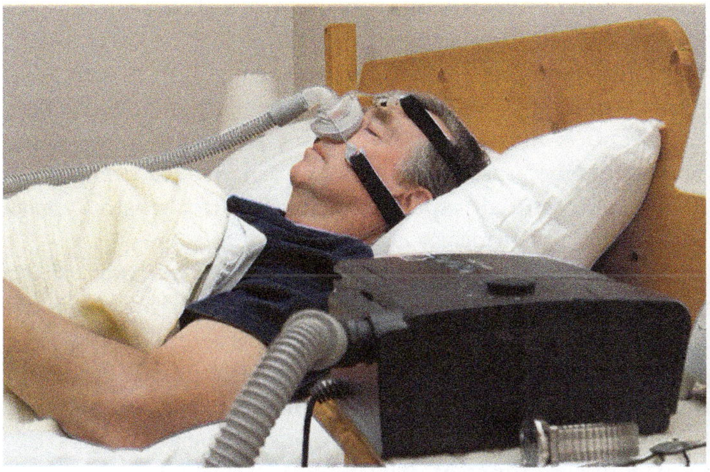

A

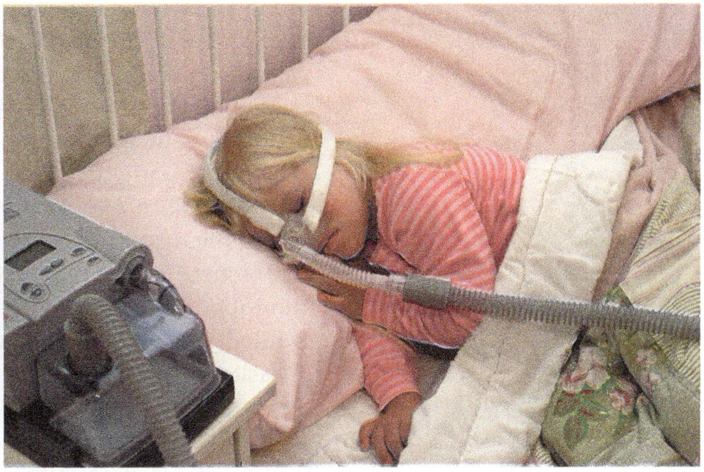

B

Tracheostomy Tubes

A ***tracheostomy*** is a surgical opening through the neck into the trachea (Figure 37-8). When the opening created is permanent, it is called a ***stoma***. A tracheostomy is usually created near the second to fourth tracheal ring. A tracheostomy tube (a short breathing tube and flange) is inserted into the airway to allow the patient to breathe through the stoma instead of through the nose and mouth. It is often called a "trach" (pronounced *trayk*) tube.

Tracheostomy tubes used by older children and adults are usually double-cannula tubes. A double-cannula tube has an inner cannula (a tube within a tube) that can be locked into place and removed periodically for cleaning. Tracheostomy tubes for young children are usually single-cannula tubes that don't have the removable inner cannula. A bag–valve mask can be connected to either type of trach tube—to the inner cannula of a double-cannula tube or directly to a single-cannula tube.

Trach tubes usually come with an obturator, which is a long "plug" that is placed inside the tube to help guide it during insertion and that also prevents material from getting into and clogging the tube during insertion. The obturator is removed after the trach tube is in place.

A tracheostomy procedure may be performed for long-term reasons in patients with neuromuscular disorders, spinal cord injuries, tumors, congenital deformities, coma, and a variety of other conditions that affect the patient's ability to breathe or maintain a patent airway. A patient with a tracheostomy tube may or may not be on a home ventilator. Tracheostomy patients who are on ventilators may be on them all the time or only when sleeping.

tracheostomy
a surgical opening in the neck into the trachea.

stoma
a surgically created permanent opening into the body, as with a tracheostomy, colostomy, or ileostomy.

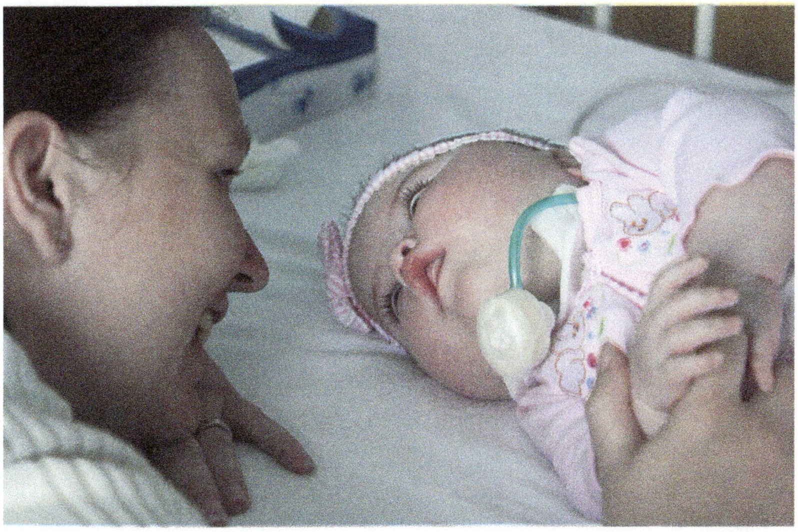

FIGURE 37-8 Infant with tracheostomy tube. *(© Life in View/Science Source)*

Tracheostomy patients range from newborns to the very elderly. A patient with a tracheostomy may or may not be able to speak, depending on the patient's condition. Some are able to speak by covering the tracheostomy tube briefly and making use of a speaker valve attached to the tube or an electronic box applied to the larynx. Do not make assumptions about whether a patient with a tracheostomy can speak.

Problems associated with tracheostomy tubes include displacement and obstruction. Displacement is relatively rare, and is more commonly associated with very young patients or patients with altered mental status. Caregivers frequently have been taught how to replace a tube, but this can be difficult especially when the tracheostomy tract where the tube is inserted has been newly surgically created.

Tracheostomy tube obstruction typically occurs when a buildup of mucus forms in the tube. Obstructions can be cleared by simple suctioning, and most caregivers are trained to perform this skill. Obstructions are sometimes more severe, however, and occasionally necessitate replacement of the tube. Because the tube bypasses the upper airway's function of warming, filtering, and humidifying inspired air, suctioning of the tube is often required routinely. Sometimes this procedure is even needed every few hours. This is especially common during times of distress, in the first few weeks after tube insertion, or if the patient has an infection. Other problems include infection around the stoma and a higher risk of routine viral and bacterial respiratory infections leading to respiratory distress.

Patients with tracheostomies require extensive care, and their caregivers are given substantial training. Caregivers should be very familiar with the procedures used to suction the tube. They should also know how to change and replace the tracheostomy tube since it needs to be regularly cleaned. Although these procedures are outside the scope of practice for most EMTs, you may find yourself in a situation where you need to prompt caregivers to take these actions to address an emergency. Always follow local protocols.

EMT Assessment and Transport. Carefully assess the tracheostomy tube for any blockage, and clear it (under protocol or by having caregivers perform this). To clear a blockage, carefully insert a whistle-tip catheter (a soft, flexible catheter used to suction tracheostomy or endotracheal tubes) into the stoma. (See Figure 37-9.) Determine the correct depth of insertion by measuring the suction tubing against the length of the obturator, which is the same length as the trach tube itself. You will usually be able to find the obturator among the patient's tracheostomy supplies. If you can't locate the obturator for measurement, stop inserting the suction catheter when you feel resistance. Suction as the catheter is being withdrawn, using a twisting motion as it is slowly removed. The patient may "buck" (jump or jerk a little) during this procedure.

If the patient requires further suctioning (indicated by visible or audible mucus), insert the suction tip into a container of sterile water to remove any mucus left in the catheter, then repeat. The patient on a ventilator may need to be ventilated by a bag–valve mask between suctionings. During transport, the patient should be positioned with head slightly elevated to allow for mucus drainage.

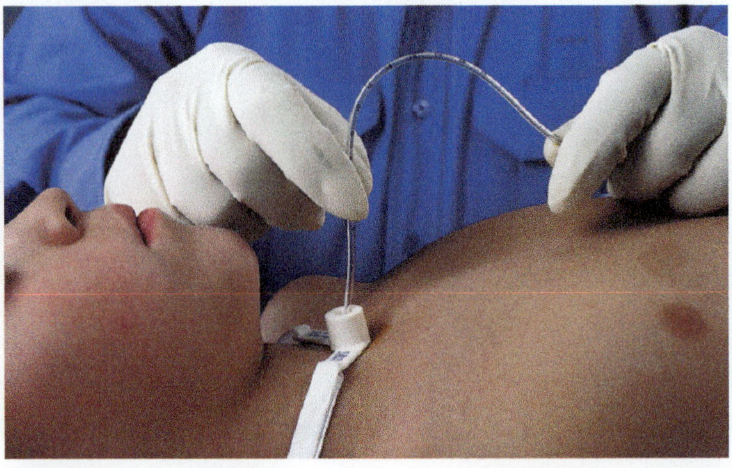

FIGURE 37-9 Suctioning a tracheostomy tube.

Home Ventilators

A ***ventilator*** is a device that breathes for a patient. A home ventilator weighs anywhere from several pounds to more than twenty pounds, and can range from the size of this textbook to the size of a desktop computer. It is programmed to take over the functions of inhalation, exhalation, timing, and rate of breathing. Although dependent on the ventilator for breathing, the patient may still lead an active life.

ventilator
a device that breathes for a patient.

The ventilator is attached to a ribbed tube called a ventilator circuit, which may come in various lengths, that enters the trachea. The tube from the ventilator may be attached to a plastic or metal port (called a cannula) that enters through a stoma in the neck. It may also be attached to an endotracheal tube through the mouth.

The patient on a home ventilator may call EMS for a variety of problems with the device. As with a tracheostomy tube, mucous plugs and secretions develop that require suctioning, and the patient may develop infections or respiratory distress. In addition, the home ventilator depends on AC power, so power failures may be cause for concern. Ventilators do have backup batteries that generally last an hour or more.

Home ventilators are tailored with settings that are the most comfortable for the patient. In the case of a mechanical failure, or during transport of the patient, a bag–valve–mask (BVM) device can take over the function of the ventilator. During this procedure, you should adjust the rate, volume, and pressure of the BVM to the patient's comfort level. This can often be accomplished with guidance from the patient or the caregivers. If the patient or caregivers are unable to provide guidance, you should observe for adequate chest rise and improving skin color.

EMT Assessment and Transport. To address an emergency involving a home ventilator, consider the memory aid **DOPE**:

- **D—Displacement.** Has the tracheostomy tube been displaced? This can be determined by observing for chest rise during ventilation, looking for subcutaneous air around the site of the tracheostomy, or assessing placement in the same way you would when assisting with endotracheal intubation. For example, you might be asked to listen with a stethoscope for lung sounds on both sides of the chest and to attach capnography to confirm the presence of exhaled CO2. If the tube has been displaced, a family member or caregiver may be able to replace it.
- **O—Obstruction.** Is the tracheostomy tube obstructed? Is there a mucous plug? This may be visible or audible, but it can also be recognized by a failure to achieve chest rise during ventilation. If an obstruction is suspected, it may be reasonable to attempt suctioning (if protocol allows) or enlist a caregiver to provide the intervention. Some obstructions will require the tube to be replaced. A caregiver can be prompted to take this action.
- **P—Pneumothorax/Pneumonia.** Patients on a ventilator are at risk for developing a pneumothorax. This can be identified by listening to lung sounds. (A pneumothorax will present as diminished or absent lung sounds on one side.) Other findings include unequal chest rise, signs of hypoxia, and shock. A pneumothorax is a true emergency. Initiate rapid transport and intercept with ALS if possible. Pneumonia is an acute infection of the lung tissue itself. Pneumonia can be a life-threatening infection, especially in patients with a compromised respiratory system and chronic underlying respiratory diseases.
- **E—Equipment.** Occasionally, a ventilator emergency will simply be the result of a mechanical or electrical failure of the ventilator itself. The first action you should take in a ventilator emergency is to remove the circuit and attempt to ventilate the patient with a BVM. This step can rule out equipment failure, but it also can rule out tube displacement and obstruction. While a team member ventilates, a second can assist caregivers with troubleshooting the ventilator device. Is there a power failure? Can it be plugged in or have its batteries replaced? Is the circuit clear? Occasionally, with long circuits, the problem may be as simple as a bed wheel's running over the tubing. If a caregiver is unavailable, simply continue to ventilate the patient and initiate transport.

Not all ventilator situations are emergencies. In many cases, you may be managing a ventilated patient for other reasons. While caring for a patient with a home ventilator, ensure that the ventilator tube does not have any buildup of mucus, and suction as needed. During transport, it may be easier to use a BVM while moving the patient to the ambulance, depending on the location and situation (e.g., stairs or with a heavy patient). If you use a BVM at any point, ensure that it is the appropriate size for the patient and that it is connected to oxygen. If the patient has a tracheostomy tube and the BVM does not fit the tube attachment, use the face mask from the BVM to cover the stoma and secure the mask to provide a good seal against the neck, then ventilate as normal. Some ventilated patients may also be able to be ventilated traditionally (by mouth) if you simply seal the opening in the trachea with a gloved hand or occlusive dressing.

If the ventilator is left attached to the patient, firmly affix it to the stretcher. Secure the ventilator to prevent movement in the ambulance during transport. Consider transport time versus battery life and plug the ventilator into the ambulance's inverter if available. If a BVM will be used during transport, obtain extra help so you can continue to provide assessment and care.

Cardiac Devices

Implanted Pacemakers and Cardiac Defibrillators

A patient may have an implanted pacemaker or automatic implanted cardiac defibrillator. These devices are both designed to respond to potentially lethal electrical rhythm changes in the heart.

pacemaker
a device implanted under the skin with wires implanted into the heart to modify the heart rate as needed to maintain an adequate heart rate.

A ***pacemaker*** is a small device implanted under the skin, with wires attached to the heart. The pacemaker is designed to prevent the heart rate from becoming too slow. Early pacemakers were set at a fixed rate, but modern pacemakers are "rate responsive"—that is, they detect what the patient is doing and modify the heart rate accordingly. For example, if the patient is moving around and performing an action, a sensor will detect this and increase the rate to allow for the activity. In addition, if the breathing rate increases, the pacemaker will increase the heart rate as well. The pacemaker delivers a series of low-energy pulses at set intervals to stimulate the heart to beat at a faster rate. These pulses are not felt by the patient and cannot be detected on the skin or felt by providers. The pacemaker does not squeeze the heart or fix damaged muscle; rather, it helps regulate the timing of each beat.

automatic implanted cardiac defibrillator (AICD)
a device implanted under the skin of the chest to detect any life-threatening dysrhythmia and deliver a shock to defibrillate the heart.

Like a pacemaker, an ***automatic implanted cardiac defibrillator (AICD)*** is placed under the skin with wires inserted into the heart. The AICD varies in size from slightly larger than a 9-volt battery to the size of a wallet. It is usually implanted in the upper left chest area, although occasionally it may be implanted in the area of the left upper quadrant of the abdomen. It is generally palpable through the skin. The AICD senses when a patient develops a life-threatening cardiac rhythm and delivers an electrical shock to the heart to restore a normal electrical rhythm. The energy developed by an AICD is far less than is delivered by an automated external defibrillator (AED) and poses no risk to the provider who might be in contact with the patient when the AICD fires.

Point of View

"I went to school with a guy who got into a motorcycle crash. He was hurt pretty bad. He had an injury to his spine that put him in a wheelchair and on a ventilator. I think about him from time to time. When I became an EMT and started transporting patients, it really got me thinking. What if he ever needed an ambulance?

"The logistics of either taking the ventilator or ventilating him with a BVM is probably scarier to him than it is to me. But it is pretty intimidating to me too, let me tell you. I'd do it. But I'd be nervous.

"Do you think it's normal to feel that way?"

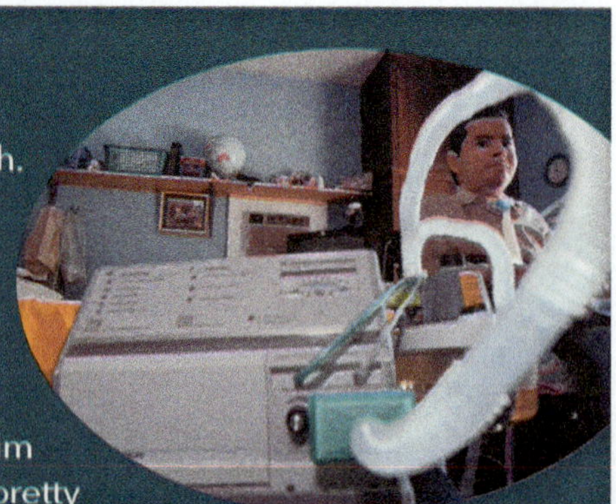

(Jim Slosiarek/Journal Times/AP Images)

The implanted defibrillator is designed to detect life-threatening cardiac rhythms (ventricular fibrillation and ventricular tachycardia). Newer models may have a pacemaker feature built in as well. The AICD delivers a single shock when a life-threatening rhythm is detected. This shock is often very painful to the patient, and is generally rated as a 6 on a 1-to-10 pain scale. If the single shock does not correct the rhythm or if the rhythm returns, other shocks will be delivered, one at a time, until the dysrhythmia is resolved, or the machine is turned off. The AICD can be turned off only by a special magnet and generally in only a hospital setting.

NOTE: *The occurrence of an AICD shock is often very upsetting to the patient. Be prepared to provide emotional support.*

Although muscle twitches may be seen on the patient, providers and caregivers will not be shocked or harmed if the AICD shocks while they are touching the patient. The AICD is not dangerous if it shocks when the patient is wet. Patients are generally instructed to call their doctor if they feel fine after a shock. However, if they have any symptoms such as dizziness, chest pain, shortness of breath, or not feeling well, or if they are shocked more than twice in any 24-hour period, they are instructed to go to the hospital or call EMS.

The functioning of pacemakers and AICDs can be affected by certain electromagnetic and radio frequency signals, so people with these devices should not stand still in the doorway of a business with an electronic anti-theft device or stand still in a walk-through metal detector (although walking through either of these without stopping is not harmful). Stereo speakers and mobile telephones should not be held against a pacemaker or AICD device. In addition, electric motors (as in power tools) and gas-powered tools (such as chainsaws and snowblowers) must be kept at least 6 inches away from the AICD or pacemaker when it is running.

Most patients who have one or both of these devices have had a significant cardiac medical history. They may be on multiple medications and may carry wallet cards or wear bracelets stating that they have one of these devices in use.

EMT Assessment and Transport. Depending on the nature of the call and chief complaint, the EMT may request ALS transport for a patient with a pacemaker or AICD device. A patient who merely has a pacemaker as part of his medical history may not need ALS, but if the pacemaker is malfunctioning, or if an AICD has discharged, this patient is a high-risk cardiac patient and should be treated as such with appropriate oxygenation and frequent reassessment. If the patient goes into cardiac arrest, CPR and an AED are indicated. AED pads should be placed so that they do not cover any implanted device. Although the patient may have received internal defibrillation from the patient's device, the presence of an ongoing cardiac arrest state means that more aggressive treatment is needed.

Wearable Defibrillators

An AICD is a permanently implanted device. Certain patients who are at risk for sudden death from cardiac dysrhythmias but who, for medical reasons, do not have an implanted AICD may be prescribed a ***wearable cardioverter defibrillator (WCD)***. The LifeVest®, manufactured by ZOLL, is the only commercially available WCD. Like an AICD, the device activates and delivers shocks when it senses a rapid life-threatening dysrhythmia. The device alerts a patient with audible, visible, and tactile alerts prior to delivering a treatment shock, and thus allows a conscious patient to delay the treatment by simultaneously pressing two response buttons (Figure 37-10). The LifeVest® will warn bystanders with both a siren alert and voice command instructing them not to interfere. CPR can be performed while the patient is wearing the LifeVest® WCD as long as it is not issuing a voice command that says otherwise. Follow your local protocols as to when to perform CPR and when to remove the LifeVest® and use your AED during a cardiac arrest. If removal of the LifeVest® is indicated, disconnect the battery pack first.

wearable cardioverter defibrillator (WCD) an external defibrillator worn by a patient to detect any rapid life-threatening dysrhythmia and deliver a shock to defibrillate the heart.

Ventricular Assist Devices

A ***ventricular assist device***, or *VAD*, is an implanted mechanical pump that takes over for the pumping action of one and sometimes two of the ventricles of the heart. These devices are typically used to support a patient who has severe heart failure and is awaiting heart transplant.

ventricular assist device a battery-powered mechanical pump implanted in the body to assist a failing ventricle in pumping blood.

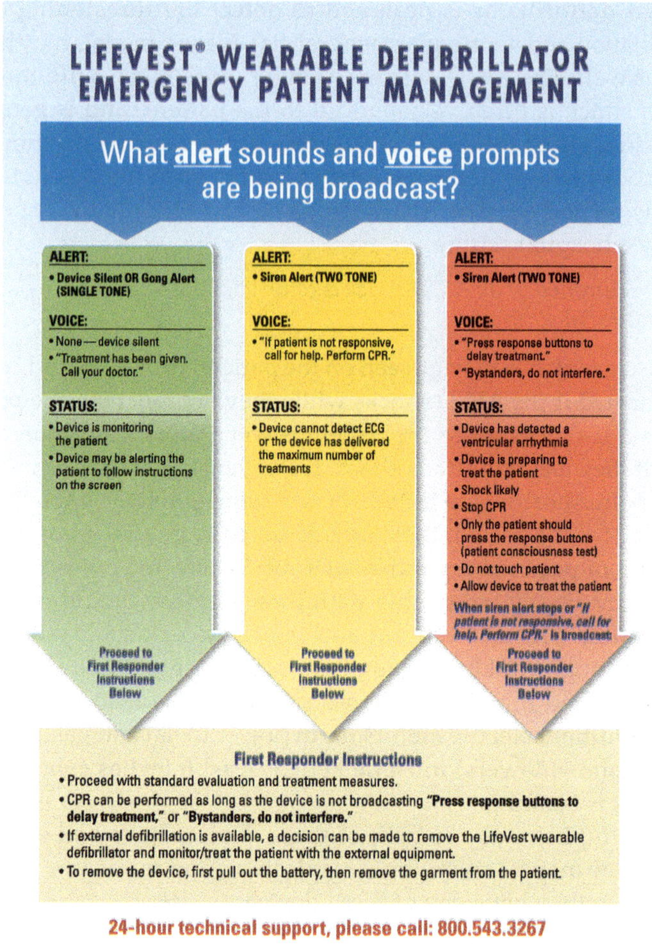

FIGURE 37-10 First responder information about LifeVest. *(Zoll LifeVest)*

The VAD moves blood from the ventricle through an inserted tube to a pump implanted in the abdomen, where the blood is pressurized and sent back to the circulatory system. A tube typically extends from the VAD through the abdominal wall to an external pump battery and control panel.

Problems that may be associated with VADs are infection, air leakage, and battery failure. All require rapid transport to a hospital.

EMT Assessment and Transport. The patient with a VAD will have an external battery pack that may be the size of a small backpack or briefcase (Figure 37-11). This should be carefully secured and prevented from tugging on the attached tubing. Failures of the battery system should first be addressed by attempting to plug the unit into an AC source in the home, inverter in an ambulance, or alternate battery pack. This will repower the system and allow functioning of the pump. If the pump itself fails, a hand or foot pump is sometimes included with the system as a backup. The pump must be squeezed for each beat of the heart. Heart transplant centers will generally provide training to local EMS personnel if someone in the community has a VAD. The training is specific to the model used by local patients.

VAD patients present unique assessment challenges, as the smooth motion of the mechanical pump does not always generate a pulse. Assessment of circulatory function generally starts by ensuring the pump is running. Typically, it creates a distinct sound as it pumps. Circulation is also judged by assessment of the patient. Mental status and skin color are reasonable indicators of how well the VAD is working. Failure of a VAD may result in cardiac arrest. If a device has truly failed, as indicated by lack of power or absence of the sound of the pump functioning, CPR may be indicated. It is generally preferable to first attempt to reengage the VAD by restoring power or by troubleshooting following manufacturer's recommendations, but if that fails, you should begin chest compressions. Follow local protocol.

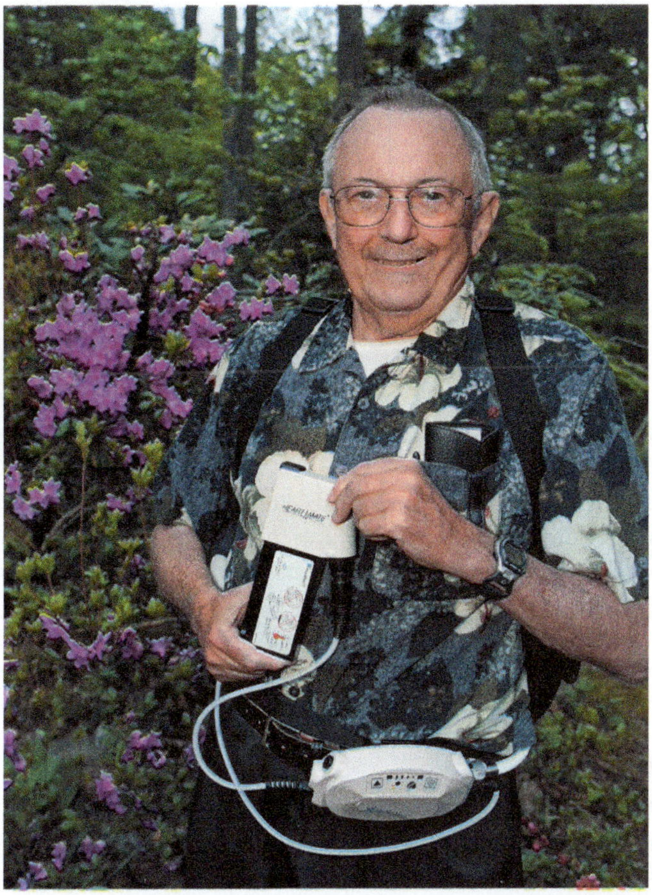

FIGURE 37-11 This patient holds one of the two batteries that powers his implanted left ventricular assist device (LVAD). The LVAD's controller is attached to his belt. *(George Widman/AP Images)*

Gastrourinary Devices

Feeding Tubes

A ***feeding tube*** is used in patients who are unable to feed themselves or can't swallow. It may be used short-term (during recovery from surgery) or long-term (for chronic conditions). A feeding tube is most commonly seen in one of two forms: a nasogastric tube or a gastric tube.

feeding tube
a tube used to provide delivery of nutrients to the stomach. A nasogastric feeding tube is inserted through the nose and into the stomach; a gastric feeding tube is surgically implanted through the abdominal wall and into the stomach.

A *nasogastric tube (NG-tube)* is a long tube inserted through the nose into the stomach that can be used to deliver nutrients. In addition, the device can be used in emergency departments and by some ALS providers to suction out the stomach's contents—for example, in the case of certain overdoses, or to introduce medications. The NG-tube is generally taped to the patient's nose or cheek to prevent the tube from dislodging. A *gastrostomy tube (G-tube)* is a feeding tube surgically implanted through the abdominal wall and into the stomach (Figure 37-12). It is used to provide longer-term nutrient delivery than would be provided by an NG-tube. The G-tube is held in place by a balloon inside the stomach. It can also be used by hospital personnel to drain stomach contents. Some feeding tubes are placed through the abdominal wall, directly into the small intestine. For example, a jejunostomy tube (*J-tube*) is placed into the jejunum section of the small intestine.

Common problems with both NG-tubes and G-tubes include dislodgement, infection at the site of insertion, and clogging that prevents nutrients from being provided to the patient. All of these conditions warrant transport and evaluation in a hospital setting.

EMT Assessment and Transport. Ensure that the feeding tube is secured with tape to the patient's body before transport. If protocols allow and nutrients are being administered during transport, keep the nutrient source higher than the level of the NG-tube or G-tube and hang it like an IV bag. Although the tube is not pressurized when nutrients are not being administered, the protective end cap should be placed on the tube to prevent leakage. If a tube has been dislodged, do not attempt to replace it. In certain circumstances,

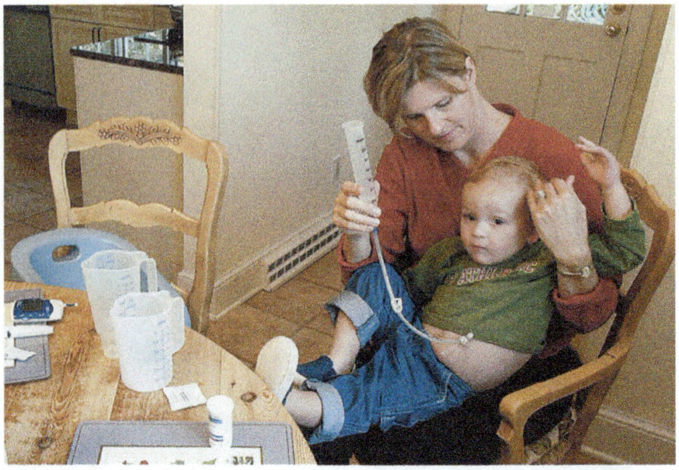

FIGURE 37-12 In her home kitchen, this mother is administering a liquid cornstarch solution to her child through an implanted gastric feeding tube. The child has a rare disease that requires him to ingest cornstarch every four hours to avoid seizures and hospitalization. *(David T. Foster III/The Charlotte Observer/AP Images)*

the family may have attempted or may be able to replace the tube themselves. However, if this is not possible, simply cover the opening in the abdomen with an occlusive dressing and transport. If the patient has recently completed the administration of nutrients, it may be recommended that the patient remain in a seated position, or at least in a position of no less than 30-degree recline, for 30–60 minutes following the feeding session. Life-threatening priorities may make this impossible, but this positional requirement should be accommodated when appropriate.

Urinary Catheters

urinary catheter
a tube inserted into the bladder through the urethra to drain urine from the bladder.

A ***urinary catheter*** is used for patients who have lost the ability to urinate or the ability to control when they urinate. Most commonly seen are indwelling Foley catheters; other types include the externally applied condom catheter. Most catheters are inserted into the bladder through the urethra and use a balloon to hold the tubing in place. The external tubing is connected to a collection bag (Figure 37-13), which may be a bag strapped to a leg or a larger drainage bag, called a down drain, that may hang on the side of a patient's bed. Patients with leg bags are generally those who are more active than patients with down drains, as the leg bag may be hidden under clothing when the patient is in public.

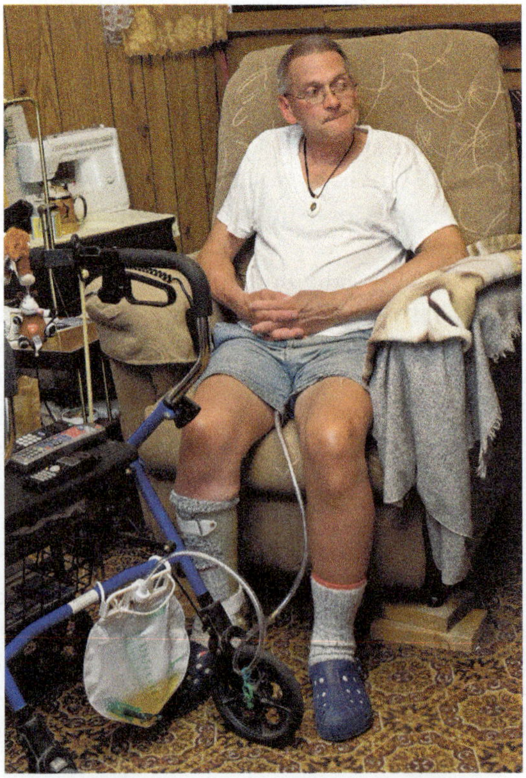

FIGURE 37-13 This patient has a urinary catheter that is connected to a collection bag.

Common problems EMTs see with urinary catheters include infection, blockages causing lack of urinary output, discoloration of urine, and dislodgement of the catheter.

EMT Assessment and Transport. During transport, keep the catheter bag lower than the level of the patient (but not on a floor), and use care not to damage the bag with a stretcher or lifting device. Document and report any discoloration of the urine or any odors from the urine itself. Drainage bags should be emptied when they are one-third to one-half full. EMTs may want caregivers to empty the bag before transport to prevent overfilling, which will cause backflow into the bladder. Some patients are required to keep track of their total urine output every day, so document the amount emptied.

Ostomy Bags

As an EMT, you may also encounter a patient who has an ***ostomy bag***, also called an *ostomy pouch*. An ostomy bag is connected to the site of a colostomy or an ileostomy. A colostomy or ileostomy is the result of a surgery that brings a section of the intestine through the abdominal wall to divert the flow of stool away from the normal path to the rectum. An ostomy may be necessary because of a medical condition such as Crohn's disease or ulcerative colitis, or because a patient has cancer, especially colon cancer. An ostomy bag is usually attached to the patient's leg, and often will not be visible under clothing. Common problems include infection at the stoma site; blockage; and, in some cases, dislodgement.

ostomy bag
an external pouch that collects fecal matter diverted from the colon or ileum through a surgical opening (colostomy or ileostomy) in the abdominal wall.

EMT Assessment and Transport. Use care to prevent breakage or dislodgement as a result of rough handling when moving a patient with an ostomy bag.

Dialysis

A patient who requires ***dialysis*** has renal failure. In this disorder, the kidneys are unable to remove the buildup of toxins that occurs with the metabolism of daily life. Patients with renal failure also have difficulty maintaining fluid balance and can be challenged with low- or high-volume states. Dialysis takes over some of the functions the kidneys typically perform. It removes toxins, filters the blood, and helps regulate fluid levels in the body. There are two forms of dialysis: hemodialysis and peritoneal dialysis.

dialysis
the process of filtering the blood to remove toxic or unwanted wastes and fluids.

Hemodialysis is performed by attaching the patient to an external machine called a *dialyzer*. The procedure is usually performed at a dialysis center, although home units do exist. Hemodialysis requires the use of large needles and tubing to remove and return the blood. The needles are inserted into a site where an artery has been surgically connected to a vein: an arteriovenous (A-V) fistula. These fistulas are most commonly found on the forearm of the patient but can sometimes be found in the lower leg. Because fistulas essentially create a large blood vessel, they are vulnerable to external trauma. Bleeding from a fistula site can be massive and difficult to control. Other complications encountered with patients on hemodialysis include infection at the site of external dialysis catheters. Hemodialysis patients are also prone to hypovolemia, particularly in the period immediately following dialysis. Syncope and episodes of low blood pressure are common.

Peritoneal dialysis requires a permanent catheter that is implanted through the patient's abdominal wall and into the peritoneal cavity. Several liters of a specially formulated dialysis solution are run into the abdominal cavity, where they will remain for roughly two hours to absorb the waste products from the body (via the peritoneal lining), and ultimately are drained back into the dialysis bag to be discarded. Peritoneal dialysis can be performed at home. Common complications encountered with patients on peritoneal dialysis include dislodging of the catheter and infection in the peritoneal cavity (peritonitis), which results in the normally clear dialysis fluid turning cloudy. If you encounter patients on peritoneal dialysis who believe that they have a peritoneal infection based on a color change in their drained fluid, bring the suspicious bag of fluid with these patients to the hospital to allow testing of the fluid.

Review the chapter *Hematologic and Renal Emergencies* for a more complete discussion of dialysis.

EMT Assessment and Transport. Do not take a blood pressure on any arm with an A-V shunt, fistula, or graft, as this can cause damage that requires surgical repair.

If a shunt, graft, or fistula ruptures, significant blood loss (500 mL or more per minute) will occur very quickly. In the case of a bleeding shunt, stop the bleeding by direct pressure. In the case of a fistula or graft bleed, which may be indicated by significant swelling under the skin at the site, apply direct pressure. *Do not* release the pressure until advised by a physician to do so because there is a high likelihood of the high pressure bleeding dislodging clots that are forming. In all cases of bleeding from a shunt, fistula, or graft, the patient should be treated for shock, transported, and carefully monitored.

Central IV Catheters

central IV catheter a catheter surgically inserted for long-term delivery of medications or fluids into the central circulation.

Sometimes a patient you encounter will have a ***central IV catheter***. A patient who receives frequent IV therapy, such as with chemotherapy, antibiotics, or total parenteral nutrition, may have one of a variety of such catheters. Inserted in a hospital through surgery or under radiography, central IV catheters prevent patients from having to endure multiple needlesticks in their arms. Central IV catheters are usually inserted via a surgical venous puncture to introduce medications or fluids into the central circulation. A common problem with central IV catheters is infection.

One form of central IV catheter is the *peripherally inserted central catheter (PICC) line*, which has an external tube slightly larger than IV tubing. The catheter is inserted into a peripheral vein, then threaded into the central circulation. A PICC line is often found inserted into the patient's arm.

Another form of central IV catheter is a *central venous line*, which may be inserted through a subclavian, jugular, or femoral vein. Central venous lines carry a variety of brand names, such as a Groshong®, a Hickman®, or a Broviac® catheter. These catheters may have one, two, or three external IV tubes that are attached to the patient's chest.

Finally, a central IV catheter may be in the form of an *implanted port* that can be felt under the skin. This port has no external tubing, and a special needle called a Huber is required to access this port (Figure 37-14). Brand names for these catheters include Port-a-Cath® and Mediport®.

FIGURE 37-14 Central IV catheters. *(Photos: Vadym Zaitsev/Shutterstock)*

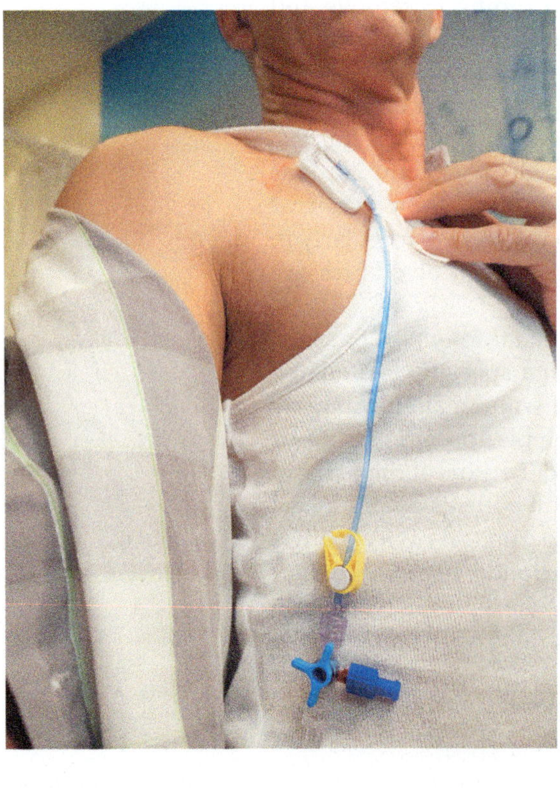

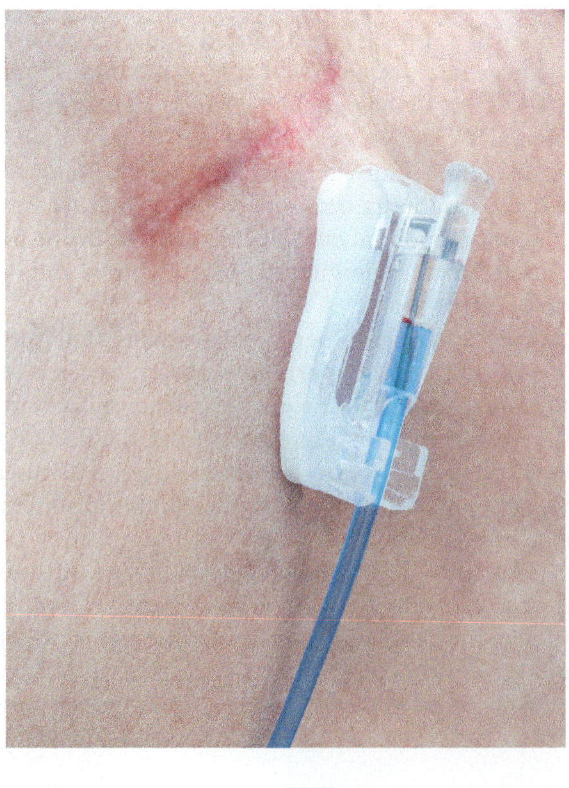

EMT Assessment and Transport. In most cases, neither the EMT nor a family caregiver will use a central IV catheter to administer medications to the patient or for any other purpose. Use of a central IV catheter is usually restricted to hospital personnel. However, awareness of the presence of a central IV device is important for the EMT, who must exercise caution to avoid any tugging or contamination of the catheter site.

You should not place an AED pad over a central line catheter (whether external or implanted), as the catheter will reduce conduction during defibrillation. Simply offset the pad to one side, above, or below the catheter.

You should also have a high index of suspicion for sepsis and septic shock in patients with indwelling catheters. Central lines are a direct route for microbes to enter the body and account for a large portion of the infections that lead to septic shock. For more information on sepsis, review the chapter *Infectious Diseases and Sepsis.*

Ventriculoperitoneal (VP) Shunts

A ventriculoperitoneal shunt is a drainage device that runs from the brain to the abdomen or to the atrium of the heart to relieve excess cerebrospinal fluid. These devices are common in children with special health care needs. There may be a palpable reservoir on the side of the skull. If the shunt malfunctions, pressure inside the skull will rise, causing an altered mental status. An altered mental status may also be caused by an infection. These patients can be prone to seizures and respiratory compromise.

EMT Assessment and Transport. Emergencies in shunt patients can arise from either the shunt or routine conditions not associated with the shunt. Manage medical problems as you would in any other patient. Manage airways and prevent hypoxia. Transport the patient to an appropriate facility and consult medical control for specific instructions.

Physical Impairments

Patients who call EMS may have a variety of impairments that affect their hearing, sight, or speech. When one of these senses has been adversely affected or removed, you should take extra care and time to help the patient adjust. It is important to remember, however, that these impairments do *not* necessarily affect the patient's ability to think. Each limitation requires different approaches and considerations when you are assessing and treating the patient.

Although hearing loss is more common in the elderly than in younger persons, it is not restricted to the older patient. Approach each patient individually, and ascertain the patient's abilities. Not all patients with hearing loss can read lips, and in most cases, yelling or slowing down your speech will only make matters worse. One of the easiest ways to communicate with a patient with hearing loss is to write your questions and explain your actions on a piece of paper. Many dispatch centers and communities also have TDD/TTY phones and may be able to relay information through these devices.

NOTE: *TDD/TTY stands for* telecommunication device for the deaf/teletypewriter. *The system consists of a keyboard, display screen, and modem connected to an analog telephone line. The user can type in a message and receive a response that is displayed on the screen.*

Impairments to sight can be partial or complete. Determine if the patient has poor vision or no vision. Blind patients might not use lights in their home or might not notice lights that have burned out. It is good practice for the EMT to always carry a small flashlight, even during the day. Patients may know the layout of their home very well, and rely on the layout's being consistent, so if anything is moved for transport of the patient, be sure to return it to its original position. If the patient has a guide dog, federal law allows for the patient to bring the dog along in an ambulance, unless the dog is a direct threat to others (for example, if it is barking or growling).

A patient who is unable to speak (i.e., aphasic) may need to write answers to your questions, use a TDD/TTY phone, or have a computer that speaks the words he types.

Many elderly persons contend with difficulty walking or standing, but problems with gait and balance can occur at any age. Carefully assist people who have such disabilities, and make sure to bring along any helping devices they want to have with them, such as

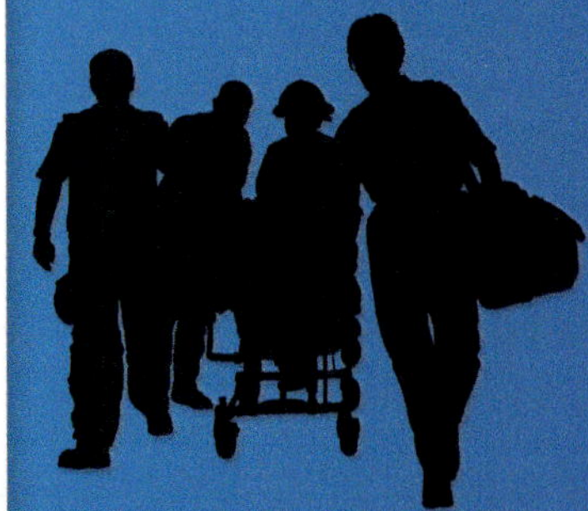

Think Like an EMT

EMTs Need to Know

Patients with special needs pose challenges for EMTs at all levels. For each of the following situations, explain how you would handle it and where you might turn for help or advice.

1. You are treating an unresponsive diabetic patient when you notice he has an insulin pump. You believe you should turn it off but are not sure how.
2. You are treating a patient who has just performed peritoneal dialysis at home. She complains of excruciating pain with even the least movement.
3. You are called for a possible respiratory infection in a child. You arrive to find that the patient has a trach and a ventilator. You are not sure how to transport the ventilator.

a cane, a walker, or braces. Patients in wheelchairs may be difficult to assess completely, as they may be unable to stand or turn for complete physical assessment. If a patient in a wheelchair is moved to a stretcher, ensure that the wheelchair either safely accompanies the patient or is secured from theft or loss.

EMT Assessment and Transport. Approach and treat each patient with one or more physical impairments by providing whatever extra assistance is required. Carefully assess to determine if an impairment is the patient's baseline or if it is a new problem (for example, a person suffering a stroke who has lost the ability to speak). Determine patients' comfort levels and any abilities or tools they use to compensate. During care, carefully explain all of your actions and treatments. Bring any devices the patient uses, such as a walker, a hearing aid, glasses, speech computer, or other items to help communicate with hospital staff, and make the environment more comfortable. If the patient has a wheelchair, consider the use of a wheelchair van if one is available.

CORE CONCEPT
How to recognize and deal with cases of abuse and neglect

Abuse and Neglect

Keep in mind that patients with special challenges can be more vulnerable to physical or sexual abuse, exploitation, and neglect because of their dependence on others. This vulnerable population can include children and adults, especially the elderly. Be alert to this possibility during your scene size-up, history taking, and assessment. Stories that are inconsistent with injuries, multiple injuries in various stages of healing, repeated injuries, and caregivers' indifference to the patient should bring to mind the possibility of abuse or neglect. As with any suspected case of abuse or neglect, do not make accusations. Do your best to get the patient out of the environment, and report your suspicions according to the requirements of your jurisdiction (see the chapter *Medical, Legal, and Ethical Issues*)—at a minimum to the receiving physician.

CORE CONCEPT
How to deal with issues of child abuse and neglect, and with children with special needs

Child Abuse and Neglect

Although the number of known child abuse cases is large, the real number is even larger than the statistics indicate. Experts believe that for every abused child seen by the emergency department or family physician, there are many more unreported cases who never receive care.

Child abusers are mothers, fathers, sisters, brothers, grandparents, stepparents, babysitters, and other caregivers. They are white-collar workers, blue-collar workers, the rich, and the poor. There is no distinction as to race, creed, ethnicity, or economic background.

Child abuse can take several different forms, often occurring in combination:

- Psychological (emotional) abuse
- Neglect
- Physical abuse
- Sexual abuse

What constitutes neglect is a serious legal question. If a child goes without proper food, shelter, clothing, supervision, treatment of injuries and illnesses, a safe environment, or love, the effects surely will be seen but will seldom directly trigger an emergency call. Physical and sexual abuse are the problems likely to be seen by EMTs. If signs of neglect are observed in the course of a call, they should also be reported to the receiving physician and proper authorities in the event that the child is not transported.

Physical and Sexual Abuse

Abusers inflict almost every imaginable kind of injury and maltreatment. Physically abused children—often called "battered" children—are beaten with fists, hairbrushes, electric cords, pool cues, pots and pans, and almost any other object that can be used as a weapon. They are intentionally burned with hot water, steam, open flames, cigarettes, and other thermal sources. Battered children might be severely shaken, thrown into their cribs or down steps, pushed out of windows and over railings, and even pushed from moving cars.

Sexual abuse ranges from adults exposing themselves to children to sexual intercourse or sexual torture. Often, cases in which sexual abuse results in serious physical injury are reported to the authorities. However, some cases—especially those in which only emotional injury or minor physical injury was done—are not reported, and therefore they are difficult to estimate.

Patient Assessment

Physical Abuse

In cases of physical abuse of children, you might find (Figure 37-15):

- Slap marks, bruises, abrasions, lacerations, and incisions of all sizes and with shapes matching the item used. You may see wide welts from belts, a looped shape from cords, or the shape of a hand from slapping. You may find swollen limbs, split lips, black eyes, and loose or broken teeth. Often the injuries are to the back, legs, and arms.
- Broken bones are common, and all types of fractures are possible. Many battered children have multiple fractures, often in various stages of healing, or have fracture-associated complications.
- Head injuries are common, with concussions and skull fractures being reported. Closed head injuries occur to many infants and small children who have been severely shaken.
- Abdominal injuries include ruptured spleens, livers and lungs lacerated by broken ribs, internal bleeding from blunt trauma and punching, and lacerated and avulsed genitalia.
- Bite marks showing the teeth size and pattern of the abuser's mouth may be present.
- Burn marks that are small and round from cigarettes; "glove" or "stocking" burn marks from dipping in hot water; burns on buttocks and legs (the creases behind the knees and at the thighs are protected when flexed and may be spared burns during forced lower extremity immersion; and demarcation burns in the shape of an iron, stove burner, or other hot utensil are frequently found.
- Indications of shaking an infant include a bulging fontanelle due to increased intracranial pressure from the bleeding of torn blood vessels in the brain, unconsciousness, and typical signs and symptoms of head and brain injuries. Injuries to the central nervous system from shaken baby syndrome are among the most lethal child abuse injuries.

FIGURE 37-15 Child abuse injuries: (A) Bruised buttocks on a child. (B) Cord-whip injury on a teenager. *(Photo A: © Janet M. Gorsuch, RN, MS, CRNP. Photo B: Courtesy of Akron Children's Hospital)*

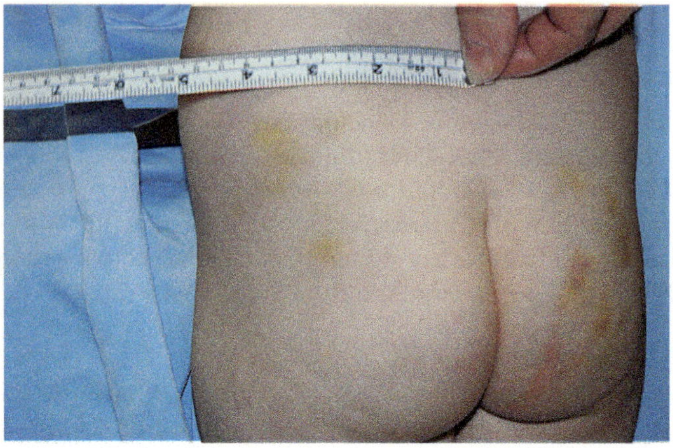

A

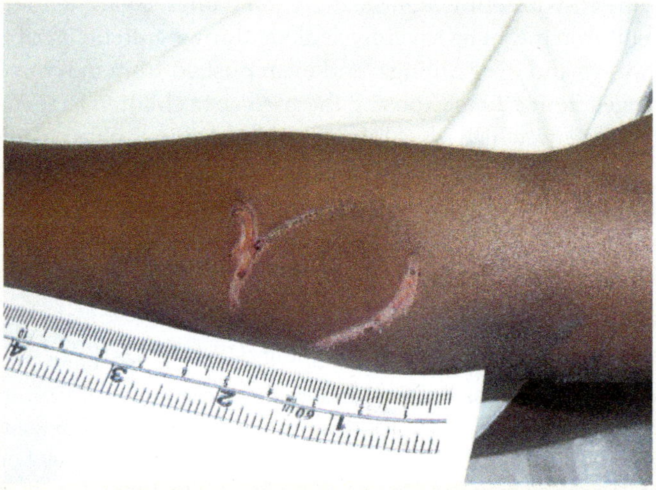

B

Sometimes you will treat an injured child and never consider abuse, especially if the child relates well with the parents and there appears to be a strong bond between them. In other cases, there can be certain indications that abuse may be occurring in or outside the home, with the family feeling they must not admit to the problem. Be on the alert for:

- Repeated responses to provide care for the same child or children in a family. Remember that in areas with many hospitals, you may see the child more frequently than any one hospital.
- Indications of past injuries. This is one reason you must do a physical examination and remove articles of clothing. Pay special attention to the child's back and buttocks.
- Poorly healing wounds or improperly healed fractures. It is extremely rare for a child who has had a fracture and who has been given proper orthopedic care to show angulations and large "bumps" and "knots" of bone at the "healed" injury site.
- Indications of past burns or fresh bilateral burns. Children seldom put both hands on a hot object or touch the same hot object again. (True, some do—this sign is only an indication, not proof.) Some types of burns are almost always linked to

child abuse, such as cigarette burns to the body and burns to the buttocks and lower extremities that result from the child being dipped in hot water.

- Many different types of injuries to both sides, or to the front and back, of the body. This gains even more importance if the adults on the scene keep insisting that the child "falls a lot."
- Unusual behavior from the child. The child may seem afraid to tell you how the injury occurred. The child may seem to expect no comfort from the parents, or may have little or no apparent reaction to pain.
- The parent or caregiver at the scene who does not wish to leave you alone with the child, tells conflicting or changing stories, overwhelms you with explanations of the cause of the injury, or faults the child. These should arouse your suspicions and cause you to more carefully assess the situation.

Pay attention to the adults as you treat the child:

- Do they seem inappropriately unconcerned about the child?
- Do they have trouble controlling their anger?
- Do you feel that at any moment there may be an emotional explosion?
- Do any of the adults appear to be in a deep state of depression?
- Are there indications of alcohol or drug abuse?
- Do any of the adults speak of suicide or seeking mercy for their unhappy children?

Although parents or caregivers might have called for help for the child, they may be reluctant to provide a history of the injury and might refuse transport. Take note of any parents who refuse to have their child sent to the nearest hospital or to a hospital where the child has been seen before. This may indicate fear of the staff's remembering, or seeing a record of, past injuries. (You cannot transport without parental consent; however, you may be able to convince the parents the child needs to be seen by a doctor because of certain signs and symptoms that are "difficult to determine" in the field.) Be the child's advocate, but do not accuse the parent.

Patient Assessment

Sexual Abuse

Rearrange or remove clothing only as necessary to determine and treat injuries. This will help preserve evidence where possible. Examine the genitalia only if there is obvious injury, or the child tells you of a recent injury. The child may be hysterical, frightened, or withdrawn and unable to give you a history of the incident. Be calm and as reassuring as possible. The following are common signs of sexual abuse:

- Obvious signs of sexual assault, including burns or wounds to the genitalia
- Any unexplained genital injury, such as bruising, lacerations, or bloody discharge from genital orifices (openings)
- Seminal fluid on the body or clothes, or other discharges associated with sexually transmitted diseases
- In rare cases, children may tell you they were sexually assaulted.

Remain professional and control your emotions. Protect the child from embarrassment. Say nothing that may make children feel they are to blame for the sexual assault. (Many believe that they are.) It is also important that you remain calm and composed to ensure that you do not tip off the potential abuser to your suspicions because the potential abuser may refuse to allow you to continue to care for the child, thus creating a situation that may further endanger the child.

Patient Care

Patient with Physical or Sexual Abuse

Fundamental Principles of Care

There are few moments where the specific nature of your dispatch will indicate physical and sexual abuse. More often, these signs and symptoms are identified through the routine interaction and general assessment of the patient. That means all EMTs must be constantly vigilant to find any indication of abuse. We have the unique opportunity and the solemn responsibility of going into places and interacting with people that other branches of the health care system will never have. In many cases, EMS represents the only entry point into the social service system. Although medical interventions will always take priority, we should never forget to constantly look after those who need our help the most.

Emergency care for physical or sexual abuse includes the following steps:

- Dress and provide other appropriate care for injuries as necessary.
- Preserve evidence of sexual abuse if it is suspected.
- Discourage the child from going to the bathroom (for both defecation and urination).
- Give nothing to the patient by mouth.
- Do not have the child wash or change clothes.
- Transport the child.

NOTE: *By law, you must plainly and clearly report to the medical staff any finding or suspicion regarding possible physical or sexual abuse.*

It may be difficult, but remember that the parent or caregiver needs help as well. Your actions, response, and concern directed toward suspected abusers can help them recognize their problem and may encourage them to seek therapy and rehabilitation. Also bear in mind that your suspicions may be unfounded. Not every injury to a patient is the result of abuse (Figure 37-16). Suspicions should be aroused not by individual injuries but by patterns of injuries and behavior.

FIGURE 37-16 Skin findings that mimic abuse. (A) Child with lesions of impetigo infection. (B) Child with rash from *Candida* infection ("diaper rash"). *(Photos A and B: © David Effron, MD)*

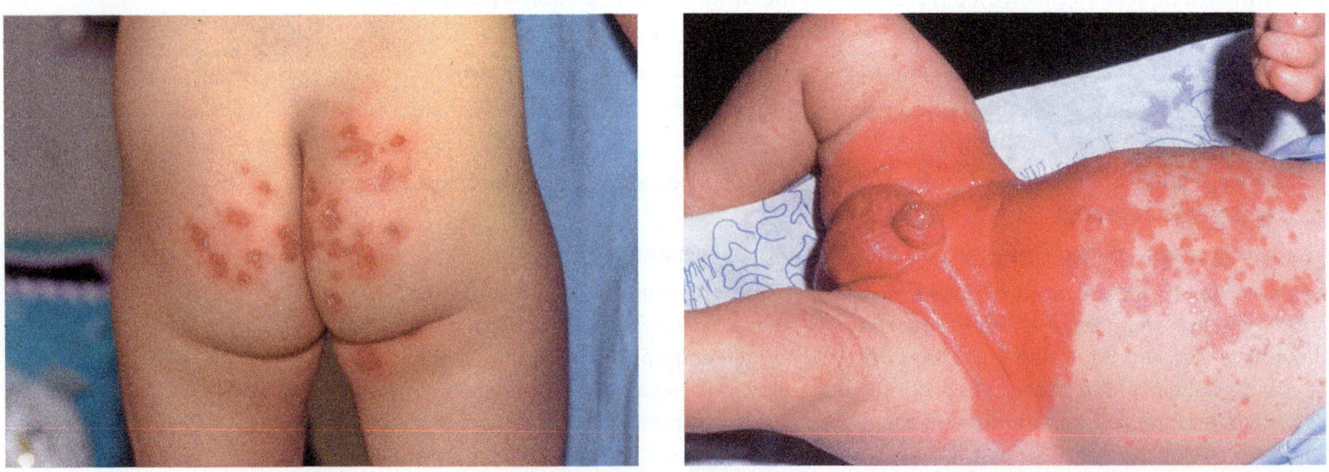

A B

Elder Abuse and Neglect

Elder abuse and neglect have occurred for many years but have only recently received the attention they deserve. There are essentially three ways in which elders can be abused or neglected: physically, psychologically, and financially. Physical abuse includes pushing, shoving, hitting, or shaking of an older person. It occasionally includes sexual abuse. Physical neglect includes improper feeding, inadequate support resulting in poor hygiene, or inadequate medical care. Psychological abuse and neglect include threats, insults, or ignoring an older person ("the silent treatment"). Financial abuse and neglect include exploitation or misuse of an older person's belongings or money.

Detecting elder abuse and neglect can be difficult. Don't automatically assume that an injury is the result of a simple fall, even though falls are common among the frail elderly. Evaluate any injury in this age group with an eye toward recognizing signs of abuse or neglect. Many states have laws that require the reporting of such suspicions. Be aware of the laws in your state and of local protocols and take whatever actions you are permitted to take to help the victim of abuse.

Adult Abuse

So far we have discussed very specific populations in the context of abuse and neglect. In many cases, pediatrics and geriatrics are specific, legally defined protected groups. However, many other types of patients can suffer abuse and neglect. Just as in child abuse situations, dependent adults frequently fall victim to the harm and neglect of caregivers. Dependent adults include patients with developmental disabilities, physical challenges, or other situations that require them to depend on others for day-to-day care. Because of their vulnerable state, it is not uncommon for them to suffer from physical and emotional abuse or neglect, and also from abandonment and even financial or material exploitation. The approach to recognizing abuse in these patients is much like that for recognizing child or elder abuse. Do not make assumptions, but be ever vigilant to identify potentially harmful actions and situations. Important clues will come not only from physical signs of harm or neglect, but also by examining scene clues (cleanliness, the presence of food, etc.) and caregiver interaction.

Specific warning signs include:

- Unexplained absence of caregivers or potentially harmful periods of abandonment
- Signs of hunger, malnourishment, or improper toilet routine, or other signs of neglect
- Improper or unusual interactions with caregivers
- Caregiver interference with assessment, treatment, or transport.

Adult-abuse situations can be challenging, as specific laws and reporting mandates differ from state to state. It will be important for you to review local social service resources and, when in doubt, to involve law enforcement.

Role of the EMT in Cases of Suspected Abuse or Neglect

Remember that you are charged with providing emergency care for any injured patient. You are not a police officer, court investigator, social worker, or judge. Gather information from the caregiver away from the patient, without expression of disbelief or judgment. Talk with the patient separately about how an injury occurred. As you assess the patient and provide appropriate care, control your emotions and hold back accusations. Do not indicate to the caregivers or others at the scene that you suspect abuse or neglect. Do not ask the patient if there has been abuse. Doing so when others are around could produce stress too great for the patient to handle.

If you are suspicious about the MOI, transport the patient even though the severity of injury may not warrant such action.

In some states, EMTs are mandated reporters; they are required by law to report suspicions of child, elder, and in some cases adult abuse or neglect. Most often, reporting means contacting your state's social service reporting hotline. Often, just notifying hospital personnel or law enforcement about your suspicions is not enough. Be familiar with your state laws. Even if reporting possible abuse or neglect is not a legal requirement in your state, it is a professional obligation. As an EMT, you may be the only advocate an abused patient has. Be conscientious.

Past responses can be checked and future responses noted in case a pattern develops to indicate possible abuse. However, even when talking to your partner, the hospital staff, the police, and your superiors, use the terms *suspected* and *possible*. Always be objective and report only the facts. Avoid generalizations and assumptions. Do not call someone an abuser. Keep in mind that the courts can deal harshly with those who provide patient care and then violate the confidentiality of the patient, the family, and the home. Rumors about abuse may, in the long run, cause mental or physical harm to your patient.

Always remember that your suspicions might not be correct. Even when you see something that concerns you, stay open to the possibility that what you suspect might not be what has happened.

Intimate Partner Violence

Intimate partner violence, also known as domestic violence or abuse, is a pattern of violent or coercive behavior that one uses to gain and maintain power and control over an intimate partner. Domestic violence is never an isolated incident. Abusers use a series of tactics to hold power and control over their victims. These tactics can be physical, emotional, economic, or sexual. Intimate partner violence can affect people regardless of race, age, gender, income, educational status, sexual orientation, or gender identity.

As an EMT, it is not uncommon to see the same patient for abuse-related issues multiple times, and it may be frustrating to see a victim be abused and return to the abuser. However, people stay in abusive relationships for a multitude of reasons. Sometimes it is financial. Some victims simply do not have the means to leave. Sometimes it is emotional. Some victims fear being stigmatized as a victim. But too often, it is simply about safety, as the highest risk to a victim is at the time of leaving. In other words, victims may be staying simply because they know their lives will be at risk if they leave. It is important to know that most people eventually do leave, and your interaction can be an important means to offering that victim help. Remember that isolation is an important tactic of abusers. As a result, EMS may be the most sophisticated form of medical care the patient has access to and perhaps the only outlet to social service referral. Your ability to point the victim to intimate partner violence advocacy groups may be essential to ending the cycle of violence.

Recognizing intimate partner violence is not simple. Occasionally, the situation will be clear; the victim may report it, or law enforcement may request EMS after discovering injuries. More often, intimate partner violence is less overt. Remember that this form of abuse is about power and control and that isolation and secrecy are common tactics. Physical injuries can be obvious, but often only occur after other subtle tactics of control fail. Assessment of the patient who has experienced intimate partner violence should ideally be done away from the partner and/or any children. Patients who have experienced intimate partner violence are more likely to be truthful with you if they feel safe. Your assessment should look for injuries but remember there are many other signs of intimate partner violence. Other signs include:

- Fear by the victim of talking to EMS or law enforcement
- Reluctance to accept treatment or transport
- Obvious isolation of the victim (inability or difficulty contacting EMS, friends, or other family)
- Delays in seeking treatment
- History that does not match injuries or injury patterns

- Unusual interaction with the victim's partner or family, including the suspected perpetrator's attempts to interfere with assessment or treatment, attempts to deny access to the victim, conflicting history, or unusual attention (overwatching) of your interaction with the victim

If faced with suspected intimate partner violence, take care of medical issues first. Remember that you may be the only medical care this victim will ever have access to. Although transport may be warranted, it is not uncommon for victims to refuse. Be aware that the refusal may represent important safety planning by the victim. Take care not to be judgmental or accusatory in your interactions.

Familiarize yourself with your local intimate partner violence advocacy organization and be ready to make a referral, even if it's the tenth time you've responded to this address. This advocacy can represent a vitally important connection to the outside world and can be an important means to ending the violence. You should be sincere in your interactions. Some helpful points to make to victims include:

- Letting victims know that there are organizations in their community that can help. It is best to have the contact numbers ready.
- Noting that services are free and confidential
- Stating that local intimate partner violence projects have 24-hour toll-free hotlines staffed by people who care.

Although these points may seem obvious to you, batterers frequently use lies and deception to further isolate their victims.

As with any form of abuse, it is important to leave the investigation to law enforcement. You can be vital, however, in documenting statements the patient makes to you on scene. Document objectively and state facts, not opinions. This documentation can be as important to the potential investigation as it is to your medical care of the patient.

Human Trafficking

Human trafficking is the exploitation of a person for the purpose of compelled labor or a commercial sex act through the use of force, fraud, or coercion. It is modern-day slavery, occurring in every state in the United States, and is a crime under U.S. federal law. The two primary forms are sex trafficking and labor trafficking. Trafficking victims are of every gender, age, ethnicity, socioeconomic background, and nationality. Human trafficking is the fastest-growing criminal industry worldwide. In the United States, reports of human trafficking rose 35.7 percent in 2016 compared with the previous year. It is a crime of low risk and high profits fueled by the demand for cheap goods and commercial sex. Aside from being one of the greatest social injustices of our time, human trafficking is a public health issue, and exposes victims to serious health risks such as physical abuse, malnutrition, untreated injuries, sexually transmitted infections, unsafe abortions, substance addiction, and mental health issues. One way that traffickers maintain control over their victims is through isolation. However, 88 percent of trafficking victims will have contact with a health care provider while being trafficked, with as many as 68 percent of these encounters occurring in the emergency department. EMTs can be a powerful force in the fight against human trafficking. As first responders, EMTs can directly observe environmental situations and interactions that other health care providers do not have access to. The EMT first must understand that human trafficking exists, and what it is. EMTs should know the common indications of human trafficking and the appropriate questions to ask in order to obtain more information. In doing so, EMTs can use their unique position to recognize possible instances of human trafficking. If trafficking is suspected, law enforcement should be immediately and discreetly notified.

The following are some classic clinical presentations found in trafficking victims, as published by the U.S. Department of Homeland Security as part of the Blue Campaign:

- Bruises in various stages of healing caused by physical abuse
- Scars, mutilations, or infections due to improper medical care
- Urinary difficulties, pelvic pain, pregnancy, or rectal trauma caused from working in the sex industry

- Chronic back, hearing, cardiovascular, or respiratory problems as a result of forced manual labor in unsafe conditions
- Poor eyesight and/or eye problems due to dimly lit work sites
- Malnourishment and/or serious dental problems
- Disorientation, confusion, phobias, or panic attacks caused by daily mental abuse, torture, and culture shock

While physical findings may indicate a human trafficking situation, important clues may also be found in the scene survey and in the social interactions of those on the scene. Consider the following red flags for potential human trafficking situations:

- Is the patient accompanied by another person who seems controlling?
- Does person accompanying the patient insist on giving information/talking?
- Does the patient have trouble communicating due to a language/cultural barrier?
- Are the patient's identification documents (e.g., passport, driver's license) being held or controlled by someone else?
- Does the patient appear submissive or fearful?
- Is the patient inadequately dressed for the situation/work the patient does?
- Are there security measures designed to keep the patient on the premises?
- Does the patient live in a degraded, unsuitable place or share sleeping quarters?
- Is the patient suffering from classical presentations found in trafficking victims?

Treat medical issues first. Like other victims of abuse, human trafficking victims may have limited access to medical care, and your interventions may be the only level of the health care system they are exposed to.

Remember that human trafficking is a criminal act perpetrated by sophisticated and often dangerous criminals. Always consider scene safety. You should not disclose your suspicions of human trafficking to the victim or to anyone on scene. Doing so can not only escalate the danger on a scene, but it can also significantly impair the ability of law enforcement to investigate and prosecute the human traffickers. It is not your responsibility to investigate or interrogate anyone regarding human trafficking. Report your suspicions immediately to law enforcement and consider utilizing local or national human trafficking–reporting resources. The National Human Trafficking Hotline phone number is 1 (888) 373-7888. Always follow local protocol regarding reporting steps. As in intimate partner violence, complete your run documentation with objectivity and remember the importance of any patient statements or scene clues. Your information may be a vital component of an ongoing investigation.

Chapter Review

Key Facts and Concepts

- Patients with special challenges include those who are homeless or living in poverty, are very obese, have sensory impairments, are terminally ill, have developmental disorders, and/or are technology-dependent.
- A disability is a condition that interferes with a person's ability to engage in everyday activities, such as working or caring for oneself.

- Although patients with special challenges may require EMS for problems related to their disabilities or chronic conditions, do not assume that this is the only reason you were called for a particular patient. These patients may have the same medical emergencies (an anaphylactic reaction to a new medication, for example) as more routine patients.
- It is critical for EMTs to treat patients who have special challenges with empathy and respect.
- The homeless, poor, and very obese are at increased risk of health problems.
- When dealing with a patient who has autism, use the ABCS: *awareness* (that ASD patients behave and react differently from most patients), *basic* (keep instructions, questions, treatments, and the environment simple), *calm* (be calm and patient; don't lose your temper, yell, or try to force the patient), and *safety* (as much as possible, interact with patients in their familiar surroundings, where they feel safe).
- Patients with special challenges, their families, and their caregivers are often very knowledgeable about the patients' needs and the function of their special equipment. As much as possible, rely on their expertise and involve them in the patients' care.

Key Decisions

- What is the patient's problem today? Is it a complication of the disability or chronic condition, or is this a new and unrelated problem?
- Must any special equipment remain with the patient during transport, or can it stay behind? In either case, what steps are necessary to prepare the patient for transportation?
- How knowledgeable is the patient or the family or caregiver about the situation? What information and assistance can any of them provide to make the situation easier?
- If the patient has a disability that impairs communication, what is the best way to communicate?

Chapter Glossary

autism spectrum disorders (ASD) developmental disorders that affect, among other things, the ability to communicate, report medical conditions, self-regulate behaviors, and interact with others.

automatic implanted cardiac defibrillator (AICD) a device implanted under the skin of the chest to detect any life-threatening dysrhythmia and deliver a shock to defibrillate the heart.

bariatrics the branch of medicine that deals with the causes of obesity as well as its prevention and treatment.

central IV catheter a catheter surgically inserted for long-term delivery of medications or fluids into the central circulation.

continuous positive airway pressure (CPAP) a device worn by a patient that blows oxygen or air under constant low pressure through a tube and mask to keep airway passages from collapsing at the end of a breath.

dialysis the process of filtering the blood to remove toxic or unwanted wastes and fluids.

disability a physical, emotional, behavioral, or cognitive condition that interferes with a person's ability to carry out everyday tasks, such as working or caring for oneself.

feeding tube a tube used to provide delivery of nutrients to the stomach. A nasogastric feeding tube is inserted through the nose and into the stomach; a gastric feeding tube is surgically implanted through the abdominal wall and into the stomach.

obesity a condition of having too much body fat, defined as a body mass index of 30 or greater.

ostomy bag an external pouch that collects fecal matter diverted from the colon or ileum through a surgical opening (colostomy or ileostomy) in the abdominal wall.

pacemaker a device implanted under the skin with wires implanted into the heart to modify the heart rate as needed to maintain an adequate heart rate.

stoma a surgically created opening into the body, as with a tracheostomy, colostomy, or ileostomy.

tracheostomy a surgical opening in the neck into the trachea.

urinary catheter a tube inserted into the bladder through the urethra to drain urine from the bladder.

ventilator a device that breathes for a patient.

ventricular assist device a battery-powered mechanical pump implanted in the body to assist a failing left ventricle in pumping blood to the body.

wearable cardioverter defibrillator (WCD) an external vest worn by a patient to detect any life-threatening dysrhythmia and deliver a shock to defibrillate the heart.

Preparation for Your Examination and Practice

Short Answer

1. List several advanced medical devices you might find when responding to patients with special challenges at home.
2. What health problems are associated with obesity?
3. If a tracheostomy tube is blocked, describe a method of clearing the blockage, if your protocols allow.
4. If a ventilator that a patient relies on to breathe malfunctions, what life support care should you perform?
5. What are some specific health problems associated with homelessness?

6. List and briefly describe the "ABCS" for dealing with a patient who has autism.
7. If a patient cannot hear or cannot speak, describe several methods that might facilitate communication with the patient.

Thinking and Linking

Patients with special needs can pose a number of challenges in assessment and management. This exercise combines material you have learned in this chapter with material from previous chapters. Decide how you would handle each of the following situations.

1. Your patient is a 2-year-old girl having a seizure on only one side of her body. Her father tells you she was born without a corpus callosum, the band of fibers that connects the left and right sides of the brain. Describe how you will assess and manage the patient. What are some questions you should ask the parents to ensure the patient gets the best care?
2. Your patient is a 30-year-old woman whom you estimate to weigh approximately 600 pounds. She is in her second-floor apartment, which she has not left for more than a year. There is no elevator. What resources do you need to get the patient out of her apartment and to the hospital? What are your considerations in moving and transporting the patient?
3. Your patient is a 45-year-old man who receives continuous ambulatory peritoneal dialysis. When you arrive, the patient is allowing fluid to be drained from his abdomen into a collection bag. How should you determine the best way to manage the patient's dialysis process during transport?
4. Your patient is a 12-year-old boy with a severe developmental disability. His teacher says his nose began bleeding and she has not been able to stop it. The patient is frightened of you. He is kicking and screaming, and refuses to let you near him. How would you handle this situation?

Critical Thinking Exercises

A call to a patient with special needs may require some creative problem solving. Describe how you would handle each of the following situations, and explain your reasoning.

1. You are called to respond to a patient who has an arteriovenous (A-V) fistula that is used during his triweekly visits to the dialysis center. The patient presents as pale, sweaty, anxious, and almost incoherent. Could the cause of his condition be related to the A-V fistula? How might you determine if this is the case? What actions should you take?
2. You are called to a nursing home to transport a 79-year-old patient who had a severe stroke 6 months ago. She has a feeding tube in place, a colostomy bag, and a urinary catheter. Today she is presenting with a fever, a heart rate of 120, respirations of 24, and a blood pressure of 100/60. What are your primary concerns with this patient? What are your considerations for dealing with her feeding tube, colostomy bag, and urinary catheter?
3. Think back to your training in basic life support (BLS). What BLS training might you draw upon to help you deal with a patient with special needs whose life-sustaining equipment has malfunctioned?
4. Your patient is a paraplegic, paralyzed from the waist down after a vehicle collision. She called EMS today because she thinks she has pneumonia. She lives alone and has a service dog that assists her. She insists that she must take the dog with her. How should you handle this situation?
5. Your patient is a 10-year-old girl with autism who does not speak. She has fallen from a chair she was standing on, and seems to have injured her ankle. When she sees you coming in, she becomes visibly terrified. How can you best assess and treat this child?

Pathophysiology to Practice

The following questions are designed to assist you in gathering relevant clinical information and making accurate decisions in the field.

1. What risk factors do the homeless and poor have for developing serious health problems? Why might patients in this group be less able to compensate for illness and injury?
2. What is the difference between congenital and acquired diseases? What are examples of each?
3. Why might a patient who is paralyzed be more prone to bedsores, pneumonia, and other infections?

Street Scenes

You answer a call for a young girl who has an issue with her tracheostomy tube. Dispatch tells you 18-month-old Amber's parents left her in the care of her Aunt Dorothy for a day. Dorothy is familiar with Amber's tracheostomy but has not had any experience with anything going wrong. Unfortunately, something went wrong. Late in the afternoon, Amber experienced a fever and began to look a little gray. That's when Dorothy called EMS.

Your initial impression as you enter Amber's room is that she is alert but in some respiratory distress, with cyanosis around the lips. When you examine her tracheostomy, you see that there is a small amount of mucus coming from her trach tube. Her radial pulse is rapid and weak.

Street Scene Questions

1. **What is this patient's priority?**
2. **What additional information do you need to treat the patient?**

Next to Amber you see several small soft suction catheters. You remove one from the package, attach it to your suction device, measure the length to insert by comparing it with the obturator on the table next to the patient, and suction some mucus out of her trach tube. Amber's color begins to improve. Your partner tells you the patient's pulse is 128 and her respiratory rate is 44.

Street Scene Questions

3. How should you reassess the patient?
4. What equipment should you take to the hospital with Amber?

You listen to Amber's breathing through her trach tube and no longer hear the gurgling sounds that were initially audible. She is moving air well. Although her color is better than when you found her, she appears pale and still in some respiratory distress, although less than before you suctioned her. Amber's pulse oximeter reading has increased from 85 percent to 91 percent. You gather Amber's "ready to go" bag with her medical records and Emergency Information Form as you prepare her for transport. You administer high-concentration oxygen and suction her trach tube a few more times on the trip to the emergency department.

Later, Amber's parents call your station to thank you for what you did. Amber has a respiratory infection that is responding well to treatment. Dorothy was very impressed with your calm professionalism, and the entire family is very grateful.

7 SECTION

Operations

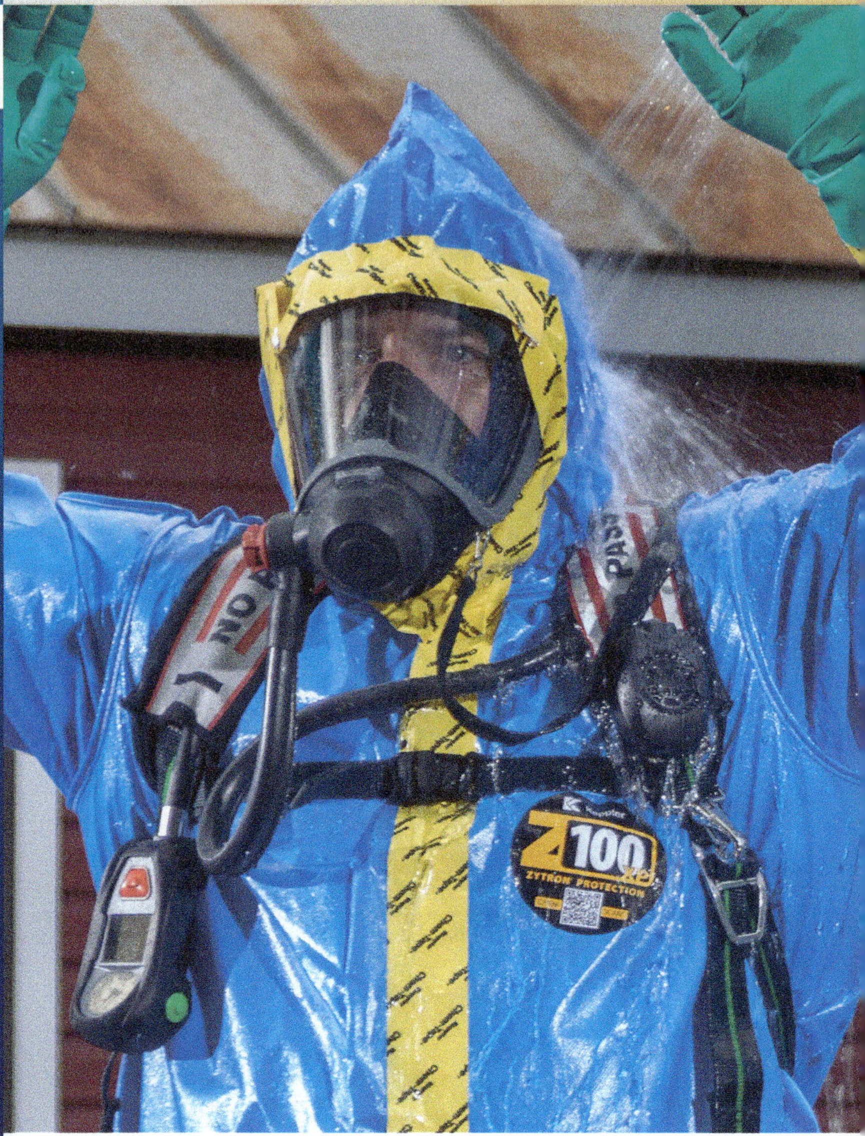

This module deals with EMS operations and organization, both for the day-to-day conduct of your job as an EMT and for certain special situations.

Chapter 38, *EMS Operations*, will lead you through the sequence of tasks before, during, and after an ambulance call. Chapter 39, *Hazardous Materials, Multiple-Casualty Incidents, and Incident Management*, covers emergencies that involve large numbers of patients and those that involve hazardous materials, with emphasis on the Incident Management System. Chapter 40, *Highway Safety and Vehicle Extrication*, discusses how to remain safe at a scene where you are exposed to traffic, as well as the EMT's responsibilities during patient extrication. Finally, Chapter 41, *EMS Response to Terrorism*, discusses kinds of terrorist attacks that may involve an EMS response, and considerations and techniques for ensuring your own self-protection when an act of terrorism may have been involved.

EMS Operations

38

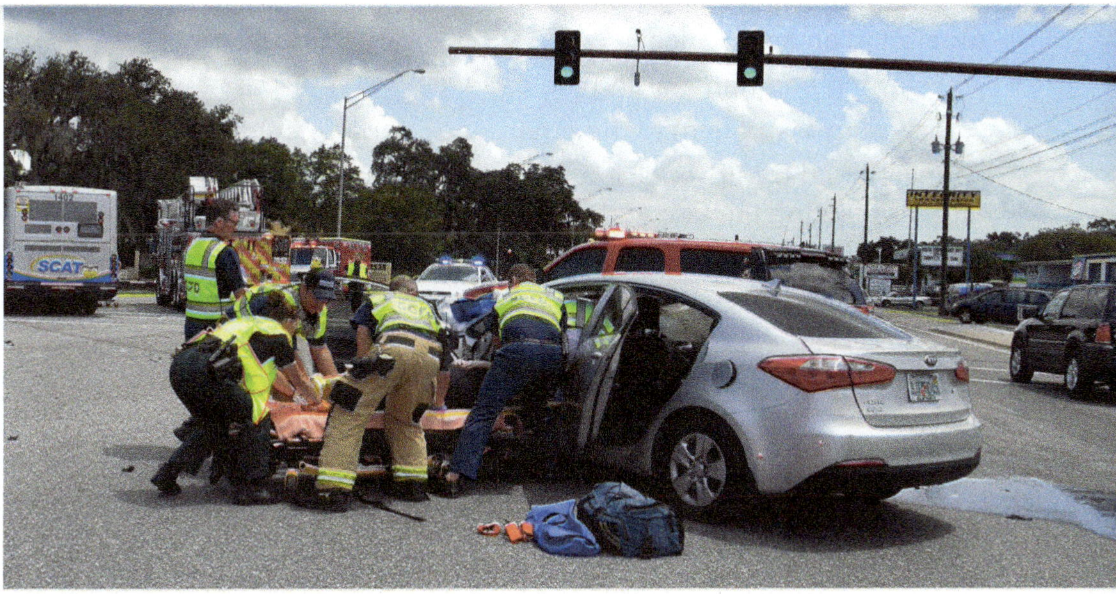

(© Ed Effron)

Related Chapters

The following chapters provide additional information related to topics discussed in this chapter:

- **1** Introduction to Emergency Medical Services
- **2** Well-Being of the EMT
- **3** Lifting and Moving Patients
- **11** Scene Size-Up
- **12** Primary Assessment
- **15** Secondary Assessment
- **17** Communication and Documentation
- **39** Hazardous Materials, Multiple-Casualty Incidents, and Incident Management
- **40** Highway Safety and Vehicle Extrication
- **41** EMS Response to Terrorism

Standard

EMS Operations (Principles of Safely Operating a Ground Ambulance; Air Medical)

Competency

Applies knowledge of operational roles and responsibilities to ensure patient, public, and personnel safety.

Core Concepts

- Phases of an ambulance call
- Preparation for a call
- Operating an ambulance
- Transferring and transporting the patient
- Transferring the patient to the emergency department staff
- Terminating the call, replacing and exchanging equipment, and cleaning and disinfecting the unit and equipment
- When and how to use air rescue

Outcomes

After reading this chapter, you should be able to:

38.1 Summarize the circumstances that must be attended to in order to ensure your ambulance is prepared for calls. (pp. 1144–1151)

- State the relationship between the type of ambulance and the ability to be best prepared for response.
- Recognize where to find lists of required equipment and supplies for EMT ambulances.
- Given a set of equipment and supply items, identify whether the items are required for ambulances.
- Recognize the components of the daily ambulance inspection for which EMTs are responsible.
- Describe the inspection of the patient compartment supplies and equipment.

38.2 Summarize the processes of receiving and responding to EMS calls. (pp. 1151–1152)

- Explain the information you should receive from emergency medical dispatch about a call.
- State the EMTs' process in acknowledging that they have received and are responding to the call.

38.3 Outline the concepts of professional emergency vehicle operations. (pp. 1153–1158)

- Recognize the attitudes and actions needed to safely operate an ambulance.
- Apply general concepts of emergency vehicle operations law to driving the ambulance.
- Outline the proper uses of the ambulance's warning devices.
- Identify conditions that affect the efficiency and safety of operating the ambulance.
- Compare the benefits and drawbacks of using a global positioning system (GPS) in navigation.

38.4 Summarize the actions responders must take to protect the safety of themselves and the patient at a highway incident. (pp. 1158–1159)

- Explain hazards associated with highway response.
- List actions EMTs must take to improve scene safety when responding to a highway scene.

38.5 Summarize the EMT's actions in preparing patients for and transporting them to the hospital. (pp. 1159–1165)

- Evaluate characteristics of the patient and scene to select a proper means of transporting the patient to the ambulance.
- Explain what it means to package the patient for transport.
- Describe the EMT's actions while preparing the patient for transport.
- Describe the EMTs actions during transportation of the patient.

38.6 Summarize the EMT team's responsibilities in terminating the call and preparing for the next call. (pp. 1166–1171)

- Outline the steps to be taken at the hospital, including transfer of the patient to hospital staff.
- Describe steps needed to prepare the ambulance for another call.
- Outline the steps to be taken en route back to quarters to ensure your ambulance is available for another call.
- Outline the steps to be taken once you arrive back in quarters to ensure that all aspects of your ambulance are fully prepared for another response.

38.7 Summarize considerations in requesting and interacting with air rescue units. (pp. 1171–1173)

- Outline reasons for considering a call for an air rescue unit.
- State the information required to initiate an air medical response.
- Differentiate between landing zones that are correctly prepared and those that are not.
- State procedures for approaching a helicopter in the landing zone.

Your responsibilities may differ somewhat depending on the type of EMS agency you join. However, most nonmedical operational responsibilities include the following five phases:

- Preparing for the ambulance call
- Receiving and responding to a call
- Transferring the patient to the ambulance
- Transporting the patient to the hospital
- Terminating the call

Preparing for the Ambulance Call

CORE CONCEPT
Phases of an ambulance call

CORE CONCEPT
Preparation for a call

The modern ambulance has come a long way from its primitive beginnings. Far more than just a means of transport, today's ambulance is a well-equipped and efficiently organized mobile prehospital emergency department and communications unit. It is one of the most important modes for people to access emergency health care in the United States.

The U.S. Department of Transportation has issued specifications for Type I, Type II, and Type III ambulances (Figure 38-1). Because of the extra equipment now placed on ambulances for specialty rescue, advanced life support, and hazardous materials operations, their gross vehicle weight has been easily exceeded in some communities. This has necessitated introduction of a medium-duty truck chassis built for rugged durability and large storage and work areas. As needs evolve, ambulance standards will also continue

FIGURE 38-1 Four types of ambulances: (A) Type I, (B) Type II, (C) Type III, (D) medium duty; and (E) a specialty response vehicle.

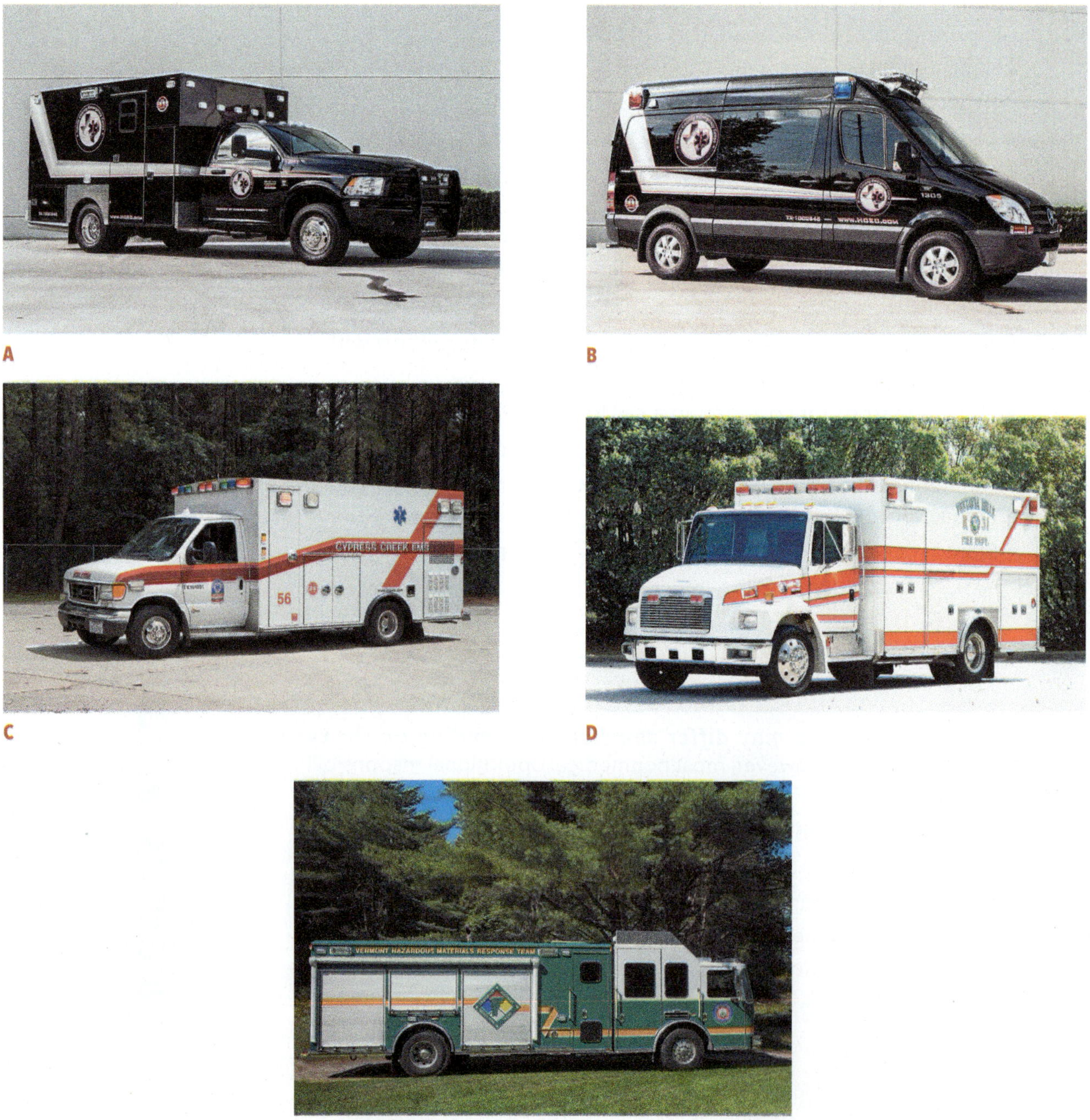

to evolve. Currently the standards are not without controversy, and revisions are under consideration by several different EMS-related authorities. At the time of this printing, many states still use the Federal Specification KKK-A-1822(F) standards (more commonly referred to as "K-Specs"). Some states use the newer National Fire Protection Association Standard 1917 for Automotive Ambulances.

Ambulance Supplies and Equipment

If an ambulance does not have the proper equipment for patient care and transportation, it is just a ride to the hospital. In fact, an ambulance without proper equipment may have its agency cited and fined a considerable amount of money by a state EMS regulatory agency. In addition, the EMS personnel responsible may find themselves cited and fined. Table 38-1 lists recommendations of the American College of Surgeons, the American College of Emergency Physicians, the National Association of EMS Physicians, and the American Academy of Pediatrics. EMS services are regulated in most states, and each state has a list of equipment required to be carried by EMS response units. Refer to your state or regional office for your specific regulations and an equipment list. (*Text continues on page 1148.*)

TABLE 38-1 Recommended Equipment for Basic Life Support Ambulances

RECOMMENDED EQUIPMENT FOR BASIC LIFE SUPPORT AMBULANCES	
A. Ventilation and airway equipment	**1.** Portable and fixed suction apparatus with a regulator (per federal specifications; see Federal Specification KKK-A-1822F reference) • Wide-bore tubing, rigid pharyngeal curved suction tip; tonsillar and flexible suction catheters, 6F-16F are commercially available (Be equipped with one between 6F and 10F and one between 12F and 16F.) **2.** Portable oxygen apparatus capable of metered flow with adequate tubing **3.** Portable and fixed oxygen supply equipment • Variable flow regulator **4.** Oxygen administration equipment • Adequate-length tubing; transparent mask (adult and child sizes), both nonrebreathing and valveless; nasal cannulas (adult and child sizes) **5.** Bag-valve-mask (manual resuscitator) • Hand-operated, self-reexpanding bag; adult (>1,000 mL) and child (450–750 mL) sizes with oxygen reservoir/accumulator; valve (clear, disposable, operable in cold weather); and mask (adult, child, infant, and neonate sizes) **6.** Airways • Nasopharyngeal (16F-34F; adult and child sizes) • Oropharyngeal (sizes 0-5; adult, child, and infant sizes) **7.** Pulse oximeter with pediatric and adult probes **8.** Saline drops and bulb suction for infants
B. Monitoring and defibrillation	All ambulances should be equipped with an automated external defibrillator (AED) unless staffed by advanced life support (ALS) personnel who are carrying a monitor/defibrillator. The AED should have pediatric capabilities, including child-sized pads and cables.
C. Immobilization devices	**1.** Cervical collars • Rigid for children ages 2 years or older; child and adult sizes (small, medium, large, and other available sizes) **2.** Head immobilization device (not sandbags) • Firm padding or commercial device **3.** Lower extremity (femur) traction devices • Lower extremity, limb-support slings, padded ankle hitch, padded pelvic support, traction strap (adult and child sizes) **4.** Upper and lower extremity immobilization devices • Joint-above and joint-below fracture (adult and child sizes), rigid support constructed with appropriate material (cardboard, metal, vacuum, wood, or plastic) **5.** Impervious backboards (long, short; radiolucent preferred) and extrication devices • Short (extrication, head-to-pelvis length) and long (transport, head-to-feet length), with at least three appropriate restraint straps (chin strap alone should not be used for head immobilization) and with padding for children and handholds for moving patients

(continued)

TABLE 38-1 Recommended Equipment for Basic Life Support Ambulances (*continued*)

RECOMMENDED EQUIPMENT FOR BASIC LIFE SUPPORT AMBULANCES	
D. Bandages	**1.** Commercially packaged or sterile burn sheets **2.** Triangular bandages • Minimum two safety pins each **3.** Dressings • Sterile multitrauma dressings (various large and small sizes) • ABDs (abdominal pads), 10″ × 12″ (25 × 30.5 cm) or larger • 4″ × 4″ (10 × 10 cm) gauze sponges or suitable size **4.** Gauze rolls • Various sizes **5.** Occlusive dressing or equivalent • Sterile, 3″ × 8″ (8 × 20 cm) or larger **6.** Adhesive tape • Various sizes (including 1″ and 2″ [2.5 and 5 cm]) hypoallergenic • Various sizes (including 1″ and 2″ [2.5 and 5 cm]) adhesive **7.** Arterial tourniquet (commercial preferred)
E. Communication	Two-way communication device between EMS provider, dispatcher, and medical direction
F. Obstetric kit (Commercially packaged are available.)	**1.** Kit (separate sterile kit) • Towels, 4″ × 4″ (10 × 10 cm) dressing, umbilical tape, sterile scissors or other cutting utensil, bulb suction, clamps for cord, sterile gloves, blanket **2.** Thermal absorbent blanket and head cover, aluminum foil roll, or appropriate heat-reflective material (enough to cover newborn)
G. Miscellaneous	**1.** Sphygmomanometer (pediatric and adult regular- and large-size cuffs) **2.** Adult stethoscope **3.** Length-based or weight-based tape or appropriate reference material for pediatric equipment sizing and drug dosing based on estimated or known weight **4.** Thermometer with low-temperature capability **5.** Heavy bandage or paramedic scissors for cutting clothing, belts, and boots **6.** Cold packs **7.** Sterile saline solution for irrigation (1-liter bottles or bags) **8.** Flashlights (two) with extra batteries and bulbs **9.** Blankets **10.** Sheets (minimum four), linen or paper, and pillows **11.** Towels **12.** Triage tags **13.** Disposable emesis bags or basins **14.** Disposable bedpan **15.** Disposable urinal **16.** Wheeled cot (conforming to national standard at the time of manufacture) **17.** Folding stretcher **18.** Stair chair or carry chair **19.** Patient care charts/forms **20.** Lubricating jelly (water-soluble)
H. Infection control (Latex-free equipment should be available.)	**1.** Eye protection (full peripheral glasses or goggles, face shield) **2.** Face protection (for example, surgical masks per applicable local or state guidance) **3.** Gloves, nonsterile (Must meet NFPA 1999 requirements found at http://www.nfpa.org/.) **4.** Coveralls or gowns **5.** Shoe covers **6.** Waterless hand cleanser, commercial antimicrobial (towelette, spray, liquid) **7.** Disinfectant solution for cleaning equipment **8.** Standard sharps containers, fixed and portable **9.** Disposable trash bags for disposing of biohazardous waste **10.** Respiratory protection (for example, N-95 or N-100 mask–per applicable local or state guidance)

TABLE 38-1 Recommended Equipment for Basic Life Support Ambulances (*continued*)

RECOMMENDED EQUIPMENT FOR BASIC LIFE SUPPORT AMBULANCES	
I. Injury-prevention equipment	1. All individuals in an ambulance need to be secured with appropriate restraints. (There is currently no national standard for transport of uninjured children.) 2. Protective helmet 3. Fire extinguisher 4. Hazardous material reference guide 5. Traffic signaling devices (reflective material triangles or other reflective, nonigniting devices) 6. Reflective safety wear for each crew member (Must meet or exceed ANSI/ISEA performance Class II or III if working within the right of way of any federal-aid highway. Visit http://www.reflectivevest.com/federalhighwayruling.html for more information.)
Optional Basic Equipment This section is intended to assist EMS providers in choosing equipment that can be used to ensure delivery of quality prehospital care. Use should be based on local resources. The equipment in this section is not mandated or required.	
A. Optional equipment	1. Glucose meter (per state protocol) 2. Elastic bandages • Nonsterile (various sizes) 3. Mobile phone 4. Infant oxygen mask 5. Infant self-inflating resuscitation bag 6. Airways • Nasopharyngeal (12Fr, 14Fr) • Oropharyngeal (size 00) 7. Alternative airway devices (for example, a rescue airway device such as the King Airway or laryngeal mask airway) as approved by local medical direction 8. Alternative airway devices for children (Few alternative airway devices that are FDA-approved have been studied in children. Those that have been studied, such as the LMA, have not been adequately evaluated in the prehospital setting.) 9. Neonatal blood pressure cuff 10. Infant blood pressure cuff 11. Pediatric stethoscope 12. Infant cervical immobilization device 13. Pediatric backboard and extremity splints 14. Topical hemostatic agent 15. Appropriate CBRNE PPE (chemical, biological, radiological, nuclear, explosive personal protective equipment), including respiratory and body protection 16. Applicable chemical antidote auto-injectors (at a minimum for crew members' protection; additional for patient treatment based on local or regional protocols; appropriate for adults and children)
B. Optional basic life support medications	1. Albuterol 2. EpiPens 3. Oral glucose 4. Nitroglycerin (sublingual tablet or paste) 5. Aspirin 6. Naloxone
C. Interfacility transport	Additional equipment may be needed by ALS and BLS prehospital care providers who transport patients between facilities. Transfers may be done to a lower or higher level of care, depending on the specific need. Specialty transport teams, including pediatric and neonatal teams, may include other personnel such as respiratory therapists, nurses, and physicians. Training and equipment needs may vary depending on the skills needed during transport of these patients. There are excellent resources available that provide detailed lists of equipment needed for interfacility transfer, such as the *American Academy of Pediatrics Guidelines for Air and Ground Transport of Neonatal and Pediatric Patients*.

(*continued*)

TABLE 38-1 Recommended Equipment for Basic Life Support Ambulances (*continued*)

Appendix: Extrication Equipment

Adequate extrication equipment must be readily available to the EMS responders but is more often found on heavy rescue vehicles than on the primary responding ambulance. In general, the devices or tools used for extrication fall into several broad categories: disassembly, spreading, cutting, pulling, protective, and patient-related. The following is necessary equipment that should be available either on the primary response vehicle or on a heavy rescue vehicle.

A. Disassembly tools	**1.** Wrenches (adjustable) **2.** Screwdrivers (flat- and Phillips-head) **3.** Pliers **4.** Bolt cutter **5.** Tin snips **6.** Hammer **7.** Spring-loaded center punch **8.** Axes (pry, fire) **9.** Bars (wrecking, crow) **10.** Ram (4-ton)
B. Spreading tools	**1.** Hydraulic jack/spreader/cutter combination cutting tools **2.** Saws (hacksaw, fire, windshield, pruning, reciprocating) **3.** Air-cutting gun kit
C. Pulling tools/devices	**1.** Ropes/chains **2.** Come-along **3.** Hydraulic truck jack **4.** Air bags
D. Protective devices	**1.** Reflectors/flares **2.** Hard hats **3.** Safety goggles **4.** Fireproof blanket **5.** Leather gloves **6.** Jackets/coats/boots
E. Miscellaneous	**1.** Shovel **2.** Lubricating oil **3.** Wood/wedges **4.** Generator **5.** Floodlights

NOTE: Local extrication needs may necessitate additional equipment for water, aerial, or mountain rescue.
Source: Adapted from American College of Surgeons, Committee on Trauma; American College of Emergency Physicians; National Association of EMS Physicians; American Academy of Pediatrics.

Compare the items listed in Table 38-1—and lists of equipment required by your state or region—with the inventory of your ambulance. Learn where each item is stored, what every item's purpose is, and when it should be used. If the item is a mechanical device, also learn how it works and how it should be maintained.

Ensuring Ambulance Readiness for Service

As a professional rescuer, you are expected by the public and your organization to be ready when an emergency occurs. Therefore, you must be sure that you, your vehicle, and your equipment are ready to respond. Most services require that an inspection of the vehicle and equipment be conducted at the start of every shift to ensure readiness. Inspection of the vehicle and equipment is typically tracked by a checklist. The checklist and inspection process are an important part of recordkeeping for many different EMS services and may be a critical component of an investigation process.

Do a brief shift report with the off-going crew if possible. Ask if they experienced any problems with either the ambulance or its equipment during their shift. If there was a problem described by the off-going crew, make sure to communicate that to a shift supervisor and thoroughly document the stated problem. Perform a thorough bumper-to-bumper inspection of the ambulance (Scan 38-1) using the checklist provided by your service. There

SCAN 38-1 Inspecting the Ambulance

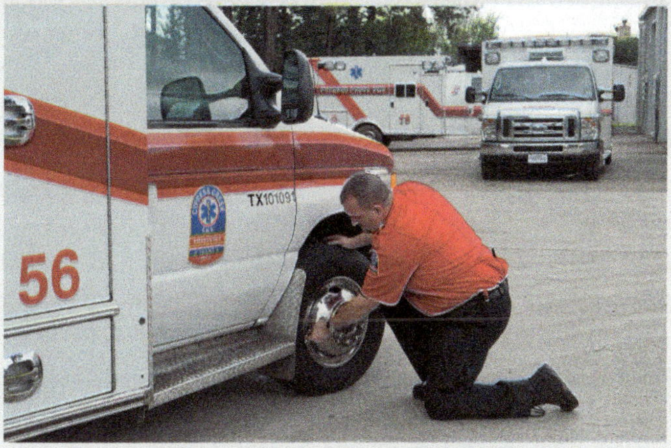

1. Check the ambulance body, wheels, tires, and windshield wipers.

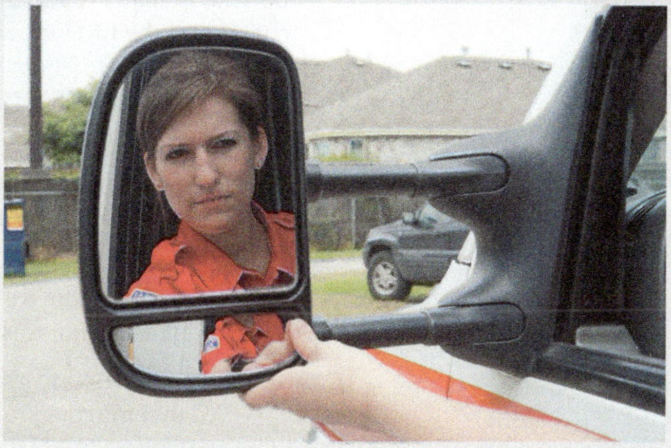

2. Check the windows, doors, and mirrors.

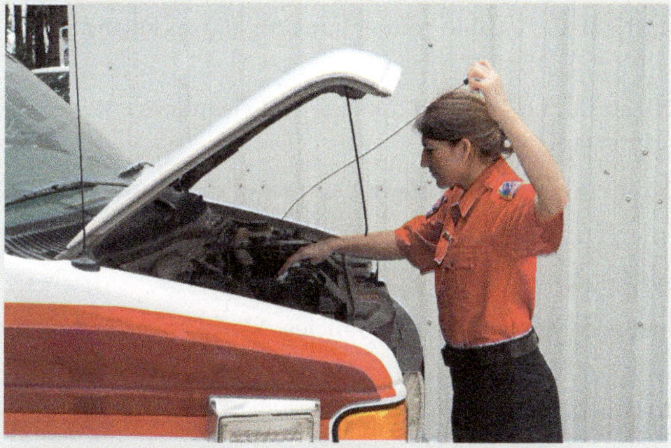

3. Check under the hood.

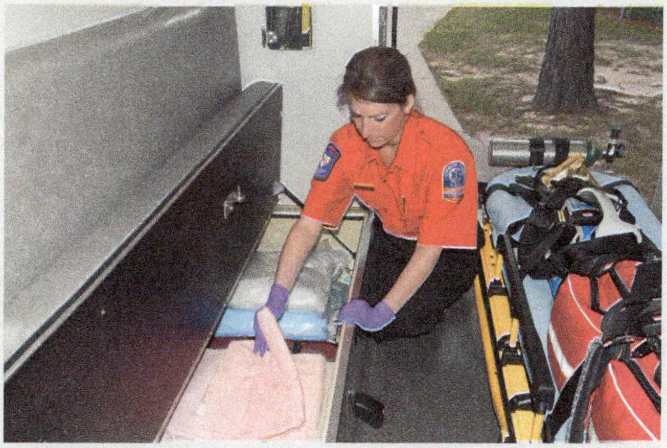

4. Check the interior surfaces and upholstery.

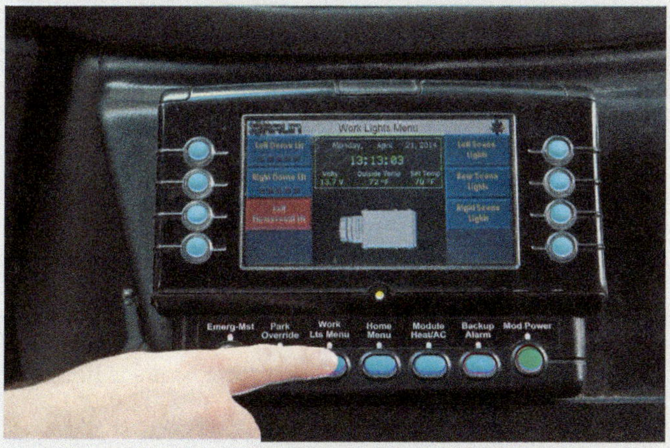

5. Check the dash instruments and communications equipment.

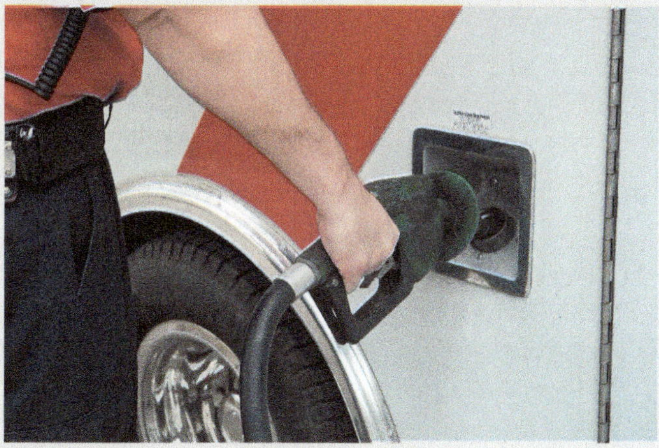

6. Check the fuel level and refuel as needed.

are usually two components to the inspection: a vehicle component and an equipment component. In many cases, the EMT assigned to be the driver completes the vehicle component check, and the EMT crew leader completes the medical equipment check.

Ambulance Inspection, Engine Off

The following inspection steps can be taken while the ambulance is in quarters:

1. Inspect the body of the vehicle. Report any damage that may be evident. Indicate past damage that has not been repaired.
2. Inspect the wheels and tires. Check for damaged or worn wheel rims and tire sidewalls. Check the tread depth. Use a pressure gauge to ensure that all tires are properly inflated. Do not forget to inspect the inside rear tires and their air pressure as well.
3. Inspect the windows and mirrors. Look for broken glass and loose or missing parts. See that mirrors are clean and properly adjusted for maximum visibility.
4. Check the operation of every door and all latches and locks.
5. Check the level of the fluids: oil, coolant, windshield wiper, brake, and transmission fluids.
6. Check the battery. Inspect the battery cable connections for tightness and signs of corrosion.
7. Inspect the interior surfaces and upholstery for damage and cleanliness. Wipe down the steering wheel with disinfectant.
8. Check the windows for operation. See that the interior surface of each window is clean.
9. Test the horn, siren, and emergency lights.
10. Adjust the driver's seat and ensure the seat belts are operational.
11. Check the fuel level. Refuel according to agency policies. Many agencies specify a minimum fuel level.

    NOTE: *Allow the engine to cool before removing any pressure caps.*

Ambulance Inspection, Engine On

The next steps require you to start the engine. Pull the ambulance from quarters if engine exhaust fumes will be a problem. Some agencies may use an exhaust-removal system. Set the parking brake, put the transmission in park, and have your partner chock the wheels before undertaking the following steps:

1. Check the dash-mounted indicators to see if any light remains on to indicate a possible problem with oil pressure, engine temperature, or the vehicle's electrical system.
2. Check dash-mounted gauges for proper operation.
3. Depress the brake pedal. Note whether pedal travel seems correct or excessive. Check air pressure as needed.
4. Test the parking brake. Move the transmission lever to a drive position. Replace the lever to the park position as soon as you are sure that the parking brake is holding.
5. Turn the steering wheel from side to side.
6. Check the operation of the windshield wipers and washers. The glass should be wiped clean without streaking each time the blades move.
7. Turn on the vehicle's warning lights. Have your partner walk around the ambulance and check each flashing and revolving light for operation. Turn off the warning lights.
8. Turn on the other vehicle lights. Have your partner walk around the ambulance again, this time checking the headlights (high and low beams), turn signals, four-way flashers, brake lights, reverse lights, side and rear scene-illumination lights, and box marker lights.

9. Check the operation of the heating and air conditioning equipment in both the driver's compartment and the patient compartment. This is also a good time to check the on-board suction if the engine is running.
10. Operate the communications equipment. Test portable as well as mobile radios and any cellular telephone communications.
11. If your unit is equipped with a back-up camera, make sure that the camera is not damaged and is clean from debris, and that the image on the driver's screen is clear.
12. Return the ambulance to quarters. While you are backing up, have your partner note whether the backup alarm is operating (if the vehicle is so equipped).

Inspection of Patient Compartment Supplies and Equipment

Shut off the engine and complete your inspection by checking the patient compartment and all exterior cabinets:

1. Using your checklist, conduct a detailed inspection and inventory of the equipment and supplies.
2. Check treatment supplies, interior equipment, and exterior equipment. Items should not only be identified; they should also be checked for completeness, condition, and operation. Check the pressure of oxygen cylinders. Test oxygen and ventilation equipment for proper operation. Examine rescue tools for rust and dirt. Operate battery-powered devices to ensure that the batteries have a proper charge. Some equipment, such as the AED, may require additional testing. See that an item-by-item inspection of everything carried on the ambulance is done, with findings recorded on the inspection report.
3. When you are finished, complete the inspection report. Correct any deficiencies. Replace missing items. Make your supervisor aware of any deficiencies that cannot be immediately corrected.
4. Finally, clean the unit for infection control and appearance. Use only approved cleaning and disinfecting materials. Maintaining the ambulance's appearance enhances your organization's image in the public's eye while also inspiring confidence in your role. EMTs who take pride in their work show it by taking pride in the appearance of their ambulance.

If a call comes in while you are performing your vehicle check, take the call and finish the check when you return to service. An exception would be if any essential equipment were missing. In that case, report your ambulance as "out of service" until the critical items have been replaced, allowing for another, properly equipped ambulance to be dispatched.

Receiving and Responding to a Call

In many areas of the country, a person needs only to dial 911 to access ambulance, fire, or police services 24 hours a day. A trained Emergency Medical Dispatcher (EMD) records information from callers, decides which service is needed, and alerts that service to respond. (Always say "nine-one-one" when talking to community or school groups. Children cannot find "eleven" on the phone dial or keypad.)

Role of the Emergency Medical Dispatcher

Many cities and communication centers train and certify Emergency Medical Dispatchers (EMDs) based on the medical priority system. This system originated in 1979 through the leadership of Jeffrey Clawson, MD. An EMD is trained to perform the following tasks:

- Ask questions of the caller and assign a priority to the call.
- Provide prearrival medical instructions to callers, and information to crews.

- Dispatch and coordinate EMS resources.
- Coordinate with other public safety agencies.

When answering a call for help, the EMD obtains as much information as possible about the situation that may help the responding crew. The questions the EMD should ask are:

1. **What is the exact location of the patient?** The EMD must ask for the house or building number and the apartment number, if any. It is important to ask for the street name with the direction designator (e.g., North, East), the nearest cross street, the name of the development or subdivision, and the exact location of the emergency.
2. **What is your call-back number?** (Enhanced 911 will show the number.) "Stay on the line. Do not hang up until I [the EMD] tell you to." In life-threatening situations, after the units have been dispatched, the EMD will offer instructions to the caller for the caller or others on the scene to follow until the units arrive. It is also important for the caller to stay on the line in case a question arises about the location that was given.
3. **What's the problem?** This will provide the chief complaint. It will help the EMD decide which line of questioning to follow and the priority of the response to send.
4. **How old is the patient?** Most ambulances are set up to respond to the scene with a pediatric kit if the patient is a child rather than an adult. If prearrival CPR instructions are given, it will be necessary to distinguish whether the person is an infant, a child, or an adult.
5. **What's the patient's sex?** Ask this if it is not obvious from the information given.
6. **Is the patient conscious?** An unconscious patient is a higher response priority.
7. **Is the patient breathing?** If the patient is conscious and breathing, the EMD will often ask many additional questions relative to the chief complaint to determine the appropriate level of response; for example, Emergency Medical Responders, EMTs, or ambulances may respond "cold" (at normal speed) or "hot" (an emergency, lights-and-siren mode). If the patient is not breathing, or the caller is not sure whether the patient is breathing, the EMD will dispatch the maximum response and begin the appropriate prearrival instructions for a nonbreathing patient, which may also involve telephone CPR if the patient does not have a pulse.

If the call is for a traffic collision, a series of key questions must be asked to help determine the priority and amount of response. With thorough questioning of the caller, it may be possible for the EMD to appropriately dispatch one unit "hot" and backup units "cold," which in turn may help reduce emergency-vehicle collisions. Thorough questioning also allows the EMD to determine if an entrapment and/or fire situation is imminent, to dispatch the appropriate apparatus.

This is how an EMD might dispatch an ambulance to the location of a sick person:

> MEDCOM to Ambulance 641 and Medic 640, respond Priority 1 to a 60-year-old unconscious female with breathing difficulty. The location is the bus station on Route 9 at the intersection with Kunker Road. Time now is 1745 hours.

The EMD may repeat the message to minimize any question as to its content and to ensure the ambulance has received the call. Many EMS systems have the responding crew repeat the address back to the dispatch center, to confirm the correct address and make sure that the message is placed on the dispatch recording.

Some computer-based dispatch systems have the EMS crew acknowledge the call by a specific keystroke on the computer. The computer may also provide directions to the scene in conjunction with a global positioning system (GPS). An exact 911 street address is very helpful when using GPS.

Operating the Ambulance

Even if you will only occasionally be driving an ambulance, you may be mandated to attend emergency vehicle operator training, which has both classroom and in-vehicle road sessions. This training adds to your skill set and decreases the chance of collision and liability for you and your agency.

CORE CONCEPT
Operating an ambulance

Being a Safe Ambulance Operator

To be a safe ambulance operator, you should:

- Be physically fit. You should not have any impairment that prevents you from operating the ambulance or any medical condition that might disable you while driving.
- Be mentally fit, with your emotions under control. The judgment of someone operating an ambulance should not be compromised by the excitement of lights and sirens.
- Be able to perform under stress.
- Have a positive attitude about your ability as a driver but not be an unreasonable risk taker.
- Be tolerant of other drivers. Always keep in mind that people react differently when they see an emergency vehicle. Accept and tolerate the bad habits of some drivers. This will help you avoid "road rage."

Some additional safety tips include:

- Never drive while under the influence of alcohol, illicit or recreational drugs such as marijuana or cocaine, antihistamines that cause drowsiness, or tranquilizers.
- Never drive while taking prescription medications that can impair your ability to operate a motor vehicle. These same medications also affect your ability to treat patients. Your agency should have a standard operating guideline or other policy regarding what medications warrant this warning and how long after the last dose is deemed safe to drive.
- Never drive with a suspended license.
- Always wear your glasses or contact lenses if required for driving.
- Evaluate your ability to drive based on personal stress, illness, fatigue, or sleepiness. Energy drinks should be used with caution. Drinking these beverages when you are tired or sleepy may make you feel more awake, but you may still have reduced reaction times and other negative consequences of prolonged fatigue.

Understanding the Law

Every state has statutes that regulate the operation of emergency vehicles. Emergency vehicle operators are generally granted certain exemptions with regard to speed, parking, passage through traffic signals, and direction of travel. However, the laws also state that if an emergency vehicle operator does not drive with due regard for the safety of others, the driver of that emergency vehicle must be prepared to suffer the consequences, such as tickets, lawsuits, or even time in jail.

The following list contains some points typically included in laws regulating ambulance operation:

- An ambulance operator must have a valid driver's license and may be required to complete a training program and/or an additional endorsement to the operator's driver's license.
- Privileges granted under the law to the operators of ambulances apply when the vehicle is responding to an emergency or is involved in the emergency transport of a sick or injured person. When the ambulance is not on an emergency call, the laws that apply to the operation of nonemergency vehicles also apply to the ambulance. The source of many citizen complaints is the unsafe operation of ambulances during nonemergency operations.

- Even though certain privileges are granted during an emergency, the exemptions granted do not provide immunity to the operator in cases of reckless driving or disregard for the safety of others.
- Privileges granted during emergency situations apply only if the operator uses warning devices in the manner prescribed by law. Typically, this means operation of the warning/emergency lighting systems as well as of the siren.

Most statutes allow emergency vehicle operators to:

- Park the vehicle anywhere if it does not damage personal property or endanger lives.
- Proceed past red stop signals, flashing red stop signals, and stop signs. Some states require that emergency vehicle operators come to a full stop, then proceed with caution. Other states require only that an operator slow down and proceed with caution.
- Exceed the posted speed limit as long as life and property are not endangered. Some states will place limitations in miles per hour over the posted limit (e.g., 10–15 miles an hour over the posted speed limit).
- Pass other vehicles in no-passing zones after properly signaling, ensuring the way is clear, and taking precautions to avoid endangering life and property. This does not include passing a school bus with its red lights flashing. Wait for the bus driver to clear the children and turn off the red lights of the bus.
- With proper caution and signals, disregard regulations that govern direction of travel and turning in specific directions.

If you ever become involved in an ambulance collision, the laws will be interpreted by the court based on two key issues: (1) Did you use due regard for the safety of others? and (2) Was it, to the best of your knowledge, a true emergency? The requirement of due regard actually sets a higher standard for drivers of emergency vehicles than for other drivers. This is why an investigation by a district attorney or grand jury, as well as one by your ambulance service, is not uncommon following a collision.

Most states reserve the emergency mode of operation for a true emergency, defined as one in which the best information available to you is that loss of life or limb is possible. When dispatched to a call, there is often not much information to go on, so a "collision" will get an emergency response. However, once you arrive and find that your patient is stable with no life-threatening injuries or conditions, it is no longer a true emergency. A lights-and-siren, high-speed response to the hospital in such a situation would be inappropriate. Advising other responding units of this type of information is very important as soon as you understand the particular situation.

The exemptions described here are just examples of those often granted to ambulance operators. Do not assume that they are granted in your state. Obtain a copy of your state's rules and regulations, and carefully study them.

Using the Warning Devices

Safe emergency vehicle operation can be achieved when proper use of warning devices is coupled with sound emergency and defensive driving practices. Studies show that some drivers do not see or hear an ambulance until it is within 100 feet, so never let the lights and siren give you a false sense of security.

The Siren. Although the siren is the most commonly used audible warning device, it is also the most misused. Consider the effects that sirens have on other motorists, patients in ambulances, and ambulance operators themselves:

- The continuous sound of a siren may cause a sick or injured person to suffer increased fear and anxiety, and the patient's condition may worsen as stress builds up.
- Ambulance operators themselves are affected by the continuous sound of a siren. Tests have shown that inexperienced ambulance operators tend to increase their driving speeds from 10 to 15 miles per hour while continually sounding the siren. In some

cases, operators using a siren were unable to negotiate curves that they could pass through easily when not sounding the siren. Sirens also affect hearing, especially if used for long periods with the siren speaker over the cab. The best placement for the speaker is in the vehicle grill.

Many states have laws that regulate the use of audible warning signals. In areas where there are no statutes, ambulance organizations usually create their own policies. If your organization does not, you may find the following suggestions helpful:

- Use the siren sparingly and only when you must. Some states require use of the siren at all times when the ambulance is responding in the emergency mode. Others require it only when the operator is exercising any of the exemptions discussed earlier.
- Never assume that all motorists will hear your siren. Buildings, trees, and dense shrubbery may block siren sounds. Soundproofing keeps outside noises from entering vehicles, and in-vehicle sound systems also decrease the likelihood that an outside sound will be heard.
- Always assume that some motorists will hear your siren but ignore it.
- Be prepared for the erratic maneuvers of other drivers. Some drivers panic when they hear a siren.
- Do not pull up close to a vehicle and then sound your siren. This may cause the driver to jam on his brakes, and you may be unable to stop in time. Use the horn when you are close to a vehicle ahead.
- Never use the siren indiscriminately, and never use it to scare someone or just to get someone's attention.

The Horn. The horn is standard equipment on all ambulances. Experienced operators find that the judicious use of the horn often clears traffic as quickly as the siren. The guidelines for using a siren apply to the horn as well.

Visual Warning Devices. Whenever the ambulance is on the road, night or day, the headlights should be on. This increases the vehicle's visibility to other drivers. In some states, headlights are now required of all vehicles in low-visibility conditions or whenever the windshield wipers are in use. Alternating flashing headlights should be used only if they are attached to secondary headlamps. In most states, it is illegal to drive at night with one headlight out. In some states, the use of the alternating flashing headlights at night is prohibited.

The large lights on the outermost corners of the ambulance patient compartment box should flash together in unison, rather than alternating. This helps the driver who is approaching from a distance identify the full size of your vehicle. There are several available types of lights on ambulances, including rotating lights, flashing lights, strobe lights, and light-emitting diode (LED) lights. When planning the lighting package of an ambulance, check the research before making your decision. In general, it is wisest for the package to combine different types of lights in strategic places rather than just featuring one type of lighting system.

Four-way flashers and directional signals should not be used as emergency lights. Doing so can be confusing to the public, as well as being illegal in some states. Drivers expect a vehicle with four-way flashers on to be traveling at a very slow speed. In addition, the flashers may disrupt the function of the directional signals.

When the ambulance is in the emergency response mode, either en route to the scene or to the hospital with a high-priority patient, all the emergency lights should be used. The vehicle should be easily seen from 360 degrees.

Speed and Safety

You are often told to drive in a slow and careful manner. At this point, you may be thinking something like "How will I ever get a seriously ill or injured person to a hospital if I poke along?" We are not suggesting that you "poke along." However, we do suggest you drive with these facts in mind:

- Excessive speed increases the probability of a collision.
- Speed increases stopping distance, reducing the chance of avoiding a hazardous situation.

Remember that the laws in most states excuse you from obeying certain traffic laws only in a true emergency and only with due regard for the safety of others. Except in these circumstances, obey speed limits, stoplights and stop signs, yield signs, and other laws and posted limits. Approach intersections with caution, avoid sudden turns, and always signal lane changes and turns properly. Be sure that the ambulance driver and all passengers wear seat belts whenever the ambulance is in motion.

Escorted or Multiple-Vehicle Responses

When the police provide an escort for an ambulance, there are additional hazards. Too often, the inexperienced ambulance operator follows the escort vehicle too closely and is unable to stop when the lead vehicle brakes hard. Also, inexperienced operators may assume that other drivers know their vehicle is following the escort. In fact, other drivers will often pull out in front of the ambulance just after the escort vehicle passes.

Because of the dangers involved with escorts, most EMS systems recommend no escorts unless the operator is not familiar with the location of the patient (or hospital) and must be given assistance from the police.

The dangers in multiple-vehicle responses can be the same as those generated by escorted responses, especially when the responding vehicles travel in the same direction close together. A great danger also exists when two vehicles approach an intersection at the same time. They may fail to yield for each other, and other drivers may yield for the first vehicle but not the second. Obviously great care must be used at intersections during multiple-vehicle responses.

Factors That Affect Response

During one 20-year period tracked by The National Highway Traffic Safety Administration and reported at 222.ems.gov, there were about 1500 ground ambulance collisions and 2600 people injured annually, including 33 fatalities! Surprisingly, most ambulance collisions take place in seemingly safe conditions (dry roads, clear weather conditions, and daylight hours). Many occur in intersections. In addition, an ambulance response can be affected by several factors:

- **Day of the week.** Weekdays usually have the heaviest traffic, because people are commuting to and from work. In resort areas, weekend traffic may be heavier.
- **Time of day.** In major employment centers, traffic over major roads tends to be heavy in all directions during commuting hours.
- **Weather.** Adverse weather conditions reduce safe driving speeds and, thus, increase response times. A heavy snowfall can temporarily prevent any response at all. Be careful to lengthen your following distance whenever there is decreased traction on the road because of inclement weather.
- **Road maintenance and construction.** Traffic can be seriously impeded by road construction and maintenance activities. Be aware of area road construction, and plan responses as needed.
- **Railroads.** There are more than a quarter-million grade crossings in the United States where traffic is often blocked by long, slow freight trains. Some communities may use a secondary response system on the other side of train tracks that split the town in half.

- **Bridges and tunnels.** Traffic over bridges and through tunnels slows during rush hours. Collisions—including ambulance collisions—tend to occur when drivers forget that bridges freeze before roadways.
- **Schools and school buses.** The reduced speed limits in force during school hours slow the flow of vehicles. An emergency vehicle should never pass a stopped school bus with its red lights flashing. Wait for the school bus driver to signal you to proceed by turning off the lights. Emergency vehicles attract children, who may venture out into the street to see them. The operator of every emergency vehicle should slow down when approaching a school or playground. Obey the directions given by school crossing guards.

Getting There: Navigating to the Scene

Many EMS services have GPS navigation installed in their emergency vehicles (Figure 38-2). This is an excellent tool for navigation to emergency scenes and hospitals. However, there is still no substitute for an intimate knowledge of the response area. Often, GPS suggests a route that may not be possible because of recent road construction or other changes in the area. GPS devices can also be a significant distraction! Be careful about attempting to operate the GPS while driving. Driving while distracted increases the chance of a crash.

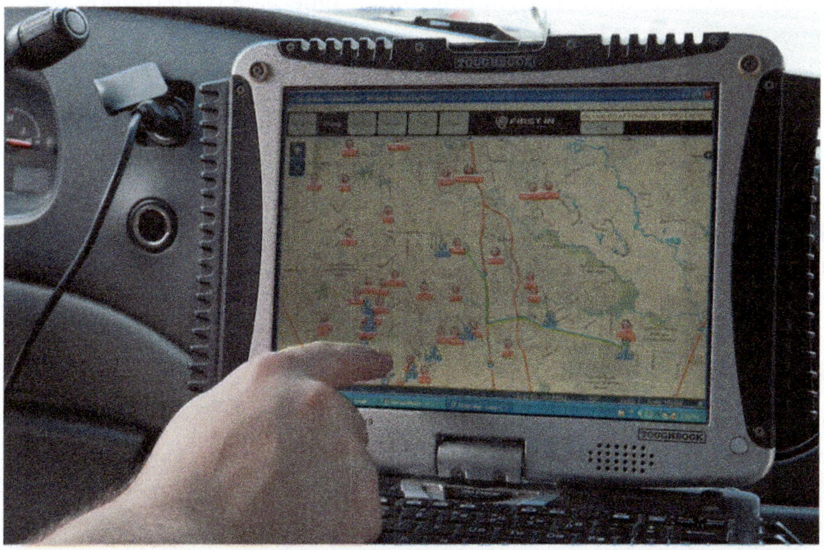

FIGURE 38-2 A GPS device is an excellent tool for navigation to emergency scenes and hospitals.

Point of View

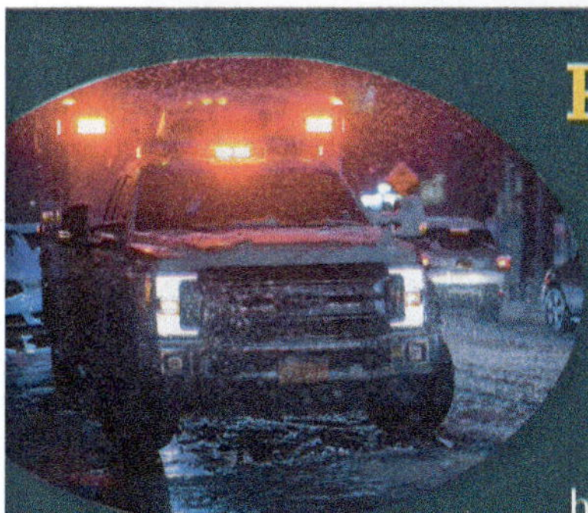

(Michelle_C/Shutterstock.)

"I never realized when I started doing EMS that I'd have to drive in the same stuff that is causing all the crashes.

"We were called for a three-car collision on Highway 17, a road on the outskirts of the city. With the snow that was building up, it took us a good fifteen white-knuckled minutes to get out there. We drove carefully and most of the time at less than half the speed we would have used to get there on a clear day. People were sliding all over the road. We just had to tell ourselves we wouldn't do any good if we didn't get there.

"When we did get to the scene, we had to be very careful parking so someone didn't hit us. A trooper and a fire engine were parked between our back door and the traffic. We were only at the scene for about five minutes when a car spun out of control and almost hit the trooper's car. Crazy.

"You don't have snow days in EMS like you had in school. That's for sure! C'mon, spring."

Obtain detailed maps of your service area. Hang one map in quarters, and place another in the ambulance. Even if you have GPS navigation, check the maps before you leave for a call. If you get lost while responding to a call, turn off your emergency lights and siren and pull over. Recheck the map and recheck the GPS. Call the EMD on the radio and obtain additional instructions.

Response Safety Summary

The following list summarizes important points about how to make a safe response.

- Minimize lights-and-siren "hot" responses. Remember: Driving with lights and siren involves high risk.
- Wear your seat belts.
- Know where you are going before you respond. Use GPS and check the maps. Be familiar with your response area.
- Come to a complete stop at intersections.
- Don't be a distracted driver. Have the crew leader operate the radio, siren, GPS, computer, and other devices.
- Don't eat or drink when responding under emergency conditions. Pay complete attention to the task at hand.
- Don't listen to music, text, talk on mobile phones, or indulge in any other distracting activities. Pay 100 percent attention to safe driving.

"I always wear my protective gear at a crash. When you get to the danger, it is too late to go back and put it on. Do it right the first time."

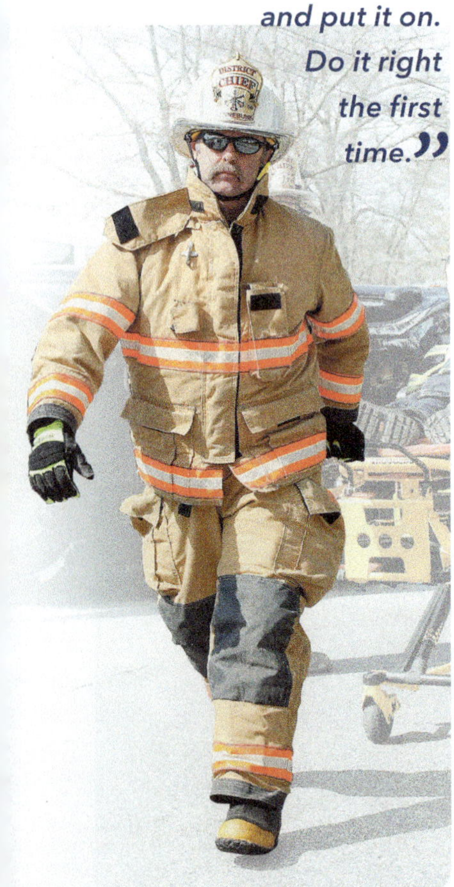

(© Daniel Limmer)

Safety at Highway Incidents

Operation at highway incidents exposes EMTs to significant danger. EMTs, firefighters, and police officers are injured and killed every year while operating at the scenes of highway incidents. The following are some tips for improving the safety of highway operations. (There will be a more thorough discussion of safety at highway incidents in the chapter *Highway Safety and Vehicle Extrication*.)

Keep Unnecessary Units and People off the Highway. If you are not the primary or first-arriving unit, stay off the highway. Park or stage your unit near the on-ramp until the first unit has sized up the incident and determined the resources needed. You don't want to expose people to any more risk than necessary when working on the highway. *The more vehicles and people gathered, the greater the risk.*

Avoid Crossovers Unless a Turn Can Be Completed without Obstructing Traffic. Crossovers on limited-access highways involve high risk. Consider avoiding this maneuver if possible. It may be safer to go to the next off-ramp and change directions on busy highways or during peak traffic hours.

Protect the Scene if Yours Is the First Unit On Scene. The first unit on scene blocks the incident by parking the apparatus in a manner that protects the incident. The apparatus is placed to block the crash from traffic by using the vehicle as a barrier. The best vehicle for this is a fire truck because of its size and weight. Ideally, ambulances should be parked in a safe loading area (Figure 38-3).

The EMT should conduct a scene size-up, then transmit an arrival report, canceling or requesting additional resources as needed. To avoid overcrowding the site, cancel any apparatus that is not needed. (*Remember: The more vehicles and people gathered, the greater the risk.*)

Wear Your PPE. If there is no extrication in progress, wear an ANSI-approved safety vest and a helmet. If extrication is indicated, then you should wear full turnout clothing. In these instances, EMS workers should match the level of protection being worn by the extrication personnel.

FIGURE 38-3 Park the ambulance properly at the scene of a collision.

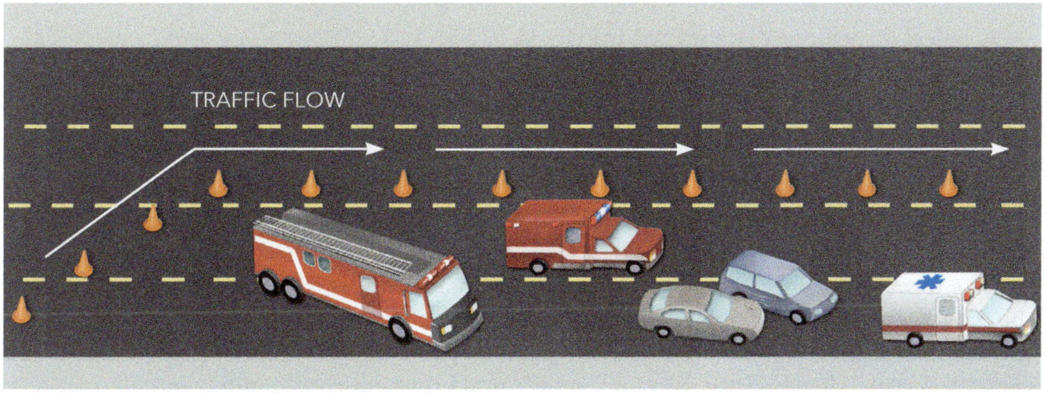

Place Cones/Flares and Reduce Emergency Lighting. Place cones/flares strategically to warn and direct traffic around the incident. Remember that response lights can blind approaching drivers and increase scene risks. Consider reducing emergency lighting to prevent blinding motorists. Avoid using flares if engine fluids or fuel is leaking nearby.

Unit Placement Is Important! Consider crash-scene preservation when placing apparatus. Avoid driving over debris and skid marks because the police consider these to be crime scene evidence. If extrication is necessary, leave room for placing rescue vehicles that will be needed to do the extrication. Prevent anyone from blocking the egress of ambulances, and try to keep all ambulances facing in the same direction.

Try to keep the ambulance on the same side of the road as the incident. It is very dangerous to carry stretchers across lanes of moving traffic. Do not have emergency personnel cross the road in traffic. (Review Figure 38-3).

Backing Up. As an operator of an emergency vehicle, you should avoid backing up, if possible, especially during emergencies. There are large blind spots in your mirrors and a danger of striking a pedestrian, an object, or another vehicle. If you must back up, position someone at the rear of the ambulance as a spotter to guide the backing process (Figure 38-4).

Transferring the Patient to the Ambulance

CORE CONCEPT
Transferring and transporting the patient

On most ambulance runs, you will be able to reach sick or injured people without difficulty, assess their condition, carry out emergency care procedures where they are lying, and transfer them to the ambulance. At times, however, dangers at the scene or the priority of patients will dictate moving a patient before assessment and emergency treatments can be completed.

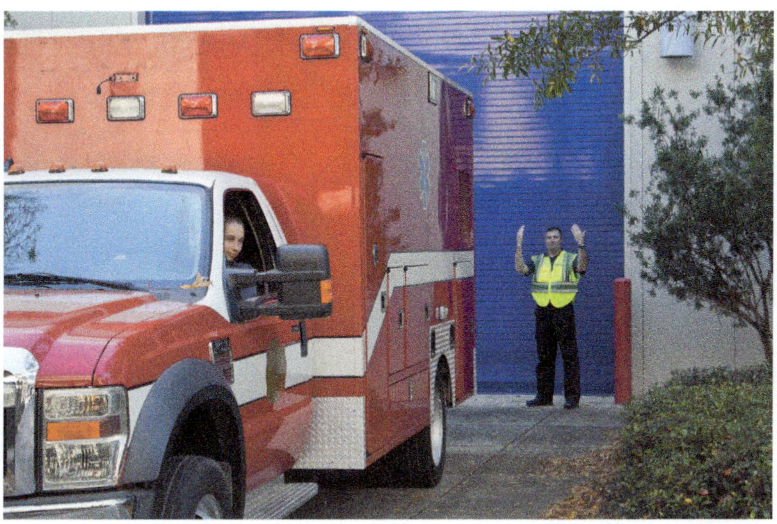

FIGURE 38-4 Use a spotter to help guide the ambulance when backing up. *(© Steve Salengo)*

Transfer to the ambulance is accomplished in four steps, regardless of the complexity of the operation:

1. Select the proper patient-carrying device.
2. Package the patient for transfer.
3. Move the patient to the ambulance.
4. Load the patient into the ambulance.

The wheeled ambulance stretcher is the most commonly used device for transferring the patient to the ambulance.

The term *packaging* refers to the sequence of operations required to ready the patient to be moved and to combine the patient and the patient-carrying device into a unit ready for transfer. A sick or injured patient must be packaged so the condition is not aggravated. You must complete all necessary care for wounds and other injuries, stabilize impaled objects, and check all dressings and splints before placing a patient on the patient-carrying device. The properly packaged patient is covered and secured to the patient-carrying device.

When packaging severely ill or injured patients, packaging is a balance between expedience and function. Patients should be firmly secured to transport devices and backboards so they will not fall or worsen their current condition in any way. Yet packaging must be done quickly and efficiently to get patients promptly and safely to the hospital.

Covering a patient helps to maintain body temperature, prevents exposure to the elements, and provides privacy (Figure 38-5). A single blanket, or perhaps just a sheet, may be all that is required in warm weather. A sheet with blankets should be used in cold weather. When practical, cuff the blankets under the patient's chin, with the top sheet outside. Do not leave sheets and blankets hanging loose. Tuck them under the mattress at the foot and sides of the stretcher. In wet weather, place a plastic cover over the blankets during transfer, removing it once you are in the ambulance, to prevent overheating. In cold or wet weather, cover the patient's head, leaving the face exposed.

A patient-carrying device should have a minimum of three straps for holding the patient securely. The first strap should be at the chest level, the second at hip or waist level, and the third on the lower extremities. Sometimes there is a fourth strap if two are crossed at the chest.

Some stretchers have straps that act as a harness and restrain the upper body (Figure 38-6). By combining over-the-shoulder straps with encircling straps, the patient is more securely held on the stretcher in the event of a collision. If your stretcher has this type of harness, make sure to use it each time. If you are involved in a collision and this type of restraint system is applied improperly, the EMS crew can be held responsible for the patient's injuries.

FIGURE 38-5 This patient is packaged for cold, wet conditions.

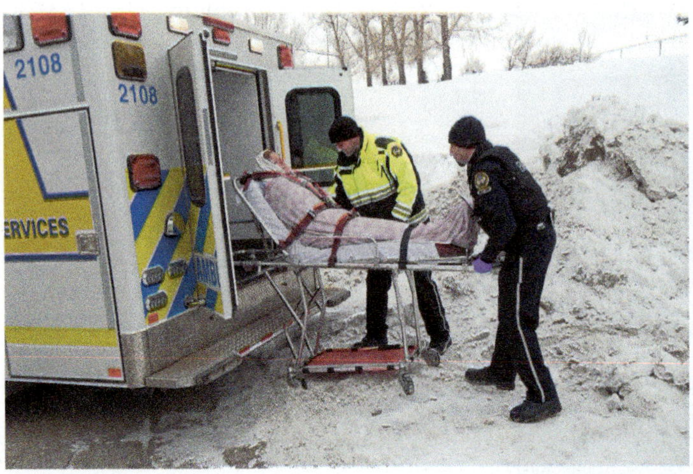

FIGURE 38-6 Stretcher straps that act as a harness secure and restrain the patient's upper body.

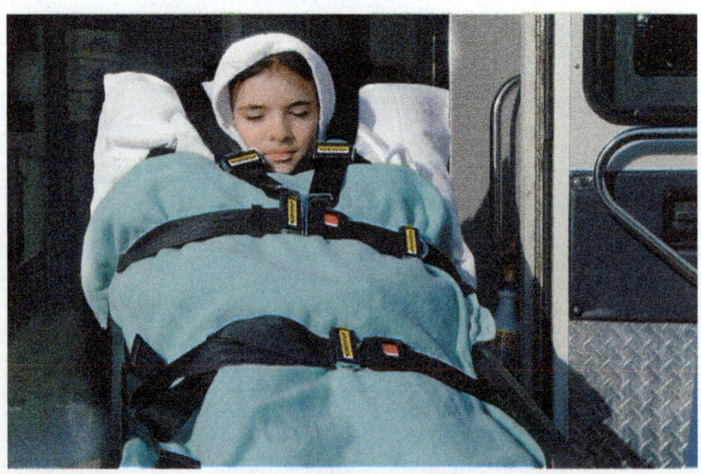

Think Like an EMT

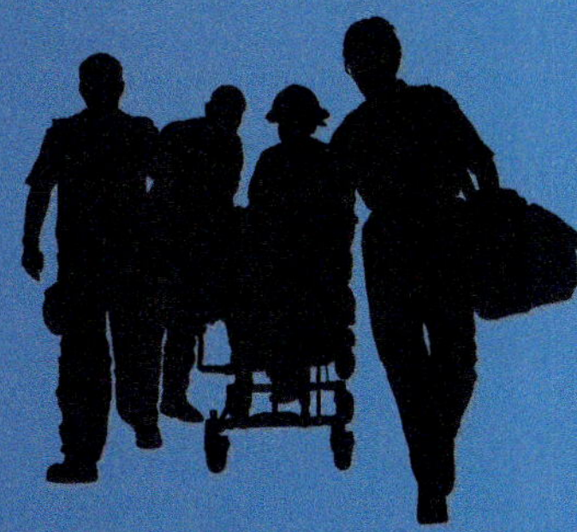

Arriving Safely

Although most of this text has discussed treating the patient at the scene, your response and vehicle placement are important aspects of your responsibilities at a call. Proper vehicle placement ensures that you and the vehicle are safe and that the vehicle's contents are available to you in a convenient location. For each of the following situations, explain where you would park the ambulance if you were first arriving:

1. You are called to a railroad car derailment.
2. You are called to a collision on the interstate. An engine company and trooper are parked at the scene, blocking oncoming traffic.
3. You are called to a scene involving domestic violence. Police are not yet on the scene.

All patients, including those receiving CPR, must be secured to the patient-carrying device before transfer to the ambulance. If your patient is not on a carrying device such as a spine board but instead is just on the ambulance stretcher, some states, as a matter of policy, require shoulder harnesses that secure the patient to the stretcher, to prevent sliding forward in case of a short stop.

Much has been said about protecting the patient from a possible ambulance collision, but the EMT in the patient compartment is actually at greater risk. The patient is secured to the stretcher and obtains some safety benefit from that. Most of the time, however, the EMT is unsecured and vulnerable in the event of a collision. When traveling in an ambulance, you should remain seated, wearing a seat belt or harness when possible. Although it isn't always possible to remain seated, avoid unnecessary movement during emergency response and transport.

Unsecured equipment turns into projectiles upon collision, threatening both the patient and EMT. Always ensure that all equipment in the patient compartment (e.g., oxygen cylinders, kits) has been secured.

Transporting the Patient to the Hospital

Transport involves more than just driving to the hospital. A series of tasks must be undertaken from the time a patient is loaded into the ambulance until the patient's care is transferred to hospital personnel.

Preparing the Patient for Transport

The following activities may be required to prepare patients for transport once they are in the ambulance:

- **Continue your assessment.** Make sure that conscious patients are breathing without difficulty once you have positioned them on the stretcher. Make sure that any patient unconscious with an airway in place has an adequate air exchange once in position for transport.
- **Secure the stretcher in place in the ambulance.** Always ensure that patients are safe during the trip to the hospital. Before closing the door, and certainly before signaling the ambulance operator to move, make sure that the cot is securely in place. Patient compartments are equipped with a locking device that prevents the wheeled

stretcher from moving about while the ambulance is in motion. Failure to engage the locking device fully at both ends of the stretcher can have disastrous consequences once the ambulance is in motion.

- **Position and secure the patient.** During transfer to the ambulance, patients must be firmly secured to a stretcher. This does not mean that patients must be transported in that position. Positioning in the ambulance should be dictated by the nature of the illness or injury.
  - If not transferred to the ambulance in that position, shift any unconscious patient who has no potential spine injury or a patient with an altered mental status into the recovery position (lying on one side). This will promote maintenance of an open airway and drainage of fluids.
  - Remember that the head and foot ends of the ambulance stretcher can be raised. Patients with breathing difficulty and no possibility of spinal injury may be more comfortable being transported in a sitting position.
  - Patients with a potential spinal injury must remain immobilized on the long spine board, with patient and board together being secured to the stretcher. If resuscitation is required, patients must remain supine, with constant monitoring of the airway and suctioning equipment ready. If resuscitation is not required, an unresponsive patient and spine board can be rotated as a unit and the board propped on the stretcher so the patient is on one side, allowing fluids and vomitus to drain from the mouth.
- **Adjust the security straps.** Security straps applied when patients are being prepared for transfer to the ambulance may tighten unnecessarily by the time they are loaded into the patient compartment. Adjust the straps so they still hold the patient safely in place but are not so tight that they interfere with circulation or respiration or cause pain.
- **Prepare for respiratory or cardiac complications.** If the patient is likely to develop cardiac arrest, position a short spine board or CPR board underneath the mattress prior to starting on the trip. Then, if arrest does occur, time will not be wasted locating and positioning the board. Riding on a hard board may not be comfortable, but temporary discomfort is better than permanent injury or even death from delayed resuscitation.
- **Loosen constricting clothing.** Clothing may interfere with circulation and breathing. Loosen ties and belts, and open any clothing around the neck. Straighten clothing that is bunched under safety straps. Remember that clothing bunched at the crotch may be painful. Before you do anything to rearrange the patient's clothing, however, explain what you are going to do and why.
- **Load a relative or friend who must accompany the patient.** Consider the following guidelines if your service does not prohibit the transport of a relative or friend with a patient: First, encourage the person to seek alternative transportation if available. If there is just no other way the relative or friend can get to the hospital, allow the person to ride in the operator's compartment—not in the patient's compartment where the relative or friend may interfere with patient care. Make certain the person buckles the seat belt. If an uninjured child must come along, bring the family's child car seat and use it.
- **Load personal effects.** If a purse, briefcase, overnight bag, or other personal item is to accompany the patient, make sure it is properly secured in the ambulance. If you load personal effects at the scene of a collision, be sure to tell a police officer what you are taking. Follow policies and fill out forms, if any, required by your local system for safeguarding personal effects.
- **Talk to your patient.** Apprehension often increases once a sick or injured person is loaded in an ambulance. The patient is held down by straps. is in a strange, confined space, and may be suddenly separated from family members and friends. Maintaining a conversation with the patient helps allay fears and concerns, builds patient rapport, and simply helps pass the time.

- **Avoid letting patients sit on the bench or airway seat.** Unless it's a multiple-casualty incident or there is some other extenuating circumstance, patients belong on the stretcher. Simply put, it's the safest place for them to be. If a patient suddenly becomes uncooperative and wants to jump out of a moving vehicle or assault the EMT, the stretcher and restraints will slow this down and might even avert a tragedy.

When you are satisfied that the patient is ready, signal the operator to begin the trip to the hospital. If this is a high-priority patient, most of the preparation steps—loosening clothing, checking bandages and splints, reassuring the patient, even vital signs—can be done en route rather than delaying transport.

Caring for the Patient en Route

Having at least one EMT in the patient compartment is considered minimum staffing for an ambulance, although having two is preferred. Seldom will you be able to merely ride along with your patient. You may have to undertake a number of activities en route:

- **Notify the hospital.** Most EMS services radio the hospital with a patient report.
- **Continue to provide emergency care as required.** If life support efforts were initiated prior to loading the patient into the ambulance, they must be continued during transport to the hospital. Maintain an open airway, resuscitate, administer to the patient's needs, provide emotional support, and do whatever else is required, including updating your findings from the primary patient assessment.
- **Use safe practices during transport.** In most cases, the patient packaging and preparation will be completed prior to loading. En route to the hospital, vitals may need to be repeated, the patient has to be tended to, and the hospital must be called on the radio. Remain seat-belted as much as possible. If a crash occurs, being belted improves your chances of survival and helps reduce injuries. Stow any unnecessary equipment, because equipment can become projectiles in a crash. Probably the most important safety consideration is this: *Is it really necessary to transport this patient with lights and siren on?* When you are running "hot," the chances of a crash significantly increase. In most EMS systems, true emergencies needing a "hot" ride to the hospital constitute less than 5 percent of all transports. Don't use lights and siren for the drive to the hospital unless it is a life-or-death situation!

Pediatric Note

Remember that a toy such as a teddy bear can do much to calm a frightened child. Many ambulance units carry a sanitized, soft or padded, brightly colored toy just for these occasions. It is difficult at best to get information from a young child whose parents have been injured and transported in another ambulance. Small children do not, as a rule, carry identification.

When transporting a child, remember that you are a complete stranger in a hostile environment. The collision scene, confusion, noise, injuries, possible pain, disappearance of a parent, EMTs caring for injuries, and attempts to gather information all create a terrifying experience for a child. The presence of a female EMT or female police officer may be helpful because sometimes young children feel more comfortable talking to a woman. A smile and a calm, reassuring tone of voice are things that cannot be learned from a textbook, yet they may be the most critical care needed by the frightened child.

- **Compile additional patient information.** If the patient is conscious, and emergency care efforts will not be compromised, record the patient information. Compiling information during the trip to the hospital serves two purposes. First, it allows you to complete your report. Second, supplying information temporarily refocuses the patient's mind away from current problems. Remember, however, that this is not an interrogation session. Ask your questions in a friendly yet professional manner.
- **Continue assessment and monitor vital signs.** Keep in mind that vital sign changes indicate a change in a patient's condition. For example, an unexplained increase in pulse rate may signify deepening shock. Record vital signs and be prepared to report changes to an emergency department staff member as soon as you reach the medical facility. Reassess vital signs every 5 minutes for an unstable patient, and every 15 minutes for a stable patient.
- **Notify the receiving facility.** Transmit patient assessment and management information. Provide your estimated time of arrival.

Transferring the Patient to the Emergency Department Staff

CORE CONCEPT

Transferring the patient to the emergency department staff

You should take the following steps to ensure that the patient transfer to the care of emergency department personnel is accomplished smoothly and without incident. Brief as it may be, the transfer is a crucial step during which your primary concern must be the continuation of patient-care activities. The steps of the transfer are illustrated in Scan 38-2.

- **In a routine admissions situation or when an illness or injury is not life-threatening, check first to see what is to be done with the patient.** If emergency department activity is particularly hectic, it might be better to leave your patient in the relative security and comfort of the ambulance while your operator determines where the patient is to be taken. Otherwise, the patient may be subjected to distressing sights and sounds and perhaps be in the way. (If you do leave the patient in the ambulance, make sure an EMT remains with the patient at all times.) *Under no circumstances should a nonemergency patient be wheeled into a hospital, placed in a bed, and left!* This is vital for you to remember. Unless you transfer care of your patient directly to a member of the hospital staff, you may be open to a charge of abandonment.

  Staff members may be treating other seriously ill and injured persons, so suppress any urge to demand attention for your patient. Simply continue emergency care measures until someone can assume responsibility for the patient. When properly directed, transfer the patient to a hospital stretcher.
- **Assist emergency department staff as required and provide a verbal report.** Stress any changes in the patient's condition that you have observed.
- **As soon as you are free from patient-care activities, prepare the prehospital care report.** Remember, the job is not over until the paperwork is complete. Find a quiet spot and complete your prehospital care report (PCR).
- **Transfer the patient's personal effects.** If a patient's valuables or other personal effects were entrusted to your care, transfer them to a responsible emergency department staff member. Some services have policies that involve obtaining a written receipt from emergency department personnel as protection from a charge of theft. Make sure to document any transfer of patient belongings.
- **Obtain your release from the hospital.** This task is not as formal as it sounds. Simply ask the emergency department nurse or physician if your services are still needed. In rural areas where not all hospital services are available, it may be necessary to transfer a seriously ill or injured person to another medical facility. If you leave and have to be recalled, the patient will lose valuable time.

SCAN 38-2 Transferring the Patient

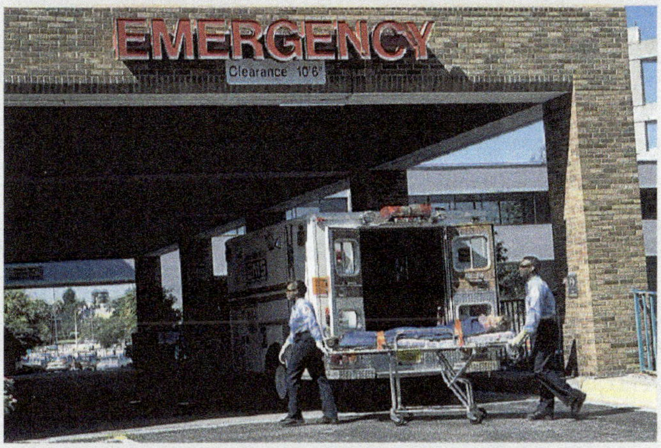

1. Transfer the patient as soon as possible. Stay with the patient until transfer is complete.

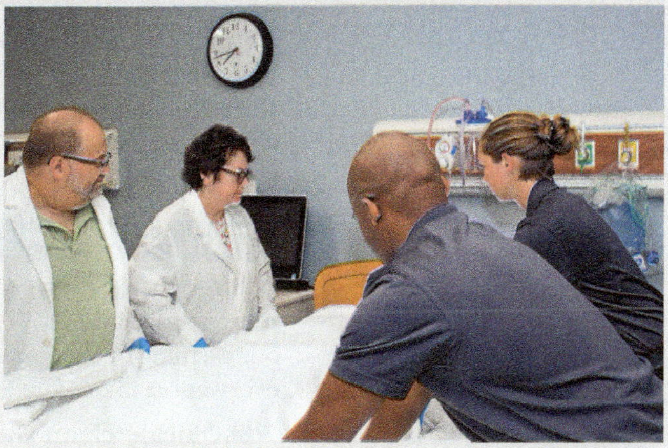

2. Assist the emergency department staff as required. *(© Steve Salengo)*

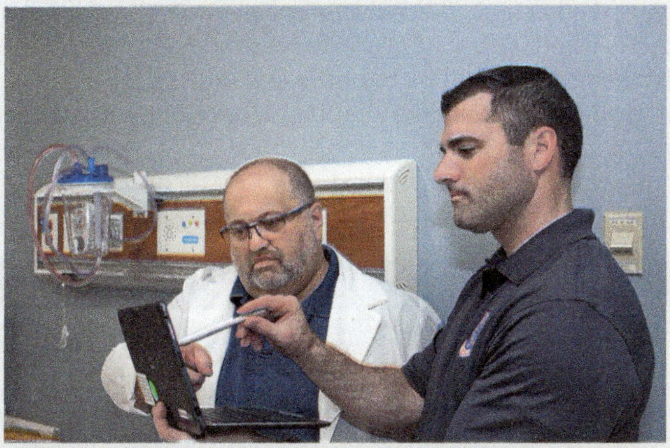

3. Provide a verbal report and a prehospital care report (PCR). *(© Steve Salengo)*

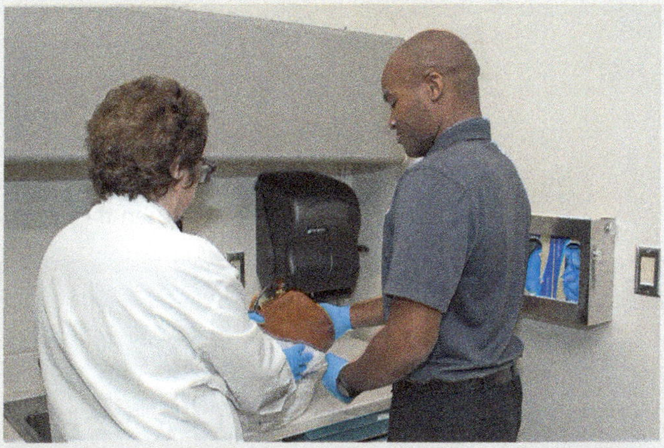

4. Transfer the patient's personal effects. *(© Steve Salengo)*

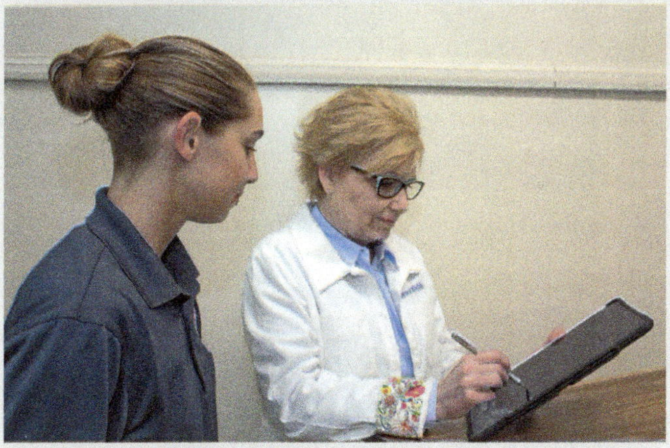

5. Obtain your release from the hospital (if applicable). Obtain any additional patient paperwork and signatures as required. *(© Steve Salengo)*

Terminating the Call

CORE CONCEPT
Terminating the call, replacing and exchanging equipment, and cleaning and disinfecting the unit and equipment

An ambulance run is not really over until the personnel and equipment that comprise the prehospital emergency care–delivery system are ready for the next response. The functions of EMTs in this final phase of activity include more than just changing the stretcher linen and cleaning the ambulance. A number of tasks must be accomplished at the hospital, during the return to quarters, and after arrival at the station.

At the Hospital

While still at the hospital, the ambulance crew should begin preparing the ambulance to respond to another call. Time, equipment, and space limitations sometimes preclude vigorous cleaning of the ambulance while it is parked at the hospital. However, you should make every effort to prepare the vehicle quickly for the next patient (Scan 38-3):

1. **Quickly clean the patient compartment while taking appropriate Standard Precautions.** Follow biohazard-disposal procedures according to your agency's OSHA exposure-control plan. Examples of biohazards are contaminated dressings and used suction catheters.
   - Clean up blood, vomitus, and other body fluids that may have soiled the floor. Wipe down any equipment that has been splashed. Place disposable towels used to clean up blood or body fluids directly into a red biohazard bag.
   - Remove and dispose of trash such as bandage wrappings, open but unused dressings, and similar items.
   - Sweep away caked dirt that may have been tracked into the patient compartment. When the weather is inclement, mop up water and mud from the floor.

SCAN 38-3 Activities at the Hospital

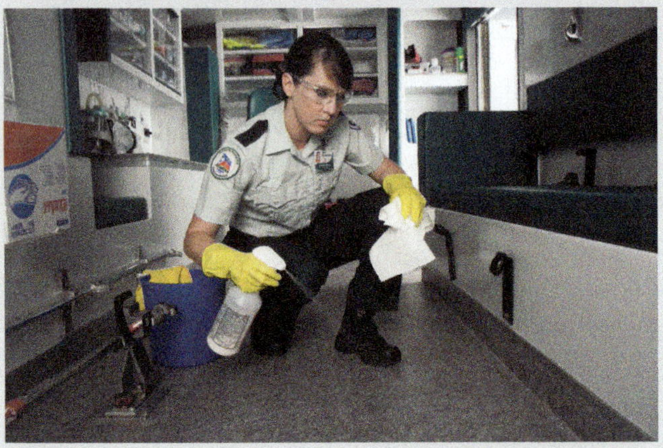

1. Clean the ambulance interior.

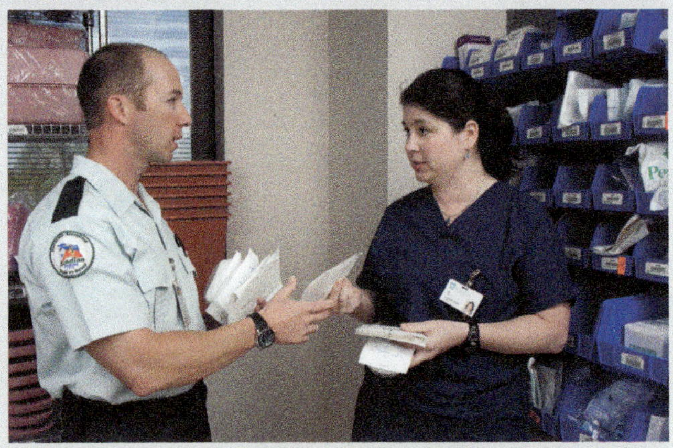

2. Replace disposable equipment per local protocols.

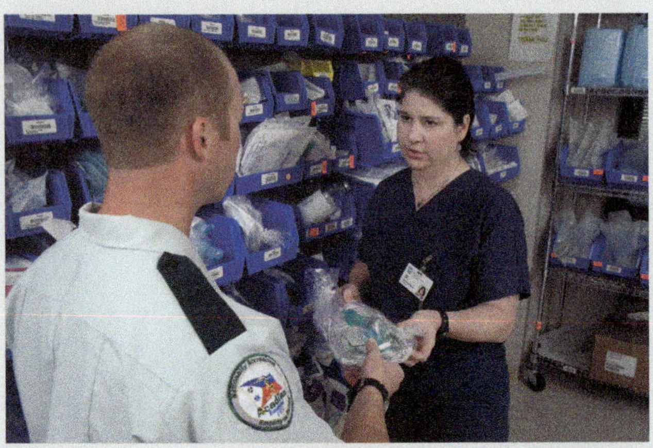

3. Replace airway equipment per local protocols.

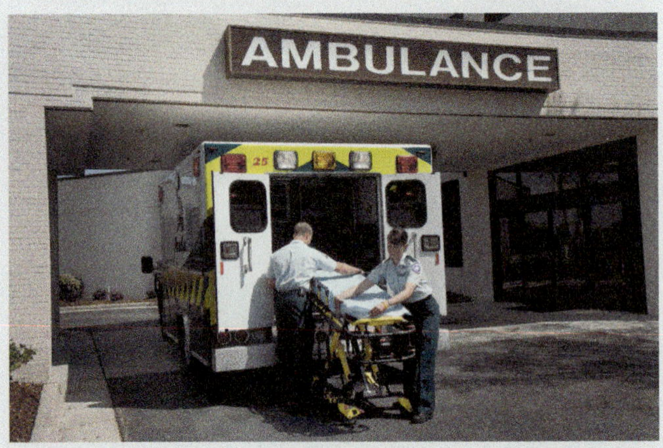

4. Clean and make up the ambulance stretcher with fresh linens.

- Bag dirty linens or blankets to be laundered.
- Use a deodorizer to neutralize odors of vomit, urine, and feces. Various sprays and concentrates are available for this purpose.

2. **Prepare respiratory equipment for service.**
   - Clean and properly disinfect nondisposable, reusable parts of respiratory-assist and inhalation-therapy devices to keep them from becoming reservoirs of infectious agents that could contaminate the next patient. Disinfect the suction unit.
   - Place used disposable items in a plastic bag and discard them. Replace with new disposable items.
3. **Replace expendable items.**
   - If you have a supply-replacement agreement with the hospital, replace used expendable items from hospital storerooms on a one-for-one basis—such as sterile dressings, bandaging materials, towels, disposable oxygen masks, disposable gloves, sterile water, and oral airways. Do not abuse this exchange program. Keep in mind that the constant abuse of a supply-replacement program usually leads to its discontinuation. At the very least, abuse places a strain on ambulance–hospital relations.
   - If your agency has its own stock-replacement policy, make sure to keep track of what has been used and what is needed upon return to the station.
4. **Exchange equipment according to your local policy.**
   - Exchange items such as splints and spine boards. Several benefits are associated with an equipment exchange program: Exchange of items eliminates the need to subject patients to injury-aggravating movements just to recover equipment. It allows crews not to be delayed at the hospital. It also enables ambulances to return to quarters fully equipped for the next response.
   - When equipment is available for exchange, quickly inspect it for completeness and operability. Parts are sometimes lost or broken when an immobilizing device is removed from a patient.
   - If you do find that a piece of equipment is broken or incomplete, notify someone in authority so that the device can be repaired or replaced.
5. **Make up the ambulance cot.** The following procedure is one of many that can be used to make up a wheeled ambulance stretcher:
   - Raise the stretcher to the high-level position if possible, to make the procedure easier. The stretcher should be flat, with the side rails lowered and straps unfastened.
   - Remove unsoiled blankets and pillows and place them on a clean surface.
   - Remove all soiled linen and place it in the designated receptacle.
   - Clean the mattress surface with an appropriate EPA-approved, low-level disinfectant unless there is visible blood. Blood should be cleaned up using a 1:100 bleach/water solution or a high-level disinfectant solution.
   - Center the bottom sheet on the mattress and open it fully. If a full-sized bedsheet is used, first fold it lengthwise before placing it on the stretcher.
   - Tuck the sheet under each end of the mattress; form square corners, and tuck them under each side.
   - Place a disposable pad, if one is used, on the center of the mattress.
   - Fully open the blanket. If a second blanket is used, open it fully and match it to the first blanket. This task should be done with an EMT at each end of the stretcher.
   - Open a top sheet in the same way, placing it on top of the blanket. Fold the blanket(s) and top sheet together lengthwise to match the width of the stretcher, folding one side first and then the other.
   - Tuck the foot of the folded blanket(s) and sheet under the foot of the mattress.
   - Tuck the head of the folded blanket(s) and sheet under the head of the mattress.
   - Place the slip-covered pillow lengthwise at the head of the mattress and secure it with a strap.
   - Buckle the safety straps and tuck in excess straps.
   - Raise the side rails.

NOTE: *A neatly prepared stretcher inspires confidence. Do not use stained linen, even though it might be clean. Always make the presentation of your stretcher a matter of personal and professional pride.*

The stretcher is now ready for the next patient. It must be reemphasized that this is one of many techniques for preparing a wheeled ambulance stretcher for service. Whatever the method, it should meet the following objectives:

- Prepare for the next call as soon and as quickly as possible.
- Store all linens, blankets, and pillows neatly on the stretcher.
- Fold or tuck all linens and blankets so they will be contained within the stretcher frame.
- Place the stretcher back into the ambulance.
- Replace any nondisposable patient-care items.
- Check for equipment left in the hospital.

En Route to Quarters

When heading back to quarters, your emphasis should be on a safe return. An ambulance operator might practice every suggestion for safe vehicle operation while en route to the hospital, then totally disregard those suggestions during the return to quarters. Defensive driving must be a full-time effort. Do not forget that the driver and all passengers must wear seat belts.

1. **Radio the EMD.** Let the EMD know that you are returning to quarters and that you are available (or not available) for service. Valuable time is lost if an EMD has to locate and alert a backup ambulance when the EMD does not know that a ready-for-service unit is on the road. Be sure that you notify the EMD if you stop and leave the ambulance unattended for any reason during the return to quarters.
2. **Air out the ambulance if necessary.** If the patient just delivered to the hospital has an airborne communicable disease, or if it was not possible to neutralize disagreeable odors while at the hospital, make the return trip with the windows of the patient compartment partially open, weather permitting. If the unit has sealed windows, use the air-conditioning or ventilating system (do not set on recirculate) to air out the patient compartment.
3. **Refuel the ambulance.** Local policy usually dictates the frequency with which an ambulance is refueled. Some services require the operator to refuel after each call regardless of the distance traveled. In other services, the policy is to refuel when the gauge reaches a certain level. At any rate, the fuel should be at such a level that the ambulance can respond to an emergency and get to the hospital without fear of running out of fuel.

In Quarters

When you return to quarters, a number of activities need to be completed before the ambulance is ready for another call and can be placed back in service (Scan 38-4).

With the emphasis today on protection from infectious diseases, you need to take every precaution to protect yourself. It is essential that you follow your agency's OSHA exposure-control plan. Always wear gloves when handling contaminated linen, cleaning the equipment, handling the respiratory equipment, and cleaning the ambulance interior. (There may be many hidden nooks and crannies where the patient's blood or body fluids could be gathered.)

Once in quarters, you are ready to complete the cleaning and disinfecting chores.

1. **Place contaminated linens in a biohazard container and noncontaminated linens in a regular hamper.**
2. **As necessary, clean any equipment that touched the patient.** Brush stretcher covers and other rubber, vinyl, and canvas materials clean; then wash them with soap and water.
3. **Clean and disinfect used nondisposable respiratory-assist and inhalation therapy equipment.**
   - Disassemble the equipment so all surfaces are exposed.
   - Fill a large plastic container with the cleaning solution outlined in your service's infection control plan.

SCAN 38-4 Terminating Activities in Quarters

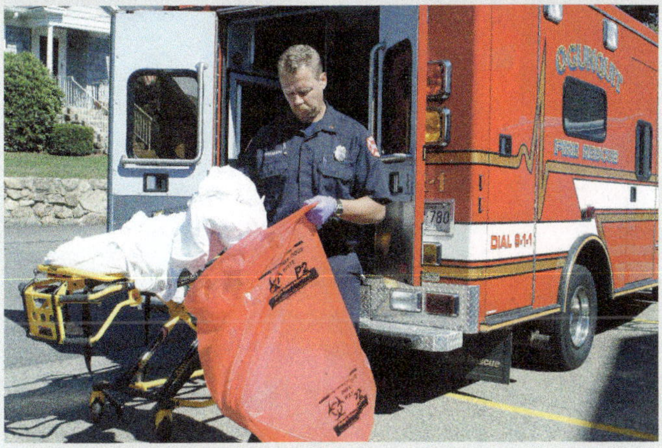

1. Place contaminated linens in a biohazard container, and noncontaminated linens in a regular hamper.

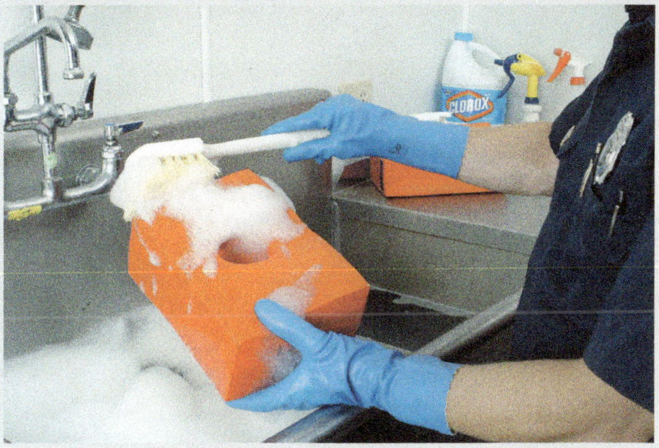

2. Remove and clean patient-care equipment as required.

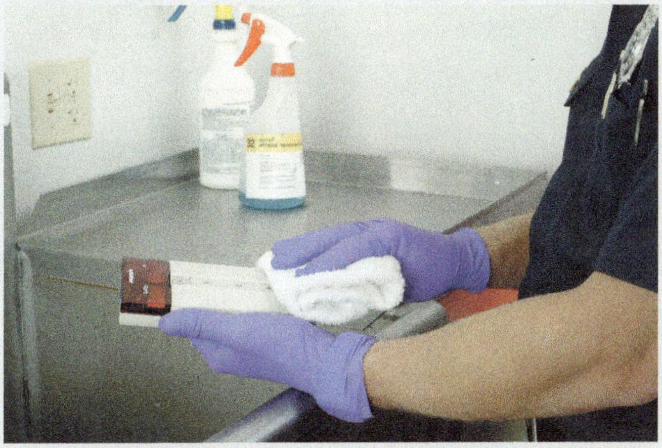

3. Clean and sanitize respiratory equipment as required.

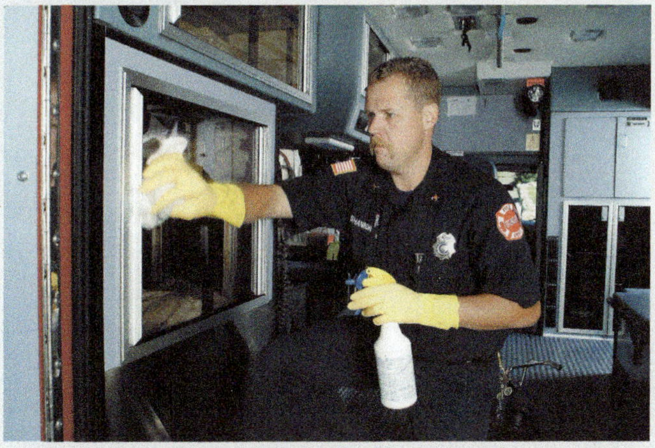

4. Clean and sanitize the ambulance interior as required. Use germicide on devices or surfaces that were in contact with blood or other body fluids.

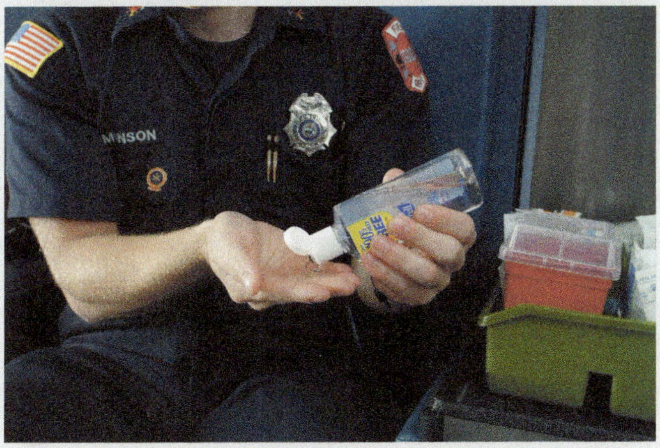

5. Sanitize your hands. Thoroughly wash with soap and water if available and change soiled clothing. Do this first if exposed to a communicable disease.

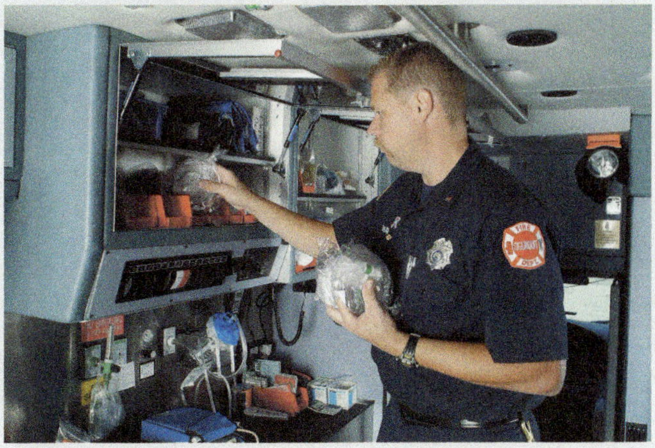

6. Replace expendable items as required.

(continued)

SCAN 38-4 Terminating Activities in Quarters (*continued*)

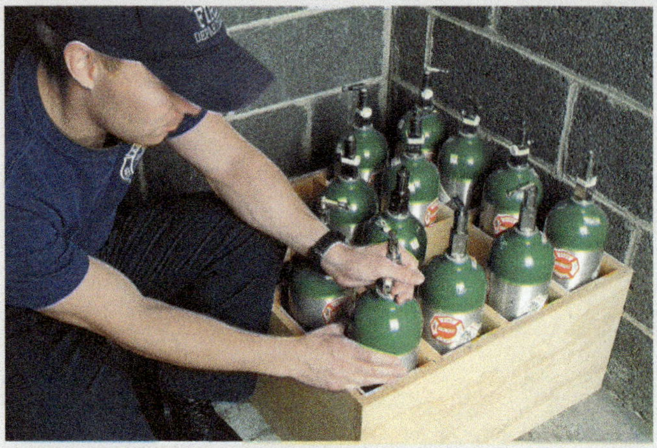

7. Replace oxygen cylinders as necessary.

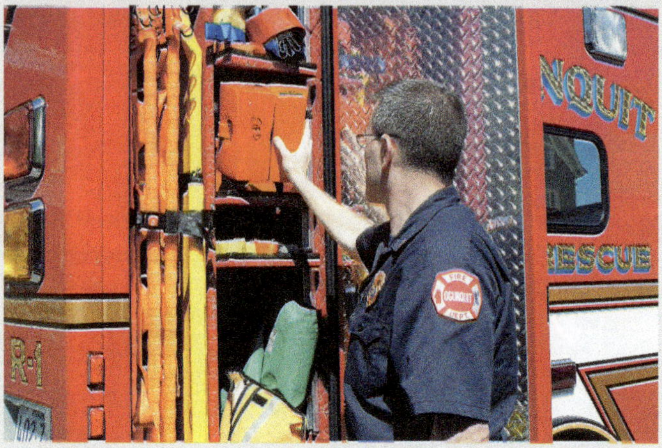

8. Replace patient-care equipment as needed.

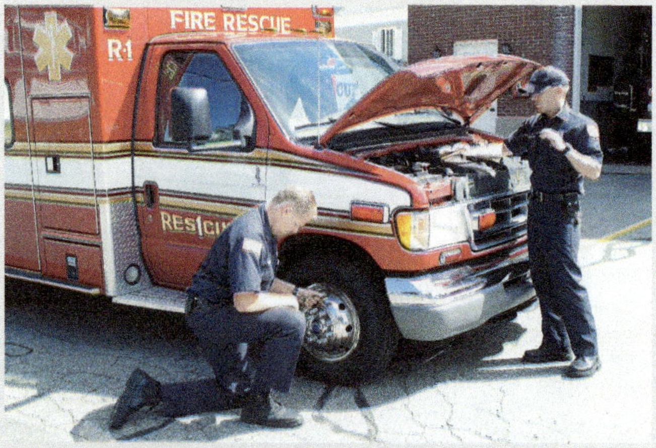

9. Maintain the ambulance as required. Report problems that will take the vehicle out of service.

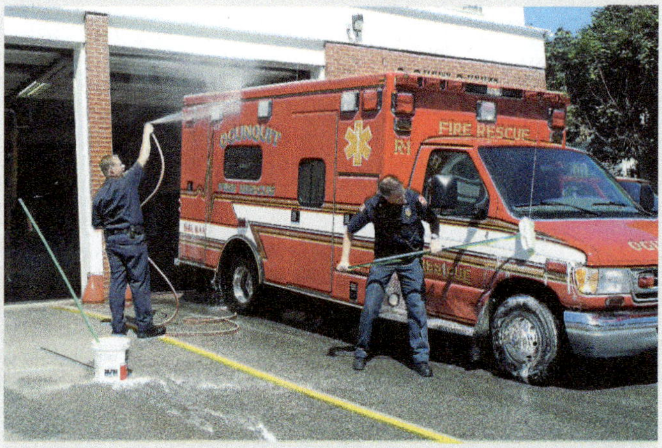

10. Clean the ambulance exterior as needed.

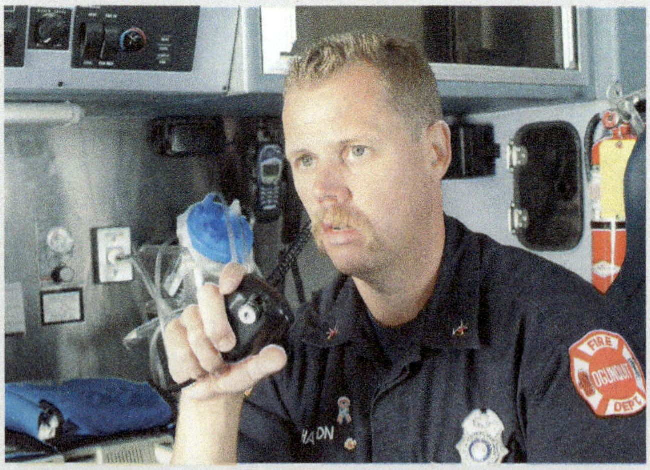

11. Report the unit ready for service.

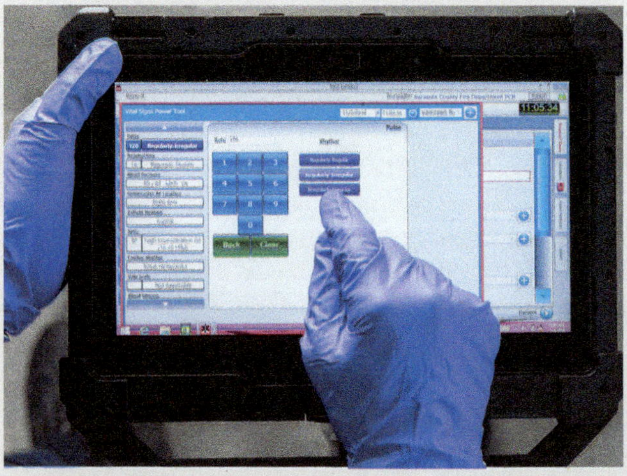

12. Complete any unfinished report forms as soon as possible.

- Clean the inner and outer surfaces with a suitable brush. Inner surfaces can be cleaned with a small bottle brush, whereas outer surfaces can be cleaned with a hand or nail brush. Make sure all encrusted matter is removed.
- Rinse the items with tap water.
- Soak the items in an EPA-approved germicidal solution. An inhalation therapist at a local hospital can suggest a germicide suitable for respiratory equipment.

Follow directions for dilution, safe handling, and soaking time. Gloves are recommended when using most germicides.
- After the prescribed soaking period, hang the equipment in a well-ventilated, clean area, and allow it to dry for 12–24 hours.

4. **Clean and sanitize the patient compartment.** Use an EPA-approved germicide to clean any fixed equipment or surfaces contacted by the patient's body fluids.
5. **Prepare yourself for service.**
   - Wash thoroughly, paying attention to the areas under your fingernails. Remember that contaminants can collect there and become a source of infection not only to you but also to the persons you touch.
   - Change soiled clothes. Clean contaminated clothing as soon as possible, especially if you were exposed to someone with a communicable disease. It is a good policy to bring a spare uniform to work, and each EMS agency should have a washer and dryer. It is against OSHA regulations for blood- or body fluid–soiled clothes to be taken home to be washed.
6. **Replace expendable items.** Exchange them with items from the unit's storeroom.
7. **Replace or refill oxygen cylinders.** Do this in accordance with your service's procedures.
8. **Replace patient-care equipment.**
9. **Carry out postoperation vehicle-maintenance procedures as required.** If you find something wrong with the vehicle, correct the problem or make someone in authority aware of it.
10. **Clean the vehicle.** A clean exterior lends a professional appearance to an ambulance. Check for broken lights, glass and body damage, door operation, and other parts that may need repair or replacement.
11. **Complete your paperwork.** Complete any unfinished report forms as soon as possible, and report the unit ready for service.

Air Rescue

In some circumstances, it is best for a patient to be transported by an air rescue helicopter (Figure 38-7) or fixed-wing aircraft. The following are some considerations for use of this kind of transport. Since geographic and other circumstances—as well as the availability of such transport—will vary in different localities, follow your local protocols.

CORE CONCEPT
When and how to use air rescue

When to Call for Air Rescue

Air rescue may be required for any of the following reasons:

- **Operational reasons.** Operational reasons for air rescue include: (1) to speed transport to a distant trauma center or other special facility, (2) when extrication of a high-priority patient is prolonged and air rescue can speed transport, and (3) when a patient must be rescued from a remote location that can be reached by helicopter only. Follow your local protocols.
- **Clinical reasons.** Medical reasons for air rescue primarily affect patients who are high-priority for rapid transport—for example, a patient:
  - In shock
  - With a Glasgow Coma Scale total of less than 10
  - With a head injury and altered mental status
  - With chest trauma and respiratory distress
  - With penetrating injuries to the body cavity
  - With an amputation proximal to the hand or foot
  - With extensive burns
  - With a serious mechanism of injury
  - Who is post–cardiac arrest with a pulse.

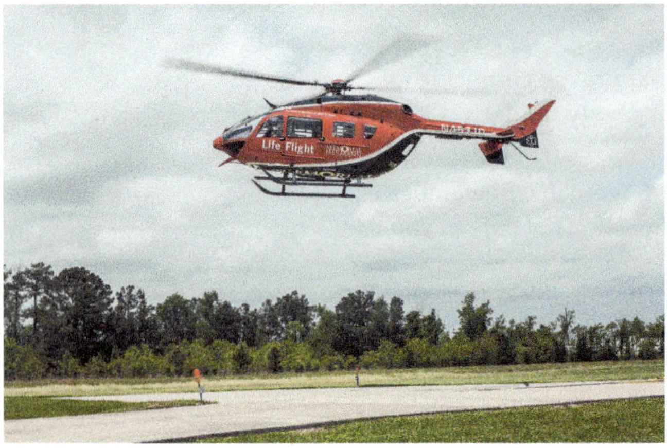

FIGURE 38-7 Patients are sometimes transported by air rescue helicopter.

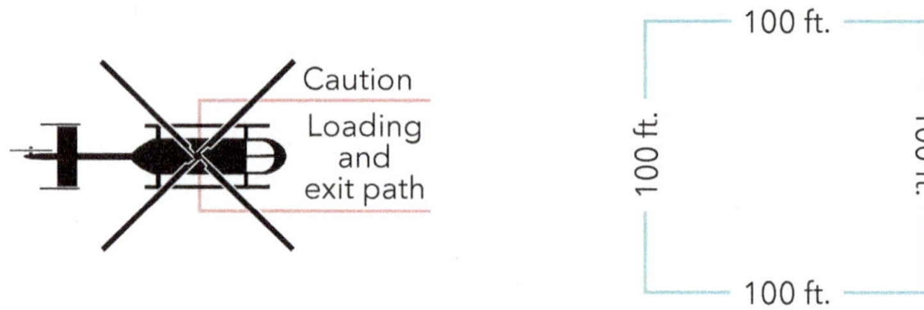

FIGURE 38-8 Helicopter landing zone.

Patients with certain medical conditions may also be flown by helicopter. Cardiac patients requiring catheterization or surgery, stroke patients, and those patients requiring hyperbaric oxygen treatment (e.g., after carbon monoxide poisoning) are examples of medical patients who may be flown by air. In many cases, you will transport these patients to your local hospital for stabilization, and the helicopter will transfer the patient from one hospital to another. Cardiac-arrest patients are usually not transported by air rescue unless they are hypothermic. Follow your local protocols.

How to Call for Air Rescue

In some areas, air rescue may be called for by any law enforcement, fire, or EMS command officer at the scene of an incident. In addition, as an EMT, you may radio dispatch or get medical direction for advice if you think such a service is needed. When calling an air rescue service, give your name and callback number; your agency name; the nature of the situation; the exact location, including crossroads and major landmarks; and the exact location of a safe landing zone. If you have the ability to provide GPS coordinates, provide them. Follow your local protocols.

How to Set up a Landing Zone

A helicopter requires a landing zone, or LZ, approximately 100 feet by 100 feet (approximately 30 large steps on each side [about 30 meters by 30 meters]) on ground that has a slope of less than 8 degrees. The landing zone and approach/departure path should be clear of wires, towers, vehicles, people, and loose objects (Figure 38-8). The landing zone should be marked with one flare in an upwind position. During night operations, *never* shine a light into the pilot's eyes during landing or takeoff, or while the aircraft is running on the ground. Also consider that some aeromedical systems extend the size of their landing zone (e.g., 125 feet by 125 feet [38 meters by 38 meters]). Keep emergency lights on. Many aeromedical services offer ground safety courses and landing zone coordinator training. Consider requesting assistance from law enforcement and fire agencies as needed.

Describe the landing zone to the air rescue service:

- **Terrain.** "The landing zone is located on top of a hill." "The landing zone is located in a valley."
- **Major landmarks.** "There is a river (major highway, factory, water tower) to the north (east, west, south) of the landing zone."
- **Estimated distance to nearest town.** "The landing zone is approximately 12 miles west of Centerville."
- **Other pertinent information.** "There are wires on the east side of the landing zone." "There is a deep ditch to the west." "Winds are out of the north–northeast at about 10 miles per hour."

How to Approach a Helicopter

Do not approach a helicopter unless escorted by the flight personnel. Allow the helicopter crew to direct the loading of the patient. Stay clear of the tail rotor at all times. Keep all traffic and vehicles 100 feet (30 meters) or more distant from the helicopter. Do not smoke within 200 feet (60 meters) of the aircraft. Be aware of the danger areas around helicopters, as shown in Scan 38-5. *Never* walk around the tail rotor area.

SCAN 38-5 Danger Areas Around Helicopters

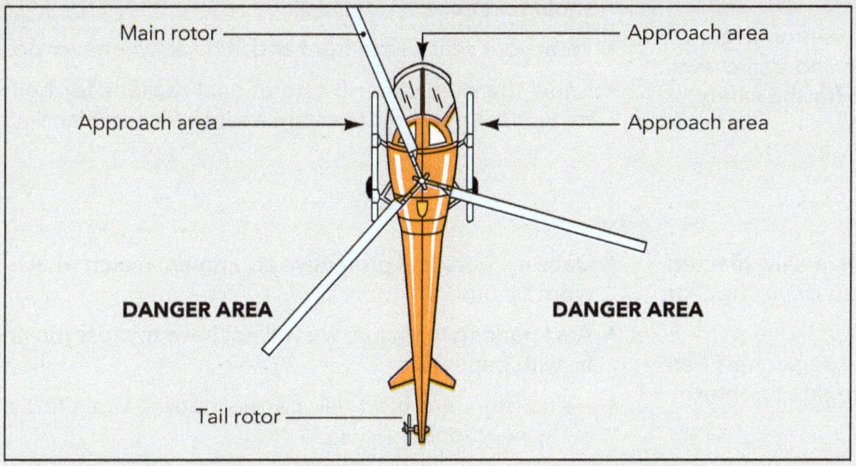

(A)

A. The area around the tail rotor is extremely dangerous. A spinning rotor cannot be seen.

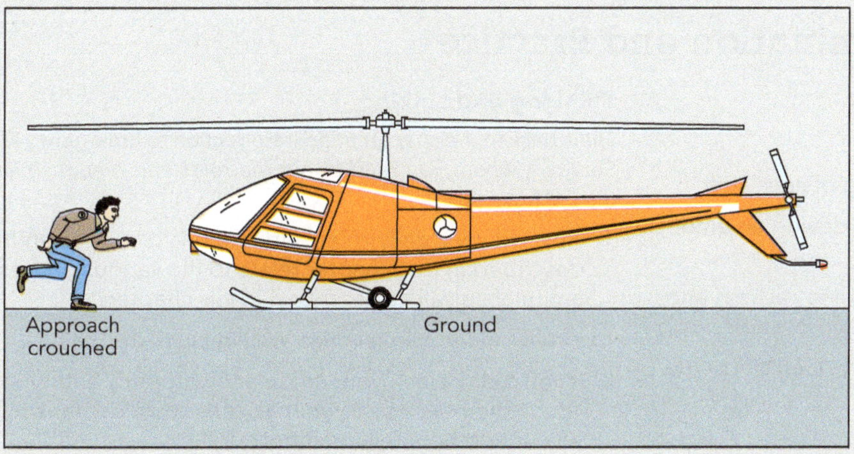

(B)

B. A sudden gust of wind can cause the main rotor of a helicopter to dip to a point as close as 4 feet (1.2 meters) from the ground. Always approach a helicopter in a crouch when the rotor is moving.

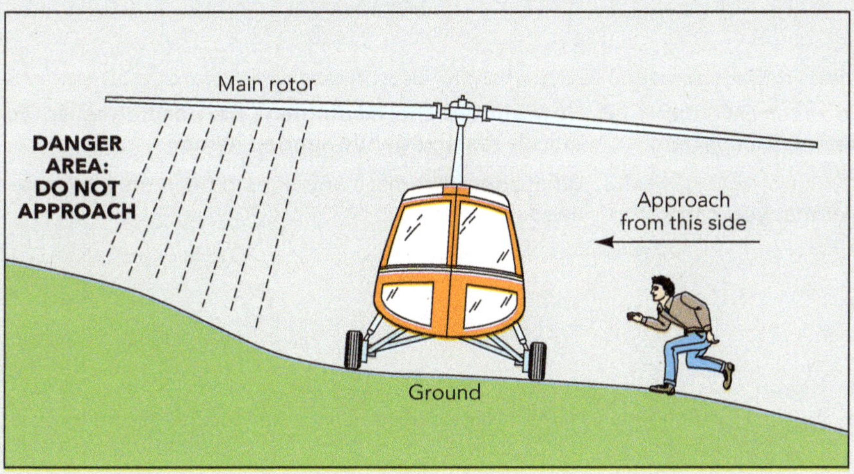

(C)

C. Approach the aircraft from the downhill side when a helicopter is parked on a hillside.

Chapter Review

Key Facts and Concepts

- Inspect the vehicle to ensure it is complete and critical items can be easily located.
- A "hot" response means using lights and siren. Hot responses involve high risk. A "cold" response means no lights or siren. Cold responses decrease risk.
- The laws in most states allow the driver of an emergency vehicle running "hot" to break some vehicle and traffic laws. However, it must be done with due regard for the safety of others.
- Pay attention! Do not text, make phone calls, drink beverages, or be in any way distracted while driving.
- Secure all gear. It can become a projectile in a crash!
- Don't let your patient become a projectile. Use the stretcher shoulder straps.
- Wear your seat belt in front and in back (whenever possible).
- Know the medical and operational reasons for helicopter transport. Know how to set up a safe helicopter landing zone.

Key Decisions

- Does this patient have a true emergency adversely affected by time? How will this affect my decision to drive "hot" or "cold" to the hospital?
- How can I park to best protect the scene and personnel? Can I create a safe zone from traffic? Is the scene safe to enter?
- Does my personal protective equipment match what is being worn by others?
- Am I parking to ensure we will not have to cross moving traffic with patients?
- Helicopters are high-risk transportation. Does this patient really need one?

Preparation for Your Examination and Practice

Short Answer

1. List the five phases of an ambulance call.
2. List activities you perform at the beginning of each shift.
3. List three ways to prevent collisions when driving an emergency vehicle.
4. What types of stretcher straps are essential to restrain and prevent a patient from becoming a projectile in a collision?
5. Describe the steps that should be followed when air rescue is required.

Thinking and Linking

Think back to the chapter titled Introduction to Emergency Medical Services, *where you read about the roles and responsibilities of the EMT.*

1. How do your daily roles and responsibilities as an EMT as described in that chapter relate to the various phases of an ambulance call as described in this chapter?

Think back to the chapter titled Well-Being of the EMT.

2. If you didn't clean your ambulance properly and blood was left on the bench seat, what disease could be transmitted to you or another crew member?

Critical Thinking Exercises

Organizing your equipment is a key part of your job as an EMT. The purpose of this exercise will be to consider how best to manage the equipment you will need at the emergency scene.

1. What equipment should you include in a kit that you carry to the scene?
2. How should the equipment be positioned so you can quickly reach urgently needed items?
3. What special items, if any, should be in the kit to meet local needs?

Street Scenes

You receive a Priority 1 call. "Ambulance 19, respond to 1901 Greentop Road for a report of a cardiac arrest." You acknowledge, get into the ambulance, and buckle up. Your partner does the same and turns on the red lights and siren. The dispatcher tells you that there is no additional information from the caller and you will be the first unit to arrive. You know it will be a long response because the call is at the far end of your district, and you feel pressured to hurry. As you approach an intersection, your partner changes the siren from wail to yelp and goes through without slowing down. "That light was red," you tell him. He doesn't respond, and keeps driving at the same speed. When he starts to weave through traffic, you suggest an alternative route to avoid the approaching rush hour congestion.

Street Scene Questions

1. When operating an ambulance using the red lights and siren, what precautions do you need to take?
2. How can speed affect the safety of ambulance operation?
3. What driving techniques might be used to make driving to this scene safer?

All of a sudden, a car comes out of a driveway and into your path. Your partner hits the brakes, performs an evasive move, and just misses the other vehicle. You notice that a box of tissues and a stethoscope landed on the floor in the patient compartment. "What would have happened if I had been back there with a patient?" you ask. Your partner finally realizes he is driving too fast and slows down. At the next intersection, he slows down even more and makes sure that traffic has come to a stop before going through. During the rest of the response, you focus on preparing for your arrival on the scene.

You have decided to load all your equipment on the stretcher and wheel it to the front door as soon as the ambulance is parked. As you pull up to the scene, your partner finds a good spot to park where the ambulance will not create a hazard. He leaves the warning lights on for visibility.

Your patient is in his bedroom, sitting on his bed, and greets you as you approach. You immediately ask him why EMS was called. "My wife called because I passed out. It's happened before but my doctor isn't sure what causes it." Your partner radios dispatch that the patient is alert and that another unit is not needed. You assess the patient, obtain a patient history, and get a set of vital signs. The patient is alert and oriented, his pulse is 82 with a blood pressure of 130/82, respirations are 20, and skin is unremarkable. The patient says that he takes a medication because his cholesterol is "way up there." The patient's wife reports that he was sitting in a chair and slumped over. She did not see any seizure activity. He did not respond to verbal stimulus, so she moved him to the floor. He regained consciousness within 2 minutes.

Street Scene Questions

4. What should you do first for patient care?
5. What information should you provide to the dispatcher?

The patient consents to transport to the hospital for further evaluation. You move him by stair chair from the bedroom to the stretcher. You place the patient on the stretcher and fasten all the safety straps. You place the stretcher into the ambulance compartment and, after it is in the bracket, you recheck to make sure it is properly secured. Your partner puts the stair chair away in its compartment and asks what the priority is to the hospital. "Priority 2," you answer. "Based on the assessment, there is no need to use the red light and siren."

39

Hazardous Materials, Multiple-Casualty Incidents, and Incident Management

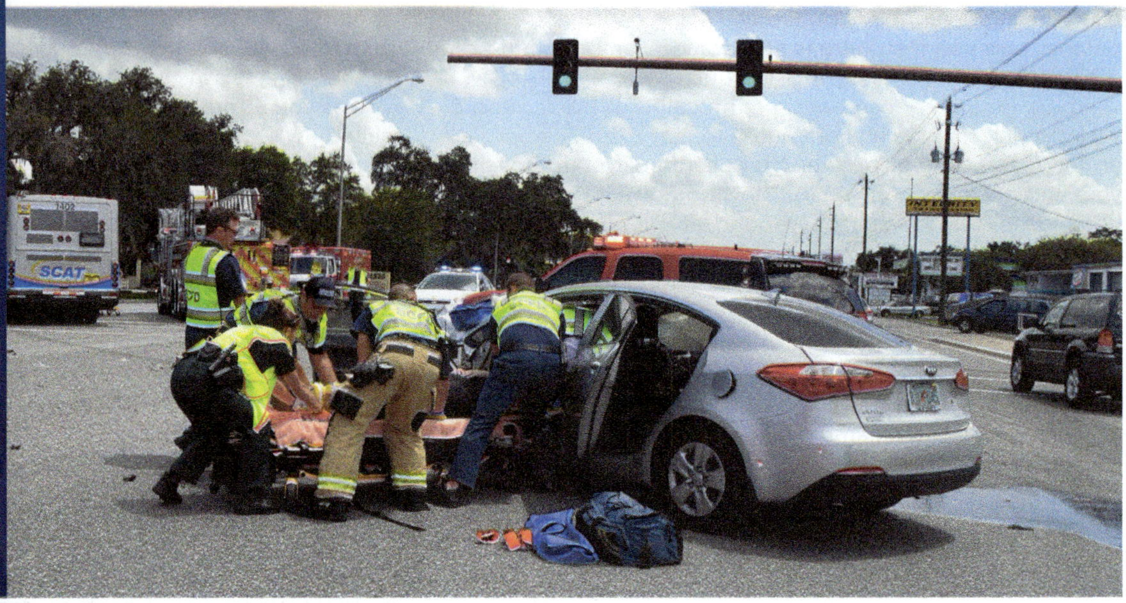

(© Ed Effron)

Related Chapters

The following chapters provide additional information related to topics discussed in this chapter:

Standard

EMS Operations (Incident Management; Multiple-Casualty Incidents; Hazardous Materials)

Competency

Applies knowledge of operational roles and responsibilities to ensure patient, public, and personnel safety.

Core Concepts

- How to identify and take appropriate action in a hazardous materials incident
- How to identify a multiple-casualty incident
- The Incident Command System
- Triage considerations

- Transportation and staging logistics
- Psychological aspects of multiple-casualty incidents

Outcomes

After reading this chapter, you should be able to:

39.1 Summarize concepts related to hazardous materials. (pp. 1178–1180)

- Describe the features of a hazardous material.
- Compare the federal legislation guiding the regulation of hazardous materials and the response to hazardous materials incidents.
- Explain the potential for hazardous materials incidents.
- Compare levels of hazardous materials training with the responsibilities for response at the scene of a hazardous materials incident.

39.2 Summarize the EMT's responsibilities with respect to hazardous materials incident scene management. (pp. 1180–1186)

- Recognize indications of a potential hazardous materials incident.
- Explain the process of controlling the scene.
- Identify ways an EMT can identify the substance involved in a hazardous materials incident.
- Explain the information a first-arriving EMT team at a hazardous materials incident will need to provide to a resource agency to get advice.

39.3 Summarize the EMT's roles in the treatment of others at the scene of a hazardous materials incidents. (pp. 1186–1192)

- Describe the process of rehabilitation operations.
- Describe the process of caring for injured and contaminated patients.
- Describe the processes for decontamination.

39.4 Summarize concepts related to multiple-casualty incidents. (pp. 1192–1199)

- Identify the primary feature that makes an event a multiple-casualty incident.
- Recognize the desirable characteristics of a disaster plan.
- Explain situations that have an increased likelihood of creating a mass-casualty incident.
- Identify ways for increasing the effectiveness of response to mass-casualty incidents.
- Outline the Incident Command System (ICS) structure and functions.
- Describe how to set up Incident Command if your ambulance is first on the scene at a multiple-casualty incident.
- Explain the potential psychological impacts on multiple-casualty incident (MCI) survivors and responders.

39.5 Summarize the EMS branch functions within the ICS structure. (pp. 1200–1210)

- Apply triage criteria to a variety of MCI patient portrayals.
- Outline the selection of triaged patients for secondary triage and treatment.

- Identify the relationship between the staging area and transport area at an MCI.
- Recognize the role of the staging and transportation supervisors in maintaining an organized approach to the MCI.
- Compare communication with hospitals in an MCI with routine EMS communication with hospitals.

Key Terms

cold zone, *1181*

Command, *1194*

decontamination, *1188*

disaster plan, *1192*

hazardous material (HAZMAT), *1178*

hot zone, *1181*

Incident Command, *1195*

Incident Command System (ICS), *1194*

multiple-casualty incident (MCI), *1192*

National Incident Management System (NIMS), *1194*

single incident command, *1195*

staging area, *1209*

staging supervisor, *1209*

surge capacity, *1210*

transportation supervisor, *1209*

treatment area, *1209*

treatment supervisor, *1209*

triage, *1201*

triage area, *1209*

triage supervisor, *1201*

triage tag, *1205*

unified command, *1195*

warm zone, *1181*

You have already learned how to deal with many situations in which an individual patient needs emergency care. However, you also need to know what to do if you are called to the scene of an explosion, an airline crash, a multiple-vehicle pileup, an earthquake, the aftermath of a tornado, or some other situation in which there are many known or potential patients. Although you are not trained to deal with all the complexities of such emergencies, you must be able to recognize them and call for the appropriate assistance. This chapter offers the essentials that every EMT should know about special operations involving multiple patients and/or hazardous materials.

Hazardous Materials

CORE CONCEPT

How to identify and take appropriate action in a hazardous materials incident

Hazardous materials (HAZMATs) are everywhere, and EMS frequently responds to incidents involving them. Because many incidents begin as routine EMS calls, it will be up to you to recognize a HAZMAT situation early, call in the appropriate resources, be familiar with your local plan for management of a hazardous material incident, and understand your role in such an incident. Understanding your role in a HAZMAT incident will help you be much more effective as well as assist you in maintaining a safe response action for all personnel involved.

According to the U.S. Department of Transportation (DOT), a ***hazardous material (HAZMAT)*** is "any substance or material in a form which poses an unreasonable risk to health, safety, and property when transported in commerce." Hazardous materials may also be found in storage areas both in large venues (warehouses) and small venues (residential homes). One of the undesirable aspects of our modern world is the growing number of such materials (Table 39-1). The DOT estimates that over 800,000 HAZMAT shipments occur daily in the United States. Hazardous materials are used for the manufacture of products and can also be the waste products of manufacturing. Even though safety procedures have been established and are followed for the most part, accidents involving hazardous materials do occur. Hazardous material incidents are especially likely to take place at factories, along railroads, and on local, state, and federal highways.

hazardous material (HAZMAT) any substance or material in a form that poses an unreasonable risk to health, safety, and property when transported in commerce or kept in storage at a warehouse, port, depot, or railroad facility.

TABLE 39-1 Examples of Hazardous Materials

MATERIAL	POSSIBLE HAZARD
Benzene (benzol)	Toxic vapors; can be absorbed through the skin; destroys bone marrow
Benzoyl peroxide	Fire and explosion
Carbon tetrachloride	Damages internal organs
Cyclohexane	Explosive; eye and throat irritant
Diethyl ether	Flammable and can be explosive; irritant to eyes and respiratory tract; can cause drowsiness or unconsciousness
Ethyl acetate	Irritates eyes and respiratory tract
Ethylene chloride	Damages eyes
Ethylene dichloride	Strong irritant
Heptane	Respiratory irritant
Hydrochloric acid	Respiratory irritant; exposure to high concentration of vapors can produce pulmonary edema; can damage skin and eyes
Hydrogen cyanide	Highly flammable; toxic through inhalation or absorption
Methyl isobutyl ketone	Irritates eyes and mucous membranes
Nitric acid	Produces a toxic gas (nitrogen dioxide); skin irritant; can cause self-ignition of cellulose products (e.g., sawdust)
Organochlorides (e.g., chlordane, DDT, dieldrin, lindane, methoxychlor)	Irritates eyes and skin; fumes and smoke toxic
Perchloroethylene	Toxic if inhaled or swallowed
Silicon tetrachloride	Water-reactive to form toxic hydrogen chloride fumes
Tetrahydrofuran (THF)	Damages eyes and mucous membranes
Toluol (toluene)	Toxic vapors; can cause organ damage
Vinyl chloride	Flammable and explosive; listed as a carcinogen

As an EMT, you will be highly skilled in emergency care. However, without specialized training, you are essentially a layperson when it comes to hazardous materials. Special training is required to understand HAZMATs, to work at the scene of incidents involving these materials, and to render the scene safe. You cannot judge the state of a container or the probability of explosion without the benefit of such training. Do not assume that you can use safety equipment unless you are trained in the care, field testing, and use of the equipment. With HAZMAT incidents, you may be able to do nothing more than stay a safe distance away from the scene until expert help arrives. That may seem counterintuitive, but you cannot care for those affected by the incident if you are not kept safe.

Training Required by Law

Two federal agencies—the Occupational Safety and Health Administration (OSHA) and the Environmental Protection Agency (EPA)—have developed regulations to deal with the increasing frequency of HAZMAT emergencies. These regulations are meant to enhance the knowledge, skills, and safety of emergency response personnel, as well as to bring about a more effective response to HAZMAT emergencies. The regulations are described in the OSHA publication *29 CFR 1910.120—Hazard Communication Standard (2012)*. This replaces the previous standard, which had been adopted in 1994. (CFR stands for "Code of Federal Regulations.")

This chapter provides an introduction to the elements found in the revised *CFR 1910.120 Hazard Communication Standard*.

According to the regulations, employers are responsible for determining, providing, and documenting the appropriate level of training for each employee. Training is required for "all employees who participate, or who are expected to participate, in emergency response to hazardous substance accidents." When you work for an emergency response agency, expect to participate in and be held to these training standards. Take time to learn as much as you can via continuing education and mandatory in-service sessions, as hazardous materials constantly change. It is a very dynamic environment.

OSHA's Hazardous Waste Operations and Emergency Response (HAZWOPER) standards identify five levels of training:

1. **First Responder Awareness.** Rescuers at this level are likely to witness or discover a hazardous-substance release. They are trained only to recognize the problem and initiate a response from the proper organizations.
2. **First Responder Operations.** This level of training is for those who initially respond to releases or potential releases of hazardous materials to protect people, property, and the environment. They stay at a safe distance, keep the incident from spreading, and protect others from any exposures.
3. **Hazardous Materials Technician.** This level is for rescuers who actually plug, patch, or stop the release of a hazardous material. A minimum number of hours of training is required.
4. **Hazardous Materials Specialist.** This level of rescuer is expected to have a more directed or specific knowledge of the various substances that the rescuer may be called upon to contain. This role allows the specialist to act as a site liaison with federal, state, local, and other government authorities with regard to site activities.
5. **On-Scene Incident Commander.** This level of rescuer implements the Incident Command System (ICS) and all applicable emergency response plans to control and manage a HAZMAT incident.

Most of the training levels outlined by OSHA have a fire service focus. EMS responders should be trained to the awareness level and perhaps the operations level but in different skills. Responding to this difference, the National Fire Protection Association has published Standard #473, which deals with competencies for EMS personnel at hazardous material incidents.

Regardless of agency affiliation, as an EMT, you play an important role. You are usually among the first on the scene for all types of HAZMAT calls. Your initial decisions and actions lay crucial groundwork for the remainder of the incident; this is a great deal of responsibility. Maintaining proficiency with hazardous materials in your specific response role is very important.

Responsibilities of the EMT

Your responsibilities as an EMT at a hazardous material incident include recognizing that a HAZMAT incident exists, calling in appropriate resources, controlling the scene, and identifying the substance.

Recognize a HAZMAT Incident

Whether HAZMAT incidents are very obvious or very subtle, you must quickly recognize one for what it is. It helps to be aware of the locations where HAZMATs are likely. These include highways where incidents involve common carriers, trucking terminals, chemical plants or places where chemicals are used, on delivery trucks, agriculture and garden centers, railways, and laboratories. Don't get caught by surprise by not being aware during your response. The EMT can be the key early communicator of a hazardous material incident.

Every community has chemical hazards. Identification starts with awareness and knowledge of what exists in the community. Spend some time with local police and fire agencies and learn about or develop preincident plans for common hazardous materials.

Local emergency management agencies often have joint hazardous material training sessions and exercises. Take time to participate in these types of sessions and learn how to work with other public safety providers.

When you arrive at a potential incident as an EMT, you must restrain your natural impulse to take action. Never assume the scene is safe. After the initial patients, EMTs are the most likely to become injured or killed because they tend to quickly react. Therefore, assess the situation first. Take a command position and stay a safe distance from the site before you take action. Once a HAZMAT is recognized, only those personnel trained to the technician level and equipped with the proper personal protective equipment should enter the immediate site. All patients leaving the site of the incident should be considered contaminated until proven otherwise. It may be your responsibility as the EMT to assist in guaranteeing that any patient to be transported to a medical facility is thoroughly decontaminated. This is important, as a contaminated patient could contaminate and shut down an ambulance or even an emergency room.

Control the Scene

Your primary concerns at the scene of a hazardous material incident are your safety and the safety of your crew, the patient, and the public. If you arrive first at the scene of a HAZMAT incident, establish a "danger zone" and a "safe zone." Keep all people out of the danger zone and try to convince them to leave the immediate area. Stay in the safe zone until expert help arrives and makes other areas safe to enter. Advise the subsequent responding units of the dangers you have observed as they arrive after you.

The safe zone should be on the same level as and upwind from the incident site. Avoid being downhill, in case there are flowing liquids or gases that are burning or otherwise unsafe. Avoid low-lying areas, in case fumes are escaping and hanging close to the ground. Avoid being downwind of the scene, so you will not be in the path of escaping gases or heated air. Also be aware that a sewer system can rapidly spread hazardous materials over a large area. Having public utilities agencies on the scene can be a substantial help to emergency response personnel and command staff.

Call for the help you will need. The support services required at the scene of a hazardous material incident may include fire services, special rescue personnel, local or state HAZMAT experts, and law enforcement personnel for crowd control. If the incident has taken place at an industrial site or along a railway, the company experts in hazardous materials need to be notified. Don't forget the private stakeholders in such incidents. Much of this can be initiated by a single call to your dispatcher.

Implement your agency's Incident Management System. Establish Command and maintain that role until you are relieved by someone higher in the chain of command. Maintain the Incident Management System until you are relieved, or until the incident is taken care of and you are released.

The situation should be prevented from becoming worse. Establish a perimeter, evacuate people if necessary, and direct bystanders to a safe area. It cannot be overemphasized that EMTs should not risk personal safety by initiating rescue attempts. Emergency response resources can be overwhelmed when the rescuers themselves have to be rescued.

While help is on the way, establish control zones. Isolate the ***hot zone*** (the area of contamination or the area of danger). Establish a decontamination corridor (area where patients will be decontaminated) in the ***warm zone***, an area immediately adjacent to the hot zone. Equipment and other emergency rescuers should be staged in the next adjacent area—the ***cold zone***. Station yourself in the cold zone.

hot zone
area immediately surrounding a HAZMAT incident; extends far enough to prevent adverse effects outside the zone.

warm zone
area where personnel and equipment decontamination and hot zone support take place; it includes control points for the access corridor and, thus, assists in reducing the spread of contamination.

cold zone
area where the Incident Command post and support functions are located.

Identify the Substance

As a responding EMT, you may be the first to recognize that a hazardous material situation exists. For example, you may answer a call to a business where four employees are ill after being in the warehouse. Whenever there are multiple medical patients, think HAZMAT (and remember not to make yourself a patient as well).

You must make a safe attempt to identify the hazardous material and assess the severity of the situation. Until that is done, it will be difficult to determine the risk to the public, rescuers, patients, and the environment. You must try to find out what the substance is and what its properties and dangers might be; whether or not there is imminent danger of the contamination spreading; what you can hear, see, and smell; how many patients are involved; and if there is any danger of secondary contamination from the patients. (Secondary contamination occurs when a contaminated person makes contact with someone who previously was noncontaminated).

Because it is not safe to approach the scene, you must obtain information indirectly or from a distance. Ways of obtaining information safely may include the following:

- **Use binoculars to look for identifying signs, labels, or placards from a safe distance** (Figure 39-1). In many cases there will be a colored placard (Figure 39-2) on the storage container, vehicle, tank, or railroad car.

NOTE: *Do not approach the scene to obtain this information.*

- **Search for placards.** A commonly used placarding system is the National Fire Protection Association (NFPA) 704 System. It uses numerical and color coding to show the type and degree of health hazard, fire hazard, reactivity, and specific hazard contained within a fixed facility (Figure 39-3).

  Diamond-shaped placards used in the transportation of dangerous goods not only show the hazard class, such as "explosives," "flammable gas," or "poison"; they also bear a division number that provides more specific information on the material, as shown in Table 39-2. In addition, a four-digit identification number may appear on the placard itself or on a panel near the placard. Older placards are usually orange and have an identification number preceded by the letters *UN* or *UA*. Your dispatcher may have access to the name of the material through this identification number.

NOTE: *Studies by the now-defunct Office of Technology Assessment have shown that some states reported that 25 percent to 50 percent of identification placards are incorrect. These same studies indicated that many shipping documents also were inaccurate or incomplete. In all cases, try to confirm materials/products via as many different information sources as possible (e.g., driver of a freight truck, railroad operator, originating warehouse, and so on).*

- **Look for labels.** The DOT requires that packages, storage containers, and vehicles containing hazardous materials bear labels or placards with markings that identify the nature of the contents. Pictograms are required as of June 1, 2015. These are part of the new Hazard Communication Standard, and align labels with the UN Globally Harmonized System (GHS) for labeling dangerous chemicals. You may also see the signal word "WARNING" or "DANGER." *Warning* is used for less severe hazards, and *Danger* is used for more severe hazards (Figure 39-4).

FIGURE 39-1 Binoculars will allow a visual inspection of the hot zone from a safe distance. A pair should be available in each emergency response vehicle.

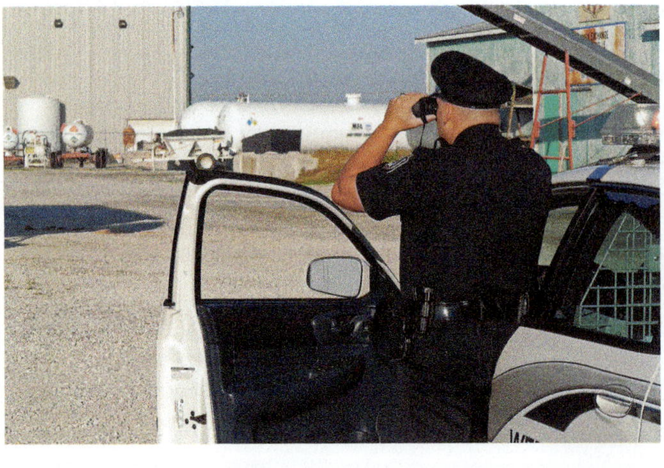

FIGURE 39-2 Vehicles carrying hazardous materials are required to display placards that communicate the nature of their cargo. Emergency Response Guides (ERGs) should be available in each emergency vehicle.

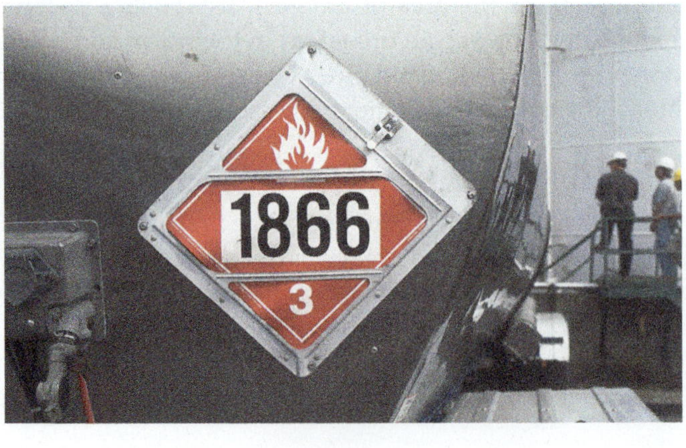

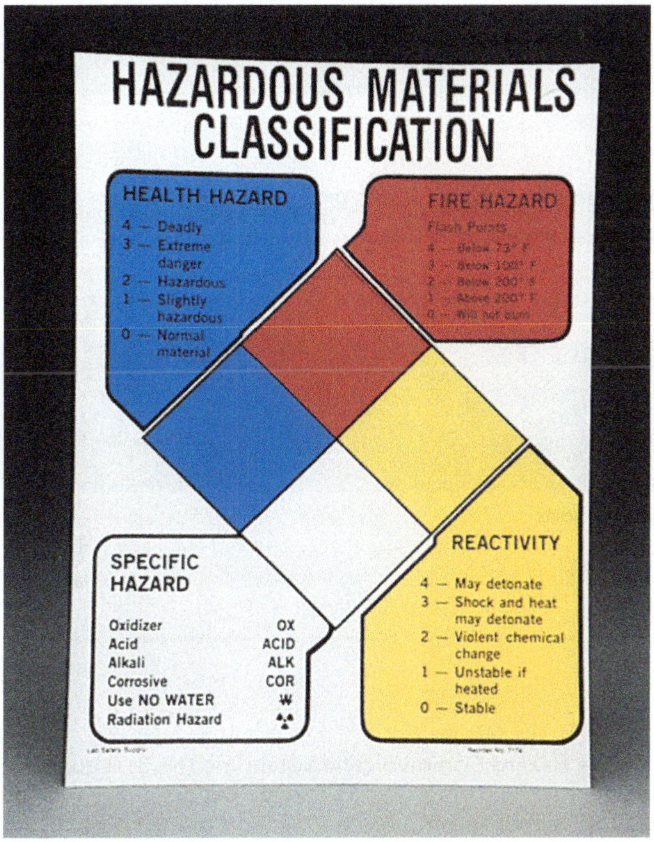

FIGURE 39-3 This is the key to the National Fire Protection Association (NFPA) 704 System of numeric and color codes to hazardous materials.

TABLE 39-2 Hazard Classification System

CLASS 1–EXPLOSIVES	
Division 1.1	Explosives with a mass explosion hazard
Division 1.2	Explosives with a projection hazard
Division 1.3	Explosives with predominantly a fire hazard
Division 1.4	Explosives with no significant blast hazard
Division 1.5	Very insensitive explosives; blasting agents
Division 1.6	Extremely insensitive detonating articles
CLASS 2–GASES	
Division 2.1	Flammable gases
Division 2.2	Nonflammable, nontoxic, compressed gases
Division 2.3	Gases toxic by inhalation
Division 2.4	Corrosive gases
CLASS 3–FLAMMABLE LIQUIDS AND COMBUSTIBLE LIQUIDS	
CLASS 4–FLAMMABLE SOLIDS; SPONTANEOUSLY COMBUSTIBLE MATERIALS; AND DANGEROUS-WHEN-WET MATERIALS	
Division 4.1	Flammable solids
Division 4.2	Spontaneously combustible materials
Division 4.3	Dangerous-when-wet materials

(continued)

TABLE 39-2 Hazard Classification System (*continued*)

CLASS 5—OXIDIZERS AND ORGANIC PEROXIDES	
Division 5.1	Oxidizers
Division 5.2	Organic peroxides
CLASS 6—TOXIC MATERIALS AND INFECTIOUS SUBSTANCES	
Division 6.1	Toxic materials
Division 6.2	Infectious substances
CLASS 7—RADIOACTIVE MATERIALS	
CLASS 8—CORROSIVE MATERIALS	
CLASS 9—MISCELLANEOUS DANGEROUS GOODS	
Division 9.1	Miscellaneous dangerous goods
Division 9.2	Environmentally hazardous substances
Division 9.3	Dangerous wastes

FIGURE 39-4 As of June 1, 2015, the Hazard Communication Standard (HCS) requires pictograms on labels to alert users of the chemical hazards to which they may be exposed. Each pictogram consists of a symbol on a white background framed within a red border, and represents a distinct hazard or hazards. The pictogram on the label is determined by the chemical hazard classification. *(Occupational Safety and Health Administration, U.S. Department of Labor,* https://www.osha.gov/Publications/HazComm_QuickCard_Pictogram.html*)*

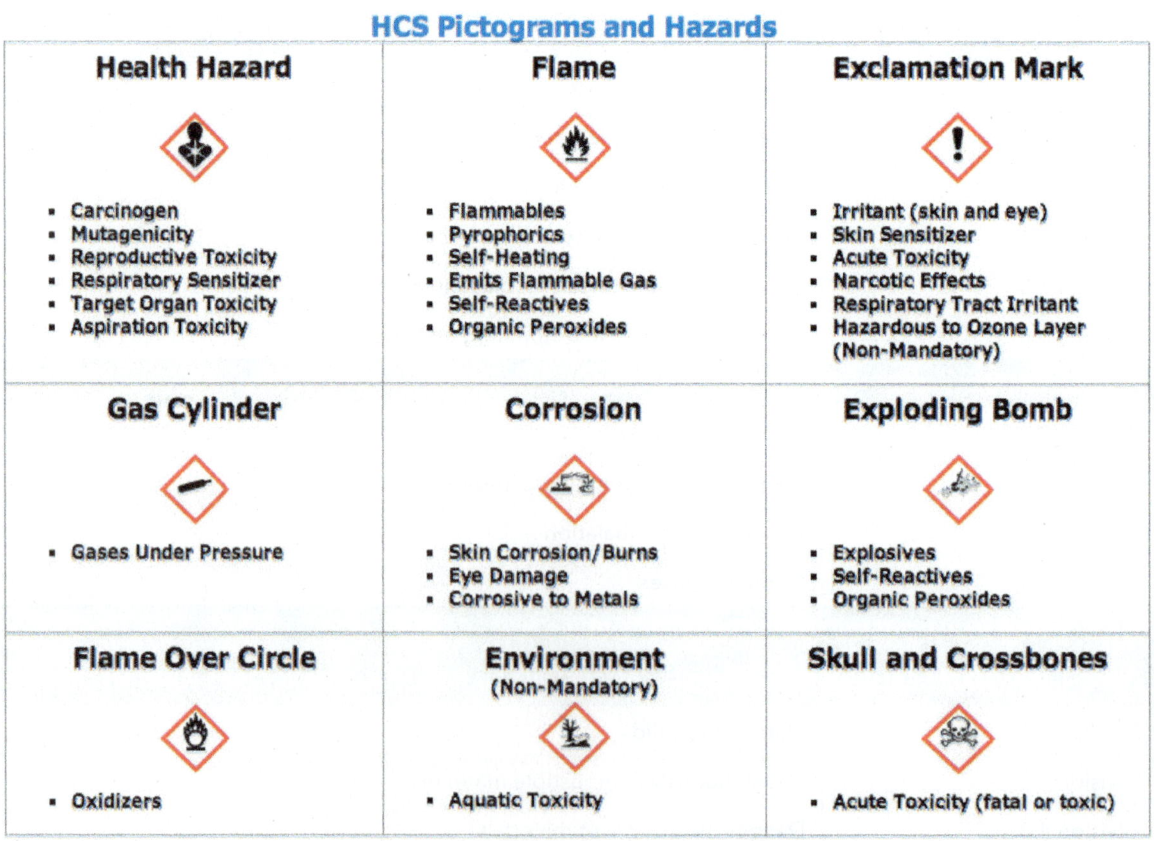

- **Check invoices, bills of lading (trucks), and shipping manifests (trains).** If you can safely obtain them, these documents will identify the exact substance being transported, the exact quantity, its place of origin, and its destination.
- **Review safety data sheets (SDSs).** Safety data sheets (SDSs), formerly called material safety data sheets (MSDSs), must be provided on hazardous materials by all manufacturers. These sheets must be maintained at the work site by the employer and must be available to all employees, on the grounds that employees working with hazardous materials have a right to know about them. If you can safely obtain these sheets, they generally name the substance, its physical properties, fire and explosion hazard information, health hazard information, and emergency first aid treatment.
- **Interview workers or others leaving the hot zone.** These people may be good sources of information about the substance involved. Vehicle drivers, plant and railroad personnel, and perhaps even bystanders may be able to tell you the name of the hazardous material. Workers at a manufacturing site often understand very well what chemicals are used, the processes, and their reactions. However, note that workers may identify a substance by its trade name and not realize that it is a mixture of many chemicals.

EMTs are expected to understand some of the common substance-identifying systems available and to make a preliminary identification based on this information. On the basis of this preliminary information, you can obtain advice about what initial actions should be taken at the scene from your dispatcher, a hazardous material expert, or one of the following sources:

- **Emergency Response Guidebook (ERG)** (Figure 39-5). This essential booklet, published by the DOT, Transport Canada, and the Secretariat of Communications and Transportation of Mexico, provides the names of chemicals and concise but thorough descriptions of the actions that should be taken in case of a HAZMAT emergency. Be sure to have the latest edition in your vehicle at all times. This guidebook is also now available as a smartphone app.

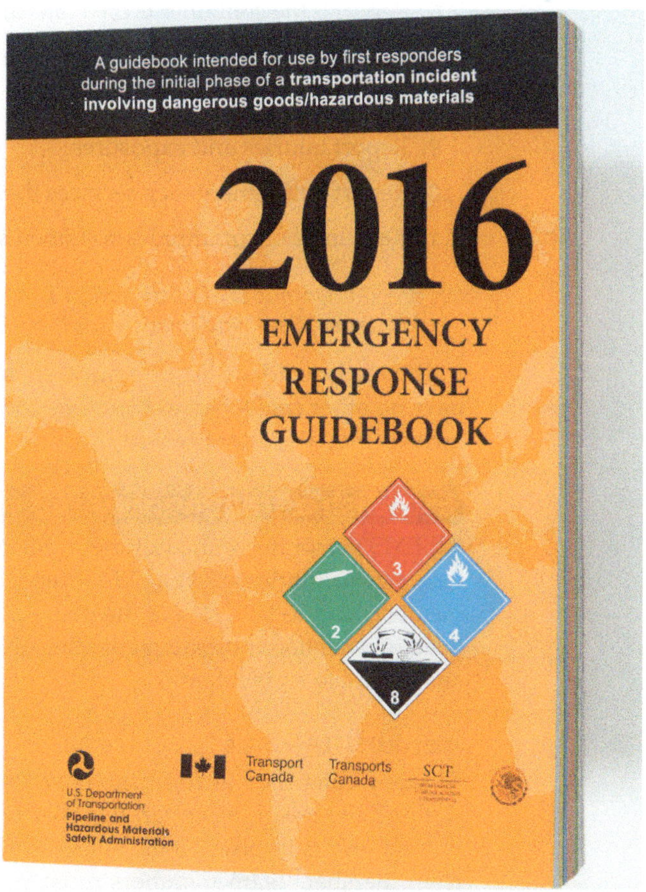

FIGURE 39-5 Have the latest edition of the *Emergency Response Guidebook* in your vehicle at all times.

- **Chemical Transportation Emergency Center (CHEMTREC).** This group, established in Washington, D.C., is a service of the Chemical Manufacturers Association. They can provide your dispatcher or you with information about the hazardous material through a 24-hour toll-free telephone number for the United States and Canada, which is 800-424-9300. For calls originating elsewhere and for collect calls, the number is 703-527-3887. When you call, keep the line open, so changes at the scene can be reported to CHEMTREC and the center staff can confirm that they have contacted the shipper or manufacturer. CHEMTREC staff will be able to direct you as to your initial course of action.
- **CHEM-TEL, Inc.** This emergency response communication service can be reached 24 hours a day at 800-255-3924 in the United States and Canada. For calls originating elsewhere or collect calls, use 813-979-0626.
- **A current list of state and federal radiation authorities.** These organizations provide information and technical assistance on handling incidents involving radioactive materials. The list is maintained by both CHEMTREC and CHEM-TEL, Inc.
- **Regional poison control centers.** This source is often overlooked during a hazardous material situation. Using their reference and medical resources, they can provide essential guidance in the decontamination and treatment of patients affected by hazardous materials.

When you call one of the previously named sources for advice, do the following:

1. Give your name, agency, and callback number.
2. Explain the nature and location of the problem.
3. Report the identification number(s) of the material(s) involved, if there is a safe way for you to obtain this information.
4. Give the name of the carrier, shipper, manufacturer, consignee, and point of origin.
5. Describe the container type and size.
6. Report if the container is on a rail car, on a truck, in open storage, or in housed storage.
7. Estimate the quantity of material transported and released.
8. Report local conditions (e.g., the weather, terrain, and proximity to schools or hospitals).
9. Report injuries and exposures.
10. Report local emergency services that have been notified.
11. Keep lines of communication open at all times.

NOTE: *Do not take hasty action because you think you have identified the nature of the substance. Seek and follow expert advice. Do only what you have been trained to do.*

If there is no identification number, and no one knows what is being carried, you may have no other choice but to wait for experts to arrive at the scene. When a HAZMAT team arrives, they will identify and deal with the unknown substances.

Establish a Treatment Area

All EMS personnel and equipment must be staged in the cold zone. EMS personnel have two responsibilities at a HAZMAT incident: to monitor and rehabilitate the HAZMAT team members and to take care of the injured. These two distinct responsibilities should be outlined in a standard operating guideline that personnel can refer to during training, response, and arrival to an incident.

Rehabilitation Operations

To safely enter the hot zone, the HAZMAT team members must wear chemical-protective clothing and breathing apparatus. Wearing this protective equipment for prolonged periods of time results in physiologic stress and impairs normal heat regulation of the HAZMAT team member. Team members must be carefully monitored prior to, during, and after emergency operations (Figure 39-6). This is done to make sure that their condition does not

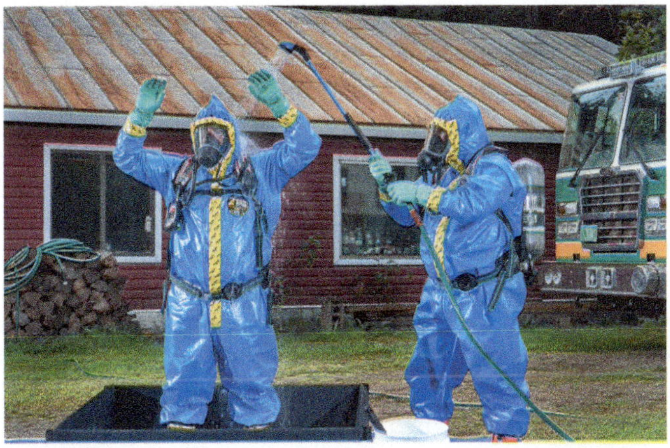

FIGURE 39-6 HAZMAT teams have prescribed methods for decontamination and removal of HAZMAT suits.

deteriorate to a point where safety or the integrity of the operation is jeopardized. To address this need, you should establish an area of operations called rehabilitation (rehab). Although the rehab area supervisor might not be an EMS provider, all rehab operations must include EMTs, advanced EMTs, and/or paramedics.

The characteristics of the rehab area should include the following:

- Located in the cold zone
- Protected from weather extremes (i.e., shielded from rain or snow, and staged in a warm area in a cold environment, or in a cool area in a warm environment)
- Large enough to accommodate multiple rescue crews
- Easily accessible to EMS units
- Free from exhaust fumes
- Allows for rapid reentry into the emergency operation

While suiting up in chemical-protective equipment, HAZMAT team members should have their baseline vital signs taken. When the HAZMAT team members show signs of fatigue, or when they have had 45 minutes of work time, they are typically sent to rehab. As soon as possible after exit from the hot zone, reassess their vital signs, including blood pressure, heart rate, and oral temperature. Vital sign parameters will vary based on local guidelines. Team members who display an elevated heart rate (usually greater than 110 beats per minute) or any elevation in body temperature will require ongoing medical reassessments in the rehab area until pulse and temperature return to baseline. Always follow your local protocols and consult medical direction. All preentry and postexit vitals should be documented on a flow sheet.

In addition to medical monitoring, rehab should be set up for hydration, rest, and in some cases nourishment of HAZMAT team members. Proper hydration and rehydration are important elements in preventing heat stress and promoting optimal physical performance. Follow local protocols for the volumes and types of oral rehydration solution to be used in rehab. Coffee and caffeinated beverages should be avoided because they promote dehydration. The National Fire Protection Association 1584 *Standard on the Rehabilitation Process for Members during Emergency Operations and Training Exercises* provides a comprehensive overview of rehab operations.

When incidents will be of extended duration, some type of nourishment may be provided in rehab. Foods low in sodium and saturated fats are recommended. Bananas, apples, oranges, and other fruits are excellent for fast nourishment. In cold environments, soups and stews are more easily eaten and digested than sandwiches.

Care of Injured and Contaminated Patients

Hazardous material or terrorist incidents (see the chapter *EMS Response to Terrorism*) involve civilians and/or other public safety providers. Prompt, safe, and effective decontamination procedures are essential to protect against or reduce the effects of exposure to both patients and other public safety providers. Decontamination is performed to protect citizens, personnel, equipment, and the environment from the harmful effects of the contaminants.

decontamination
a chemical and/or physical process that reduces or prevents the spread of contamination from persons or equipment; the removal of hazardous substances from employees and their equipment to the extent necessary to preclude foreseeable health effects.

The NFPA defines ***decontamination*** as a chemical and/or physical process that reduces or prevents the spread of contamination from persons or equipment. According to OSHA, decontamination is the removal of hazardous substances from employees and their equipment to the extent necessary to preclude foreseeable health effects.

EMTs must work with Incident Command and HAZMAT team members to determine the most appropriate course of action. The decision whether to stay at the scene and decontaminate or to begin evacuation must be made after careful consultation with CHEMTREC, the poison control center, and other reference sources.

In the decontamination (decon) corridor in the warm zone, the HAZMAT team will decontaminate HAZMAT team members and any patients rescued. EMS is responsible for setting up the medical treatment area in the cold zone to receive decontaminated patients. Unless EMS personnel are trained to the HAZMAT technician level or higher, they must remain in the cold zone.

The field decon process is designed to remove contaminants and deliver a relatively "clean" patient to EMS personnel for care and transportation (Figure 39-7). However, there is a chance of secondary contamination from patients to EMS personnel. It is important that EMS personnel work closely with the decon officer and consult with medical direction on both treatment and appropriate protection during transportation.

FIGURE 39-7 An example of a field decontamination process.

9-Station Decontamination Procedure

STEPS	
Station 1. Rescuers enter decon areas and mechanically remove contaminants from victims. Tools are dropped in tool drop area. Rescuers are in SCBA and protective clothing. **Proceed to Station 2.**	Remove Contaminants Tool Drop
Station 2. *Gross Decontamination*: Victims and rescue personnel are showered and/or scrubbed by decon personnel. Dilution is conducted inside diked area. Victims may be transported directly to Station 6. **Proceed to Station 6.**	Gross Decon
Station 3. *Protective Clothing Removal*: Rescuers remove protective clothing, clothing is isolated and labeled for later disposal. Clothing is placed on contaminated side. **Proceed to Station 4.**	PPC Removal
Station 4. *SCBA Removal*: Rescue personnel remove and isolate their SCBA. If re-entry is necessary, personnel don new SCBA from noncontaminated side. **Proceed to Station 5.**	SCBA Removal
Station 5. *Personal Clothing Removal*: All clothing and personal items are removed. Victims who have not been undressed are undressed here. All clothing and personal items are isolated in plastic bags and labeled for later disposal. **Proceed to Station 6.**	Personal Clothing Removal
Station 6. *Body Washing*: Full body washing is performed using soft scrub brushes or sponges and soap or mild detergent. Cleaning tools are bagged for later disposal. **Proceed to Station 7.**	Body Washing
Station 7. *Dry Off*: Towels and sheets are used to dry off. Rescuers and victims are dressed in clean clothes. Towels/sheets are bagged for later disposal. **Proceed to Station 8.**	Dry Off
Station 8. *Medical Assessment*: Rapid patient assessment is conducted by rescuers. Necessary stabilization procedures are accomplished. **Proceed to Station 9.**	Medical Assessment
Station 9. *Transport*: Transfer of patient to hospital for medical attention or to recovery areas for rest and observation.	Transport

The following points are important when treating and transporting HAZMAT patients:

- Field-decontaminated patients are not completely "clean." Chemicals that pose a risk of secondary contamination to rescuers sometimes settle in hard-to-clean areas of the body. These areas are typically the scalp/hair, groin, buttocks, armpits, and between fingers and toes.
- Personal protective equipment or clothing (PPE/PPC) is needed to prevent secondary contamination of rescuers. EMS personnel may need to wear PPE such as Tyvek coveralls and booties to prevent contamination and exposure. They may also need to wear a double layer of gloves. Often nitrile or neoprene is best, because these are more resistant to chemicals than are standard latex or vinyl gloves. Consult with the decon officer to determine if your PPE is suitable or if they have more appropriate PPE.
- Protect vehicles from contamination. In the decon process, patients are washed and are usually dripping wet. Since they cannot be completely decontaminated in the field, some of their water runoff could contaminate an emergency vehicle. To prevent this, the water runoff must be contained by either placing the patient in a disposable decontamination pool or covering the inside of an ambulance with plastic. Follow your agency's standard operating guidelines.
- Consider used equipment as disposable. When an item such as a long board, splint, blood pressure cuff, or stethoscope is used, it might not be able to be decontaminated and may require disposal. Many EMS systems have plans/logistical considerations for this kind of situation.
- Structural firefighting clothing is not designed or recommended for use when working in hazardous material environments. If personnel in firefighting gear encounter a hazardous chemical environment, they should take precautions to minimize the chance of contamination.

When treating a contaminated patient is unavoidable, it is crucial to identify the hazardous material. Follow the treatment instructions given in the *Emergency Response Guidebook* or by the poison control center.

Four types of patients are encountered by EMTs:

- Uninjured and not contaminated
- Injured and not contaminated
- Uninjured and contaminated
- Injured and contaminated

If you are confronted with contaminated patients prior to the arrival of the HAZMAT team, do the following:

1. Take precautions appropriate to the substance as listed in the *Emergency Response Guidebook*. This usually means isolation from the substance. Be sure to use PPE similar to what you would use for splash protection from bloodborne pathogens.
2. Follow the first aid measures listed in the *Emergency Response Guidebook* and other care interventions recommended by poison control if safe to do so.
3. Manage the patient's critical needs. Do not forget to manage the A-B-Cs.
4. If treatment calls for irrigation with water, remember that water only dilutes most substances; it does not neutralize them. Cut the patient's clothing off and irrigate the patient's body with large amounts of water. Try to contain the runoff. If possible, use tepid or warm water to prevent hypothermia. Try to avoid flushing contaminants directly into open wounds. Pay particular attention to areas such as patches of dense body hair, ear canals, the navel, fingernails, the groin, and the armpits. Use disposable equipment whenever possible. Discard it later.
5. After treating the patient, decontaminate yourself. Your clothing may need to be disposed of.

Remember that the severity of any poisoning depends on the substance, route of entry, dosage, and duration of contact. Immediate emergency care measures as listed in the *Emergency Response Guidebook* may decrease the severity of the poisoning and save lives. Whenever possible, the entire decontamination process should be carried out by qualified personnel from the HAZMAT team before the EMT touches the patient.

Contaminated personnel (injured or not) pose a secondary contamination risk and should be decontaminated prior to leaving the scene. If scene decontamination is not performed, patients must be decontaminated at an appropriate hospital decon site before they enter the emergency department.

Phases of Decontamination

The two major phases of decontamination are gross decontamination and secondary decontamination. (There is usually a third or tertiary decontamination phase, but it generally occurs at a medical facility, and may involve such processes as sterilization or debridement.)

Gross decontamination is the removal or chemical alteration of the majority of the contaminant. It must be assumed that some residual contaminant will always remain on the host after gross decontamination. This residual contamination can cause cross-contamination.

Secondary decontamination is the alteration or removal of most of the residual product contamination. It provides a more thorough decontamination than the gross effort. However, some contaminant may still remain attached to the host.

Mechanisms for Decontamination

There are seven common mechanisms for performing decontamination. They are:

- **Emulsification.** This is the production of a suspension of ordinarily immiscible (unmixable)/insoluble materials using an emulsifying agent such as a surfactant, soap, or detergent.
- **Chemical reaction.** This is a process that neutralizes, degrades, or otherwise chemically alters the contaminant. Normally a chemical reaction does not ensure that all hazards have been eliminated, and reaction procedures can be both difficult and dangerous to perform. Chemical reaction is therefore not recommended for use on living tissue.
- **Disinfection.** This is a process that removes the biologic (etiologic) contamination hazards as the disinfectant destroys microorganisms and their toxins.
- **Dilution.** This is a process that simply reduces the concentration of the contaminant. It is most commonly used for substances that are miscible (mixable)/soluble. Huge quantities of solvent may be required to dilute even small volumes of some solute contaminants.
- **Absorption and adsorption.** This is the penetration of a liquid or gas into another substance. An example is water soaking into a sponge.
- **Removal.** This is the physical process of removing contaminants by pressure or vacuum. Most efforts involve the use of water, though solids can be removed with brushes and wipes; even air can be used.
- **Disposal.** This is the aseptic removal of a contaminated object from a host, after which the object is disposed of. (*Aseptic* means using sterile instruments and/or otherwise preventing the spread of the contaminant.)

Decontamination Procedures

The objectives of the responders assigned to decontamination are to:

- Determine the appropriate level of protective equipment based on materials and associated hazards.
- Properly wear and operate in PPE.

- Establish an operating time log.
- Set up and operate the decontamination line.
- Prioritize the decontamination of patients according to a triage system.
- Perform triage in PPE.
- Be able to communicate while in PPE.

A basic list of equipment required for decontamination includes:

- Buckets
- Brushes
- Decontamination solution
- Decontamination tubs
- A dedicated water supply
- Tarps or plastic sheeting
- A containment vessel for water runoff
- A pump to transfer wastewater from decontamination tubs to a containment vessel
- An A-frame ladder (to reach the top of the responder's suit)
- Appropriate-level PPE for responders performing decontamination.

Decontamination for Patients Wearing PPE. Take the following steps to decontaminate a patient who is wearing PPE:

1. Rinse, starting at the head and working down.
2. Scrub the suit with a brush, starting at the head and working down. Pay special attention to heavily contaminated areas (e.g., hands, feet, and the front of the suit).
3. Rinse again, starting at the head and working down.
4. Assist the patient in removing PPE.
5. Contain the runoff of hazardous wastewater.

Decontamination for Patients Not Wearing PPE. The decontamination of patients not wearing PPE proceeds in a different manner. As always, the first and foremost consideration is responder safety. If responders are incapacitated, they are unable to help others.

You should use a public address system to direct ambulatory patients to a decontamination line. This provides a rapid form of triage. Note that patients who may have been involved in an explosion incident may have loss of hearing; you may have to use hand signals or use large signs to communicate your commands. Patients should be instructed to begin decontamination by removing their clothing. Have people remove shoes, socks, jewelry, watches, and other items that trap materials against the skin. They should also remove contact lenses as soon as possible. Double-bag their clothing for disposal or decontamination later. Valuables and identification should be bagged and may (based on hazards) be carried by the patients.

Next, the patients should receive a 2- to 5-minute water rinse. Solid or particulate contaminants should be lightly brushed off (dry decontamination) as completely as possible prior to washing (wet decontamination). Viscous liquid contaminants (including vesicants, which are blistering agents) should be blotted off prior to washing. If the material is water-reactive, it must be brushed off prior to the application of water. Rinsing is done as needed to flush remaining chemicals that may react with the moisture of the skin and eyes. You should also use an appropriate decontamination solution.

Washing and rinsing should start at the head to reduce contamination on or near the nose, mouth, ears, and eyes. After removal of patient's contact lenses, the eyes should be irrigated. Open wounds should be irrigated starting from the area nearest to the body core and working outward. You may use plastic wrap to isolate the wound once it has been cleaned. Use a low-water-pressure system to avoid aggravating soft-tissue injuries and to avoid overspray and splashing. A low-pressure system will also help prevent the creation of an aerosol out of dry product.

During decontamination, patients should be given some type of cover for modesty and protection from the elements. Protection from hypothermia should be a consideration.

Although not strictly a form of self-protection, decon is vital to prevent, reduce, and remove contamination for both responders and patients.

Multiple-Casualty Incidents

multiple-casualty incident (MCI)
any medical or trauma incident involving multiple patients.

CORE CONCEPT
How to identify a multiple-casualty incident

A ***multiple-casualty incident (MCI)***—or, in some areas, a multiple-casualty situation (MCS)—is an event that places a great demand on EMS equipment and personnel resources. The number of patients required before an MCI can be declared varies in practice. Some jurisdictions will declare an MCI for as few as three patients, on the grounds that practice with smaller-scale incidents will help EMTs prepare for larger ones. Other jurisdictions reserve the MCI designation for five, seven, or more patients (Figure 39-8). The most common MCI is an automobile collision with three or more patients. You will likely respond to many incidents with three to fifteen potential patients. Incidents with large-scale casualties are rare and apt to be "once in a career" events.

The important ingredient in defining an MCI is that, for whatever reason, the EMS system's ability to respond to the situation is challenged or hampered *by the situation itself*. For any MCI plan to be effective, it must be flexible and expandable enough to be used from small, three-patient incidents to large-scale incidents of fifteen or more patients. In other words, the plan for "the big one" should be a logical extension of the same plan used to manage smaller incidents.

"Multiple casualties can be stressful. Do what you learned. Follow the plan."

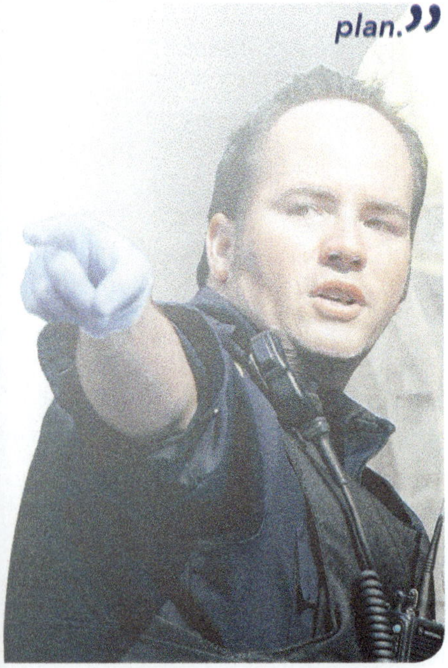

(Kevin Link/Science Source)

Multiple-Casualty Incident Operations

Though the principles of managing small- and large-scale MCIs are generally the same, large-scale MCIs unfold over a longer period of time and require greater support from outside agencies. Well-trained and practiced EMTs can usually cope with a small-scale MCI pretty well. However, experience has shown that even the best-trained EMTs have a difficult time managing an incident of greater magnitude.

One way to minimize the operating difficulties of a large-scale MCI is for every EMT to be familiar with the local ***disaster plan***.

disaster plan
a predefined set of instructions for a community's emergency responders.

A disaster plan is a predefined set of instructions that tells a community's various emergency responders what to do in specific emergencies (Figure 39-9). Although no disaster plan can address every problem that could arise, there are several features common to every good disaster plan. The disaster plan should be:

- **Written to address the events that are conceivable for a particular location** (e.g., Kansas needs to plan for tornadoes, not hurricanes).
- **Well publicized.** Each emergency responder should be familiar with the plan and how it is to be put into operation.
- **Realistic.** The plan must be based on the actual availability of resources.
- **Rehearsed.** Experience has proven that the only way to get a plan to work correctly is to exercise it and, in so doing, work out the unforeseen "bugs."

It is beyond the scope of this text to teach you how to write a disaster plan or even to impart enough knowledge for you to be in charge of a disaster operation. However, it is important to introduce basic information about your potential roles in such an incident. Knowing that these resources exist will be important as you enter the profession.

FIGURE 39-8 Multiple-casualty incidents may range from small to large. (A) A car crash with as few as three to five patients will be declared a multiple-casualty incident by many EMS jurisdictions. (B) In this bus crash, all passengers were triaged, and forty-four patients were transported to area hospitals. *(Photo A: © Ed Effron; Photo B: Mark Ide/Science Source)*

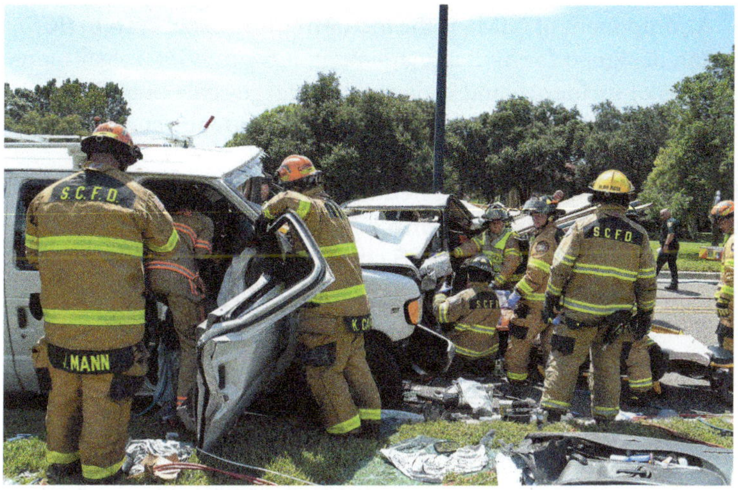

A

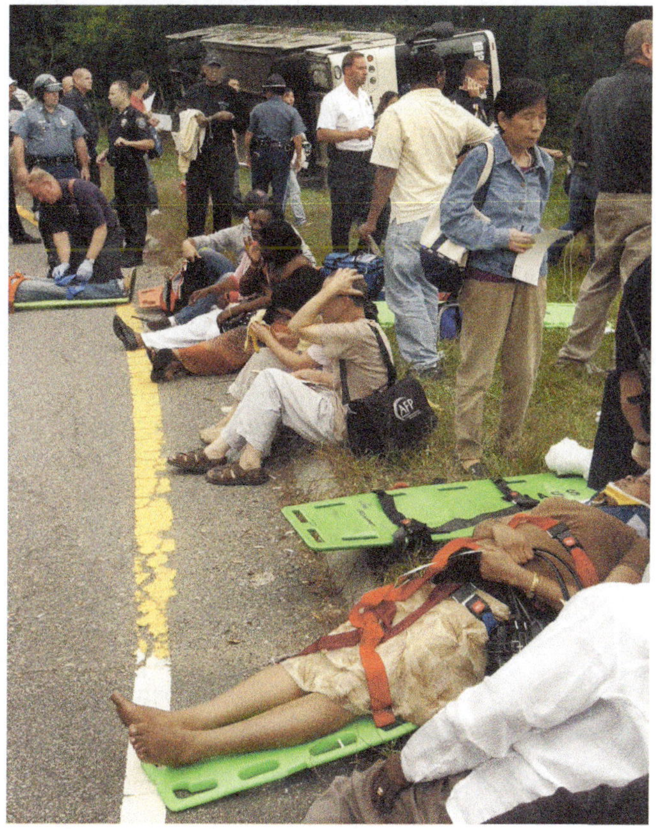

B

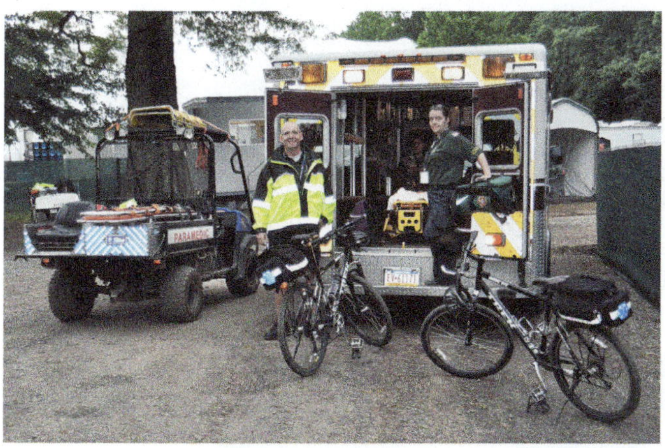

FIGURE 39-9 Mass gatherings, such as sporting events, usually require an EMS presence to deal with individual emergencies. This bike crew and "gator" vehicle were standing by at a U.S. Open golf tournament. However, mass gatherings also have the potential to suddenly become large-scale MCIs if, for example, someone sets off a bomb, or the grandstands collapse. *(© Edward T. Dickinson, MD)*

National Incident Management System (NIMS) the management system used by federal, state, and local governments to manage emergencies in the United States.

Incident Command System (ICS) a subset of NIMS designed specifically for management of multiple-casualty incidents.

CORE CONCEPT

The Incident Command System

Command the first on the scene to establish order and initiate the Incident Command System.

Incident Command System

By federal declaration, the ***National Incident Management System (NIMS)*** is the management system used by federal, state, and local governments to manage emergencies in the United States (Figure 39-10). A component of NIMS is the ***Incident Command System (ICS)***. Although not specifically a plan designed for MCI management, ICS provides a clear management framework for all types of incidents, and especially for large-scale ones. In addition, it is mandated by law for the management of some types of incidents, such as those involving hazardous materials.

ICS originated in California, where it was designed as a management plan to handle large-scale firefighting operations involving multiple agencies and jurisdictions. As a flexible tool for managing people and resources, ICS components include Command, Operations, Logistics, Planning, and Finance. The most commonly used components are Command and Operations. Many incidents require only these two functions.

Command

Command, which must be established at all incidents, involves a person who assumes responsibility for overall incident management. This individual stays in the position of Command unless that function is transferred to another person or until the incident is brought to a conclusion.

ICS considers the manageable span of control to be between three to seven people. As the MCI escalates and becomes more complex, the number of people and span of control become too large for one person to manage effectively. At this point, Command designates people to handle the specific functions needed to manage the incident. These *sections* include:

- Operations
- Planning
- Logistics
- Finance

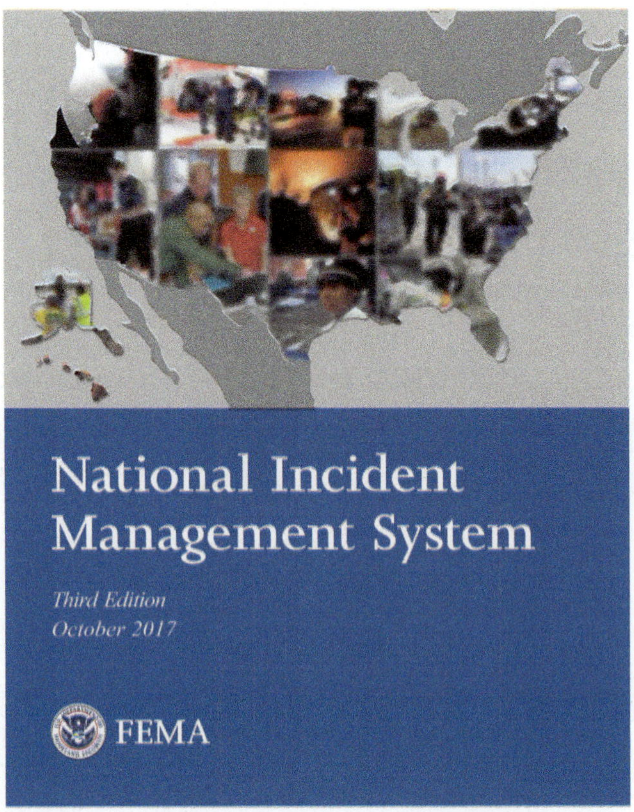

FIGURE 39-10 The National Incident Management System (NIMS) is mandated by the Federal Emergency Management Agency (FEMA). *(National Incident Management System, FEMA, Department of Homeland Security)*

Command assumes all incident management functions except those that Command may delegate to someone else. Unless an incident is very complex, the most common function designated is Operations.

Two methods of Command defined under NIMS are single incident command and unified command. In ***single incident command***, a single agency controls all resources and operations. In many communities, for example, EMS is managed by fire services. Accordingly, single incident command is often used at fire and rescue incidents, with the Incident Commander provided by the fire service (Figure 39-11A). However, if police agencies have major involvement, if there is a separate EMS provider, or if other agencies are involved, ***unified command*** is more appropriate (Figure 39-11B). In unified command, several agencies work independently but cooperatively, rather than one agency exercising control over the others. In most communities, unified command is the best way to manage resources. It recognizes that large-scale incidents tend to be complex and that the right agency must take the lead at the right time, with Command officers from all agencies cooperating.

single incident command command organization in which a single agency controls all resources and operations.

unified command command organization in which several agencies work independently but cooperatively.

Command Functions

Initially, ***Incident Command*** is assumed by the most senior member of the first emergency service on the scene. Very often this will be an EMS unit. Depending on jurisdiction, laws, or protocols, Incident Command may be transferred later to another individual, or may be continued by whoever established it.

Incident Command the person or persons who assume overall direction of a large-scale incident.

Two modes or phases of action must then be undertaken: scene size-up/triage and organization/delegation. First, Command and the crew do an initial scene size-up, start the triage process, and call for backup. While waiting for help, initial triage is completed, and Command gets ready for arriving resources, beginning to construct an *incident action plan (IAP)*.

When reinforcements arrive, there are two options for the person who initially assumed Command: Continue to be in Command or transfer Command to someone of higher rank. In a unified system, Incident Command would be assumed cooperatively by the Command of each service. Command is positioned at a location close enough to allow observation of the scene but secure enough to permit management of incoming resources and communication with others. In a unified command system, EMS, Police, and Fire Command establish one

FIGURE 39-11 (A) A single incident command organization. (B) A unified command organization.

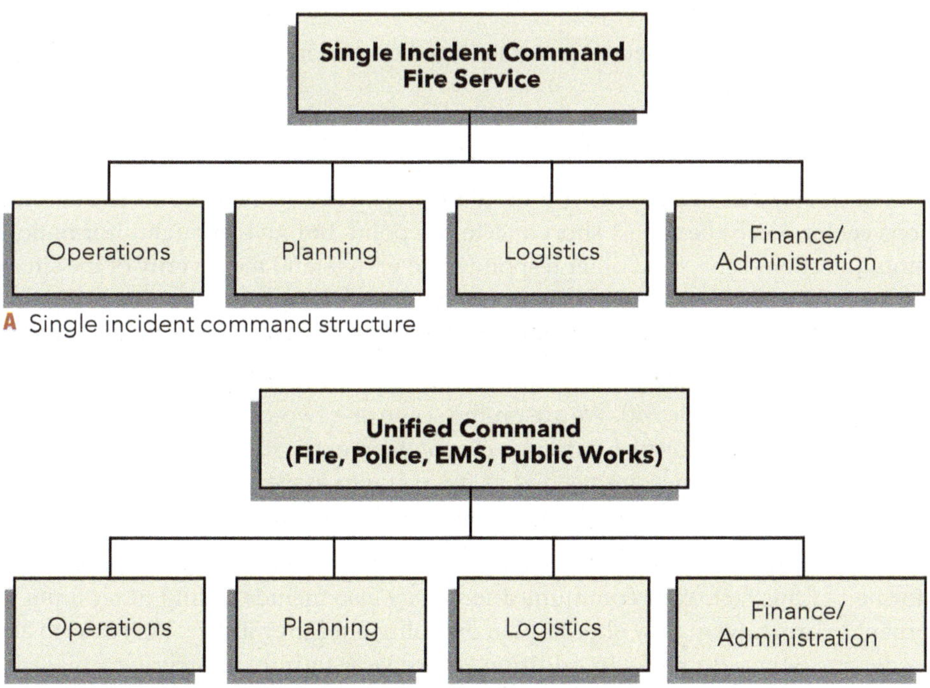

A Single incident command structure

B Unified command structure

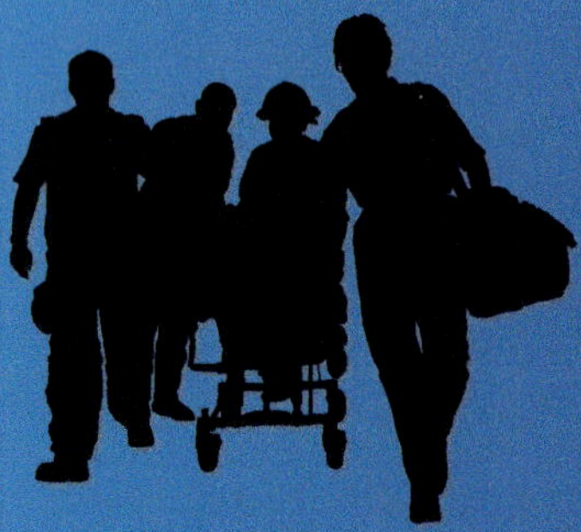

Think Like an EMT

We Have *How Many* Patients?

One of the key elements of this chapter is handling the multiple-casualty incident. The concepts that were described in the *Scene Size-Up* chapter return here with increased importance. For each of the following scenarios, determine what resources you would call for in your initial report to the dispatcher.

1. You are called to a shopping mall for "sick people." You arrive to find dozens of people standing outside the mall, coughing and rubbing their eyes. Looking around the parking lot, you see hundreds of cars.
2. You arrive at a motor-vehicle crash in which two cars collided at an intersection with considerable force. One patient has been ejected. Three others don't appear to be moving.
3. You are treating a woman in her home for flulike symptoms. You notice that her husband and one child are also sick. You check on another child sleeping in the same residence and find that he won't wake up.

field command post together and stay there. The command post should be clearly marked. In single incident command mode, one person acts as Command, and EMS would typically be a group under the Operations section.

Scene Size-Up

Size up the scene by making a sweep to determine what needs must be met:

1. Arrive at the scene and establish Incident Command. Put on the proper identification.
2. Do a quick walk through the scene (or, if it is a HAZMAT scene, observe from a safe distance) and assess the number of patients, hazards, and degree of entrapment. Identify the number of patients, including the "walking wounded"; apparent priority of care; need for extrication; number of ambulances needed; other factors affecting the scene and corresponding resources needed to address them; and areas where resources can be staged.
3. Get as calm and composed as possible to radio in an initial scene report and call for additional resources.

Communications

Once scene size-up has been done, you should make an initial scene report to the communications center. Keep the report short and to the point, but give enough information for the communications center and other responders to understand the severity of the situation and react accordingly. Give yourself a unique Command name to distinguish yourself and your incident location from other personnel and incidents that may be using the same radio system. Example:

> MEDCOM, this is Medic 640. We are on the scene of a two-car collision with severe entrapment of four Priority 1 patients. Dispatch an extrication unit and four paramedic ambulances. Police are needed at the scene to assist with traffic and crowd control. Medic 640 is assuming Franklin Avenue Command.

If the disaster plan is to be put into operation, it is critical that other responding units be informed of this fact. Your communications may also include telling other units what equipment to bring, what they should plan on doing once they arrive, how best to access the scene, and where to park. In addition, make sure to inform arriving units of any hazards that may be present.

As help begins to arrive, control of on-scene communication is important. Once units arrive, as much face-to-face communication as possible should be used, especially between Command and Command's direct subordinates. This will help to reduce radio channel crowding. If you feel you are getting too tied up in radio communications, designate a radio aide.

Basically, the flow of communications at the scene should correspond to the organizational chart being used. Accordingly, the only unit talking to the communications center and requesting resources is Command. The only ones who talk to Command are those directly subordinate to Command. All others talk only to the officer or supervisor they are assigned to. These mandates should be addressed in your standard operating guidelines, and are collectively known as the "chain of command."

Organization

Getting organized early and aggressively is very important. You must have a plan to deploy resources when they arrive. In addition, you must decide which subordinate officers will be needed and where resources will be placed. A common mistake is to underestimate the resources that will be needed. New patients not found during scene size-up have a way of appearing. Think big! Order big! Put resources in the staging area if they are not needed right away (Figure 39-12). In urban/suburban incidents, backup can be fast and overwhelming. If you do not think about supply and staging areas early, you take the chance of being overrun. Remember, you can always turn units around relatively easily, rather than needing them and not having them.

It is important to prevent "freelancing." Freelancing is uncoordinated or undirected activity at the scene. Given the opportunity, most rescuers will arrive on the scene and begin setting their own priorities. Effective command can help prevent this problem. When Command is established early, people and crews are assigned to tasks as they arrive. Freelancing can be a cause of line-of-duty injuries (LODI) and line-of-duty deaths (LODD).

It is helpful to have some personal tools to help get organized. For example, many organizations have distilled the major points of their plans into a "tactical worksheet" they can use in the field. With enough use, the plan can become committed to memory (Figure 39-13).

Scene Management

The senior person on the first-arriving EMS unit will likely assume Incident Command (known simply as Command). This person will establish a command post to oversee the incident's medical aspects and the safety of all personnel, designate area supervisors, and work closely with the fire and police commanders. On larger incidents, Command may have a *command staff* which includes a public information officer, a liaison officer, and a safety officer.

It is important to keep uninjured people from becoming injured. This will probably require restricting access to the scene to only those personnel performing triage (explained later in this text), extrication from wreckage, and patient care. As resources arrive at the scene, police officers or safety officers may take over this function.

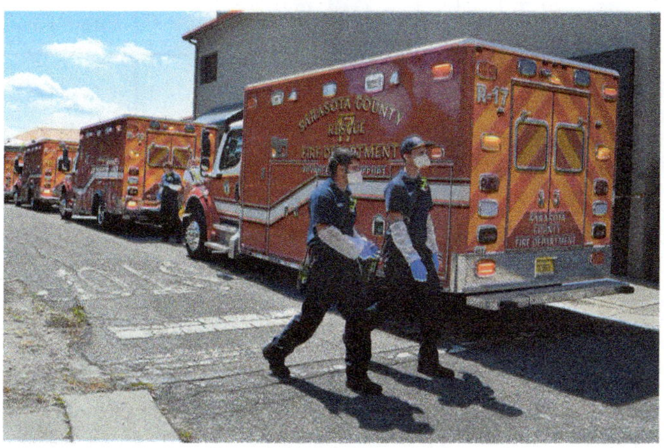

FIGURE 39-12 Ambulance staging. *(© Ed Effron)*

FIGURE 39-13 An example of an incident tactical worksheet.

INCIDENT TACTICAL WORKSHEET

Location ____________

Med. Command ____________

_____ Establish unified command with fire & police
_____ Place 2 cones on command vehicle

_____ Put bib on
_____ Designate triage officer

_____ Advise inbound units where to stage
_____ Advise crews to stay with units until given instructions
_____ Advise units to switch to EMS Admin., 265 or 715

LEVEL 1 *(3-10 Patients)*

- ___ Declare MCI
- ___ EMS All Call
- ___ Request # of Units Needed
- ___ Cover Town/Sr. Medic Act 615
- ___ Roll Call Hospitals
- ___ Transport Officer?

(2-5 Amb. Needed)

LEVEL 2 *(11-25 Patients)*

- ___ Declare MCI
- ___ EMS All Call
- ___ Request # of Units Needed
- ___ Cover Town/Sr. Medic Act 615
- ___ Roll Call Hospitals
- ___ Get Mutual Aid Units
- ___ Designate Treatment Officer
- ___ Designate Transport Officer
- ___ Designate Staging Officer
- ___ REMO MD to Scene
- ___ Consider Rehab & CISD

(6-13 Amb. Needed)

LEVEL 3 *(over 25 Patients)*

- ___ Declare MCI
- ___ EMS All Call
- ___ Request # of Units Needed
- ___ Cover Town/Sr. Medic Act 615
- ___ Roll Call Hospitals
- ___ Get Mutual Aid Units
- ___ Designate Treatment Officer
- ___ Designate Transport Officer
- ___ Designate Staging Officer
- ___ REMO MD to Scene
- ___ Request Bus to Scene

(over 13 Amb. Needed)

FIRE

- ___ Assess # of Units Needed
- ___ EMS All Call Req. 619
- ___ Designate Triage
- ___ Set Up Rehab at Air Bank
- ___ Use 619 as ALS Unit

RESCUE

- ___ Establish Perimeter
- ___ Request Speciality Units
- ___ Triage Officer Handles Inner Circle

HAZMAT

- ___ Req. # of Units Needed
- ___ EMS All Call
- ___ Est. Command in Cold Zone
- ___ Designate Triage
- ___ Identify Agent
- ___ Research Decontamination
- ___ Research Med.
- ___ Medical Baseline Assessment of Team
- ___ Don Protective Barriers
- ___ Assist With Decontamination
- ___ Rehabilitate

HOSPITAL ROLL CALL	AMCH	St. PETERS	MEMORIAL	VA	ELLIS	St. CLARE'S	LEONARD	St. MARY'S	SAMARITAN
CAN TAKE									
# PATIENTS SENT									

 # OF PATIENTS BY PRIORITY

1 (Red)	2 (Yellow)	3 (Green)	0 (Black)	TOTALS

UNITS RESPONDING

620 621 622 ____ ____
630 631 632 ____ ____
640 641 642 ____ ____
650 651 652 ____ ____
610 611 605 ____ ____
TSU-1 TSU-2 ____ ____
619 ___ ___ ____ ____
Guild. ___ ___ ____ ____
CPHM ___ ___ ____ ____
Albany ___ ___ ____ ____
Mohawk ___ ___ ____ ____
Empire ___ ___ ____ ____

UNITS IN STAGING

620 621 622 ____ ____
630 631 632 ____ ____
640 641 642 ____ ____
650 651 652 ____ ____
610 611 605 ____ ____
TSU-1 TSU-2 ____ ____
619 ___ ___ ____ ____
Guild. ___ ___ ____ ____
CPHM ___ ___ ____ ____
Albany ___ ___ ____ ____
Mohawk ___ ___ ____ ____
Empire ___ ___ ____ ____

Point of View

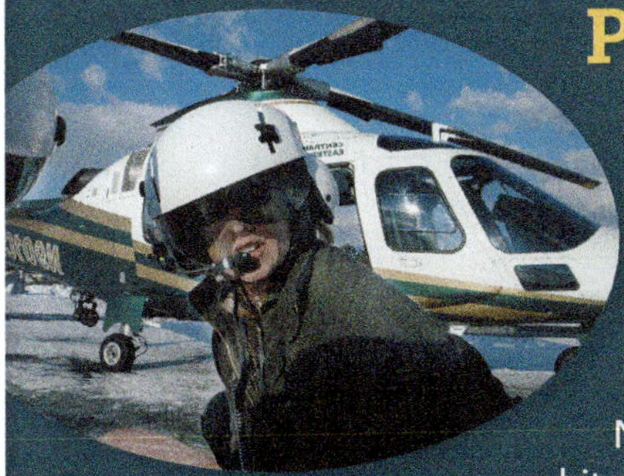

"You know how you figure if you ever get into a car crash, it'll be a fender bender? Not me. I had to do it big. Real big.

"I was on the freeway, coming over the crest of a hill. Fortunately, I was going slow enough so I was able to stop just before a big wreck on the other side. There must've been ten or twelve cars all over the road. Sounds like I did good, right? Nope. The tractor trailer behind me couldn't stop fast enough. He hit me so hard, he pushed me into the car in front of me and then into three others. Squished my little car like an accordion.

"While that was really the pits, I never realized that there would be injured people all over the place. I mean, this road was littered with crashed cars and injured people. When the rescue people finally got to my car, they tied a red ribbon around my wrist and put a red sticker on my windshield. I was starting to feel bad. I asked an EMT what the red meant. He smiled at me very nicely and said, 'You'll be heading out first.'

"'OK, great,' I thought. Things were getting a little fuzzy. Then I saw spacemen heading my way. They had helmets on. They took me to a helicopter. I couldn't believe it. I thought maybe I was hallucinating, but sure enough, they loaded me in and flew me to the gosh-darned hospital.

"Too bad I couldn't have flown that helicopter to work and missed that whole crash thing. I'd probably still have my spleen!"

Psychological Aspects of MCIs

CORE CONCEPT
Psychological aspects of multiple-casualty incidents

During MCIs, EMTs often encounter another, frequently overlooked condition: psychologically stressed patients. Although they may outwardly exhibit few signs of injury or emotional stress, people involved in MCIs have been subjected to devastating circumstances with which they are normally unprepared to cope. Proper early management of the psychologically stressed patient can support later treatment and help ensure a faster recovery.

Adequately managing a patient during an MCI may require you to administer "psychological first aid." This may take the form of talking with a terrified parent, child, or witness. You should not attempt to engage in psychoanalysis, and should not say things that are untrue in an attempt to calm a patient. However, a caring, honest demeanor can reassure a patient, as will listening to the patient and acknowledging any fears and problems. Often this is all the patient will need.

Patients are not the only ones subject to emotional stress during a multiple-casualty incident; emergency responders are as well. It is very important that you understand that large-scale or horrific MCIs (Figure 39-14 and Figure 39-15) may affect rescuers as much as, if not more than, nonrescuers. Many jurisdictions have stress debriefing counselors available for responders after the event. It is important for the responder to be vigilant for unhealthy behaviors brought about by stressful events.

EMTs who become emotionally incapacitated should be treated as patients and removed to an area where they can rest without viewing the scene. These patients must be monitored by an EMS provider until a clinically competent provider can take over. These EMTs should not be allowed to return to duty. They should be evaluated by a trained professional who can properly assess psychological health.

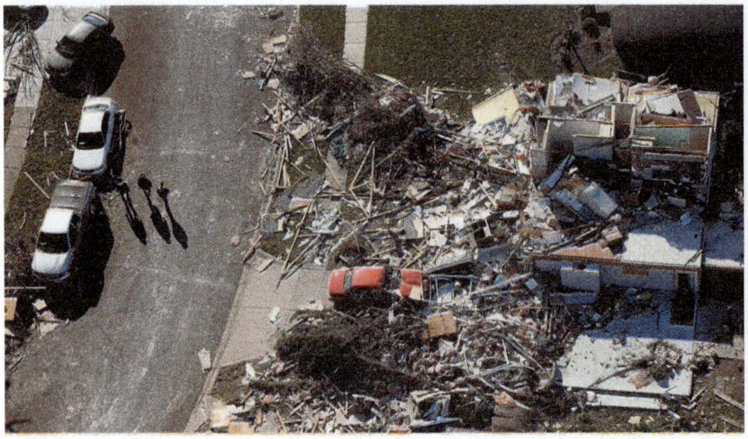

FIGURE 39-14 A tornado can cause great devastation.
(Charles Rex Arbogast/AP Images)

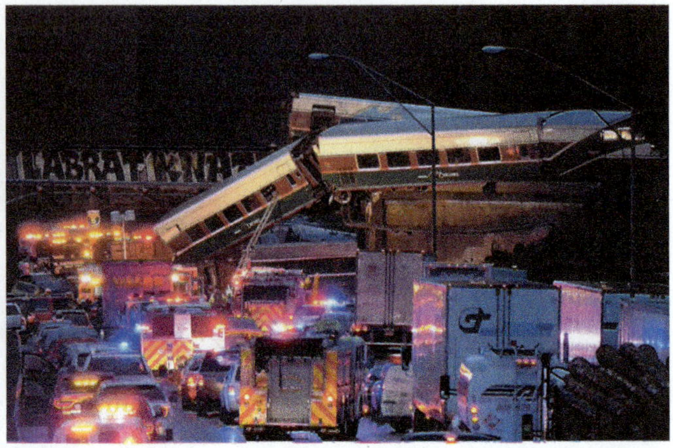

FIGURE 39-15 A train wreck can cause multiple casualties.
(Alex Milan Tracy/Sipa USA/Newscom)

EMS Branch Functions

Under NIMS, in a very large and complex multiple-casualty incident, EMS will function as a branch under the Operations section. For smaller MCIs, the EMS worker who has assumed Incident Command may be able to handle all aspects of management without delegating tasks to others. However, as an incident increases in size and complexity, additional staff and area supervisors will be needed (Figure 39-16, Figure 39-17, and Figure 39-18). The EMS branch generally includes the following:

- Extrication strike teams (in cases of entrapment)
- Staging area
- Triage area
- Treatment area
- Transportation area
- Rehabilitation area

Individuals and agencies on the scene will be assigned particular roles in one or more areas. Most systems use brightly colored reflective vests that can be worn over protective clothing to make each incident role easy to identify. Any EMT arriving at the scene at this time would be expected to report to an area supervisor for assignment of specific duties. Once assigned a specific task, the EMT should complete the task and report back to the area supervisor.

FIGURE 39-16 An organization for a small incident.

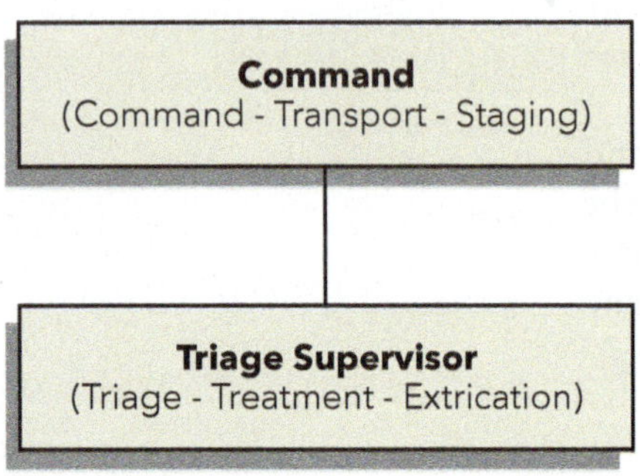

FIGURE 39-17 An organization for a medium-sized incident.

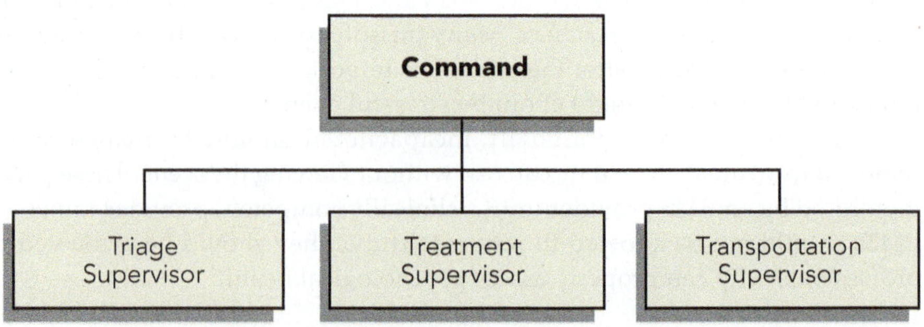

FIGURE 39-18 An organization for a major incident.

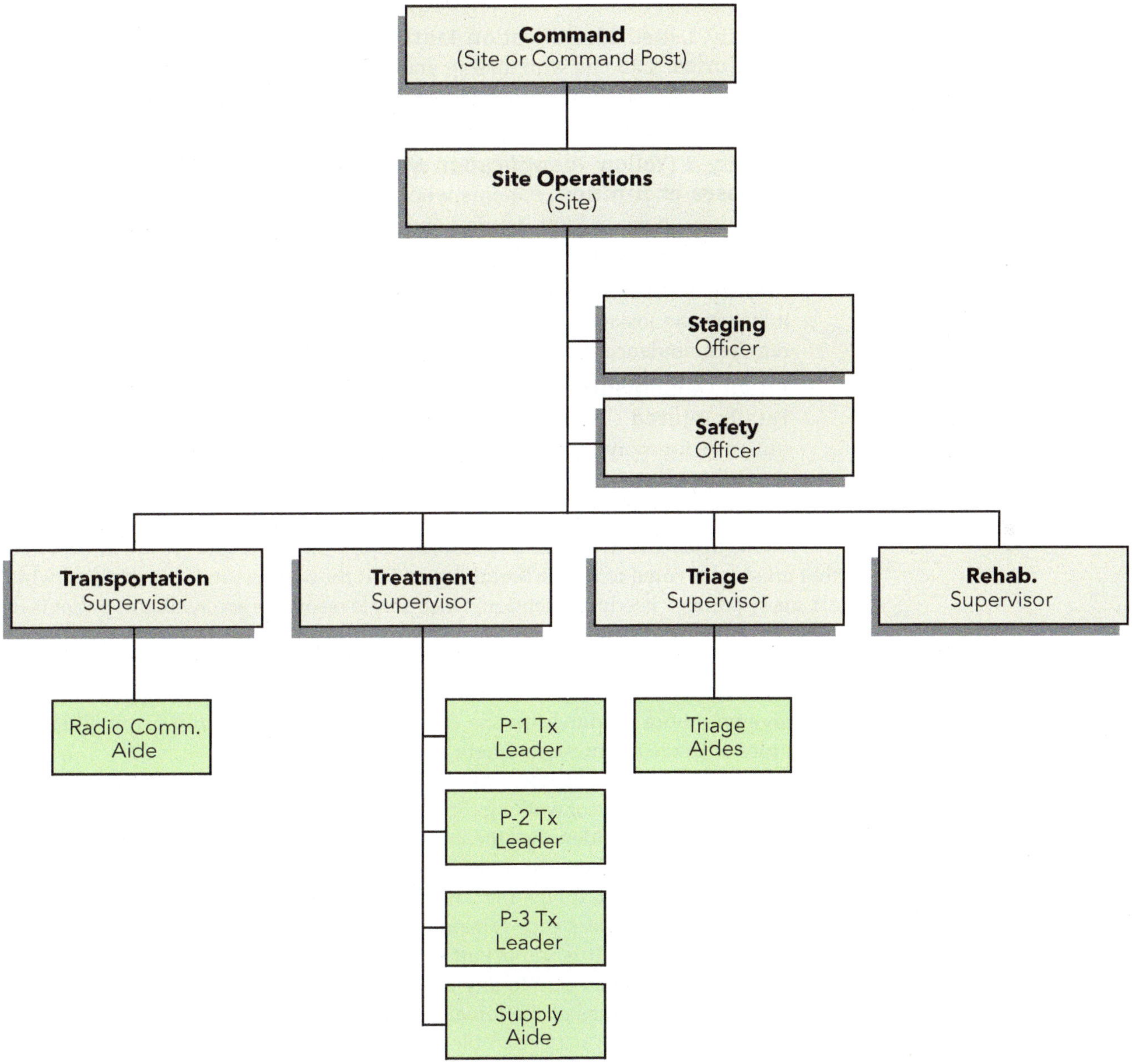

Triage

Once organization has been established, the next task is to quickly assess all the patients and assign each a priority for receiving emergency care or transportation to definitive care. This process is called ***triage***, which comes from a French word meaning "to sort." The most knowledgeable EMS provider becomes the ***triage supervisor***. The triage supervisor calls for additional help (if needed), assigns available personnel and equipment to patients, and remains at the scene to assign and coordinate personnel, supplies, and vehicles.

triage
the process of quickly assessing patients at a multiple-casualty incident and assigning each a priority for receiving treatment; from a French word meaning "to sort."

triage supervisor
the person responsible for overseeing triage at a multiple-casualty incident.

Primary Triage

When faced with more than one patient, your goal must be to afford the greatest number of people the greatest chance of survival. To accomplish this goal, you must provide care to patients according to the seriousness of illness or injury while keeping in mind that spending a lot of time trying to save one life may prevent a number of other patients from receiving the treatment they need. *It may help to think of the entire scene as one big "body."*

CORE CONCEPT
Triage considerations

To properly triage a group of patients, you should quickly classify each patient into one of four groups:

- **Priority 1 (Red Identification Marker): Treatable Life-Threatening Illnesses or Injuries.** Patients with airway and breathing difficulties, uncontrolled or severe bleeding, decreased mental status, severe medical problems, shock (hypoperfusion), and/or severe burns.
- **Priority 2 (Yellow Identification Marker): Serious but Not Life-Threatening Illnesses or Injuries.** Patients who have burns without airway problems; major or multiple bone or joint injuries; and/or back injuries with or without spinal cord damage. These patients generally need ambulance transport.
- **Priority 3 (Green Identification Marker): "Walking Wounded."** Patients with minor musculoskeletal injuries or minor soft-tissue injuries. The patients might not require ambulance transport.
- **Priority 4 (Sometimes Called Priority 0) (Black Identification Marker): Dead or Fatally Injured.** Examples include patients with exposed brain matter, cardiac arrest (no pulse for more than 20 minutes, excluding patients with cold-water drowning or severe hypothermia), decapitation, severed trunk, or incineration. For large incidents, patients in respiratory arrest may fall under this priority.

Patients in arrest are considered Priority 4 (or 0) when resources are limited. The time that must be devoted to rescue breathing or CPR for one person is not justified when there are many patients needing attention. Once ample resources are available, patients in arrest may become Priority 1.

How triage is performed depends on the number of injuries, the immediate hazards to personnel and patients, and the location of backup resources. Local operating procedures will give you more guidance on the exact method of triage for a given situation. Basic principles of triage are presented here.

The first triage cut can be done rapidly by using a bullhorn, PA system, or loud voice to direct all patients capable of walking (Priority 3) to move to a particular area. This has a twofold purpose. It quickly identifies the individuals who have an airway and circulation, and it physically separates them from patients who will generally need more care. You might call out "If you can walk, follow me!" while leading them to the area.

You must rapidly assess each remaining patient, stopping only to secure an airway or stop profuse bleeding. It is important that you not develop "tunnel vision"—spending time rendering additional care to any one patient and thus failing to identify and correct life-threatening conditions of the remaining patients. If Priority 3 patients are nearby and well enough to help, they may be employed to assist you by maintaining an airway or direct pressure on bleeding wounds of other patients. (In this situation, you should provide the appropriate PPE.) Priority 3 patients who have been reluctant to leave ill or injured friends or relatives may be permitted to stay near them, where they can be of possible help later, especially in situations of language differences.

Once all patients have been assessed and treated for airway and breathing problems and severe bleeding, more-thorough treatment can be initiated. You will need to render care to the patients who are most seriously injured or ill but who stand the best chance of survival with proper treatment. This requires treating all the Priority 1 patients first, Priority 2 patients next, and Priority 3 patients last. Priority 4 patients do not receive treatment unless no other patients are believed to be at risk of dying or suffering long-term disability if their conditions go unattended.

Usually patients will be immobilized on backboards, if necessary, and carried by "runners" to the appropriate secondary sector (as described later in this text). Extensive treatment does not occur at the incident site, since it is in a hazard zone and could impede rescue and initial treatment of other patients.

START

The START method of triage (Figure 39-19) was developed by the Newport Beach, California, Fire Department and Hoag Hospital, also in Newport Beach. *START* stands for *Simple Triage and Rapid Treatment*. The foundation of the system is the speed, simplicity, and consistency of its application. It relies on some simple commands and the following physiologic parameters, which can be remembered by the mnemonic *RPM*:

Respiration
Pulse
Mental Status

START triage is intended to be completed in about 30 seconds per patient.

Begin by asking all patients who can walk to get up and go to a collection point, such as an ambulance or a building. Since those who can do this are . . .

- Conscious
- Able to follow commands
- Able to walk

FIGURE 39-19 START triage.

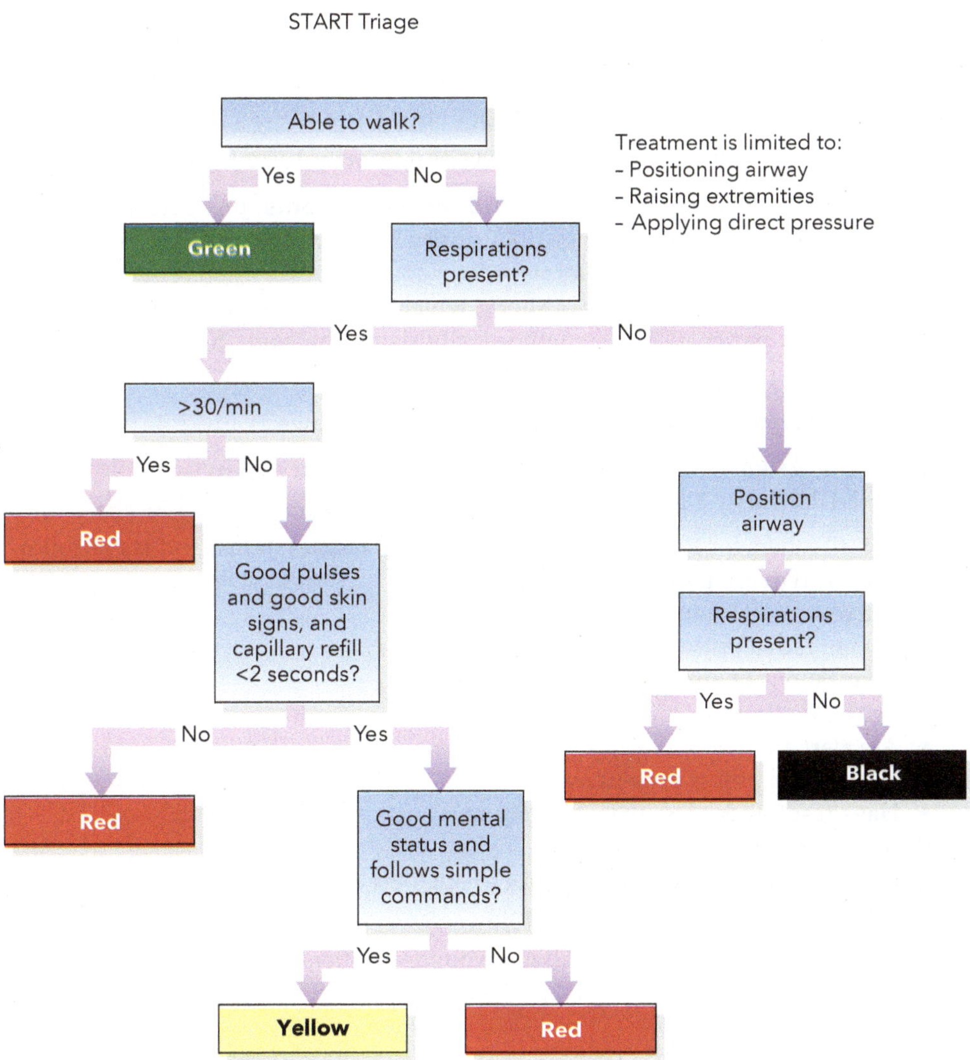

. . . they obviously are perfusing their brain, are breathing, have a pulse, and have a nervous system that is currently working. All of these patients are considered to be Priority 3 (*green tag*) patients for right now. (They are often called the "walking wounded.") This also leaves people at the site who are unable to hear, walk, or follow commands and are the Priority 1, 2, or 4 (0) patients. Among these patients, you must now focus your attention on those who are likely to be of higher priority.

Start making your triage sweep methodically by avoiding patients who are obviously conscious. The only three treatments provided during START triage are to:

- Open an airway and insert an oropharyngeal airway.
- Apply pressure to bleeding.
- Elevate an extremity.

Assess Respiration (Breathing Status) First. If the patient is *not breathing* and your attempts to open the airway do *not* start breathing, tag the patient as a Priority 4 (*black tag*) patient. If the patient *starts breathing* after the airway is opened, then tag as a Priority 1 (*red tag*). Is the patient breathing more than 30 times per minute? If so, tag the patient as a Priority 1 (*red tag*) patient. Is the patient breathing fewer than 30 times per minute? If so, go to the next step.

Assess Radial Pulse Second. If the patient is *unresponsive, not breathing*, and has *no pulse*, tag the patient as a Priority 4 (*black tag*) patient. If the patient is *breathing* but has *no radial pulse*, tag as a Priority 1 (*red tag*) patient. If the patient is *breathing* and *has a pulse, good skin signs*, and *capillary refill less than 2 seconds*, go to the next step.

Assess Level of Consciousness (Mental Status) Third. If *alert*, tag as a Priority 2 (*yellow tag*) patient. If there is any *altered mental status*, tag as a Priority 1 (*red tag*) patient.

Now Retriage the Priority 3 "Walking Wounded" Patients. Just because they could initially walk does not mean some of the Priority 3 patients do not have serious medical conditions and might not deteriorate! Many could have an altered mental status, be bleeding, and have significant signs of shock, which could cause them to be recategorized as higher-priority patients. Move methodically using the same START assessment of (1) respiration, (2) pulse, and (3) mental status.

A START Summary. A quick summary of START is as follows:

1. Order the walking wounded to some type of temporary collection point. They are considered **Priority 3 (*green*)** for now.
2. Assess all others for RPM (respiration, pulse, and mental status) and tag as follows:
   Priority 1 (red) are patients who have:
   - Altered mental status or . . .
   - Absent radial pulse or . . .
   - Respirations of greater than 30/minute

   Priority 2 (yellow) are patients who:
   - Are alert and . . .
   - Have radial pulses present and . . .
   - Have respirations less than 30/minute

   Priority 4 (black) are patients who:
   - Are not breathing (after an attempt to open the airway) or . . .
   - Have no pulse and are not breathing
3. Retriage all **Priority 3 (green)** walking wounded patients.

Patient Identification

By now, it should be clear that a system will be required to group and identify patients by treatment priority. A widely used system is to color-code patients according to their priority. The START system, discussed previously, is one example of a color-coding system. Where

Priority 1 is red; Priority 2 is yellow; Priority 3 is green; and Priority 4 is black. Other systems' color codes may be slightly different.

Since different localities have different systems, it is important that you know and understand the system used in your area. It is equally important that different services in the same region use the same coding system. This is because many MCIs are multiple-agency events. If each agency were to use a different system, there would be no way to correctly coordinate the order in which patients were to receive care. Training sessions and emergency management–related exercises can help alleviate coding system problems. Follow your agencies' standard operating guidelines.

As you move among patients to conduct initial triage, you should affix a ***triage tag*** to each patient, indicating the priority group to which that patient has been assigned. Triage tags are color-coded and may have space in which limited medical information can be recorded (Figure 39-20, Figure 39-21, and Figure 39-22). As the situation allows, try to get as much pertinent medical history as you can on your patients. This will help you monitor for changes in patient status, especially deterioration situations.

triage tag
color-coded tag indicating the priority group to which a patient has been assigned.

There are some local variations of the triage tag. Some use adhesive-backed colored shipping labels. Others use colored surveyor's tape or duct tape to classify patients. Surveyor's tape can be quickly tied on as an armband. Duct tape will stick to just about anything in any kind of weather. For this reason, it is particularly useful in an MCI setting. It is also useful to have a laundry marker or wax pencil handy for wet conditions, when a standard pen or pencil will not write well. Creativity is a valuable trait to have during an MCI event.

Whatever system you use, it is vital that the color coding be easily located and identified. When properly performed, this coding allows another rescuer to quickly identify which treatment group patients belong to and to institute treatment in that manner. Always be mindful that a patient's status can change and that an MCI event can last for hours, if not days.

SALT

SALT (*Sort, Assess, Lifesaving Interventions, Treatment/Transport*) is another method used at MCIs that is gaining popularity and acceptance in EMS systems (Figure 39-23). SALT was developed by a workgroup convened by the National Association of EMS Physicians with funding from the Centers for Disease Control and Prevention. SALT, along with the Model Uniform Core Criteria (MUCC) for Mass Casualty Triage, provides another framework that EMS providers can use at MCIs.

SALT uses a *forward movement* of patients, based on priority, while moving them *away* from the incident. Patients are moved forward to a casualty collection point. This is an area where they can be sorted and prioritized for further forward movement to treatment areas and transport to hospitals, if appropriate.

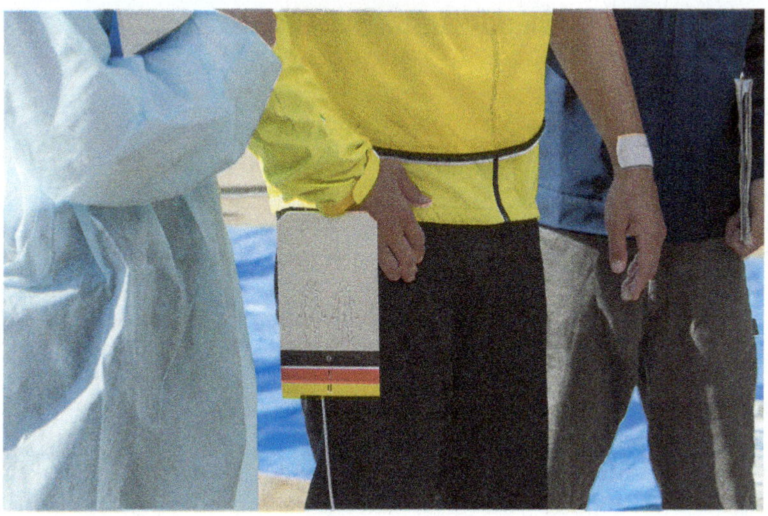

FIGURE 39-20 The triage tag indicates the priority group to which that patient has been assigned. *(HikoPhotography/ Shutterstock)*

FIGURE 39-21 Triage tag (front and back) used to identify Priority 1, 2, 3, and 0 patients.

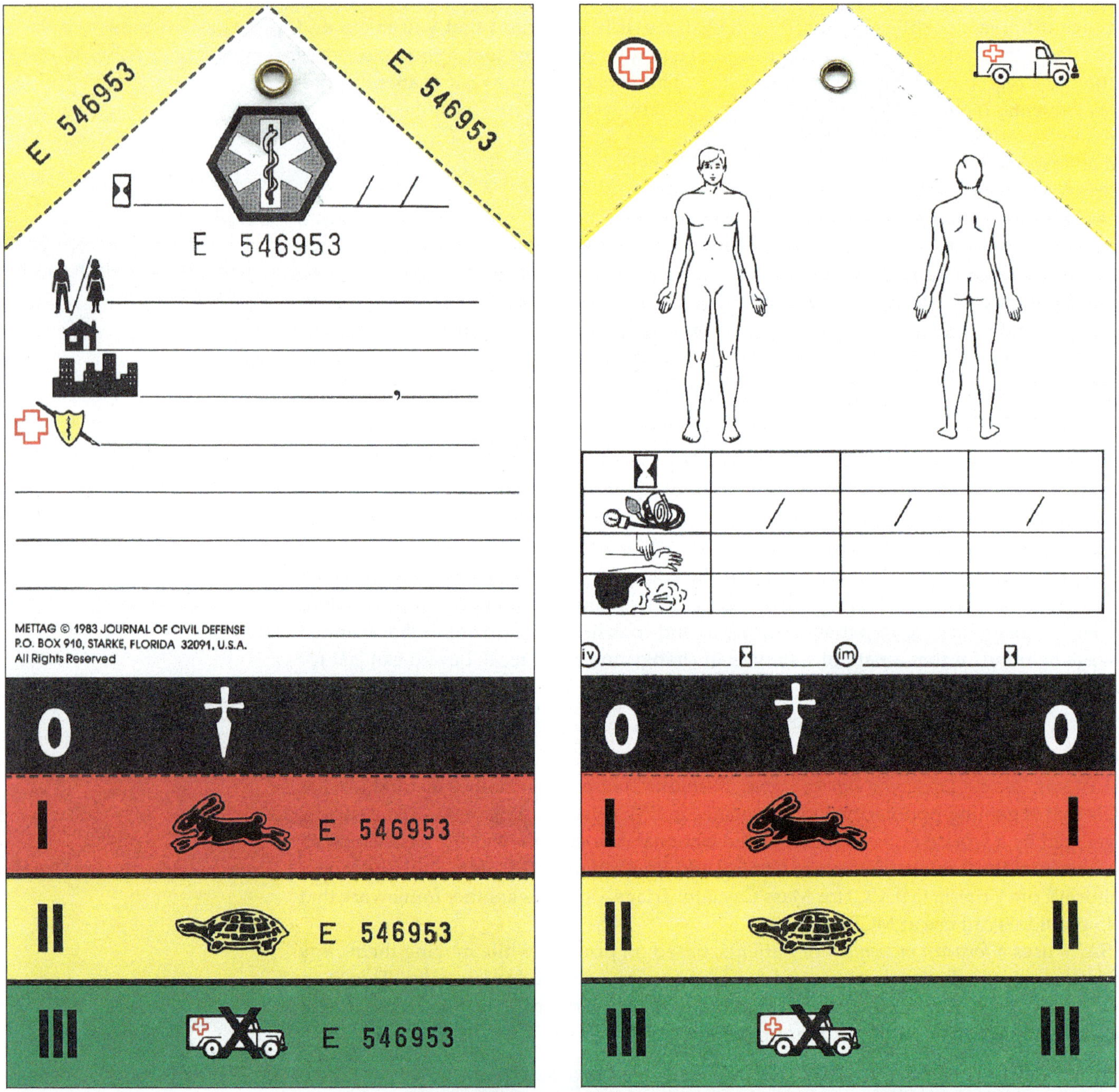

Sort. SALT begins with the Sort function. Announce, in a loud voice or through a loudspeaker, "If you can hear me and can walk, move to [the safe area]." Note that these patients will typically be your lowest assessment and treatment priority. Next, for the patients who remain in place, say, "If you need help, wave your arm or move your leg." Patients who can follow commands and have purposeful movement but cannot walk or move themselves are typically a higher priority for assessment and treatment. Finally, those who are still and who have not walked or waved are typically patients with the highest assessment and treatment priority.

Assessment and Lifesaving Interventions. Assessment and lifesaving interventions are performed next and occur at the same time. Once you assess and identify a life threat, you should provide a lifesaving intervention, provided that it will not take longer than 1 minute and will not require you (or another EMS provider) to stay with the patient

FIGURE 39-22 EMS disaster tag (front and back).

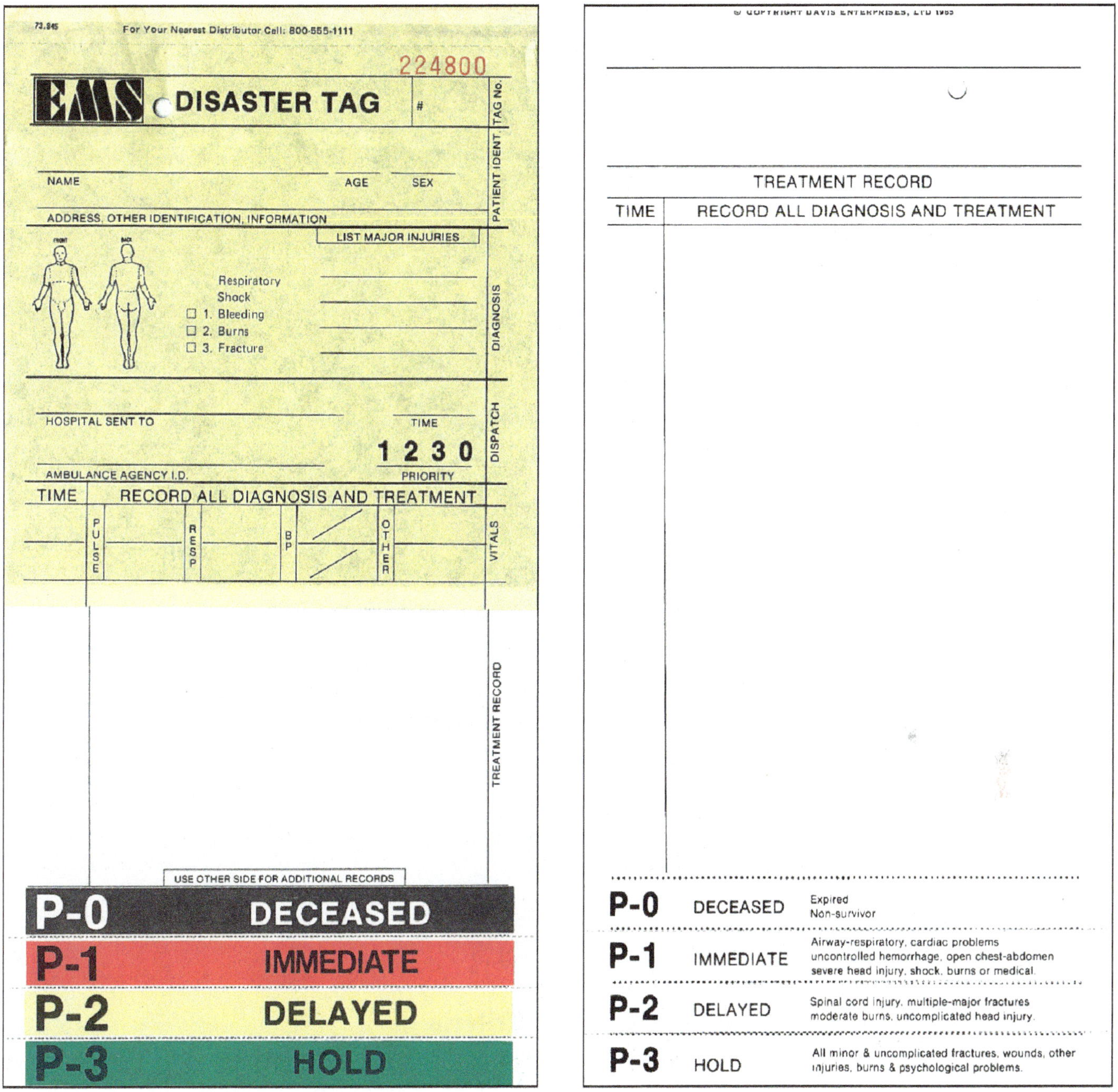

afterward. An example of an intervention an EMT would perform is applying a tourniquet to a patient with a severe hemorrhage.

Remember to keep moving! You must maintain forward movement of yourself, fellow EMS providers, and patients under the SALT system. Provide lifesaving interventions immediately, then move on to the next patient. As you assess and provide lifesaving interventions, you will categorize or tag patients by priority, then move them forward to the casualty collection point.

Treatment/Transport. As patients receive triage tags, they should move forward (or be moved forward) to a casualty collection point. From there, patients continue to move forward (or be moved forward) to a treatment area and eventually to an ambulance for transport to a receiving hospital.

FIGURE 39-23 Flow of patient triage with SALT method.

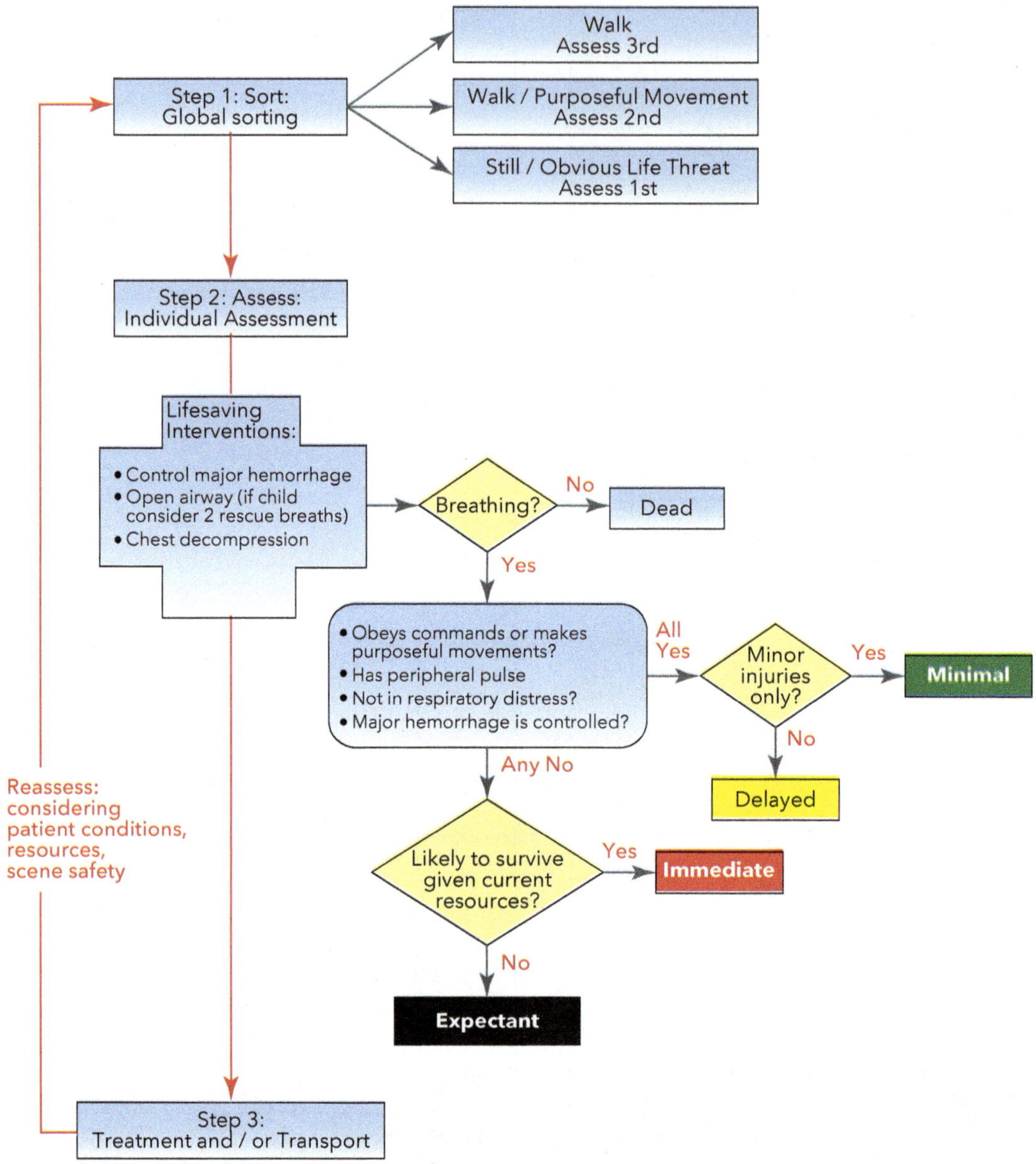

SALT and MUCC Triage Criteria

Immediate (color code red): Patients with severe injuries who are likely to survive with treatment are tagged as Immediate. Assess the following:

- Does the patient have a peripheral pulse?
- Is the patient not in respiratory distress?
- Is hemorrhage controlled?
- Does the patient follow commands or make purposeful movements?

A patient with a "no" answer to any of these questions but who is likely to survive should be tagged as Immediate. Immediate patients should be moved forward to the casualty collection point first.

Delayed (color code yellow): Patients with serious injuries that will require eventual forward movement but are not tagged as Immediate are tagged as Delayed. Assess the following:

- Does the patient have a peripheral pulse?
- Is the patient not in respiratory distress?
- Is hemorrhage controlled?
- Does the patient follow commands or make purposeful movements?

A patient with a "yes" response to all of these with a significant injury (such as a long bone fracture) should be tagged as Delayed.

Minimal (color code green): Patients with minor injuries should be tagged as Minimal. Most Minimal patients should have moved forward during the Sort phase.

Dead (color code black): Patients with injuries incompatible with life or without spontaneous respirations are triaged as Dead (or Deceased). Assess the following:

- Is an adult patient not breathing after EMT opens the airway?
- Is a child patient not breathing after EMT opens the airway and give two breaths?

Patients tagged Dead (or Deceased) are those for whom you answered one of the above questions "yes." They do not move forward from the point of injury to the casualty collection point, but remain in place.

Expectant (color code gray): Patients who are unlikely to survive given the available resources should be tagged as Expectant. These patients should receive treatment and other resources only after the Immediate patients have been moved forward. An example would be a patient with a severe burn covering nearly the total body surface area.

Crew rest rotations, as possible, will be very important for long-duration MCIs. Crew rest periods will both decrease the incidence of mistakes and assist in maintaining the long-term psychological health of crew members.

Secondary Triage and Treatment

As more personnel arrive at the incident scene, they should be directed to assist with the completion of initial triage. If triage has been completed, these EMTs can initiate treatment. It is very important that the EMT report into the correct command structure to keep the EMT from freelancing. Resources may be thin, especially early in the MCI event; every EMT counts.

Secondary triage is generally performed at a patient collection point, or ***triage area***, from which patients are assigned to treatment groups.

Patients are physically separated into treatment groups based on their priority level as designated by a triage tag. Some systems call for vehicles to carry red, yellow, and green tarps, which are used to designate these areas. An area to which triaged patients are removed is referred to as a ***treatment area***. Each treatment area should have its own ***treatment supervisor***, an EMT responsible for overseeing the triage and treatment within that area. The treatment supervisor should retriage the patients in that area to determine the order in which they will receive treatment. Secondary triage is important to ensure that patients are treated and transported according to their priority.

During secondary triage, it may be necessary to recategorize a patient whose condition has deteriorated or improved, or who was incorrectly triaged. That patient should be designated to a higher- or lower-priority group than was originally medically warranted. This will necessitate moving the patient to the proper treatment area as resources permit. Some systems use a different disaster tag during secondary triage on which more detailed information about the patient can be recorded. (Review Figure 39-22.)

The treatment-area EMTs will need supplies and equipment from the ambulances such as bandages, blood pressure cuffs, and oxygen.

triage area
the area where secondary triage takes place at a multiple-casualty incident.

treatment area
the area in which patients are treated at a multiple-casualty incident.

treatment supervisor
person responsible for overseeing treatment of patients who have been triaged at a multiple-casualty incident.

CORE CONCEPT
Transportation and staging logistics

Transportation and Staging Logistics

Once patients have been properly assessed and triaged, and once treatment for the patients has been initiated according to their priority, consideration must be given to the order in which the patients will be transported to a hospital. Again, this is done according to triage priority.

It is advisable to have a ***staging area*** from which ambulances can be called to transport patients. The staging area will be the responsibility of the ***staging supervisor***, who must keep track of the ambulance vehicles and personnel. In large-scale incidents, the staging supervisor may need to arrange for certain human needs, such as rest rooms, meals, and rotation of crews.

No ambulance should proceed to a treatment area unless requested by the ***transportation supervisor*** and directed by the staging supervisor. The staging supervisor is responsible for communicating with each treatment area regarding the number and priority of the patients in that area. This information can then be used by the transportation supervisor to arrange for transport of patients from the scene to the hospital in the most efficient way.

staging area
the area where ambulances are parked and other resources are held until needed.

staging supervisor
person responsible for overseeing ambulances and ambulance personnel at a multiple-casualty incident.

transportation supervisor
person responsible for communicating with sector officers and hospitals to manage transportation of patients to hospitals from a multiple-casualty incident.

It is vital that no ambulance transport any patient without the approval of the transportation supervisor, since the transportation supervisor is responsible for maintaining a list of patients and the hospitals to which they are transported. This information is relayed from the transportation supervisor to each receiving hospital. (In a large-scale incident, the transportation officer may actually have an aide who does nothing but speak to hospitals.) In this way the hospitals know what to expect and receive only the patients they are capable of handling. It is critical that the EMTs on the ambulance comply with the instructions of the transportation supervisor. Failure to do so may result in patients being transported to the wrong facilities. During an MCI, it is very important that the transportation officer knows about the local hospitals' capabilities. Taking too many patients to one hospital could overwhelm that hospital's capability to treat them. Overwhelming a hospital's ***surge capacity*** could bring about poor outcomes.

surge capacity
a measurable representation of ability of a medical facility to manage a sudden influx of patients. It is dependent on a variety of variables, including the number of open beds, physical space, supplies, staff, and any special considerations (such as contaminated or contagious patients).

Once an ambulance has completed its run to a hospital, it will probably be directed to return to the staging area, perhaps bringing needed supplies, to await its next instructions from the staging supervisor.

Communicating with Hospitals

It is important that receiving hospitals be alerted to the nature of the MCI or disaster as soon as the magnitude of the incident is known. This allows the hospitals to call in additional personnel or to clear beds as necessary to accept the anticipated number of patients. The hospitals have their own disaster management plans and will set those in motion once contacted about the MCI event.

Because radio communication channels will be heavily used, the transportation officer, not individual EMTs, should communicate with the hospitals. This will keep unnecessary radio usage to a minimum. It will also ensure that the proper information is recorded at both ends of the ambulance ride. In large-scale MCIs, it is not necessary to give a patient report for each patient, since the treating and transporting EMTs will most likely be different and there will generally be too many patients to allow EMTs to give a good patient radio report under the circumstances. In these instances the hospital may be told only basic information—for example, that they are receiving a Priority 1 patient with respiratory problems.

Chapter Review

Key Facts and Concepts

- Maintain a high index of suspicion and awareness. Many HAZMAT incidents start out as routine EMS calls.
- The biggest problem in most HAZMAT incidents is identifying the offending substance. Look for the shipping placard and the SDS. Use the *Emergency Response Guide* to help determine your initial actions. Be aware that the shipping placard and records may not be correct.
- Remember hot zone/warm zone/cold zone. Once you realize it's a HAZMAT incident, get to the cold zone and call for help.
- Keep responders in rehab until they are rested and hydrated, and their vitals return to normal.
- Patients who have been "decontaminated" almost always still have some contamination.
- Patients being transported must be cared for by competent EMS responders with Operations-level training and equipment.
- Practice your MCI plan and procedure at small incidents, as this will make managing larger ones easier.
- NIMS and Incident Management are the national standard for incident management.
- Learn and practice START triage essentials.
- Be alert for signs of stress after incidents, and seek help as necessary.

Key Decisions

- What is the hazardous substance? What risk does it pose to me, the other rescuers, and the public?
- Does anyone need immediate evacuation?
- If a patient has some contamination, can we safely start decontamination?
- Is this incident at a level where I should institute the Incident Management System?
- Should I start using triage tags?
- What additional resources should I call for?

Chapter Glossary

cold zone area where the Incident Command post and support functions are located.

Command the first on the scene to establish order and initiate the Incident Command System.

decontamination a chemical and/or physical process that reduces or prevents the spread of contamination from persons or equipment; the removal of hazardous substances from employees and their equipment to the extent necessary to preclude foreseeable health effects.

disaster plan a predefined set of instructions for a community's emergency responders.

hazardous material (HAZMAT) any substance or material in a form that poses an unreasonable risk to health, safety, and property when transported in commerce or kept in storage at a warehouse, port, depot, or railroad facility.

hot zone area immediately surrounding a HAZMAT incident; extends far enough to prevent adverse effects outside the zone.

Incident Command the person or persons who assume overall direction of a large-scale incident.

Incident Command System (ICS) a subset of the National Incident Management System (NIMS) designed specifically for management of multiple-casualty incidents.

multiple-casualty incident (MCI) any medical or trauma incident involving multiple patients.

National Incident Management System (NIMS) the management system used by federal, state, and local governments to manage emergencies in the United States.

single incident command command organization in which a single agency controls all resources and operations.

staging area the area where ambulances are parked and other resources are held until needed.

staging supervisor person responsible for overseeing ambulances and ambulance personnel at a multiple-casualty incident.

surge capacity a measurable representation of ability of a medical facility to manage a sudden influx of patients. It is dependent on a variety of variables including the number of open beds, physical space, supplies, staff, and any special considerations (such as contaminated or contagious patients).

transportation supervisor person responsible for communicating with sector officers and hospitals to manage transportation of patients to hospitals from a multiple-casualty incident.

treatment area the area in which patients are treated at a multiple-casualty incident.

treatment supervisor person responsible for overseeing treatment of patients who have been triaged at a multiple-casualty incident.

triage the process of quickly assessing patients at a multiple-casualty incident and assigning each a priority for receiving treatment; from a French word meaning "to sort."

triage area the area where secondary triage takes place at a multiple-casualty incident.

triage supervisor the person responsible for overseeing triage at a multiple-casualty incident.

triage tag color-coded tag indicating the priority group to which a patient has been assigned.

unified command command organization in which several agencies work independently but cooperatively.

warm zone area where personnel and equipment decontamination and hot zone support take place; it includes control points for the access corridor and thus assists in reducing the spread of contamination.

Preparation for Your Examination and Practice

Short Answer

1. List the information contained in an initial report of a hazardous material incident.
2. Explain how to identify a hazardous material and how to obtain information about that material.
3. Describe the general assessment and emergency care of a patient with a hazardous material injury.
4. Describe the major components and benefits of an Incident Management System.
5. Define the basic role of the EMT at a multiple-casualty incident.
6. Explain why patients are assigned priorities during triage.
7. Identify four priority categories of triage.

Thinking and Linking

Think back to the chapter titled Well-Being of the EMT, *and link information from that chapter with information from this chapter as you consider the following situations:*

1. At an MCI, one EMT, who was among the first to arrive and has been working at peak level ever since, looks really tired. As Incident Commander, you ask if she wants a break. She says she is fine and doesn't need a break. What should you do?

2. Several weeks after working an MCI, you start having trouble sleeping, are having trouble concentrating, and find you are snapping at your family and coworkers. You realize the symptoms may be related to that MCI but figure you'll get over it. Right? Wrong? What should you do?

Critical Thinking Exercises

When you are first on scene at a possible multiple-casualty incident with possible hazardous material involvement, what should you do? The purpose of this exercise will be to think through your actions at such an incident.

- Your call is to a motor-vehicle collision with an unknown number of injuries. As your unit approaches the scene, you see that three cars and downed wires are involved. You get a whiff of gasoline as you pass by. The drivers are visible in each vehicle—one appears to be conscious, and the other two are bent forward or slumped back. There are passengers visible in two vehicles, one or more of whom may need extrication. How should you proceed?

Street Scenes

It's raining hard, and there's a loud noise on the station PA system, with the dispatcher saying "Ambulances Alpha 2, Alpha 5, Bravo 1, and Charlie 10, respond to a three-car motor-vehicle crash at the intersection of Avenues A and B. Unknown how many occupants. Timeout of 1933 hours." You turn to your partner and say, "This call is only about ten blocks away. We should be the first on scene." As you head toward the scene, you are notified by dispatch that the police are on scene and report a total of nine occupants. Additional ambulances are being dispatched.

You and your partner agree that you will establish Incident Command and he will do triage. "Dispatch, Bravo 1 is on scene and establishing Incident Command." The first thing you do is put on the Command bib for identification. Your partner puts on the triage bib and takes triage tags to check on the cars' occupants. You briefly tell the police officer you are Incident Command. The officer informs you that the captain is responding, has three units handling traffic control, and has also requested heavy rescue from the fire department in case extrication is needed.

With flashlight in hand, and while trying to keep the rain out of your eyes, you perform a scene size-up. You realize that you need a place to stage the other ambulances for easy access and so they don't get blocked in. You see a location and quickly share your idea with the police officer, who agrees and who tells the police units to make sure that area is accessible for the ambulances. You call dispatch on the radio using the identifier "Incident Command" and ask that they instruct all responding ambulances to stage in the parking lot of a nearby insurance company.

Street Scene Questions

1. As Incident Command, what are some of the things you need to do?
2. What information do you expect first from the triage officer?
3. How will you decide which patients go to which hospitals?

Your partner advises you that three patients are Priority 1, five are Priority 2, and one is Priority 3. You radio dispatch with this information. You are told that a canvass of local hospitals has already been done and that the trauma center can handle all Priority 1 patients. The other patients can be divided among the other three area hospitals. You ask that someone call the trauma center back to confirm that they will be getting three patients and notify the other hospitals will be getting two each.

You then ask dispatch to tell you how many ambulances have been dispatched. You are informed there are a total of five. Remembering that one of the ambulances is yours, you request two more ambulances. Two of the dispatched ambulances are on scene and parked in the staging area. You tell them to each take a Priority 1 patient. The next arriving ambulance is assigned to the last Priority 1 patient. You ask the triage officer if some of the Priority 2 or 3 patients can be doubled up, which seems appropriate for four of the patients.

Street Scene Questions

4. Is there a need for a safety officer on this scene?
5. How should patient information be transmitted to the hospitals?
6. What information should you be sharing with Police Command and Fire Command?

The fire captain tells you that his crew has disconnected the batteries of all the vehicles and will stand by to assist with extrication. Access has been gained to all patients using hand tools. You ask if his safety officer can continue in that role until all the patients are off the scene.

The first ambulance is loaded and en route to the trauma center. The second will shortly be en route. You advise these crews to notify the hospital directly but tell them to keep the transmissions short.

The last Priority 1 patient is out of the car, and you tell the triage supervisor that the other hospitals get two patients each. He should coordinate this with crews and tell them to call the patient information directly in to the hospital.

Within 30 minutes of the call notification, every patient is en route to a hospital. You let Police and Fire Command know. Your partner looks at you and says, "Not bad for someone who looks like a drowned rat."

Highway Safety and Vehicle Extrication

40

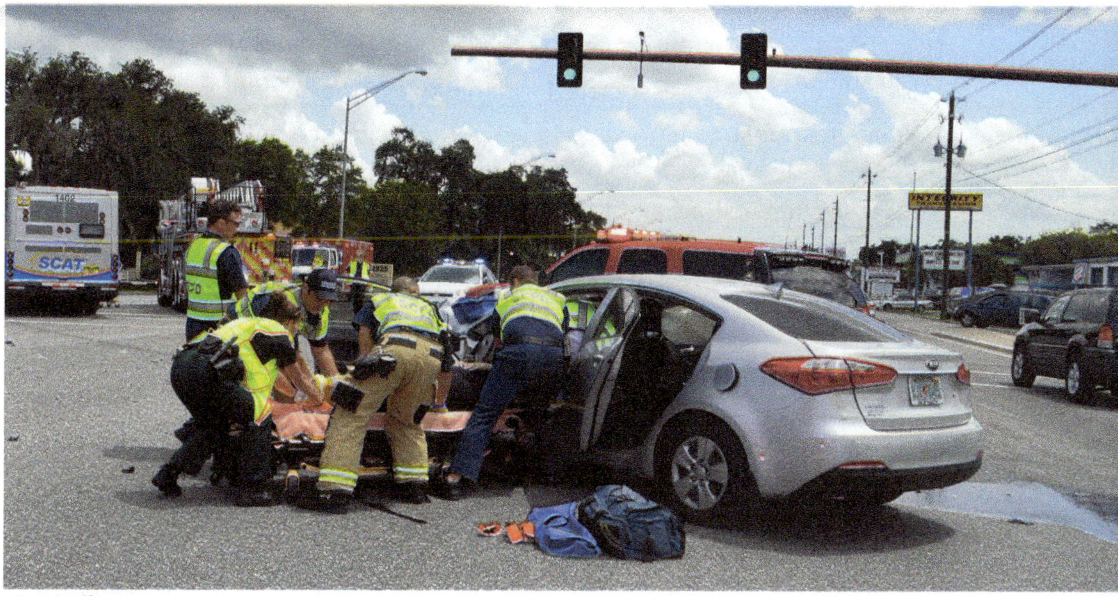

(© Ed Effron)

Related Chapters

The following chapters provide additional information related to topics discussed in this chapter:

2 Well-Being of the EMT
11 Scene Size-Up
39 Hazardous Materials, Multiple-Casualty Incidents, and Incident Management

Standard

EMS Operations (Vehicle Extrication)

Competency

Applies knowledge of operational roles and responsibilities to ensure patient, public, and personnel safety.

Core Concepts

- How to position emergency apparatus to create a safe work zone at a highway emergency
- How to recognize and manage hazards at the highway rescue scene
- How to stabilize a vehicle
- How to gain access to the patient in a crashed vehicle
- How to disentangle a patient from a crashed vehicle

Outcomes

After reading this chapter, you should be able to:

40.1 Summarize concepts of highway emergency operations. (pp. 1214–1219)

- Identify the hazards associated with highway emergency operations.
- Relate response to highway scenes to the incidence of line-of-duty deaths (LODD).
- Describe the actions an EMT should take at a highway scene if that EMT's ambulance is the first-arriving vehicle.
- Explain the reason for establishing Incident Command as the first-arriving unit on the scene of a highway emergency.
- Recognize the guidelines for effective placement of traffic control cones or flares.
- Outline the safety actions all EMTs should take at the scene of highway operations.

40.2 Summarize the concepts of vehicle extrication operations. (pp. 1219–1240)

- Compare the EMT's role as a team member in an extrication with that of trained rescue personnel performing the extrication procedures.
- Recognize the general steps rescuers will take in performing extrication procedures.
- Describe steps to avoid injury from damaged vehicles and structures at the scene of highway emergency operations.
- Identify safety precautions for occupants who will be inside the car during extrication procedures.
- Identify equipment that can help EMTs access a damaged vehicle while awaiting response of an extrication team.
- Describe the features of commonly used approaches to extrication.

At least ten types of specialty rescue teams may be available in a community, depending on the community's hazards. Each specialty requires a significant amount of additional training over and above your EMT course. These specialties include vehicle rescue, water rescue, ice rescue, high-angle/low-angle rescue, hazardous material response, trench rescue, dive rescue, backcountry or wilderness rescue, farm rescue, and confined-space rescue. Training that is available in each of these specialties often depends on the types of emergency responses that might be required in your community.

The focus of this chapter is the EMT's role at the scene of a vehicle collision where extrication of the patient is required, since this is the most common type of rescue across the United States (Figure 40-1).

Highway Emergency Operations

One of the greatest hazards emergency responders face today is oncoming traffic at highway incidents. Drivers are in quiet cars with distractions that can range from mobile phones to onboard video players. Distracted drivers pose a great risk to everyone operating at a highway incident. It requires a team effort of police, fire, and EMS to ensure a work area that is

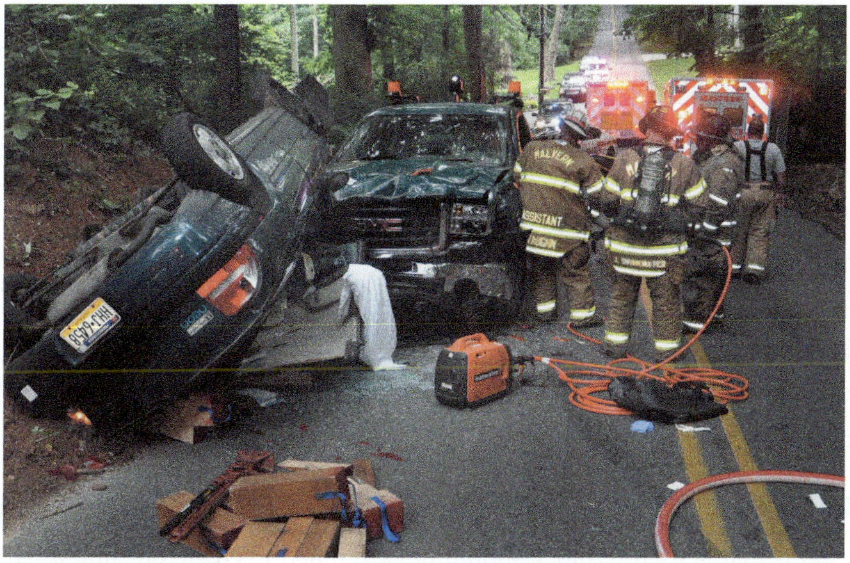

FIGURE 40-1 A vehicle collision where extrication of the patient is required is the most common type of rescue across the United States. *(© Edward T. Dickinson, MD)*

as safe as possible from as many hazards as possible. EMTs are not typically in charge of highway incidents but play a key role because they are called to treat the injured who are likely to be entrapped in wreckage.

The care of the injured and safety of the responders are both high priorities at a highway incident. Responding agencies and personnel need to be aware of their responsibilities in this hazardous environment. To achieve these goals, the following factors are important:

- EMS response should be limited to only the staff and vehicles needed to accomplish the mission and should not expose more people than necessary to the risks of highway operations.
- The first-arriving unit should institute "blocking" to protect the work area. Because of its size and weight, fire apparatus is preferred for this purpose.
- If it is necessary to block lanes of traffic, vehicles should be cleared as quickly as possible, so the flow of traffic can return to normal. However, if scene safety dictates blocking lanes of traffic, blocking should be maintained until response and extrication tasks are completed.

CORE CONCEPT

How to position emergency apparatus to create a safe work zone at a highway emergency

Initial Response

On limited-access highways, only the primary or first-due units should proceed directly to the scene. The first unit arriving must establish Incident Command immediately. Units sent for backup should stage off the highway until they are requested to the scene. This requires coordination between dispatch and responding units as well as preexisting response protocols and standard operating guidelines.

The first-arriving units should:

- Establish Command and confirm the exact location of the incident with the dispatch center.
- Use apparatus to institute "upstream blocking" of the scene to protect the work area. Although fire apparatus is ideal, as already noted, any first-arriving unit can institute blocking. If fire apparatus responds subsequently, they can be placed behind the lighter units.
- Ensure that rescue trucks (police or EMS) arriving to perform extrication are positioned downstream of the initial blocking vehicle.

Congestion at incidents is a big problem. To minimize scene congestion, units should park facing the same direction and remain in single file, if possible. Again, larger units should provide upstream blocking, whereas Command and EMS units should be downstream in the "safe zone." This response ideal is a dynamic one, as specialized situations such as fire will necessitate redirecting assets. Responding units need to exercise extreme caution in performing turnarounds on limited-access highways. These should be done only when a turn can be completed without obstructing the flow of traffic in either travel direction or when all traffic movement has stopped.

EMS personnel should avoid parking their units and conducting ambulance loading on the side that is across traffic flow from the side where the crashed vehicle or vehicles are located. Unless a roadway is completely shut down, EMS crews should avoid crossing over lanes of traffic on foot, especially when they are trying to move patients. Doing so is extremely dangerous. Whenever possible, park downstream from the crash in a safe zone created by blocking from upstream apparatus.

NOTE: *In 2012, according to estimates compiled by officials with the Hampton Roads Transportation Planning Organization in Virginia, 120 police officers, 83 firefighters, 21 emergency medical services personnel, and 34 tow operators were killed in line-of-duty deaths (LODD) nationwide.*

Positioning Blocking Apparatus

The apparatus that is used to block should be positioned to create one-and-a-half to two lanes of blockage (Figure 40-2). This will usually create a large enough work zone. The driver of the apparatus must also consider preservation of the crash scene and must avoid running over road debris or crash evidence. Incapacitation of an ambulance could seal the fate of the victim of a critical multivehicle crash.

Ideal blocking placement has the fire apparatus positioned at an angle, with its working side toward the work zone to protect the crew. The front wheels are rotated away from the incident. In the event that a motorist strikes the engine, the engine will be a barrier. If the engine is pushed by the striking vehicle on impact, the unit will move away from the work zone. Some incidents may require more than one piece of blocking apparatus.

It is important to leave space in the area immediately next to the crash to position vehicle extrication units (Figure 40-3). Ambulances, command vehicles, and other units should be positioned downstream from the crash. Positioning units in this manner allows for safer patient loading and rapid departure from the scene.

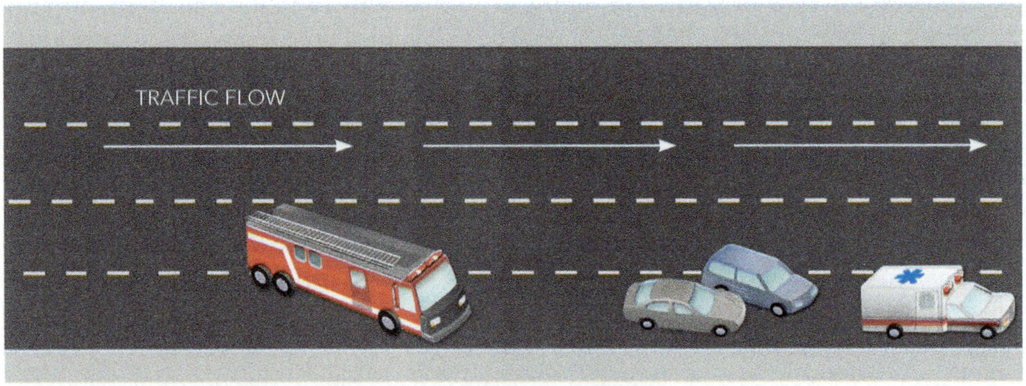

FIGURE 40-2 Blocking with no extrication.

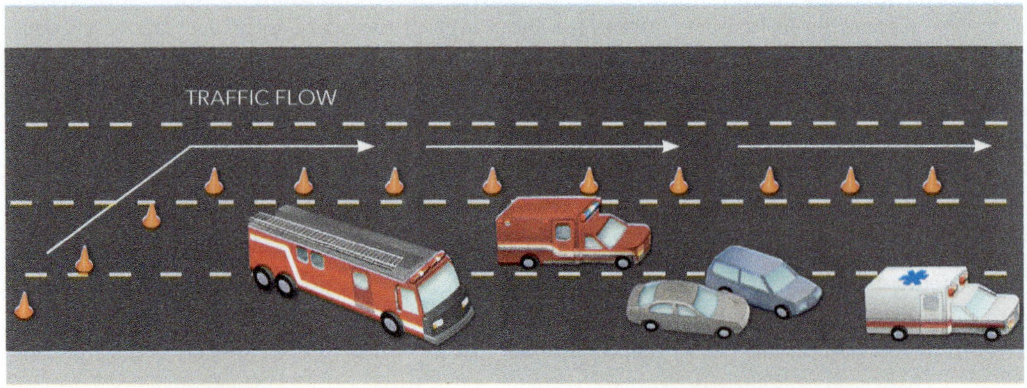

FIGURE 40-3 Blocking with placement of a rescue truck.

Exiting the Vehicle Safely

Responders who are exiting apparatus are at high risk of being struck by a passing vehicle. They should always exit into the safe zone, if possible, after checking to be sure that traffic has stopped. Be sure everyone in the responding vehicle is communicating, looking out for traffic, and monitoring when it is safe to exit the unit.

Being Seen and Warning Oncoming Traffic

Before exiting the vehicle, all responders should be in full protective clothing or, at a minimum, ANSI-approved safety vests and helmets (Figure 40-4), The ANSI Class 2 traffic vest became a federal mandate in 2009 as 23 CFR Part 634 (Worker Visibility). It applies to all workers on public access roadways, regardless of whether they are public safety personnel or construction workers.

To help slow oncoming traffic, flares, traffic cones, or other devices should be placed to channel traffic away from the incident and establish a safe work zone. Cones and/or flares should be placed on an angle across the road and around the site (Scan 40-1). Some apparatus have amber flashing directional arrows to direct traffic that should be activated to assist in alerting oncoming traffic.

If it is necessary to channel traffic around a curve, hill, or ramp, the first cone or flare must be placed before the hill or curve. The intent is to warn oncoming traffic of a hazard ahead. The rest of the cones, as already noted, should be placed diagonally across the lanes and around the work zone.

Night Operations

At night, headlights or flashing lights can temporarily blind drivers who are approaching an emergency scene, preventing them from seeing emergency workers. In this circumstance, reflective safety vests become ineffective. Therefore, drivers of emergency apparatus parked at highway incidents should turn off vehicle headlights. In addition, they should shut off any white response lighting that could blind oncoming drivers. The regulations for the correct lighting combinations for emergency vehicles can be referenced in the National Fire Protection Agency 1901 standard. NFPA 1901: *Standard for Automotive Fire Apparatus* outlines the lighting packages required for emergency vehicles that will be used to transport emergency personnel to the scene of an emergency.

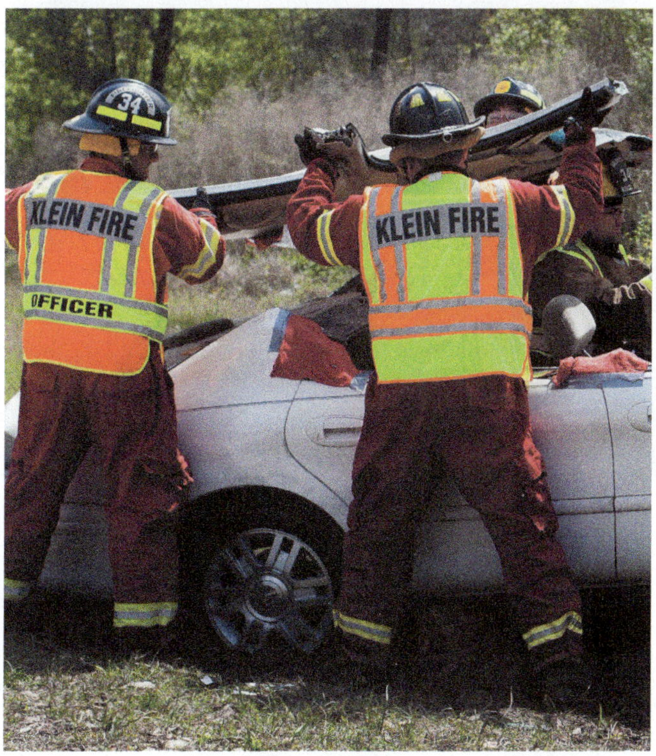

FIGURE 40-4 An EMT wears a highly visible vest when working in or near traffic.

The best combination of lights to provide maximum visibility is:

- Red/amber warning lights—on
- Headlights—off
- Fog lights—off
- Traffic directional boards operating

SCAN 40-1 Positioning Cones or Flares to Control Traffic

POSTED SPEED (MPH/KPH)	STOPPED DISTANCE FOR THAT SPEED (FEET/METERS)		DISTANCE TO ADD FOR POSTED SPEED (FEET/METERS)		DISTANCE OF THE FARTHEST WARNING DEVICE (FEET/METERS)
20 mph/32 kph	50 feet/15 meters	+	20 feet/6 meters	=	70 feet/21 meters
30 mph/48 kph	75 feet/23 meters	+	30 feet/9 meters	=	105 feet/32 meters
40 mph/64 kph	125 feet/38 meters	+	40 feet/12 meters	=	165 feet/50 meters
50 mph/80 kph	175 feet/53 meters	+	50 feet/14 meters	=	225 feet/67 meters
60 mph/97 kph	275 feet/84 meters	+	60 feet/18 meters	=	335 feet/102 meters
70 mph/112 kph	375 feet/114 meters	+	70 feet/21 meters	=	445 feet/135 meters

Cones or flares are positioned according to a formula that includes the stopping distance for the posted speed plus a margin of safety. *The stopping distance for large trucks is greater than for cars*, so flares on truck routes should extend beyond the distances shown above.

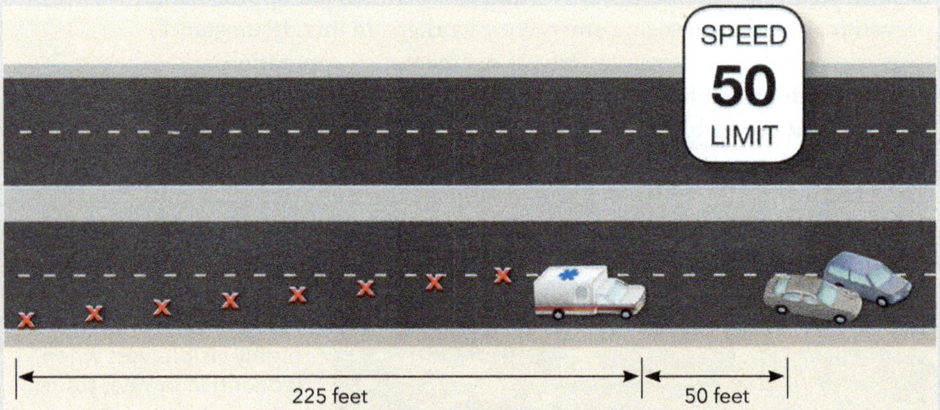

Cones or flares positioned on a straight road. Approaching vehicles are moved into the correct lane before they reach the edge of the danger zone.

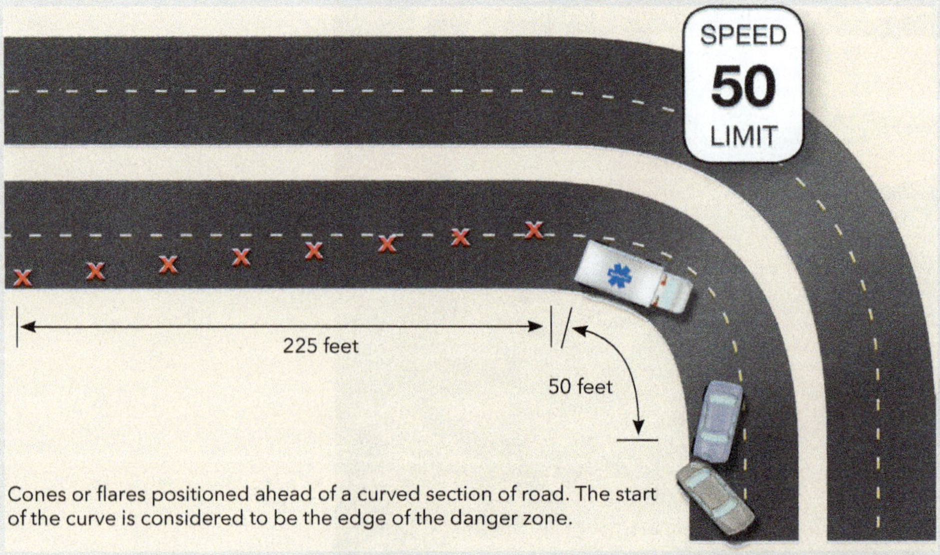

Cones or flares positioned ahead of a curved section of road. The start of the curve is considered to be the edge of the danger zone.

SCAN 40-1 Positioning Cones or Flares to Control Traffic (*continued*)

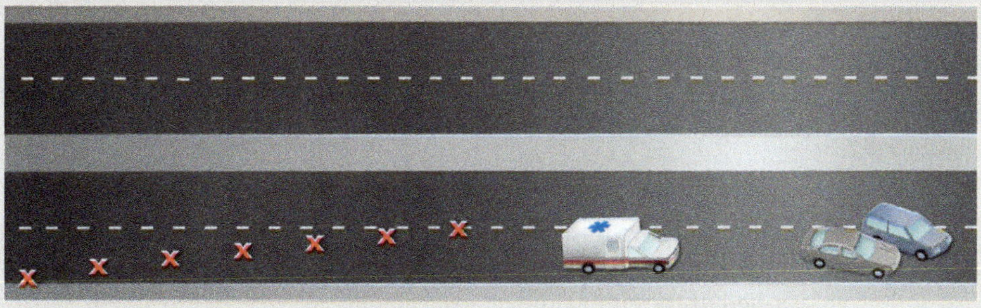

Cones or flares positioned on a hill. The flares slow approaching vehicles and make them turn into the correct lane before they reach the top of the hill.

Vehicle Extrication

Extrication is the process by which entrapped patients are rescued from vehicles, buildings, tunnels, or other places. There are 10 phases of the extrication or rescue process that you, as an EMT, should understand and understand the safe manner of performing:

1. Preparing for rescue
2. Sizing up the situation
3. Recognizing and managing hazards
4. Stabilizing the vehicle prior to entering
5. Gaining access to the patient
6. Providing primary patient assessment and a rapid trauma assessment
7. Disentangling the patient
8. Immobilizing and extricating the patient from the vehicle
9. Providing assessment, care, and transport to the most appropriate hospital
10. Terminating the rescue

As an EMT, you are responsible for the medical component of the rescue process; others are responsible for the mechanical or physical components. As you carry out your responsibilities, attention to safety must be your highest priority—to help minimize the potential for injury to yourself and the other rescuers as well as any additional injury to your patient. Although you might never personally perform disentanglement, it is important for you to understand the rescue process so you can keep your patient informed and anticipate any dangerous steps in the extrication action plan.

Preparing for Rescue

Modern rescue is a sophisticated process. It requires preparation that is a combination of training, practice, and the right protective gear and tools. New vehicle types and configurations are rolled out yearly. Imagine the transition to hybrid, electric-, propane-, and hydrogen-powered vehicles. Each brings a particular challenge to extrication crews. As previously noted, training and practice for specific types of rescue, including vehicle rescue, will be above and beyond your basic EMT course. The availability of such training will depend to a great extent on the kinds of rescues most likely to be required in your area. The kinds of protective gear and tools that should be available for vehicle rescue will be discussed throughout this chapter.

Sizing Up the Situation

As you arrive on the scene of a vehicle crash, it is important to conduct a good size-up to evaluate hazards and assess the need for additional resources. This is initially done by observing the scene through the windshield as you approach. Quickly determine how

"If you arrive first at a highway incident, park to protect the work area and establish Incident Command."

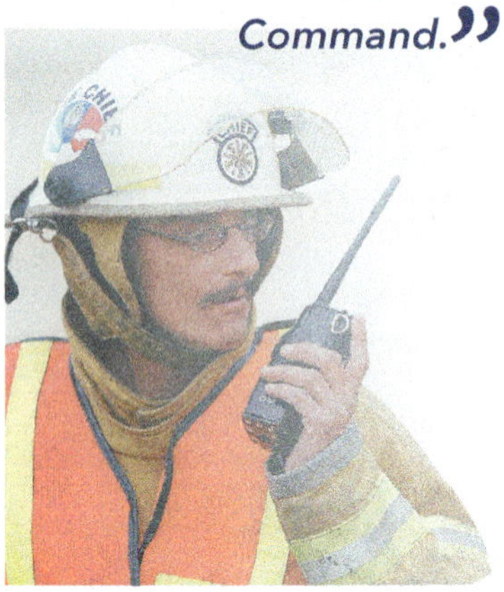

(Kevin Link/Science Source)

many patients are involved, their priority, and the mechanisms of injury. Will additional ambulances be needed? If so, call them right away. You can always cancel them if they are not actually needed. It is better to call an additional unit and turn it around when not needed rather than not to call it and discover later that it was needed. What is the extent of the patient's entrapment? Conduct an initial triage sweep and, using START triage (as was explained in the chapter *Hazardous Materials, Multiple-Casualty Incidents, and Incident Management*), sort and tag the patients as soon as possible.

During scene size-up, you must be able to assess extrication needs well enough to communicate with the extrication team and anticipate what they will be doing. Effective rescue requires a balance of medical and mechanical skills, with the right amount of each applied at the right time.

During all of this, you will keep in mind that the most seriously injured patients must reach the hospital or trauma center for lifesaving surgery as quickly as possible. As the EMT, you must plan how you can begin emergency care and initiate transport as rapidly as possible.

Although a low-priority trauma patient has time for elective packaging and more time-consuming elective extrication procedures, a critical patient does not. For example, a stable patient complaining of neck pain has the time for careful short spine board or vest immobilization, whereas a high-priority trauma patient cannot afford the time this may take. Rapid extrication to a long spine board, taking 2 minutes, may be more appropriate for this patient. The patient's medical needs must always drive the process of extrication and patient care. The principles of spinal stabilization remain the same regardless of whether the patient is low- or high-priority, but the requirements for speed of removal will dictate the specific technique you use.

Recognizing and Managing Hazards

CORE CONCEPT

How to recognize and manage hazards at the highway rescue scene

As explained in the following sections, some collision-related hazards must be managed, if not eliminated, even before any attempt is made to reach injured persons in damaged vehicles. Fire and unsafe electrical threats are two common types of collision-related hazards.

Protective Gear for EMS Responders

At a crash, any personnel who are working in the "inner circle"—that is, the area immediately around and including the vehicle—should wear full protective turnout gear to avoid being injured. At a minimum, the emergency responder needs to consider wearing head, eye, hand, and foot protection when working in a hazardous area such as a motor-vehicle accident. If the emergency responder will have direct patient contact, then Standard Precautions must be considered as well. Your agency should have a policy on what personal protective equipment (PPE) will be required for each hazard scenario.

Protective gear is important. Get your own if your service does not provide it (most states require it on ambulances) ***and use it***! Consider reviewing the following National Fire Protection Association standards when purchasing protective gear and uniforms: NFPA 1951 (USAR Protective Equipment), NFPA 1973 (Gloves for Structural Firefighting), and NFPA 1975 (Station/Work Uniforms).

EMS personnel have a wide selection of PPE available to them. Until recently, most PPE was designed for structural firefighting and not for rescue/EMS operations. Today rescuers have a wide variety of compact, lightweight helmets with integral eye protection. Eye protection is as important as any other personal protective intervention that an EMT can use. There are now PPE garments designed for urban search and rescue (USAR) operations that are ideal for EMS. They are lightweight and breathable, and provide protection from flame, fluids, and common chemicals. This is in stark contrast to firefighter PPE, which is designed with greater insulation to provide protection from heat/flame. As a result, firefighter PPE is much heavier and bulkier.

Additional safety considerations have evolved, designed to protect emergency personnel during transport. For example, although a standard seat belt and shoulder strap are effective restraint devices for the front seat driver and passenger, such devices were never

Think Like an EMT

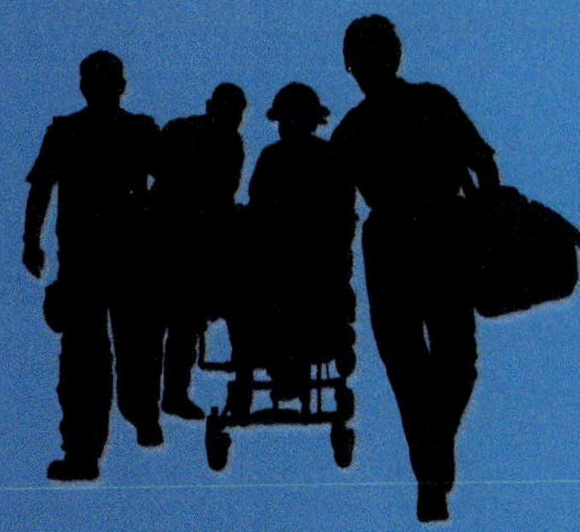

When Minutes Count, Decisions Matter

Patient priority is an important consideration in rescue operations. More time is available to gain access to a stable patient than to an unstable one who needs quick transport. Scene decisions are based both on the type of entrapment and on the patient's condition. Your responsibility as an EMT is to represent the patient's needs in the rescue effort. For each patient described here, determine whether the extrication must be done quickly because the patient is unstable or if more time is available.

1. Your patient was involved in a head-on crash. The patient is unresponsive with a rapid pulse.
2. Your patient was driving a car that was rear-ended with minor-to-moderate damage. She is alert and oriented. Her pulse is 80; respirations are 16. The car's frame has shifted, so none of the doors will open.
3. Your patient was a front-seat passenger who was thrown into the back seat. You can reach only the patient's upper body, but you find a rapid pulse and clammy skin. The patient is alert and talking with you.

well adapted to the medical crew in the patient compartment. More recent development of specialized harnesses has made crew restraint systems more effective in the patient compartment, reducing injuries to providers during collisions. (Figure 40-5).

Working in Traffic. As discussed at the beginning of this chapter, being struck by a vehicle while working in traffic is a major hazard facing the EMT. Since 2009, federal highway

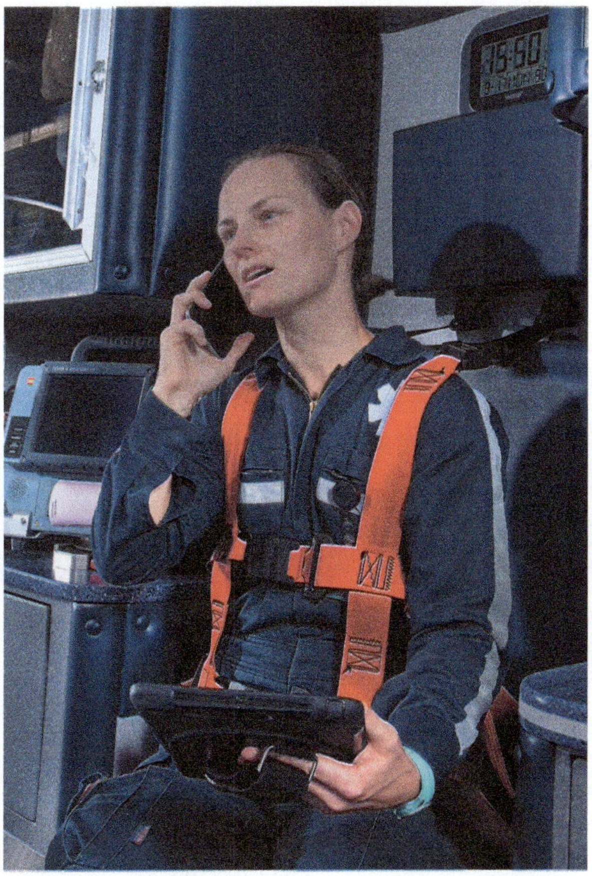

FIGURE 40-5 EMT in harness during transport.

FIGURE 40-6 EMTs working in traffic should be dressed for both daytime and nighttime visibility. (A) EMTs dressed for daytime visibility. (B) The same clothing in approaching headlights at night.

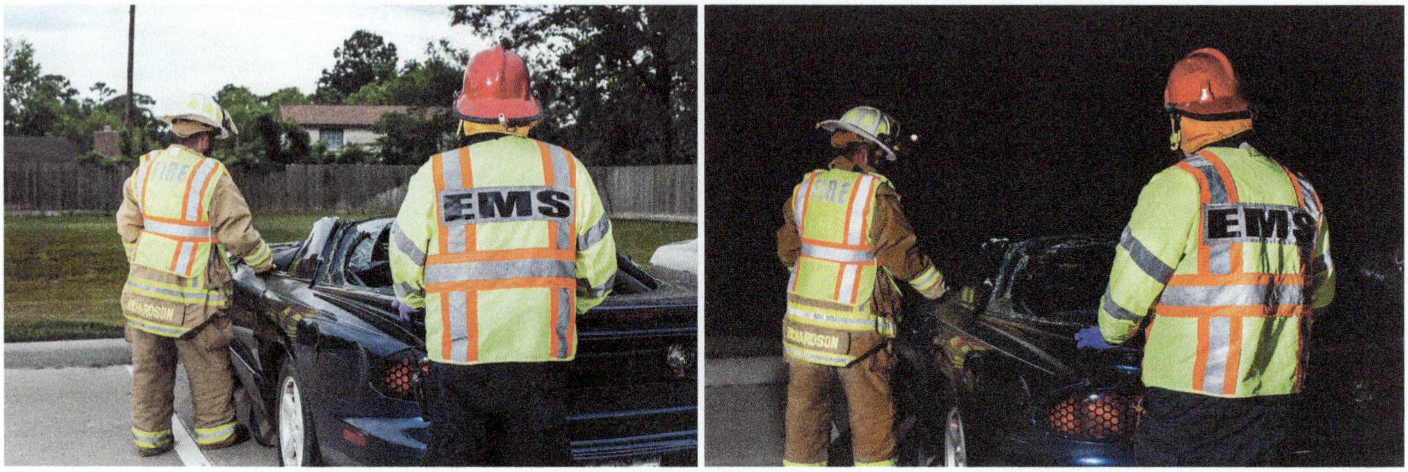

A B

standards have required that all emergency responders wear ANSI safety vests when working in highway operations. To enhance safety, they should also wear helmets. The Occupational Safety and Health Administration (OSHA) may impose fines if responders do not wear appropriate safety vests or specific rescue/extrication-related equipment on an emergency scene.

Safety vests greatly enhance both day and night visibility, giving rescuers added protection because motorists can see them. The best way to understand this is to study Figure 40-6, which shows clothing with reflective elements in daytime and nighttime settings.

During Extrication Operations. When extrication is in progress at a motor-vehicle collision, the rescuer has an increased exposure to flame, glass, fluids, and sharp objects. The best practice is to wear EMS or firefighter turnout clothing, including a helmet and eye protection (Figure 40-7).

Matching the Level Others Are Wearing. One of the easiest ways to determine the correct PPE is to look at what other workers in the industry are doing and match their level of PPE. A typical construction site is a hard hat job. In other words, workers there are required to wear a hard hat and safety glasses. Therefore, the rescuer too should wear that level of PPE. The highway level of PPE is a hard hat and safety vest, and at extrications, one should wear full turnouts.

Helmets. Wearing effective head protection is essential. One good piece of headgear that offers adequate protection is a rescue helmet that meets NFPA 1951 Standards for USAR PPE. Many EMTs prefer a model that does not have a rear brim, which can be awkward

FIGURE 40-7 Full turnout gear should be worn at an extrication.

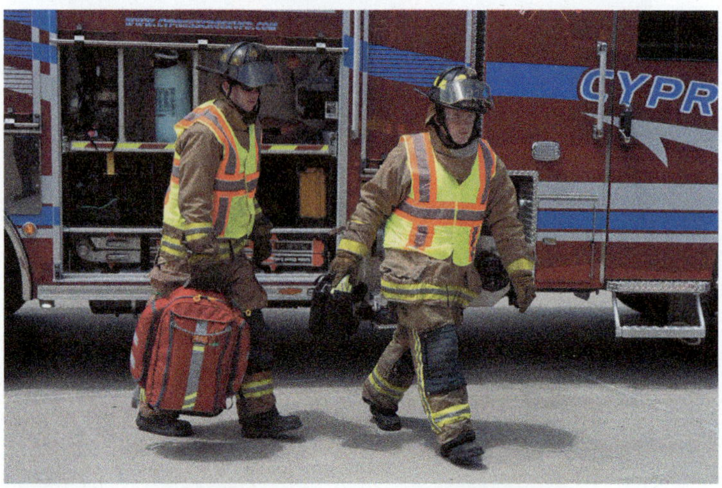

in tight spaces. Helmets with rear brims designed for fire suppression are also effective, and many EMTs prefer to use that type of PPE instead. All helmets should be brightly colored with reflective stripes and lettering to make the wearer visible both day and night and should display the Star of Life on each side to identify the wearer as an EMS provider. The helmet should also indicate the wearer's level of training to make scene management easier when many EMS and rescue units are on hand. Local protocols and standard operating guidelines may also assist in selecting specific helmet-related or PPE uniform–related identifiers for EMS, rescue, and fire service personnel.

Eye Protection. Eye protection is vital. ***Hinged plastic helmet shields do not provide adequate protection***; flying particles can strike the eyes from underneath or from the side. Protection is best provided by safety goggles with a soft vinyl frame that conforms to the face and provides indirect venting to keep them fog-free, or safety glasses with large lenses and side shields.

Hand Protection. Because EMTs stick their hands into all sorts of unfriendly places, every EMT should have optimal hand protection. Good protection is afforded by wearing disposable vinyl or other synthetic gloves underneath either firefighter's gloves or leather gloves.

Firefighter's gloves will protect your hands from a variety of sharp, hot, cold, and dangerous surfaces. They are bulky but can be worn in most rescue situations. If greater dexterity is needed, you can wear intermediate-weight leather gloves. Fabric garden or work gloves are too thin to offer adequate protection.

Body Protection. An EMT will often protect head, eyes, and hands but leave the body virtually unprotected. Light shirts or nylon jackets should never be allowed inside the inner circle, because they do little to protect the EMT from jagged metal, broken glass, or flash fires.

Good upper-body protection is offered by wearing either a short or mid-length turnout coat that meets OSHA requirements. A heavy-duty EMS or rescue jacket can be used to protect you from bad weather and minor injury. As with helmets, bright colors and reflective material will help make your jacket more visible.

Good lower-body protection can be provided by wearing either turnout pants with cuffs wide enough to pull over work shoes or fire-resistant trousers or jumpsuits. Serious consideration should be given to wearing high-top, steel-toe work shoes with extended tops to protect the ankles.

In this day and age, ballistics protection may be an important consideration. Body armor may offer the emergency responder added protection in situations where there could be a threat of violence. If ballistics protection is considered, the response agency must work with local law enforcement to use this equipment. It is very important that all responders understand their roles in violent situations and that all response agencies work together to ensure the highest level of safety for all those involved.

Safeguarding Your Patient

When your patients have been injured in a collision, it is your responsibility to see to it that further injuries are not inflicted during the rescue operation. You can minimize the chance of such additional injuries by shielding the patient and exercising care. The following items can be used to protect the patient from heat, cold, flying particles, and other hazards:

- *An aluminized rescue blanket* offers protection from bad weather and, to a degree, from flying particles. A paper blanket does not afford this protection; it merely hides the patient's view of the debris that is about to strike the patient.
- *A lightweight, vinyl-coated paper tarpaulin* can protect the patient from bad weather.
- *A wool blanket* should be used to protect the patient from cold. Cover the wool blanket with an aluminized blanket or a salvage cover whenever glass must be broken near a patient since glass particles are just about impossible to remove from wool blankets.
- *Short and long spine boards* can shield a patient from contact with tools and debris.

- *Hard hats, safety goggles, industrial hearing protectors, disposable dust masks, and thermal masks* (in cold weather—and unless the patient has airway or breathing problems, or is on oxygen) will protect a patient's head, eyes, ears, and respiratory passages.
- *Emotional support for the patient* might not be a specific PPE-related component, but the EMT should recognize that verbal communication and compassion for the conscious patient who is entrapped will be of significant benefit.

Managing Traffic

Collisions almost always produce traffic problems. Often the wreckage blocks lanes of traffic. Even if it does not, backups are caused when curious drivers slow down to "rubberneck," or stare at, the scene. Rescuers, firefighters, and police usually handle traffic control. However, what if the ambulance EMTs are responding alone, or ahead of other emergency service units?

Obviously personal safety, rescue, and emergency care have priority. However, an ambulance crew should still initiate basic traffic control (when conditions render this possible), channeling vehicles past the scene. Remember to be extremely watchful and careful when you work to control traffic to be sure that you are not struck by an approaching or passing vehicle.

Your ambulance and its warning lights will serve as the first form of traffic control. However, you should position other warning devices as soon as possible. Bad weather, darkness, vegetation, and curved or hilly roadways may keep approaching motorists from seeing your ambulance soon enough to safely stop.

Using Flares for Traffic Control. Although some argue that flares are unsafe, when used properly, they are still a good device for warning motorists of dangerous conditions. Moreover, several dozen flares can be carried behind the front seat of an ambulance, whereas battery-powered flashing lights—an alternative to flares—take up valuable compartment space.

Review Scan 40-1, which shows the proper positioning of cones or flares at collision scenes, including a straight road, a curved road, and a hill. Keep in mind that the stopping distance for large trucks is much greater than for cars. When the road carries truck traffic, extend the flare strings beyond the distances shown.

Remember the following points when you place flares:

- Look for and avoid spilled fuel, dry vegetation, and other combustibles before you ignite and position flares, especially at a road edge.
- Do not throw flares out of moving vehicles.
- Position a few flares at the edge of the danger zone as soon as the ambulance is parked. They will supplement the ambulance warning lights.
- Take a handful of flares and walk (carefully) toward oncoming traffic.
- Position the flares every 10 feet (3 meters), if possible, to channel vehicles into an unblocked lane. (Do not turn your back to traffic while placing flares.)
- If the collision has occurred on a two-lane road, position flares in both directions.
- Be careful when lighting the flare. The flare should be held away from your body and ignited in a motion away from your body.
- Never use a flare as a traffic wand; flares can spew molten phosphorous, which can cause third-degree burns to the skin.

Supplemental Restraint Systems: Airbags

Auto airbag systems have revolutionized automobile safety. Manufacturers emphasize that airbags are not designed to replace seat belts but rather to be used in conjunction with seat belts; consequently, airbags are often referred to as *supplemental restraint systems (SRS)*. Airbags are designed to inflate on impact, dissipate kinetic energy, and minimize trauma to the body. During rescue, it is important to see if an airbag has deployed.

Witnesses may have noticed "smoke" inside the vehicle during airbag deployment. This is not actually smoke but rather dust from the cornstarch or talcum used to lubricate the bag as well as from the seal and particles within the bag. The powder may contain sodium hydroxide, which can irritate the skin. For this reason, it will be important to wear protective gloves and eyewear when you gain access to the passenger compartment. It also will be important to protect the patients from getting additional dust in their eyes or wounds. Experts recommend that the EMT lift a deployed airbag and examine the steering wheel and dash, which may reveal if the patients struck any of these areas with enough energy to damage them.

One hazard to watch for is an airbag that remains undeployed after a crash. If an airbag deploys during the extrication process, it can seriously injure rescuers. To disable the airbags, the battery must be disconnected. Disconnecting the power will cause the system to power off in 2–3 minutes, depending on the type of system. *Some vehicles may take up to 30 minutes to deactivate, but most vehicles take 1 minute or less. Although disconnecting the battery will significantly lower the chance of accidental deployment, it does not make it 100 percent safe.* Keep in mind that just turning off the ignition might not disable the system, because most systems operate independently of the ignition.

Energy-Absorbing Bumpers

Most cars are equipped with 5-mile-per-hour bumpers designed to absorb low-speed front- and rear-end collision forces. If the bumpers were involved in the collision, you may notice that the bumper's shock absorber system is compressed, or "loaded." Never stand in front of a loaded bumper. If it springs out and strikes your knees, it could cause serious injury. Some rescuers chain the shock absorber to prevent an uncontrolled release. A safe practice is to place yourself diagonally (at an oblique angle) or perpendicularly to the bumpers. Care must also be taken if the energy-absorbing bumpers are in close proximity to a fire. In some cases, the high heat has caused these types of bumpers to release. The emergency responder should approach these vehicles at a 45-degree angle (not head-on) if there is going to be an attempt at either fire suppression or patient care.

Spectators

Spectators do more than just create problems for passing motorists. If allowed to wander freely, they will close in on the wreckage just to get a better view. In fact, they may get so close that they interfere with rescue and emergency care efforts. Rescue squads, police, and fire units have personnel and equipment for crowd control; ambulances usually do not. However, an EMT can usually initiate some crowd-control measures. If local policies permit it, ask for assistance from one or more responsible-looking bystanders. Ask the persons you recruit to keep the spectators away from the danger zone. Give them a roll of barricade tape if you have one. Be sure not to put the recruited personnel in unsafe positions such as near spilled fuel or an unstable vehicle. Be aware that if you ask a civilian bystander for assistance, you may be held liable for injury to the bystander or the patient. Be circumspect in your decision, and be sure that you will be able to defend your action to demonstrate why this intervention was essential at the time.

Electrical Hazards

Electricity poses many dangers at vehicle-collision scenes. When there is an electrical hazard, establish a danger zone and a safe zone. The danger zone should be entered only by individuals responsible for controlling the hazard, such as power company personnel or specialty rescue. The safe zone should be sufficiently far away to ensure that an arcing or moving wire could not possibly injure any of the rescue personnel or bystanders.

Keep in mind the safety points in the following list. Many have to do with taking precautions around conductors. A conductor is a wire or any other object or material that will carry electricity.

- High voltages are not as uncommon on roadside utility poles as people often think. In some areas, wood poles support conductors of as much as 500,000 volts.

- Assume that the entire area is extremely dangerous. Conductors may have touched and energized any part of the system, including electrical, telephone, cable TV, and other wires supported by the utility pole; guy wires; ground wires; the pole itself; the ground surrounding the pole; and nearby guard rails and fences. Assume that severed or displaced conductors may be touching and energizing every wire and conductor at the highest voltage present. Dead wires may be reenergized at any moment. Energized conductors may arc to the ground. Keep overzealous bystanders and untrained civilians away from these hazards.
- Ordinary protective clothing does not protect against electrocution.

Remembering these points and the following procedures may keep you alive at the scene of a collision where unconfined electricity is a hazard.

Broken Utility Pole with Wires Down. A broken utility pole with wires down is very dangerous. You probably cannot work safely in the area until a power company representative assures you that the power is off and the scene is safe. You must remember that if downed wires are still energized, electricity will be flowing in all directions. Treat all downed wires as live until an electrical professional has confirmed that the wires have been de-energized. If you discover that a utility pole is broken and wires are down:

- Park the ambulance outside the danger zone.
- Before you leave the ambulance, be sure that no portion of the vehicle, including the radio antenna, is contacting any sagging conductors.
- Order spectators and nonessential emergency service personnel from the danger zone. Use perimeter tape to set up a large safety zone.
- Discourage occupants of the collision vehicle from leaving the wreckage; keep them calm and reassured.
- Prohibit traffic flow through the danger zone.
- Determine the number of the nearest pole you can safely approach, and ask your dispatcher to advise the power company of the pole number and its location. Advise dispatch to instruct the power company that this is an emergent situation that requires an appropriate response.
- Do not attempt to move downed wires. Metal implements will, of course, conduct electricity, but even implements that might not appear to be conductive, such as tools with wood handles or natural fiber ropes, may have a high moisture content that will conduct electricity and can electrocute a well-intentioned rescuer.
- Stand in a safe place until the power company cuts the wires or disconnects the power.

Be especially careful when approaching a collision located in a dark area such as a rural roadside at night. As you walk from the ambulance, sweep the area ahead of you, to each side and overhead, with the beam of a powerful hand light. An energized conductor may be dangling just at head level. If you discover that a wire is down, leave the area immediately and notify the power company.

Sometimes, especially in wet weather, a phenomenon known as *ground gradient* may provide your first clue that a wire is down. Voltage is greatest at the point where a conductor touches the ground, then diminishes with distance from the point of contact. That distance may be several inches or many feet. Being able to recognize and respond properly to energized ground can save your life.

Stop your approach immediately if you feel a tingling sensation in your legs and lower torso. This sensation means that you are on energized ground. Current is entering one foot, passing through your lower body, and exiting through your other foot. If you continue, you risk being electrocuted! *Move immediately opposite to your present direction, using exactly the instructions that follow.*

Turn 180 degrees and shuffle away from the danger area, allowing no break in contact between your feet and the ground. This technique helps prevent your body from completing a circuit with energized ground, which can cause electrocution. (A circuit is a circular path for electrical flow, such as up one leg, down the other, and through the ground. Hopping on one leg or keeping your feet together creates a straight path rather than a circular circuit, and may prevent electrocution.)

Broken Utility Pole with Wires Intact. Even if wires are intact, a broken utility pole is still dangerous. Wires that are still holding up the pole can break at any time, dropping the pole and wires onto the scene. If you arrive to find such a situation:

- Park the ambulance outside the danger zone.
- Notify your dispatcher of the situation.
- Stay outside the danger zone until power company representatives can de-energize the conductors and stabilize the pole.
- Keep spectators and other emergency service personnel out of the danger zone.

Damaged Pad-Mounted Transformer. When electrical cables run underground, the transformer may be mounted on a pad above ground (Figure 40-8). When an aboveground pad-mounted electrical transformer is struck and damaged, it poses a serious threat. In such a situation:

- Request an immediate power company response.
- Do not touch either the transformer case or a vehicle touching it, and warn other emergency service personnel not to touch it either.
- Stand in a safe place until the power company de-energizes the transformer.
- Keep spectators out of the danger zone.

Vehicle Fires

When you find a vehicle on fire, always request the response of firefighting apparatus. Do not assume that someone else has called the fire department. In fact, fire apparatus should always stand by during vehicle extrication. Dispatch protocols and standard operating guidelines should have these types of responses as common practice.

Extinguishing a vehicle fire is the responsibility of persons who are trained and equipped for the job: firefighters. However, if the vehicle is occupied, it may become necessary to take action. If the vehicle is unoccupied, it may be best to monitor the fire for extension and wait for fire crews. If action must be taken, there are some measures trained EMTs can take when they arrive before fire units (Scan 40-2). Please keep in mind that the following recommendations for the suppression of a vehicle fire is for standard combustible engines only. There are many alternative-fuel vehicles on the road today. Those hazards will be discussed a little later in this chapter.

For small fires, a 15- or 20-pound (6- or 9-kg) class A:B:C dry chemical fire extinguisher can extinguish virtually anything that may be burning in a vehicle, including upholstery,

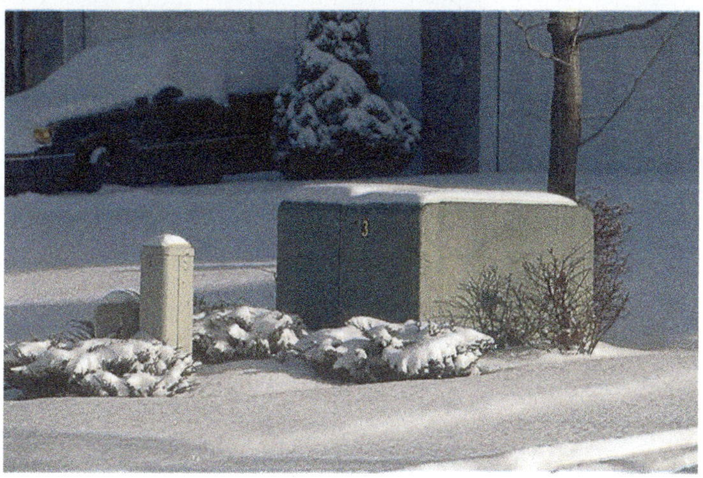

FIGURE 40-8 A pad-mounted transformer, if damaged, poses a serious threat.

SCAN 40-2 Extinguishing Fires in Collision Vehicles

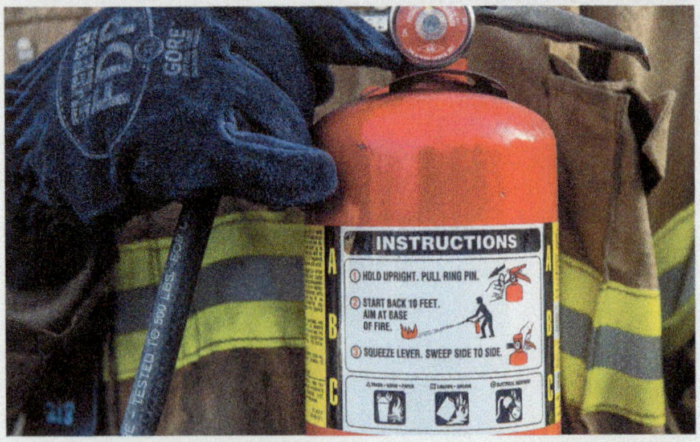

Markings that identify an extinguisher that can be used for Class A, B, and C fires.

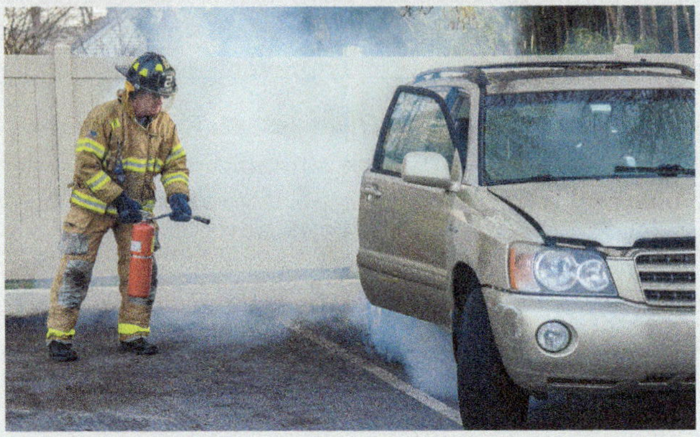

Approach the vehicle from a safe direction with proper protective equipment.

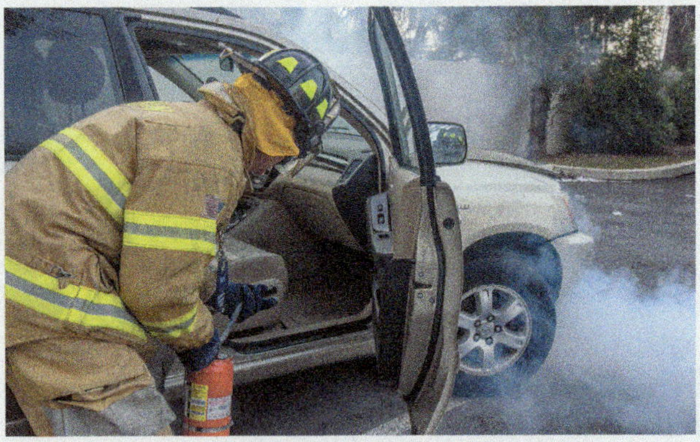

Extinguishing a fire under the dash. Care must be taken not to fill the vehicle's interior with a cloud of agent.

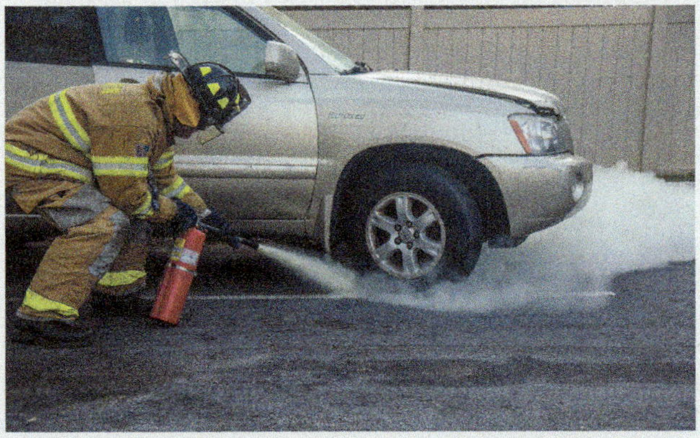

Extinguishing fuel burning under a vehicle. Flames are swept away from the vehicle.

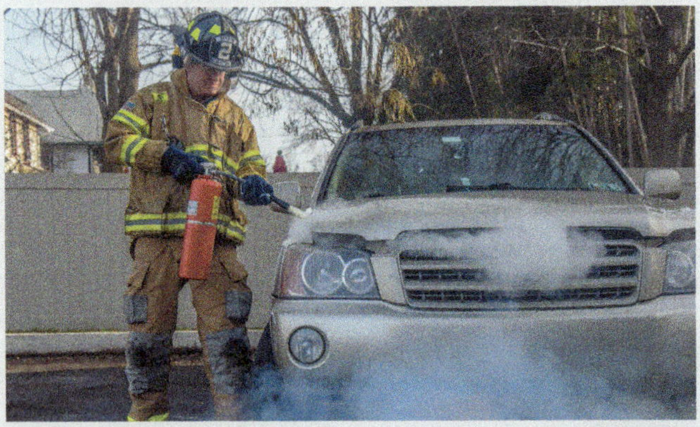

Extinguishing a fire in the engine compartment when the hood is partially open.

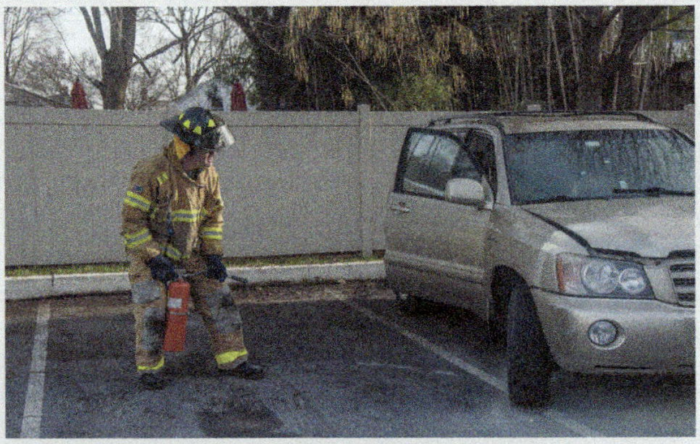

After using the extinguisher, observe from a safe location to make sure the fire is fully out.

fuel, and electrical components. Only burning magnesium and other flammable metals cannot be extinguished by an A:B:C extinguisher. Before you try to put out a fire, always put on a full set of protective gear.

Fire in the Engine Compartment. If the hood is fully open, stand close to an A-post (front roof-supporting post) of the vehicle and, if possible, with your back to the wind to guard against the agent's blowing back into your face or entering the passenger compartment. (Dry chemical extinguishing agents irritate respiratory passages and may contaminate open wounds.) Then sweep the extinguisher across the base of the fire with short bursts. Use no more than necessary to extinguish the fire. You will need what is left if there is a subsequent flare-up.

If the hood is open to the safety latch, do not raise the hood higher; leave it where it is. This will help to restrict airflow and deprive the fire of oxygen. Direct the agent through any opening to the engine compartment: between hood and fender, around the grill, under a wheel well, or through a broken headlamp assembly. Again, use no more agent than is needed.

If the hood is closed tight, let the fire burn under the closed hood, leaving its extinguishment to the fire department, and continue to get the patients out of the vehicle. The firewall should protect the passenger area long enough to get the patients out of the vehicle, using emergency moves. It is important to note that if resources are immediately available, a rapid extrication modality should be employed on the patient(s).

Fire in the Passenger Compartment or Trunk. If the fire is under the dash, or in upholstery or other combustibles, carefully apply the agent directly to the burning material. Apply sparingly to avoid creating a cloud of powder that may be harmful to occupants. If there is fire in the trunk, as with fire under a closed hood, leave extinguishment to the fire department and continue working to get patients out of the vehicle. Please note that burning materials in a vehicle are among most dangerous, posing an immediate danger to life and health. EMTs must be mindful of this and take as many protective measures as possible to protect their own and their patients' well-being and safety.

Fire under the Vehicle. Using a portable unit to extinguish burning fuel under a vehicle may be an exercise in futility when the spill is large. However, when people are trapped in the vehicle, you may feel the urge to try. Attempt to sweep the flames from under the passenger compartment as you apply the agent. If you do extinguish the fire, be sure that sources of ignition are then kept away. The vehicle's own catalytic converter (usually found in the area under the front passenger's feet) can be an ignition source since its temperature can reach more than 1200 degrees Fahrenheit (649 degrees Celsius).

Truck Fires. An A:B:C extinguisher can also be used to combat truck fires. Be aware, however, that burning truck tires are especially dangerous. Flames can quickly spread to the vehicle's body and its cargo, or the tires can blow apart when heated by fire. *Never* stand directly in front of a truck wheel when there is a fire; instead, approach from a 45-degree angle.

> **NOTE:** *At times, you will find that fuel is leaking from a damaged vehicle but is not on fire. If you discover that a fuel tank is leaking, call for fire department response. The fire department will be able to address the hazard through vapor suppression and absorption of the fuel. Furthermore, they will be ready to address any suppression needs. The decision to continue the rescue effort should be governed by your perception of the danger. You should not be expected to continue rescue operations if gasoline is pooled under the vehicle or flowing toward a source of ignition. Warn spectators away from flowing fuel. Do not use flares near spilled fuel or in the path of flowing fuel. Watch where you park your vehicle, as your ambulance's catalytic converter can easily ignite spilled fuel or other combustibles.*

Disabling a Vehicle's Electrical System

Many rescue units routinely disable the electrical system of each collision vehicle by cutting a battery cable. Unless gasoline is pooled under a vehicle or undeployed airbags need to be disabled, cutting the battery out of the electrical system may not only be a waste of time; it may actually hinder the rescue operation. Remember that many cars have electrically powered door locks, window operators, and seat-adjustment mechanisms. Being able to lower a window rather than breaking it eliminates the likelihood of spraying occupants with glass. Being able to operate door locks may eliminate the need to force doors open. And being able to operate a powered seat can create space in front of an injured driver.

If there is a reason to disrupt the electrical system, disconnect the negative cable from the battery. In this way you will not be likely to produce a spark that can drop onto spilled fuel or ignite battery gases. Such a spark can be created when the positive cable is pulled away from the battery terminal or when a tool touches a metal component while in contact with the positive terminal or cable.

Alternative-Fuel Vehicles. The vehicles on the road today have come a long way from the standard combustion engine that was prevalent in vehicles in past decades. Gone are the days of strictly gasoline and diesel engines in our cars and trucks. Today we have a variety of new alternative-fuel vehicles that the emergency responder must be aware of. Each of these types of vehicle offers a unique set of challenges for both rescue and fire suppression. Some of the alternative fuels on the road today are as follows:

- Biodiesel
- Flex fuel
- Natural gas
- Propane
- Hydrogen
- Solar
- Battery
- Hybrid—a combination of different forms of energy

Safety has to be paramount whenever one of these types of vehicles is encountered. Hazards can range from extremely flammable gases to high voltage, so the emergency responder must be aware of the hazards that may be presented. While emergency responders are not expected to be experts in each new fuel system, they must be aware that they exist, and understand that it may be best not to intervene if responder safety is going to be a concern.

When these types of vehicle are involved in a collision, the emergency responder must take a few key steps in order to maintain a safe working environment for both the responder and patient. First and foremost is to turn the vehicle to the off position. While this may sound obvious, many newer cars do not even use a key. Proximity ignition systems use a keyless entry device, or fob; therefore there might not be a key to insert or remove from the dashboard. If this is the case, the emergency responder should try to obtain the ignition fob and place it far away from the vehicle, to ensure that the ignition will not be accidentally turned on.

Another hazard with electric and hybrid vehicles is that the engine may appear to be in the off mode but not be. These types of vehicle do not have combustion engines, so the emergency responder might not hear the motor running. As previously stated, it is important to ensure that the vehicle is in the off mode and that the transmission is secured in the park mode. Location of the battery system could also be a problem with these types of vehicle. Many vehicle manufacturers place the battery systems outside of the engine compartment.

Flammable gases such as natural gas and propane have become popular fuels for automobile manufacturers. Compressed natural gas and liquefied natural gas are popular fuels in both public and commercial vehicle fleets. Natural gas is a relatively stable fuel, which makes it a safe fuel alternative. It is nontoxic and has a limited flammable range. Its ignition temperature, which is approximately 1,100°F (593°C), is actually much greater than that of gasoline. Natural gas has a vapor density that makes it lighter than air, so if it is released, it will dissipate easily in air.

Propane is another fuel that is gaining popularity. It can be found in many applications that the rescuer may encounter in over-the-road transportation. Many of the same hazards found with natural gas are prevalent with propane. However, propane has a vapor density that is heavier than air, so it tends to sink and may cause a problem with pooling gases in low-lying areas, especially in colder weather.

As battery technology improves, electric vehicles have been gaining popularity. These types of vehicles offer a unique set of challenges for the emergency responder. Electric vehicles are equipped with battery packs that provide power to the engine and controls. Many of these systems are high-voltage as opposed to the 12-volt systems in many traditional vehicles. Depending on the automobile manufacturer, the emergency responder may encounter different types of battery systems. Common batteries used in electric vehicles include lead acid batteries, nickel metal hydride batteries, and lithium ion batteries. Some common issues that can be associated with each battery type are as follows:

- **Lead Acid Batteries**
  - May generate corrosive gases when heated.
  - Crushed batteries may spill corrosive electrolyte.
  - If burning, lead acid batteries should be extinguished with CO_2, dry chemical, or foam.
- **Nickle Metal Hydride Batteries**
  - Nickle metal hydride batteries may react with organic chemicals.
  - Contact with other metals may produce flammable hydrogen gas.
  - If burning, a Class D fire extinguisher should be used.
- **Lithium Ion Batteries**
  - Lithium ion can be highly reactive.
  - Lithium ion batteries tend to be small, which will increase the energy capacity.
  - If burning, lithium ion batteries should be extinguished with CO_2 or dry chemical.
  - The battery pack is high-voltage, so it should not be penetrated.

Stabilizing a Vehicle

CORE CONCEPT
How to stabilize a vehicle

Unstable collision vehicles pose a hazard to rescuers and patients alike. Scan 40-3 shows methods for stabilizing a vehicle involved in a collision.

NOTE: *Rescuers often fail to stabilize a collision vehicle because it appears to be stable. Rather than taking the chance of incorrectly "reading" a collision vehicle's stability—and having the vehicle move during rescue, with disastrous results—you should consider any collision vehicle from which patients need to be extricated to be unstable, and act accordingly.*

If your ambulance is equipped with stabilization equipment, you should attend a formal vehicle rescue course that includes basic stabilization procedures taught by a qualified instructor. If the ambulance is not equipped for stabilization procedures or if you are not trained, stand by until a rescue unit has stabilized the vehicle, even if roof posts are intact and the vehicle appears to be stable. Malpractice attorneys have specialists (consultants) trained in rescue who investigate rescue-specific operations for motor-vehicle collisions, as they are often a substantial revenue-producing event in litigation. Use good common sense, and these legal interventions can be mitigated.

The information on vehicle stabilization that follows is intended only to help you understand the process that trained personnel will be following. It is not a substitute for formal training in stabilization procedures.

Vehicle on Its Wheels

A collision vehicle that is upright on four inflated tires looks stable. However, it is easily rocked up and down, side to side, and back and forth on its suspension as rescuers climb into and over it. These motions can seriously aggravate occupants' injuries. First, if rescuers have access to the inside of the vehicle, they should make sure the engine is turned off, the vehicle is in park, the keys are removed from the ignition, and the parking brake is set.

SCAN 40-3 Stabilizing Vehicles Involved in a Collision

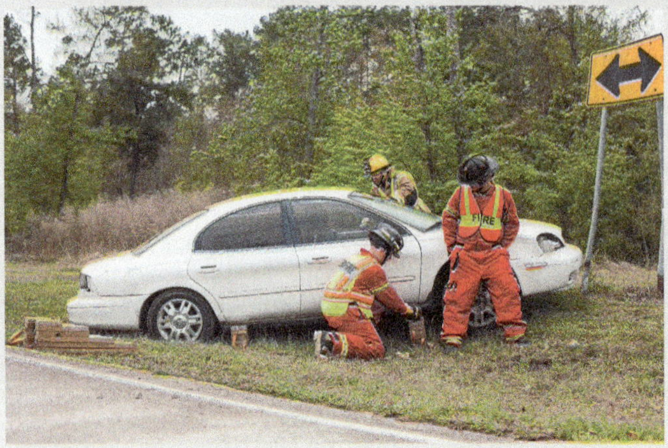

Stabilizing a car on its wheels with cribbing while patient contact is initiated.

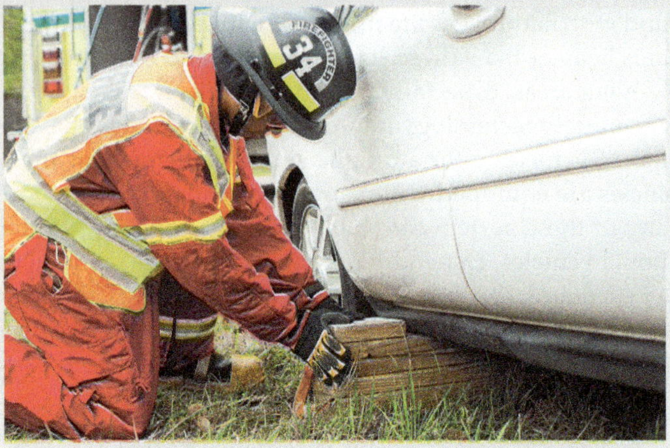

Placing a step chock. Keep hands clear of the vehicle while placing the chock.

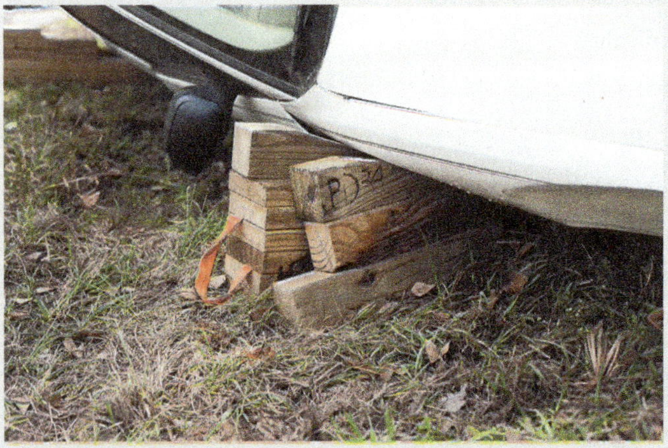

A vehicle on its side stabilized with cribbing.

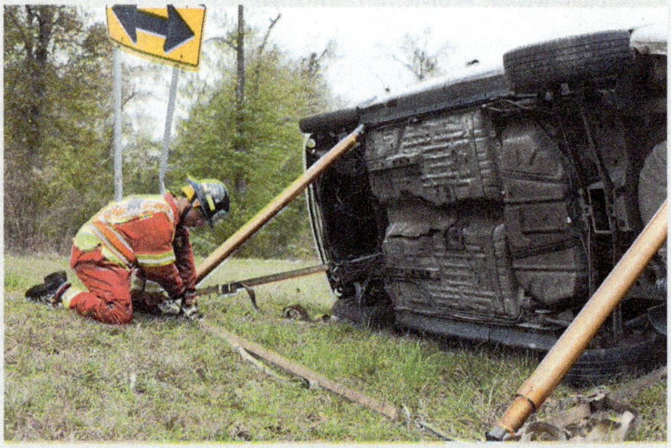

A vehicle on its side stabilized with struts. For maximum stability, it may be best to place cribbing on one side, struts on the other.

These are very important steps, because with hybrid or electric vehicles, the rescuer may not hear an engine running even when the vehicle is still in a run mode and the transmission is engaged. The best method of stabilizing a vehicle on its wheels is by using three step chocks—one on each side and a third under the front or back of the vehicle. Deflating the tires so the vehicle rests on the chocks is a common practice among many rescue services across the country. It is important to follow your local protocols in this regard.

Whenever significant "tool work" must be done to extricate patients, such as door or roof removal,—tires may be deflated (if necessary to further stabilize the vehicle) by pulling the valve stems from their casing with pliers. Slashing the tires is an inappropriate technique for deflating tires. A police officer should be told the tires have been deflated, so investigators will not think that the tires are flat as a result of the collision. Record that you have deflated the tires in your documentation. In fact, record as much as you can about the extrication process in your ambulance call report.

NOTE: *Tires do not need to be deflated in all crashes–only in situations where significant "tool work," such as door or roof removal, must be done to extricate a patient or patients.*

A list of the equipment that can be carried to stabilize a vehicle and gain access appears in Table 40-1. Selected items are shown in Figure 40-9. If the ambulance is not equipped with step chocks, a degree of stabilization can be accomplished by placing wheel chocks or 2″ × 4″ (5 cm × 10 cm) cribbing in front of and behind two tires on the same side.

TABLE 40-1 Supplies and Equipment for Vehicle Stabilization and Gaining Access

QUANTITY	ITEM
10	2″ × 4″ × 8″ (5 cm × 10 cm × 20 cm) cribbing
10	4″ × 4″ × 18″ (10 cm × 10 cm × 45 cm) cribbing
4	Step chocks
6	Wood wedges
2	Vehicle wheel chocks
100 feet (30.5 meters)	Nylon $^1/_2$″ (1.25 cm) utility rope
2 sets	Struts
1	Door-and-window kit with hand tools
1	Pair, battery pliers
1	12″ (30 cm) adjustable wrench
1	3- or 4-pound (1.4- to 1.8-kg) drilling hammer
1	Spring-loaded center punch
2	Hacksaws with spare blades
1	10″ (25 cm) locking-type pliers
1	10″ (25 cm) water-pump pliers
Several	12″ to 15″ (30 cm to 38 cm) flat prybars
1	8″ (20 cm) flat-blade screwdriver
1	12″ (30 cm) flat-blade screwdriver
1	Spray container of power steering fluid as a lubricant
1	Flathead ax
1	Glas-Master windshield saw
1	Combination forcible-entry tool, such as a Halligan or Biel tool
500 feet (152 meters)	Perimeter tape

FIGURE 40-9 (A) Heavy rescue equipment for vehicle extrication. (B) Pry bar.

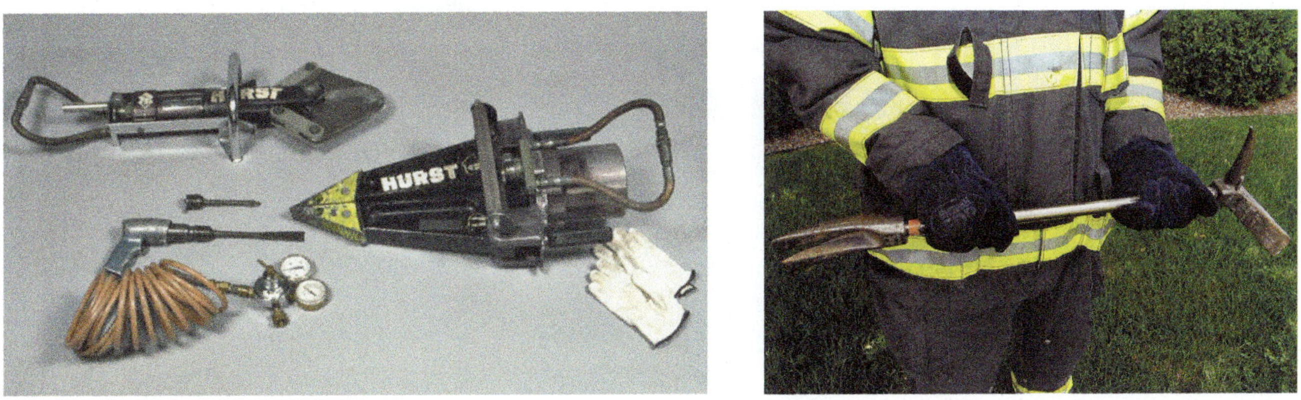

A

B

If a car has rolled over several times and has come to rest on its wheels, the roof might be crushed, which can preclude access through windows. In this case, the roof may need to be raised before doors can be opened, or the roof can be removed.

NOTE: *When placing cribbing, never kneel on both knees. Always squat so you can quickly move away from the vehicle if you have to. Once the vehicle is stabilized, if a door must be opened, tie it in the fully open position before you try to crawl inside.*

Vehicle on Its Side

When a vehicle is on its side, spectators will often attempt to push it back onto its wheels. They fail to realize that this movement may injure the vehicle's occupants, possibly severely. If this occurs before your arrival, document it. Instead, the vehicle should be stabilized on its side. If the vehicle is on its side, do not attempt to gain access before it is stabilized using ropes, stabilization struts, and/or cribbing. Although a car on its side may appear stable, simply climbing onto one side in an attempt to open a door may cause the vehicle to drop onto its roof or wheels. Moreover, you can be trapped under the vehicle when it topples, and the patient(s) inside the vehicle could suffer more injuries.

A person who will act as a safety guide or safety officer can be placed at each end of the vehicle to "feel" the vehicle's movement and quickly warn the rescuers who are placing cribbing, struts, or ropes to get back if the vehicle begins to fall over. Some services will deploy two ropes looped around the same wheel in both directions so personnel can temporarily hold the vehicle stable while placing struts and/or cribbing. There are many ways to stabilize a vehicle on its side, from using manpower alone to using hydraulic rams and pneumatic jacks. The objective is to increase the number of contacts with the ground, to make the vehicle on its side more stable. Safety officers have saved many lives and countered many injuries for EMS and the fire service in these situations. Their job is one that is underappreciated but highly valuable.

Vehicle on Its Roof

If the vehicle is resting on its roof, roof posts are intact (Figure 40-10), and the vehicle appears stable, it may be tempting to try to reach the vehicle's occupants by gaining access through window or door openings immediately and without stabilizing the vehicle. However, if the posts collapse, as is often the case when the windshield integrity has been broken, the vehicle may come crashing down and injure the EMT who is attempting to climb into the vehicle or who has an arm in a window opening. It can also cause more injuries to the patient, including critical or even fatal injuries.

You must wait to gain access until the rescue crew has stabilized the vehicle. This is usually accomplished by building a box crib with square-cut lumber (4 × 4s [10 cm × 10 cm]) under the vehicle.

FIGURE 40-10 Car posts. *(3DMI/ Shutterstock)*

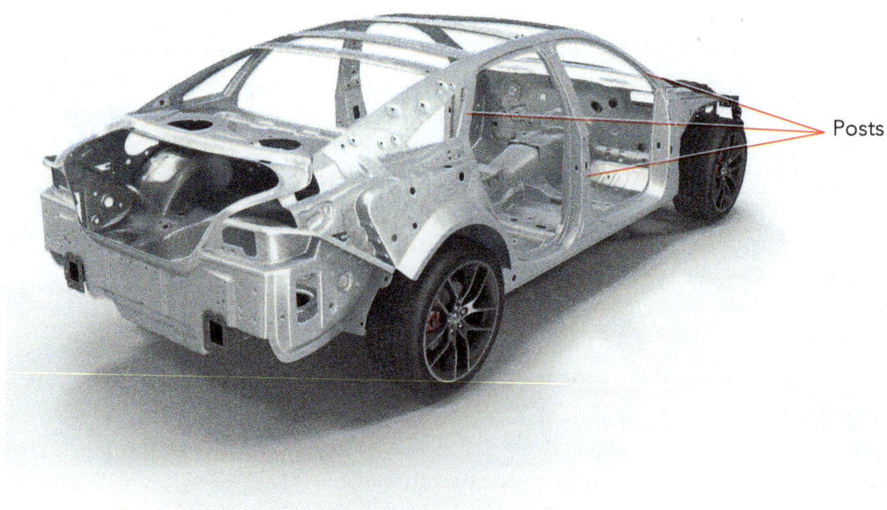

A vehicle on its roof is likely to be in one of four positions:

- Horizontal, with the roof crushed flat against the vehicle's body and both the trunk lid and hood contacting the ground
- Horizontal, resting entirely on the roof, with space between the hood and the ground and space between the trunk lid and the ground
- Front end down, with the front edge of the hood contacting the ground and the rear of the car supported by the C-posts (rear posts)
- Front end up, with the trunk lid contacting the ground and much of the weight of the vehicle supported by the A-posts (front posts)

If the vehicle is tilted with the engine—which is the heaviest part of the vehicle—on the ground and the trunk in the air, it can often be stabilized by using two step chocks upside down under the trunk.

When the roof is crushed flat against the body, as when all the roof posts have collapsed, the car is essentially a steel box resting on the ground with the occupants completely trapped inside. Unless the vehicle is on a hill or perched precariously on debris or another vehicle, this is the one time when stabilization is unnecessary. The structure is rigid. In such a situation, it may be impossible to gain access through a window, a door, or the roof. However, it may be possible to cut through the floor pan and have an EMT either crawl inside, if the opening is big enough or the EMT small enough, or reach through the opening to touch and offer emotional support to the occupants until rescue personnel can lift or open the vehicle.

If the vehicle is unstable and cannot be safely approached by an EMT, get as close as you safely can so you can talk or signal to the occupants to reassure them that help is on its way and begin getting an idea of their condition.

Remember that when the vehicle is found in any of the previously described positions, it should be considered unstable and must be stabilized by trained personnel prior to entry by an EMT.

Gaining Access

CORE CONCEPT
How to gain access to the patient in a crashed vehicle

Why does a car door not fly open in a crash? The answer is the Nader pin (named for Ralph Nader, the consumer advocate who lobbied for the device), a case-hardened pin in an automobile door. In a collision, the cams in the door locks grasp the pin to keep the door from flying open, preventing occupants from being thrown from the vehicle. All cars sold in the United States since 1966 have been equipped with the Nader pin.

The Nader pin is a safety device, since being thrown from a vehicle (ejection) is far more dangerous than being kept inside during a crash. The main complicating factor now with ejections is not wearing a seat belt. However, the Nader pin does make gaining access to vehicle occupants more difficult. Prior to the device, rescue personnel could open a door with a crowbar. Subsequently, rescuers had to start using a hydraulic spreader to peel the cams off the pins. Ironically, safety features designed to keep occupants inside wrecked vehicles were keeping rescuers out! Each new safety improvement to vehicles created a new challenge to rescue personnel.

Vehicle rescue training became a complicated business, and rescuers were asked to learn dozens of techniques, some of which could be used on only certain models of cars. The need for effective but simplified procedures became evident. The next few sections will describe a procedure that has been developed to meet this need.

Simple Access

First remember that, as an EMT, your responsibility is not to rescue the vehicle but to rescue the patient. You will usually assume that an occupant or occupants of the vehicle have sustained life-threatening injuries and that at least one EMT needs to gain quick access to the patient, even while rescuers are working to gain a more wide-open access, create exits, and disentangle occupants.

After the vehicle is stable enough for you to approach it safely, check to see if a door can be opened or if an occupant of the vehicle can roll down a window or unlock a door. ("Try before you pry!") Such ordinary ways of getting into the vehicle are known as simple access. Many EMTs have been humbled by not being able to open a car door and beginning a mechanical extrication process, then having another EMT or responder open the opposite door without a problem. Common sense can easily overcome an adrenaline rush.

Complex Access

If simple access fails, you may need to use tools or special equipment to break a window and gain access even while the rescue crew is dismantling the vehicle for extrication of the occupants (Figure 40-11). When tools or equipment are used for this purpose, the process is known as *complex access*.

All automotive glass is one of two types: laminated or tempered. Windshields and some side and rear van and truck windows are laminated safety glass—two sheets of plate glass bonded to a sheet of tough plastic like a glass-and-plastic sandwich. Most passenger car side and rear windows are tempered glass. They are very resilient, but when they do break, rather than shattering into sharp fragments, they break into small, rounded pieces.

You will usually try to gain access through a side or rear window as far as possible from the passengers. Use a spring-loaded center punch against a lower corner to break the glass (Figure 40-12). Punch out finger holds in the top of the window, and use your gloved fingers to pull fragments away from the window.

A flathead ax is usually required to break through a windshield. This can also be done very quickly using a Glas-Master® or similar saw (Figure 40-13). Although a windshield is usually not broken to gain access, the rescue squad may need to remove it if they plan to displace the dash or steering column, or remove the roof. Before breaking the windshield, cover the passengers with aluminized rescue blankets or tarps if possible. Avoid the use of hospital-style blankets that will allow the tiny slivers of glass to pass through and come in contact with the patient. Making verbal contact with the patient(s) and providing emotional support is very important in this type of situation. Imagine having your vision restricted and being covered by a tarp while you are injured and trapped in a vehicle.

Once you gain an entry point, at least one EMT who is properly dressed in adequate PPE should crawl inside the vehicle and immediately begin the primary assessment and rapid trauma assessment, as well as manual cervical stabilization. Do not forget to explain what is going on and provide emotional support by talking to and reassuring the patient that everything that can be done is being done. Access holes are usually small, so do not be tempted to pull a patient out of an access hole prior to spinal immobilization.

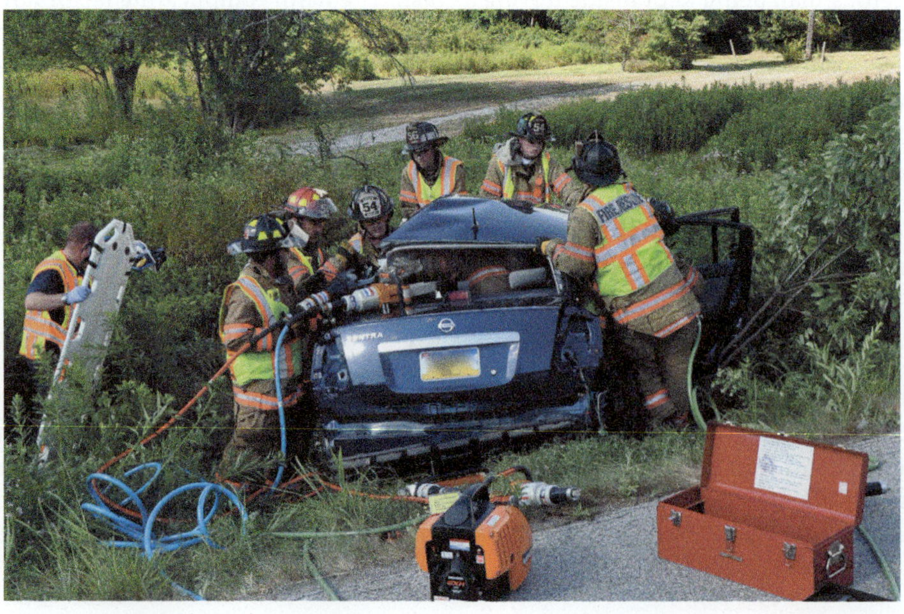

FIGURE 40-11 Complex access involves the use of tools and equipment to reach and extricate the patient. *(© Edward T. Dickinson, MD)*

FIGURE 40-12 Using a spring-loaded center punch to break the window glass.

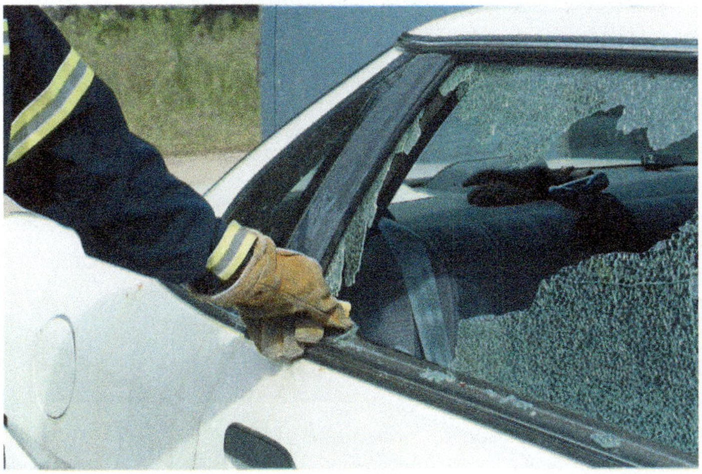

FIGURE 40-13 A Glas-Master® saw can aid in windshield removal.

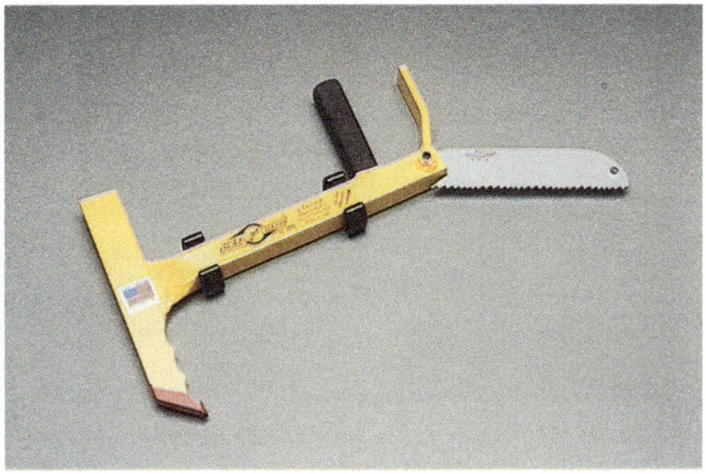

Disentanglement: A Three-Part Action Plan

CORE CONCEPT

How to disentangle a patient from a crashed vehicle

In most instances EMTs will not be directly involved in disentanglement other than to act as the patient's advocate and be the EMT inside the vehicle. However, it is helpful to understand the plan for complex access that may be used by rescue personnel to free the trapped patient.

The following is a description of a three-part procedure that can be accomplished by fire, rescue, and EMS personnel with the appropriate equipment. The procedure is not vehicle-specific; it can be used on virtually any car or truck. Furthermore, the procedure does not include a lot of techniques that require special equipment. Personnel can be trained in a short course. Most important to EMS personnel, there is no need to fill several compartments of the ambulance with rescue equipment.

Steps One and Two: Gain Access by Disposing of Doors and the Roof. For more than twenty-five years, emergency service personnel have been trained to carry out a progression of procedures to reach the occupants of a wrecked vehicle: First try the doors; if that fails, unlock and unlatch the doors by nondestructive or destructive means; when all else fails, gain access through window openings. However, this multipart procedure is time-consuming and requires a number of tools.

A quicker and far more efficient procedure is first to dispose of the doors, then to dispose of the roof as soon as hazards have been controlled and the vehicle is stable. Disposing of the doors and roof has four benefits:

1. It makes the interior of the vehicle accessible. EMS personnel can stand beside or climb into the vehicle and pursue emergency care efforts while rescuers carry out disentanglement procedures.
2. It creates a large exit through which an occupant can be quickly removed when a life-threatening injury exists, or when fire or another hazard is threatening the operation.
3. It provides fresh air and helps cool off the patient when heat is a problem.
4. Quick access to a critical patient can improve survivability and reduce disability.

Scan 40-4 illustrates procedures for removing the doors and roof using hydraulic tools. If no hydraulic rescue tool is available, these procedures can be accomplished with ordinary hacksaws and a spray container of lubricant.

NOTE: *After roof posts are cut and/or doors removed, ensure that all sharp edges are covered with appropriate protection to avoid injury to the rescuers and the patient.*

SCAN 40-4 Disposing of the Doors and Roof

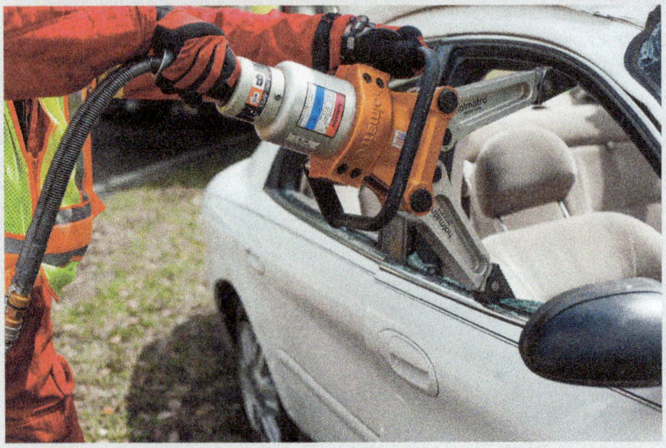

1. Displace the door to expose hinges, and move the door away from the patient compartment.

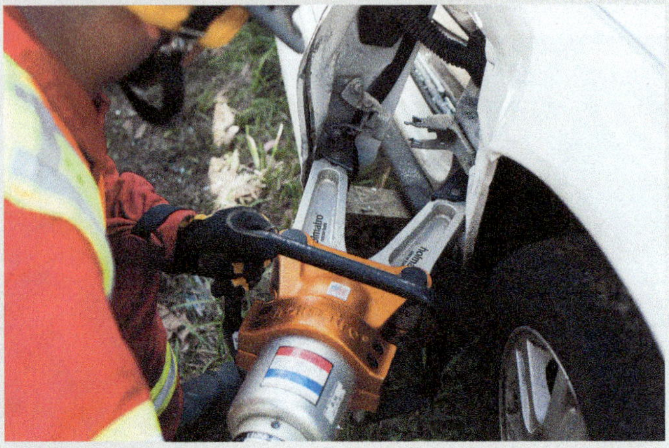

2. Remove the door.

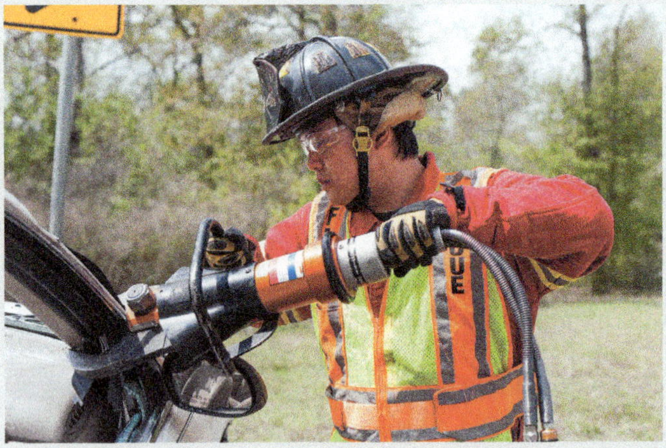

3. Cut the A-post (front roof supporting post) to begin roof removal.

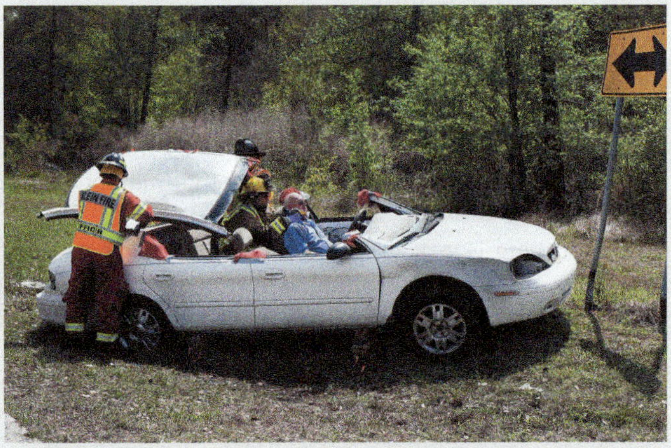

4. With B- and C-posts (center and rear supporting posts) cut, roll the roof away while a rescuer enters the rear seat to stabilize the patient's head and neck.

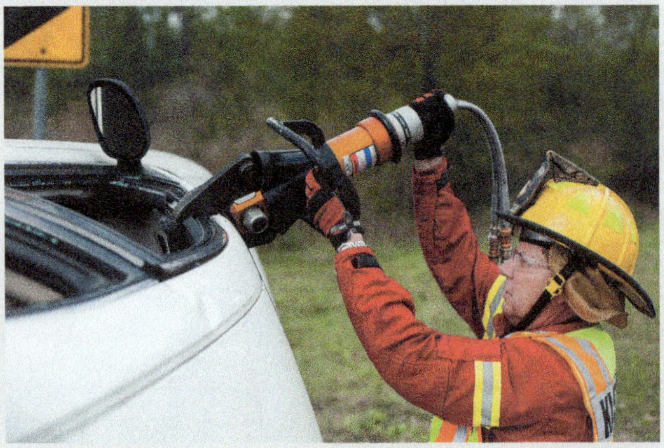

5. For a vehicle on its side, cut the posts.

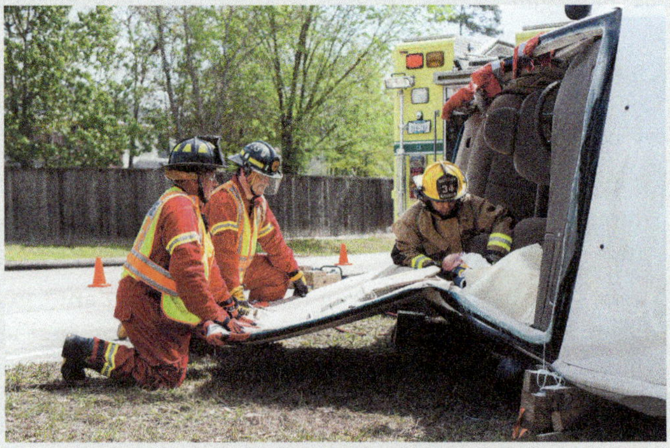

6. Remove the roof to expose and extricate the patient.

Step Three: Disentangle Occupants by Displacing the Front End. Most vehicle rescue training courses include procedures for displacing or removing seats, dash assemblies, steering wheels, steering columns, and pedals. A quicker and more efficient way to disentangle an injured driver and/or passenger from these mechanisms of entrapment is to displace the entire front end of the vehicle. Although the task sounds difficult, it is not. Scan 40-5 illustrates a procedure for displacing the front end of a passenger car with a hydraulic rescue tool. A dash displacement can also be accomplished with heavy-duty jacks and hacksaws.

If the steering wheel hub is large and rectangular, the car probably has an airbag or airbags (the passenger-side bag being in the glove compartment area). If the bags have not deployed, they are not likely to deploy now unless extrication involves displacing the dash or steering wheel. If such displacement is to be done, airbag manufacturers recommend following these guidelines:

- Disconnect the battery cables, starting with the negative terminal. Remember that the airbag may deploy, as vehicles and their electrical systems are different and at times will vary with respect to eliminating electrical discharge to the system.
- Avoid placing your body or objects against an airbag module or in its path of deployment. (Even after disconnecting the battery cables, a slight electrical charge capable of deploying an airbag remains.)

SCAN 40-5 Displacing the Front End of A Car

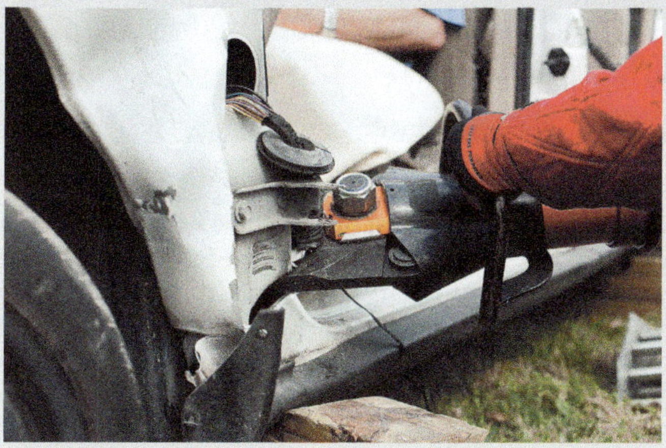

1. Make cuts for the spreader tool.

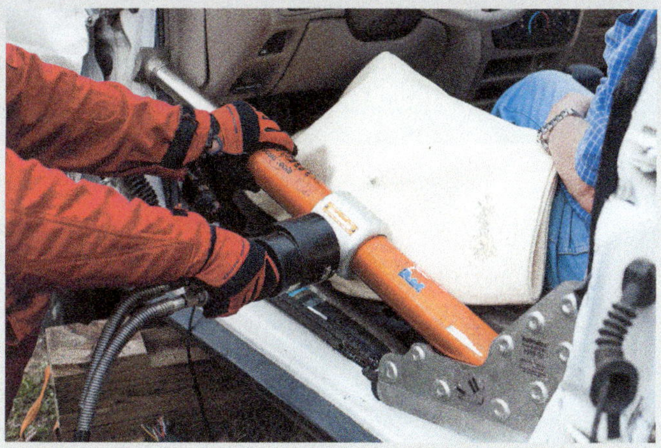

2. Use the spreader to roll back the dash.

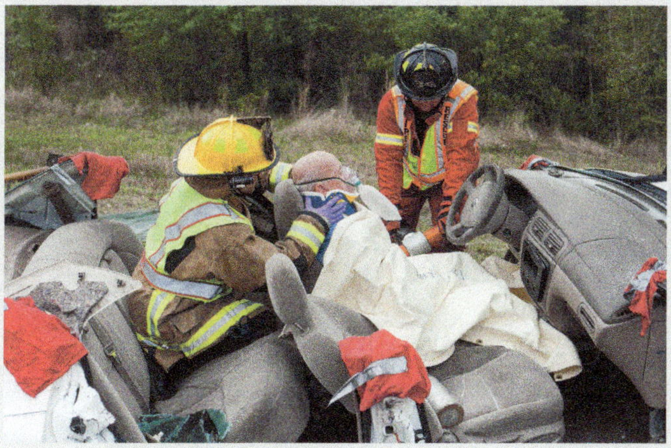

3. Displace the dashboard to gain access to the patient.

- Do not displace or cut the steering column until the system has been fully deactivated.
- Do not cut or drill into an airbag module.
- Do not apply heat in the area of the steering wheel hub.

Point of View

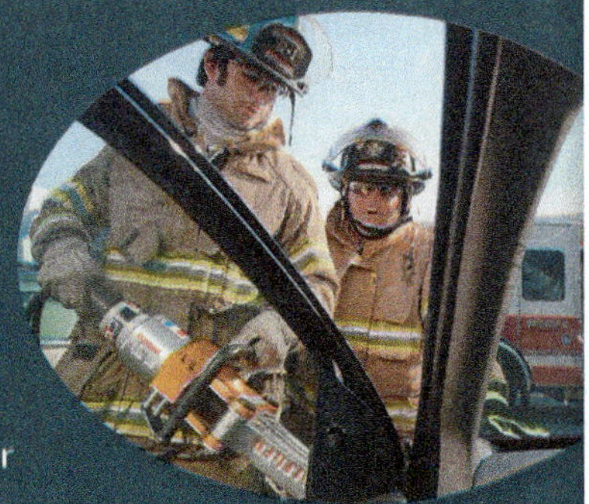

"I was driving along, minding my own business, when a truck pulled out from a side street in front of me. It was a horrible crash. I can still hear the loud crunch and breaking glass. I should say I can still feel it. It was awful. My airbags went off. I was sitting in a cloud of dust.

"I tried to get out and I couldn't. The door wouldn't open. Then I noticed that my ankle was killing me. My foot was wedged under the gas pedal.

"I was upset. OK, I was freaking out. In fact, I was pretty irrational when the ambulance got there. They tried to calm me down and told me the fire department was on the way to get me out. I was getting calmer until I saw and heard those giant whatchamacallits they were going to use to cut–yes, cut–me out. Then they put a blanket over me so I'd be safe. I was never claustrophobic–until then. I don't mean to be a whiner, but that really shook me!

"They got me out of the car on a board and into the ambulance, but by the time I got to the hospital, I was shaking and spent. What an ordeal. I don't want to imply for a minute that the EMTs and firefighters were any less than professional. They were great. But let me tell you, that was a day I don't ever want to live through again."

You may wonder, must the three-part procedure just described be used for all extrication operations? Must the three procedures always be accomplished in the same order? Must these procedures always be used? Not at all. In some cases, it may be necessary only to force a door open to reach a single patient and create an exit for removal. In other cases, it may be prudent to open doors before disposing of the roof, or to dispose of the roof before displacing the doors. In still other situations, there may be no need to displace the front end of a collision vehicle.

The extent to which you, as an EMT, will participate in vehicle rescue procedures depends on the role your EMS unit plays in vehicle rescue and whether or not your ambulance arrives ahead of fire and rescue units. The main purpose for the EMT to know extrication procedures is to incorporate them into the patient care plan.

Chapter Review

Key Facts and Concepts

- Remember, highway operations are *high-risk*. Take these precautions:
  - Wear high-visibility garments.
  - Position the ambulance for blocking until fire apparatus arrives. Then position ambulances "downstream" in the safe zone.
  - Reduce lighting that may blind passing drivers.
  - Avoid crossing traffic lanes with patients.
- Scene size-up is key. How many patients are there? What is the triage status? Are additional resources needed?
- Protect yourself. Look out for:
  - Traffic
  - Undeployed airbags (Disconnect the battery to deactivate the airbag system.)
  - Loaded bumpers
  - Sharp metal.
- Match the level of PPE being worn by other public safety responders.
- Ensure scene safety:
  - If wires are down, keep spectators back! If wires are over an occupied car, don't allow the occupants to exit until the power company deactivates the wires.
  - Make sure the vehicle is stable! Be sure it won't roll away or tip over.
- First try simple means to gain access.
- Protect your patient during the extrication process.

Key Decisions

- What is the best access to the scene for my unit? Is my unit needed on the limited-access highway? Do we have standard operating guidelines or dispatch protocols for that contingency?
- What level of PPE and what high-visibility garments do I need at this scene? How might I be an advocate for these garments if we do not have them?
- If I am first in, where should I park the apparatus?
- How many patients are there? What are the triage priorities? What are the immediate resources?
- Can patients be accessed and extricated by simple means?
- Does the battery need to be disconnected?
- Does the vehicle need to be stabilized? If so, what is the most efficient and time-expedient way for the type of patient I have?

Preparation for Your Examination and Practice

Short Answer

1. Your EMS unit is first to arrive on the scene of a high-speed collision on a busy highway that involved multiple vehicles. What initial actions should you take?
2. What gear should be worn at the scene of a highway incident to improve your visibility to others?
3. What gear should be worn during a vehicle extrication?
4. What must be done to deactivate automobile airbags?
5. You have arrived at a crash, and all the doors look jammed. What steps should you take to gain access? In what order?
6. Do you know what rescue resources are in your jurisdiction that you might call for?

Thinking and Linking

Think back the chapter Hazardous Materials, Multiple-Casualty Incidents, and Incident Management, *and link information from that chapter with information from this chapter as you consider the following situations:*

1. One of the vehicles involved in a highway crash is a tanker that is now leaking some unidentified substance. What steps are required at this scene that would not be necessary at a "simple" two-car crash?
2. The highway crash you are dispatched to is a seven-car pile-up. Your unit is first on scene. What steps are required that would differ from those for crashes involving one car striking a tree?

Critical Thinking Exercises

Rescue scenes require decision making of a type that more typical calls may not require. The purpose of this exercise will be to consider how you might make decisions specific to a rescue scene.

1. From your knowledge of your own community, which of the 10 types of rescue specialty teams are needed, and who provides the service? Do you or your dispatch agency know how to contact them for response in a timely manner? Have you trained together so you understand each other's roles?
2. After considering the safety of yourself and others, what should be your primary goal at the scene of a vehicle collision?

Street Scenes

You're on the scene of a one-car crash into a telephone pole. You position the ambulance about 50 feet behind the crash site with warning lights on, and both you and your partner put on full turnout gear, including helmets, gloves, eye protection, and reflective vests.

To control traffic, your partner places flares over a 200-foot (71-meter) section leading to the scene. You look around to make sure there are no wires in the area and none on the vehicle. The scene appears to be safe. You go to the patient, notice the passenger side is intruded 2 feet (0.6 meter), and see only one occupant, the driver. Two wheels of the vehicle are up on the sidewalk, and the car appears to be unstable. You identify yourself to the occupant but don't get a response. Next, you try to open the door, but it is jammed. You decide the car must have spun around, as you observe more damage on the driver's side of the vehicle. You advise dispatch that heavy rescue is needed.

Street Scene Questions

1. What are the scene-safety issues that you need to address?
2. What techniques should you consider for extrication?

Heavy rescue has an ETA of 10 minutes. The patient isn't responding, so you and your partner agree that entry is needed now. First you put chocks at the wheels to make sure the car doesn't shift. Next, you pick a spot on the window that seems to place the patient at lowest risk, use a punch, and start removing glass. Once inside, you observe that your patient is a male about 30 years old with snoring respirations. You perform a primary assessment and find he is responsive to only painful stimuli. The snoring respirations stop when you move his jaw forward and manually stabilize his head and neck, but his breathing remains irregular. You administer oxygen, and you suspect that you may need to start assisting respirations. At that moment, heavy rescue arrives, and you report the scene status and patient condition.

Street Scene Questions

3. Should rapid extrication be considered for this patient?
4. Describe assessment for this patient.

The lieutenant of heavy rescue tells you he will handle the battery disconnect and have his crew check to see if more cribbing is needed for vehicle stability. You maintain an airway and manual stabilization of the patient from inside the vehicle while your partner applies a cervical collar and leaves to prepare the backboard. Rescue is able to pop a door open and allow full access to the patient. You are just about to say that the patient is clear when you see his foot is caught under a pedal. You tell the lieutenant from heavy rescue about the patient's trapped foot, and his crew sets up a small hydraulic jack. You make sure the patient is protected.

Once the foot is free, you and your partner decide that a rapid extrication is the best approach, and move the patient to the board. When the patient is outside the vehicle, your partner is able to perform a rapid trauma assessment while you maintain manual stabilization. He checks the chest, and it seems OK. (The patient was wearing a seat belt.)

The patient's respiration rate is about 28 and slightly irregular; ventilatory assistance is not needed yet. His pulse is 90 and regular. The patient is secured to the board and taken to the ambulance for further assessment and transport to the hospital. Considering the damage to the vehicle, you're surprised that the only injuries you find are a bump on the left side of the patient's head and a swollen left ankle. By the time you get to the hospital, the patient is responding to verbal stimuli.

Later that day, you are curious about this patient, and call the hospital. The charge nurse tells you the patient suffered only a concussion and a bruised ankle and that he will stay overnight for observation.

EMS Response to Terrorism

41

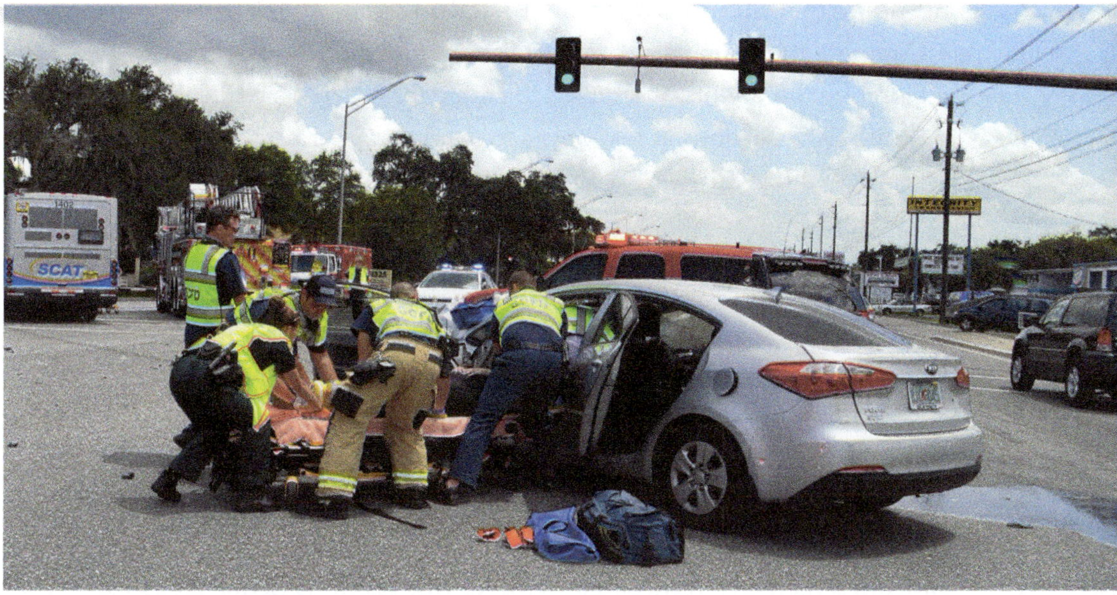

(© Ed Effron)

Related Chapters

The following chapters provide additional information related to topics discussed in this chapter:

- **2** Well-Being of the EMT
- **11** Scene Size-Up
- **30** Soft-Tissue Trauma
- **39** Hazardous Materials, Multiple-Casualty Incidents, and Incident Management

Standard

EMS Operations (Terrorism and Disaster)

Competency

Applies knowledge of operational roles and responsibilities to ensure patient, public, and personnel safety during terrorism situations.

Core Concepts

- Types of terrorism and examples of terrorist tactics and doctrine
- How to identify the type of threat posed by a terrorist event
- Use of time/distance/shielding for protection at a terrorist event
- How to respond to and deal with threats from a terrorist event
- Applying strategy, tactics, and countermeasures at a terrorist event
- Self-protection and safety awareness at a terrorist event

Outcomes

After reading this chapter, you should be able to:

41.1 Summarize concepts of terrorism. (pp. 1245–1253)

- Compare the features of domestic and international terrorism.
- Describe the agents often used to create terrorism incidents.
- Relate EMT's actions in responses to incidents of terrorism to the terrorist's frequent goal of including arriving public safety personnel as targets.
- Describe EMT actions that anticipate the presence of multiple devices or terrorists.
- Identify events and structures that are at higher risk for terrorist attacks.
- Recognize the importance of specific dates in the risk for terrorist attacks.
- Give examples of on-scene indications of a potential terrorist attack.
- Describe the potential harms posed when certain agents are weaponized and disseminated.
- Name basic principles to apply during terrorism incidents.

41.2 Explain the general considerations associated with specific types of weapons used in terrorist events. (pp. 1253–1258)

- Identify the harms associated with chemical agents.
- Describe self-protection against chemical agent exposure.
- Identify the harms associated with biologic agents.
- Describe self-protection against biologic agent exposure.
- Identify the harms associated with radiologic/nuclear incidents.
- Describe self-protection measures associated with radiologic/nuclear incidents.
- Identify harms associated with explosives.
- Describe self-protective measures associated with explosives.

41.3 Explain the specific considerations associated with chemical agents of terrorism. (pp. 1258–1261)

- Give examples of the impact of each of the characteristics of a chemical agent—physical, volatility, chemical, and toxicologic—that can impact the severity and spread of exposure.
- Describe actions of each other classifications of chemical agents: choking, vesicating, cyanides, nerve agents, and riot-control agents.
- Relate signs and symptoms to the possibility of nerve agent exposure.
- Relate the availability of nerve agent antidotes to the limitations in their use.
- Given a variety of hazardous material scenarios, utilize the DOT emergency guidebook to make initial decisions about establishing evacuation and work zones.

41.4 Explain the specific considerations associated with biologic agents of terrorism. (pp. 1261–1269)

- Discern between the use of living organisms and the use of toxins produced by the organisms in terms of harms caused.
- Identify the features of biologic weapons that influence their potential for use in terrorism attacks.

- Recognize specific biologic agents of concern for high potential for mass harm in terrorism attacks.
- Identify sources of information for guidance on the correct response to specific exposures.

41.5 Explain the specific considerations associated with radiologic/nuclear agents of terrorism. (pp. 1269-1270)

- Compare sources of radiation that may be used in terrorism attacks.
- Outline the progressive nature of the impact of radiation on the tissues as the dose of radiation increases.

41.6 Explain specific considerations associated with terrorism events using incendiary and explosive devices. (pp. 1270-1272)

- Identify additional risks beyond heat that may be associated with the use of incendiary devices.
- Describe the impact of blast injuries on various regions of the body.

41.7 Explain the roles of strategies and tactics in guiding the response to terrorism events. (pp. 1272-1279)

- Prioritize the outcomes desired by the use of an Incident Command System at a hazardous materials incident.
- Defend the priority of EMT protection first–before other actions.
- Size up the scene to determine the presence of clues to a possible terrorist event.

Key Terms

contamination, *1256*
dissemination, *1258*
domestic terrorism, *1246*
exposure, *1255*
international terrorism, *1246*
multiple devices, *1249*
permeation, *1256*
rem, *1270*
routes of entry, *1255*
secondary devices, *1249*
strategies, *1272*
tactics, *1272*
terrorism, *1246*
weaponization, *1259*
weapons of mass destruction (WMD), *1248*
zoonotic, *1265*

Terrorism is nothing new on the planet. Its history dates back hundreds of years, to the Dark Ages. Just since the early 1900s, there have been thousands of bombings and incendiary devices used for terrorist purposes. Of course, EMS has had a prominent part in responding to violent acts since the inception of EMS in the early 1970s across the world.

Since the terrorist attacks on the United States of September 11, 2001, the role of emergency responders has been redefined. Emergency services provided by EMS, fire rescue, and law enforcement are now defined by the U.S. government as one of five parts of the National Critical Infrastructure–the infrastructure considered to be critical to the continued operation of our nation. Those roles are being better developed for each public safety profession. EMS is moving forward as a major asset for such events, and its capabilities are being better defined and revised. The revised fire service role (for those fire service agencies that have EMS responsibilities) is being better defined and reshaped also.

EMS is a key part of the public safety net, the support network that ensures the safety and health of our citizens. Thus, the evolution of EMS involves not only improvements in emergency medical care but a constant refinement of the response mission as well. EMS performs not only a public safety role, but also a public health role in these types of events.

Defining Terrorism

terrorism
the unlawful use of force or violence against persons or property to intimidate or coerce a government, the civilian population, or any segment thereof, in furtherance of political or social objectives (FBI definition). *See also* domestic terrorism; international terrorism.

The U.S. Department of Justice's Federal Bureau of Investigation (FBI) defines ***terrorism*** as "the unlawful use of force or violence against persons or property to intimidate or coerce a government, the civilian population or any segment thereof, in furtherance of political or social objectives."

CORE CONCEPT
Types of terrorism and examples of terrorist tactics and doctrine

Two types of terrorism are commonly noted as occurring in the United States: domestic terrorism and international terrorism. After the coordinated September 11, 2001, terrorist attacks in New York, Washington, D.C., and western Pennsylvania, the U.S. Department of Homeland Security (DHS) inaugurated color codes to indicate current threat levels. Because this system was used constantly regardless of the threat level, it was found to cause the public to ignore elevated threat levels when they occurred, which was the exact opposite of its intended purpose. In 2011, the Homeland Security Advisory System (HSAS) was retired and a more responsive system was established (Figure 41-1). The National Terrorism Advisory System (NTAS) was implemented by DHS to serve as the nation's alert system. Rather than the color coding of the former HSAS to display generalized threat levels, the NTAS operates by providing specific and detailed information to the public. This information can be disseminated to the American public through multiple delivery methods, including personal email and text messages. More information regarding the NTAS, including an email sign-up for notifications, can be found at the DHS website, www.dhs.gov.

Domestic Terrorism

domestic terrorism
terrorism directed against one's own government or population. *See also* terrorism; international terrorism.

Domestic terrorism involves groups or individuals whose terrorist activities are directed at their own government or population. Domestic terrorism in the United States, as well as in other countries, is changing somewhat, with a trend away from structured organizations to a fragmented, leaderless phenomenon in which individuals or small groups act independently in planning and executing their attacks. However, it should be anticipated that this trend may move back toward better organized schemes in the future. A range of motivations can fuel domestic terrorist groups or individuals.

Until recently, Americans thought of terrorism as something usually perpetrated by persons of foreign birth, not living in the United States but coming to the United States from somewhere else for the purpose of committing terrorist acts. More recently, we are becoming aware that some American citizens have been or are becoming radicalized, either falling under the deliberate influence of foreign groups or, in some cases, becoming sympathetic with those domestic extremist groups and seeking them out, desiring to join in their causes, and willing to become terrorists themselves.

Some American would-be terrorists are indoctrinated overseas in terrorist training camps; for example, the "shoe bomber," who attempted to blow up an American Airlines flight in 2001, as well as the man who attempted to detonate a car bomb in Times Square in 2010 were Americans trained in other countries to carry out acts against the United States. Others, such as the Tsarnaev brothers who bombed the Boston Marathon in 2013 (Figure 41-2), may have been radicalized via the internet, with the older of the two possibly receiving some training in terrorist tactics while visiting family members abroad. Radicalization is also a growing phenomenon among prison populations in the United States.

Domestic terrorist groups or individuals can be fueled by a range of motivations. A wide variety of domestic terrorist groups and individuals have been identified, including environmental terrorists; antigovernment militias; racial-hate groups; and groups with extreme political, religious, or other philosophies or beliefs. These groups may or may not be influenced by foreign interests; they may be radicalized by extremist groups within the country.

International Terrorism

international terrorism
terrorism that is purely foreign-based or directed. *See also* terrorism; domestic terrorism.

International terrorism involves groups or individuals whose terrorist activities are purely foreign-based and/or directed by countries or groups outside the targeted country, or whose activities cross national boundaries. As already noted with regard to domestic terrorism, a

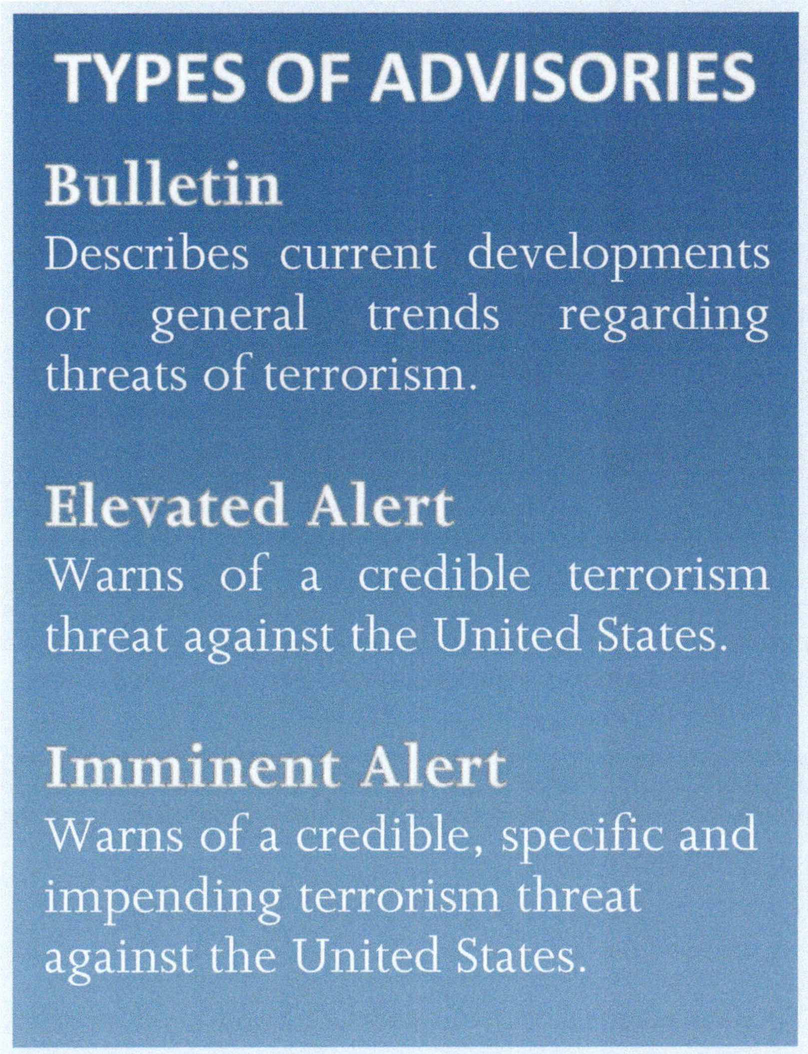
TYPES OF ADVISORIES
Bulletin
Describes current developments or general trends regarding threats of terrorism.
Elevated Alert
Warns of a credible terrorism threat against the United States.
Imminent Alert
Warns of a credible, specific and impending terrorism threat against the United States.

A

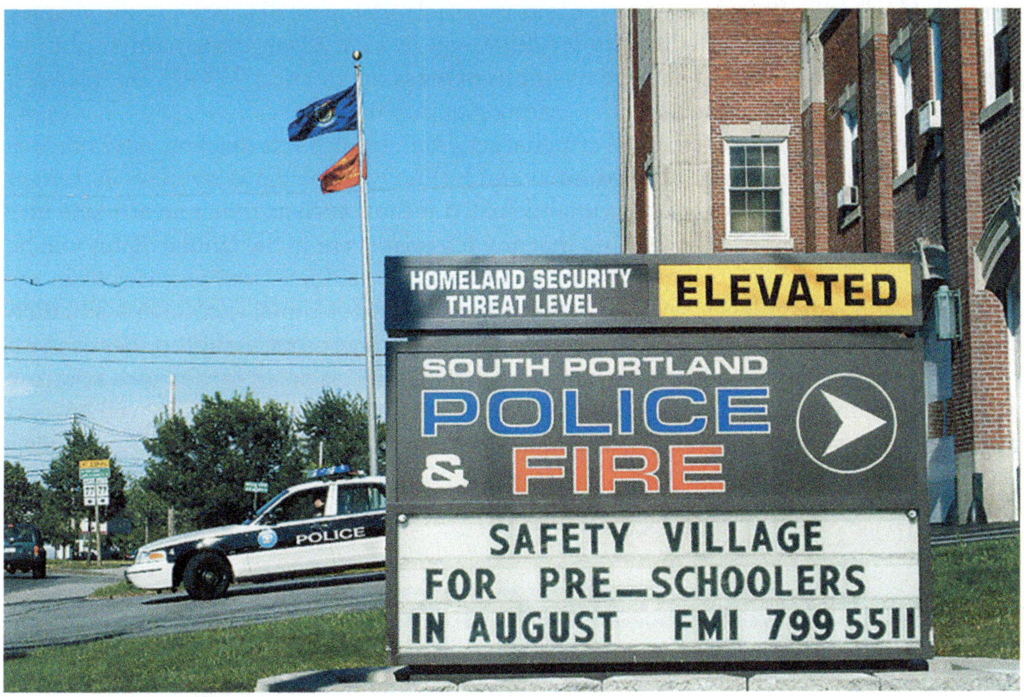
HOMELAND SECURITY THREAT LEVEL
ELEVATED
SOUTH PORTLAND
POLICE
& FIRE
SAFETY VILLAGE
FOR PRE_SCHOOLERS
IN AUGUST FMI 799 5511
POLICE

B

FIGURE 41-1 (A) NTAS alert categories. (B) Yellow elevated level shown at Portland, Maine, police and fire building.
(Photo A: *National Terrorism Advisory System Bulletin available in https://www.dhs.gov/sites/default/files/publications/15_1214_ntas_sample_bulletin.pdf)*

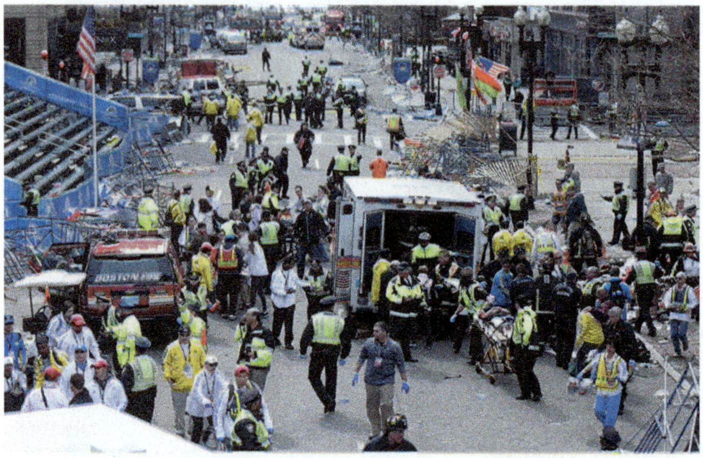

FIGURE 41-2 The bombing of the Boston Marathon in 2013 was perpetrated by two young men who may have become radicalized partly via the internet. *(Charles Krupa/AP Images)*

trend in international terrorism is the shift from well-organized, state-sponsored localized groups to loosely organized, international networks of terrorists.

These networks may be loosely connected or may have incredibly complex organizational constructs. Individuals and groups have increasingly turned to a variety of sources of funding, including private sponsorship, drug trafficking, crime, and illegal trade. Much of the funding comes from people in the United States via money-laundering schemes, drug trafficking, or even donations.

weapons of mass destruction (WMD) weapons, devices, or agents intended to cause widespread harm and/or fear among a population.

Types of Terrorism Incidents

In addition to armed attacks, incidents of terrorism may involve what are often called the *CBRNE* agents:

Chemical

Biologic

Radiologic

Nuclear

Explosive

"When you respond to any kind of terrorist incident, you are going to see an event of a scope and duration unlike anything you have ever seen before."

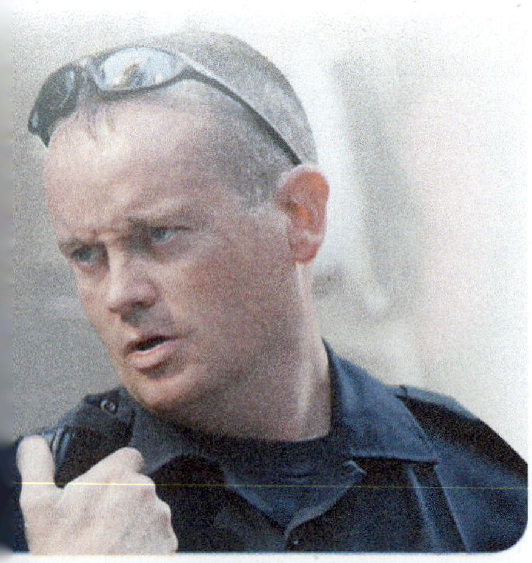

(Kevin Link/Science Source)

The CBRNE agents are considered to be technologic hazardous agents—a broad field, of which HAZMATs (the types of hazardous materials that were discussed in the chapter *Hazardous Materials, Multiple-Casualty Incidents, and Incident Management*) are a subcategory. The CBRNE agents, often called ***weapons of mass destruction (WMD)***, are intended to cause widespread harm and/or fear among a population.

Terrorism incidents can encompass criminal activities. In such acts as arson, environmental crime, and industrial sabotage, criminal and technologic incidents overlap. Terrorism can be committed by conventional or unanticipated means, such as flying an airplane into a building. The EMT must bear in mind that any terrorist event in the United States will be considered a crime scene, bringing in many different law enforcement agencies from the local, state, and federal levels. When EMS and fire service personnel encounter a situation that arouses suspicion of criminal acts, reporting these to the appropriate authorities can be a very important terrorism countermeasure. Although the FBI, as noted earlier, uses a narrow definition of terrorism, EMS has responsibilities for violent incidents that go well beyond that limited scope. This chapter will principally cover terrorism involving CBRNE agents.

Terrorism and EMS

Emergency Medical Responders as Targets

Emergency medical responders are often the principal targets of a terrorist attack, as will be discussed in more detail later in this chapter. Responders must stay alert and never assume the incident scene is safe until this is verified by appropriate agencies or authorities.

Point of View

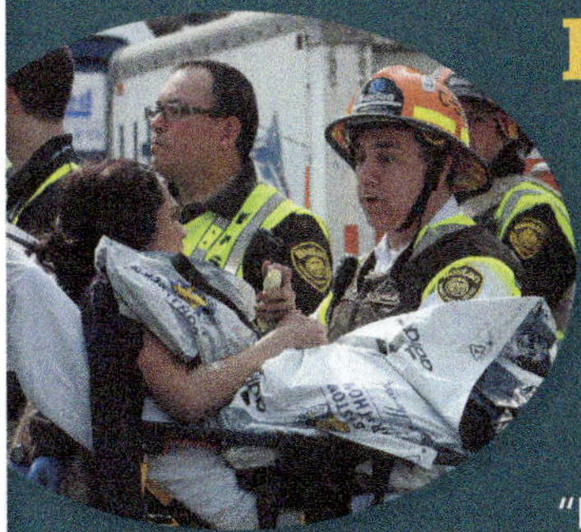

(Jeremy Pavia/AP Images)

"When you take your EMT class, you learn about a lot of things. You even learn about what to do at multiple-casualty incidents.

"I had some minor MCIs in my early days. Car crashes with five patients, a fire with a lot of smoke inhalation. But nothing could prepare me—no class and no experience—for the real 'big one': a terrorist incident.

"I'm not going to tell stories. All I can say is that sometimes things are of a magnitude that you can't even conceive until you are there. You are a small cog in a big wheel. You feel like you are both so small in a big incident and yet so important for being there. The injuries and specific things you see actually become secondary to the hugeness of it all.

"It was tough. It was enormous. It was mass humanity and mass confusion at the same time. It'll happen again somewhere. It may happen to you. It will be tough, but you'll be glad you were there to do your job. Someone has to."

Responders must weigh the threat or risk of their actions against the benefit of their actions. This is true at all emergency scenes, of course, but even more true at the scene of a terrorist attack.

NOTE: *Always remember: The EMS provider's safety is the most important consideration when responding to a potential terrorist incident. The responder who gets hurt cannot help others.*

Identify the Threat Posed by the Event

CORE CONCEPT
How to identify the type of threat posed by a terrorist event

EMS response to a terrorist event is complicated. You may be dealing with a hazardous material or mass-casualty incident, using recognized protocols such as the HAZMAT procedures and Incident Management System discussed in the chapter *Hazardous Materials, Multiple-Casualty Incidents, and Incident Management*. A terrorist incident, however, may involve two additional factors that all responders will have to take into account: deliberate targeting of responders and crime scene considerations.

Terrorists have a history of using ***multiple devices*** and/or booby traps to target emergency responders. In January 1997, a bomb went off outside an Atlanta family-planning clinic. One hour after the initial detonation, a second bomb went off close to the point where the Incident Command post had been established, which resulted in several injuries to responders and could have caused deaths. Imagine if the second bomb at the Boston Marathon in 2013 had detonated 1–2 minutes after the first one instead of seconds later. The results could have been much more catastrophic. A related term is ***secondary devices***, referring to those intended to harm those who respond to the initial attack; however, emergency response planners prefer the term *multiple devices* because it is more likely to make first responders aware of and prepared for the possibility of one or more destructive events following the first one.

multiple devices
destructive devices, such as bombs, including both those used in the initial attack and those placed to be activated after an initial attack and timed to injure emergency responders and others who rush in to help care for those targeted by an initial attack. *See also* secondary devices.

secondary devices
destructive devices, such as bombs, placed to be activated after an initial attack and timed to injure emergency responders and others who rush in to help care for those targeted by an initial attack. *See also* multiple devices.

If the incident is a potential act of terrorism, it is also a crime scene. Although there will be similarities between terrorist events and nonterrorist mass-casualty incidents (such as major transportation collisions and HAZMAT incidents), crime scene considerations—such as the need to preserve evidence and the need to guard against further criminal activity—will complicate responder operations.

Regardless of the mechanism or motive behind an incident, responders should remain focused on reducing the impact of the event as efficiently and safely as possible. Whether dealing with a terrorist or a nonterrorist event, all responders should follow their agency's established operating guidelines. All responders on the scene should operate under an

Incident Command System and use some type of staff-personnel accountability system that is compatible with those used by all participating agencies.

Although recognizing suspicious incidents may be difficult, being alert to clues, surroundings, and events will greatly assist in identification. Clues such as the *OTTO* signs, discussed in the following sections will help with this process:

Occupancy or location

Type of event

Timing of the event

On-scene warning signs

Occupancy or Location

The following types of occupancy or location are sometimes targeted by terrorists or extremists. A call to such a location should make the responding crew especially alert to the possibility that the emergency may be related to a terrorist attack:

- **Symbolic and historical targets.** These include targets that represent some organization or event that is particularly offensive in the minds of an extremist individual or group. Examples may include:
  - Government buildings (including the Washington Monument, the U.S. Capitol, and the like)
  - The Statue of Liberty
  - The Liberty Bell
  - The Wall Street Financial District

  The World Trade Center (Figure 41-3), with its great height and location at the financial hub of New York City, became such a target twice, in 1993 and again, disastrously, on September 11, 2001.
- **Public buildings or assembly areas.** These areas provide the opportunity for attention-getting mass casualties. Some of these public buildings are also symbolic targets, so the terrorist can cause massive casualties and link the owner/operator of the building or assembly area with danger in the minds of the public. These targets include shopping malls, convention centers, entertainment venues, sporting arenas, and tourist destinations.
- **Controversial businesses.** These businesses usually have a history of attracting the enmity of extremist groups. Family-planning clinics, nuclear facilities, animal-research facilities, car dealerships, large-scale commercial developments perceived to be adversely affecting the environment, and furriers all fall into this category.
- **Infrastructure systems.** These operations are necessary for the continued functioning of our society. Major cities are full of targets such as bridges, power plants, phone companies, water-treatment plants, mass transit, and hospitals. Attacks on any of these have the potential to disrupt entire regions and cost hundreds of millions of dollars to correct.

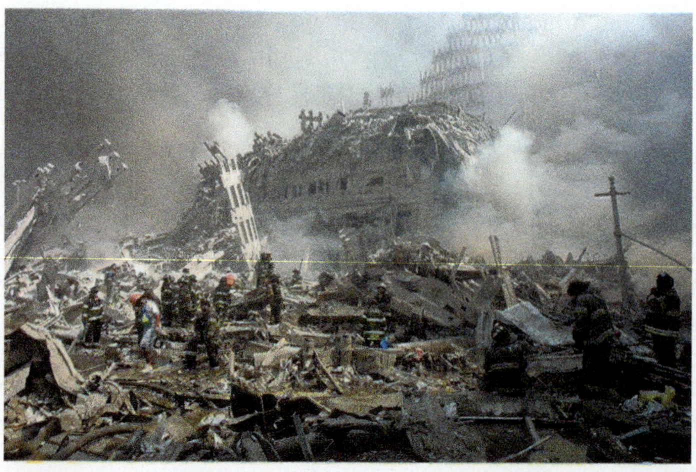

FIGURE 41-3 The Twin Towers of the World Trade Center in New York City were destroyed and thousands were killed on September 11, 2001, when terrorists flew hijacked jetliners into the famous skyscrapers. *(Shawn Baldwin/AP Images)*

Type of Event

Certain types of events should raise your awareness of possible terrorist involvement. In general, they can be categorized as follows:

- **Explosions and/or incendiaries.** These are among the favorite weapons of terrorists. Any bombing or suspicious fire may raise suspicions of terrorist involvement, especially when combined with a previously listed type of location or occupancy.
- **Incidents involving firearms.** These should always be treated as suspicious. If they occur in conjunction with other indicating factors, such as a sniper attack or taking of hostages in a mall, terrorism is a definite possibility.
- **Nontrauma mass-casualty incidents.** These incidents have occurred as the arsenal of terrorism increases in sophistication. When large numbers of victims are generated without obvious (physical) injury but with symptoms of illness, you may suspect terrorist involvement.

Timing of the Event

For many years to come, April 19 will be a day around which government facilities operate at a heightened state of security awareness. It is the anniversary of both the fire at the Branch Davidian compound in Waco, Texas, and the bombing of the Alfred P. Murrah building in Oklahoma City, and so has become a rallying point for antigovernment extremists. National holidays are also possible target dates. In addition, foreign terror organizations may carry out attacks on certain anniversary dates.

Aside from significant anniversaries and holidays, events that occur on specific days of the week and at certain times of day are worth treating with suspicion. A fire in a subway tunnel at the height of rush hour might be aimed at harming a large number of people and alarming the public, and may indicate terrorism.

On-Scene Warning Signs

When you arrive on the scene, you should always watch for signs that you are dealing with a suspicious incident. Unexplained patterns of illness or deaths can be attributed to chemical, radiologic, or biologic agents. Some of these substances have recognizable odors and/or tastes. Unexplained signs and symptoms of skin, eye, or airway irritation may be linked to chemical contamination, as may unexplained vapor clouds, mists, and plumes.

Always remain on the lookout for chemical containers, spray devices, or lab equipment in unusual locations. Watch for items or containers that appear out of place at unusual incidents, as they might contain a secondary device. Large fires, spot fires, and fires of unusual behavior may also arouse suspicion, as can anything that appears abnormal for a given incident scene. Early recognition of suspicious signs and early reporting of these observations by the first responding agencies can mean the difference between an ineffective and an effective mitigation of the event.

Recognize the Harms Posed by the Threat

To implement self-protection measures, you must first understand the types of harm to which you can be exposed. These types of harm—Thermal, Radiologic, Asphyxiation, Chemical, Etiologic, Mechanical, and Psychological—can be categorized using the acronym *TRACEM-P*.

The TRACEM-P Harms

- **Thermal harm.** This refers to harm caused by either extreme heat, such as that generated by burning liquids or metals, or extreme cold from cryogenic materials, such as liquid oxygen. Radiant heat can melt protective clothing and other equipment if an individual is too near the heat source.
- **Radiologic harm.** This refers to danger from alpha particles, beta particles, or gamma rays, which are generally produced by sources such as nuclear fuels, by-products of nuclear power production, or nuclear bombs. Figure 41-4 shows the relative penetrating power of the three types of radiation.

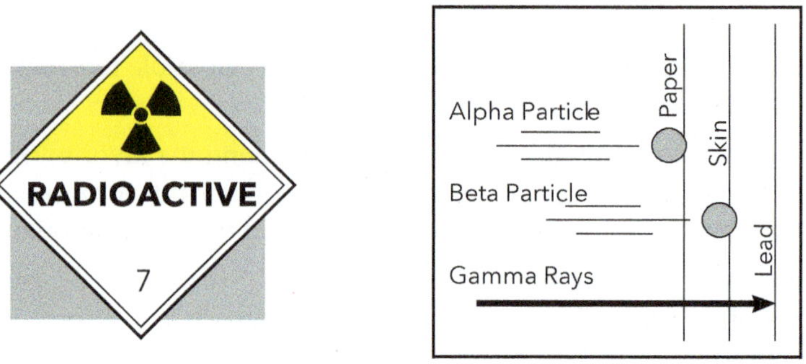

FIGURE 41-4 (*Left*) Radioactivity is the United States Department of Transportation's Hazard Class 7. (*Right*) The relative penetrating power of alpha, beta, and gamma radiation.

- **Asphyxiation.** This is caused by a lack of oxygen in the atmosphere. One common cause of this is heavier-than-air gases such as argon, carbon dioxide, or chemical vapors in a confined space. Extremely dusty situations such as the site of the World Trade Center towers' collapse create additional problems. An oxygen level of 19.5 percent is required for normal breathing.
- **Chemical harm.** This harm is posed by toxic or corrosive materials. These can include acids such as sulfuric acid, caustics such as lye, and chemical toxins ranging from cyanides to nerve agents.
- **Etiologic harm.** Etiology concerns the causes of disease—whether it comes from disease-causing organisms such as bacteria and viruses or toxins derived from living organisms.
- **Mechanical harm.** This is any sort of physical trauma, such as gunshot wounds, slip-trip-and-fall injuries, and injury from bomb fragments or shrapnel.
- **Psychological harm.** This can, of course, result from any violent or traumatic event. Terrorist events are designed to create fear, invoke panic, reduce faith in government, and (as the name indicates) cause terror. In fact, psychological harm is generally the purpose of a terrorist attack. Responders and patients will be subject to posttraumatic stress and survivor guilt. These effects may occur during or right after the event, or may manifest themselves at a much later time.

Professional counseling is available to responders in many local communities. Identify your resources for professional counseling through your agency before an event occurs.

Time/Distance/Shielding

CORE CONCEPT
How to respond to and deal with threats from a terrorist event

Protection of the EMT is based on avoiding or minimizing exposure through the principles of time, distance, and shielding.

- **Time.** Minimize your time at a dangerous scene, such as a crime scene or a HAZMAT scene. Spend the shortest amount of time possible in the dangerous area or exposed to a hazardous material, a biologic agent, or radiation. An example of using time constraints would be executing rapid entries to perform reconnaissance or rescue. The less time you spend in the affected area, the less likely you are to become injured. Minimizing the time you spend in the affected area will also reduce your chances of contaminating a crime scene.
- **Distance.** Maximize your distance from the hazard area or the projected hazard area. One example of using distance would be avoiding contact by following the recommended guidelines regarding hazardous materials in the current edition of the *Emergency Response Guidebook*. You can determine the safe distances from vehicles suspected of containing explosives from the recommendations in *Vehicle Bomb Explosion Hazard and Evacuation Distance Tables*, obtainable from the federal Bureau of Alcohol, Tobacco, Firearms, and Explosives (Figure 41-5).
- **Shielding.** Use appropriate shielding to address specific hazards. Shielding can consist of vehicles, buildings, fire-protection clothing, HAZMAT suits, positive pressure

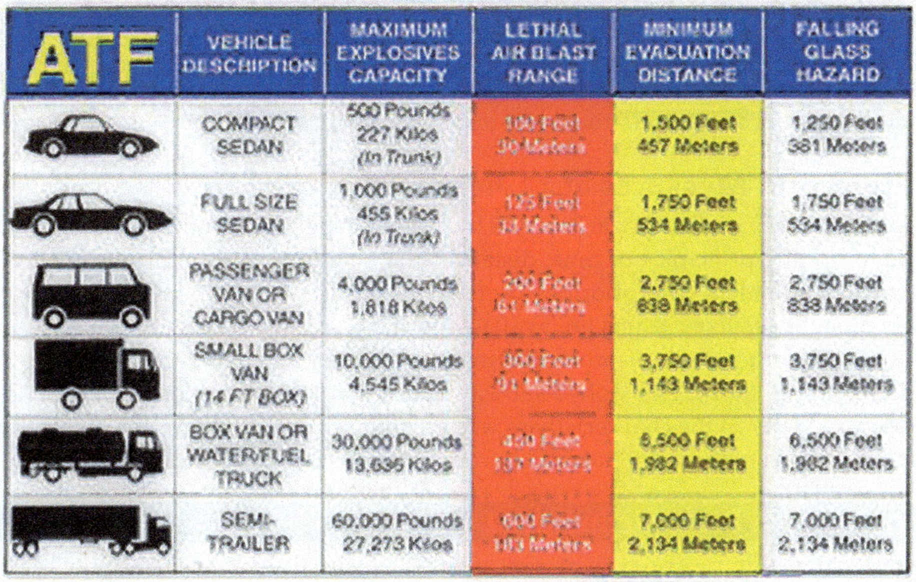

ATF	VEHICLE DESCRIPTION	MAXIMUM EXPLOSIVES CAPACITY	LETHAL AIR BLAST RANGE	MINIMUM EVACUATION DISTANCE	FALLING GLASS HAZARD
	COMPACT SEDAN	500 Pounds 227 Kilos (In Trunk)	100 Feet 30 Meters	1,500 Feet 457 Meters	1,250 Feet 381 Meters
	FULL SIZE SEDAN	1,000 Pounds 455 Kilos (In Trunk)	125 Feet 38 Meters	1,750 Feet 534 Meters	1,750 Feet 534 Meters
	PASSENGER VAN OR CARGO VAN	4,000 Pounds 1,818 Kilos	200 Feet 61 Meters	2,750 Feet 838 Meters	2,750 Feet 838 Meters
	SMALL BOX VAN (14 FT BOX)	10,000 Pounds 4,545 Kilos	300 Feet 91 Meters	3,750 Feet 1,143 Meters	3,750 Feet 1,143 Meters
	BOX VAN OR WATER/FUEL TRUCK	30,000 Pounds 13,636 Kilos	450 Feet 137 Meters	6,500 Feet 1,982 Meters	6,500 Feet 1,982 Meters
	SEMI-TRAILER	60,000 Pounds 27,273 Kilos	600 Feet 183 Meters	7,000 Feet 2,134 Meters	7,000 Feet 2,134 Meters

FIGURE 41-5 Vehicle Bomb Explosion Hazard and Evacuation Distance Tables. *(Source: U.S. Department of the Treasury Bureau of Alcohol, Tobacco, Firearms, and Explosives, http://www.libertyreferences.com/atf-vehicle-bomb-and-explosion-hazard-evacuation-distance-tables.shtml)*

self-contained breathing apparatus, and personal protective equipment (PPE). Also consider the vaccinations recommended by your service to provide immunization against specific diseases. Always remember that a vehicle does not provide adequate protection from explosive devices.

Responders should use all three forms of protection whenever possible. Just because you feel properly shielded does not mean that you can spend excessive time in close proximity to a contaminated site.

Responses to Terrorist Incidents

The following sections will cover the TRACEM-P harms for the CBRNE terrorism categories. The TRACEM-P harms that are not listed are not relevant to the CBRNE category (chemical, biologic, radiologic/nuclear, explosive) that is being discussed. In each CBRNE category, each harm listed is identified as primary or secondary for that specific type of agent.

CORE CONCEPT
Use of time/distance/shielding for protection at a terrorist event

Responses to a Chemical Incident

Chemical incidents can include many classes of hazardous materials. Materials can be inhaled, ingested, absorbed, or injected. These materials can include industrial chemical or warfare-type agents.

NOTE: *It is important to obtain a weather report from the dispatch center when responding to suspected chemical incidents to ensure you approach upwind from any potential airborne chemicals. Find out if your dispatch agency has this type of capability.*

Types of Harm from Chemical Incidents

The following types of harm can result from chemical incidents:

- **Thermal harm.** This is a secondary harm, since many chemical reactions create heat. The chemicals involved may also be flammable.
- **Asphyxiation.** This is a secondary harm, and is possible because some chemical reactions may deplete oxygen or create gases that displace oxygen.
- **Chemical harm.** This is the primary harm, and it includes a wide variety of effects such as corrosivity and reactivity. Chemical harm may also have a several systemic effects that may attack the central nervous system, cardiovascular system, respiratory system, and other body systems.
- **Mechanical harm.** This is a secondary harm that must be taken into account because corrosive chemicals such as strong acids can weaken structural elements.

- **Psychological harm.** This is a secondary harm. Many individuals will react emotionally to a possible chemical exposure. This type of response can happen at the scene, immediately afterward, or sometime well after the event. Responders who are overcome emotionally should be removed/escorted from the scene and provided psychological assistance after the situation is managed appropriately.

Self-Protection Measures at a Chemical Incident

Because of the wide variety of hazards posed by chemical agents, responders should always take care to use the principles of time, distance, and shielding to minimize exposure. At any incident, responders who prioritize protective measures can help limit exposure and contamination. Specialized teams are available in most areas to deal with chemical incidents. It is important to use self-protection measures including respiratory protection and protective clothing. In the 1995 Tokyo subway attack involving the chemical nerve agent sarin (discussed later in the chapter), there was secondary contamination of a rescuer who performed CPR on a patient and later died from the exposure.

Responses to a Biologic Incident

A biologic incident (Figure 41-6) will present as either a focused emergency or a public health emergency. A focused emergency is a situation in which a potential or actual point of origin or source of a disease is located (such as a single case, or a small and localized number of cases, of a disease) and attempts are made to prevent or minimize damage and spread. A public health emergency manifests itself as a sudden demand on the public health infrastructure with no apparent explanation for the occurrence. Causative agents may be bacteria, viruses, or toxins. These agents may cause harm by being inhaled or ingested into the body.

- **Bacteria.** These single-celled organisms can grow in a variety of environments. Dangers to humans come from two directions: disease-causing bacteria growing in the human body and bacteria that grow outside of the body but produce toxins that may pose a danger. (*Rickettsia* are sometimes classified as a genus of bacteria, and sometimes as organisms that share characteristics of both bacteria and viruses. Like bacteria, they can be destroyed by antibiotics. Like viruses, they can live and multiply only inside cells. They cause diseases such as Q fever and typhus. In the remainder of this chapter, *Rickettsia* will be grouped with bacteria.) Anthrax, a bacterium, has been the weapon of choice in several American bioterrorist events.
- **Viruses.** These are the smallest known entities capable of reproduction. They grow only inside of living cells, and cause those cells to produce additional viruses. Viruses cannot be treated with antibiotics.

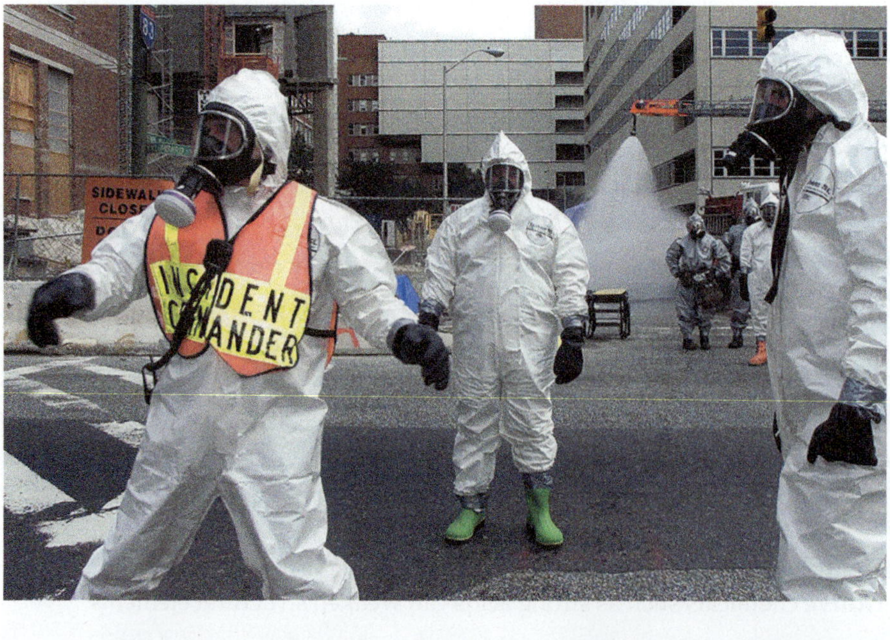

FIGURE 41-6 In Baltimore, a specialized team trains to handle a bioterrorism incident. The Incident Commander is to the left. *(Alex Dorgan-Ross/AP Images)*

- **Toxins.** These are poisons produced by living organisms. The organisms may be bacteria, fungi, flowering plants, insects, fish, reptiles, or mammals. Often toxins are distilled from plant material. For example, the extremely potent toxin ricin is distilled from the castor bean plant. A tiny drop of ricin can be deadly. The FBI has disrupted terrorist attempts to use ricin, such as a 2009 event in Las Vegas, Nevada, in which a police officer was sickened by secondary contamination from ricin at a crime scene.

Critical Information about Biologic Incidents

What Is an Exposure? ***Exposure*** equals the *dose* or the *concentration* of the agent multiplied by *time* (the duration of the exposure).

exposure
the dose or concentration of an agent multiplied by the time, or duration.

- **Doses.** Depending on the substance, these can be measured in either milligrams (mg) or micrograms (mcg) per kilogram of body weight. *Biological doses* are measured in fractions of micrograms per kilogram of body weight.
- **Concentration.** The concentration of an agent is measured in parts per million.

NOTE: *If you reduce the dose, concentration, or time near the agent, you will reduce the exposure.*

Remember that infectious dose data are standardized. They are typically based on a 150-pound (70-kilogram) male in good health. Individuals who fall below these parameters may become infected at lower doses. Examples include the elderly, who are often in poor health, and young children, whose body weight is less than 150 pounds.

Four Major Routes of Entry. ***Routes of entry*** are critical concepts that must be understood prior to studying individual WMD agents. Exposures occur through "routes" or pathways into the body. Biologic agents can enter the body through four routes:

routes of entry
pathways into the body, generally by absorption, ingestion, injection, or inhalation.

1. Absorption (skin contact)
2. Ingestion (mouth)
3. Injection (needles or projectiles)
4. Inhalation (breathing)

Biologic agents seldom enter the body through *the skin*. The exception is T2 mycotoxins, which can be absorbed through the skin. Factors that affect skin absorption are:

- Injury to the skin
- Skin temperature/blood flow
- Higher concentration = greater exposure
- Area with more hair = more exposure
- Length of exposure
- Type of agent

Ingestion is a common route to infection. Ingestion includes swallowing biologic agents in food or drink or accidentally swallowing the agent by itself. One highly likely way to become infected is to eat or drink before completing decontamination procedures.

Injection or puncturing can be accidental or purposeful. Vectors (such as mosquitoes or fleas) can carry biologic agents from one host to another. Personnel can become infected with biologic agents by accidentally injecting themselves through improper handling of a needle or puncturing themselves with a jagged piece of debris. Common routes for biologic infection are:

- Vector (a disease-carrying organism)
- Jagged glass or metal
- A syringe
- A high-pressure device

Inhalation has the potential to cause more biologic agent infection than any other route of exposure, provided the particle is small enough to reach the lower respiratory tract. The degree of infection is based on:

- Rate of breathing
- Depth of breathing

Decontamination after inhalation is only psychologically beneficial.

contamination
contact with or presence of a material (contaminant) that is present where it does not belong and that is somehow harmful to persons, animals, or the environment.

What Is Contamination? ***Contamination*** is caused by contact with or presence of a *contaminant*, which is material that is present where it does not belong and that is somehow harmful to persons, animals, or the environment. As contaminants, biologic agents may be in solid, liquid, or aerosol form. Dealing with each of these requires a different set of skills and operations.

Things that can be contaminated include:

- Hard and soft surfaces
- Skin and hair
- Clothing

Exposure versus Contamination. Exposure occurs when a substance is taken into the body through one of the routes of exposure. Contamination occurs when a substance clings to surface areas of the body or clothing.

permeation
the movement of a substance through a surface or, on a molecular level, through intact materials; penetration, or spreading.

Clothing and other materials can become *permeated* with a contaminant. ***Permeation*** is the movement of a substance through a surface or, on a molecular level, through intact materials. In general, it means penetration, or spreading. However, biologic agents can usually be washed out of clothing. In most cases, clothing and PPE can be reused after decontamination. The removal of clothing removes most of the contamination. It is important to ensure that a patient's dignity is protected during the decontamination operation. Many services carry extra Tyvek suits or a box of oversized trash bags to cover patients whose clothing has been removed.

Types of Harm from Biologic Incidents

The following types of harm can result from biologic incidents:

- **Chemical harm.** This could be a secondary hazard—for example, at the scene of a clandestine laboratory.
- **Etiologic harm.** This is the primary type of harm. These materials are classified as Class 6 Hazardous Materials (Poison) by the U.S. Department of Transportation.
- **Mechanical harm.** This is a possible secondary hazard where explosives have been used to disperse the agent.
- **Psychological harm.** This is a secondary harm. Just the thought of possible exposure to or contamination by a biologic agent can cause stress, even if the person has not actually come in contact with the agent. Many people will contact 911 and/or report to emergency departments and health care outlets with the thought that they may be infected from an agent. This can cause depletion of resources and hospital/health care surge, but those suffering this kind of psychological harm must receive care regardless of whether they have suffered physical harm.

Self-Protection Measures at a Biologic Incident

Take care to limit exposure and contamination if a biologic incident is suspected. PPE provides a shield to isolate a person from the hazards that can be encountered at an incident. Such equipment includes both personal protective clothing and respiratory protection. Adequate PPE should protect the respiratory system, skin, face, hands, feet, head, and body.

Limiting exposure and contamination can be accomplished by responders prioritizing protective measures at any incident. It is important to get as much information as possible to be prepared for what you are going into. The order of protection priorities should be:

- Self-protection (*Respiratory protection is the priority.* Always protect yourself first. You don't need to become one more patient at the scene.)
- Using the buddy system
- Availability of rapid intervention teams
- Civilian protection (Moving civilians to an area of refuge may be their best protection.)

Responses to a Radiologic/Nuclear Incident

As rogue nations continue to acquire and sell nuclear technology, the possibility of a nuclear detonation cannot be dismissed. Small nuclear devices known as "suitcase bombs" were developed during the Cold War and remain in stockpiles with the potential to fall into the wrong hands. A more practical possibility is the use of a radiologic dispersion device that would involve the use of a conventional explosive containing radiologic material, such as medical waste or low-level radioactive sources. Such a device is commonly called a "dirty bomb." Spreading of radioactive materials might also be accomplished by sabotaging or attacking a nuclear power facility.

Identifying a nuclear incident may be difficult because radiation cannot be detected by the senses. Furthermore, symptoms of radiologic exposure are generally delayed for hours or days. Exposure to radiation can, however, be treated if it is diagnosed early.

Types of Harm from Radiologic/Nuclear Incidents

The following types of harm can result from radiologic/nuclear incidents:

- **Thermal harm.** This is a primary harm from a nuclear explosion.
- **Radiologic harm.** This is the primary danger from radiologic materials. Because of the nature of the materials, this will represent an ongoing hazard, the scope of which will be determined only when the amount and identity of the substance involved are ascertained. Radiologic exposure is generally more dangerous to children, pregnant women, and the elderly. The first signs and symptoms are often nausea, vomiting, and diarrhea.
- **Chemical harm.** This secondary harm is a concern because many radiologic substances are also chemical hazards. This is an area often overlooked by responders who are concentrating on radiation effects.
- **Mechanical harm.** This is a primary harm from a nuclear explosion.
- **Psychological harm.** This is a secondary harm. As in all terrorist incidents, a sudden traumatic occurrence can cause immediate or delayed emotional or psychological reactions.

Self-Protection Measures at a Radiologic/Nuclear Incident

Time, distance, and shielding are the mainstays of self-protection at a radiologic incident. The use of radiologic detection equipment is the best method of determining whether your self-protection measures are appropriate and effective.

As noted in the following section, *all* explosive incidents should be treated as potential disseminations of radiologic (or biologic or chemical) materials. This will ensure you take the appropriate protective measures, even before the nature of the explosion can be ascertained. In addition, review the information on decontamination procedures in the chapter *Hazardous Materials, Multiple-Casualty Incidents, and Incident Management*.

NOTE: *Keep in mind that a bombing may have been a suicide bombing, and one of the bomb victims may be the bomber. For this reason, request that law reinforcement officers search all patients at the scene for weapons prior to transport. If a bomb is found on a person, immediately evacuate all persons from the area and cordon it off for response by explosives ordnance detail personnel.*

Responses to an Explosive Incident

Explosive incidents can involve a wide variety of devices, from small pipe bombs to large vehicle bombs. An incident may involve an attack against a fixed target or against a group of people, such as emergency responders. The incident may be an isolated event or may involve secondary devices, booby traps, or suicide bombers.

The materials involved will always include some form of explosive. However, as noted earlier, the detonation may also be designed to disperse biologic, chemical, or radiologic materials. The explosive may be improvised or commercially manufactured. The bomb itself may be equipped with switches or controls that can be activated by light, pressure, movement, or radio transmissions, including cellular phones . For this reason, untrained personnel should never attempt to handle or neutralize an unexploded device. Always assume a device to have remote-detonation capability.

Explosives are categorized as high-order explosives (HE) or low-order explosives (LE). HE explosives produce a defining supersonic overpressurization shock wave. Examples of HE explosives include TNT, C-4, Semtex, nitroglycerin, dynamite, and ammonium nitrate fuel oil (ANFO). LE explosives create a subsonic explosion and lack the overpressurization wave produced by HE explosives. Examples of LE explosives include pipe bombs, gunpowder, and most pure petroleum-based bombs, such as Molotov cocktails or aircraft used as guided missiles. HE and LE explosives cause different injury patterns (see Figure 30-13 blast injuries). Bombs and explosives have been and probably will continue to be the weapons used most frequently by terrorists, along with small arms fire such as high-capacity handguns and assault-style weapons (e.g., AK-47s).

Types of Harm from Explosive Incidents

The following types of harm can result from explosive incidents:

- **Thermal harm.** This is a primary hazard to those exposed to the heat generated by the detonation. It is usually not an ongoing risk unless unexploded materials are present.
- **Asphyxiation.** This is a potential secondary harm, because of the possibility of extremely dusty conditions that can aerosolize a variety of toxins, such as asbestos.
- **Chemical hazards.** These hazards are created as a result of the explosive reaction either from chemicals already present at the detonation site or if chemicals have been included in the device for dispersal.
- **Mechanical harm.** This is another primary harm typically seen at bombing incidents. It can result from blast overpressure, shock waves, and penetrating injury from fragmentation. (Review Blast Injury Patterns later in this chapter and information on types of blast injuries in the chapter *Soft-Tissue Trauma.*)
- **Psychological harm.** This secondary harm often results, as happens in any violent incident. A stunned response could last seconds or minutes, causing individuals to "freeze" and be temporarily unable to think or act. Delayed reaction shows up later in the form of posttraumatic stress.

Self-Protection Measures at an Explosive Incident

With explosive incidents, the responder needs both preblast and postblast protection. *Preblast* is defined as that portion of operations that occurs after a written or verbal warning is received but before an explosion takes place. *Postblast* refers to operations occurring after at least one detonation has occurred.

Dissemination and Weaponization

dissemination spreading.

It is important to be familiar with the potential methods for ***dissemination*** of CBRNE materials, particularly chemical, biologic, and radiologic/nuclear agents. Responders also must not forget that many industrial materials can be used just as effectively as military agents.

The Respiratory Route

The most effective and most common means of dissemination is to enable the material to enter through the respiratory tract. As you have learned in the respiratory care sections of this text, the respiratory tract has a vast and delicate surface area that is exposed to the outside environment through respiration. The deeper into the passageways of the lungs that a terrorist can "place" a harmful material and the longer the material remains there, the more effective it will be.

The passageways of the respiratory system become smaller and smaller as they progress deeper into the lungs. Particulates, gases, and vapors will be trapped and held at various levels based on factors such as the size of the particles, the depth and rate of respiration, and whether the material is water- or lipid- (nonwater-) soluble.

Other routes of exposure, as discussed in the following text, can be harmful, even lethal. However, remember that the most effective means of achieving mass casualties is to have the materials enter the body through respiration.

Other Routes

Other means of dissemination depend upon the agent used. For example, the effectiveness of the ingestion, or alimentary, route of exposure depends on whether the agent can survive the stomach's acidic environment. Many bacteria cannot live in low-pH conditions, although others can. An example of a bacteria that can live in low-pH conditions would be anthrax, a bacterium that can survive for long periods of time and in harsh environments as dormant spores. (Anthrax can infect a person through contact with the skin, ingestion, or inhalation—inhalation being the most lethal route.)

Some have raised concerns over terrorists' ability to contaminate a domestic water supply as an ingestion route of exposure. Processes such as dilution, filtration, and chlorination greatly reduce this potential threat. In addition, the fact that only 1 percent of a domestic water supply is consumed through ingestion further reduces the potential effectiveness of this means of dissemination.

The dermal, or percutaneous, route of exposure (through the skin) is very effective with the blister agents, or vesicants, but less effective with many of the biologic agents. Nerve agents with an organophosphate base, such as sarin, soman, or taban, easily penetrate the skin and cause systemic effects. Only a few biologic materials are dermally active, because healthy, intact skin provides an excellent barrier. The use of vectors such as fleas to disseminate biologic agents (e.g., bubonic plague) presents significant logistical difficulties to the terrorist and is therefore not likely to be a readily selected means of dissemination.

Some bacterial and many viral agents can be disseminated effectively by human-to-human contact. With such agents, especially when there is a delayed incubation period, it is possible to infect a large population prior to detection. These factors are of particular concern with smallpox, pneumonic plague, and viral hemorrhagic fevers, to name a few.

Weaponization

In summary, ***weaponization*** of *most* of the agents we will discuss is most effective when targeted through the inhalation route. If the terrorists can get the materials into a respirable form—that is to say, in particles no more than approximately 3–5 microns in diameter—they can achieve the greatest number of casualties. Such airborne dissemination can be created by applying various forms of energy to the material. Energy such as heat would cause a liquid to evaporate faster, resulting in a higher airborne concentration. Explosives or sprayers could also be used to aerosolize and disseminate the materials.

weaponization packaging or producing a material, such as a chemical, biologic, or radiologic agent so that it can be used as a weapon–for example, by dissemination in a bomb detonation or as an aerosol sprayed over an area or introduced into a ventilation system.

Characteristics of CBRNE Agents

Characteristics of the various CBRNE agents (chemical, biologic, radiologic/nuclear, and explosive) are discussed in the following sections.

Chemical Agents

Chemical Agent Considerations

Physical Considerations. Known agents cover the whole range of physical properties. Under various ambient conditions, their physical state may be gaseous, liquid, or solid. Their vapor pressures vary from high to negligible. Their vapor densities vary from slightly lighter than air to considerably heavier. The range of odors varies from none to highly pungent or characteristic. They may be soluble or insoluble in water. These varied physical properties affect the agent's behavior in the field with respect to such considerations as vapor hazard, persistency, and possible means of decontamination.

Volatility Considerations. Agents that have a low boiling point and high vapor pressure tend to be nonpersistent; that is, they will evaporate more readily. Evaporation presents good news and bad news. The bad news is that the more volatile (easily evaporable) a material, the greater the airborne concentration that will be released. The good news is that the more volatile a material, the less time it will remain on a surface area. Agents that have a high boiling point (and therefore a lower vapor pressure) tend to be more persistent.

Chemical Considerations. The only general characteristic of the known chemical agents is that they are sufficiently stable to survive dissemination and transport to the site of their action. However, their inherent reactivity and stability can widely vary. Some chemically reactive agents naturally lose their potency at a rapid rate, whereas other less-reactive agents require, for example, bleach solutions to inactivate them. Solid adsorbents (e.g., Fuller's earth) are also very effective decontaminants.

Toxicologic Considerations. Keep in mind that not all individuals of a species react in the same way to a given amount of agent. Some are more or less sensitive as a result of various factors, including genetic background, race, and age. The route of entry can also influence the effect. Toxicologic studies estimate the potential biologic effects of chemical agents by different routes of entry. The physical properties of the materials may alter the toxicologic effects and the response of the affected system.

SLUDGEM

Some nerve agents act on the parasympathetic nervous system. For example, the enzyme acetylcholinesterase is inhibited by the nerve agent and fails to break down the neurotransmitter acetylcholine. This causes an overstimulation of the parasympathetic nervous system and a specific set of signs and symptoms.

SLUDGEM is a mnemonic used to remember the signs and symptoms of nerve agent poisoning. The letters stand for:

Salivation—due to stimulation of the salivary glands

Lacrimation—due to stimulation of the lacrimal glands

Urination—due to relaxation of the internal sphincter muscle of the urethra

Defecation—due to relaxation of the anal sphincter

GI upset—changes to smooth muscle tone in the GI tract

Emesis—vomiting because of GI system effects

Miosis—abnormal contraction of the pupils

Classifications of Chemical Agents

Chemical weapons can be classified broadly in the following manner:

- **Choking agents.** These predominately respiratory irritants can be found not only as weaponized materials but also as commonly encountered industrial chemicals. Many of these common industrial chemicals are classified as simple asphyxiants, such as chlorine.

- **Vesicating agents (blister agents).** These agents cause chemical changes in the cells of exposed tissues almost immediately on contact. However, in many cases, the effects are not felt or realized until hours after the exposure.
- **Cyanides.** Formerly referred to as "blood agents," these actually have no impact on the blood. They work by preventing the use of oxygen within the body's cells, and therefore are cellular asphyxiants.
- **Nerve agents.** These agents inhibit an enzyme that is critical to proper nerve transmission, allowing the parasympathetic nervous system to run out of control. Many agencies carry nerve agent antidote kits for their emergency response personnel (Figure 41-7). Many of these nerve agents are stronger versions of common pesticides from the organophosphate family, and are easily absorbed through the skin. Most have a smell of petroleum and have a milky off-white color. They produce the signs and symptoms that make up the mnemonic SLUDGEM.
- **Riot-control agents.** These agents include irritating materials and lacrimators (tear-flow increasers). The effects of these materials seldom last more than several minutes after exposure has ended, although pepper spray can trigger asthmatic reactions. Riot-control agents such as mace, pepper spray, and CS gas have the ability to trigger respiratory distress in people with a history of asthma. These agents are effective crowd-control/crowd-dispersal countermeasures; however, the EMT must recognize the effectiveness of these agents and take appropriate precautions if working within the area of use.

Biologic Agents

Biologic agents are defined as microorganisms or toxins that can cause disease processes. Most commonly the biologic agents are bacteria, viruses, or toxins, and a wide variety of biologic agents are of concern as possible agents of terrorism. Virtually any biologic material can be weaponized and disseminated; some are just more effective than others.

It is important to understand the differences between a bacterium, a virus, and a toxin. The differences can influence the ease of manufacture as well as the availability of antidotes and, to some extent, their effectiveness. Some characteristics of the three were noted earlier in the chapter. Additional characteristics are discussed in the following text.

A *bacterium* is a small, free-living microorganism. "Free-living" means that it can live outside of a host cell. Many bacteriologic agents respond to antibiotic therapies and, for the most part, are treatable conditions if detected early enough. The EMT should be on alert for fever, nausea, vomiting, and diarrhea of a sudden onset or in a normally healthy person. Multiple patients in the same area in a short period of time are often an indicator of an acute poisoning of a population. Normal flu or seasonal illnesses have a period of spread that is much slower. In addition, an illness usually travels from one person to another. In contrast, multiple people may be exposed to a biologic agent all at once, and therefore may display the same signs and symptoms in a short period of time.

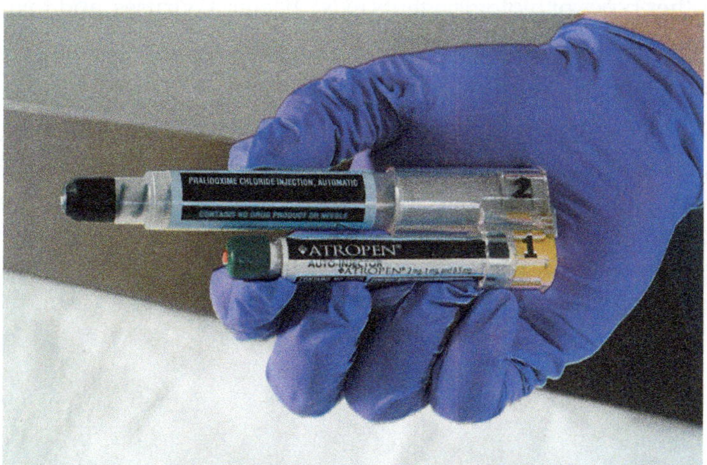

FIGURE 41-7 Many emergency response agencies provide nerve agent antidote kits to their personnel.

TABLE 41-1 Biologic Agent Quick Reference Guide *(continued on facing page)*

DISEASE (CLASS)	ROUTE OF INFECTION	INCUBATION PERIOD/ONSET TIME	HUMAN-TO-HUMAN TRANSMISSION
		BACTERIA	
Anthrax (bacterium)	S, D, R	1-6 days	No, except for cutaneous infection
Cholera (bacterium)	D, DC	1-5 days	Rare
Plague, bubonic (bacterium)	V, R	2-10 days	High
Plague, pneumonic (bacterium)	V, R	2-3 days	High
Q fever (bacterium)	V, R	2-10 days	Rare
Tularemia (bacterium)	V, R, D	2-10 days	No

V = vector, R = respiratory, D = digestive, DC = direct human-to-human contact, S = skin

A *virus* is an organism that requires a host cell inside which to live and reproduce; thus, it is intimately dependent on the cell that it infects. The diseases that viruses produce generally do not respond to antibiotics, which cannot reach them inside their host cells. However, some may be responsive to the few antiviral compounds that exist.

In contrast to bacteria and viruses, *toxins* are not living organisms. Simply put, a toxin is a poisonous chemical compound that is produced by or derived from a living organism. The producing organism could be a plant, an animal, or a microorganism. Examples include ricin, which is derived from the castor bean; mycotoxins, which are produced by fungi; and the botulinum toxin, which is produced by the bacterium *Clostridium botulinum*, which is considered to be one of the deadliest toxins on the planet.

Although other types of biologic agents exist, bacteria, viruses, and toxins are the most common.

Biologic Agent Considerations

The biologic weapons of greatest concern are listed in Table 41-1. As you review this table, note that the primary concern for all of the biologic agents is personal protection if the agent is transmitted from human to human. The role of EMS in patient care and treatment will be primarily supportive in nature, as most bacteria agents and many of the viral agents have treatment regimens.

Regardless of whether the agent is a bacterium, a virus, or a toxin, there are certain features that influence their potential for use as weapons. They are:

- Infectivity
- Virulence
- Toxicity
- Incubation period

TABLE 41-1 Biologic Agent Quick Reference Guide *(continued)*

SIGNS AND SYMPTOMS	DECONTAMINATION OR INFECTION CONTROL PROCEDURES	PREHOSPITAL CARE
	BACTERIA	
Fever, malaise, and mild chest discomfort, followed by severe respiratory distress with difficulty breathing, sweating, stridor (harsh breathing sounds), and cyanosis (bluish skin color); shock and death within 36 hours of severe symptoms.	Universal body decon with low-pressure, soap-and-water wash, then 0.5 percent hypochlorite solution, then second soap-and-water wash.	Supportive according to local protocols.
Range of no symptoms to severe symptoms with sudden onset, vomiting, abdominal distension, and pain with little or no fever followed rapidly by diarrhea. Fluid loss can exceed 10 liters per day.	Enteric precautions, soap-and-water washes, and a hypochlorite solution for equipment. Personal contact rarely causes infection.	Supportive care directed at rapid fluid replacement.
High fever, chills, malaise, tender lymph nodes (buboes), which may progress to infection throughout the bloodstream, with spread to the central nervous system, lungs, and elsewhere.	Isolation precautions, secretion, and lesion (open sore or skin infection) precautions. Use of soap and water for personnel decon; use heat, UV rays, or disinfectants for equipment.	Supportive care and respiratory and circulatory support.
High fever, chills, headache, coughing up blood, and blood poisoning, with rapid progression to breathing difficulty, stridor (harsh breathing sounds), and cyanosis (bluish skin color); death is due to respiratory failure or circulatory collapse.	Strict isolation precautions. Use of soap and water for personnel decon, or heat, UV rays, and disinfectants for equipment.	Supportive care and respiratory and circulatory support.
Fever, cough, and sharp chest pain.	Use of soap and water or a weak 0.5 percent hypochlorite solution.	Supportive care.
Local ulcer and regionally enlarged lymph nodes that may develop into abscesses, fever, chills, headache, and malaise. Signs include fever, headache, malaise, discomfort behind the breastbone, weight loss, and nonproductive cough.	Secretion and lesion precautions, strict isolation not required; use of heat or disinfectants renders the organism harmless.	Supportive care.

(continued)

- Transmissibility
- Lethality
- Stability

Unique to many of these biologic agents, and distinct from their chemical counterparts, is the ability to multiply over time and actually increase their effect. Therefore, biologic material that can readily replicate itself has a greater potential to be transmitted from person to person. The potential epidemiologic impacts of such a biologic weapon are obvious.

These factors are discussed in more detail in the following list.

- **Infectivity.** The infectivity of an agent reflects the relative ease with which the microorganisms involved establish themselves in a host species. Pathogens with high infectivity cause disease with relatively few organisms, whereas those with low infectivity require a larger number. High infectivity does not necessarily mean that the symptoms and signs appear more quickly or that the illness will be more severe. Instead, it simply means that it takes only a small number of organisms to produce symptoms, regardless of timing or severity.
- **Virulence.** An agent's virulence reflects the relative severity of the disease produced by a microorganism. Different strains of the same microorganism may cause diseases of different severity.
- **Toxicity.** An agent's toxicity reflects the relative severity of the illness or incapacitation produced by a toxin.
- **Incubation period.** A sufficient number of microorganisms or a sufficient quantity of toxin must penetrate the body to produce infection (the infective dose) or intoxication (the intoxicating dose). Infectious agents then must multiply (replicate) to produce

TABLE 41-1 Biologic Agent Quick Reference Guide *(continued on facing page)*

DISEASE (CLASS)	ROUTE OF INFECTION	INCUBATION PERIOD/ONSET TIME	HUMAN-TO-HUMAN TRANSMISSION
TOXINS			
Botulinum (toxin)	D, R	24 hours to several days	No
Ricin (toxin)	D, R	24-72 hours	No
Staphylococcal enterotoxin B (SEB) (toxin)	D, R	4-6 hours	No
Trichothecene mycotoxins (T2) (toxin)	R, S, DC, D	Minutes to hours	Yes
VIRUSES			
Smallpox (virus)	R, S, DC	10-12 days	High
Venezuelan equine encephalitis (VEE) (virus)	R, V	2-6 days	Low
Viral hemorrhagic fevers (VHFs) (virus)	DC, V, R	3-21 days	Moderate

V = vector, R = respiratory, D = digestive, DC = direct human-to-human contact, S = skin

disease. The time between exposure and the appearance of symptoms is known as the incubation period. This is governed by many variables, including the initial dose, virulence, route of entry, rate of replication, and host immunologic factors. The incubation period could be hours, days, or weeks.

- **Transmissibility.** Some biologic agents can be transmitted directly from person to person. Indirect transmission (for example, via vectors, such as insects) may be a significant means of spread as well. In the context of biologic warfare casualty management, the relative ease with which an agent is passed from person to person (its transmissibility) constitutes the principal concern.
- **Lethality.** Lethality reflects the relative ease with which an agent causes death in a susceptible population. We can quantify a material's relative lethality by determining its "lethal dose" or "lethal concentration" (LD or LC, respectively).
- **Stability.** The viability of a biologic agent is affected by various environmental factors, including temperature, relative humidity, atmospheric pollution, ultraviolet light, and sunlight. A quantitative measure of stability is an agent's decay rate (e.g., "aerosol decay rate").

Additional factors that may influence the suitability of a microorganism or toxin as a biologic weapon include ease of production, stability when stored or transported, and ease of dissemination.

TABLE 41-1 Biologic Agent Quick Reference Guide *(continued from facing page)*

SIGNS AND SYMPTOMS	DECONTAMINATION OR INFECTION CONTROL PROCEDURES	PREHOSPITAL CARE
	TOXINS	
Drooping eyelids, weakness, dizziness, dry mouth and throat, blurred vision and double vision, impaired speech, hoarseness, and difficulty swallowing, followed by symmetrical descending paralysis and respiratory failure.	0.5 percent hypochlorite solution and/or soap and water.	Aggressive respiratory support, and supportive care for other symptoms.
Weakness, fever, cough, and fluid in the lungs 18–24 hours postexposure, followed by severe respiratory distress and death from lack of blood oxygen in 36–72 hours.	0.5 percent hypochlorite solution and/or soap and water.	Supportive care with aggressive airway management. Volume replacement of gastrointestinal fluid loss.
Sudden onset, with fever, chills, headache, muscle pain, and nonproductive cough. Some may develop respiratory distress and pain behind the breastbone. If ingested, nausea, vomiting, and diarrhea may occur.	0.5 percent hypochlorite solution and/or soap and water.	Supportive care directed at respiratory support.
Skin pain, itching, redness, blisters, tissue death, nose and throat pain, nasal discharge, sneezing, cough, breathing difficulty, wheezing, chest pain, coughing up blood, lack of muscle coordination, shock, and death.	Soap and water, after clothing has been removed. Eye exposure: copious saline irrigation.	Supportive care directed at respiratory and circulatory support.
	VIRUSES	
Malaise, fever, chills, vomiting, headache, and backache; 2–3 days later, sores which develop into pus-filled blisters, more abundant on face and extremities.	Strict quarantine with respiratory isolation for a minimum of 16–17 days following exposure for all contacts. Patients are infectious until all scabs heal.	Supportive care.
Sudden onset, with malaise, spiking fever, chills, severe headache, intolerance of light, and muscle pains. Nausea, vomiting, cough, sore throat, and diarrhea may follow.	Standard Precautions; infectious through mosquito bites.	Pain relievers for headache and muscle pain, anticonvulsants, and respiratory support.
Fever, easy bleeding, purplish beneath-the-skin hemorrhage spots, low blood pressure, shock, swelling, malaise, muscle pain, headache, vomiting, and diarrhea.	Decon with hypochlorite or phenolic disinfectants. Use Standard Precautions.	Supportive care directed at respiratory and circulatory support.

Bacteria

As noted earlier, bacteria are single-celled organisms that can grow in a variety of environments. Like the cells of the human body, they have an internal cytoplasm surrounded by a rigid cell wall. Unlike human body cells, they lack an organized nucleus or other intracellular structures. They can reproduce independently, but they require a host to provide food and other support. To obtain this, they bind to the outsides of host cells in the body.

For purposes of weaponization, bacteria are relatively easy to grow, reproduce, and spread.

Anthrax. Anthrax is a naturally occurring ***zoonotic*** disease (a disease that can move through the animal–human barrier) found commonly in livestock. As carriers of anthrax, cattle, sheep, and horses can infect humans naturally, particularly those who handle the hair, wool, hides, or excrement of infected animals.

zoonotic able to move through the animal-human barrier; transmissible from animals to humans.

The most common human form of anthrax seen in natural cases is the cutaneous form of anthrax, which is also known as *woolsorter's disease*. This condition is found in those persons who have had open sores or lacerations contaminated with anthrax spores during the handling of hides or shearing of wool.

Anthrax also can be transmitted by contaminated meat. However, this is extremely rare, because cooking the meat will destroy the anthrax. If transmitted in this way, the gastrointestinal form of anthrax is seen.

As noted earlier, anthrax can survive the acids of the stomach when so many other biologic agents will not readily survive the ingestion route of exposure. Anthrax is a *sporulating bacterium*. Simply put, sporulating (spore-producing) bacteria create a hard, seedlike shell over themselves that makes them very resistant to breakdown by UV light and other insults. Therefore, areas contaminated by anthrax can remain contaminated for long periods of time. This is why special sporicidal soaps are best used as decontamination materials.

The form of anthrax that is of greatest concern is the inhalational form. If anthrax can be aerosolized in small enough particles (3–5 microns in diameter) so they can be inhaled and retained in the deeper portions of the respiratory tract, then this form of anthrax can be transmitted by the respiratory route. This form of anthrax is very lethal.

With all forms of anthrax, antibiotic therapy works well to counteract the effects, provided that antibiotics are given early enough in the disease process. The problem with inhalational anthrax, however, is that it commonly presents with nonspecific respiratory symptoms, and might not be recognized as anthrax. Therefore, the start of antibiotic administration may be delayed and, if it is not started before the "anthrax eclipse," such therapy may have little benefit. The eclipse is a brief, 12- to 39-hour period during the disease process in which recovery seems to be occurring and the patient feels much better. However, shortly after the eclipse, the symptoms return and death follows in 2–3 days.

Cholera. Outbreaks of cholera typically are seen in developing nations, particularly those without effective sanitary systems. This gastroenteritic agent is more incapacitating than it is lethal if proper care is rendered.

Essentially, cholera is a diarrheal disease caused by the bacterium *Vibrio cholera*. This bacterium readily multiplies within the small intestines and releases an enterotoxin that causes the intestines to release large volumes of fluids, causing severe diarrhea and a characteristic "rice water" stool. Death generally occurs from the secondary effects of severe dehydration and electrolyte imbalances.

Proper supportive care aimed at correcting these dehydration-related problems and the use of oral rehydration salts and antibiotics is generally very effective. From a personal protection standpoint, responders should avoid direct contact with bodily fluid and excrement. Otherwise, incidence of human-to-human transmission is low.

Plague. We know it best as the "Black Death" of the Middle Ages, which was a naturally occurring form of the plague. The plague bacterium (*Yersinia pestis*) is a zoonotic bacterium carried by rats and ground squirrels. It is transmitted to humans by fleas.

In this naturally occurring infection of the human, the plague begins as the bubonic form (*bubo-* referring to a swollen or enlarged lymph node), primarily in the legs. With lack of treatment, it progresses to the systemic form, which develops into the highly contagious pneumonic plague. Pneumonic plague is the primary syndrome seen if plague is aerosolized and inhaled, whereas bubonic plague is seen first in natural occurrences or if weaponized via vectors such as fleas.

The incubation period for plague is 2–10 days, depending on the form. The pneumonic form has an incubation period of as little as 2–3 days. As with many aerosolized biologic weapons, the initial symptoms are fever, weakness, and nonspecific respiratory symptoms. As the pneumonia rapidly progresses, bloody sputum, severe dyspnea (breathing difficulty), and cyanosis (bluish skin color) are found. Definitive diagnosis can be made only by laboratory tests and is impossible to determine in the field.

Since the pneumonic form is highly transmissible from human to human by aerosolized droplets generated by coughing, respiratory precautions are indicated. Field care consists of self-protection and supportive treatment of the patient. Again, antibiotics are required, and are most effective if started within 24 hours of the onset of the pneumonic form.

Q Fever. Q fever is a zoonotic rickettsial disease caused by *Coxiella burnetii*. The natural disease results from exposure to domestic livestock. Q fever in spore form can withstand harsh environments and remain viable for months. As a biologic weapons agent, Q fever is similar to anthrax.

The incubation period for Q fever is about 10–20 days, with uneventful recovery as a rule. It has multiple symptoms, including fever, chills, and headache. Q fever pneumonia is a frequent complication. Other symptoms can include sweating, malaise, fatigue, loss of appetite, and weight loss. The fatality rate is low.

Q fever is diagnosed through serology testing. Other laboratory findings might not be helpful, due to the difficulty in isolating rickettsia. Treatment consists of antibiotics and support therapy.

Tularemia. Tularemia is a zoonotic disease caused by *Francisella tularensis* (a gram-negative bacillus). It is also known as rabbit fever or deer fly fever. Natural exposure to tularemia is usually from the bites of infected animals, deer flies, ticks, or mosquitoes. Tularemia has been weaponized in aerosol form.

The symptoms of tularemia include fever, headache, and weight loss. A patient may have respiratory symptoms, substernal discomfort, and a nonproductive cough. Pneumonia may also be present. Natural tularemia has a mortality rate of 5 percent to 10 percent.

Tularemia is diagnosed by laboratory serology. The treatment of tularemia is with antibiotics with appropriate support therapy. Isolation is not required.

Toxins

As discussed earlier, toxins are not living organisms but rather chemical compounds produced by living organisms. Toxins, including botulinum toxin, shiga toxin, shellfish toxin, and ricin, are some of the most deadly compounds known.

Toxins are not volatile—that is, they do not vaporize or aerosolize without the application of energy such as from an explosive. In addition, most toxins are not dermally active, so intact skin provides an effective barrier. (An exception is the T2 mycotoxin, which is derived from a fungus.) Since toxins do not replicate themselves, they are not human-to-human transmissible. The best method of weaponization varies with the particular toxin. As examples, botulinum is best disseminated through ingestion, whereas the T2 mycotoxin is most effective when aerosolized.

Botulinum. The botulinum toxin is one of the deadliest compounds known. It has an LD50 (lethal dose for 50 percent of the test population) of 0.001 mcg/kg, or 0.1 mcg for a 100-kg (220-pound) human. By weight, botulinum is 15,000–100,000 times more toxic than the nerve agents.

Ricin. Ricin is a potent protein toxin that is derived from the beans of the castor plant. Ricin has gained a lot of attention in recent years, because some groups in the United States have manufactured the material with the specific intent of killing law enforcement officers and public officials. In addition, the recipe for ricin has been published (along with others) on the internet and in various books. Around the world, assassinations as well as nonterrorist murder attempts have occurred using ricin.

The major effect of ricin is to interrupt the body's protein-manufacturing process at the cellular level by altering the RNA needed for proper proteins. This results in cellular death and necrosis, or tissue death. Ricin is readily available and easily made. It is very effective by any route of exposure, and is most effective through inhalation. The patient will present with symptoms characteristic of the route of exposure. Treatment is supportive, depending on the route of exposure.

Staphylococcal Enterotoxin B (SEB). SEB is a toxin that most commonly affects the gastrointestinal tract, when ingested, to produce a form of food poisoning. After aerosolization and inhalation, SEB produces a potentially deadly syndrome.

As with most of the biologic toxins, the respiratory form normally presents in the early stages with fever, general weakness, and nonspecific respiratory symptoms. Later, fevers ranging from 103°F to 106°F (39°C to 41°C), retrosternal chest pain (pain behind the breastbone), and pulmonary edema (fluid in the lungs) may be seen. Severe cases can be fatal, but more often SEB, especially after ingestion, is incapacitating in nature. Treatment is supportive, and no specific antitoxin is available.

Trichothecene Mycotoxins (T2). Trichothecene mycotoxins (T2) are produced from fungal metabolism (usually molds). T2 is soluble in water, is heat-resistant, and can penetrate intact skin. Natural trichothecene has caused moldy corn toxicosis in animals. There is suspicion that some groups have weaponized T2.

The symptoms of T2 exposure include weight loss, vomiting, diarrhea, weakness, dizziness, hypotension, and shock. The onset of illness occurs within hours of exposure, and death occurs within 12 hours. There is currently no vaccine for T2 exposure. Skin decontamination is recommended using soap and water or hypochlorite. These solutions remove the toxin but do not neutralize it.

The treatment for T2 exposure is based on the symptoms. Ascorbic acid has been proposed to reduce lethality. Dexamethasone has also been shown to reduce lethality. Superactive activated charcoal will adsorb the remaining toxin and reduce lethality for ingested T2 poisons.

Viruses

Viruses are the simplest microorganisms and are obligatory intracellular parasites—that is, they replicate only inside host cells. In contrast to human body cells—which contain a nucleus, the nucleic acids DNA and RNA, and various structures necessary for life and reproduction—a virus contains only one nucleic acid, either DNA or RNA.

A virus replicates by attaching itself to a host cell, then penetrating the cell with its own genetic code, whether DNA or RNA. The viral genetic code then instructs the host cell to produce the necessary components to allow the virus to replicate. During this process, the host cell might then release the virus or might be destroyed.

Since the replication of a virus depends on a complicated process using host cells, it is not easy to manufacture viruses in large quantities. A terrorist organization trying to grow them would have to meet significant logistical demands. The organization would need to have well-educated personnel and be very well financed compared with those attempting to make weapons using either bacteria or biologic toxins. Therefore, although possible, the weaponization of a virus is less likely than the weaponization of a bacterium or toxin.

Smallpox. In 1980, the World Health Organization (WHO) declared the smallpox virus eradicated worldwide through immunization efforts. The last eight cases of smallpox occurred in the United States in 1949. The last documented case of smallpox anywhere in the world occurred in 1978 in Birmingham, England, when the virus accidentally escaped its containment and infected and killed an unimmunized medical photographer.

Today there are only two known repositories of the virus: The Centers for Disease Control and Prevention (CDC) in Atlanta, Georgia, and the Russian equivalent, Vector, in Novizbresk, Russia. However, clandestine stockpiles may exist in other parts of the world. If they exist, we do not know their extent or location.

Immunization against smallpox in the United States stopped in the 1970s, and those immunizations given had an effective duration estimated at only 10 years. Therefore, the majority of U.S. citizens today have no immunity to the virus.

Smallpox is a highly contagious disease with an incubation period that averages 12 days. Early signs and symptoms include acute-onset fever, weakness, headache, backache, and vomiting. This is followed in 2–3 days by the development of a rash and chickenpox–like blisters starting in the area of the mouth, throat, and face, which spread to the hands and forearms. Although the blisters also form on the trunk of the body, they are more prominent on the face and extremities than are the blisters found in chickenpox (an important diagnostic distinction). The patient should be considered contagious until all of the scabs separate from the skin. The mortality rate for smallpox in the unvaccinated patient is 30 percent.

Transmission of smallpox occurs by respiratory droplets, therefore requiring respiratory isolation. Furthermore, a strict 17-day quarantine is required for any person in contact with a smallpox patient.

Encephalitis. Encephalitis (inflammation of the brain) has numerous forms: eastern, western, St. Louis, and others. The weaponization concern is the Venezuelan Equine Encephalitis, or VEE. This zoonotic disease is, as the name indicates, endemic to the geographical region of Venezuela. An outbreak of this form of encephalitis must be closely scrutinized.

Naturally occurring encephalitis is a disease found in birds and wild animals. It is transmitted to horses and humans by mosquitoes. Thus, any naturally occurring VEE outbreak should be associated with an outbreak in animals. If only humans are infected with VEE, without the corresponding effects on indigenous animals, then the potential for an unnatural occurrence should be investigated.

Since encephalitis causes swelling of the brain, the patient will present with neurologic symptoms. VEE onset is sudden, with fever and the profound central nervous system effects of headache, photophobia (intolerance of light), and altered consciousness.

It is estimated that 90 percent to 100 percent of persons exposed to VEE are susceptible to its effects. However, because the fatality rate is 1 percent or less, VEE is far more likely to be incapacitating than lethal. Human-to-human transmission is possible, so people should take appropriate body substance precautions, including respiratory protection (HEPA or N-95 respirator) in the case of any patient with a productive cough.

The Viral Hemorrhagic Fevers (VHFs). The names of these diseases are commonly heard and, in the public's perception, are associated with deadly diseases. VHF is a classification of a group of diseases that includes ebola, dengue fever, Marburg, lassa fever, and many more. What these diseases have in common are their effects. Caused by viruses, they change the clotting characteristics of the blood and the permeability of the capillaries. This results in systemic hemorrhage and liquefaction of solid organs, all in association with a fever (hence the name *viral hemorrhagic fevers*).

These highly contagious and highly lethal diseases present with a rapid onset of fever, weakness, and easy bruising and bleeding. Many times, the effects can be seen first in the sclera of the eyes (the fibrous tissue covering the "whites" of the eyes). In this area, bleeding and leaking of the capillaries may be easily observed. This is then followed by the involvement of all mucous membranes.

The method of transmission to humans varies as much as the number of diseases included in the classification of viral hemorrhagic fevers. Contact with blood and other secretions is definitely a mode. The respiratory portal of entry is even more likely. Therefore, Standard Precautions and aggressive respiratory precautions must be taken. With few exceptions, there are no vaccines and no cures, and the use of antiviral therapies has met with only limited success. The field treatment of patients will be directed to preventing the spread of the disease and providing supportive care and treatment for hypovolemia (decreased blood pressure caused by capillary permeability and hemorrhage). Depending on the disease, the mortality rate will range between 5 percent and 90 percent. An intravenous serum is available to treat many strains of VHF.

Radioactive/Nuclear Devices

Potential Scenarios

When considering the possibility of a terrorist organization using a nuclear weapon, four potential scenarios should be evaluated: (1) the use of a military nuclear weapon; (2) the use of an improvised nuclear weapon; (3) the use of a "dirty bomb," or radiologic dispersal device; and (4) the sabotage of a nuclear facility.

Military Nuclear Devices. Although not unheard of, it is highly unlikely that any terrorist organization could both (1) successfully obtain a military nuclear device and (2) successfully deploy and activate the device without detection by intelligence-gathering agencies. In addition, the potential of a retaliatory response by the United States (or any other nation with nuclear weapons) is a powerful deterrent.

Improvised Nuclear Devices. It's a common belief that the basic information needed to construct a nuclear device is easily obtained. This might very well be the case. However, knowing how to construct the device to the exacting specifications necessary to make it work is another issue. In addition, the physical act of assembling the weapon—that is, placing the radioactive material into the device without the proper shielding—would expose the individual to unsurvivable levels of radiation. Even if all of these obstacles could be overcome, the intelligence community more than likely would detect the acquisition of the prerequisite materials and information before the device could be constructed.

Radiologic Dispersal Device (RDD) or "Dirty Bomb." An RDD is any device that disseminates a radioactive material—for example, a conventional bomb that spreads a radioactive substance upon exploding. This is a more likely scenario than the previous two possibilities listed, which involve using an actual atom-splitting nuclear bomb. However, an RDD

TABLE 41-2 Systemic Effects of Rem Dosages

STARTING DOSE	SYSTEM AFFECTED	EFFECTS
150 rem*	Blood	• Suppression of the blood-forming characteristics of the bone marrow • Opportunistic diseases after the white blood cells die and are not replaced (7 days) • Anemia as red blood cells die off (in approximately 30 days) • Clotting difficulties as platelets are not replaced (30–60 days)
500 rem	Gastrointestinal system	• Death of the tissues of the gastrointestinal (GI) tract • Nausea and vomiting with profound fluid loss • Hypovolemia (fluid loss) and shock • Prognosis is poor if symptom onset is within 2 hours of the exposure
1,000 rem	Central nervous system	• Damage to the vascular bed of the central nervous system (CNS) • Results in cerebral edema (swelling of the brain) and profound CNS effects (headaches, blurred vision, strokelike symptoms, and death) • Prognosis is poor for radiologic exposures with CNS effects

** rem = roentgen equivalent (in) man; a measure of radiation dosage*

poses many of the same logistical problems in getting the radioactive material out of its containment and into the device without killing oneself. And if we as emergency responders learn to regard every explosive incident as a potential dissemination means for radioactive materials (as well as for chemical and biologic materials), we can use very readily available detection equipment to confirm or rule out the presence of radioactive materials. Medical waste, radiologic cameras, and sources from industrial processes such as food sterilization are all common sources for radiologic materials that can cause injury.

Sabotage. From the standpoint of nuclear terrorism, the most likely scenario is the sabotage of an existing facility. However, nuclear power plants within the United States are highly hardened facilities. With close regulation, the security at these facilities can be tightened significantly if intelligence-gathering activities indicate credible threats. Furthermore, the checks and balances and redundant safety measures used at such plants make it very difficult for an act of sabotage to occur without being detected in advance. More likely targets are the less hardened, small-scale facilities such as those found in universities.

None of this is to say that there is no potential for an act of nuclear terrorism. However, the possibility of success is limited.

Effects of Radiation

If a terrorist were to use a radiologic material, three body systems would be most severely affected: the blood-forming system (specifically the bone marrow), the gastrointestinal system, and the central nervous system. These effects and the ***rem*** (roentgen equivalent [in] man, a measure of radiation dosage) dose necessary to produce each of them are summarized in Table 41-2.

rem
roentgen equivalent (in) man; a measure of radiation dosage.

Incendiary Devices

The use of incendiary devices by terrorists is more plausible than the use of nuclear devices. Obviously, it is not hard to obtain or initiate items such as Molotov cocktails; propane bombs; or even small, shaped charges on existing storage containers of flammable gases or liquids. In addition, the terrorist may elect to initiate the weapon with complicated chemical, electronic, or mechanical initiation devices. In these cases, the impacts of the initiation items themselves must be considered (chemicals, radios, or remote control devices for toys or models).

Specialized teams are generally available to deal with incendiary devices. These teams are often affiliated with the military or with law enforcement agencies (Figure 41-8). Since even seemingly small devices can cause considerable damage, know how to contact the agency that is responsible for dealing with incendiary devices in your area.

FIGURE 41-8 (A) A specialized truck contains equipment for handling explosives, including (B) a robot that can be rolled out to deactivate an explosive device, allowing crew members to remain at a safe distance.

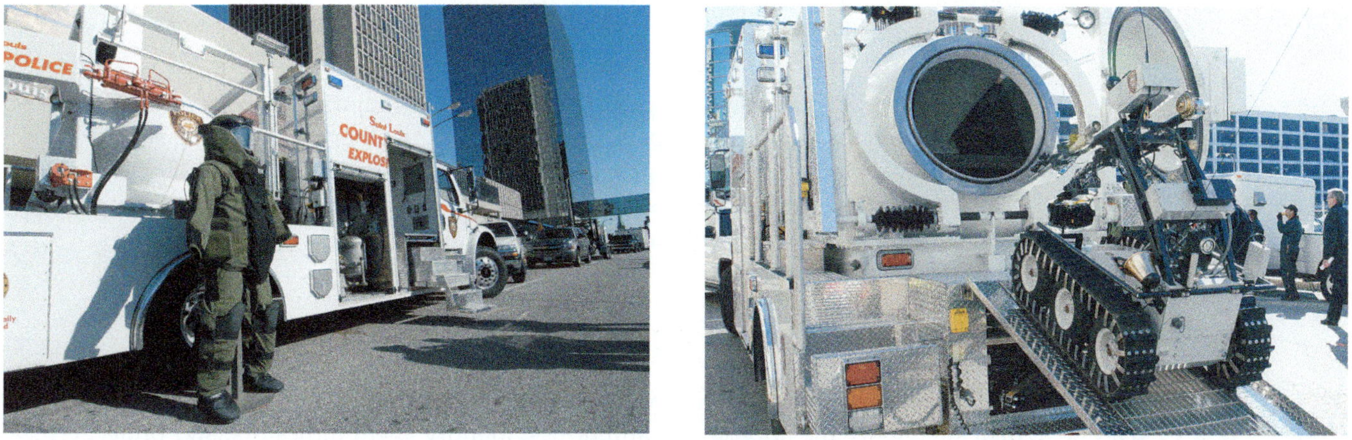

A B

Blast Injury Patterns

Review the information on blast injuries in the chapter *Soft-Tissue Trauma*. Primary and secondary blast injuries create specific injury patterns. There are two mechanisms: a high-energy (HE) overpressurization—usually a blast wave—and a low-energy (LE) blast wind. Parts of the body that are especially vulnerable to blast injuries are the lungs, ears, abdomen, and brain.

Lung Injury

"Blast lung" is a direct consequence of the HE overpressurization wave, and the most common cause of death. It is the most common fatal primary blast injury among initial survivors. Signs of blast lung are usually present at the time of primary assessment or triage, but they have been reported as late as 48 hours after the explosion. Blast lung is characterized by three signs: apnea, bradycardia, and hypotension (cessation or pauses in breathing, slow heart rate, and low blood pressure, respectively). Blast lung should be suspected for anyone with breathing difficulty, cough, coughing up blood, or chest pain following blast exposure.

Ear Injury

Primary blast injuries of the auditory system cause significant injury but are easily overlooked. Injury is dependent on the ear's orientation to the blast. The rupture of the tympanic membrane is the most common injury to the middle ear. Signs of ear injury are usually present at the time of primary assessment and should be suspected for anyone presenting with hearing loss, ringing in the ears, or bleeding from the external canal. It should be noted that many of these victims will not be able to hear you provide evacuation and/or treatment directions when you arrive on scene. Hand signals or preprinted index cards may be effective means of communicating with these patients.

Abdominal Injury

Gas-containing sections of the GI tract are most vulnerable to primary blast effects, which can cause immediate rupture of the large or small intestines, hemorrhage, mesenteric shear injuries, solid organ lacerations, and testicular rupture. Blast abdominal injury should be suspected in anyone exposed to an explosion who has abdominal pain, nausea, vomiting of blood, testicular pain, unexplained hypovolemia, or any findings suggestive of an acute abdomen. Clinical findings may be absent until the onset of complications hours or days later.

Brain Injury

Primary blast waves can cause concussions or mild traumatic brain injury (MTBI) without a direct blow to the head. Consider the patient's proximity to the blast, particularly when given complaints of headache, fatigue, poor concentration, lethargy, depression, anxiety, insomnia, or other constitutional symptoms. The symptoms of concussion and posttraumatic stress disorder can be similar. Many patients exposed to high-energy primary blast waves are not salvageable.

Treatment for Blast Injuries

The treatment for patients who incur thermal and blast injuries from these weapons is no different from the treatment for patients exposed to any other thermal or blast injury. Local protocols must be followed. As appropriate, follow your system's HAZMAT and multiple-casualty incident procedures, as discussed in the chapter *Hazardous Materials, Multiple-Casualty Incidents, and Incident Management*.

Strategy and Tactics

CORE CONCEPT

Applying strategy, tactics, and countermeasures at a terrorist event

EMS responders should understand how to apply tactical considerations to isolate the incident site, notify the appropriate authorities, identify agent indicators, and protect critical assets. The DOT *Emergency Response Guidebook* provides additional information for the common terrorist weapons:

- Nerve agents (Guide #153)
- Blister agents (Guide #153)
- Blood agents (Guides #117, 119, 125)
- Choking agents (Guides #124, 125)
- Irritant agents (riot control) (Guides #153, 159)

Use of an Incident Command System was discussed in the chapter *Hazardous Materials, Multiple-Casualty Incidents, and Incident Management*.

Priorities for responders are:

- Life safety
- Incident stabilization
- Protection of property

Additional critical asset considerations include:

- Responders
- Responders' equipment
- Organizational function continuity

strategies broad general plans designed to achieve desired outcomes.

tactics specific operational actions to accomplish assigned tasks.

Strategies are broad general plans designed to achieve desired outcomes. ***Tactics*** are specific operational actions responders take to accomplish their assigned tasks. This section will discuss tactics for:

- Isolation
- Notification
- Identification
- Protection

Isolation

Initial Considerations

Approaching the site of an act of terrorism (which is also a criminal event) presents unique challenges to the EMS responder. To effectively implement scene control and ensure public safety, emergency responders must quickly and accurately evaluate the incident area and determine the severity of danger. Once the magnitude of the incident is realized, attempts to isolate the danger can begin. Establishing control (work) zones early will enhance public protection and facilitate medical treatment.

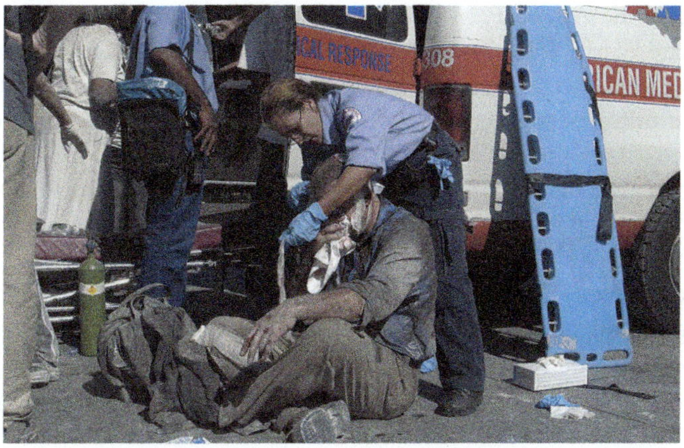

FIGURE 41-9 Panicked, contaminated people can overwhelm the best efforts of first-arriving responders when response resources are limited. *(Amy Sancetta/AP Images)*

Initially, when response resources are limited, isolating the hazard area and controlling a mass exodus of panicked and contaminated people will likely overwhelm the best efforts of first-arriving responders (Figure 41-9). Responders must use all available resources effectively and efficiently to prepare the scene for ongoing operations.

Responders must be aware that terrorists may still be lurking nearby, waiting for responders to arrive. In fact, as noted earlier, the responders could be the actual targets. Terrorists may also be among the injured. If this is suspected, initial scene control will likely be delayed and dictated by law enforcement activities. Making sure to follow Incident Command directions and not "freelance" is of paramount importance. First responders are not used to considering that their scenes are fraught with people who wish to hurt them; this possibility must be kept in mind.

As in all hazardous situations, self-protection is a top priority. A responder who becomes a patient only adds to the burden on available resources. Responders must anticipate the potential for multiple hazard locations.

Responders may have to define outer and inner operational perimeters. There may be several hazards within the outer perimeter that must be isolated, especially when patients are scattered throughout the boundaries of the incident, or when there have been multiple targets that contain dangers.

Controlling the scene, isolating hazards, and attempting to conduct controlled evacuations will be resource-intensive and require law enforcement personnel. Inordinate security may be needed for the event, so responders should request additional assistance early.

After a bombing, access to the scene may be limited due to rubble or debris. Police activity may also interfere with establishing access and exit avenues for EMS operations. Another problem may involve large numbers of contaminated patients and would-be rescuers moving in and out of the exclusion zone in an uncontrolled manner. In chemical, biologic, and radiologic/nuclear incidents, secondary contamination is a major risk.

Establishing Perimeter Control

Law enforcement agencies should establish perimeter control at terrorist incidents by following recognized methods or standard operating procedures. Maintaining control of the perimeter may be difficult due to the design of the terrorist or panic among the patients.

Responders need to recognize and evaluate dangers critical to implementing perimeter control. Adequate evaluation of potential harm will guide decisions and considerations for setting standoff distances or establishing work zones. To perform this task efficiently and effectively, responders should first take time to perform an adequate size-up of the situation.

When initially determining your operating perimeter, it is better to overestimate the size of the perimeter than to underestimate. Once you establish a perimeter, it is often easier to reduce than to increase the perimeter after operations are set up. Depending on the size and complexity of the incident, you may need to divide the boundaries or identify them as having outer and inner perimeters.

The *outer perimeter*, the most distant control point or boundary of the incident, is used to restrict all public access to the incident. For example, the outer perimeter established after the bombing of the Alfred P. Murrah Federal Building in Oklahoma City enclosed 20 square blocks. The World Trade Center footprint was more than 16 acres, with the perimeter encompassing all of lower Manhattan. The *inner perimeter* (or hot zone) isolates known hazards within the outer perimeter. It is often used to control movement of responders. Inner perimeters are established when several suspicious parcels are sighted. The locations of these items are isolated until such time as specialists have rendered the area safe.

Several types of terrorist incidents may require outer and inner perimeter controls. Incidents involving improvised explosive devices should always have responders thinking about multiple devices. Use inner perimeters to control access to any suspicious area. In cases involving chemical or biologic dispersion devices, you may need to use inner perimeters to isolate areas highly suspected of contamination as well as of possible multiple devices. In cases of radioactive contamination, inner perimeters may be necessary to isolate possible areas of contamination until specialists with radiation meters have determined the actual level of danger to responders.

Perimeter Control Factors

Perimeter control may be influenced by a variety of factors. These factors should all be considered and weighed in relation to each other when attempting to determine the next course of action.

The amount and types of resources on hand will provide a rough estimate of what is possible to accomplish. The capability of available resources must also be considered. People should not attempt actions beyond their training. The ability of the resources to self-protect is a related factor. No matter how well trained personnel are, if they are unable to properly protect themselves, they cannot function in a hazardous environment. The size and configuration of the incident, as well as the stability of the scene, will also come into play.

These factors are the same whether you are dealing with a noncriminal hazardous material incident or a terrorist attack.

NOTE: *Never lose sight of the fact that the behavior of a material is not determined by whether the release was accidental or deliberate.*

Notification

In a terrorism event, it is critical that appropriate response and support agencies (at local, state, and federal levels) be notified. Notification is usually required by established directives, procedures, or statutes. The appropriate agencies and points of contact should be noted in local EMS or emergency management plans.

It is not the on-scene EMT's responsibility to perform notification functions. Notification is usually done by a dispatch center or emergency operations center. However, an initial radio report by an EMT is often the "trigger event" that starts the notification process. For example, notification that a possible improvised explosive device (IED) is involved generates a notification of federal law enforcement agencies.

Identification

Identify any indicators of a particular agent. Note the presence of any chemical containers or lab materials, especially those that seem out of place at the site or for which safety data sheets or shipping manifests are missing. Observe placards and labels on storage tanks or vehicles from a safe distance with binoculars. Obtain the correct spelling of any chemical or biologic agent. Consult your current edition of the *Emergency Response Guidebook*. Contact a poison control center or a CHEMTREC or CHEM-TEL hotline, as appropriate, to help identify and deal with the substance. (Review the chapter *Hazardous Materials, Multiple-Casualty Incidents, and Incident Management* with regard to hazardous material incidents.)

If there is an unusual pattern or incidence of illness, document the numbers of patients involved, their signs and symptoms, and any other relevant information, including pertinent negatives (for example, the absence of an obvious cause for the outbreak). Transmit this information to the appropriate authorities.

Protection

Protection of critical assets is an important function in terrorism or other criminal incidents. EMS critical assets include people, vehicles, and equipment/supplies. An applicable military term is *force protection*. Force protection means that EMS forces are protected to ensure mission accomplishment.

Effective protection requires a partnership between EMS responders and security agencies (e.g., law enforcement, private security, and National Guard units). Security agencies provide protection through perimeter protection, entry control, and traffic control.

EMTs are not armed or trained in security protection; they do not directly engage in security operations. As an EMT, your protection responsibilities include the following:

- Make an initial scene size-up to determine security threats. Always consider the possibility of multiple devices.
- Request protection (read: security) via radio as soon as practical.
- Establish vehicle staging and triage/treatment areas in protected locations.
- Advise EMS Command about protection/security concerns.
- Immediately report suspicious people or activities.

Decontamination

NFPA 473 lists as a competency for EMS personnel "Gross Decontamination. The initial phase of the decontamination process during which the amount of surface contamination is significantly reduced. This phase can include mechanical removal and initial rinsing."

Review the information on decontamination procedures in the chapter *Hazardous Materials, Multiple- Casualty Incidents, and Incident Management*.

Self-Protection at a Terrorist Incident

CORE CONCEPT

Self-protection and safety awareness at a terrorist event

At this point, it is a good idea to review and reinforce what you have learned about protecting yourself in the event that you are called to respond to a terrorist incident.

Protect Yourself First

As always, remember that if you, the EMT, are injured, you cannot help anyone else. For self-protection, you can rely mostly on what you already know about multiple casualty incidents, the Incident Management System, personal protective equipment (PPE), crime scenes, hazardous material incidents, and decontamination procedures. Scene size-up and situational awareness are important reassessments in a response to a potential terrorist incident. For example:

- Are patients displaying signs and symptoms of hazardous substance exposure?
- Are there unconscious patients with minimal or no trauma?
- Are there patients exhibiting SLUDGEM signs/seizures?
- Is there blistering, reddening of skin, discoloration, or skin irritation?
- Are the patients having difficulty breathing?

It is important to look for physical indicators and other outward warning signs. When responding, consider if there is evidence of the following:

- Medical mass casualties or fatalities with minimal or no trauma
- Responder casualties
- Dead animals and vegetation
- Unusual odors, color of smoke, or vapor clouds

A few elements may be involved in a terrorist incident that would not necessarily be involved in the usual range of EMS calls. These include the fact that emergency medical responders are often targets, that an unusual incidence or pattern of illness may result from a deliberately disseminated biologic agent that cannot immediately be identified, and that an explosive device may have been detonated not only for the purpose of causing physical damage but also to spread chemical, biologic, or radiologic agents.

How to Protect Yourself

Given the wide range of possible agents and devices that can be used in terrorist attacks, how can you best protect yourself? Review the following guidelines, summarized from the text of this chapter.

Recognize a Possible Terrorist Event

Remember the OTTO clues that should arouse suspicion of terrorist involvement:

- Occupancy or location (a place or business that terrorist groups might target)
- Type of event (perhaps one with large crowds)
- Timing (a national holiday or an anniversary date important to terrorist organizations)
- On-scene clues (chemical containers or other out-of-place items, or an unexplained pattern of illness)

Don't Rush In!

When terrorist involvement is possible (for example, at a bombing or explosion):

- Wait until the appropriate authority says the scene is safe to enter.
- Follow your Incident Command protocols.
- Wear appropriate PPE.
- Beware of possible multiple explosive devices or booby traps.
- Search all patients for explosives or weapons—or wait for police to do so—since a suicide bomber may be one of the patients. If an explosive device is found, immediately evacuate the area.

Understand the TRACEM-P Harms

Understand what kind of harm is most likely to result from any given type of terrorist weapon or agent, and focus your self-protective measures accordingly. The TRACEM-P harms are:

- Thermal
- Radiologic
- Asphyxiation
- Chemical
- Etiologic (disease-causing)
- Mechanical
- Psychological

Time, Distance, and Shielding

These three elements—time, distance, and shielding—can be put to use to reduce exposure to every type of terrorist agent. Don't forget to use all three when possible.

The following paragraphs will summarize the likely TRACEM-P harms, as well as appropriate time/distance/shielding measures, for each type of CBRNE (chemical, biologic, radiologic/nuclear, explosive) agent.

At a Chemical Incident

Chemical harm is the primary potential harm. Keep exposure *time* to a minimum. (For example, rotate teams for short periods; decontaminate yourself as quickly as possible.) Remain at a *distance*, outside the contaminated area, unless trained and equipped to enter it. *Shield* yourself by wearing protective clothing and respiratory protection, such as self-contained breathing apparatus (SCBA).

At a Biologic Incident

Etiologic harm is the primary potential harm—that is, the possibility of contracting the disease yourself. Limit exposure and contamination. Keep exposure *time* at a minimum, except as needed to assess and treat patients. Promptly take recommended decontamination measures. (Review Table 41-1.) Stay at a *distance* from contaminated areas as much as possible. *Shield* yourself by keeping recommended vaccinations and inoculations up to date and by wearing clothing and equipment that protects your skin, face, hands, feet, head, body, and respiratory system (for example, a HEPA or N-95 mask).

At a Radiologic/Nuclear Incident

Radiologic harm is the primary potential harm, with potential *thermal harm* and *mechanical harm* as well if an explosive device was involved. Limit your *time* in the contaminated area. Local protocols should define your exact time limits for exposure. Follow your local decontamination procedures promptly after any exposure. Remain at a *distance* from the contaminated area unless you are trained and equipped to enter it. *Shield* yourself behind structures or materials that are impervious to penetration by alpha, beta, and gamma radiation. (Review Figure 41-4.)

At an Explosive Incident

Thermal and *mechanical harms* are the primary potential harms at an explosive incident. *Etiologic harm* is possible if the device was used to disperse biologic agents; *chemical harm* is possible if used to disperse chemical agents. If an explosion has already occurred, limit the *time* you spend in the hazardous area, since the possibility exists of multiple explosions or attacks on emergency medical responders. For the same reasons, remain at a *distance* from the scene until authorities declare it safe to enter. *Shield* yourself by wearing proper turnout gear, including hard hat, protective gloves, fire-protection clothing, or other equipment as necessary for a scene where structural collapse has occurred or may occur. Also wear PPE appropriate for a chemical, biologic, or radiologic incident if there is any possibility that the explosive device was used to disperse such agents.

Resources

The EMT should be aware of resources that may be utilized during any type of multiple casualty incident (MCI), especially if it was a *chemical, biologic, radiologic/nuclear* or *explosive* terrorist incident. The *Strategic National Stockpile* (SNS) is a nationally available stockpile of pharmaceuticals and medical supplies to be used when local resources are used up due to a national disaster or terrorist incident. This stockpile was created in 1999 and delivers essential disaster medical supplies to communities requesting aid. The Strategic National Stockpile is managed by the Office of the Assistant Secretary for Preparedness and Response (ASPR) in the U.S. Department of Health and Human Services. For further regarding the EMT's role and responsibilities during a multiple casualty incident, consult the chapter *Hazardous Materials, Multiple-Casualty Incidents, and Incident Management.*

Future Trends

As society changes, the EMT must not only be familiar with established and identified threats as described previously but must anticipate new threats and their impact on emergency medical response (Figure 41-10). The following are terrorist trends and anticipated threats which the EMT must familiarize themselves with to remain current and proficient. As the response environment is constantly evolving, this list is by no means all-encompassing.

Active Shooter/Mass Shooting Incidents. The Federal Bureau of Investigation defines an *active shooter* as "an individual actively engaged in killing or attempting to kill people in a populated area." While such incidents can have political motivations, there is also the possibility that these incidents may not be attributable to terrorism. Regardless of the shooter's motivations, an active shooter/mass shooting incident has the potential to be a *multiple casualty incident*. The response to such an incident will have emergency medical

FIGURE 41-10 Terrorist events. (A) Parkland, Florida, school shooting. (B) Las Vegas shooting. (C) Headlines about Las Vegas shooting. (D) Pipe bomb threat. *(Photo A: John McCall/Sun Sentinel/TNS/Newscom.* Photo B: *David Becker/Gettyimages.* Photo C: *CBW/ Alamy Stock Photo.* Photo D: *MARK MAKELA/REUTERS/Newscom.)*

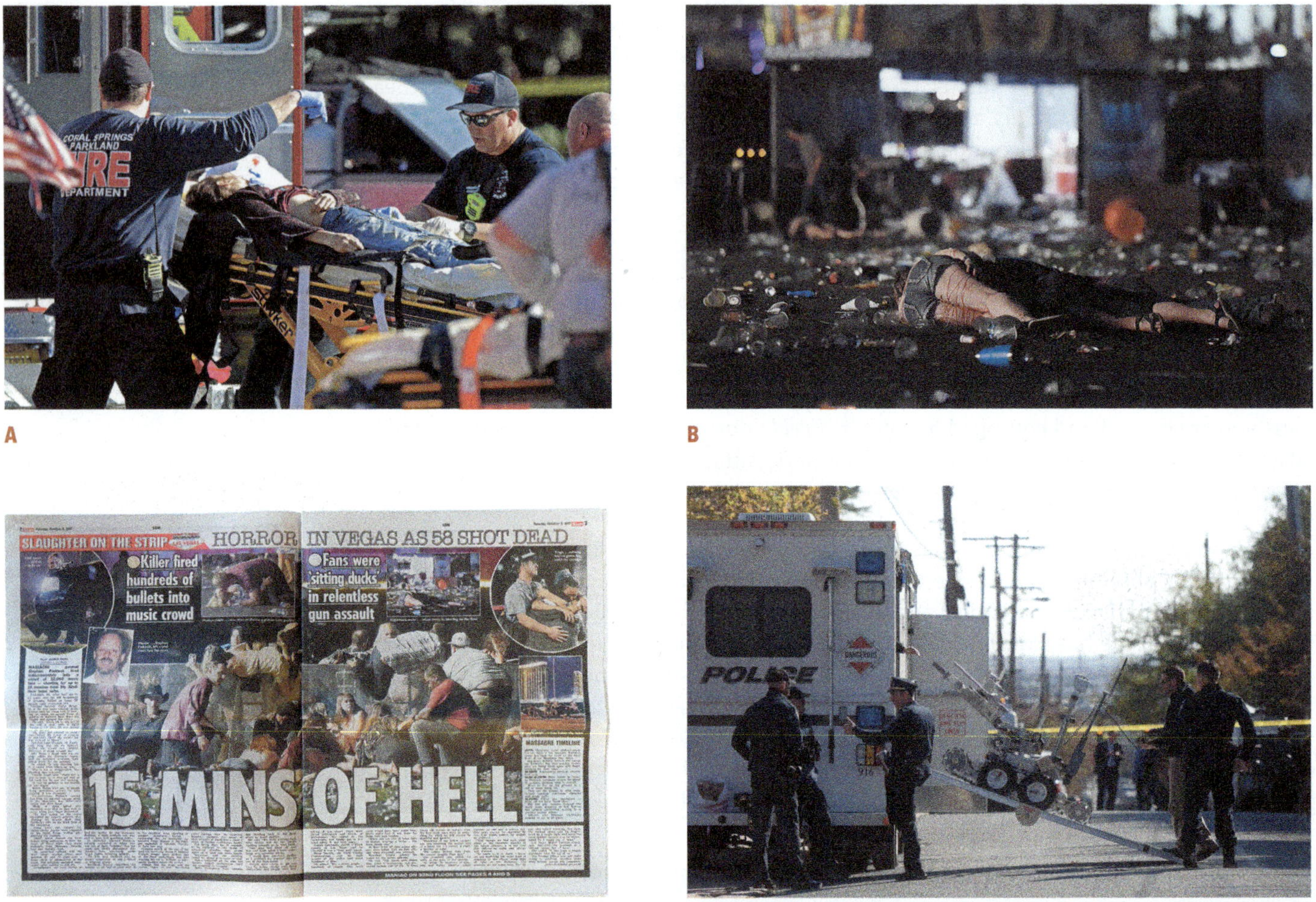
CORAL SPRINGS PARKLAND
SLAUGHTER ON THE STRIP
HORROR IN VEGAS AS 58 SHOT DEAD
Killer fired hundreds of bullets into music crowd
Fans were sitting ducks in relentless gun assault
15 MINS OF HELL

A B C D

providers partnered with law enforcement. Joint training exercises with law enforcement prior to such events are key to successful mitigation of these types of incident. In May 2018, the NFPA (National Fire Protection Association)—along with a consortium of national responders from many disciplines, including law enforcement—released NFPA 3000. NFPA 3000 is a consensus document which outlines best practices for training and mitigation of active shooter/hostile event response (ASHER). For further information regarding the EMT's role and responsibilities at a multiple casualty incident, consult the chapter *Hazardous Materials, Multiple-Casualty Incidents, and Incident Management*.

Cyberterrorism. The EMT must be aware that computer and data systems, while essential to health care, can pose a liability and danger if compromised. Hospital systems have been shown to be vulnerable to computer crimes. Regardless of whether these incidents are politically motivated, the damages to health care systems can be disastrous. A cyberattack in 2018 resulted in a hospital system paying a ransom to the attackers to unlock their computers. This is on top of the damage to the hospital's reputation and potential risk for identity theft that patients now face. In addition to entire health care systems, medical devices themselves have been shown to be vulnerable to hacking. Such devices as pacemakers and insulin pumps have been shown to be vulnerable to unauthorized computer hacks, which can jeopardize patient safety. While this is beyond the scope of this text to discuss in detail, the EMT can help safeguard against such attacks by practicing safe handling of patient health information (PHI). Refer to chapter *Medical, Legal, and Ethical Issues*, Box 4-1 The Privacy Rule of the Health Insurance Portability and Accountability Act (HIPAA), for further regarding the EMT's role in protecting PHI.

Use of Drugs of Abuse as Chemical Weapons. The EMT must be aware that many drugs of abuse also hold the potential to be used as chemical weapons if disseminated properly. With increased abuse of narcotics, one such opioid (a synthetic opiate) has become prevalent and popular owing to its potency. Fentanyl is a potent and legitimate medication used to alleviate pain or in anesthesia. However, it also has a high potential for abuse, owing both to its availability and to its potency. This potency also makes it ideal as a potential chemical weapon if it were to be disseminated properly. In 2002, such a compound was used by Russian forces against terrorists who had taken 750 hostages. Unfortunately, 117 of the hostages died from exposure to the compounds. The EMT must be aware that drugs of abuse can be used by terrorists as chemical weapons, potentially resulting in a multiple casualty incident. For further information regarding the EMT's role and responsibilities at a multiple casualty incident, consult the chapter *Hazardous Materials, Multiple-Casualty Incidents, and Incident Management*. For further information regarding drugs of abuse, consult the chapter *Poisoning and Overdose Emergencies*.

Think Like an EMT

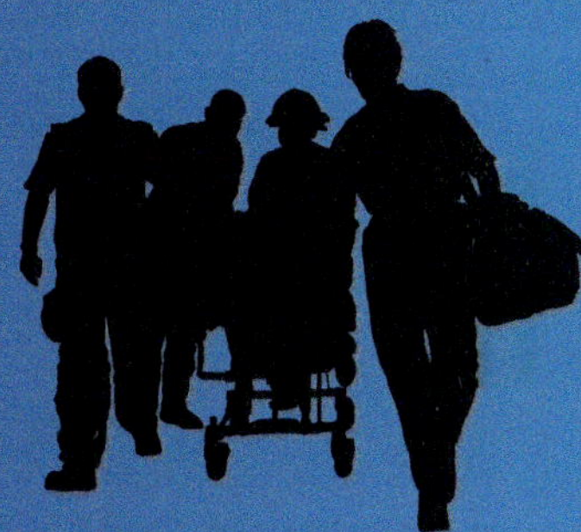

It Could Happen to You . . .

Terrorism can come from many sources and on many scales–from local to nationwide. Your safety from a number of hazards is vital. In each situation, explain what hazards you may suspect and how to keep yourself safe. It is the most important decision you can make.

1. You are called to respond with the police and fire department to an office complex where a worker opened an envelope containing white powder.
2. There was an explosion in a downtown office complex. You respond with the police and fire department to treat patients from the blast.

Chapter Review

Key Facts and Concepts

- There have been terrorist attacks throughout history. However, since the events of September 11, 2001, the modern world has been a different place because of the threat of terrorism.
- There are many different types of agents and weapons that can be used by terrorists. *CBRNE* is used to remember the different types. *TRACEM-P* is used to remember the types of hazards posed by these agents.
- You must be sure to protect yourself from terrorist attacks as well as secondary attacks that are designed to injure or kill rescuers and further the physical and psychological impact of the attack.

Key Decisions

- Is this a terrorist incident or a potential terrorist incident?
- What type of agent is being used?
- Am I in danger from the initial attack or from secondary attacks?
- How can I best protect myself from danger and hazards?
- How do I fit into the incident response plan for this incident?

Chapter Glossary

contamination contact with or presence of a material (contaminant) that is present where it does not belong and that is somehow harmful to persons, animals, or the environment.

dissemination spreading.

domestic terrorism terrorism directed against one's own government or population. *See also* terrorism; international terrorism.

exposure the dose or concentration of an agent multiplied by the time, or duration.

international terrorism terrorism that is purely foreign-based or -directed. *See also* terrorism; domestic terrorism.

multiple devices destructive devices, such as bombs, including both those used in the initial attack and those placed to be activated after an initial attack and timed to injure emergency responders and others who rush in to help care for those targeted by an initial attack. *See also* secondary devices.

permeation the movement of a substance through a surface or, on a molecular level, through intact materials; penetration, or spreading.

rem roentgen equivalent (in) man; a measure of radiation dosage.

routes of entry pathways into the body, generally by absorption, ingestion, injection, or inhalation.

secondary devices destructive devices, such as bombs, placed to be activated after an initial attack and timed to injure emergency responders and others who rush in to help care for those targeted by an initial attack. *See also* multiple devices.

strategies broad general plans designed to achieve desired outcomes.

tactics specific operational actions to accomplish assigned tasks.

terrorism the unlawful use of force or violence against persons or property to intimidate or coerce a government, the civilian population, or any segment thereof, in furtherance of political or social objectives (FBI definition). *See also* domestic terrorism; international terrorism.

weaponization packaging or producing a material, such as a chemical, biologic, or radiologic agent, so it can be used as a weapon—for example, by dissemination in a bomb detonation, or as an aerosol sprayed over an area or introduced into a ventilation system.

weapons of mass destruction (WMD) weapons, devices, or agents intended to cause widespread harm and/or fear among a population.

zoonotic able to move through the animal–human barrier; transmissible from animals to humans.

Preparation for Your Examination and Practice

Short Answer

1. List and briefly describe the five most common types of terrorism incident.
2. What are multiple devices? What precautions should be taken by an EMT regarding multiple devices?
3. List several types of events that should trigger an EMT's suspicion of possible terrorism involvement.
4. List the seven types of harm that can result from a terrorism incident and the seven-letter acronym for these types of harm.
5. Briefly discuss the concept of time, distance, and shielding.
6. Discuss several self-protection measures for biologic incidents.
7. Discuss the tactics for isolation, notification, identification, and protection.

Thinking and Linking

Think back to the chapter Hazardous Materials, Multiple-Casualty Incidents, and Incident Management, *and link the information on multiple-casualty incidents, HAZMATs, and decontamination from that chapter with information in this chapter as you consider the following situation:*

- Multiple medic units are called to a "possible mass-casualty incident" at the main airport terminal. The first-arriving unit reports that there is a mass exodus of people from the terminal. Many of the patients have some type of fluid with an unusual odor on their clothing. They are clearly contaminated with an unknown substance. What immediate actions should be taken? What protection measures are critical? What decontamination procedures should be implemented?

Critical Thinking Exercises

When responding to a terrorist incident, remember that dangers to the responders may be as great as the dangers for the initial victims of the attack. The purpose of this exercise will be to consider how you might respond to such an incident.

1. You respond to an explosion in a crowded public market. Your supervisor tells you to wait before entering. You see injured people all around and wonder why you aren't allowed in to help. Why would you be held back?
2. You are one of a group of EMTs treating a group of patients that may have been exposed to a nerve agent in a public transportation system. You notice one, then another, of the EMTs you are working with develop an altered mental status. What should you do?
3. You are picking up a friend at the bus station when you notice a man acting suspiciously. The man turns away every time a police officer or employee walks by. He has a large wheeled suitcase, which he pushes into a crowd. Then he runs away. What should you do? What possible terrorist weapons would fit in the suitcase? Which is the more important consideration: the person's physical appearance or the pattern of behavior?

Street Scenes

So far, it's been a slow Wednesday afternoon for your unit, Medic 15. At 14:45, things change. The dispatcher announces, "Medic 15, Engine 11, respond to 5565 Baypoint Boulevard at the Conference Center construction site, worker down from unknown injuries." You and your partner suspect some type of construction injury. One minute later, the dispatcher states, "Medic 15, Engine 11, additional information, two more workers are down; we are now receiving multiple calls."

Your partner reminds you that the Conference Center project was vehemently opposed by the Environmental Life Movement (ELM) because the site was on previously protected wetlands.

On arrival, you are met by the construction manager. He is extremely emotional, and says, "There's guys collapsing all over the place. We noticed a funny smell; then it got hard to breathe."

Street Scene Questions

1. What are the indicators that this may be a suspicious incident?
2. What steps should be taken to isolate the area?
3. What steps should be taken to identify a possible mechanism of injury?
4. Identify the critical personal protection issues on this scene.

You follow your service's HAZMAT and multiple casualty incident procedures and wait in the cold zone while a rescue team with HAZMAT suits and self-contained breathing apparatus brings the construction workers out from the toxic environment, and the decon team conducts decontamination procedures. With proper personal protection in place, you then perform assessment/triage, treatment, and transport.

Officials suspect that the cause of the incident was a deliberate–rather than an accidental–release of a toxic agent, but the exact substance involved and its source are still under investigation. As an EMT on the scene, expect to be interviewed by multiple law enforcement investigators asking you what you observed and what you did during your time at the event.

Street Scenes

At 03:30, your medic unit responds to a "car fire with possible injuries." The dispatcher reminds you that the location is near the headquarters of Stop American Imperialism, an organization that opposes the United States' involvement in the Middle East and other parts of the world. A group called Patriots United is suspected of recently vandalizing the storefront from which Stop American Imperialism operates.

You and Engine 15 simultaneously arrive. There is a car on fire in a dead-end alley. You can't see a patient or a bystander, so you stand by while the engine pulls a line into the alley. Suddenly the engine crew stops and retreats. The lieutenant states, "We see some type of wire stretched across the alley!"

Street Scene Questions

1. What are the indicators that this is a suspicious incident?
2. What protection precautions should be initiated–and by whom?
3. Discuss the proper notification procedures. What support agencies are required on this scene?

The incident turns out to be not a simple car fire or collision but, instead, a bombing. The alley where the car was bombed runs directly behind the Stop American Imperialism storefront, and the bombed-out car is registered to one of that organization's leaders. Neither he nor anyone else was in the car when it was bombed, so officials believe the bombing was intended to lure emergency responders to the scene, where they would be killed or injured by the secondary device, a trip-wired booby trap. Investigators are following various clues at the scene, including components of the bomb device, to track down the perpetrators.

Appendix A

Basic Cardiac Life Support Review

Some EMT students learned cardiopulmonary resuscitation (CPR) before they began their EMT courses. Others learn it in their EMT courses. This section reviews the elements of CPR in accordance with the American Heart Association's *2015 Guidelines for Cardiopulmonary Resuscitation and Emergency Cardiovascular Care*.

Before Beginning Resuscitation

When a patient's breathing and heartbeat stop, *clinical death* occurs. This condition may be reversible through CPR and other treatments. However, when the brain cells die, *biological death* occurs. This usually happens within 10 minutes of clinical death, and it is not reversible. In fact, brain cells will begin to die after 4 to 6 minutes without fresh oxygen supplied from air breathed in and carried to the brain by circulating blood. *Cardiopulmonary resuscitation (CPR)* consists of the actions you take to revive a person–or at least temporarily prevent biological death–by keeping the person's heart and lungs working.

Although you may perform CPR alone for a short period, at some point you will work with other EMS and health care providers. An essential element of success in any resuscitation effort is *teamwork*. Rescuers perform many tasks during a resuscitation effort, and to be successful, they must work together in a coordinated, organized, and efficient manner. Many of these tasks are time sensitive and quite specific in how they must be performed, so working together is vital. This is especially true because many things happen simultaneously when the resuscitation effort is proceeding well. A team leader must be knowledgeable about resuscitation techniques, skilled in patient assessment, and clear in his or her directions to the team. Communication among members of the team must be accurate and timely to give the patient the best chance of revival.

Another element of successful resuscitation efforts is the ability to tailor the approach to the patient based on the circumstances. A patient who was submerged under water will receive the same general sequence of assessment steps as a patient who suddenly collapsed at home, but the specifics of treatment may be quite different. A good team adapts its approach to the apparent cause of a cardiac arrest. Table A-1 lists the initial steps in basic life support resuscitation, including assessing the patient, activating EMS, positioning the patient, and ensuring an open airway.

Assessing the Patient

Patient assessment is crucial. Initiate resuscitation after determining that the patient needs it. The required assessments are often described as determining unresponsiveness, breathlessness, and pulselessness–or the ABCs (airway, breathing, and circulation). As Table A-1 shows, these categories overlap, and treatment might not occur in A-B-C sequence. For example, a patient in cardiac arrest should receive chest compressions before rescue breaths (i.e., C-A-B sequence).

Determining Unresponsiveness

When you encounter a patient who has collapsed, your first action is to determine unresponsiveness. Tap or gently shake the patient (being careful not to move a patient with possible spinal injury) and shout, "Are you OK?" The patient who is able to respond does not require cardiopulmonary resuscitation.

If the adult patient is unresponsive, immediately activate EMS unless the patient's condition is likely caused by a problem other than heart disease (e.g., submersion, injury, or drug overdose). If the patient is a child or an infant, activate EMS after 2 minutes of resuscitation unless you have reason to think the patient's condition is caused by heart disease.

Determining Breathlessness

The American Heart Association no longer recommends a separate step of "look, listen, and feel" for breathing. This takes time that delays compressions. Make a quick scan of the patient for signs of life or breathing (e.g., purposeful moving, chest wall movement). At the same time, check the pulse. You will still be able to look for signs of breathing while you are checking the pulse. The patient who is breathing adequately does not require resuscitation. Gasps are not effective breaths.

If the patient is not breathing but definitely has a pulse, provide two ventilations (as explained later).

Determining Pulselessness

At the same time that you evaluate breathing, determine pulselessness by feeling for the carotid artery in an adult or a child or the brachial artery in an infant. The adult patient who has a pulse does not require chest compressions. If an infant or child has a pulse slower than 60 beats per minute, begin CPR (ventilations and chest compressions).

If the patient has a pulse but is not breathing, provide rescue breathing (artificial ventilations). Even experienced providers sometimes have difficulty evaluating the presence of a pulse, so unless you definitely feel a pulse in the adult patient, begin chest compressions.

Assessing in A-B-C or C-A-B Sequence

Assessments of the ABCs are included in the steps just described. Keep the ABCs in mind throughout every patient encounter, whether or not resuscitation is under way. If the answer to any of the ABC questions that follow is no, take the appropriate steps to correct the situation.

Is the patient's *airway* open?

Is the patient *breathing*?

Does the patient have *circulation* of blood (a pulse)?

TABLE A-1 Basic Life Support Steps

ASSESSMENT	SPECIAL CONSIDERATIONS
• As you approach the patient, observe for signs of life: rise and fall of the chest, moaning, wheezing, coughing, or other sounds or movements.	• If the patient has signs of life, proceed in **A-B-C sequence**. Open the **Airway** with the head-tilt, chin-lift method; then evaluate **Breathing** and **Circulation**.
• When you reach the patient, assess for unresponsiveness by tapping the patient on the shoulder and shouting.	• Consider whether the patient may have a spine injury and require the jaw-thrust method.
• Palpate the carotid pulse at the same time that you put your head close to the patient's mouth to observe more closely for chest movement and listen for sounds of breathing.	• In an infant, check the brachial pulse.
MANAGEMENT	**SPECIAL CONSIDERATIONS**
• For adults, if there are no signs of life and no pulse (or questionable pulse), activate the emergency response system if not already done and, if there is no AED available, proceed in **C-A-B sequence**. Administer 30 **Chest compressions**.	• Tailor your actions to the cause of the patient's condition and the resources available. If there is reason to believe the patient arrested because of a respiratory problem (e.g., drowning or overdose), make ventilations a higher priority. If more than one rescuer is available, work in a coordinated fashion to perform actions simultaneously or as efficiently as possible.
• Open the **Airway** with the head-tilt, chin-lift method, and restore **Breathing** by giving two ventilations. • If a child or infant has a pulse but it is less than 60, begin ventilations and compressions.	• Children and infants usually arrest because of respiratory, not cardiac, problems. • If the patient may have a spine injury, use the jaw-thrust method.
• Repeat the cycle of 30:2 compressions to ventilations.	• If the patient may have a spine injury, use the jaw-thrust method. • If a pulse is present but breathing is absent or abnormal, ventilate the patient at the rate appropriate for the patient's age.

Keep in mind that the proper treatment will not necessarily occur in A-B-C order. If the patient appears lifeless and has no pulse, the above steps should be performed in C-A-B order with chest compressions performed before rescue ventilations.

Activating EMS

If you have assistance, the other person should call 911 or otherwise activate the EMS system as soon as a patient collapses or is discovered in collapse. The quicker a defibrillator can reach the patient, the greater the patient's chances of survival.

If you are alone, you will have to determine whether to activate EMS immediately or to initiate 2 minutes of resuscitation before EMS activation. In most cases, 2 minutes of resuscitation before activating EMS is recommended for children and infants, but immediate activation of EMS is recommended for adults. However, there are some instances mentioned below that indicate a different approach.

With an adult, first determine unresponsiveness, pulse, and breathing (as described earlier), and activate EMS before returning to the patient to initiate the next steps. Cardiac arrest in an adult is likely to be the result of a disturbance of the heart's electrical activity that will require defibrillation, so getting defibrillation equipment to the patient takes precedence over starting CPR. When cardiac arrest is probably not the result of a disturbance of the heart's electrical activity, however (e.g., submersion, injury, or drug overdose), it is more important to perform rescue breathing, so you would perform CPR briefly before activating EMS.

If the patient is a child or an infant, perform 2 minutes of resuscitation before activating EMS. Children and infants generally have healthy hearts, and cardiac arrest in these patients is likely to have resulted from respiratory arrest. In this situation, rescue breathing is more likely to be helpful, and defibrillation are less likely to help. If the child has heart disease, however, cardiac arrest is more like that of an adult. In this instance, calling for a defibrillator is more important than performing rescue breathing.

So generally, for children and infants, perform 2 minutes of resuscitation before activating EMS, and for adults activate EMS before performing rescue breathing.

Positioning the Patient

When you have determined that the patient is unresponsive and have activated EMS, then do what you can to position the patient in a supine position (on the back). This may require helping the patient onto the floor or stretcher or onto his or her back if the patient was found in another position. If you have reason to suspect that the patient was injured, you or a helper must support the neck and hold the patient's head still and in line with the spine while you are moving, assessing, and providing care for the patient.

Opening the Airway

Most airway problems are caused by the tongue. As the head tips forward, the tongue may slide into the airway, especially when the patient is lying on his or her back. When the patient is unconscious, the risk of airway problems is worsened because unconsciousness causes the tongue to lose muscle tone and the muscles of the lower jaw (to which the tongue is attached) to relax.

Two procedures can help to correct the position of the tongue and thus open the airway. These procedures are the head-tilt, chin-lift maneuver and the jaw-thrust maneuver.

Head-Tilt, Chin-Lift Maneuver

The head-tilt, chin-lift maneuver (Figure A-1) provides for maximum opening of the airway. It is useful on all patients who need assistance in maintaining an airway or breathing. It is one of the best methods for correcting obstructions caused by the tongue. However, since it involves changing the position of the head, the head-tilt, chin-lift maneuver should only be used on a patient whom you can be quite sure has not suffered a spinal injury.

Follow these steps to perform the head-tilt, chin-lift maneuver:

1. Once the patient is supine, place one forehead, on the forehead and the fingertips of the other hand under the bony area at the center of the patient's lower jaw.
2. Tilt the head by applying gentle pressure to the patient's forehead.
3. Use your fingertips to lift the chin and support the lower jaw. Move the jaw forward to a point where the lower teeth are almost touching the upper teeth. Do not compress the soft tissues under the lower jaw, which can press and close off the airway.
4. Do not allow the patient's mouth to close. To provide an adequate opening at the mouth, you may need to use the thumb of the hand supporting the chin to pull back the patient's lower lip. For your own safety (to prevent being bitten), do not insert your thumb into the patient's mouth.

Jaw-Thrust Maneuver

The jaw-thrust maneuver (Figure A-2) is most commonly used to open the airway of an unconscious patient or one with suspected head, neck, or spinal injuries.

Follow these steps to perform the jaw-thrust maneuver:

1. Carefully keep the patient's head, neck, and spine aligned, moving the patient as a unit into the supine position.
2. Kneel at the top of the patient's head. For greater comfort, you might rest your elbows on the same surface the patient is lying on.
3. Reach forward and gently place one hand on each side of the patient's lower jaw, at the angles of the jaw below the ears.
4. You can help to stabilize the patient's head by using your wrists or forearms.
5. Using your index fingers, push the angles of the patient's lower jaw forward.
6. You may need to retract the patient's lower lip with your thumb to keep the mouth open.
7. Do not tilt or rotate the patient's head. *Remember: The purpose of the jaw-thrust maneuver is to open the airway without moving the head or neck.*

NOTE: *The jaw-thrust maneuver is the only widely recommended procedure for use on patients with possible head, neck, or spinal injuries.*

FIGURE A-1 The head-tilt, chin-lift maneuver, side view. Inset photo shows EMT's fingertips under the bony area at the center of patient's lower jaw.

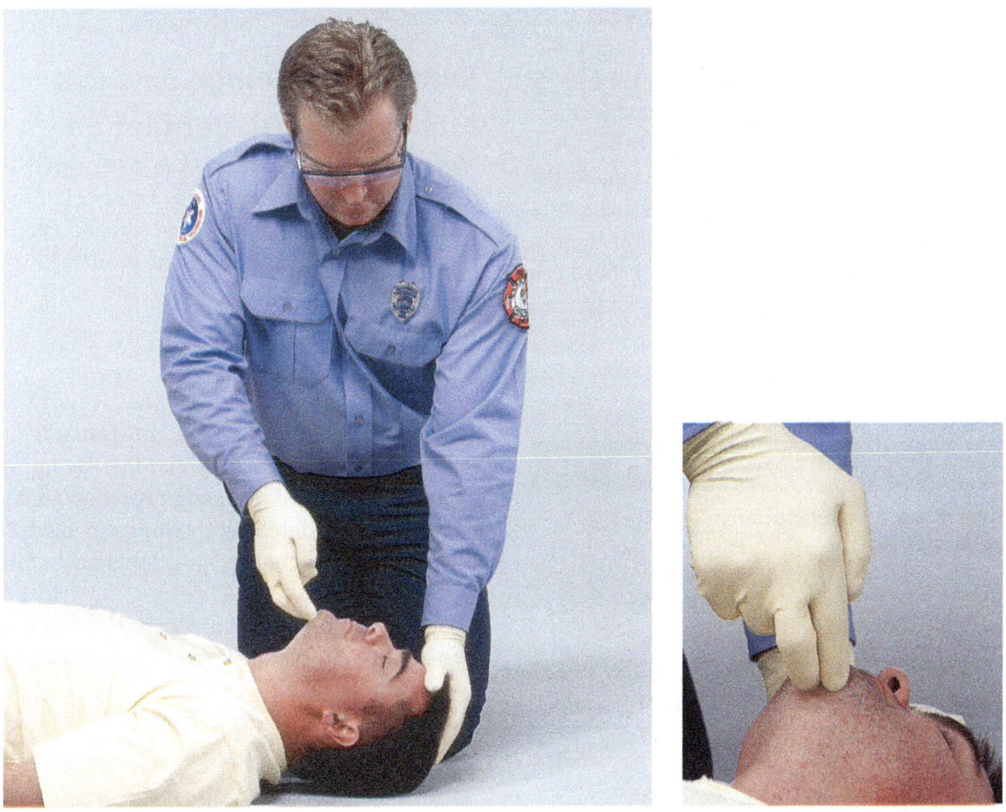

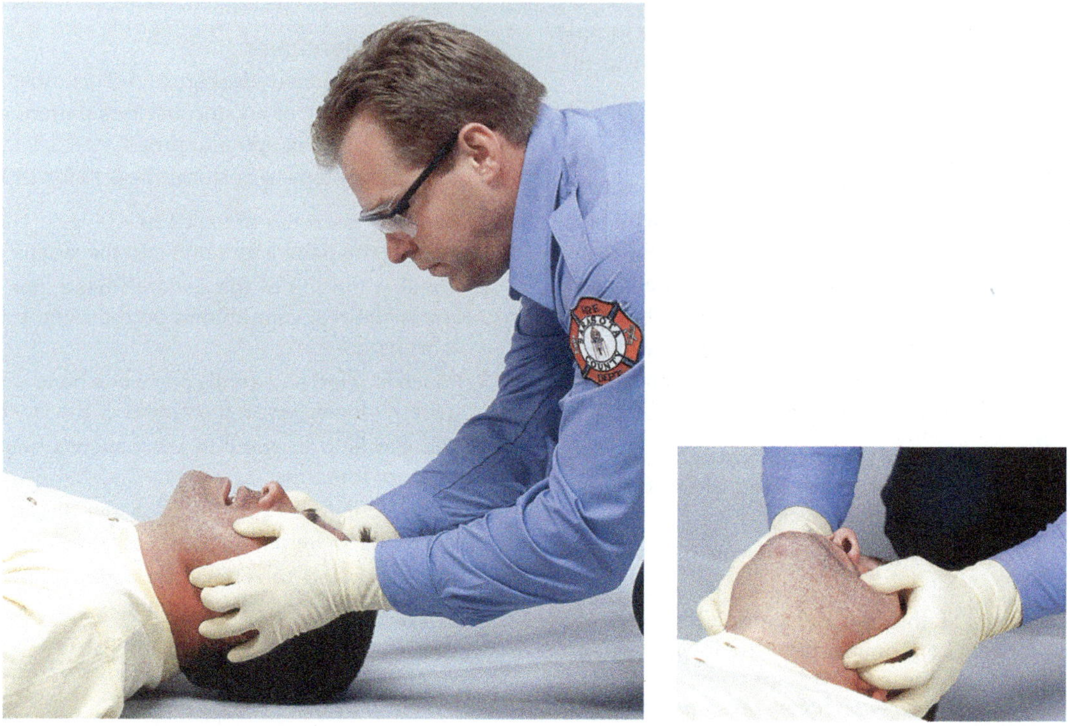

FIGURE A-2 The jaw-thrust maneuver, side view. Inset photo shows EMT's finger position at angle of jaw, just below the ears.

Initial Ventilations and Pulse Check

The reason most apneic (nonbreathing) adults are not breathing is that the heart stopped. You will see very few adults with a pulse but with no breathing. Oxygen is often still in the patient's bloodstream. Since this is so common, you should start CPR with chest compressions, not ventilations, under ordinary circumstances. When the cause of the cardiac arrest is respiratory in nature, it may be reasonable to take a different approach and start with ventilations. In this case, deliver 2 breaths, each delivered over 1 second and of sufficient volume to make the chest rise (Table A-2). If the first breath is unsuccessful, reposition the patient's head before attempting the second breath. If the second ventilation is unsuccessful, assume that there is a foreign-body airway obstruction and perform airway clearance techniques (as described later).

TABLE A-2 Rescue Breathing

	ADULT	CHILD	INFANT
Age	Puberty and older	1 yr-puberty	Birth-1 yr
Ventilation duration	1 sec	1 sec	1 sec
Ventilation rate	10-12 breaths/min	12-20 breaths/min	12-20 breaths/min

If initial ventilations are successful, you have confirmed an open airway. If the patient has no pulse, begin chest compressions with ventilations (as described later under "CPR"). If the patient has a pulse but breathing is absent or inadequate, perform rescue breathing.

Rescue Breathing

Mouth-to-Mask Ventilation

Mouth-to-mask ventilation is performed using a pocket face mask with a one-way valve. The pocket face mask is made of soft, collapsible material and can be carried in your pocket, jacket, or purse. The steps of mouth-to-mask ventilation are illustrated in Scan A-1.

Gastric Distention

Rescue breathing can force some air into the patient's stomach, causing the stomach to become distended. This may indicate that the airway is blocked, that there is improper head position, or that the ventilations being provided are too large or too quick to be accommodated by the lungs or the trachea. This problem is seen more frequently in infants and children but can occur with any patient.

A slight bulge is of little worry, but major distention can cause two serious problems. First, the air-filled stomach reduces lung volume by forcing the diaphragm upward. Second, regurgitation (the passive expulsion of fluids and partially digested

SCAN A-1 Mouth-To-Mask Ventilation

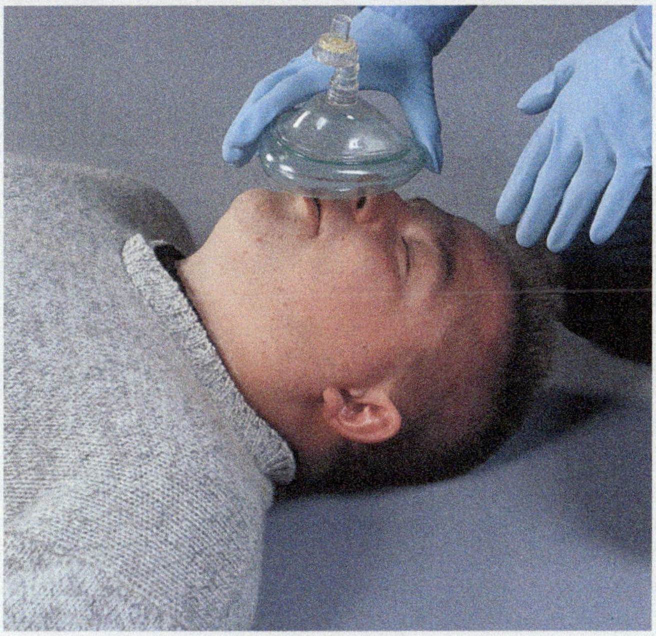

1. Position the patient and prepare to place the mask.

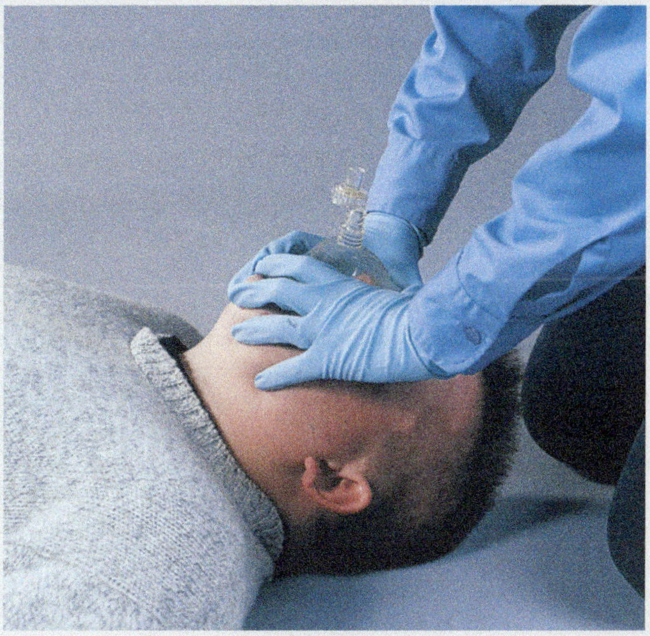

2. Seat the mask firmly on the patient's face.

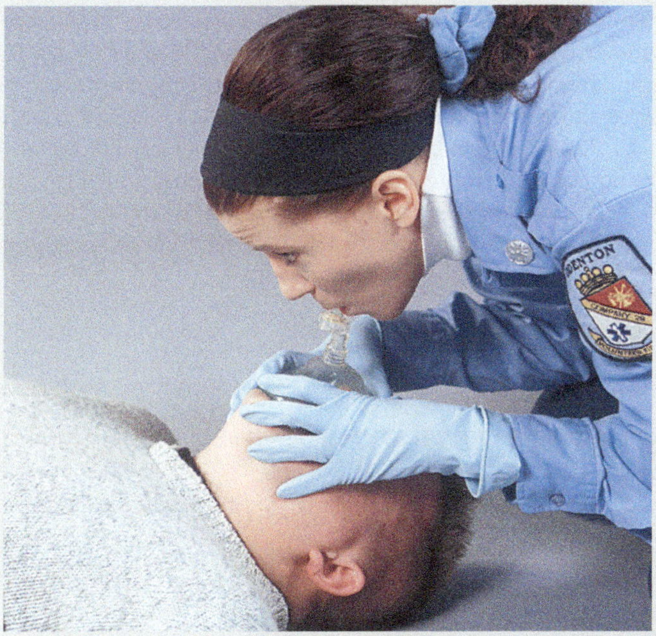

3. Open the patient's airway, and watch the chest rise as you ventilate through the one-way valve.

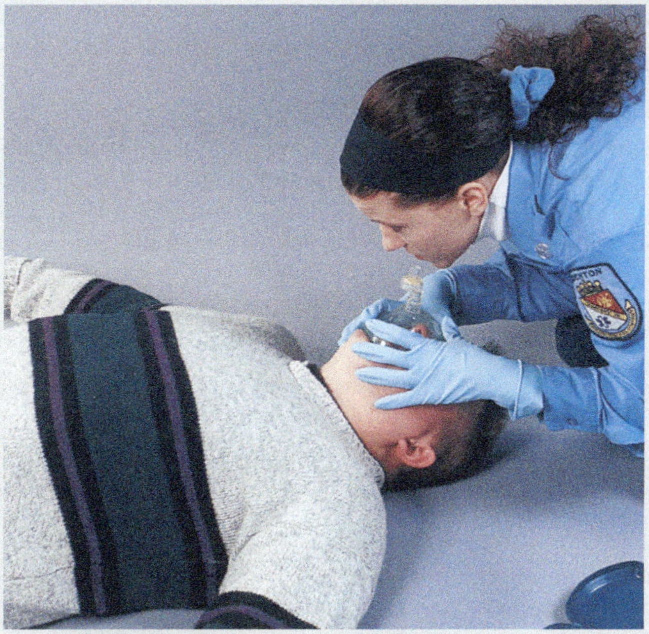

4. Watch the patient's chest fall during exhalation. Ventilate the adult patient 10–12 times a minute and a child or infant 12–20 times a minute. If the pocket mask has an oxygen inlet, provide supplemental oxygen.

foods from the stomach into the throat) or vomiting (the forceful expulsion of the stomach's contents) is a strong possibility. This could lead to additional airway obstruction or aspiration of vomitus into the patient's lungs. When this happens, lung damage can occur and a lethal form of pneumonia may develop.

The best way to avoid gastric distention, or to avoid making it worse once it develops, is to position the patient's head properly, to avoid ventilations that are too forceful and too quickly delivered, and to limit the volume of ventilations delivered. The volume delivered should be limited to the size breath that causes the chest to rise. This is why it is so important to watch the patient's chest rise as each ventilation is delivered and to feel for resistance to your breaths.

When gastric distention is present, be prepared for vomiting. If the patient does vomit, roll the entire patient onto one side. (Turning just the head may allow for aspiration of vomitus as well as aggravation of any possible neck injury.) Manually stabilize the head and neck as you roll the patient. Be prepared to clear the patient's mouth and throat of vomitus with gauze and gloved fingers. Apply suction if you are trained and equipped to do so.

Recovery Position

Patients who resume adequate breathing and pulse after rescue breathing or CPR and who do not require immobilization for possible spinal injury are placed in the recovery position. The recovery position allows for drainage from the mouth and prevents the tongue from falling backward and causing an airway obstruction.

The patient should be rolled onto one side. This should be done moving the patient as a unit, not twisting the head, shoulders, or torso. The patient may be rolled onto either side; however, it is preferable to have the patient facing you so monitoring and suctioning may be more easily performed.

If the patient does not have sufficient respirations to support life, the recovery position must not be used. Place the patient supine and assist ventilations.

CPR

Checking for Circulation

Before beginning CPR, you should confirm that the patient is pulseless. In an adult or child (not an infant), check the carotid pulse (Figure A-3). While stabilizing the patient's head and maintaining the proper head tilt, use your hand that is closer to the patient's neck to locate the "Adam's apple" (the prominent bulge in the front of the neck). Place the tips of your index and middle fingers directly over the midline of this structure. Slide your fingertips to the side of the patient's neck closer to you. Keep the palm side of your fingertips against the patient's neck. Feel for a groove between the Adam's apple and the muscles located along the side of the neck. Very little pressure needs to be applied to the neck to feel the carotid pulse. Keep in mind that laypeople are taught not to check for a pulse but to look for signs of circulation: normal breathing, coughing, or movement. In an infant, check for a brachial pulse (Figure A-4). If the adult patient is pulseless, begin CPR. If an infant or child has a pulse slower than 60 beats per minute, begin CPR (ventilations and chest compressions).

To provide chest compressions, place the patient supine on a hard surface and compress the chest by applying downward pressure with your hands. This action causes an increase of pressure inside the chest and possible actual compression of the heart itself, one or both of which force the blood out of the heart and into circulation. When pressure is released, the heart refills with blood. The next compression sends this fresh blood into circulation, and the cycle continues.

How to Perform CPR

CPR is a method of artificial breathing and circulation. When natural heart action and breathing have stopped, you must provide an artificial means to oxygenate the blood and keep it in circulation. This is accomplished by providing chest compressions and ventilations.

CPR can be done by one or by two rescuers. All of the information under "Providing Chest Compressions" and "Providing Ventilations" applies to both one-rescuer and two-rescuer CPR. Specific information about each type of CPR follows under

FIGURE A-3 Check the carotid pulse to confirm circulation.

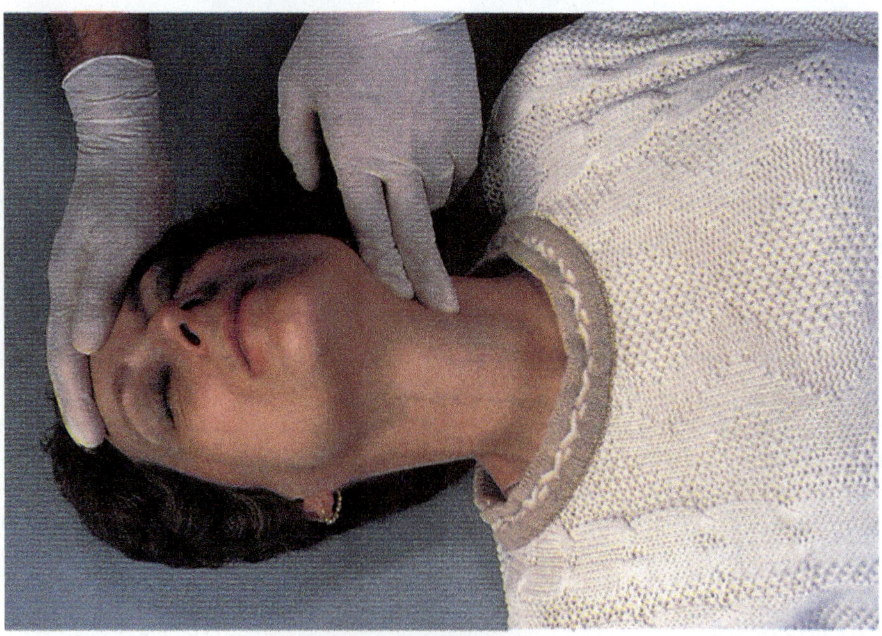

FIGURE A-4 For infants, determine circulation by feeling for a brachial pulse. *(© Daniel Limmer)*

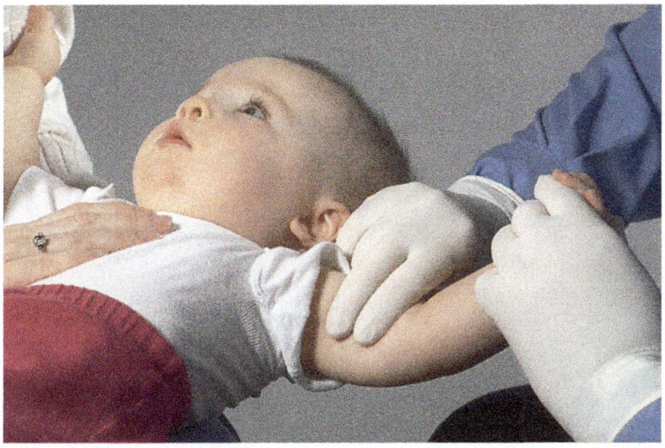

"One-Rescuer and Two-Rescuer CPR." Scan A-2 and Scan A-3 can help you follow and review these procedures as they are described below. These procedures are for an adult patient. Procedures for infants and children will be described later.

NOTE: *Do not initiate CPR on any adult who has a pulse.*

Providing Chest Compressions

After you have placed the patient supine on a hard surface and your hands are properly positioned on the CPR compression site:

1. Place the heel of your hand on the sternum between the nipples. Put your other hand on top of the first with your fingers interlaced. Straighten your arms and lock your elbows. You must not bend the elbows when delivering or releasing compressions.
2. Make certain that your shoulders are directly over your hands (directly over the patient's sternum). This will allow you to deliver compressions straight down onto the site. Keep both of your knees on the ground or floor.
3. Deliver compressions STRAIGHT DOWN with enough force to depress the sternum of a typical adult 2 to 2.4 inches (5-6 cm).
4. Fully release pressure on the patient's sternum, but *do not* bend your elbows and *do not* lift your hands from the sternum, which can cause you to lose correct positioning of your hands. Your movement should be from your hips. Compressions should be delivered in a rhythmic, not a "jabbing," fashion. *The amount of time you spend compressing should be the same as the time for the release*. This is known as the 50:50 rule: 50 percent compression, 50 percent release.

Providing Ventilations

Ventilations are given between sets of compressions. The mouth-to-mask techniques described earlier for rescue breathing are used.

One-Rescuer and Two-Rescuer CPR

Scan A-3 shows the techniques of one-rescuer CPR and two-rescuer CPR for the adult patient and describes compression rates and ratios for CPR on adults, children, and infants. The AHA recommends using a BVM for two-rescuer BLS.

CPR Techniques for Children and Infants

The techniques of CPR for children and infants are essentially the same as those used for adults. However, some procedures and rates differ when the patient is a child or an infant. (If younger than 1 year of age, the patient is considered an infant. Between 1 year and puberty, the patient is considered a child. Past the age of puberty, adult procedures apply to the patient. Keep in mind that the size of the patient can also be an important factor. A very small 10-year-old who has reached puberty may have to be treated as a child.)

SCAN A-2 Locating the CPR Compression Site

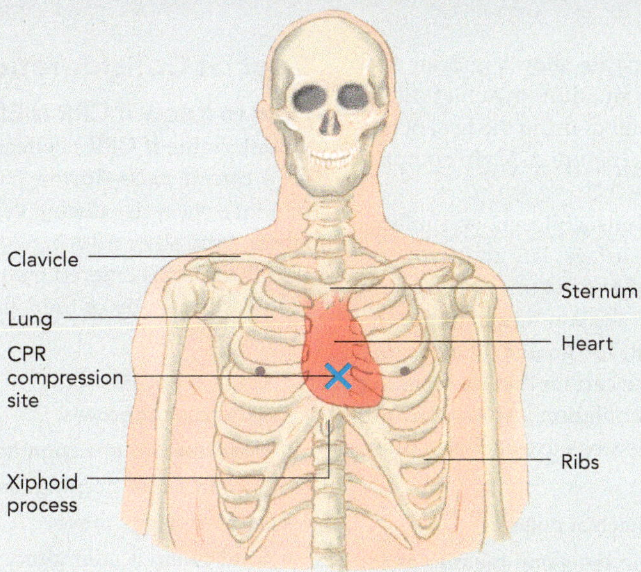

The compression site for CPR is on the sternum midway between the nipples. The preferred method for trained health care providers is outlined in steps 1 to 4 under "Providing Chest Compressions."

SCAN A-3 CPR Summary–Adult Patient

ONE RESCUER	FUNCTIONS	TWO RESCUERS
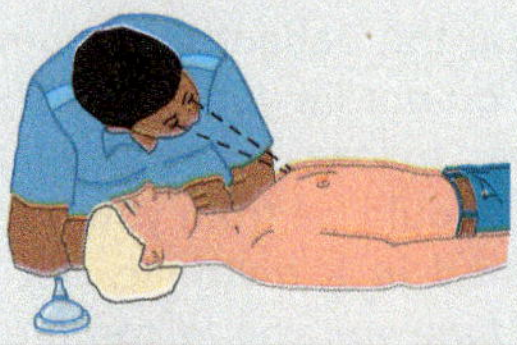	• Establish unresponsiveness • Position patient • If there's no response, call 911 • Call for an AED	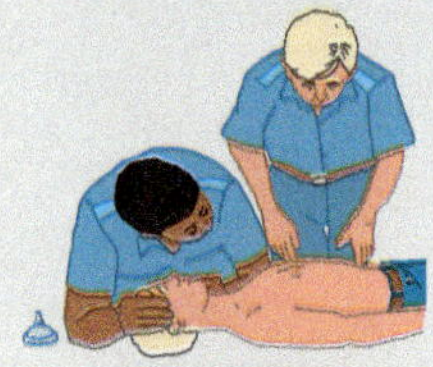
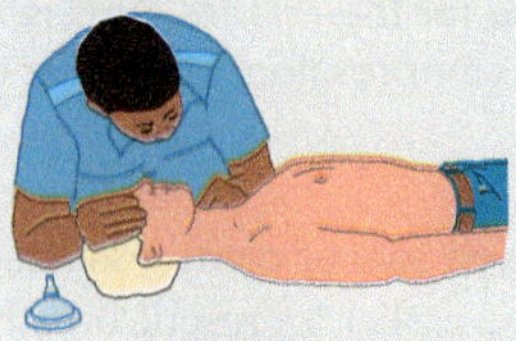	• Check carotid pulse and breathing . . . (5–10 seconds) If no pulse . . . • Begin chest compressions	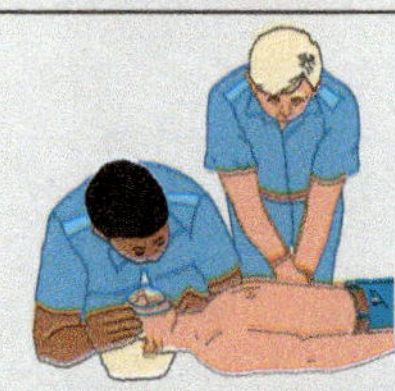
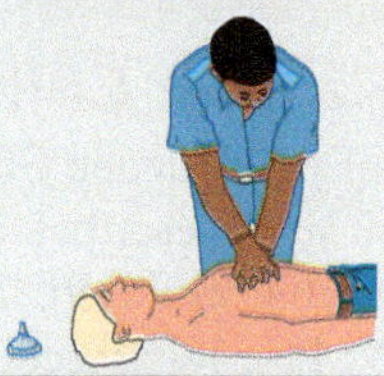	**DELIVER COMPRESSIONS** 2–2.4 inches (5–6 cm) 100–120/min	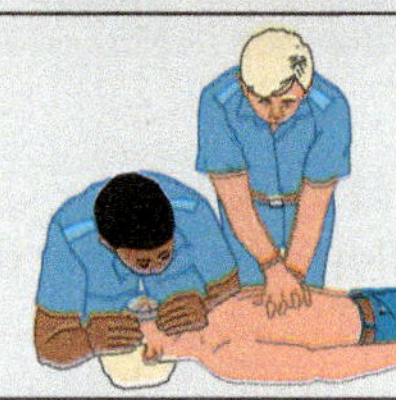
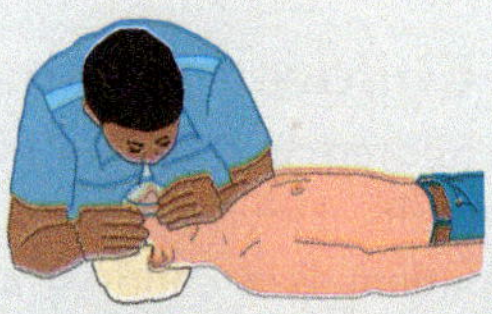	**DELIVER VENTILATIONS** Compression ventilation ratio 30:2	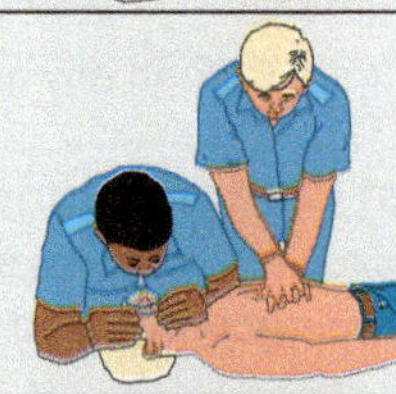
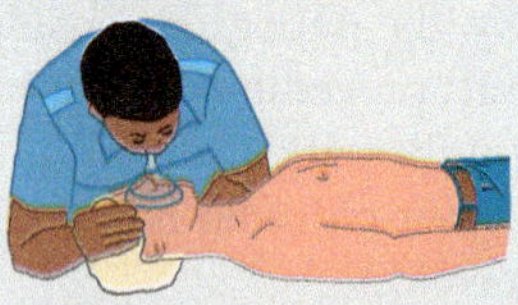	• Continue compressions and ventilations • Limit pulse checks • Switch every 5 cycles to prevent fatigue **CONTINUE PERIODIC ASSESSMENT**	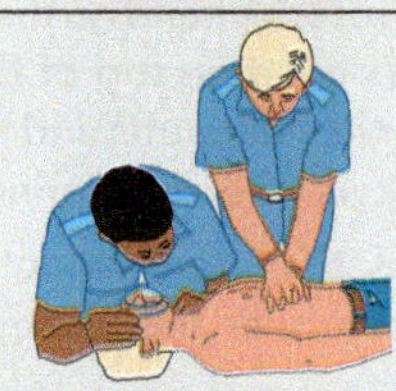

NOTE: Wear gloves and use either a pocket mask with one-way valve or bag–valve mask

The techniques of CPR for an infant are shown in Scan A-4. For a child, CPR is conducted as for an adult, the chief difference in procedure being the hand position–using the heel of one or two hands–for chest compressions (Figure A-5). To compare adult, child, and infant CPR, see Table A-3.

When CPR must be performed, adults, children, and infants are placed on their backs on a hard surface. For an infant, the hard surface can be the rescuer's hand or forearm. For an infant or a child, use the head-tilt, chin-lift or the jaw-thrust maneuver, but apply only a slight tilt for an infant. Too great a tilt may close off the infant's airway; however, make certain that the opening is adequate. (Note chest rise during ventilation.) Always be sure to support an infant's head. Take these steps to establish a pulse in an infant or a child:

- *For an infant*, you should use the brachial pulse.
- *For a child*, determine circulation in the same manner as for an adult.

Special Considerations in CPR

How to Know if CPR Is Effective

To determine if CPR is effective, *if possible have someone else feel for a carotid pulse* during compressions and watch to see the patient's chest rise during ventilations. *Listen for exhalation of air*, either naturally or during compressions, as additional verification that air has entered the lungs.

In addition, any of the following indications of effective CPR may be noticed:

- Pupils constrict.
- Skin color improves.
- Heartbeat returns spontaneously.
- Spontaneous, gasping respirations are made.
- Arms and legs move.
- Swallowing is attempted.
- Consciousness returns.

SCAN A-4 Infant CPR

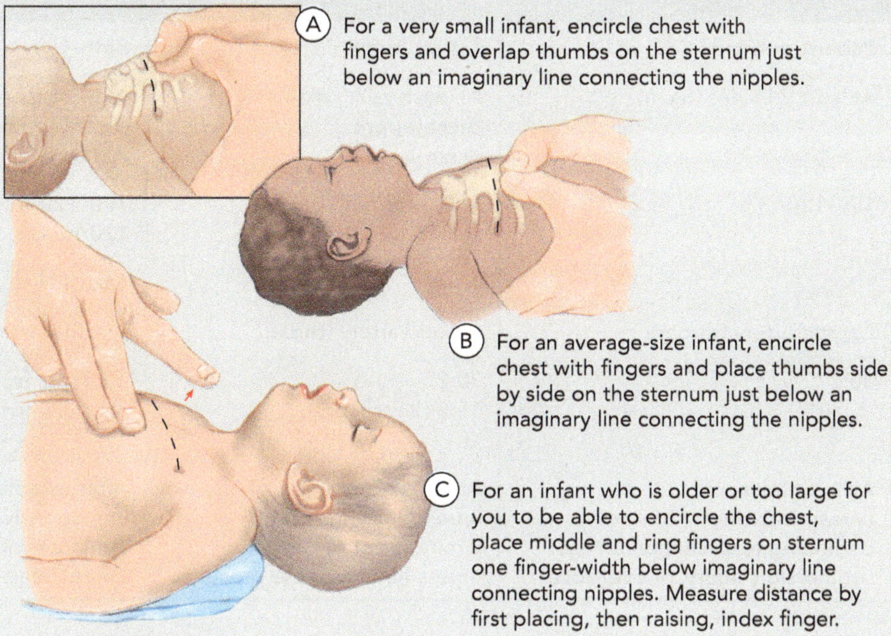

Position fingers for chest compressions according to the age and size of the infant. The two-thumbs-encircling-hands method is preferred when two rescuers are present.

FIGURE A-5 Performing chest compressions on a child.

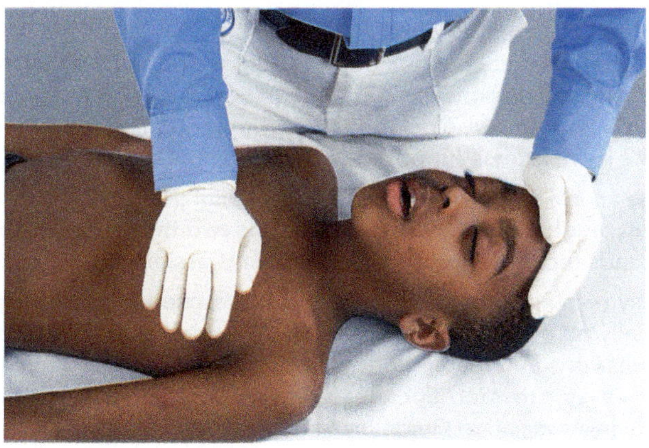

Interrupting CPR

Once you begin CPR, you may interrupt the process for no more than 10 seconds to check for pulse and breathing or to reposition yourself and the patient.

In addition to these built-in interruptions, you may interrupt CPR to:

- Move a patient onto a stretcher.
- Move a patient down a flight of stairs or through a narrow doorway or hallway.
- Move a patient into or out of the ambulance.
- Suction to clear vomitus or airway obstructions.
- Allow for defibrillation or advanced cardiac life support measures to be initiated.
- Assess the patient for signs of life when taking over CPR from someone else.
- Switch positions to minimize fatigue. (When practical, no one on the team should compress the chest for more than 2 minutes at a time. Compressing the chest is very tiring, and rescuers are poor judges of when their compressions are no longer deep enough or fast enough.)

Whenever you must interrupt compressions, it is very important that you do it quickly to minimize the amount of time during which the patient is not circulating blood. When CPR is resumed, begin with chest compressions rather than with ventilations.

When Not to Begin or to Terminate CPR

As discussed earlier, CPR should not be initiated when you find that the patient–even though unresponsive and perhaps not breathing–does have a pulse. Usually, of course, you will perform CPR when the patient has no pulse. *However, there are special circumstances in which CPR should not be initiated even though the patient has no pulse:*

- **Obvious mortal wounds.** These include decapitation, incineration, a severed body, and injuries that are so extensive that CPR cannot be effectively performed (e.g., severe crush injuries to the head, neck, and chest).
- **Rigor mortis.** This is the stiffening of the body and its limbs that occurs after death, usually within 4–10 hours.

TABLE A-3 CPR for Adults, Children, and Infants

	ADULT	CHILD	INFANT
Age	Puberty and older	1 yr-puberty	Birth-1 yr
Compression depth	At least 2 inches (5 cm)	At least 1/3 AP diameter of chest (approximately 2 inches [5 cm])	At least 1/3 AP diameter of chest (approximately 1 1/2 inches [4 cm])
Compression rate	100-120/min	100-120/min	100-120/min (newborn 120/min)
Each ventilation	1 sec	1 sec	1 sec
Pulse check location	Carotid artery (throat)	Carotid artery (throat)	Brachial artery (upper arm)
One-rescuer CPR compressions-to-ventilations ratio	30:2	30:2 15:2 (2 rescuers)	30:2 (alone) 15:2 (2 rescuers) 3:1 (newborn)
When working alone: Call 911 or emergency dispatcher	After establishing unresponsiveness–before beginning resuscitation unless submersion, injury, or overdose	After establishing unresponsiveness and 2 minutes of resuscitation unless heart disease present	After establishing unresponsiveness and 2 minutes of resuscitation unless heart disease present

- **Obvious decomposition.**
- **A line of lividity.** Lividity is a red or purple skin discoloration that occurs when gravity causes the blood to sink to the lowest parts of the body and collect there. Lividity usually indicates that the patient has been dead for more than 15 minutes unless the patient has been exposed to cold temperatures. Using lividity as a sign requires special training.
- **Stillbirth.** CPR should not be initiated for a stillborn infant who has died hours prior to birth. This infant may be recognized by blisters on the skin, a very soft head, and a strong disagreeable odor.
- **Valid advance directive or Do Not Resuscitate (DNR) order.**

In all cases, if you are in doubt, seek a physician's advice. Once you have started CPR, you must continue to provide CPR until:

- Spontaneous circulation occurs. (Then provide rescue breathing as needed.)
- Spontaneous circulation and breathing occur.
- Another trained rescuer can take over for you.
- You turn care of the patient over to a person with a higher level of training.
- You are too exhausted to continue.
- You receive a "no CPR" order from a physician or other authority per local protocols.
- There are three criteria that have been extremely accurate in determining when it is reasonable to stop CPR without missing anyone who has a chance of survival:
    1. The arrest was not witnessed by EMS personnel or first responders.
    2. There has been no return of spontaneous circulation (patient regains a pulse) after three rounds of CPR and rhythm checks with an automated external defibrillator (AED).
    3. The AED did not detect a shockable rhythm and did not deliver any shocks.

If you turn the patient over to another rescuer, this person must be trained in basic cardiac life support.

The Trained Health Care Provider versus the Lay Provider

As an EMT, you will be regarded as a "trained health care provider" with regard to CPR. The training you receive is more in-depth than a lay rescuer or bystander might receive. The course for people who wish to learn CPR and have no medical background differs from the training an EMT receives in the following ways:

- Lay rescuers are not trained to check for a pulse before beginning compressions in CPR. If the patient is not breathing and does not otherwise respond (breathing, cough, or movement), the lay rescuer is supposed to begin compressions.
- As an EMT, you will be taught additional techniques that are not taught to lay rescuers, such as the two-thumbs-encircling-hands technique for two-rescuer compression in infants.
- Lay rescuers may be reluctant to do rescue breathing, especially on a stranger. Also, coordinating and timing both compressions and respirations is likely to be beyond the abilities of a lay provider. For these reasons, the current American Heart Association Guidelines recommend that the lay rescuer perform compressions without respirations.

It is possible for you to come upon a bystander performing CPR and see some of these differences in practice. If you ask the bystander, "Does the patient have a pulse?" the bystander might not have checked (and in fact was not required to do so).

Remember that performing CPR is quite stressful for the layperson or bystander. In many cases CPR will be performed by a member of the patient's family. It is important to be supportive and use a nonjudgmental tone about the efforts undertaken by the layperson or bystander.

Clearing Airway Obstructions

Not every airway problem is caused by the tongue (the situation in which you would use the head-tilt, chin-lift maneuver or the jaw-thrust maneuver, described earlier, to open the airway). The airway can also be blocked by foreign objects or materials.

These can include pieces of food, ice, toys, or vomitus. This problem is often seen with children and with patients who have abused alcohol or other drugs. It also happens when an injured person's airway becomes blocked by blood or broken teeth or dentures.

Airway obstructions are either partial or complete. Partial and complete obstructions have different characteristics that may be noted during assessment, and each type has a different procedure of care. It is important to understand the differences between partial and complete obstructions and the correct care for each.

Mild Airway Obstruction

Conscious patients trying to indicate airway problems will usually point to their mouth or hold their neck. Many do this even when a partial obstruction does not prevent speech. Ask patients if they are choking, or ask if they can speak or cough. If they can, then the obstruction is mild.

Ask the conscious patient with an apparent mild airway obstruction to cough. A strong and forceful cough indicates enough air is being exchanged. Continue to encourage the patient to cough in the hope that such action will dislodge and expel the foreign object. *Do not* interfere with the patient's efforts to clear the obstruction by means of forceful coughing.

In cases where the patient has an apparent mild airway obstruction but cannot cough, or has a very weak cough where the patient is blue or gray or shows other signs of poor air exchange, treat the patient as if there were a severe airway obstruction, as described below.

Severe Airway Obstruction

Be alert for signs of a severe airway obstruction in the conscious or unconscious patient:

- *The conscious patient* with a severe airway obstruction will try to speak but will not be able to. This patient will also not be able to breathe or cough, and sometimes will display the distress signal for choking by clutching the neck between thumb and fingers.
- *The unconscious patient* with a severe airway obstruction will be in respiratory arrest. When ventilation attempts are unsuccessful, it becomes apparent that there is an obstruction.

Abdominal Thrusts

The use of abdominal thrusts to clear a foreign body from the airway of an adult or child (not an infant) patient is performed as follows:

For the conscious adult or child (not an infant) who is standing or sitting

1. Make a fist and place the thumb side of this fist against the midline of the patient's abdomen between waist and rib cage. Avoid touching the chest, especially the area immediately below the sternum.
2. Grasp your properly positioned fist with your other hand and apply pressure inward and up toward the patient's head in a smooth, quick movement. Deliver rapid thrusts until the obstruction is relieved.

For the unconscious adult or child (not an infant) or for a conscious patient who cannot sit or stand, or if you are too short to reach around the patient to deliver thrusts

Place the patient in a supine position and begin CPR. Every time you open the airway, look in the mouth for an object. If, and only if, you see an object, remove it by sweeping your fingers in the patient's mouth from one side to the other.

If the obstruction is not relieved after a series of five thrusts, reassess your position and the patient's airway. If the patient is unconscious and the obstruction is visible, remove it. Attempt to ventilate the patient and, if unsuccessful, repeat the series of thrusts. Repeat the sequence until the obstruction is relieved.

Chest Thrusts

Chest thrusts are used in place of abdominal thrusts when the patient is in the late stages of pregnancy, or when the patient is too obese for abdominal thrusts to be effective. The use of chest thrusts to relieve an airway obstruction is described below.

For the conscious adult who is standing or sitting

1. Position yourself behind the patient and slide your arms under the armpits so you encircle the chest.
2. Form a fist with one hand, and place the thumb side of this fist on the midline of the sternum about 2-3 finger widths above the xiphoid process. This places your fist on the lower half of the sternum but not in contact with the edge of the rib cage.
3. Grasp the fist with your other hand, and deliver chest thrusts directly backward toward the spine until the obstruction is relieved.

For the unconscious adult

1. Place the patient in a supine position.
2. Perform CPR. Every time you open the airway, look in the mouth for an object. If, and only if, you see an object, remove it by sweeping your fingers in the patient's mouth from one side to the other.

Airway Clearance Sequences

Table A-4 lists sequences of procedures to use in the event of a severe airway obstruction or a mild airway obstruction. Note that, as discussed earlier, you should activate the EMS system as soon as unresponsiveness is determined, before carrying out the remainder of the airway clearance procedures.

Airway clearance procedures are considered to have been effective if any of the following happens:

- Patient reestablishes good air exchange or spontaneous breathing.
- Foreign object is expelled from the mouth.
- Foreign object is expelled into the mouth, where it can be removed by the rescuer.
- Unconscious patient regains consciousness.
- Patient's skin color improves.

If a person has only a mild airway obstruction and is still able to speak and cough forcefully, do not interfere with attempts to expel the foreign body. Carefully watch, however, so you can immediately provide help if this partial obstruction becomes a complete one.

Procedures for a Child or Infant

The procedure for clearing a foreign body from the airway of a child is very similar to that used for an adult. The airway clearance procedure for an infant uses a combination of back blows and chest compressions as shown in Scan A-5.

TABLE A-4 Airway Clearance Sequences

	ADULT	CHILD	INFANT
Age	Puberty and older	1 year–puberty	Birth–1 year
Conscious	Ask, "Are you choking?" Abdominal thrust maneuver until obstruction is relieved or patient loses consciousness	Ask, "Are you choking?" Abdominal thrusts until obstruction is relieved or patient loses consciousness	Observe signs of choking (small objects or food, wheezing, agitation, blue color, not breathing). Series of 5 back blows and 5 chest thrusts
Unconscious	Establish unresponsiveness. If alone, call for help. Then open airway. Attempt to ventilate. If unsuccessful, perform CPR. Remove visible objects (no blind sweeps).	Establish unresponsiveness. Open airway. Attempt to ventilate. If unsuccessful, perform CPR. Remove visible objects (no blind sweeps). After 2 minutes, call for help if alone.	Establish unresponsiveness. Open airway. Attempt to ventilate. If unsuccessful, perform CPR. Remove visible objects (no blind sweeps). After 2 minutes, call for help if alone.

SCAN A-5 Clearing the Airway–Infant

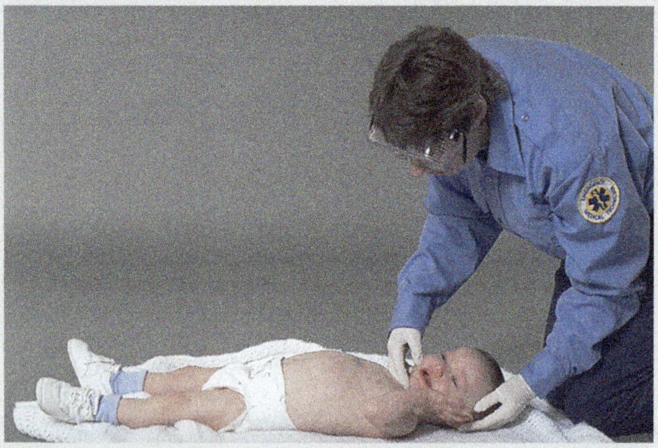

1. Recognize and assess for choking. Look for breathing difficulty, ineffective cough, and lack of strong cry.

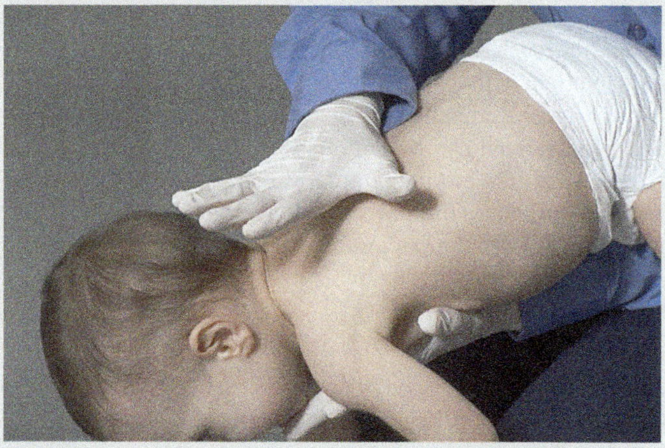

2. Give up to 5 back blows . . .

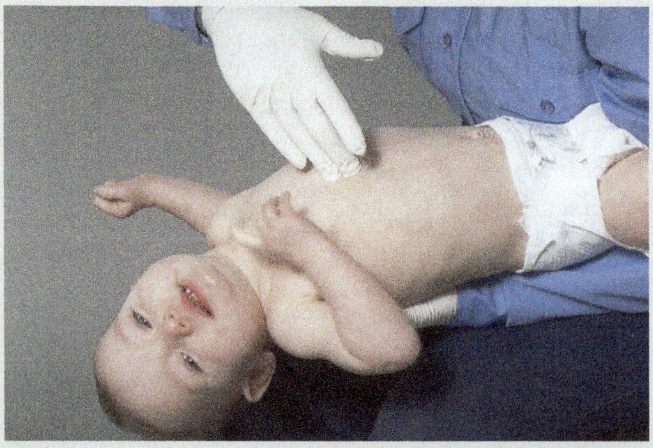

3. . . . and 5 chest compressions, alternating back blows and chest compressions until the obstruction is relieved.

NOTE: *If the infant becomes unresponsive, immediately start CPR by performing 30 chest compressions. (Do not do a pulse check.)*

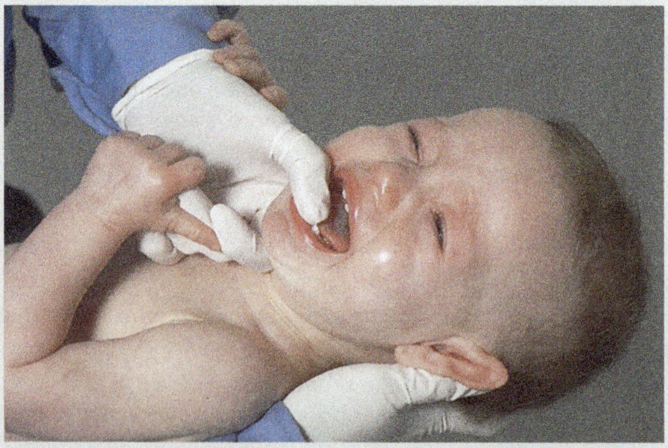

4. If the infant is unresponsive after 30 chest compressions (or if the 5 back blows and 5 chest compressions have not cleared the obstruction in a responsive infant), open the airway and look for a foreign body. If you see one, remove it. (Never do blind finger sweeps.) Attempt 2 breaths and continue alternating chest compressions and ventilations until the obstruction is relieved. If you are working alone, after 2 minutes, activate the EMS system and continue airway clearance and ventilation efforts. Transport as quickly as possible.

For both a child and an infant, a major difference from adult procedures is:

- If the child or infant becomes unconscious, send someone else to activate the EMS system. If no one else is available, wait until you have either relieved the obstruction or you have attempted the airway obstruction sequence for 2 minutes.

Applying ECG Electrodes

An electrocardiogram (ECG) provides data on the heart's electrical activity. In the field, it is used to alert EMS personnel to life-threatening rhythm disturbances. Interpretation of an ECG has traditionally been a paramedic skill. However, to save time on calls, you may be asked to assist. Make sure that you review the ECG equipment (Figure A-6). You should know how to turn on the monitor, how to record an ECG strip, how to change the battery, and how to change the roll of ECG paper. (These are the things that most often need to be done while the paramedic is involved with the patient.)

You also may be asked to carry out four steps in the process of applying the electrodes:

1. Turn on the ECG monitor.
2. Plug in the monitoring cables or "leads."
3. Attach the monitoring cables to the electrodes.
4. Apply the electrodes to the patient's body.

Become familiar with the electrodes used by the paramedics with whom you work. There are two types: monitoring electrodes (with smaller pads) and combination monitoring/defibrillator electrodes (with larger pads). The one most commonly used by paramedics is the monitoring electrode.

If you are asked to apply monitoring electrodes to the patient's body, you will need three or four (depending on the device)–each one giving a different "view" of the heart's electrical activity. First prepare the patient's skin. The best connection is on dry, bare skin, so it may be necessary to shave excessive hair and dry the area. Use a washcloth to remove oil from the skin and consider using an antiperspirant on patients with very sweaty skin. Become familiar with the monitoring configuration (where to place the electrodes) used by ALS personnel in your system. The most common setup is placing the negative (white) electrode under the center of the right clavicle, the positive (red) electrode on the left lower chest, and the ground remaining electrode under the center of the left clavicle or the right lower chest (Figure A-7A).

FIGURE A-6 Check the ECG monitor/defibrillator.

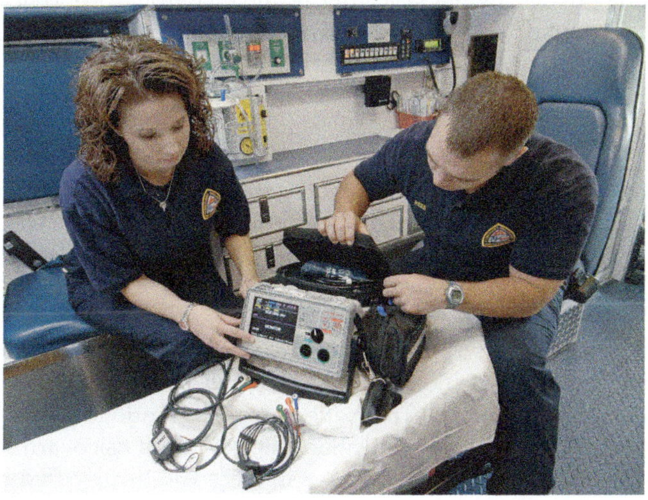

The abbreviations on the cables that attach to the electrodes are LA, RA, LL, and RL, for left arm, right arm, left leg, and right leg. Some ALS providers prefer the electrodes to be placed on the actual extremities (Figure A-7B) rather than on the corresponding portion of the torso. Procedures for this vary, so follow the directions from the ALS provider you are assisting or the protocols of your EMS system.

ALS and many BLS systems have moved toward the routine use of a 12-lead ECG in the field. These machines usually provide a computerized interpretation of the patient's cardiogram that can easily be transmitted to the emergency department via cellular phone. A 12-lead ECG is used to assist in the diagnosis of an acute myocardial infarction (AMI). In the case of an AMI, "time is muscle." As the clock ticks, more and more heart muscle becomes dysfunctional and finally dies in

FIGURE A-7 (A) The most common positioning of electrodes for an ECG is shown here. Become familiar with the monitoring configuration used by ALS personnel in your system. (B) Some ALS providers prefer placing electrodes on the extremities.

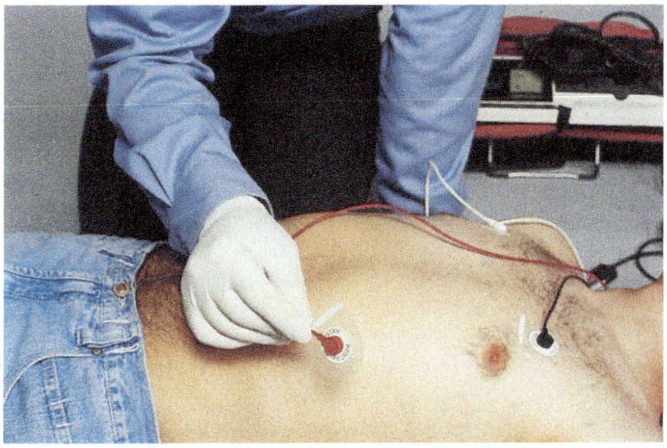

A

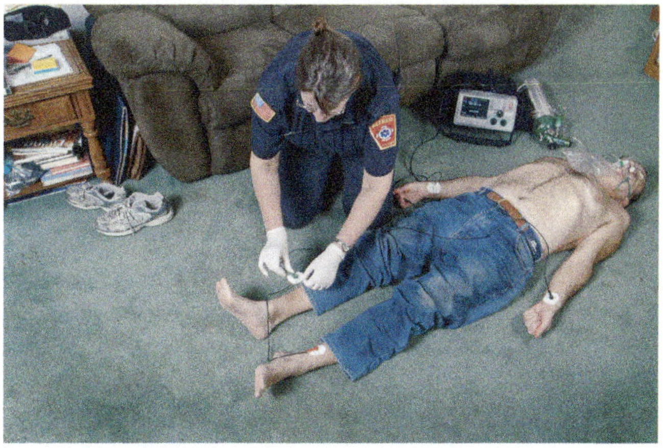

B

the absence of oxygenated blood. With field diagnosis of AMI made possible by the 12-lead ECG, the time from AMI to hospital treatment with drugs or procedures to break up the clots causing the AMI can be reduced.

If 12-lead ECG monitors are used in your system, ask the paramedics to review the lead placement with you, as this is slightly more complex than the simple three electrodes you may be used to. Figure A-8 demonstrates lead placement for the 12-lead ECG and shows the 12-lead electrodes in place.

Post–Cardiac Arrest Care

In the event that your cardiac arrest patient has a return of spontaneous circulation (ROSC) (i.e., a pulse), there are several things you should do. This patient is in a precarious position and will need all of your attention. There is a high risk of arresting again, so leave the AED pads in place and be prepared to defibrillate again.

Unless you were able to defibrillate within a minute or two after the cardiac arrest, the patient will probably remain unconscious and will need respiratory support. The patient may breathe less frequently than a normal patient, so judge the adequacy and rate of breathing to determine your next steps. If the patient's breathing is inadequate, ventilate or assist ventilations with oxygen. If respirations are adequate, administer sufficient oxygen to maintain an oxygen saturation of at least 94%.

Monitor the patient's pulse frequently, at least every 30 seconds or so if that is practical. Since you will probably be providing ventilation, it may be difficult to tell if the patient has gone back into cardiac arrest. If you are not sure whether the patient has a pulse, look for other signs of circulation, such as movement. Do not mistake gasping agonal respirations for adequate breathing. If you are not sure, ventilate, compress the chest, and have the AED check the rhythm.

ALS can be helpful not only in caring for the patient but also in determining the transport destination. When there is a choice of hospitals, it is important to go to one that has the specialized facilities and staff necessary to care for a patient who is recovering from cardiac arrest.

The issue of how much oxygen to administer to patients who were in cardiac arrest but now have a spontaneous pulse is a potentially complicated one. Ideally, if the patient is perfusing sufficiently for you to get a pulse oximeter reading, you should reduce the amount of oxygen the patient is getting to attain an oxygen saturation reading between 95 percent and 100 percent. This is a significant challenge in a moving ambulance with limited staff and many other tasks to perform for an unstable patient. If you can do this without sacrificing other important steps, do so in accordance with local protocols. Do not allow the patient to become hypoxic, however. If you must make a choice, it is better to overoxygenate the patient than to underoxygenate the patient.

FIGURE A-8 (A) 12-lead ECG lead placement. (B) 12-lead electrodes in place.

Lead V_1 The electrode is at the fourth intercostal space just to the right of the sternum.
Lead V_2 The electrode is at the fourth intercostal space just to the left of the sternum.
Lead V_3 The electrode is at the line midway between leads V_2 and V_4.
Lead V_4 The electrode is at the midclavicular line in the fifth interspace.
Lead V_5 The electrode is at the anterior axillary line at the same level as lead V_4.
Lead V_6 The electrode is at the midaxillary line at the same level as lead V_4.

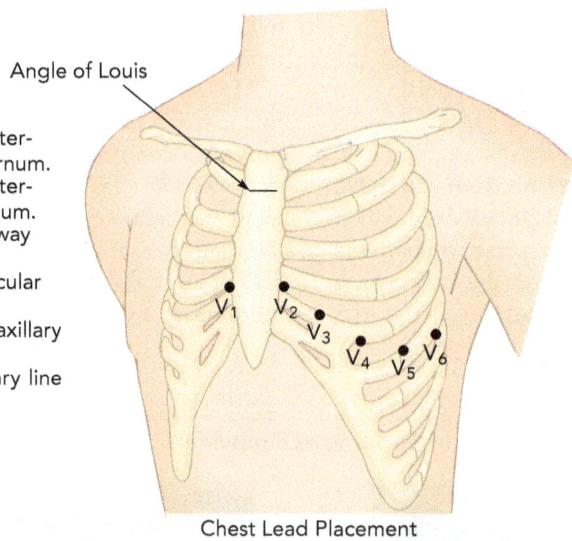

A

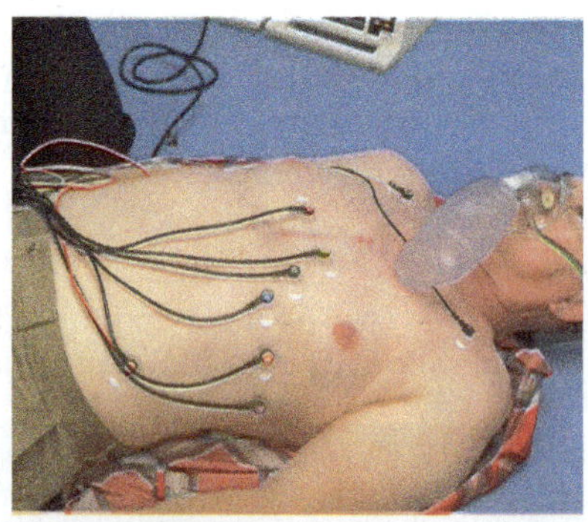

B

Medical Terms

As an EMT, you will probably never have to use more than a few medical terms in the course of your prehospital emergency care activities, and most of them will probably deal with parts of the body. Physicians and nurses prefer EMTs to speak in common layperson language rather than medical terms. However, if you are an avid reader, much of what you read is likely to be freely sprinkled with medical terms; if you cannot translate them, you may not understand what you are reading.

Medical terms are composed of words, roots, combining forms, prefixes, and suffixes, as explained in the chapter *Medical Terminology*.

Following are lists of standard medical terms and word parts.

Direction of Movement, Position, and Anatomical Posture

The following terms are used to denote direction of movement, position, and anatomical posture:

abduction movement away from the body's midline.

adduction movement toward the body's midline.

afferent conducting toward a structure.

anterior the front surface of the body.

anterior to in front of.

caudad toward the tail.

cephalad toward the head.

circumduction circular movement of a part.

craniad toward the cranium.

deep situated remote from the surface.

distal situated away from the point of origin.

dorsal pertaining to the back surface of the body.

dorsiflexion bending backward.

efferent conducting away from a structure.

elevation raising a body part.

extension stretching, or moving, jointed parts into or toward a straight condition.

external situated outside.

flexion bending, or moving, jointed parts closer together.

inferior situated below.

internal situated inside.

laterad toward the side of the body.

lateral situated away from the body's midline.

lateral rotation rotating outward away from the body's midline.

left lateral recumbent lying horizontal on the left side.

mediad toward the midline of the body.

medial situated toward the body's midline.

medial rotation rotating inward toward the body's midline.

palmar concerning the inner surface of the hand.

peripheral away from a central structure.

plantar concerning the sole of the foot.

posterior pertaining to the back surface of the body.

posterior to situated behind.

pronation lying face downward or turning the hand so the palm faces downward or backward.

prone lying horizontal, facedown, and flat.

protraction pushing forward, such as happens with the mandible.

proximal situated nearest the point of origin.

recumbent lying horizontal, generally speaking.

retraction drawing back, such as happens with the tongue.

right lateral recumbent lying horizontal on the right side.

rotation turning around an axis.

superficial situated near the surface.

superior situated above.

supination lying face upward or turning the hand so the palm faces forward or upward.

supine lying horizontal, flat on the back, and faceup.

ventral the front surface of the body.

Planes

A plane is an imaginary flat surface that divides the body into sections.

coronal or frontal plane an imaginary plane that passes through the body from side to side and divides it into front and back sections.

midsagittal plane an imaginary plane that passes through the body from front to back and divides it into equal right and left halves.

sagittal plane an imaginary plane parallel to the midsagittal plane. It passes through the body from front to back and divides the body into right and left sections.

transverse plane an imaginary plane that passes through the body and divides it into upper and lower sections.

Word Parts

*In this list, prefixes are generally followed by a hyphen (**ambi-**). Combining forms have a slash and a vowel following the root (**arthr/o**). Suffixes are generally identified by a preceding hyphen (**-emia**).*

a- (not, without, lacking, deficient) *afebrile*, without fever.

ab- (away from) *abduct*, to draw away from the midline.

abdomin/o (abdomen) *abdominal*, pertaining to the abdomen.

-able, -ible (capable of) *reducible*, capable of being reduced (as with a fracture).

ac- (to) *acclimate*, to become accustomed to.

acou (hear) *acoustic*, pertaining to sound or hearing.

acr/o (extremity, top, peak) *acrodermatitis*, inflammation of the skin of the extremities.

acu (needle) *acupuncture*, the Chinese practice of piercing specific peripheral nerves with needles to relieve the discomfort associated with painful disorders.

ad- (to, toward) *adduct*, to draw toward the midline.

aden/o (gland) *adenitis*, inflammation of a gland.

adip/o (fat) *adipose*, fatty; fat (in size).

aer/o (air) *aerobic*, requiring the presence of oxygen to live and grow.

af- (to) *afferent*, conveying toward.

ag- (to) *aggregate*, to crowd or cluster together.

-algesia (painful) *hyperalgesia*, overly sensitive to pain.

-algia (painful condition) *neuralgia*, pain that extends along the course of one or more nerves.

ambi- (both sides) *ambidextrous*, able to perform manual skills with both hands.

ambl/y (dim, dull, lazy) *amblyopia*, lazy eye.

amphi-, ampho- (on both sides, around both) *amphigonadism*, having both testicular and ovarian tissues.

amyl/o (starch) *amyloid*, starchlike.

an- (without) *anemia*, a reduced volume of blood cells.

ana- (upward, backward, excess) *anaphylaxis*, an unusual or exaggerated reaction of an organism to a substance to which it becomes sensitized.

andr/o (man, male) *android*, resembling a man.

angi/o (blood vessel, duct) *angioplasty*, surgery of blood vessels.

ankyl/o (stiff) *ankylosis*, stiffness.

ant-, anti- (against, opposed to, preventing, relieving) *antidote*, a substance for counteracting a poison.

ante- (before, forward) *antecubital*, situated in front of the elbow.

antero- (front) *anterolateral*, situated in front and to one side.

ap- (to) *approximate*, to bring together; to place close to.

apo- (separation, derivation from) *apoplexy*, sudden neurologic impairment due to a cardiovascular disorder.

-arium, -orium (place for something) *solarium*, a place for the sun.

arteri/o (artery) *arteriosclerosis*, thickening of the walls of the smaller arteries.

arthri/o (joint, articulation) *arthritis*, inflammation of a joint or joints.

articul/o (joint) *articulated*, united by joints.

as- (to) *assimilate*, to take into.

at- (to) *attract*, to draw toward.

audi/o (hearing) *audiometer*, an instrument to test the power of hearing.

aur/o (ear) *auricle*, the flap of the ear.

aut/o (self) *autistic*, self-centered.

bi- (two, twice, double, both) *bilateral*, having two sides; pertaining to two sides.

bio (life) *biology*, the study of life.

blephari/o (eyelid) *blepharitis*, inflammation of the eyelid.

brachi/o (upper arm) *brachialgia*, pain in the upper arm.

brady- (slow) *bradycardia*, an abnormally slow heart rate.

bronch/o (larger air passages of the lungs) *bronchitis*, inflammation of the larger air passages of the lungs.

bucc/o (cheek) *buccal*, pertaining to the cheek.

cac/o (bad) *cacosmis*, a bad odor.

calc/o (pebble) *calculus*, an abnormal, hard inorganic mass such as a gallstone.

calcane/o (heel) *calcaneus*, the heel bone.

calor/o (heat) *caloric*, pertaining to heat.

cancr/o (cancer) *cancroid*, resembling cancer.

capit/o (head) *capitate*, head-shaped.

caps/o (container) *capsulation*, enclosed in a capsule or container.

carcin/o (cancer) *carcinogen*, a substance that causes cancer.

cardi/o (heart) *cardiogenic*, originating in the heart.

carp/o (wrist bone) *carpal*, pertaining to the wrist bone.

cat-, cata- (down, lower, under, against, along with) *catabasis*, the stage of decline of a disease.

-cele (tumor, hernia) *hydrocele*, a confined collection of water.

celi/o (abdomen) *celiomyalgia*, a pain in the muscles of the abdomen.

-centesis (perforation or tapping, as with a needle) *abdominocentesis*, surgical puncture of the abdominal cavity.

cephal/o (head) *electroencephalogram*, a recording of the electrical activity of the brain.

cerebr/o (cerebrum) *cerebrospinal*, pertaining to the brain and spinal fluid.

cervic/o (neck, cervix) *cervical*, pertaining to the neck (or cervix).

cheil/o, chil/o (lip) *cheilitis*, inflammation of the lips.

cheirio, chir/o (hand) *cheiralgia*, pain in the hand.

chlor/o (green) *chloroma*, green cancer, a greenish tumor associated with myelogenous leukemia.

chol/e (bile, gall) *choledochitis*, inflammation of the common bile duct.

chondr/o (cartilage) *chondrodynia*, pain in a cartilage.

chrom/o, chromat/o (color) *monochromatic*, being of one color.

chron/o (time) *chronic*, persisting for a long time.

-cid- (cut, kill, fall) *insecticide*, an agent that kills insects.

circum- (around) *circumscribed*, confined to a limited space.

-cis- (cut, kill, fall) *excise*, to cut out.

-clysis (irrigation) *enteroclysis*, irrigation of the small intestine.

co- (with) *cohesion*, the force that causes various particles to unite.

col- (with) *collateral*, secondary or accessory; a small side branch such as a blood vessel or nerve.

col/o (colon, large intestine) *colitis*, inflammation of the colon.

colp/o (vagina) *colporrhagia*, bleeding from the vagina.

com- (with) *comminuted*, broken or crushed into small pieces.

con- (with) *congenital*, existing from the time of birth.

contra- (against, opposite) *contraindicated*, inadvisable.

cor/e, core/o (pupil) *corectopia*, abnormal location of the pupil of the eye.

cost/o (rib) *intercostal*, between the ribs.

crani/o (skull) *cranial*, pertaining to the skull.

cry/o (cold) *cryogenic*, that which produces low temperature.

crypt/o (hide, cover, conceal) *cryptogenic*, of hidden or unknown origin.

cyan/o (blue) *cyanosis*, bluish discoloration of the skin and mucous membranes.

cyst/o (urinary bladder, cyst, sac of fluid) *cystitis*, inflammation of the bladder.

cyt/o (cell) *cytoma*, tumor of the cell.

-cyte (cell) *leukocyte*, white cell.

dacry/o (tear) *dacryorrhea*, excessive flow of tears.

dactyl/o (finger, toe) *dactylomegaly*, abnormally large fingers or toes.

de- (down) *descending*, coming down from.

dent/o (tooth) *dental*, pertaining to the teeth.

derm/o, dermat/o (skin) *dermatitis*, inflammation of the skin.

dextr/o (right) *dextrad*, toward the right side.

di- (twice, double) *diplegia*, paralysis affecting like parts on both sides of the body.

dia- (through, across, apart) *diaphragm*, the partition that separates the abdominal and thoracic cavities.

dipl/o (double, twin, twice) *diplopia*, double vision.

dips/o (thirst) *dipsomania*, alcoholism.

dis- (to free, to undo) *dissect*, to cut apart.

dors/o (back) *dorsal*, pertaining to the back.

-dynia (painful condition) *cephalodynia*, headache.

dys- (bad, difficult, abnormal, incomplete) *dyspnea*, labored breathing.

-ectasia (dilation or enlargement of an organ or part) *gastrectasia*, dilation (stretching) of the stomach.

ecto- (outer, outside of) *ectopic*, located away from the normal position.

-ectomy (the surgical removal of an organ or part) *appendectomy*, surgical removal of the appendix.

electr/o (electric) *electrocardiogram*, the written record of the heart's electrical activity.

-emia (condition of the blood) *anemia*, a deficiency of red blood cells.

en- (in, into, within) *encapsulate*, to enclose within a container.

encephal/o (brain) *encephalitis*, inflammation of the brain.

end-, endo- (within) *endotracheal*, within the trachea.

ent-, ento- (within, inner) *entopic*, occurring in the proper place.

enter/o (small intestine) *enteritis*, inflammation of the intestine.

ep-, epi- (over, on, upon) *epidermis*, the outermost layer of skin.

erythr/o (red) *erythrocyte*, a red blood cell.

esthesia (feeling) *anesthesia*, without feeling.

eu- (good, well, normal, healthy) *euphoria*, an abnormal or exaggerated feeling of well-being.

ex- (out of, away from) *excrement*, waste material discharged from the body.

exo- (outside, outward) *exophytic*, to grow outward or on the surface.

extra- (on the outside, beyond, in addition to) *extracorporeal*, outside the body.

faci/o (face, surface) *facial*, pertaining to the face.

febr/i (fever) *febrile*, feverish.

-ferent (bear, carry) *efferent*, carrying away from a center.

fibr/o (fiber, filament) *fibrillation*, muscular contractions due to the activity of muscle fibers.

-form (shape) *deformed*, abnormally shaped.

-fugal (moving away) *centrifugal*, moving away from a center.

galact/o (milk) *galactopyria*, milk fever.

gangli/o (knot) *ganglion*, a knotlike mass.

gastr/o (stomach) *gastritis*, inflammation of the stomach.

gen/o (come into being, originate) *genetic*, inherited.

-genesis (production or origin) *pathogenesis*, the development of a disease.

-genic (giving rise to, originating in) *cardiogenic*, originating in the heart.

gloss/o (tongue) *glossal*, pertaining to the tongue.

glyc/o (sweet) *glycemia*, the presence of sugar in the blood.

gnath/o (jaw) *gnathitis*, inflammation of the jaw.

gnos/o (knowledge) *prognosis*, a prediction of the outcome of a disease.

-gram (drawing, written record) *electrocardiogram*, a written record of the heart's electrical activity.

-graph (an instrument for recording the activity of an organ) *electrocardiograph*, an instrument for measuring the heart's electrical activity.

-graphy (the recording of the activity of an organ) *electrocardiography*, the method of recording the heart's electrical activity.

gynec/o (woman) *gynecologist*, a specialist in diseases of the female genital tract.

hem/a, hem/o, hemat/o (blood) *hematoma*, a localized collection of blood.

hemi- (one-half) *hemiplegia*, paralysis of one side of the body.

hepat/o (liver) *hepatitis*, inflammation of the liver.

heter/o (other) *heterogeneous*, from a different source.

hidr/o, hidrot/o (sweat) *hidrosis*, excessive sweating.

hist/o (tissue) *histodialysis*, the breaking down of tissue.

hom/o, home/o (same, similar, unchanging, constant) *homeostasis*, stability in an organism's normal physiological states.

hyal/o (glass) *hyaline*, glassy, transparent.

hydr/o (water, fluid) *hydrocephalus*, an accumulation of cerebrospinal fluid in the skull with resulting enlargement of the head.

hyper- (beyond normal, excessive) *hypertension*, abnormally high blood pressure.

hypn/o (sleep) *hypnotic*, that which induces sleep.

hypo- (below normal, deficient, under, beneath) *hypotension*, abnormally low blood pressure.

hyster/o (uterus, womb) *hysterectomy*, surgical removal of the uterus.

-iasis (condition) *psoriasis*, a chronic skin condition characterized by lesions.

iatr/o (healer, physician) *pediatrician*, a physician who specializes in children's disorders.

-id (in a state, condition of) *gravid*, pregnant.

idio- (peculiar, separate, distinct) *idiopathic*, occurring without a known cause.

il- (not) *illegible*, cannot be read.

ile/o (ileum) *ileitis*, inflammation of the ileum.

ili/o (ilium) *iliac*, pertaining to the ilium.

im- (negative prefix) *immature*, not mature.

in- (in, into, within) *incise*, to cut into.

infra- (beneath, below) *infracostal*, below a rib, or below the ribs.

inter- (between) *intercostal*, between two ribs.

intra- (within) *intraoral*, within the mouth.

intro- (within, into) *introspection*, the contemplation of one's own thoughts and feelings; self-analysis.

ir/o, irid/o (iris) *iridotomy*, incision of the iris.

ischi/o (ischium) *ischialgia*, pain in the ischium.

-ismus (abnormal condition) *strabismus*, deviation of the eye that a person cannot overcome.

iso- (same, equal, alike) *isometric*, of equal dimensions.

-itis (inflammation) *endocarditis*, inflammation within the heart.

kerat/o (cornea) *keratitis*, inflammation of the cornea.

kinesi/o (movement) *kinesialgia*, pain upon movement.

labi/o (lip) *labiodental*, pertaining to the lip and teeth.

lact/o (milk) *lactation*, the secretion of milk.

lal/o (talk) *lalopathy*, any speech disorder.

lapar/o (flank, abdomen, abdominal wall) *laparotomy*, an incision through the abdominal wall.

laryng/o (larynx) *laryngoscope*, an instrument for examining the larynx.

lept/o (thin) *leptodactylous*, having slender fingers.

leuc/o, leuk/o (white) *leukemia*, a malignant disease characterized by the increased development of white blood cells.

lingu/o (tongue) *sublingual*, under the tongue.

lip/o (fat) *lipoma*, fatty tumor.

lith/o (stone) *lithotriptor*, an instrument for crushing stones in the bladder.

-logist (a person who studies) *pathologist*, a person who studies diseases.

log/o (speak, give an account) *logospasms*, spasmodic speech.

-logy (study of) *pathology*, the study of disease.

lumb/o (loin) *lumbago*, pain in the lumbar region.

lymph/o (lymph) *lymphoduct*, a vessel of the lymph system.

-lysis (destruction) *electrolysis*, destruction (of hair, for example) by passage of an electric current.

macr/o (large, long) *macrocephalous*, having an abnormally large head.

malac/o (a softening) *malacia*, the morbid softening of a body part or tissue.

mamm/o (breast) *mammary*, pertaining to the breast.

-mania (mental aberration) *kleptomania*, the compulsion to steal.

mast/o (breast) *mastectomy*, surgical removal of the breast.

medi/o (middle) *mediastinum*, middle partition of the thoracic cavity.

mega- (large) *megacolon*, an abnormally large colon.

megal/o (large) *megalomaniac*, a person impressed with his own greatness.

-megaly (an enlargement) *cardiomegaly*, enlargement of the heart.

melan/o (dark, black) *melanoma*, a tumor composed of darkly pigmented cells.

men/o (month) *menopause*, cessation of menstruation.

mes/o (middle) *mesiad*, toward the center.

meta- (change, transformation, exchange) *metabolism*, the sum of the physical and chemical processes by which an organism survives.

metr/o (uterus) *metralgia*, pain in the uterus.

micr/o (small) *microscope*, an instrument for magnifying small objects.

mon/o (single, only, sole) *monoplegia*, paralysis of a single part.

morph/o (form) *morphology*, the study of form and shape.

multi- (many, much) *multipara*, a woman who has given two or more live births.

my/o (muscle) *myasthenia*, muscular weakness.

myc/o, mycet/o (fungus) *mycosis*, any disease caused by a fungus.

myel/o (marrow, also often refers to spinal cord) *myelocele*, protrusion of the spinal cord through a defect in the spinal column.

myx/o (mucous, slimelike) *myxoid*, resembling mucus.

narc/o (stupor, numbness) *narcotic*, an agent that induces sleep.

nas/o (nose) *oronasal*, pertaining to the nose and mouth.

ne/o (new) *neonate*, a newborn infant.

necr/o (corpse) *necrotic*, dead (when referring to tissue).

nephr/o (kidney) *nephralgia*, pain in the kidneys.

neur/o (nerve) *neuritis*, inflammation of nerve pathways.

noct/i (night) *noctambulism*, sleepwalking.

norm/o (rule, order, normal) *normotension*, normal blood pressure.

null/i (none) *nullipara*, a woman who has never given birth to a child.

nyct/o (night) *nycturia*, excessive urination at night.

ob- (against, in front of, toward) *obturator*, a device that closes an opening.

oc- (against, in front of, toward) *occlude*, to obstruct.

ocul/o (eye) *ocular*, pertaining to the eye.

odont/o (tooth) *odontalgia*, toothache.

-oid (shape, form, resemblance) *ovoid*, egg shaped.

olig/o (few, deficient, scanty) *oligemia*, lacking in blood volume.

-oma (tumor, swelling) *adenoma*, tumor of a gland.

onych/o (nail) *onychoma*, tumor of a nail or nail bed.

oo- (egg) *ooblast*, a primitive cell from which an ovum develops.

oophor/o (ovary) *oophorectomy*, a surgical removal of one or both ovaries.

ophthalm/o (eye) *opthalmic*, pertaining to the eyes.

-opsy (a viewing) *autopsy*, postmortem examination of a body.

opt/o, optic/o (sight, vision) *optometrist*, a specialist in adapting lenses for the correcting of visual defects.

or/o (mouth) *oral*, pertaining to the mouth.

orch/o, orchid/o (testicle) *orchitis*, inflammation of the testicles.

orth/o (straight, upright) *orthopedic*, pertaining to the correction of skeletal defects.

-osis (process, an abnormal condition) *dermatosis*, any skin condition.

oste/o (bone) *osteomyelitis*, inflammation of bone or bone marrow.

ot/o (ear) *otalgia*, earache.

ov/i, ov/o (egg) *oviduct*, a passage through which an egg passes.

ovari/o (ovary) *ovariocele*, hernia of an ovary.

pachy- (thicken) *pachyderma*, abnormal thickening of the skin.

palat/o (palate) *palatitis*, inflammation of the palate.

pan- (all, entire, every) *panacea*, a remedy for all diseases, a "cure-all."

para- (beside, beyond, accessory to, apart from, against) *paranormal*, beyond the natural or normal.

path/o (disease) *pathogen*, any disease-producing agent.

-pathy (disease of) *osteopathy*, disease of a bone.

-penia (an abnormal reduction) *leukopenia*, deficiency in white blood cells.

peps/o, pept/o (digestion) *dyspepsia*, poor digestion.

per- (throughout, completely, extremely) *perfusion*, the passage of fluid through the vessels of an organ.

peri- (around, surrounding) *pericardium*, the sac that surrounds the heart and the roots of the great vessels.

-pexy (fixation) *splenopexy*, surgical fixation of the spleen.

phag/o (eat) *phagomania*, an insatiable craving for food.

pharyng/o (throat) *pharyngospasms*, spasms of the muscles of the pharynx.

phas/o (speech) *aphasic*, unable to speak.

phil/o (like, have an affinity for) *necrophilia*, an abnormal interest in death.

phleb/o (vein) *phlebotomy*, surgical incision of a vein.

-phobia (fear, dread) *claustrophobia*, a fear of closed spaces.

phon/o (sound) *phonetic*, pertaining to the voice.

phor/o (bear, carry) *diaphoresis*, profuse sweating.

phot/o (light) *photosensitivity*, abnormal reactivity of the skin to sunlight.

phren/o (diaphragm) *phrenic nerve*, a nerve that carries messages to the diaphragm.

physi/o (nature) *physiology*, the science that studies the function of living things.

pil/o (hair) *pilose*, hairy.

-plasia (development, formation) *dysplasia*, poor or abnormal formation.

-plasty (surgical repair) *arthroplasty*, surgical repair of a joint.

-plegia (paralysis) *paraplegia*, paralysis of the lower body, including the legs.

pleur/o (rib, side, pleura) *pleurisy*, inflammation of the pleura.

-pnea (breath, breathing) *orthopnea*, difficult breathing except in an upright position.

pneum/o, pneumat/o (air, breath) *pneumatic*, pertaining to the air.

pneum/o, pneumon/o (lung) *pneumonia*, inflammation of the lungs with the escape of fluid.

pod/o (foot) *podiatrist*, a specialist in the care of feet.

-poiesis (formation) *hematopoiesis*, formation of blood.

poly- (much, many) *polychromatic*, multicolored.

post- (after, behind) *postmortem*, after death.

pre- (before) *premature*, occurring before the proper time.

pro- (before, in front of) *prolapse*, the falling down or sinking of a part.

proct/o (anus) *proctitis*, inflammation of the rectum.

pseud/o (false) *pseudoplegia*, hysterical paralysis.

psych/o (mind, soul) *psychopath*, one who displays aggressive antisocial behavior.

-ptosis (abnormal dropping or sagging of a part) *hysteroptosis*, sagging of the uterus.

pulmon/o (lung) *pulmonary*, pertaining to the lungs.

py/o (pus) *pyorrhea*, copious discharge of pus.

pyel/o (renal pelvis) *pyelitis*, inflammation of the renal pelvis.

pyr/o (fire, fever) *pyromaniac*, compulsive fire setter.

quadri- (four) *quadriplegia*, paralysis of all four limbs.

rach/i (spine) *rachialgia*, pain in the spine.

radi/o (ray, radiation) *radiology*, the use of ionizing radiation in diagnosis and treatment.

re- (back, against, contrary) *recurrence*, the return of symptoms after remission.

rect/o (rectum) *rectal*, pertaining to the rectum.

ren/o (the kidneys) *renal*, pertaining to the kidneys.

retro- (located behind, backward) *retroperineal*, behind the perineum.

rhin/o (nose) *rhinitis*, inflammation of the mucous membranes of the nose.

-rrhage (abnormal discharge) *hemorrhage*, abnormal discharge of blood.

-rrhagia (hemorrhage from an organ or body part) *menorrhagia*, excessive uterine bleeding.

-rrhea (flowing or discharge) *diarrhea*, abnormal frequency and liquidity of fecal discharges.

sanguin/o (blood) *exsanguinate*, to lose a large volume of blood either internally or externally.

sarc/o (flesh) *sarcoma*, a malignant tumor.

schiz/o (split) *schizophrenia*, any of a group of emotional disorders characterized by bizarre behavior (erroneously called split *personality*).

scler/o (hardening) *scleroderma*, hardening of connective tissues of the body, including the skin.

-sclerosis (hardened condition) *arteriosclerosis*, hardening of the arteries.

scoli/o (twisted, crooked) *scoliosis*, sideward deviation of the spine.

-scope (an instrument for observing) *endoscope*, an instrument for the examination of a hollow body, such as the bladder.

-sect (cut) *transect*, to cut across.

semi- (one-half, partly) *semisupine*, partly, but not completely, supine.

sept/o, seps/o (infection) *aseptic*, free from infection.

somat/o (body) *psychosomatic*, both psychological and physiological.

son/o (sound) *sonogram*, a recording produced by the passage of sound waves through the body.

spermat/o (sperm, semen) *spermicide*, an agent that kills sperm.

sphygm/o (pulse) *sphygmomanometer*, a device for measuring blood pressure in the arteries.

splen/o (spleen) *splenectomy*, surgical removal of the spleen.

-stasis (stopping, controlling) *hemostasis*, the control of bleeding.

sten/o (narrow) *stenosis*, a narrowing of a passage or opening.

stere/o (solid, three-dimensional) *stereoscopic*, a three-dimensional appearance.

steth/o (chest) *stethoscope*, an instrument for listening to chest sounds.

sthen/o (strength) *sthenometer*, an instrument for measuring muscular strength.

-stomy (surgically creating a new opening) *colostomy*, surgical creation of an opening between the colon and the surface of the body.

sub- (under, near, almost, moderately) *subclavian*, situated under the clavicle.

super- (above, excess) *superficial*, lying on or near the surface.

supra- (above, over) *suprapubic*, situated above the pubic arch.

sym-, syn- (joined together, with) *syndrome*, a set of symptoms that occur together.

tachy- (fast) *tachycardia*, a very fast heart rate.

-therapy (treatment) *hydrotherapy*, treatment with water.

therm/o (heat) *thermogenesis*, the production of heat.

thorac/o (chest cavity) *thoracic*, pertaining to the chest.

thromb/o (clot, lump) *thrombophlebitis*, inflammation of a vein due to a blood clot.

-tome (a surgical instrument for cutting) *microtome*, an instrument for cutting thin slices of tissue.

-tomy (a surgical operation on an organ or body part) *thoracotomy*, surgical incision of the chest wall.

top/o (place) *topographic*, pertaining to special regions (of the body).

trache/o (trachea) *tracheostomy*, an opening in the neck that passes to the trachea.

trans- (through, across, beyond) *transfusion*, the introduction of whole blood or blood components directly into the bloodstream.

tri- (three) *trimester*, a period of three months.

trich/o (hair) *trichosis*, any disease of the hair.

-tripsy (surgical crushing) *lithotripsy*, surgical crushing of stones.

troph/o (nourish) *hypertrophic*, enlargement of an organ or body part due to an increase in the size of cells.

ultra- (beyond, excess) *ultrasonic*, beyond the audible range.

uni- (one) *unilateral*, affecting one side.

ur/o (urine) *urinalysis*, examination of urine.

ureter/o (ureter) *ureteritis*, inflammation of a ureter.

urethr/o (urethra) *urethritis*, inflammation of the urethra.

vas/o (vessel, duct) *vasodilator*, an agent that causes dilation of blood vessels.

ven/o (vein) *venipuncture*, surgical puncture of a vein.

ventr/o (belly, cavity) *ventral*, relating to the belly or abdomen.

vesic/o (blister, bladder) *vesicle*, a small fluid-filled blister.

viscer/o (internal organ) *visceral*, pertaining to the viscera (abdominal organs).

xanth/o (yellow) *xanthroma*, a yellow nodule in the skin.

xen/o (stranger) *xenophobia*, abnormal fear of strangers.

xer/o (dry) *xerosis*, abnormal dryness (as of the mouth or eyes).

zo/o (animal life) *zoogenous*, acquired from an animal.

ILLUSTRATIONS

Anatomy and Physiology

Skeletal System

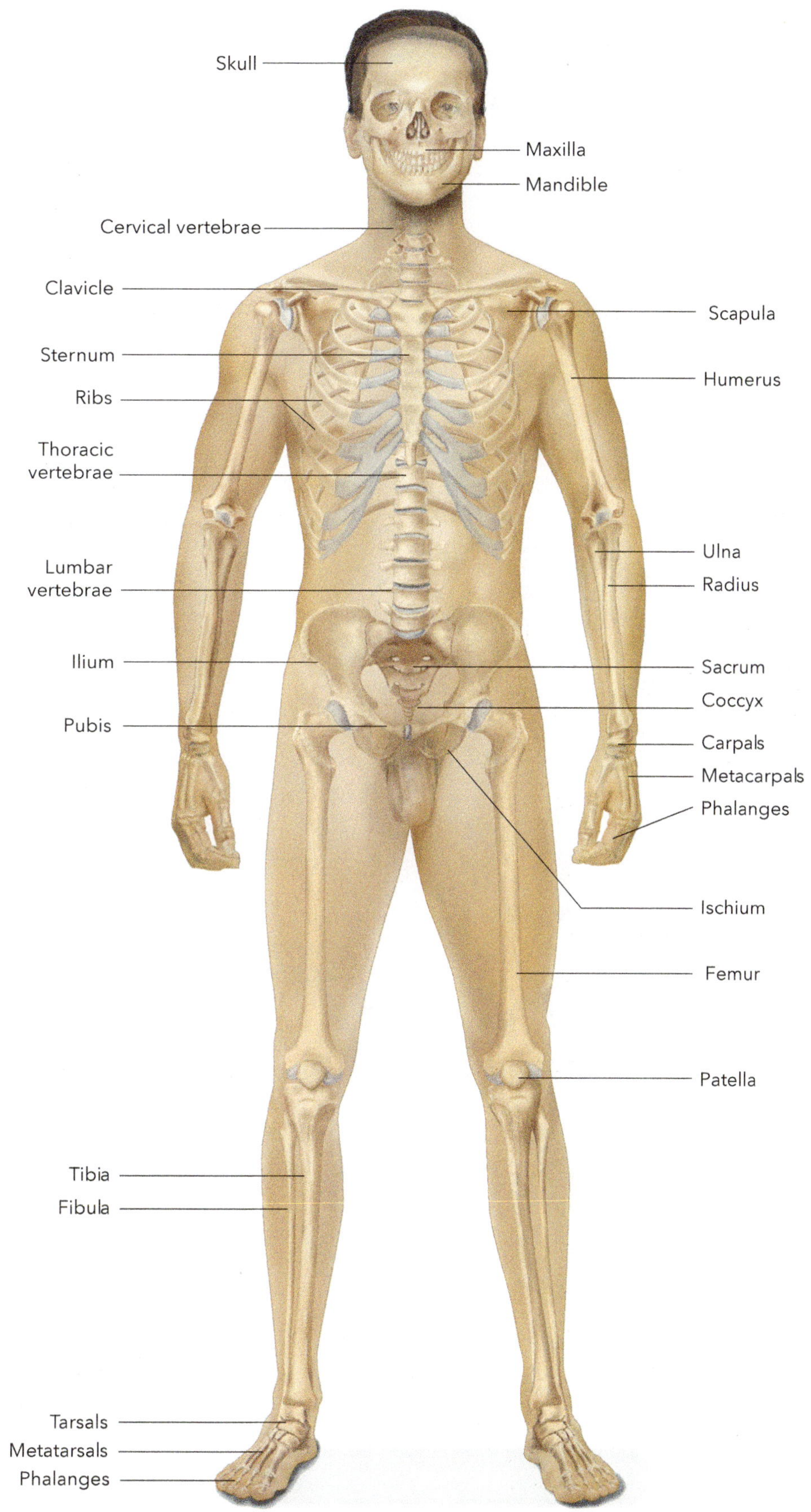

Muscular System

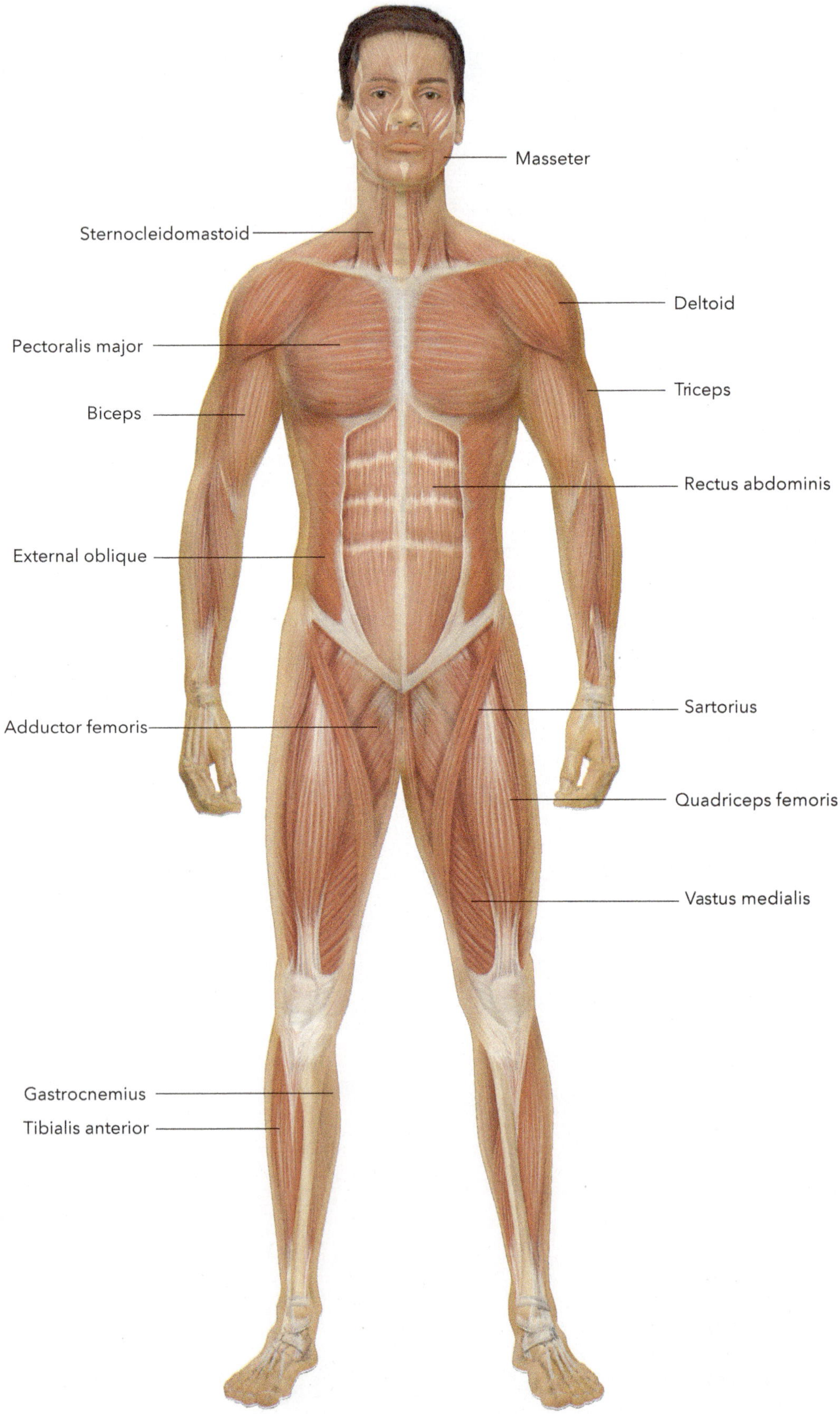

Respiratory System

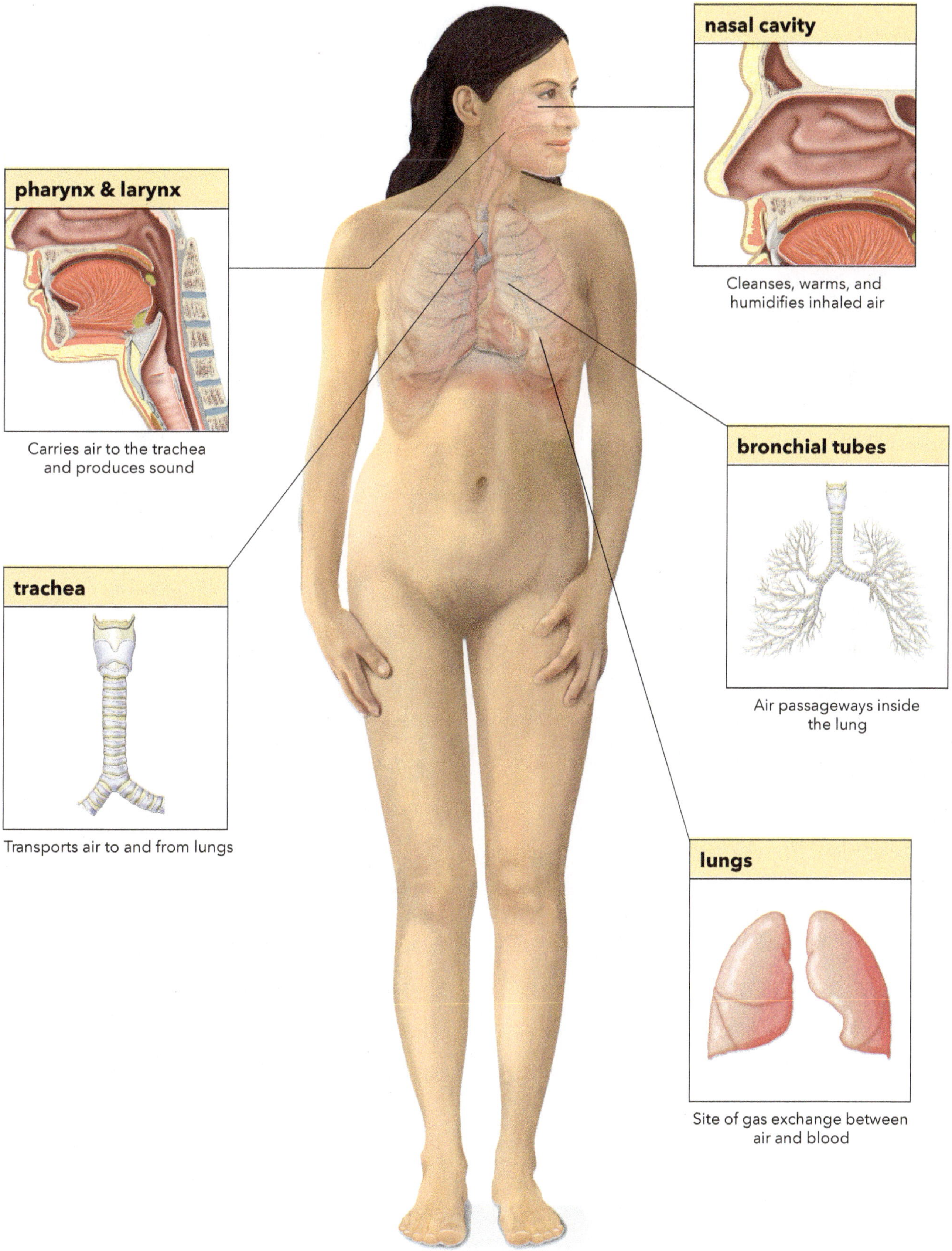

Cardiovascular System

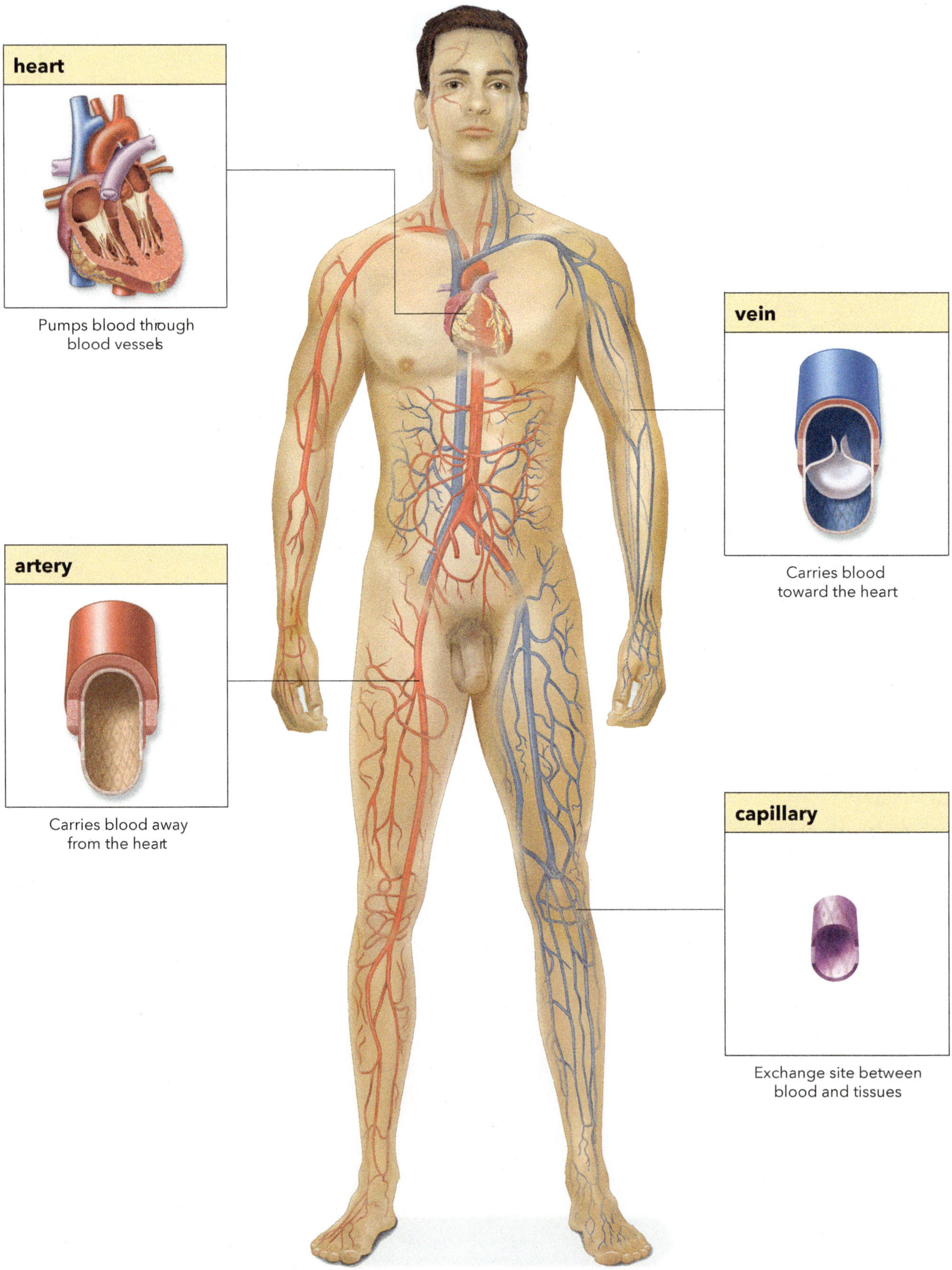

Nervous System

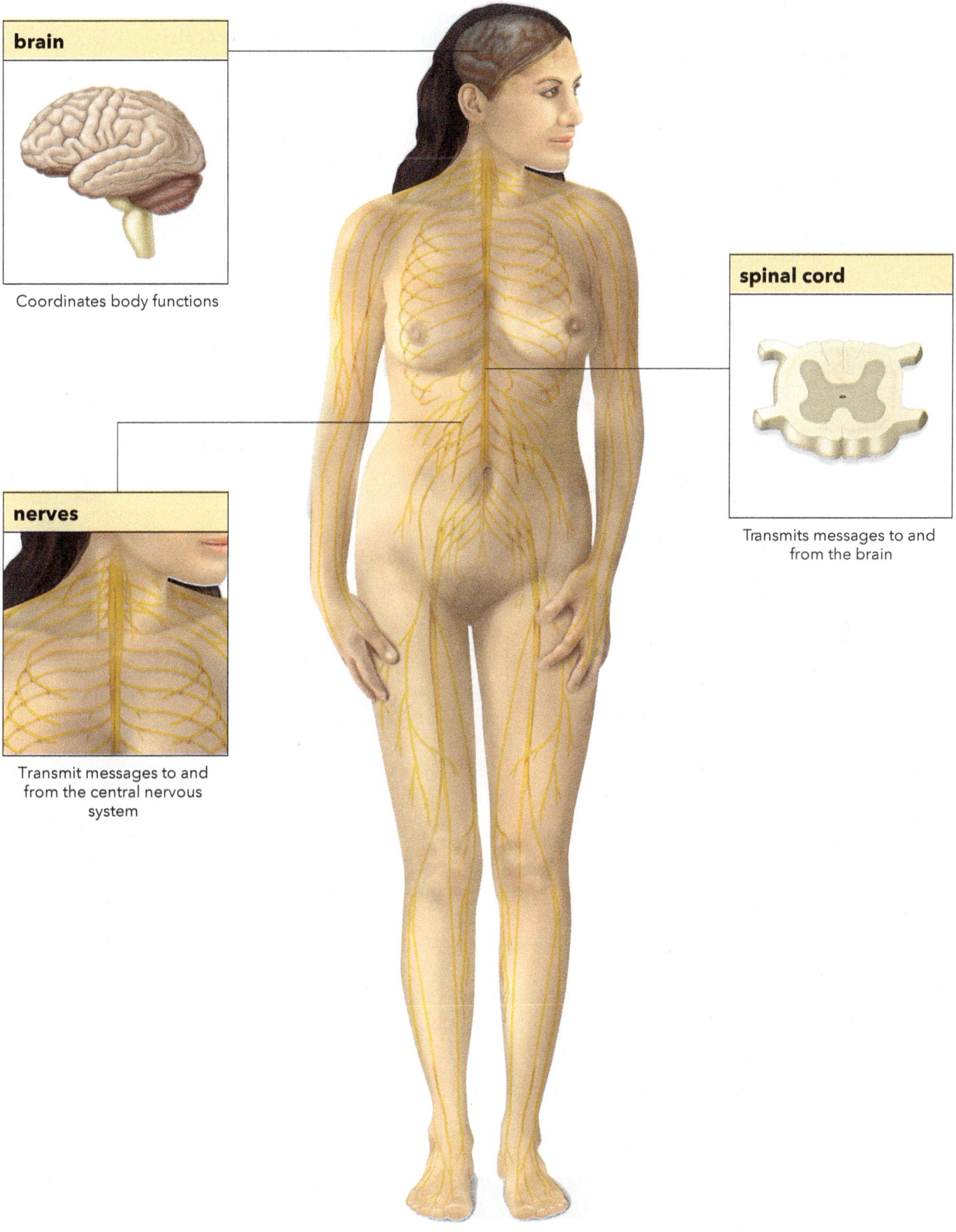

Digestive System

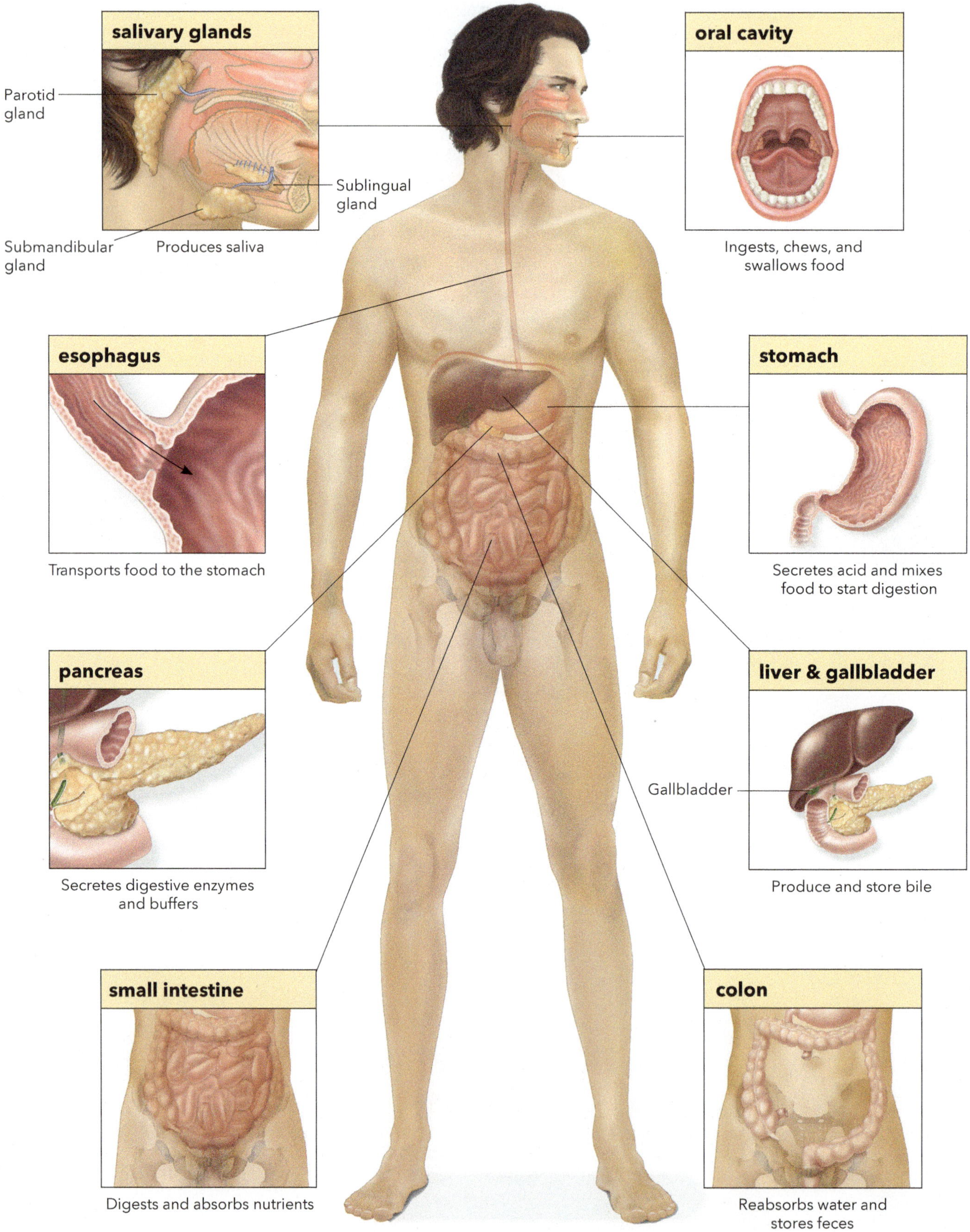

Integumentary System

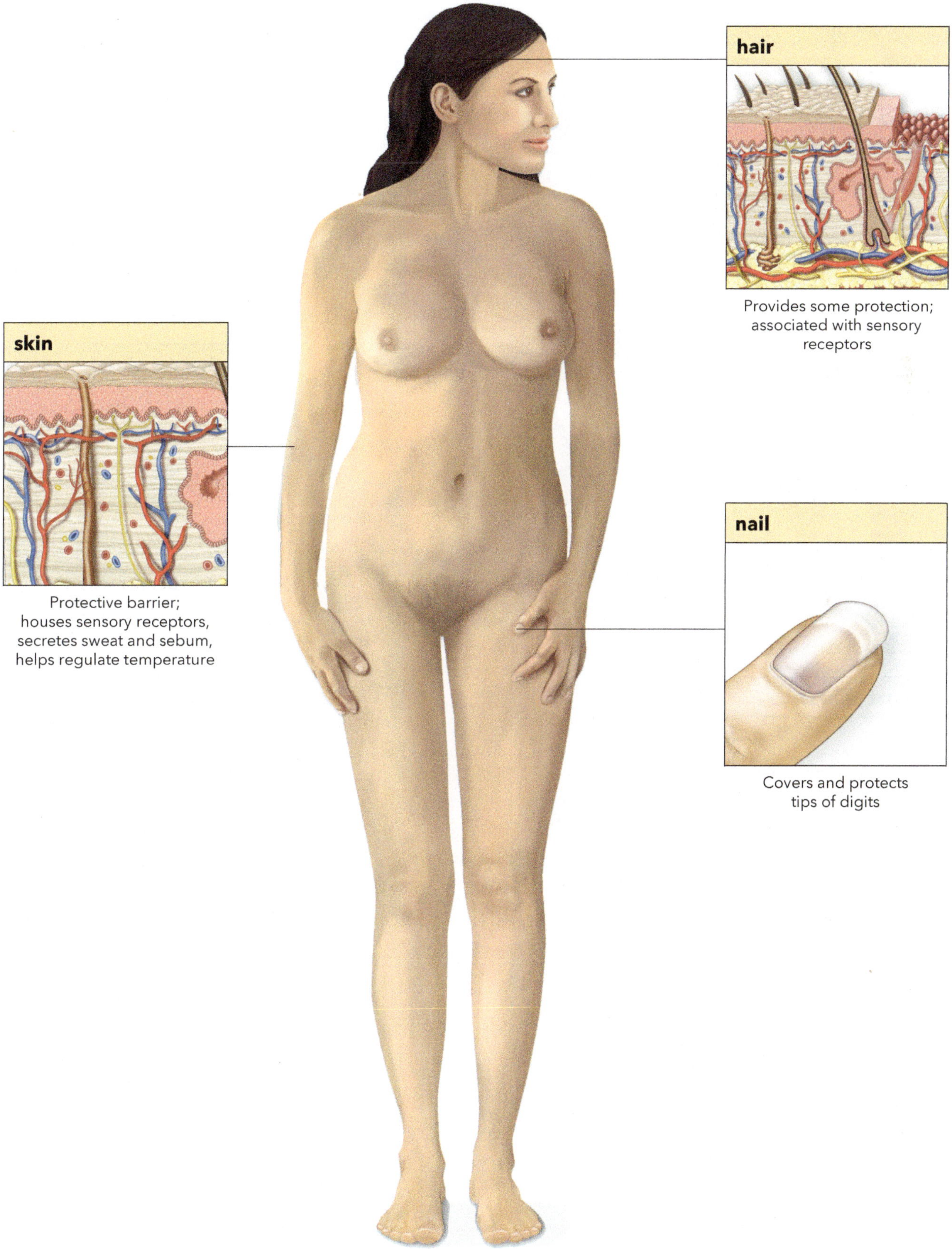

Endocrine System

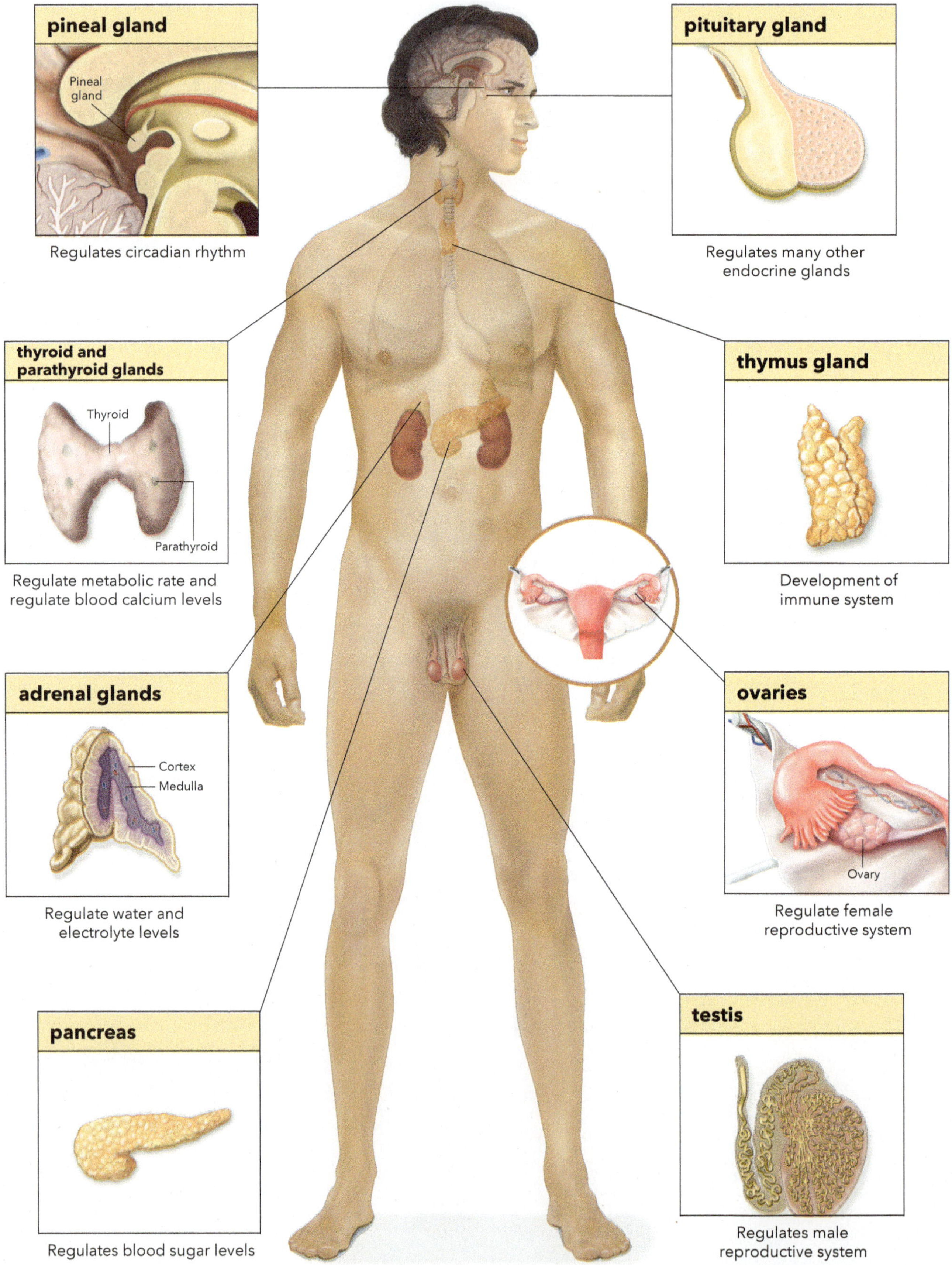

Renal System

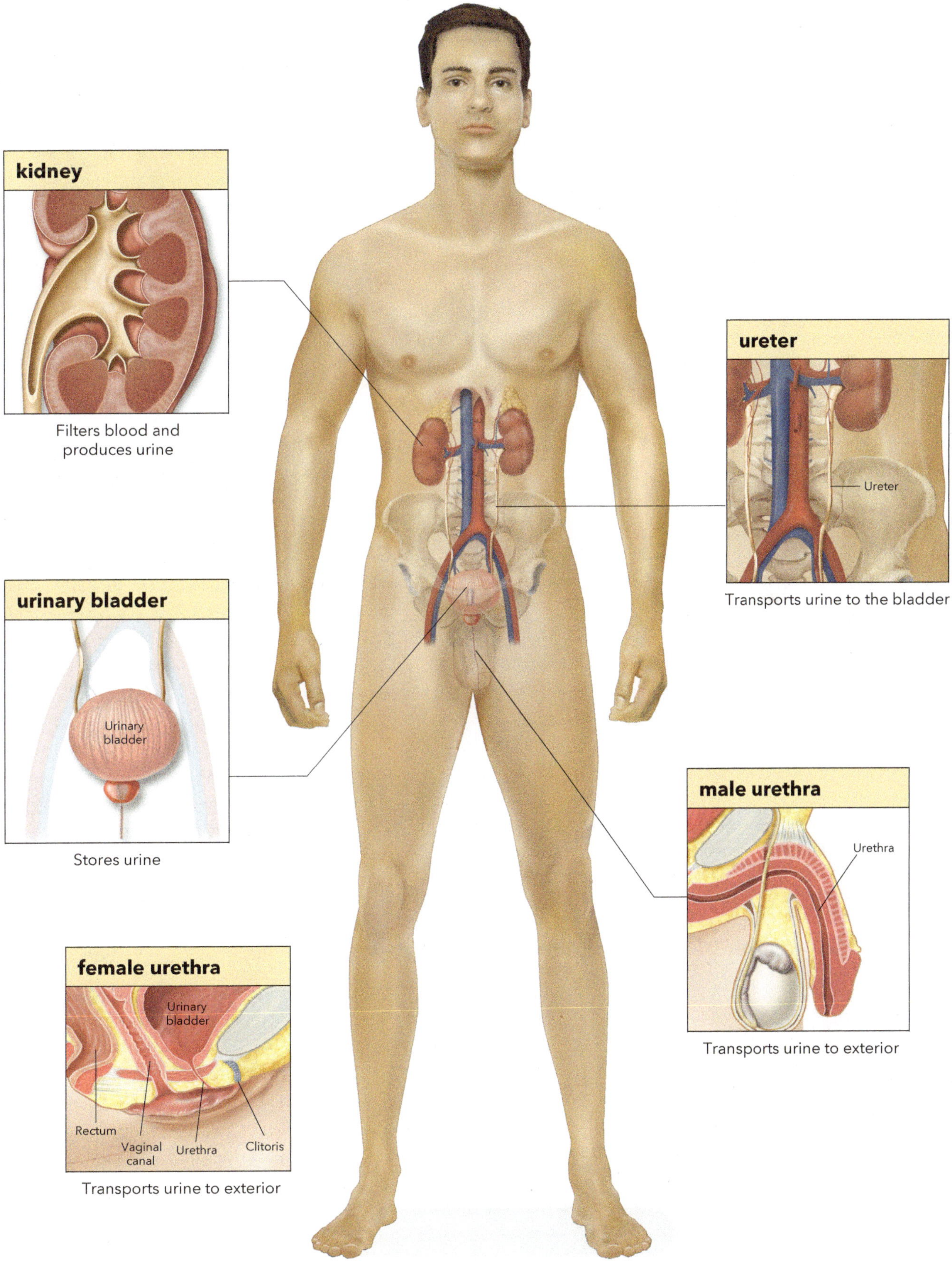

Male Reproductive System

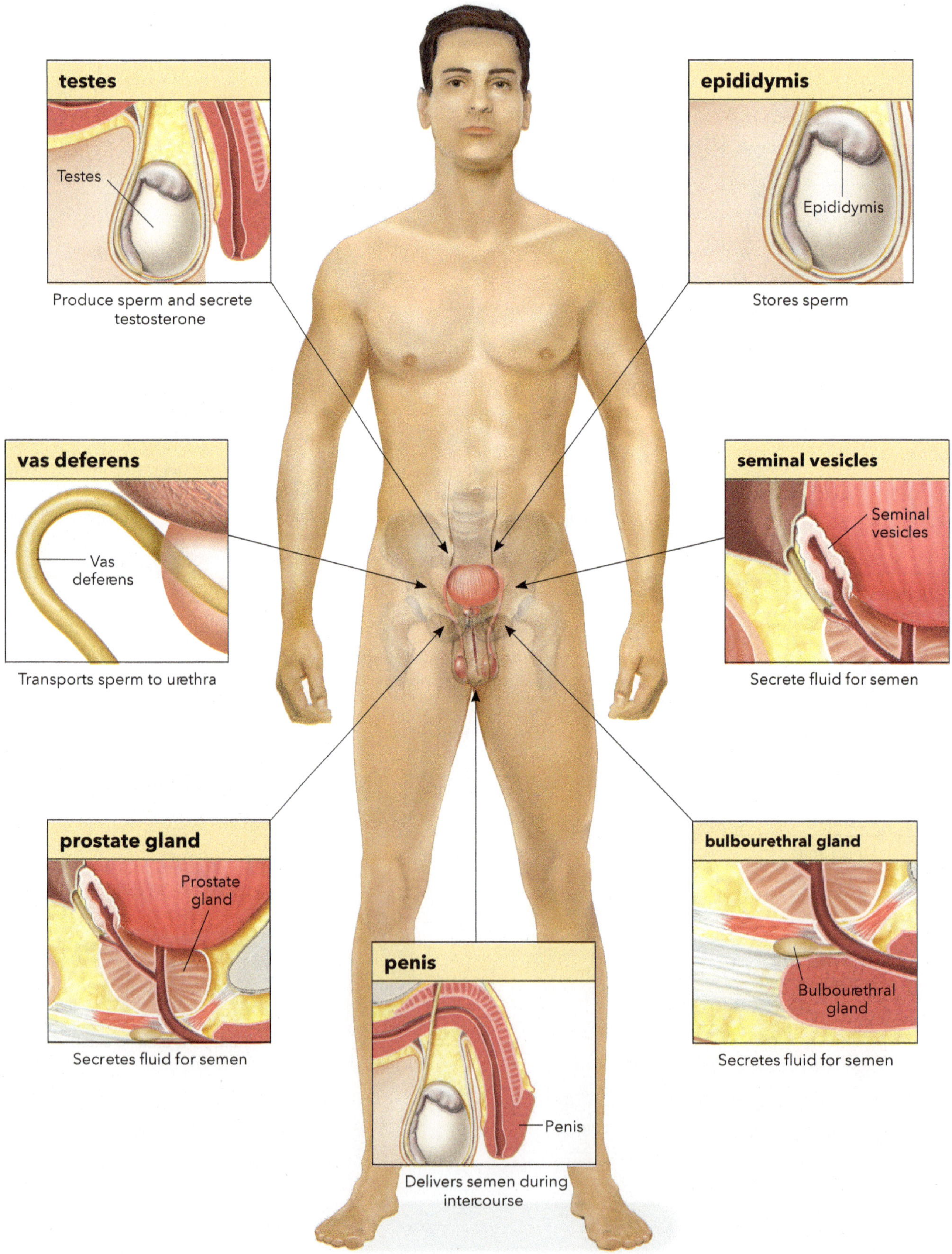

Female Reproductive System

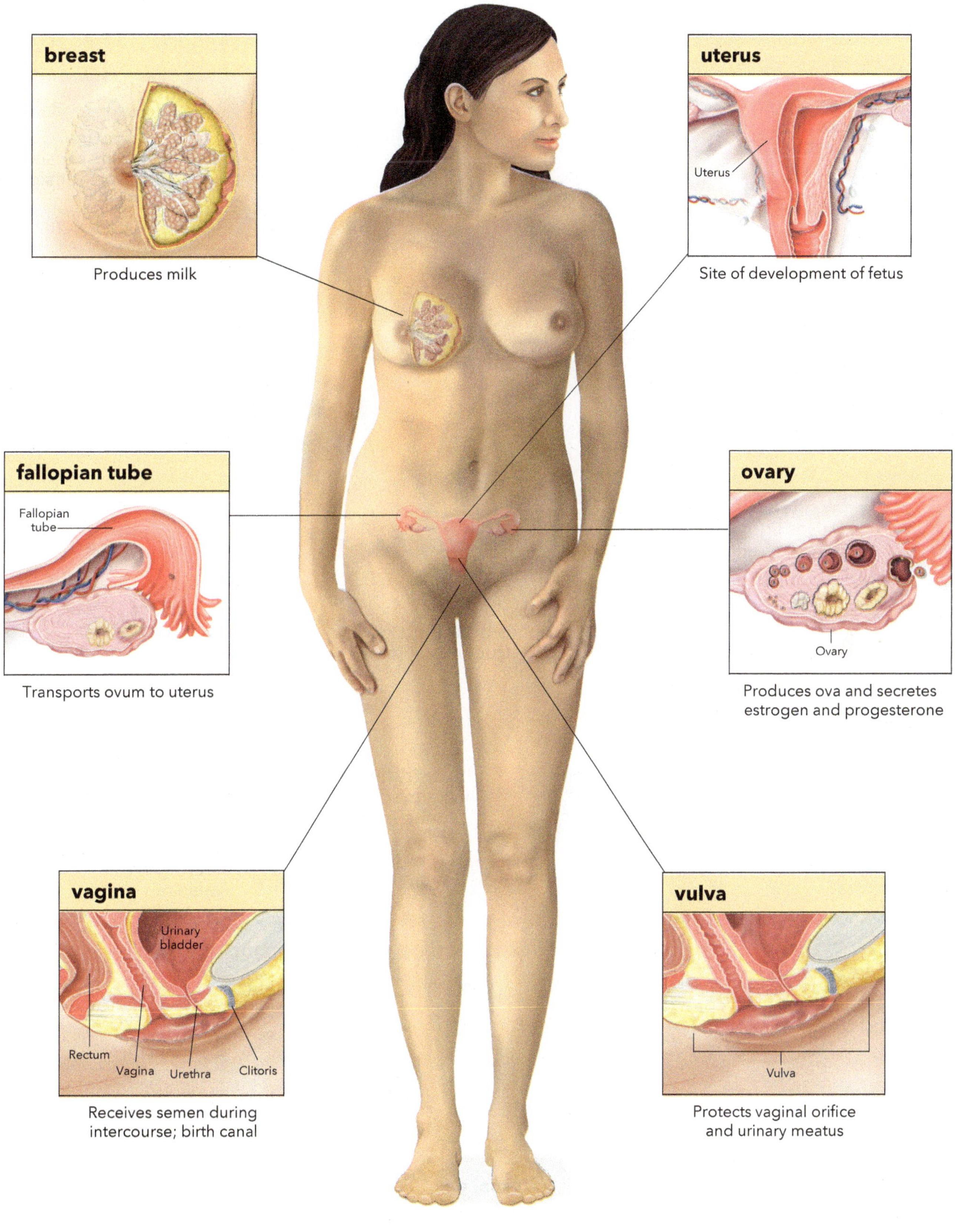

Special Senses

The Eye

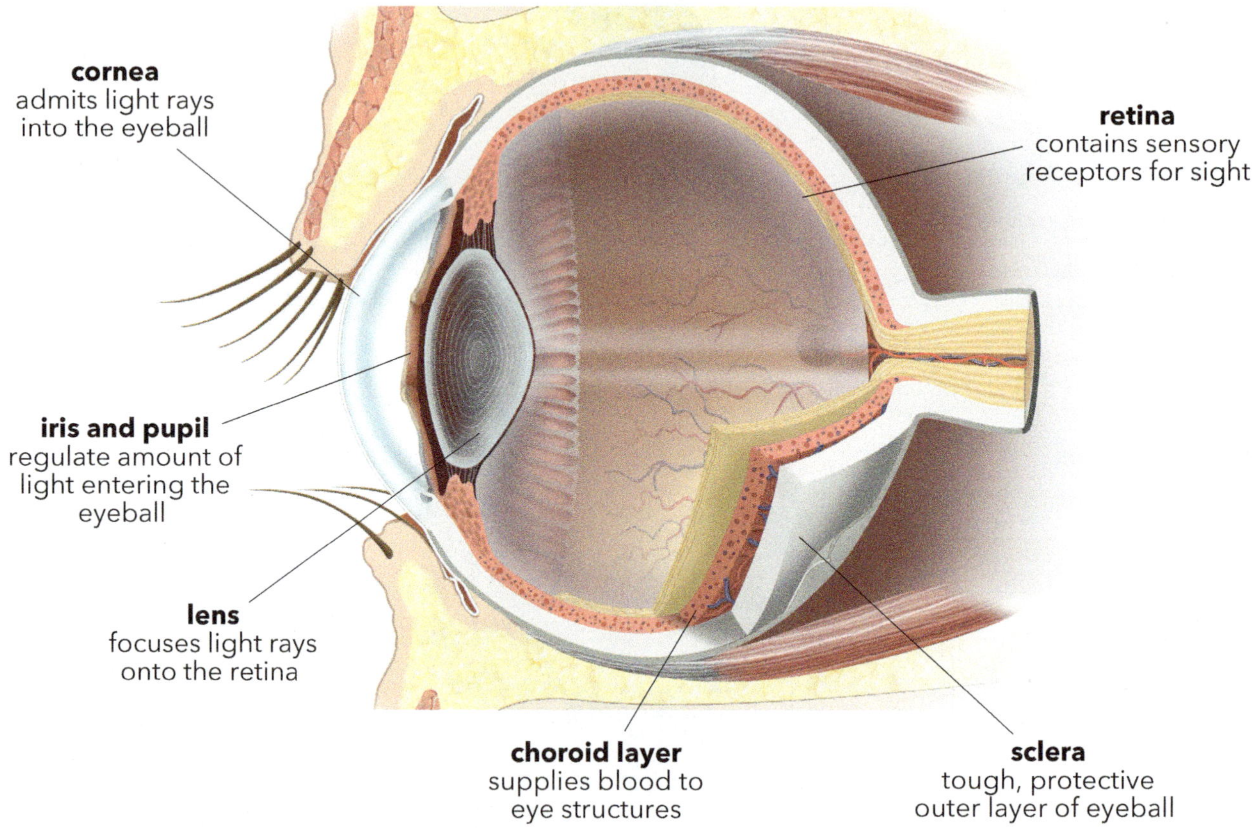

The Ear

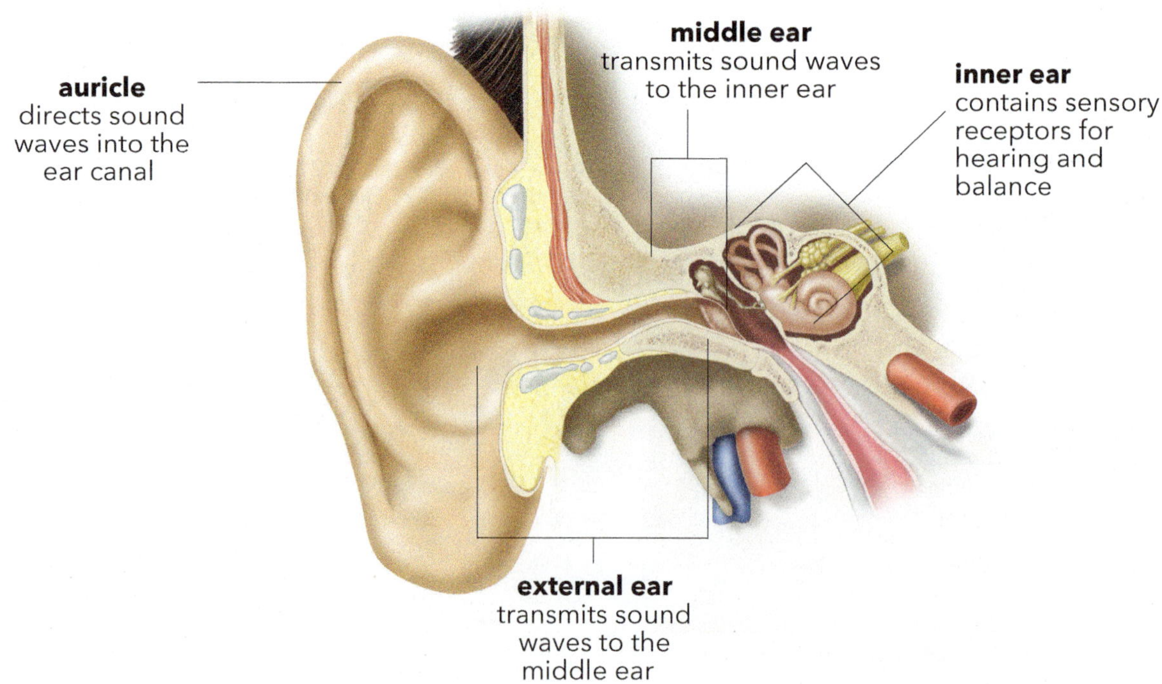

Answer Key

The following are text questions and answers/discussion suggestions for Think Like an EMT, a feature within the narrative, and for end-of-chapter Short Answer questions, Critical Thinking Exercises, Pathophysiology to Practice questions, and Street Scene questions.

CHAPTER 1 Introduction to Emergency Medical Services

Think Like an EMT—A Key Concept

1. There are several pieces of information you must gather to determine which hospital is most appropriate for your patient. For example, is the patient requesting transport to a particular hospital because his physician practices there? Whenever possible, try to make provisions for patient choice. Or is the patient's condition too unstable to bypass a closer facility in favor of a hospital a little farther away? In many cases your local jurisdiction will have specific policies or guidelines that direct patient transport and hospital destination. These policies often include provisions for transporting patients to specialty centers such as burn and trauma centers. Hospitals are increasingly specializing in managing certain areas of care, such as cardiac and stroke emergencies, thus transport to these facilities should always be considered under the direction of local policy or medical control.
2. Rendering care to your patient, especially something invasive such as medication administration, requires the completion of a comprehensive physical assessment and patient history in conjunction with understanding how these findings relate to the patient's medical or traumatic emergencies. Understanding the risks and benefits of the treatment you provide and basing your decisions on the facts and evidence revealed during your assessment of the patient will help you develop a treatment plan that meets the needs of the patient without doing harm.

Short Answer

1. The components of the EMS system are 911 and Emergency Medical Dispatchers, Emergency Medical Responders, EMTs (all levels) and ambulances, emergency department, and other hospital units.
2. Special designations of hospitals include trauma centers, burn centers, pediatric care centers, cardiac centers, and stroke centers. EMT students should become familiar with those available in their region; asking your EMT instructor what they are is a good place to start.
3. The four national levels of EMS training and certification are Emergency Medical Responder (EMR), Emergency Medical Technician (EMT), Advanced Emergency Medical Technician (AEMT), and Paramedic.
4. The roles and responsibilities of the EMT include personal safety, and safety for the crew, patient, and bystanders; working with other public safety professionals; patient assessment; patient care; lifting and moving; transport; transfer of care; patient advocacy; and promotion of public health and safety.
5. Some of the desirable personal and physical attributes of the EMT include being in good health and able to lift and carry up to 125 pounds; having good eyesight and hearing; being able to clearly communicate in written and oral forms; and being pleasant, sincere, cooperative, resourceful, a self-starter, emotionally stable, able to lead, and neat and clean. Additionally the EMT should be of good moral character, be in control of any personal habits that may detract from patient care, and consistently be nonjudgmental and fair to all patients.
6. Quality improvement is a process of continual self-review with the purpose of identifying and correcting aspects of the system that require improvement.
7. The difference between on-line and off-line medical direction is that in on-line medical direction, the on-duty physician gives orders directly to the EMT by telephone or radio. In off-line medical direction, the EMT carries out written standing orders from the Medical Director.

Critical Thinking Exercises

1. The desirable personal traits that EMTs should strive to exemplify include a pleasant, sincere, and cooperative attitude around patients and customers. Being able to step up as a leader and remain emotionally stable during stressful situations is important. Effective listening and communication skills are essential if you want to be successful in the health care industry. Because your patients come from such a diverse population of different cultures and backgrounds–many of which may be different from your own–it is critical that you are open-minded and nonjudgmental of your patients and the people you care for. You can strive to incorporate these traits into your everyday care by thinking about them daily and approaching each patient (regardless of the circumstances) with the same attitude.
2. You can continually refresh your knowledge and skill performance by taking advantage of conferences, seminars, lectures, classes, videos, and demonstrations. The EMT can take advantage of online web-based learning when working in remote locations. Additionally, EMTs can review literature and study evidence-based research that pertains to emergency care.

Street Scene Questions

1. Chuck Hartley should involve the new EMT in all aspects of the job. For example, a new EMT should help check the ambulance and equipment at the start of the shift. Chuck should also provide an explanation of operating procedures, such as the standing orders under which they operate. In other words, new EMTs need to know what is expected of them if they are to perform as expected.
2. Chuck exhibits numerous unprofessional behavior characteristics, such as an unkempt uniform, telling the new EMT to sit until he is needed, failure to introduce himself to the patient, using insulting or derogatory terms such as "hon" in addressing the patient, loudly criticizing the new EMT in front of others, and dismissal of patient concerns, such as instructing her to "tell it to the doctor."
3. The characteristics you should expect from someone providing initial field training might include the following:
   - Good communication skills
   - Neat and well-kept appearance
   - Polite and courteous behavior, both with other EMTs and with patients
   - Willingness to explain the job
   - Understanding the needs of a new EMT (empathy)
   - Good patient skills
   - Willingness to act as a team player
4. Susan Miller came to work in a well-pressed uniform. She expressed an obvious interest in and memory of the new EMT and communicated job expectations in a clear manner. She set an example by providing an orientation to the ambulance, equipment, and EMS agency procedures. She made the new intern a part of the call and provided numerous examples of professional patient care. She monitored actions taken by the new EMT, making every effort not to belittle the person.
5. Susan establishes a good professional standard and served as a role model for the EMT to follow. The student intern will have a much more positive experience in that type of learning environment.
6. There are many personal traits that you should work to develop as a professional EMT, such as always striving to be pleasant, sincere, cooperative, neat, respectful, and a good listener.

CHAPTER 2 Well-Being of the EMT

Think Like an EMT—Standard Precautions

1. through 5. For discussion: The EMT should be able to anticipate similar situations that would necessitate these and other Standard Precautions.

Short Answer

1. Acute stress happens suddenly, as might be seen after handling a serious pediatric call or a major catastrophe. Delayed stress, otherwise known as Posttraumatic stress disorder (PTSD) is a stress reaction that occurs to a person days, months, or even years from the inciting event. Finally, cumulative stress reaction, or burnout, is not triggered by a single critical incident but instead results from sustained, recurring low-level stressors–possibly in more than one aspect of one's life–and develops over a period of years.
2. Some situations that may cause stress for an EMT include multiple-casualty incidents, emergencies involving infants and children, severe injuries, abuse and neglect, the death of a coworker, or personal situations unrelated to work.
3. eSCAPe is a conceptual way to deal with posttraumatic stress. The lowercase "**e**'s" at the beginning and end of the word stand for *every patient* and *every time*. **S** reminds us that social support is important to avoid feelings of isolation. **C** is a reminder to give choices to patients so they have a sense of control. **A** stands for anticipating events for the patient to reduce anxiety. **P** stands for helping the patient to plan and organize. The eSCAPe process can be used with fellow EMTs as well, lessening the impact of emotional trauma.
4. The different stages or responses a person may exhibit when confronted with death and dying include: denial–the patient denies the fact that he is dying; anger–the patient becomes angry about the situation; bargaining–the patient tries to postpone death, even if only briefly; depression–the patient is sad or in despair over things left undone; and acceptance–the patient is ready to die. Understanding what the families and the patients go through can help EMTs deal with the stress they feel as well as their own emotions during this time, so they can provide the best care possible to the patient and/or family.
5. Examples of personal protective equipment include: protective gloves–used whenever assessing a patient to protect from blood, mucous, secretions, controlled bleeding, suctioning, artificial ventilation, and CPR; eye protection–used with splashing, spattering, or spraying body fluids; masks–used with infections spread by airborne droplets (such as measles); and gowns–used with arterial bleeding and childbirth.

Critical Thinking Exercises

Unless you stay safe yourself, you will not be able to help your patient and you may suffer serious injury–or die. Retreat to a safe place and call for a response by law enforcement. Approach the patient only when law enforcement informs you the scene is safe. It is important for the EMT to always realize that no matter how serious the situation may seem, the first priority is to care for oneself and keep at a safe distance until authorized to enter the scene by police.

Pathophysiology to Practice

1. Common colds, viruses, and influenza are typically spread by tiny droplets when an infected person breathes, coughs, or sneezes on or near you. These "bugs" (otherwise known as pathogens) can also be transmitted by touching something contaminated, then touching your nose or eyes.
2. The body's response to stress is to activate the sympathetic nervous system. This causes an increased heart rate, increased respiratory rate and dilated bronchial passages, and an increased blood pressure. All of this is part of the body's compensatory mechanism to handle the stress. Although the stress response can be beneficial in the short order, long term or continued stress can start to have a detrimental effect on one's body and mind.
3. The difference between good stress (eustress) and bad stress (distress) on the body often comes down to one's own resistance and ability to cope with stress. Stress impacts different people differently; for example, two EMTs on the same call may have opposite responses. More simply, the stress of jogging two miles will obviously have a much different impact on the body than the cumulative stress of running back-to-back multiple-casualty incidents.

Street Scene Questions

1. It's essential for you to wear protective gloves on this call because the patient has bad facial injuries that may bring you into contact with blood and other body fluids. Gloves help minimize possible exposure to bloodborne pathogens. Intact skin can offer some protection in case of accidental exposure. In this case, however, you are aware of a partially healed cut on the hand, making the potential risk of exposure even greater if no gloves are worn.
2. Occupational injuries and exposures often don't seem like a big deal–until they happen to you. Don't underestimate the devastating effects of occupational exposure, especially the possibility of transferring a disease to family members and/or fellow EMS workers. In addition, occupational exposure can cause considerable anxiety as EMTs wait to determine if they have actually contracted the disease, especially because during this time they will often take powerful prophylactic medications with significant side effects.
3. Anytime a potential exposure occurs, it is critical to immediately notify your supervisor. This is not the time to hide the incident or minimize what occurred. Supervisory personnel are typically trained to manage just these situations and determine the extent of the exposure. It is always better to be safe than sorry, which may include an occupational evaluation at the emergency department, physical examination, and baseline blood tests.
4. The anxiety of waiting for test results is often the worst part of an occupational exposure. This anxiety can lead to a strained marital relationship as your family will be justifiably concerned if you could somehow infect them, and tension with coworkers can develop from an inability to talk about the situation, out of either fear or embarrassment.
5. Hand washing is a first-line defense against infection. Even though you wear gloves, you must still wash your hands after your gloves are removed. In fact, it is recommended that the EMT wash their hands before an emergency, use hand sanitizer after removing your gloves, and then wash your hands with soap and water as soon as it is possible to.
6. At a minimum, all EMTs should have two sets of gloves and eye protection immediately available. Wear the gloves and eye protection on every patient encounter. The second pair of gloves can be used if you notice a hole in your first pair, or the first pair rips during patient contact. Gowns and additional protective gear (masks, etc.) may be necessary depending on your assessment of the situation and should be readily available on the ambulance.

CHAPTER 3 Lifting and Moving Patients

Think Like an EMT—Choosing a Patient-Carrying Device

1. A patient complaining of severe respiratory distress in an upstairs back bedroom should probably be moved by a stair chair unless his difficulty breathing is so severe that he can't sit up or he requires ventilation. In those situations, a Reeves-type stretcher is a better option.
2. A patient thrown from an ATV several hundred yards into the woods has likely suffered a significant mechanism of injury and should be placed on a long spine board (i.e. backboard). The patient should be fully secured with spinal motion restriction precautions taken. Then, the "packaged" patient can be placed in a Stokes (wire frame) basket for extrication.
3. The patient would most likely placed and secured on a long spine board (or a "backboard"), with full spinal motion restrictions taken prior to movement. Some EMS systems may have protocol which indicates to remove the patient from the backboard before transport, and secure the patent to the stretcher. Others may recommend transport with the patient on the backboard. The ultimate decision is made at the local level, but the EMT should use techniques and equipment that gets the patient safely from his location of injury to the ambulance.
4. An unresponsive medical patient found down in a narrow hallway would likely benefit from rapid extrication using a Reeves-type device, allowing two EMTs to carry the patient out of the hallway to the stretcher. A stair chair may also be an option you can employ to move the patient based on the dynamics of the building you are in.

Short Answer

1. Body mechanics is the proper use of the body to facilitate lifting and moving. Principles of body mechanics include:
   - Position your feet properly, shoulder width apart.
   - When lifting, use your legs, not your back, to do the lifting.
   - When lifting, never twist or attempt to make any moves other than the lift.
   - When lifting with one hand, do not compensate by tilting your body in the opposite direction while walking.
   - Keep the weight as close to your body as possible.
   - When carrying a patient on stairs, use a stair chair instead of a stretcher whenever possible.
2. A number of situations may require the emergency move of a patient, including when the scene is hazardous, when care of life-threatening conditions requires repositioning, such as putting a patient on a hard surface to perform CPR. Finally, when other patients must be reached for immediate treatment, such as moving the driver out of a wrecked vehicle so you can reach a critically injured patient inside the car.
3. Lifts include the extremity lift, the direct ground lift, the draw-sheet method, and the direct carry method. Drags include the shoulder drag, the foot drag, the "fireman's drag," the incline drag, the clothes drag, and the blanket drag.
4. A long-axis drag is a drag from the shoulders of the patient that causes the remainder of the body to assume its natural anatomical position, with the spine and all limbs in normal alignment. This emergency move minimizes or prevents aggravation of a spinal injury.

Critical Thinking Exercises

1. A patient who has fallen 18 feet with suspected spinal injuries should be lifted and moved with a long spine board, during which the patient should have complete spinal motion restriction techniques employed.
2. A patient with chest pain and no spine injury who lives on an upper floor of a building with no elevator should be moved with a stair chair. This is the safest way to remove him from the building. Caution should be exercised by the EMTs since they are using stairs, and always remain in constant verbal contact with the patient to help alleviate any fears of this type of move.
3. A patient found in an environment where there is risk of immediate explosion should be moved emergently with a shoulder drag. This will allow the EMT to begin rendering care at a location which is not a risk for injury.

Street Scene Questions

1. Remove the patient from the vehicle by applying a cervical collar after conducting the necessary neurologic exams. Then the patient should be rotated in the seat and placed onto a long spine board for movement.
2. When using extrication devices, keep in mind that they can have a negative impact on the patient's airway or breathing and can cause significant patient discomfort. The cervical collar should not be applied too tightly and board straps should not restrict the patient's respirations.
3. The key to moving any patient, especially in an extrication, is a well-coordinated team effort. The EMT providing manual cervical spine motion restriction is responsible for announcing all the moves. For example, this EMT might say, "Slide the patient onto the long board on the count of three." The crew must continually monitor the patient, especially the A-B-Cs and any change in the level of consciousness. A quick neurologic exam should be done both before and after the move.
4. In this scenario, the equipment included a cervical collar, a long spine board, straps, head immobilizer, stretcher, and stretcher-locking device. The equipment was selected based on the mechanism of injury and for maximum patient safety to protect against possible neck or spinal injury.
5. Current practice is that the long spine board should be used as a short-term transportation device to remove a patient from the immediate scene to the stretcher, rather than for long-term immobilization. Long-term immobilization on a rigid backboard may cause breathing problems and unnecessary discomfort for the patient.
6. By the time the patient reaches the hospital, the EMTs will have moved the patient five times. 1) They rotated the patient onto the long spine board. 2) They transported the patient on the backboard to a stretcher at the ambulance. 3) They removed the patient from the backboard and onto the wheeled stretcher for transport to the hospital. 4) Once at the hospital, they removed the wheeled stretcher from the ambulance and transported the patient into an exam room. 5) In the exam room, the EMTs transferred the patient from the EMS wheeled cot to a hospital bed.

CHAPTER 4 Medical, Legal, and Ethical Issues

Think Like an EMT—Ethical Dilemmas

1. Overhearing a colleague admit to a serious clinical error means that you have an ethical responsibility to tell the truth about what you heard. If this event isn't reported, harm could come to the patient. While reporting fellow EMTs is not popular, it might be possible to talk to the provider who made the mistake and encourage him to tell the

truth rather than having you bring it to light. Ultimately, the paramedic likely needs additional education on drug calculations or drug administration and will not receive help if no one is aware of the error.

2. First, driving with any alcohol in your system should be avoided at all cost. However, attempting to provide care while you are intoxicated, even if there is not a lot of alcohol in your system, is still a recipe for disaster. Considering the alcohol content of the drinks and how long ago you had them will help to determine if you are intoxicated. Some recommend not stopping if you have consumed any alcohol. How would you feel as a patient if you smelled alcohol on the breath of an EMT treating you?
3. A patient is telling you a suspicious story. Unfortunately, you have no way of knowing if the patient is even telling the truth. Most would recommend reporting this to the police. Follow your local guidelines and protocols and consider discussing this concern with your supervisor to learn how the EMS system handles these types of concerns.

Short Answer

1. The difference between expressed and implied consent is significant because a patient offering expressed consent is an adult who is mentally competent, has the capacity to make decisions, is informed of the risks associated with the care the patient is about to receive, and is conveying a conscious decision to receive the care. In implied consent, patients are typically unconscious or incapacitated in some way such that you must assume they would agree to be treated if they were conscious.
2. A finding of negligence requires that all of the following circumstances be proved: The EMT had a duty to the patient (duty to act); the EMT did not provide the standard of care (committed a breach of duty); and by not providing the standard of care, the EMT caused harm to the patient (proximate causation). The harm can be physical or psychological.
3. Your first priority is always patient care, but it is still possible to preserve evidence and minimize your impact on the scene during the course of your actions. It is important to prioritize patient care, as the patient may have life-threatening injuries. However, your actions within the scene should be as controlled as possible and still preserve good patient care, so that any evidence that may be present is still usable by the police. Additionally, doing a scene size-up will provide you with information to give to law enforcement, especially if you were the first person on scene. Whenever possible and appropriate, work closely with law enforcement.
4. If an EMT has initiated care and then leaves a patient without ensuring the patient has been turned over to someone with equal or higher training, it constitutes abandonment. The fact that this patient was left in a hospital bed doesn't matter; there must still be a transfer of care to a person (not to a location).
5. Leaving a copy of the patient care report on the bulletin board at the station for everyone to review is a violation of the HIPAA law. Any information you obtain about a patient's history, condition, or treatment is considered confidential and must not be shared with anyone else. Sharing the information with another caregiver involved with the continuing care of the patient (such as the nurse receiving the patient at the hospital) is allowed, but tacking a run report up on a bulletin board for all crews (and potentially visitors at the station) to see is illegal.

Critical Thinking Exercises

1. This may not fit the strict definition of "duty to act" because you were not officially dispatched to this call and it is not in your primary EMS response area. However, you still have a moral and ethical obligation to render aid, since you are on duty and you are trained providers. In general, if you follow your conscience and provide care, you will incur less liability than if you do not act. Always follow your local protocols and laws. For this specific situation, contact your dispatchers so they can notify local EMS and police about the accident.
2. Think back to your care of the patient and your actions on the call. Were the actions of your crew so obviously responsible for the patient's death that a lawsuit is in order? Does *res ipsa loquitur* apply? If not, evaluate your care and actions on the call against the tests of negligence: (1) Did you have a duty to act? (2) Did you provide the standard of care or commit a breach of duty? (3) If you failed to provide the standard of care, did your actions cause harm to the patient (also known as proximate causation)? In order for negligence to be proven, all factors must apply.
3. A critical decision such as withholding CPR should not be made based on hearsay; it should be made based on a legal document. Without the actual DNR present, you should continue CPR and consider making contact with medical direction for further guidance.

Street Scene Questions

1. Radio transmissions can be easily monitored by a curious public, so you should share over the radio only information that is directly related to immediate care. In this particular situation, the presence of infectious disease has no direct bearing on the care steps initiated in the field. As a result, the hospital staff does not need to be notified at the time of the radio report.
2. All patient information should be treated as confidential and should not be released except with written permission, to continue care of the patient, or upon request by legal subpoena. It's very simple: It's the law and you must abide by it.
3. The fact that the patient has AIDS is definitely part of her medical history and should be shared, discreetly, with the staff member receiving the patient at the hospital. Keep in mind that if this very private information about the patient becomes public against her wishes, it may impact more than just her treatment. There are many areas where AIDS discrimination still occurs in employment and housing.

4. Informing all of the hospital staff of the patient's condition is highly inappropriate, and the patient's condition is irrelevant, because infection control precautions should be the standard in any medical institution and should not rely on information supplied by an EMT. You assume every patient you encounter has the potential to be an occupational exposure and so you approach every patient encounter the same: with Standard Precautions.
5. Sharing the patient's health history with other EMS providers constitutes a breach of patient confidentiality. Not only is this action inappropriate, but sharing information may carry some legal consequences, especially if it has a negative impact on the patient.
6. The principles of patient confidentiality can be described very simply: If there is not a need to know, then don't share it. In other words, if a colleague is not directly involved in patient care, then that colleague has no need to know anything about the patient or the patient's information. This standard applies to personnel at the hospital, fire department, police department, and of course members of the public and media. It is your professional responsibility to protect the patient's information from breach of confidentiality. Failure to do so could mean civil and criminal penalties.

CHAPTER 5 Medical Terminology

Short Answer

1. The following anatomical terms are defined as:
   - Medial: toward the midline of the body
     Lateral: to the side, away from the midline of the body
   - Anterior: the front of the body or body part
     Posterior: the back of the body or body part
   - Proximal: closer to the torso
     Distal: farther away from the torso
2. Two prefixes that mean "below" are *brady-* and *hypo-*.
3. Two suffixes that mean "pertaining to" are *-ac* and *-al*.
4. *Prone* means lying on the abdomen. *Supine* means lying on the back.
5. The midaxillary line extends vertically from the center of the armpit through the ankle.
6. The abdominal quadrants are formed by imaginary horizontal and vertical lines drawn through the navel to form right upper, left upper, right lower, and left lower quadrants.
7. *Palmar* refers to the palm of the hand.

Critical Thinking Exercises

The patient has a laceration on his lateral left arm originating at his shoulder and extending distally to his elbow. He has another laceration on the medial aspect of his left arm just proximal to the wrist. He has an open, angulated mid-shaft injury to the left femur with the bone ends protruding through the skin overlying his left leg.

Street Scene Questions

1. Knowledge of medical terminology helps you to form and recall concepts of the patient's anatomy. This knowledge will also help guide your assessment and care and will be the basis of a correctly worded oral report on the patient's condition during transport.
2. The patient feels pain in the center of his chest.
3. Pain in the left upper quadrant is located above the belly button (navel).
4. The upper part of the humerus, the long bone of the upper arm, is injured and possibly broken.
5. There is a penetrating soft tissue wound to the left axilla.
6. Breath sounds are present to the right thorax only, breath sounds on the left are absent.

CHAPTER 6 Anatomy and Physiology

Think Like an EMT—Identifying Possible Areas of Injury

1. A patient who has fractured the bones of the arm just above the wrist has likely broken the radius and ulna.
2. Located in the upper left quadrant of the abdomen, the spleen is a solid organ that is often injured in blunt trauma and can cause severe internal bleeding.
3. The large bone in the thigh is the femur. Because this is the largest bone in the body, blood loss can be significant and can exceed 1 liter.

Short Answer

1. The musculoskeletal system functions to give the body shape, to protect vital internal organs, and the joints are formed in such a way that with muscular contraction, it allows for body movement.
2. The five divisions of the spine and their locations are:
   - Cervical: neck (supports the head)
   - Thoracic: upper back (ribs attached to each vertebra)

- Lumbar: lower back (bears the majority of the body's weight)
- Sacral: posterior pelvis (forms the posterior portion of the pelvic bone)
- Coccyx: distal spine (originates from the sacral region)

3. During inhalation, the muscles of the rib cage and the diaphragm contract. The diaphragm lowers, and the ribs move upward and outward, which expands the chest and creates a negative pressure inside the chest cavity that pulls air into the lungs. During exhalation, the intercostal muscles and the diaphragm relax. The ribs move downward and inward, while the diaphragm rises, causing the chest to decrease in size and positive pressure to build inside the chest cavity, which pushes air out of the lungs.
4. The four places where a peripheral pulse may be palpated are the radial artery, brachial artery, carotid artery, and femoral artery. It can also be felt at the popliteal fossa, dorsalis pedis, and posterior tibial locations.
5. The central nervous system is composed of the brain and the spinal cord. The brain receives information from the body and, in turn, sends impulses to different areas of the body to respond to internal and external changes. The spinal cord rests within the spinal column and stretches from the brain to the lumbar vertebrae. Nerves branch from each part of the cord and reach throughout the body. The peripheral nervous system consists of two types of nerves: sensory and motor. The sensory nerves pick up information from throughout the body and transmit it to the spinal cord and brain. The motor nerves carry messages from the brain to the body. Finally, the 12 pairs of cranial nerves, which originate on the brain, are also considered to be part of the peripheral nervous system. Some cranial nerves may be motor or sensory only. Other cranial nerves carry both sensory and motor innervation.
6. The functions of the skin participates in include protection, water balance, temperature regulation, excretion, and shock absorption.

Critical Thinking Exercises

The wound at the nipple level and mid-clavicular line is likely to affect the heart and lungs. The wound to the right upper quadrant may affect the liver, gallbladder, and kidney. The wound to the center of the left upper quadrant may affect the tip of the liver, kidney, pancreas, spleen, and possibly the stomach or intestines.

Street Scene Questions

1. Knowledge of the patient's anatomy will help guide your assessment and care. The mechanism of injury will point to anatomic locations of potential injury. Understanding underlying structures will help you predict the potential damage and its severity. Understanding airway anatomy and physiology will help you manage the airway better. Pediatric anatomy will also have to be considered, as there are many anatomical differences between a child and an adult such as a proportionally larger tongue than an adult (which may occlude the airway) or proportionately larger heads in infants/children, which further strain the cervical vertebrae and can allow for easier head/brain injuries.
2. When assessing the child's abdomen, be alert for signs of internal bleeding such as bruising, puncture wounds, abdominal guarding or rigidity, pain, and tenderness.
3. The child's decreased mental status is significant. He also had an airway problem that you corrected. Furthermore, his abdominal assessment points to additional underlying injuries and the potential for internal bleeding.
4. Altered mental status can have many causes. It could be caused by internal bleeding from the abdomen or it could be a traumatic brain injury. Consider also other fractures and wounds associated with high-energy trauma.

CHAPTER 7 Principles of Pathophysiology

Think Like an EMT—Why is Her Heart Beating Rapidly?

This scenario serves as a reminder of how calling on your knowledge of pathophysiology can help you as you consider not only what the patient's physical findings are (including vital signs) but also what may be going on inside the patient's body to cause these findings. It allows you to develop an index of suspicion about what the injuries may be and how they can present . . . such as finding tachycardia from a possible internal bleed.

Short Answer

1. Metabolism is the conversion of glucose and other nutrients into energy in the form of adenosine triphosphate (ATP), which is the energy the cells of the body need to operate normally. Necessary components to the creation of ATP include oxygen and glucose.
2. Three types of respiratory dysfunction are disruption of respiratory control, disruption of pressure in the thorax, and disruption of lung tissue. Disruption of respiratory control occurs when the brain fails to appropriately control breathing. Without regulatory messages being sent, breathing can cease or become ineffective. Disruption of pressure occurs when the integrity of the chest cavity is broken and air passes in and out through the chest wall. This interferes with the pressure changes necessary to move air in and out through the glottic opening and often causes lung collapse. Disruption of lung tissue occurs when lung tissue

is displaced or destroyed by disease or mechanical force. Injured or diseased tissue cannot exchange oxygen and carbon dioxide.

3. Dilation and constriction of blood vessels help maintain the necessary pressure in the cardiovascular system to ensure the tissues of the body are being perfused adequately. The changes in vascular tone give the body the capability to adapt either to changes in the volume of circulating blood or to changes in the amount of blood being pumped by the heart.

4. Cardiac output is the amount of blood pumped by the heart each minute. Components include stroke volume (how much blood is pumped per beat) and heart rate (how many times the heart beats per minute). Written as a formula, it is expressed as $CO = SV \times HR$.

5. The body compensates for cardiopulmonary challenges in predictable ways. Commonly, the autonomic nervous system engages the fight-or-flight mechanism of its sympathetic arm. This causes blood vessels to constrict and the heart to beat faster and stronger. The sympathetic nervous response also causes pupils to dilate and the skin to sweat. Chemoreceptors in the brain and blood vessels sense increasing carbon dioxide and hypoxia, and stimulate the respiratory system to breathe faster and deeper to eliminate more carbon dioxide from the blood. Signs and symptoms of these sympathetic changes include increased pulse and respirations, delayed capillary refill, narrowing pulse pressure, and pale skin. Pupils may be dilated, and the patient may be sweaty even in cool environments.

Critical Thinking Exercises

1. The chest injury caused the lung to collapse. This led to a significant impairment of gas exchange at the alveolar level–a V/Q mismatch where blood was being delivered to the lungs, but the collapsed alveoli could not be ventilated so oxygen did not reach the bloodstream. Blood cells could not pick up oxygen; as a result, cells became hypoxic. Without oxygen, aerobic metabolism could not be fueled, so cells began to switch to anaerobic metabolism, which creates large amounts of acids that can further damage cellular function.

2. The respiratory system delivers oxygen from room air to the bloodstream and removes carbon dioxide from the body. The circulatory system delivers oxygen and glucose to the cells and removes the hydrogen acids and carbon dioxide for elimination. The blood vessels dilate and constrict to provide sufficient pressure in the cardiovascular system to move blood, and the blood components carry the oxygen and glucose to each tissue cell and remove waste products.

Pathophysiology to Practice

1. With a damaged heart, the body's ability to compensate by managing cardiac output is impaired. Cardiac injuries can limit the ability to change heart rate and stroke volume and therefore limit increases in cardiac output. If the cardiac output cannot be maintained, then blood pressure will drop and tissues may not be properly perfused.

2. A patient with a loss of tone in the blood vessels would lose the ability to control pressure within the cardiovascular system, so the person could not adapt to blood loss by vasoconstriction. Furthermore, excessive dilation of blood vessels can drop blood pressure leading to inadequate tissue perfusion and shock.

3. Red blood cells carry oxygen. A deficit in the number of these cells disrupts the body's ability to move sufficient levels of oxygen in the cardiovascular system. In times of challenge, an oxygen transporting deficit may seriously affect the body's ability to compensate. A loss of red blood cells also limits the body's ability to remove waste products such as carbon dioxide from the tissues. This can also be damaging to the tissues. Ultimately this will contribute to hypoperfusion and death.

Street Scene Questions

1. You will want to know how long his problem has been going on. Does he have any history of GI-related problems such as ulcers or other types of GI bleeding? Does he have any other medical problems or take any medications?

2. His fast heart rate and pale skin point to compensated shock. With the history he has presented, this person has the potential to be critically ill, and if the shock continues to progress, he is at risk for death.

3. This person has no radial pulse because the pressure in the cardiovascular system is very low, likely from blood volume loss. His heart rate has increased to compensate for the decrease in cardiac output and blood pressure. The respiratory rate has increased to help compensate for tissue hypoxia caused by the poor perfusion.

4. The low blood pressure was predictable based on the weak radial pulse and tachycardia.

5. This person's low blood pressure is likely caused by internal bleeding in the GI tract. Clues that indicate this diagnosis include the dark stools, the tender abdomen, and the findings of shock.

6. ALS should be contacted. Advanced personnel can administer intravenous fluid to help increase cardiovascular volume, which in turn can increase tissue perfusion.

CHAPTER 8 Lifespan Development

Think Like an EMT—Determining if Vital Signs Are Normal

1. A 3-year-old boy who is groggy with a pulse of 60/minute is abnormal. He should be alert and active with a pulse of 70-120/minute.
2. A 65-year-old man describing a feeling of "skipping heartbeats" and a pulse of 130/minute is abnormal. A normal rate for his age is around 70/minute. He may be suffering from one of any number of fast heart rhythms.
3. A 42-year-old man who fell off a curb and hurt his ankle with a respiratory rate of 16 is normal.
4. A 77-year-old woman complaining of dizziness with a pulse of 56/minute is likely abnormal. A normal heart rate for her age is 70/minute. However, further assessment of her other vital signs (blood pressure, etc.) will give you a clearer impression of her condition.
5. A 3-month-old baby with a respiratory rate of 30 is normal, as the expected range is 30-60/minute for an infant up to 6 months of age.

Short Answer

1. The following descriptions fit with the following age groups:
   - Decreased metabolism: late adulthood (61 years and older)
   - Toilet trained: toddler (average age 28 months)
   - Empty nest syndrome: middle adulthood (41-60 years)
   - Noticeable development of external sex organs: adolescence (13-18 years)
   - Rooting reflex: infant (birth to 1 year)
   - Self-destructive behaviors common: adolescence (13-18 years)
   - Peak physical condition: early adulthood (19-40 years)
   - Twilight years: late adulthood (61 years and older)
2. Your ability to communicate with younger patients will depend on their stage of development. An infant is often perfectly charming, compliant, and willing to cooperate. However, as children develop separation anxiety and fear of strangers, your approach will have to be more delicate. Later, among the adolescent age group, kids strive for independence. Body image and privacy are big concerns. Most adolescents want you to treat them as adults yet still want to fully indulge in the comforts of childhood.

Critical Thinking Exercises

A 16-year-old girl hesitant to open up or answer your questions in front of her friends is not unusual. Kids go through an often painful process of discovering their own identities during their adolescent years and don't want to risk embarrassing themselves in front of their peers. Body image is a great concern at this point in life, and eating disorders can also be an issue. The patient has become sexually mature by this age and may be sexually active. Try to overcome her hesitancy by limiting or removing bystanders. If a female crew member is available to conduct the interview and assessment, the patient may feel more comfortable offering information to her.

Pathophysiology to Practice

1. After suffering a mechanism of injury like the one described, the patient's elevated heart rate is likely due to the excitement of the incident and the stimulation of the patient's sympathetic nervous system, which causes a faster heart rate and higher blood pressure. There is no way to know whether the patient might have suffered internal injuries or bleeding, based solely on a heart rate, without performing a further assessment.
2. Knowing what medications a patient is taking can help determine a patient's preexisting medical conditions. It's often through your questions about the patient's medications that you get much of your history about illnesses and conditions the patient has had in the past. A common medication is insulin. If a patient takes insulin, even most laypersons know that the patient has diabetes.

Street Scene Questions

1. Children who are 3 or 4 years old are expected to cling fiercely to their mothers, especially in a stressful and traumatic incident such as this. Children at this age fear separation from their parents, and the incident has most likely magnified his fears all the more. Thus, this would be an expected sign from the patient in this situation.
2. Given the patient's level of anxiety, you should use a very gentle approach and calm voice with the patient. Even with a gentle approach, kids at this age seldom tolerate being strapped down and placed on a long spine board. Make sure you have plenty of help, and try to limit how many people talk to the child at once. Be sure the patient's mother is allowed to stay with him at all times.
3. The patient's mother is key to your successful management of this patient. By keeping her calm and involved in his care, you will, in turn, help keep the patient calm and cooperative. Make sure she understands that you are doing everything possible to help her son and make him comfortable. If at all possible, avoid separating the mother and son.

4. All of his vital signs appear to be normal for a patient of this age.
5. Many caregivers carry a quick reference card with them that lists normal vital sign ranges for different ages. They may even have an app they access on their smart phone.
6. Keep it very basic, and explain what you plan to do prior to doing it. Avoid surprises and never lie to the patient or "sugarcoat" things; if you do, you will lose his trust. Telling a child that something won't hurt when it will actually be painful is the surest way to create an uncooperative patient for the rest of your transport. Be truthful without scaring him, and provide lots of encouragement for his bravery. And again, enlist the mother as much as possible in helping the patient understand what is going on to him and around him.

CHAPTER 9 Airway Management

Think Like an EMT—Will the Airway Stay Open?

1. The 16-year-old asthma patient's airway will not likely stay open. Although asthma is primarily a breathing problem, his attack is leading to a decrease in mental status, which threatens his airway.
2. The 72-year-old female patient's airway will likely stay open unless her condition significantly worsens. Her problem is likely a breathing issue and not related to her airway. She may be critical as a result of her pneumonia, but at this moment, her airway is stable.
3. The 35-year-old male patient's airway is seriously threatened. His position and drooling indicate a difficulty keeping his airway open and are classic signs of edema as a result of an infection in the larynx. This patient has a high probability of losing his airway.
4. The 16-month-old's barking cough indicates an upper airway issue and certainly concerns you. However, in small children the subglottic edema that causes the seal-like bark is often well tolerated and might not truly threaten the airway. On the other hand, there are some children who do not tolerate this well at all. If this is the case, this infection can significantly threaten the airway. Observe these children for signs of adequate oxygenation, and assess on a case-by-case basis.

Short Answer

1. The main structures of the airway are the mouth, nose, tongue, nasopharynx, oropharynx, hypopharynx, epiglottis, glottis, trachea, bronchi, bronchioles, and alveoli.
2. Airway care is typically the highest priority because without a patent airway, oxygenation and ventilation cannot occur. Lack of oxygenation will quickly lead to patient death. In fact all efforts, however heroic, will be doomed to defeat if the patient does not have an adequate airway.
3. Signs of an inadequate airway include no air movement, choking, stridor, snoring, and gurgling.
4. The head-tilt, chin-lift maneuver should be used to open the airways of patients who are not at risk of spinal injury. This maneuver moves the head and neck and, therefore, violates the in-line neutral position that may be necessary to maintain in a patient with a suspected spinal injury. The jaw-thrust maneuver should be used on patients with the potential for spinal injury, as it theoretically does not move the neck.
5. Airway adjuncts help maintain an open airway by displacing the tongue anterior so it does not occlude the oropharynx and may also elevate the epiglottis to allow a channel for air to move into the trachea and lungs. Suctioning removes liquids and loose substances from the airway to prevent them from obstructing air movement and to prevent aspiration of these into the lower airway and lungs.

Critical Thinking Exercises

1. This patient needs immediate airway intervention, including suctioning, positioning, and potentially the insertion of an airway adjunct. Further treatment will include positive pressure ventilation and probably advanced life support assistance. First, though, the airway should be suctioned before determining if positive pressure ventilation is needed.
2. Stridor indicates a partially obstructed airway at the level of the glottis and epiglottis. Your immediate concern is the threat of the airway occluding completely. Rapid transport is necessary and ALS intercept if possible.
3. Snoring respirations indicate turbulent airflow through the partially occluded airway, most commonly by the tongue. In an injured or ill patient, it generally indicates a decreased capability to maintain the airway as consciousness decreases. Corrective actions include positioning the head, opening the airway manually, and potentially inserting an airway adjunct.

Pathophysiology to Practice

1. The signs of a partially obstructed airway include difficulty breathing, difficulty speaking, stridor, snoring, choking, gurgling, and coughing.
2. An altered mental status can impact the patient's airway because as mental status decreases, control of the muscles that keep the airway open can be impaired. The loss of

tone in these muscles can lead to the epiglottis falling back and obstructing the glottic opening and the tongue to fall into the back of the oropharynx. Altered mental status can also cause a loss of the gag reflex. Without this protective reflex, patients are at risk for aspiration.

3. Neck trauma can immediately impact the airway by disrupting pathways and destroying structures, but it might also threaten long-term patency by causing swelling to occur in the airway passages. This swelling can obstruct the movement of air.

Street Scene Questions

1. Once safety has been ensured and you have donned your personal protective equipment, the first patient care priorities are to establish responsiveness and, if necessary, open the airway and check for breathing.
2. For an unconscious person, you should be prepared to open the airway, potentially to suction or insert an airway, to support breathing if it is found to be inadequate, and to begin CPR if the patient is found to be pulseless.
3. Necessary equipment should include personal protective equipment, airway management tools such as suction and airway adjuncts, and ventilation support devices such as a bag-valve mask and supplemental oxygen.
4. After determining the scene is safe, you should immediately assess the airway and breathing. After those have been assessed and treated, you should perform a pulse check. Consider also a scene assessment to determine the mechanism of injury.
5. In an unresponsive person, you should first open the airway manually, then "look, listen, and feel" for air movement. Look at the chest for rise and fall; listen for the sounds of air movement; feel for air moving and for the rise of the chest. If the airway has any abnormal sounds, immediately correct that as appropriate. If breathing is found to be inadequate, then support that function by initiating positive pressure ventilation with a BVM device attached to oxygen.
6. The patient should be rapidly turned on his side (if it is safe to do so) to allow gravity to assist with clearing fluid from his airway. You should then employ suction to further clear any remaining vomit.
7. Because of the possibility of spinal injuries, the patient's airway should be opened with a jaw-thrust maneuver. Consider using an airway adjunct such as an NPA or OPA to help maintain the airway.

CHAPTER 10 Respiration and Artificial Ventilation

Think Like an EMT—Oxygen or Ventilation?

1. A patient found on the floor with no pulse or respirations must be immediately ventilated with a bag-valve mask and high-concentration oxygen.
2. A 14-year-old patient with a fractured femur and strong but mildly rapid pulse and respirations is likely experiencing significant pain. The patient certainly does not need ventilation but may need oxygen based on the EMT's assessment of the patient's oxygenation status and pulse oximeter finding.
3. A 64-year-old alert patient with chest pain and stable vital signs needs oxygen administration if he is hypoxic or suspected of being hypoxic.
4. A 78-year-old COPD patient with rapid, shallow respirations who is no longer oriented should be manually ventilated with high-concentration oxygen to ensure the patient's tidal volume can be improved with each manual respiration. Because the patient is still somewhat awake, the ventilations should be "timed" with his spontaneous attempts at ventilation so as not to agitate the patient and produce gastric insufflation (air pushed into the stomach).

Short Answer

1. Signs of respiratory distress include rapid respirations, accessory muscle use, anxiety, pursed-lip breathing, and sitting in the tripod position. In the case of respiratory distress, the patient should have a relatively normal pulse oximetry and have a relatively normal mental status, as increased respiratory efforts are meeting the metabolic needs of the body. This is generally treated with oxygen therapy.
2. Signs of respiratory failure include all the signs of respiratory distress plus signs that the body is no longer compensating for the respiratory challenge. These signs include altered mental status, dropping pulse oximetry level, cyanosis, slowing/irregular respirations, and respiratory fatigue. The treatment for this is positive pressure ventilation with oxygen supplementation.
3. The techniques of artificial ventilation are:
   - Mouth-to-mask: Connect oxygen to the inlet on the mask, and run at 15 liters per minute. Place yourself at the head of the patient and position the mask on the patient's face. Hold the mask firmly in place while maintaining head tilt. Take a breath and exhale into the mask port or one-way valve at the top of the mask port with just enough volume to make the chest rise. Remove your mouth from the port, and allow for passive exhalation.
   - BVM: Position yourself at the patient's head and establish an open airway. Suction and insert an airway adjunct as necessary. Select the correct size mask for the patient. Position the mask on the patient's face. Form a *C* around the ventilation port with your thumb

and index finger. Use the middle, ring, and little fingers under the patient's jaw to hold the jaw firmly to the mask. With your other hand, squeeze the bag once every five seconds, causing the patient's chest to rise. Release pressure on the bag, and let the patient passively exhale.

4. If only a lone rescuer is present, he or she will need to perform all the tasks of BVM ventilation. With two rescuers, however, one person will hold the mask seal on the patient's face with two hands while the other squeezes the bag. For a patient with suspected trauma, the provider holding the mask must simultaneously perform a jaw-thrust maneuver. For a patient with no suspected trauma, the head-tilt, chin-lift maneuver may be used to open the airway.
5. Under normal circumstances, the body contracts the diaphragm and expands the chest cavity to create a negative pressure and "pull" air in through the glottic opening and into the lungs. Artificial ventilation, such as BVM ventilation, relies on positive pressure to "push" air into the lungs.
6. Any condition that causes hypoxia will benefit from supplemental oxygen. Such conditions could include bronchospasm, acute pulmonary edema, and shock. Hypoxic patients who are breathing adequately most commonly benefit from high-concentration oxygen delivered through a nonrebreather (NRB) mask, but in some cases, these patients may not tolerate high-concentration rates. In cases where patients will not tolerate an NRB mask, lower-flow delivery devices such as a nasal cannula may be a better choice. Some EMS systems may also allow providers to use alternative devices such as Venturi masks, or to titrate the level of oxygen administration based on patient condition and oxygen levels. (Always follow local protocols.)

Critical Thinking Exercises

1. After donning personal protective equipment and ensuring the scene is safe, the EMT should open this patient's airway and, if necessary, support it with an airway adjunct and suctioning as appropriate. Her altered mental status, slow respiratory rate, and cyanosis all point to respiratory failure. This patient needs immediate respiratory assistance with a bag-valve mask device and supplemental oxygen.
2. At a minimum, this patient needs immediate supplemental oxygen. Further assessment will be necessary to identify respiratory failure, but his inability to speak and position certainly point to at least impending failure. If your assessment identifies further indications of respiratory failure, then immediate artificial ventilation is necessary.
3. Although this patient may just be anxious after the motor-vehicle crash, a thorough assessment must be completed to ensure the fast rate is not due to an injury. Rapid respiratory rates can indicate inadequate breathing, but further assessment will be necessary to identify respiratory failure. The information provided (i.e., she is walking around, is alert, and has normal skin color) seems to indicate that at this time the patient is not in respiratory failure and will likely not need artificial ventilations.

Pathophysiology to Practice

1. To identify the respiratory status of a patient, both oxygenation and ventilation must be assessed. Mental status, skin color, and pulse oximetry all can be used to assess oxygenation. Listening to lung sounds, observing respiratory effort, and looking for accessory muscle use help assess ventilation as well. If no deficits in oxygenation or ventilation are noted during these assessments, the patient is breathing adequately. Any deficits with either element point to inadequate breathing and respiratory failure.
2. A breathing patient may need artificial ventilation if breathing is deemed to be inadequate. Signs include altered mental status, cyanosis, slowing or irregular respirations, absent alveolar ventilation as evidenced by lung auscultation, and respiratory fatigue.
3. When using a bag-valve mask, watch for chest rise to ensure adequate volume initially. Additionally, listening to breath sounds over the alveolar regions of the lungs will let you know that the ventilations are sufficient to oxygenate the alveoli.

Street Scene Questions

1. After donning personal protective equipment and ensuring scene safety, you gather a general impression and then complete a primary assessment. If problems are found, immediate treatment must be initiated.
2. The essential elements of assessing this patient's breathing include observing his effort and mental status; assessing his skin color; listening to his chest for air movement and unusual lung sounds; and obtaining a pulse oximetry reading.
3. Immediate treatment will likely include supplemental high-concentration oxygen. It may also be important to assist this patient with his inhaler (if protocols allow). Assessment may also indicate respiratory failure. As such, you should be prepared to provide artificial ventilations while ensuring the airway remains patent.
4. The breathing is not adequate. Fatigue, cyanosis, and difficulty speaking all point to respiratory failure, as do the periods of slowed and irregular breathing.
5. This patient requires artificial ventilations immediately. You should attempt to time your ventilations with the patient's spontaneous efforts (as long as they are present) to help avoid gastric insufflation and subsequent vomiting.

CHAPTER 11 Scene Size-Up

Think Like an EMT—Should I or Shouldn't I?

1. The possibility that there might be an explosion is an initial, serious, and very legitimate concern. You would have to think how long it would be before help was likely to arrive and judge how advanced the fire was at this point. You would look to see whether the person was seriously trapped (perhaps requiring mechanical extrication) or whether it appeared the person could be pulled from the vehicle. Safety from traffic at the scene would be a potential concern as well. If you decided you would attempt an approach, you would need to be prepared to leave again if forced to do so for your own safety.
2. You would first take cover and call 911. From your place of cover, you could then attempt to determine whether the scene was still dangerous. You would observe whether the man on the ground appeared to be a victim of the scene or a participant in it. This might affect your decision about whether to approach the person who was down before law enforcement arrived and secured the scene.
3. First, you would call for help, likely by contacting dispatch on your portable radio. Next, you might approach the scene cautiously to determine whether the perpetrator had left the scene. After this you would consider assessing and assisting the woman who was stabbed. If however, anything about the scene concerns you, your best approach is not to approach.
4. The first consideration would be to determine the extent of injury and call for assistance. In addition to the bleeding, could there have been injury to the neck or spine? If so, stabilization would be important. If possible, you would create a barrier with a clean cloth between your hands and the blood, and provide pressure to stop the bleeding.

Think Like an EMT—Determining Areas of Concern at the Scene

1. Conditions are icy, which means there is potential for the truck to slip further into the ditch. You should avoid placing yourself in a position where you could be caught under the truck should it tip more to the right. Other traffic could slip in the same icy part of the road as the truck, which means increased danger for EMT personnel. Barriers and flags need to be established as quickly as possible to protect workers at the scene and oncoming traffic. You should scout for any damage to utility poles or downed electrical lines in the vicinity. The contents of the truck are unknown, and may be of personal harm if they become dislodged. This is crucial to establish in case there is danger of leakage or explosion. The driver of the vehicle is at an angle to the road. This may make extrication more difficult, especially if there is risk of spinal injury.
2. Collisions on interstate highways require police support and/or blocking vehicles to establish a safe corridor to check on the victims due to the speed of surrounding traffic. Another ambulance should be called to the scene to help with victims of the crash. Angle of impact will determine what injury patterns are most likely, so this should be noted in scene size-up.
3. This scene could be caused by use of a weapon or weapons. Your first task is to assess for safety, your own and others'. Find a safe spot from which you can view the scene and determine what is going on and how many people may be involved. You would immediately call for police support. Once they clear the scene, then EMS can enter and start patient care.
4. The first and most important task here is to move residents, bystanders and yourself a safe distance from a potential explosion. Ensure that police have been called to the scene. Assist anyone from the home to a safe staging area. Alert dispatch so they can summon the appropriate support of the fire department and utilities department to handle the potential gas leak.
5. The distance of the fall and the landing area (bushes, grass, concrete) are crucial factors to determine. The patient's position can be seen from a distance and will likely give clues to potential spinal or extremity injuries. Also be aware that the patient may have fallen due to a collapse of the construction site or the scaffolding being used. At all construction sites, the EMT should be alert for collapse.

Short Answer

1. In the case of leaking gasoline or a vehicle fire, consider the danger zone to be 100 feet in all directions from the wreckage. Park outside the danger zone, upwind, and uphill if possible. Avoid gutters, ditches, and gullies that can carry fuel to the ambulance. Do not use flares. Use orange traffic cones during daylight and reflective triangles at night. In the case of hazardous materials, check with a hazardous materials reference to determine the danger zone. In all cases, park upwind. Park uphill if liquid is flowing, but on the same level if there are gases that may rise. Park behind a natural or an artificial barrier whenever possible. In the case of downed power lines, consider the danger zone as the area in which people or vehicles might be contacted by energized wires if the wires pivoted around their points of attachment.
2. Indicators of violence or potential violence include fighting or loud voices, weapons visible or in use, signs of alcohol or drug use, unusual silence, evidence of a struggle at the scene (broken furniture, glass, etc.), and knowledge of prior violence at this address.

3. Protective gloves–routine patient assessment, controlled bleeding, suctioning, artificial ventilation, CPR. Eye protection–splashing, spattering, or spraying body fluids. Masks–infections spread by airborne droplets. N-95 or HEPA respirator–diseases spread by airborne particles such as tuberculosis.
4. Injuries to bones and joints are common following falls and vehicle collisions. Burns are common injuries from fires and explosions. Penetrating soft-tissue injuries can be associated with gunshot wounds and altercations. Blast injuries could include burns, punctures/penetrations, and falls.
5. Potential sources of information about the nature of the patient's illness include the patient, family members, and bystanders at the scene. Also assess the scene for things like medications, garbage cans or commodes containing vomitus, or oxygen concentrators.
6. There are countless scenarios where both medical and trauma calls can tax the available resources and prompt you to summon additional assistance. Whether the situation involves lifting a large patient, assessing or transporting multiple patients, or calling resources with additional training (ALS or law enforcement), it's important to be proactive and call early whenever possible.

Critical Thinking Exercises

First, make certain the police have secured the scene before you enter it. If you fail to do so, you could easily find yourself and your partner hostages or shooting victims. Once the scene is secure, you will proceed with normal scene size-up steps: Take Standard Precautions. Confirm the mechanism of injury (reported to be a gunshot in this case). Establish the number of patients. (There might be several shooting victims or persons injured by falls or other actions, or even a person suffering a heart attack from the stress of the event.) Decide whether more resources are needed to handle the call.

Pathophysiology to Practice

1. A patient with stab wounds to the lower anterior and posterior ribs would have wounds to the internal organs as follows:
   - A penetrating injury to the area of the lower left lateral ribs could puncture any of the organs in the left quadrants, including the spleen, intestines, and pancreas.
   - A penetrating injury to the area of the lower right lateral ribs could puncture any of the organs in the right quadrants, including the liver, intestines, pancreas, and gallbladder.
   - A penetrating injury to the posterior side of the patient on either side is more likely to penetrate either of the kidneys. Depending on the length of the penetrating object, other organs (listed above) may be impacted as well.
2. If the patient were able to protect himself somewhat by lying in a fetal position, he might be able to shield the liver, spleen, intestines, pancreas, and gallbladder. However, the kidneys are more likely to be exposed to penetrating trauma because of their location on the posterior side.

Street Scene Questions

1. Issues might include a quick check for the number of patients, identification/confirmation of the mechanism of injury, rapid assessment to determine the severity of injuries, need for additional resources, and so on. The placard on the side of the truck also needs to be identified to determine the contents of the truck and the potential need for a special hazmat team.
2. Although the crew has donned protective gear and made efforts to limit traffic hazards, they must wait until the vehicles are stabilized and the placard is identified before safely approaching the patients.
3. Standard Precautions should include, at a minimum, disposable gloves and eye protection–especially because of the high probability of cuts and open wounds from this type of collision.
4. The second ambulance should be parked in a staging area that is upwind from the scene and at a safe distance. Safeguards should also be taken so the ambulance is away from moving traffic and has an easy means of egress after the patient is loaded.
5. The patients need to be properly covered and protected during the extrication process. Also, a member of the crew should remain with the patients to calm their fears, answer questions, and monitor their status.
6. You can help ensure the patient safely gets from the scene to the ambulance by considering whether the ambulance should be moved closer to the patient to facilitate loading. Also consider using appropriate equipment to move the patient to the ambulance safely.

CHAPTER 12 Primary Assessment

Think Like an EMT—Determining Priority

1. A responsive patient with difficulty breathing while sitting up is high priority.
2. A man who "passed out" at a wedding and is still unresponsive is high priority due to his altered mental status.

3. A responsive child who got her foot caught in bike spokes and may have broken her foot is lower priority.
4. A responsive patient who describes severe pain in his abdomen is high priority.
5. A patient who only moans and appears to have ingested alcohol is high priority due to his change in mental status and possible inability to protect his own airway.

Short Answer

1. When forming a general impression of a patient, look at the patient's environment, whether the suspected problem is medical or trauma, whether there are any mechanisms of injury, and the patient's age and sex. Overall, you should form the general impression by looking, listening, and smelling. It is gathered through direct observation and through your feelings and intuition.
2. Assess the patient's mental status using AVPU as follows:
   - Alert–Patients who are awake and can answer your questions correctly. Patients who are oriented to person can tell you their name. Patients who are oriented to place can say where they are. Patients who are oriented to time can tell you the day, date, and time.
   - Verbal–If the patient appears to have a depressed level of consciousness, appears asleep when you arrive, or does not take note of your approach, determine if the patient responds to verbal stimuli such as talking or shouting. If patients do respond by opening their eyes or somehow responding to you appropriately, then they are said to be "alert to verbal stimuli".
   - Painful–If the patient does not respond to verbal stimuli, determine if the patient responds to painful stimuli by pinching a toe, ear, or squeezing the trapezius muscle between the neck and the shoulder.
   - Unresponsive–The patient is not spontaneously alert, nor will they respond to verbal or painful stimuli.
3. Assess airway breathing and circulation as follows:
   - Airway–If the patient is talking or crying, the airway is open. If the airway is not open, if the patient is not alert, or if the patient is breathing noisily, open the airway by using the jaw-thrust maneuver for trauma patients and the head-tilt, chin-lift maneuver for medical patients. Suction the airway as needed for fluid and insert an airway adjunct such as an OPA or NPA as appropriate. If the airway is blocked, perform the Heimlich maneuver or back blows and chest thrusts until the airway is cleared.
   - Breathing–If the patient is not alert, use the technique you learned in CPR class to listen, look, and feel for breathing. Perform rescue breathing if necessary, and implement the use of a BVM device with oxygen supplementation as soon as possible. If the patient is breathing, count the breathing rate. If a conscious patient is breathing at a rate of less than 8 breaths per minute or more than 24 breaths per minute, administer oxygen using a nonrebreather mask.
   - Circulation–Take the patient's pulse. Start with the radial pulse in adults and the brachial pulse in infants. If you cannot feel these peripheral pulses, check the carotid pulse. If the pulse is absent at the radial and carotid locations, administer CPR and apply an automated external defibrillator. Check for bleeding, and control any major bleeding. Check the skin for temperature, moisture, and color. Warm, pink, dry skin indicates good circulation. Pale, cool, and moist skin indicates poor circulation.
4. The C-A-B approach puts the "C" (circulation/compressions) step of primary assessment before the "A" and "B" (airway and breathing) steps. The CAB approach is performed only on apparently lifeless patients with no breathing or with agonal breathing, and involves an immediate pulse check and initial compressions when the pulse is absent.
5. A-B-C is the traditional approach to the patient in the primary assessment. It is performed on most patients you encounter in this sequence: airway, breathing, circulation. Whenever a deficit is noted in the airway, breathing, or circulation components, the EMT should immediately support that lost function.
6. The statement that the order of interventions depends on the patient's condition and number and priority of conditions means that "ABC" is a mnemonic to remind you of the three main things you must assess and treat, as necessary, during the primary assessment. However, "ABC" does *not* indicate the *order* in which you must do these steps. For example, a patient with vomit in the airway would be suctioned first. A patient with arterial bleeding would get bleeding control first. You will consider the A-B-Cs on every call, but the order may differ depending on the patient's needs.
7. The statement "Multiple EMTs can accomplish multiple priorities simultaneously" means that when there are two or more EMTs or other trained personnel on scene, many tasks can be carried out at the same time. This is often the case. For example, one EMT could initiate spinal motion restriction procedures while another suctioned the patient. In another call, one EMT could control bleeding while the other EMT opened the airway.
8. Making a priority decision means determining whether a patient has a life-threatening condition, which makes them a priority that requires immediate transport to the hospital.
9. A trauma patient needs spinal motion restriction precautions of the head and spine during the primary assessment if so indicated. To further protect the spine should the patient have an airway occlusion, a jaw-thrust maneuver should be used rather than the head-tilt, chin-lift maneuver. An unresponsive patient or one with respiratory distress meeting hypoxic criteria needs high-concentration oxygen by nonrebreather mask or bag-valve mask if breathing inadequately and transport as a high-priority patient. In fact, any level of responsiveness below that of "alert" may indicate the possibility of a life-threatening problem.

Critical Thinking Exercises

In the first section, questions 1-3 ask you to state whether the patient's priority is stable, potentially unstable, or unstable.

1. One might be inclined to minimize this patient's condition because of where he was found–outside a bar–and simply assume he's intoxicated. But that is very risky. At this point, you only know that he has been unconscious and that better control of his airway has improved his condition. His condition remains unstable.
2. Although the patient's A-B-Cs are fine and she is alert, her skin signs are a big concern. In addition, your intuition is telling you something is wrong. Caregiver intuition can be one of your best diagnostic tools in patient assessment. This patient is potentially unstable.
3. Assuming the patient's A-B-Cs are fine and her level of hydration is normal, this patient is stable.

In the second section, questions 1-6 ask you to decide, for each patient, which portion of the primary assessment should be performed first (i.e., C-A-B approach or A-B-C approach).

1. For a patient who is unresponsive with arterial bleeding from his neck: Begin with bleeding control. This bleeding will be fatal in a very short time. You will learn later in the text how to apply an occlusive dressing.
2. For a patient with a broken ankle and no other apparent injury: This patient doesn't appear to have major issue to the airway, breathing, or circulation components. Do a quick but thorough check of the A-B-Cs to be sure nothing is overlooked.
3. For a patient who is not moving and does not appear to be breathing: This patient would first receive a pulse check. In the absence of a pulse, begin compressions.
4. For a patient who tells you she has severe difficulty breathing: For this patient, take an A-B-C approach to check the airway, then position her appropriately. Administration of oxygen or ventilation (as required) would occur next. Once completed with airway and breathing, then proceed to circulation and a pulse check.
5. For a patient who has ingested too much alcohol and is vomiting: Treat the airway first. Suctioning and positioning will be necessary if the patient has an altered mental status and can't control his airway.
6. For a patient who is doubled over and screaming because of abdominal pain: The screaming indicates that the airway is patent and he is moving air in and out. As part of a thorough airway check, you will need to make sure there has been no vomiting that would require suctioning. This patient also likely has a pulse, but you should check the rate and the patient's skin color, temperature, and condition to assess for possible shock from internal bleeding.

Pathophysiology to Practice

1. Unless the level of consciousness improved drastically, administering oxygen would not in itself lead you to change an unresponsive patient's priority. All unresponsive patients should be considered unstable, high-priority patients.
2. Because the patient's family is most familiar with his normal mental status, it is important to gather the history from them. This patient is considered a stable, lower-priority patient until you can determine what abnormal behavior prompted the call for help today.
3. Be sure to take Standard Precautions. First, always scan the scene to determine whether it is safe to approach. Because you are alone in the middle of the street, you do not have the benefit of a partner or someone else helping to watch traffic or other hazards for you. Without first taking these precautions, you could become part of the scene yourself. Next, form a general impression to determine how serious the patient's condition is, and call for additional resources to help. If available, enlist a bystander to assist with manual spinal motion restriction of the patient's head and neck until you can complete full precautions. Assess the patient's mental status and his A-B-Cs. If during the primary assessment you discover any life-threatening conditions, perform the appropriate interventions immediately. In this case the patient has gurgling respirations, and his airway should be cleared in whatever way is possible. There may not be much more you can do until more help arrives, but remember the saying: "The most important things you can do for your patients are in the A-B-Cs."

Street Scene Questions

1. While rapidly determining responsiveness, you should perform manual spinal motion restriction precautions according to your protocol, followed by an assessment of the A-B-Cs.
2. To help maintain spinal motion restriction, the jaw-thrust maneuver is the most appropriate method for opening the airway. It accomplishes two objectives–opening the airway by bringing the tongue and jaw forward while at the same time maintaining in-line manual cervical spine motion restriction in case the spine has been injured.
3. The level of responsiveness is VERBAL because the patient is responding to a verbal stimulus.
4. Primary assessment should always follow the same general steps: Form a general impression, assess mental status, assess airway, assess breathing, assess circulation, and determine priority. The cause of Joey's seizures might confirm whether he has a medical condition, but you must still identify any immediate life-threatening conditions, correct them, then decide on the patient's priority for immediate transport or further on-scene interventions. Remember that if the steps in primary assessment are not followed consistently and systematically, it is very possible to overlook and neglect to manage a life-threatening situation.
5. The patient should be positioned on his side (sometimes referred to as the *recovery position*) if there is no possibility

of spinal injury. This will promote fluid drainage from his mouth should he vomit or have heavy secretions. If spinal trauma is suspected, and spinal motion restriction precautions have been taken, and the patient is now supine on a long board, then the patient should be suctioned frequently by the EMT.

6. The status of the patient was downgraded because of his improved mental status.

CHAPTER 13 Vital Signs and Monitoring Devices

Think Like an EMT—Solving Assessment Problems

1. First, observe the ease with which the patient speaks. If he speaks long (six-plus-word) sentences without having to catch his breath, the patient is experiencing minimal distress. You can wait a short time for him to stop talking or tell him you'll need him to be quiet so you can listen to his lungs (or heart) while you are really counting respirations through the stethoscope. If patients are aware you are counting their breaths, the results may not be accurate.
2. Obtain the blood pressure from the other arm once you move the patient to a transportation device and into a more open area. Remember that you will have other indicators, including mental status, pulse, respirations, and skin color, which are a significant part of the patient picture and will let you know how well the patient is perfusing.
3. In a patient with a serious mechanism of injury, in the absence of a radial pulse, you should next go to the carotid artery to check the pulse. Look for other signs of life as well, including movement, moaning, or respiratory effort. If a patient was responsive and you cannot feel a pulse in one wrist, you should check the pulse at her other wrist as you can be certain she has a pulse if she is conscious. If, however, the patient with a serious medical condition has no radial nor carotid pulse, you should initiate CPR.

Short Answer

1. Vital signs traditionally measured in EMS are respiration; pulse; skin color, temperature, and condition (plus capillary refill in infants and children); pupils; and blood pressure.
2. Vital signs should be taken more than once because the patient's condition may change while in your care. You should repeat vital signs on stable patients every 15 minutes. You should repeat vital signs on unstable patients every 5 minutes. Repeat vital signs after every medical intervention or if there is an sudden change in the patient's condition or mental status.

Critical Thinking Exercises

1. If you are attempting to assess for a radial pulse and cannot find one, do not spend more than a couple of seconds searching for the pulse location before checking the other arm or another artery, such as the brachial or carotid artery.
2. If you ever question a blood pressure reading, whether the reading came from a blood pressure monitor or was measured by auscultation from another caregiver, always repeat the procedure manually in the other arm, or wait one minute first if using the same arm.
3. Nail polish can cause an inaccurate reading on a pulse oximeter. (Blue nail polish actually gives the most inaccurate readings.) One option is to carry acetone wipes to quickly remove the nail polish from the patient's fingernail before attaching the device. Remove any artificial nail. If the nail is too thick or it is not possible to remove the polish or an artificial nail, you may try attaching a probe to the patient's toe or earlobe. Occasionally, a different probe may be needed for different body locations.

Pathophysiology to Practice

1. Remember that the heart fills during diastole, and the faster the heart rate, the shorter the diastolic filling time which means the chambers of the heart will fail to completely fill with blood before contracting, leading to poor blood flow from the ventricles and weaker pulses felt in the periphery.
2. The sympathetic nervous system and the hormone epinephrine work to combat blood loss by constricting blood vessels. This causes more blood from the periphery, such as the skin, to be shunted toward the core of the body, such as the heart and lungs, where it is needed the most. Skin appears pale and sweaty because of the vasoconstrictive properties of epinephrine.
3. The diastolic pressure is the pressure that remains in the arteries when the left ventricle relaxes and refills. Chronically high pressures during this relaxation phase, also known as diastolic hypertension, obviously increase the stress and wear on cardiac structures and put the patient at much greater risk for heart disease, stroke, and kidney disease.

Street Scene Questions

1. After determining scene safety, your primary concern is assessment of the A-B-Cs. In the case of Ms. Alvarez, the airway is patent, but her breathing is a little rapid. This finding warrants further assessment and at least the consideration of administering supplemental oxygen.
2. Vital signs obtained for any patient include number of respirations per minute (including quality), pulse rate per minute (including quality), blood pressure, skin color, and temperature, as well as an evaluation of the pupils.

3. Because Ms. Alvarez is complaining of abdominal pain, questions during the patient interview should be aimed at determining the quality and severity of the pain, the length of time the patient has experienced the pain, what the pain "feels like," and what, if anything, brought on the pain. Also ask about any symptoms that may have started before the abdominal pain such as dizziness, diarrhea, constipation, trouble breathing, and so on.
4. In addition to evaluating the patient's pain, ask if Ms. Alvarez has had previous episodes of the condition and whether she has seen a doctor for this (or any) condition. If so, find out what the doctor has said about the condition. Inquire about any medications she might be taking for the abdominal pain or for any other medical conditions.
5. Yes, another set of vital signs should be taken. A patient with rapid respirations and signs and symptoms suggesting possible abdominal bleeding (as evidenced by her blood pressure) should have vital signs taken approximately every 5 minutes.
6. In a calm manner, give the patient an honest appraisal of the vital signs and assessment findings. Point out possible consequences of refusing transport. If the patient still expresses an unwillingness to go to the hospital, you should contact medical direction and perhaps request the patient's permission to contact her personal physician. Also, if you have been unable to convince the patient to go to the hospital, another member of the crew might try to convince her to change her mind, or if any family member is on scene, they too can be very effective at getting a patient to change their mind about transport.

CHAPTER 14 Principles of Assessment

Think Like an EMT—Critical Thinking and Decision Making

The feature in this opening segment of the chapter does not call for answers but rather states why a successful secondary assessment relies on solid clinical judgment and critical thinking. Students may want to discuss this statement before proceeding with the rest of the chapter.

Short Answers

1. Critical thinking is an analytic process that can help someone think through a problem in an organized and efficient manner. It is thinking that is reflective, reasonable, and focused on deciding what to do in a particular situation. It involves the use of facts, principles, theories, and other pieces of information.
2. Different clinicians have different levels of training and experience, time, technology, and other resources. All clinicians begin with the same basic approach though: Gather information, consider possibilities, and reach a conclusion. How they implement these steps, however, varies significantly. The emergency physician and the EMT are similar in that they both work under certain time constraints, must quickly rule out or treat immediate threats to life, and focus much of their questioning and assessment on ruling out the worst-case scenario. When settling on a differential diagnosis, they primarily differ in the number of tools and tests available to them. Emergency physicians have many more tools available, allowing them to focus on a significantly larger number of possible diagnoses compared with EMTs, not to mention the thousands of additional hours of training and clinical exposure physicians have compared to personnel working in the prehospital environment.
3. "Search satisfying" means that once you find what you are looking for, you stop looking for other causes or possibilities of the condition, or even a coexisting problem. In practice, this translates into a situation where if you suspect something is causing the problem and have the slightest inkling you might be right, you may fail to look for a secondary diagnosis that may be complicating things. An example may be having an unresponsive patient and attributing it to IV drug use when you find needle tracks on the arm, but overlooking that the patient is also diabetic and could be experiencing a hypoglycemic episode. "Confirmation bias" is somewhat similar and means that a clinician looks for evidence to support a particular diagnosis they already have in their mind. In doing so, the clinician might overlook evidence that refutes or reduces the probability of that diagnosis. So while the first error is one in not recognizing multiple problems may exist, the second problem is not ensuring that the assumed problem is the actual one.
4. To obtain a history of present illness from a patient with chest pain, use OPQRST:
   - Onset–What were you doing when the pain started?
   - Provocation–Can you think of anything that might have triggered this pain?
   - Quality–Can you describe the pain for me?
   - Radiation–Where exactly is the pain? Does it seem to spread anywhere, or does it stay right here?
   - Severity–How bad is the pain?
   - Time–When did the pain start? Has it changed at all since it started?

Critical Thinking Exercises

1. A 52-year-old man complaining of chest pain while at work who is alert and oriented first needs a calm approach, especially since he tells you he thinks it may "just be stress." Form a general impression, and conduct a quick primary assessment. Use the OPQRST memory aid to gather a history. From a critical thinking perspective, you might ask yourself:
   - Does this patient have an obvious problem, or do I need to think more critically?

- What other information should I get to confirm or refute the working diagnosis?
- How specific does my field diagnosis have to be to decide the best treatment?

2. A 67-year-old man who is now unresponsive after acting unusually in front of his wife, developing slurred speech, and complaining of an odd feeling in his arm needs an immediate intervention to manage his airway. An unresponsive patient is not likely able to manage his own airway and breathe effectively. While assuring his airway and assessing the rest of his A-B-Cs, you should gather history information from his wife and ask yourself these questions from a critical thinking perspective:
   - Have I addressed all potential life threats first before going on with the assessment and diagnostic process?
   - Does this patient have an obvious problem, or do I need to think more critically?
   - Are there other causes besides the obvious one for this patient's condition?
   - How specific does my field diagnosis have to be to decide the best treatment?
   - What is the best thing I can do for the patient *right now*?
3. An 18-year-old snowboarder who took a fall and thinks he may have broken his ankle mostly needs to be directed to remain still while you conduct a full trauma assessment. Determine the mechanism of injury and the likelihood of any other injuries or the need for spinal motion restriction precautions. From a critical thinking perspective, ask yourself:
   - Does this patient have an obvious problem, or do I need to think more critically?
   - What other information should I get to confirm or refute the working diagnosis?
   - Could there be other injuries his clothing, or the cold ambient weather be masking?
4. A 41-year-old woman with difficulty breathing and pain when she breathes in deeply needs reassurance and a methodical assessment and history gathering. Because she is anxious, she needs a calm approach. The early administration of supplemental oxygen, if indicated, may help reduce her anxiety. From a critical thinking perspective, ask yourself:
   - Have I addressed life threats first before beginning the assessment and diagnostic process?
   - Does this patient have an obvious problem, or do I need to think more critically?
   - What other information should I get to confirm or refute the working diagnosis?
   - How specific does my field diagnosis have to be to decide the best treatment?
   - What is the best thing I can do for the patient right now?

Street Scene Questions

1. Once the primary assessment is complete, proceed with a secondary assessment to assess the patient's mental status, check for any pain or discomfort (using the OPQRST memory aid), and consider using the Cincinnati Prehospital Stroke Scale, or another approved scale, to predict if a stroke is the cause of his findings.
2. Mr. Ronson could be having a diabetic emergency, a neurologic emergency such as a CVA or TIA, or a cardiac emergency such as a heart attack or hypertensive crisis.
3. Knowing the medications patients are taking can often tell you a lot about their history and the illnesses they're being treated for. You might also be able to determine when the patient last took his medication for his diabetic condition. The presence of high blood pressure medicine reinforced hypertension, which is a leading cause of stroke, and the high cholesterol medicine also suggests that cardiovascular disease is likely to be present.
4. You should complete a full primary and secondary assessment along with an assessment of his mental status and any pain or discomfort. Use the Cincinnati Prehospital Stroke Scale or another system approved scale to assess for predictive signs of stroke.
5. This patient should be considered potentially unstable until you can gather more information. Transport should be expedited until you can rule out the possibilities that he is having a stroke, heart attack, or serious diabetic emergency. Most likely, he should be emergently transported so he can receive diagnostic imaging and a full cardiovascular workup at the hospital to definitively determine the cause(s) of his findings.
6. You should call for an ALS intercept anytime the patient needs an ALS intervention such as intravenous dextrose or advanced airway control.

CHAPTER 15 Secondary Assessment

Think Like an EMT—Challenges in History Gathering

1. Listening is important, especially when the patient is talkative, but you may eventually need to focus the history or transport will be delayed. Redirecting the patient politely with phrases such as "I see, but I need to focus on why you called today. Can you tell me about ..." may help.
2. At times the EMT may have to question the patient in more privacy, especially with sensitive topics. To help negotiate this delicate situation, you could ask the question while the parents aren't in the room or when bringing the patient out to the ambulance. It may be possible to have a parent leave

the room to get something (medications or the patient's coat) so you can ask the question privately.

3. In this case, the patient's behavior may be due to his medical condition. His family may be the best source of information. If he can answer, he may do so very slowly, so giving a little time (but not so much as to cause delay in treatment) may help. Also, remember that a patient with a depressed mental status may not give the most correct answers.

4. While ensuring your safety, get down to the patient's level and attempt to establish rapport. Talk slowly and quietly. Ask questions that are easy to answer (e.g., ask the patient's name) to see if the patient is oriented enough to respond.

Mid-Chapter Review

Short Answer

1. In medical patients, unlike trauma patients, there are not many external sources of information about what is wrong with the patient. For medical emergencies, the most important source of information about the problem is usually what the patient can tell you. So when the patient is awake and responsive, obtaining the patient's history comes first.

2. For the responsive medical patient, the first step of your secondary assessment is talking with the patient to obtain the history of the present illness and the past medical history, followed by performing the physical exam and gathering the vital signs. Your differentials come more often from what the patient tells you and less often from the physical exam findings. In the unresponsive medical patient, the process is turned around. Because you cannot obtain a history from the patient, you will begin with a rapid physical assessment and collection of baseline vital signs to develop differentials. After these procedures, you will gather as much of the patient's history as you can from any bystanders or family members who may be present.

Critical Thinking Exercises

1. Put your hand on his shoulder and say: "I know you are concerned about your father. You can help him by trying to calm down and answer a few questions for me about his medical history. Take a few deep breaths. Good. You look calmer. Are you ready to answer my questions?"

2. Continue to talk to him for a few minutes about unrelated matters. Then say, "Sir, although I'm really enjoying our conversation. I really need to get refocused on why you called EMS so we can best care for you. So I need you to answer a few questions for me related to the problem you're having today. OK?"

Pathophysiology to Practice

Nicotine present in tobacco products causes increased blood pressure and heart rate, decreased oxygen to the heart, increased blood clotting, and damage to cells that line coronary arteries and other blood vessels. A person's risk of heart attack greatly increases with the number of cigarettes the person smokes. People who smoke a pack of cigarettes a day have more than twice the risk of heart attack as nonsmokers. About 30 percent of all deaths from heart disease in the United States are directly related to cigarette smoking.

Street Scene Questions

1. The patient presents with difficulty breathing, rapid respirations, and a rapid pulse. Until you can assess her condition further, you should consider her a high-priority patient as she may rapidly deteriorate with delayed or inefficient care.

2. You should take a baseline set of vitals, as indicated in the opening part of the scenario. After eliminating any immediate life threats, you should begin to gather a history of the present illness, focusing on questions that pertain to the condition cited by the patient. Administer supplemental oxygen per protocol, assess for its effect on the patient, and check the patient's pulse oximetry reading (if available).

3. Since this is a medical patient, you should ask the OPQRST questions and then specific questions about her previous medical history. Of particular importance is the use of an inhaler or other medications that are commonly prescribed to asthma patients.

4. Signs and symptoms of a worsening condition might include a decrease in the patient's the level of consciousness, more labored breathing, use of accessory muscles, tripod positioning, increased difficulty talking (e.g., one-to-two word answers), a respiratory rate that is either too fast or too slow, a diminishing pulse oximeter reading, and increased patient anxiety. Signs and symptoms of an improving condition might include a "normal" respiration rate (e.g., little or no distress), the ability to talk in complete sentences, an alert mental state, absence of cyanosis, and a normal or improved oxygen saturation reading on the pulse oximeter.

Think Like an EMT—Rapid Trauma or Focused Exam?

1. A patient who was found ejected from a vehicle in a rollover collision should receive a rapid trauma exam–even if there appears to be only minor injuries–due to the significant mechanism of injury.
2. A patient who tripped and possibly broke his wrist will receive a focused exam as long as the mechanism of injury doesn't indicate that additional injury is likely. For example, if the patient hit his head during the fall and is now disoriented, he would receive spinal motion restriction precautions and a rapid trauma assessment.
3. A patient with minor neck pain from a motor-vehicle accident with a major mechanism of injury will receive a rapid trauma exam due to the significant mechanism of injury. Spinal motion restriction precautions may also be warranted based upon local protocol.
4. A patient who fell six feet, lost consciousness, and broke an ankle should receive a rapid trauma exam. This may seem like a borderline situation because a fall of six feet may not match standards for significant mechanism of injury in an adult. However, the loss of consciousness should alert you to potentially serious problems and cause you to be vigilant and complete a rapid trauma exam. You can always slow down if the patient is found to be stable.

Chapter Review: Secondary Assessment of the Trauma Patient

Short Answer

1. A rapid trauma assessment is performed on patients with a severe mechanism of injury, or those patients who have sustained trauma and have injuries that have made them a high priority patient (disturbances to the airway, breathing, or circulatory components or an acute change in mental status) based on the primary assessment.
2. The steps for the rapid trauma assessment included assessment of the head, neck, chest, abdomen, pelvis, extremities, and posterior of the body to detect additional signs and symptoms of injury before you depart the scene for the hospital.
3. The EMT should perform a detailed physical exam on trauma patients who did not sustain a significant mechanism of injury and do not present with any disturbances to the airway, breathing, and circulatory components (or change in mental status), as determined by the primary survey. The steps of the detailed physical exam include an assessment of the head, neck, chest, abdomen, pelvis, extremities, and posterior of the body to detect signs and symptoms of injury. It differs from the rapid trauma assessment only in that it also includes examination of the face, ears, eyes, nose, and mouth during the examination of the head.

Critical Thinking Exercises

1. A patient who fell three stories and is currently bleeding into his airway requires an immediate intervention to correct a life-threatening condition. Bleeding into the airway must be corrected before any further assessment can be completed. In fact, if the airway is not patent, it will doom all other care interventions to failure and the patient to death. Continue suctioning until your partner returns to provide more help. Notify ALS for backup or intercept while enroute.
2. Manage these situations as follows:
   - Cut finger: Although the cut is bleeding profusely, a cut to a finger is not a significant mechanism of injury. Unless you are unable to control the bleeding with direct pressure and other normal methods, you can complete on-scene assessment and initiate care before transporting the patient.
   - Schoolyard shooting: This is a significant mechanism of injury given it is a shooting. Additionally, a significant blood loss has already taken place and caused unknown internal injuries to the patient. This further underscores the significance of the mechanism. Because she is able to speak, assume that her airway and breathing are adequate, at least for the moment. Immediately apply direct pressure to control the bleeding, administer oxygen by nonrebreather mask, provide spinal motion restriction precautions as indicated by local protocol, and transport her expeditiously, providing ongoing monitoring and any needed additional care en route. Contact ALS for intercept while enroute.
   - Unconscious on sidewalk: There is no way to know the cause of this patient's condition. Quickly ensure adequate airway and breathing, provide oxygenation or ventilation as needed, provide spinal motion restriction precautions as indicated by local protocol, and transport without spending additional time at the scene, monitoring the patient's condition en route. Notify ALS for backup or intercept while enroute.

Pathophysiology to Practice

Lungs produce audible sounds that you can auscultate through a stethoscope whenever air rushes in and out of the lung structures: the lung tubing (bronchi and bronchioles), and the air sacs (alveoli). If a lung collapses, such as in a pneumothorax, air cannot move through these structures, and so it fails to resonate with audible sounds.

Street Scene Questions

1. The patient is suffering from multiple traumas. The A-B-Cs are the first priority while providing manual spinal motion restriction precautions (based on protocol). The first treatment priority is securing the airway and ensuring adequate respirations (breathing). Due to facial injuries, you must make sure that mucus, blood, and/or teeth are not causing airway obstructions. You should vigilantly suction as needed and, if necessary, turn the patient on his side to allow for drainage. Next, you should apply an occlusive dressing over the stab wound to the anterior chest. You should also provide the patient with high-concentration oxygen and, if necessary, assist ventilation. Watch for the potential development of a tension pneumothorax throughout the call. This is a high-priority patient and you should notify dispatch to send an ALS unit to your scene or to meet you enroute as appropriate.
2. The patient needs rapid transport to a trauma center rapidly given his injuries. After managing the airway and breathing, and controlling any external bleeding, you should package the patient for immediate transport to the hospital, preferably a Level I trauma center if there is one available.
3. You should take a baseline set of vital signs as soon as possible. Because the patient has a serious mechanism of injury, vitals should be retaken every 5 minutes.
4. The patient seems to have developed difficulty breathing. You should remove the corner of the dressing, have the patient exhale if possible, then reseal the dressing to deal with this probable tension pneumothorax. Raising a corner of the occlusive dressing provides some relief. If this is successful, you should then continue to monitor the patient. Be prepared to assist ventilations.
5. The A-B-Cs remain the first priority. However, as time and patient conditions permit, the secondary assessment should include a complete and methodological head-to-toe survey for any other injuries that may be hidden, unnoticed, or slow to progress.

CHAPTER 16 Reassessment

Think Like an EMT—Trending Vital Signs

1. A multiple-trauma patient who fell 15 feet with a dropping blood pressure and increasing heart rate is likely deteriorating.
2. A 64-year-old female patient who fell and is complaining of hip pain demonstrates vitals that are returning towards normal.
3. A 19-year-old female with lower-extremity injuries who shows a dropping blood pressure and increasing heart rate is likely deteriorating.

Short Answer

1. The four steps of reassessment are:
   - Repeat the primary assessment: Reassess the patient's mental status. Maintain an open airway. Monitor the breathing for rate and quality. Reassess the pulse for rate and quality. Monitor skin color and temperature. Reestablish patient priorities based upon the findings.
   - Repeat and record the vital signs, interpreting them against the patient's condition.
   - Repeat the history and physical exam, specifically chief complaints and injuries.
   - Check interventions: Ensure adequacy of oxygen delivery and artificial ventilation if being provided. Ensure management of bleeding, and check that all other interventions are having the desired effect.
2. By documenting the findings, the EMT can note any changes in the patient's condition, adjust treatment, or begin new treatment. Trending is evaluating and recording changes in a patient's condition, such as slowing respirations or rising pulse rate, that may show improvement or deterioration over time, and that can be shown by documenting repeated assessments.

Critical Thinking Exercises

If your reassessment turns up these findings, intervene as follows:

1. Gurgling respirations: Immediately suction the patient's airway.
2. Bag on nonrebreather mask collapses completely when patient inhales: Increase the liter flow of oxygen being delivered to the patient so the bag does not collapse completely during each inhalation.
3. Snoring respirations: Open or reposition the airway manually.

Pathophysiology to Practice

Asthma is an obstructive disease resulting from the small bronchioles in the lungs contracting and becoming narrowed while overproduction of mucus further obstructs airflow. This results in air becoming trapped in the distal airways and alveoli and normal gas exchange, especially the exchange of oxygen with the bloodstream, diminishes. Even though your patient's breathing rate may not be affected yet by her asthma attack, the amount of oxygen she's carrying in her blood has been reduced. Measuring the blood oxygen level (SpO_2) with a pulse oximeter tells you how much oxygen is attached to hemoglobin on her red blood cells. Those red blood cells may not have enough oxygen to keep oxygenating her brain, heart, and other tissues. If the SpO_2 number is low, you can help her system facilitate better gas exchange by providing supplemental oxygen.

Street Scene Questions

1. Patients who are less than alert (who are responding to only verbal or painful stimuli) may have difficulty maintaining their airways. These patients may be positioned in such a manner as to occlude their airways through a partial blockage by the tongue—a condition that can be resolved by repositioning. Also, with less-than-alert patients, you need to be prepared for suctioning as well. You may also need to move these patients into a position that will facilitate drainage, such as the lateral recovery position. Any patient who is unresponsive or poorly responsive must be monitored constantly. Be prepared to reposition the patient as needed and intervene with airway adjuncts such as OPAs (oropharyngeal airways) or NPAs (nasopharyngeal airways) as necessary to control the airway. Have suctioning equipment immediately available.
2. At this point, you should complete a history of the present illness. Questions might include the following: Has the patient had a similar condition in the past? Is the patient taking any blood pressure medication or blood thinners? If so, what is the medication? Is the patient compliant in taking it? In specifically questioning the husband, you might ask: "When was the last time you saw your wife?" "Was she manifesting any of the current signs or symptoms at that point, such as trouble walking, slurred speech, or obvious facial drooping?" In specifically questioning the patient, you might ask: "Are you having any trouble breathing?" "Are you in any pain?"
3. Reassessment includes continually monitoring the patient's airway and breathing, circulation status, and any changes in her level of consciousness. Periodically reassess the patient's speech, and observe for facial drooping. Reassess the patient's pupils and vital signs every 5 minutes. Periodically reevaluate changes in movement, strength, and sensation in all extremities.

CHAPTER 17 Communication and Documentation

Think Like an EMT—Communication Challenges

1. The emergency medical responders may be busy with a critical patient, they may have forgotten, they could be in danger, or their portable radio may not work or be able to reach the closest tower. Call them on your radio, and ask for an update. If unable to, ask your dispatcher to try and contact them.
2. Advise the hospital that the patient has apparently ingested a large quantity of alcohol. (Never assume this is the only problem.) Advise of his current level of responsiveness (the patient responds to painful stimuli by withdrawing), and note that his level of responsiveness has varied since patient contact. Recontact the hospital if the patient's condition worsens, so the hospital staff can prepare.
3. Depending on time and resources, you could step away from the chaotic scene to eliminate background noise and try again. Be sure you are talking slowly and clearly. If it appears to be a radio problem, ask the dispatcher if he heard the transmission. If so, he could advise the hospital by radio or phone for you.
4. By stating "The patient is nonverbal, but his eyes are open and he localizes pain by looking where painful stimulus is applied," you have painted a picture of the patient's mental status.

Think Like an EMT—Choosing How and What to Document

1. Only information that is medically relevant should be documented. For example, if the patient is addicted to drugs, it may be pertinent to note whether the patient admitted to or denied alcohol or drug use prior to this incident. Alcohol or drug use may also make a patient incapable of providing consent or making an informed patient refusal. Use objective (factual) statements rather than subjective (opinion) statements in your documentation. Use terms such as *patient stated* before noting subjective information and put quotes around the words or statements so that anyone reading the report will know the source.
2. You are always allowed to review the call report or PCR before you testify in court or appear in a deposition. This is a legal document that records your observations and actions at the call. It will refresh your memory and will not cause bias or interference with the legal proceedings. Additionally, everyone who is involved with the case will by then have also reviewed the PCR, so you should also.
3. Cases such as those involving child, elder, and sexual abuse exempt providers from any HIPAA privacy requirements associated with a report *to appropriate authorities* and *relevant health care providers*. As a matter of fact, many states specifically provide immunity from lawsuits for those who report these suspected incidents in good faith.

Short Answer

1. The steps of a medical radio report are:
   - Unit identification and level of provider ("Memorial Hospital, this is Community BLS Ambulance 6 en route to your location...")
   - Estimated time of arrival ("... with a 15-minute ETA.")
   - Patient's age and sex ("We are transporting a 68-year-old male patient ...")
   - Chief complaint ("... who complains of pain in the abdomen.")
   - Brief, pertinent history of the present illness ("Onset of pain was 2 hours ago and is accompanied by slight nausea but no vomiting.")
   - Major past illnesses ("The patient has a history of high blood pressure, Crohn disease, and arthritis.")
   - Mental status ("Patient is alert and oriented, never lost consciousness.")
   - Baseline vital signs ("Vital signs are pulse 88, regular and full; respirations 20 and unlabored; skin normal; and blood pressure 134 over 88.")
   - Pertinent findings of the physical exam ("Our exam revealed tenderness in both upper abdominal quadrants. They were not rigid on palpation.")
   - Emergency medical care given ("For care, we have placed the patient in a position of comfort.")
   - Response to emergency medical care ("The level of pain has not changed during our care. Mental status has remained unchanged. Vital signs are basically unchanged.")
   - If your system requires, or if you have questions, contact medical direction. ("Does medical direction have any orders?")
2. Effective interpersonal communication with patients should include these qualities:
   - Use eye contact.
   - Be aware of your position and body language.
   - Use language the patient can understand.
   - Be honest.
   - Use the patient's proper name.
   - Listen attentively and carefully.
3. Subjective information is that which is from an individual point of view–the patient, bystanders, even the EMT (e.g., patient says, "I feel like I've got the flu.", or "I am really nauseated."). Objective information is that which is observable, measurable, and verifiable (e.g., vital signs). A pertinent negative is something that is not present but that is important to note (e.g., "The patient states that her chest pain does not radiate.", or "The patient fell down 12 steps but denies head, neck, or back pain.").
4. The narrative report (or patient care report) should be written in such a way that it is clear, legible, and complete as this is the only record the emergency department staff will have regarding the patient's presentation and what care was provided by EMS. The EMT should avoid the use of codes or unusual abbreviations as these may not be familiar to the emergency department staff and may create confusion. They should always use correct spelling, clear writing, and complete statements. Written reports that are unclear to the staff may cause harmful errors in patient care and make it difficult for the quality improvement team to conduct reviews.
5. Important steps to take and important items to document when a patient is refusing care or transportation to the hospital include:
   - Try again to persuade the patient to go to a hospital. Consider having a family member assist you in this task if one is available.
   - Ensure the patient is able to make a rational, informed decision (e.g., not under the influence of alcohol or other drugs or illness/injury effects).
   - Inform the patient why the patient should go and what may happen to the patient if not.
   - Consult medical direction as directed by local protocols.
   - If the patient still refuses, document any assessment findings and emergency medical care given, and have the patient sign a refusal form.
   - Have a family member, police officer, or bystander sign the form as a witness. If the patient refuses to sign the refusal form, have a family member, police officer, or bystander sign the form verifying that the patient refused to sign.

Critical Thinking Exercises

1. The correct sequence for a medical radio report is indicated by the numbers in parentheses that precede the information items:
   - (5) Complaining of chest pain radiating to the shoulder
   - (3) 56 years old
   - (13) Oxygen applied at 2 liters per minute via nasal cannula
   - (9) Alert and oriented
   - (4) Female patient
   - (7) Came on 20 minutes ago while mowing the lawn.
   - (8) History of high blood pressure and diabetes
   - (2) ETA 20 minutes
   - (10) Pulse 86, respirations 22, skin cool and moist, blood pressure 110/66, SpO_2 96 percent
   - (14) Oxygen relieved the pain slightly.
   - (6) Denies difficulty breathing.
   - (15) You are requesting orders from medical direction.
   - (1) You are on Community BLS Ambulance 4.
   - (11) Lung sounds equal on both sides
   - (12) Placed in a position of comfort
2. A sample narrative might say: 56 y.o. female c/o chest pain radiating to the shoulder. Onset 20 minutes prior to our arrival while mowing lawn. Physical exam: alert and oriented, BP 110/66, pulse 86, resp. 22, SpO_2 96 percent, skin cool and moist, lungs equal bilaterally, denies dyspnea. History: HTN and diabetes. Treatment: O_2 2 lpm via nasal cannula, placed in POC. Response: some pain relief with O_2. Information included in the

written report is generally more comprehensive since radio reports are meant to highlight the important data. For example, some elements of the detailed physical examination would not have been part of the radio report. Additionally, only the written report will become part of the patient's medical records associated with this emergency, so it should be as thorough and comprehensive as possible.

Street Scene Questions

1. The following information should be included in a prehospital care report: run data (agency name, unit number, date, times, run call number, names and certification levels of crew members); patient data (nature of call, mechanism of injury, location of patient, treatment, signs and symptoms, baseline vitals, level of consciousness, history of present illness, care administered and the effects of each care step, changes in the patient's condition throughout the call, insurance and billing information); and narrative (objective and pertinent subjective information, pertinent negatives).
2. An accurate and thorough prehospital care report is important because the document not only is included in the patient's permanent medical record but is often used as a legal document in civil and criminal cases. In addition, the data from the PCR is used for administrative purposes, education, and quality improvement. Noting the patient has complaints to his left foot and was not properly restrained also illustrates why the injuries existed, and reduces the likelihood that the EMT's care contributed to any problems as they were documented as present prior to EMS arrival.
3. Having your partner review your prehospital care report before submitting it is a great way to ensure it gets completed effectively. It is always possible to overlook information or to see situations from a personal perspective. After all, both of you were present on the call and it's important to have consensus about what occurred.
4. All copies of the prehospital care report must be the same and must accurately reflect the care rendered. If the version of events in the medical record were to differ from a version located at the provider or EMS agency, legal questions could arise about the care provided to the patient.

CHAPTER 18 General Pharmacology

Think Like an EMT—We Are Really Close to the Hospital. Should I Give Aspirin?

Absolutely. The one medication that has been found to reduce mortality in the event of a myocardial infarction (heart attack) is aspirin. The sooner it is administered, the sooner it begins to take effect. As long as protocols allow and there are no medical reasons to avoid administration, you should definitely give the aspirin. Remember that although transport is an important part of your job, EMS was conceived with the idea of bringing therapy to the patient. Aspirin therapy is just one such example.

Think Like an EMT—ALS Is on the Way. Should I Assist the Patient with Her Inhaler?

Yes, you should assist with the administration of the inhaler. Although ALS is close, early administration of bronchodilator medications such as albuterol is important to the overall success of treatment. The arriving paramedics may carry bronchodilators, but even in the 5–8 minutes you wait, your patient may progress to a stage of respiratory distress that will be less responsive to the medications the paramedics carry. Your immediate actions may dictate how effective early treatments are. Always follow local protocols, but remember that you have been granted those protocols for important reasons.

Think Like an EMT—How or Whether to Assist with Medications

1. If you are on scene with a patient experiencing cardiac-type chest pain and he suggests that he take some of his wife's prescription of nitroglycerin, tell him that it is contraindicated. The patient has not been screened for other drug interactions and may be taking a medication that might negatively interact with the nitroglycerin. Consider contacting medical control.
2. A diabetic patient who responds only to loud stimuli and is very sleepy is unlikely to be able to control her own airway, control her oral secretions, and swallow properly. Administering oral glucose, which is the consistency of thick pancake syrup, will only further compromise the patient's ability to breathe effectively if it causes an airway occlusion. Oral glucose is limited to patients who can self-administer it and swallow well.
3. A COPD patient breathing 48 times per minute with shallow tidal volume is in moderate to severe distress. Administering his prescribed inhaler may improve your delivery of oxygen to the patient and could provide temporary relief to the patient until he can be further evaluated in the emergency department. However, it is important to remember that if the patient is breathing too shallowly, the effectiveness of the medication may be hampered because it may not reach the portions of the patient's lungs where it would properly exert its action.

Short Answer

1. Aspirin, oxygen, oral glucose, and in many EMS systems naloxone, are medications that are often carried on ambulances and may, in certain circumstances with proper protocol approval, be administered by an EMT.
2. Bronchodilator inhalers, nitroglycerin, and epinephrine auto-injectors are medications for which EMTs can commonly assist with patient administration.
3. Other forms of medications are powder, liquids, gels, sublingual sprays, and inhaled gases.
4. On-line medical direction implies speaking directly to a physician, as in calling a doctor on the radio from an emergency scene. An example of online medical direction would be to request permission to assist a patient with the administration of their inhaled bronchodilator. Off-line medical direction indicates physician involvement "behind the scenes," such as in the development of written guidelines and protocols that the EMT would follow in most situations. An example of this would be the automatic administration of oxygen via nasal cannula to a patient with chest pain and a pulse oximeter reading less than 95%.
5. Medications may be administered orally, sublingually, inhaled, injected, instilled onto the nasal mucosa for absorption (intranasally), or even absorbed through the skin.

Critical Thinking Exercises

Although nitroglycerin may be helpful for chest pain, administering medication that was not specifically prescribed to the patient is never a good idea. You should thank the family member for being willing to help, but you should not administer the non-prescribed medication. To do so is operating outside your scope of practice.

Pathophysiology to Practice

Reassessment should include repeating the primary assessment and vital signs. Certain medications will cause predictable side effects (for example, epinephrine causes an increased heart rate and nitroglycerin often reduces the blood pressure), but in general you should look for any signs of improvement or deterioration in the patient's condition.

Street Scene Questions

1. Additional patient history questions might include:
   - How long has the pain been going on?
   - Have you ever had this pain before?
   - Do you have any medical history?
   - Do you take any medications?
   - When was your last meal?
2. Nitroglycerin might be helpful if the patient has it prescribed to him. Depending on your local protocols, you may need to contact medical direction before making the decision. Be sure to assess blood pressure before administering nitroglycerin; ask the patient if they take any erectile dysfunction medications. Always consider the five rights of medication administration before administering it.
3. Assessing the patient's vital signs before administering a medication is essential. Nitroglycerin, especially, can cause a drop in the patient's blood pressure, so it is very important to ensure the patient's pressure is not already too low before giving the medication.
4. You want to know that the medication is prescribed to the patient, that it is not expired, and that the correct dose can be safely administered.
5. When administering nitroglycerin in tablet form, one tablet should be placed under the patient's tongue until it dissolves. The tablet should not be chewed or swallowed. When administering the spray, do not shake the canister before use; hold it upright, ask the patient to open his mouth and elevate his tongue, and then press the button once with your index finger while aiming at the sublingual area. Ask the patient to close his mouth and avoid swallowing.
6. Vital signs should be reassessed shortly after administration and every 5 minutes thereafter.

CHAPTER 19 Respiratory Emergencies

Think Like an EMT—Administering a Prescribed Inhaler

1. A 14-year-old patient with difficulty breathing and a history of asthma will benefit from the use of an inhaler. Always follow local protocols and medical direction for use of medications.
2. Do not use the inhaler, because it isn't prescribed to the patient. In addition, wheezes may be present in conditions other than asthma. Furthermore, there is no indication provided thus far that even indicates that the wheezes in the patient are from the same disease process as the wheezes experienced by her daughter.
3. Although the inhaler is indicated for the patient's asthma, it won't do much good here, because the patient isn't breathing adequately. The reason you don't hear wheezes is that she isn't breathing deeply or strongly

enough to move air through the constricted airways. The medication in the inhaler won't get deep into the lungs, where it is needed to exert its action. Instead, ventilate the patient with a BVM connected to oxygen, transport promptly, and request an ALS intercept if available in your area.

Short Answer

1. All patients (adults, children, and infants) who become hypoxic will see an increase in their respiratory rate initially. Sensors in the brainstem and the aortic arch constantly detect how much oxygen is being carried in the blood. If it is too low, signals from the brain are sent to breathing muscles to increase the respiratory rate in an attempt to better oxygenate the blood as it passes by the alveoli.
2. The effect of hypoxia on the patient's pulse rate may vary depending on the patient's age. In an adult, hypoxia will increase the heart rate, cardiac output, and blood pressure. This is due to the direct stimulation of the sensors in the aorta that detect low oxygen levels in the bloodstream. The goal is to increase cardiac output in an attempt to better perfuse the lungs with blood so oxygen transfer can occur. In children and infants however (the younger - the more prominent), the heart rate often falls sharply to become very slow (bradycardic) from hypoxia.
3. Signs of inadequate breathing include a breathing rate excessively above or below normal; irregular rhythm; diminished, unequal, or absent breath sounds; extremely labored or increased respiratory effort; use of accessory muscles (may be pronounced in infants and children and involve nasal flaring, seesaw breathing, grunting, and retractions between the ribs and above the clavicles and sternum); and shallow respiratory depth.
4. A patient in heart failure can also suffer from bronchoconstriction and wheezes. If bronchoconstriction is apparent and the patient's physician has prescribed the inhaler's use during such a situation (however unlikely that may be), then it is indicated and the EMT can assist with the administration per protocol. It is important to note that the medication will have the side effect of increasing heart rate, so be sure to monitor vital signs and limit repeated doses of the medication.
5. Differences between adult and child/infant respiratory systems include:
   - Mouth and nose–In general, all structures are smaller and more easily obstructed in children than in adults.
   - Pharynx–Infants' and children's tongues take up proportionally more space in the mouth than do adults'.
   - Trachea–The trachea is narrower and obstructed more easily by swelling; it is also softer and more flexible. Like other cartilage in the infant and child, the cricoid cartilage is less developed and less rigid.
   - Diaphragm–The chest wall is softer; infants and children tend to depend more heavily on the diaphragm for breathing.
6. Signs and symptoms of breathing difficulty include altered level of consciousness, dizziness, fainting, restlessness, anxiety, confusion, combativeness, cyanosis, straining neck and facial muscles, tightness in the chest, straining intercostal muscles, numbness or tingling in the hands and feet, flaring nostrils, pursed lips, coughing, crowing, high-pitched barking, respiratory noises such as wheezing or rattling, and the patient's sitting in a tripod position.

Critical Thinking Exercises

1. A 45-year-old male with severe difficulty breathing, rapid rate of respirations, shallow breaths, minimal chest expansion, and difficulty speaking has <u>inadequate</u> breathing. Reasoning: The rapid, shallow breaths and minimal chest expansion do not permit adequate filling of the alveoli of the lungs for oxygen and carbon dioxide transfer.
2. A 65-year-old female with a normal rate, regular rhythm of respirations, good chest expansion, and slightly labored breathing is breathing <u>adequately</u>. Reasoning: Although the patient perceives that she is having trouble breathing, the normal rate and rhythm and good chest expansion indicate that her respirations are presently able to fill the alveoli of her lungs and ensure adequate oxyenation.
3. A drowsy 3-year-old patient with retractions, nasal flaring, and a rapid rate of respiration is breathing <u>inadequately</u>. Reasoning: The patient's muscle retractions and nasal flaring indicate that the child is working very hard to draw air into her lungs. The rate is too fast to permit adequate filling of the alveoli. The child's drowsiness is an alarming sign of hypoxia.

Pathophysiology to Practice

1. Yes, a patient can develop pulmonary edema without developing peripheral edema. Depending on how the patient is positioned most of the time, as with lying down, edema may not form in the lower extremities. In addition, if the pulmonary edema is acute–if it has developed quickly and not chronically–peripheral edema will not be a component of the illness as it takes a longer amount of time to develop.
2. The expiratory phase will be prolonged because asthma is an obstructive disease where air becomes trapped in the alveoli because of bronchoconstriction and excessive mucus production. During exhalation, the patient must exhale more forcefully because of the stale, trapped air taking longer to exit the lungs through the constricted and obstructed airways.
3. The SpO_2 simply measures the amount of oxygen being carried on red blood cells in the bloodstream; this is just one measure of what's going on in the body. The patient may be in moderate to severe distress and yet be showing a "normal" pulse oximetry reading because the body is able to maintain

normal oxygenation at the expense of heightened respiratory effort. There are also some conditions, such as a low body temperature or low acid level in the body, that cause oxygen to stay attached to red blood cells instead of oxygenating tissues, leading to hypoxia even though the pulse oximeter shows a normal reading. This is why you must assess the whole patient–all vital signs, including the SpO_2 reading.

For each of these patients, the following conditions are most likely:

1. **(C)** A 10-year-old patient is more likely to have asthma. The other respiratory diseases do not affect children.
2. **(B)** An 82-year-old patient who recently discovered she can't sleep lying down is most likely experiencing heart failure. Her "nocturnal dyspnea" or inability to lie flat while sleeping is likely due to fluid accumulating in her lungs during sleep.
3. **(A)** A 76-year-old patient who reports difficulty breathing with fever and increased mucus production is likely suffering from a COPD disorder. This disease is characteristic of increased mucus production.
4. **(B)** A patient who has had a prior heart attack with difficulty breathing who reports gaining 5 pounds in the past 2-3 days is likely suffering from heart failure and an accumulation of fluids due to a weakened heart.
5. **(A)** A very skinny elderly man who is constantly on a nasal cannula at 2 liters per minute at home is likely suffering from a chronic disease such as COPD.
6. **(C)** A 35-year-old man who has difficulty breathing while playing racquetball is likely suffering an asthma attack, given the sudden onset and no history of other chronic illnesses.

Street Scene Questions

1. As with any patient, you should protect the airway and evaluate the patient's breathing. Make sure the airway is clear, and provide ventilations as necessary. Although the patient is speaking, the tongue or secretions could still be a potential problem.
2. You should ask the husband the questions in a SAMPLE history, except for "E" (event). You should elicit that part of the history from the neighbor. Examples of questions you might ask the neighbor include: "What type of activity was Mrs. Bartolone performing at the onset of her breathing problem?" "When did you first observe the episode?" "What posture was the patient in at that time?" "Was her breathing fast or slow?" "Could she speak in complete sentences?" "Was she working to breathe?" "Was her breathing noisy?" "Did you notice any peculiar skin color–especially around the lips?"
3. The medical history reveals that Mrs. Bartolone had to be intubated and placed on a ventilator during an episode 6 months earlier. This information, coupled with the patient's long smoking history, indicates that you should consider her a high priority as her ventilatory status may rapidly diminish.
4. The patient should receive high-concentration oxygen, since her normal 2 liters per minute are obviously insufficient in this situation.
5. No, the patient is not a good candidate for use of an inhaler as her breathing is too shallow and her mental status is deteriorating and she may no longer be able to be coached on how to properly use the inhaler. Signs and symptoms in the scenario indicate that the patient is in immediate need of oxygen which should be attached to the BVM device.
6. This patient should be considered a high priority, with lights and siren for transport to the hospital given her medical history, changes in mental status, and deteriorating pulmonary function.

CHAPTER 20 Cardiac Emergencies

Think Like an EMT—Meeting Sublingual Nitroglycerin Criteria

1. You should not give nitroglycerin to this 84-year-old patient with chest pain. The drug might make his low blood pressure even lower, which would be harmful to him.
2. You should give nitroglycerin to this 68-year-old patient. He has a history of cardiac problems, he is having chest pain, and his blood pressure is high enough.
3. This patient is trickier to determine than the first two. The confounding factor is that the pain is atypical (in his "stomach"), especially when compared with what he experienced with a prior heart attack, although the pain could still have a cardiac origin. His first nitroglycerin spray didn't work. His vital signs are still within acceptable limits. Get a more detailed history and contact medical direction for additional advice. If for some reason you are unable to contact medical direction, since upper abdominal pain in a patient at risk for heart disease is considered an "angina equivalent," you would be justified in providing nitroglycerin and treating the pain as presumed cardiac pain.

Short Answer

1. Best positions for the following patients are:
    a. For the patient with difficulty breathing and blood pressure 100/70, a sitting-up position as long as the patient tolerates it. If he becomes hypotensive, complains of dizziness, or has diminished mental status, lay the patient back as much as needed.
    b. For the patient with chest pain and blood pressure of 180/90, sitting up is an appropriate position if the patient tolerates it.
2. Contraindications for the administration of aspirin are allergy, gastrointestinal bleeding, and history of asthma.

3. Contraindications for the administration of nitroglycerin are hypotension, allergy, or recent use of an erectile dysfunction medication.
4. Signs and symptoms indicating pulmonary edema are respiratory distress, crackles, pink frothy sputum, a history of heart failure, and having a prescription for one or more heart failure medications.

Critical Thinking Exercises

1. This question asks you to describe the role that 12-lead ECG plays in your local system of care and whether EMTs use this assessment tool. Answers may vary, but fundamentally if the 12 lead is obtained prehospitally and transmitted to the hospital, the hospital then has more time to prepare for the patient's arrival, to include having EMS transport the patient directly to the coronary catheterization suite (in some hospital systems)
2. If the nearest hospital does not have the capability to perform interventional cardiology procedures such an emergency angioplasty or coronary artery stent placement to treat the acute MI, it may be appropriate to bypass that hospital for one that does. Always follow local or regional destination protocols that determine appropriate facilities in such situations. In cases where the destination preference is less clear, contact medical direction for additional guidance.

Pathophysiology to Practice

1. The patient with central chest pain radiating to his back, a "bubble" on a blood vessel in his chest, and normal vital signs most likely has an aortic aneurysm. If the aneurysm ruptures, the chance of survival is low, and if the blood is unable to clot because of aspirin, that would decrease the chance of survival even more. Nitroglycerin is not indicated for an aortic dissection. If in doubt, contact medical direction for advice regarding nitroglycerin for this patient, and if it is advised, monitor his blood pressure to be sure it does not drop too much.
2. This patient with CHF has run out of his "water pills," has gained weight, has awakened short of breath, and needs to be propped up on two pillows. Because he stopped taking the pill that helps him eliminate excess fluid, he now has too much fluid in his circulatory system for his heart to handle, and the excess fluid is leaking out of his blood vessels. When he is upright during the day, that fluid is likely to leak into his abdominal cavity and/or lower legs. At night, when he lies flat, the capillaries surrounding the alveoli of his lungs leak fluid into the lungs, which causes shortness of breath.

Street Scene Questions

1. The equipment you should take to the side of every potential cardiac patient includes the following: nonrebreather mask, portable oxygen tank, a nasal cannula, a suction unit, equipment to take vital signs, a defibrillator (AED) in case of cardiac arrest, and a bag-valve mask with oxygen reservoir. A stair chair may also be listed in this situation because the patient is on the second floor of the apartment complex.
2. The patient's ongoing and worsening chest pain and shortness of breath suggest acute coronary syndrome.
3. The assessment information you need to obtain next would be a set of vital signs and a history. Data you solicit should include the following: any relevant medical history, current treatment by a physician, prescribed medications (particularly nitroglycerin), and presence of an implanted device (pacemaker or defibrillator)(use the SAMPLE mnemonic aid to help in gathering this information). In addition, you should ask the patient about the signs and symptoms that led her to summon EMS. Using the OPQRST model for her complaints, you might ask these questions:
    - **O**nset: Was the onset of the complaint sudden or slow?
    - **P**rovocation: What was the patient doing when the symptoms started? Does anything cause the pain to lessen or intensify?
    - **Q**uality: Can the patient describe what the pain feels like?
    - **R**adiation: Where does she feel the pain? Does it radiate to other parts of the body such as the neck or arms?
    - **S**everity: How would she rate her pain on a scale of 1–10? Has the severity of the pain changed after the administration of nitroglycerin and/or oxygen?
    - **T**ime: How long has the patient had these particular signs and symptoms they are complaining of today?
4. For this patient, whose symptoms suggest acute coronary syndrome, initiate transport and obtain a 12-lead ECG if protocol and equipment allows. Make appropriate notifications to activate the cardiac system of care and, if they are prescribed for the patient and approved by medical direction, help administer aspirin and/or nitroglycerin. Diligently monitor the patient for acute changes in status. Convey any changes to the hospital and the ALS intercept unit.

CHAPTER 21 Resuscitation

Think Like an EMT—Is Your Patient Really in Cardiac Arrest?

1. The 77-year-old patient does not need chest compressions. She is in extreme respiratory distress and definitely in a peri-arrest state. However, she still has a palpable carotid pulse at 130/min. She does need positive pressure ventilations.

2. The 1-month-old patient will not be helped by chest compressions. Limb rigidity and lividity (pooling of blood) indicate the patient died some time ago. Resuscitation is not an option.
3. The 8-month-old patient requires immediate chest compressions. She is not responsive, is apneic, and has no brachial pulse. She is in cardiac arrest.

Short Answer

1. Cardiac arrest is indicated by unresponsiveness, apnea, and absence of a palpable pulse.
2. The appropriate depth of chest compression is 2 inches (5 cm) for adults and children after puberty. For infants and prepubescent children, it is one-third the anterior-posterior depth of the chest, or 1.5 inches (3.8 cm).
3. Three safety measures to keep in mind when using an AED are to ensure the patient is not in a wet location, to dry the skin before attaching the pads, and to step back clear of the patient before the shock is given.
4. Steps for AED are as follows: Turn on the AED; apply pads as indicated to the patient's chest; clear the patient when indicated, so the device can analyze the patient's status; if advised, press the button to administer a shock; immediately resume CPR; perform CPR for 2 minutes (five cycles), unless the patient wakes up, moves, or begins to breathe; follow AED prompts.

Critical Thinking Exercises

1. The question asks you to evaluate the system where you work with respect to the chain of survival: links that are strong and links that need work. Answers will vary, depending on the particular system where you are working or studying. Initially, use your EMT instructor as a resource regarding who to speak with to obtain relevant information to answer this question.
2. The question asks how successful your system is in resuscitating patients from cardiac arrest. Answers will vary, depending on the particular system where you are working or studying. Again, use your EMT instructor as a resource to help direct you where to find the relevant information.

Pathophysiology to Practice

1. The patient is likely suffering from commotio cordis, which is life threatening ventricular fibrillation following blunt force chest trauma. As ventricular fibrillation is a life-threatening dysrhythmia. His heart is not pumping any oxygenated blood to the cells of his heart or brain. These organs are rapidly dying. Use of an AED and CPR are priority treatments for this patient.
2. This patient is likely hypothermic and should be transported for rewarming while resuscitation is ongoing. Hypothermia may change the ability to defibrillate (depending on local protocols). Airway and breathing will be a priority (as will CPR and defibrillation), as the patient is likely hypoxic.

Street Scene Questions

1. The team needs to first confirm cardiac arrest. Is she truly unresponsive? Is she breathing? Is there a pulse? The team leader should step in to assume assessment and care and first ensure that the patient is apneic, pulseless, and in cardiac arrest. Given the circumstances, cardiac arrest is very likely, so it may also be reasonable to direct your team to quickly move the patient to the firm surface of the floor and begin chest compressions if no pulse is found.
2. Quality chest compressions and rapid defibrillation.
3. You should consider the triangle of life. One provider at the head to manage airway and ventilations, one provider at the patient's side to perform chest compressions, and another provider on the other side of the patient to attach the AED. The two additional providers could be used for ALS procedures (if their scope of practice allowed) or could assist with compressions, ventilations, and patient movement as needed.
4. The patient's gasping is probably an agonal respiration. Unless there is an associated improvement in the patient, you should continue with the normal steps of resuscitation.
5. The team should switch compressors and immediately resume CPR. The airway manager might consider adding an airway adjunct. You should coordinate ALS and prepare for the next analyzation in 2 minutes.

CHAPTER 22 Diabetic Emergencies and Altered Mental Status

Think Like an EMT—The Sweet Taste of Success

1. This patient appears to be responsive and likely able to protect her airway. Her altered mental status and diabetic history round out the facts needed to decide glucose is appropriate at this time.
2. Although this patient has a diabetic history, there is nothing that says his seizure is related to his diabetes (as opposed to his head injury). In addition, his mental status isn't alert enough to administer an oral medication for fear

of possible aspiration. If he comes out of his seizure and becomes alert, you can obtain a further history.

3. Although this patient was involved in a collision, a diabetic emergency may have caused it. His altered mental status and diabetic history are enough to administer the glucose. Ensure that he is able to control his own airway before administering the oral glucose.

Short Answer

1. Signs of a diabetic emergency include altered mental status, seizures, pale skin, diaphoresis, tachycardia, rapid breathing, frequent urination, and increased thirst.
2. A history of diabetes can be obtained most easily by questioning the patient, family, or other bystanders familiar with the patient. Other indicators include medic alert bracelets; medications such as insulin or oral antidiabetics; and the presence of syringes, glucose meters, and/or an insulin pump.
3. After scene safety is ensured, treatment of a diabetic emergency must include a thorough assessment. Treat immediate life threats such as airway or breathing issues, and attempt to determine if the emergency is the result of hyper- or hypoglycemia (if possible). If you cannot make this determination, or if the patient is hypoglycemic, consider administering oral glucose if the patient has an intact airway and can control oral secretions. Oral glucose will replenish absent sugar stores in the bloodstream and potentially reverse hypoglycemia.
4. Unless local protocols dictate otherwise, baseline vitals should be obtained prior to administration of any medication.
5. Treatment of a patient with a seizure should include protection from trauma related to the seizure by moving them off any furniture and protecting their head. Additionally, maintain the airway and breathing support necessary, use supplemental oxygen per protocol, and perform thorough assessment to possibly identify the cause of the seizure.
6. For either a conscious or an unconscious stroke patient, conduct a thorough assessment that includes identification of when the stroke began. Care for a conscious stroke patient should include reassuring the patient, monitoring the airway, and administering oxygen according to local protocol. Transport the conscious stroke patient in a semi-sitting position. Care for an unconscious stroke patient should include maintaining an open airway and providing high-concentration oxygen and ventilatory support as needed. For transport, the unconscious stroke patient should be positioned lying on the affected side. Transport any stroke patient to a hospital with the capabilities to manage a stroke patient or as guided by local stroke care protocols.
7. Care for dizziness and/or syncope should include supplemental oxygen per protocol, a request for ALS assistance, laying the patient supine, and loosening tight clothing.

Critical Thinking Exercises

Oral glucose is not appropriate in an unconscious patient as they may aspirate on it. Contact ALS, support the airway and breathing if necessary, provide supplemental oxygen according to protocol, and initiate transport.

Pathophysiology to Practice

1. A seizure associated with hypoxia may be identified in the primary assessment. Disturbances to the airway and breathing make hypoxia a likely etiology. Consider also events leading up to the seizure as well. Did the patient have trouble breathing or choke? If the patient seized secondary to epilepsy, the presence of this disease is typically identified through gathering the patient history. Does the patient have a history of seizures? Do they take any antiseizure medications?
2. The history should reveal an event such as choking or severe respiratory distress that would cause hypoxia or a history of epilepsy (or multiple seizures over a period of years, which would indicate epilepsy even if the patient has not been diagnosed with epilepsy). Vital signs assessment that includes SpO_2 readings would indicate whether the patient's blood oxygen level is low (below 95 percent for mild hypoxia, below 90 percent for severe hypoxia). The history and physical assessments would also help to pinpoint other possible causes of a seizure, such as stroke, head trauma, toxic exposure or ingestion, hypoglycemia, infection, heat exposure, or pregnancy. Some seizures, including those associated with epilepsy, are of unknown origin.

Street Scene Questions

1. Every patient deserves a thorough patient assessment, particularly a patient with an altered mental status of a yet unknown cause.
2. Scene safety is always the first concern, but immediately following safety is the concern for primary assessment-related problems. Always rule out issues with the A-B-Cs first.
3. Many medical problems and traumatic injuries can make a patient seem intoxicated. Brain injuries, stroke, diabetic emergencies, and seizures can all make patients act as if they were drunk.
4. Patient assessment should be consistent in most situations, and certainly should not be based solely on a brief visual inspection and conversation as your partner just did. In this

situation, many etiologies could be at fault for the altered mental status so you should be extremely thorough in your assessment. If you discover more information, your assessment may be adjusted based on any newfound clues indicating possible trauma, diabetes, stroke, or alcohol abuse, or even a toxic exposure.

5. Obtaining a previous medical history may be difficult in an altered or uncooperative patient. Try asking questions. If that is not possible, consider taking clues from the scene such as presence of a medic alert bracelet or patient medications.
6. Any patient with an altered mental status is a high priority. Changes in mental status can indicate critical life threats. ALS is certainly warranted here. Given ALS response to your location, it may be a better idea to have them intercept with you while enroute to the hospital.

CHAPTER 23 Allergic Reactions

Think Like an EMT—Allergic Reaction or Anaphylaxis?

For the patients described below, allergic reaction or anaphylaxis is indicated by their presentation as follows:

1. A patient with a history of allergic reactions to bee stings reporting that she feels her throat "closing up" after a bee sting is likely starting to have an anaphylactic reaction because of the impending compromise of her airway. She needs immediate intervention.
2. A patient reports his skin is "just itching all over" is likely having an allergic reaction to something. Because there is no respiratory distress, or signs or symptoms of shock, you would not consider this anaphylaxis.
3. A patient who has an "allergy" to dairy products and reports only a stomach upset and diarrhea is likely having an allergic reaction. Because there is no respiratory distress, or signs or symptoms of shock, you would not consider this anaphylaxis.
4. A patient who is allergic to peanuts and has swelling of the face and neck, difficulty breathing, and a rapid pulse is likely having anaphylaxis because of the difficulty breathing and the tachycardia can also indicate a shock finding. This patient needs immediate intervention.
5. A patient who is allergic to penicillin, accidentally took a medication containing penicillin, is reporting dizziness, and has stable vital signs is likely having an allergic reaction only. Because there is no respiratory distress or signs or symptoms of shock, you would not consider this anaphylaxis.

Short Answer

1. The indications for the administration of an epinephrine auto-injector include the following: Patient exhibits the signs of an anaphylactic reaction, medication is prescribed for the patient by a physician, and medical direction authorizes its use for the patient.
2. Some of the more common causes of allergic reactions include:
   - Insect bites and stings from bees, yellow jackets, and wasps
   - Foods such as nuts, eggs, shellfish, and milk
   - Plants such as poison ivy, poison oak, and plant pollen
   - Medications such as penicillin and other antibiotics
   - Other irritants such as dust, chemicals, soaps, and makeup
3. Signs and symptoms of an anaphylactic reaction involving the skin, respiratory system, and cardiovascular system might include:
   - Skin: itching; hives; red skin; swelling of the face; warm, tingling feeling in the face, mouth, chest, feet, and hands
   - Respiratory system: tightness in the throat or chest; cough; rapid breathing; labored, noisy breathing; hoarseness, muffled voice, or loss of voice; stridor; wheezing
   - Cardiovascular system: increased heart rate, decreased blood pressure, poor peripheral perfusion

Critical Thinking Exercises

1. This patient does not have respiratory or circulatory compromise, but he may be headed in that direction. Presently his vital signs and adequate breathing indicate this is not the time to give epinephrine. However, the nature of shellfish allergies is that they can become severe, so the EMT should perform repeated assessments on the patient, looking for a worsening reaction. This is a good case to report to medical direction for advice.
2. This is not an anaphylactic reaction, and may not be an allergy. Some patients have nausea and vomiting as a side effect of pain pills. As such, epinephrine is not appropriate at this time. Transport the patient and observe her in case signs of allergic reaction do develop.
3. This is a prime candidate for the epinephrine auto-injector. He has signs of impending airway compromise and early shock. Follow local protocols to give the medication.

Pathophysiology to Practice

Any patients who are awake, whether they are experiencing an anaphylactic reaction or an anxiety attack, will experience similar effects from the administration of epinephrine. Remember that it's a very powerful drug that's primarily used to try to save the lives of patients in cardiac arrest. Because epinephrine mimics many effects of the sympathetic nervous system, administering it in a conscious patient is very risky because it can cause anxiety, difficulty breathing, rapid heart rate, palpitations, sweating, headache, nausea and vomiting, dizziness, and high blood pressure. However, you consider these side effects to be "acceptable trade-offs" when a patient is having anaphylaxis, because of the life-threatening nature of the condition and the effectiveness of epinephrine in treating it. Administering epinephrine to a patient having an anxiety attack is a significant–and reportable–drug error.

Street Scene Questions

1. Mr. Meeker is showing signs and symptoms of an anaphylactic reaction. He is using accessory muscles to breathe, and his face and neck look flushed. In addition, he cannot speak in complete sentences, which further demonstrates ventilatory involvement. He seems potentially unstable and needs to be monitored closely for what may be a life-threatening condition.
2. He obviously has an allergy to hornet stings. Physiologically, his immune system's antibodies are responding, but they are getting way out of hand. The overreaction of his immune system is causing histamine and other chemicals to be dumped into the bloodstream. This causes blood vessels to dilate, his blood pressure to fall, and many of his tissues to swell, including those in the lungs (bronchioles and larger airways) and the tissues surrounding his airway (glottis opening, epiglottis, and oral structures). Additional manifestations include thick mucus produced in the airways, and he might develop urticaria (hives).
3. From the information gathered thus far, it appears that Mr. Meeker is developing severe respiratory distress, which could, in turn, lead to respiratory failure and arrest. Even if he gets definitive care (an injection of epinephrine), he will probably need ventilatory support and supplemental oxygen.
4. The patient needs immediate control of his airway and breathing by administration of high-concentration oxygen through a bag-valve mask. Monitor the patient for shock, and arrange for quick ALS intercept or rapid transport to the nearest hospital. If your EMS system carries EpiPens, contact medical direction to determine if it should be administered.

CHAPTER 24 Infectious Diseases and Sepsis

Think Like an EMT—What's Going On?

1. Chickenpox causes intense itching, but the patient's normal appearance and behavior, as well as the lack of a fever, suggest an environmental cause of his rash, such as a reaction to a new laundry detergent.
2. These signs and symptoms sound like a typical case of influenza. Although it is more common during the winter months, influenza can occur at any time of year. A viral upper respiratory infection (a "cold") is more gradual in onset and does not typically cause a high fever. To differentiate this from meningitis, you might ask if light hurts the patient's eyes and if touching the chin to the chest is painful.
3. A homeless person is at risk for a number of diseases, including tuberculosis, pneumonia, and influenza. You might ask him if he's had night sweats and weight loss, which would be more likely with TB and less likely (but not impossible) with pneumonia or influenza. There are so many potential causes of this patient's condition that you may not be able to narrow them down. The most important actions to take in this situation are to protect yourself from infectious respiratory diseases and to treat the patient for shortness of breath.

Short Answer

1. The following is a list of SIRS criteria:
   - Temperature lower than 96.8° Fahrenehit (36° Celsius) or higher than 101° Fahrenheit (38.3° Celsius)
   - Heart rate over 90
   - Respiratory rate greater than 20
   - Systolic blood pressure less than 90 mmHg in patients who are suspected of septic shock
   - New-onset altered mental status or worsened mental status compared with normal in patients who are suspected of septic shock
2. The body systems that are the most common sources of sepsis are the pulmonary system, gastrointestinal system, genitourinary system, and central nervous system.
3. The incubation period is the time from exposure to development of the first symptoms. The transmissible period (also called the infectious period) is when the patient can spread the disease to others.
4. The answer to whether you have had the vaccinations you need to take care of patients without getting sick yourself is an individual one. As a health care worker, you have a duty to protect yourself and the public by being up-to-date on immunizations. As an EMT, you will likely have to provide proof of current immunizations, and the EMS service may require additional immunizations.
5. Hepatitis A is passed by the fecal-oral route, whereas hepatitis B and C are passed through blood, cerebrospinal fluid, amniotic fluid, and sex (semen and vaginal fluids). Symptoms of hepatitis A, B, and C include fever, nausea, vomiting, abdominal pain, loss of appetite, malaise, and jaundice, although some patients show no symptoms, especially with hepatitis C. Hepatitis A is usually not severe. Hepatitis B and C can lead to very severe illness, though not everyone becomes symptomatic. Hepatitis A usually clears up and has no long-lasting effects, but hepatitis B and C can lead to chronic illness and liver cirrhosis or liver

cancer. Hepatitis A and B can be prevented by vaccination and using Standard Precautions. There is no vaccine against hepatitis C, so prevention rests on the use of Standard Precautions. There is no specific treatment for hepatitis A and B, but there are approved treatments for hepatitis C that can eradicate the virus from the body.

6. Symptoms of meningococcal meningitis include headache, nausea, vomiting, photophobia, nuchal rigidity (stiff neck), fever, and rash. The rash consists of petechiae that do not blanch when you press on them. They do not blanch because the petechiae are caused by pinpoint hemorrhages under the skin.

Critical Thinking Exercises

Take care of the 2-year-old as you would any child with respiratory distress, but make sure to explain to both the child and the parents what you are doing and why. Once the patient is stabilized, take a moment to talk with the parents and explain that this sounds like a viral upper respiratory infection known as croup, and the barking cough makes the condition seem worse than it is. Determine if they have any other concerns, and do your best to address them.

Pathophysiology to Practice

Ask the patient to touch his chin to his chest. If he is unable or it is extremely painful to do so (a sign known as nuchal rigidity), this is likely a sign of meningeal irritation and signifies an urgent need for additional assessment and management in the emergency department.

Street Scene Questions

1. The genitourinary system is one of the most common locations for a source of sepsis. The length of the urethra in males ordinarily makes it difficult for microorganisms to invade the bladder from the external environment, but when a urinary catheter remains in place for an extended period, an infection becomes much more likely. This infection can easily grow into sepsis.
2. Three: heart rate over 90 (his is 92), respiratory rate greater than 20 (his is 22), and new-onset altered mental status. The SIRS criteria he doesn't meet are abnormal temperature and hypotension.
3. The patient now meets only one of the criteria, altered mental status, but he is very close to meeting the criteria for heart rate, respiratory rate, and temperature.
4. You should alert the hospital that this patient merits a sepsis alert. A patient's vital signs naturally fluctuate slightly, and the changes you detected in the second set are so small that they may very well reflect that normal variation. Another set of vital signs will probably give you a more accurate picture of any trend.

CHAPTER 25 Poisoning and Overdose Emergencies

Think Like an EMT—Administer Naloxone?

1. A 24-year-old male who is found unresponsive with a pulse and a normal respiratory rate is unlikely to have overdosed with a narcotic medication, given his respiratory rate. Narcotics cause the respirations to be depressed, and if this patient did overdose with enough narcotics to cause unresponsiveness, then the respiratory rate would also be slower.
2. The 56-year-old female has likely overdosed on a narcotic medication, given her altered mental status and the slow respiratory rate. As such, the use of naloxone would be justified.
3. A 44-year-old male found in cardiac arrest (no pulse or respirations) should not receive naloxone initially. Rather, he should be expediently treated with CPR and defibrillation as warranted. During this time, it may be advantageous to contact medical direction to determine if naloxone administration would be appropriate.
4. A 72-year-old female who is cyanotic around her lips and moans to painful stimuli should initially be ventilated and oxygenated to ensure her altered mental status is not from hypoxia. Following this, if the mental status and respiratory status does not improve, contact medical direction to consider the administration of naloxone.
5. Although this 18-year-old male admits to drug use, he currently still has a normal mental status and respirations. As such, the use of naloxone would not be warranted at this time. Although the administration of the medication would not harm the patient, if he did use the drug it apparently is not in his system yet, and you would not want the naloxone to wear off prematurely.

Think Like an EMT—Find the Clues

1. Look for prescription bottles and nonprescription meds. Look throughout the house, including the kitchen, bedroom, refrigerator, and bath. Check garbage cans for empty containers, and the toilet for vomitus. Look for loose pills anywhere in the house. Be sure to ask the patient what he took and what medications he knows of around the house.

2. After ensuring your safety and getting the patient extricated from the hazardous environment, you should attempt to determine how long the patient was in the garage with the car running. You may get this information from the patient (if he is conscious) or from family or neighbors.
3. Look for any chemicals the patient may have been using in the garden, however do not become overcome by the same thing that overcame the patient. Look around the garden, in garages or sheds, and even in garbage cans for chemical containers.

Short Answer

1. Poison can be ingested, inhaled, absorbed, and injected into the body.
2. The sequence of assessment steps in cases of poisoning is: Detect and immediately treat life-threatening problems in the primary assessment, gather a patient history and vital signs during the secondary assessment, consult medical direction as appropriate, and transport the patient with all containers and labels from the substance. Reassess the patient en route.
3. Gather the following information about a poisoning case before contacting medical direction:
   - What substance was involved?
   - When did the exposure occur?
   - How much was ingested?
   - Over how long a period did the ingestion occur?
   - What interventions have the patient, family, or well-meaning bystanders taken?
   - What is the patient's estimated weight?
   - What effects is the patient experiencing from the ingestion?
4. Emergency care steps for an ingested poisoning include gathering whatever information is available about the poison and contacting medical direction on the scene or en route. Administer activated charcoal as instructed by medical direction and position the patient for vomiting. Have suction equipment readily available, and never discard vomitus until it can be inspected by the receiving facility personnel or physician.
5. Emergency care steps for an inhaled poisoning include safely removing the patient from the source of the poison, establishing an open airway, and inserting an OPA or NPA if needed. Administer oxygen as appropriate to maintain SpO2 at or above 95%. Gather the patient's history, take vital signs, expose the chest for auscultation, contact medical direction, and initiate emergency transport. Emergency care steps for an absorbed poisoning include safely removing the patient from the source of the poison while avoiding your own cross-contamination. Always brush powders from the patient first, being careful not to abrade the patient's skin. Remove contaminated clothing. Irrigate with clear water for at least 20 minutes while catching contaminated water and disposing of it safely. Contact medical direction and initiate transport.

Critical Thinking Exercises

You will need to convince the patient that he needs to be transported because the toxic exposure may take longer to manifest itself. While doing so, prevent the patient from brushing at his jeans. Making sure that you are wearing protective gloves, brush off as much of the powder that remains on his hands and other body areas as possible. *Do not* try to rinse contaminated areas with water or any other "neutralizing" substance. Remove the patient's jeans and any other clothing or jewelry that might be contaminated with the pesticide. Transport him immediately, bringing along the pesticide container and its labels.

Pathophysiology to Practice

1. The poison control center's information that rattlesnake venom primarily affects the cardiovascular system should help you anticipate signs and symptoms you may see in the patient, such as a rapid, weak pulse; a low blood pressure; skin color changes; and weakness. These bites tend to be very painful when they first occur, and symptoms develop quickly. The patient will need to be transported to the hospital.
2. The poison control center's information that coral snake venom primarily affects the nervous system should help you anticipate signs and symptoms in the patient such as blurred vision, confusion, headache, slurred speech, numbness, paralysis, and coma. These bites may be painless at first, and major symptoms may not develop for hours. That's why these patients should always be further evaluated in the emergency department even when they might describe feeling fine right after the bite.

Street Scene Questions

1. Sample questions might include: "Do you have the original container?" "Do you know how much oil was previously in the lamp?" "Did you see your child drink the oil?" "What clues convinced you that she actually swallowed the oil?" "When do you think your daughter might have drunk the oil?" "Have you provided any treatment for your daughter?" "Has your daughter vomited?" "How much did she vomit?" "Did you save the vomit?"
2. Signs and symptoms for this substance can vary, depending on a number of factors, such as the weight of the patient, amount ingested, stomach contents, and whether or not the patient has vomited. Determine the level of consciousness, complete a primary survey and establish a set of vitals. Observe skin color and temperature. As with any patient, it is important to ensure that the child can maintain her own airway and breathing. Monitor for changes that

might alert you to the seriousness of the poisoning. Check the patient's pupils to determine whether they are equal and reactive; some poisons cause the pupils to constrict or dilate. The pupils may or may not react to light. Remember that seizure activity can also occur with an ingested poison.

3. Most of the care should be focused on the A-B-Cs. Consider the need for immediate transport. Depending on local or state protocols, contact poison control en route to the hospital. Because the ingested substance is a petroleum-based product, neither the use of activated charcoal nor syrup of ipecac is indicated. The lamp, or at least some of the oil, should be transported to the hospital along with the patient.
4. Consider contacting poison control, and discuss supportive care with medical direction. Remember that your local, state, and regional protocols will determine many of your actions here.

CHAPTER 26 Abdominal Emergencies

Think Like an EMT—Assessing a Patient with Abdominal Pain

1. For all patients with abdominal pain, you should get a history of oral intake as well as a history of recent vomiting, urination, and bowel movements. Females should also be asked about their obstetric and gynecologic history and the possibility of pregnancy. You will also perform a physical examination, including palpation of the abdominal quadrants.
2. You have the oral intake history, but ask specifically about recent bowel and bladder activity. Palpate the abdomen. Ask about vomiting and fever.
3. As with the first two questions, ask about vomiting and recent bowel and bladder activity, to include if there have been any changes to bowel/bladder activity. Determine the oral intake. Palpate the abdomen.

Short Answer

1. Some of the signs and symptoms seen with abdominal distress are nausea, vomiting, and diarrhea; pain with palpation and guarding; distention and bloating; discoloration of the abdomen; vomiting blood or coffee grounds-like emesis; black, tarry stools; tearing pain that radiates around to the back; and shock.
2. Visceral pain is pain coming from the organs that typically have fewer nerve endings. Visceral pain may vary in presentation. If the pain is intermittent, crampy, or colicky, it often comes from hollow organs of the abdomen. Pain that is dull and persistent often originates from solid organs of the abdomen. Parietal pain, as the name implies, arises from the parietal peritoneum, the lining of the abdominal cavity–thus, it is often referred to as peritoneal tenderness. Because of its more widespread and efficient nerve endings, pain originating from the parietal peritoneum is easier to locate and describe than pain from the visceral organs. It is described as sharp and localized, and it may change with body position. Visceral pain may arise in a patient complaining of abdominal pain and constipation who has a small bowel obstruction. Parietal pain may be seen with patients who have internal abdominal bleeding or an abdominal abscess that is irritating the peritoneal lining of the abdomen.
3. The treatment of a patient with abdominal pain is largely supportive. Treat the A-B-Cs, administer supplemental oxygen as necessary, place the patient in a position of comfort, and transport promptly. As part of the reassessment during transport, you should monitor vital signs.
4. The abdominal quadrants are the right upper quadrant (RUQ), left upper quadrant (LUQ), right lower quadrant (RLQ), and left lower quadrant (LLQ). The quadrants are determined by dividing the abdomen into four equal parts with imaginary lines drawn both vertically and horizontally through the umbilicus (the navel). The right and left sides of the quadrants are the patient's right and left.

Critical Thinking Exercises

Use the OPQRST memory aid to build a complete picture of the patient's present illness. Ask questions about each of the OPQRST factors (e.g., Onset - Did the pain originate suddenly or gradually? Provocation/Palliation–What makes the pain better or worse? Quality–Can you describe what the pain is like? Region/Radiation–Can you point to where you feel the pain?, Does the pain radiate elsewhere? Severity - How severe is the pain on a 1-10 scale? Time - How long have you been having this abdominal pain?). Then continue questioning the patient about the rest of his past medical history, or SAMPLE history (allergies, medications, pertinent past history, last oral intake, and events leading to the emergency). If the patient is female, you would also ask questions about the patient's menstrual cycle and possible vaginal bleeding, and other questions that might indicate a possible ectopic pregnancy. This patient would probably be most comfortable by lying on her side with her knees drawn up.

Pathophysiology to Practice

Elderly patients with abdominal pain must be carefully assessed, since research has shown they are up to nine times more likely to die than younger patients with the same cause of the abdominal pain. Compared with younger patients, elderly patients are more likely to present with life-threatening internal bleeding from causes such as gastrointestinal bleeding and abdominal aortic aneurysm. GI bleeding can occur anywhere from the esophagus to the rectum and may be gradual or acutely massive. These patients often develop signs of profound hypoperfusion. They may also have blood in their vomitus or bowl. Abdominal aortic aneurysm (AAA) is a ballooning or weakening in the wall of the aorta as it passes through the abdomen. Blood can leak from this weakened vessel wall, the affected area may grow larger or even suddenly rupture open. This is a surgical emergency and requires prompt transportation to an appropriate hospital.

Street Scene Questions

1. This patient seems to be showing signs of a medical emergency. Her skin color is pale and sweaty, she is breathing rapidly, and her pulse is fast. You should consider this patient unstable based on this information and prepare for rapid intervention and transport.
2. The symptoms reportedly came on suddenly. The rapid breathing, fast pulse, and pale and sweaty skin are initial clues that this patient has a potential medical emergency, and these signs are consistent with shock (hypoperfusion). Consider requesting ALS intervention unless transporting directly to the hospital will take less time.
3. The vomit can provide a number of important pieces of information for the hospital. Some of the helpful information is quantity; contents; presence of blood; and presence of coffee grounds-looking material, indicative of digested blood.
4. This patient may require IV therapy to replace the fluid and possible blood loss. Also, if she has a breathing emergency that requires a protected airway (and you are unable to perform endotracheal intubation), then ALS will be able to protect the airway, if necessary, and prevent aspiration if the patient vomits again.
5. This patient seems to be having a potentially life-threatening event that requires definitive care, possibly surgery, and/or blood replacement. It is important to get her to a hospital rapidly with ALS interventions started as early as possible.
6. Yes, the patient seems to be in compensated shock at present, and possibly to be deteriorating into decompensated shock. She has a rapid pulse, pale and sweaty skin, and her breathing is becoming rapid. She also has findings consistent with internal bleeding. The patient's blood pressure may be dropping. (We don't know her baseline normal, given the medication she is taking.)
7. It is always important to take notice of something as significant as a "mini-stroke." Also note that she is taking blood pressure medication; this may be the reason for her low blood pressure readings. The aspirin she is taking may also be responsible for abdominal bleeding as it can damage the mucosal lining of the stomach, and it can contribute to slow clotting of blood.
8. The patient should be placed in a position of comfort. Additional pain will cause more discomfort and aggravate her condition to the point where vital signs will become affected and your ability to complete a reassessment will also be affected. A key factor to consider is if the patient is going to vomit again, or keeps vomiting. In this case, consider transporting the patient in a recovery position to help with draining of vomitus from the mouth.

CHAPTER 27 Behavioral and Psychiatric Emergencies and Suicide

Think Like an EMT—Psych Condition or Hidden Medical Condition?

1. In this case a stroke or diabetic emergency could cause similar symptoms. Obtain a history from the patient, and observe for medical alert identification. If you have the ability to perform blood glucose measurement, do so. A stroke scale may be helpful if the patient is cooperative. A history of brain injury or other cause of altered mental status should be explored.
2. Alcohol may have caused the emergency, but it isn't the only potential cause. Perform a thorough history and a blood glucose measurement. Stroke isn't as likely in a 21-year-old. Consider drug use in addition to alcohol use and diabetes. Also look for evidence of brain injury or seizure history.
3. Depression won't normally cause aggressive behavior. Dementia or Alzheimer's may. Look for a history of this as well as compliance with her medications. Look for evidence of seizure, head injury, or diabetes. You may not be able to perform a stroke scale, but observe for signs of asymmetry in speech or for movement that is new to the patient.

Short Answer

1. A number of medical conditions can alter a person's mental status and behavior, including low blood sugar, lack of oxygen, inadequate blood to the brain or stroke, brain trauma, mind-altering substance abuse, excessive cold, excessive heat, and psychological conditions.
2. A number of methods will help calm a patient suffering from a behavioral or psychiatric emergency. Always speak slowly and calmly. Use a calm and reassuring tone. Listen to the patient, and rephrase statements back to the patient to ensure you are hearing information correctly and to let the patient know that you are listening actively. Do not be judgmental, no matter what the patient may say. Show compassion, not pity. Use positive body language; avoid crossing your arms or looking disinterested. Acknowledge the patient's feelings. Do not enter the patient's personal space; instead, stay at least 3 feet away.

3. Some of the signs and symptoms of behavioral or psychiatric emergency include panic or anxiety; unusual appearance, disordered clothing, and poor hygiene; agitated or unusual activity; unusual speech patterns or inability to carry on a coherent conversation; and reports of unusual or abnormal sounds or smells.
4. When your scene size-up reveals that it is too dangerous to approach a patient, *always* call for the police or fire department as appropriate, and wait for them to clear the scene. Do not leave the patient alone. Instead, if possible, try to talk to the patient from a safe distance.
5. A number of factors can help you assess a patient's risk for suicide, including previous threats of suicide; depression; high current or recent stress levels; previous attempts at suicide; a suicide plan; recent emotional trauma; age (those 15–25 and over 40 are at greater risk); alcohol and drug abuse; and apparent "sudden improvement" from depression.
6. Answers will vary depending on your state laws. In most states patients cannot be transported against their will without a legal document or psychiatric hold authorizing the transport. In some cases these can be signed only by a judge; in other cases they can be signed by law enforcement and physicians. Generally, though, if patients present with a clear-and-present danger of hurting themselves (or others in the process), then transport should be considered.

Critical Thinking Exercises

1. This could be a case of excited delirium, a very dangerous situation in which a patient will act extremely agitated or psychotic. This situation is thought to be due to drug intoxication or elevated temperature. The patient will suddenly cease struggling; often within minutes, the patient begins breathing inadequately and subsequently dies. Meanwhile, law enforcement and rescuers think the patient finally just "calmed down" and may fail to reassess. Always be alert for this sequence of events, and monitor the patient closely throughout the call. Have plenty of help, plan your activities, and always place the patient supine.
2. Be aware of your state laws regarding involuntary restraint and transportation of minors. Most states have laws that allow patients to be transported against their will if they are a danger to themselves or others. If the parents do not give permission to transport the patient, it will be helpful to contact medical direction and call for a law enforcement response for the safety of yourself, the patient, and the parents, and to help avoid liability problems if you attempt transport on your own. During transport, be acutely aware of the patient and his behavior, noting any findings that may indicate he is about to become violent towards you.
3. Whether or not someone "thinks" the patient is just seeking attention is completely irrelevant. Statistics show that a person who has attempted suicide in the past is more likely to commit suicide than one who has not. This patient must be assessed and transported. Given how the patient "attempted" suicide, you will need to constantly assess and reassess the A-B-Cs, recheck mental status and vitals, support any lost function, and do so while keeping yourself and your partner safe.

Pathophysiology to Practice

1. A patient with an imbalance in blood sugar can cause the rapid onset of erratic and hostile behavior that has nothing to do with the patient's psychological health. It's simply a matter of having too little or too much sugar available in the patient's blood.
2. A patient with head trauma can experience vast personality changes ranging from irritability to irrational behavior, as well as altered mental status, amnesia, or confusion.
3. A lack of oxygen (hypoxia) can cause restlessness, confusion, and altered mental status. The brain is a very sensitive organ that needs a constant supply of oxygen to function effectively and remain stable.

Street Scene Questions

1. Your first and foremost concern is scene safety. If the scene is known to be unsafe or if the patient is believed to have violent tendencies, you should not even get close to the scene until law enforcement officials have secured it. Remember that you cannot provide care if you become hurt. In fact, if you become injured in this type of situation, the event is compounded by the need to summon other units. Be safe! Be cautious!
2. In this case, scene safety should be handled by the appropriate law enforcement agency. Police officers are trained and equipped to handle these situations. As indicated in the scenario, you should make sure that all EMS personnel and bystanders are in a safe area in case the patient exits the building prior to the arrival of police officers. You should then await and follow law enforcement directives.
3. You should approach the patient after police declare the scene safe. In addition, a police officer might need to remain in the area until everybody is confident that the patient will not attempt to harm himself or others. In this scenario, you decide to approach after the police clear the scene, without a partner, in order to minimize patient agitation. However, a police officer remains in the area. In some cases a police officer might accompany EMS personnel to the hospital. If needed, physical restraints are used cautiously and only in select situations after contact with medical direction.
4. Rules for approaching a patient with a behavior disorder include:
   - Identify yourself.
   - Speak slowly and clearly.
   - Listen to the patient.

- Do not be judgmental.
- Use positive body language.
- Acknowledge the patient's feelings.
- Do not enter the patient's personal space.
- Be alert to the patient's emotional status.

5. Safety guidelines for dealing with agitated patients include:
   - Be alert and remain concerned with scene safety.
   - Treat life-threatening problems during the primary survey.

   Remember that some medical or traumatic injuries may mimic behavioral emergencies.
   - Be prepared to spend time talking with the patient.
   - Encourage the patient to discuss the problem; then listen.
   - Never play along with visual or auditory hallucinations.
   - If it appears that it might help, involve a family member or friend.
   - Consider physical restraints only as a last resort. If used, make every attempt not to cause additional harm to the patient. Pay very close attention to airway and breathing throughout the entire transport to the hospital.
6. Yes, all patients need to be assessed. In cases of behavioral emergencies, you should never assume the absence of an underlying medical or trauma-related condition. If behavioral patients will cooperate, you have an ethical and legal responsibility to take a full set of vital signs and to conduct a physical examination of the patient. During this time, don't underestimate how important communication skills are in the management of behavioral emergencies.

CHAPTER 28 Hematologic and Renal Emergencies

Think Like an EMT—Should You Request Advanced Life Support?

1. A 29-year-old patient with sickle cell anemia and severe pain in his arms and chest could be suffering from acute chest syndrome. Chest syndrome is characterized by shortness of breath and chest pain associated with hypoxia when blood vessels in the lungs become blocked. This patient will benefit from an ALS treatment and transport.
2. A 42-year-old patient who recently completed his peritoneal dialysis and complains of severe abdominal pain that is worsened by movement likely does not require an ALS transport unless he develops priority signs and symptoms. He may have developed an infection or infiltration of his peritoneum or catheter. He still requires transport and evaluation in the emergency department.
3. A 55-year-old female who refused to leave her house to go to her hemodialysis appointments and now complains of severe difficulty breathing, tachycardia, and anxiety definitely needs ALS intervention because of her priority signs and symptoms. She may be suffering from an electrolyte imbalance or kidney failure; the patient could even go into ventricular fibrillation or another lethal rhythm.
4. A 37-year-old sickle cell anemia patient complaining of extreme fatigue likely does not need an ALS transport as long as he does not develop signs of acute chest syndrome, high fever, hypoperfusion, or stroke. He should still be transported to the emergency department for evaluation.

Short Answer

1. Sickle cell anemia is an inherited disease in which patients have a genetic defect in their hemoglobin that results in an abnormal structure of the red blood cells, which causes them to block blood flow through the vessels during times of stress or hypoxia.
2. Patients with sickle cell disease have red blood cells composed of defective hemoglobin that causes the cells to lose their ability to have a normal shape and compressibility. Instead of normal, doughnut-shaped red blood cells, sickle cell patients have red blood cells that resemble a sickle, or crescent, when observed under a microscope. During times of stress or hypoxia, these misshapen red blood cells move throughout the bloodstream, where they can become clogged in capillaries and organs because of their shape and lack of compressibility. This is known as *sludging*.
3. Chronic renal failure patients on hemodialysis must have specialized intravascular access sites established to allow for their frequent dialysis treatments. These sites are the surgical connection between an artery and a vein, known as a fistula. Because arteries maintain a much higher pressure than do veins, the site will create turbulent blood flow across the fistula. The palpable vibration of this turbulent blood flow is known as a "thrill."
4. In hemodialysis, patients are connected to a dialysis machine that pumps their blood through specialized filters to remove toxins and excess fluid. This is almost always completed in a local or regional dialysis center. Peritoneal dialysis, in contrast, is typically completed at home. Patients have a permanent catheter implanted through the abdominal wall and into the peritoneal cavity. Several liters of a specially formulated dialysis solution are then infused into the abdominal cavity and left in place for several hours, where it absorbs waste material and excess fluid; then the fluid is drained back out of the abdomen and into the bag and discarded.
5. Patients who miss a dialysis appointment are at risk for fluid and toxin buildup in their system. This can manifest with symptoms similar to heart failure. These patients may develop shortness of breath, peripheral and pulmonary edema, and even cardiac rhythm disturbances from electrolyte abnormalities.

Critical Thinking Exercises

1. It is critical that patients with end-stage renal disease maintain their regularly prescribed schedule of dialysis. Their kidneys simply have no other way of balancing fluids and electrolytes and removing toxins. Missing even a single treatment can be deadly for some patients, who could very quickly develop pulmonary edema and shortness of breath.
2. Unfortunately, it can be very easy to classify patients as "drug seekers" when you encounter so many different individuals complaining of pain and seeking relief. However, doing so in this case is irresponsible. Reviewing the pathophysiology of sickle cell disease should prompt you to remember that these patients can develop severe pain in their arms, legs, chest, and/or abdomen due to sludging of sickled red blood cells in the capillaries. This is known as sickle cell pain crisis. These patients need supplemental oxygen and transportation to the hospital where they will likely receive IV fluids and pain medication. During transport, monitor for signs of inadequate breathing, hypoperfusion, and stroke symptoms.

Pathophysiology to Practice

1. A patient with sickle cell disease who starts to show signs and symptoms of stroke is a huge concern. Because sickled cells are more likely to become blocked–or to sludge–in capillaries and organs throughout the bloodstream, the risk of stroke in these patients is greatly increased. This patient should be transported to a designated stroke center if available.
2. Patients with sickle cell disease eventually lose normal function of their spleen. This organ is extremely vascular, filters a large percentage of blood, and has infection-fighting functions. Because sickled red blood cells become sludged here, the spleen is severely damaged and fails to perform its function of fighting infections. This places these patients at a higher risk for severe, life-threatening infections than those with normal splenic function.

Street Scene Questions

1. Initially you should complete a primary assessment of the patient and evaluate her mental status. Ask the staff members what the patient's normal level of consciousness is and how her presentation today differs from her norm. Carefully assess the airway for patency, breathing for adequacy, and circulation for good perfusion markers. The patient's color is not good, so get the pulse oximeter attached.
2. The history of the patient's dialysis is significant because any patient with end-stage renal disease has the potential to develop complications with the neurologic, respiratory, and cardiovascular systems due to fluid overload, electrolyte abnormalities, and toxic waste buildup in the bloodstream, as well as an increased risk of infection.
3. You should complete a full set of vital signs and a secondary assessment. Listen to her lungs. Test the patient's blood sugar if your local protocols allow it. Because the patient is not really following your commands appropriately, you should assess her for stroke by using a stroke scale.
4. The patient's condition may well be related to her dialysis. Because the patient has difficulty breathing and some wet-sounding lung sounds, you should be concerned about pulmonary edema and congestive heart failure. Furthermore, she also has peripheral edema that points towards fluid overload.
5. Given the patient's deteriorated mental status and respiratory impairment, it is in the patient's best interest to be transported to the hospital, where she can be treated for the pulmonary edema and further evaluated by an emergency department physician. Although she will still need dialysis, the hospital will be able to provide it. If the staff on the scene disagree with your decision, you can always contact medical direction, run the situation by them, and follow their guidance about where to transport the patient.

CHAPTER 29 Bleeding and Shock

Think Like an EMT—No Pressure, No Problem

1. You should expedite this patient because of the potential for internal injuries, such as injuries to the chest or lungs. Since his vitals are elevated, he is anxious, and the skin is cool and moist, this could be a serious situation indicating early shock.
2. Just because the bleeding is from hemorrhoids doesn't mean the patient isn't in shock. Her appearance screams shock as evidenced by pale and sweaty skin, and her feeling of wanting to pass out when she stands up indicates orthostatic hypotension.
3. The patient hasn't lost enough blood to have shock. Your bigger concerns are if the patient can't maintain his airway because of blood flow and whether the head injury is a concern. Right now, there doesn't seem to be a big rush, but he needs transport.

Short Answer

1. The three main blood vessels and the bleeding that might present from each are:
   - Arteries: Arterial bleeding is often rapid, spurting with each heartbeat, profuse, and bright red.
   - Veins: Venous blood is usually characterized by a steady flow, can be quite heavy, and is usually dark red or maroon in color.
   - Capillaries: Capillary bleeding is usually slow, oozing, and red (though not as bright as arterial blood).
2. The patient care steps for external bleeding include performing a scene size-up, taking Standard Precautions, applying direct pressure to the wound, and administering oxygen if hypoxia is suspected. If hemostatic dressings are available, they can be applied, using a gloved hand to provide pressure. If bleeding fails to stop, you may need to consider a tourniquet placement. The patient should be assessed and treated for shock.
3. Perfusion is defined as the supply of oxygen to, and removal of wastes from, the body's cells and tissues as a result of the flow of blood through the capillaries. Hypoperfusion is the body's inability to adequately circulate blood to the body's cells to supply them with oxygen and nutrients and inadequate removal of wastes, similar to what occurs in shock.
4. Signs and symptoms of shock include altered mental status; pale, cool, and clammy skin; nausea and vomiting; and vital sign changes (increased pulse, increased respirations, decreasing blood pressure, and narrow pulse pressure). Late signs of shock include thirst, dilated pupils, and cyanosis around the lips and nail beds. The causes of the shock findings are a combination of increasing sympathetic tone and decreasing intravascular volume from the blood loss.
5. The three major types of shock and their causes are:
   - Cardiogenic shock, caused by inadequate pumping of blood by the heart
   - Distributive shock, caused by uncontrolled dilation of blood vessels due to anaphylactic, neurogenic, or septic causes
   - Obstructive shock, caused by obstructed blood flow from the heart due to conditions such as cardiac tamponade, pulmonary embolism, or tension pneumothorax.

   The overall term *hypovolemic shock* simply means an insufficient volume in the circulatory system.
6. Managing shock specifically entails maintaining an open airway, administering oxygen, controlling any external bleeding, keeping the patient warm, and transporting the patient in a supine position.

Critical Thinking Exercises

The mechanism of injury suggests the possibility of internal bleeding. Vitals indicate that shock may be starting. Obviously, the first step is to take Standard Precautions. Spinal motion restriction precautions should be employed based on local protocol. Treat for shock by maintaining the airway, providing supplemental oxygen as appropriate, assisting with ventilations (if necessary), controlling any external bleeding, keeping the patient warm, and providing immediate transport.

Pathophysiology to Practice

Bleeding does not necessarily need to be present for shock to have occurred. Some medications cause vasodilation, leading to decreased venous return and, hence, decreased cardiac output. Some medications, such as aspirin and warfarin, can cause severe internal bleeding when taken in excess. Bleeding does not necessarily need to be present for shock to have occurred. Shock can also occur from an overdose of medications such as beta blockers (labetalol, propranolol) and high blood pressure medications (Norvasc, captopril).

Street Scene Questions

1. The fact that the patient has sustained some type of traumatic injury makes him a candidate for high-priority treatment. Even so, the EMS providers still need to perform some kind of primary assessment to determine such information as level of responsiveness, breathing, and signs of internal bleeding, which are potential problems with trauma.
2. In addition to the mechanism of injury, you will want assessment information such as vital signs (respiration rate, pulse, blood pressure, and skin color). The arriving EMTs might also ask about bruising or discoloration over the injured area, as these are important signs of possible internal bleeding.
3. Yes, the mechanism of injury is important. In the case of a trauma patient, the mechanism of injury can help determine the location, type, and severity of injuries sustained.
4. Treatment priorities depend on the A-B-Cs. Because you suspect internal bleeding, rapid transport is indicated. You should consider administration of supplemental oxygen according to protocol and attempt to keep the patient warm and remain alert to signs of shock.
5. Vital signs should be taken every 5 minutes to determine changes in the patient's condition since he is a high priority patient. In cases of internal bleeding, you can expect that the pulse rate will increase and become threadier. You can also expect the respiratory rate to become more rapid and increasingly labored. The patient's skin will grow paler and more moist. As the signs and symptoms of shock (hypoperfusion) intensify, you can expect dilated pupils, delayed capillary refill time (which is not always a reliable indicator), and cyanosis around the lips and nail beds. The detailed assessment may reveal tenderness in the left upper abdominal quadrant.

CHAPTER 30 Soft Tissue Trauma

Think Like an EMT—Burns By the Numbers

1. This patient's burns are 45 percent superficial.
2. This patient's burns are approximately 3 percent partial thickness.
3. This patient's burns are 45 percent partial thickness (around the legs, front and back, so 18 + 18) + 9 percent full thickness (arms).

Short Answer

1. The types of closed soft-tissue injuries are contusions, hematomas, and crush injuries.
2. The types of open soft-tissue injuries are abrasions, lacerations, punctures, avulsions, amputations, and crush injuries.
3. An object impaled in the cheek should only be removed if it has already gone through the inside surface of the cheek, both the entrance and exit of the object is visualized, and the object can be easily pulled out in the same direction that it entered. If this cannot be done, the object should be stabilized in place.
4. The three classifications (depths) of burns are:
   - Superficial burn–a burn that involves only the epidermis The skin is typically red and painful.
   - Partial thickness burn–a burn in which the epidermis is burned through and the dermis is damaged The burn site will be reddened, painful, and moist, and blisters will be present.
   - Full thickness burn–a burn in which all the layers of the skin are damaged, the burned tissue may be painless, and the overlying eschar is typically hard or firm to the touch.
5. The difference between a dressing and a bandage is that a dressing is placed directly on a wound and a bandage holds a dressing in place. Dressings must always be sterile as they go against an open wound, while bandages need not be sterile (although often they are).
6. The qualities of an effective bandage are that it should hold a dressing snugly in place and cover all four of its edges but not restrict blood supply. If a bandage is too loose, it will slip around and bleeding can still occur from beneath it. Indications that a bandage is too tight can include pain, pale or cyanotic skin, cold skin, numbness, and tingling.

Critical Thinking Exercises

It's not uncommon to arrive on scene to find a patient bandaged up like this by well-meaning bystanders. However, *you* are the definitive care provider. As the EMS professional, you need to view all of the patient's wounds with your own eyes. Failure to do so could cause you to miss something or fail to control bleeding properly. Do not make the mistake of arriving at the hospital without having assessed the severity of every potential injury and wound. If the patient is unstable and needs to be expedited, do not delay transport, but rather assess the wounds en route. This is the only way to know how much the patient is bleeding and which wounds need your direct attention or intervention. In this case, as you carefully remove the dressing and bandage, you should be prepared to apply direct pressure immediately if you see a significant amount of bleeding. Once you have inspected the wound, rebandage it.

Pathophysiology to Practice

When caring for a burn patient, always think beyond the burn. Try to determine any mechanism of injury that might have occurred with the burn incident. If the patient has decreased blood pressure or other signs of shock, always assume the potential of other serious injuries and sources of bleeding because the shock that accompanies significant burns does not manifest typically till hours after the incident. Thus, any shock findings that occur right after a burn could actually be from concurrent trauma or blood loss. Attempt to determine the patient's problem through standard assessment techniques of physical exam and history gathering.

Street Scene Questions

1. The patient seems alert and appears to have walked to the present location after her injury. She has an open airway and is breathing without any obvious distress. Judging from the blood-soaked towel, the immediate focus of care is on "C," or circulation.
2. Until further assessment, the patient might be assigned low-priority transport. However, she has the potential to lose a significant amount of blood, and you should be ready to upgrade the patient's priority as necessary.
3. The bleeding must be controlled if it is not. You should apply direct pressure with a sterile dressing. If necessary, you can consider a tourniquet proximal to the injury if bleeding remains uncontrolled. Once the bleeding is controlled, you should assess pulses, motor ability, and sensation in the injured arm. You should also administer supplemental oxygen as appropriate, keep the patient warm, and observe for signs of shock.
4. A suspicion of alcohol consumption should not interfere with your assessment and treatment. You must obtain a set of vitals and the patient's history. Based on the pool of blood on the patio and the lack of motion of the patient's finger, the patient appears to have the potential to become

unstable. You should consider upgrading her priority from "low" to "high" because of these findings.

5. You must monitor the bleeding and stabilize the patient's arm with some type of splinting device or sling. You should take vital signs every 15 minutes if she is still prioritized as stable, or every 5 minutes if she is upgraded to a high priority patient. In either instance, compare subsequent vitals the baseline set of vitals. You should then reassess motor function and sensation as well. Because of the potential for shock, the patient should be kept warm and perhaps be placed on the cot with her legs elevated.

CHAPTER 31 Chest and Abdominal Trauma

Think Like an EMT—What's the Likely Cause?

1. Because the patient has diminished lung sounds on one side and describes sharp pain that changes when he breathes, it's likely that he has suffered a collapsed lung (pneumothorax). This can occur spontaneously in patients of any age, including during physical activity such as jogging.
2. Absent lung sounds on one side of the chest, accompanied by distended neck veins and hypotension following penetrating trauma, are likely indications of development of a tension pneumothorax. If the injury was just to the heart and caused cardiac tamponade, the patient would still have the distended neck veins and hypotension, but breath sounds would be clear and equal. The pulmonary and cardiovascular findings in this patient point to a tension pneumothorax as the most likely injury.
3. A patient who was shot in the chest near the fourth intercostal space with hypotension, distended neck veins, narrowing pulse pressure, and normal lung sounds on both sides of the chest is likely developing a cardiac tamponade. The sac surrounding the heart may have been penetrated by the bullet and is filling with blood or fluid, compressing the heart. This increases venous congestion and causes the distended neck veins and hypotension. Since the lungs were not injured, breath sounds are normal.

Short Answer

1. Signs and symptoms of a flail chest include paradoxical movement of the chest cavity during spontaneous breathing, difficulty breathing, a palpable area of instability to the chest wall, and pain at the injury site. Signs of shock and hypoxia are likely.
2. The difference between a pneumothorax and a tension pneumothorax is one of pressure. A pneumothorax occurs when air enters the chest cavity, causing collapse of a lung. In a tension pneumothorax, the air trapped in the chest cavity can build up such pressure that it collapses the lung on that side and puts pressure on the heart, great blood vessels, and the unaffected lung on the other side. This can reduce the ability of the heart and lungs to pump and oxygenate blood. Typically breath sounds will be absent on the injured side and diminished on the opposite side.
3. Care for a penetrating wound to the chest should include maintaining the patient's airway and providing ventilatory and circulatory support, if needed. Initially the EMT should seal the open chest wound as quickly as possible, even by using a gloved hand if necessary. Subsequently, the EMT would apply an occlusive dressing (depending on local protocols, sealed on all four sides or with a flutter valve), administer supplemental oxygen based on protocol, provide care for shock, and transport as soon as possible.
4. Care for an open abdominal wound should include keeping the airway open, staying alert for vomiting, placing the patient supine with legs flexed at the knees, administering supplemental oxygen per protocol, providing care for shock, constantly monitoring vital signs, and transporting as soon as possible. Never give the patient anything by mouth. Cover an open abdominal wound with evisceration by soaking a sterile dressing with sterile saline and placing the moist dressing over the wound. Additionally, apply an occlusive dressing over the moist dressing and treat the patient for shock.

Critical Thinking Exercises

Absent breath sounds on the side of the injury may indicate a collapsed lung (pneumothorax) progressing into a tension pneumothorax. The nail also may have damaged a major blood vessel or the heart itself. If the occlusive dressing you applied is sealed on all four sides, air building up in the chest cavity will have no way to escape and can cause lung collapse and increased pressure on the heart. In accordance with local protocols or online medical direction, pick up a corner of the dressing to let air escape while the patient is exhaling. Maintain a patent airway. Administer oxygen per protocol, care for shock, and transport as quickly as possible. Provide basic life support (ventilations or CPR) if necessary. Request ALS intercept if available and if it will not delay the patient's arrival at the hospital.

Pathophysiology to Practice

1. Blunt trauma to the chest always carries with it the potential of damage to underlying structures as well as flail chest. However, oxygenation and ventilation of the patient are critical to her survival. If her breathing is becoming shallow or more difficult, you must assist her breathing with supplemental oxygen via bag-valve-mask device. Be careful

in tracking or assisting her inhalations, as there is always a possibility that aggressive assisted ventilations might cause a pneumothorax or convert a simple pneumothorax to a tension pneumothorax. However, without knowing the extent of her injuries from the blunt trauma, providing her ventilatory assistance is the priority right now.

2. Blunt trauma to the lower rib area has the potential to injure solid organs such as the liver on the right and spleen on the left. Both organs are very vascular. Depending on the amount of force exerted, these organs can bleed profusely or may actually just ooze blood undetected until orthostatic hypotension becomes apparent.

Street Scene Questions

1. Your general impression of the patient is that he is already exhibiting poor skin signs and guarding his chest due to pain. Because the mechanism of injury and impact were on his side of the vehicle, you should be concerned about blunt-force chest and abdominal trauma.
2. Until you can assess him further, his skin signs and breathing difficulty should give you concern. He is potentially unstable, and you should consider him a high-priority patient at this point.
3. Once you know the scene is safe to enter and you've taken Standard Precautions, you may need to initiate spinal motion restriction precautions based on local protocol. If the patient has findings consistent with hypoxia, initiate supplemental oxygen per protocol. Try to continue assessing the patient while you work with the fire department to safely extricate the patient from the vehicle.
4. The patient remains a high priority because his radial pulse is weak and rapid. The pain he is describing on his left side could mean he has suffered damage to one of the very vascular organs in that area, such as the spleen, or even may have suffered an underlying pulmonary injury.
5. Complete spinal motion restriction precautions as appropriate, and continue to reassess the patient. Try listening to lung sounds again when you can get into the quieter environment of the ambulance. If one is readily available nearby, the patient should be transferred to an Advanced Life Support ambulance. However, transport should not be delayed. The patient meets the criteria to be transported to a trauma center, which can provide the most optimal care for the patient.

CHAPTER 32 Musculoskeletal Trauma

Think Like an EMT—Sticks and Stones May Break My Bones, but Trauma Centers Save Me

1. A local hospital is acceptable for this patient as long as the head injury isn't more severe than the suspected fracture. If his mental status and vitals stay within normal limits, a trauma center may not be necessary. When in doubt, radio the hospital for medical direction.
2. A long backboard as a body splinting device and transport to a trauma center are appropriate for this patient. He has multiple fractures with an altered mental status and vitals that indicate shock is progressing. Transport expeditiously and continue assessment and care enroute.
3. This patient doesn't have major complaints, but his mechanism of injury is significant and vital signs demonstrate shock is progressing. This patient needs transported to a trauma center. Put your patient on a long backboard for whole body splinting, and initiate transport immediately while providing additional care enroute.

Short Answer

1. Bones are hard, semi-rigid, complex structures composed of calcium and protein fibers. Bones are covered by a strong, white fibrous material called periosteum, through which the blood vessels and nerves pass as they enter and leave the bone. They are the body's framework, providing support and protection for the internal organs. They store salts and metabolic materials and are a site of red blood cell production. Bones may be classified according to shape; they include long bones, flat bones, short bones, and irregular bones. With the muscles, ligaments, and tendons, they play a major part in the body's ability to move.
2. The signs and symptoms of musculoskeletal injury are pain and tenderness; deformity or angulation; grating or crepitus; swelling/edema; bruising/contusions; exposed bone ends through the overlying skin; joints becoming locked and not moving; and nerve and blood vessel compromise.
3. Take and maintain all Standard Precautions. Perform the primary assessment. After life-threatening conditions have been addressed, all patients with a painful, swollen, or deformed extremity must be splinted. For a low-priority (stable) patient, splint before transport. For a high-priority (unstable) patient, immobilize the whole body on a long spine board; then initiate transport rapidly and continue assessment and care enroute. If appropriate, cover open wounds with sterile dressings, assess PMS before and after immobilization, elevate the extremity while preserving stability, and apply a cold pack to the area to help reduce swelling. Injured long bones should be realigned using manual traction, then splinted. Injured joints should be splinted in the position found unless the distal extremity is cyanotic or lacks pulses, in which case the EMT can attempt to place the joint in a normal anatomic position once to see if the distal pulse returns.

4. Long bones with angulated and deformed injuries should be realigned to anatomic position to restore effective circulation to the distal extremity and to fit it into a splint. This process may also help to decrease bleeding from the bone as well.
5. The basic principles of splinting are as follows: Expose the area and control bleeding before splinting. Assess pulses, motor abilities, and sensation before and after splinting. Align long-bone injuries with gentle traction if there is severe deformity. Splint to immobilize the injury site and adjacent joints. Choose a splinting method based on the severity of the patient's condition and priority decision. Pad splints for patient comfort. If possible, splint patients before moving them. If the patient is unstable, don't waste time splinting.
6. Some of the hazards of splinting include neglecting other life-threatening conditions; applying the splint so tightly that soft tissues are compressed and injury is caused to adjacent nerves, blood vessels, and muscles; and applying the splint so loosely or inappropriately that further soft-tissue injury occurs from bone/joint movement.
7. The basic splints carried on ambulances include rigid splints, formable splints, and traction splints. The splint chosen depends on the bone/joint that is injured.

Critical Thinking Exercises

1. Assessment findings that indicate that a patient with a musculoskeletal injury is in shock, or is progressing into shock, include vital sign changes (such as tachycardia, narrowed pulse pressure, rapid breathing, and hypotension); altered mental status; pale, cool, or clammy skin; and nausea and vomiting.
2. Identifying a patient with a rapid pulse and anxiety from *pain* versus a patient with a rapid pulse and anxiety from *shock* really comes down to your ability to conduct a thorough assessment and differentiate between patients who are stable and patients who are unstable. The patient in shock may have the additional signs and symptoms of narrowed pulse pressure or low systolic blood pressure; altered mental status; and pale, cool, and clammy skin. Other signs of shock include thirst, dilated pupils, and cyanosis around the lips and nail beds.

Pathophysiology to Practice

1. Bones can cause shock because they are living, vascular structures that contain a rich supply of blood. A bone fracture can interrupt millions of tiny blood vessels innervating the bone tissue, leading to significant bleeding. For example, a fracture of the femur can lead to 1,000 mL of blood loss or more. In addition, broken bone ends can move around and damage surrounding tissues, even puncturing the overlying skin, causing additional bleeding.
2. When distal circulation is compromised or shut down, tissues beyond the injury become starved for oxygen and die, not unlike a blood vessel being occluded during a stroke or heart attack. The broken long bone(s) of extremities must be repositioned to ensure circulation is established in the distal limb. The patient may have a few moments of pain during the maneuver, but this intervention may mean saving the limb and preventing amputation.
3. There are many cases when bones might fracture yet present without obvious deformity. Examples include greenstick fractures and comminuted fractures. In some cases a bone might not be displaced when fractured. This is why you should splint all suspected musculoskeletal fractures.

Street Scene Questions

1. Because the patient appears stable, this patient is probably a low priority. This priority could change after a complete assessment, however; it's always possible the patient may have some internal bleeding at the injury location.
2. Perform a secondary assessment and obtain the history and vital signs. Ask the patient about allergies, medications, and her last meal. Given this information, the EMT can continue to treat the patient appropriately.
3. Signs and symptoms of a broken long bone include pain and tenderness, deformity or angulation, grating (crepitus), swelling/edema, bruising/contusions, exposed bone ends through the overlying skin, and distal nerve and/or blood-vessel compromise. When assessing a patient with a possible musculoskeletal injury, consider assessing the six Ps: pain, pale skin, pulses diminished, paresthesia (a tingling sensation), pressure, and paralysis.
4. The major concern with this type of injury is possible nerve, vessel, or muscle damage at and below the injury site. As part of the assessment, take the following steps: Evaluate pedal pulses, look at skin color, feel for temperature, check capillary refill in the foot, ask the patient to move her foot and toes, and see if the patient can feel someone touch her toes and foot. Any deficit noted should be documented in the PCR.
5. After assessing the patient, splint the injury, making sure the procedure is done with as little movement as possible while ensuring that the injury is aligned properly. The entire leg should be secured to immobilize the joint above and below the injury site. Be sure to apply padding as appropriate and then reassess vitals as well as pulses, motor function, and sensation below the injury site. Monitor the injury enroute to ensure that additional problems from splinting do not occur.

CHAPTER 33 Trauma to the Head, Neck, and Spine

Think Like an EMT—More than a Pain in the Neck

1. If the patient appears to have pain (even if she denies it) and she consents to care, she should have spinal motion restriction precautions used. Sometimes the shock of the crash masks the pain temporarily, and patients may not realize they are injured.
2. The head injury and significant mechanism of injury indicate that spinal motion restriction precautions should be taken prior to transport.
3. Without a significant mechanism of injury, complaint of pain, or distracting condition evident, the patient doesn't require spinal motion restriction precautions to be taken.

Short Answer

1. The two components of the central nervous system are the brain and spinal cord. Messages from all over the body travel up the spinal cord and are received by the brain, which decides how to respond to changing conditions both inside and outside the body by sending stimuli messages down the spinal cord and out to the body. Thus, the spinal cord functions as a relay between body and the brain.
2. Determining possible skull or brain injury can be very difficult. Therefore, you should always assume skull or brain injury when indicated by a relevant mechanism of injury. Signs of brain injury can include visible skull fragments, altered mental status, deep laceration or severe bruising to the head, depression or deformity of the skull, severe pain at the site of a head injury, Battle sign (late sign), raccoon eyes (late sign), one eye that appears sunken, bleeding or clear fluid from the ears or nose, personality changes, Cushing reflex, irregular breathing patterns, temperature changes, blurred or multiple-image vision, impaired hearing or ringing in the ears (tinnitus), equilibrium problems, forceful vomiting, motor posturing, paralysis on one side of the body, seizure activity, and deteriorating vital signs.
3. Appropriate treatment for a patient with a possible head or brain injury includes taking Standard Precautions. Use the jaw-thrust maneuver to open and maintain the patient's airway. Monitor changes in breathing and support any lost function with a BVM and oxygen. Apply a cervical collar and provide spinal motion restriction precautions. Control the patient's bleeding if needed. Keep the patient at rest. Monitor vital signs every 5 minutes. Talk to the conscious patient, providing emotional support. Dress and bandage open wounds. Manage the patient for shock. Transport promptly and consider ALS backup or intercept en route to a trauma center.
4. Any of the following mechanisms of injury will support a suspicion of a spine injury: if a patient was involved in a motor-vehicle or motorcycle collision; was struck by a vehicle; fell to the ground from a height; received blunt trauma to the spine or above the clavicles; sustained penetrating trauma to the head, neck, or torso; was involved in a diving accident; was found hanging by the neck; or was found unconscious due to trauma.
5. The appropriate care for a patient with a possible spine injury includes providing spinal motion restriction precautions . Apply a cervical collar while maintain manual spinal motion restriction until fully secured to a long backboard. Do not forget, however, that you may simultaneously be treating loss of function to the airway, breathing, and circulatory components of the body if the patient is severely injured. Reassess sensory and motor function in all four extremities both before and after immobilization.

Critical Thinking Exercises

1. This may be neurogenic shock. Injuries to the thoracic or lumbar spine can prevent impulses from the sympathetic nervous system from reaching the body as they normally would. As a result, the heart rate is typically not found to be rapid, the blood pressure may be lowered from an absence of vasoconstriction, the pulses may feel bounding, and the skin may be warm and dry.
2. Targeted hyperventilation in cases of severe head injuries may be used by ALS providers in certain situations while monitoring the end-tidal CO_2 levels ($ETCO_2$). However, uncontrolled hyperventilation as being done by your partner can reduce blood perfusion to the brain and worsen the brain injury. You should immediately instruct your partner to ventilate appropriately at a rate of 10-12/minute.
3. Go to the patient, identify yourself, and seek consent for treatment. Due to the mechanism of injury, assume the possibility of injuries to the head and spine. Initiate manual spinal motion restriction precautions for the head and neck. Assess the A-B-Cs rapidly. Quickly assess the sensory and motor function in all four extremities. After assessing the head and the neck, apply a cervical collar while maintaining manual stabilization. Apply the appropriate immobilization device. Administer high-concentration oxygen as protocol indicates. Reassess sensory and motor function in all four extremities. Control any bleeding and dress and bandage open wounds. Keep the patient at rest. Manage the patient for shock, even if shock is not present. Reassure the patient. Monitor vital signs every 5 minutes and initiate transport.

Pathophysiology to Practice

Nipple level is innervated by T4.

Navel is innervated by T10.

Little finger is innervated by C8.

Big toe is innervated by S1.

Street Scene Questions

1. The patient appears to be unconscious, with a head injury and possible spinal injury. The oozing from the head seems to be from an abrasion but merits closer assessment in case it is an indication of a more significant injury, such as an open skull fracture. Because of the mechanism of injury and the patient's lack of consciousness, the teenager should be considered a high priority for transport.
2. After donning your PPE for spinal precautions, assessment and protection of the A-B-Cs are always the top priority. To accomplish these tasks, first establish manual spinal motion restriction of the head and neck. Manage the patient's airway and breathing components as necessary, and scan the body for and treat any major bleeds. After confirming the source of bleeding from the head abrasion, treat it as appropriate but keep pressure to a minimum if a skull fracture is suspected. Establish and monitor the patient's level of consciousness. Take a baseline set of vitals and get a history from the patient, bystanders, and mother (when she arrives). Place the patient on a long spine board, securing the torso first, then the head. Use the appropriate equipment to secure the head in place. Initiate transport, consider ALS backup or intercept. En route, reassess the patient's vital signs and level of responsiveness and repeat your primary assessment.
3. A good way of monitoring changes in the level of responsiveness is to ask the patient to repeat the number that he was previously told. If he can't remember the number, repeat it and ask him to recall it a minute or two later. Another method might be to ask the patient age-appropriate questions, such as his birthday, favorite cartoons or TV shows, his name, and so on. The purpose is to ascertain the level of alertness and any changes for the better or worse. It is important to become familiar with the neurologic assessment method used in your area, and important that local hospitals understand this tool. For example, if your EMS system uses the Glasgow Coma Scale (GCS), ensure the receiving hospitals understand the "scoring" system. The same holds true for AVPU. Evaluation tools have limited effectiveness if they can't be used to communicate information on the patient's neurologic status.

CHAPTER 34 Multisystem Trauma

Think Like an EMT—Determining Criticality

1. The patient's presentation is a stable one, and the injury sustained is likely not life-threatening. Transportation to a local hospital is appropriate as long as the patient remains stable en route.
2. The boy's deteriorating mental status is the most alarming issue. The potential for brain injury should point you in the direction of prompt transport to the trauma center.
3. This woman has trauma to her extremities–and possibly to her uterus. This is a serious condition and the trauma center is the prudent choice, but consult medical direction first. The obstetric surgery capabilities at the local hospital may be warranted.

Short Answer

1. You should consider a number of factors when determining whether to perform an intervention on the scene or en route to the hospital. Life-threatening injuries related to the A-B-Cs of primary assessment must be taken care of immediately, regardless of the time it takes to do so. Basically, perform those interventions that, if not done at once, could impact patient outcome (e.g., permanent disability or death). Such interventions usually include any procedure required to open the airway (such as suctioning), support ventilations, and control external bleeding. In addition, spinal motion restriction precautions as protocol indicates should also be employed on scene. All other interventions should be evaluated against the time it takes to complete them, given it may delay transport.
2. Interventions to complete prior to transport for a critical trauma patient include suctioning the airway, inserting an oral or nasal airway, restoring a patent airway by sealing a sucking chest wound, ventilating with a bag-valve-mask device, administering high-concentration oxygen, controlling bleeding, performing CPR and utilizing the AED, and performing spinal motion restriction procedures.
3. The decision to bypass a closer hospital in favor of a more distant trauma center is based on local, regional, or state protocols. Specialized trauma centers can usually provide the definitive treatment required by the patient with multiple injuries. A Level I trauma center will have surgical specialists available 24 hours a day and can provide lifesaving interventions immediately on the patient's arrival.
4. Although a fractured femur is a severe injury, it becomes a lesser priority if the patient does not have a patent airway or needs ventilatory support. Life-threatening conditions related to the A-B-Cs must come first. In addition, if application of a traction splint will result in a *significant* delay in transport and if the patient is a high priority, then splinting might be postponed so the patient can receive definitive care at a trauma center or hospital. Remember to treat the whole patient and avoid distraction by a single injury—even if the injury is as serious as a fractured femur. In other words, interventions must be prioritized while keeping in mind the importance of the "golden hour."

Critical Thinking Exercises

Despite what your partner thinks, this patient has vital signs trending towards shock, suffered a significant mechanism of injury, and complains of pain in his chest, where he could easily develop any number of life-threatening conditions. The patient meets criteria to go to a trauma center based on the mechanism of injury and perhaps on anatomic criteria. His vital signs might still be adequate to the point of not strictly meeting physiologic criteria–but only barely. The patient should go to a trauma center.

Pathophysiology to Practice

1. Geriatric patients must be prioritized higher because they tend not to compensate for shock as effectively as the rest of the population, and they commonly have comorbidities such as hypertension, cardiac disease, or pulmonary diseases that can complicate treatment.
2. Any penetrating injury, especially penetrating abdominal trauma, is considered a surgical emergency and should be prioritized higher and transported to a hospital with 24-hour surgical capabilities (i.e., trauma center).
3. Patients taking anticoagulants should be prioritized higher because the blood-clotting mechanism will be diminished. If they have either internal or external bleeding, it will be harder to control and stop and can subsequently lead to hypovolemia much faster.
4. Patients with amputations necessitate higher priority because they require prompt surgical intervention to realize the best chance for recovery of the reattached limb.

Street Scene Questions

1. The collision appears to be a high-impact crash involving two vehicles–a full-size pickup truck and a compact car. At least two patients are slumped over inside the smaller vehicle, and fluid is draining from under the engine, which can become a hazard to you. The scene must be secured for a number of reasons–a potentially unstable vehicle, an unknown (and possibly hazardous) fluid leak, high-speed traffic, curious onlookers, and so on. Heavy extrication equipment may be required, and the patients might be high priority, based on the mechanism of injury (high-speed collision).
2. Additional resources might include police units to control the traffic, heavy rescue for extrication, a fire department crew to handle the leaking fluid, and additional ambulances (depending on the severity of the injuries and the final number of patients).
3. The female passenger should be transported before the driver, if possible. Unlike the driver, who was found conscious but dazed, the passenger appears motionless at first. Although responsive to verbal stimuli, she is highly agitated, suggesting possible brain injury. Her airway is clear, but she exhibits slightly labored and shallow breathing. Patient complaints of right arm pain indicates a possible fracture. The patient's radial pulse (strong and rapid) and skin (warm and dry) suggest that her body may be compensating for some blood loss (although the signs do not yet point to a critical situation). The patient is also unrestrained, which means easier removal than the fully restrained driver. Finally, remember not to discount the driver of the pickup truck, even though he is ambulatory and reports no immediate life threats. Make sure he is reassessed again by your crew or an incoming crew.
4. Given the mechanism of injury and the primary assessment findings listed in the preceding answer, you might conclude that the passenger has sustained multiple-system trauma and requires rapid transport to the nearest trauma center and/or hospital. This decision necessitates rapid extrication.
5. Examples of critical interventions include initiation of spinal motion restriction precautions, assurance of an open airway, rapid extrication based on local protocols, supporting lost function to the breathing if respirations are inadequate, a rapid neurologic assessment (for pain, sensation, and movement) both before and after extrication, placement and securing of the patient to a long spine board, ongoing monitoring of the airway, suctioning and application of high-concentration oxygen as necessary, immobilization of the right arm (possibly enroute to the hospital), and reassessment (vitals every 5 minutes). Consider ALS backup or intercept during transport to a trauma center.
6. If you have not already taken a baseline set of vitals, do so now (to monitor changes in the patient's condition). Although the patient is alert only to verbal stimuli, you can still gather a partial history. For example, you might question the husband or driver of the pickup truck and take down information on the patient's medical alert bracelet. Perform a focused head-to-toe assessment, paying close attention to lung sounds, tenderness, and signs/symptoms of head trauma (fluid from the nose and ears, deformity, sluggish/nonreactive pupils). Try to elicit information pertinent to the pregnancy, which should be communicated to medical direction and the receiving hospital as soon as possible.
7. Local, regional, or state protocols usually establish guidelines for transport to a trauma center or hospital. Medical direction, if available, can advise you on the most appropriate action. As previously stated, the assessment findings indicate rapid transport to a trauma center, if available, within an appropriate time frame.

CHAPTER 35 Environmental Emergencies

Think Like an EMT—Safety First

1. The patient is several hundred feet out in the water. This is a long distance to swim. Even if you can swim out there, the patient might inadvertently pull you under. Call for help and look for a way to safely rescue the swimmer.
2. Someone has fallen through the ice, and the obvious risk is the one you should be worried about: you and the others breaking through and falling in as well. Clear the ice of all onlookers. Call for help. Look for devices such as ropes or sticks that can be used for a rescue.
3. If there are reports that someone has already been bitten by a snake, then the snake (or other snakes) might still be around, especially around the rocks. The patient should be moved to a clearing where both you and the patient will have lesser chance of further bites.

Short Answer

1. Active rewarming may be permitted if the patient is alert and responsive, medical direction orders it, and transport time will be great. Passive rewarming is always permitted for any patient with a lowered body temperature.
2. Situations in which a patient may be suffering from hypothermia in addition to another condition include alcohol ingestion, underlying illness, overdose or poisoning, major trauma, outdoor resuscitation, lying on a tile floor in an air conditioned environment following a fall, and decreased ambient temperature.
3. Initially the skin of the affected area appears white and waxy. As the condition progresses to actual freezing, the skin turns mottled or blotchy, and the color turns from white to grayish yellow, finally changing to grayish blue. Swelling and blistering may occur during the rewarming process.
4. A patient suspected of having a heat emergency with moist, pale, and cool skin should be managed as follows:
   - Remove the patient to a cooler environment.
   - Administer oxygen.
   - Remove clothing and cool the patient by fanning.
   - Put the patient in a supine position, keeping the patient at rest.
   - If the patient is responsive and not nauseated, give the patient water.
   - Apply moist towels over muscle cramps.
   - Transport.
5. A patient suspected of having a heat emergency with hot, dry skin should be managed as follows:
   - Remove the patient to the ambulance and run the air conditioner on high.
   - Remove the patient's clothing; apply cool packs to the neck, groin, and armpits. Fan aggressively.
   - Administer oxygen.
   - Transport immediately.
6. The proper care for a patient with a snakebite includes:
   - Call medical direction.
   - Treat for shock and conserve body heat.
   - Keep the patient calm.
   - Control bleeding at the bite marks, if any. Clean the fang marks with soap and water.
   - Remove jewelry on the bitten extremity.
   - Immobilize the bitten extremity, perhaps using a splint.
   - Apply light constricting bands above and below the bite if ordered to do so by medical direction.
   - Transport and continually monitor the patient's vital signs.

Critical Thinking Exercises

1. A patient who is not alert will not be able to take warm fluids. Transporting a patient in this condition by snowmobile may be too risky and needs to be weighed against the risks of staying on scene and performing passive rewarming. If there is any nearby house or building that could offer shelter and warmth, consider moving the patient there while additional help is summoned.
2. A patient suffering from a heat emergency who exhibits hot skin rather than cool skin is in serious trouble. The body's temperature-regulating mechanism has failed; therefore, the body can no longer rid itself of excessive heat by the mechanism known as sweating (hence the hot, dry skin). This is sometimes known as heat stroke. Normally, temperature is regulated by a number of mechanisms, including perspiration and evaporative heat loss. However, if the patient begins to exhibit hot skin–whether dry or moist–the potential for a true emergency exists. The implications are that the patient can suffer brain injury, seizures, and other medical emergencies if the core temperature is not lowered quickly.
3. As you first observe the scene of the capsized boat, you must immediately take a number of things into consideration, including your own safety and the safety of the others who have started swimming out to the site. Without delay, conduct a scene size-up to include the following:
   - Check for scene safety. If you are not a trained rescuer in water safety, it is probably not prudent for you to attempt the rescue. You won't be any good to those at the scene if you become a victim yourself.
   - Take Standard Precautions if possible.
   - Try to determine the mechanism of injury.
   - Try to determine the number of patients. You should probably include the people swimming out to the boat who are acting as rescuers, since they may become victims themselves.

- Decide what resources you want to request. Since you are at a public lake and others are around (and screaming), you may not be the only one calling for help. Think quickly about how you want to frame your report before making the call. Aside from asking for additional help, think also about the equipment you might need, including oxygen, backboards, and blankets, and water rescue.

Pathophysiology to Practice

1. Altered mental status results when the electrical system of the brain malfunctions. This occurs when the body temperature falls to about 92°F (33°C), which indicates hypothermia. Rapid active rewarming in these patients can cause serious cardiac and circulatory complications. Therefore, an altered mental status in a patient who may be hypothermic is a contraindication to active rewarming. Passive rewarming is indicated instead during transport, and active rewarming will be initiated by the emergency department.
2. About 65 percent of the body's cooling mechanisms involve the skin. When the skin is hot, you know that the cooling mechanisms have failed and the patient is in serious condition. He must be cooled rapidly and aggressively to prevent long-term neurologic damage and death.

Street Scene Questions

1. Besides the obvious (A-B-Cs), you should suspect hypothermia as well as other underlying problems such as malnutrition or untreated medical conditions. Because of the patient's situation, he is at risk of pneumonia and respiratory infections as well as medical conditions suggested by the signs and symptoms (stroke, trauma from a fall, and so on).
2. Basically, the patient needs complete primary and secondary assessments. As with all patients, assess the A-B-Cs, make sure the patient's airway remains open and breathing is adequate, and consider the use of supplemental oxygen. Briefly ensure that there is no major bleeding. Once the primary assessment is complete and immediate care is initiated, take a complete set of baseline vital signs. Because the patient was found outside on a cold night, he needs to be assessed for hypothermia. Try to determine the patient's orientation to time and place and other items in a past medical history. You should use a detailed head-to-toe survey to determine whether the patient has other medical problems or has sustained a traumatic fall.
3. Active rewarming in the field is not recommended given his altered mental status. However, you can initiate passive rewarming. For example, remove all the patient's wet clothing and wrap the patient in one or more blankets. Consider a thermal (space) blanket as an outer shell. The patient's head should be covered to prevent additional heat loss. Unless recommended by medical direction and/or local protocols, do not apply hot packs or administer warm fluids in the prehospital setting. The exceptions include rare cases of long or delayed transport time, and then only with approval from medical direction. Reassess the patient frequently because, even with passive warming, an unresponsive patient or a patient suffering from extreme hypothermia can deteriorate rapidly.
4. Take the patient's vital signs as often as every 5 minutes. Given the findings, he is considered a priority patient. Realize that the more hypothermic the patient, the harder it is to take vital signs. Heart rate and respirations can fall below normal, but the patient may still sustain the rate and respirations needed to survive. When a person becomes hypothermic, the body can sometimes survive neurologically intact for a significant period of time after vital signs have become depressed.
5. Hypothermic patients should be handled gently. Rough handling can result in ventricular fibrillation. Always keep a defibrillator (AED) close to the patient throughout transport. In fact, it may be a good idea to apply the AED pads during transport so that they are on and ready should you need to use the AED (follow local protocol).

CHAPTER 36 Obstetric and Gynecologic Emergencies

Think Like an EMT—My Baby Won't Wait!

1. This baby is coming–and quickly as evidenced by the close contractions, crowning, and urge to push. Additionally since this is her fourth child, the birthing process will likely be much quicker. Prepare for delivery at the scene.
2. This baby will likely wait. Ask the mother about feeling the need to push and if she feels as if she must move her bowels. In the absence of either of these, you should make it to the hospital. Typically, the labor of the first birth is the longest as compared to a pregnant female's subsequent children.
3. Transport this patient. Since there has been no significant change over 8 hours despite the presence of labor contractions, there may be a problem with birthing. Given no signs of imminent delivery, transport is the correct decision.

Short Answer

1. The anatomical structures associated with pregnancy are:
   - The ovaries: Produce the ova, or egg, that will be fertilized by the male.
   - The fallopian tubes: Transport the ova to the uterus and are the typical site of fertilization.
   - The uterus: the muscular structure that houses the fetus during pregnancy
   - The placenta: the vascular organ that perfuses and nourishes the fetus during pregnancy within the uterus
   - The vagina: the birth canal

2. The three stages of labor are:
   - Stage 1: start of contractions to full dilation of the cervix
   - Stage 2: full dilation of the cervix to birth of the fetus
   - Stage 3: birth of the fetus to expulsion of the placenta
3. Prepare the mother for delivery by controlling the scene and the mother's privacy. Ask bystanders to leave. In addition to gloves, put on a gown, cap, mask, and eye protection. Place the mother on the floor, elevate the buttocks with a blanket or pillow, and have the mother lie with her knees drawn up and spread apart. Use sterile sheets or towels to drape the area and position the obstetric kit within easy reach.
4. To resuscitate a newly born infant, the baby should initially be dried, warmed, and stimulated. If that is not enough, administer supplemental oxygen. Positive pressure ventilation and chest compressions follow immediately if other initial measures are unsuccessful.
5. Complications of delivery include breech presentations such as a foot, a hand, or the buttocks presenting first. Prolapsed cord occurs when the umbilical cord presents prior to the baby; a nuchal cord occurs when the cord is wrapped around the baby's neck.
6. Predelivery emergencies include eclampsia, where seizures occur, and abruptio placentae, where the placenta prematurely detaches from the uterine wall, causing massive internal bleeding. Placenta previa is another problem that occurs when the placenta blocks the birth canal (at the cervix); it can cause vaginal bleeding and harm the presenting fetus.

Critical Thinking Exercises

Because the patient does not have the urge to push or move her bowels, and because she is not crowning, there is likely time to transport her to the hospital (although clearly individual circumstances may dictate different plans). Consider also the fact that this is her first pregnancy, which typically takes longer to progress.

Pathophysiology to Practice

1. Vital sign changes that occur with pregnancy include the following: Respirations typically increase slightly, blood pressure drops slightly (but can be high with certain pregnancy related emergencies), and the pulse generally increases.
2. Shock may be more difficult to recognize, as vital signs that typically indicate early compensation (fast pulse and increased respirations) may already be present under the normal circumstances of pregnancy. The EMT will have to be alert to other signs of deterioration.
3. The severity of vaginal bleeding may be assessed by asking the patient how many pads she has needed to use in the last measure of time (i.e., last hour, last 12 hours, last day). While external hemorrhage is never good, an equal or greater concern is the internal bleeding that may be occurring concurrently. The EMT should always assume the worst, that the mother has lost or is still continuing to lose a significant amount of blood. This assumption of the worst will underscore the importance of rapid assessment, treatment, and transport.
4. The priorities of assessing and treating a neonate include maintaining warmth while assuring airway, breathing, and circulation. The EMT should always recall the "inverted pyramid" of neonatal resuscitation when managing a newborn.

Street Scene Questions

1. Once safety has been assured, the first priority is to make contact with the patient and assess the status of what sounded like an imminent delivery.
2. You should request ALS, since assistance in treating what may be multiple patients is never a bad idea. Depending on the condition of the mother and the newborn, airway management, intravenous fluids, and ALS medications may be warranted.
3. In addition to the traditional SAMPLE history, ask the patient how far along the pregnancy is, whether she has received prenatal care from an obstetrician, whether there have been any problems with the pregnancy, whether there has been any problem with previous deliveries, and whether the mother has any medical problems.
4. Immediate care for the newborn should include suctioning of the mouth and nose, drying of the skin, warming, and stimulating.
5. Important maternal care includes providing emotional support, monitoring for excessive hemorrhage, and assessing vital signs. Allowing the baby to begin breast feeding may also help the uterus to contract and stop bleeding.

CHAPTER 37 Emergencies for Patients with Special Challenges

Think Like an EMT—EMTs Need to Know

1. The patient's family is the first place to look for answers because they are most likely familiar with the device. You may also contact medical direction for advice. Fortunately, though, many devices have an obvious switch to turn them off with, if that should be the case.
2. In this case the patient may be the best source of information. Although you should be considerate of the pain she is in and realize that she may become angry with you for having to answer questions while in pain, she will be the best source to answer your questions about how dialysis works

and also to give you information on how best to move her while not causing undue additional pain.

3. The parents or visiting health care workers are the best source of information, especially with technology dependent children. Since health care workers aren't always present, parents are commonly trained in operation and troubleshooting the devices. If the ventilator can't be transported, transport the patient without it and ventilate the patient through the trach tube en route with an appropriate-sized BVM at the appropriate rate. Be sure to alert the hospital that you are about to arrive with a patient who needs a ventilator.

Short Answer

1. The following are advanced medical devices that may be found in homes of patients with special challenges:
   - Respiratory devices
     - Continuous positive airway pressure (CPAP)
     - Tracheostomy tube
     - Home ventilator
   - Cardiac devices
     - Implanted pacemaker
     - Automatic implanted cardiac defibrillator (AICD)
     - Left ventricular assist device (LVAD)
   - Gastro-urinary devices
     - Nasogastric (NG) tube
     - Gastric tube (G-tube)
     - Urinary catheters
     - Ostomy bags
     - Peritoneal dialysis
   - Central IV catheters
     - Peripherally inserted central catheter (PICC) lines
     - Central venous lines (Groshong®, Hickman®, Broviac®)
     - Implanted port (Port-a-Cath®, Mediport®)
   - Devices to assist in instances of physical impairment
     - TDD/TTY phone
     - Computer that speaks words
     - Cane, walker, or brace
     - Wheelchair
2. Obesity is associated with an increased risk for cancer, diabetes, hypertension, heart attack, stroke, liver and gallbladder disease, arthritis, sleep apnea, musculoskeletal problems, and respiratory problems.
3. To clear a blockage in a tracheostomy tube, carefully insert a whistle-tip suction catheter. Determine the correct depth of insertion by measuring the suction tubing against the length of the obturator, which is the same length as the trach tube itself. If you can't locate the obturator for measurement, stop insertion of the catheter when you feel resistance. Suction as the catheter is being withdrawn, using a twisting motion as it is slowly removed. If the patient requires further suctioning (indicated by visible or audible mucus), insert the suction tip into a container of sterile water to remove any mucus left in the catheter and then repeat the suctioning process. A patient on a ventilator may need to be ventilated by BVM between suctioning.
4. In the case of a mechanical failure, or during transport of the patient, a bag-valve-mask device can take over the function of the ventilator. During this procedure, you should adjust the rate, volume, and pressure of the BVM to the patient's comfort level. This can be done with guidance from the patient. If the patient can't provide guidance, observe for adequate chest rise and improving skin color. (**Note:** *If the BVM does not fit the tube attachment, use the face mask from the BVM to cover the stoma, secure the mask to provide a good seal against the neck, and ventilate as normal.*)
5. Homelessness can be associated with mental health problems, malnutrition, substance abuse, HIV/AIDS, tuberculosis, bronchitis and pneumonia, environmental emergencies, wounds, and skin infections.
6. A mnemonic to use when dealing with patients who have autism is A-B-C-S: awareness, basic, calm, and safety. These mean:
   - **A**wareness: Be aware that ASD patients behave and react differently from most patients.
   - **B**asic: Keep instructions, questions, treatments, and the environment simple.
   - **C**alm: Be calm and patient; don't lose your temper, yell, or try to force the patient.
   - **S**afety: As much as possible, interact with patients in familiar surroundings where they feel safe.
7. The first thing that should be done when approaching the patient is to determine the patient's ability to hear and/or speak. If a patient with hearing loss can read lips, then use this approach. If not, then communicate by writing questions and information on a piece of paper. TDD/TTY phones, if available, can be used to relay information. These approaches will also work for patients who are unable to speak. In addition, some patients who are aphasic (unable to speak) may have a computer that speaks words they type into the device. If family is available, they may provide insight into how best to communicate with the patient. They may also assist you in communicating with the patient.

Critical Thinking Exercises

1. The fistula may be ruptured, causing significant blood loss, which is indicated by swelling at the site. Apply direct pressure and do not release it until advised by a physician to do so. There may e a chance for the patient to develop an infection at the site from repeated injections during dialysis. This patient's presentation could be from the development of sepsis. Should this be the case, support any lost function to the A-B-Cs and contact ALS.
2. The patient's signs, symptoms, and circumstances likely indicate an infection that may be leading to septic shock. The initial patient-care concerns are the airway, breathing,

oxygenation, and circulation. The nursing home staff can assist you in preparing the feeding tube, colostomy bag, and urinary catheter for transport. The urinary catheter bag can be temporarily placed at the patient's level to move her but should be positioned lower than the patient during transport.

3. If an airway or ventilation device has failed, provide an open airway (use suction as necessary) and use a bag-valve-mask device to ventilate. If a pacemaker or AICD has failed, provide CPR and use the AED as indicated by the patient's condition.
4. If at all possible, you must allow the dog to accompany the patient. You may refuse only if the dog is a threat to you or others.
5. Understanding that this young patient has autism, think about how you can implement the *A-B-C-S* mnemonic. First, simply have an *awareness* that the patient will likely react differently than most. Second, keep your instructions and questions *basic* and your treatment simple. Third, be as *calm* as possible and avoid adding to the patient's level of anxiety. Finally, try to keep the patient in an environment that is *safe* and comfortable, preferably a place she recognizes and is used to.

Pathophysiology to Practice

1. The homeless and poor may be malnourished, might live in unsanitary conditions, and may not have been able to seek help for health problems early in their progression. Medical problems in the homeless typically exist longer before any attempts to treat them are made, and treatment of homeless people is often inconsistent or nonexistent. So, homeless patients typically decompensate easily and more quickly given their current medical problem.
2. A congenital condition is one that is present at birth, such as certain heart defects. An acquired disease occurs after birth and may be the result of exposure to an infectious disease, another medical condition, or trauma. Acquired diseases include AIDS and atherosclerotic heart disease.
3. The lack of sensation means that the patient cannot feel pain associated with excess pressure on the skin or with developing sores. If not properly cared for, the patient might not be moved often enough to relieve pressure on the tissues to prevent development of bedsores. Weakness of the chest muscles can impair the cough reflex, making it difficult to clear infectious material from the airway, resulting in respiratory infections. Finally, since paralyzed patients may have tubes inserted into their body (for example a urinary catheter), the presence of the tubes increases their risk for infections, especially if these tubes and devices are not cared for properly.

Street Scene Questions

1. The A-B-Cs are the first concern with regard to the care and treatment of this patient. Ensure the patient has a patent airway, and assess for problems with positioning or mucus blockage. The airway must be checked and monitored, with corrective action taken as necessary. Regarding breathing, the patient needs oxygen immediately. Be prepared to assist with ventilations if needed. If ALS is not immediately available, then consider prompt transport. This patient should be treated as a high priority.
2. After the initial exam, perform the history and physical exam. Ask the patient's aunt about Amber's past medical history. If possible, determine the onset of the problem, including whether it was sudden or gradual, and solicit any associated observations made by the caregiver. Information about the facility that normally treats Amber may allow you to contact them directly, if needed, for guidance.
3. Continue to reassess the patient's airway, respiratory status, skin color, and pulse. The use of a pulse oximeter will allow you to trend her saturation level, which could provide you with useful information.
4. If Amber has special equipment that you cannot provide (such as extra suction catheters in the appropriate size), you should take them with you. Ask the aunt whether the parents left instructions about equipment that needs to accompany Amber.

CHAPTER 38 EMS Operations

Think Like an EMT—Arriving Safely

1. Park uphill and upwind at potential chemical incidents, such as a train wreck. You must also be aware of the risk of explosion (e.g., a propane-powered car) and park a significant distance away until the hazards are dealt with. If this be the case, have the fire department bring you the patients in a safe zone.
2. Park past the collision. On an interstate scene, you should have a blocking vehicle (e.g., a fire engine or highway department barricade truck) between you and traffic still traveling in the same direction in the lane. By parking past the scene, you will be able to load the patient with the safety of the blocking vehicles behind you.
3. Stage out of sight from the residence and far enough away that any dangerous persons won't come from the scene to you. Drive to the scene only when advised the police have secured it. Also, as you approach, the police may direct you where to park in case the outside location is also a crime scene.

Short Answer

1. The five phases of an ambulance call are:
   - Preparing for the ambulance call
   - Receiving and responding to a call
   - Transferring the patient to the ambulance
   - Transporting the patient to the hospital
   - Terminating the call
2. At the beginning of each shift, spend the time to be sure that you, your vehicle, and your equipment are ready to respond. Talk with the off-going crew, get a brief shift report, and learn about any issues that might have come up with the ambulance or equipment during their shift. Complete a thorough bumper-to-bumper inspection of the ambulance using a checklist provided by your service, during which you will inspect the vehicle and the equipment.
3. There are a number of very effective ways to reduce your chances of having a collision when driving an emergency vehicle. Come to a complete stop at intersections against a red light or stop sign, minimize lights-and-siren responses whenever possible, and become familiar with your response area, so you know where you're going when you receive an emergency dispatch. In addition, work to minimize all possible distractions when driving. Leave the radio communications, navigation, and mapping to your partner if you are driving, and avoid eating, drinking, talking on the cell phone, or listening to music during an emergency response.
4. A patient-carrying device should have a minimum of three straps for holding the patient securely. The first strap is placed at chest level, the second strap is placed at hip or waist level, and the third strap is placed around the lower extremities. Sometimes there is a fourth strap if two are crossed at the chest. Newer stretchers also have two upper straps that come over the shoulder and clasp at the chest to act as a harness to restrain the upper body with a rapid deceleration of the ambulance.
5. Using air-rescue resources comes with some critical responsibilities for those responders on the scene. They must ensure a safe environment upon which the aircraft can land and relaunch. Prior to the arrival of the aircraft, set up a landing zone:
   - The landing zone should be a minimum of 100 feet by 100 feet on a flat surface that is clear of wires, towers, vehicles, people, and loose objects that might fly up when the aircraft lands. (Responders often underestimate the power of the helicopter's down force, or "rotor wash.") Once a site has been chosen, place one flare in an upwind position to allow the pilot to judge wind direction. During night operations, keep emergency lights on and shine headlights onto the landing zone (never skyward toward the pilot). One word of caution: the use of flares in fields may cause a fire; be sure this does not happen.
   - Once the helicopter has landed, approach the aircraft only when escorted by flight personnel, and allow the helicopter crew to direct the loading of the patient. It is critical that all personnel be aware of their positions with regard to the tail rotor of the aircraft and avoid this area at all times. This important information varies from location to location. Your instructor will provide information on resources in your jurisdiction.

Critical Thinking Exercises

1. Equipment contained within a kit that should be available to carry onto a scene includes:
   - Two-way radio
   - Portable oxygen
   - Oxygen administration equipment, BVM, airways, and masks
   - Pulse oximeter
   - Medications (those approved by medical direction)
   - Automatic external defibrillator (AED)
   - Dressings, gauze, bandages, tape, cold packs, and burn sheets
   - Blood pressure cuff, stethoscope, shears, flashlight, blanket, towels, triage tags
   - Infection-control equipment such as exam gloves, eye protection, face protection, gowns, shoe covers, and N-95 or N-100 masks.
2. Items that are retrieved regularly (such as the blood pressure cuff, stethoscope, and oxygen masks) for routine calls should be placed in a bag or "jump kit" in the vehicle near the rear or side door (or on top of the stretcher) so, upon arrival on the scene, your crew can exit the vehicle, retrieve the bag(s), and enter the scene quickly with the most essential equipment in hand. Equipment that is used infrequently (such as the obstetric kit, traction splint, burn sheets, and immobilization equipment) can be placed inside the vehicle in a more secure location where they can be retrieved under those special circumstances that require them.
3. Special items that may be dictated by local requirements include:
   - Advanced or alternative airways
   - Glucose meter
   - Specialized pediatric equipment such as smaller blood pressure cuffs, stethoscopes, spinal immobilization equipment, and oxygen masks and airways
   - Medications such as oral glucose, albuterol, nitroglycerin, and auto-injector EpiPens
   - Specialty equipment related to specific interfacility transfer work
   - Cellular telephone.

Street Scene Questions

1. The first precaution is to make sure the vehicle has had a proper "preflight" check to ensure everything is in safe working order. Next, the driver needs to get into the driver's seat with a "safety mindset" and drive defensively, which means driving cautiously and anticipating what other motorists will do. The driver must also drive with "due

regard" for the safety of others. Although the laws may grant special privileges to emergency vehicle drivers, they don't excuse a driver from negligence. Guidelines to keep in mind when operating an ambulance include:

- Control your speed and be mindful of road conditions.
- Stop at stop signs and traffic signals.
- Avoid driving with lights and sirens unless it is absolutely necessary.
- Unless the patient is critical, drive to the hospital "cold."
- Remember that the patient and EMTs in the patient compartment need a smooth ride.
- Remember that even with lights and sirens, motorists may not see or hear the ambulance in time. Drive accordingly.

2. Most medical conditions will not be adversely affected by an additional few minutes. It's often said that 95 percent of EMS responses do not require speed or lights and siren, so slow down. Ask yourself this: Is it really worth taking all this risk for a patient with a minor injury or illness to save a few minutes when the patient might wait in the ED for a few hours? "Hot" responses typically save only a few minutes. Is this really necessary?
3. Slow down and stop at intersections. Drive defensively, "cover the brake," and be prepared to stop! Most ambulance crashes occur at intersections, so proceed through them with great caution. Proceeding through a traffic signal without stopping is very risky and likely to cause a crash. After the call, in this specific situation, have a conversation with the driver about stopping at intersections and slowing down. In addition, have the driver let you operate the siren so he can concentrate on the driving.
4. Make sure the scene is safe, carry in the equipment needed for a possible cardiac arrest along with the jump-kit, take Standard Precautions, and begin with the A-B-Cs.
5. Give the dispatcher an arrival report. The patient is alert, breathing, and in minimal distress. Advise whether other resources should be canceled, upgraded, or downgraded in their response. A good arrival report informs the dispatcher and responding units of the true nature of an incident.

CHAPTER 39 Hazardous Materials, Multiple-Casualty Incidents, and Incident Management

Think Like an EMT—We Have *How Many* Patients?

1. Activate your MCI plan. Based on the fact that you see "dozens" of people, you may be looking at 25-plus patients, and more may still be inside. This is a large-scale multiple-casualty incident and must be treated as such. It is a bigger issue than simply calling for additional ambulances. This will require prolonged operations and resources. Be sure the HAZMAT team is activated.
2. Assume that you will need an ambulance and crew for each of the four critical patients. You may also need to call for fire department response for extrication or personnel assistance, as well as law enforcement to control the traffic and bystanders.
3. With this many people in the same home with similar illnesses, the concern may be a carbon monoxide poisoning situation. Assume that there are four patients–and you and your crew may now also fall into the patient category. Exit the building, taking the patients with you if possible. Immediately call for additional ambulances and the fire department.

Short Answer

1. When giving an initial report of a hazardous material incident, be sure to alert the dispatcher to the fact that you are dealing with a HAZMAT incident and to request appropriate support services. Try to identify the hazardous materials by using binoculars to look for identifying signs, labels, or placards and compare them to information found in the Emergency Response Guidebook. If possible, try to report:
   - The material involved
   - Wind direction
   - Safe staging location
   - The number of fire and HAZMAT resources you think you will need
   - Who has information on the substance involved, such as SDS.
2. The biggest challenge in dealing with a HAZMAT situation is in identifying the substance accurately. The most complicated situations can often involve unknown substances or chemicals. To help mitigate this, when chemicals are involved in transportation, transporting vehicles are required to have placards that can be referenced in the yellow Emergency Response Guidebook. This not only helps identify the substance but also guides the medical care, evacuation, and emergency actions. Buildings may use the NFPA 704 system, which can advise responders about the flammability, danger, and reactivity of the substances inside. The real gold standard, however, is for the building owner, shipper, or keeper of the substance to provide responders with the SDS, or safety data sheet. In this situation, the HAZMAT team may have to do extensive work to determine the substance involved.
3. Care of a patient with a hazardous-material injury always starts with a scene size-up, scene safety, and the A-B-Cs. In a HAZMAT situation, the critical determination is whether the patient poses a risk of secondary contamination to the rescuers. Any patient with a hazardous-material injury must be fully decontaminated by a qualified HAZMAT team before being turned over to the EMS personnel, regardless of the severity of the medical condition.

4. The major components and benefits of the Incident Command System are interoperability between responding agencies, clear lines of authority, and a management structure conducive to managing a large incident.
5. Overall, the roles of EMS in a multiple-casualty incident are handling triage, treatment, and transportation. The role of the first-arriving EMTs is to initiate the agency's incident management plan. Establish Command, complete a scene size-up, give an arrival report to dispatch, request or cancel resources, and begin triage-treatment-transportation activities.
6. Assigning priorities during triage allows limited resources to focus efforts on patients with the greatest needs. The process is focused on saving lives by first putting effort into the patients who have the most serious injuries but who, with proper care, are expected to survive. This gives the greatest number of people the greatest chance of survival.
7. The four priority categories of triage are:
   - Priority-1 (RED)–treatable life-threatening conditions
   - Priority-2 (YELLOW)–serious but non-life-threatening conditions
   - Priority-3 (GREEN)–walking wounded
   - Priority-4 or 0 (BLACK)–dead or expected to die

Critical Thinking Exercises

Establish a perimeter around the danger area and keep people out. Radio an arrival report to dispatch and request additional resources such as the power company, fire department, extrication, police, and additional EMS units. Put on personal protective equipment, and position your vehicle to protect the scene and create a safe working area. This should be performed in a manner consistent with your local procedures.

Street Scene Questions

1. Given the complexity of the scene, it's important to "unify" the Command with both police and fire service supervisors when they arrive. Another approach might be to transfer overall Incident Command to either police or fire. This may allow EMS to better focus on the tactics needed for triage-treatment-transportation. However, when first on the scene and Command is established:
   - Put on an ICS bib, and use ICS radio identifiers.
   - Size up the incident.
   - Give an arrival report to dispatch.
   - Develop a mental incident action plan.
   - Request any additional resources needed.
   - Determine how responding units will be used when they arrive.
   - Position/stage the resources.
   - Assign tactical roles such as extrication, treatment, and transportation.
2. The triage officer is responsible for reporting back on exactly how many patients there are and their priority levels and ensuring patients have been properly tagged by priority: RED, YELLOW, GREEN, or BLACK.
3. Depending on the number of EMS system resources available, this could be deemed a major incident. Once the number of patients and their priorities are known, dispatch should call the hospitals and determine how many patients each hospital can take by priority. In an urban area, it may be possible to distribute the patients to multiple hospitals. In rural settings, all the patients may be transported to the same hospital. In either case, notify the hospital(s) early to allow the staff as much time as possible to prepare for the surge of patients that will be arriving.
4. There is always a need for a safety officer, especially in this case. There are wires down, a fuel spill, a fire hazard, extrication, and multiple casualties. If there isn't a dedicated person to assume the role of safety officer, then Command must assume that function.
5. The method by which information is transmitted during an MCI depends on the local EMS system. Some systems limit radio traffic by relaying minimal information through dispatch to the hospital. Other systems establish a direct link and call the hospitals from the scene. It's important to understand how your local/regional procedures for MCI management work so you can follow them effectively.
6. Cooperation with fire and police is essential. Coordinate resource requests to minimize radio traffic and dispatch overload. Share overall incident action plans and tactical objectives.

CHAPTER 40 Highway Safety and Vehicle Extrication

Think Like an EMT—When Minutes Count, Decisions Matter

1. A patient involved in a head-on crash who is unresponsive with a rapid pulse is an unstable patient and requires a quick extrication.
2. A patient who was rear-ended, is alert, and is oriented with stable vital signs is a stable patient with time available for the extrication.
3. A patient thrown from the front to the backseat during a collision who has a rapid pulse and clammy skin is an unstable patient and requires a quick extrication.

Short Answer

1. Your responsibility is the scene size-up, which involves scanning the scene for hazards, estimating the number of patients, degree of entrapment, vehicle instability, and any risks to the rescuers posed by traffic. Although the EMS focus should be on triage, treatment, and transportation, all ICS roles must be carried out by the first-arriving EMTs if establishing Command. Whoever establishes Command must maintain it until it can be transferred to another agency or a higher-ranking official.
2. ANSI-approved Class 2 safety vests and helmets should be worn at the scene of a highway incident to improve your visibility to others.
3. EMS or firefighter turnout clothing, including a helmet, heavy gloves, and eye protection, should be worn during a vehicle extrication. Match the protective gear worn by others at the scene.
4. To deactivate the automobile air bags, disconnect the battery - disconnect the negative (black) terminal first.
5. First try simple access methods such as opening the door or rolling down a window. If those are unsuccessful, use complex access methods involving tools such as a spring-loaded punch, axes, or saws designed for window glass to gain access to your patient or patients. If you need to break a glass, try not to break the one next to the patient if you are trying to gain initial entry. Protect patients from breaking/broken glass as best possible.
6. Research resources available in your local area. Resources will vary - but likely include police and fire at a minimum.

Critical Thinking Exercises

1. Types of rescue specialty teams include vehicle rescue, water rescue, ice rescue, high-angle rescue, hazardous material response, trench rescue, dive rescue, backcountry or wilderness rescue, farm rescue, and confined-space rescue. One or more of these may be active in your area, depending on the characteristics of your community. It is the responsibility of all involved to coordinate training exercises of mock disasters so that when one occurs, and they inevitably will, the system as a whole will run as smoothly as possible.
2. After considering the safety of yourself and others, your primary goal at the scene of a vehicle collision is assessment and care of the patient.

Street Scene Questions

1. Scene safety issues deal with both seen and unseen hazards. Although vehicle instability is an obvious safety issue for both the patient and the rescuers, you should suspect possible gasoline leaks and/or problems with the vehicle's electrical system. The first and foremost concerns are checking for any leaking fluids, particularly gasoline, and stabilizing the vehicle. You might also consider disconnecting the battery.
2. Once the vehicle is stabilized, you should look for the safest way of accessing the patient, making sure to safeguard both yourself and the injured driver. Before breaking a window, always confirm that it's necessary because the door on the less damaged side of the vehicle may still be operable. If a window must be broken, make every effort to protect the patient from shards of glass, perhaps by using padding or insulating material for protection, or by initially breaking a window on the opposite side of the vehicle.
3. Yes, rapid extrication should be considered. Based on the primary assessment of snoring respirations and level of responsiveness (response to only painful stimuli), the patient is unstable and thus a high priority.
4. The assessment follows in ABC order. The snoring respirations must be corrected. In most cases this will require a jaw-thrust maneuver (in a trauma patient) to move the tongue forward while a second EMT applies a cervical collar. Next, evaluate the patient's respirations. At the very least, this patient should receive high-concentration oxygen by nonrebreather mask. Be prepared to assist ventilations with a bag-valve mask with supplemental oxygen. Next, check the patient's circulation for external hemorrhage and overt signs and symptoms of internal bleeding. Also check the peripheral and central pulse. Because this is a trauma patient, you should then initiate a head-to-toe assessment in accordance with the extrication procedure. Once this is completed, obtain a set of vital signs. A SAMPLE history can be taken if the patient regains consciousness.

CHAPTER 41 EMS Response to Terrorism

Think Like an EMT—It Could Happen to You . . .

1. Do not enter the area, based on what you learned from dispatch. Instead, wait for the HAZMAT team to bring decontaminated patients to you. Do not allow contaminated patients or rescuers into your ambulance; do not take contaminated patients to the hospital.
2. From dispatch information, it would be hard to tell if the explosion was terrorism or not. Either way, do not enter the area until it has been secured for stability and absence of additional undetonated explosive devices. Terrorists may place secondary devices designed to harm rescuers.

Short Answer

1. The five most common types of terrorist incidents are chemical, biologic, radiologic, nuclear, and explosive. A chemical event usually entails a gaseous material released into the atmosphere. This substance has properties that are very toxic or potentially fatal when inhaled. A biologic substance is a bacterium, virus, or toxin that can cause immediate illness or death, or a substance that can take time to incubate, making people sick in the process. A radiologic event is when radiologic material is released into the atmosphere. Depending on a number of factors, such as proximity, quantity of the material, and potency, it can have an immediate and/or long-range impact on humans or animals. Nuclear devices can be very similar to radiologic devices but may have the added concern of incendiary potential to do immediate harm to a large area, depending on the device's size. An explosive device, such as a bomb, can cause injury from the initial explosion as well as the secondary damage caused by destruction from the explosion. In addition, these devices sometimes contain materials (e.g., nails) that are shot into the area of the explosion and can also cause harm.
2. *Multiple devices* is a term used when there is more than one destructive device used in a terrorist attack. Usually one device detonates initially, and a secondary device (or multiple devices) are staged to detonate at a later point in time, with the intent of injuring more responders. For example, a device may be set off inside a building, and multiple others may be set to explode in an area where people might congregate after exiting the building. EMS responders need to be alert to the fact that in a terrorist event, there may be more than one device. Scene safety, including being alert to this fact, is a priority. Responders must try to stay clear of the area until it is deemed safe. When establishing staging and triage areas, make sure these areas have been secured and, if necessary, guarded during the entire event.
3. Some of the types of events that should trigger the EMT to be suspicious are those taking place at or near symbolic and historical targets, public buildings or places of assembly, controversial businesses, and infrastructure systems.
4. The seven types of harm from an incendiary system are thermal, radiologic, asphyxiation, chemical, etiologic, mechanical, and psychological. The acronym for these is TRACEM-P.
5. The concepts of time, distance, and shielding suggest you minimize the time you are in the area of possible risk at a dangerous scene, maximize the distance from the hazardous area, and use as much shielding as possible, whether it be in the form of a vehicle, a structure, or use of specialized protective clothing and protective breathing apparatus. The more shielding, the better, so utilize multiple methods whenever available.
6. Distance can be a helpful protection measure for biologic incidents. The farther away from the immediate area of danger, the better. (Also pay attention to wind direction.) Use of appropriate protective equipment may be another effective protection technique, particularly if a responder intends to get near or within the contaminated area. This may include use of specialized protective breathing equipment. Limiting the time in the contaminated area should also be a consideration.
7. *Isolation* can take on many forms at an incident where terrorism is suspected. Make sure emergency responders and civilians don't get hurt by a secondary device; permit only those who have a need to be there and are wearing proper protective gear to enter the perimeter. This also allows for control in an area that is apt to be very chaotic. *Notification* is alerting the appropriate agencies that there is an event. Many times EMS is one of the first to arrive at an act of terrorism. Notifying additional resources and specialized response units needs to occur quickly. *Identification* refers to the agent or material that might be involved. This is important information for protecting responders and making decisions on the types of protective equipment and barriers that are required. In addition, knowing the agent will help in determining how to handle decontamination. Therefore, determining what agents are involved needs to be a priority. *Protection* is done to shield critical assets from additional harm and damage. Responders must first ensure that they are protected. Once that is done, they must try to protect vehicles, equipment, and supplies.

Critical Thinking Exercises

1. The scene may not have been deemed safe yet. Emergency medical responders are often principal targets of terrorist attacks, and it is possible that law enforcement and/or the fire department is canvasing the scene to ensure there is no secondary device planted somewhere that might injure EMS responders.
2. Treating patients exposed to a nerve agent is delicate work as it is, but to see your own colleagues potentially become victims themselves is terrifying. Stop what you are doing, evacuate immediately, request help for your colleagues, and report to the HAZMAT team for decontamination and treatment.
3. The ethnic background of the suspicious man is really irrelevant, since many past terrorist incidents on American soil have been the responsibility of U.S. citizens. However, this gentleman appears and his behavior is very suspicious, and your intuition tells you something is wrong. You should definitely report your observations immediately to the nearest authority, since a suitcase could easily conceal any of the CBNRE agents intended to cause widespread harm to the traveling public.

Street Scene Questions (#1)

1. Indicators that this may be a suspicious incident include the multiple casualties, a "funny smell," and the historical knowledge that a radical group that has opposed construction.
2. The area should immediately have a perimeter established, for which law enforcement (or possibly the fire department) takes the primary responsibility. This process should also include determining inner and outer perimeters. Notify

other responding units of the danger in the area, and instruct them not to enter.

3. Attempt to determine the mechanism of injury by starting with the initial clues of the smell, numerous victims, and symptoms of the victims. Ask the construction manager if there is any construction material that might cause these symptoms. See if there is a container that may have markings that can be called in to CHEMTREC for possible identification of the substance. If no container can be identified, then study the signs/symptoms of the ill/injured for possible clues that can be provided to Poison Control, which is a good resource for identification and specific cases. At a bare minimum, it is obvious that in this scene a substance has become airborne and that the poison, given the rapidity of onset, was most likely inhaled.
4. Those who need to be in the inner perimeter (hot zone) need to have full protective equipment (specifically rated for HAZMAT), which includes proper protective breathing apparatus. Until the substance is identified and specific hazards and risks are known, nobody should enter without proper personal protective equipment (PPE).

Street Scene Questions (#2)

1. The first indicator that this is a suspicious event is the location of the incident (headquarters of a militant group). The next is that the fire is in a dead-end alley, which limits the means of ingress and egress. Another is the wire that is observed stretched across the alley, which may well be a "trip wire" for some type of device.
2. All people involved should retreat from the immediate area to a safe distance and shield themselves. Until the possible secondary device (wire across the alley) is deactivated by experts, the scene remains dangerous and unsafe. Another possibility is that there is an explosive device in the car.
3. The first support agency is the police, who will establish a perimeter and protect civilians and responders. (That role might belong to the fire department, so know your local resources.) Then, experts in explosive devices are needed to deactivate the device(s). Certain federal law enforcement agencies may also be needed to investigate.

Glossary

911 system a system for telephone access to report emergencies. A dispatcher takes the information and alerts EMS or the fire or police department as needed. *Enhanced 911* also identifies the caller's phone number and location automatically.

abandonment leaving a patient after care has been initiated and before the patient has been transferred to someone with equal or greater medical training.

A-B-Cs airway, breathing, and circulation.

abdominal quadrants four divisions of the abdomen used to pinpoint the location of a pain or injury: the right upper quadrant (RUQ), the left upper quadrant (LUQ), the right lower quadrant (RLQ), and the left lower quadrant (LLQ).

abortion spontaneous (miscarriage) or induced termination of pregnancy.

abrasion (ab-RAY-zhun) a scratch or scrape.

abruptio placentae (ab-RUPT-si-o plah-SENT-ta) a condition in which the placenta separates from the uterine wall; a cause of prebirth bleeding.

absorbed poisons poisons that are taken into the body through unbroken skin.

acetabulum (AS-uh-TAB-yuh-lum) the pelvic socket into which the ball at the proximal end of the femur fits to form the hip joint.

acromioclavicular (ah-KRO-me-o-klav-IK-yuh-ler) **joint** the joint where the acromion and the clavicle meet.

acromion (ah-KRO-me-on) **process** the highest portion of the shoulder.

activated charcoal a substance that adsorbs many poisons and prevents them from being absorbed by the body.

active rewarming application of an external heat source to rewarm the body of a hypothermic patient.

acute coronary syndrome (ACS) a blanket term used to represent any symptoms related to lack of oxygen (ischemia) in the heart muscle. Also called *cardiac compromise*.

acute myocardial infarction (AMI) (ah-KUTE MY-o-KARD-e-ul in-FARK-shun) the condition in which a portion of the myocardium dies as a result of an occlusion; often called a heart attack by laypersons.

adolescence stage of life from 13 to 18 years.

advance directive a DNR order; instructions written in advance of an event.

aerobic (air-O-bik) **metabolism** the cellular process in which oxygen is used to metabolize glucose. Energy is produced in an efficient manner, with minimal waste products.

afterbirth the placenta, membranes of the amniotic sac, part of the umbilical cord, and some tissues from the lining of the uterus that are delivered after the birth of the baby.

agonal breathing irregular, gasping breaths that precede apnea and death.

air embolism gas bubble in the bloodstream. The plural is *air emboli*. The more accurate term is *arterial gas embolism (AGE)*.

airway the passageway by which air enters and leaves the body. The structures of the airway are the nose, mouth, pharynx, larynx, trachea, bronchi, and lungs.

allergen something that causes an allergic reaction.

allergic reaction an exaggerated immune response.

alveolar ventilation the amount of air that reaches the alveoli.

alveoli (al-VE-o-li) the microscopic sacs of the lungs where gas exchange with the bloodstream takes place.

amniotic (am-ne-OT-ik) **sac** the "bag of waters" that surrounds the developing fetus.

amputation (am-pyu-TAY-shun) the surgical removal or traumatic severing of a body part, usually an extremity.

anaerobic (AN-air-o-bik) **metabolism** the cellular process in which glucose is metabolized into energy without oxygen. Energy is produced in an inefficient manner, with many waste products.

anaphylaxis (an-ah-fi-LAK-sis) a severe or life-threatening allergic reaction in which the blood vessels dilate, causing a drop in blood pressure, and the tissues lining the respiratory system swell, interfering with the airway. Also called *anaphylactic shock.*

anatomic position the standard reference position for the body in the study of anatomy. In this position, the body is standing erect, facing the observer, with arms at the sides and the palms of the hands forward.

anatomy the study of body structure.

anemia deficiency in the normal number of red blood cells in the circulation.

aneurysm (AN-u-rizm) the dilation, or ballooning, of a weakened section of the wall of an artery.

angina pectoris (AN-ji-nah [or an-JI-nah] PEK-to-ris) signs of acute coronary syndrome (usually chest pain) occurring when blood supply to the heart is reduced and a portion of the heart muscle is not receiving enough oxygen.

angulated fracture a fracture in which the broken bone segments are at an angle to each other.

anterior the front of the body or body part.

antidote a substance that will neutralize the poison or its effects.

aorta (ay-OR-tah) the largest artery in the body. It transports blood from the left ventricle to begin systemic circulation.

apnea (Ap-ne-ah) the absence of breathing.

appendix a small tube located near the junction of the small and large intestines in the right lower quadrant of the abdomen, the function of which is not well understood. Its inflammation, called appendicitis, is a common cause of abdominal pain.

arterial bleeding bleeding from an artery, which is characterized by bright red blood that is often spurting, profuse, and difficult to control.

arteriole (ar-TE-re-ol) the smallest kind of artery.

artery any blood vessel carrying blood away from the heart.

artificial ventilation the use of positive pressure to force air or oxygen into the lungs when a patient has stopped breathing or has inadequate breathing. Also called *positive pressure ventilation*.

asphyxial (ass-FIX-ial) **cardiac arrest** a cardiac arrest caused by systemic hypoxia, typically due to a respiratory disorder or shock.

aspirin a medication used to reduce the clotting ability of blood to prevent and treat clots associated with myocardial infarction.

assault placing a person in fear of bodily harm.

asystole (ay-SIS-to-le) a condition in which the heart has ceased generating electrical impulses. Commonly called *flatline*.

ataxic (AY-taks-ic) **respirations** a pattern of irregular and unpredictable breathing commonly caused by brain injury.

atomizer a device attached to the end of a syringe that atomizes medication (turns it into very fine droplets).

atria (AY-tree-ah) the two upper chambers of the heart. There is a right atrium (which receives unoxygenated blood returning from the body) and a left atrium (which receives oxygenated blood returning from the lungs). *Singular* atrium.

aura a sensation experienced by a seizure patient right before the seizure, which might be a smell, sound, or general feeling.

auscultation (os-kul-TAY-shun) listening. A stethoscope is used to auscultate for characteristic sounds.

autism spectrum disorders (ASD) Developmental disorders that affect, among other things, the ability to communicate, report medical conditions, self-regulate behaviors, and interact with others.

automatic implanted cardiac defibrillator (AICD) a device implanted under the skin of the chest to detect any life-threatening dysrhythmia and deliver a shock to defibrillate the heart.

automatic transport ventilator (ATV) a device that provides positive pressure ventilations. It includes settings designed to adjust ventilation rate and volume, is portable, and is easily carried on an ambulance.

automaticity (AW-to-muh-TISS-it-e) the ability of the heart to generate and conduct electrical impulses on its own.

autonomic (AW-to-NOM-ik) **nervous system (ANS)** the division of the peripheral nervous system that controls involuntary motor functions.

AVPU a memory aid for classifying a patient's level of responsiveness or mental status. The letters stand for **A**lert, **V**erbal response, **P**ainful response, **U**nresponsive.

avulsion (ah-VUL-shun) the tearing away or tearing off of a piece or flap of skin or other soft tissue. This term also may be used for an eye pulled from its socket or a tooth dislodged from its socket.

bag-valve mask (BVM) a handheld device with a face mask and self-refilling bag that can be squeezed to provide artificial ventilations to a patient. It can deliver air from the atmosphere or oxygen from a supplemental oxygen supply system.

bandage any material used to hold a dressing in place.

bariatric having to do with patients who are significantly overweight or obese.

bariatrics the branch of medicine that deals with the causes of obesity as well as its prevention and treatment.

base station setup with two-way radios at a fixed site, such as a hospital or dispatch center.

battery causing bodily harm to or restraining a person.

behavior the manner in which a person acts.

behavioral emergency when a patient's behavior is not typical for the situation; when the patient's behavior is unacceptable or intolerable to the patient, the patient's family, or the community; or when a patient may harm self or others.

bilateral on both sides.

bladder the round, saclike organ of the renal system used as a reservoir for urine.

blood pressure the pressure caused by blood exerting force against the walls of blood vessels. Usually arterial blood pressure (the pressure in an artery) is measured. There are two parts: *diastolic blood pressure* and *systolic blood pressure*.

blood pressure monitor a machine that automatically inflates a blood pressure cuff and measures blood pressure.

blunt-force trauma injury caused by a blow that does not penetrate the skin or other body tissues.

body mechanics the proper use of the body to facilitate lifting and moving and to prevent injury.

bonding formation of a close relationship through frequent association.

bones hard but flexible living structures that provide support for the body and protection to vital organs.

brachial (BRAY-key-al) **artery** the artery of the upper arm; the site of the pulse checked during infant CPR.

brachial (BRAY-key-al) **pulse** the pulse felt in the upper arm.

bradycardia (BRAY-duh-KAR-de-uh) a slow pulse; any pulse rate below 60 beats per minute.

Braxton-Hicks (braks-tun-hiks) **contractions** irregular prelabor contractions of the uterus.

breech presentation when the baby's buttocks or both legs appear first during birth.

bronchi (BRONG-ki) the two large sets of branches that come off the trachea and enter the lungs. There are right and left bronchi. *Singular* bronchus.

bronchoconstriction (BRON-ko-kun-STRIK-shun) the contraction of smooth muscle that lines the bronchial passages that results in a decreased internal diameter of the airway and increased resistance to airflow.

buffer system a system that helps manage the pH of the body to maintain it at a normal level.

calcaneus (kal-KAY-ne-us) the heel bone.

capillaries (KAP-i-lair-e) thin-walled, microscopic blood vessels where the oxygen/carbon dioxide and nutrient/waste exchange with the body's cells takes place.

capillary bleeding bleeding from capillaries, which is characterized by a slow, oozing flow of blood.

cardiac arrest a state in which the heart is no longer pumping blood.

cardiac compromise *See* acute coronary syndrome.

cardiac conduction system a system of specialized muscle tissues that conducts electrical impulses that stimulate the heart to beat.

cardiac muscle specialized involuntary muscle found only in the heart.

cardiac output the amount of blood ejected from the heart in one minute (heart rate · stroke volume).

cardiogenic shock shock, or lack of perfusion, brought on not by blood loss but by the heart's inadequate pumping action. It is often the result of a heart attack (MI) or congestive heart failure.

cardiopulmonary resuscitation (CPR) actions taken to revive a person by keeping the person's heart and lungs working.

cardiovascular (KAR-de-o-VAS-kyu-ler) **system** related to the system made up of the heart (cardio) and the blood vessels (vascular); the *circulatory system*.

cardiovascular system the heart and the blood vessels.

carotid (kah-ROT-id) **arteries** the large neck arteries, one on each side of the neck, that carry blood from the heart to the head.

carotid (kah-ROT-id) **pulse** the pulse felt along the large carotid artery on either side of the neck.

carpals (KAR-pulz) the wrist bones.

cartilage tough tissue that covers the joint ends of bones and helps to form certain body parts, such as the ear.

cell phone a phone that transmits through the air instead of over wires, so the phone can be transported and used over a wide area.

cellular respiration the exchange of oxygen and carbon dioxide between cells and circulating blood.

central IV catheter a catheter surgically inserted for long-term delivery of medications or fluids into the central circulation.

central nervous system (CNS) the brain and spinal cord.

central neurogenic hyperventilation a pattern of rapid and deep breathing caused by injury to the brain.

central pulses the carotid and femoral pulses, which can be felt in the central part of the body.

cerebrospinal (suh-RE-bro-SPI-nal) **fluid (CSF)** the fluid that surrounds the brain and spinal cord.

cervix (SUR-viks) the lower neck of the uterus at the entrance to the birth canal.

chain of survival a metaphor that describes the key elements of cardiac arrest management. Each link in the chain describes a different but interconnected intervention; when combined, these interventions offer optimal care.

chemoreceptors (kee-mo-re-cept-erz) chemical sensors in the brain and blood vessels that identify changing levels of oxygen and carbon dioxide.

Cheyne (CHAY-ne) **-Stokes breathing** a distinct pattern of breathing characterized by quickening and deepening respirations followed by a period of apnea.

chief complaint the statement (usually in the patient's own words) that describes the symptoms or concern associated with the primary problem the patient is having; in emergency medicine, it is the reason the patient calls EMS.

clavicle (KLAV-i-kul) the collarbone.

closed extremity injury an injury to an extremity with no associated opening in the skin.

closed wound an internal injury with no open pathway from the outside.

closed-ended question a question requiring only a "yes" or "no" answer.

coagulopathy loss of the normal ability to form a blood clot with internal or external bleeding.

cold zone area where the Incident Command post and support functions are located.

combining form a word root with an added vowel that can be joined with other words, roots, or suffixes to form a new word.

Command the first on the scene to establish order and initiate the Incident Command System.

comminuted fracture a fracture in which the bone is broken in several places.

commotio cordis (com-mo-shee-o cord -iss) a cardiac arrest dysrhythmia caused by acute blunt force trauma to the chest.

communicable diseases diseases that can be passed from one individual to another, either through direct contact or contact with secretions from an infected person.

compartment syndrome injury caused when tissues such as blood vessels and nerves are constricted within a space, as from swelling or from a tight dressing or cast.

compensated shock period when the patient is developing shock but the body is still able to maintain perfusion.

compound a word formed from two or more whole words.

compression fraction the amount of time chest compressions are being performed compared with the total time of patient contact.

concussion mild closed head injury without detectable damage to the brain. Complete recovery is usually expected, but effects may linger for weeks, months, or even years.

conduction the transfer of heat from one material to another through direct contact.

confidentiality the obligation not to reveal information obtained about a patient except to other health care professionals involved in the patient's care or under subpoena or in a court of law or when the patient has signed a release of confidentiality.

consent permission from the patient for care or other action by the EMT.

constrict (kon-STRIKT) get smaller.

contamination contact with or presence of a material (contaminant) that is present where it does not belong and that is somehow harmful to persons, animals, or the environment; introduction of dangerous chemicals, disease, or infectious materials.

continuous ambulatory peritoneal dialysis (CAPD) a gravity exchange process for peritoneal dialysis in which a bag of dialysis fluid is raised above the level of an abdominal catheter to fill the abdominal cavity and lowered below the level of the abdominal catheter to drain the fluid out.

continuous cycler-assisted peritoneal dialysis (CCPD) a mechanical process for peritoneal dialysis in which a machine fills and empties the abdominal cavity of dialysis solution.

continuous positive airway pressure (CPAP) a form of noninvasive positive pressure ventilation (NPPV) consisting of a mask and a means of blowing oxygen or air into the mask to prevent airway collapse or to help alleviate difficulty breathing.

contraindications (KON-truh-in-duh-KAY-shunz) specific signs or circumstances under which it is not appropriate and may be harmful to administer a drug to a patient.

contusion a bruise; in brain injuries, a bruised brain caused when the force of a blow to the head is great enough to rupture blood vessels.

convection carrying away of heat by currents of air, water, or other gases or liquids.

coronary (KOR-o-nar-e) **arteries** blood vessels that supply the muscle of the heart (myocardium).

coronary artery disease (CAD) diseases that affect the arteries of the heart.

cranium (KRAY-ne-um) the bony structure making up the forehead, top, back, and upper sides of the skull.

crepitation (krep-uh-TAY-shun) the grating sound or feeling of broken bones rubbing together.

cricoid (KRIK-oid) **cartilage** the ring-shaped structure that forms the lower portion of the larynx.

crime scene the location where a crime has been committed or any place that evidence relating to a crime may be found.

critical incident stress management (CISM) a comprehensive system that includes education and resources to prevent stress and to deal with stress appropriately when it occurs.

crush injury an injury caused when force is transmitted from the body's exterior to its internal structures. Bones can be broken; muscles, nerves, and tissues can be damaged, causing internal bleeding. In extreme cases where the torso is compressed, internal organs such as the stomach or urinary bladder can be ruptured, causing internal bleeding and allowing digested food or urine to spread into the abdominal cavities.

danger zone the area around the wreckage of a vehicle collision or other incident within which special safety precautions should be taken.

dead air space air that occupies the space between the mouth and alveoli but that does not actually reach the area of gas exchange.

decompensated shock period when the body can no longer compensate for low blood volume or lack of perfusion. Late signs such as decreasing blood pressure become evident.

decompression sickness a condition resulting from nitrogen trapped in the body's tissues, caused by coming up too quickly from a deep, prolonged dive. A symptom of decompression sickness is "the bends," or deep pain in the muscles and joints.

decontamination the removal or cleansing of dangerous chemicals and other dangerous or infectious materials from employees and their equipment to preclude foreseeable health effects.

defibrillation delivery of an electrical shock to stop the fibrillation of heart muscles and restore a normal heart rhythm.

dehydration (de-hi-DRAY-shun) an abnormally low amount of water in the body.

dermatome (DERM-uh-tohm) an area of the skin that is innervated by a single spinal nerve.

dermis (DER-mis) the inner (second) layer of skin, rich in blood vessels and nerves, found beneath the epidermis.

detailed physical exam an assessment of the head, neck, chest, abdomen, pelvis, extremities, and posterior of the body to detect signs and symptoms of injury. It differs from the rapid trauma assessment only in that it also includes examination of the face, ears, eyes, nose, and mouth during the examination of the head.

diabetes mellitus (di-ah-BEE-tez MEL-i-tus) also called *sugar diabetes* or just *diabetes*, the condition brought about by decreased insulin production or the inability of the body cells to use insulin properly. The person with this condition is a diabetic.

diabetic ketoacidosis (di-ah-BET-ic KEY-to-as-id-DO-sis) **(DKA)** a condition that occurs as the result of high blood sugar (hyperglycemia), characterized by dehydration, altered mental status, and shock.

diagnosis a description or label for a patient's condition that assists a clinician in further evaluation and treatment.

dialysis the process by which toxins and excess fluid are removed from the body by a medical system independent of the kidneys.

diaphoresis (DI-uh-for-EE-sis) sweating; condition of cool, pale, and moist/sweaty skin.

diaphragm (DI-uh-fram) the muscular structure that divides the chest cavity from the abdominal cavity; a major muscle of respiration.

diastolic (di-as-TOL-ik) **blood pressure** the pressure remaining in the arteries when the left ventricle of the heart is relaxed and refilling.

differential diagnosis a list of potential diagnoses compiled early in the assessment of the patient.

diffusion a process by which molecules move from an area of high concentration to an area of low concentration.

digestive system system by which food travels through the body and is digested or broken down into absorbable forms.

dilate (DI-late) get larger.

dilution (di-LU-shun) thinning down or weakening by mixing with something else. Ingested poisons are sometimes diluted by drinking water or milk.

direct carry a method of transferring a patient from bed to stretcher, during which two or more rescuers curl the patient to their chests, then reverse the process to lower the patient to the stretcher.

direct ground lift a method of lifting and carrying a patient from ground level to a stretcher in which two or more rescuers kneel, curl the patient to their chests, stand, then reverse the process to lower the patient to the stretcher.

disability a physical, emotional, behavioral, or cognitive condition that interferes with a person's ability to carry out everyday tasks, such as working or caring for oneself.

disaster plan a predefined set of instructions for a community's emergency responders.

dislocation the disruption or "coming apart" of a joint.

dissemination spreading.

distal farther away from the torso.

distention (dis-TEN-shun) a condition of being stretched, inflated, or larger than normal.

distributive shock hypoperfusion due to a lack of blood vessel tone. Blood vessel dilation leads to decreased pressure within the circulatory system.

do not resuscitate (DNR) order a legal document, usually signed by both patient and physician, which states that the patient has a terminal illness and does not wish to prolong life through resuscitative efforts.

domestic terrorism terrorism directed against one's own government or population. *See also* terrorism; international terrorism.

dorsal referring to the back of the body or the back of the hand or foot. A synonym for *posterior*.

dorsalis pedis (dor-SAL-is PEED-is) **artery** artery supplying the foot, lateral to the large tendon of the big toe.

downers depressants, such as benzodiazepines, that depress the central nervous system, and which are often used to bring on a more relaxed state of mind.

draw-sheet method a method of transferring a patient from bed to stretcher by grasping and pulling the loosened bottom sheet of the bed.

dressing any material (preferably sterile) used to cover a wound that will help control bleeding and prevent additional contamination.

drop report (or transfer report) an abbreviated form of the PCR that an EMS crew can leave at the hospital when there is not enough time to complete the PCR before leaving.

drowning the process of experiencing respiratory impairment from submersion/immersion in liquid, which may result in death, morbidity (illness or other adverse effects), or no morbidity.

duty to act an obligation to provide care to a patient.

dyspnea (DISP-ne-ah) shortness of breath; labored or difficult breathing.

dysrhythmia (dis-RITH-me-ah) a disturbance in heart rate and rhythm.

early adulthood stage of life from 19 to 40 years.

eclampsia (e-KLAMP-se-ah) a severe complication of pregnancy that produces seizures and is very dangerous to the infant and mother.

ectopic (ek-TOP-ik) **pregnancy** implantation of the fertilized egg outside the body of the uterus, occurring in the fallopian tube (oviduct), cervix, or abdominopelvic cavity.

edema (eh-DEE-muh) swelling associated with the movement of water into the interstitial space.

electrolyte (e-LEK-tro-lite) a substance that, when dissolved in water, separates into charged particles.

embolism (EM-bo-lizm) blockage of a vessel by a clot or foreign material brought to the site by the blood current.

embryo (EM-bree-o) the baby from fertilization to eight weeks of development.

endocrine (EN-do-krin) **system** system of glands that produce chemicals called hormones that help to regulate many body activities and functions.

end-stage renal disease (ESRD) irreversible renal failure to the extent that the kidneys can no longer provide adequate filtration and fluid balance to sustain life; survival with ESRD usually requires dialysis.

enteral (EN-tur-al) referring to a route of medication administration that uses the gastrointestinal tract, such as swallowing a pill.

epidermis (ep-i-DER-mis) the outer layer of the skin.

epiglottis (EP-i-GLOT-is) a leaf-shaped structure that prevents food and foreign matter from entering the trachea.

epilepsy (EP-uh-lep-see) a medical condition that causes seizures.

epinephrine (EP-uh-NEF-rin) a hormone produced by the adrenal glands. As a medication, it constricts blood vessels and dilates respiratory passages, and is used to relieve severe allergic reactions.

ethical regarding a social system or social or professional expectations for applying principles of right and wrong.

evaporation the change from liquid to gas. When the body perspires or gets wet, evaporation of the perspiration or other liquid into the air has a cooling effect on the body.

evidence-based techniques techniques or practices that are supported by scientific evidence of their safety and efficacy, rather than merely on supposition and tradition.

evisceration (e-vis-er-AY-shun) an intestine or other internal organ protruding through a wound in the abdomen.

exchange one cycle of filling and draining the peritoneal cavity in peritoneal dialysis.

excited delirium bizarre and/or aggressive behavior, shouting, paranoia, panic, violence toward others, insensitivity to pain, unexpected physical strength, and hyperthermia, usually associated with cocaine or amphetamine use. Also called *agitated delirium*.

exhalation (EX-huh-LAY-shun) a passive process in which the intercostal (rib) muscles and the diaphragm relax, causing the chest cavity to decrease in size and air to flow out of the lungs; also call expiration.

expiration *See* exhalation.

exposure the dose or concentration of an agent multiplied by the time, or duration.

expressed consent consent given by adults who are of legal age and are mentally competent to make a rational decision with regard to their medical well-being.

extremities (ex-TREM-i-teez) the portions of the skeleton that include the clavicles, scapulae, arms, wrists, and hands (upper extremities) and the pelvis, thighs, legs, ankles, and feet (lower extremities).

extremity lift a method of lifting and carrying a patient in which one rescuer slips hands under the patient's armpits and grasps the wrists, while another rescuer grasps the patient's knees.

fallopian (fu-LO-pe-an) **tube** the narrow tube that connects the ovary to the uterus. Also called the *oviduct*.

feeding tube a tube used to provide delivery of nutrients to the stomach. A nasogastric feeding tube is inserted through the nose and into the stomach; a gastric feeding tube is surgically implanted through the abdominal wall and into the stomach.

femoral (FEM-o-ral) **artery** the major artery supplying the leg.

femur (FEE-mer) the large bone of the thigh.

fetus (FE-tus) the baby from eight weeks of development to birth.

fibula (FIB-yuh-luh) the lateral and smaller bone of the lower leg.

FiO_2 fraction of inspired oxygen; the concentration of oxygen in the air we breathe.

flail chest fracture of two or more adjacent ribs in two or more places that allows for free movement of the fractured segment.

flowmeter a valve that indicates the flow of oxygen in liters per minute.

foramen magnum (FOR-uh-men MAG-num) the opening at the base of the skull through which the spinal cord passes from the brain.

Fowler position a sitting position.

fracture (FRAK-cher) any break in a bone.

full thickness burn a burn in which all the layers of the skin are damaged. There are usually areas that are charred black or areas that are dry and white. Also called a *third-degree burn*.

gag reflex vomiting or retching that results when something is placed in the back of the pharynx. This is tied to the swallow reflex.

gallbladder a sac on the underside of the liver that stores bile produced by the liver.

general impression impression of the patient's condition that is formed on first approaching the patient, based on the patient's environment, chief complaint, and appearance.

generalized seizure a seizure that affects both sides of the brain.

glottic opening the level of the vocal cords that defines the boundary between the upper and lower airways.

glucose (GLU-kos) a form of sugar, the body's basic source of energy.

Good Samaritan laws a series of laws, varying by state, designed to provide limited legal protection for citizens and some health care personnel when they are administering emergency care.

greenstick fracture an incomplete fracture.

hallucinogens (huh-LOO-sin-uh-jens) mind-affecting or mind-altering drugs that act on the central nervous system to produce excitement and distortion of perceptions.

hazardous material (HAZMAT) any substance or material in a form that poses an unreasonable risk to health, safety, and property when transported in commerce or kept in storage at a warehouse, port, depot, or railroad facility.

hazardous material incident the release of a harmful substance into the environment.

head-tilt, chin-lift maneuver a means of correcting blockage of the airway by the tongue by tilting the head back and lifting the chin. Used when no trauma or injury is suspected.

heart failure (HF) the failure of the heart to pump blood with normal efficiency; also known as *congestive heart failure (CHF)*.

hematoma (hem-ah-TO-mah) a swelling caused by the collection of blood under the skin or in damaged tissues as a result of an injured or broken blood vessel. In a head injury, a collection of blood within the skull or brain.

hemorrhage (HEM-o-rej) bleeding, especially severe bleeding.

hemorrhagic (HEM-or-AJ-ik) **shock** shock resulting from blood loss.

hemostatic (HEM-o-STAT-IK) **agents** substances applied as powders, dressings, gauze, or bandages to open wounds to stop bleeding.

herniation (her-ne-AY-shun) pushing of a portion of the brain downward toward the foramen magnum as a result of increased intracranial pressure.

HIPAA the Health Insurance Portability and Accountability Act, which includes the Privacy Rule protecting the privacy of patient-specific health care information and providing the patient with control over how this information is used and distributed.

history of the present illness or injury (HPI) information gathered regarding the symptoms and nature of the patient's current concern; the events and or mechanism leading up to the current problem.

hives red, itchy, possibly raised blotches on the skin that often result from allergic reactions; also known as urticaria.

hot zone area immediately surrounding a HAZMAT incident; extends far enough to prevent adverse effects outside the zone.

humerus (HYU-mer-us) the bone of the upper arm, between the shoulder and the elbow.

humidifier a device connected to the flowmeter to add moisture to the dry oxygen coming from an oxygen cylinder.

hydrostatic (HI-dro-STAT-ik) **pressure** the pressure within a blood vessel that tends to push water out of the vessel.

hyperglycemia (HI-per-gli-SEE-me-ah) high blood sugar.

hypersensitivity an exaggerated response by the immune system to a particular substance.

hyperthermia (HI-per-THURM-e-ah) an increase in body temperature above normal, which is a life-threatening condition in its extreme.

hypoglycemia (HI-po-gli-SEE-me-ah) low blood sugar.

hypoperfusion inability of the body to circulate adequate blood to the body's cells to supply them with oxygen and nutrients. A life-threatening condition. Also called *shock*. *See also* perfusion.

hypothermia (HI-po-THURM-e-ah) generalized cooling that reduces body temperature below normal, which is a life-threatening condition in its extreme.

hypovolemic (HI-po-vo-LE-mik) **shock** shock resulting from blood or fluid loss.

hypoxia (hi-POK-se-uh) an insufficiency of oxygen in the body's tissues.

ilium (IL-e-um) the superior and widest portion of the pelvis.

implied consent the consent it is presumed patients or their parents or guardians would give if they could, such as for an unconscious patient or a child whose parents cannot be contacted when care is needed.

in loco parentis literally 'in place of a parent,' indicating a person who may give consent for care of a child when a parent is not present or able to give consent.

Incident Command the person or persons who assume overall direction of a large-scale incident.

Incident Command System (ICS) a subset of NIMS designed specifically for management of multiple-casualty incidents.

index of suspicion awareness that there may be injuries.

indications specific signs or circumstances under which it is appropriate to administer a drug to a patient.

induced abortion expulsion of a fetus as a result of deliberate actions taken to terminate the pregnancy.

infancy stage of life from birth to 1 year of age.

infectious diseases diseases that can be spread by bacteria, viruses, and other microbes.

inferior away from the head, usually compared with another structure that is closer to the head (e.g., the lips are inferior to the nose).

ingested poisons poisons that are swallowed.

inhalation (IN-huh-LAY-shun) an active process in which the intercostal (rib) muscles and the diaphragm contract, expanding the size of the chest cavity and causing air to flow into the lungs; another term for inspiration.

inhaled poisons poisons that are breathed in.

inhaler a spray device with a mouthpiece that contains an aerosol form of a medication that a patient can spray into the airway.

injected poisons poisons that are inserted through the skin—for example, by needle, snake fangs, or insect stinger.

inspiration (IN-spuh-RAY-shun) *See* inhalation.

insulin (IN-suh-lin) a hormone produced by the pancreas or taken as a medication by many people with diabetes.

international terrorism terrorism that is purely foreign-based or directed. *See also* terrorism; domestic terrorism.

interventions actions taken to correct or manage a patient's problems.

intracranial (IN-truh-KRAY-ne-ul) **pressure (ICP)** pressure inside the skull.

involuntary muscle muscle that responds automatically to brain signals but cannot be consciously controlled.

ischemia (is-KEEM-e-ah) an insufficient supply of oxygenated blood to an area of the body.

ischium (ISH-e-um) the lower, posterior portions of the pelvis.

jaw-thrust maneuver a means of correcting blockage of the airway by moving the jaw forward without tilting the head or neck. Used when trauma or injury is suspected to open the airway without causing further injury to the spinal cord in the neck.

joints places where bones articulate, or come together.

jugular (JUG-yuh-ler) **vein distention (JVD)** bulging of the neck veins.

kidneys organs of the renal system used to filter blood and regulate fluid levels in the body.

labia (LAY-be-uh) soft tissues that protect the entrance to the vagina.

labor the three stages of the delivery of a baby that begin with the contractions of the uterus and end with the expulsion of the placenta.

laceration (las-uh-RAY-shun) a cut; in brain injuries, a cut to the brain.

large intestine the muscular tube that removes water from waste products received from the small intestine and moves anything not absorbed by the body toward excretion from the body.

larynx (LAIR-inks) the voice box.

late adulthood stage of life from 61 years and older.

lateral to the side, away from the midline of the body.

liability being held legally responsible.

libel false, injurious information in written form.

ligaments tissues that connect bone to bone.

lightening the sensation of the fetus moving from high in the abdomen to low in the birth canal.

limb presentation when an infant's limb protrudes from the vagina before the appearance of any other body part.

liver the largest organ of the body, which produces bile to assist in breakdown of fats and assists in the metabolism of various substances in the body.

local cooling cooling or freezing of particular (local) parts of the body.

lungs the organs where exchange of atmospheric oxygen and waste carbon dioxide takes place.

lymphatic (lim-FAT-ik) **system** the system composed of organs, tissues, and vessels that helps to maintain the fluid balance of the body and contributes to the body's immune system.

malar (MAY-lar) the cheekbone. Also called the *zygomatic bone*.

malleolus (mal-E-o-lus) protrusion on the side of the ankle. The *lateral malleolus*, at the lower end of the fibula, is seen on the outer ankle; the *medial malleolus*, at the lower end of the tibia, is seen on the inner ankle.

mandible (MAN-di-bul) the lower jawbone.

manual stabilization using one's hands to prevent movement of a patient's head and neck until a cervical collar can be applied.

manual traction the process of applying tension to straighten and realign a fractured limb before splinting. Also called *tension*.

manubrium (man-OO-bre-um) the superior portion of the sternum.

maxillae (mak-SIL-e) the two fused bones forming the upper jaw.

mechanism of injury a force or forces that may have caused injury.

meconium staining amniotic fluid that is greenish- or brownish-yellow rather than clear, caused by fetal defecation; a possible indication of maternal or fetal distress during labor.

medial toward the midline of the body.

medical direction oversight of the patient-care aspects of an EMS system by the Medical Director. Direction can be either off-line or on-line.

Medical Director a physician who assumes ultimate responsibility for the patient-care aspects of the EMS system.

medical patient a patient with one or more medical diseases or conditions.

mental status level of responsiveness.

metabolism (meh-TAB-o-lizm) the cellular function of converting nutrients into energy.

metacarpals (MET-uh-KAR-pulz) the hand bones.

metatarsals (MET-uh-TAR-sulz) the foot bones.

midaxillary (mid-AX-uh-lair-e) **line** a line drawn vertically from the middle of the armpit to the ankle.

midclavicular (mid-clah-VIK-yuh-ler) **line** the line through the center of each clavicle.

middle adulthood stage of life from 41 to 60 years.

midline an imaginary line drawn down the center of the body, dividing it into right and left halves.

minute volume the amount of air breathed in during each respiration multiplied by the number of breaths per minute.

miscarriage *See* spontaneous abortion.

mobile radio a two-way radio that is used or affixed in a vehicle.

mons pubis soft tissue that covers the pubic symphysis; area where hair grows when a woman reaches puberty.

moral regarding personal standards or principles of right and wrong.

Moro reflex a response to being startled in which the infant throws out both arms, spreads the fingers, then grabs with fingers and arms.

multiple birth when more than one baby is born during a single delivery.

multiple devices destructive devices, such as bombs, including both those used in the initial attack and those placed to be activated after an initial attack and timed to injure emergency responders and others who rush in to help care for those targeted by an initial attack. *See also* secondary devices.

multiple trauma more than one serious injury.

multiple-casualty incident (MCI) any medical or trauma incident involving multiple patients.

multisystem trauma one or more injuries that affect more than one body system.

muscles tissues that can contract to allow movement of a body part.

musculoskeletal (MUS-kyu-lo-SKEL-e-tal) **system** the system of bones and skeletal muscles that support and protect the body and permit movement.

naloxone an antidote for narcotic overdoses.

nasal (NAY-zul) **bones** the bones that form the upper third, or bridge, of the nose.

nasal cannula (NAY-zul KAN-yuh-luh) a device that delivers low concentrations of oxygen through two prongs that rest in the patient's nostrils.

nasopharyngeal (NAY-zo-fah-RIN-jeul) **airway** a flexible breathing tube inserted through the patient's nostril into the pharynx to help maintain an open airway.

nasopharynx (NAY-zo-FAIR-inks) the area directly posterior to the nose.

National Incident Management System (NIMS) the management system used by federal, state, and local governments to manage emergencies in the United States.

nature of the illness what is medically wrong with a patient.

negligence a finding that there was failure to act properly in a situation in which there was a duty to act, that needed care as would reasonably be expected of the EMT was not provided, and that harm was caused to the patient as a result.

neonate (NEE-oh-nate) a newly born infant or an infant less than 1 month old.

nervous system the system of brain, spinal cord, and nerves that governs sensation, movement, and thought.

neurogenic shock hypoperfusion caused by a spinal cord injury that results in systemic vasodilation and nerve paralysis.

neurotransmitters chemicals within the body that transmit a message in the brain from the distal end of one neuron to the proximal end of the next neuron.

nitroglycerin (NYE-tro-GLIS-uh-rin) a drug that helps to dilate the coronary vessels that supply the heart muscle with blood.

nonrebreather (NRB) mask a face mask-and-reservoir bag device that delivers high concentrations of oxygen. The patient's exhaled air escapes through a valve and is not rebreathed.

obesity a condition of having too much body fat, defined as a body mass index of 30 or greater.

obstructive shock a term commonly used to describe the different conditions that block the flow of blood and cause hypoperfusion.

occlusion (uh-KLU-zhun) blockage, as of an artery, by fatty deposits.

occlusive dressing any dressing that forms an airtight seal.

off-line medical direction standing orders issued by the Medical Director that allow EMTs to give certain medications or perform certain procedures without speaking to the Medical Director or another physician.

on-line medical direction orders from the on-duty physician given directly to an EMT in the field by radio or telephone.

open extremity injury an extremity injury in which the skin has been broken or torn through from the inside by an injured bone, or from the outside by something that has caused a penetrating wound with associated injury to the bone.

open wound an injury in which the skin is interrupted, exposing the tissue beneath.

open-ended question a question requiring more than just a "yes" or "no" answer.

opioids a class of drugs that affects the nervous system and changes many normal body activities. Their legal use is for the relief of pain. Illicit use is to produce an intense state of relaxation.

OPQRST a memory aid in which the letters stand for questions asked to get a description of the present illness: onset, provocation, quality, region/radiation, severity, time.

oral glucose (GLU-kos) a form of glucose (a kind of sugar) given by mouth to treat an awake patient (who is able to swallow) with an altered mental status and a history of diabetes.

orbits the bony structures around the eyes; the eye sockets.

organ donor a person who has completed a legal document that allows for donation of organs and tissues in the event of death.

oropharyngeal (OR-o-fah-RIN-jeul) **airway** a curved device inserted through the patient's mouth into the pharynx to help maintain an open airway.

oropharynx (OR-o-FAIR-inks) the area directly posterior to the mouth.

ostomy bag an external pouch that collects fecal matter diverted from the colon or ileum through a surgical opening (colostomy or ileostomy) in the abdominal wall.

ovaries egg- and hormone-producing organs within the female reproductive system.

ovulation (ov-U-LA-shun) the phase of the female reproductive cycle in which an ovum is released from the ovary.

oxygen a gas commonly found in the atmosphere. Pure oxygen is used as a medication to treat any patient whose medical or traumatic condition may cause the patient to be hypoxic, or low in oxygen.

oxygen cylinder a cylinder filled with oxygen under pressure.

oxygen saturation (SpO_2) the ratio of the amount of oxygen present in the blood to the amount that could be carried, expressed as a percentage.

pacemaker a device implanted under the skin with wires implanted into the heart to modify the heart rate as needed to maintain an adequate heart rate.

palmar referring to the palm of the hand.

palmar reflex a grasping reflex in which an infant grabs onto a finger placed in the infant's palm.

palpation touching or feeling. A pulse or blood pressure may be palpated with the fingertips.

pancreas a gland located behind the stomach that produces insulin and juices that assist in digestion of food in the duodenum of the small intestine. The pancreas also functions as part of the endocrine system.

paradoxical (pair-uh-DOCK-si-kal) **motion** movement of a part of the chest in the opposite direction to the rest of the chest during respiration.

parenteral (pair-EN-tur-al) referring to a route of medication administration that does not use the gastrointestinal tract, such as with an intravenous medication.

parietal pain a localized, intense pain that arises from the parietal peritoneum, the lining of the abdominal cavity.

partial rebreather mask a face mask and reservoir oxygen bag with no one-way valve to the reservoir bag, so some exhaled air mixes with the oxygen; used in some patients to help preserve carbon dioxide levels in the blood to stimulate breathing.

partial seizure a seizure that affects only one part or one side of the brain.

partial thickness burn a burn in which the epidermis (first layer of skin) is burned through and the dermis (second layer) is damaged. Burns of this type cause reddening, blistering, and a mottled appearance. Also called a *second-degree burn*.

passive rewarming covering a hypothermic patient and taking other steps to prevent further heat loss and help the body rewarm itself.

past medical history (PMH) information gathered regarding the patient's health problems in the past.

patella (pah-TEL-uh) the kneecap.

patent (PAY-tent) open and clear; free from obstruction.

patent airway an airway (passage from nose or mouth to lungs) that is open and clear and will remain open and clear without interference to the passage of air into and out of the body.

pathogens the organisms that cause infection, such as viruses and bacteria.

pathophysiology (path-o-fiz-e-OL-o-je) the study of how disease processes affect the function of the body.

patient outcomes the long-term survival of patients.

pedal edema accumulation of fluid in the feet or ankles.

peer reviewed submitted to a professional journal and reviewed by several of the researcher's peers.

pelvis the basin-shaped bony structure that supports the spine and is the point of proximal attachment for the lower extremities.

penetrating trauma injury caused by an object that passes through the skin or other body tissues.

penis the organ of male reproduction responsible for sexual intercourse and the transfer of sperm.

perfusion (per-FEW-zhun) the supply of oxygen to and removal of wastes from the cells and tissues of the body as a result of the flow of blood through the capillaries.

perineum (per-i-NE-um) the surface area between the vagina and anus.

peripheral nervous system (PNS) the nerves that enter and exit the spinal cord between the vertebrae, the 12 pairs of cranial nerves that travel between the brain and organs without passing through the spinal cord, and all of the body's other motor and sensory nerves.

peripheral pulses the radial, brachial, posterior tibial, and dorsalis pedis pulses, which can be felt at peripheral (outlying) points of the body.

peritoneum the membrane that lines the abdominal cavity (the *parietal peritoneum*) and covers the organs within it (the *visceral peritoneum*).

peritonitis bacterial infection within the peritoneal cavity.

permeation the movement of a substance through a surface or, on a molecular level, through intact materials; penetration, or spreading.

personal protective equipment (PPE) equipment that protects the EMS worker from infection and/or exposure to the dangers of rescue operations.

phalanges (fuh-LAN-jiz) the toe bones and finger bones.

pharmacodynamics (FARM-uh-KO-die-nam-ICS) the study of the effects of medications on the body.

pharmacology (FARM-uh-KOL-uh-je) the study of drugs, their sources, their characteristics, and their effects.

pharynx (FAIR-inks) the area directly posterior to the mouth and nose. It is made up of the oropharynx and the nasopharynx.

Physician's Order for Life-Sustaining Treatment (POLST) physician order that states not only the patient's wishes regarding resuscitation attempts but also the patient's wishes regarding artificial feeding, antibiotics, and other life-sustaining care if the patient is unable to state those desires later.

physiology the study of body function.

placenta (plah-SEN-tah) the organ of pregnancy where exchange of oxygen, nutrients, and wastes occurs between a mother and fetus.

placenta previa (plah-SEN-tah PRE-vi-ah) a condition in which the placenta is formed in an abnormal location (low in the uterus and close to or over the cervical opening) that will not allow for a normal delivery of the fetus; a cause of excessive prebirth bleeding.

plane a flat surface formed when slicing through a solid object.

plantar referring to the sole of the foot.

plasma (PLAZ-mah) the fluid portion of the blood.

plasma oncotic (PLAZ-ma on-KOT-ik) **pressure** the pull exerted by large proteins in the plasma portion of blood that tends to pull water from the body into the bloodstream.

platelets components of the blood; membrane-enclosed fragments of specialized cells.

pneumothorax air in the chest cavity.

pocket face mask a device, usually with a one-way valve, to aid in artificial ventilation. A rescuer breathes through the valve when the mask is placed over the patient's face. It also acts as a barrier to prevent contact with a patient's breath or body fluids. It can be used with supplemental oxygen when fitted with an oxygen inlet.

poison any substance that can harm the body by altering cell structure or functions.

portable radio a handheld two-way radio.

positional asphyxia inadequate breathing or respiratory arrest caused by a body position that restricts breathing.

positive pressure ventilation *See* artificial ventilation.

posterior tibial (TIB-ee-ul) **artery** artery supplying the foot, behind the medial ankle.

posterior the back of the body or body part.

postictal (post-IK-tul) **phase** the period of time immediately following a tonic-clonic seizure in which the patient goes from full loss of consciousness to full mental status.

power grip gripping with as much hand surface as possible in contact with the object being lifted, all fingers bent at the same angle, and hands at least 10 inches apart.

power lift a lift from a squatting position with weight to be lifted close to the body, feet apart and flat on the ground, body weight on or just behind the balls of the feet, and the back locked in. The upper body is raised before the hips. Also called the *squat-lift position*.

preeclampsia (pre-e-KLAMP-se-ah) a complication of pregnancy in which the woman retains large amounts of fluid and has hypertension, and which may progress to eclampsia.

prefix word part added to the beginning of a root or word to modify or qualify its meaning.

premature infant any newborn weighing less than 5½ pounds (2½ kg) at birth or born before the thirty-seventh week of pregnancy.

preschool age stage of life from 3 to 5 years.

pressure dressing a bulky dressing held in position with a tightly wrapped bandage, which applies pressure to help control bleeding.

pressure regulator a device connected to an oxygen cylinder to reduce cylinder pressure so it is safe for delivery of oxygen to a patient.

priapism (PRY-ah-pizm) persistent erection of the penis that may result from spinal injury and some medical problems.

primary assessment the first element in a patient assessment; steps taken for the purpose of discovering and dealing with any life-threatening problems. The six parts of primary assessment are: (1) forming a general impression, (2) assessing mental status, (3) assessing airway, (4) assessing breathing, (5) assessing circulation, and (6) determining the priority of the patient for treatment and transport to the hospital.

priority the decision regarding the need for immediate transport of the patient versus further assessment and care at the scene.

prolapsed umbilical cord when the umbilical cord presents first and is squeezed between the vaginal wall and the baby's head.

prone lying facedown.

protocols lists of steps, such as assessments and interventions, to be taken in different situations. Protocols are developed by the Medical Director of an EMS system.

proximal closer to the torso.

pubis (PYOO-bis) the medial anterior portion of the pelvis.

pulmonary air embolism a blockage in the blood circulation of the lung caused by a blood clot or air bubble.

pulmonary (PUL-mo-nar-e) **artery** the vessel that carries deoxygenated blood from the right ventricle of the heart to the lungs.

pulmonary edema accumulation of fluid in the lungs.

pulmonary respiration the exchange of oxygen and carbon dioxide between the alveoli and circulating blood in the pulmonary capillaries.

pulmonary vein vessel that carry oxygenated blood from the lungs to the left atrium of the heart.

pulse the rhythmic beats that are felt through the skin and that are caused as waves of blood move through and expand the arteries.

pulse oximeter an electronic device for determining the amount of oxygen carried in the blood, known as the oxygen saturation or SpO_2.

pulse quality the rhythm (regular or irregular) and force (strong or weak) of the pulse.

pulse rate the number of pulse beats per minute.

pulseless electrical activity (PEA) a condition in which the heart's electrical rhythm remains relatively normal, yet the mechanical pumping activity fails to follow the electrical activity, causing cardiac arrest.

puncture wound an open wound that tears through the skin and destroys underlying tissues. A *penetrating puncture wound* can be shallow or deep. A *perforating puncture wound* has both an entrance and an exit wound.

pupil the black center of the eye.

pyelonephritis an infection that begins in the urinary tract and ascends up the ureter into the kidney.

quality improvement a process of continuous self-review with the purpose of identifying and correcting aspects of the system that require improvement.

radial artery artery of the lower arm; the artery felt when taking the pulse at the thumb side of the wrist.

radial (RAY-de-ul) **pulse** the pulse felt at the wrist.

radiation sending out energy, such as heat, in waves into space.

radius (RAY-de-us) the lateral bone of the forearm.

rapid trauma assessment a rapid assessment of the head, neck, chest, abdomen, pelvis, extremities, and posterior of the body to detect signs and symptoms of injury.

reactivity (re-ak-TIV-uh-te) in the pupils of the eyes, reacting to light by changing size.

reassessment a procedure for detecting changes in a patient's condition. It involves four steps: repeating the primary assessment, repeating and recording vital signs, repeating the physical exam, and checking interventions.

recovery position lying on the side. Also called *-lateral recumbent position*.

red blood cells components of the blood. They carry oxygen to and carbon dioxide away from the cells.

referred pain pain that is felt in a location other than where the pain originates.

rem roentgen equivalent (in) man; a measure of radiation dosage.

renal failure loss of the kidneys' ability to filter the blood and to remove toxins and excess fluid from the body.

renal system the body system that regulates fluid balance and the filtration of blood. Also called the *urinary system*.

repeater a device that picks up signals from lower-power radio units, such as mobile and portable radios, and retransmits them at a higher power. It allows low-power radio signals to be transmitted over longer distances.

reproductive system the body system that is responsible for human reproduction.

res ipsa loquitur a Latin term meaning 'the thing speaks for itself.'

resilience toughness; an ability to recover quickly from difficult situations.

respiration (RES-pir-AY-shun) the diffusion of oxygen and carbon dioxide between the alveoli and the blood (pulmonary respiration) and between the blood and the cells (cellular respiration); the act of breathing in and out.

respiratory arrest when breathing completely stops.

respiratory distress increased work of breathing; a sensation of shortness of breath.

respiratory failure the inadequacy of breathing to the point where oxygen intake or the ventilation removal of carbon dioxide is not sufficient to support life.

respiratory (RES-puh-ruh-tor-e) **quality** the normal or abnormal (shallow, labored, or noisy) character of breathing.

respiratory (RES-puh-ruh-tor-e) **rate** the number of breaths taken in one minute.

respiratory (RES-puh-ruh-tor-e) **rhythm** the regular or irregular spacing of breaths.

respiratory (RES-pir-ah-tor-e) **system** the system of nose, mouth, throat, lungs, and muscles that brings oxygen into the body and expels carbon dioxide. Also called the *pulmonary system*.

reticular (ruh-TIK-yuh-ler) **activating system (RAS)** series of neurologic circuits in the brain that control the functions of staying awake, paying attention, and sleeping.

retroperitoneal space the area posterior to the peritoneum, between the peritoneum and the back.

return of spontaneous circulation (ROSC) the heart beating again after successful resuscitation.

root foundation of a word that is not a word that can stand on its own.

rooting reflex a reflex response in which a hungry infant automatically turns toward the stimulus when the cheek or one side of the mouth is touched.

routes of entry pathways into the body, generally by absorption, ingestion, injection, or inhalation.

rule of nines a method for estimating the extent of a burn. For an adult, each of the following areas represents 9 percent of the body surface: the head and neck, each upper extremity, the chest, the abdomen, the upper back, the lower back and buttocks, the front of each lower extremity, and the back of each lower extremity. The remaining 1 percent is assigned to the genital region.

rule of palm a method for estimating the extent of a burn. The palm and fingers of the patient's own hand, which make up about 1 percent of the body's surface area, are compared with the patient's burn to estimate its size.

"safe haven" law a law that permits a person to drop off an infant or child at a police, fire, or EMS station or to deliver the infant or child to any available public safety personnel. The intent of the law is to protect children who may otherwise be abandoned or harmed by parents who are unable or unwilling to care for them.

SAMPLE a memory aid in which the letters stand for elements of the past medical history: signs and symptoms, allergies, medications, pertinent past history, last oral intake, and events leading to the injury or illness.

scaffolding building on what one already knows.

scapula (SKAP-yuh-luh) the shoulder blade.

scene size-up steps taken when approaching the scene of an emergency call: checking scene safety, taking Standard Precautions, noting the mechanism of injury or nature of the patient's illness, determining the number of patients, and deciding what, if any, additional resources to call for.

schizophrenia a chronic mental disorder that affects how a person thinks, feels, and behaves. People with severe or untreated schizophrenia may seem like they have lost touch with reality.

school age stage of life from 6 to 12 years.

scope of practice a set of regulations and ethical considerations that define the scope, or extent and limits, of the EMT's job.

secondary devices destructive devices, such as bombs, placed to be activated after an initial attack and timed to injure emergency responders and others who rush in to help care for those targeted by an initial attack. *See also* multiple devices.

seizure (SEE-zher) a sudden change in sensation, behavior, or movement. The most severe form of seizure produces violent muscle contractions called convulsions.

sepsis a life-threatening condition resulting from an abnormal and counterproductive response by the body that causes damage to tissues and organs. The body overreacts and secretes substances that, instead of helping, hurt cells, tissues, and organs.

shock the body's inability to circulate blood adequately to the body's cells to supply them with oxygen and nutrients, which is a life-threatening condition. Also known as *hypoperfusion*.

sickle cell anemia (SCA) an abnormally low number of RBCs in the circulation due to sickle cell disease.

sickle cell disease (SCD) an inherited disease in which patients have a genetic defect in their hemoglobin that results in an abnormal structure of the red blood cell.

side effect any action of a drug other than the desired action.

sign something regarding the patient's condition that you can see.

single incident command command organization in which a single agency controls all resources and operations.

skeleton the bones of the body.

skin the layer of tissue between the body and the external environment.

skull the bony structure of the head.

slander false, injurious information stated verbally.

small intestine the muscular tube between the stomach and the large intestine, divided into the duodenum, the jejunum, and the ileum, that receives partially digested food from the stomach and continues digestion. Nutrients are absorbed by the body through its walls.

sphygmomanometer (SFIG-mo-mah-NOM-uh-ter) the cuff and gauge used to measure blood pressure.

spinal motion restriction a procedure for limiting movement of the head, neck, and spine when spinal injury is possible or likely

spinous (SPI-nus) **process** the bony bump on a vertebra.

spleen an organ located in the left upper quadrant of the abdomen that acts as a blood filtration system and a reservoir for reserves of blood.

spontaneous abortion when the fetus and placenta deliver before the 20th week of pregnancy; commonly called a *miscarriage*.

sprain the stretching and tearing of ligaments.

staging area the area where ambulances are parked and other resources are held until needed.

staging supervisor person responsible for overseeing ambulances and ambulance personnel at a multiple-casualty incident.

standard of care for an EMT providing care for a specific patient in a specific situation, the care that would be expected to be provided by an EMT with similar training when caring for a patient in a similar situation.

Standard Precautions a strict form of infection control that is based on the assumption that all blood and other body fluids are infectious; also known as Standard Precautions.

standing orders a policy or protocol issued by a Medical Director that authorizes EMTs and others to perform particular skills in certain situations.

status epilepticus (STAY-tus or STAT-us ep-i-LEP-ti-kus) a prolonged seizure or situation when a person suffers two or more convulsive seizures without regaining full consciousness.

sternum (STER-num) the breastbone.

stillborn born dead.

stoma (STO-ma) a surgically created permanent opening into the body, as with a tracheostomy, colostomy, or ileostomy.

stomach muscular sac between the esophagus and the small intestine where digestion of food begins.

strain muscle injury resulting from overstretching or overexertion of the muscle.

strategies broad general plans designed to achieve desired outcomes.

stress a state of physical and/or psychological arousal to a stimulus.

stretch receptors sensors in blood vessels that identify internal pressure.

stroke a condition of altered function caused when an artery in the brain is blocked or ruptured, disrupting the supply of oxygenated blood or causing bleeding into the brain. Formerly called a *cerebrovascular accident (CVA)*.

stroke volume the amount of blood ejected from the heart in one contraction.

subcutaneous (SUB-ku-TAY-ne-us) **layers** the layers of fat and soft tissues found below the dermis.

sucking reflex a reflex in which stroking a hungry infant's lips causes the infant to start sucking.

suctioning (SUK-shun-ing) use of a vacuum device to remove blood, vomitus, and other secretions or foreign materials from the airway.

sudden cardiac arrest a cardiac arrest occurring due to the abrupt onset of a dysrhythmia.

sudden death a cardiac arrest that occurs within 2 hours of the onset of symptoms. The patient may have no prior symptoms of coronary artery disease.

suffix word part added to the end of a root or word to complete its meaning.

superficial burn a burn that involves only the epidermis, the outer layer of the skin. It is characterized by reddening of the skin and perhaps some swelling. A common example is a sunburn. Also called a *first-degree burn*.

superior toward the head (e.g., the chest is superior to the abdomen).

supine hypotensive syndrome dizziness and a drop in blood pressure caused when the mother is in a supine position and the weight of the uterus, infant, placenta, and amniotic fluid compress the inferior vena cava, reducing return of blood to the heart and cardiac output.

supine lying on the back.

surge capacity a measurable representation of ability of a medical facility to manage a sudden influx of patients. It is dependent on a variety of variables, including the number of open beds, physical space, supplies, staff, and any special considerations (such as contaminated or contagious patients).

symptom something regarding the patient's condition that the patient tells you.

syncope (SIN-ko-pee) fainting.

systemic vascular resistance (SVR) the pressure in the peripheral blood vessels that the heart must overcome to pump blood into the system.

systolic (sis-TOL-ik) **blood pressure** the pressure created in the arteries when the left ventricle contracts and forces blood out into circulation.

tachycardia (TAK-uh-KAR-de-uh) a rapid pulse; any resting pulse rate above 100 beats per minute in an adult.

tactics specific operational actions to accomplish assigned tasks.

tarsals (TAR-sulz) the ankle bones.

tearing pain sharp pain that feels as if body tissues are being torn apart.

telemetry the process of sending and receiving data wirelessly.

temperament the infant's nature or personality, especially in terms of responding to the environment.

temporal (TEM-po-ral) **bones** bones forming part of the sides of the skull and the floor of the cranial cavity.

temporomandibular (TEM-po-ro-mand-DIB-yuh-lar) **joint** the movable joint between the mandible and the temporal bone, also called the TMJ.

tendons tissues that connect muscle to bone.

tension pneumothorax a type of pneumothorax in which air accumulation puts pressure on the heart and vena cava and causes shock.

terrorism the unlawful use of force or violence against persons or property to intimidate or coerce a government, the civilian population, or any segment thereof, in furtherance of political or social objectives (FBI definition). *See also* domestic terrorism; international terrorism.

testes (TES-tees) the male organs of reproduction used for the production of sperm and hormones.

thorax (THOR-ax) the chest.

thrill a vibration felt on gentle palpation, such as that which typically occurs within an arterial-venous fistula.

thrombus (THROM-bus) a clot formed of blood and plaque attached to the inner wall of an artery or vein.

thyroid (THI-roid) **cartilage** the wing-shaped plate of cartilage that sits anterior to the larynx and forms the Adam's apple.

tibia (TIB-e-uh) the medial and larger bone of the lower leg.

tidal volume the volume of air moved in one cycle of breathing.

toddler phase stage of life from 12 to 36 months.

tonic-clonic (TON-ik-KLON-ik) **seizure** a generalized seizure in which the patient loses consciousness and has jerking movements of paired muscle groups.

torso the trunk of the body, or the body without the head and the extremities.

tort a civil, not a criminal, offense; an action or injury caused by negligence from which a lawsuit may arise.

tourniquet (TURN-i-ket) a device used for bleeding control that constricts all blood flow to and from an extremity.

toxin a poisonous substance secreted by bacteria, plants, or animals.

trachea (TRAY-ke-uh) the "windpipe"; the structure that connects the pharynx to the lungs.

tracheostomy (tray-ke-OS-to-me) a surgical incision through the neck and into the trachea held open by a metal or plastic tube.

tracheostomy mask a device designed to be placed over a stoma or tracheostomy tube to provide supplemental oxygen.

traction splint a splint that applies constant pull along the length of a lower extremity to help stabilize the fractured bone and to reduce muscle spasm in the limb. Traction splints are used primarily on femoral shaft fractures.

transportation supervisor person responsible for communicating with sector officers and hospitals to manage transportation of patients to hospitals from a multiple-casualty incident.

trauma patient a patient suffering from one or more physical injuries.

trauma score a system of evaluating trauma patients according to a numerical rating system to determine the severity of the patient's trauma.

treatment area the area in which patients are treated at a multiple-casualty incident.

treatment supervisor person responsible for overseeing treatment of patients who have been triaged at a multiple-casualty incident.

trending changes in a patient's condition over time, such as slowing respirations or rising pulse rate, that may show improvement.

triage the process of quickly assessing patients at a multiple-casualty incident and assigning each a priority for receiving treatment; from a French word meaning "to sort."

triage area the area where secondary triage takes place at a multiple-casualty incident.

triage supervisor the person responsible for overseeing triage at a multiple-casualty incident.

triage tag color-coded tag indicating the priority group to which a patient has been assigned.

trust versus mistrust concept developed from an orderly, predictable environment versus a disorderly, irregular environment.

ulna (UL-nah) the medial bone of the forearm.

umbilical (um-BIL-i-kal) **cord** the fetal structure containing the blood vessels that carry blood to and from the placenta.

unified command command organization in which several agencies work independently but cooperatively.

unilateral limited to one side

universal dressing a bulky dressing.

untoward (un-TORD) **effect** an effect of a medication in addition to its desired effect that may be potentially harmful to the patient.

uppers stimulants such as cocaine and methamphetamine that affect the central nervous system and excite the user.

ureters (YER-uh-terz) the tubes connecting the kidneys to the bladder.

urethra (you-RE-thra) tube connecting the bladder to the vagina or penis for excretion of urine.

urinary catheter a tube inserted into the bladder through the urethra to drain urine from the bladder.

uterus (U-ter-us) the muscular abdominal female organ where the fetus develops; the womb.

V/Q match ventilation/perfusion match. This implies that the alveoli are supplied with enough air and that the air in the alveoli is matched with sufficient blood in the pulmonary capillaries to permit optimum exchange of oxygen and carbon dioxide.

vagina (vuh-JI-na) the female organ of reproduction used both for sexual intercourse and as a passageway from the uterus for the fetus.

valve a structure that opens and closes to permit the flow of a fluid in only one direction.

vein any blood vessel returning blood to the heart.

venae cavae (VE-ne KA-ve) the superior vena cava and the inferior vena cava. These two major veins return blood from the body to the right atrium. *Singular* vena cava.

venom a toxin (poison) produced by certain animals, such as snakes, spiders, and some marine life forms.

venous bleeding bleeding from a vein, which is characterized by dark red or maroon blood and a steady, easy-to-control flow.

ventilation the process of moving gases (oxygen and carbon dioxide) into and out of the pulmonary circulation; also, artificial provision of breaths.

ventilator a device that breathes for a patient.

ventral referring to the front of the body. A synonym for *anterior*.

ventricles (VEN-tri-kulz) the two lower chambers of the heart. There is a right ventricle (which sends oxygen-poor blood to the lungs) and a left ventricle (which sends oxygen-rich blood to the body).

ventricular assist device a battery-powered mechanical pump implanted in the body to assist a failing ventricle in pumping blood.

ventricular tachycardia (ven-TRIK-u-ler tak-i-KAR-de-uh) **(V-tach)** a condition in which the heartbeat is quite rapid; if rapid enough, ventricular tachycardia will not allow the heart's chambers to fill with enough blood between beats to produce blood flow sufficient to meet the body's needs.

Venturi mask a face mask-and-reservoir bag device that delivers specific concentrations of oxygen by mixing oxygen with inhaled air.

venule (VEN-yul) the smallest kind of vein.

vertebrae (VERT-uh-bray) the 33 bones of the spinal column (singular *vertebra*).

visceral pain a poorly localized, dull, or diffuse pain that arises from the abdominal organs, or viscera.

vital signs outward signs of what is going on inside the body, including respiration; pulse; skin color, temperature, and condition (plus capillary refill in infants and children); pupils; and blood pressure.

volatile chemicals vaporizing compounds, such as cleaning fluid, that are breathed in by the abuser to produce a "high."

voluntary muscle muscle that can be consciously controlled.

warm zone area where personnel and equipment decontamination and hot zone support take place; it includes control points for the access corridor and, thus, assists in reducing the spread of contamination.

water chill chilling caused by conduction of heat from the body when the body or clothing is wet.

watt the unit of measurement of the output power of a radio.

weaponization packaging or producing a material, such as a chemical, biologic, or radiologic agent so that it can be used as a weapon–for example, by dissemination in a bomb detonation or as an aerosol sprayed over an area or introduced into a ventilation system.

weapons of mass destruction (WMD) weapons, devices, or agents intended to cause widespread harm and/or fear among a population.

wearable cardioverter defibrillator (WCD) an external defibrillator worn by a patient to detect any rapid life-threatening dysrhythmia and deliver a shock to defibrillate the heart.

white blood cells components of the blood. They produce substances that help the body fight infection.

wind chill chilling caused by convection of heat from the body in the presence of air currents.

xiphoid (ZI-foid) **process** the inferior portion of the sternum (breastbone).

zoonotic able to move through the animal–human barrier; transmissible from animals to humans.

zygomatic (ZI-go-MAT-ik) **arches** the bones that form the structure of the cheeks.

Index

f after page number indicates figures; *t* stands for tables.

B

C

J

K

L

M

Q

R

S

T

U

V